Community and Public Health Nursing

Promoting the Public's Health

Community and Public Health Nursing

Promoting the Public's Health

Ninth Edition

Cherie Rector, PhD, RN, PHN
Professor Emeritus
Department of Nursing
California State University, Bakersfield
Bakersfield, California

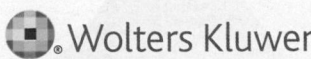

. Wolters Kluwer

Philadelphia • Baltimore • New York • London
Buenos Aires • Hong Kong • Sydney • Tokyo

Publisher: Julie Stegman
Senior Acquisitions Editor: Christina C. Burns
Development Editor: Shana Murph
Production Project Manager: David Orzechowski
Design Coordinator: Terry Mallon
Illustration Coordinator: Jennifer Clements
Manufacturing Coordinator: Karin Duffield
Prepress Vendor: SPi Global

Ninth edition

9 8 7 6 5 4 3

Printed in China

Library of Congress Cataloging-in-Publication Data
Names: Rector, Cherie L., editor.
Title: Community and public health nursing : promoting the public's health / [edited by] Cherie
  Rector.
Other titles: Community & public health nursing.
Description: 9th edition. | Philadelphia : Wolters Kluwer, [2016] | Preceded by Community &
  public health nursing : promoting the public's health / [edited by] Judith Ann Allender, Cherie
  Rector, Kristine D. Warner. 8th ed. c2014. | Includes bibliographical references and index.
Identifiers: LCCN 2016028226 | ISBN 9781496349828
Subjects: | MESH: Community Health Nursing | Public Health Nursing | Nurse's Role | Health
  Promotion | United States
Classification: LCC RT98 | NLM WY 108 | DDC 610.73/43—dc23 LC record available at https://
  lccn.loc.gov/2016028226

LWW.com

To my husband, my children, and my grandchildren—they make it all worthwhile!
This book is dedicated to them and to my parents and my sisters who always
encouraged me to keep learning, growing, and believing.

—Cherie Rector

ACKNOWLEDGMENTS

It saddened me that I was unable to continue to work with my dear friend and colleague Dr. Cherie Rector on the ninth edition of this textbook. Her unwavering devotion to public health nursing practice, research, and nursing education has been an inspiration to me over the past decade. Cherie and her team of contributors reflect the best that our specialty practice has to offer. I join her in encouraging all of you to consider practicing in the community at some point in your career. There is no better way to make real and lasting changes to the health and welfare of the public, whether it is locally, nationally, or in the international arena. I would also like to express my gratitude to Dr. Judy Allender. It was she who first gave me the opportunity to join her as a contributor in the sixth edition and to team with Cherie as a coauthor for the seventh and eighth editions. Her mentorship in public health nursing education provided the opportunity for me to share with so many students my passion for this specialty and my belief that there is not a finer career than serving as a PHN.

Kristine D. Warner, PhD, MPH, RN
Assistant Dean and Managing Director
MEPN Program
University of California, San Francisco
San Francisco, California

Despite this being the ninth edition of this textbook, it remains a work in progress. Feedback from nursing students and faculty, as well as from working public health nurses, continues to be reflected in this edition of the book. It is hoped that this textbook meets the needs of students and faculty, and continuing comment and reaction is always welcome.

The contributors, both continuing and new to this edition, have worked diligently, and gratitude is owed for sharing their expertise and knowledge. It is also important to acknowledge the work of past contributors whose words may still be found in some form in this ninth edition. I am especially grateful to have worked with Dr. Kristine Warner on the last two editions of this book and appreciate the thought and insight she has always brought to this project. I would also like to acknowledge the work of Dr. Judy Allender, who first gave me the opportunity to contribute to the fifth and sixth editions of this textbook, and then to work with Kris Warner as coauthors on the past two editions.

Editors Shana Murph, Jennifer Forestieri and Christina Burns, as well as the administrative staff at Wolters Kluwer, have worked tirelessly, and their efforts are greatly appreciated. Natalie Silver, who helped with photos/permissions and APA references, was a valuable member of the team on this edition. I thank her for her efforts and her quick turnarounds.

It would have been impossible to complete this edition without the love and support (not to mention patience) of family, friends, and close colleagues. It is my hope that this textbook may spark an interest in nursing students to explore public health nursing and join us in this great specialty area of nursing!

Cherie Rector, PhD, RN, PHN
Professor Emeritus
Department of Nursing
California State University, Bakersfield
Bakersfield, California

ABOUT THE AUTHOR

Dr. Cherie Rector is a native Californian and an Emeritus Professor in the Department of Nursing at California State University, Bakersfield. While there she served as lead faculty in community health nursing, Director of the School Nurse Credential Program and the RN to BSN Program, helping to develop and revise curriculum in those areas. She also served in an administrative position as Director of Allied Health and the Disabled Students Program at College of the Sequoias. She has also been the Coordinator of the School Nurse Credential Program and the RN to BSN Program at California State University, Fresno, overseeing curriculum development in those areas. Undergraduate teaching areas have included community health nursing, foundations/health assessment, health teaching, and leadership; graduate courses have consisted of community health nursing, research, vulnerable populations, family theories, interprofessional development, and school nursing. She has served as a consultant to school districts and hospitals in the areas of child health, research and evidence-based practice, and has served on various state, local, and national boards and in leadership roles in professional nursing organizations. Over the course of her career, Dr. Rector has practiced in community health and school nursing settings and in acute care neonatal nursing. Her grants, research, publications, and presentations have focused largely on child and adolescent health, school nursing, public health nursing, nursing education, and disadvantaged students. She earned an associate degree in nursing from College of the Sequoias and a bachelor of science in nursing degree from the Consortium of the California State Universities, Long Beach. She completed a master's degree in nursing (Clinical Nurse Specialist, Community Health) and a school nurse credential from California State University, Fresno. Her PhD in educational psychology is from the University of Southern California. She is an active member of the American Public Health Association, the Western Institute of Nursing, and the Association of Community Health Nursing Educators. Dr. Rector and her husband have three grown sons, eight grandsons, and three granddaughters.

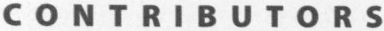

CONTRIBUTORS

Sheila Adams-Leander, RN, PhD
Associate Professor
Milwaukee School of Engineering
  University
Milwaukee, Wisconsin
Chapter 5

Peggy H. Anderson, DNP, MS, RN
Associate Teaching Professor
Brigham Young University College of
  Nursing
Provo, Utah
Chapter 22

Barbara Blake, RN, PhD ACRN,
  FAAN
Professor
Kennesaw State University
Kennesaw, Georgia
Chapter 23

Anne Bongiorno, PhD, APHN-BC
Associate Professor
State University of New York,
  Plattsburgh
Plattsburgh, New York
Chapter 4

Bonnie Callen, PhD, RN, PHCNS-BC
Associate Professor (Retired)
University of Tennessee, Knoxville
Knoxville, Tennessee
Chapter 24

Beverly A. Dandridge, MSN, FNP,
  MSAJS, CCHP
CAPT, USPHS Commissioned Corps
USPHS Commissioned Corps Liaison
Department of Homeland Security
Washington, District of Columbia
Chapters 17 and 30

Janna L. Dieckmann, PhD, RN
Associate Professor
University of North Carolina at
  Chapel Hill
Chapel Hill, North Carolina
Chapter 26

Rebecca Doughty, MN, RN, PhD(c)
Director of Health Services
Spoken Public Schools
Spokane, Washington
Chapter 30

Mary Ann Drake, PhD, RN, CNE
Professor
Webster University
St. Louis, Missouri
Chapter 18

Naomi Ervin, PhD, RN, PHCNS-BC,
  FNAP, FAAN
Adjunct Professor
Madonna University
Livonia, Michigan
Chapter 25

Deborah S. Finnell, DNS, PHMHP-BC,
  CARN-AP, FAAN
Associate Professor
Johns Hopkins School of Nursing
Baltimore, Maryland
Chapter 27

MAJ Lakisha N. Flagg, DrPH, MS,
  CPH, APHN-BC
Chief, Army Public Health Nursing
Brooke Army Medical Center
Joint Base San Antonio
  Fort Sam Houston, Texas
Chapter 15

Ezra C. Holston, PhD, RN
Assistant Professor
University of Tennessee, Knoxville
Knoxville, Tennessee
Chapter 19

Barbara Joyce, PhD, RN, CNS,
  ANEF
Associate Professor
Helen and Arthur E. Johnson Beth-El
  College of Nursing & Health
  Sciences
University of Colorado at Colorado
  Springs
Colorado Springs, Colorado
Chapter 20

Betty C. Jung, MPH, RN, MCHES
Program Director
Public Health Expertise Network of
  Mentors (PHENOM)
Adjunct Lecturer
Southern Connecticut State
  University
New Haven, Connecticut
Chapter 7

Katherine Laux Kaiser, PhD, RN,
  PHCNS-BC
Professor
University of Nebraska Medical
  Center, College of Nursing
Omaha, Nebraska
Chapter 21

Mary Lashley, PhD, RN, PHNCS-BC
Professor
Towson University
Towson, Maryland
Chapter 28

Angelique Lawyer, MSN, MPH,
  APHN-BC, RN
*Nurse Consultant, Chief Surgeon's
  Office*
National Guard Bureau
Arlington, Virginia
Chapter 31

Jeanne M. Leffers, PhD, RN, FAAN
Professor Emeritus
University of Massachusetts, Dartmouth
North Dartmouth, Massachusetts

Karin L. Lightfoot, PhD, MSN,
  RN-BC, PHN
Assistant Professor
California State University, Chico
Chico, California
Chapters 8 & 14

Colleen Marzilli, PhD, DNP, MBA,
  RN-BC, CCM, APHN-BC, CNE
Assistant Professor
The University of Texas at Tyler
Tyler, Texas
Chapter 10

Debra J. Millar, MSN, RN, APHN-BC
Assistant Professor
California State University, Stanislaus
Turlock, California
Chapters 12 and 16

Mary Ellen Miller, PhD, RN, APHN-BC
Associate Professor
Director, Bridging the Gaps Lehigh
  Valley Affiliate
DeSales University
Center Valley, Pennsylvania
Chapter 31(Lead)

Margaret Oot-Hayes, PhD, RN
Professor
Regis College
Weston, Massachusetts
Chapter 30

Judith M. Paré, PhD, RN
Dean, School of Nursing and
* Behavioral Sciences*
Becker College
Worcester, Massachusetts
Chapter 29

Carol Pochron, MSN, RN
Adjunct Professor
DeSales University
Center Valley, Pennsylvania
Chapter 31

Cherie Rector, PhD, RN, PHN
Professor Emeritus
Department of Nursing
California State University,
  Bakersfield
Bakersfield, California
Chapters 1, 2, and 29

Annmarie Donahue Samar, PhD,
  PHCNS-BC, NEA-BC, RN
Professor
Framingham State University
Framingham, Massachusetts
Chapter 10

Lisabeth M. Searing, PhD, RN
Assistant Professor
Illinois Wesleyan University
Bloomington, Illinois
Chapter 6

Bryan W. Sisk, RN, BSN, MPH
Associate Director Patient Care
* Services*
Nurse Executive
Central Texas Veterans Health Care
  System
Temple, Texas
Veteran's Content Expert
* Contributor*

Susan M. Swider, PhD, APHN-BC,
  FAAN
Professor, Department of Community,
* Systems and Mental Health Nursing*
Program Director, DNP in Advanced
* Public Health Nursing and*
* Leadership to Enhance Population*
* Health Outcomes*
Rush University College of Nursing
Chicago, Illinois
Chapter 13

Gloria Ann Jones Taylor, PhD, RN
Professor
Kennesaw State University
Kennesaw, Georgia
Chapter 23

Dana Todd, PhD, APRN
Associate Professor
Murray State University
Murray, Kentucky
Chapters 3, 11, and 21

Kristine D. Warner, PhD, MPH, RN
Assistant Dean and Managing
* Director*
MEPN Program
University of California, San Francisco
San Francisco, California
Chapter 2

Robin M. White, PhD, MSN, RN
Assistant Professor
University of Tampa
Tampa, Florida
Chapter 29

Elizabeth Wright, MSN, RN
Assistant Professor of Nursing
Indiana Wesleyan University
Marion, Indiana
Chapter 32

Marjory D. Williams, PhD, RN
Associate Chief Nursing Service,
* Education and Research*
Central Texas Veterans Health Care
  System
Temple, Texas
Veteran's Content Expert Contributor

CONTRIBUTORS TO PREVIOUS EDITION

Elizabeth M. Andal, PhD, MSN,
  APRN-BC, FAAN
Mental Health Service Consultant
Las Vegas, Nevada
Chapter 27

Margaret Avila, PhD, PHN, RN/NP
Assistant Professor
California State University, Los Angeles
Los Angeles, California
Chapter 29

Lydia C. Bourne, BSN, RN, MA, PHN
Principal, Bourne & Associates
Legislative Advocate
El Macero, California
Chapter 13

Paula Dorhout, RN, MSN,
  APHN-BC
Southeast Region Nursing Director
Children's Medical Services
West Palm Beach, Florida
Chapter 10

Marie P. Farrell, EdD, MPH,
  RN, ACC
Professor
Human and Organizational
  Development
Fielding Graduate University
Santa Barbara, California
Chapter 16

Sheila Holcomb, EdD, RN, MSN, PHN
School Nurse
Walnutwood High School
Rancho Cordova, California
Chapter 20

Roberta Lavin, PhD, APRN
Chair and Professor
Clarke University
Dubuque, Iowa
Captain (Retired)
U.S. Public Health Service
Washington, District of Columbia
Chapter 17

Barbara B. Little, DNP, MPH, RN,
  APHN-BC
Associate Professor
Florida State University, College of
  Nursing
Tallahassee, Florida
Chapter 10

Eileen Lukes, PhD, RN, COHN-S,
  CCM, FAAOHN
Health Services Manager
Boeing Company
Mesa, Arizona
Chapter 31

Erin D. Maughan, RN, PhD,
  APHN-BC
Director of Research
National Association of School
  Nurses
Silver Spring, Maryland
Chapter 30

Barbara J. Polivka, PhD, RN
*Professor and Shirley B. Powers
    Endowed Chair in Nursing
    Research*
University of Louisville School of
    Nursing
Louisville, Kentucky
Chapter 4

Cherie Rector, PhD, RN, PHN
Professor Emeritus
Department of Nursing
California State University,
    Bakersfield
Bakersfield, California
*Chapters 1, 4, 5, 6, 10, 15, 21, 22,
    24, 25, and 29*

Bassam M. Salemeh, PhD
Instructor
Microbiology and Biology
Antelope Valley College
Lancaster, California
Chapter 7

Phyllis G. Salopek, MSN, FNP
Assistant Professor
California State University, Chico
Chico, California
Chapter 19

Joann E. Smith, PhD, RN, APHN, CNE
Assistant Professor
Howard University
Washington, District of Columbia
Chapter 22

Karen Smith-Sayer, MSN, RN, PHN
Public Health Nurse
CA Department of Corrections
Pelican Bay State Prison
Crescent City, California
Chapter 8

Sharon S. Strand, MSN, PHN, RN-BC
Health Specialist
Mountain States Early Head Start
Coeur d'Alene, Idaho
Chapter 29

Mary E. Summers, PhD, MSN, RN,
    PHN
Professor Emeritus
Sacramento State University
Sacramento, California
Chapter 12

Rose Utley, PhD, RN, CNE
Professor
Missouri State University
Springfield, Missouri
Chapter 31

Kristine D. Warner, PhD, MPH, RN
Professor
Director ASBSN Program
California State University, Stanislaus
Stockton, California
Chapters 2, 3, 7, 11, 12, 14, 19, and 32

Joyce Zerwekh, EdD, RN
Emeritus Professor of Nursing
Concordia University
Portland, Oregon
Chapter 32

REVIEWER LIST

Pamela Ark, PhD, RN
BSN Director, Associate Professor
Tennessee State University
Nashville, Tennessee

Barbara Blackford, MSN, RN-CNE
Assistant Professor
Marian University
Indianapolis, Indiana

Anne Bongiorno, PhD, APHN-BC,
    CNE
Associate Professor
SUNY Plattsburgh Department of
    Nursing
Plattsburgh, New York

Diane Bridge, EdS, MSN, RN
Assistant Professor
School of Nursing
Liberty University
Lynchburg, Virginia

Adelita Cantu, PhD, RN
Associate Professor
University of Texas Health Science
    Center San Antonio
San Antonio, Texas

Toni Chops, MS, RN, CNE
Assistant Professor
Mt. Carmel College of Nursing
Columbus, Ohio

Cathleen Colleran-Santos, DNP, RN
*Associate Professor of Nursing/Program
    Coordinator of RN-BSN Program*
Curry College
Milton, Massachusetts

Charlene Douglas, PhD
*Associate Professor/Coordinator for
    Community Health Nursing*
George Mason University
Fairfax, Virginia

Rose Marie Fowler-Swarts, MSN,
    BSN, RN
Assistant Professor
University of Central Missouri
Warrensburg, Missouri

Connie Wallace Hazzard, EdD, MSN,
    RN, PMHCNS-BC, BSN
Assistant Professor
Nebraska Methodist College
Omaha, Nebraska

Denise Isibel, DNP, MSN, BSN, RN
Senior Lecturer
Old Dominion University
Williamsburg, Virginia

Michelle Kluka, MSN, RN
Visiting Instructor
Oakland University School of Nursing
Rochester, Michigan

Dana Manley, PhD, APRN
Associate Professor
Murray State University
Benton, Kentucky

Bette Mariani, PhD, RN
Assistant Professor
Villanova University College of
    Nursing
Villanova, Pennsylvania

Ruth McDermott-Levy, PhD, RN
Associate Professor
Villanova University
Villanova, Pennsylvania

Lori M. Metzger, PhD, NP-C, MSN,
    CRNP, RN-BC
Assistant Professor
Bloomsburg University
Bloomsburg, Pennsylvania

Geraldine Moore, Ed, MSN, RN
Professor
Molloy College
Rockville Centre, New York

Patti Moss, MSN, RN
Assistant Professor
Lamar University
Bridge City, Texas

PREFACE

Barbara Spradley began the first edition of this book in 1981, and the ninth edition of *Community and Public Health Nursing: Promoting the Public's Health* continues to provide undergraduate nursing students with an introduction to public health and population-focused nursing in the community. Nursing in community settings may include sites such as public health departments, schools, correctional facilities, community-based organizations, churches and parishes, as well as industrial or business settings. Although most newly graduated nurses plan to work in hospital and acute care settings, especially since the bulk of their education has been focused toward that end, it is still important to provide a solid grounding in public and community health nursing. That content is what distinguished university-prepared nurses from hospital or diploma nurses early on, and it remains an important area of practice. Knowledge of public health nursing provides new nurses with a broader focus of patient care (e.g., families, aggregates, communities, populations, and not just individual patients). Even though a new graduate may choose to work in a hospital setting, it is still important for the nurse discharging the patient to have an understanding of the patient's unique circumstances and how to best join with the patient and their family in working to prevent further illness and promote better health. To help students better understand the "whole" patient, throughout this book, students are provided with examples and information that will broaden their knowledge of patients and enable them to provide more effective nursing care—wherever they may choose to be employed. Population-focused tools and interventions are needed in acute care, as infection rates continue to rise and nurse-sensitive outcome indicators are closely monitored. Nonpayment for medical errors or early hospital readmissions is becoming the norm, and nurses are involved in quality improvement and patient safety at all levels of practice and in all practice settings.

In the process of learning about public health nursing, it is hoped that a spark may be lit in those nursing students interested in this nursing specialty and its rich history. Public health nurses often work in a more autonomous practice setting and can have a real impact on the general health status of their communities through large-scale interventions and political advocacy. Nurses working in the community are important role models for social justice and are on the front line of communicable disease prevention and control.

The purpose of this book is to give undergraduate students a solid, basic grounding in public health nursing practice and to introduce them to key populations with whom they may work in the community setting, as well as important public health principles. Entry-level public health nurses may also find it a helpful resource as they begin to familiarize themselves with their unique practice settings and target populations. The nexus of public health nursing lies in the application of public health principles along with nursing science and practice skills in order to promote health, prevent disease, and protect at-risk populations. Throughout this book, the term *community health nurse* is used interchangeably with *public health nurse* as a description of the practitioner who does not simply "work in the community" (i.e., is physically located outside the hospital setting, in the community), but rather one who has a focus on nursing and public health science that informs their community-based, population-focused nursing practice.

NEW TO THIS EDITION

This edition reflects a continuing effort to try to keep this textbook user-friendly for nursing students, who are entering the world of public health nursing for the first time. The goal is to write in an accessible style with little use of jargon or long passages of dry narrative. Also, a more conversational quality is sought, and the use of examples or features that highlight student, client, practitioner, and instructor perspectives on common issues and problems is used to make this new area more familiar to students. Pertinent examples and case studies are used throughout the book to convey real-life situations and interventions in order to aid students in applying the concepts and principles of public health nursing practice. Storytelling has been shown to be very effective in nursing education, as Patricia Benner and others have noted. These client stories (case studies) can greatly influence learning, especially as the student strives to grasp the art and skill of working with clients in a community setting. The goal of this book is also to provide the most accurate, pertinent, and current information for students and nursing faculty. Experts in various fields and specialty areas of public health nursing, including Homeland Security and the military, as well as veteran's health, have contributed to this edition, in an effort to provide a balanced and complete product. With the addition of over 35 contributors from across the country and countless reviewers, the content reflects a broad spectrum of views and expertise. However, it has been carefully edited to make this a cohesive textbook with a shared commentary.

New Content

- QSEN: Focus on Quality—feature highlights quality and safety concepts in applicable chapters. These include QSEN (Quality and Safety Education for Nurses) concepts related to environmental health and disasters, patient-centered care (family/community; empowerment), teamwork/collaboration (communication; system barriers), EBP/QI/ethics, and data (i.e., tracking the homeless).
- Population-Focus—this feature helps refocus student attention to chapter concepts from a population-focused viewpoint. Although chapter content often contains population-based information, in some chapters, an additional focus on population is needed. Current case studies or examples of effective population-based interventions help make the concept of population-based health more evident and understandable to students.
- LGBT content has been incorporated throughout the text and in some features in an effort to help nursing students to better comprehend and address the needs of this population.
- Veterans Health content has also been the focus of some features (e.g., Case Files, Perspectives), critical thinking activities, and has been added to chapter content in order to better explore this population and the PHN role in serving them.

New Organization

For the ninth edition, population-focused public health nursing and *Healthy People 2020* goals and objectives have been emphasized throughout the text, and additional case studies, perspectives, and examples of evidence-based practice have been added. More visual interest, with photos and new graphics highlighting written content, is incorporated into this edition. Chapter and unit organization is similar, but additional content has been added where needed and some content moved to *thePoint*.

Unit I, Foundations of Community Health Nursing, covers fundamental principles and background about public health nursing. Chapter 1 discusses basic public health concepts of health, illness, wellness, community, aggregate, population, interprofessional collaboration, and levels of prevention. Leading Health Indicators are introduced in this chapter, along with *Healthy People 2020* goals and objectives. In Chapter 2, public health nursing's rich and meaningful history is explored, along with social influences that have shaped our current practice. New features, highlighting PHN examples during different historical phases have been added, along with new photos. Educational preparation and the roles and functions of public health nursing are discussed in both Chapters 2 and 3. Core Public Health Functions are described in Chapter 3, and common settings for public health nursing are introduced, along with the roles of community health nurses, and QUAD Council PHN Competencies. Chapter 4 considers values, ethical principles, and decision making unique to this nursing specialty. Quality and safety are also introduced. Evidence-based practice and research principles relating to community health nursing are discussed, along with the nurse's role in utilizing current research. Community-based

participatory research is highlighted. Cultural principles are defined, and the importance of cultural diversity and sensitivity in public health nursing are explained in Chapter 5, as well as cultural assessment and folk remedies. Several cultural groups are highlighted.

Unit II, Public Health Essentials for Community Health Nursing, covers the structure of public health within the health system infrastructure and introduces the basic public health tools of epidemiology, communicable disease control, and environmental health. Chapter 6 examines the economics of health care and compares U.S. outcomes with those of other countries, while also discussing the implications of the Affordable Care Act and the impact of health care reform on community health nursing. It also examines official health agencies and their organizational structures, as well as types of health insurance, and landmark legislation and policies related to public health. Different methods of epidemiologic investigation and research are explored in Chapter 7, along with the PHN's role in epidemiology. Population-focused communicable disease control, immunization programs, and communicable disease investigation are covered in Chapter 8. Important environmental health concepts and assessments are included in Chapter 9, along with public health nursing's role in researching and intervening to promote a healthier environment for all. Prevention is emphasized and an ecological approach is used to address issues of environmental health and safety.

Unit III, Community Health Nursing Toolbox, includes common tools used by the public health nurse to ensure effective practice. Chapter 10 covers communication, collaboration, working with groups, contracting with clients, and the use of informatics and health technology in community health nursing. Big Data, EHRs, mobile health, and GIS, among other technologies, are examined, and examples of technology applications are provided. Health promotion is the focus of Chapter 11, with an emphasis on helping clients and aggregates achieve behavioral change through the application of the levels of prevention, as well as educational and theoretical models. In Chapter 12, the focus is on planning and developing community health programs including the contribution of the QSEN project to community/public health nursing practice. Designing interventions and evaluating outcomes, along with social marketing approaches and grant funding, are examined. Chapter 13 concludes this unit with an explanation of the public health nurse's role in political advocacy and policy making, highlighting examples of PHN and community involvement in addressing policy issues.

Unit IV, The Community as Client, further expands the focus of the public health nurse. Chapter 14 examines common theories and models used in public health nursing practice, with examples of application to practice. Chapter 15 applies the nursing process to communities as clients (contrasted to individual patient focus in acute care). Different types of assessments are discussed, along with sources of data, community diagnoses, and community development. Global health and international nursing are considered in Chapter 16. International agencies, NGOs, and various foundations, along with global health problems/practices, are discussed and are highlighted by real-life case examples and perspectives.

Preparedness is examined in Chapter 17, with a closer look at disasters, terrorism, and war. The public health nurse's role in emergency preparedness, disaster management, preventive measures against terrorism, and *Healthy People 2020* objectives are also included in this chapter, along with triage and QSEN considerations during mass casualty incidents and disasters.

Unit V, The Family as Client, introduces the family as an aggregate, and Chapter 18 provides theoretical frameworks to promote healthy families and help nurses to better understand and work with families experiencing dysfunction. Applying the nursing process to families, completing family health assessments, and making home visits are covered in Chapter 19. Helpful tools are provided, and case studies help to emphasize concepts. In Chapter 20, family violence, including child, spousal/intimate partner, and elder abuse, is examined. Other violence affecting families, such as rape, homicide, suicide, and community violence, is also included, along with effective prevention strategies, assessments, interventions, and resources.

Unit VI, Promoting and Protecting the Health of Aggregates with Developmental Needs, provides information about client groups as often aggregated by public health departments. Chapter 21 covers common issues, concerns, and interventions for maternal child clients and their infants (e.g., adolescent pregnancy, risk factors, health services for mothers and infants through preschool). Health problems affecting children and adolescents (e.g., diabetes, asthma, injuries, communicable disease, substance abuse, preventive programs) are examined in Chapter 22, and the prevention and health promotion concerns of adult women and men are highlighted in Chapter 23, along with the PHN's role. Unique issues facing the older client can be found in Chapter 24 (e.g., common myths, preventive measures, health services, end-of-life care). These chapters build upon the content presented in Unit V, and describe public health nursing efforts with these select population groups.

Unit VII, Promoting and Protecting the Health of Vulnerable Populations, deals with how to best address the needs of the most vulnerable among us. In Chapter 25, the concept of vulnerability is addressed along with theoretical frameworks and effective methods of working with vulnerable clients and populations. In Chapter 26, clients with chronic illnesses and disabilities are discussed, along with the role of the community health nurse working with these clients. Federal legislation and national organizations serving those with disabilities and chronic illnesses are also highlighted. Chapter 27 covers clients and populations with behavioral health problems, such as mental health issues and substance abuse, and provides screening, intervention, and referral resources for PHNs. The homeless population is addressed in Chapter 28, along with factors contributing to homelessness and the role of the community health nurse. Chapter 29 addresses the unique challenges of rural, migrant, and urban populations. It also explores issues of social justice, medically underserved populations, and frontier nursing.

Unit VIII, Settings for Community Health Nursing, examines public and private settings in more depth. Practice options in government-sponsored agencies, such as state and local public health departments, public schools, correctional facilities, and the U.S. Public Health Service are described in Chapter 30. Nurse-led health centers, faith-based nursing, occupational health, and entrepreneurship are included in Chapter 31, which focuses on private agency opportunities for PHNs. These chapters provide overviews of a number of practice options available to both new and experienced nurses. Finally, the important roles of home health and hospice/palliative care nursing, especially given our aging population, are discussed in Chapter 32.

Features of the Text

The ninth edition of *Community and Public Health Nursing: Promoting the Public's Health* includes key features from previous editions as well as new features.

Features continued from previous editions include the following:

- **Evidence-Based Practice**—this feature incorporates current research examples and how they can be applied to public/community health nursing practice to achieve optimal client, aggregate, and population outcomes.
- **From the Case Files**—presentation of a scenario/case study, often with student-centered, application-based questions. Emphasizing nursing process, students are challenged to reflect on assessment and intervention in typical, yet challenging, examples of public health nursing practice.
- **Levels of Prevention Pyramid** boxes enhance understanding of the levels of prevention concepts, basic to community health nursing. Each box addresses a chapter topic, describes nursing actions at each of the three levels of prevention, and is unique to this text in its complexity and comprehensiveness.
- *Healthy People 2020*—highlights pertinent goals and objectives to promote health and is applied to specific populations or problems noted in each of the chapters. Where appropriate, mid-term or 2010 evaluations are included in the text.
- **Voices From the Community/Student Voices/ Perspectives**—this feature is included in most chapters and provides stories (viewpoints) from a variety of sources. The perspective may be from a nursing student, a novice or experienced public health nurse, a faculty member, a policy maker, or a client. These short features are designed to promote critical thinking, help students reflect on commonly held misconceptions about public/community health nursing, and recognize the link between skills learned in this specialty practice and other practice settings, especially acute care hospitals.
- **What Do YOU Think?**—brief features, scattered throughout the text, used to provoke thought or stir discussion on subject matter that is often unique to public health. Much like an instructor would stop and ask a thought question during lecture, these features encourage the reader to pause and more deeply consider an issue.
- **Learning Objectives** and **Key Terms** sharpen the reader's focus and provide a quick guide for mastering the chapter content.
- **Summary**—includes highlights at the end of each chapter, providing an overview of material covered and serving as a review for study.

- **References** at the end of each chapter provide classic sources, current research, and a broad base of authoritative information for furthering knowledge on each chapter's subject matter.
- **Activities to Promote Critical Thinking**—this feature is provided at the close of each chapter and is designed to challenge students, promote critical thinking and application of chapter content, as well as active involvement in solving community health problems. Internet activities, small group work, and interviews with clients or key community informants or experts are often included.
- **Additional Assessment Tools** are provided throughout the chapters. They are added to enhance assessment skills with individuals, families, or aggregates/populations.

thePoint®

Community and Public Health Nursing: Promoting the Public's Health, ninth edition, has ancillary resources designed with both students and instructors in mind, available on Web site: thePoint®

- Guided Lecture Notes and PowerPoint Presentations
- Student Quiz Bank
- Journal Articles
- Assignments, Discussion Topics, Case Studies, and Pre-Lecture Quizzes
- Test Generator
- Learning Objectives
- Image Bank

COMPREHENSIVE, INTEGRATED DIGITAL LEARNING SOLUTIONS

We are delighted to introduce an expanded suite of digital solutions to support instructors and students using *Community and Public Health Nursing: Promoting the Public's Health*, ninth edition. Now for the first time, our textbook is embedded into two integrated digital learning solutions—one specific for prelicensure programs and the other for postlicensure—that build on the features of the text with proven instructional design strategies. To learn more about these solutions, visit http://www.nursingeducationsuccess.com/ or contact your local Wolters Kluwer representative.

Lippincott CoursePoint

Our prelicensure solution, Lippincott CoursePoint, is a rich learning environment that drives course and curriculum success to prepare students for practice. Lippincott CoursePoint is designed for the way students learn. The solution connects learning to real-life application by integrating content from *Community and Public Health Nursing* with video cases, interactive modules, and evidence-based journal articles. Ideal for active, case-based learning, this powerful solution helps students develop higher-level cognitive skills and asks them to make decisions related to simple-to-complex scenarios.

Lippincott CoursePoint for Community and Public Health Nursing features:

- Leading content in context: Digital content from *Community and Public Health Nursing: Promoting the Public's Health*, ninth edition, is embedded in our Powerful Tools, engaging students and encouraging interaction and learning on a deeper level.
- The complete interactive eBook features annual content updates with the latest evidence-based practices and provides students with anytime, anywhere access on multiple devices.
- Full online access to Stedman's Medical Dictionary for the Health Professions and Nursing ensures students work with the best medical dictionary available.
- Powerful tools to maximize class performance: Additional course-specific tools provide case-based learning for every student:
- Video Cases help students anticipate what to expect as a nurse, with detailed scenarios that capture their attention and integrate clinical knowledge with community and public health concepts that are critical to real-world nursing practice. By watching the videos and completing related activities, students will flex their problem-solving, prioritizing, analyzing, and application skills to aid both in NCLEX preparation and preparation for practice.

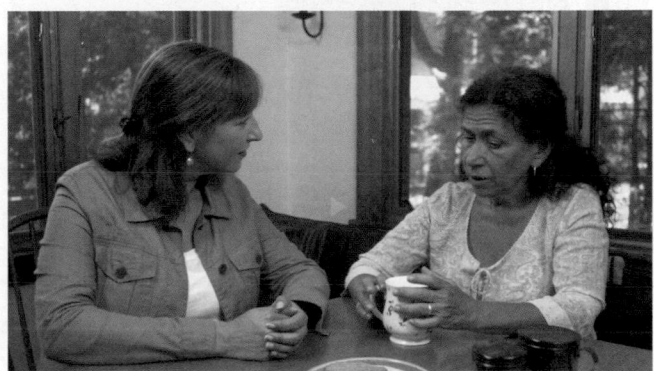

- Interactive Modules help students quickly identify what they do and do not understand, so they can study smartly. With exceptional instructional design that prompts students to discover, reflect, synthesize, and apply, students actively learn. Remediation links to the digital textbook are integrated throughout.
- Curated collections of journal articles are provided via Lippincott NursingCenter, Wolters Kluwer's premier destination for peer-reviewed nursing journals. Through integration of CoursePoint and NursingCenter, students will engage in how nursing research influences practice.
- Data to measure students' progress: Student performance data provided in an intuitive display lets instructors quickly assess whether students have viewed interactive modules and video cases outside of class, as well as see students' performance on related NCLEX style quizzes, ensuring students are coming to the classroom ready and prepared to learn.

To learn more about Lippincott CoursePoint, please visit www.nursingeducationsuccess.com/coursepoint

Lippincott
RN to BSN
Online

Lippincott RN to BSN Online: Nursing Research is a postlicensure solution for online and hybrid courses, marrying experiential learning with the trusted content in *Community and Public Health Nursing*, ninth edition.

Built around learning objectives that are aligned to the BSN Essentials and QSEN nursing curriculum standards, every aspect of Lippincott RN to BSN Online is designed to engage, challenge, and cultivate postlicensure students.

- Self-paced interactive modules employ key instructional design strategies—including storytelling, modeling, case-based and problem-based scenarios—to actively involve students in learning new material and focus students' learning outcomes on real-life application.

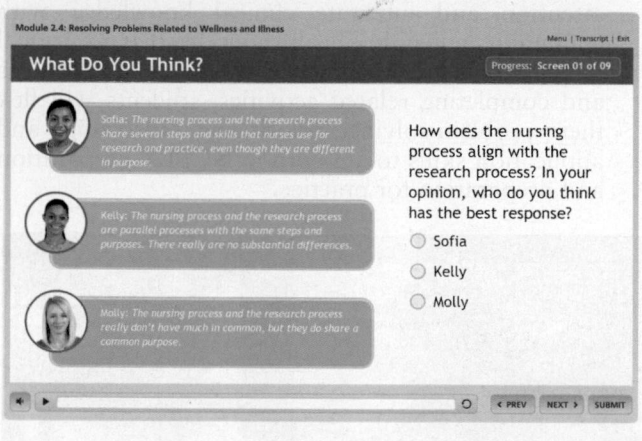

- Pre- and postmodule assessments activate students' existing knowledge prior to engaging with the module and then assess their competency after completing the module.
- Discussion board questions create an ongoing dialogue to foster social learning.
- Writing and group work assignments hone students' competence in writing and communication, instilling the skills needed to advance their nursing careers.
- Collated journal articles acquaint students to the body of nursing research ongoing in recent literature.
- Case study assignments, including unfolding cases that evolve from cases in the interactive modules, aid students in applying theory to real-life situations.
- Best Practices in Scholarly Writing Guide covers APA formatting and style guidelines.

Used alone or in conjunction with other instructor-created resources, Lippincott RN to BSN Online adds interactivity to courses. It also saves instructors time by keeping both textbook and course resources current and accurate through regular updates to the content.

To learn more about Lippincott RN to BSN Online, please visit http://www.nursingeducationsuccess.com/nursing-education-solutions/lippincott-rn-bsn-online/

CONTENTS

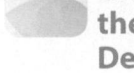

Community and Public Health Nursing

Promoting the Public's Health

FOUNDATIONS OF COMMUNITY HEALTH NURSING

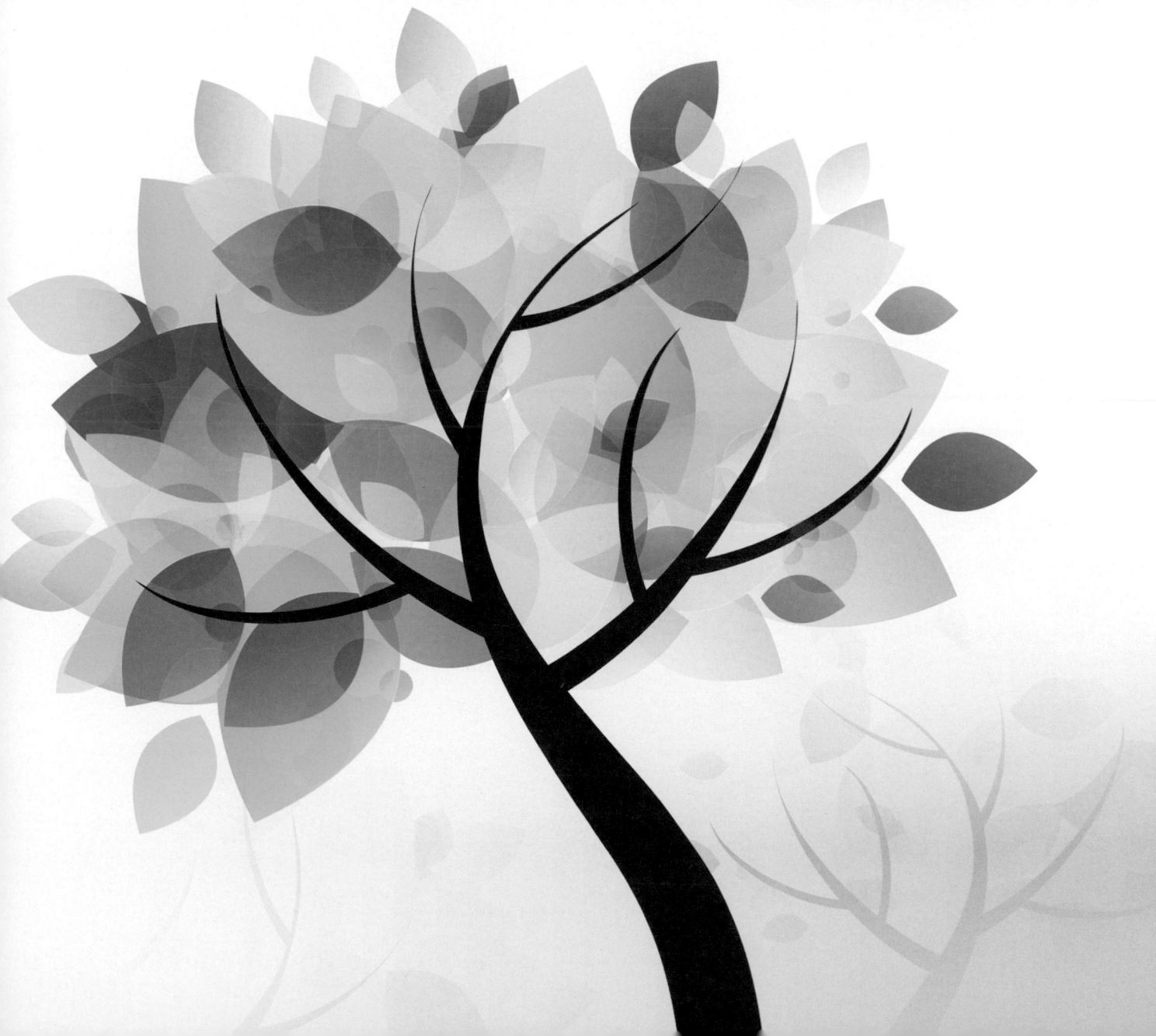

The Journey Begins: Introduction to Community Health Nursing

"For a community to be whole and healthy, it must be based on people's love and concern for each other."

—*Millard Fuller* (1935–2009), Founder, Habitat for Humanity

KEY TERMS

Aggregate
Collaboration
Community
Community health
Community health nursing
Continuous needs
Epigenetics

Episodic needs
Genomics
Geographic community
Global health
Health
Health continuum
Health literacy

Health promotion
Illness
Leading health indicators
Pharmacogenomics
Population
Population focused
Primary prevention

Public health
Public health nursing
Secondary prevention
Self-care
Self-care deficit
Tertiary prevention
Wellness

LEARNING OBJECTIVES

Upon mastery of this chapter, you should be able to:

- Define community health and distinguish it from public health.
- Explain the concept of community.
- Diagram the health continuum.
- Name 3 of the 10 leading health indicators.
- Discuss ways that public health nursing (PHN) practice is linked to acute care nursing practice.
- Discuss the two main components of community health practice (health promotion and disease prevention).
- Differentiate among the three levels of prevention.
- Describe the eight characteristics of community health nursing.

Opportunities and challenges in nursing are boundless and rapidly changing. You have spent a lot of time and effort learning how to care for individual patients in medical–surgical and other acute care–oriented nursing specialties. Now you are entering a unique and exciting area of nursing–community/public health.

As one of the oldest specialty nursing practices, public health nursing offers unique challenges and opportunities. A nurse entering this field will encounter the complex challenge of working with populations rather than just individual clients and the opportunity to carry on the heritage of early public health nursing efforts with the benefit of modern sensibilities. There is the challenge of expanding nursing's focus from the individual and family to encompass communities and the opportunity to affect the health status of populations. There also is the challenge of determining the needs of populations at risk and the opportunity to design interventions to specifically address their needs. There is the challenge of learning the complexities of a constantly changing health care system and the opportunity to help shape service delivery. Public health nursing is community based and, most importantly, it is population focused. Operating within an environment of rapid change and increasingly complex challenges, this nursing specialty holds the potential to shape the quality of community health services and improve the health of the general public.

You have provided nursing care in familiar acute care settings for the very ill, both young and old, but always with other professionals at your side. You have worked as part of a team, in close proximity, to welcome a new life, reestablish a client's health, or comfort someone toward a peaceful death. Now, you are being asked to leave that familiar acute care setting and go out into the community—into homes, schools, recreational facilities, work settings, parishes, and even street corners that are commonplace to your clients and unfamiliar to you. Here, you will find few or no monitoring devices, charts full of laboratory data, or professional and allied health workers at your side to assist you. You will be asked to use the nontangible skills of listening, assessing, planning, teaching, coordinating, evaluating, and referring. You will also draw on the skills you have learned throughout your acute care setting experiences (e.g., behavioral health nursing, women's, children's, adult health nursing) and begin to "think on your feet" in new and exciting situations. Often, your practice will be solo, and you will need to combine creativity, ingenuity, intuition, and resourcefulness along with these skills. You will be providing care not only to individuals but also to families and other groups in a variety of settings within the community. Talk about boundless opportunities and challenges! (See Perspectives: Student Voice.)

You may feel that this is too demanding. You may be anxious about how you will perform in this new setting. But perhaps, just perhaps, you might find that this new area is a rewarding kind of nursing—one that constantly challenges you, interests you, and allows you to work holistically with clients of all ages, at all stages of illness and wellness, one that absolutely demands the use of your critical thinking skills. And you may decide, when you finish your public health nursing course, that you have found your career choice. Even if you are not drawn away from acute care nursing, your community health nursing experience will give you a deeper understanding of the people for whom you provide care—where and how they live, the family and cultural dynamics at play, and the problems they will face when discharged from your care. You will

also discover myriad community agencies and resources to better assist you in providing a continuum of care for your clients. Finding out begins with understanding the concepts of community and health.

This chapter provides an overview of the basic concepts of community and health, the components of public health practice, and the salient characteristics of contemporary public health nursing practice, so that you can enter this specialty area of nursing in concert with its intentions. The opportunities and challenges of community health nursing will become even more apparent as the chapter progresses. The discussion of the concepts and theories that make public health nursing an important specialty within nursing begins with the broader field of community health, which provides the context for public health nursing practice.

COMMUNITY HEALTH

Human beings are social creatures. All of us, with rare exception, live out our lives in the company of other people. An Eskimo lives in a small, tightly knit community of close relatives; a rural Mexican may live in a small village with hardly more than 200 members. In contrast, someone from New York City might be a member of many overlapping communities, such as professional societies, a political party, a religious group, a cultural society, a neighborhood, and the city itself. Even those who try to escape community membership always begin their lives in some type of group, and they usually continue to depend on groups for material and emotional support. Communities are an essential and permanent feature of the human experience.

The communities in which we live and work have a profound influence on our collective health and well-being (Muth, 2015). How can community green spaces influence obesity rates in children? A research example may provide some clues. In a population-based study of schoolchildren, researchers in Spain found 11% to 19% lower levels of obesity and overweight, as well as less excessive screen time (TV and gaming), in residential areas that had surrounding green

PERSPECTIVES STUDENT VOICE

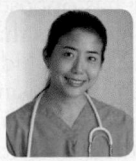

I was really terrified when I got to my community health rotation and found that I had to go to people's homes and knock on their doors! I was going to graduate in a few months, and I felt really comfortable in the hospital.... I knew the routines and the machines well. Now, I had to actually find houses and apartments in an area of the city I would normally never venture into! And it wasn't clear to me what I was supposed to do! I didn't have much equipment—a baby scale, a blood pressure cuff, a stethoscope, a thermometer, and a paper tape measure—that was all! I was told to go visit this 16-year-old mother who had a 4-month-old baby and to monitor the baby's progress. I don't even have children! What can I tell her? And, besides, she is a teenager who "knows it all." My clinical instructor told me to "build a relationship with her" and to "gain trust and rapport." That is hard to do when you are scared to death! I was afraid of her responses, of being out in that part of the city alone, and of trying to answer questions without anyone there to turn to. But I wanted to get through nursing school, so I drove over there and knocked on her door. I was shocked to see the condition of the apartment building in which she lived—peeling paint, loud music, trash everywhere, and strange characters at every turn. When she answered the door, she seemed uninterested—or maybe a little defensive. I told her who I was and why I was there, and she motioned me inside and pointed toward the baby, propped up on the tattered couch. I spent the next 15 weeks visiting Anna and her baby: weighing and measuring the baby, doing a Denver II and sharing the results with Anna, helping her schedule appointments for immunizations, listening to Anna's story of abuse and abandonment, and realizing that what I was doing was actually exciting and rewarding. By the end of my rotation, I was truly going to miss Anna and little José! He always smiled at me, and I enjoyed "playing" with him as I instructed her about baby-proofing her apartment, finding resources for food and clothing, and getting birth control. We even talked about how she could finish high school. I thought about Anna and José occasionally, when young mothers would bring their babies into the emergency department, where I worked after graduation. I learned from my community health nursing rotation that I needed to look beyond the bravado of a teenage mother and try to "connect" with her in order to assure that she would follow through with the antibiotics and antipyretics we were prescribing for her baby's dangerously high fever and serious infection. A year and a half after I graduated, one day when it had been particularly hectic but was now calming down, I glanced up to see Anna and José. She looked so relieved to see me! She was frantic with worry about the serious burn José had on his right hand. The other nurses were mumbling about "child abuse" and how "irresponsible teen mothers always were." I learned that Anna had left José with a neighbor for an hour while she visited a nearby high school to see about getting her GED. The older neighbor was not used to dealing with a busy toddler, and she had left the handle of a pan of refried beans where José could reach it. The team treated José's burn, and I gave Anna instructions for follow-up care. The bond we had developed was still there. She trusted me, and I knew that she would follow through with the instructions. I also knew that the other nurses who were making comments about her did not know Anna's circumstances. I feel that I am a more effective ER nurse because of the things I learned in community health. Someday, when I get tired of the hospital, I may try working as a public health nurse. You never know!

Courtney, Age 25

---

spaces (Dadvand et al., 2014). From the beginning, people have attempted to create healthier communities. Here are three recent examples:

- Before the historic Surgeon General's Report on Smoking and Health, it was common to see people smoking on television, at work, in restaurants, and even in physician offices (CDC, 2011; Kanarek et al., 2011). Since that report linked tobacco to disease and death more than 40 years ago, much has changed in our living spaces. In most states, it is now uncommon to see smoking in public places, and smokers are often relegated to outdoor smoking areas. With the assistance of the Master Settlement Agreement negotiated by state attorneys general and the tobacco industry in 1999, $206 billion has been given to states to promote smoking cessation; create smoke-free environments in the workplace, restaurants, and bars; and develop antismoking public information campaigns; however, during times of budget deficit, some funds were used to balance state budgets (Clark,

Sparks, McDonald, & Dickerson, 2011). Along with policy changes and settlements, public awareness has been raised about the harmful effects of secondhand smoke (Kroon, Corelli, Roth, & Hudmon, 2013). However, smoking still causes around 443,000 deaths annually in the United States, and by 2030, it is expected that 10 million people around the world will die annually because of smoking (Clark et al., 2011). Smokers tend to suffer diseases of old age on average 12 years earlier than do nonsmokers, and they also appear physically older (McEwen & Grothier, 2014). Although total U.S. consumption of tobacco products has dropped from 20.9% in 2005 to 17.8% in 2013, and many states have been successful in implementing strategies suggested by the Centers for Disease Control and Prevention (CDC) (e.g., raising prices of tobacco products, enacting laws for smoke-free public spaces, limiting tobacco advertising while utilizing antismoking campaigns, limiting access to tobacco vending machines or sales to minors, smoking cessation programs and hotlines), more needs to be done in order to reach the *Healthy People 2020* goal of adult cigarette smokers at or below 12% (Jamal et al., 2014). The Surgeon General has recommended further strategies (e.g., lowering nicotine content to nonaddictive levels, placing even greater restrictions on sales of products, and banning some categories of tobacco products completely) (Jamal et al., 2014). Even though 56% of Americans now report that they would like to make smoking in public places illegal, 19% generally oppose an outright ban on smoking, leaving a toehold for tobacco companies to promote the individual's right to choose smoking over the public's right to the health benefits of banning tobacco (Gallup, 2014). Vaping or using e-cigarettes is now being similarly banned in some areas (Moore, Chang, & Larson, 2014).

- More than 26 million American children and adults live with asthma. Evidence of a connection between asthma attacks and community environments has been demonstrated both in the United States and abroad (Iqbal, Oraka, Chew, & Flanders, 2014). Inner-city children have been shown to demonstrate higher rates of asthma, and research has shown strong allergic reactions, especially to rat and cat allergens (Rao et al., 2015). Public health officials note chronic environmental factors as a possible cause for increased asthma cases: pollution from high-traffic areas, secondhand smoke in homes, as well as poor living conditions characterized by dust mites, mold, industrial air pollution, mouse and cockroach droppings, and animal dander. However, research completed at Johns Hopkins University in 2015 counters that claim. Researchers examined records for 23,065 children living in 5,853 census tracts and found asthma prevalence of 12.9% for inner-city children and 10.6% for those living outside of inner cities. When they statistically adjusted for age, gender, region, and race/ethnicity, there was no statistical difference found. They noted that poverty increased the risk of asthma for children (Keet et al., 2015). For 2015, the city named "asthma capital" of the United States was Memphis, Tennessee (Asthma and Allergy Foundation of America [AAFA], 2015). Many of the asthma capitals were in the South, largely owing to the lack of smoke-free legislation in many tobacco-producing states, along with poor air quality and high pollen counts. To further make the case for a connection between environment and asthma, the 1996 Olympics in Atlanta brought an unexpected benefit: a 42% reduction in asthma-related emergency room visits. With the Olympic congestion downtown, Atlanta restricted traffic and thus improved air quality. The same outcomes were experienced with the Beijing Olympics. Internationally, Singapore also noticed a reduction in emergency room visits for asthma after it restricted automobile traffic in its central business district (Li, Wang, Zhang, Lin, & Yang, 2011).

- In a local effort to address the problem of childhood obesity, Santa Clara County—where one in four children are obese or overweight—passed an ordinance that sets standards for toys included with children's restaurant meals. It simply requires that the meals that include the toys meet basic nutritional standards. It does not ban toys. However, the fast food industry has opposed this effort, as they spend over $360 million on toys that encourage kids and parents to purchase 1.2 billion kids' meals annually. Second only to television advertising targeted to children, the toys given away with kids' meals are a substantial expenditure by the fast food industry. And interestingly, 10 of 12 meals with the highest calorie levels were found to include toys—indicating that these toys are used to market meals to children that may promote obesity (Public Health Institute, 2010). So, lawmakers counter that toys should only be used as an incentive for kids to purchase meals with lower sugar, sodium, fat, and calories; a model ordinance is now available on the Web for other communities to access (Change Lab Solutions, 2015). The community of Santa Clara, and later San Francisco, California, took a stand to improve their environment in order to address a serious health problem that is affecting their population.

Systems theory, advanced by biologist Ludwig von Bertalanffy in the 1940s and modified by Ross Ashby in the 1950s, proposes that systems are open that there is interaction between systems and their environment (European Meeting on Cybernetics and Systems Research [EMCSR], 2012). As systems theory reminds us that a whole is greater than the sum of its parts, the health of a community is more than the sum of the health of its individual citizens. A community that achieves a high level of wellness is composed of healthy citizens, functioning in an environment that protects and promotes health. Public health, as a specialty of nursing practice, seeks to provide organizational structure, a broad set of resources, and the collaborative activities needed to accomplish the goal of an optimally healthy community.

When you work in hospitals or other acute care settings, your primary focus is the individual patient. Patients' families are often viewed as ancillary. Public health, however, broadens the view to focus on families, aggregates, communities, and populations. The community becomes the recipient of service, and health becomes the product. Viewed from another perspective, public health is concerned with the interchange between population groups and their total environment and with the impact of that interchange on collective health. The narrow view of the solitary patient, so common in acute care nursing, is expanded to encompass a much wider vista.

Although many believe that health and illness are individual issues, evidence indicates that they are also community issues and that the world is a community. The spread of the human immunodeficiency virus (HIV) pandemic (nationally and internationally) is a dramatic and tragic case in point, having spread across the globe with 35 million people in 2013 living with HIV/AIDS and an additional 2.1 million new infections annually (AIDS. gov, 2014). Sadly, approximately 19 million do not know that they are infected with the virus. Other community, national, and global concerns include the rising incidence and prevalence of tuberculosis, second in infectious deaths only to HIV/AIDS (World Health Organization [WHO], 2015a), the serious international public health problem of cardiovascular disease (American Heart Association, 2015), the rise in antibiotic resistance that has led to calls for global treaties to combat resistant strains (Hoffman et al., 2015), terrorism, and pollution-driven environmental hazards. Whereas the United States and other developed nations continue to fight rising rates of obesity, many countries in Africa battle malnutrition and starvation. Communities can influence the spread of disease, provide barriers to protect members from health hazards, organize ways to combat outbreaks of infectious disease, and promote practices that contribute to individual and collective health (American Nurses Association [ANA], 2013; County Health Rankings, 2015; Institute of Medicine [IOM], 2002).

Many different professionals work in community health to form a complex team. The city planner designing an urban renewal project necessarily becomes involved in community health. The social worker providing counseling about child abuse or working with adolescent substance abusers is involved in public or community health. A physician treating clients affected by a sudden outbreak of hepatitis and assisting public health epidemiologists and PHNs to find the source is engaged in public health practice. Prenatal clinics, meals for the elderly, genetic counseling centers, and educational programs for the early detection of cancer all are part of the public health effort.

The professional nurse is an integral member of this team, a linchpin and a liaison between physicians, social workers, government officials, and law enforcement officers. Public health nurses work in every conceivable kind of community agency, from a state public health department to a community-based advocacy group. Their duties range from examining infants in a well-baby clinic to teaching elderly stroke victims in their homes to planning community and population-focused interventions (e.g., marketing campaigns to reduce tobacco use) to carrying out epidemiologic research or engaging in health policy analysis and decision-making. Despite its breadth, however, public health nursing is a specialized practice. It combines all of the basic elements of professional clinical nursing with public health and community practice. Together, we will examine the unique contribution made by community health nursing to our health care system.

Community health and public health share many features. Both are organized community efforts aimed at the promotion, protection, and preservation of the public's health. Historically, as a practice specialty, public health has been associated primarily with the efforts of official or government entities—for example, federal, state, or local tax-supported health agencies that target a wide range of health issues. In contrast, private health efforts or nongovernmental organizations (NGOs), such as those of the American Lung Association or the American Cancer Society, work toward solving selected health problems. The latter augments the former. Currently, community health practice encompasses both approaches and works collaboratively with all health agencies and efforts, public or private, which are concerned with the public's health. In this text, community health practice refers to a focus on specific, designated communities. It is a part of the larger

PERSPECTIVES
PUBLIC HEALTH NURSING INSTRUCTOR

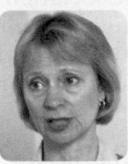

When I first introduce the topic of public health, I ask students "Why do people end up in the hospital?" Many of them give the usual answers—"They need surgery," "They get in accidents," and the like. Then, I tell them the *Story of Jason*:

"Why is Jason in the hospital? (Because he has a bad infection in his leg.)

But why does he have an infection? (Because he has a cut on his leg and it got infected.) But why does he have a cut on his leg? (Because he was playing in the junkyard next to his apartment building and there was some sharp, jagged steel there that he fell on.)

But why was he playing in a junkyard? (Because his neighborhood is kind of run-down. A lot of kids play there, and there is no one to supervise them.)

But why does he live in that neighborhood? (Because his parents can't afford a nicer place to live.)

But why can't his parents afford a nicer place to live? (Because his Dad is unemployed and his Mom is sick.)

But why was his Dad unemployed? (Because he doesn't have much education and he can't find a job.) But why…?"

And they suddenly become more aware of the complex social and economic issues that affect health (Public Health Agency of Canada, 1999. *Toward a Healthy Future: Second Report on the Health of Canadians*, p. vii.).

public health effort and recognizes the fundamental concepts and principles of public health as its birthright and foundation for practice.

In the IOM's landmark publication, *The Future of the Public's Health* (1998), the mission of public health is defined simply as "fulfilling society's interest in assuring conditions in which people can be healthy" (p. 7). (See Perspectives: Public Health Nursing Instructor.) Winslow's classic 1920 definition of **public health** still holds true and forms the basis for our understanding of community health in this text:

> Public health… is the science and art of preventing disease, prolonging life, and promoting health and efficiency through organized community efforts for the sanitation of the environment, the control of communicable infections, the education of the individual in personal hygiene, the organization of medical and nursing services for the early diagnosis and preventive treatment of disease, and the development of the social machinery to insure everyone a standard of living adequate for the maintenance of health (Clinton County Health Department, n.d., para. 1).

More recent and concise definitions of public health include "an effort organized by society to protect, promote, and restore the people's health" (Last, 2014, p. 1) and "the health of the population as a whole rather than medical health care, which focuses on treatment of the individual ailment" (LMAS District Health Department, n.d., para. 1). A Web site sponsored by the Association of Schools of Public Health with support from Pfizer Public Health, *What Is Public Health?* (ASPH, 2015), provides some interesting videos and information about this topic and also proffers this definition:

> Public health protects and improves the health of individuals, families, communities, and populations locally and globally (para. 1).
>
> The public health field confronts global health issues, such as improving access to health care, controlling infectious disease, and reducing environmental hazards, violence, substance abuse, and injury (para. 3).
>
> Public health professionals focus on preventing disease and injury by promoting healthy lifestyles. (para. 2).

The core public health functions have been delineated as assessment, policy development, and assurance. These are discussed in more detail in Chapter 3.

Given this basic understanding of public health, the concept of community health can be defined. **Community health** is the identification of needs, along with the protection and improvement of collective health, within a geographically defined area.

One of the challenges public health practice faces is to remain responsive to the community's health needs. As a result, its structure is complex; numerous health services and programs are currently available or will be developed. Examples include health education, family planning, accident prevention, environmental protection, immunization, nutrition, early periodic screening and developmental testing, school programs, mental health services, occupational health programs, and the care of vulnerable populations. The Department of Homeland Security, for example, is a community health and safety agency developed in the aftermath of the terrorist attacks on New York City and Washington, DC, on September 11, 2001.

Community health practice, a part of public health, is sometimes misunderstood. Even many health professionals think of community health practice in limiting terms such as sanitation programs, health clinics in poverty areas, or massive public awareness campaigns to prevent communicable disease. Although these are a part of its ever-broadening focus, community health practice is much more. To understand the nature and significance of this field, it is necessary to more closely examine the concept of community and the concept of health.

THE CONCEPT OF COMMUNITY

The concepts of community and health together provide the foundation for understanding community health. Broadly defined, a community is a collection of people who share some important feature of their lives. In this text, the term **community** refers to a collection of people who interact with one another and whose common interests or characteristics form the basis for a sense of unity or belonging. It can be a society of people holding common rights and privileges (e.g., citizens of a town), sharing common interests (e.g., a community of farmers), or living under the same laws and regulations (e.g., a prison community). The function of any community includes its members' collective sense of belonging and their shared identity, values, norms, communication, and common interests and concerns (Anderson & McFarlane, 2015). Some communities—for example, a tiny village in Appalachia—are composed of people who share almost everything. They live in the same location, work at a limited type and number of jobs, attend the same churches, and make use of the sole health clinic with its visiting physician and nurse. Other communities, such as members of Mothers Against Drunk Driving (MADD) or the community of professional nursing organizations, are large, scattered, and composed of individuals who share only a common interest and involvement in a certain goal. Although most communities of people share many aspects of their experience, it is useful to identify three types of communities that have relevance to community health practice: geographic, common interest, and health problem or solution. Unit 4 contains more in-depth information about the community as client.

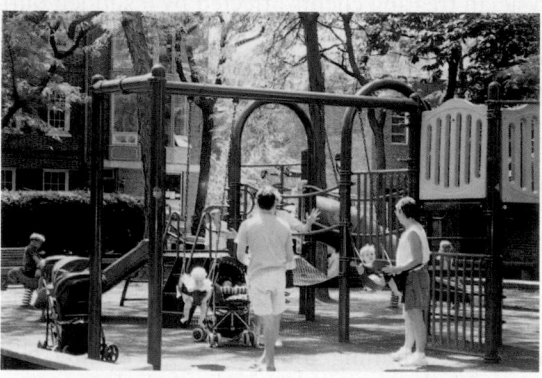

Geographic Community

A community often is defined by its geographic boundaries and thus is called a **geographic community**. A city, town, or neighborhood is a geographic community. Consider the community of Hayward, Wisconsin. Located in northwestern Wisconsin, it is set in the north woods environment, far removed from any urban center and in a climatic zone characterized by extremely harsh winters. With a population of approximately 2,300, it is considered a rural community. The population has certain identifiable characteristics, such as age and sex ratios, and its size fluctuates with the seasons: summers bring hundreds of tourists and seasonal residents. Hayward is a social system as well as a geographic location. The families, schools, hospital, churches, stores, and government institutions are linked in a complex network. This community, like others, has an informal power structure. It has a communication system that includes gossip, the newspaper, the "co-op" store bulletin board, and the radio stations. In one sense, then, a community consists of a collection of people located in a specific place and is made up of institutions organized into a social system.

Local communities such as Hayward vary in size. A few miles south of Hayward lay several other communities, including Northwoods Beach and Round Lake;

these three, along with other towns and isolated farms, form a larger community called Sawyer County. If a nurse worked for a health agency serving only Hayward, that community would be of primary concern; however, if the nurse worked for the Sawyer County Health Department, this larger community would be the focus. A public health nurse employed by the State Health Department in Madison, Wisconsin, would have an interest in Sawyer County and Hayward, but only as part of the larger community of Wisconsin.

Frequently, a single part of a city can be treated as a community. Cities are often broken down into *census tracts*, or neighborhoods. In Seattle, for example, the district near the waterfront forms a community of many transient and homeless people. In New York City, the neighborhood called Harlem is a community, as is the Haight-Ashbury district of San Francisco.

In community health, it is useful to identify a geographic area as a community. A community demarcated by geographic boundaries, such as a city or county, becomes a clear target for the analysis of health needs. Available data, such as morbidity and mortality figures, can augment assessment studies to form the basis for planning health programs. Media campaigns and other health education efforts can readily reach intended audiences. Examples include distributing educational information on safe sex, self-protection, the dangers of substance abuse, or where to seek shelter from abuse and violence. A geographic community is easily mobilized for action. Groups can be formed to carry out intervention and prevention efforts that address needs specific to that community. Such efforts might include more stringent policies on day care, shelters for battered women, work site safety programs in local hazardous industries, or improved sexuality education in the schools. Furthermore, health actions can be enhanced through the support of politically powerful individuals and resources present in a geographic community.

On a larger scale, the world can be considered as a global community. Indeed, it is very important to view the world this way. Borders of countries change with political upheaval. Communicable diseases are not aware of arbitrary political boundaries. A person can travel around the world in <24 hours, and so can diseases. Children starving in Africa affect persons living in the United States. Political uprisings in the Middle East have an impact on people in Western countries. Floods or tsunamis in Southeast Asia or volcano eruptions in Iceland have meaning for other national economies. The world is one large community that needs to work together in order to ensure a healthy today and a healthier and safer tomorrow. **Global health** has become a dominant phrase in international public health circles. Globalization raises an expectation of health for all, for if good health is possible in one part of the world, the forces of globalization should allow it elsewhere and everyone then enjoys the benefits (InterAction, 2013). Governments need to work together to develop a broader base for international relations and collaborative strategies that will place greater emphasis on global health security. We learn more about global health issues and the global community in Chapter 16.

Common-Interest Community

A community also can be identified by a common interest or goal. A collection of people, even if they are widely scattered geographically, can have an interest or goal that binds the members together. This is known as a *common-interest community*. The members of a church in a large metropolitan area, the members of an international nursing professional organization, and families who have lost members to suicide are all common-interest communities. Sometimes, within a certain geographic area, a group of people may develop a sense of community by promoting their common interest. Disabled individuals scattered throughout a large city may emerge as a community through a common interest in promoting adherence to federal guidelines for wheelchair access, parking spaces, toilet facilities, elevators, or other services for the disabled. The residents of an industrial community may develop a common interest in air or water pollution issues, whereas others who work but do not live in the area may not share that interest. Communities form to protect the rights of children, stop violence against women, clean up the environment, promote the arts, preserve historical sites, protect endangered species, develop a smoke-free environment, or provide support after a crisis. The kinds of shared interests that lead to the formation of communities vary widely.

Common-interest communities whose focus is a health-related issue can join with community health agencies to promote their agendas. A group's single-minded commitment is a mobilizing force for action. Many successful prevention and health promotion efforts, including improved services and increased community awareness of specific problems, have resulted from the work of common-interest communities. MADD is one example. In 1980, after a repeat drunk-driving offender killed her 13-year-old daughter Cari, Candace Lightner gathered with a group of outraged mothers at a restaurant in Sacramento, California. Across the country, another mother was soon touched by a similar tragedy. Cindi Lamb's five-and-a-half-month-old infant daughter became a quadriplegic at the hands of a repeat drunk driver. Within a short time, the two women joined forces to form MADD, and 2 years later, President Ronald Reagan organized a Presidential Task Force on drunk driving and invited MADD to participate. With media attention and perseverance, MADD quickly grew to over 100 chapters across the United States and Canada and worked to establish a federal legal minimum drinking age and standard blood alcohol levels of 0.08%, as well as to defend sobriety checkpoints before the Supreme Court. The National Highway Transportation and Safety Administration credited MADD when they released the 1994 figures showing a 30-year low in alcohol-related traffic deaths. Even though our U.S. numbers have dropped considerably, still, in 2013, over 10,000 people were killed and almost 300,000 injured by drunk drivers. MADD now claims more than 3 million members worldwide and is one of the largest and most successful common-interest organizations (MADD, 2015). Similar dangers exist with texting and driving, but the common-interest community has not yet solidified behind this cause as with MADD. About one third of drivers between 18 and 64 admit to texting while driving, and 341,000 accidents in 2013 resulted from texting while driving. Forty-six states ban texting while driving, but much still needs to be done (Schumaker, 2015).

Community of Solution

A type of community encountered frequently in community health practice is a group of people who come together to solve a problem that affects all of them. The shape of this community varies with the nature of the problem, the size of the geographic area affected, and the number of resources needed to address the problem. Such a community has been called a *community of solution.* For example, a water pollution problem may involve several counties whose agencies and personnel must work together to control upstream water supply, industrial waste disposal, and city water treatment. This group of counties forms a community of solution focusing on a health problem. In another instance, several schools may collaborate with law enforcement and health agencies, as well as legislators and policy makers, to study patterns of substance abuse among students and design possible preventive approaches. The boundaries of this community of solution form around the schools, agencies, and political figures involved. Figure 1–1 depicts some communities of solution related to a single city.

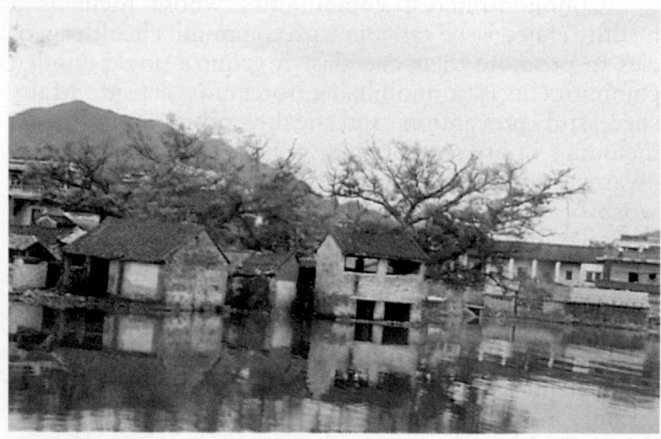

In recent years, communities of solution have formed in many cities to attack the spread of HIV/AIDS and have worked with community members to assess public safety and security and create plans to make the community a safer place in which to live. Public health agencies, social service groups, schools, and media personnel have banded together to create public awareness of dangers that are present and to promote preventive behaviors (e.g., childhood obesity). The 1967 Folsom Report recognized that community problem solving is often hampered by the very administrative and political entities and structures that should be helping. Instead, they often create "barriers to communication and compromise," and thus communities of solution must step in (Griswold, Lesko, & Westfall, for the Folsom Group, 2013, p. 232). More integration of health services (e.g., acute care, ambulatory, community care) to create better value and streamlined services, creation of larger networks, opportunities for partnerships, recognition of existing barriers and environmental hazards, better

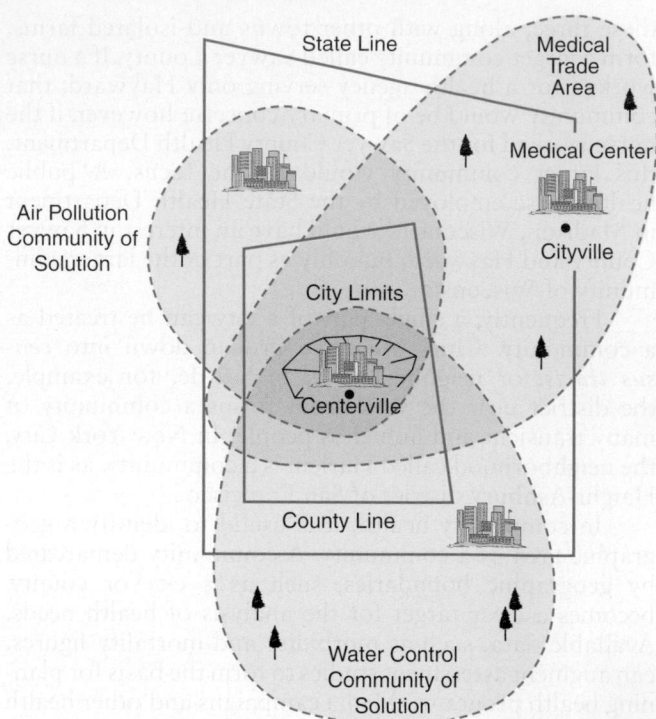

FIGURE 1–1 A city's communities of solution. State, county, and city boundaries (*solid lines*) may have little or no bearing on health solution boundaries (*dashed lines*).

coordination between community partners and governmental authorities, and sharing of technology and knowledge are all critical components in communities of solution. One example is HeartBeat Connections, a community of solution in a rural area, that acknowledged the most common barriers for clinical cardiovascular disease prevention (e.g., lack of follow-up, lack of time) and organized an interprofessional team using telephone outreach to manage medications and provide counseling and education. They also integrated medical care and public health by connecting clients to farmers' markets, fitness facilities, weight management classes, and other community resources. Another program examined social determinants of health in an inner-city area of Milwaukee to create a chronic disease management program located in food pantries. Nurse-led teams of community health workers and faith-based volunteers focused on clients with high cholesterol, hypertension, and diabetes (Griswold et al., 2013). A community of solution is an important conduit for change in community health.

Populations and Aggregates

The three types of communities just discussed underscore the meaning of the concept of community: in each instance, a collection of people chose to interact with one another because of common interests, characteristics, or goals. The concept of population has a different meaning. In this text, the term **population** refers to all of the people occupying an area or to all of those who share one or more characteristics. In contrast to a community, a *population* is made up of people who do not necessarily interact with one another and do not necessarily share a sense of belonging to that group. A population may be defined geographically, such as the population of the United States or a city's population. This designation of a population is useful in community health for epidemiologic study and for collecting demographic data for purposes such as health planning. A population also may be defined by common qualities or characteristics, such as the elderly population, the homeless population, or a particular racial or ethnic group. In community health, this meaning becomes useful when a specific group of people (e.g., homeless individuals) is targeted for intervention; the population's common characteristics (e.g., the health-related problems of homelessness) become a major focus of the intervention.

In this text, the term *aggregate* refers to a mass or grouping of distinct individuals who are considered as a whole and who are loosely associated with one another. It is a broader term that encompasses many different-sized groups. Both communities and populations are types of aggregates. The aggregate focus, or a concern for groupings of people in contrast to individual health care, becomes a distinguishing feature of community health practice. Community health nurses may work with aggregates such as pregnant and parenting teens, elderly adults with diabetes, or gay men with HIV/AIDS. Unit 6 discusses public health nursing with aggregates and Unit 7 discusses vulnerable populations.

Most registered nurses (RNs) in the United States work in hospitals (56% in 2013), revealing a similar percentage in 2004. These nurses most often work with individuals, not aggregates or communities. However, over 14% of RNs work in public or community health and home health settings and have a greater focus on families and communities (Budden, Zhong, Moulton, & Cimiotti, 2013). With health care reform legislation, the nursing workforce in public health, home visitation programs, and nurse-managed health centers is being expanded, and grant funding for nursing faculty and advanced practice nurses is more readily available (American Nurses Association [ANA], 2014). Dr. David Satcher, former U.S. Surgeon General, has remarked:

> Nurses have always been ahead of their time in their focus on prevention and health promotion. As we move toward a more balanced health system with more focus and support for health promotion and disease prevention, the role of nurses will be more significant than ever before. (Delack, 2010)

Because of public health nursing's focus on communities, aggregates, and families, new nursing and health care delivery systems may be developed that are more gainful and effective in preventing health problems that require expensive hospitalizations.

Community health workers, including community health nurses, need to define the community targeted for study and intervention: Who are the people who comprise the community? Where are they located, and what are their characteristics? A clear delineation of the community or population must be established before the nurse can assess needs and design interventions. The complex nature of communities also must be understood. What are the characteristics of the people in terms of age, gender, race, socioeconomic level, and health status? How does the community interact with other communities? What is its history? What are its resources? Is the community undergoing rapid change, and, if so, what are the changes? These questions, as well as the tools needed to assess a community for health purposes, are discussed in detail in Chapter 15.

THE CONCEPT OF HEALTH

Health, in the abstract, refers to a person's physical, mental, and spiritual state; it can be positive (as being in good health) or negative (as being in poor health). Optimal health is defined in a seminal article by a well-known health care consultant as "a dynamic balance of physical, emotional, social, spiritual, and intellectual health" (O'Donnell, 2009, p. iv). In a classic article from 1997, Sarrachi describes health as a "basic and universal human right" (p. 1409). The World Health Organization (WHO) offers a positive explanation of health as "a state of complete physical, mental, and social wellbeing and not merely the absence of disease or infirmity" (WHO, 2015b, para. 1). Our understanding of the concept of health builds on this classic definition. **Health**, in this text, refers to a holistic state of well-being, which includes soundness of mind, body, and spirit. Community health practitioners place a strong emphasis on **wellness**, which includes this definition of health, but also incorporate the capacity to develop a person's potential to lead a fulfilling and productive life—one that can be measured in terms of *quality of life*. Today, our health is greatly affected by the lifestyles we lead, the preventive measure we take, and the risk behaviors in which we engage (Chong, Tsunaka, Tsang, Chan, & Cheung, 2011). An individual's behavioral risk factors, such as smoking, physical inactivity, or substance abuse, can be assessed through the use of various interview techniques and questionnaires or surveys (Anderson et al., 2014; Humeniuk et al., 2011). The Behavioral Risk Factor Surveillance Survey, the Youth Risk Behavior Survey, Jackson's Smoking Susceptibility Scale, and the Physical Activity and Nutrition Behaviors Monitoring Form are some examples.

There is an increasing awareness of the strong relationship of health to environment. This is not a new concept. Almost 150 years ago, Florence Nightingale explored the health and illness connection with the environment. She believed that a person's health was greatly influenced by ventilation, noise, light, cleanliness, diet, and a restful bed (Leffers, McDermott-Levy, Smith, & Sattler, 2014). She laid down simple rules about maintaining and obtaining "health," which were written for laywomen caring for family members to "put the constitution in such a state as that it will have no disease" (Nightingale, 1859/1992, preface). The "built environment" is a concept under study by public health and other professionals, as it is well documented that the man-made structures and surroundings in a community (e.g., highways and bike paths, parks and open spaces, public buildings, and housing developments) have an impact on the health of individuals and populations (CDC, 2016a; Hystad et al., 2014; Trowbridge & Schmid, 2013). Environment's relationship to health is discussed in more detail in Chapter 9.

In some cultures, health is viewed differently. Some see it as the freedom from and absence of evil. Illness may be seen as punishment for being bad or doing evil (Galanti, 2013). Many individuals come from families in which beliefs regarding health and illness are heavily influenced by religion, superstition, folk beliefs, or "old wives' tales." This is not unusual, and encountering such beliefs when working with various groups in the community is common. Chapter 5 explores these beliefs more thoroughly for a better understanding of how health beliefs influence every aspect of a person's life, as well as principles of transcultural nursing in the community.

Prerequisites for health were outlined in the WHO (2015b) as "peace, shelter, education, food, income, a stable eco-system, sustainable resources, social justice, and equity" (para. 4). Although health is widely accepted as desirable, the nature of health is often ambiguous. Consumers and providers often define health and wellness in different ways. To clarify the concept for nurses who are considering community health practice, the distinguishing features of health are briefly characterized here; the implications of this concept for professionals in the field can then be examined more fully.

The Health Continuum: Wellness–Illness

Society suggests a polarized or "either/or" way of thinking about health: either people are well or they are ill. Yet, wellness is a relative concept, not an absolute, and **illness** is a state of being *relatively* unhealthy. The study of factors affecting health and illness is known as epidemiology, and it is discussed in Chapter 7. There are many levels and degrees of wellness and illness, from a robust 75-year-old woman who is fully active and functioning at an optimal level of wellness to a 75-year-old man with end-stage renal disease whose health is characterized as frail. Someone recovering from pneumonia may be mildly ill, whereas a teenaged boy with functional limitations because of episodic depression may be described as mildly well.

The continuum, however, can change. The Human Genome Project, begun in 1990 and completed in 2003, ushered in the genomic era of health care. This project has the potential to move the health continuum toward greater health. *Genomics*, the identification and plotting of human genes and the study of the interaction of genes with each other and the environment, is beginning to alter how we view and treat disease. Intervention services can be individually designed based on genetic findings, and client lifestyle modifications may be recommended from birth—a very powerful type of preventive health care. In the last 10 years, specific genes for about 3,000 mendelian (monogenic) diseases have been discovered, and genetic links between over 900 gene locations and complex traits (multigenic) diseases have been established (Green, Guyer, & National Human Genome Research Institute, 2011). **Pharmacogenomics** can now, in limited fashion, permit the design of drugs tailored to a person's genetic makeup or to a targeted disease. For example, we now have "rapid genomic analysis" of tumors in a relatively quick period of time (days, not months) and are able to determine the

"molecular taxonomy" of the disease along with which treatment is most effective in fighting specific breast cancers (Green et al., 2011, p. 209). This has also shown promise with brain tumors (Carey, 2015). Currently, those with a family history of breast and ovarian cancer are encouraged to look into genetic counseling and testing for BRCA 1/2 mutations, and individuals diagnosed with colon cancer have genetic counseling and testing options to determine if their cancer is an hereditary form called Lynch syndrome. These innovations are already credited with saving lives (U.S. Department of Health and Human Services [USDHHS], 2016b). We may soon be able to identify individuals who may have adverse reactions to medications, based upon their genetic susceptibility, and could create "epigenetic test panels for obesity" (Cordero, Li, & Oben, 2015, p. 361; Green et al., 2011). Already, hundreds of biotech products are in clinical trials, some involving the connection between genetics, microbes, and disease (Furusawa, Horinouchi, Hirasawa, & Shimizu, 2013). The capacity for this new age of health care will be a reality over the next decade, and we must guard against limiting access to this type of care and permitting further disenfranchisement of vulnerable populations while safeguarding information, protecting human subjects, and assuring ethical oversight (Green et al., 2011). Ethical issues such as this will be discussed in more detail in Chapter 4.

Other innovations in **epigenetics**, the study of human gene activity changes not involving alterations in DNA that can be passed from one generation to the next, may be even more astounding. Epigenetic marks can turn genes off and on and help explain why "environmental factors like diet, stress, and prenatal nutrition can make an imprint on genes... passed from one generation to the next" (Cloud, 2010, para. 8); there is some evidence that a substantial component of risk for metabolic disease (e.g., adult obesity) has a basis in prenatal development (Godfrey et al., 2011). Lifestyle choices like overeating, smoking, and drug use may influence genes that affect obesity and longevity, for instance, to be more strongly or weakly expressed. Drugs have already been developed for some epigenetic marks (e.g., blood malignancies, tumors), and this area of science holds promise in discovering why, for instance, autism is more frequently found in boys or why one twin develops asthma when the other does not. The Human Epigenome Project has begun but will take much more time and technological advances in order to achieve success than the Human Genome Project did. Leaders in the field of epigenetics estimate that it will be another decade before we will be able to determine "how one person's epigenome differs from another" (Powledge, 2015, para. 11).

Because health involves a range of degrees from optimal health at one end to total disability or death at the other (Fig. 1–2), it often is described as a continuum. This **health continuum** applies not only to individuals but also to families and communities. A nurse might speak of a *dysfunctional family*, meaning one that is experiencing a relative degree of illness or altered functioning; or a healthy family might be described as one that exhibits many wellness characteristics, such as effective communication and conflict resolution, as well as the ability to

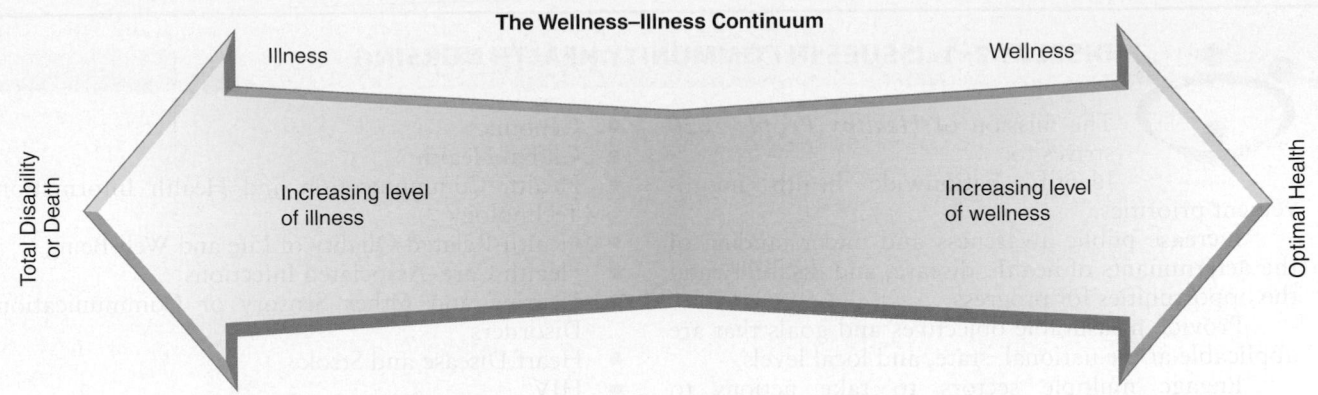

The level (degree) of illness increases as one moves toward total disability or death; the level of wellness increases as one moves toward optimal health. This continuum shows the relative nature of health. At any given time a person can be placed at some point along the continuum.

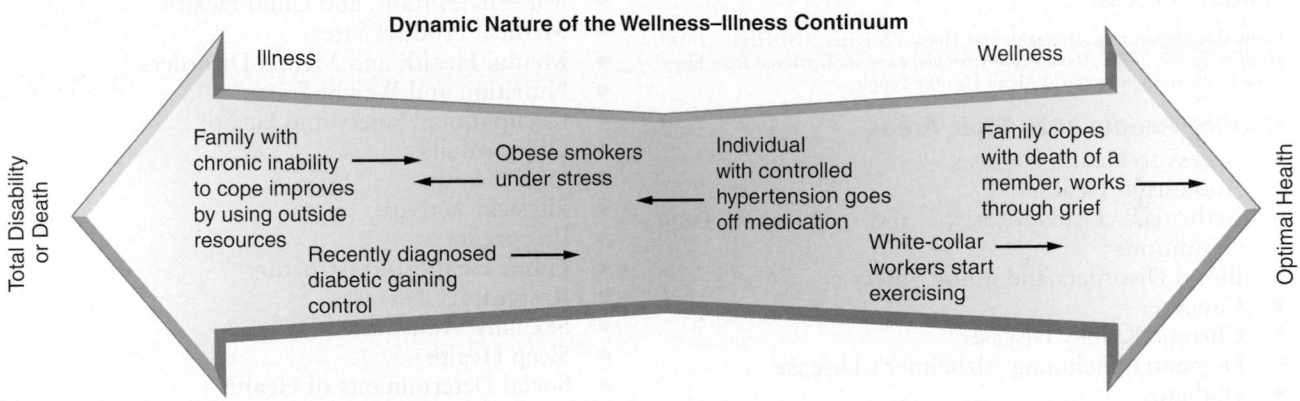

A person's relative health is usually in a state of flux, either improving or deteriorating. This diagram of the wellness-illness continuum shows several examples of people in changing states of health.

FIGURE 1–2 The health continuum.

effectively work together and use resources appropriately. More information on families is included in Unit 5.

Likewise, a community, as a collection of people, may be described in terms of degrees of wellness or illness. The health of an individual, family, group, or community moves back and forth along this continuum throughout the lifespan. Healthy people make healthy communities and a healthy society. The Declaration of Alma Ata, which took place in 1978, noted that health is a "fundamental human right" and that the level of health must be raised for all countries in order for any society to improve their health (WHO, 2015c, para. 2).

By thinking of health relatively, as a matter of degree, the scope of nursing practice can be broadened to focus on preventing illness or disability as well as promoting wellness. Traditionally, most health care has focused on treatment of acute and chronic conditions at the illness end of the continuum. Gradually, the emphasis is shifting to focus on the wellness end of the continuum, as outlined in the government document, *Healthy People 2020* (U.S. Department of Health and Human Services [USDHHS], 2016a). This effort aims to improve the health of American citizens by establishing objectives and benchmarks that can be monitored over time. There have been Healthy People objectives for 2000, 2010, and now

for 2020. The four overarching goals of *Healthy People 2020* are to:

- Attain high-quality, longer lives free of preventable disease, disability, injury, and premature death
- Achieve health equity, eliminate disparities, and improve the health of all groups
- Create social and physical environments that promote good health for all
- Promote quality of life, healthy development, and healthy behaviors across all life stages (para. 5)

These goals overarch the 42 topics and objectives (see Display 1–1). The objectives are stated in measurable terms that specify targeted incidence and prevalence changes and address age, gender, and culturally vulnerable groups along with improvement in public health systems. Progress toward the *Healthy People 2010* objectives has been mixed, with the final report noting that out of 969 original objectives, only 733 had reliable sources of data tracking. Of those final 733 objectives, 23% met or exceeded targets, 48% moved toward the target, 5% showed no change, and 24% actually moved away from the target (CDC, 2013). Whereas our life expectancy has improved and childhood immunization rates have risen, with some advancement toward reducing racial

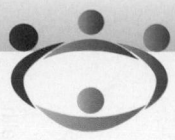

DISPLAY 1-1   ISSUES IN COMMUNITY HEALTH NURSING

The mission of *Healthy People 2020* strives to:

Identify nationwide health improvement priorities.

Increase public awareness and understanding of the determinants of health, disease, and disability and the opportunities for progress.

Provide measurable objectives and goals that are applicable at the national, state, and local levels.

Engage multiple sectors to take actions to strengthen policies and improve practices that are driven by the best available evidence and knowledge

Identify critical research, evaluation, and data collection needs.

From U.S. Department of Health and Human Services (USDHHS). (2016). *Healthy People 2020: About healthy people, para. 4.* Retrieved from http://www.healthypeople.gov/2020/About-Healthy-People).

Healthy People 2020 Topic Areas

- Access to Health Services
- Adolescent Health
- Arthritis, Osteoporosis, and Chronic Back Conditions
- Blood Disorders and Blood Safety
- Cancer
- Chronic Kidney Disease
- Dementia, including Alzheimer's Disease
- Diabetes
- Disability and Health
- Early and Middle Childhood
- Educational and Community-Based Programs
- Environmental Health
- Family Planning
- Food Safety

- Genomics
- Global Health
- Health Communication and Health Information Technology
- Health-Related Quality of Life and Well-Being
- Health Care–Associated Infections
- Hearing and Other Sensory or Communication Disorders
- Heart Disease and Stroke
- HIV
- Immunization and Infectious Diseases
- Injury and Violence Prevention
- Lesbian, Gay, Bisexual, and Transgender Health
- Maternal, Infant, and Child Health
- Medical Product Safety
- Mental Health and Mental Disorders
- Nutrition and Weight Status
- Occupational Safety and Health
- Older Adults
- Oral Health
- Physical Activity
- Preparedness
- Public Health Infrastructure
- Respiratory Diseases
- Sexually Transmitted Diseases
- Sleep Health
- Social Determinants of Health
- Substance Abuse
- Tobacco Use
- Vision

From U.S. Department of Health and Human Services (USDHHS). (2016). *Healthy People 2020: Topics & objectives.* Retrieved from http://www.healthypeople.gov/2020/topicsobjectives2020/default

---

and ethnic disparities, our rates of obesity and diabetes have risen well beyond baseline levels from the previous decade (CDC, 2013). The **leading health indicators** for *Healthy People 2020*, an outcomes metric for measuring progress toward national public health goals, are found in Display 1–2.

Community health practice ranges across the entire health continuum; it always works to improve the degree of health in individuals, families, groups, and communities. In particular, community health practice emphasizes the promotion and preservation of wellness and the prevention of illness or disability. *Healthy People 2010* and *Healthy People 2020* emphasize that the health of an individual is linked to the health of the larger community and that this larger community's health is related to the health of the corresponding state and ultimately our nation (Barile et al., 2013).

Community characteristics of health have been described by the Centers for Disease Control as health-related quality of life indicators. Early descriptions included such things as rates of poverty and unemployment, levels of high school education and severe work

disability, mortality rates, and the proportion of adolescent births (Kanarek et al., 2000). However, even what most people would consider lifestyle choices (e.g., dietary patterns leading to obesity, reduced levels of physical activity, smoking, alcohol consumption) can be strongly influenced by environmental factors. Canada has examined such factors as income distribution, life stress, body mass index (BMI) and dietary practices, smoking and alcohol use, unemployment rate, leisure time physical activity, number of health professionals, as well as the total health expenditures in their list of health indicators (Public Health Agency, 2013). The *Community Health Status Indicators Project* provides county-level reports related to such things as infectious and chronic diseases, health-related quality of life, behavioral risk factors, vulnerable populations, causes of death, births, and summary measures of health and health disparities (Kanarek, Tsai, & Stanley, 2011). How does the United States compare to other developed countries on population health indicators? (See Chapter 6 for details.) *Partnerships to Improve Community Health* and *Racial and Ethnic Approaches to Community Health (REACH)* are programs designed

DISPLAY 1–2 LEADING HEALTH INDICATORS

The leading health indicators are used to measure the health of the nation. There are 26 indicators arranged under 12 general topics. Each of the leading health indicators has one or more objectives from *Healthy People 2010* associated with it. As a group, the leading health indicators reflect the major health concerns in the United States, and progress toward the goals derived from these will be assessed during the 2010–2020 time period. The leading health indicators were selected on the basis of their ability to motivate action, the availability of data to measure progress, and their importance as public health issues. The federal consumer health information Web site, www.healthfinder.gov, is a good starting point for more information on these topics. The Progress Update is available for download at www.healthypeople.gov.

Access to Health Services
- Increase the proportions of persons with health insurance (AHS-1.1).
- Increase the proportion of persons who have a usual primary provider (AHS-3).

Clinical Preventive Services
- Increase the proportion of adults who receive a colorectal cancer screening based on the most recent guidelines (C-16).
- Increase the proportion of adults with hypertension whose blood pressure is under control (HDS-12).
- Reduce the proportion of the diabetic population with an A1c value >9% (D-5.1).
- Increase the proportion of children aged 19 to 35 months who receive the recommended doses of DTaP, polio, MMR, Hib, hepatitis B, varicella, and PCV vaccines (IID-8).

Environmental Quality
- Reduce the number of days the Air Quality Index (AQI) exceeds 100 (EH-1).
- Reduce the proportion of children exposed to secondhand smoke (TU-11.1).

Injury and Violence
- Reduce fatal injuries (IVP-1.1).
- Reduce homicides (IVP-29).

Maternal, Infant, and Child Health
- Reduce all infant deaths (MICH-1.3).
- Reduce total preterm births (MICH-9).

Mental Health
- Reduce the suicide rate (MHMD-1).
- Reduce the proportion of adolescents who experience major depressive episodes (MDEs) (MHMD-41).

Nutrition, Physical Activity, and Obesity
- Increase the proportion of adults who meet current federal physical activity guidelines for aerobic physical activity and muscle strengthening activity (PA-2.4).
- Reduce the proportion of adults who are obese (NWS-9).
- Reduce the proportion of children and adolescents who are considered obese (NWS-10.4).
- Increase total vegetable intake for persons aged 2 years and older (NWS-15.1).

Oral Health
- Increase the proportion of children, adolescents, and adults who visited the dentist in the past year (OH-7).

Reproductive and Sexual Health
- Increase the proportion of sexually active females aged 15 to 44 years who received reproductive health services in the past 12 months (FP-7.1).
- Increase the knowledge of serostatus among HIV-positive persons (HIV-13).

Social Determinants
- Increase the proportion of students who graduate with a regular diploma 4 years after starting ninth grade (AH-5.1).

Substance Abuse
- Reduce the proportion of adolescents using alcohol or any illicit drugs during the past 30 days (SA-13.1).
- Reduce the proportion of adults engaging in binge drinking during the past 30 days (SA-14.3).

Tobacco
- Reduce the number of adults who are current cigarette smokers (TU-1.1).
- Reduce the number of adolescents who smoked cigarettes in the past 30 days (TU-2.2).

From U.S. Department of Health and Human Services (USDHHS). (2016). *Healthy People 2020: Leading health indicators topics.* Retrieved from http://www.healthypeople.gov/2020/leading-health-indicators/2020-LHI-Topics

to focus on population-based interventions and participatory approaches to improve the health of local communities (CDC, 2016b). They provide resources and support for local communities to address the preventable risk factors related to chronic disease, such as poor diet, tobacco use, excessive use of alcohol, and physical inactivity (Largo-Wight, 2011). A healthy community environment is defined as one that "encompasses aspects of human health, disease, and injury that are determined or influenced by factors in the overall environment"; it is important to note the interplay between health and the environment, not just "how health is affected by the direct pathological impacts of various chemical, physical, and biological agents, but also by factors in the broad

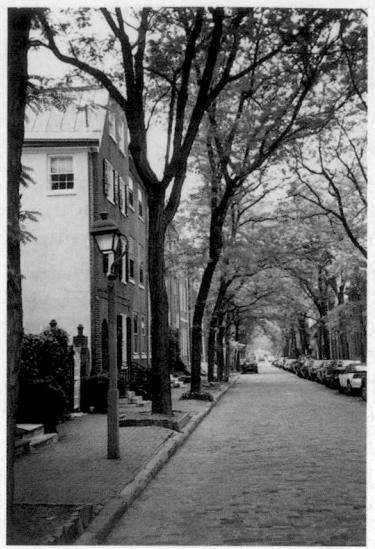

What do *you* think?

Life expectancy has risen 40 years since 1900, yet only 7 years of this growth can be attributed to disease care improvements. The remainder of the gain is the result of improvements in prevention and environmental health (e.g., clean water, improved sanitation). Do you think there is a direct link between your health and your environment?

physical environments" (e.g., urban development, housing, transportation, agriculture, industry) (CDC, 2014, para. 4).

Another description of a healthy community, first described by Cottrell (1976) as a *competent community*, is one in which the various organizations, groups, and aggregates of people making up the community do at least four things:

1. They collaborate effectively in identifying the problems and needs of the community.
2. They achieve a working consensus on goals and priorities.
3. They agree on ways and means to implement the agreed-on goals.
4. They collaborate effectively in the required actions.

Healthy communities and healthy cities impact the health of their populations and vice versa. In the 1980s, the WHO initiated the *Healthy Cities* movement to improve the health status of urban populations. A healthy city is defined as "one that is continually creating and improving those physical and social environments and expanding those community resources that enable people to mutually support each other in performing all functions of life and in developing their maximum potential" (WHO, 2015e, para. 1). The 10 key components of a healthy city are listed in Display 1–3. How many of these are found in your city or community?

Health as a State of Being

Health refers to a state of being, including many different qualities and characteristics. An individual might be described in terms such as energetic, outgoing, enthusiastic, beautiful, caring, loving, and intense. Together, these qualities become the essence of a person's existence; they describe a state of being. Similarly, a specific geographic community, such as a neighborhood, has many characteristics. It might be characterized by the terms congested, deteriorating, unattractive, dirty, and disorganized. These characteristics suggest diminishing degrees of vitality. A third example might be a population, such as workers involved in a massive layoff, who band together to provide support and share resources to effectively seek new employment. This community shows signs of healthy adaptation and positive coping.

Health involves the total person or community. All of the dimensions of life affecting everyday functioning determine an individual's or a community's health, including physical, psychological, spiritual, economic,

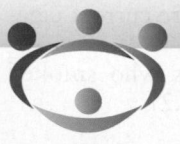

DISPLAY 1–3 QUALITIES OF A HEALTHY COMMUNITY

- Equity (lack of disparities)
- A strong economy and employment opportunities (lack of poverty)
- Education
- Health care and preventive health services
- A stable, sustainable ecosystem and environment
- Inclusive, equitable, and broad community participation
- Employ environmental strategies
- Engage multisector participation
- The capacity to assess and address their own health concerns
- Collaboration between partners

- Housing/Shelter
- Civic engagement
- Healthy public policy
- Access to healthy food
- Safety
- Opportunities for active living
- Transportation
- Empowered population
- Healthy child development
- Use data to guide and measure efforts

From Health Resources in Action. (2013, July 25). *Defining healthy communities.* Boston, MA: Author. Retrieved from http://www.hria.org/uploads/catalogerfiles/defining-healthy-communities/defining_healthy_communities_1113_final_report.pdf

and sociocultural experiences. All of these factors must be considered when dealing with the health of an individual or community. The approach should be holistic. A client's placement on the health continuum can be known only if the nurse considers all facets of the client's life, including not only physical and emotional status but also the status of home, family, and work.

When considering an aggregate or group of people in terms of health, it becomes useful for intervention purposes to speak of the "health of a community." With aggregates as well as individuals, health as a state of being does not merely involve that group's physical state but also includes psychological, spiritual, and socioeconomic factors. As an example, the health of the Gulf Coast region is yet to be fully determined after a massive oil-drilling spill in the Gulf of Mexico that has caused losses in fishing, tourism, and wetlands storm protection as a result of the worst oil spill in U.S. history. In 2015, 5 years after the spill, an $18.7 billion settlement was reached (Naylor, 2015). The true impact—including long-term health effects—is hotly contested and will not be known for years. It is another serious blow to this region affecting population health. This oil spill comes 5 years after hurricane Katrina made landfall on the Gulf Coast in August 2005. Widespread damage occurred after the deadliest hurricane since the 1920s with over 80% of the city underwater, and then, only 26 days later, hurricane Rita (the fourth most intense Atlantic hurricane on record) hit near the Texas–Louisiana border causing over $150 billion in damages (Plyer, 2015). The Centers for Disease Control (CDC) estimated that more than 200,000 people converged on evacuation centers, and the country watched in anguish as the Federal Emergency Management Agency (FEMA) struggled to meet the emergency needs of the survivors. Over one million people were displaced and over a million housing units were damaged across the Gulf Coast (Plyer, 2015). At the same time, over 1,800 deaths were attributed to Katrina, and the survivors were left with many physical, emotional, and social difficulties. There were hundreds of chemical and petroleum spills in the Katrina aftermath, and health problems related to contact with polluted water (e.g., rashes, asthma, nausea). Mold exposure was another environmental hazard, and the temporary housing trailers provided to survivors were found to have high levels of formaldehyde (three times the average household exposure) causing residents to have nosebleeds, respiratory problems, skin rashes, and headaches (Anthamattan & Hazen, 2011). We examine disaster and bioterrorism as it relates to community health nursing in Chapter 17.

Subjective and Objective Dimensions of Health

Health involves both *subjective* and *objective* dimensions; that is, it involves both how people feel (subjective) and how well they can function in their environment (objective). Subjectively, a healthy person is one who feels well and who experiences the sensation of a vital, positive state. Healthy people are full of life and vigor, capable of physical and mental productivity. They feel minimal discomfort and displeasure with the world around them. Again, people experience varying degrees of vitality and

well-being. The state of feeling well fluctuates. Some mornings we wake up feeling more energetic and enthusiastic than we do on other mornings. How people feel varies day by day, even hour by hour; nonetheless, how they feel overall is a strong indicator of their overall state of health.

Health also involves the objective dimension of ability to function. A healthy individual or community carries out necessary activities and achieves enriching goals. Unhealthy people not only feel ill but they are limited, to some degree, in their ability to carry out daily activities. Indeed, levels of illness or wellness are measured largely in terms of ability to function (Junehag, Asplund, & Svedlund, 2014). A person confined to bed is labeled sicker than an ill person managing self-care. A family that meets its members' needs is healthier than one that has poor communication patterns and is unable to provide adequate physical and emotional resources. A community actively engaged in crime prevention or in policing of industrial wastes shows signs of healthy functioning. The degree of functioning is directly related to the state of health (see Perspectives: Voices From the Community).

The ability to function can be observed. A man dresses and feeds himself and goes to work. Despite financial exigencies, a family nourishes its members through a supportive emotional climate. A community provides adequate resources and services for its members. These performances, to some degree, can be regarded as indicators of health status.

The actions of an individual, family, or community are motivated by their values. Some activities, such as walking and taking care of personal needs, are functions valued by most people. Other actions, such as bird watching, volunteering to help a charity, or running, have more limited appeal. In assessing the health of individuals and communities, the community health nurse can observe people's ability to function but also must know their values, which may contrast sharply with those of the professional. The influence of values on health is examined more closely in Chapter 4.

The subjective dimension (feeling well or ill) and the objective dimension (functioning) together provide a clearer picture of people's health. When they feel well and demonstrate functional ability, they are close to the

PERSPECTIVES
VOICES FROM THE COMMUNITY

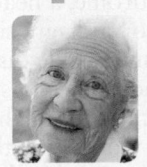

I never thought much about being healthy or not, now that you ask. I keep busy, I cook like I'm expecting company, I have a good appetite. I really think all these so-called healthy things people suggest are fads, just so someone can get rich—like tofu and low fat this and that. Don't give me margarine, only butter, . . . and skim milk, it's like drinking water! I work in my garden, I read, and I eat fresh foods, and don't talk to me about my smoking, it's the one pleasure I have left.

—Bettie, age 81

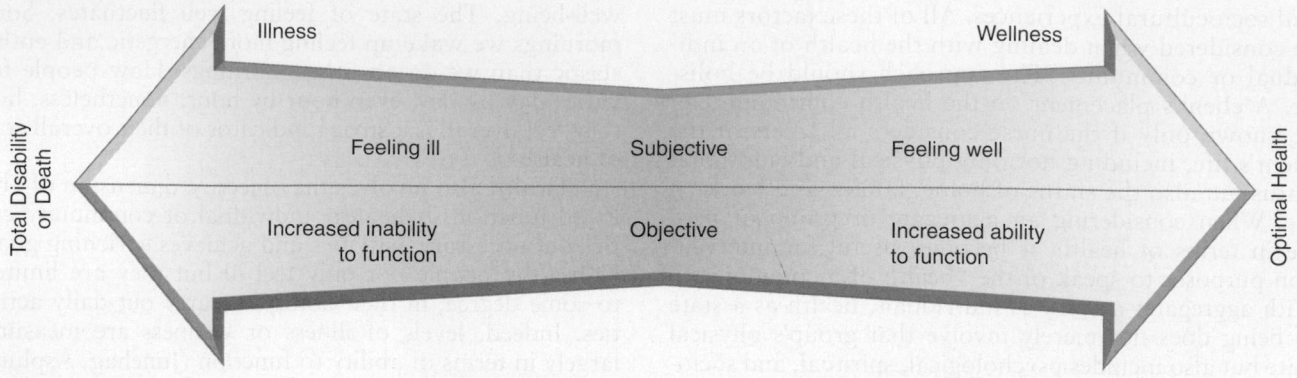

FIGURE 1–3 Subjective and objective views of the wellness–illness continuum.

wellness end of the health continuum. Even those with a disease, such as arthritis or diabetes, may feel well and perform well within their capacity. These people can be considered healthy or closer to the wellness end of the continuum. Figure 1–3 depicts the relationships between the subjective and objective views of health.

Continuous and Episodic Health Care Needs

Community health practice encompasses populations in all age groups with birth to death developmental health care needs. These **continuous needs** may include, for example, assistance with providing a toddler-proof home or establishing positive toilet-training techniques, help in effectively dealing with the progressive emancipation of preteens and teenagers, anticipatory guidance for reducing and managing the stress associated with retirement, or help coping with the death of an aged parent. These are developmental events experienced by most people, and they represent typical life occurrences. The community health nurse has the skills to work at the individual, family, and group level to meet these needs. On an individual and family level, a home visit may be the appropriate place for intervention. If the nurse sees that the community has many young and growing families, and several families have similar developmental issues, a class for mothers and babies, parents and teenagers, or pre-retirement adults may be formed to meet weekly at the library or health clinic waiting room. In these instances, the nurse works with groups ranging from small to large.

In addition, populations may have a one-time, specific, negative health event, such as an illness or injury that is not an expected part of life. These **episodic needs** might derive from the birth of an infant with Down's syndrome, a head injury incurred from an automobile crash, or a diagnosis of HIV/AIDS, tuberculosis, or another communicable disease. For instance, in 2014, the CDC raised its response level for the Ebola outbreak in West Africa to its highest alert status. Two Americans who were working with patients there had contracted Ebola and were treated in the United States with an experimental medication (Mundell, 2014). Months later, a nurse in Texas contracted Ebola from her patient who had traveled to West Africa. The patient died, but the nurse survived (McLaughlin & Yan, 2015). See more on communicable diseases in Chapter 8.

In a given day, the community health nurse may interact with clients having either continuous or episodic health care needs, or both. For example, when can parents expect a child with Down's syndrome to begin toilet training? How do middle-aged adults, planning their retirement and preparing for the death of an aged parent, deal with their adult child's AIDS diagnosis? Complex situations such as these may be positively influenced by the interaction with and services of the community health nurse.

COMPONENTS OF COMMUNITY HEALTH PRACTICE

Community health practice can best be understood by examining two basic components—promotion of health and prevention of health problems. The levels of prevention are a key to community health practice.

Promotion of Health

Promotion of health is recognized as one of the most important components of public health and community health practice. **Health promotion** includes all efforts that seek to move people closer to optimal well-being or higher levels of wellness. Nursing, in particular, has a social mandate for engaging in health promotion (Pender, Murdaugh, & Parsons, 2014). Health promotion programs and activities include many forms of health education—for example, teaching the dangers of drug use, demonstrating healthful practices such as regular exercise, and providing more health-promoting options such as heart-healthy menu selections. Community health promotion, then, encompasses the development and management of preventive health care services that are responsive to community health needs. Wellness programs in schools and industry are examples. Demonstration of such healthful practices as eating nutritious foods and exercising more regularly often is performed and promoted by individual health workers. In addition, groups and health agencies that support a smoke-free environment, encourage physical fitness programs for all ages, or demand that food products be properly labeled underscore the importance of these practices and create public awareness.

The goal of health promotion is to raise levels of wellness for individuals, families, populations, and communities (WHO, 2015d). Community health efforts accomplish this goal through a three-pronged effort to:

1. Increase the span of healthy life for all citizens
2. Reduce health disparities among population groups
3. Achieve access to preventive services for everyone

Specifically, in the 1980s, the U.S. Public Health Service published the Surgeon General's Report, *Healthy People*, and continued with *Promoting Health, Preventing Disease: 1990 Health Objectives for the Nation* and *Healthy People 2000*. The third set of health objectives for the nation, *Healthy People 2010* (CDC, 2015), built on the previous two decades of success in Healthy People initiatives. These documents provide guidance for promoting health as a nation. *Healthy People 2020* carries on this tradition.

The Surgeon General's Report provided vision and an agenda for significantly reducing preventable death and disability nationwide, enhancing quality of life, and greatly reducing disparities in the health status of populations. It emphasized the need for individuals to assume personal responsibility for controlling and improving their own health destiny. It challenged society to find ways to make good health available to vulnerable populations whose disadvantaged state placed them at greater risk for health problems. Finally, it called for an intensified shift in focus from treating preventable illness and functional impairment to concentrating resources and targeting efforts that promote health and prevent disease and disability. The Institute of Medicine's 2001 report, *The Future of the Public's Health in the 21st Century*, notes that the majority of health care spending, "as much as 95%," focuses on "medical care and biomedical research," whereas evidence suggests that "behavior and environment are responsible for over 70% of avoidable mortality" and that health care is only one of many "determinants of health" (p. 2).

The implications of this national agenda for health have far-reaching consequences for persons engaged in health care. For centuries, health care has focused on the illness end of the health continuum, but health professionals can no longer justify concentrating most of their efforts exclusively on treating the sick and injured. We now live in an age when it is not only possible to promote health and prevent disease and disability, but it is our mandate and responsibility to do so. (For more on health promotion, see Chapter 11.)

Prevention of Health Problems

Prevention of health problems constitutes a major part of community health practice. Prevention means anticipating and averting problems or discovering them as early as possible in order to minimize potential disability and impairment. It is practiced on three levels in community health: primary prevention, secondary prevention, and tertiary prevention (Pacala, 2015). These concepts recur throughout the chapters of this text, in narrative format and in the Levels of Prevention Pyramids, because they are basic to community health nursing. Once the differences among the levels of prevention are recognized, a sound foundation on which to build additional community health principles can be developed.

Primary prevention obviates the occurrence of a health problem; it includes measures taken to keep illness or injuries from occurring. It is applied to a generally healthy population and precedes disease or dysfunction. Examples of primary prevention activities by a public health nurse include providing childhood vaccinations; encouraging elderly people to install and use safety devices (e.g., grab bars by bathtubs, hand rails on steps) to prevent injuries

from falls; teaching young adults healthy lifestyle behaviors, so that they can make them habitual behaviors for themselves and their children; or working through a local health department in consultation with a school district to help control and prevent communicable diseases such as rubeola, poliomyelitis, or varicella by providing regular immunization programs and vaccine oversight.

Primary prevention involves anticipatory planning and action on the part of community health professionals, who must project themselves into the future, envision potential needs and problems, and then design programs to counteract them so that they never occur. A community health nurse who instructs a group of overweight individuals on how to follow a well-balanced diet while losing weight is preventing the possibility of nutritional deficiency (see Levels of Prevention Pyramid). Educational programs that teach safe sex practices or the dangers of smoking and substance abuse are other examples of primary prevention. In addition, when the community health nurse serves on a fact-finding committee exploring the effects of a proposed toxic waste dump on the outskirts of town, the nurse is concerned about primary prevention. The concepts of primary prevention and planning for the future are foreign to many social groups, who may resist on the basis of conflicting values. The Parable of the Dangerous Cliff (Display 1–4) illustrates such a value conflict. How often does our nation put an ambulance at the bottom of the cliff? How cost-effective is that approach?

Secondary prevention involves efforts to detect and treat existing health problems at the earliest possible stage, when disease or impairment is already present. Hypertension and cholesterol screening programs in many communities help to identify high-risk individuals and encourage early treatment to prevent heart attacks or stroke. Other examples are encouraging breast and testicular self-examination, regular mammograms, and Pap smears for early detection of possible cancers and providing skin testing for tuberculosis (in infants at 1 year of age and periodically throughout life, with increasing frequency for high-risk groups). Secondary prevention attempts to discover a health problem at a point when intervention may lead to its control or eradication. This is the goal behind testing of water and soil samples for contaminants and hazardous chemicals in the field of community environmental health. It also prompts community health nurses to watch for early signs of child abuse in a family, emotional disturbances among widows, or alcohol and drug abuse among adolescents.

Tertiary prevention attempts to reduce the extent and severity of a health problem to its lowest possible level, so as to minimize disability and restore or preserve function. Examples include treatment and rehabilitation of persons after a stroke to reduce impairment, postmastectomy exercise programs to restore functioning, and early treatment and management of diabetes to reduce problems or slow their progress. The individuals involved have an existing illness or disability whose impact on their lives is lessened through tertiary prevention. In community health, the need to reduce disability and restore function applies equally to families, groups, communities, and individuals. Many groups form for rehabilitation and offer support and guidance for those recuperating from some physical or mental disability. Examples include

LEVELS OF PREVENTION PYRAMID

SITUATION: Poor nutritional habits and inactivity are leading to obesity among children and adults and greater incidence of type 2 diabetes.

GOAL: Using the three levels of prevention, negative health conditions are avoided, or promptly diagnosed and treated, and population health is improved.

TERTIARY PREVENTION

Rehabilitation	Primary Prevention	
	Health Promotion and Education	*Health Protection*
• If diabetic, encourage weight, blood pressure, and cholesterol maintenance, along with good glucose control to prevent complications of diabetes. • Reassess data to determine effectiveness of interventions.	• Teach children and families the importance of maintaining a healthy weight through proper diet and exercise. Promote awareness of dangers of obesity and diabetes through use of PSAs and billboards.	• Provide weight loss support. • Provide access to periodic health care to check A_1C levels and foot and eye exams.

SECONDARY PREVENTION

Early Diagnosis	Prompt Treatment
• Encourage weight loss in obese populations to prevent development of type 2 diabetes. Provide screening programs for high-risk groups. • Refer clients with high glucose or other problems (e.g., hypertension, high cholesterol) to primary care provider or diabetes clinics.	• Initiate educational and incentive programs to improve dietary practices. • Teach clients (individuals or families) on a one-to-one basis to modify dietary practices and activity levels.

PRIMARY PREVENTION

Health Promotion and Education	Health Protection
• Provide nutrition educational programs to promote awareness at schools, work sites, etc. • Encourage restaurants and schools to offer healthy menu items. • Recommend nutrition classes offered at neighborhood centers or health care facilities	• Promote physical fitness, nutritional, and wellness activities. • Work with local entities to reduce easy access to sodas, tax high-calorie foods, and provide easier access to fresh fruits and vegetables, as well as provide bike paths and walking clubs.

Alcoholics Anonymous, halfway houses for psychiatric patients discharged from acute care settings, ostomy clubs, and drug rehabilitation programs. In broader community health practice, tertiary prevention is used to minimize the effects of an existing unhealthy community condition. Examples of such prevention are insisting that businesses provide wheelchair access, warning urban residents about the dangers of a chemical spill, and recalling a contaminated food or drug product. When a community experiences a disaster such as an earthquake, a fire, a hurricane, or even a terrorist attack, preventing injuries among the survivors and volunteers during rescue is another example of tertiary prevention—eliminating additional injury to those already experiencing a tragedy.

Health assessment of individuals, families, and communities is an important part of all three levels of preventive practice. Health status must be determined to anticipate problems and select appropriate preventive measures. Community health nurses working with young parents who themselves have been victims of child abuse can institute early treatment for the parents to prevent abuse and foster adequate parenting of their children. If the assessment of a community reveals inadequate facilities and activities to meet the future needs of its growing senior population, agencies and groups can collaborate to develop the needed resources.

Health problems are most effectively prevented by maintenance of healthy lifestyles and healthy environments. To these ends, community health practice directs many of its efforts to providing safe and satisfying living and working conditions, nutritious food, and clean air and water. This area of practice includes the field of preventive medicine, which is a population-focused, or community-oriented, branch of medical practice that incorporates public health sciences and principles (American Board of Medical Specialties, n.d.).

DISPLAY 1–4 PARABLE OF THE DANGEROUS CLIFF

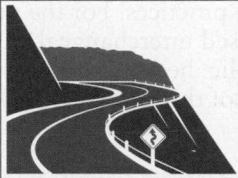 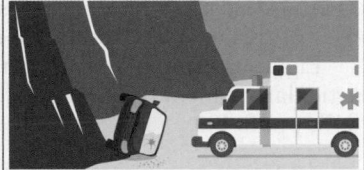

Twas a dangerous cliff, as they freely confessed,

Though to walk near its crest was so pleasant;
But over its terrible edge there has slipped
  A duke, and full many a peasant.
The people said something would have to be done
  But their projects did not at all tally.
Some said, "Put a fence around the edge of the cliff";
  Some, "an ambulance down in the valley."
The lament of the crowd was profound and was loud,
  As their hearts overflowed with their pity;
But the cry of the ambulance carried the day
  As it spread through the neighboring city.
A collection was made to accumulate aid
  And the dwellers in highway and alley
Gave dollars or cents not to furnish a fence
  But "an ambulance down in the valley."
"For the cliff is all right if you're careful," they said.
  "And if folks ever slip and are dropping,
It isn't the slipping that hurts them so much
  As the shock down below when they're stopping."
So for years (we have heard), as these mishaps occurred,

Quick forth the rescuers sally,
To pick up the victims who fell from the cliff,
  With the ambulance down in the valley.
Said one in his plea, "It's a marvel to me
  That you'd give so much greater attention
To repairing results than to curing the cause;
  You had much better aim at prevention.
For the mischief, of course, should be stopped at its source,
  Come neighbors and friends, let us rally.
It is far better sense to rely on a fence
  Than an ambulance down in the valley."
"He is wrong in his head," the majority said;
  "He would end all our earnest endeavor.
He's a man who would shirk this responsible work,
  But we will support it forever.
Aren't we picking up all, just as fast as they fall, and
  giving them care liberally?
A superfluous fence is of no consequence,
  If the ambulance works in the valley."
The story looks queer as we've written it here,
  But things oft occur that are stranger.
More humane, we assert, than to care for the hurt,
  Is a plan for removing the danger.
The very best plan is to safeguard the man,
  And attend to the thing rationally;
To build up the fence and try to dispense
  With the ambulance down in the valley.
Better still! Cut down the hill!

Adapted from Malins, J. (1896). Fence or ambulance? *Journal of Education, 76*(11), 291.

CHARACTERISTICS OF COMMUNITY HEALTH NURSING

As a specialty field of nursing, community health nursing adds public health knowledge and skills that address the needs and problems of communities and aggregates and focuses care on communities and vulnerable populations. Public health nursing is grounded in both public health science and nursing science, which makes its philosophical orientation and the nature of its practice unique. It has been recognized as a subspecialty of both fields. Recognition of this specialty field continues with a greater awareness of the important contributions made by community health nursing to improve the health of the public.

Knowledge of the following elements of public health is essential to community health nursing (ANA, 2013; Swider, Krothe, Reyes, & Cravetz, 2013):

- Priority of preventive, protective, and health-promoting strategies over curative strategies (see Chapters 11 and 12)
- Means for measurement and analysis of community health problems, including epidemiologic concepts and biostatistics (see Chapter 7)

- Influence of environmental factors on aggregate health (see Chapter 9)
- Principles underlying management and organization for community health, because the goal of public health is accomplished through organized community efforts (see Chapter 15)
- Public policy analysis and development, along with health advocacy and an understanding of the political process (see Chapter 13)

Confusion over the meaning of "community health nursing" arises when it is defined only in terms of where it is practiced. Because health care services have shifted from the hospital to the community, many nurses in other specialties now practice in the community. Examples of these practices include home health care, community mental health, geriatric nursing, long-term care, and occupational health. Although community health nurses today practice in the same or similar settings, the difference lies in applying the public health principles to large groups and communities of people—or having a population focus (Fig. 1–4). For nurses moving into this field of nursing, it requires a shift in focus—from individuals to a broader focus on aggregates and populations. Nursing and other theories undergird its practice (see Chapter 14),

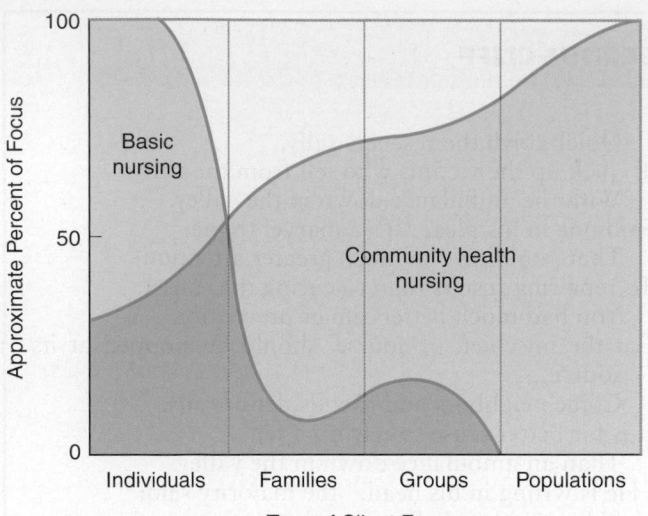

FIGURE 1–4 Difference in client focus between basic nursing and community health nursing.

and the nursing process (incorporated in Chapters 15 and 19) is one of its basic tools (see the levels of prevention discussed earlier).

Community health nursing, then, as a specialty of nursing, combines nursing science with public health science to formulate a community-based and population-focused practice (Anderson & McFarlane, 2015). "Public health nursing practice focuses on population health through continuous surveillance and assessment of the multiple determinants of health with the intent to promote health and wellness; prevent disease, disability, and premature death; and improve neighborhood quality of life" (ANA, 2013, p. 2) (see Display 1–5). For instance, community health nurses are nursing when their concern for homeless individuals sleeping in a park leads to development of a program providing food and shelter for this population. Community health nurses are nursing when they collaborate to institute an HIV/AIDS education curriculum in the local school system. When they assess the needs of elderly people in retirement homes to ensure necessary services and provide health instruction and support, they are, again, nursing. They utilize primary, secondary, and tertiary interventions that are evidence-based and develop programs and services that help achieve health for all.

During the first 70 years of the 20th century, community health nursing was known as **public health nursing.** The PHN section of the American Public Health Association's (2013) definition of a public health nurse is someone who promotes and protects the health of populations and who is prepared at the baccalaureate level. The later title of community health nursing was adopted to better describe where the nurse practices. For the purposes of this text, the terms are used interchangeably.

Eight characteristics of public health nursing are particularly salient to the practice of this specialty (ANA, 2013, pp. 8–9):

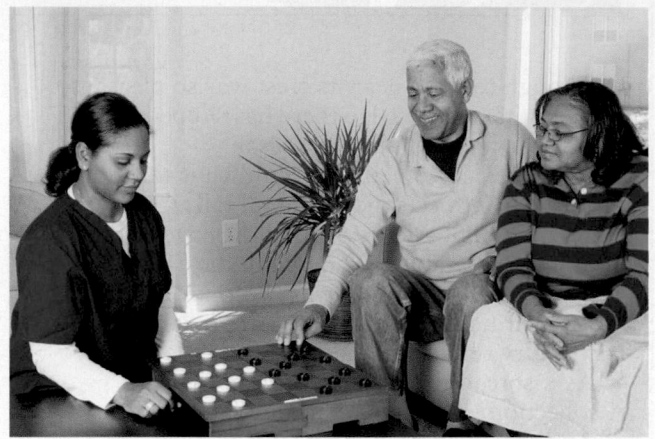

1. The client or "unit of care" is the population.
2. The primary obligation is to achieve the greatest good for the greatest number of people or the population as a whole.
3. Public health nurses collaborate with the client as an equal partner.
4. Primary prevention is the priority in selecting appropriate activities.
5. Public health nursing focuses on selecting strategies that create healthy environmental, social, and economic conditions in which populations may thrive.
6. A public health nurse is obligated to actively identify and reach out to all who might benefit from a specific activity or service.
7. Optimal use of available resources and creation of new evidence-based strategies are necessary to assure the best overall improvement in the health of the population.

DISPLAY 1–5 THE DEFINITION AND PRACTICE OF PUBLIC HEALTH NURSES

Public health nursing is the practice of promoting and protecting the health of populations using knowledge from nursing, social, and public health sciences (para. 2).

Key characteristics of practice include (1) a focus on the health needs of an entire population, including inequities and the unique needs of subpopulations; (2) assessment of population health using a comprehensive, systematic approach; (3) attention to multiple determinants of health; (4) an emphasis on primary prevention; and (5) application of interventions at all levels—individuals, families, communities, and the systems that impact their health (para. 4).

The baccalaureate degree in nursing (BSN) is recommended for entry-level public health nurses (para. 12).

From American Public Health Association (APHA) Public Health Nursing Section. (2013). *The definition and practice of public health nursing.* Washington, DC: APHA.

8. Collaboration with other professions, populations, organizations, and stakeholder groups is the most effective way to promote and protect the health of people.

Population Focused

The central mission of public health practice is to improve the health of population groups. Community health nursing shares this essential feature: it is **population focused**, meaning that it is concerned for the health status of population groups and their environment. A population may consist of the elderly living throughout the community or of Middle Eastern refugees clustered in one section of a city. It may be a scattered group with common characteristics, such as people at high risk of developing heart disease or battered women living throughout a county. It may include all people living in a neighborhood, district, census tract, city, state, or province. Community health nursing's specialty practice serves populations and aggregates of people.

Working with individuals and families as aggregates has been common for community health nursing; however, such work must expand to incorporate a population-oriented focus, a feature that distinguishes it from other nursing specialties. Basic nursing focuses on individuals, and community health nursing focuses on aggregates, but the many variations in community needs and nursing roles inevitably cause some overlap.

A population-oriented focus requires the assessment of relationships. When working with groups and communities, the nurse does not consider them separately but rather in context—that is, in relationship to the rest of the community. When an outbreak of hepatitis occurs, for example, the community health nurse does more

than just work with others to treat it. The nurse tries to stop the spread of the infection, locate possible sources, and prevent its recurrence in the community. As a result of their population-oriented focus, community health nurses seek to discover possible groups with a common health need, such as expectant mothers or groups at high risk for development of a common health problem (e.g., obese children at risk for type 2 diabetes, victims of child abuse). Community health nurses continually look for problems in the environment that influence community health and seek ways to increase environmental quality. They work to prevent health problems, such as promoting school-based education about nutrition and physical activity or exercise programs for groups of seniors.

The Greatest Good for the Greatest Number of People

A population-oriented focus involves a new outlook and set of attitudes. Individualized care is important, but prevention of aggregate problems in community health nursing practice reflects more accurately its philosophy and benefits more people. The community or population at risk is the client (see Display 1–6). Furthermore, because community health nurses are concerned about several aggregates at the same time, service will, of necessity, be provided to multiple and overlapping groups. The ethical theory of *utilitarianism* promotes the greatest good for the greatest number. Further discussion of ethical principles in community health nursing can be found in Chapter 4.

Clients as Equal Partners

The goal of public health, "to increase quality and years of healthy life and eliminate health disparities" (CDC, 2013, para. 1), requires a partnership effort. Just as

---

DISPLAY 1–6 PARABLE OF THE TREES: POPULATION-FOCUSED PRACTICE

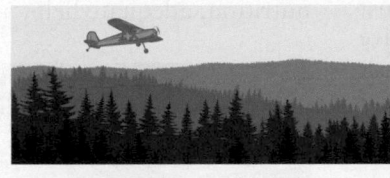 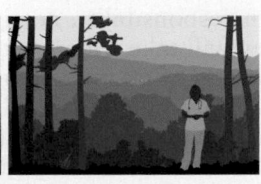

There were once two sisters who inherited a large tract of heavily forested land from their grandmother. In her will, the grandmother stipulated that they must preserve the health of the trees. One sister studied tree surgery and became an expert in recognizing and treating diseased trees. She also was able to spot conditions that might lead to problems and prevent them. Her work was invaluable in keeping single or small clusters of trees healthy. The other sister became a forest ranger. In addition to learning how to care for individual trees, she studied the environmental conditions that affected the well-being of the forest. She learned the importance of proper ecologic balance between flora and fauna and the impact of climate, geography,

soil conditions, and weather. Her work was to oversee the health and growth of the whole forest. Although she spent time walking through the forest assessing conditions, her aerial view from their small plane was equally important for spotting fires, signs of disease, or other potential problems. Together, the sisters preserved a healthy forest.

Nursing also has tree surgeons and forest rangers. Various nursing specialties, like the tree surgeons, serve the health needs of individuals and families. Community health nurses, like the forest rangers, study and address the needs of populations. Both are needed and must work together to ensure healthy communities.

learning cannot take place in schools without student participation, the goals of public health cannot be realized without consumer participation. Community health nursing's efforts toward health improvement go only so far. Clients' health status and health behavior will not change unless people accept and apply the proposals (developed in collaboration with clients) presented by the community health nurse.

Public health nurses can encourage individuals' participation by promoting their autonomy rather than permitting a dependency. For example, elderly persons attending a series of nutrition or fitness classes can be encouraged to take the initiative and develop health or social programs on their own. Independence and feelings of self-worth are closely related. By treating people as independent adults, with trust and respect, community health nurses help promote self-reliance and the ability to function independently. Autonomy is an important objective of public health, as is equality (Owens & Cribb, 2013).

Frequently, consumers are intimidated by health professionals and are uninformed about health and health care. They do not know what information to seek and are hesitant to act assertively. For example, a migrant worker brought her 2-year-old son, who had symptoms resembling those of scurvy, to a clinic. Recognizing a vitamin C deficiency, the physician told her to feed the boy large quantities of orange juice but gave no further explanation. Several weeks later, she returned to the clinic, but the child was much worse. After questioning her, the nurse discovered that the mother had been feeding the child large amounts of an orange soft drink, not knowing the difference between that beverage and orange juice. Obviously, the quality of care is affected when the consumer does not understand and cannot participate in the health care process. **Health literacy**, or the ability to "obtain, process, and understand basic health information and services needed to make appropriate health decisions," is an important concept that is discussed more fully in Chapter 10 (Eberle, 2014, para. 1).

When people believe that their health, and that of the community, is their own responsibility, not just that of health professionals, they will take a more active interest in promoting it. The process of taking responsibility for developing one's own health potential is called **self-care**. As people maintain their own lives, health, and well-being, they are engaging in self-care. Some examples of self-care activities at the aggregate level include building safe playgrounds, developing teen employment opportunities, and providing senior exercise programs.

When people's ability to continue self-care activities drops below their need, they experience a **self-care deficit**. At this point, nursing may appropriately intervene. However, nursing's goal is to assist clients to return to or reach a level of functioning at which they can attain optimal health and assume responsibility for maintaining it (Alligood, 2014; Berbiglia, 2011; Breiddal, 2012). To this end, community health nurses foster their clients' sense of responsibility by treating them as adults capable of managing their own affairs. Nurses can encourage people to negotiate health care goals and practices, develop their own programs, contact their own resources (e.g., support groups, transportation services), identify and implement

lifestyle changes that promote wellness, and learn ways to monitor their own health.

When planning for the health of communities, for example, partnerships must be established and the values and priorities of the community incorporated into program planning, data collection and interpretation, and policymaking. More information on program planning is given in Chapter 12.

Prioritizing Primary Prevention

In community health nursing, the promotion of health and prevention of illness are a first-order priority. Less emphasis is placed on curative care. Some corrective actions always are needed, such as cleanup of a toxic waste dump site, stricter enforcement of day care standards, or home care of the disabled; however, community health best serves its constituents through preventive and health-promoting actions (Anderson & McFarlane, 2015; USDHHS, 2016a). These include services to mothers and infants, prevention of environmental pollution, school health programs, senior citizens' fitness classes, and "workers' right-to-know" legislation that warns against hazards in the workplace.

Another distinguishing characteristic of community health nursing is its emphasis on positive health, or wellness (Anderson & McFarlane, 2015). Medicine and acute care nursing have dealt primarily with the illness end of the health continuum. With the potentials of genomics and epigenetics becoming reality, the wellness end of the continuum will come into greater focus. In contrast, community health nursing always has had a primary charge to prevent health problems from occurring and to promote a higher level of health. For example, although a community health nurse may assist a population of new mothers in the community with postpartum fatigue and depression, the nurse also works to prevent such problems among women of childbearing age by developing health education programs, establishing prenatal classes, and encouraging proper rest and nutrition, adequate help, and stress reduction.

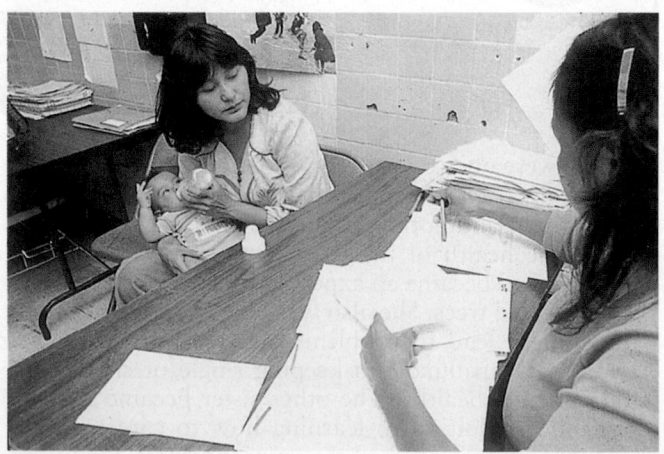

Community health nurses concentrate on the wellness end of the health continuum in a variety of ways. They teach proper nutrition or family planning, promote immunizations among preschool children, encourage regular physical and dental checkups, assist with starting exercise classes or physical fitness programs, and promote healthy interpersonal relationships. Their goal is to help the community reach its optimal level of wellness.

This emphasis on wellness changes the role of community health nursing from a reactive to a proactive stance. It places a greater responsibility on community health nurses to find opportunities for intervention. In clinical nursing and medicine, individual patients seek out professional assistance because they have health problems. They present their problems to the health care practitioner for diagnosis and treatment. Public health nurses, in contrast, seek out potential health problems in the community. They identify high-risk groups and institute preventive programs. They watch for early signs of child neglect or abuse and intervene when any occur, often long before a request for help is made. They look for possible environmental hazards in the community, such as smoking in public places or lead-based paint in older housing units, and work with appropriate authorities to correct them. A wellness emphasis requires taking initiative and making sound judgments, which are characteristics of effective community health nursing.

Selecting Strategies That Create Healthy Conditions in Which Populations May Thrive

With our population focus, it is prudent for public health nurses to design interventions for the whole community, not limiting it to only those individuals seeking service, or only the poor and vulnerable, but promoting the health of entire populations and working to prevent "disease, injury and premature death" (ANA, 2013, p. 3). Advocacy for our clients (individuals, families, aggregates, communities, or populations) is an essential function of public health nursing. We want to create healthy environments for our clients so that they can thrive and not simply survive, and we do this by having a proactive stance toward trends in health care and society, ever changing public concerns, and work with policy and legislative activities (ANA, 2013). More information about health advocacy and policymaking is provided in Chapter 13.

Actively Reaching Out

We know that some clients are more prone to develop disability or disease because of their vulnerable status (e.g., poverty, no access to health care, homeless). Outreach efforts are needed to promote the health of these clients and to prevent disease. In acute care and primary health care settings, like emergency rooms or physician offices, clients come to you for service. However, in community health, nurses must focus on the whole population—not just those who come to us for services—and seek out clients wherever they may be (ANA, 2013). Like Lillian Wald and her Henry Street Settlement, community health nurses must learn about the populations they serve and be willing to search out those most at risk. You can learn more about the rich history of community/public health nursing in Chapter 2. Chapters 25 through 29 cover vulnerable populations.

Optimal Use of Available Resources

It is our duty to wisely use the resources we are given. For most public health agencies, budgets are critically stressed. Tertiary health care uses up the greatest percentage of our health care dollar, leaving decreased funds for primary and secondary services (IOM, 2002; McClellan & Rivlin, 2014), and challenging economic times lead to deep budget cuts at state and local levels. The use of documented evidence as a basis for community health nursing practice promotes more efficient and cost-effective strategies in health promotion (ANA, 2013). It is vital that community health nurses ground their practice in research (see Chapter 4) and use that information to educate policy makers about best practices (see Chapter 13). Utilizing personnel and resources effectively and prudently will pay off in the long run.

Interprofessional Collaboration

Community health nurses must work in cooperation with other team members, coordinating services and addressing the needs of population groups. This interprofessional **collaboration** among health care workers, other professionals and organizations, and clients is essential for establishing effective services and programs. Individualized efforts and specialized programs, when planned in isolation, can lead to fragmentation and gaps in health services. For example, without collaboration, a well-child clinic may be started in a community that already has a strong Early and Periodic Screening and Developmental Testing (EPSDT) program, yet community prenatal services may be nonexistent. Interprofessional collaboration is important in individualized practice, because nurses need to plan with the client, family, physician, social worker, physical therapist, teacher, or counselor and must keep them informed of the client's health status; however, it is an even greater necessity when working with population groups, especially those from vulnerable or at-risk segments.

Effective collaboration requires team members who are strong individuals, with various areas of expertise, and who can make a commitment to team goals. Community health nurses who think and act interdependently make a great contribution to the team effort. In appropriate situations, community health nurses also function autonomously, making independent judgments. Collaboration involves working with members of other professions on community advisory boards and health planning committees to develop needs assessment surveys and to contribute toward policy development efforts. In addition to partnering with the population, other groups the public health nurse collaborates with include:

- Academic and research institutions
- Businesses and industries
- Community organizations, coalitions, and advocacy groups
- Community service agencies such as schools, law enforcement, urban planning, and emergency response
- Faith-based organizations
- Health care providers and facilities
- Legislative, regulatory, and policy-making bodies
- Local, state, and federal public health organizations

- Members of the public health team, such as epidemiologists, social workers, health promotion specialists, nutritionists, environmental health workers, and health educators (ANA, 2013, p. 15).

Interprofessional collaboration requires clarification of each team member's role, a primary reason for community health nurses to fully understand the nature of their practice. When planning a city-wide immunization program with a community group, for example, community health nurses need to explain the ways in which they might contribute to the program's objectives. They can offer to contact key community leaders, with whom they have established relationships, to build community acceptance of the program. They can share their knowledge of the public's preference about times and locations for the program. They can meet with various local agencies and organizations (e.g., health insurance companies, local hospitals) to gain financial support. They can help to organize and give immunizations, and they can influence planning for follow-up programs. Another component includes development of policies to promote and protect the health of clients. Meeting with local legislators and providing testimony to local, state, and national bodies are common methods of ensuring enactment of effective health policies. Public

health nurses can join with others to promote legislation to mandate helmets for cyclists, ban sugar-laden beverages in school vending machines, or provide funding for specific community-based programs. Collaboration is discussed further in Chapter 10.

Client participation is promoted when people serve as partners on the health care team. An aim of community health nursing is to collaborate *with* people rather than do things *for* them. As consumers of health services are treated with respect and trust, confidence and skill in self-care are gained. Thus, promoting their own health and that of their community as their contribution to health programs becomes increasingly valuable. The consumer perspective in planning and delivering health services makes those services relevant to consumer needs. Community health nurses encourage the involvement of health care consumers by soliciting their ideas and opinions, by inviting them to participate on health boards and committees, and by finding ways to promote their participation in decisions affecting their collective health. By assessing the needs of community, based partly upon the population's perceptions, the public health nurse can discover the most pressing health needs and work toward more effective interventions. Community assessment and intervention are explored in depth in Chapter 15.

SUMMARY

Community health nursing has opportunities and challenges to keep the nurse interested and involved in a community-focused career for a lifetime. Community health is more than environmental programs and large-scale efforts to control communicable disease. It is defined as the identification of needs and the protection and improvement of collective health within a geographically defined area. To comprehend the nature and significance of community health and to clarify its meaning for the specialty practice of community health nursing, it is important to understand the concepts of community and of health.

A *community*, broadly defined, is a collection of people who share some common interest or goal. Three types of communities were discussed in this chapter: geographic, common-interest, and health problem-solving communities. Sometimes, a community such as a neighborhood, city, or county is formed by geographic boundaries. At other times, a community may be identified by its common interest; examples are a religious community, a group of migrant workers, or citizens concerned about air pollution. A community also is defined by a pooling of efforts by people and agencies toward solving a health-related problem.

Health is an abstract concept that can be understood more clearly by examining its distinguishing features. First, people are neither sick nor well in an absolute sense but have levels of illness or wellness. These levels may be plotted along a continuum ranging from optimal health to total disability or death. This is known as the *health continuum*. A person's state of health is dynamic, varying from day to day and even hour to hour.

Second, health is a state of being that includes all of the many characteristics of a person, family, or community, whether physical, psychological, social, or spiritual. These characteristics often indicate the degree of wellness or illness of an individual or community and suggest the presence or absence of vitality and well-being.

Third, health has both subjective and objective dimensions: the subjective involves how well people feel; the objective refers to how well they are able to function. Most often, functional performance diminishes dramatically toward the illness end of the health continuum.

Fourth, health care needs can be either continuing, as in developmental concerns that occur over a person's lifetime, or episodic, occurring unexpectedly once or twice in a lifetime. Community health nursing deals with continuing needs, whereas episodic needs are more often managed in acute care settings.

Community health practice incorporates the elements of promotion of health and prevention of health problems.

The eight important characteristics of community health practice are the client is the population; the primary obligation is to achieve the greatest good for the greatest number of people; working with clients as equal partners; primary prevention is the priority; focus on strategies that create healthy environmental, social, and economic conditions; actively identify and reach out to all who might benefit; make optimal use of available resources and create new evidence-based strategies; and collaborate with a variety of professions, populations, organizations, and other stakeholders to promote and protect the health of populations (ANA, 2013).

ACTIVITIES TO PROMOTE CRITICAL THINKING

1. Identify a community of people about whom you have some knowledge. What makes it a community? What characteristics do this group of people share? Work on this activity in a group of peers or family members. Do they think as you do? Is there a difference between the views of family members and those of nursing student peers?
2. Select three populations for whom you have some concern, and place each group on the health continuum. What factors influenced your decision?
3. Describe three preventive actions (one primary, one secondary, and one tertiary) that might be taken to move each of your selected populations closer to optimal wellness.
4. Select a current health problem and identify the three levels of prevention and corresponding activities in which you as a community health nurse would engage at each level.
5. Discuss how you might implement one health promotion effort with each of your selected populations.
6. Browse the Internet for community health nursing research articles that focus on levels of prevention. Find one focusing on each level. For those involved in the articles focusing on secondary and tertiary prevention, what could you as a community health nurse have done to keep the clients at the primary level of prevention?
7. Place yourself on the health continuum. What factors influenced your decision?
8. Using the eight characteristics of community health nursing outlined in this chapter, give examples of how a community health nurse might demonstrate meeting each characteristic.

REFERENCES

AIDS.gov. (2014). *Global statistics: The global HIV/AIDS epidemic.* Retrieved from https://www.aids.gov/hiv-aids-basics/hiv-aids-101/global-statistics/

Alligood, M. R. (2014). *Nursing theorists and their work.* St. Louis, MO: Elsevier Mosby.

American Board of Medical Specialties. (n.d.). *Preventive medicine.* Author. Retrieved from https://www.theabpm.org/aboutus.cfm

American Heart Association (AHA). (2015). AHA statistical update. *Circulation, 131,* e29–e322. doi: 10.1161/CIR.0000000000000152.

American Nurses Association (ANA). (2013). *Public health nursing: Scope and standards of practice* (2nd ed.). Silver Springs, MD: Author.

American Nurses Association (ANA). (2014). *Health care reform. Health care transformation: The Affordable Care Act and more.* Retrieved from http://www.nursingworld.org/MainMenuCategories/Policy-Advocacy/HealthSystemReform/AffordableCareAct.pdf

American Public Health Association (APHA) Public Health Nursing Section. (2013). *The definition and practice of public health nursing.* Washington, DC: APHA.

Anderson, A. S., Macleod, M., Mutrie, N., Sugden, J., Dobson, H., Treweek, S., ... Wyke, S. (2014). Breast cancer risk reduction—Is it feasible to initiate a randomized controlled trial of a lifestyle intervention programme (ActWell) within a national breast-screening programme? *International Journal of Behavioral Nutrition and Physical Activity, 11*, 156. doi: 10.1186/s12966-014-0156-2. Retrieved from http://www.ijbnpa.org/content/11/1/156#abs

Anderson, E. T., & McFarlane, J. (2015). *Community as partner: Theory and practice in nursing* (7th ed.). Philadelphia, PA: Lippincott Williams & Wilkins.

Anthamattan, P., & Hazen, H. (2011). *An introduction to the geography of health.* New York, NY: Routledge.

Association of Schools of Public Health (ASPH). (2015). *Discover: What is public health?* Retrieved from http://www.aspph.org/discover/

Asthma and Allergy Foundation of America (AAFA). (2015). *2015 asthma capitals: The most challenging places to live with asthma.* Retrieved from www.asthacapitals.com

Barile, J. P., Reeve, B. B., Smith, A. W., Zack, M. M., Mitchell, S. A., Kobau, R., ... Thompson, W. W. (2013). Monitoring population health for Healthy People 2020: Evaluation of the NIH PROMIS(R) global health, CDC Healthy Days, and satisfaction with life instruments. *Quality of Life Research, 22*(6), 1201–1211.

Berbiglia, V. A. (2011). The self-care deficit nursing theory as a curriculum conceptual framework in baccalaureate education. *Nursing Science Quarterly, 24*(2), 137–145.

Breiddal, S. M. (2012). Self-care in palliative care: A way of being. *Illness, Crisis & Loss, 20*(1), 5–17.

Budden, J. S., Zhong, E. H., Moulton, P., & Cimiotti, J. P. (2013). Highlights of the National Workforce Survey of Registered Nurses. *Journal of Nursing Regulation, 4*(2), 5–14.

Carey, B. (2015). Brain tumor's genetic makeup critical in treatment, research finds. *Brain in the News: The Dana Foundation, 22*(6), 1–2.

Centers for Disease Control and Prevention (CDC). (2011). Smoking in top-grossing movies—United States, 2010. *Morbidity and Mortality Weekly Review (MMWR), 60*(27), 909–913.

Centers for Disease Control and Prevention (CDC). (2013). *Healthy People 2010: Final report.* Retrieved from http://www.cdc.gov/nchs/healthy_people/hp2010/hp2010_final_review.htm

Centers for Disease Control and Prevention (CDC). (2014). *About healthy places.* Retrieved from http://www.cdc.gov/healthyplaces/about.htm

Centers for Disease Control and Prevention (CDC). (2015). *Healthy People 2010.* Retrieved from http://www.cdc.gov/nchs/healthy_people/hp2010.htm

Centers for Disease Control and Prevention (CDC). (2016a). *Designing and building healthy places.* Retrieved from http://cdc.gov/healthyplaces/

Centers for Disease Control and Prevention (CDC). (2016b). *Division of Community Health (DCH): Making healthy living easier.* Retrieved from http://www.cdc.gov/nccdphp/dch/programs/index.htm

Change Lab Solutions. (2015). *Model ordinance for toy giveaways at restaurants.* Retrieved from http://changelabsolutions.org/publications/healthier-toy-giveaway-meals

Chong, C. S., Tsunaka, M., Tsang, H. W., Chan, E. P., & Cheung, W. M. (2011). Effects of yoga on stress management in healthy adults: A systematic review. *Alternative Therapies in Health & Medicine, 17*(1), 32–38.

Clark, T. T., Sparks, M. J., McDonald, T. M., & Dickerson, J. D. (2011). Post-tobacco Master Settlement Agreement: Policy and practice implications for social workers. *Health & Social Work, 36*(3), 217–224.

Clinton County Health Department. (n.d.). *A definition of public health.* Retrieved May 15, 2010 from http://www.clintoncountygov.com/departments/health/print_page/aboutus.pdf

Cloud, J. (2010, January 6) *Why DNA isn't your destiny.* Retrieved from http://www.time.com/time/printout/0,8816,1951968,00.html#

Cordero, P., Li, J., & Oben, J. A. (2015). Epigenetics of obesity: Beyond the genome sequence. *Current Opinion in Clinical Nutrition & Metabolic Care, 18*(4), 361–366.

Cottrell, L. S. (1976). The competent community. In B. H. Kaplan, R. N. Wilson, & A. H. Leighton (Eds.), *Further explanations in social psychiatry* (pp. 195–209). New York, NY: Basic Books.

County Health Rankings. (2015). *County health rankings and roadmaps: A healthier nation, county by county.* Retrieved from http://www.countyhealthrankings.org/

Dadvand, P., Villanueva, C. M., Font-Ribera, L., Martinez, D., Basagana, X., Belmonte, J., ... Nieuwenhuijsen, M. J. (2014). Risks and benefits of green spaces for children: A cross-sectional study of associations with sedentary behavior, obesity, asthma, and allergy. *Environmental Health Perspectives, 122,* 1329–1335.

Delack, S. (2010). An apple a day. *NASN School Nurse, 25*(6), 255.

Eberle, M. (2013). *Health literacy.* Retrieved from https://nnlm.gov/outreach/consumer/hlthlit.html

European Meeting on Cybernetics and Systems Research (EMCSR). (2012, March 22). *Looking back ... Systems Theory and Ludwig von Bertalanffy.* Retrieved from http://emcsr.net/looking-back-systems-theory-and-ludwig-von-bertalanffy/

Furusawa, C., Horinouchi, T., Hirasawa, T., & Shimizu, H. (2013). Systems metabolic engineering: The creation of microbial cell factories by rational metabolic design and evolution. *Advanced in Biochemical Engineering & Biotechnology, 131,* 1–23.

Galanti, G. (2013). *Caring for patients from different cultures* (5th ed.). Philadelphia, PA: University of Pennsylvania Press.

Gallup Poll. (2014, July 30). *Americans favor ban on smoking in public, but not total ban.* Retrieved from http://www.gallup.com/poll/174203/americans-favor-ban-smoking-public-not-total-ban.aspx?version=print

Godfrey, K. M., Sheppard, A., Gluckman, P. D., Lillycrop, K. A., Burdge, G. C., McLean, C., ... Hanson, M. A. (2011). Epigenetic gene promoter methylation at birth is associated with child's later adiposity. *Diabetes, 60*(5), 1528–1534.

Green, E. D., Guyer, M. S.; National Human Genome Research Institute. (2011). Charting a course for genomic medicine from base pairs to bedside. *Nature, 470,* 204–213.

Griswold, K. S., Lesko, S. E., & Westfall, J. M.; for the Folsom Group. (2013). Communities of solution: Partnerships for population health. *Journal of the American Board of Family Medicine, 26*(3), 232–238.

Hoffman, S. J., Outterson, K., Rottingen, J. A., Cars, O., Clift, C., Rizvi, Z., ... Zorzet, A. (2015). An international legal framework to address antimicrobial resistance. *Bulletin of the World Health Organization, 93,* 66.

Humeniuk, R., Ali, R., Babor, T., Souza-Formigoni, M. L., de Lacerda, R. B., Ling, W., ... Vendetti J. (2011). A randomized controlled trial of a brief intervention for illicit drugs linked to the Alcohol, Smoking and Substance Involvement Screening Test (ASSIST) in clients recruited from primary health-care settings in four countries. *Addiction, 107,* 957–966.

Hystad, P., Davies, H. W., Frank, L., Van Loon, J., Gehring, U., Tamburic, L., & Brauer, M. (2014). Residential greenness and birth outcomes: Evaluating the influence of spatially correlated built-environment factors. *Environmental Health Perspectives, 122*(10), 1095–1102.

Institute of Medicine. (1998). *The future of public health.* Washington, DC: National Academy Press.

Institute of Medicine. (2002). *The future of the public's health in the 21st century.* Washington, DC: National Academy Press.

InterAction. (2013). *Global health: Investing in our future.* Washington, DC: Author.

Iqbal, S., Oraka, E., Chew, G., & Flanders, W. D. (2014). Association between birthplace and current asthma: The role of environment and acculturation. *American Journal of Public Health, 104*(51 Suppl. 1), S175–S182.

Jamal, A., Agaku, I. T., O'Conor, E., King, B. A., Kenemer, J. B., & Neff, L. (2014, November 28). Current cigarette smoking among adults—United States, 2005–2013. *Morbidity and Mortality Weekly Review (MMWR), 63*(47), 1108–1112.

Junehag, L., Asplund, K., & Svedlund, M. (2014). Perceptions of illness, lifestyle and support after an acute myocardial infarction. *Scandinavian Journal of Caring Sciences, 28*(2), 289–296.

Kanarek, N., Sockwell, D., Jia, H., Reese, S., Owen, P., Bender, B., ... Futa, M. (2000). Community indicators of health-related quality of life: United States, 1993–1997. *Morbidity and Mortality Weekly Report (MMWR), 49*(13), 281–285.

Kanarek, N., Tsai, H. L., & Stanley, J. (2011). Health ranking of the largest US counties using the community health status indicators peer strata and database. *Journal of Public Health Management and Practice, 17*(5), 401–405.

Keet, C. A., McCormack, M. C., Pollack, C.E., Peng, R. D., McGowan, E., & Matsui, E. C. (2015). Neighborhood poverty, urban residence, race/ethnicity, and asthma: Rethinking the inner-city asthma epidemic. *Journal of Allergy and Clinical Immunology, 135,* 655–662.

Kroon, L. A., Corelli, R. L., Roth, A. P., & Hudmon, K. S. (2013). Public perceptions of the ban on tobacco sales in San Francisco pharmacies. *Tobacco Control, 22*(6), 369–371.

Largo-Wight, E. (2011). Cultivating healthy places and communities: Evidenced-based nature contact recommendations. *International Journal of Environmental Health Research, 21*(1), 41–61.

Last, J. M. (2014). *Public health*. Retrieved from http://dx/doi.org/10.1036/1097-8542.556300 (http://www.accessscience.com/content/public-health/556300)

Leffers, J., McDermott-Levy, R., Smith, C. M., & Sattler, B. (2014). Nursing education's response to the 1995 Institute of Medicine Report: Nursing, health, and the environment. *Nursing Forum, 49*(4), 214–224.

Li, Y., Wang, W., Zhang, X., Lin, W., & Yang, Y. (2011). Impact of air pollution control measures and weather conditions on asthma during the 2008 Summer Olympic Games in Beijing. *International Journal of Biometerology, 53*(4), 547–554.

LMAS District Health Department. (n.d.). *Definition of public health*. Retrieved from http://lmasdhd.org/index.php?page=public-health

McClellan, M., & Rivlin, A. (2014). *Improving health while reducing cost growth: What is possible? Health Policy Issue Brief*. Washington, DC: The Brookings Institute.

McEwen, A., & Grothier, L. (2014). Smoking cessation: The heart of the matter. *Nurse Prescribing, 12*(2), 93–99.

McLaughlin, E. C., & Yan, H. (2015). *Texas nurse who contracted Ebola sues hospital company*. Retrieved from http://www.cnn.com/2015/03/02/us/nina-pham-hospital-lawsuit/

Moore, I., Chang, H., & Larson, K. (2014, April 19). *Los Angeles E-cigarette ban takes effect*. Retrieved from http://www.nbclosangeles.com/news/local/Less-Than-24-Hours-Before-the-E-Cig-Ban-Takes-Effect-255825081.html

Mothers Against Drunk Driving (MADD). (2015). *Campaign to eliminate drunk driving*. Retrieved from http://www.madd.org/drunk-driving/

Mundell, E. J. (2014, August 7). *CDC raises Ebola outbreak response to highest alert level*. Retrieved from http://consumer.healthday.com/general-health-information-16/emergencies-and-first-aid-news-227/cdc-raises-ebola-outbreak-response-to-highest-alert-status-690572.html

Muth, N. D. (2015). Zip code trumps genetic code in determining health. *IDEA Fitness Journal*, 31–37.

Naylor, B. (2015, July 15). *BP to pay $18.7 billion to settle Gulf Coast oil spill claims*. Retrieved from http://www.npr.org/sections/thetwo-way/2015/07/02/419429262/bp-to-pay-18-billion-to-settle-gulf-coast-oil-spill-claims

Nightingale, F. (1859/1992). *Notes on nursing: What it is, and what it is not [Commemorative edition]*. Philadelphia, PA: Lippincott Williams & Wilkins.

O'Donnell, M. P. (2009). Definition of health promotion 2.0: Embracing passion, enhancing motivation, recognizing dynamic balance, and creating opportunities. *American Journal of Health Promotion, 24*(1), iv.

Owens, J., & Cribb, A. (2013). Beyond choice and individualism: Understanding autonomy for public health ethics. *Public Health Ethics, 6*(3), 262–271.

Pacala, J. (2015). Tools of prevention. *Merck Manuals Online Library*. Retrieved from http://www.merckmanuals.com/home/fundamentals/prevention/tools-of-prevention

Pender, N. J., Murdaugh, C., & Parsons, M. A. (2014). *Health promotion in nursing practice* (7th ed.). Upper Saddle River, NJ: Prentice-Hall.

Plyer, A. (2015, August 28). *Facts for features: Katrina impact*. http://www.datacenterresearch.org/data-resources/katrina/facts-for-impact/

Powledge, T. M. (2015, February 24). *Epigenetics and disease: What it takes to get on the long road ahead*. Retrieved from http://www.geneticliteracyproject.org/2015/02/24/epigenetics-and-disease-what-it-takes-to-get-on-the-long-road-ahead/

Public Health Agency of Canada. (2013). *What makes Canadians healthy or unhealthy?* Retrieved from http://www.phac-aspc.gc.ca/ph-sp/determinants/determinants-eng.php#defining

Public Health Institute. (2010, May 7). *Santa Clara county toy law allows incentives for healthy food*. Retrieved from http://www.phi.org/news_events/news-viewRelease.cfm?pressReleaseID=196&year=2010

Rao, D. R., Sordillo, J. E., Kopel, L. S., Gaffin, J. M., Sheehan, W. J., Hoffman, E., … Phipatanakul, W. (2015). Association between allergic sensitization and exhaled nitric oxide in children in the School Inner-City Asthma Study. *Annals of Allergy, Asthma & Immunology, 114*, 250–260.

Sarrachi, R. (1997). The World Health Organization needs to reconsider its definition of Health. *British Medical Journal, 314*, 1409–1410.

Schumaker, E. (2015, June 8). *Ten statistics that capture the dangers of texting and driving*. Retrieved from http://www.huffingtonpost.com/2015/06/08/dangers-of-texting-and-driving-statistics_n_7537710.html

Swider, S., Krothe, J., Reyes, D., & Cravetz, M. (2013). The Quad Council practice competencies for public health nursing. *Public Health Nursing, 30*(6), 519–536.

Trowbridge, M. J., & Schmid, T. L. (2013). Built environment and physical activity promotion: Place-based obesity prevention strategies. *Journal of Law, Medicine, & Ethics, 41*(Suppl. 2), 46–51.

U.S. Department of Health and Human Services (USDHHS). (2016a). *Healthy people 2020: About healthy people*. Retrieved from http://healthypeople.gov/2020/about/default.aspx

U.S. Department of Health and Human Services (USDHHS). (2016b). *Healthy People 2020: Genomics*. Retrieved from http://www.healthypeople.gov/2020/topics-objectives/topic/genomics

U.S. Department of Health and Human Services (USDHHS). (2016c). *Healthy People 2020. Leading health indicators*. Retrieved from http://www.healthypeople.gov/2020/LHI/default.aspx

World Health Organization (WHO). (2015a). *Healthy cities*. Retrieved from http://www.who.int/healthy_settings/types/cities/en/

World Health Organization (WHO). (2015b). *Health*. Retrieved from http://www.who.int/trade/glossary/story046/en/

World Health Organization (WHO). (2015c). *WHO called to return to the Declaration of Alma Ata*. Retrieved from http://www.who.int/social_determinants/tools/multimedia/alma_ata/en/

World Health Organization (WHO). (2015d). *The Ottawa Charter for health promotion*. Retrieved from http://www.who.int/healthpromotion/conferences/previous/ottawa/en/

World Health Organization (WHO). (2015e). Media centre: Tuberculosis. *Fact sheet No. 104*. Retrieved from http://www.who.int/mediacentre/factsheets/fs104/en/#

thePoint: Everything You Need to Make the Grade!

thePoint® Visit http://thePoint.lww.com/Rector9e for selected readings, study aids for all learning styles, and more!

CHAPTER 2

History and Evolution of Community Health Nursing

"Our basic idea was that the nurse's peculiar introduction to the patient and her organic relationship with the neighborhood should constitute the starting point for a universal service to the region. We considered ourselves best described by the term 'public health nurses.'"

—**Lillian Wald** (1867–1940), Pioneer of Public Health Nursing

KEY TERMS

Causal thinking
Community-based nursing
Consumption

District nursing
Frontier nursing service
Henry street settlement

Industrial nursing
Nightingale model
Tenement

Visiting nurse association

LEARNING OBJECTIVES

Upon mastery of this chapter, you should be able to:

- Describe the four stages of community health nursing's development.
- Recognize the contributions of selected nursing leaders throughout history to the advancement of community health nursing.
- Analyze the impact of societal influences on the development and practice of community health nursing.
- Explore the academic and advanced professional preparation of community health nurses.

You just left the home of a client who is concerned about a new family that just moved into the building where she lives. This family of six lives in an apartment with barely enough room for two. After years in this neighborhood, you are well aware of the high rents charged for apartments with peeling paint, rodents, and garbage all around the buildings. Your client is concerned that the young mother looks "worn out" and coughs all the time. She said she tried to help, but the family doesn't speak much English. She describes four young children all under the age of about 5. She's never seen the husband, but you know that most of the men in this neighborhood leave early in the morning to try to get some day work, so you are not surprised. You thank her for the information and assure your client that you will do what you can to help her new neighbors. You start thinking about how you will prepare for the visit to the family who doesn't even expect you. At the top of your planning list is trying to find someone who speaks their language; you only know a few words. You suspect without even seeing the mother what the cough means, although you hope you are wrong. Then you think about the four young children living so close together and creating so much work for a woman who isn't well. The husband may want to help his wife more, but if he doesn't work, they don't have money to pay rent and buy food. You wonder if he has the cough too.

As you read this scenario, what picture comes to mind? What language did this family speak? What disease did this young mother most likely have? Now, think about when this event might have occurred. If you thought this was a current scenario, it certainly could be, but this scenario was actually set in the early 1900s. This family emigrated from Greece and had not yet mastered the English language. The mother likely had **consumption** (the common name for tuberculosis at that time). Because birth control information was not available to most women, the mother was unable to effectively space out her pregnancies. The filthy and overcrowded housing, termed **tenements,** was typical of the time. The husband found work as a laborer where he could. Few social services were available—if there was no work, there was no food for the family, and no money to pay the rent. The family came to America with the hope of a new start, but what they found was in many ways worse than what they had left. At least at home in Greece, they had family and friends to count on; here, they were alone. There were others from Greece who lived in the neighborhood, but it wasn't the same support system as every person was struggling to survive. Life was hard, and they worried most about their children, wondering what the future could hold for them.

Public health nurses in the early 20th century had to deal with many of the same issues we face today. We thought that tuberculosis was a disease of the past; now clients with multidrug-resistant strains are becoming alarmingly more common. Poverty, communicable diseases, poor housing, lack of social services, and limited access to family planning information remain as challenges to improving the health of our populations. As a community health nurse, you will be facing similar challenges to those faced by nurses of the past. As Abrams and Hays (2013) remind us, public health nursing practice is dynamic and "the problems of public health emerge and recycle in both new and familiar ways" (p. 475). History may not seem to be exciting, but without it, we often fail to see patterns and learn from the past mistakes. The occasionally misquoted saying by George Santayana (1863–1952), "Those who cannot remember the past

are condemned to repeat it," serves to caution us not to "forget" our heritage (Wikiquote, 2016, para. 3). As you read through this chapter, think about how public health nursing practice today has been shaped by the hard work of those nurses who went before.

This chapter examines the international roots of community health nursing as a specialty, exploring the historical and philosophical foundations that undergird the dynamic nature of its practice. The chapter traces community health nursing's rich historical development, highlighting the contributions of several nursing leaders and examining the global societal influences that shaped early and evolving community health nursing practice. The final section of the chapter describes the academic and advanced professional preparation required of public health nurses today. Nursing's past influences its present, and both guide its future in the 21st century.

HISTORICAL DEVELOPMENT OF COMMUNITY HEALTH NURSING

Before the nature of public health nursing can be fully grasped or its practice defined, it is necessary to understand its roots and the factors that shaped its growth over time. Public health nursing is the product of centuries of growth and adaptation. Its practice has adapted to accommodate the needs of a changing society, yet it has always maintained its initial goal of improved population health. Community health nursing's development, which has been influenced by changes in nursing, public health, and society, can be traced through several stages. This section examines these stages.

The history of public health nursing, since its recognized inception in Europe and more recently in America, encompasses continuing change and adaptation (Donahue, 2011). The historical record reveals a professional nursing specialty that has been on the cutting edge of innovations in public health practice and has provided leadership to public health efforts. A summary of public health nursing made in the early 1900s still holds true:

It is precisely in the field of the application of knowledge that the public health nurse has found her great opportunity and her greatest usefulness. In the nationwide campaigns for the early detection of cancer and mental disorders, for the elimination of venereal disease, for the training of new mothers, and the teaching of the principles of hygiene to young and old; in short, in all measures for the prevention of disease and the raising of health standards, no agency is more valuable than the public health nurse (Central Hanover Bank and Trust Company, Department of Philanthropic Information, 1938, p. 8)

In tracing the development of public health nursing and, later, community health nursing, the leadership role has been clearly evident throughout its history. Nurses in this specialty have provided leadership in planning and developing programs, in shaping policy, in administration, and in the application of research to community health.

Four general stages mark the development of public/community health nursing: (1) the early home care nursing stage, (2) the district nursing stage, (3) the public health nursing stage, and (4) the community health nursing stage. See Chapter 1 for a more complete discussion of the interchangeable terms *public health nurse* and *community health nurse*. In the course of the historical evolution of this specialty, there was a definite shift in thinking about the focus of practice, resulting in the broader use of the term *community health nurse*. However, the discussion that follows is about the practice emphasis, not the title. There are nurses in practice who use the title public health nurse, in addition to those called community health nurses; the term community/public health nurse has been widely accepted as depicting the generalist practice in this specialty (Callen et al., 2010). The title public health nurse is used, not just for those working in public health agencies but also those working in many diverse community settings where population-focused nursing occurs (Kulbok, Thatcher, Park, & Meszaros, 2012). Whether by custom, preference, or established employment title, nurses call themselves by many professional titles. It is important to recognize that the work of the nurse is, as it always has been, to improve the health of the community.

Early Home Care Nursing (Before Mid-1800s)

The prototype of **community-based nursing** can be seen within the historical development of home care nursing. For many centuries, female family members and friends tended the sick at home. In fact, in 1837, Farrar reminded women, "You may be called upon at any moment to attend upon your parents, your brothers, your sisters, or your companions" (p. 57). The focus of this care was to reduce suffering and promote healing.

The Origins of Early Nursing

The early roots of home care nursing began with religious and charitable groups; even emergency care was provided. In 1244, a group of monks in Florence, Italy, known as the Misericordia, provided first aid care for accident victims on a 24-hour basis. Another example is the Knights Hospitallers, who were warrior monks in Western Europe. They protected and cared for pilgrims on their way to Jerusalem (Pugh, 2001). During the

1500s, the Spanish nurse Bernardino de Obregon and his congregation provided both care of the ill and specialized nursing training at "houses of approval" (Jesús & Martínez, 2010, p. 27). These and other men's contributions to the early practice of nursing have been long overlooked. Further, the lack of attention to these early works "perpetuates the notion of men nurses as anomalies" (Evans, 2004, p. 321).

Medieval times saw the development of various institutions devoted to the sick, including hospitals and nursing orders. In England, the Elizabethan Poor Law, written in 1601, provided medical and nursing care to the poor and disabled. St. Frances De Sales organized the Friendly Visitor Volunteers in the early 1600s in France. This association was directed by Madame de Chantel and assisted by wealthy women who cared for the sick poor in their homes (Dolan, 1978). In 1617, St. Vincent de Paul started the Sisters of Charity in Paris, France. This organization was composed of nuns and lay women dedicated to serving the poor and needy. The ladies and sisters, under the supervision of Mademoiselle Le Gras in 1634, promoted the goal of teaching people to help themselves as they visited the sick in their homes. In their emphasis on preparing nurses and supervising nursing care, as well as determining causes and solutions for clients' problems, the Sisters of Charity laid a foundation for modern community health nursing (Bullough & Bullough, 1978).

Unfortunately, the years that followed these accomplishments marked a serious setback in the status of nursing and care of the sick. From the late 1600s to the mid-1800s, the social upheaval after the Reformation caused a decline in the number of religious orders, with subsequent curtailing of nursing care for the sick poor. Babies continued to be delivered at home by self-declared midwives, who generally had little or no training. Most midwives in the 14th to the 17th century were women "of a mature age, married or widowed with grown-up children," and they learned the skill of midwifery from experience or apprenticeship working with a veteran midwife (Kontoyannis & Katsetos, 2011, p. 32). Concern over high maternal mortality rates prompted efforts to better prepare midwives and medical students. One midwifery program began in Paris in 1720, and, in 1741, Dr. William Smellie organized a midwifery program in London (Bullough & Bullough, 1978). Licenses were available, but fees were often high. When long labors resulted in fetal death, midwives called in barber-surgeons who used "hooks, knives, or crockets" to remove the dead fetus (Kontoyannis & Katsetos, 2011, p. 33). A 17th century birth was "women's business," and when the midwife arrived, the husband left the room, which was described as "dark and warm." The midwife performed an internal exam to determine the degree of cervical dilation, after applying "fresh butter or other oils" to her hand; she then worked to "stretch the opening" and applied "various sweet oils or lubricants ...to the perineal area... to encourage softening and relaxation of the tissues" (Kontoyannis & Katsetos, 2011, p. 33). How does that compare to current practice?

The Industrial Revolution created additional problems; among them were epidemics, high infant mortality, occupational diseases and injuries, and increasing mental illness in both Europe and America. Hospitals were built in larger cities, and dispensaries were developed to provide greater access to physicians. However, disease was rampant; mortality rates were high; and institutional conditions, especially in prisons, hospitals, and "asylums" for the insane, were deplorable. The sick and afflicted were kept in filthy rooms without adequate food, water, cover, or care for their physical and emotional needs (Bullough & Bullough, 1978). Reformers such as John Howard, an Englishman who investigated the spread of disease in hospitals in 1789, revealed serious needs that would not be addressed until much later (Bullough & Bullough, 1978; Kalisch & Kalisch, 2004). It would take another 64 years and the seminal work of John Snow with the London cholera epidemic of 1853 to link a water pump with the transmission of the disease (Ramsey, 2006). The germ theory proposed by Louis Pasteur in 1862 dispelled many myths of the time, including the miasmic theory of disease (Fealy, McNamara, & Geraghty, 2010). The term miasma referred to "bad air" and was attributed as the cause of illness not "germs." The work of these early scientists would bring attention to the need for changes in the care of the sick as well as the prevention of illness.

During this same period, Dorothea Dix brought attention to the plight of the mentally ill from abuse and neglect in U.S. jails and almshouses. In what was arguably one of the first social research efforts in the United States, she presented her firsthand accounts of the terrible situations she found to the legislatures of Massachusetts, New York, New Jersey, and Pennsylvania (Reddi, 2005). Through her efforts, there was an almost 10-fold increase in the number of mental institutions, and the overall care of the mentally ill improved. Although not trained as a nurse, Dix would in later years oversee the Union Army female nurses prior to resuming her efforts with the mentally ill.

Although few in number, both Catholic and Anglican religious nursing orders continued the work of caring for the sick poor in their homes. For example, in 1812, the Sisters of Mercy organized in Dublin to provide care for the sick at home. With the status of women at an all-time low, often only the least respectable women pursued nursing. In 1844, in his novel *Martin Chuzzlewit*, Charles Dickens (1910) portrayed the nurse Sairey Gamp (Fig. 2–1) as an unschooled and slovenly drunkard, reflecting society's view of nursing at the time (Dolan, Fitzpatrick, & Herrmann, 1983). It was in the midst of these deplorable conditions and in response to them that Florence Nightingale began her work.

The Early Nightingale Years

Much of the foundation for modern community health nursing practice was laid through Florence Nightingale's remarkable accomplishments (Fig. 2–2). She has been referred to as a reformer, a reactionary, and a researcher who developed the "secular profession of nursing in the 19th century" (Abrams & Hays, 2013, p. 475; Palmer, 2001). Born in 1820 into a wealthy English family, her extensive travel, excellent education—including training at the first school for nurses in Kaiserswerth, Germany—and determination to serve the needy resulted in major reforms and improved status for nursing. Her work during the Crimean War (1854–1856) with the wounded in Scutari

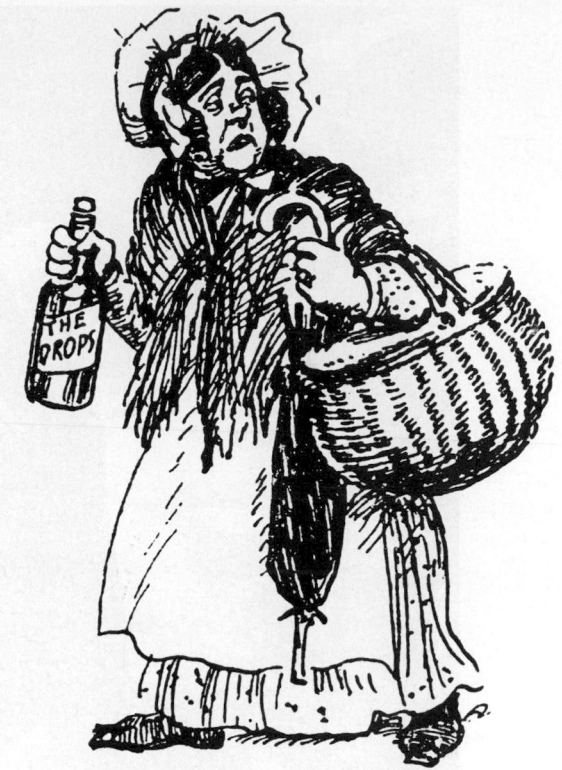

FIGURE 2–1 Sairey Gamp.

is well documented (Florence Nightingale Museum Trust, 1997; Lee, Clark, & Thompson, 2013; Woodham-Smith, 1951). Conditions in the military hospitals during the war were unspeakable. Thousands of sick and wounded men lay in filth, without beds, clean coverings, food, water, or laundry facilities. Florence Nightingale organized competent nursing care and established kitchens and laundries that resulted in hundreds of lives saved. Her work further demonstrated that capable, holistic nursing intervention could prevent illness and improve the health of a population at risk—precursors to modern community health nursing practice (Hogan, 2015). Nightingale's subsequent work reforming health in the military was supported by implementation of another public health strategy: the use of biostatistics. Through meticulously gathered data and statistical comparisons, Miss Nightingale demonstrated that military mortality rates, even in peacetime, were double those of the civilian population because of the terrible living conditions in the barracks. She promoted five essential components to optimal health and healing—pure air and water, efficient drainage, cleanliness, and adequate lighting. This work led to important military reforms and prioritization of hygiene (Lee et al., 2013). Even during World War II, British nurses were still fighting disease and unsanitary conditions as they worked with civilian victims of typhus epidemics—once again bringing Nightingale's work to the forefront (Brooks, 2013).

Miss Nightingale's concern for populations at risk included a continuing interest in the population of the sick at home. Her book, *Notes on Nursing: What It Is, and What It Is Not*, published in England in 1859, was written

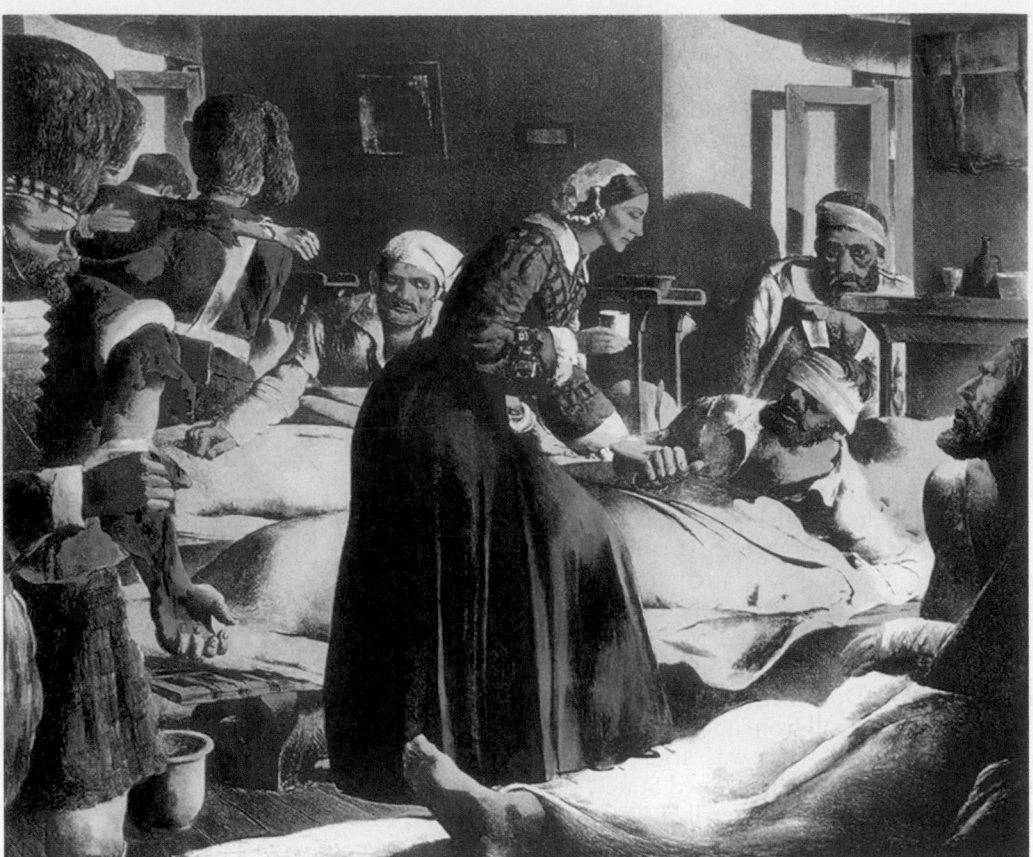

FIGURE 2-2 Florence Nightingale's concern for populations at risk, as well as her vision and successful efforts at health reform, provided a model for community health nursing today.

to improve nursing care in the home. It was also during this period that Nightingale clarified nursing as a woman's occupation (Evans, 2004). This gender distinction in nursing was due more to the culture of the times than as a direct exclusion of men from the practice; it was consistent with social norms of that period. Florence Nightingale also became a skillful lobbyist for health care reform. Her exemplary influence on English politics and policy improved the quality of existing health care and set standards for future practice. Furthermore, she demonstrated how population-focused nursing works (Lee et al., 2013).

In her work to help establish the first nonreligious school for nurses in 1860 at St. Thomas Hospital in London, she promoted a standard for proper education and supervision of nurses in practice, known as the **Nightingale Model**. Principles she wrote about in *Notes on Nursing* relate directly to her early education and the notions held by Hippocrates in ancient Greece, which she had studied for years. Specifically, her concern with the environment of patients, the need for keen observation, the focus on the whole patient rather than the disease, and the importance of assisting nature to bring about a cure all reflect Hippocrates' teachings (Nightingale, 1859/1969; Palmer, 2001).

Another great nurse and healer in her own right was Mary Seacole (1805–1881), who has been called the "Black Nightingale." She was the daughter of a Scottish soldier and a well-respected "doctress" who practiced Creole or Afro-Caribbean medicine in Jamaica and began helping her mother at an early age. Married only briefly

to Edwin Seacole, her husband died in 1844. Spending many years developing her skills, she helped populations who experienced tropical diseases, especially cholera, in Central America, Panama, and the Caribbean. She attempted, through many formal channels, to join Florence Nightingale in Scutari, but was rejected again and again. Undaunted, she went to the Crimea on her own to open a hotel for sick and convalescing soldiers, where she met Miss Nightingale and many of the troops she had cared for in Jamaica. Many of the military commanders sought her out for her knowledge of healing, and she was affectionately known by the troops as "Mother Seacole." After the war and into her old age, she continued to provide nursing care in London and when visiting Jamaica. She focused her caregiving among high-risk clients of the day and did so in an innovative, entrepreneurial manner unique for women, especially for women of color in the 1800s (National Geographic Education Staff, 2013). Her autobiography *Wonderful Adventures of Mrs. Seacole in Many Lands* was published in 1857 and became a best seller, providing much needed financial support for Mary Seacole (National Geographic Education Staff, 2013; Stanley, 2007). W.H. Russell Esq. wrote in the introduction "...I trust that England will not forget one who nursed her sick, who sought out her wounded to aid and succour them, and who performed the last offices for some of her illustrious dead" (Seacole, 1857). United Kingdom (UK) and Jamaican stamps were issued in her honor, and her portrait hangs in the National Portrait Gallery (UK) (National Geographic Education Staff, 2013) (see Display 2–1).

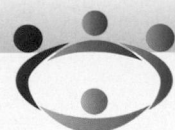

DISPLAY 2–1 TWENTY YEARS IN HISTORY: 1845 TO 1865

1845	Dorothea Dix addresses the New Jersey and Pennsylvania legislatures regarding abuse and neglect of the mentally ill.
1848	The first women's rights convention in the United States is held in Seneca Falls, New York.
1849	Harriet Tubman escapes from slavery and will lead many slaves to freedom through the Underground Railroad.
1850	Florence Nightingale begins nursing training at the Institute of St. Vincent de Paul in Alexandria, Egypt.
1854	Florence Nightingale cares for the injured in the Crimean War.
1855	Mary Seacole establishes a boarding house to care for sick and injured soldiers in the Crimea.
1857	Ellen Ranyard pioneers the first "district nursing" program in England.
1860	Florence Nightingale's *Notes on Nursing: What It Is, and What It Is Not* is published.
1861	Civil War embroils the country until 1865.
	Harriet Tubman serves as an unpaid nurse to wounded civilians and soldiers. Dorothea Dix is placed in charge of all female nurses in Union military hospitals.
1865	Sojourner Truth serves as a nurse for the Freedman's Relief Association during Reconstruction in Washington, DC.

District Nursing (Mid-1800s to 1900)

Nightingale's Continued Influence

The next stage in the development of community health nursing was the formal organization of visiting nursing or **district nursing**. In 1859, William Rathbone, an English philanthropist, became convinced of the value of home nursing as a result of private care given to his wife. He employed Mary Robinson, the nurse who had cared for his wife, to visit the sick poor in their homes and teach them proper hygiene to prevent illness. The need was so great that it soon became evident that more nurses were needed. In 1861, with Florence Nightingale's help and advice, Rathbone opened a training school for nurses connected with the Royal Liverpool Infirmary and established a visiting nurse service for the sick poor in Liverpool. Florence Lees, a graduate of the Nightingale School, was appointed first Superintendent-General of the District Nursing System (Hughes, 1902; Mowbray, 1997). As the service grew, visiting nurses were assigned to districts in the city—hence the name, district nursing. The names of these nurses were entered into a central roll, and they were known as "Queen's Nurses," as Queen Victoria recognized the benefits of this program for her people and was a supporter (Hughes, 1902, p. 344). Subsequently, other British cities also developed district nursing training and services. An example is the Nurse Training Institution for district nurses, founded in Manchester in 1864 and the work done by Ellen Ranyard and others in London (Prochaska, 1980/2003). Privately financed, the nurses were trained and then "dispensed food and medicine" to the sick poor in their homes; they were "closely supervised by various middle and upper class women who collected the necessary supplies" (Bullough & Bullough, 1978, p. 143).

Although Florence Nightingale is best remembered for her professionalization of nursing, she had a full understanding of the need for community health nursing. This was documented in her writings and recorded conversations:

- Hospitals are but an intermediate stage of civilization. At present, hospitals are the only place where the sick poor can be nursed, or, indeed often the sick rich. But the ultimate object is to nurse all sick at home (Nightingale, 1876).
- The aim of the district nurse is to give first-rate nursing to the sick poor at home (Nightingale, 1876 [cited in (Mowbray, 1997, p. 24)]).
- The health visitor must create a new profession for women (conversation with Frederick Verney, 1891 [cited in (Mowbray, 1997, p. 25)]).

For years, Miss Nightingale studied the social and economic conditions of India (Nightingale, 1864). The plight of the poor and ill in India led her to become involved with Frederick Verney in a pioneering "health at home" project in England in 1892. She wrote a series of papers on the need for "home missioners" and "health visitors," endorsing the view that prevention was better than cure, and set up training courses in 1980 for "sanitary visitors," later known as "health visitors" who taught families about cleanliness in the home, food preparation, and hygiene (Mowbray, 1997; Wright, 2011, p. 304).

Home Visiting Takes Root

In the United States, the first community health nurse, Frances Root, hired by the Women's Branch of the New York Mission in 1877, pioneered home visits to the poor in New York City. District nursing associations were founded in Buffalo in 1885 and in Boston and Philadelphia in 1886 (Display 2–2). These district associations served the sick poor exclusively, because patients

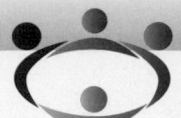

DISPLAY 2-2   TWENTY YEARS IN HISTORY: 1873 TO 1893

1873	First Nightingale model nursing school established in the United States at Bellevue Hospital.
1877	Francis Root—First Public Health Nurse hired by the Women's Branch of the New York Mission.
1878	Woman Suffrage Amendment is introduced in the U.S. Congress.
1879	Mary Eliza Mahoney becomes the first African American to graduate from an American nursing school.
1881	American Red Cross established by Clara Barton and associates becoming its first president.
1885	Visiting Nurse Association established in Buffalo, New York.
1886	Visiting Nurse Associations established in Philadelphia and Boston.
1893	Lillian Wald and Mary Brewster organized a visiting nurses service for the poor in New York, which would be named the Henry Street Settlement in 1906. *American Society of Superintendents of Training Schools for Nursing* founded by Isabel Adams Hampton Robb (later renamed the National League for Nursing).

with enough money had private home nursing care. However, the English model with its standards for visiting nurses' education and practice, established in 1889 under Queen Victoria, was not followed in the United States. Instead, visiting nursing organizations sprang up in many cities without common standards or administration. Twenty-one such services existed in the United States in 1890 (Bullough & Bullough, 1978; Kalisch & Kalisch, 2004).

Although district nurses primarily cared for the sick, they also taught cleanliness and wholesome living to their patients, even during that early period. For example, the Boston program, founded by the Women's Educational Association, "emphasized the teaching of hygiene and cleanliness, giving impetus to what was called instructive district nursing" (Bullough & Bullough, 1978, p. 144). This early emphasis on prevention and "health nursing" became one of the distinguishing features of district nursing and, later, of public health nursing as a specialty.

The work of district nurses in the United States focused mostly on the care of individuals. District nurses recorded temperatures and pulse rates and gave simple treatments to the sick poor under the immediate direction of a physician. They also instructed family members in personal hygiene, diet and healthful living habits, and the care of the sick. The problems of early home care patients in the United States were numerous and complex. Thousands of European and eastern European immigrants filled tenement housing in the poorest and most crowded slums of the large coastal cities during the late 1800s. Inadequate sanitation, unsafe and unhealthy working conditions, and language and cultural barriers added to poverty and disease. Nursing educational programs at that time did not prepare district nurses to cope with their patients' multiple health and social problems.

The sponsorship of district nursing changed over time. Early district nursing services in both England and the United States were founded by religious organizations. Later, sponsorship shifted to private philanthropy. Funding came from contributions and, in a few instances, from fees charged to patients on an ability-to-pay basis. Finally, visiting nursing began to be supported by public money. An early example occurred in Los Angeles where, in 1898, a nurse was hired as a city employee, making Los Angeles the first city in the United States to establish "municipal nursing" (Brainard, 1922). Although one form of funding dominated, all three types of financing continued to exist, as they still do. Although the government was beginning to assume more responsibility for the public's health, most district nursing services during this time remained private.

In England, the establishment of "health visitors" in poor areas of London began early in the 19th century. These health care providers enhanced the English model of health visitor/district nurse/midwife as the backbone of the primary health care system in the second half of the 1800s. "The impact of early health visiting was clearly shown by the halving of infant mortality in the areas within two years" (Beine, 1996, p. 59). The main focus of the health visitor's work was giving advice to poor mothers and teaching hygiene to prevent infant diarrhea (Beine, 1996).

Public Health Nursing (1900 to 1970)

By the beginning of the 20th century, district nursing had broadened its focus to include the health and welfare of the general public, not just the poor. This new emphasis was part of a broader consciousness about public health. Robert Koch's demonstration that tuberculosis was communicable led the Johns Hopkins Hospital to hire a nurse, Reba Thelin, in 1903, to visit the homes of tuberculosis patients. Her job was to ensure that patients followed prescribed regimens of rest, fresh air, and proper diet and to prevent possible infection (Sachs, 1908). A growing sense of urgency about the interrelatedness of health conditions and the need to improve the health of all people led to an increased number of private health agencies. These agencies supplemented the often-limited work of government health departments. By 1910, new federal laws made states and communities accountable for the health of their citizens.

Nurses Making a Difference

Around 1900, Jessie Sleet was hired by the Charity Organization Society's (COS) tuberculosis committee as a temporary district nurse in New York City (Mosley, 2007). Her position called for her to visit the city's Black community, which was ravaged by the disease. Jessie Sleet had been trained at the Provident Hospital in Chicago (a hospital for Black patients), which had a nurse's training program for Black women. Credited as the first Black public health nurse, Ms. Sleet was not eagerly accepted by the COS membership, but they agreed in the hope that the Black community would eventually accept her. She was so successful in her efforts that, 1 year later, the society hired her as a permanent employee (Mosley, 2007). Jessie Sleet was a pioneer in early community health nursing practice and forged the way for many others. Display 2–3 outlines other historical events during those intervening years.

As specialized programs such as infant welfare, tuberculosis clinics, and venereal disease control were developed, there was an increased demand for nurses to work in these areas (Fig. 2–3). As Bullough and Bullough (1978, p. 143) commented, "Although the hospital nursing school movement emphasized the care of the sick, a small but growing number of nurses were finding employment in preventive health care." In 1900, there were an estimated 200 public health nurses. By 1912, that number had grown to 3,000 (Gardner, 1936). This was an important development: "it brought health care and health teaching to the public, gave nurses an opportunity for more independent work, and helped to improve nursing education" (Bullough & Bullough, 1978, p. 143).

The role of the district nurse expanded during this stage. Lillian D. Wald (1867–1940), a leading figure in this expansion, first used the term *public health nursing* to describe this specialty (Ruel, 2014). District nurses, while caring for the sick, had pioneered in health teaching, disease prevention, and promotion of good health practices. Now, with a growing recognition of familial and environmental influences on health, public health nurses broadened their practice even more. Nurses working outside of the hospital increased their knowledge and skills in specialized areas such as tuberculosis, maternal and child health, school health, and mental disorders (Fig. 2–4).

Lillian Wald's contributions to public health nursing were enormous. A graduate of the New York Hospital Training School, she started teaching home nursing but quickly changed to a career of social reform and nursing activism (Christy, 1970). Appalled by the conditions of an immigrant neighborhood in New York's Lower East Side, she and a nurse-friend, Mary Brewster, started the **Henry Street Settlement** in 1893 to provide nursing and welfare services. The Lower East Side was home to many poor Irish, Italian, Jewish, and Chinese immigrants, and the Henry Street Visiting Nurse Service visited many sick children and families in their homes. One of the worst periods of depression occurred during this time, and the nurses supplied individuals and families with ice for keeping food fresh and also meals, medicine, and sterilized milk. They also made referrals to hospitals and clinics, as needed, and "emphasized the human dignity of even the poorest" tenement families (Fee & Bu, 2010, p. 1206). Wald's books, *The House on Henry Street* (1915) and *Windows of Henry Street* (1934), portray her work and views on public health nursing. Nurses supervised visits conducted through her organization; this was in contrast to earlier models, in which lay boards administered nursing services, and actual care was supervised

---

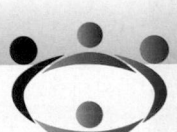

DISPLAY 2-3 TWENTY YEARS IN HISTORY: 1894 TO 1914

1894	Mary Adelaide Nutting appointed Superintendent of the Johns Hopkins School of Nursing—under her leadership, the curriculum was expanded from 2 to 3 years and limited the number of hours students could work.
1895	Vermont Marble Company forms the Industrial Nursing Service to care for sick employees and their families.
1897	First meeting of the *Nurses Associated Alumnae of the United States and Canada* that in 1911 would be renamed the American Nurses Association.
1898	Spanish American War leads to outbreak of Yellow Fever among solders.
1900	Jessie Sleet Scales becomes the first African American public health nurse in United States.
1902	New York City Board of Education hires Lina Rogers Struthers as a school nurse and begins the first public school nurse program in the county.
1905	American Red Cross receives Congressional Charter.
1906	Pure Food and Drug Act (prohibits misbranding and adulteration of drugs).
1909	Metropolitan Life Insurance Company provides first insurance reimbursement for visiting nursing care.
1910	Public Health Nursing program instituted at Teacher's College, Columbia University.
1912	National Organization for Public Health Nursing formed, with Lillian Wald as the first President.
1914	Margaret Sanger publishes the monthly newsletter *The Woman Rebel* to promote contraception and is charged with distributing illegal "birth control" information.

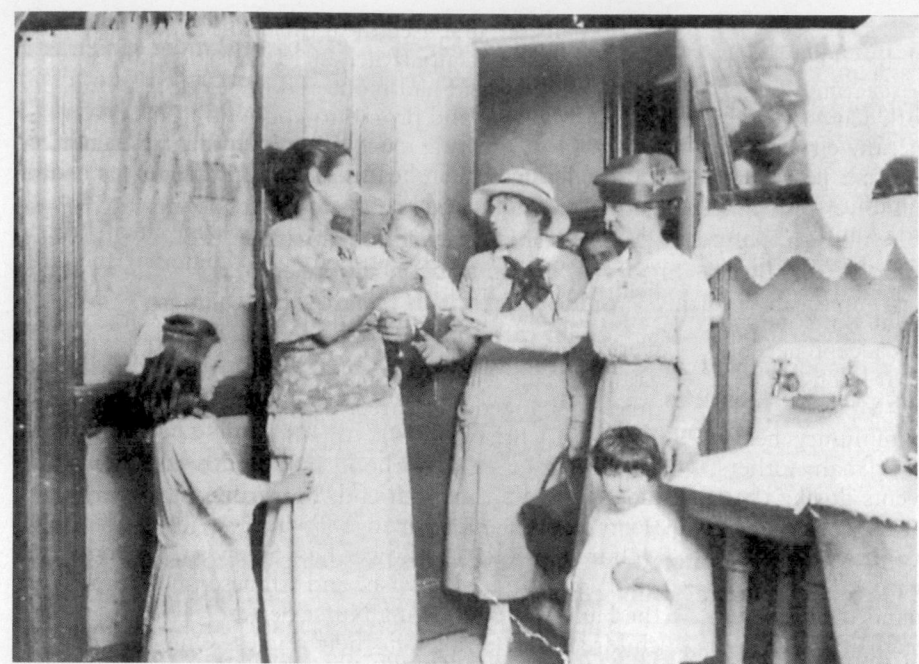

FIGURE 2–3 This photo depicts an early public health nurse, carrying her bag of equipment and supplies, at a regular home visit in the late 1800s. Physical and psychological care, as well as health lessons, were provided to families.

by laypersons. It was during these early years that Wald asked Jessie Sleet to recommend another Black nurse for service at the settlement (Mosley, 2007). Miss Sleet recommended her schoolmate Miss Elizabeth Tyler, a graduate of the Freedmen's Hospital Training School for Nurses (Washington, DC). In 1906, Miss Tyler became the first Black nurse hired at the Henry Street Settlement; she would not be the last, as the number steadily grew

(Fee & Bu, 2010). This was no small event in the progress of public health nursing and was a clear demonstration of Lillian Wald's commitment to social change.

Wald's Growing Influence

The work done at the Henry Street Settlement showed clearly that nursing could reduce illness-caused employee absenteeism. She demonstrated this in her early work

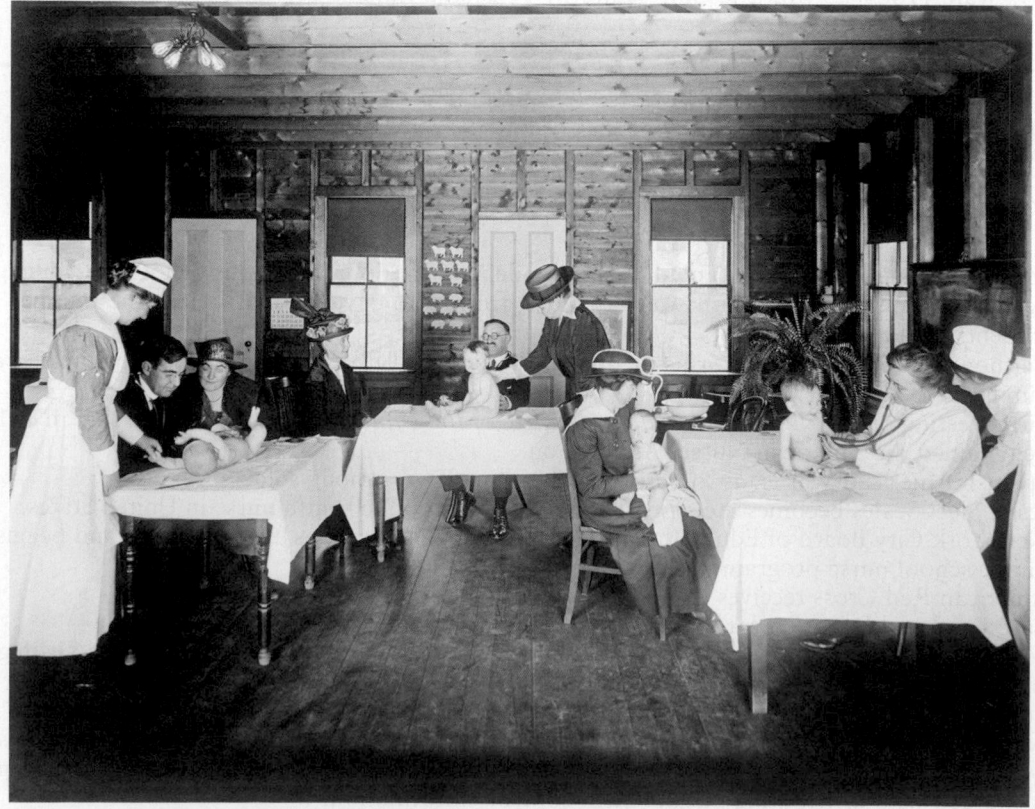

FIGURE 2–4 Well baby clinic in Framingham, Massachusetts (1920).

with the city of New York. She would use this success to address the issue of childhood illness and school absenteeism (Bullough & Bullough, 1978; Hawkins & Watson, 2010). In the early 1900s, medical inspectors sent home approximately 15 to 20 children per day from each school in New York City for health-related reasons. However, no one followed up with them to make sure that they were properly treated and returned to school. Wald suggested that placing nurses in the schools would allow for follow-up on recurring cases and home visits during the periods of exclusion. She argued that the nurses could supplement the work done by local physicians, who occasionally examined the children. Offering the services of one nurse for 1 month, Wald hoped to demonstrate how effective a school nurse could be. The work done by this first school nurse, Lina Rogers Struthers, was a resounding success (Kalisch & Kalisch, 2004). One year after this initial experiment, the number of children sent home from the New York City schools had dropped dramatically. By September 1903, only 1,000 children needed to be excluded (compared with 10,000 one year earlier); this was a nearly 10-fold reduction. As a result, the New York Board of Health hired dozens of nurses to work at the schools becoming the first school nursing program in the country; by 1905, 44 nurses covered 181 public schools (Hawkins & Watson, 2010; Vessey & McGowen, 2006). In 1917, Lina Rogers Struthers would go on to author the first textbook for school nurses *The School Nurse: A Survey of the Duties and Responsibilities of the Nurse in the Maintenance of Health and Physical Perfection and the Prevention of Disease Among School Children.* See Chapter 30 for current information about school nursing. See Perspectives for an early school nurse's experience (Figs. 2–5 and 2–6).

Just 6 years after her efforts with the New York City schools, Wald embarked on another visionary path. In 1909, she convinced the Metropolitan Life Insurance Company that nurse intervention could reduce death rates (Hamilton, 2007; Hawkins & Watson, 2003). In collaboration with the Henry Street Settlement, the company organized the Visiting Nurse Department and provided services to policyholders in a section of Manhattan (see Display 2–3). The success of this program resulted in expansion to other parts of the city and to 12 other eastern cities within 1 year. By 1912, the company had organized 589 Metropolitan nursing centers and, when possible, contracted with local Visiting Nurses Associations, although they also hired their own nurses (Kalisch & Kalisch, 2004; Ruel, 2014).

The legendary accomplishments of Lillian Wald reflect her driving commitment to serve needy populations. Through her efforts, the New York City Bureau of Child Hygiene was formed in 1908 and the Children's Bureau at the federal level in 1912. Wald's emphasis on illness prevention and health promotion through health teaching and nursing intervention, as well as her use of epidemiologic methodology, established these actions as hallmarks of public health nursing practice. She promoted rural nursing and family-focused nursing and encouraged improved coursework at the Teachers

PERSPECTIVES
LILLIAN "TOMMY" FULLER

Lillian Fuller was born in 1902, the only girl in a family of seven children living in rural Minnesota. Thus, she was nicknamed "Tommy." She grew up in Mountain Iron, a boomtown for iron mining and lumber companies for several decades. The town was owned by the mining company and surrounded by large ore pits; her family lived in a tar-papered house near saloons, bordellos, and the local jail. As a senior in high school, she decided that she wanted to be a nurse, but remembering the Dickens' character, Sairey Gamp, her family sent her to a college in St. Paul. She later prevailed and attended a hospital nursing school in Chicago, where she spent some time with the Chicago Visiting Nurse Association (VNA), under Edna L. Foley (a colleague of Lillian Wald). She worked with "crippled children" in four schools in the Hull-House district, where she met Jane Addams (the founder of social work). She arranged social services and physiotherapy for children in the Infantile Paralysis Aftercare program until she graduated from nursing school in 1925. She continued to work for the VNA until 1933, when she returned to Mountain Iron and took a nursing position with the Works Progress Administration (WPA)—a depression-era program to help unemployed individuals find jobs. She did a health census of her community for the WPA for a fee of $100. The next year, she worked as a half-time school nurse at the Mountain Iron School for $65 a month. She utilized the public health model of school nursing, as she was taught, and did the usual eye testing, first aid, checking for head lice, and taking care of rashes, stomachaches, colds, and accidents. She had medications on hand (even morphine), as the nearest hospital was five miles away, and she was thought of as the local health care authority as there was often no physician available. Because she was so well known in the community, she was able to initiate sex education programs in the schools and began a Future Nurses Club. In the summers, she worked as a camp nurse; the first year, there was a polio epidemic that cost the life of one of the counselors and sickened two of the campers. After many years of diligent service "Tommy" finally retired from school nursing in 1967, about the time that the first public health nurse practitioners were graduating from a new program in Colorado. She continued to provide service to the community, visiting sick elderly and lobbying for removal of an abandoned iron "tipple" or waste dump. A senior housing unit was eventually built on the site. Her practice spanned an important period in nursing: from early VNA service, working with colleagues of Lillian Wald, to a school nursing practice on the Iron Range of Minnesota where she often practiced independently and was an advocate for her children, families, and community. We can learn much from her life and service.

From Hawkins, J. W., & Watson, J. C. (2010). School nursing on the Iron Range in a public health nursing model. Public Health Nursing, 27(6), 571–578.

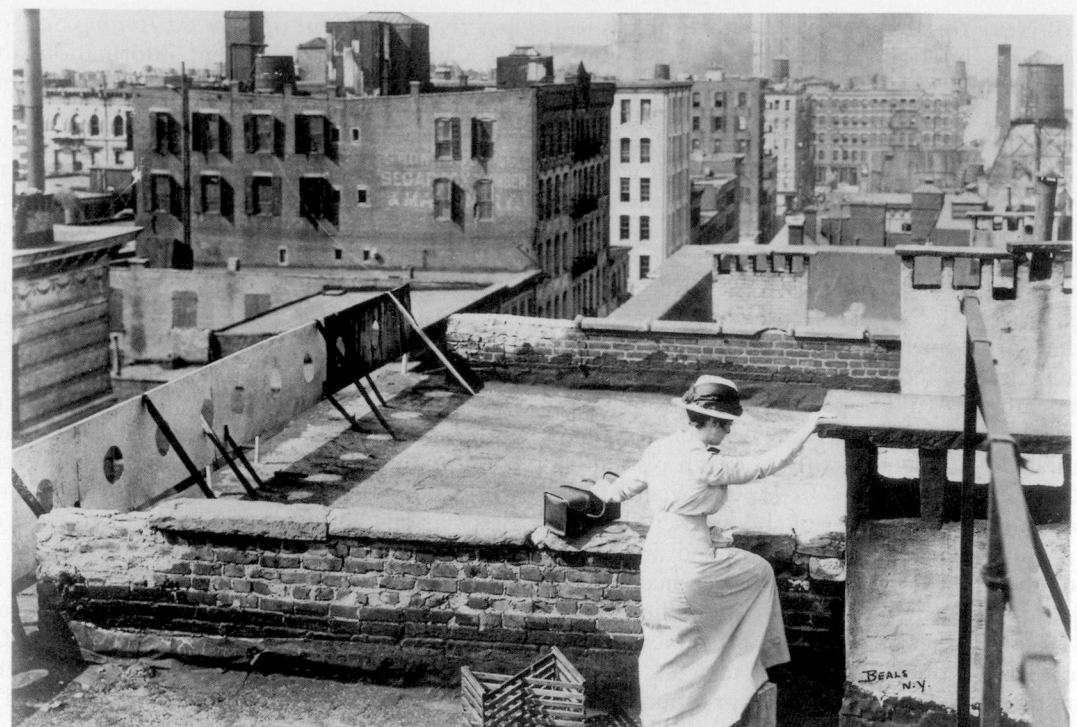

FIGURE 2–5 Lillian Wald climbing on rooftops in New York City. Used with permission of Visiting Nurse Service of New York.

College of Columbia University (New York) to prepare public health nurses for practice. Through her work and influence with the legislature to establish health and social policies, improvements were made in child labor and pure food laws, tenement housing, parks, city recreation centers, immigrant handling, and teaching of mentally handicapped children. In 1912, she helped to found and was first president of the National Organization for Public Health Nursing (NOPHN), an organization that set standards and guided public health nursing's further development and impact on public health (Christy, 1970; Feld, 2008). Her exemplary accomplishments truly reflect a concern for populations at risk. They further demonstrate how nursing leadership, involvement in policy formation, and use of epidemiology led to improved health for the public.

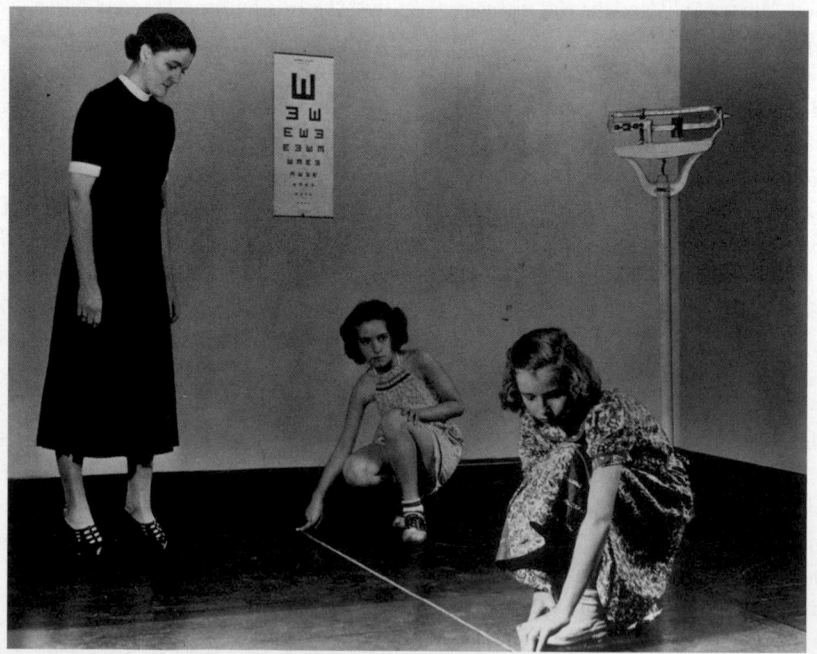

FIGURE 2–6 Students helping school nurse determine correct distance for eye exams (around 1935).

Another Nurse—Another Problem

During the same period that Lillian Wald and her contemporaries were working to alleviate the suffering caused by disease and poverty, another nurse, Margaret Sanger, began a different battle. Sanger, who was born in 1879, had seen her own mother die at the age of 48 after a long struggle with tuberculosis. Her 18 pregnancies undoubtedly contributed to her both contracting the disease and eventually succumbing to it. After her mother's death, she was accepted at White Plains Hospital as a nursing probationer (Ruffing-Rahal, 1986). Later, as a visiting nurse, Sanger was prevented by the Comstock Act of 1873 from providing any information on contraception to the women she cared for (Baker, 2011; Draper, 2006). She knew, as did many others, that the affluent and educated in American society were the only ones to have reliable contraception. Even discussing the topic was prohibited, placing increased pressure on the poor and uneducated women who were most in need of this basic information. In 1912, Sanger watched helplessly as a 28-year-old mother of three died from abortion-induced septicemia. "A few months earlier, during a similar crisis, this woman had begged Sanger for the "secret" of preventing future pregnancy" (Ruffing-Rahal, 1986, pp. 247–248). In 1916, Sanger openly offered birth control information in the Brownsville section of Brooklyn. Ten days after opening the first birth control clinic in America, Sanger was arrested, and the clinic was closed. But, later attempts were more successful (Baker, 2011). This was not the first, nor would it be her last encounter with the legal system (see Display 2–4). Her open defiance of a law that she saw as unjust eventually resulted in the formation of the International Planned Parenthood Federation (Fig. 2–7).

Call the Midwife

In Great Britain, midwifery continued to be in demand. This was especially true among the working class during the post–war period of the 1950s and 1960s. With

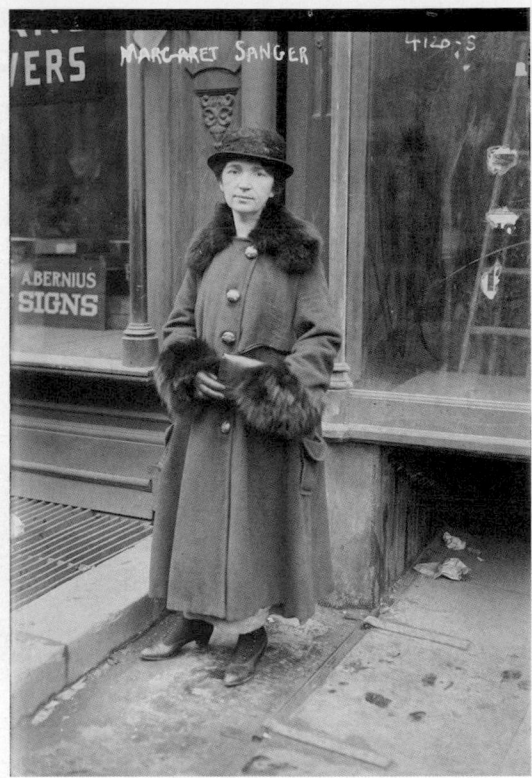

FIGURE 2–7 Margaret Sanger, thought to be standing in front of her birth control clinic.

London's East End as the backdrop, the popular PBS/BBC series, *Call the Midwife*, depicts the work of midwives during that time period (Stevens, 2013). At that time, there were over 10,000 midwives and district nurses in England, many traveling to home visits on bicycles, who provided education on nutrition, food safety, and care of infants and children, as well as home health care for injured workers and their usual duties of delivering babies.

DISPLAY 2–4 TWENTY YEARS IN HISTORY: 1917 TO 1937

1917	United States entry into World War I.
	The 18th Amendment is passed by Congress (ushering in Prohibition).
1918	U.S. Public Health Service establishes Division of Public Health Nursing to aid the war effort.
	World War I Armistice.
	Worldwide influenza epidemic begins.
	Frances Reed Elliott becomes the first African American nurse accepted into the American Red Cross Nursing Service.
1919	19th Amendment passed by Congress.
1920	Women vote for the first time in a presidential election.
1921	Margaret Sanger founds the American Birth Control League to distribute contraception information.
1925	Frontier Nursing Service established.
1929	Stock Market crash (beginning of the Great Depression).
1933	18th Amendment repealed (Prohibition ends).
1935	Passage of the Social Security Act.
1937	Birth control information now legal in all but two states (Massachusetts and Connecticut).

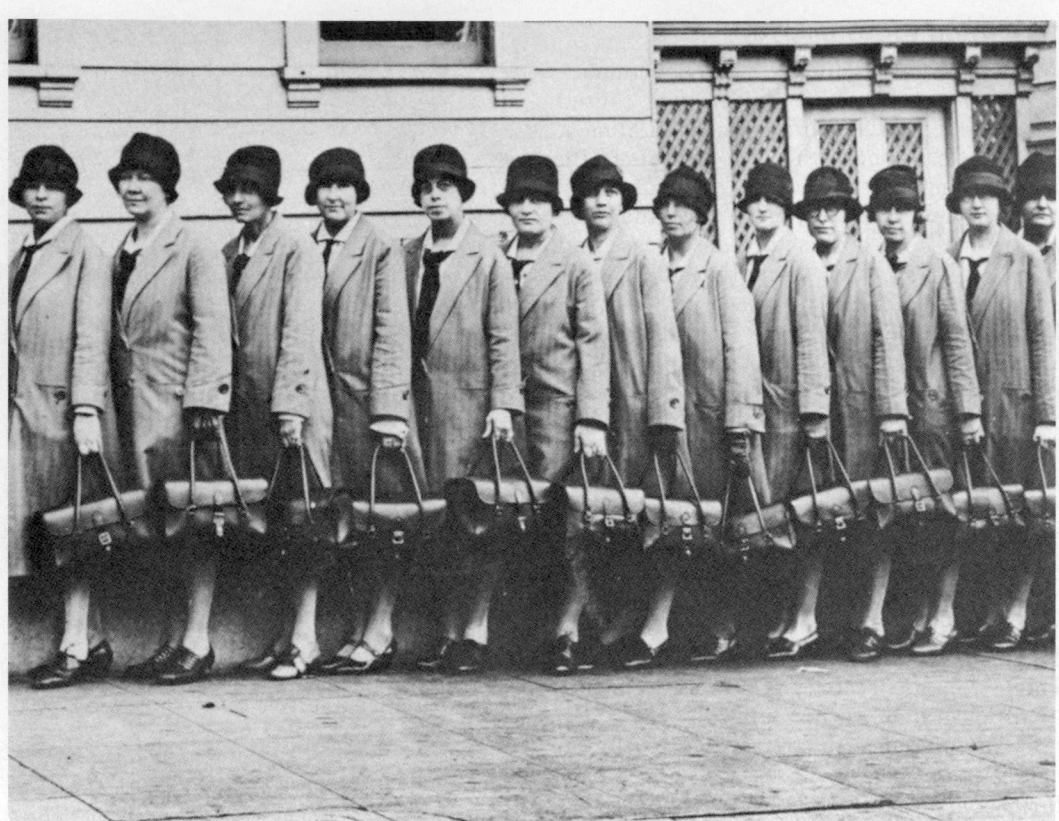

FIGURE 2–8   Public health nurses—with uniforms, bags, and sensible walking shoes. (Photograph courtesy of Visiting Nurses and Hospice of San Francisco.)

During this period of public health nursing, as a result of the influence of Lillian Wald and other nursing leaders, the family began to emerge as a unit of service (Fig. 2–8). The multiple problems faced by many families impelled a trend toward nursing care generalized enough to meet diverse needs and provide holistic services. There was also a call for specialization in some densely populated areas where tuberculosis, infant care, and school children were a primary concern (Brainard, 2012; King, 2011; Ruel, 2014). Public health nurses gradually gained more autonomy in such areas as home care and instruction of good health practices to families and community groups. Some examples include population work with children and families affected by polio and the subsequent mass immunization clinics after a vaccine was developed, as well as a single PHN's experience providing care to those living in an isolated outpost on Kodiak Island, Alaska, during an outbreak of tuberculosis-related pneumonia (Carter, 2001; Curtis, 2008). Their collaborative relationships with other community health providers grew as the need to avoid gaps and duplication of services became apparent. One example of an innovative program was the East Harlem Nursing and Health Service that operated between 1928 and 1941. It's territory was 87 city blocks that housed 112,000 mostly Italian immigrants and Italian Americans; most of the men were factory workers, trades-men, and laborers, and the families, especially the infants, had higher mortality rates than those for New York City overall (D'Antonio, 2013). They offered "integrated family services," with interdisciplinary and independent public health nurses practicing in tandem with other professionals who specialized in nutrition, mental health, social work, and education. A goal was to directly affect the "process of family building" and address the social determinants of health that devastated families during the Great Depression. With federal funding available, Mayor LaGuardia promoted public health nursing, along with hospital construction and neighborhood health centers. A shift from home births to hospital deliveries was dramatic—from 85% in 1927 having babies at home with midwives to 65% in 1934 having babies delivered by physicians in hospitals. This, along with the failure to attain financial sustainability as required by their major funder, the Rockefeller Foundation, led to the demise of this innovative public health program (D'Antonio, 2013). Out of necessity, public health nurses began keeping better records of their services and continued home visiting for those in need. They also responded to population health needs, as more individual care was now available at hospitals and health centers. See From the Case Files: New York City PHNs and the 1918 Influenza Pandemic.

Another form of public health nursing, **industrial nursing**, also expanded during the early 1900s. J. & J. Colmans of Norwich, England, hired Philippa Flowerday Reid, the first known industrial nurse, in 1878. Her job was to assist the company physician and to visit sick employees and their families in their homes. In the United States, the Vermont Marble Company was first to begin a nursing service in 1895, and other companies followed soon after. By 1910, 66 firms in the United

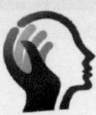

From the Case Files I

New York City PHNs and the 1918 Influenza Pandemic

The 1918 influenza pandemic caused over 40 million deaths worldwide and 675,000 U.S. deaths. The country was at war (World War I), and the American Red Cross, the U.S. Public Health Service, and health care workers were stretched thin. The epidemic began in New York City with three cases during mid-September, 1918. It spread quickly and crossed social class and income boundaries; within a few days, there were 31 new cases reported (Keeling, 2009). Cities across the Eastern seaboard requested assistance, and a coordinated plan for a decentralized response was set in place. Lillian Wald, who directed the Henry Street visiting nurses, had weathered epidemics on the Lower East Side of New York City before and quickly responded to this new, even more virulent threat. When making home visits, nurses found "whole families were ill…without anyone to give them the simplest nursing care" (Keeling, 2009, p. 2735). One person described "People, desperate in their need watched from windows and doorways for the nurse. They surrounded her on the street, imploring her to go in six directions at once" (Geister, 1957, October, pp. 583–584). Wald noted almost 500 calls for nursing services to patients with influenza and pneumonia in the "first four days of October" and that nurses were instructed to wear masks but "31 out of….170 had succumbed to influenza" (Keeling, 2009, p. 2736). The Nurses' Emergency Council was organized for a citywide response, led by Lillian Wald who requested that all who employed nurses allow them to work in caring for those afflicted by the epidemic. With this central structure, duplication of services was avoided, and quicker services could be provided. Wald requested automobiles for the visiting nurses to help them travel more quickly and carry "linens, pneumonia jackets, and quarts of soup"; the nurses started work early every morning and went out again at 4 PM to check on cases reported later each day (Keeling, 2009, p. 2737). They finished rounds around midnight, only to start again early the next morning. In Harlem, a nurse reported on a family of seven—the mother has influenza, "the father has lobar pneumonia, two children have measles and bronchopneumonia, and one child is only four weeks old," noting that they had no care until their case was reported to the VNA. This was a common situation across the city. As the epidemic began to subside, the Nurses' Emergency Council discontinued central services on the 6th of November, and the Henry Street nurses opened postinfluenza clinics to address the follow-up needs of families. There were almost 11,000 deaths from influenza and almost 10,000 deaths from pneumonia reported in New York City over the 2-month period of the epidemic. All that the nurses could provide was comfort care—clean linens, bed baths, fluids, and monitoring. There was little help from the federal level of government, and private, philanthropic, and religious organizations worked together with local government and nursing agencies to combat the deadly epidemic.

How do you think your city or county would respond to a new pandemic threat similar to the one in 1918? How would PHNs be involved?

From Keeling, A. W. (2009). "When the city is a great field hospital": The influenza pandemic of 1918 and the New York City nursing response. Journal of Clinical Nursing, 18, 2732–2738.
Geister, J. (1957, October). The flu epidemic of 1918. Nursing Outlook, 5, 582–584.

States employed nurses. During World War I, the number of industrial nurses greatly increased with the recognition that nursing service reduced worker absenteeism (Bullough & Bullough, 1978). Early industrial nursing was the forerunner of modern occupational and environmental health nursing. See Chapter 31 (Fig. 2–9).

During this stage, the institutional base for much of public health nursing shifted to the government. By 1955, 72% of the counties in the continental United States had local health departments. Public health nursing constituted the major portion of these local health services and emphasized health promotion, as well as care for the ill at home (Scutchfield & Keck, 2009). Some of the district nursing services, known as **visiting nurse associations** (VNAs), remained privately funded and administered, offering their own home nursing care. In some places, city or county health departments joined administratively and financially with VNAs to provide a combination of services, such as home care of the sick and health promotion to families. The Red Cross offered public health nursing services from 1912 to 1951. The first incarnation was the Rural Nursing Services headed by Fannie Clement, and the Town and Country Nursing Service was organized and provided both rural areas and cities with nursing services. Jane A. Delano was the director of the Red Cross during this time. The final incarnation was the Red Cross Public Health Nursing Service, and the earliest service of Philadelphia Red Cross Society nurses was to Johnstown flood victims. The Red Cross provided public health nursing services to families of soldiers during both World Wars (Ramsay, 2012).

Rural public health nursing, which had already been organized around 1900 in Great Britain, Germany, and Canada, also expanded in the United States (see Chapter 29). Initially, starting in 1912, rural nursing was privately financed and largely administered through the Red Cross and the Metropolitan Life Insurance Company, but responsibility had shifted to the government by the 1940s (Bullough & Bullough, 1978). An innovative example of rural nursing was the **Frontier Nursing Service**,

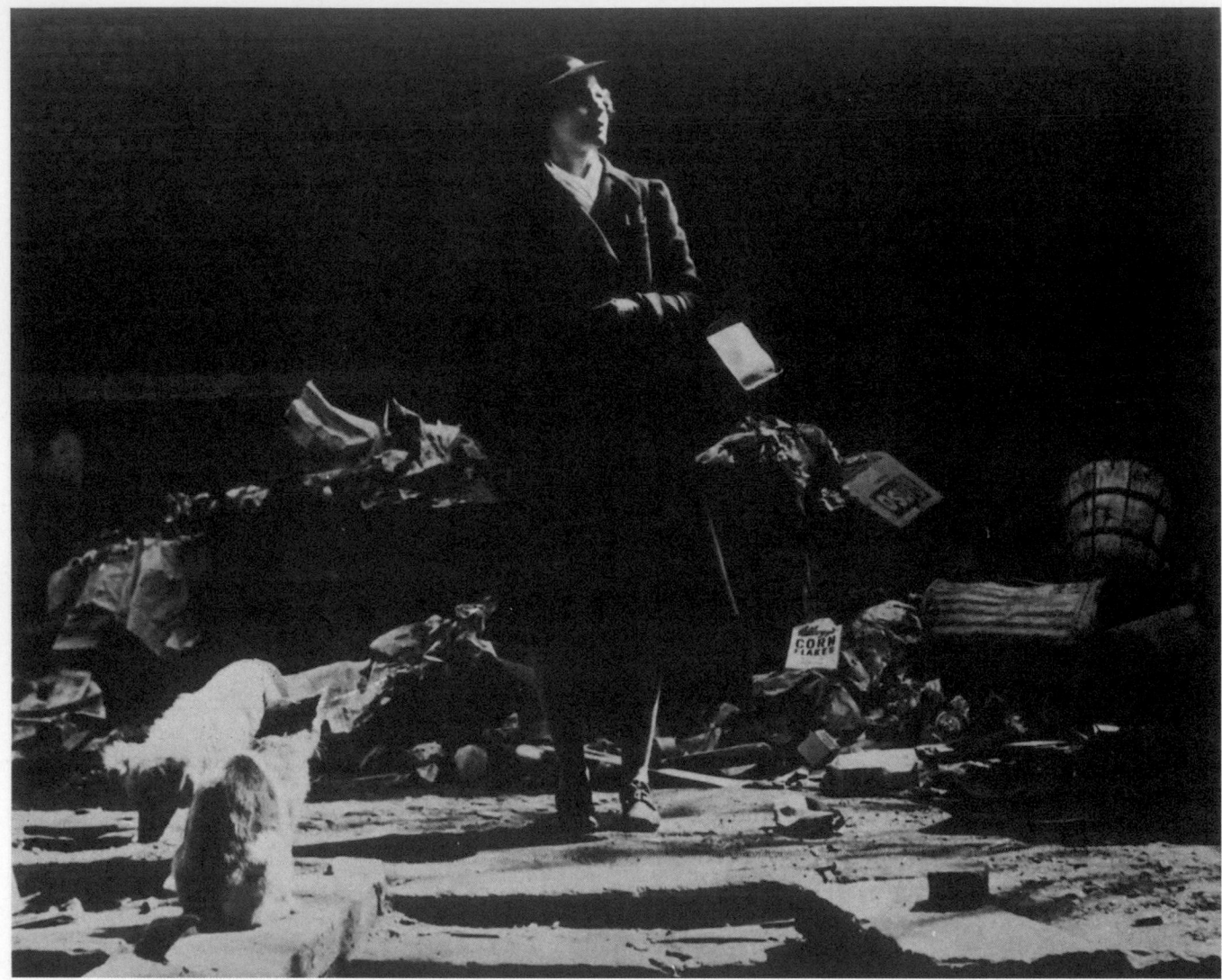

FIGURE 2–9   A PHN, wearing an overcoat, hat, and carrying a nurses' bag, stands in front of a pile of trash as she makes her way through a neighborhood.

which was started by Mary Breckenridge (1881–1965) in 1925, to serve mountain families in Kentucky. From six outposts, nurses on horseback visited remote families to deliver babies and provide food and nursing services. The work was hard, but rewarding; it combined general public health nursing and midwifery (January, 2009). Over the years, the service has expanded to provide medical, dental, and nursing care. The Frontier Nursing Service continues today, with its remarkable accomplishments of reducing mortality rates and promoting health among this disadvantaged population, as the parent holding company for the Frontier School of Midwifery and Family Nursing. It is the largest nurse–midwifery program in the United States. In addition, Mary Breckinridge Healthcare, Inc. consists of a home health agency, two outpost clinics, one primary care clinic, and the Kate Ireland Women's Healthcare Clinic (Simpson, 2000). For more on rural nursing and the Frontier Nursing Service, see Chapter 29. See Perspectives: Roaming Through the Hills with the PHN.

This public health nursing stage was characterized by service to the public, with the family targeted as a primary unit of care. Official health agencies, which placed greater emphasis on disease prevention and health promotion, provided the chief institutional base (Fig. 2–10).

Nurses in Military Service

Since Florence Nightingale's service to the British soldiers during the Crimean War, nurses have continued to provide service during wartime. Women served in many capacities (nurses, cooks, seamstresses) during the Revolutionary war. Clara Barton, famous for founding the American Red Cross, volunteered her services during the Civil War, as did about 20,000 women of different races and classes (D'Antonio, 2010). Some nursing graduates were contracted to serve during the Philippine American War and in the Spanish American War at the turn of the 20th century.

In 1901, the Army Nurse Corps was established, and in 1908, the Navy Nurse Corps was added (Lineberry, 2013). During World War I, many new graduates responded to the pleas of the Red Cross for nurses to care for the sick and wounded and entered the Army Nurse Corps. At the

PERSPECTIVES
ROAMING THROUGH THE HILLS WITH THE PHN

As a state nursing supervisor, I visit PHNs during a typical week providing services in rural Virginia. The first PHN's territory consisted of a mountainous area, with winding, often muddy roads. Our first visit was made on horseback: "The road straight up the mountain was winding and lovely and way below in a gorge ran a stream" on our way to Star-Chapel School (Webb, 2011, p. 291). After traveling by horseback all day, we crossed a final stream to reach a house that backed up to the mountain; "the stream dashing over the rocks at the front door" where we were invited to spend the night (p. 292). The family was eager to help the nurse who had cared for others during the 1918 flu epidemic. At the school, we checked the children, and the PHN talked to them about how to prevent disease and the importance of personal hygiene. We visited two more schools on the way back home. In the southwest corner of the state, I visited another PHN, and we traveled 30 miles by logging train, which seemed to be "balanced on the peak of a mountain top" to visit a small, isolated town that desperately wants a nurse to visit schoolchildren and families (p. 292). In another county, the PHN visits with a girl who is recovering from meningitis, and her mother brags that she wants a clean glass and washes her hands now before she eats every

meal. We then travel to a log cabin where mothers and children meet every week, and the PHN weighs babies and provides health pamphlets and talks about "babies, screening houses, homemade ice boxes," and other topics of interest (p. 293). The women cook gingerbread and make hot cocoa in an old stone fireplace there. We later visited a rundown camp and saw many women "each with three to eight children hanging on their skirts," and a 14-year-old who stopped dipping snuff, as the nurse advised (p. 293). The nurse had promised her a prize, and she proudly claimed it. The PHN talked with a 12-year-old girl who refused to go to school and found that the reason was that she couldn't see, and her eyes were hurting. The mother agreed that she needed to see a specialist, but the girl would not agree to this unless her father made her go. The PHN was disappointed to see a 4-year-old, who had agreed to stop chewing tobacco, come by to visit her with a cigarette in his mouth! Our state needs many more PHNs, and we are budgeting the money for services, but we don't have enough nurses who are willing to do this type of rural pioneer nursing. It can be very rewarding.

From Webb, B. (2011). Roaming through Virginia with the public health nurse. Public Health Nursing, 28(3), 291–293. Reprint of 1920 article.

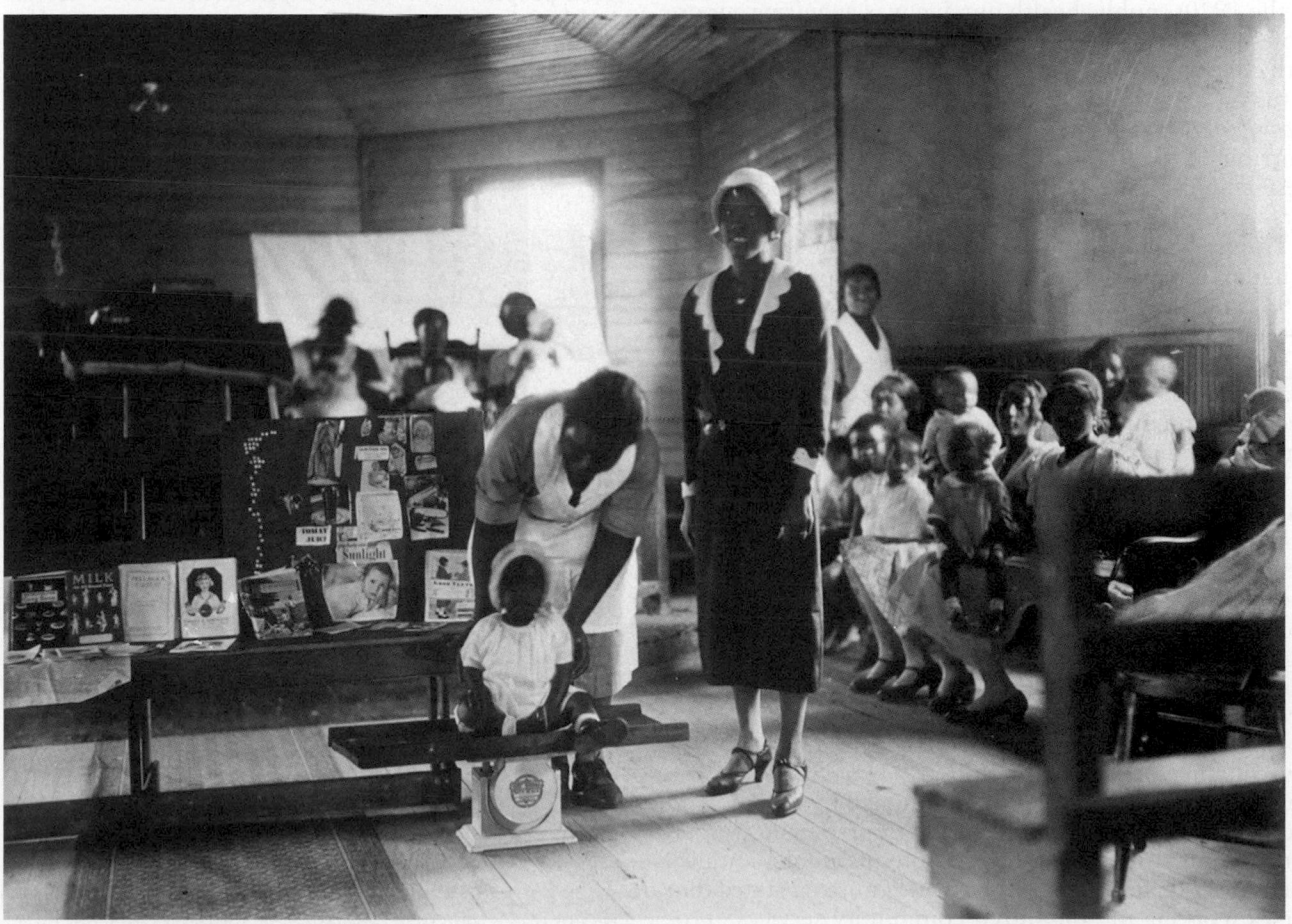

FIGURE 2–10 Preschool child is weighed by African American nurse at an improvised baby station and child health clinic set up in a church.

start of World War II, the Red Cross called for 50,000 nurses to join the armed services (Lineberry, 2013). In 1945, President Franklin D. Roosevelt "desegregated nursing in the U.S. Armed Forces" (D'Antonio, 2010, p. 132). Earlier, in 1942, the Cadet Nurse Corps was created to feed the demand for nurses during World War II, but military nurses didn't receive permanent commissioned officer status until 1947 (Robinson, 2009). About 74,000 nurses served during the second world war, and some ended up behind enemy lines, in combat, and as Japanese prisoners of war (Lineberry, 2013). Using educational benefits of the G.I. Bill, military nurses returning from World War II were sometimes limited because of enforced freshman quotas for women, as male veterans were given preference until 1952 (Barnum, 2011). However, schools of public health reported increased enrollment by returning military nurses in programs preparing them for public health nursing. This specialty practice provided them with more autonomy and a more independent practice than hospital nursing (Barnum, 2011).

In 2011, 18% of the over 2.2 million active military personnel were females (National Public Radio, 2011). Not all female military personnel are nurses and not all military nurses are females. See more on publicly-funded settings for nurses, including the U.S. Public Health Service, in Chapter 30.

The Profession Evolves

By the 1920s, public health nursing was acquiring a more professional stature, in contrast to its earlier association with charity. Nursing as a whole was gaining professional status as a science, in addition to being an art. National nursing organizations began to form during this stage and contributed to nursing's professional growth. The first of these emphasized establishing educational standards for nursing. Called the American Society of Superintendents of Training Schools for Nurses in the United States and Canada, it was started by Isabel Hampton Robb in 1893, and later became known as the National League of Nursing Education in 1912. This was the forerunner of the National League for Nursing (NLN), which was established in 1952 (Ellis & Hartley, 2012). In 1890, a meeting of nursing leaders at the World's Fair in Chicago initiated an alumnae organization of 10 schools of nursing to form the National Associated Alumnae of the United States and Canada in 1896, which was created to promote nursing education and practice standards. In 1899, the group was renamed the Nurses' Associated Alumnae of the United States and Canada. Canada was excluded from the title in 1901, because New York, where the organization was incorporated, did not allow representation from two countries. In 1911, the organization went through a final name change to the American Nurses' Association (ANA), while Canadian nurses formed their own nursing organization (Ellis & Hartley, 2012). As mentioned previously, NOPHN, founded by Lillian Wald and Mary Gardner, brought together nurses who worked in the community setting to promote the public's health. Their 1929 definition of public health nursing stated that nurses working in "organized community services" provided care to the "individual, family, and community" in order to correct "defects," prevent disease, and promote

health and that duties also "may include skilled care of the sick in their homes" (Abrams, 2004, p. 507). In 1931, NOPHN developed "general and specialized objectives" regarding work with individuals, families, and communities (Abrams, 2004, p. 507). In 1949, the organization outlined 12 functions of skilled public health nurses working in the community setting:

> Maternity, infancy, preschool, school, and adult health services; morbidity, communicable diseases, tuberculosis, syphilis and gonorrhea; orthopedic; industrial; and mental hygiene (Abrams, 2004, p. 508).

The organization also began adopting the term community health nursing as a less "restrictive" view that incorporated a greater focus on scientific advances in health care that involved changing the behavior of individuals, compared to public health nursing that focused primarily on population health and environmental control of communicable diseases and sanitation (Abrams, 2004, p. 508). In 1952, NOPHN merged with the NLN. These three organizations, in particular, strengthened ties between nursing groups and improved nursing education and practice (Figs. 2–11 and 2–12).

As nursing education became increasingly rigorous, collegiate programs began to include public health as essential content in basic nursing curricula. The first collegiate program with public health content to be accredited by the NLN began in 1944 (National Organization for Public Health Nursing, 1944; Display 2–5). Previously,

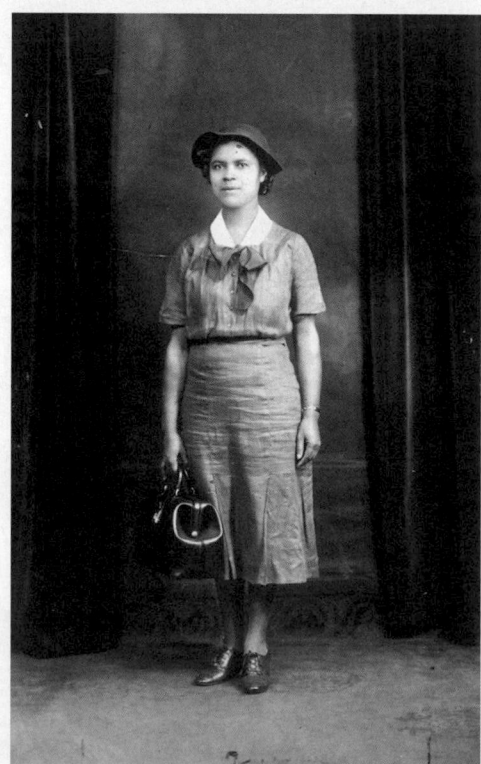

FIGURE 2–11 Ethel May Jones, an African American public health nurse who was employed as a midwife/teacher by a State Board of Health, is shown dressed in her uniform and carrying her bag.

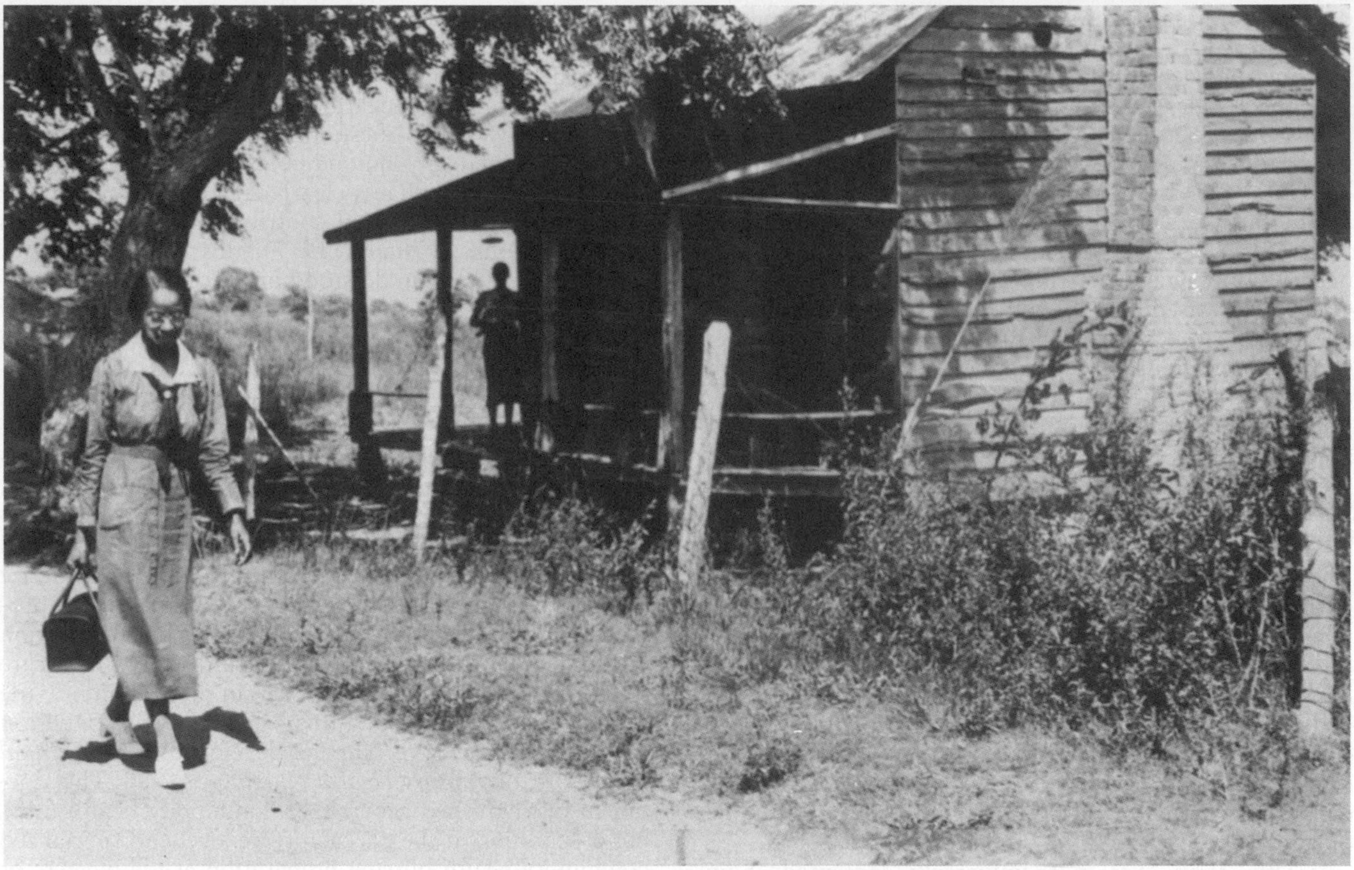

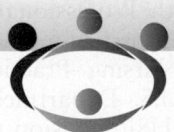

FIGURE 2–12 An African American public health nurse walks pass a rural wooden house.

DISPLAY 2–5 TWENTY YEARS IN HISTORY: 1941 TO 1961

1941	United States enters into World War II.
1943	Cadet Nursing Corps Program established, providing federal funding for academic nursing education in exchange for work in "essential nursing services."
1944	First basic program in nursing accredited as including sufficient public health content.
	Public Health Service Act authorizes qualified nurses to be commissioned in the U.S. Public Health Service.
1945	World War II ends.
	United Nations votes to establish the World Health Organization.
1946	Hill-Burton Act approved—shift to hospital-based care with federal funding of hospitals and medical centers.
	Communicable Disease Center established (forerunner of the Centers for Disease Control and Prevention).
1949	Lucile Petry Leone becomes the Chief Nurse Officer of the Public Health Service, the first nurse, and the first woman to achieve flag rank in the Public Health Service or military.
1950	United States involved in Korean Conflict (this ends in 1953).
1954	Brown vs. Board of Education—Landmark Supreme Court decision prohibits racial segregation in public schools.
1955	Introduction of the Salk Polio vaccine.
1956	Health Amendments Act provided funds to support public health nurse advanced training.
1961	The Peace Corps is founded.
	United States enters into the Vietnam War.

only postgraduate courses in public health nursing had been offered for nurses choosing this specialty. Adelaide Nutting had developed the first such course in 1912, at Teachers College in New York, in affiliation with the Henry Street Settlement. A group of agencies met in 1946 to establish guidelines for public health nursing, and by 1963, public health content was required for NLN accreditation in all baccalaureate degree level nursing programs (Kulbok & Glick, 2014). The nurse practitioner (NP) movement, starting in 1965 at the University of Colorado, was initially a part of public health nursing and emphasized primary health care to rural and underserved populations. The number of educational programs to prepare NPs increased, with some NPs continuing in public health and others moving into different clinical areas (Hawkins & Watson, 2010).

Community Health Nursing (1970 to the Present)

The emergence of the term *community health nursing* heralded a new era. By the late 1960s and early 1970s, while public health nurses continued their work, many other nurses who were not necessarily practicing public health were based in the community. Their practice settings included community-based clinics, doctors' offices, worksites, and schools. To provide a label that encompassed all nurses in the community, the ANA and others called them community health nurses. Display 2–6 provides examples of significant events in mid-1960s to early 1980s.

This term was not universally accepted, however, and many people—including nurses and the general public—had difficulty distinguishing community health nursing from public health nursing. For example, nursing education, recognizing the importance of public health content, required course work in public health

---

DISPLAY 2–6 TWENTY YEARS IN HISTORY: 1965 TO 1985

1965   Medicare and Medicaid are established.
1969   National Environmental Policy Act provides first coordinated oversight effort.
1972   Social Security Administration allows Medicare coverage for those <65 years with long-term chronic disease and end-stage renal disease.
1973   U.S. military troops leave South Vietnam. Roe vs. Wade—Landmark Supreme Court decision legalizes abortion.
1977   Global smallpox eradication achieved.
1978   Drug-resistant TB reported in Mississippi.
1979   *Healthy People: The Surgeon General's Report on Health Promotion and Disease Prevention* released.
1985   Red Cross Blood Services begin testing for HIV antibody.

---

for all baccalaureate students. This meant that graduates were expected to incorporate public health principles such as health promotion and disease prevention into nursing practice, regardless of their sphere of service. Consequently, some questioned whether public health nursing retained any unique content. Although leaders such as Carolyn Williams clearly stated that community health nursing's specialized contribution lay in its focus on populations (Williams, 1977), this concept did not appear to be widely understood or practiced.

Confusion also arose regarding the question of whether community health nursing was a generalized or a specialized practice. Graduates from baccalaureate nursing programs were inadequately prepared to practice in public health; their education had emphasized individualized and direct clinical care and provided little understanding of applications to populations and communities. By the mid-1970s, various community health nursing leaders had identified knowledge and skills needed for more effective community health nursing practice (Roberts & Freeman, 1973). These leaders valued promoting the health of the community, but both education and practice continued to emphasize direct clinical care to individuals, families, and groups in the community (de Tornyay, 1980). Reflecting this view, the ANA's Division of Community Health Nursing developed *A Conceptual Model of Community Health Nursing* in 1980. This document distinguished generalized community health nursing preparation at the baccalaureate level and specialized community health nursing preparation at the masters or postgraduate level. The generalist was described as one who provides nursing service to individuals and groups of clients while keeping "the community perspective in mind" (American Nurses Association, Community Health Nursing Division, 1980, p. 9).

To distinguish the domains of community and public health nursing, in 1984, the U.S. Department of Health and Human Services, Bureau of Health Professionals, Division of Nursing, convened a Consensus Conference on the Essentials of Public Health Nursing Practice and Education in Washington, DC (U.S. Department of Health and Human Services [USDHHS], Division of Nursing, 1984). This group concluded that *community health nursing* was the broader term, referring to all nurses practicing in the community, regardless of their educational preparation. *Public health nursing*, viewed as a part of community health nursing, was described as a generalist practice for nurses prepared with basic public health content at the baccalaureate level and a specialized practice for nurses prepared in public health at the master's level or beyond. For a public health nursing viewpoint, see Perspectives: Nursing Instructor and the Public Health Nursing Bag (Fig. 2–13).

Finally, confusion also arose regarding the changing roles and functions of community health nurses. Accelerated changes in health care organization and financing, technology, and social issues made increasing demands on community health nurses to adapt to new patterns of practice. Many new kinds of community health services appeared. Hospital-based programs reached into the community. Private agencies proliferated, offering home care and other community-based services. Other

PERSPECTIVES
NURSING INSTRUCTOR AND THE PUBLIC HEALTH NURSING BAG

When I was a nursing student, I shadowed a public health nurse on her visits for a day. She carried the standard PHN bag, a rectangular flat-topped black leather bag with long handles on both sides; she seemed to be a magician, as she continued to pull things out of her bag during the home visit to a very poor migrant family living in a small rural farm labor camp. She had a folded newspaper in the back pocket of her bag, and she carefully unfolded it and placed her bag on top of it. She pulled out a small bottle of liquid soap and a few paper towels, and washed her hands at the kitchen sink as she asked the mother about her concerns and questions. She weighed and measured the newborn (scale carried in the trunk of her car; disposable paper tape and paper barrier for scale from her bag) and performed a brief exam (stethoscope and supplies from her bag). She gave the mother a card with information on birth control and the location/hours of the health department clinic. The mother was worried about the 2-year-old being fussy and not wanting to eat and asked the nurse to check her for a sore throat. The nurse pulled out a tongue depressor and an otoscope to check the child's ears and throat. Ear tips were cleaned with alcohol swabs from her bag, and trash was properly disposed of. She reported to the mom that the little girl had no current signs of an infection, but to watch for her and go to the clinic if she felt that things got worse. The mother also expressed concern about her 4-year-old, thinking that he may not be "ready for school" in the fall, so the nurse pulled Denver testing supplies out of her bag and assessed the child. She talked to the mother about developmentally appropriate activities for the child and pulled a sticker from her bag to reward the 4-year-old for "playing games" with her and the 2-year-old for complying with the brief exam. When the visit was over, the PHN had cleaned and put everything (but the baby scale) carefully back into place in her bag (e.g., stethoscope, otoscope, supplies); she picked it up and folded the newspaper with the "dirty" side inward, and she was ready for the next visit.

You may or may not be using the PHN bag in your nursing program today. Only about one third of nursing schools responding to a 2009 survey reported that they used the traditional PHN bag in their clinical courses (Aaltonen et al., 2009). But, the bag is still very

functional, and it has a rich history. You can see early photos of Lillian Wald carrying a PHN bag over the tenement rooftops in New York City. Zarbock (1996) noted that PHNs for many decades have provided care in the home from the depths of the small, black public health nursing bag. Abrams (2009) noted that the bag was needed for carrying "supplies that were required in a home but which would not have been available" (p. 106). Common supplies in the 1930s included bottled green soap, Vaseline, alcohol, shaving cream, oral and rectal thermometers (glass), tongue depressors, safety pins, applicators, hand lotion, and various glass supplies (e.g., medicine droppers, connectors, tips). Rubber supplies included catheters and rectal tubes. Dressings, towels, and other linens, along with an apron, masks, and cord ties, were also included. A folder for health forms, notes, pamphlets, maps, pencils, pens, and a notebook were also carried. If the local medical society approved, the nurse might also include a stethoscope and sphygmomanometer. Sometimes, newspapers and a cap and gown were needed in cases where contamination was an issue (NOPHN, 1939). Aseptic technique was used, with the inside of the bag considered clean, and all bottles either washed in hot water or sterilized before being returned to the bag after use. For decades, bag technique was taught in nursing schools. If possible, the bag was placed on a chair rather than the floor, and newspapers were used as a barrier if needed. A waste bag could be made out of folded newspapers, and the PHN had to wash her hands before reaching into the bag for supplies (NOPHN, 1939). Abrams (2009) notes that the bag was a "symbol of authority and respect" and that it often served as "a teaching tool" as the nurse demonstrated good hygiene when working with families. Many families and communities became familiar with the "public health nurse carrying her black bag"—which became both a symbol and a tool (p. 109).

I am proud to carry the little black bag that embodies such a rich history.

Holly, Public Health Nursing Instructor

From Aaltonen, P., Richards, E. L., Webster, K., & Davis, L. (2009). Use of the public health nursing bag in the academic setting. *Public Health Nursing*, 26(1), 88–94; Abrams, S. E. (2009). The public health nursing bag as tool and symbol. *Public Health Nursing*, 26(1), 106–109.

community health professionals assumed responsibilities that traditionally had been the domain of public health nursing. For example, some school counselors in Oregon began coordinating home visits previously done by school nurses, and health educators (who were part of a more recently developed discipline) took over large segments of client education. Social workers, too, provided services that overlapped with community health nursing roles. Health educators, counselors, social workers, epidemiologists, and nutritionists working in community health came prepared with different backgrounds and emphases

in their practice. Their contributions were and still are important. Their presence, however, forced community health nurses to reexamine their own contribution to the public's health and incorporate stronger interdisciplinary and collaborative approaches into their practice (see "Levels of Prevention Pyramid").

The debate over these areas of confusion continued through the 1980s, and some issues remain unresolved. Still, the direction in which public health and community health nursing must move remains clear: to care *for*, not simply *in*, the community. Public health nursing

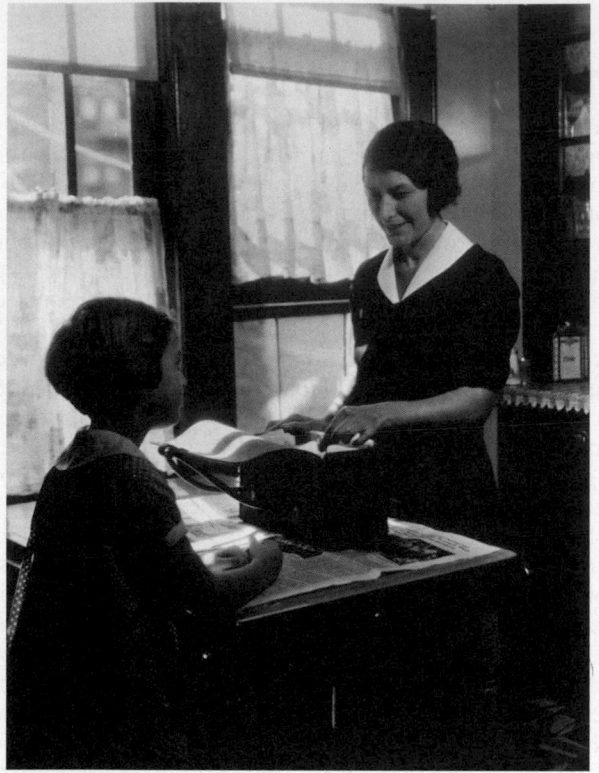

FIGURE 2–13 A PHN on a home visit. The nurse is removing something from her bag in preparation for an examination as a little girl watches.

continues to mean the synthesis of nursing and the public health sciences applied to promoting and protecting the health of populations. Community health nursing, for some, refers more broadly to nursing in the community.

In this text, the term *community health nursing* is used synonymously with *public health nursing* and refers to specialized, population-focused nursing practice, which applies public health science and nursing science. A possible distinction between the two terms might be to view community health nursing as a beginning level of specialization and public health nursing as an advanced level. A position paper sponsored by the Association of Community Health Nursing Educators (ACHNE) emphasized the use of the title, public health nurse, as the "unique ecological focus on population health" and the "synergy of the nursing, social, and public health sciences" (Levin et al., 2008, p. 179). Clarification and consensus on the meaning of these terms may help to avoid misconceptions and misuse and are explored more fully in Chapter 3. Whichever term is used to describe this specialty, the fundamental issues and defining criteria remain the same:

- Are populations and communities the target of practice?
- Are the nurses prepared in public health and engaging in public health practice?

As public/community health nursing continues to evolve, many signs of positive growth are evident. Community health nurses are carving out new roles for themselves in primary health care. Collaboration and interdisciplinary teamwork are recognized as crucial to effective community nursing. Practitioners work through many kinds of agencies and institutions, such as senior citizen centers, ambulatory services, mental health clinics, and family planning programs. Community needs assessment, documentation of nursing outcomes, program evaluation, quality improvement, public policy formulation, and community nursing research are high

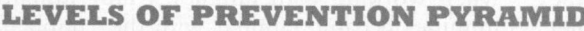
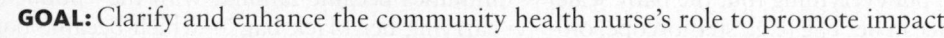

LEVELS OF PREVENTION PYRAMID

GOAL: Clarify and enhance the community health nurse's role to promote impact

TERTIARY PREVENTION

- Promote increasing influence of the nurse through an expanded role in service delivery
- Minimize the impact of community misunderstandings of the nurse's role through education

SECONDARY PREVENTION

- Promote aggregate-level interventions
- Foster nurse involvement on community boards and other political groups

PRIMARY PREVENTION

- Participate in policy formation
- Be politically active
- Assist in acquiring funding for community health programs
- Conduct research on health and nursing outcomes to enhance evidence-based practice
- Collaborate with the news media to publicize current public health issues

priorities. This field of nursing is assuming responsibility as a full professional partner in community health.

Internationally, community health nursing services are well established in England, Scandinavia, the Netherlands, and Australia. Services, however, are relatively underdeveloped in France and Ireland. Furthermore, relatively few professional nurses are working in the community in central and Eastern Europe and in Russia. Ivanov and Paganpegara (2003) note that changes have occurred in nursing education subsequent to the collapse of the Soviet Union, but they have not included content in public health nursing. Moreover, the concepts of health promotion and health education are not well understood, with the vast majority of health care provided at the tertiary level. It is concerning that modernization in many countries has not included expansion of public health services in general and community health nursing more specifically. A study in Turkey found that public health nursing education needed to be strengthened and updated (Kadioglu, Albayrak, & Esin, 2013).

For countries in the European Union, new public health nursing competencies form the basis of revised core educational modules that are focused on upgrading public health nursing and promoting better health for individuals and populations (Danielson, Krogerus-Therman, Sivertsen, & Sourtzi, 2005). A comparative study of public health nursing preparation in Canada and European Union countries found that varied practice environments and educational practices led to inconsistencies in preparation as well as involvement in policy making and leadership in PHN practice (Hemingway, Aarts, Koskinen, Campbell, & Chassé, 2012). In the United Kingdom, dual programs for nursing and health visitors (public health nursing) are encouraged and have been shown to increase the number of nurses who go into health visiting or public health nursing (Drennan, Porter, & Grant, 2013).

In many of the most populated regions of the world—such as China, Africa, and India—volunteers, lay providers, and paraprofessionals often provide the bulk of community health services. In Thailand, nursing has moved from hospital-based training to university-based education, with an increased professionalization of nursing (Thaweeboon, Peachpansri, Pochanapan, Senachack, & Pinyopasakul, 2011). In Taiwan, a call was issued for high school graduation as a minimum requirement for college nursing program entrance, along with revised curriculum content that bases teaching approaches on the public health needs of an increasingly older and chronically ill population (Yeh, Chao, & Chao, 2012). Ayandiran, Irinoye, Olayiwola, and Mtshali (2013) chronicled the "long and tortuous journey" of nursing education reforms in Nigeria to improve nursing practice by promoting evidence-based practice and critical thinking (p. 7). They call for meaningful use of distance learning technologies to provide access to all nurses. A survey of 150 Nigerian nurses found that most nurses valued continuing professional education, but wanted online courses and a means for utilizing this as a way to move up the career ladder. However, currently, no monitoring or evaluation methods are in place to fully determine the impact of continuing education on nursing competence or outcomes for patients (Nsemo, John, Etifit, Mgbekem, & Oyira, 2013). As they continue to make progress toward improved nursing practice and outcomes, a survey noted that Nigerian public health nurses found that the use of standardized nursing languages in charting improved documentation (Odutayo, Olaogun, Oluwatosin, & Ogunfowokan, 2013).

In 1978, a joint World Health Organization and the United Nations Children's Fund International Conference in Alma-Ata, in the Soviet Union, adopted a declaration on primary health care as the key to attaining the goal of health for all by the year 2000. At this conference, delegations from 134 governments agreed to incorporate the concepts and principles of primary health care in their health care systems to reach this goal (World Health Organization, 1978; 2016). This was adopted by the World Health Assembly and endorsed by the United Nations General Assembly in 1981. On paper, at least, everyone acknowledged the crucial need for nurses to be involved in reaching this goal. In practice, support has not been forthcoming in many countries. Policy makers and the public still need to be educated to realize that nursing's most effective contributions to the overall health of the population are based in the community.

Table 2–1 summarizes the most important changes that have occurred during community health nursing's four stages of development. It shows these changes in terms of focus, nursing orientation, service emphasis, and institutional base.

Table 2-1 Development of Community Health Nursing

Stages	Focus	Nursing Orientation	Service Emphasis	Institutional Base (Agencies)
Early home care (before mid-1800s)	Sick poor	Individuals	Curative	Lay and religious orders
District nursing (1860–1900)	Sick poor	Individuals; preventive	Curative; beginning of	Voluntary; some government
Public health nursing (1900–1970)	Needy public	Families	Curative; preventive	Government; some voluntary
Emergence of community health nursing (1970–present)	Total community	Populations; illness prevention	Health promotion; practice	Many kinds; some independent

SOCIETAL INFLUENCES ON THE DEVELOPMENT OF COMMUNITY HEALTH NURSING

Many factors have influenced the growth of community health nursing. To better understand the nature of this field, the forces that began and continue to shape its development must be recognized. Six are particularly significant: advanced technology, progress in causal thinking, changes in education, demographic changes and the role of women, the consumer movement, and economic factors.

Advanced Technology

Advanced technology has contributed in many ways to shaping the practice of community health nursing. For example, technologic innovation has greatly improved health care, nutrition, and lifestyle and has resulted in an increase in life expectancy. Consequently, community health nurses direct an increasing share of their effort toward meeting the needs of the elderly population and addressing chronic conditions. The advances in technology in the home can be life altering, as we now have advances in genetics and genomics, less invasive surgical and diagnostic techniques, electronic health records, and 3-D printing of human tissues and organs (Huston, 2013). For example, the use of social media can enable the community health nurse to reach an even broader audience. Duggan and Smith (2014) found that 73% of U.S. adults use social media and about half are active on several networking sites. PatientsLikeMe is an example of consumer Web sites that permits individuals to "monitor their disease, treatments, and self-reported experiences" (Jackson, Fraser, & Ash, 2014, para. 7). They can also choose to share information with researchers and other patients with similar symptoms or diseases.

Despite the benefits, with any type of information sharing, there is always the risk of inaccurate information being disseminated. Online access to health information can provide a critical link to information for all individuals, especially isolated elderly persons, but it is important to recognize that not all Web sites are reputable. It is critical for the community health nurse to carefully check any Web sites that are recommended for clients. And, it is important for clients to access only reputable sites and participate in discussion groups that utilize a facilitator or moderator. Technology is also helpful in monitoring health, such as smartphone apps or devices that track diet, exercise, and sleep. Public health nurses can use technology to promote social media campaigns for disease prevention and foster healthy habits. Social media can have a downside, as cyber bullying and a potential for invasion of privacy exist (Jackson et al., 2014).

Advanced technology has been a strong force behind industrialization and urbanization. Population density leads to many health-related problems, particularly the spread of disease and increased stress. As people travel and relocate, they are separated from families and traditional support systems; technology such as Skype and social media such as Facebook help keep them connected.

Finally, innovations in communications and computer technology have shifted America from an industrial society to more of an "information economy." Our economy is built on information—the production and marketing of knowledge—making it global and active around-the-clock. Community health nurses now are in the business of information distribution, and they use computer technologies to enhance the efficiency and effectiveness of their services. Geographic information systems (GIS) is an example of emerging computer technology that the community health nurse can use to design and evaluate population-focused programs (Callen et al., 2010). GIS technology can be a valuable tool for many purposes, including examining health disparities and outbreaks of disease and for determining health priorities within a community (Rababah, Curtis, & Drew, 2014). This spatial software permits nursing research and epidemiologic studies examining the association between stressful environmental exposures and preterm birthrates for African American mothers (Bloch, 2011). GIS is also helpful in public health nursing as a tool for program planning and determining accessibility of community services (Carlson, York, & Primomo, 2011).

Telenursing, telehealth, and nursing informatics are part of our professional activities as community health nurses. We communicate by e-mail, use computer-based applications to enhance education among peers and with clients, and utilize electronic health records and billing programs. We have the ability to remotely visit our clients, and we regularly videoconference on smartphones, tablets, and laptops. We can even take a "bird's-eye" view of the distribution of service providers and chronic disease clusters in a community through the use of GIS technology. Access to information is increasing, and the use of the information is limitless. The emerging difficulty is how to manage the sheer volume of information and still meet the needs of our communities. See Chapter 10.

Community health nurses, as well as nurses in all areas of the profession, are developing skills with informatics and various forms of technology. The Technologies Informatics Guiding Education Reform (TIGER) encourages this integration of technology into nursing practice (Jackson et al., 2014).

Progress in Causal Thought

Relating disease or illness to its cause is known as **causal thinking** in the health sciences. Progress in the study of causality, particularly in epidemiology, has significantly affected the nature of community health nursing (Fos & Fine, 2000; Thomas & Weber, 2001). The *germ theory* of disease causation, established in the late 1800s, was the first real breakthrough in control of communicable disease. At that time, it was established that disease could be spread or transmitted from patient to patient or from nurse to patient by contaminated hands or equipment. Nurses incorporated the teaching of cleanliness and personal hygiene into basic nursing care.

A second advance in causal thinking was initiated by the tripartite view that called attention to the interactions among a causative agent, a susceptible host, and the environment. This information offered PHNs new ways to control and prevent health disorders (Galea, Riddle, & Kaplan, 2010). For example, nurses could decrease the vulnerability of individuals (hosts) by teaching them healthier lifestyles. They could instigate measles vaccination programs as a means of preventing the organism (agent) from infecting children. They could promote proper disinfection of a neighborhood swimming pool (environment) to prevent disease.

Further progress in causal thinking led to the recognition that not just one single agent but many factors—a multiple causation approach—contribute to a disease or health disorder, as well as health inequalities (Raphael, 2012). A food poisoning outbreak that is associated with a restaurant might be caused not only by the *Salmonella* organism but also by improper food handling and storage, lack of adherence to minimum food preparation standards, and lack of adequate health department supervision and enforcement (see Chapter 7). A chronic condition such as coronary heart disease can be related to other kinds of multicausal factors such as heredity, diet, lack of exercise, smoking, and personal and work stress.

Community health nurses can control health problems by examining all possible causes and then attacking strategic causal points. Efforts to prevent human immunodeficiency virus (HIV)/AIDS provide a dramatic case in point. Contact reporting, condom use, protection of health workers serving patients infected with the HIV, screening for HIV infection, and public education about HIV/AIDS were most helpful at the start of the epidemic as an example of a multifaceted approach. Once antiretroviral medications became available, public health nurses visited vulnerable HIV/AIDS clients and provided much needed social support and monitoring of medication compliance, as well as additional education (Kelly, Hartman, Graham, Kallen, & Giordano, 2014). Daily or monthly nursing visits and nurse observation of prophylactic HIV medication among high-risk injection drug users in Thailand improved medication adherence and lowered HIV infection risk (Martin et al., 2015).

Current causal thinking has led to a broader awareness of unhealthy conditions; in addition to disease, problems such as accidents and environmental pollution are major targets of concern. Work-related stress, environmental hazards, chemical food additives, and alcohol and nicotine consumption during pregnancy are all examples of concerns in community health nursing practice.

Nursing's contribution to public health adds a further application to causal thinking. That is, nursing seeks to identify and implement the causes, or contributing factors, of wellness. Community health nurses do more than prevent illness; they seek to promote health. By conducting research and applying evidence-based practice findings, community health nurses promote health-enhancing behaviors. Nurses promote healthier lifestyle practices such as eating healthy diets, exercising, and maintaining social support systems; promote healthy conditions in schools and worksites; and designing meaningful activities for children, adolescents, adults, and the elderly (Kulbok et al., 2012).

Changes in Education

Changes in education, especially those in nursing education, have had an important influence on community health nursing practice. Education, once an opportunity for a privileged few, has become widely available; it is now considered a basic right and a necessity for a vital society. When people's understanding of their environment grows, an increased understanding of health usually is involved. For the community health nurse, health teaching has steadily assumed greater importance in practice. For the learner, education has led to more responsibility. As a result, people believe that they have a right to know and question the reasons behind the care they receive. Community health nurses have shifted from planning for clients to collaborating with clients.

Education has had other effects. Scientific inquiry, considered basic to progress, has created a dramatic increase in knowledge. The wealth of information relevant to community health nursing practice means that nursing students have more content to assimilate, and practicing community health nurses have to make greater efforts to keep abreast of knowledge in their field. In contrast to earlier times, when nurses were trained to work as apprentices in hospitals or health agencies and to follow orders perfunctorily, today's educational programs, including continuing education, prepare nurses to think for themselves in the application of theory to practice. Evidence-based practice is emphasized, and students implement projects based upon best evidence and community values (Kulbok et al., 2012; Milbrath & DeGuzman, 2015). Environmental health issues have come to the forefront. Leffers, McDermott-Levy, Smith, and Sattler (2014) examined the response of nursing education to the 1995 Institute of Medicine report on *Nursing, Health, and the Environment*. They noted that the Alliance of Nurses for Healthy Environments, a group of public health nurses and others committed to promoting environmental health issues, was instrumental in making progress in this area of nursing education. The Henry Street Consortium (Schaffer et al., 2010), the Quad Council (Swider, Krothe, Reyes, & Cravetz, 2013), and the American Nurses Association (2013) have all updated public health nursing competencies and standards of practice, and others have sought to clarify competencies in family planning public health nursing (Hewitt, Roye, & Gebbie, 2014). Olson Keller, Strohschein, and Schaffer (2011) have described the synthesis of public health and nursing beliefs, values, and practice in their document, "Cornerstones of Public Health Nursing." Rush University evaluated and revised their graduate curriculum for advanced practice clinical nurse specialist in public/community health nursing to match outcome competencies of the Quad Council competencies for second-tier manager/specialist roles (Swider et al., 2006); others have provided teaching and learning strategies for baccalaureate degree programs that offer entry-level public health nursing courses (Callen et al., 2013).

Public health professionals, including public health nurses, are often members of interdisciplinary teams, highlighting the need for more interprofessional educational opportunities for all helping profession students (Uden-Holman, Curry, Benz, & Aquilino, 2015). Population-level simulations regarding poverty and other issues help to bring serious problems to life for nursing students (Yang, Woomer, Agbemenu, & Williams, 2014). But, due to diminishing public health budgets, finding appropriate clinical placements for public health nursing students can be challenging, and innovative solutions for clinical placements are often required (Young, Acord,

Schuler, & Hansen, 2014). Poor utilization of public health nursing credentialing exams, often due to a perceived lack of value/reward or recognition in the workplace or a lack of knowledge about the exams, has caused issues with availability of these exams (American Nurses Credentialing Center [ANCC], 2016; Bekemeier, 2009; Doutrich & Dotson, 2012; Little, Vandenhouten, & DeVance-Wilson, 2013).

While baccalaureate nursing degree programs provide public health nursing coursework, graduate-level programs in community/public health nursing have been on the decline since the 1996 release of the AACN document, *Essentials of Master's Education for Advanced Practice Nursing*, defining advanced practice nursing as only those specialties that require graduate coursework in advanced physical assessment, pathophysiology, and pharmacology and focusing on provision of care to individuals. In 2006, the Doctorate of Nursing Practice degree was approved. Some instruction in population health is required; however, the curriculum does not easily match the needs of advanced public health nurses (Canales & Drevdahl, 2014; Swider et al., 2009; Swider, Levin, & Kulbok, 2015). While Duffy, McCullagh, and Lee's (2015) assessment of the need for advanced practice public health nurses in Michigan showed promising results, this may not be true in other areas.

In 2014, 55% of RNs had a bachelor's degree or higher; this is short of the 80% recommended by 2020 in the Institute of Medicine (IOM) report, *The Future of Nursing: Leading Change, Advancing Health* (American Nurses Association, 2014; IOM, 2011). More advanced degrees were also promoted in this report and the need for barriers to be removed so that nurses could "practice to the full extent of their education and training" (IOM, 2011, p. 4). Working "as full partners" with many other professionals, nurses should be involved in "redesigning health care" and implementing evidence-based practice to improve patient outcomes and nursing practice (p. 4). With health care reform, a paradigm shift from illness care to wellness and health promotion is taking place. Disease prevention and promotion of wellness and health are important areas of focus for public health nurses, and a population focus is an important component of health care reform. Care coordinators, who can help individuals better manage their chronic illnesses and promote more effective use of health care resources, are also part of health care reform (Kunic & Jackson, 2013). All of these changes have an impact on nursing education. In this new health care system, there is a strong need to focus on learning to work effectively as team members, systems approaches to care, and understanding of new payment structures that reward innovation, efficiency, safety, and quality, rather than waste and inefficiency (Buerhaus et al., 2012; Chard, 2013).

Community health nursing has always required a fair measure of independent thinking and self-reliance; now, community health nurses need skills in such areas as population assessment, policy making, political advocacy, research, management, collaborative functioning, global health, human diversity, as well as information and health care technology (Callen et al., 2010, 2013; Kulbok et al., 2012). As the result of expanding education, public health nurses have had to reexamine their practice, sharpen their knowledge and skills, and clarify their roles.

Demographic Changes and the Role of Women

The changing demographics in the United States and the changing role of women have profoundly affected community health nursing. In the 20th century, the Women's Rights movement made considerable progress; women achieved the right to vote and gained greater economic independence by moving into the labor force (see Displays 2–2 and 2–4). In 2014, over 140 million people were employed in nonfarm positions in the United States, marking a recovery from the 2007–2009 Great Recession with average weekly hours and wages both increasing (U.S. Department of Labor, Bureau of Labor Statistics, 2015). Our current labor force is "older, more racially and ethnically diverse, and composed of more women" (Toosi, 2012, p. 43). The total labor force is projected to grow more slowly (e.g., 1% over the 2010 to 2020 time period), with 53% males and 47% females by 2020.

Nursing has historically been a predominantly female profession. In 2012, there were 2.9 million active registered nurses and over 3.8 million expected by 2025 (USDHHS, 2014). Nationally, the average age of the RN workforce is 50, with 53% of RNs over the age of 50; between 2010 and 2013, 11% of licenses issues were to males. Although most nursing schools remain full and many have a waiting list, the number of nurses staying active in their profession is dwindling. Those remaining in the profession are "graying" and retiring. Added to this is the aging population of nursing faculty, which raises concern over meeting the increased demand for nurses in the coming decade.

Salaries for nurses compare favorably with those for other workers who have 4 years of education in fields other than health care, such as education, human services (e.g., social work), and business. When compared with other workers in the health care field, however, nurses generally do not fare as well. For example, among the 2,655,020 practicing RNs in the United States in 2015, the median salary was $67,490. In comparison, the median salary for physical therapists was $84,020; for dental hygienists, it was $72.330; and for occupational therapists, it was $80,150 (U.S. Department of Labor, Bureau of Labor Statistics, 2016).

Changing demographics, such as shifting patterns in immigration, varying numbers of births and deaths, and a rapidly increasing population of elderly persons, affect community health nursing planning and programming efforts. Monitoring these changes is essential for relevant and effective nursing services. Equally important is a diverse and representative workforce in nursing. The 2013 findings of the National Sample Survey of Registered Nurses indicated that the vast majority of nurses (83%) specifying a racial background selected White (non-Hispanic). Approximately 6% identified as Asian and 6% as Black/African American; Hispanic/Latino comprised 3%, and only 2% of nurses declared Native American/Alaskan Native, or Native Hawaiian/Other Pacific Islander (1% respectively). An additional one percent stated "Other" (Budden, Zhong, Moulton, & Cimiotti, 2013). Currently, about 15% of nurses work in public health or community settings (e.g., corrections, school nursing, occupational nursing, home health, public/community health agencies). Increased racial and ethnic representation in community health nursing is essential and remains one of the major challenges facing the profession in the coming years.

Although the diversity of career options and employment opportunities for women has been a positive social factor, these gains have impacted the number of women entering nursing. As a profession, nursing's contributions and status have improved, but its ability to compete with careers offering higher pay and status remains problematic. Changes resulting from the women's movement continue. Nurses still struggle for equality—equality of recognition, respect, and autonomy, as well as job selection, equal pay for equal work, and equal opportunity for advancement in the health field. If community health nurses are to influence the field of community health, they need status and authority equal to that of their colleagues. This step requires nurses to demonstrate their competence and learn to be assertive in assuming roles as full professional partners. The women's movement has contributed to community health nursing's gains in assuming leadership roles, but a need for greater influence and involvement remains for all nurses.

The Consumer Movement

The consumer movement has also affected the nature of community health nursing. Consumers have become more aggressive in demanding quality services and goods; they assert their right to be informed about goods and services and to participate in decisions that affect them regardless of sex, race, or socioeconomic level. This movement has stimulated some basic changes in the philosophy of community health nursing. Health care consumers are viewed as active members of the health team rather than as passive recipients of care. They may contract with the community health nurse for family care or group services, represent the community on the local health board, or act as ombudsmen by serving as representatives or advocates for their community constituents (e.g., to investigate

complaints and report findings to protect the quality of care in a local nursing home). This assumption of consumers' responsibility for their own health means that the community health nurse often supplements clients' services, rather than primarily supervising them (Hagel, Keith, Brown, Samoylova, & Hoversten, 2015).

The consumer movement has also contributed to increased concern for the quality of health services, including a demand for more humane, personalized health care. Dissatisfied with fragmented services offered by an array of health workers, consumers seek more comprehensive, coordinated care (Marjoua & Bozic, 2012). For example, senior citizens in a high-rise apartment building need more than a series of social workers, nutritionists, recreational therapists, nurses, and other callers ascertaining a variety of specific needs and starting a variety of separate programs. Community health nurses seek to provide holistic care by collaborating with others to offer more coordinated, comprehensive, and personalized services—a case management approach. The 2015 Gallup Poll is an example of the current attention given to the opinions of consumers and is discussed in Display 2–7. In this poll, nursing is the most highly rated profession with respect to honesty and ethics; not a bad position to be in.

Economic Forces

Myriad economic forces have affected the practice of public health nursing. Unemployment and the rising cost of living, combined with mounting health care costs, resulted in greater numbers of people carrying little or no health insurance. With limited or no access to needed health services, these populations are especially vulnerable to health problems and further economic stress. Health care reform, or the Affordable Care Act, was enacted to address this problem, but it is not a panacea (see Chapter 6). Other economic forces affecting public health nursing are changing health care financing patterns; decreased federal, state, and local subsidies of public health programs; and pressures for health care cost containment (see Chapter 6; Display 2–8). The 2012 Institute of Medicine report, *For the Public's Health:*

DISPLAY 2–7 NURSES RANK HIGHEST IN HONESTY AND ETHICAL STANDARDS

Nurses are again at the top of the list, according to a Gallup Poll taken in 2015. When asked how they would rate the honesty and ethical standards of members of various professions, Americans rated nurses highest. Each year, a random sample of American rates select professions on a five-point scale ranging from "very high" to "very low." Since being added to the list in 1999, nurses have been at the top of the list each year except 2001, when firefighters took the No. 1 spot. The four lowest professions in 2015 were car salespeople, telemarketers, and members of Congress at 8%, and lobbyists at 7%. Here are the results for the top ten scoring professions:

Profession	Percentage
Nurses	85%
Pharmacists	68%
Medical doctors	67%
High school teachers	60%
Police officers	56%
Clergy	45%
Funeral directors	44%
Accountants	39%
Journalists	27%
Bankers	25%

From Gallup. (2015). *Honesty/ethics in professions*. Retrieved from http://www.gallup.com/poll/1654/honesty-ethics-professions.aspx

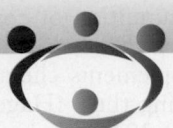

DISPLAY 2–8 TWENTY YEARS IN HISTORY: 1986 TO 2006

1986	*Standards of Community Health Nursing Practice* published by ANA.
	National Center for Nursing Research created at the National Institutes of Health.
1990	*Healthy People 2000: National Health Promotion and Disease Prevention Objectives.*
1991	Elizabeth Dole becomes the first woman president of the American Red Cross since Clara Barton.
1993	National Center for Nursing Research becomes the National Institute of Nursing Research.
1996	*Health Insurance Portability and Accountability Act* (HIPPA) signed into law.
	Food and Drug Administration issues restrictive regulations for cigarettes and smokeless tobacco.
1997	Oregon legalizes Death With Dignity, allowing terminally ill patients to end their lives with self-administered lethal injection.
1999	*Scope and Standards of Public Health Nursing Practice* published by ANA.
	Targeted drug therapies for some cancers introduced (Herceptin, TyKerb).
2000	*Healthy People 2010: Understanding and Improving Health.*
	Draft sequencing of human genome completed and released to public.
2001	September 11 attacks result in over 3,000 deaths in New York City, Washington, and Pennsylvania.
2002	Hormone replacement therapy linked to increased risk of heart attack, blood clots, stroke, and breast cancer.
2003	War in Iraq begins.
	Worldwide epidemic of Severe Acute Respiratory Syndrome (SARS).
2006	Medicare Part D Prescription Drug benefit implemented.
	Public Health Nursing: Scope and Standards of Practice published by ANA.
	HIV-cocktail drug, Atripla, and HPV vaccine, Gardasil, approved by FDA.

Investing in a Healthier Future, notes that a large amount of this nation's disease burden is preventable and that health care reforms to access, quality, and payment systems are not sufficient to improve our health and level of health care expenditures. Population-based health interventions are needed, along with universal coverage and addressing system inefficiencies and waste. Changes in how funding is allocated to local and state public health departments, along with a "dedicated, stable, and long-term financing structure" for communities and an infrastructure for federal research to promote prevention strategies, implement programs, and determine comparative effectiveness of interventions (p. 11).

Global economic forces also influence community health nursing practice. As the United States experiences increasing interdependence with foreign countries for trade, investment, and production of goods, the population has experienced a growing mobility and increased immigration, particularly among Hispanic and Asian groups. Refugees from wars and uprisings are also seeking asylum. Under these conditions, the spread of communicable diseases poses a serious threat, as do problems associated with unemployment and poverty. Furthermore, the fastest-growing sector of the job market is in technical fields, which require new or retrained workers, and these jobs frequently are accompanied by health problems related to the stresses of ever-changing technology and financial and competitive pressures to produce.

Community health nursing has responded to these economic forces in several ways. One is by assuming new roles, such as health educators in industry or case managers for government and privately sponsored programs for the elderly. Another is by directly competing with other community health service providers, particularly in such areas as ambulatory care or home care. Still another is by developing new programs and service emphases. Elder daycare, respite care, drug prevention projects, mentoring programs for pregnant/parenting adolescents, programs for the homeless, lifestyle intervention clinics, and working with social workers to meet the health needs of foster children are a few examples of the response by public health nursing to the changing community needs created by demographic and economic forces (Nymberg & Drenvenhorn, 2015; Schaffer & Mbibi, 2014; Schneiderman, 2008). Yet another PHN response has been to develop new revenue-generating services, such as workplace wellness or health-screening programs, to augment depleted budgets. Economic factors continue to play a significant role in shaping community health nursing practice. Yet, public health nurses continue to be resourceful in finding ways to foster the community's optimal health while adapting to changing economic conditions (Fig. 2–14).

PREPARATION FOR COMMUNITY HEALTH NURSING

The demands of community health nursing practice are significant, as described in Chapter 1, and are elaborated elsewhere in this textbook. The daily routine of

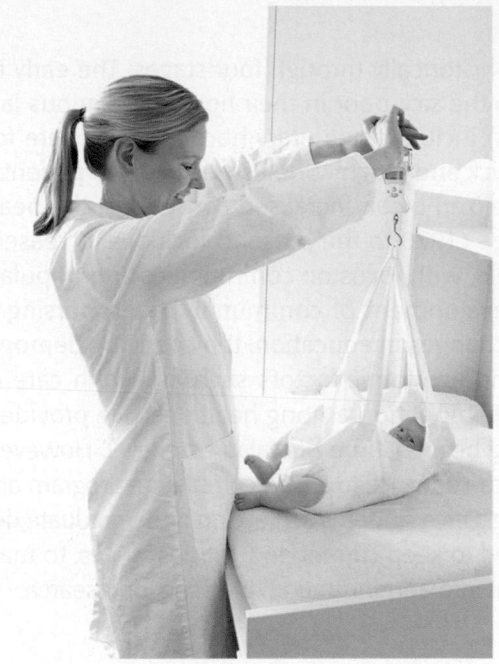

FIGURE 2–14 Community Health Nurse weighing a baby.

the public health nurse may include organizing a flu clinic for seniors in the community, making home visits, giving a presentation on playground safety at a parent–teacher meeting, participating in a team meeting about a population-focused grant, answering telephone calls, and charting. All of the skills learned in a basic bachelor's degree nursing program are needed. Furthermore, larger public health nurse roles also include service on community advisory boards, grant writing for new programs, or participation in or presentation of in-service programs. Academic preparation for this role is necessary, as is continuous professional development, and this training must meet the requirements of both employers and, in many instances, state regulations. While associate degree nursing programs do not specifically entail public health nursing coursework, RN to BSN completion programs are available and provide the coursework needed for PHN certification in most states. Continuing education is encouraged and may be required in your state. To move up into supervisory or leadership roles, or as advanced practice nurses (e.g., nurse practitioners working in women's health or well-child clinics), graduate-level education is needed (Display 2–9).

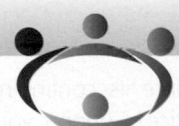 **DISPLAY 2–9 TWENTY YEARS IN HISTORY: 2008 AND BEYOND**

2008   Barack Obama elected President; first African American to hold this position.
2009   *Essentials of Baccalaureate Nursing Education for Entry Level Community/Public Health Nursing* published by the Association of Community Health Nursing Educators, Education Committee.
       H1N1 swine outbreak declared a national emergency with over 22 million American's contracting the disease and 4,000 deaths.
2010   *Patient Protection and Affordable Care Act* signed and includes federal funding for nurse–family home visitation programs such as the Nurse Family Partnership to improve maternal/child health.
       Grant funding approved for existing school-based clinics as well as new construction.
       Institute of Medicine publishes the *Future of Nursing: Leading Change, Advancing Health*.
2011   *The Future of Nursing: Leading Change, Advancing Health*, an Institute of Medicine report was released.
       Healthy People 2020 released.
       Medicare reimbursement to Certified Nurse-Midwives increased from 65% to 100% of the Physician Fee Schedule.
       National Health Service Corps (NHSC) hires over 10,000 additional nurses and other health care professionals.
2012   *Patient-Centered Outcomes Research Institute (PCORI)* established, with two recognized nurse leaders/researchers serving on the Board of Governors and Methodology Committee.
       Institute of Medicine publishes *For the Public's Health: Investing in a Healthier Future*.
2013   Under *Affordable Care Act*, grants and scholarships expanded for nursing and other health professionals.
       ANA publishes second edition of *Public Health Nursing: Scope and Standards of Practice*.
2014   *Advanced Nursing Education Grant* program funded to expand the number of nurses in advanced nursing education and practice.
       Nursing Education and Loan Repayment Program expanded to include up to 85% of loan forgiveness for registered nurses, advanced practice nurses, and faculty members working a minimum of 2 years in either critical shortage areas or accredited schools of nursing.
2015   Right-to-Die legislation for terminally ill patients enacted in California.

From American Nurses Association. (2014, June 18). *Healthcare transformation: The Affordable Care Act and more.* Retrieved from http://nursingworld.org/MainMenuCategories/Policy-Advocacy/HealthSystemReform/AffordableCareAct.pdf

SUMMARY

The specialty of community health nursing developed historically through four stages. The early home care stage (before the mid-1800s) emphasized care to the sick poor in their homes by various lay and religious orders. The district nursing stage (mid-1800s) included voluntary home nursing care for the poor by specialists or "health nurses" who treated the sick and taught wholesome living to patients. The public health nursing stage (1900–1970) was characterized by an increased concern for the health of the general public. The community health nursing stage (1970 to the present) includes increased recognition of community health nursing as a specialty field, with focus on communities and populations.

Six major societal influences have shaped the development of community health nursing. They are advanced technology, progress in causal thinking, changes in education, the changing demographics and role of women, the consumer movement, and economic factors such as health care costs, access, limited funds for public health, and increased competition among health service providers.

Academic preparation for community health nursing begins at the baccalaureate level. However, students beginning at the diploma or associate degree level can advance to a BSN completion program and are then prepared to enter this challenging specialty in nursing. Once students achieve an undergraduate degree, completion of additional educational programs is required to keep current and, in most states, to maintain licensure, advance in practice opportunities, or branch out into administration, teaching, or research.

ACTIVITIES TO PROMOTE CRITICAL THINKING

1. Select one societal influence on the development of community health nursing and explore its continuing impact. What other events are occurring today that shape community health nursing practice? Support your arguments with documentation. Use the Internet to find your documentation.
2. Search the Web for information about a historical public health nursing leader. Using this information, determine how this practitioner might deal with current population-based issues such as HIV/AIDS, sexually transmitted diseases, obesity, or child neglect and abuse.
3. Read a historical article about early public health nursing experiences (e.g., January, 2009 article or Curtis, 2008 article listed in the References). Compare these experiences with your public health clinical experiences today. What are the most striking similarities and differences?
4. Assume that you have been asked to make a home visit to a 75-year-old man, living alone, whose wife recently died. Besides assessing his individual needs, what additional factors should you consider for assessment and intervention that would indicate an aggregate or population-focused approach? What self-care practices might you promote? How would you provide health education to your client?
5. Interview a public health nursing director or supervisor to determine what population-based programs are offered in your locality. Explore nursing's role in the assessment, development, implementation, and evaluation of these programs. Discuss with the director how community health nurses might expand their population-focused interventions.
6. Find information about advanced nursing degrees that may be available locally or online. Compare your findings with other classmates' findings. Which specialty areas are of interest to you?

REFERENCES

Aaltonen, P., Richards, E. L., Webster, K., & Davis, L. (2009). Use of the public health nursing bag in the academic setting. *Public Health Nursing, 26*(1), 88–94.

Abrams, S. E. (2004). From function to competency in public health nursing, 1931 to 2003. *Public Health Nursing, 21*(5), 507–510.

Abrams, S. E. (2009). The public health nursing bag as tool and symbol. *Public Health Nursing, 26*(1), 106–109.

Abrams, S. E., & Hays, J. C. (2013). On the shoulders of younger giants public health nursing moves forward. *Public Health Nursing, 30*(6), 475–476.

American Nurses Association. (2013). *Public health nursing: Scope and standards of practice* (2nd ed.). Silver Spring, MD: Author.

American Nurses Association. (2014). *The nursing workforce 2014: Growth, salaries, education, demographics, and trends.* Retrieved from http://www.nursingworld.org/MainMenuCategories/ThePracticeofProfessionalNursing/workforce/Fast-Facts-2014-Nursing-Workforce.pdf

American Nurses Association, Community Health Nursing Division. (1980). *A conceptual model of community health nursing* (Publication No. CH-10 2M 5/80). Kansas City, MO: Author.

American Nurses Credentialing Center (ANCC). (2016). *ANCC Certification Center*. Retrieved from http://www.nursecredentialing. org/certification.aspx#specialty

Ayandiran, E. O., Irinoye, O. O., Olayiwola, F. J., & Mtshali, N. G. (2013). Education reforms in Nigeria: How responsive is the nursing profession? *International Journal of Nursing Education Scholarship, 10*(1), 1–8.

Baker, J. H. (2011). *Margaret Sanger: A life of passion*. New York, NY: Hill and Wang.

Barnum, N. C. (2011). Public health nursing: An autonomous career for World War II nurse veterans. *Public Health Nursing, 28*(4), 379–386.

Beine, J. (1996). Changing with the times. *Nursing Times, 92*(48), 59–62.

Bekemeier, B. (2009). Nurses' utilization and perception of the community/public health nursing credential. *American Journal of Public Health, 99*(5), 944–949.

Bloch, J. R. (2011). Using geographical information systems to explore disparities in preterm birth rates among foreign-born and US-born Black mothers. *Journal of Obstetric, Gynecologic, and Neonatal Nursing, 40*(5), 544–554.

Brainard, A. M. (1922). *The evolution of public health nursing*. Philadelphia, PA: W. B. Saunders Company.

Brainard, A. M. (2012). The many sided opportunity of field nursing. *Public Health Nursing, 29*(3), 283–285.

Brooks, J. (2013). Nursing typhus victims in the Second World War, 1942–1944: A discussion paper. *Journal of Advanced Nursing, 70*(7), 1510–1519.

Budden, J. S., Zhong, E. H., Moulton, P., & Cimiotti, J. P. (2013). Highlights of the National Workforce Survey of Registered Nurses. *Journal of Nursing Regulation, 4*(2), 5–14.

Buerhaus, P. I., DesRoches, C., Applebaum, S., Hess, R., Norman, L. D., & Donelan, K. (2012). Are nurses ready for health care reform? A decade of survey research. *Nursing Economics, 30*(6), 318–329.

Bullough, V., & Bullough, B. (1978). *The care of the sick: The emergence of modern nursing*. New York, NY: Neale, Watson.

Callen, B., Block, D., Joyce, B., Lutz, J., Brown-Schott, N., & Smith, C. M. (2010). Essentials of baccalaureate nursing education for entry-level community/public health nursing. *Public Health Nursing, 27*, 371–382.

Callen, B., Smith, C. M., Joyce, B., Lutz, J., Brown-Schott, N., & Block, D. (2013). Teaching/learning strategies for the Essentials of Baccalaureate Nursing Education for entry-level community/public health nursing. *Public Health Nursing, 30*(6), 537–547.

Canales, M. K., & Drevdahl, D. J. (2014). Community/public health nursing: Is there a future for the specialty? *Nursing Outlook, 62*(6), 448–458.

Carlson, T., York, S., & Primomo, J. (2011). The utilization of geographic information systems to create a site selection strategy to disseminate an older adult fall prevention program. *Social Science Journal, 48*(1), 159–174.

Carter, K. F. (2001). Trumpets of attack: Collaborative efforts between nursing and philanthropies to care for the child crippled with polio 1930 to 1959. *Public Health Nursing, 18*(4), 253–261.

Central Hanover Bank and Trust Company, Department of Philanthropic Information. (1938). *The public health nurse*. New York, NY: National Organization for Public Health Nursing.

Chard, R. (2013). The personal and professional impact of the Future of Nursing report. *AORN Journal, 98*(3), 273–280.

Christy, T. W. (1970). Portrait of a leader: Lillian D. Wald. *Nursing Outlook, 18*(3), 50–54.

Curtis, M. (2008). Stricken village. *Public Health Nursing, 25*(4), 383–386.

D'Antonio, P. (2010). *American nursing: A history of knowledge, authority, and the meaning of work*. Baltimore, MD: Johns Hopkins University Press.

D'Antonio, P. (2013). Cultivating constituencies: The story of the East Harlem Nursing and Health Service, 1928–1941. *American Journal of Public Health, 103*(6), 988–996.

Danielson, E., Krogerus-Therman, I., Sivertsen, B., & Sourtzi, P. (2005). Nursing and public health in Europe—A new continuous education programme. *International Nursing Review, 52*, 32–38.

de Tornyay, R. (1980). Public health nursing: The nurse's role in community-based practice. *Annual Review of Public Health, 1*, 83.

Dickens, C. (1910). *Martin Chuzzlewit*. New York, NY: Macmillan.

Dolan, J. A. (1978). *Nursing in society: A historical perspective*. Philadelphia, PA: W. B. Saunders.

Dolan, J. A., Fitzpatrick, M. L., & Herrmann, E. K. (1983). *Nursing in society: A historical perspective* (15th ed.). Philadelphia, PA: W. B. Saunders.

Donahue, M. P. (2011). *Nursing the finest art: An illustrated history* (3rd ed.). Maryland Heights, MO: Mosby Elsevier.

Doutrich, D., & Dotson, J. W. (2012). The future of the population-focused, public health clinical nurse specialist. *Nursing Clinics of North America, 47*(2), 305–313.

Draper, L. (2006). Working women and contraception: History, health, and choices. *AAOHN Journal, 54*, 317–324.

Drennan, V. M., Porter, E. M., & Grant, R. L. (2013). Graduates from dual qualification courses, registered nurse and health visitor: A career history study. *Nurse Education Today, 33*, 925–930.

Duffy, S. A., McCullagh, M., & Lee, C. (2015). Future of advanced practice public health nursing education. *Journal of Nursing Education, 54*(2), 102–107.

Duggan, M., & Smith, A. (2014). *Social media update 2013*. Washington, DC: Pew Research Center.

Ellis, J. R., & Hartley, C. L. (2012). *Nursing in today's world: Trends, issues, and management* (10th ed.). Philadelphia, PA: Wolters Kluwer Health/Lippincott Williams & Wilkins.

Erwin, P. C., & Brownson, R. C. (2017). *Scutchfield & Keck's principles of public health practice* (4th ed.). Boston, MA: Cengage Learning.

Evans, J. (2004). Men nurses: A historical and feminist perspective. *Journal of Advanced Nursing, 47*, 321–328.

Farrar, E. W. (1837). *The young lady's friend—By a lady*. Boston, MA: American Stationer's Co.

Fealy, G. M., McNamara, M. S., & Geraghty, R. (2010). The health of hospitals and lessons from history: Public health and sanitary reform in the Dublin hospitals, 1858–1898. *Journal of Clinical Nursing, 19*, 3468–3476. doi: 10.1111/j.1365-2702.2010.03475.x.

Fee, E., & Bu, L. (2010). The origins of public health nursing: The Henry Street Visiting Nurse Service. *American Journal of Public Health, 100*(7), 1206–1207.

Feld, M. N. (2008). *Lillian Wald: A biography*. Chapel Hill, NC: University of North Carolina Press.

Florence Nightingale Museum Trust. (1997). *The Florence Nightingale Museum's school visit pack*. London, UK: Author.

Fos, P. J., & Fine, D. J. (2000). *Designing health care for populations: Applied epidemiology in health care administration*. San Francisco, CA: Jossey-Bass.

Galea, S., Riddle, M., & Kaplan, G. A. (2010). Causal thinking and complex system approaches in epidemiology. *International Journal of Epidemiology, 39*(1), 97–106.

Gardner, M. S. (1936). *Public health nursing* (3rd ed.). New York, NY: Macmillan.

Geister, J. (1957, October). The flu epidemic of 1918. *Nursing Outlook, 5*, 582–584.

Hagel, J., Keith, J., Brown, J. S., Samoylova, T., & Hoversten, S. D. (2015, February 18). *A consumer-driven culture of health: The path to sustainability and growth*. Retrieved from http://dupress.com/articles/future-of-us-health-care/

Hamilton, D. (2007). The cost of caring: The Metropolitan Life Insurance Company's visiting nurse service, 1909–1953. In P. D'Antonio, E. D. Baer, S. D. Rinker, & J. E. Lynaugh (Eds.), *Nurses' work: Issues across time and place* (pp. 141–164). New York, NY: Springer Publishing Company.

Hawkins, J. W., & Watson, J. C. (2003). Public health nursing pioneer: Jane Elizabeth Hitchcock 1863–1939. *Public Health Nursing, 20*(3), 167–176.

Hawkins, J. W., & Watson, J. C. (2010). School nursing on the Iron Range in a public health nursing model. *Public Health Nursing, 27*(6), 571–578.

Hemingway, A., Aarts, C., Koskinen, L., Campbell, B., & Chassé, F. (2012). A European Union and Canadian review of public health nursing preparation and practice. *Public Health Nursing, 30*(11), 58–69.

Hewitt, C. M., Roye, C., & Gebbie, K. M. (2014). Core competency model for the family planning public health nurse. *Public Health Nursing, 31*(5), 472–479.

Hogan, D. (2015 September). Public health nursing: A rich history. *The Florida Nurse, 10*.

Hughes, A. (1902). The origin, growth, and present status of district nursing in England. *American Journal of Nursing, 2*(5), 337–345.

Huston, C. (2013). The impact of emerging technology on nursing care: Warp speed ahead. *Online Journal of Issues in Nursing, 18*(2), Manuscript 1. Retrieved from http://nursingworld.org/

MainMenuCategories/ANAMarketplace/ANAPeriodicals/ OJIN/TableofContents/Vol-18-2013/No2-May-2013/Impact-of-Emerging-Technology.html

Institute of Medicine (IOM). (2011). *The future of nursing: Leading change, advancing health*. Washington, DC: National Academies Press.

Institute of Medicine (IOM). (2012). *For the public's health: Investing in a healthier future*. Washington, DC: National Academies Press.

Ivanov, L. L., & Paganpegara, G. (2003). Public health nursing education in Russia. *Journal of Nursing Education, 42*, 292–295.

Jackson, J., Fraser, R., & Ash, P. (2014). Social media and nurses: Insights for promoting health for individual and professional use. *Online Journal of Issues in Nursing, 19*(3), Manuscript 2. Retrieved from http://nursingworld.org/MainMenuCategories/ANAMarketplace/ ANAPeriodicals/OJIN/TableofContents/Vol-19-2014/No3-Sept-2014/ Insights-for-Promoting-Health.html

January, A. M. (2009). Friday at the Frontier Nursing Service. *Public Health Nursing, 26*(2), 202–203.

Jesús, M., & Martínez, A. C. (2010). *The houses of approval of the nurses Obregones in the Spain of the 16th century: Precedents of our schools of nursing*. Abstract presented at the International Perspectives in the History of Nursing, Royal College of Nursing, London, England.

Kadioglu, H., Albayrak, S., & Esin, M. N. (2013). Public health nursing education in Turkey: A national survey. *International Nursing Review, 60*, 536–542.

Kalisch, P. A., & Kalisch, B. J. (2004). *American nursing: A history* (4th ed.). Philadelphia, PA: Lippincott Williams & Wilkins.

Keeling, A. W. (2009). "When the city is a great field hospital": The influenza pandemic of 1918 and the New York City nursing response. *Journal of Clinical Nursing, 18*, 2732–2738

Kelly, J. D., Hartman, C., Graham, J., Kallen, M. A., & Giordano, T. P. (2014). Social support as a predictor of early diagnosis, linkage, retention, and adherence to HIV care: Results from the STEPS study. *Journal of the Association of Nurses in AIDS Care, 25*(5), 405–413.

King, M. G. (2011). Four responsibilities of the tuberculosis nurse, circa 1919. *Public Health Nursing, 28*(5), 469–472.

Kontoyannis, M., & Katsetos, C. (2011). Midwives in early modern Europe (1400–1800). *Health Science Journal, 5*(1), 31–36.

Kulbok, P. A., & Glick, D. F. (2014). "Something must be done!" Public health nursing education in the United States from 1900 to 1950. *Family & Community Health, 37*(3), 170–178.

Kulbok, P. A., Thatcher, E., Park, E., & Meszaros, P. S. (2012). Evolving public health nursing roles: Focus on community participatory health promotion and prevention. *Online Journal of Issues in Nursing, 17*(2), Manuscript 1. doi: 10.3912/OJIN.Vol17No02Man01.

Kunic, R. J., & Jackson, D. (2013). Transforming nursing practice: Barriers and solutions. *AORN Journal, 98*(3), 235–248.

Lee, G., Clark, A. M., & Thompson, D. R. (2013). Florence Nightingale—Never more relevant than today. *Journal of Advanced Nursing, 69*(2), 234–246.

Leffers, J., McDermott-Levy, R., Smith, C. M., & Sattler, B. (2014). Nursing education's response to the 1995 Institute of Medicine report: Nursing, Health, and the Environment. *Nursing Forum, 49*(4), 214–224.

Levin, P. F., Cary, A. H., Kulbok, P., Leffers, J., Molle, M., & Polivka, B. J. (2008). Graduate education for advanced practice public health nursing: At the crossroads. *Public Health Nursing, 25*(2), 176–193.

Lineberry, C. (2013, May 7). *A brief history of female nurses in the military, from the American Revolution to World War II*. Retrieved from http://www.huffingtonpost.com/cate-lineberry/history-military-nurses_b_3225854.html

Little, B., Vandenhouten, C. L., & DeVance-Wilson, C. (2013). Public health nursing certification exam on the verge of extinction? Act fast! *Public Health Nursing, 30*(2), 91–93.

Marjoua, Y., & Bozic, K. J. (2012). Brief history of quality movement in US healthcare. *Current Review of Musculoskeletal Medicine, 5*(4), 265–273.

Martin, M., Vanichseni, S., Suntharasamai, P., Sangkum, U., Mock, P. A., Leethochawalit, M., … Bangkok Tenofovir Study Group. (2015). The impact of adherence to preexposure prophylaxis on the risk of HIV infection among people who inject drugs. *AIDS, 29*(7), 819–824.

Milbrath, G. R., & DeGuzman, P. B. (2015). Neighborhood: A conceptual analysis. *Public Health Nursing, 32*(4), 349–358.

Mosley, M. O. (2007). Satisfied to carry the bag: Three black community health nurses' contributions to health care reform, 1900–1937. In P. D'Antonio, E. D. Baer, S. D. Rinker, & J. E. Lynaugh (Eds.), *Nurses' work: Issues across time and place* (pp. 65–78). New York, NY: Springer Publishing Company.

Mowbray, P. (1997). *Florence Nightingale museum guidebook*. London, UK: The Florence Nightingale Museum Trust.

National Geographic Education Staff. (2013, November 27). *Mary Seacole: Adventurer in Jamaica, Panama, and the Crimean War*. Retrieved from http://education.nationalgeographic.org/news/ mary-seacole/

National Organization for Public Health Nursing (NOPHN). (1939). *Manual of public health nursing* (3rd ed.). New York, NY: The Macmillan Company.

National Organization for Public Health Nursing (NOPHN). (1944). Approval of Skidmore College of Nursing as preparing students for public health nursing. *Public Health Nursing, 36*, 371.

Nightingale, F. (1969). *Notes on nursing: What it is, and what it is not*. London, UK: Harrison. (Original work published 1859)

Nightingale, F. (1864). *How people may live and not die in India*. London, UK: Longman, Green, Longman, Roberts, & Green.

Nightingale, F. (1876). [Letter to the editor]. *The Times* (London).

National Public Radio. (2011, June 3). *By the numbers: Today's military*. Retrieved from http://www.npr.org/2011/07/03/137536111/ by-the-numbers-todays-military

Nsemo, A. D., John, M. E., Etifit, R. E., Mgbekem, M. A., & Oyira, E. J. (2013). Clinical nurses' perception of continuing professional education as a tool for quality service delivery in public hospitals Calabar, Cross River State, Nigeria. *Nursing Education in Practice, 13*(4), 328–334.

Nymberg, P., & Drevenhorn, E. (2015). Patients' experience of a nurse-led lifestyle clinic at a Swedish health centre. *Scandinavian Journal of Caring Science*.

Odutayo, P. O., Olaogun, A. A., Oluwatosin, A. O., & Ogunfowokan, A. A. (2013). Impact of an educational program on the use of standardized nursing languages for nursing documentation among public health nurses in Nigeria. *International Journal of Nursing Knowledge, 24*(2), 108–112.

Olson Keller, L., Strohschein, S., & Schaffer, M. A. (2011). Cornerstones of public health nursing. *Public Health Nursing, 28*(3), 249–260.

Palmer, I. S. (2001). Florence Nightingale: Reformer, reactionary, researcher. In E. C. Hein (Ed.), *Nursing issues in the 21st century: Perspectives from the literature* (pp. 26–38). Philadelphia, PA: Lippincott Williams & Wilkins.

Prochaska, F. K. (2003). *Women and philanthropy in nineteenth century England*. New York, NY: Oxford University Press. (Original work published 1980)

Pugh, A. (2001). Men, monasteries, wars, and wards. (2001). *Nursing Times, 97*(44), 24–25.

Rababah, J., Curtis, A., & Drew, B. L. (2014). Informatics: Integrating a Geographic Information System into nursing research: Potentials and challenges. *Online Journal of Issues in Nursing, 19*(2). Retrieved from http://www.nursingworld.org/MainMenuCategories/ANAMarket place/ANAPeriodicals/OJIN/TableofContents/Vol-19-2014/No2-May-2014/Integrating-a-Geographic-Information-System-into-Research.html

Ramsay, A. G. (2012). The end of an era. *Public Health Nursing, 29*(4), 380–383.

Ramsey, M. A. (2006). John Snow, MD: Anaesthetist to the Queen of England and pioneer epidemiologist. *Baylor University Medical Center Proceedings, 19*(1), 24–28.

Raphael, D. (2012). *Tackling health inequalities: Lessons from international experiences*. Toronto, ON: Canadian Scholars' Press.

Reddi, V. (2005). *Dorothea Lynde Dix (1802–1887)*. Retrieved from http://www.truthaboutnursing.org/press/pioneers/dix.html

Roberts, D., & Freeman, R. (Eds.). (1973). *Redesigning nursing education for public health: Report of the conference* (Publication No. HRA 75–75). Bethesda, MD: U.S. Department of Health, Education, and Welfare.

Robinson, T. M. (2009). *Your country needs you*. Blomington, IN: Xilbris.

Ruel, S. R. (2014). Lillian Wald. *Home Healthcare Nurse, 32*(10), 597–600.

Ruffing-Rahal, M. (1986). Margaret Sanger: Nurse and feminist. *Nursing Outlook, 34*, 246–249.

Sachs, T. B. (1908). The tuberculosis nurse. *American Journal of Nursing, 8,* 597.

Schaffer, M. A., Cross, S., Olson Keller L., Nelson P., Schoon, P. M., & Henton, P. (2010). The Henry Street Consortium population-based competencies for educating public health nursing students. *Public Health Nursing, 28*(1), 78–90.

Schaffer, M. A., & Mbibi, N. (2014). Public health nurse mentorship of pregnant and parenting adolescents. *Public Health Nursing, 31*(5), 428–437.

Schneiderman, J. U. (2008). Qualitative study on the role of nurses as health case managers of children in foster care in California. *Journal of Pediatric Nursing, 23*(4), 241–249.

Scutchfield, F. D., & Keck, C. W. (2009). *Principles of public health practice.* Florence, KY: Cengage Learning.

Seacole, M. (1857). *Wonderful adventures of Mrs. Seacole in many lands.* London, England: James Blackwood Paternoster Row. Retrieved from http://digital.library.upenn.edu/women/seacole/adventures/adventures.html

Simpson, M. S. (2000). Nurses and models of practice: Then and now. *American Journal of Nursing, 100*(2), 82–83.

Stanley, D. (2007). Lights in the shadows: Florence Nightingale and others who made their mark. *Contemporary Nurse, 24*(1), 45–51.

Stevens, C. (2013, February 4). When you could call the midwife! Britain had 10,000 district nurses and midwives in the 1950s. *Daily Mail.* Retrieved from http://www.dailymail.co.uk/news/article-2272961/When-COULD-midwife-Britain-10-000-district-nurses-midwives-1950s.html

Struthers, L. R. (1917). *The School Nurse: A survey of the duties and responsibilities of the nurse in the maintenance of health and physical perfection and the prevention of disease among school children.* New York, NY: G. P. Putman's Sons.

Swider, S., Krothe, J., Reyes, D., & Cravetz, M. (2013). The Quad Council practice competencies for public health nursing. *Public Health Nursing, 30*(6), 519–536.

Swider, S., Levin, P., Cowell, J., Breakwell, S., Holland, P., & Wallander, J. (2009). Community/public health nursing practice leaders' views of the doctorate of nursing practice. *Public Health Nursing, 26*(5), 405–411.

Swider, S., Levin, P., Ailey, S., Breakwell, S., Cowell, J., ... O'Rourke, M.. (2006). Matching a graduate curriculum in public/community health nursing to practice competencies: The Rush University experience. *Public Health Nursing, 23*(2), 190–195.

Swider, S., Levin, P., & Kulbok, P. A. (2015). Creating the future of public health nursing: A call to action. *Public Health Nursing, 32*(2), 91–93.

Thaweeboon, T., Peachpansri, S., Pochanapan, S., Senachack, P., & Pinyopasakul, W. (2011). Development of the school of nursing, midwifery, and public health at Siriraj, Thailand 1896–1971: A historical study. *Nursing & Health Sciences, 13*(4), 440–446.

Thomas, J. C., & Weber, D. J. (2001). *Epidemiologic methods for the study of infectious diseases.* Oxford, UK: Oxford University Press.

Toosi, M. (2012). *Employment outlook 2010–2020: Labor force projections to 2020; a more slowly growing workforce.* Retrieved from http://www.bls.gov/opub/mlr/2012/01/art3full.pdf

Uden-Holman, T. M., Curry, S. J., Benz, L., & Aquilino, M. L. (2015). Public health as a catalyst for interprofessional education on a health sciences campus. *American Journal of Public Health, 105*(Suppl.), s104–s105.

U.S. Department of Labor, Bureau of Labor Statistics. (2015, April). *Monthly labor review: CES employment recovers in 2014.* Retrieved from http://www.bls.gov/opub/mlr/2015/article/ces-employment-recovers-in-2014-1.htm

U.S. Department of Labor, Bureau of Labor Statistics. (2016). *Occupational outlook handbook, 2016–17 edition.* Retrieved from http://www.bls.gov/ooh/healthcare/

U.S. Department of Health and Human Services (USDHHS), Division of Nursing. (1984). *Consensus conference on the essentials of public health nursing practice and education: Report of the conference.* Rockville, MD: Author.

U.S. Department of Health and Human Services (USDHHS). (2014, December). *The future of the nursing workforce: National- and state-level projections, 2012–2025.* Retrieved from http://bhpr.hrsa.gov/healthworkforce/supplydemand/nursing/workforceprojections/nursingprojections.pdf

Vessey, J. A., & McGowen, K. A. (2006). A successful public health experiment: School nursing. *Pediatric Nursing, 32*(213), 255–258.

Wald, L. D. (1915). *The house on Henry Street.* New York, NY: Holt.

Wald, L. D. (1934). *Windows of Henry Street.* Boston, MA: Little Brown.

Webb, B. (2011). Roaming through Virginia with the public health nurse. *Public Health Nursing, 28*(3), 291–293

Wikiquote. (2016). *George Santayana.* Retrieved from https://en.wikiquote.org/wiki/George_Santayana

Williams, C. A. (1977). Community health nursing: What is it? *Nursing Outlook, 25,* 250–254.

Woodham-Smith, C. (1951). *Florence Nightingale.* New York, NY: McGraw-Hill.

World Health Organization. (1978). *Primary health care: Report of the International Conference on Primary Health Care, Alma-Ata, USSR.* Geneva, Switzerland: Author.

World Health Organization. (2016). *WHO called to return to the Declaration of Alma-Ata.* Retrieved from http://www.who.int/social_determinants/tools/multimedia/alma_ata/en/

Wright, J. (2011). Public health reform and the emergence of school nursing. *British Journal of School Nursing, 6*(6), 304–305.

Yang, K., Woomer, G. R., Agbemenu, K., & Williams, L. (2014). Relate better and judge less: Poverty simulation promoting culturally competent care in community health nursing. *Nurse Education in Practice, 14*(6), 680–685.

Yeh, M. C., Chao, Y. Y., & Chao, C. (2012). Challenges and strategies for nursing education in Taiwan from a public health needs perspective. *Journal of Nursing, 59*(5), 10–15.

Young, S., Acord, L., Schuler, S., & Hansen, J. M. (2014). Addressing the community/public health nursing shortage through a multifaceted regional approach. *Public Health Nursing, 31*(6), 566–573.

Zarbock, S. F. (1996). More than squeaky blue shoes and a black bag. Home are in a rural area. *Home Care Provider, 1*(4), 205–206.

thePoint: Everything You Need to Make the Grade!

thePoint® Visit http://thePoint.lww.com/Rector9e for selected readings, study aids for all learning styles, and more!

Setting the Stage for Community Health Nursing

"One good community nurse will save a dozen policemen."

—*Herbert Hoover*

KEY TERMS

Advocate
Assessment
Assurance

Case management
Clinician
Collaborator

Educator
Leader
Manager

Policy development
Triple Aim

LEARNING OBJECTIVES

Upon mastery of this chapter, you should be able to:

- Identify the three core public health functions basic to community health nursing.
- Describe and differentiate among seven different roles of the community health nurse.
- Discuss the seven roles within the framework of public health nursing functions.
- Explain the importance of each role for influencing people's health.
- Identify and discuss factors that affect a nurse's selection and practice of each role.
- Describe seven settings in which community health nurses practice.
- Discuss the nature of community health nursing, and the common threads basic to its practice, woven throughout all roles and settings.
- Identify principles of effective nursing practice in the community.

Historically, community health nurses have engaged in many professional roles. Nurses in this professional specialty have provided care to the sick, taught positive health habits and self-care, advocated on behalf of needy populations, developed and managed health programs, provided leadership, and collaborated with other professionals and consumers to implement changes in health services. Although the practice settings may have differed, the essential goal of the community health nurse has always been a healthier community. The home certainly has been one site for practice, but so too have public health clinics, schools, factories, and other community-based locations. Today, the roles and settings of community health nursing practice have expanded even further, offering a wide range of professional opportunities. This chapter examines how the conceptual foundations and core functions of community health practice are integrated into the various roles and settings of community health nursing. It provides an opportunity to gain greater understanding about how and where community health nursing is practiced. Moreover, it will expand awareness of the many existing and future possibilities for community health nurses to improve the public's health. As you read through this chapter, think about client populations that you may have encountered in the acute care setting and consider your role with these same populations in a community setting. Perhaps you may discover a community health nursing specialty area that you never even considered.

CORE PUBLIC HEALTH FUNCTIONS

Community health nurses work as partners within a team of professionals (in public health and other disciplines), nonprofessionals, and consumers to improve the health of populations. The various roles and settings for practice hinge on three primary functions of public health: assessment, policy development, and assurance (Institute of Medicine, 1988). These functions are foundational to all roles assumed by the community health nurse and are applied at three levels of service: to individuals, to families, and to communities (see Display 3–1). Regardless of the role or setting of choice, these three essential responsibilities direct the work of all community health nurses.

Assessment

An essential first function in public health, **assessment**, means that the community health nurse must gather and analyze information that will affect the health of the people to be served. As described in Display 3–1, assessment is *the systematic collection, assembly, analysis, and dissemination of information about the health of a community*. The nurse and others on the health team need to determine health needs, health risks, environmental conditions, political agendas, and financial and other resources, depending on the individuals, community, or population targeted for intervention. Data may be gathered in many ways; typical methods include interviewing people in the community, conducting surveys, gathering information from public records (many of which are available online), and using research findings.

The community health nurse is typically both trusted and valued by clients, agencies, and private providers. Trust placed in the community health nurse can often be attributed to consistency, honesty, dependability, and an ongoing presence in the community. Although securing and maintaining the trust of others is pivotal to all nursing practice, it is even more critical when working in the community. Trust can afford a nurse access to client populations that are difficult to engage, to agencies, and to health care providers. In the capacity of trusted professional, community health nurses gather relevant client data that enable them to identify strengths, weaknesses, and needs. It is important to recognize that as difficult as it may be for the nurse to gain the trust and respect of the community, if ever lost, these attributes can be difficult if not impossible to regain.

At the community level, assessment is done both formally and informally as nurses identify and interact with key community leaders. With families, the nurse can evaluate family strengths and areas of concern in the immediate living environment and in the neighborhood. At the individual level, people are identified within the family who are in need of services, and the nurse evaluates the functional capacity of these individuals through the use of specific assessment measures and a variety of tools. Assessment of communities and families as the initial step in the nursing process is discussed more fully in Chapters 15 and 19.

Policy Development

Policy development (defined in Display 3–1) is enhanced by the synthesis and analysis of information obtained during assessment. At the community level, the nurse provides leadership in convening and facilitating community groups to evaluate health concerns and develop a plan to address those concerns. Typically, the nurse recommends specific training and programs to meet identified health needs of target populations. This is accompanied by raising the awareness of key policy makers about factors such as health regulations and budget decisions that negatively affect the health of the community (see Chapter 13). With families, the nurse recommends new programs or increased services based on identified needs. Additional data may be needed to identify trends in groups or clusters of families, so that effective intervention strategies can be used with these families. At the individual level, the nurse assists in the development of standards for individual client care, recommends or adopts risk classification systems to assist with prioritizing individual client care, and participates in establishing criteria for opening, closing, or referring individual cases.

DISPLAY 3–1 PUBLIC HEALTH NURSING WITHIN THE CORE PUBLIC HEALTH FUNCTIONS MODEL

The model includes assessment, policy development, and assurance surrounding the individual, family, and community. *Assessment* is the systematic collection, assembly, analysis, and dissemination of information about the health of a community. *Policy development* uses the scientific information gathered during assessment to create comprehensive public health policies. *Assurance* is the pledge to constituents that services necessary to achieve agreed-upon goals are provided by encouraging actions of others (private or public), requiring action through regulation, or providing service directly.

From Institute of Medicine. (1988). *The future of public health*. Retrieved from http://www.cdc.gov/nphpsp/essentialservices.html

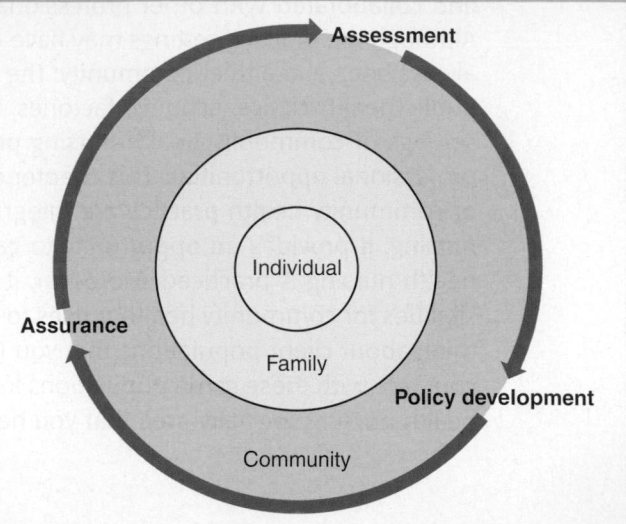

Assurance

Assurance activities—activities that make certain that services are provided—often consume most of the community health nurse's time. Community health nurses perform the assurance function at the community level when they provide services to target populations, improve quality assurance activities, maintain safe levels of communicable disease surveillance and outbreak control, and collaborate with community leaders in the preparation of a community emergency preparedness plan. In addition, they participate in outcome research, provide expert consultation, promote evidence-based practice, and provide services within the community based on standards of care.

Essential Services

To more clearly articulate the services that are linked to the core functions of assessment, policy development, and assurance, a list of 10 essential services was developed in

1994 by the Public Health Functions Steering Committee (U.S. Department of Health and Human Services [USDHHS], 1997) (see Display 3–2). This initial effort to define the service components of the core functions provided an organized service delivery plan for public health providers across the country. A model depicting the relationships between the core functions and the essential services was eventually developed (USDHHS, Office of Disease Prevention and Health Promotion, 1999). The model (Fig. 3–1) shows the types of services necessary to achieve the core functions of assessment, policy development, and assurance. It also emphasizes the circular or ongoing nature of the process. The placement of research at the center of the model is a clear indication of the high priority placed on providing scientific evidence in all areas of service delivery. Research is essential to evidence-based practice and is vital to achieving healthy communities. As you review this model, think about what types of

DISPLAY 3–2 TEN ESSENTIAL SERVICES OF PUBLIC HEALTH

1. *Monitor* health status to identify and solve community health problems.
2. *Diagnose and investigate* health problems and health hazards in the community.
3. *Inform, educate,* and *empower* people about health issues.
4. *Mobilize* community partnerships and action to identify and solve health problems.
5. *Develop policies and plans* that support individual and community health efforts.
6. *Enforce* laws and regulations that protect health and ensure safety.

7. *Link* people to needed personal health services and assure the provision of health care when otherwise unavailable.
8. *Ensure* competent public and personal health care workforces.
9. *Evaluate* effectiveness, accessibility, and quality of personal and population-based health services.
10. *Research* for new insights and innovative solutions to health problems.

From Centers for Disease Control and Prevention. (2014). *National public health performance standards: The 10 essential public health services*. Retrieved from http://www.cdc.gov/nphpsp/essentialservices.html

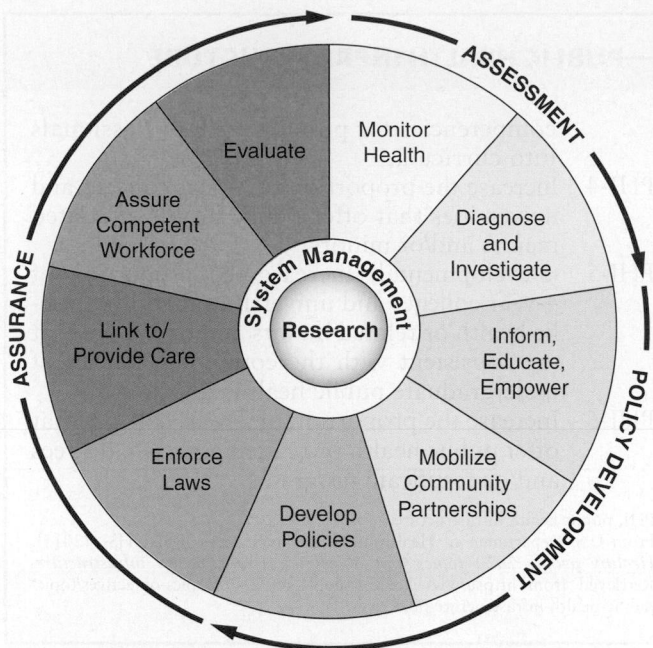

FIGURE 3–1 The core functions and 10 essential services of public health. (From Centers for Disease Control and Prevention. (2015). Retrieved from http://www.health.gov/phfunctions/public.htm)

services might be provided in each category, depending on whether you are focusing on an individual, a family, or a community. It is not necessary that the community health nurse provide each of the listed services. Working in collaboration with an interdisciplinary team, the community nurse can support the efforts of others to achieve improved health in the community. What is important is that the team members all recognize their respective roles and are working toward the same goal.

STANDARDS OF PRACTICE

In 2008, the American Association of Colleges of Nursing (AACN) published the revised *The Essentials of Baccalaureate Education for Professional Nursing Practice*. Building on the 1998 version, this document was a major step in providing clear guidelines as to what constitutes professional nursing education. Roles of beginning professional nursing practice were grouped into three broad roles: "provider of care; designer/manager/coordinator of care; and member of a profession" (AACN, 2008, p. 3). Although this document describes educational preparation in all areas of nursing practice, the link to community health nursing is quite evident. The document outlines the knowledge, skills, and attitudes seen as vital to the education of the baccalaureate nurse. Practice-focused outcomes typically associated with community health nursing are emphasized in Essential Seven: Clinical Prevention and Population Health, stressing that "health promotion and disease prevention at the individual and population level are necessary to improve population health and are important components of baccalaureate generalist nursing practice" (AACN, 2008, p. 4). This document clearly articulates the growing need to prepare nurses to assume a variety of roles in the community emphasizing that the

baccalaureate nurse "is prepared to practice with patients, including individuals, families, groups, communities, and populations across the lifespan and across the continuum of healthcare environments" (AACN, 2008, p. 4).

Community health nursing practice is further defined by specific standards developed under the auspices of the American Nurses Association (ANA) in collaboration with the Quad Council of Public Health Nursing Organizations (ANA, 2013c). The Quad Council is composed of representatives from the ANA—Council on Nursing Practice and Economics; the American Public Health Association—Public Health Nursing Section; the Association of Community Health Nursing Educators (ACHNE); and the Association of Public Health Nurses (APHN). These four organizations represent academics and professional practitioners, providing a broad spectrum of views regarding professional practice in the field of community health nursing. *Public Health Nursing: Scope and Standards of Practice* (ANA, 2013c) provides guidance as to what constitutes public health nursing and how it can be differentiated from other nursing specialties. Standards of care are consistent with the nursing process and include assessment, population diagnosis and priorities, outcomes identification, planning, implementation, and evaluation. This document is an important reference for all those practicing in the community. It provides the basis for evaluating an individual's performance in this field and is used by many employers to assess job performance.

In addition to their work on the practice standards, the ACHNE published the updated *Essentials of Baccalaureate Nursing Education for Entry-Level Community/Public Health Nursing* in 2010 (Education Committee of ACHNE). This document builds on previous versions and is consistent with both the *Essentials* document (AACN, 2008) and the scope and standards of public health nursing practice (ANA, 2013c). This document describes core professional values as well as knowledge and basic competencies. Core values of professional behavior emphasize community/population as client, prevention, partnership, healthy environment, and diversity. Building on these common values, 15 essential concepts and their related competencies are delineated including 3 newly defined essentials; communication; social justice; and emergency preparedness, response, and recovery (ACHNE, Education Committee, 2010). It is also important to recognize that an emphasis of *Healthy People 2020* is to create and support a competent public and personal health care workforce including professional competencies required for sound practice (see Display 3–3) (USDHHS, 2016a).

The community health nurse provides nursing services based on other standards developed by the ANA, such as the *Code of Ethics for Nurses with Interpretive Statements* (2015a), *Nursing's Social Policy Statement* (2010), and *Nursing: Scope and Standards of Practice* (2015b). Each of these documents provides essential information regarding sound general nursing practice. When combined with *Public Health Nursing: Scope and Standards of Practice* (ANA, 2013c), they provide the community health nurse with a clear understanding of accepted practice in this nursing specialty. The Quad Council of Public Health Nursing Organizations is comprised of the Association of Public Health Nurses (APHN), the Association of

---

DISPLAY 3-3 *HEALTHY PEOPLE 2020*—PUBLIC HEALTH INFRASTRUCTURE

Workforce Objectives

PHI-1 Increase the proportion of federal, tribal, state, and local public health agencies that incorporate core competencies for public health professionals into job descriptions and performance evaluations.

PHI-2 (Developmental) Increase the proportion of tribal, state, and local public health personnel who receive continuing education consistent with core competencies for public health professionals.

PHI-3 Increase the proportion of Council on Education for Public Health (CEPH) accredited schools of public health, CEPH-accredited academic programs, and schools of nursing (with a public health or community health component) that integrate core competencies for public health professionals into curricula.

PHI-4 Increase the proportion of 4-year colleges and universities that offer public health or related majors and/or minors.

PHI-5 (Developmental) Increase the proportion of 4-year colleges and universities that offer public health or related majors and/or minors that are consistent with the core competencies of undergraduate public health education.

PHI-6 Increase the proportion of 2-year colleges that offer public health or related associate degrees and/or certificate programs.

PHI, public health infrastructure.
From U.S. Department of Health and Human Services (USDHHS). (2015). *Healthy people 2020 topics and objectives: Public health infrastructure.* Retrieved from https://www.healthypeople.gov/2020/topics-objectives/topic/public-health-infrastructure/objectives

---

Community Health Nursing Educators (ACHNE), the Public Health Nursing Section of the American Public Health Association, and the American Nurses Association Council on Nursing Practice and Economics. The Quad Council of Public Health Nursing Organizations updated the Core Competencies for Public Health Nurses (CCPHN) in 2011. The competencies include eight domains consisting of analytic assessment skills, policy development/program planning skills, communication skills, cultural competency skills, community dimensions of practice skills, public health sciences skills, financial planning and management skills, and leadership and systems thinking skills. The competencies consist of three tiers of practice beginning with the public health nurse generalist in tier one followed by the public health nurse specialist in tier two and ending with the public health nurse administrator practice skills in tier three (Swider, Krothe, Reyes, & Cravetz, 2013). The tier one public health nursing competencies are listed in Display 3–4.

With specific standards of practice and clear competencies to achieve, the community health nurse can integrate the core functions of assessment, policy development, and assurance throughout all of the various roles and community settings of practice.

ROLES OF COMMUNITY HEALTH NURSES

Just as the health care system is continually evolving, community health nursing practice evolves to remain effective with the clients it serves. Over time, the role of the community health nurse has broadened. This breadth is reflected in the description of public health nursing from the American Public Health Association, Public Health Nursing Section (2013):

Public health nursing is a specialty practice within nursing and public health. It focuses on improving the population health by emphasizing prevention, and attending to multiple determinants of health. Often used interchangeably with community health

nursing, this nursing practice includes advocacy, policy development, and planning, which addresses issues of social justice. With a multi-level view of health, public health nursing action occurs through community applications of theory, evidence, and a commitment to health equity (para. 3).

Community health nurses wear many hats while conducting day-to-day practice. At any given time, however, one role is primary. This is especially true for specialized roles, such as that of full-time manager. This chapter examines seven major roles: clinician, educator, advocate, manager, collaborator, leader, and researcher. It also describes the factors that influence the selection and performance of those roles.

Clinician Role

The most familiar role of the community health nurse is that of clinician or care provider. The provision of nursing care, however, takes on new meaning in the context of community health practice. The **clinician** role in community health means that the nurse ensures health services are provided not just to individuals and families, but also to groups and populations. Nursing service is still designed for the special needs of clients; however, when those clients comprise a group or population, clinical practice takes different forms. It requires different skills to assess collective needs and tailor service accordingly. For instance, one community health nurse might visit elderly residents in a seniors' high-rise apartment building. Another might serve as the clinic nurse in a rural prenatal clinic that serves migrant farm workers. These are opportunities to assess the needs of entire aggregates and design appropriate services.

For community health nurses, the clinician role involves certain emphases that are different from those of basic nursing. Three clinician emphases, in particular, are useful to consider here: holism, health promotion, and skill expansion.

DISPLAY 3-4 TIER 1 PUBLIC HEALTH NURSING COMPETENCIES

Domain 1: Analytic and Assessment Skills

1. Identifies the determinants of health and illness of individuals and families, using multiple sources of data
2. Uses epidemiologic data and the ecological perspective to identify health risks for a population. Identifies individual and family assets and needs, values and beliefs, resources and relevant environmental factors
3. Identifies variables that measure health and public health conditions
4. Uses valid and reliable methods and instruments for collecting qualitative and quantitative data from multiple sources. Develops a data collection plan using appropriate technology to collect data to inform the care of individuals, families, and groups
5. Identifies sources of public health data and information. Collects, interprets, and documents data in terms that are understandable to all who were involved in the process, including communities
6. Uses valid and reliable data sources to make comparisons for assessment
7. Identifies gaps and redundancies in data sources in a community assessment through work with individuals, families, and communities
8. Applies ethical, legal, and policy guidelines and principles in the collection, maintenance, use, and dissemination of data and information
9. Describes the public health nursing applications of quantitative and qualitative data
10. Collects quantitative and qualitative data that can be used in the community health assessment process. Assesses data collected as part of the community assessment process to make inferences about individuals, families, and groups
11. Utilizes information technology to collect, analyze, store, and retrieve data related to public health nursing care of individuals, families, and groups
12. Practices evidence-based public health nursing to promote the health of individuals, families, and groups
13. Uses available data and resources related to the social determinants of health when planning care for individuals, families, and groups

Domain 2: Policy Development/Program Planning Skills

1. Identifies policy issues relevant to the health of individuals, families, and groups. Describes the structure of the public health system and its impacts on individuals, families, and groups within a population
2. Identifies the implications of policy options on public health programs and the potential impacts on individuals, families, and groups within population

3. Identifies outcomes of health policy relevant to PHN practice
4. Collects information that will inform policy decisions. Describes the legislative policy development process. Identifies outcomes of current health policy relevant to PHN practice
5. Describes the structure of the public health system. Identifies public health laws and regulations relevant to PHN practice. Provides public health nursing services in a manner consistent with laws and regulations
6. Participates as a team member in developing organizational plans to implement programs and policies
7. Participates in teams to assure compliance with organizational policies
8. Assists in the design of an evaluation plan for an individual-, family-, or community-focused program. Participates as a team member to evaluate programs to individuals, families, and groups for their effectiveness and quality
9. Understands methods and practices used to identify and access public health information for individuals, families, and groups
10. Understands that quality improvement is important to the practice of public health nursing. Participates in quality improvement teams. Describes various approaches used to improve public health processes and systems. Utilizes quality indicators and core measures to identify and address opportunities for improvement in the care of individuals, families, and groups

Domain 3: Communications Skills

1. Assesses the health literacy of the individuals, families, and groups served
2. Communicates effectively in writing, orally, and electronically. Communicates in a culturally responsive and relevant manner. Communications are characterized by critical thinking
3. Solicits input from individuals, families, and groups when planning and delivering health care
4. Utilizes a variety of methods to disseminate public health information to individuals, families, and groups within a population
5. Demonstrates presentation of targeted health information to multiple audiences at a local level, including groups, peer professionals, and agency peers
6. Communicates effectively with individuals, families, and groups and as a member of interprofessional team(s)
7. Articulates the role of public health nursing to internal and external audiences

Domain 4: Cultural Competency Skills

1. Utilizes the social and ecological determinants of health to work effectively with diverse individuals, families, and groups

(continued)

DISPLAY 3–4 TIER 1 PUBLIC HEALTH NURSING COMPETENCIES (*Continued*)

2. Uses concepts, knowledge, and evidence of the social determinants of health in the delivery of services to individuals, families, and groups. Utilizes information technology to understand the impact of the social determinants of health on individuals, families, and groups
3. Adapts public health nursing care to individuals, families, and groups based on cultural needs and differences
4. Explains factors contributing to cultural diversity
5. Articulates the benefits of a diverse public health workforce
6. Demonstrates culturally appropriate public health nursing practice with individuals, families, groups, and community members. Contributes to promoting culturally responsive work environment

Domain 5: Community Dimensions of Practice Skills

1. Utilizes an ecological perspective in health assessment, planning, and interventions with individuals, families, and groups
2. Identifies research issues at a community level. Functions effectively as a member of a community-based participatory research (CBPR) team
3. Identifies community partners for PHN practice with individuals, families, and groups
4. Collaborates with community partners to promote the health of individuals and families within the population
5. Partners effectively with key stakeholders and groups in care delivery to individuals, families, and groups
6. Participates effectively in activities that facilitate community involvement
7. Describes to individuals, families, and groups the role of government and the private and non-profit sectors in the delivery of community health services
8. Utilizes community assets and resources to promote health and to deliver care to individuals, families, and groups
9. Seeks input from individuals, families, and groups and incorporates it into plans of care
10. Supports public health policies, programs, and resources. Identifies opportunities for population-focused advocacy for individuals, families, and groups

Domain 6: Public Health Sciences Skills

1. Incorporates public health and nursing science in the delivery of care to individuals, families, and groups
2. Describes the historical foundation of public health and public health nursing

3. Describes how individual-, family-, and group-focused programs contribute to meeting the core public health functions and the 10 essential services
4. Uses basic descriptive epidemiological methods when conducting a health assessment for individuals, families, and groups
5. Interprets research relevant to public health interventions for individuals, families, and groups
6. Accesses public health and other sources of information using informatics and other information technologies
7. Identifies gaps in research evidence to guide public health nursing practice
8. Complies with the requirements of patient confidentiality and human subject protection
9. Participates in research at the community level to build the scientific base of public health nursing

Domain 7: Financial Management and Planning Skills

1. Describes the interrelationships among local, state, tribal, and federal public health and health care systems
2. Describes the structure, function, and jurisdictional authority of the organizational units within federal, state, tribal, and local public health agencies
3. Adheres to the organization's policies and procedures, including emergency preparedness and response
4. Provides data for inclusion in a programmatic budget
5. Describes the impact of budget constraints on the delivery of public health nursing care to individuals, families, and groups
6. Provides input into budget priorities
7. Provides data to evaluate care and services for individuals, families, and groups. Contributes to the evaluation plan for a program targeting individuals, families, and/or groups
8. Adapts the delivery of public health nursing care to individuals, families, and groups based on reported evaluation results
9. Provides input into the fiscal and narrative components of proposals for funding from external sources
10. Applies basic human relations and conflict management skills in interactions with peers and other health care team members
11. Utilizes public health informatics skills relative to the public health nursing care of individuals, families, and groups
12. Provides input into contracts and other agreements for the provision of services
13. Delivers public health nursing care within budgetary guidelines

---

DISPLAY 3-4 TIER 1 PUBLIC HEALTH NURSING COMPETENCIES (*Continued*)

Domain 8: Leadership and Systems Thinking Skills

1. Incorporates ethical standards of practice as the basis of all interactions with organizations, communities, and individuals. Incorporates ethical standards into all aspects of public health nursing practice
2. Applies systems theory to PHN practice with individuals, families, and groups
3. Participates with stakeholders to identify vision, values, and principles for community action
4. Identifies internal and external factors affecting PHN practice and services
5. Uses individual, team, and organizational learning opportunities for personal and professional development as a public health nurse

6. Acts as a mentor, coach, or peer advisor/reviewer for public health nursing staff. Maintains personal commitment to lifelong learning and professional development
7. Participates in quality initiatives that identify opportunities for improvement. Provides data to measure, report, and improve organizational performance
8. Adapts the delivery of public health nursing care in consideration of changes in the public health system and the larger social, political, and economic environment. Maintains knowledge of current public health laws and policies relevant to public health nursing practice

From Swider, S., Krothe, J., Reyes, D., & Cravetz, M. (2013). The Quad Council practice competencies for public health nursing. *Public Health Nursing, 30*(6), 519–536, with permission.

Holistic Practice

Most clinical nursing seeks to be broad and holistic. In community health, however, a holistic approach means considering the broad range of interacting needs that affect the collective health of the "client" as a larger system (Dossey & Keegan, 2016). Holistic nursing care encompasses the comprehensive and total care of the client in all areas, such as physical, emotional, social, spiritual, and economic. All are considered and cared for when the client is a large system, just as they should be with individual clients. The client is a composite of people whose relationships and interactions with each other must be considered in totality. Holistic practice must emerge from this systems perspective (Fig. 3–2).

For example, when working with a group of pregnant teenagers living in a juvenile detention center, the nurse would consider the girls' relationships with one another, their parents, the fathers of their unborn children, and the detention center staff. The nurse would evaluate their ages, developmental needs, and peer influences, as well as their knowledge of pregnancy, delivery, and issues related to the choice of keeping or giving up their babies. The girls' reentry into the community and their future plans for school or employment would also be considered. Holistic service would go far beyond the physical condition of pregnancy and childbirth. It would incorporate consideration of pregnant adolescents in this community as a population at risk. What factors contributed to these girls' situations, and what preventive efforts could be instituted to protect other teenagers or these teens from future pregnancies? The clinician role of the community health nurse involves holistic practice from an aggregate perspective.

Focus on Wellness

The clinician role in community health also is characterized by its focus on promoting wellness. As discussed in Chapter 1, the community health nurse provides service along the entire range of the health continuum, but especially emphasizes promotion of health and prevention of illness. Effective services include seeking out clients who are at risk for poor health and offering preventive and health-promoting services, rather than waiting for them to come for help after problems arise. The community health nurse identifies people, programs, and agencies interested in achieving a higher level of health and works with them to accomplish that goal and to sustain the expected changed behavior (Pender, Murdaugh, & Parsons, 2015). The nurse may help employees of a business learn how to live healthier lives or work with a group of people who want to quit smoking. The community health nurse may hold seminars with a men's group on enhancing fathering skills or assist a corporation with the implementation of a health promotion program. Groups and populations are identified, which may be vulnerable to certain health threats, and preventive and health-promoting programs can be designed in collaboration with the community (Pender et al., 2015). Examples include immunization of preschoolers, family planning

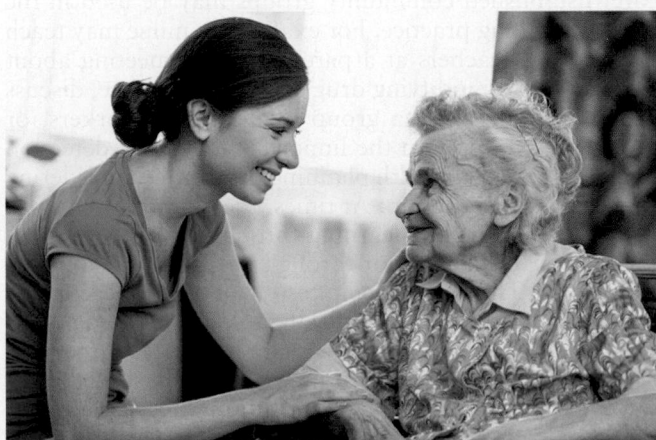

FIGURE 3–2 PHN student visiting an elderly client in her home.

programs, cholesterol screening, and prevention of behavioral problems in adolescents. Protecting and promoting the health of vulnerable populations is an important component of the clinician role and is addressed extensively in the chapters in Unit VII on vulnerable aggregates.

Expanded Skills

Many different skills are used in the role of the community health clinician. In the early years of community health nursing, emphasis was placed on physical care skills. With time, skills in observation, listening, communication, and counseling became integral to the clinician role as it grew to encompass psychological and sociocultural factors. Recently, environmental and community-wide considerations—such as problems caused by pollution, violence and crime, drug abuse, unemployment, poverty, homelessness, and limited funding for health programs—have created a need for stronger skills in assessing the needs of groups and populations and intervening at the community level. The clinician role in population-based nursing also requires skills in collaboration with consumers and other professionals, use of epidemiology and biostatistics, community organization and development, research, program evaluation, administration, leadership, and effecting change (ANA, 2013c). These skills are addressed in greater detail in later chapters.

Educator Role

A second important role of the community health nurse is that of **educator** or health teacher. Health teaching, a widely recognized part of nursing practice, is legislated through nurse practice acts in a number of states and is one of the major functions of the community health nurse (ANA, 2013c).

The educator role is especially useful in promoting the public's health for at least two reasons. First, community clients are usually not acutely ill and can absorb and act on health information. For example, a class of expectant parents, unhampered by significant health problems, can grasp the relationship of diet to fetal development. They understand the value of specific exercises to the childbirth process, are motivated to learn, and are more likely to perform those exercises. Thus, the educator role has the potential for finding greater receptivity and providing higher-yield results.

Second, the educator role in community health nursing is significant because a wider audience can be reached. With an emphasis on populations and aggregates, the educational efforts of community health nursing are appropriately targeted to reach many people. Instead of limiting teaching to one-on-one or small groups, the nurse has the opportunity and mandate to develop educational programs based on community needs that seek a community-wide impact. Community-wide anti-drug campaigns, dietary improvement programs, and improved handwashing efforts among children provide useful models for implementation of the educator role at the population level and demonstrate its effectiveness in reaching a wide audience (Bastable, 2014).

One factor that enhances the educator role is the public's higher level of health consciousness. Through plans ranging from the President's Council on Fitness, Sport and Nutrition (2016) to local antismoking campaigns, people are recognizing the value of health and are increasingly motivated to achieve higher levels of wellness. When a middle-aged man, for example, is discharged from the hospital after a heart attack, he is likely to be more interested than before the attack in learning how to prevent another. He can learn how to reduce stress, develop an appropriate and gradual exercise program, and alter his eating habits. Families with young children often are interested in learning about children's growth and development; most parents are committed to raising happy, healthy children. Health education can affect the health status of people of all ages (Pender et al., 2015). Today, in more businesses and industries, nurses promote the health of employees through active wellness education and injury prevention programs. The companies recognize that improving the health of their workers, which includes earning a living wage, means less absenteeism and higher production levels, in addition to other benefits (Kowlessar, Goetzel, Carls, Tabrizi, & Guindon, 2011; Lahiri & Faghri, 2012). Some companies even provide exercise areas and equipment for employees to use and pay for the cost of their participation or allow paid time off for exercise. See Chapter 31 for more information on occupational health nursing.

Whereas nurses in acute care teach patients with a one-on-one focus about issues related to their illness and hospitalization, community health nurses go beyond these topics to educate people in many areas. Community-living clients need and want to know about a wide variety of issues, such as family planning, weight control, smoking cessation, and stress reduction. Aggregate-level concerns also include such topics as environmental safety, sexual discrimination and harassment at school or work, violence, and drugs. What foods and additives are safe to eat? How can people organize the community to work for reduction of violence on television? What are health consumers' rights? Topics taught by community health nurses extend from personal and family health to environmental health and community organization.

As educators, community health nurses seek to facilitate client learning. Information is shared with clients both formally and informally. Nurses serve as consultants to individuals or groups. Formal classes may be held to increase people's understanding of health and health care. Established community groups may be used in the nurse's teaching practice. For example, a nurse may teach parents and teachers at a parent–teacher meeting about signs of mood-modifying drug and alcohol abuse, discuss safety practices with a group of industrial workers, or give a presentation on the importance of early detection of child abuse to a health planning committee considering funding a new program. At times, the community health nurse facilitates client learning through referrals to more knowledgeable sources or through use of experts on special topics. The nurse facilitates client self-education; in keeping with the concept of self-care, clients are encouraged and helped to use appropriate health resources and to seek out health information. The emphasis throughout the health teaching process continues to be placed on illness prevention and health promotion. Health teaching as a tool for community health nursing practice is discussed in detail in Chapter 11.

Advocate Role

The issue of clients' rights is important in health care. Every patient or client has the right to receive just, equal, and humane treatment. The role of the nurse includes client advocacy, which is highlighted in the ANA *Code of Ethics for Nurses with Interpretive Statements* (2015a) and *Nursing's Social Policy Statement* (2010). Our current health care system is often characterized by fragmented and depersonalized services, and many clients—especially the poor, the disadvantaged, those without health insurance, and people with language barriers—frequently are denied their rights. They become frustrated, confused, degraded, and unable to cope with the system on their own. The community health nurse often acts as an **advocate** for clients, pleading their cause or acting on their behalf. Clients may need someone to explain which services to expect and which services they ought to receive, to make referrals as needed, and to write letters to agencies or health care providers for them. They need someone to guide them through the complexities of the system and assure the satisfaction of their needs. This is particularly true for minorities and disadvantaged groups (Mead et al., 2013; Peek, Ferguson, Bergeron, Maltby, & Chin, 2014) (Fig. 3–3).

Advocacy Goals

Client advocacy has two underlying goals. One is to help clients gain greater independence or self-determination. Until they can research the needed information and access health and social services for themselves, the community health nurse acts as an advocate for the clients by showing them what services are available, those to which they are entitled, and how to obtain them. A second goal is to make the system more responsive and relevant to the needs of clients (Byers, 2015). By calling attention to inadequate, inaccessible, or unjust care, community health nurses can influence change (see Chapter 13).

Consider the experience of the Merrill family. Gloria Merrill has three small children. Early one Tuesday morning, the baby, Tony, suddenly started to cry. Nothing would comfort him. Gloria went to a neighbor's apartment, called the local clinic, and was told to come in the next day. The clinic did not take appointments and

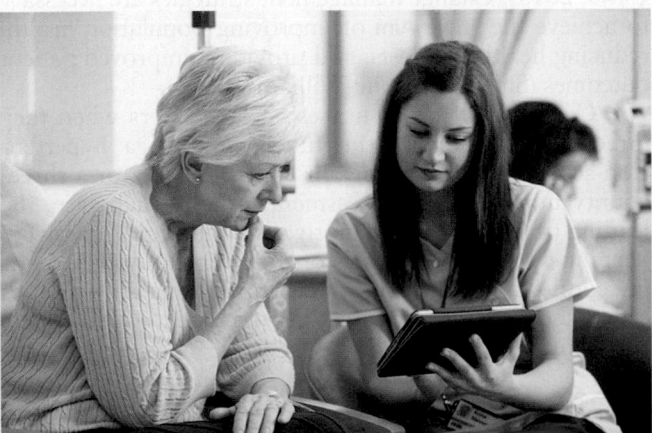

FIGURE 3–3   Like nurses working in every type of setting, PHNs are advocates for their clients.

was too busy to see any more patients that day. Gloria's neighbor reassured her that "sometimes babies just cry." For the rest of the day and night, Tony cried almost incessantly. On Wednesday, Gloria and her children made the 45-minute bus ride to the clinic and waited 3 hours in the crowded reception room; the wait was punctuated by interrogations from clinic workers. Gloria's other children were restless, and the baby was crying. Finally, they saw the physician. Tony had an inguinal hernia that could have strangulated and become gangrenous. The doctor admonished Gloria for waiting so long to bring in the baby. Immediate surgery was necessary. Someone at the clinic told Gloria that Medicaid would pay for it. Someone else told her that she was ineligible. At this point, all of her children were crying. Gloria had been up most of the night. She was frantic, confused, and felt that no one cared. This family needed an advocate.

Advocacy Actions

The advocate role incorporates four characteristic actions: being assertive, taking risks, communicating and negotiating well, and identifying resources and obtaining results.

First, advocates must be assertive. Fortunately, in the Merrill's dilemma, the clinic had a working relationship with the City Health Department and contacted Tracy Lee, a community health nurse liaison with the clinic, when Gloria broke down and cried. Tracy took the initiative to identify the Merrill's needs and find appropriate solutions. She contacted the Department of Social Services and helped the Merrill family to establish eligibility for coverage of surgery and hospitalization costs. She helped Gloria to make arrangements for the baby's hospitalization and the other children's care.

Second, advocates must take risks—go "out on a limb" if need be—for the client. The community health nurse was outraged by the kind of treatment received by the Merrill family: the delays in service, the impersonal care, and the surgery that could have been planned as elective rather than as an emergency. She wrote a letter describing the details of the Merrill's experience to the clinic director, the chairman of the clinic board, and the nursing director. This action resulted in better care for the Merrill family and a series of meetings aimed at changing clinic procedures and providing better telephone screening.

Third, advocates must communicate and negotiate well by bargaining thoroughly and convincingly. The community health nurse helping the Merrill family stated the problem clearly and argued for its solution.

Finally, advocates must identify and obtain resources for the client's benefit. By contacting the most influential people in the clinic and appealing to their desire for quality service, the nurse caring for the Merrill family was able to facilitate change.

Advocacy at the population level incorporates the same goals and actions. Whether the population is homeless people, battered women, or migrant workers, the community health nurse in the advocate role speaks and acts on their behalf. The goals remain the same: to promote clients' self-determination and to shape a more responsive system. Advocacy for large aggregates, such many with inadequate health care coverage or access to care, means changing national policies and laws (see Chapter 13). Advocacy may take the form of presenting public health nursing data to ensure that providers deliver quality services. It may mean conducting a needs assessment to demonstrate the necessity for a shelter and multiservice program for the homeless. It may mean testifying before the legislature to create awareness of the problems of battered women and the need for more protective laws. It may mean organizing a lobbying effort to require employers of migrant workers to provide proper housing and working conditions. In each case, the community health nurse works with representatives of the population to gain their understanding of the situation and to ensure their input.

Manager Role

Community health nurses, like all nurses, engage in the role of managing health services. As a **manager**, the nurse exercises administrative direction toward the accomplishment of specified goals by assessing clients' needs, planning and organizing to meet those needs, directing and leading to achieve results, and controlling and evaluating the progress to ensure that goals are met. The nurse serves as a manager when overseeing client care as a case manager, supervising ancillary staff, managing caseloads, running clinics, or conducting community health needs assessment projects. In each instance, the nurse engages in four basic functions that make up the management process. The management process, like the nursing process, incorporates a series of problem-solving activities or functions: planning, organizing, leading, and controlling and evaluating. These activities are sequential, yet they also occur simultaneously for managing service objectives (Cherry & Jacob, 2014). While performing these functions, community health nurses most often are participative managers; that is, they participate with clients, other professionals, or both to plan and implement services.

Nurse as Planner

The first function in the management process is planning. A planner sets the goals and direction for the organization or project and determines the means to achieve them. Specifically, planning includes defining goals and objectives, determining the strategy for reaching them, and designing a coordinated set of activities for implementing and evaluating them, which tends to include broader, more long-range goals (Cherry & Jacob, 2014; USDHHS, 2016a). Planning may be strategic. An example of *strategic planning* is setting 2-year agency goals to reduce teenage pregnancies in the county by 50%. Planning may be operational, which focuses more on short-term planning needs. An example of *operational planning* is setting 6-month objectives to implement a new computer system for client record keeping.

The community health nurse engages in planning as a part of the manager role when supervising a group of home health aides working with home care clients. Plans of care must be designed to include setting short-term and long-term objectives, describe actions to carry out the objectives, and design a plan for evaluating the care given. With larger groups, such as a program for a homeless population, the planning function is used

in collaboration with other professionals to determine appropriate goals for shelter and to strengthen the response to homelessness (Rogers et al., 2012). The concepts of planning with communities and families are discussed further in Chapters 15 and 19, respectively.

Nurse as Organizer

The second function of the manager role is that of organizer. This involves designing a structure within which people and tasks function to reach the desired objectives. A manager must arrange matters so that the job can be done. People, activities, and relationships have to be assembled to put the plan into effect. Organizing includes deciding on the tasks to be done, which person will do them, how to group the tasks, who reports to whom, and where decisions will be made (Cherry & Jacob, 2014). In the process of organizing, the nurse manager provides a framework for the various aspects of service, so that each runs smoothly and accomplishes its purpose. The framework is a part of service preparation. When a community health nurse manages a well-child clinic, for instance, the organizing function involves making certain that all equipment and supplies are present, required staff are hired and are on duty, and that staff responsibilities are clearly designated. The final responsibility as an organizer is to evaluate the effectiveness of the clinic. Is it providing the needed services? Are the clients satisfied? Do the services remain cost-effective? The organizer must address all of these questions.

Nurse as Leader

In the manager role, the community health nurse also must act as a **leader**. As a leader, the nurse directs, influences, or persuades others to effect change that will positively impact people's health and move them toward a goal. The leading function includes persuading and motivating people, directing activities, ensuring effective two-way communication, resolving conflicts, and coordinating the plan. Coordination means bringing people and activities together, so that they function in harmony while pursuing desired objectives. Transformational and authentic leadership is characterized by ability of leaders to inspire change and demonstrate empathy and leads to increased job satisfaction and performance (Lievens & Vlerick, 2014; Mortier, Vlerick, & Clays, 2015). Change management strategies are necessary to achieve the **Triple Aim** of improving population health, reducing healthcare costs, and providing improved patient outcomes (Shirey & White-Williams, 2015).

Community health nurses act as leaders when they direct and coordinate the functioning of a hypertension screening clinic, a weight control group, or a three-county mobile health assessment unit. In each case, the leading function requires motivating the people involved, keeping open clear channels of communication, negotiating conflicts, and directing and coordinating the activities established during planning, so that the desired objectives can be accomplished.

Nurse as Controller and Evaluator

The fourth management function is to control and evaluate projects or programs. A controller monitors the plan and ensures that it stays on course. In this function, the community health nurse must realize that plans may not proceed as intended and may need adjustments or corrections to reach the desired results or goals. Monitoring, comparing, and adjusting make up the controlling part of this function. At the same time, the nurse must compare and judge performance and outcomes against previously set goals and standards—a process that forms the evaluator aspect of this management function (Kulbok, Thatcher, Park, & Meszaros, 2012).

An example of the controlling and evaluating function is evident in a program started in several preschool day care centers. The goal of the project is to reduce the incidence of illness among the children through intensive physical and emotional preventive health education with staff, parents, and children. The two community health nurses managing the project are pleased with the progress of the classes and monitored the application of the prevention principles in day-to-day care. However, staff became busy after several weeks, and some plans were not being followed carefully. Preventive activities, such as ensuring that the children coughed into their shirtsleeve and washed their hands after using the bathroom and before eating, were not being closely monitored. Several children who were clearly sick had not been kept at home. Staff was often overlooking quiet or reserved children and not ensuring their inclusion in activities. The nurses worked with staff and parents to motivate them and get the project back on course. They held monthly meetings with the staff, observed the classes periodically, and offered one-on-one instruction to staff, parents, and children. One activity was to establish competition between the centers for the best health record, with the promise of a photograph of the winning center's children and an article in the local newspaper. Their efforts were successful.

Management Behaviors

As managers, community health nurses engage in many different types of behaviors. First described in a classic book by Mintzberg (1973), the management roles were grouped into three sets of behaviors: decision-making, transferring of information, and engaging in interpersonal relationships (Management at Work, 2016).

Decision-Making Behaviors

Mintzberg identified four types of decisional roles or behaviors: entrepreneur, disturbance handler, resource allocator, and negotiator. A manager serves in the entrepreneur role when initiating new projects. Starting a nurse-managed center to serve a homeless population is an example. Community health nurses play the disturbance handler role when they manage disturbances and crises—particularly interpersonal conflicts among staff, between staff and clients, or among clients (especially when being served in an agency). The resource allocator role is demonstrated by determining the distribution and use of human, physical, and financial resources. Nurses play the negotiator role when negotiating, perhaps with higher levels of administration or a funding agency, for new health policy or budget increases to support expanded services for clients (Management at Work, 2016). Zori, Nosek, and Musil (2010) found that nursing managers with strong critical thinking skills and open-mindedness created a more positive workplace for staff nurses.

Transfer of Information Behaviors

Mintzberg described three informational roles or behaviors: monitor, information disseminator, and spokesperson. The monitor role requires collecting and processing information, such as gathering ongoing evaluation data to determine whether a program is meeting its goals. In the disseminator role, nurses transmit the collected information to people involved in the project or organization. In the spokesperson role, nurses share information on behalf of the project or agency with outsiders (Management at Work, 2016). One effective means of information sharing is to have open, two-way communication between managers and staff that promotes teamwork (Macphee, Wardrop, Campbell, & Wejr, 2011). See Chapter 10 for more on communication.

Interpersonal Behaviors

While engaging in various interpersonal roles, the community health nurse may function as a figurehead, a leader, and a liaison. In the figurehead role, the nurse acts in a ceremonial or symbolic capacity, such as participating in a ribbon-cutting ceremony to mark the opening of a new clinic or representing the project or agency for news media coverage. In the leader role, the nurse motivates and directs people involved in the project. In the liaison role, a network is maintained with people outside the organization or project for information exchange and project enhancement (MindTools, 2015).

Management Skills

What types of skills and competencies does the community health nurse need in the manager role? Three basic management skills are needed for successful achievement of goals: human, conceptual, and technical. *Human skills* refer to the ability to understand, communicate, motivate, delegate, and work well with people (Cherry & Jacob, 2014). An example is a nursing supervisor's or team leader's ability to gain the trust and respect of staff and promote a productive and satisfying work environment. A manager can accomplish goals only with the cooperation of others. Therefore, human skills are essential to successful performance of the manager role. *Conceptual skills* refer to the mental ability to analyze and interpret abstract ideas for the purpose of understanding and diagnosing situations and formulating solutions (Zori et al., 2010). Examples are analyzing demographic data for program planning and developing a conceptual model to describe and improve organizational function. Finally, *technical skills* refer to the ability to apply special management-related knowledge and expertise to a particular situation or problem. Such skills performed by a community health nurse might include implementing a staff development program or developing a computerized management information system. See Chapter 10 on technology in PHN.

Case Management

Case management has become the standard method of managing health care in the delivery systems in the United States, and managed care organizations have become an integral part of community-oriented care. **Case management** is a systematic process by which a nurse assesses clients' needs, plans for and coordinates services, refers to other appropriate providers, and monitors and evaluates progress to ensure that clients' multiple service needs are met in a cost-effective manner. With health care reform, the importance of case management, or care coordination among an interdisciplinary team, is emphasized as a means to control costs and improve client outcomes (Families USA, 2013). As clients leave hospitals earlier, as families struggle with multiple and complex health problems, as more elderly persons need alternatives to nursing home care, as competition and scarce resources contribute to fragmentation of services, and as the cost of health care continues to increase, there is a growing need for someone to oversee and coordinate all facets of needed service (Moreo, Moreo, Urbano, Weeks, & Greene, 2014). Through case management, the nurse addresses this need in the community (Fig. 3–4).

The activity of case management often follows discharge planning as a part of continuity of care. When applied to individual clients, it means overseeing their transition from the hospital back into the community and monitoring them to ensure that all of their service needs are met. Case management also applies to aggregates (Joo & Huber, 2014). In this context, it involves overseeing and ensuring that group or population health-related needs are met, particularly for those who are at high risk of illness or injury. For example, the community health nurse may work with battered women who come to a shelter. First, the nurse must ensure that their immediate needs for safety, security, food, finances, and childcare are met. Then, the nurse must work with other professionals to provide more permanent housing, employment, ongoing counseling, and financial and legal resources for this group of women. Whether applied to families or aggregates, case management, like other applications of the manager role, uses the three sets of management behaviors and engages the community health nurse as planner, organizer, leader, controller, and evaluator.

Collaborator Role

Community health nurses seldom practice in isolation. They must work with many people, including clients, other nurses, physicians, teachers, health educators, social workers, physical therapists, nutritionists, occupational therapists, psychologists, epidemiologists, biostatisticians, attorneys, secretaries, environmentalists, city planners, and legislators. As members of the health team, community health nurses assume the role of **collaborator**, which means working jointly with others in a common endeavor, cooperating as partners. Successful community health practice depends on this multidisciplinary collegiality and leadership (Stringer et al., 2014). Everyone on the team has an important and unique contribution to make to the health care effort. As on a championship ball team, the better that all members play their individual positions and cooperate with other members, the more likely the health team is to win.

The community health nurse's collaborator role requires skills in communicating, in interpreting the nurse's unique contribution to the team, and in acting assertively as an equal partner. The collaborator role also may involve functioning as a consultant.

The following examples show a community health nurse functioning as collaborator. Three families needed to find good nursing homes for their elderly grandparents. The community health nurse met with the families, including the elderly members; made a list of desired features, such as a shower and access to walking trails; and then worked with a social worker to locate and visit several homes. The grandparents' respective physicians were contacted for medical consultation, and in each case, the elderly member made the final selection. In another situation, the community health nurse collaborated with the city council, police department, neighborhood residents, and the manager of a senior citizens' high-rise apartment building to help a group of elderly people organize and lobby for safer streets. In a third example, a school nurse noticed a rise in the incidence of drug use in her schools. She initiated a counseling program after joint planning with students, parents, teachers, the school psychologist, and a local drug rehabilitation center.

Leadership Role

Community health nurses are becoming increasingly active in the leadership role, separate from leading within the manager role mentioned earlier. The leadership role focuses on effecting change (see Chapter 11); thus, the nurse becomes an agent of change. As leaders, community health nurses seek to initiate changes that positively affect people's health. They also seek to influence people to think and behave differently about their health and the factors contributing to it. The leader recognizes the complex set of factors contributing to health outcomes and works to address those myriad factors in affecting needed change (Kulbok et al., 2012). The role of social determinants of health, such as the availability of health services and how the physical environment affects population health, is discussed in Chapter 11 in relation to health promotion of individuals and communities.

At the community level, the leadership role may involve working with a team of professionals to direct and coordinate such projects as a campaign to eliminate smoking in public areas or to lobby legislators for improved child day care facilities. When nurses guide community health decision-making, stimulate an industry's interest in health promotion, initiate group therapy,

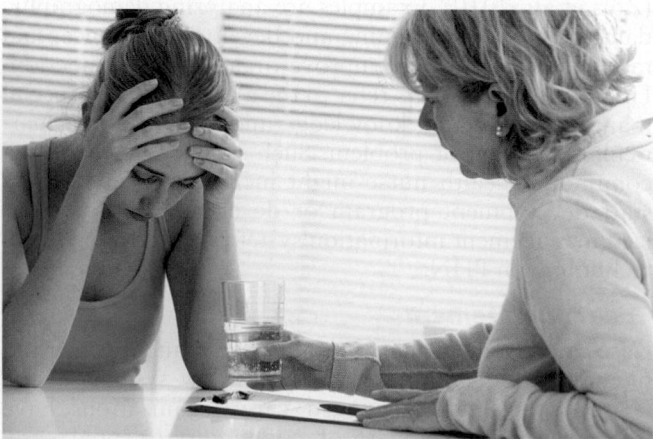

FIGURE 3–4 Community health nurses may serve as case managers for battered women and other aggregates.

direct a preventive program, or influence health policy, they assume the leadership role. For example, a community health nurse started a rehabilitation program that included self-esteem building, career counseling, and job placement to help women in a halfway house who had recently been released from prison.

The community health nurse also exerts influence through health planning. The need for coordinated, accessible, cost-effective health care services creates a challenge and an opportunity for the nurse to become more involved in health planning at all levels: organizational, local, state, national, and international. A community health nurse needs to exercise leadership responsibility and assert the right to share in health decisions (Cherry & Jacob, 2014). One community health nurse determined that there was a need for a behavioral health program in his district. He planned to implement it through the agency for which he worked, but certain individuals on the health board were opposed to adding new programs because of the cost. The nurse's approach was to gather considerable data to demonstrate the need for the program and its cost-effectiveness. He invited individual, key board members to lunch to convince them of the need. He prepared written summaries, graphs, and charts, and at a strategic time, he presented his case at a board meeting. The behavioral health program was approved and implemented.

A broader attribute of the leadership role is that of visionary. A leader with *vision* develops the ability to see what can be and leads people on a path toward that goal. A leader's vision may include long- and short-term goals. In one instance, it began as articulating the need for stronger community nursing services to an underserved population in an inner-city neighborhood served by a community health nurse. In this densely populated, tenant-occupied neighborhood, drugs, crime, and violence were commonplace. One summer, an 8-year-old boy was shot and killed. The enraged immigrant families in the neighborhood felt helpless and hopeless. The nurse visited several families, and they shared their concerns with him. The nurse felt strongly about this blighted community and offered to work with the community to effect change. He gathered volunteers from neighborhood churches, and together, they began to discuss the community's concerns. Together, they prioritized their needs and began planning to make theirs a healthy community. The nurse organized his workweek to provide health screening and education to families in the basement of a church on one morning each week. Initially, only a few families accessed this new service. In a matter of months, it became recognized as a valuable community service, and it expanded to a full day; the expanding volunteer group soon outgrew the space. The community health nurse worked closely with influential community members and the families being served. They determined that many more services were needed in this neighborhood, and they began to broaden their outreach and think of ways to provide the needed services.

Within a year, the group had written several grants to the city and to a private corporation in an effort to expand the voluntary services. The funding that they obtained allowed them to rent vacant storefront space, hire a part-time nurse practitioner, contract with the health department for additional community health nursing services, and negotiate with the local university to have medical, nursing, and social work students placed on a regular basis. The group, under the visionary leadership of the community health nurse, planned to add a one-on-one reading program for children, a class in English as a second language for immigrant families, a mentoring program for teenagers, and dental services. Even the police department had opened a substation in the neighborhood, making their presence more visible. This community health nurse's vision filled an immediate, critical need in the short term and developed into a comprehensive community center in the long term. Violence and crime diminished, and the neighborhood became a place where children could play safely.

Researcher Role

In the researcher role, community health nurses engage in the systematic investigation, collection, and analysis of data for solving problems and enhancing community health practice. But how can research be combined with practice? Although research technically involves a complex set of activities conducted by persons with highly developed and specialized skills, research also means applying that technical study to real practice situations. Community health nurses base their practice on the evidence found in the literature to enhance and change practice as needed. For example, the work of researchers over two decades supports the value of intensive home visiting to high-risk families (Glover, 2014; Olds et al., 2014). The outcomes of this research are changing practice protocol to high-risk families in many health departments today.

Research is an investigative process in which all community health nurses can become involved in asking questions and looking for solutions. Collaborative practice models between academics and practitioners combine research methodology expertise with practitioners' knowledge of problems to make public health nursing research both valid and relevant. The ongoing need for evidence-based practice is supported by *Healthy People 2020*, which stresses that the "emerging field of public health systems and services research is playing an important role in the development of this evidence base; its role should be supported and expanded over the decade, with a strong focus on translating research into practice" (USDHHS, 2016b, para. 14).

The Research Process

Community health nurses practice the researcher role at several levels. In addition to everyday inquiries, community health nurses often participate in agency and organizational studies to determine such matters as practice activities, priorities, and education of public health nurses (Gifford, Lefebre, & Davies, 2014). Some community health nurses participate in more complex research on their own or in collaboration with other health professionals (Butterfield, Hill, Postma, Butterfield, & Odom-Maryon, 2011; Wieland et al., 2011). The researcher role (at all levels) helps to determine needs, evaluate effectiveness of care, and develop a theoretic basis for community health nursing practice. Chapters 4 and 12 will explain community health research in greater detail.

Research literally means to *search again*—to investigate, discover, and interpret facts. All research in community health, from the simplest inquiry to the most complex epidemiologic study, uses the same fundamental process. Simply put, the research process involves the following steps: (1) identify an area of interest, (2) specify the research question or statement, (3) review the literature, (4) identify a conceptual framework, (5) select a research design, (6) collect and analyze data, (7) interpret the results, and (8) communicate the findings (see Chapter 4).

Investigation builds on the nursing process, that essential dynamic of community health nursing practice, using it as a problem-solving process (Burns & Grove, 2015). In using the nursing process, the nurse identifies a problem or question, investigates by collecting and analyzing data, suggests and evaluates possible solutions, and either selects a solution or rejects them all and starts the investigative process over again. In a sense, the nurse is gathering data for health planning—investigating health problems to design wellness-promoting and disease-preventing interventions for community populations.

Attributes of the Researcher Role

A questioning attitude is a basic prerequisite for good nursing practice. A nurse may have revisited a patient many times and noticed some change in her condition, such as restlessness or pallor; consequently, the nurse wonders what is causing this change and what can be done about it. In everyday practice, numerous situations challenge the nurse to ask questions. Consider the following examples:

- The local newspaper reports that another group of children has been arrested for using illegal drugs. Is there an increase in the incidence of illegal drug use in the community?
- Children attending a day care center appear to have excessive bruises on their arms and legs. What is the incidence of reported child abuse in this community? What could be done to promote earlier detection and improved reporting?
- Elderly persons are living alone and without assistance in a neighborhood. How prevalent is this situation, and what are this population's needs?
- While driving through a particular neighborhood, the nurse notices not a single playground. Where do the kids play?

Each of these questions places the nurse in the role of investigator. They demonstrate the fundamental attitude of every researcher: a spirit of inquiry. See Chapter 4 for more about research and evidence-based practice in PHN.

A second attribute, careful observation, is also evident in the examples just given. The nurse needs to develop a sharpened ability to notice things as they are, including deviations from the norm and subtle changes suggesting the need for nursing action. Coupled with observation is open-mindedness, another attribute of the researcher role. In the case of the bruises seen on day care children, a community health nurse's observations suggest child abuse as a possible cause. However, open-mindedness requires consideration of other alternatives, and as a good investigator, the nurse explores these possibilities as well.

Analytic skills also are used in this role. In the example of illegal drug use, the nurse already has started to analyze the situation by trying to determine its cause-and-effect relationships. Successful analysis depends on how well the data have been collected. Insufficient information can lead to false interpretations, so it is important to seek out the needed data. Analysis, like a jigsaw puzzle, involves studying the pieces and fitting them together until the meaning of the whole picture can be described.

Finally, the researcher role involves tenacity. The community health nurse persists in an investigation until facts are uncovered and a satisfactory answer is found. Noticing an absence of playgrounds and wondering where the children play are only a beginning. Being concerned about the children's safety and need for recreational outlets, the nurse gathers data about the location and accessibility of play areas, as well as expressed needs of community residents. A fully documented research report may result. If the data support a need for additional play space, the report can be brought before the proper authorities.

SETTINGS FOR COMMUNITY HEALTH NURSING PRACTICE

The previous section examined community health nursing from the perspective of its major roles. The roles can now be placed in context by viewing the settings in which they are practiced. The types of places in which community health nurses practice are increasingly varied and include a growing number of nontraditional settings and partnerships with nonhealth groups. Employers of community health nurses range from state and local health departments and home health agencies to managed care organizations, businesses and industries, and nonprofit organizations. For this discussion, these settings are grouped into seven categories: homes, ambulatory service settings, schools, occupational health settings, residential institutions, faith communities, and the community at large (domestic and international). This section provides a brief overview of the various settings. Chapters 30 and 31 will provide much more detail on specific roles and settings, including both public and private practice settings.

Homes

Since Lillian Wald and the nurses at the Henry Street Settlement first started their practice in 1983, the most frequently used setting for community health nursing practice was the home. In the home, all of the public health nursing roles are performed to varying degrees. Clients who are discharged from acute care institutions, such as hospitals or behavioral health facilities, are regularly referred to community health nurses for continued care and follow-up. Here, the community health nurse can see clients in a family and environmental context, and service can be tailored to the clients' unique needs (Fig. 3–5).

For example, Mr. White, 67 years of age, was discharged from the hospital with a colostomy. Doreen Levitz, the public health nurse from the county public health nursing agency, immediately started home visits. She met with Mr. White and his wife to discuss their needs as a family and to plan for Mr. White's care and adjustment to living with a colostomy. Practicing the clinician and educator roles, she reinforced and expanded on the teaching

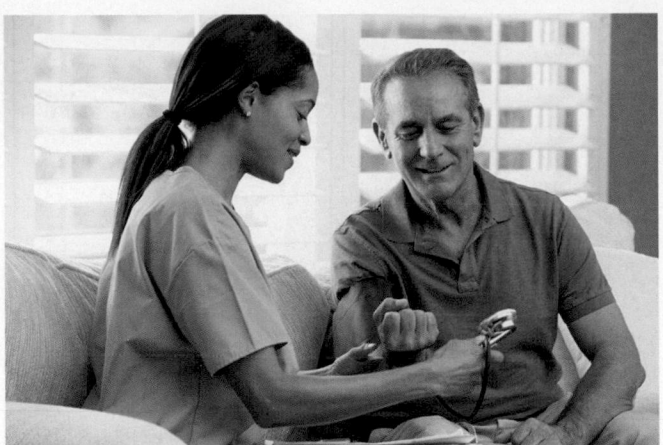

FIGURE 3-5 Public health nurses make home visits to assess and follow up with clients.

started in the hospital for colostomy care, including bowel training, diet, exercise, and proper use of equipment. As part of a total family care plan, Doreen provided some forms of physical care for Mr. White as well as counseling, teaching, and emotional support for both Mr. White and his wife. In addition to consulting with the physician and social service worker, she arranged and supervised visits from the home health aide, who gave personal care and homemaker services. She thus performed the manager, leader, and collaborator roles.

The home is also a setting for health promotion. Many community health nursing visits focus on assisting families to understand and practice healthier living behaviors. Nurses may, for example, instruct clients on parenting, infant care, child discipline, diet, exercise, coping with stress, or managing grief and loss.

The character of the home setting is as varied as the clients served by the community health nurse. In one day, the nurse may visit a well-to-do widow in her luxurious home, a middle-income family in their modest bungalow, an elderly transient man in his one-room fifth-story walk-up apartment, and a teen mother and her infant living in a group foster home. In each situation, the nurse can view the clients in perspective and, therefore, better understand their limitations, capitalize on their resources, and tailor health services to meet their needs. In the home, unlike in most other health care settings, clients are on their own "turf." They feel comfortable and secure in familiar surroundings and often are better able to understand and apply health information. Client self-respect can be promoted, because the client is host and the nurse is a guest.

Sometimes, the thought of visiting in clients' homes can cause anxiety for the nurse. This may be the nurse's first experience outside the acute care, long-term care, or clinic setting. Visiting clients in their own environment can make the nurse feel uncomfortable. The nurse may be asked to visit families in unfamiliar neighborhoods, and she must walk through those neighborhoods to locate the clients' homes. Frequently, fear of the unknown is the real fear—a fear that often has been enhanced by stories from previous nurses. This may be the same feeling as that experienced when caring for your first client, first entering the operating room, or first having a client in the intensive care unit. However, in the community, more variables exist, and basic safety measures should be used. General guidelines for safety and making home visits are covered in detail in Chapter 19. Nevertheless, the specific instructions given during the clinical experience should be followed, and everyday, commonsense safety precautions should be used.

Changes in the health care delivery system, along with shifting health economics and service delivery (discussed in Chapter 6), are changing community health nursing's use of the home as a primary setting for practice. Many local health departments are finding it increasingly difficult to provide widespread home visiting by their public health nurses. Instead, many agencies are targeting populations that are most in need of direct intervention. Examples include families of children with elevated blood lead levels, low-birth-weight babies, clients requiring directly observed administration of tuberculosis medications, and families requiring ongoing monitoring because of identified child abuse or neglect. With limited staff and limited financial resources, the highest-priority clients or groups are targeted.

With skills in population-based practice, community health nurses serve the public's health best by focusing on sites where they can have the greatest impact. At the same time, they can collaborate with various types of home care providers, including hospitals, other nurses, physicians, rehabilitation therapists, and durable medical equipment companies, to ensure continuous and holistic service. The nurse continues to supervise home care services and engage in case management. The increased demand for highly technical acute care in the home requires specialized skills that are best delivered by nurses with this expertise. Chapter 32 further examines the nurse's role in the home health and hospice settings. The ANA documents *Home Health Nursing: Scope and Standards of Practice* (2013b) and *Palliative Nursing: Scope and Standards of Practice* (ANA/Hospice and Palliative Nurses Association, 2014) offer additional insight on these specialty areas.

Ambulatory Service Settings

Ambulatory service settings include a variety of venues for community health nursing practice in which clients come for day or evening services that do not include overnight stays. A community health center is an example of an ambulatory setting. Sometimes, multiple clinics offering comprehensive services are community based or are located in outpatient departments of hospitals or medical centers. They also may be based in comprehensive neighborhood health centers. A single clinic, such as a family planning clinic or a well-child clinic, may be found in a location that is more convenient for clients, perhaps a church basement or empty storefront. Some kinds of day care centers, such as those for the physically disabled or adults with behavioral health issues, use community health nursing services. Additional ambulatory care settings include health departments (city, county, or state) and community health nursing agencies, where clients may come for assessment and referral or counseling. An increasing number of nurse-managed health centers have also been formed over the past decade, often as a community service component of schools of nursing. The mission of these centers varies, but they are typically used to enhance student clinical experiences while providing identified community needs in the areas of primary health care and health promotion (see Chapter 31).

Offices are another type of ambulatory care setting. Some community health nurses provide service in conjunction with a medical practice; for example, a community health nurse associated with a health maintenance organization sees clients in the office and undertakes screening, referrals, counseling, health education, and group work. Others establish independent practices by seeing clients in community nursing centers as well as making home visits.

Another type of ambulatory service setting includes places where services are offered to selected groups. For example, community health nurses practice in migrant camps, on tribal lands, at correctional facilities, in children's day care centers, through faith communities, in coal-mining communities, and in remote frontier areas. In each ambulatory setting, all of the community health nursing roles are used to varying degrees (see Perspectives: Student Voice).

Schools

Schools of all levels make up a major group of settings for community health nursing practice. Nurses from community health nursing agencies frequently serve private schools at elementary and intermediate levels. Public schools are served by the same agencies or by community health nurses hired through the public school system. The community health nurse may work with groups of students in preschool settings, such as Montessori schools, as well as in vocational or technical schools, junior colleges, and college and university settings. Specialized schools, such as those for the developmentally disabled, are another setting for community health nursing practice (Fig. 3–6).

Community health nurses' roles in school settings are changing. School nurses, whose primary role initially was that of clinician, are widening their practice to include more health education, interprofessional collaboration, and client advocacy. For example, one school had been accustomed to using the nurse as a first-aid provider and

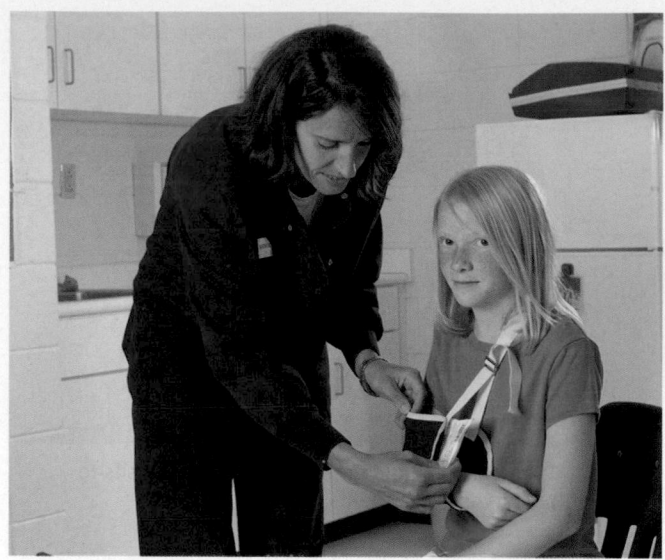

FIGURE 3–6   School nursing is another community health nursing role.

record keeper. Her duties were handling minor problems, such as headaches and cuts, and keeping track of such events as immunizations. This nurse sought to expand her practice and, after consultation and preparation, collaborated with a health educator and some of the teachers to offer a series of classes on personal hygiene, diet, and sexuality. She started a drop-in center for health counseling at the school and established a network of professional contacts for consultation and referral.

Community health nurses in school settings also are beginning to assume managerial and leadership roles and to recognize that the researcher role should be an integral part of their practice. The nurse's role with school age and adolescent populations is discussed in detail in Chapters 22 and 30. The ANA and the National Association of School Nursing have published *School Nursing: Scope and Standards of Practice* (2011), a document that provides additional information on this important specialty.

 **PERSPECTIVES STUDENT VOICE**

A GRADUATING STUDENT VIEWPOINT ON POSTGRADUATION EMPLOYMENT

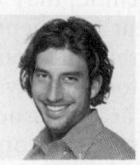 Before entering nursing school, I spent 6 years on active duty as a corpsman in the Navy. I remembered seeing some nurses who visited our hospital wearing what looked like Navy uniforms, but was told that they worked for the federal government and weren't in the Navy. I didn't think much of it until I was looking up information on the U.S. Public Health Service and the Surgeon General. Only then did it dawn on me that those nurses were part of the Commissioned Corps of the Public Health Service. I didn't even know they existed, much less what they did, so I looked around the section of the Web site dealing with nursing. It turns out that they do quite a bit—respond to disasters, provide health services to Native Americans, and even work with the federal prisons. It surprised me to find out that they hire new graduates for many of their positions. I still haven't decided what I want to do after I graduate, but I may seriously consider this option. They even have an extern program available while I'm still in school—who knows, I may be in uniform again.

Matt, Age 24

Occupational Health Settings

Business and industry provide another group of settings for community health nursing practice. Employee health has long been recognized as making a vital contribution to individual lives, the productivity of business, and the well-being of the entire nation. Organizations are expected to provide a safe and healthy work environment, in addition to offering insurance for health care. More companies, recognizing the value of healthy employees, are going beyond offering traditional health benefits to supporting health promotional efforts. Some businesses, for example, offer healthy snacks, such as fruit at breaks, and promote jogging during the noon hour. A few larger corporations have built exercise facilities for their employees, provide health education programs, and offer financial incentives for losing weight or staying well.

Community health nurses in occupational health settings practice a variety of roles. The clinician role predominated for many years, as nurses continued to care for sick or injured employees at work. However, recognition of the need to protect employees' safety and, later, to prevent their illness led to the inclusion of health education in the occupational health nurse role. Occupational and environmental health nurses also act as employee advocates, assuring appropriate job assignments for workers and adequate treatment for job-related illness or injury. They collaborate with other health care providers and company management to offer better services to their clients. They act as leaders and managers in developing new health services in the work setting, endorsing programs such as hypertension screening and weight control. Occupational health settings range from industries and factories, such as an automobile assembly plant, to business corporations and even large retail sales systems. The field of occupational health offers a challenging opportunity, particularly in smaller businesses, where nursing coverage usually is not provided. Chapter 31 more fully describes the role of the nurse serving the working adult population. The American Association of Occupational Health Nurses sets the standards for this specialty and is the exclusive publisher of the *Standards of Occupational and Environmental Health Nursing* (2012).

Residential Institutions

Any facility where clients reside can be a setting in which community health nursing is practiced. Residential institutions can include a halfway house in which clients live temporarily while recovering from drug addiction or an inpatient hospice program in which terminally ill clients live. Some residential settings, such as hospitals, exist solely to provide health care; others provide a variety of services and support. Community health nurses based in a community agency maintain continuity of care for their clients by collaborating with hospital personnel, visiting clients in the hospital, and planning care during and after hospitalization. Some community health nurses serve one or more hospitals on a regular basis by providing a liaison with the community, consultation for discharge planning, and periodic in-service programs to keep hospital staff updated on community services for their clients. Other community health nurses with similar functions are based in the hospital and serve the hospital community.

A continuing care center is another example of a residential site providing health care that may use community health nursing services. In this setting, residents usually are elderly; some live quite independently, whereas others become increasingly dependent and have many chronic health problems. The public health nurse functions as advocate and collaborator to improve services. The nurse may, for example, coordinate available resources to meet the needs of residents and their families and help safeguard the maintenance of quality operating standards. Chapter 24 discusses the community health nurse's role with elders aging in place. Chapter 32 discusses nursing services needed by clients after hospitalization through home care services or by families and clients in hospice programs. Sheltered workshops and group homes for mentally ill or developmentally disabled children and adults are other examples of residential institutions that serve clients who share specific needs.

Community health nurses also practice in settings where residents are gathered for purposes other than receiving care, where health care is offered as an adjunct to the primary goals of the institution. For example, many nurses work with camping programs for children and adults offered by religious organizations and other community agencies, such as the Boy Scouts, Girl Scouts, or the YMCA. Other camp nurses work with children and adults who have chronic or terminal illnesses, through disease-related community agencies such as the American Lung Association, American Diabetes Association, and American Cancer Society. Camp nurses practice all available roles, often under interesting and challenging conditions.

Another often-overlooked practice setting is the correctional institution. Inmates may be incarcerated both short and long term and have the same health care needs as the general public. Because of the unique nature of this population, there are typically additional health and social service needs for this population, often stemming from the reason for the incarceration in the first place (drug abuse) and that place them at increased risk for select health problems (AIDS, tuberculosis, poor nutrition, etc.). The challenge to the nurse in this setting is to provide health care in an unbiased and nonjudgmental manner within the realities of the setting. Chapter 30 discusses the role of the nurse in the correctional setting, and the ANA's *Correctional Nursing: Scope and Standards of Practice* (2013a) offers insight into this practice specialty.

Residential institutions provide unique settings for the community health nurse to practice health promotion. Clients are more accessible, their needs can be readily assessed, and their interests can be stimulated. These settings offer the opportunity to generate an environment of caring and optimal quality health care provided by community health nursing services.

Faith Communities

Faith community nursing finds its beginnings in an ancient tradition. The beginnings of community health nursing can be traced to religious orders (see Chapter 2), and for centuries, religious and spiritual communities were important sources of health care. In faith community nursing today, the practice focal point remains the faith community and the religious belief system provided by the philosophical framework. Faith community nursing may take different names such as church-based health promotion, parish nursing, or primary care parish nursing practice. Whatever the service is called, it involves a large-scale effort by the church community to improve the health of its members through education, screening, referral, treatment, and group support.

In some geopolitical communities, faith community nurses are the most acceptable primary care providers. The role of the nurse can be broad, being defined by the needs of the members and the philosophy of the religious community. However, the goal is to enhance and extend services available in the larger community, not to duplicate them.

The ANA has published standards of care for faith community nursing practice in collaboration with the Health Ministries Association, Inc. (ANA, 2012). The standards act as guidelines for faith communities that plan to offer or are offering faith community nursing services. This specialty area of practice is guided by a variety of standards set up by several groups. Together, these standards provide guidance and direction for caregiving within the faith community.

When community health nurses work as faith community nurses, they enhance accessibility to available health services in the community while meeting the unique needs of the members of that religious community, practicing within the framework of the tenets of that religion. A nurse working within a faith community must be cognizant of the basic principles and practices of the religious group served. In most situations, the nurse is a practitioner of the same religious belief system. Chapter 31 provides more detailed information about this specialty area of practice.

Community at Large

Unlike the six settings already discussed, the seventh setting for community health nursing practice is not confined to a specific philosophy, location, or building. When working with groups, populations, or the total community, the nurse may practice in many different places (Display 3–5). For example, a community health nurse, as clinician and health educator, may work with a parenting group in a church or town hall. Another nurse, as client advocate, leader, and researcher, may

---

DISPLAY 3-5 INNOVATIVE COMMUNITY HEALTH NURSING PRACTICE

In some community health nursing courses, students do not have access to an established agency such as a health department or community center from which to establish a client base. Student nurses and practicing community health nurses can provide outreach services and do case-finding in innovative settings such as these:

Settings	Clients	Roles of the Community Health Nurse
1. Senior centers when flu shots are given or commodities are distributed	Older adults	Educator, clinician, advocate
2. Outside of grocery stores, department stores, movie theaters, large pharmacies	People of all ages and families	Educator, clinician, advocate
3. At parent–teacher association (PTA) meetings, sporting events, dances, and school registration (in collaboration with school nurses)	Young adults, children, and teenagers	Educator, clinician, advocate
4. Outside of concerts, plays, the circus, etc.	People of all ages	Educator, clinician, advocate
5. Other public gatherings: farmers markets, neighborhood yard sales, etc.	People of all ages	Educator, clinician, advocate
6. Conferences or seminars	People of all ages	Leader, educator, clinician
7. "On the street"	Homeless persons, passersby, transients, low-income urban dwellers	Educator, clinician, advocate
8. Truck stops	Predominantly employed men	Educator, clinician, advocate

Leader's role—initiate, plan, strategize, collaborate, and cooperate with community groups to present programs that are focused on specific population's needs.

Educator's role—teach nutrition, stress management, safety, exercise, prevention of sexually transmitted diseases, and other men and women's health issues, child home/school/play and stranger safety, and child growth and development, and provide anticipatory guidance. Have pamphlets available to support verbal information on health and safety topics, specific diseases, social security, Medicare, and Medicaid.

Clinician's role—perform blood pressure screening, height, weight, blood testing for diabetes and cholesterol, occult blood test, hearing and vision tests, scoliosis measurements, and administration of immunizations.

Advocate's role—provide information regarding community resources as needed, cut "red tape" for those who need it, answer questions, and guide people to additional resources, such as Web sites and "800" phone numbers.

study the health needs of a neighborhood's elderly population by collecting data throughout the area and meeting with resource people in many places. Also, a nurse may work with community-based organizations such as an HIV/AIDS organization or a support group for parents experiencing the violent death of a child. Again, the community at large becomes the setting for practice for a nurse who serves on health care planning committees, lobbies for health legislation at the state capital, runs for a school board position, or assists with flood relief in another state or another country (Fig. 3–7).

Although the term "setting" implies a place, remember that community health nursing practice is not limited to a specific site. Community health nursing is a specialty of nursing that is defined by the nature of its practice, not its location, and it can be practiced anywhere. As you read through this chapter, perhaps an area of practice or a particular population captured your attention. If you are interested in tribal health, you might consider working as a U.S. Public Health Service nurse, or if you find that you are more interested in providing comprehensive health promotion programs to rural individuals, a nurse-managed health center may be of interest. Opportunities for community health nursing include the American Red Cross, state and local health

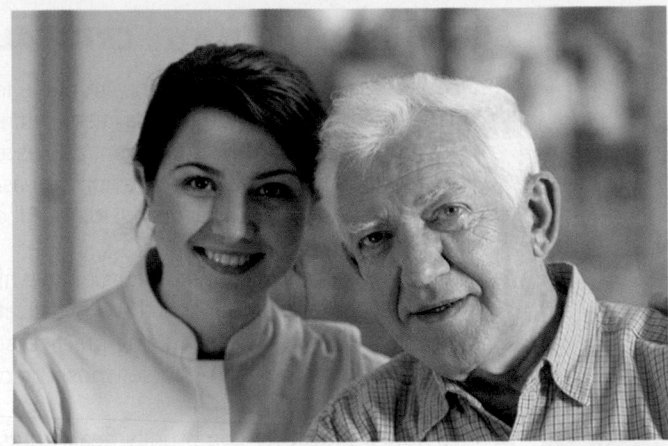

FIGURE 3–7 The community health nurse works with many different groups, including the elderly.

departments, the Peace Corps, and various international aid groups. Both private and public health agencies are actively seeking nurses with an interest in improving the health of their communities. Take some time to read over Chapters 30 and 31; perhaps you will find an opportunity that supports your professional goals.

SUMMARY

Community health nurses play many roles, including that of clinician, educator, advocate, manager, collaborator, leader, and researcher. Each role entails special types of skills and expertise. The type and number of roles that are practiced vary with each set of clients and each specific situation, but the nurse should be able to successfully function in each of these roles as the particular situation demands. The role of manager is one that the nurse must play in every situation, because it involves assessing clients' needs, planning and organizing to meet those needs, directing and leading clients to achieve results, and controlling and evaluating the progress to ensure that the goals and clients' needs are met. A type of comprehensive management of clients that has become known as *case management* is an integral part of community health nursing practice.

As a part of the manager role, the nurse must engage in three crucial management behaviors: decision-making, transferring information, and relationship building. Nurses must also use a comprehensive set of management skills: human skills that allow them to understand, communicate, motivate, and work with people; conceptual skills that allow them to interpret abstract ideas and apply them to real situations to formulate solutions; and technical skills that allow them to apply special management-related knowledge and expertise to a particular situation or problem.

There also are many types of settings in which the community health nurse may practice and in which these roles are enacted. "Setting" does not necessarily refer to a specific location or site but rather to a particular situation. These situations can be grouped into seven major categories: homes; ambulatory service settings, where clients come for care but do not stay overnight; schools; occupational health settings, which serve employees in business and industry; residential institutions such as hospitals, continuing care facilities, halfway houses, or other institutions in which people live and sleep; faith communities, where care is based on the philosophy of the religious organization; and the community at large, which encompasses a variety of expected and innovative locations.

ACTIVITIES TO PROMOTE **CRITICAL THINKING**

1. Discuss ways for a community health nurse to make service holistic and focused on wellness with
   - Preschool-age children in a day care setting
   - A group of chemically dependent adolescents
   - A group of elders living in a senior high-rise building
2. Select one public health nursing role and describe its application in meeting the needs of your friend or next-door neighbor.
3. Describe a hypothetical or real situation in which you, as a community health nurse, would combine the roles of leader, collaborator, and researcher (investigator). Discuss how each of these roles might be played.
4. If your community health nursing practice setting is the community at large, will your practice roles be any different from those of the nurse whose practice setting is the home? Why? What determines the roles played by the community health nurse?
5. Interview a practicing community health nurse and determine which roles are integral to the nurse's practice over a 1-month period. Describe the ways in which each role is enacted. How many instances of this nurse's practice were aggregate focused? In which of the settings does the nurse mostly practice? If you were a public health consultant, what suggestions might you make to expand this nurse's role into aggregate-level practice?
6. Choose one of the PHN roles or practice areas described in this chapter that may be of interest to you. Compare your choice with one or two other classmates. What drew each of you to your choice? Why?
7. Search the Internet and find two research articles on community health nursing. In what settings did the research take place? Did the nursing authors collaborate with interdisciplinary team members on this research? If so, how do you think this collaboration helped the research? If you were to conduct research in the community, would you conduct it with only nurses on the team, or would your team be interdisciplinary? Why? What would be the benefits or limits of each approach?

REFERENCES

American Association of Colleges of Nursing (AACN). (2008). *The essentials of baccalaureate education for professional nursing practice*. Washington, DC: Author.

American Association of Occupational Health Nurses. (2012). *Standards of occupational and environmental health nursing*. Pensacola, FL: Author.

American Nurses Association (ANA). (2010). *Nursing's social policy statement: The essence of the profession*. Silver Spring, MD: Nursesbooks.org.

American Nurses Association (ANA). (2011). *School nursing: Scope and standards of practice* (2nd ed.). Silver Spring, MD: Nursesbooks.org.

American Nurses Association (ANA). (2012). *Faith community nursing: Scope and standards of practice* (2nd ed.). Silver Spring, MD: Nursesbooks.org.

American Nurses Association (ANA). (2013a). *Correctional nursing: Scope and standards of practice* (2nd ed.). Silver Springs, MD: Nursesbooks.org.

American Nurses Association (ANA). (2013b). *Home health nursing: Scope and standards of practice* (2nd ed.). Silver Spring, MD: Nursesbooks.org.

American Nurses Association (ANA). (2013c). *Public health nursing: Scope and standards of practice* (2nd ed.). Silver Spring, MD: Nursesbooks.org.

American Nurses Association (ANA). (2015a). *Code of ethics for nurses with interpretive statements*. Silver Spring, MD: Nursesbooks.org.

American Nurses Association (ANA). (2015b). *Nursing: Scope and standards of practice* (3rd ed.). Silver Spring, MD: Nursesbooks.org.

American Nurses Association (ANA) and Hospice and Palliative Nurses Association (HPNA). (2014). *Scope and standards of practice: Palliative nursing, an essential resource for hospice and palliative nurses*. Silver Spring, MD: Author.

American Public Health Association. (2013). *The definition and practice of public health nursing: A statement of APHA public health nursing section*. Washington, DC: American Public Health Association.

Association of Community Health Nursing Educators (ACHNE), Education Committee. (2010). Essentials of baccalaureate nursing education for entry-level community/public health nursing. *Public Health Nursing, 27*, 371–382. doi: 10.1111/j.1525-1446.2010.00867.x.

Bastable, S. B. (2014). *Nurse as educator: Principles of teaching and learning for nursing practice* (4th ed.). Burlington, MA: Jones & Bartlett.

Burns, N., & Grove, S. K. (2015). *Understanding nursing research: Building an evidence-based practice* (6th ed.). St. Louis, MO: Saunders.

Butterfield, P. G., Hill, W., Postma, J., Butterfield, P. W., & Odom-Maryon, T. (2011). Effectiveness of a household environmental health intervention delivered by rural public health nurses. *American Journal of Public Health, 101*, S262–S270. doi: 10.2105/AJPH.2001.300164.

Byers, V. (2015). The challenges of leading change in health-care delivery from the frontline. *Journal of Nursing Management*. doi: 10.1111/jonm.12342.

Cherry, B., & Jacob, S. R. (2014). *Contemporary nursing: Issues, trends, and management* (6th ed.). St. Louis, MO: Mosby.

Dossey, B. M., & Keegan L. (2016). *Holistic nursing: A handbook for practice* (7th ed.). Burlington, MA: Jones & Bartlett Publishers.

Families USA. (2013, April). *The promise of care coordination: Transforming health care delivery*. Retrieved from http://familiesusa.org/sites/default/files/product_documents/Care-Coordination.pdf

Gifford, W., Lefebre, N., & Davies, B. (2014). An organizational intervention to influence evidence-informed decision making in home health nursing. *Journal of Nursing Administration, 44*(7/8), 395–402.

Glover, V. (2014). Maternal depression, anxiety and stress during pregnancy and child outcome: What needs to be done. *Best Practice & Research. Clinical Obstetrics & Gynaecology, 28*, 25–35.

Institute of Medicine. (1988). *The future of public health*. Washington, DC: National Academy Press.

Joo, J. Y., & Huber, D. L. (2014). An integrative review of nurse-led community-based case management effectiveness. *International Nursing Review, 61*, 14–24.

Kowlessar, N. M., Goetzel, R. Z., Carls, G. S., Tabrizi, M. J., & Guindon, A. (2011). The relationship between 11 health risks and medical and productivity costs for a large employer. *Journal of Occupational and Environmental Medicine, 53*, 468–477.

Kulbok, P. A., Thatcher, E., Park, E., & Meszaros, P. S. (2012). Evolving public health nursing roles: Focus on community participatory health promotion and prevention. *Online Journal of Issues in Nursing, 17*(2), 1.

Lahiri, S., & Faghri, P. D. (2012). Cost-effectiveness of a workplace-based incentivized weight loss program. *Journal of Occupational and Environmental Medicine, 54*(3), 371–377.

Lievens, I., & Vlerick, P. (2014). Transformational leadership and safety performance among nurses: the mediating role of knowledge-related job characteristics. *Journal of Advanced Nursing, 70*(3), 651–661.

Macphee, M., Wardrop, A., Campbell, C., & Wejr, P. (2011). The Synergy Professional Practice Model and its patient characteristics tool: A staff empowerment strategy. *Nursing Leadership, 24*(3), 42–56.

Management at Work. (2016). *Mintzberg's 10 managerial roles.* Retrieved from http://management.atwork-network.com/2008/04/15/mintzberg's-10-managerial-roles/

Mead, E. L., Doorenbos, A. Z., Javid, S. H., Haozous, E. A., Alvord, L. A., Flum, D. R., & Morris, A. M. (2013). Shared decision making for cancer care among racial and ethnic minorities: A systematic review. *American Journal of Public Health, 103*(12), 15–29.

MindTools. (2015). *Mintzberg's management roles: Identifying the roles managers play.* Retrieved from https://www.mindtools.com/pages/article/management-roles.htm

Mintzberg, H. (1973). *The nature of managerial work.* New York, NY: Harper & Row.

Moreo, K., Moreo, N., Urbano, F. L., Weeks, M., & Greene, L. (2014). Are we prepared for Affordable Care Act provisions of care coordination? Case managers' self-assessments and views on physicians' roles. *Professional Case Management, 19*(1), 18–26.

Mortier, A. V., Vlerick, P., & Clays, E. (2015). Authentic leadership and thriving among nurses: The mediating role of empathy. *Journal of Nursing Management, 24*(3), 357–365.

Olds, D. L., Kitzman, H., Knudtson, M. D., Anson, E., Smith, J. A., & Cole R. (2014). Effect of home visiting by nurses on maternal and child mortality: Results of a 2-decade follow-up of a randomized clinical trial. *JAMA Pediatrics, 168*(9), 800–806.

Peek, M. E., Ferguson, M., Bergeron, N., Maltby, D., & Chin, M. H. (2014). Integrated community-healthcare diabetes interventions to reduce disparities. *Current Diabetes Reports, 14*(3), 467–480.

Pender, N. J., Murdaugh, C. L., & Parsons, M. A. (2015). *Health promotion in nursing practice* (7th ed.). Upper Saddle River, NJ: Prentice Hall.

President's Council on Fitness, Sports and Nutrition. (2016). *About us.* Retrieved from http://fitness.gov

Rogers, E. B., Stanford, M. S., Dolan, S. L., Clark, J., Martindale, S. L. Lake, S. L., ... & Sejud, L. R. (2012). Helping people without homes: Simple steps for psychologists seeking to change lives. *Professional Psychology: Research and Practice, 43*(2), 86–93.

Shirey, M. R., & White-Williams, C. (2015). Boundary spanning leadership practices for population health. *Journal of Advanced Nursing, 45*(9), 411–415.

Stringer, M., Rajeswaran, L., Dithole, K., Hoke, L., Mampane, P., Sebopelo, S., ... Polomano, R. C. (2014). Bridging nursing practice and education through a strategic global partnership. *International Journal of Nursing Practice, 22*(1), 43–52.

Swider, S., Krothe, J., Reyes, D., & Cravetz, M. (2013). The Quad Council practice competencies for public health nursing. *Public Health Nursing, 30*(6), 519–536.

U.S. Department of Health and Human Services (USDHHS). (1997). *The public health workforce: An agenda for the 21st century.* Washington, DC: U.S. Government Printing Office.

U.S. Department of Health and Human Services (USDHHS), Office of Disease Prevention and Health Promotion. (1999). *Public health functions project.* Retrieved from http://www.health.gov/phfunctions/public.htm

U.S. Department of Health and Human Services (USDHHS). (2016a). *Healthy People 2020: About healthy people.* Retrieved from https://www.healthypeople.gov/2020/About-Healthy-People

U.S. Department of Health and Human Services (USDHHS). (2016b). *Healthy people 2020: Public health infrastructure.* Retrieved from http://healthypeople.gov/2020/topicsobjectives2020/overview.aspx?topicid=35

Wieland, M. L., Weis, J. A., Olney, M. W., Aleman, M., Sullivan, S., Millington, K., ... Sia, I. G. (2011). Screening for tuberculosis at an adult education center: Results of a community-based participatory process. *American Journal of Public Health, 101*, 1264–1267.

Zori, S., Nosek, L. J., & Musil, C. M. (2010). Critical thinking of nurse managers related to staff RNs' perceptions of the practice environment. *Journal of Nursing Scholarship, 42*(3), 305–313.

thePoint: Everything You Need to Make the Grade!

thePoint® Visit http://thePoint.lww.com/Rector9e for selected readings, study aids for all learning styles, and more!

CHAPTER 4

Evidence-Based Practice and Ethics in Community Health Nursing

"Research is formalized curiosity. It is poking and prying with a purpose."

—*Zora Neale Hurston* (1891–1960), Novelist

"We must not see any person as an abstraction. Instead, we must see in every person a universe with its own secrets, with its own treasures, with its own sources of anguish, and with some measure of triumph."

—*Elie Wiesel* from The Nazi Doctors and the Nuremberg Code

KEY TERMS

Research/Evidence-Based Practice
Community-based participatory research (CBPR)
Conceptual model
Control group
Descriptive statistics
Evidence-based practice
Experimental design
Experimental group
Generalizability
Health policy evaluation
Inferential statistics
Instrument

Integrative review
Meta-analysis
Mixed methods
Nonexperimental design
Qualitative research
Quantitative research
Quasi-experiment
Randomization
Randomized control trial (RCT)
Reliability
Research
Research utilization
Systematic review

True experiment
Validity

Ethics
Autonomy
Beneficence
Bioethics
Distributive justice
Egalitarian justice
Equity
Ethical decision-making
Ethical dilemma
Ethics
Fidelity
Instrumental values

Justice
Moral
Moral evaluations
Nonmaleficence
Respect
Restorative justice
Self-determination
Self-interest
Social justice
Terminal values
Value
Value systems
Values clarification
Veracity
Well-being

LEARNING OBJECTIVES

Upon mastery of this chapter, you should be able to:

- Discuss the concept of evidence-based practice (EBP).
- List the necessary steps in the process of EBP.
- Explain the difference between quantitative research and qualitative research.
- List the nine steps of the research process.
- Analyze the potential impact of research on community health nursing practice.
- Identify the community health nurse's role in conducting research and using research findings to improve his or her practice.

- Describe the nature of values and value systems and their influence on community health nursing.
- Articulate the impact of key values on professional decision-making.
- Discuss the application of ethical principles to community health nursing decision-making.
- Use a decision-making process with and for community health clients that incorporates values and ethical principles.

As a new student in community health nursing, you may ask, "Can I really do something to make a difference in the lives of my clients?" You may often feel shocked and discouraged by the crushing poverty and overwhelming sense of helplessness experienced by many of your clients and by the continual recurrence of substance abuse, domestic violence, job failure, and criminal activity. For the first time, you may truly confront the inequalities and injustices of our health care system. You will face many ethical dilemmas in community health nursing. You may ask, "Why should I bother to make home visits to pregnant teens? Why should I offer smoking cessation classes at the local homeless shelter? Why should I teach clients about the importance of taking their antituberculosis medications? Will it really matter?"

Recent community health nursing research validates that nursing care *does* matter and that you really *can* make a difference in the lives of your clients. For example, Nurse–Family Partnership (NFP) programs, based on research conducted by David Olds and his colleagues, are reaping results in many communities across the United States and around the world (Canadian Nurse-Family Partnership Network, 2010; Coalition for Evidence-Based Policy, 2015; Mejdoubi et al., 2013; 2015; Nurse-Family Partnership, 2011a, 2011b, 2011c, 2015; U.S. Department of Health and Human Services [USDHHS], 2011a). In a classic longitudinal study by Olds and his research team (1997), conducted with a primarily white sample in a semirural setting over a 15-year period, regular visits by public health nurses (PHNs) to poor, unmarried women and their first-born children resulted in dramatic differences when compared with similar mothers and children in a control group. Many of the women in the study were younger than 19 years of age, and nurses made an average of 9 prenatal visits and 23 child-related visits (up to age 2 years). The effects of the intervention continued for up to 15 years after the birth of the first child.

Statistically significant differences were noted in the following outcomes:

- Fewer subsequent pregnancies and an increased percentage of live births
- Longer intervals of time between first and second births
- Fewer incidences of reported child abuse and neglect
- Fewer months on public assistance and food stamps
- Fewer reported arrests and convictions of mothers
- Less impairment from alcohol or other drug use reported by mothers

In a more recent randomized 12-year follow-up study, Olds and his colleagues (2010) examined mother and child benefits when the first child turned 12. They found "no statistically significant program effects" for intimate partner violence, alcohol/drug use, arrests/incarceration, psychological distress, or placement of children in foster care (p. 419). However, in this largely African American urban sample of almost 600 participants, they did find statistical differences for:

- Longer relationships between mothers and their partners
- Decreased role impairment related to drug and alcohol use
- Greater personal sense of control

They also noted significant findings for cost savings; less government funding was spent on these participants versus control subjects on Medicaid, welfare, and food stamps (Olds et al., 2010).

A 2014 study examining data from 1,138 women compiled over two decades (1990–2011) looked at outcome measures of maternal mortality and preventable-cause child mortality rates (Olds, Kitzman, Knudtson et al., 2014). Four treatment interventions were examined. The first was simply transportation for prenatal care, the second added developmental screening for infants and toddlers to the transportation, the third included prenatal and postpartum home visiting along with transportation, and the fourth consisted of transportation, screening, pre-/postpregnancy home visiting along with infant/toddler home visiting. Findings revealed the following:

- Maternal mortality rates for both control groups (1, transportation only, and 2, transportation with child developmental screening) were higher than for those in both of the intervention groups (3, prenatal and postpartum home visiting with transportation, and 4, full home visiting with pregnant mother and infant/toddler, along with screenings and transportation). Results comparing the first two versus the last two groups were statistically significant ($p = 0.008$), indicating that the interventions were worthwhile.
- Child data, only available in groups 2 (child screening with transportation) and 4 (full intervention with transportation), revealed statistical significance for preventable-cause child mortality rate ($p = 0.04$) for those in the group with all components of the NFP (group 4).

These and other studies are powerful evidence noting the effectiveness of a program of regular community/PHN visits to this vulnerable group (USDHHS, 2011b). A classic study by the Olds research team studying pregnancy outcomes, childhood injuries, and repeated childbearing (Kitzman et al., 1997) was recognized by the National Institute of Nursing Research (National Institutes of Health, n.d.) as one of ten landmark nursing research studies.

The NFP model is based on theory and research. Olds and his colleagues have conducted repeated RCTs with different populations living in a variety of settings and contexts, over varying lengths of time (Eckenrode et al., 2010; Kitzman et al., 2010; Olds et al., 2010, 2014), and have consistently found that the NFP program:

- Improves prenatal health
- Reduces rates of subsequent pregnancies/births
- Increases intervals between births
- Increases in maternal employment
- Improves child school readiness (NFP, 2011, para. 3)

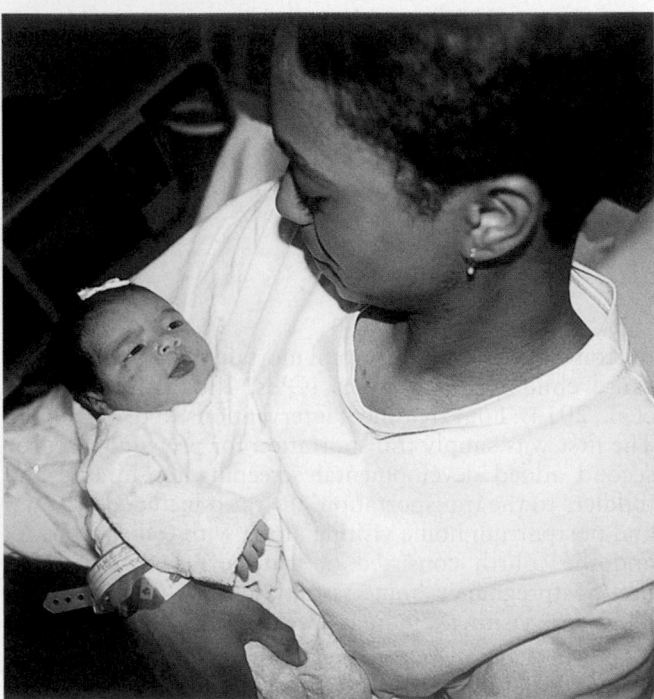

Mother–infant bonding

In a time of tight budgets, number crunchers may ask: do community health nurses really make the difference, or can less expensive health care workers also get results? An early study by Olds et al. (2004) examined differences between nurse and paraprofessional (e.g., home aides) visitation in a large, randomized study of mostly Mexican American low-income first-time mothers. At the beginning of the study, no statistical differences were noted between control and paraprofessional subjects. Two years after the end of the program, participants visited by paraprofessionals had fewer low-birth-weight babies and better results than did control subjects on measures of mastery and mental health, and their home environments were conducive to early learning. On the other hand, mothers visited by nurses showed immediate as well as long-term benefits. They had longer intervals between first and second births, there were fewer incidences of domestic violence, and their home

environments were found to be conducive to early learning. Children of those mothers had better behavioral adaptation during testing, more advanced language scores, and better executive functioning. Others have reported similar findings (Isaacs, 2008).

More current research found "no significant paraprofessional effects on emotional/behavioral problems" among children of mothers with fewer psychological means in a study comparing paraprofessionals to control group counterparts. The only statistically significant effect was on "visual attention/task switching" for 9-year-olds (Olds et al., 2014, p. 114). Those children visited by nurses were found to have

- Fewer emotional and behavioral problems overall at age 6 ($p = 0.08$)
- Fewer internalizing problems at age 9 ($p = 0.08$)
- Less dysfunctional attention at age 9 ($p = 0.07$)

When compared to control-group counterparts, nurse-visited children exhibited better receptive language at the ages of 2, 4, and 6 ($p = 0.01$), and better sustained attention at ages 4, 6, and 9 ($p = 0.006$). Olds and his fellow researchers are convinced that public/community health nurses are the key to success!

In tough budget times, state and local agencies may be hesitant to expand programs. But the costs of community health nurse visits are more than offset by the large savings in both dollars and human suffering (Olds et al., 2010). Over the years, several policy and think tank groups have done cost–benefit analyses of the NFP, all concluding that this program reaps large returns on investment. A study on "costs, outcomes, and return on investment" from NFP was funded by the Pew Center on the States and noted that Medicaid spending for a first-born child could be reduced by 8%; this translates into $12,299 in savings per family (Miller, 2012). If NFP is fully funded by Medicaid, costs are recouped by the time the child reaches age 6, and 1.4 times the cost is returned when the child reaches age 18. Food stamp costs, decrease by 9%, welfare spending by 7%, and savings in Child Protective Services, criminal justice, and special education costs can lead to savings of $18,939 per family (Miller, 2012). An earlier Brookings Institute report recommended, among other things, that the government invest $14 billion for nurse home-visiting programs to promote prenatal care and child development (Isaacs, 2007). Other policy groups have echoed their support for policy changes based upon this carefully crafted and studies intervention (NFP, 2011c). When H.R. 3590 (The Patient Protection and Affordable Care Act—"health care reform") was passed in 2010, early childhood home visitation programs were singled out as effective practices and new grant funding to states was made available to promote these programs (U.S. Congress, 2010). The original 5-year funding of the Maternal, Infant, and Early Childhood Home Visiting (MIECHV) program was due to expire at the end of 2014, but many organizations and individuals let Congress know of their support for this research-based intervention and funding was extended for 2 more years even in the face of a stagnant legislative branch of government (Schmit, Schott, Pavetti, & Matthews, 2015; NFP, 2015). Many communities have sought to institute FNP (Institute of Medicine [IOM], 2014). Dr. Olds and his colleagues (2013) have encouraged replication, using the established framework undergirding their proven results. The value of this program that provides PHNs to visit at-risk mothers and children in their homes has been validated. So, PHNs really *do* make a difference!

This evidence about the effectiveness of public health nursing visits could be gleaned only by conducting formal nursing research. Research in nursing is not a new phenomenon; Florence Nightingale is considered the earliest nurse researcher. She collected and analyzed data on the soldiers she cared for during the Crimean War (1859). She also employed principles of EBP because she sought to enhance their care by using evidence to improve her nursing practice and patient outcomes. **Research** is the systematic collection and analysis of data related to a particular problem or phenomenon. Research that is properly conducted and analyzed has the potential to yield valuable information that can affect the health of large groups of people. Indeed, it should guide our practice of community health nursing, and it often serves as the basis for changes in health care policies and programs. The Quad Council PHN Competencies include analytic assessment skills, basic public health science skills, and policy development/program planning skills that include research and EBP (2011). In the current national atmosphere of managed care and obstinately rising health care costs, the importance of valid research on how health care dollars can be spent to benefit the greatest number of people is vitally important.

EVIDENCE-BASED PRACTICE

Across many different settings, from acute to community-based care, implementation of EBP guidelines or practices has been shown to improve nursing practice and client outcomes, as well as reduce costs and standardize care (Doren et al., 2010; Stevens, 2013). But how did this more recent paradigm shift toward EBP occur? Dr. Archie Cochrane, a British epidemiologist, is widely regarded as the force behind evidence-based clinical practice in medicine (The Cochrane Collaboration, 2015). As health care has become more and more complex, we have developed "superspecialists" and increasingly advanced technology, as noted in Gawande's seminal work, *The Checklist Manifesto* (2010, p. 31). Even though we often cling to "the way we've always done it," we certainly have ample evidence of the need for a shift to EBP in health care: the IOM has been studying the issues

of health care quality and effectiveness over the 15 years or more and has called for widespread and systematic changes through their reports—*To Err Is Human: Building a Safer Health System* (IOM, 2000), *Crossing the Quality Chasm: A New Health System for the 21st Century* (IOM, 2001), and *Priority Areas for National Action: Transforming Health Care Quality* (IOM, 2003). These landmark reports draw attention to the fact that we spend billions of dollars each year researching new treatments, and more than a trillion dollars are spent annually on health care, but "we repeatedly fail to translate that knowledge and capacity into clinical practice" (IOM, 2003, p. 2). In response, the federal Agency for Healthcare Research and Quality (AHRQ) has established EBP centers across the United States and Canada. Schools of nursing, such as Arizona State University, the University of Texas Health Science Center at San Antonio, Case Western Reserve, and the University of Rochester, also have established centers for EBP.

The Future of Nursing highlights the need for nursing to work with other health professionals in "redesigning health care" by "conducting research" and improving practices through evidence-based means (IOM, 2011, pp. 7, 11). According to Melnyk and Fibneout-Overholt (2014), **evidence-based practice** in nursing means just that—systematically searching for and critically appraising and synthesizing evidence (or research findings), along with consideration of expert clinical nursing judgment and patients' wishes, in making decisions about how to care for patients or clients (see Display 4–1, Steps of Evidence-Based Practice and Fig. 4–1). Rebar, Gersch, Macnee, and McCabe (2014, p. 6) further clarify it as:

- Reviewing the best available evidence, most often the results of research
- Using the nurse's clinical expertise
- Determining the values and cultural needs of the individual
- Determining the preferences of the individual, family, and community

Olson Keller and Strohschein (2011, June 1) note that, in public health, the best available evidence includes not only that from clinical research but also from health data (e.g., immunization rates, mortality rates, health status surveys) and practice (e.g., program evaluations, reports from expert panels). Clinical reasoning is an important component in EBP. Practice knowledge of expert clinical nurses is vital to the process and efficacy

---

DISPLAY 4–1 THE STEPS OF EVIDENCE-BASED PRACTICE PROCESS

0. Cultivate a spirit of inquiry.
1. Ask the burning clinical question in PICOT format.*
2. Search for and collect the most relevant best evidence.
3. Critically appraise the evidence (i.e., rapid critical appraisal, evaluation, and synthesis)
4. Integrate the best evidence with one's clinical expertise and patient preferences and values in making a practice decision or change.

5. Evaluate outcomes of the practice decision or change based on evidence.
6. Disseminate the outcomes of the EBP decision or change.

*PICOT stands for Population/Patient Problem, Intervention, Comparison, Outcome, Time.
From Melnyk, B., & Fineout-Overholt, E. (2014). *Evidence-based practice in nursing and healthcare: A guide to best practice* (3rd ed., p. 15). Philadelphia, PA: Lippincott Williams & Wilkins, with permission.

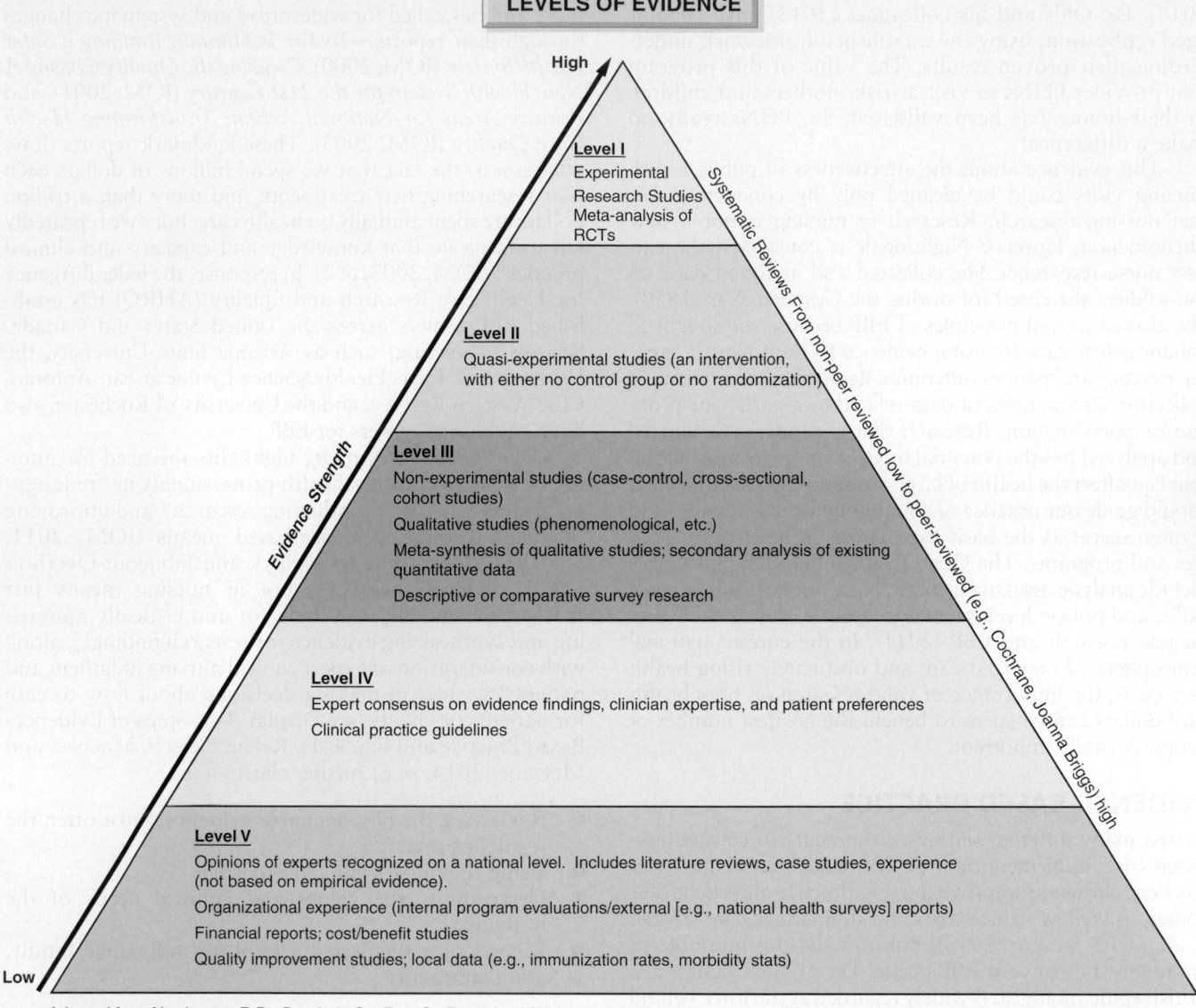

LEVELS OF EVIDENCE

High

Level I
Experimental
Research Studies
Meta-analysis of
RCTs

Level II
Quasi-experimental studies (an intervention,
with either no control group or no randomization)

Level III
Non-experimental studies (case-control, cross-sectional,
cohort studies)
Qualitative studies (phenomenological, etc.)
Meta-synthesis of qualitative studies; secondary analysis of existing
quantitative data
Descriptive or comparative survey research

Level IV
Expert consensus on evidence findings, clinician expertise, and patient preferences
Clinical practice guidelines

Level V
Opinions of experts recognized on a national level. Includes literature reviews, case studies, experience
(not based on empirical evidence).
Organizational experience (internal program evaluations/external [e.g., national health surveys] reports)
Financial reports; cost/benefit studies
Quality improvement studies; local data (e.g., immunization rates, morbidity stats)

Low

Evidence Strength

Systematic Reviews From non-peer-reviewed low to peer-reviewed (e.g., Cochrane, Joanna Briggs) high

Adapted from Newhouse, R.P., Dearholt, S., Poe, S., Pugh, L., & White, K. (2007) *Johns Hopkins Nursing Evidence-Based Practice Model & Guidelines.*
Indianpolis, IN: Sigma Theta Tau International; Olson keller, L., & Strohschein, S. (2011, June1). *Show me the evidence: Evidence-based public health nursing
practice.* Webinar. Handouts retrieved from http://publichealthnurses.org/images/uploads/Webinar_I_Slides_Updated.pdf; Olson Keller, L., & Strohschein, S.
(2011, June 15). *Innovations in translating evidence into practice.* Webinar. Handouts retrieved from http://publichealthnurses.org/images/uploads/
Web_II_Handout_(1).pdf

FIGURE 4–1 Levels of evidence.

of results (Lee, Johnson, Newhouse, & Warren, 2013a; Melnyk, Gallagher-Ford, Long, & Fineout-Overholt, 2014). Training programs are necessary for nurses to successfully apply EBP to their practices, in the community as well as in acute care (Black, Balneaves, Garossino, Puyat, & Qian, 2015). For those working in hospitals where quality improvement (QI) is at the forefront, it can be difficult to discern differences between EBP, research, and QI. It is helpful to consider Porter-O'Grady's (2010) view of EBP as the "integration of the best possible research" evidence with clinical knowledge and expertise, along with patient preferences and needs (p. 1). Thinking critically about practice problems is an important component of EBP. Reflecting on why we do things a particular way and critically thinking through a problem in a purposeful, systematic way are vital steps in the process. For instance,

Porter-O'Grady (2010) finds commonalities between EBP and critical thinking:

● Explore a problem.
● Address a purpose or goal.
● Make assumptions about the problem derived from an assessment of the problem and its elements.
● Clarify the problem around central concepts or key indicators.
● Access data, evidence, information, and sources to better explain the problem.
● Interpret accumulated evidence about the specific situation or problem.
● Use reasoning, processing, defining, planning, and documenting to guide subsequent actions in addressing the issue.

- Act on the problem, consistent with protocols and parameters, and assess its effect and impact, as well as the process.
- Evaluate, adjust, generalize, and apply to a broader problem set (indicative of a successful problem-solving process).

STEPS OF THE EBP PROCESS

The effective practitioner utilizes his or her clinical judgment and expertise to reflect on the practice of community health nursing and determine if safe, effective, quality, and cost-efficient care is being delivered. Problems or situations that need clarification can then be identified, and current research can be reviewed to guide needed changes in practice. Although acknowledged barriers exist, they can be overcome utilizing available resources (Grant, Stuhlmacher, & Bonte-Eley, 2012). Melnyk and Fineout-Overholt (2014, pp. 10–16) outline the steps of the EBP process as seen in Display 4–1:

0. Cultivate a spirit of inquiry.
1. Ask the burning clinical question in PICOT format (see below).
2. Search for and collect the most relevant best evidence.
3. Critically appraise the evidence for its validity, reliability, and applicability, and then synthesize that evidence.
4. Integrate the best evidence with one's clinical expertise and patient preferences and values in making a practice decision or change.
5. Evaluate outcomes of the practice decision or change based on evidence.
6. Disseminate the outcomes of the EBP decision or change.

These steps will be explored in more detail, as well as available resources and implications for public health nursing practice.

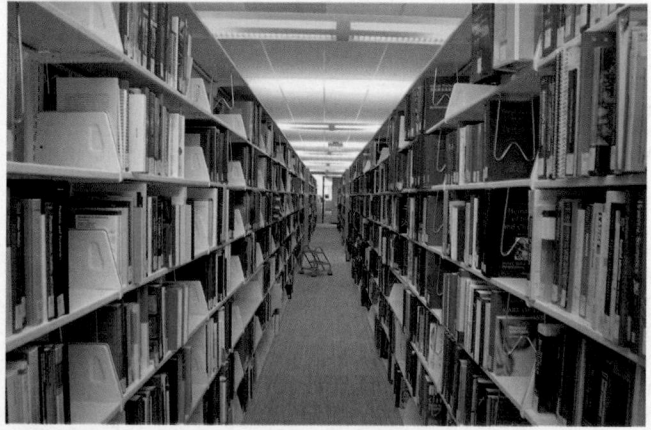

Finding evidence can be daunting in this era of information overload. (Photo courtesy of CDC Public Health Image Library.)

CULTIVATING A SPIRIT OF INQUIRY

The importance of this initial step cannot be overstated. In order for effective change to occur, current practices must be continually examined, questioned, and challenged. Individuals and organizations must be open to this cultural shift from the status quo, and it should be reflected in the agency's mission and philosophy (Melnyk & Fibneout-Overholt, 2014). There is a need for continual curiosity about how we can best conduct our practice and the evidence needed to guide our clinical decision-making; we also need to be immersed in a supportive culture that sustains this curiosity. Asking questions like "Why are we doing this?" and "Is there evidence to support this practice?" demonstrates this spirit of inquiry. Agencies that provide access to systematic reviews, evidence-based journals, and research consultants also demonstrate a commitment to this step.

ASKING THE QUESTION

What if you or your colleagues doubt the effectiveness of some method in your current nursing practice and want to find out if there is new research or evidence that may convince you to make a change? How do you begin your journey to EBP? Melnyk and others suggest that the first step to solving the problem is "asking the burning clinical question" (2014, p. 10). This question may be about client care or effective interventions, such as:

- What methods are most effective in ensuring client medication compliance with tuberculosis (TB) protocols?
- What is the best information I can give new mothers about preventing sudden infant death syndrome (SIDS)?

It could also be about systems approaches to population health:

- What is the most effective method of immunizing toddlers?
- How can PHNs better collaborate with families, physicians, and hospitals in preventing quick readmission of heart failure patients due to poor understanding and control of symptoms?

The PICOT question (see Display 4–2) is one way to develop an answerable, searchable EBP question. First, the population or problem must be specified. The Association of Women's Health, Obstetric, and Neonatal Nurses (AWHONN) asked a "burning clinical question" when they wanted to find a scientific basis for the development of standards of practice for their members regarding counseling pregnant women on smoking cessation. The project, *Setting Universal Cessation Counseling, Education, and Screening Standards* (SUCCESS), was an attempt to integrate best practices in primary care settings where women of childbearing age receive care. They did extensive searches in the Cumulative Index on Nursing and Allied Health Literature (CINAHL) and MEDLINE for research studies relating to low-birth-weight infants, effects of prenatal smoking on infants, and effects of smoking cessation intervention on premature labor and birth weight with both pregnant women and those seeking care prior to conception (Albrecht, Kelly-Thomas, Osborne, & Ogbagaber, 2011). They critically analyzed articles and found evidence of a higher incidence of many complications, including preterm labor, premature rupture of membranes, lower

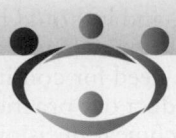

DISPLAY 4–2   PICOT: COMPONENTS OF AN ANSWERABLE, SEARCHABLE QUESTION

Term	Definition	Specific Example
Patient population/problem	The patient population or problem of interest, for example: • Age • Gender • Ethnicity • With certain disorder (e.g., hepatitis A)	For example: • Adolescent females, ages 12–20
Intervention	The intervention or range of interventions of interest, for example: • Exposure to disease • Risk behavior (e.g., smoking) • Education	For example: • Sexuality education program
Comparison intervention or issue of interest	What you want to compare the intervention against, for example: • No disease • Absence of risk factor (e.g., smoking) • Placebo or no intervention	For example: • Current practice or no intervention
Outcome	Outcome of interest, for example: • Risk of disease • Rate of occurrence of adverse outcome (e.g., death) • Accuracy of diagnosis	For example: • Unplanned pregnancies
Time	The time involved for the intervention to demonstrate an outcome, for example: • Time it takes for intervention to achieve the outcome • Time interval selected to observe the population or problem/condition	For example: • One school year (to implement curriculum)

Adapted from Melnyk, B., & Fineout-Overholt, E. (2014). *Evidence-based practice in nursing and healthcare: A guide to best practice* (3rd ed., p. 28–29). Philadelphia, PA: Lippincott Williams & Wilkins, used with permission.

birth weight and length, spontaneous abortion, and placenta previa or abruption in women using tobacco. Infants and children exposed to secondhand smoke had a higher risk for ear infections, asthma and other respiratory problems, SIDS, and learning disorders. Significant evidence suggested that this was a problem that needed to be addressed. They also concluded that health care providers could provide office-based assessments and utilize client-focused protocols. At each visit, their members are encouraged to ask women to tell them about their current smoking habit, and they implement the five A's intervention model (Ask, Advise, Assess, Assist, Arrange). If there is an indication that the client is not ready to quit smoking, the practitioner can implement the five R's (Relevance, Risks, Rewards, Roadblocks, and Repetition). This is a powerful example of taking evidence, evaluating it, and applying it to a problem that can be addressed through nursing practice and promoted by a nursing professional organization (Association of Women's Health, Obstetric and Neonatal Nurses [AWHONN], 2014).

Finding the Evidence

Melnyk and Fibneout-Overholt (2014) stress the importance of systematically searching for all relevant research on a clinical question of interest and critically analyzing the evidence. They argue that this is not merely **research utilization**, in which new interventions may be tried based on the results of one or two good studies, but true synthesis of pertinent evidence from several studies (e.g., systematic reviews of RCTs) and critical reviews of both quantitative and qualitative studies pertinent to a particular question of interest. While doing this, the nurse must keep in mind the unique needs and wants of the clients served, as well as current practice standards, guidelines, and ethical considerations. National clinical practice guidelines should be reviewed (e.g., National Guideline Clearinghouse at www.guideline.gov), and expert clinicians may be interviewed for their opinions on the problem at hand. Nurses often rely on RN peers, along with guidelines and experience with patients, rather than current evidence, and this can result in poor practice decisions because of inadequate information

(O'Leary & Mhaolrunaigh, 2012). A solid understanding of the evidence is needed.

Although expert nurses may be a good starting point in seeking evidence, clinically relevant research that is both medically sound and patient centered must be reviewed. Excellent places to begin are **integrative** or **systematic reviews** that compile all recent studies and summarize what is known about the problem or situation. The Cochrane Collaboration (www.cochrane.org) lists systematic reviews on various topics of interest to both physicians and nurses. For instance, a community health nurse working with a group of adults who have diabetes might be interested in the systematic review on the importance of exercise for clients with type 2 diabetes. An early systematic review found that those who participated in aerobic exercise had decreased body fat and triglyceride levels and improved blood sugar control (even for those who did not lose any weight). However, a later systematic review found that both aerobic and resistance exercise helped achieve control of diabetes (Yang, Scott, Mao, Tang, & Farmer, 2013). Although a community health nurse may certainly have a "hunch" that exercise is good for his or her clients, this newer systematic review of current studies provides solid evidence on which to base specific recommendations. Another review on promoting adherence to antiretroviral therapy for human immunodeficiency virus (HIV)/acquired immunodeficiency syndrome (AIDS) clients might be helpful to a PHN supervisor in designing an AIDS case management program utilizing PHNs. A systematic review of 124 studies including a large majority of RCTs done in North America, Africa, and Europe found a "large and overall strong evidence base" for five interventions: (a) cognitive-behavioral therapy (CBT), (b) education, (c) directly observed therapy (DOT), (d) treatment supporters, and (e) active reminder devices (ART) such as text messaging (Chaiyachati, Ogbuoji, Price, Suthar, Negussie, & Barnighausen, 2014, p. s199). From this evidence, a community health nurse case manager may conclude that medication compliance can be effectively ensured through development of a nurse–client relationship, group support, and focused patient education on medication management skills. Another source of systematic reviews includes the Campbell Collaboration (http://www.campbellcollaboration.org), covering education and social welfare research that may be of interest to PHNs who are examining, for instance, effective group or individual interventions such as parenting programs for teens (Barlow et al., 2011).

The AHRQ EBP centers also provide evidence reports that are easily accessible online (http://www.ahrq.gov/research/findings/evidence-based-reports/overview/index.html). Searching may be done by use of a topical index, clinical area, or health care services (e.g., bioterrorism) and technical areas (e.g., community-based participatory research [CBPR]). Other sources for systematic or integrative reviews include the following:

- Cochrane Nursing Care Field podcasts (http://cncf.cochrane.org/podcasts)
- Cochrane Public Health Group (http://ph.cochrane.org)
- *Worldviews on Evidence-Based Nursing* from Sigma Theta Tau International (www.nursingsociety.org)
- *Evidence-Based Nursing*, a British online journal (www.ebn.bmjjournals.com)

- Joanna Briggs Institute, an Australian nursing research organization (joannabriggs.org)
- The Community Guide, a CDC site for research on population health promotion (http://www.thecommunityguide.org/index.html)
- Health-Evidence Canada, a Canadian website for promoting evidence-based decision-making (http://health-evidence.ca/)
- Research and Development (RAND) Corporation research briefs (www.rand.org)

Critical Appraisal of the Evidence

Collection and critical analysis of the best evidence in the literature, like that done by AWHONN above, constitute the second and third steps in the EBP process. Systematic reviews should be carefully examined to determine validity (Thompson, Tiwari, Fu, Moe, & Buckley, 2012). You can do this by asking these types of questions:

- What was the review question? (Specific population, intervention, etc.)
- Were search strategies explained and are they reasonable?
- What were exclusion criteria/were any important, relevant studies overlooked?
- Were the studies in the review properly designed and executed (were findings valid)?
- Were there similar results found in all studies?
- How reliable are the results (only minimal bias)?
- For instance:
  - Were sample sizes large enough?
  - Were results statistically significant?
  - Were there confounding factors (e.g., outside influences that make you doubt the results; differences between groups in intervention or outcome assessment, high rates of attrition)?

It is also helpful to compare the results with previous research and clinical practice (Melnyk & Fibneout-Overholt, 2014). Qualitative research, discussed later, can also be evaluated by asking questions:

- How were study participants chosen?
- Is the data accurate and complete?
- Are the results plausible? Is it logical, consistent, and relevant?

Grids outlining levels and quality of evidence in public health nursing are available (www.publichealthnurses.org). But what if no systematic reviews are available in your area of interest? Where can you find the necessary evidence needed in order to make good practice decisions? You can look for RCTs, meta-analysis research, program evaluation studies, systematic literature reviews, or practice guidelines (see Fig. 4–1, Levels of Evidence), keeping in mind that several studies (or one or two large-scale, tightly controlled studies) are preferred.

Integrating the Evidence

Fourth, it is important to make a decision, based on your clinical expertise and knowledge of your clients' values and preferences, about incorporating this information into your practice. You can do this by asking:

- How can I apply these results to my community health nursing practice?

- Will it benefit my clients?
- Are my clients similar to the population studied?
- Do I have the necessary resources?
- Does this go against my client's values or preferences?

Evidence has shown that PHNs have been effective with different client populations in ameliorating postpartum depression, promoting awareness, and facilitating improved family functioning in families with neglected and abused children, and the benefits of the NFP for children, mothers, and families have been consistently demonstrated (Glavin, Smith, Sorum, & Ellefsen, 2010; Kobayashi, Fukushima, Kitaoka, Shimizu, & Shimmanouchi, 2014; Mejdoubi et al., 2011; NFP, 2010; Olds, Kitzman, Knudtson et al., 2014; Sierau et al., 2016). Newer research outside of public health nursing may also be applied in the community, depending upon clinical expertise and knowledge of our clients. For instance, a new area of research about treating low levels of vitamin D in the elderly found that it may reduce risk of mortality among institutionalized elderly who are at risk for falls, but it doesn't seem to reduce the rate of fractures (LeBlanc, Zakher, Daeges, & Chou, 2015). Other researchers found that for elderly females with poor renal function who are living in nursing homes, vitamin D supplements alone may not be sufficient (Terabe et al., 2012). Depending upon age group, in general, population screening for vitamin D insufficiency may be more cost-effective than universal supplementation (Lee et al., 2013b). This research might spark an interest for community health nurses to counsel adult clients attending yearly flu clinics to include this supplement in their daily regimen, especially in areas where exposure to sunlight is less prevalent.

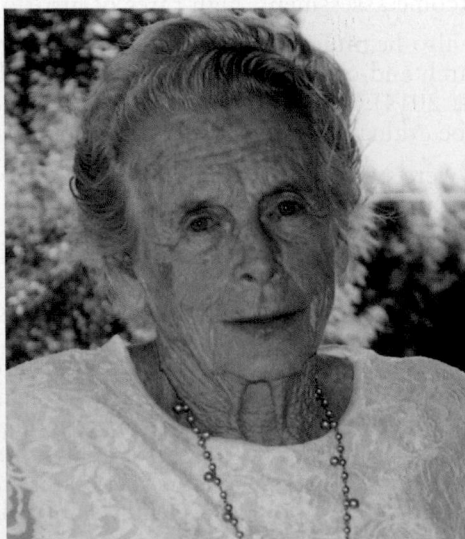

New research examines if the elderly may benefit from vitamin D supplementation.

An example of a systematic review of interest to PHNs is from the Cochrane Nursing Care Field and concerns smoking cessation. Young and Skorga (2011) produced a synopsis of a Cochrane review done by Lindson et al. in 2010 that examined 10 clinical trials for differences in success rates and adverse events between participants who abruptly quit smoking and those who utilized a more gradual reduction in smoking. Findings revealed no statistical differences between the two groups for smoking abstinence, despite types of interventions used (e.g., self-help therapy, pharmacotherapy, behavioral support). However, some of the study results were inadequate, making it impossible to conclude if there were any differences in adverse effects. Because smoking cessation is often advised for community health clients, PHNs could utilize this information to guide them to encourage either method of smoking cessation for their clients. When examining population-based strategies, The Community Guide provides task force recommendations based on systematic reviews, along with additional resources on the topic of interest. For instance, when searching the term "dental caries," community water fluoridation is recommended, as are school-based/school-linked sealant delivery programs. However, state or community sealant promotion programs are not recommended owing to insufficient evidence.

Evaluating Outcomes

The final step of the EBP process is to evaluate any practice change. For instance, if you decide to implement findings from the systematic review on HIV/AIDS medication compliance cited above, a standardized protocol of home visits and patient education by PHNs would need to be established and both baseline and postintervention data collected in order to deduce any potential positive change noted. Results can vary based on specific environment, population, implementation, and other factors. Evidence can lead you to choose a course, but evaluation of your outcomes is necessary to ensure that you have achieved the best results.

The design of an evidence-based research project represents the overall plan for carrying out the study. The overall plan guides the conduct of the study and, depending on its effectiveness, can influence investigators' confidence in their results. A major consideration in selecting a particular design is to try to control as much as possible those factors that are not included in the study but can influence the results. For example, in a classic study by Douglas, Mallonee, and Istre (1999), researchers wanted to discover the percentage of homes with functioning smoke alarms. They initially conducted a telephone survey, a commonly used method of survey research in community health, and found that 71% of households reported functioning smoke alarms. Concerned that this might be an inflated number, they conducted an on-site survey to confirm the results. After face-to-face interviews, they found that only 66% of householders reported having functioning alarms. However, when researchers actually tested the smoke alarms in those homes, only 49% were fully functioning. By having researchers actually test the smoke alarms, this design controlled for inflated results of the more commonly conducted, convenient, and economical telephone survey. Is self-report always unreliable? A classic small study of working middle-aged women revealed that self-reported weekly physical activity was strongly associated with data, indicating in this case self-report yielded reasonably reliable data (Speck & Looney, 2006). This provides evidence that the community health nurse must determine the most efficacious method of obtaining necessary data.

A more recent study examined physical activity during pregnancy and compared normal-weight and obese females (Renault et al., 2012). Baseline assessment of prepregnancy physical activity was done by questionnaire. Assessment during pregnancy was done by the use of pedometers worn for one week during every month of pregnancy. Obese participants had lower activity levels before and during pregnancy compared to normal-weight participants. Interestingly, pregnancy weight gain was higher in normal-weight participants compared to obese women. It was also lower in obese women who were noncompliant than in those who were compliant with pedometer use.

In an example of research with a specific population, researchers sought to control the variables to ensure true results. Sweet, Polivka, Chaudry, and Bouton (2014) designed and implemented an urban home-based intervention program for children with asthma. They completed pre- and postintervention assessments of asthma outcomes (e.g., symptoms, activity limitations, nighttime awakenings, use of inhalers, emergency department visits, missed days at school), caregiver quality of life (e.g., feeling helpless or frightened, missing work, awakened at night, worried about medications/side effects), asthma trigger–related household activities (e.g., smoking, using fragrance-free cleaning products), and asthma management activities (e.g., having an asthma action plan, using spacer with inhaler). At the beginning of the study, the participating families received home assessments and interventions (e.g., pest control, mold abatement) and a "Healthy Homes Action Plan" binder with a review of verbal education about ways to reduce asthma triggers around the home. This was done in an effort to provide a more consistent baseline for comparison (Sweet et al., 2014).

With another population common to PHNs, researchers knew from their review of the literature and practical experience that pregnant teens are a vulnerable population who often receive no prenatal care. Their inadequate use of resources and risk-taking behaviors often lead to premature delivery and low-birth-weight infants, as well as greater behavioral and cognitive problems of children leading to diminishing educational outcomes (Schaffer, Goodhue, Stennes, & Lanigan, 2012). The goals of the program were to refer and provide services to pregnant and parenting adolescents and children, as well as examine outcome measures of healthy births, delayed subsequent pregnancy, teens remaining in school, and improved maternal–child bonding as well as use of community resources.

Researchers sought to design a comprehensive program that included development of trust between PHN and teen participant, community outreach and coordination with schools and other agencies, utilization of a mental health curriculum, and provision of items needed to care for the infant or child (up to the age of two). Home visiting was an integral component of the program, where education about pregnancy, child development, and available community resources were stressed. Support and advocacy, along with discussion of the mental health curriculum, were also important. An evaluation of this PHN visiting program for pregnant and parenting teen in the Midwest assessed the "changes in program participants" and did not examine if the program "actually caused the changes" (p. 224). With a goal of reaching all pregnant and parenting teens, the evaluation revealed that 77% of eligible teens were referred to this program and 78% of those chose to accept services. Of those receiving 6 or more visits, 96% (vs. 90% of nonparticipants) had babies with healthy weights. For those with 10 or more visits, 76% (vs. 56% of nonparticipants) continued or graduated from school. Fewer participants had subsequent births, and more participants had safer, more supportive homes than did nonparticipants. Also, 95% had up-to-date immunizations and 97% were regularly taking their children in for well-child visits (Schaffer et al., 2012).

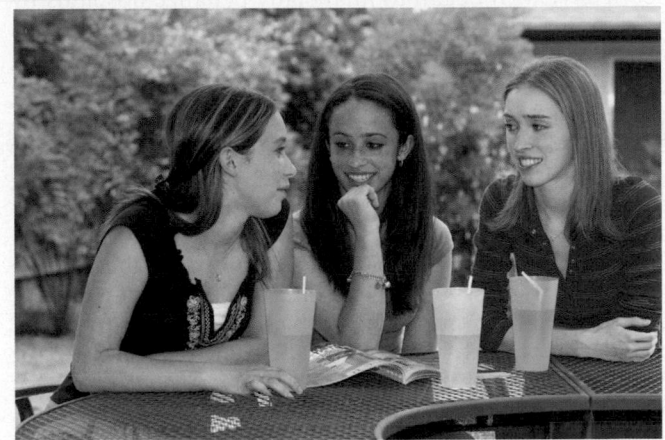

Pregnant teens

Once an intervention is developed, further research can evaluate its appropriateness and, ultimately, its effectiveness. Beyond EBP implementation, other lines of clinically based research can also be designed. The choice of research design influences the ability to generalize the results, and the attention given to the details of the study affects the value of the knowledge derived. Research done with larger numbers of participants drawn from a geographically diverse area is more complete than small-scale, exploratory studies done in an isolated area with a small, homogeneous sample. Valid tools or instruments and appropriately applied statistical methods lead to greater confidence in the results of the study.

Disseminating Outcomes

We need to share our results in order to improve the body of knowledge in public health nursing and provide studies that can be used in future systematic reviews. Often, community health nurses are required to report results to stakeholders (e.g., grant-funding agencies, local or county governing bodies). Formal reports are often required, or scorecards may be used that compare local results to state and national data. We can also share outcomes information with our colleagues locally, through informal networking, blogs, or pertinent listserv, etc. However, when EBP outcomes are shared at state and national professional meetings or through publication in peer-reviewed journals, a wider audience is reached and our knowledge based is exponentially increased.

DIFFERENCES BETWEEN EBP IMPLEMENTATION, QUALITY IMPROVEMENT, AND RESEARCH

If you have worked as a student in an acute care hospital, you have been introduced to quality or performance improvement (QI/PI) initiatives. QI/PI became even more important to health care after the IOM reports cited earlier. These approaches involve a systematic analysis of data and processes with the aim of improving the delivery of health care. Over the last decade, the National Quality Forum has endorsed over 600 quality measures, and hospitals are now required to publicly report certain quality data indicators. The Centers for Medicare and Medicaid Services (CMS) began to financially penalize hospitals by not paying for services when certain quality indicators were not met (e.g., pressure ulcers) and is now developing incentives for better quality care, such as nurse-sensitive value-based purchasing (Kavanagh, Cimiotti, Absulem, & Coty, 2012). See Chapter 6. Accrediting bodies for acute care hospitals first mandated quality care initiatives, but these are now spreading to ambulatory areas and other settings (Chassin, Loeb, Schmaltz, & Wachter, 2010). With the push for accreditation in public health agencies, this issue is becoming even more pertinent to PHNs and to public health systems with a focus on population health (Kronstadt, Beitsch, & Kaye, 2015; MacDonald, Newburn-Cook, Allen, & Reutter, 2012; Thomas, Corso, & Monroe, 2015).

The differences between QI/PI, EBP implementation, and clinical research are sometimes unclear (Conner, 2014). Melnyk and Fibneout-Overholt (2014) note that generalizability of findings is often not part of EBP project implementation because representative samples are not used. Rather, convenience samples of inpatients or clients are used to test initiatives for practice improvement. However, that distinction alone does not release nurses from gaining ethical approval (e.g., Institutional Review Board [IRB], Human Subjects Committee [HSC]). This is certainly required when disseminating results through publication or national presentations. Informed consent is another area where clear distinctions are also problematic. If you change your practice to benefit your clients, based on the best evidence and your clinical judgment/knowledge of your clients, it would be cumbersome to ask for written consent from every patient before implementing changes. It is not feasible, and it is expected that professional practice changes will be made over time without consulting clients. However, some clinical management oversight is expected in order to ensure that client rights are not violated.

One example of a QI project (or arguably an EBP implementation project) that was halted because of questions raised by the federal oversight agency for human subjects research protection is a large-scale study (67 intensive care units [ICUs] in Michigan) implementing EBP procedures to reduce catheter infection rates. The outcomes were "stunning," as it was estimated that over 1,500 lives were saved over the 18 months of the QI initiative (Gawande, 2010). However, the federal agency criticized the hospital that organized the study for dismissing the need for patient consent; it had been waived because their IRB saw it as QI and exempt. Researchers published the phenomenal results, bringing it to the attention of federal overseers. Protection of human subjects remains vitally important, and practical rules, infrastructure, and supervision within organizations can ensure that QI activities are appropriately reviewed and differentiated from clinical research. Some researchers are concerned that important research may be affected if rigid rules of consent are applied to QI studies in the same way they are in research studies (Wilfond, 2013). Stausmire (2014) provides a checklist to help nurses determine if their project falls under the auspices of an IRB (e.g., research or QI). QI is not only important in acute care settings, but public health agencies are increasingly organizing QI teams and implementing studies (Davis et al., 2014).

To effectively practice EBP implementation, community health nurses must know how to correctly compose a clinical question, find an appropriate database to search for systematic reviews or other evidence, critically review the evidence, consult practice guidelines and expert practitioners, and work with their clients to develop an appropriate plan of action. A clear understanding of basic research principles is needed to apply the principles of EBP and integrate the latest research into community health nursing practice. Evidence, in the form of systematic reviews, is most often drawn from quantitative research studies, but some public health nursing researchers also advocate the use of qualitative research in making evidence-based public health practice decisions (Martin, Kewwick, Crayton, & LeVeck, 2012; Sweet, Polivka, Chaudry, & Bouton, 2014; Weekes, Haas, & Gosselin, 2014). See Quality and Safety Education in Nursing (QSEN).

QUANTITATIVE AND QUALITATIVE RESEARCH

Scientific inquiry through research is generally pursued by means of two different approaches: quantitative research and qualitative research. Both can be part of research and EBP. **Quantitative research** concerns data that can be quantified or measured objectively. This could be as simple as counting the number of children receiving vaccination for varicella in immunization clinics during the past month and noting the number of reported cases of postvaccination complications. Fleming (2011) collected quantitative data from a school nurse database on the number and types of visits students made to school nurses' offices (total visits = 12,797). Data on visits were broken down by ethnicity and poverty level in an attempt to determine if differences existed between racial/ethnic groups and poor/not poor students who used school nursing services. Findings indicated that students who were poor regularly visited the school nurse's office, and these findings were consistent across racial/ethnic groups. Poor, black children accounted for 29% of visits and were the group using services most frequently. Most children visited the nurse for physical problems, but about 33% of poor White and Hispanic children visited the nurse for social–emotional reasons. Only 20% of Black and 10% of Asian children did this. This research gives a snapshot in time, but cannot address students' motivating factors for visits. More variables would need to be included in the study design.

QSEN—Focus on Quality: Patient-Centered Care

Recognize the patient or designee as the source of control and full partner in providing compassionate and coordinated care based on respect for patient preferences, values, and needs.

Knowledge

Integrate understanding of multiple dimensions of patient-centered care:

- Patient/family/community preferences and values
- Coordination and integration of care
- Involvement of family and friends
- Transition and continuity

Describe how diverse cultural, ethnic, and social backgrounds function as sources of patient, family, and community values.

Skills

Provide patient-centered care with sensitivity and respect for the diversity of human experiences.

Attitudes

Value seeing health care situations "through patients' eyes"; value patient's expertise with own health and symptoms; support patient-centered care for individuals and groups whose values differ from our own.

You have all dealt with individual patients in acute care settings. Some of you have also worked closely with patient families. Now, you will be widening your lens to focus on larger groups of patients (e.g., aggregates) and communities (e.g., populations). How do these QSEN competencies apply to aggregates such as mothers addicted to drugs or to population groups such as the elderly in your community?

As health care continues to evolve, nurses are being asked to shift to systems thinking, rather than just focus on an individual patient. This is how we will solve the problems with quality and safety in health care. Dolansky and Moore (2013) state that we must "broaden....problem identification from a focus on personal effort in a single situation to a focus on sequences of events with possible multiple causes for both individuals and populations" (para. 11). For example, we will not effectively address the high rates of early readmission for heart failure patients by simply checking prescriptions before discharge for an individual patient or even giving them reminder magnets to put on their refrigerators in the hope that this will help them remember to take their medications. Because many early readmissions were long ago found to often be preventable and due to inadequate discharge planning and poor follow-up/social support, among other things (Vinson, Rich, Sperry, Shah, & McNamara, 1990), hospitals are no longer being reimbursed and are seeking more innovative methods of addressing this issue.

We need to work with interdisciplinary teams to identify high-risk patients, prepare patients and their families for discharge, and then work with specialized programs that follow patients while they are at home to make sure they are weighing daily, monitoring their symptoms, and taking their medications. Early identification of potential problems and home visits by Advanced Practice Nurses (APNs) or predischarge scheduling of office visits with their medical providers has been shown to reduce 30-day readmission rates (Bradley, Curry, Horwitz, Sipsma et al., 2013). Transitional care interventions proposed by nurses (Naylor, Aiken, & Kurtzman, 2011) have demonstrated effectiveness and are proving their significance to health care reform (Stauffer, Fullerton, Fleming et al., 2011).

What other problems do you see that could benefit from a broader focus on quality and safety?

Bradley, E. H., Curry, L., Horwitz, L. I., Sipsma, H., Wang, Y., ... Krumholz, H. M. (2013). Hospital strategies associated with 30-day readmission rates for patients with heart failure. *Circulation: Cardiovascular Quality and Outcomes, 6,* 444–450.

Dolansky, M. A., Moore, S. M. (2013). Quality and Safety Education for Nurses (QSEN): The key is systems thinking. *Online Journal of Nursing, 18*(3), 1. doi: 10.3912/OJIN.Vol18No03Man01.

Naylor, M. D., Aiken, L. H., Kurtzman, E. T., Olds, D. M., & Hirschman, K. B. (2011). The care span: The importance of transitional care in achieving health reform. *Health Affairs, 30*(4), 746–754.

Stauffer, B. D., Fullerton, C., Fleming, N., Ogola, G., Herrin, J., Stafford, P. M., & Ballard, D. J. (2011). Effectiveness and cost of a transitional care program for heart failure: A prospective study with concurrent controls. *Archives in Internal Medicine, 171*(14), 1238–1243.

Vinson, J., Rich, M. W., Sperry, J. C., Shah, A. S., & McNamara, T. (1990). Early readmission of elderly patients with congestive heart failure. *Journal of the American Geriatric Society, 38*(12), 1290–1295.

Larsen and Reif (2011) provide an example of a quantitative study that includes an intervention and a control group. Because the United States is becoming increasingly diverse (see Chapter 5), the researchers wanted to find an effective method of training nursing students to more successfully work with diverse clients. They utilized the common approach of classes on culture, but added a 2- to 3-week immersion experience (living in another country/culture) for those in the intervention group. A control group did not participate in an immersion experience, but both groups were tested at baseline and again after the intervention group returned from their immersion experiences. Those who had both the classes and the immersion experience showed statistically significant posttest scores on transcultural self-efficacy and change, leading them to recommend that all nursing students be encouraged to participate in "immersion experiences to enhance transcultural competence" (p. 1). By adding the variable of immersion experiences, a greater level of transcultural effectiveness was reached.

Quantitative research is helpful in identifying a problem or a relationship between two or more variables, such as type of treatment (e.g., cultural immersion experiences) and an outcome (e.g., greater levels of transcultural self-efficacy). In so doing, quantitative studies tend to examine isolated parts of problems or phenomena and do not generally pay attention to the larger context or overall health of individuals. Quantitative research involves a reductionist tendency (i.e., focusing on the parts rather than the whole) and, if used exclusively, can limit nursing knowledge, because many of the important aspects of client services (e.g., quality of life, grieving, spirituality) cannot be measured objectively.

A more subjective or qualitative approach is needed to study those areas that need a broader focus or those that do not lend themselves to objective measurement.

Qualitative research emphasizing subjectivity asks "how" or "why." An example of this research examined mentorship provided by PHNs working with pregnant and parenting teens (Schaffer & Mbibi, 2014). Rather than just counting visits, like the previous example with school nurse visits, the researchers interviewed both PHNs and teen clients about their perceptions. PHN themes included being nonjudgmental, working from clients' strengths, meeting them where they are, sticking with them, honoring clients as persons, giving information, making referrals, and facilitating decisions. PHNs found success in the relationship with clients if teens delivered healthy babies, stayed in school/found a job, and ensured child's safety and school readiness. For the pregnant and parenting adolescent clients, the identified themes included PHN is extremely trustworthy, is part of my support network, helps me build independence, and helps me with decisions. They envisioned success as finishing school and being able to provide for their child, along with being a good role model. This information is much richer because it is not elicited from a forced-choice questionnaire; it is prompted by open-ended questions and follow-up questions in an effort to discover feelings and beliefs.

It is not uncommon to find research studies in which both quantitative and qualitative approaches are used. When both types of data are collected and analyzed (and inferences are drawn from both), this is known as **mixed methods** research (Polit & Beck, 2012). A study examining the experiences and perceptions of nurses working with elderly stroke victims at adult daycare facilities (Park & Han, 2010) used both a questionnaire and a focus group to determine the importance of services provided (skilled nursing services, functional recovery, heath counseling, referral, and supporting personal care) and the nurses' work experiences. While the survey questionnaire elicited important information about perceptions of the importance of their work, the focus group allowed nurses to more specifically discuss challenges and concerns that would not have otherwise been revealed. Concerns about policies that promoted standardized, rather than individualized, care, along with role confusion owing to the nurse's work sometimes conflicting with the duties of social workers, and the need for better education for families to provide continuity of care outside the daycare facility were some of the themes noted by researchers. This mixed method study provides a broader picture of the gaps between identified areas of "key services" and the reality of issues that need to be resolved in order to facilitate better nursing care and client outcomes (p. 267). Mixed methods are also helpful in program evaluation and can provide a more holistic vision (Polit & Beck, 2014).

Another method of analyzing research in community health uses a statistical procedure known as **meta-analysis** to evaluate the results of many similar quantitative research studies in an attempt to integrate the findings and combine the sample sizes of many small studies to obtain a single-effect measure or a summary statistic (Melnyk & Fibneout-Overholt, 2014). By combining the results of many similar studies, meta-analysis affords greater statistical power and can give the researcher a more complete general perspective, especially when research on a certain issue may seem inconclusive. An example of this type of nursing research can be found in the Cochrane Library. A meta-analysis done by Jianzhong, Ma, and Weihua (2014) sought to answer the review question, "What is the most useful strategy for communicating to consumers the effectiveness of contraceptives in preventing pregnancy?" and reviewed seven randomized controlled trials with over 4,500 female participants (p. 438). Four of the studies were from clinical sites and three from community settings. Outcome measures included knowledge of effectiveness, attitude about contraception, and choice or eventual use of a particular contraceptive method. In order for meta-analysis to be valid, studies chosen for analysis should be similar in design, participants, and methods. However, this was not the case in this study. Two trials gave participants multiple teaching sessions on contraceptives, and five trials only gave participants one session that included information on contraceptives, along with other things such as HIV. The seventh study had a control group and two intervention groups using different ways of analyzing contraceptive effectiveness. Because of the vast differences in methodologies and lack of consistent quality of the research studies, the researchers concluded that they were unable to answer their review question and determine the most useful strategy for teaching clients about contraceptive effectiveness in pregnancy prevention. They encouraged more studies and better reporting of interventions and evaluations.

UNDERSTANDING RESEARCH BASICS TO PROMOTE EBP

In order to fully integrate the principles of EBP, it is important to have a basic understanding of the research process. More in-depth information on this subject is available in nursing research texts (e.g., Polit & Beck, 2014), but a brief synopsis is provided here (see Display 4–3). EBP methods are encouraged over basic research, especially for practicing PHNs. Doctorally prepared nurses and public health professionals, in conjunction with practicing PHNs or health department staff, more often conduct traditional research studies. Problems recently identified and studied within community health nursing include the following:

- Young women's reasons to seek sexually transmitted infection screening (Backonja, Royer, & Lauver, 2014)
- Perception of barriers to immunization among parents of Hmong origin (Baker, Dang, Ly, & Diaz, 2010)
- Revealing the voices of PHNs by exploring their lived experiences (Joyce, O'Brien, Belew-LaDue, Dorjee, & Smith, 2015)
- Development of a causal model for elder mistreatment (Pickering & Phillips, 2014)

DISPLAY 4-3 STEPS IN THE RESEARCH PROCESS

All effective research follows a series of predetermined, highly specific steps, building on the previous one and providing the foundation for the eventual discussion of research findings. It is important to understand basic research principles in order to effectively implement EBP.

1. Identify an area of interest.
2. Formulate a research question or statement.
3. Review the literature.
4. Select a conceptual model.
5. Choose a research design.
6. Obtain IRB or HSC approval.
7. Collect and analyze data.
8. Interpret results.
9. Communicate findings.

Identify an Area of Interest

- The problem of interest needs *specificity* (i.e., it must be specific enough to direct the formulation of a research question). For example, concern about child safety is too broad a problem; instead, the focus could be on a narrower subject, such as the use of child restraints and car seat availability and use in a particular community.
- The problem must also be *feasible*. Feasibility concerns whether the area of interest can be examined, given available resources. For example, a statewide study of the needs of pregnant adolescents might not be practical if time or funding is limited, but a study of the same group in a given school district could be more easily accomplished.
- The *meaning* of the project and its *relevance* to nursing must also be considered, such as exploring the implications for nursing practice in the study of pregnant adolescents. The nurse's specialty influences the selection of a problem for study and also the particular perspective or approaches used. Community health nurses think in terms of the broader community; their research efforts are developed with the needs of the community or specific populations in mind.

Formulate a Research Question or Statement

- Just like the PICOT question in EBP, the research question or statement reflects the kind of information desired and provides a foundation for the remainder of the project. The manner in which the question or statement is phrased suggests the research design for the project. For example, the question "What are nurses' attitudes toward pregnant women who use methamphetamine?" determines that the design will be simple, nonexperimental, and exploratory (see later discussion). In contrast, the question "What is the effect of an educational program on nurses' attitudes toward drug-abusing pregnant women?" suggests an experiment that will evaluate changes in nurses'

attitudes toward pregnant women who abuse drugs after receiving an educational intervention. The first research question suggests a broad, open-ended conversation with nurse participants, asking them to discuss their attitudes toward pregnant women who abuse drugs, such as methamphetamine. From the data obtained, general themes and patterns will emerge, leading the researcher to some overall conclusions. The second question examines the effects that an educational program may have on nurses' attitudes about pregnant women who abuse crack cocaine, for instance. This is most likely a quantitative, evaluative study that may involve pretesting to determine the nurses' attitudes, conducting one or more classes, and then posttesting to determine whether any change occurred in attitude or beliefs.

- Good examples of research questions addressed recently by community health nurses include:
  - What are the barriers to mask wearing for Influenza-type illnesses [*variable*] among urban Hispanic households [*population of interest*] (Ferng, Wong-McLoughlin, Barrett, Currie, & Larson, 2011)?
  - Are there intentions to reduce the risk of falling again [*variable*] among older homebound women [*population of interest*] (Porter, Matsuda, & Lindbloom, 2010)?
  - What are the levels of psychological and physical abuse [*variables*] among pregnant women in a Medicaid-sponsored prenatal program [*population of interest*] (Raffo, Meghea, Zhu, & Roman, 2010)?

Review the Literature

- A traditional review of the literature consists of two phases. The first phase consists of a cursory examination of available publications related to the area of interest. Although several nursing research journals publish studies reflecting all areas of nursing practice, most specialty areas have dedicated journals. *Public Health Nursing, Family and Community Health, Journal of Community Health Nursing, American Journal of Public Health, Journal of School Health, Nursing and Health Sciences,* and *Journal of School Nursing* are some of the journals that publish studies of particular interest to community health nurses. In this phase, the investigator develops knowledge about the area of interest that is somewhat superficial but sufficient to make a decision about the value of pursuing a given topic.
- The second phase of the literature review involves an in-depth, critically evaluated search of all publications relevant to the topic of interest. The goal of this phase is to narrow the focus and increase depth of knowledge. Journal articles describing research conducted on the topic of interest provide the most important kind of information, followed

(continued)

DISPLAY 4–3 STEPS IN THE RESEARCH PROCESS (*Continued*)

by clinical opinion articles (information on the topic described by experts in the field) and books. Journal articles provide more up-to-date information than do books, and systematic investigations provide a foundation for other studies. Prior research that has already been done on the topic of interest provides a solid foundation for later replication studies.

- Criteria for compiling a good review of the literature include (a) using articles that closely relate to the topic of interest (relevancy); (b) using current articles that provide up-to-date and recent information, usually within the past 5 years (although earlier articles may be included based on their importance to the area of interest); and (c) using both primary and secondary sources. A *primary source* is a publication that appears in its original form. A *secondary source* is an article in which one author writes about another author's work; EBP systematic reviews fall into this category.

- The conclusions from the literature review become the basis for the new study's assumptions and methodology. Rather than making a "leap of knowledge," the hypothesis or research question must be created by basing assumptions on previous research studies.

Select a Conceptual Model

- In relation to research, a **conceptual model** is a framework of ideas for explaining and studying a phenomenon of interest. A conceptual model conveys a particular perception of the world; it organizes the researcher's thinking and provides structure and direction for research activities. Models are like a framework on which to "hang" concepts or variables, and they should be used to guide the design and methods for collecting research data.

- All fields of study identify their major areas of concerns or boundaries. Nursing, since the early work of Florence Nightingale, is concerned with the interaction between humans and the environment in relation to health (Blais & Hayes, 2015). Betty Neuman's Systems Model (Neuman & Fawcett, 2011) has often been used as an organizing framework for research studies in community health and acute care nursing, as well as curriculum design. Although nurse investigators frequently and successfully use conceptual models developed within other fields, the advantage of using nursing models is that they provide an understanding of the world in terms of nursing's major concerns (see Chapter 14).

Choose a Research Design

Complete descriptions of various research designs and specific methodologies are available in basic nursing research texts. For the purposes of this chapter, a few important considerations underlying design selection

are described. First, quantitative approaches use two major categories of research design: experimental and nonexperimental (or descriptive).

- **Experimental design** requires that the investigators institute an intervention and then measure its consequences. Investigators hypothesize that a change will occur as a result of their intervention, and then they attempt to test whether their hypothesis was accurate. Experimental design requires investigators to randomly assign subjects to an **experimental group** (those receiving the intervention) and a **control group** (those not receiving the intervention). This process, called **randomization**, is the systematic sorting of research subjects, so that each one has an equal probability of selection.

- Another important distinction made within the experimental category of research is between true experiments and quasiexperiments. **True experiments** are characterized by instituting an intervention or change, assigning subjects to groups in a specific manner (randomization), and comparing the group of subjects who experience the manipulation to the control group (those not receiving the intervention). **Randomized control trials** (RCTs) are generally considered the gold standard of experimental research—they are commonly used to determine the safety and efficacy of new medications or to test the effectiveness of one intervention over another, and they are a foundation of EBP (Melnyk & Fibneout-Overholt, 2014).

- **Quasi-experiments** lack one of these elements, such as the randomization of subjects. Community health nurses conduct quasi-experiments more often than true experiments because it is often difficult (and sometimes impossible) to use randomization. For instance, a nurse may conduct a nutrition education intervention with fifth grade students at a particular school. Although the nurse can have one classroom participate in the intervention and another remain the control group, he or she cannot randomly assign the children to classrooms (i.e., intervention or control). Therefore, this research would be characterized as quasi-experimental in nature.

- **Nonexperimental designs** (also called *descriptive designs*) are used in research to describe and explain phenomena or examine relationships among phenomena. Examples of this approach include examining the relationship between gender and smoking behaviors among adolescents, describing the emotional needs of families of clients with Alzheimer disease, and determining the attitudes of parents in a given community toward sex education in the schools. In each of these instances, the focus of the research is on the relationships observed or the description of what exists. Such nonexperimental designs are often the precursors of experiments.

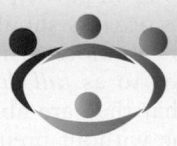

DISPLAY 4–3   STEPS IN THE RESEARCH PROCESS (*Continued*)

Obtain Institutional Review Board Approval *(see p. 16)*
Collect and Analyze Data *(see p. 16)*

Interpret Results

The explanation of the findings of a study flows from the previously formulated research plan. The findings need to be a logical conclusion, based upon the building blocks of the literature review, conceptual framework, research question, and methodology (Polit & Beck, 2014). You can't jump to a conclusion for which you have not laid a foundation. Findings need to make sense, to be reasonable and logical.

Communicate Findings

- The findings of nursing research projects need to be shared with other nurses, regardless of the studies' outcomes. Negative as well as positive findings can make a valuable contribution to nursing knowledge and influence nursing practice. Whether or not the hypothesis was verified is not the most important part of research; it is equally important to know about results that are inconclusive or not statistically significant, because this information is also necessary to build the science of nursing. For instance, in an early NFP (see beginning of this chapter) study by Eckenrode et al. (2000, 2001), researchers found that participants who received nurse home visitation during pregnancy and through the child's second birthday had significantly fewer child maltreatment reports with the mother as perpetrator or the study child as subject than did participants not receiving nurse home visitation. However, for mothers reporting more than 28 incidents of domestic violence, no significant reductions were noted. This is important information, because ongoing domestic violence may limit the effectiveness of these types of programs. A review of evidence on perinatal home visiting and intimate partner violence (Sharps, Campbell, Baty, Walker, & Bair-Merritt, 2008) concluded that those programs that add "specific intimate partner violence interventions" may be able to demonstrate reductions in violence along with improvements in infant and maternal health (p. 480). In future work, researchers need to elicit more information about domestic violence when trying to evaluate the effectiveness of this type of intervention.

- The research report should include the key elements of the research process. The research problem, methodology used, results of the study, and the investigators' conclusions and recommendations are presented. Whether investigators are presenting their findings verbally or writing for publication, they need to discuss the implications of their findings for nursing practice (Polit & Beck, 2014).

- Implementation of a diabetes prevention program in public housing communities (Whittemore, Rosenberg, Gilmore, Withey, & Breault, 2014)
- An intervention study of the expectations and self-efficacy of African American parents who discuss sexuality with their adolescent sons (Weekes, Haas, & Gosselin, 2014)
- A rural African American faith community's solutions to depression disparities (Bryant, Haynes, Kim Yeary, Greer-Williams, & Hartwig, 2014)
- Factors associated with increased HPV vaccine use in rural-frontier U.S. states (Lai, Ding, Bodson, Warner, & Kepka, 2016)
- The impact of an urban home-based intervention program on child asthma outcomes (Sweet et al., 2014)
- Policy implications of hospital nurse staffing and public health emergency preparedness (McHugh, 2010)
- Socioeconomic factors affecting infant sleep-related deaths in St. Louis (Hogan, 2014)

Each of these problem areas provides direction for the formulation of related research questions. Clear research questions, thorough review of the literature, human subjects protection, and a sound research design are factors to consider when evaluating the results of studies for incorporation into your practice.

A research question is a starting point for both traditional research and EBP methods. While somewhat similar in purpose (to answer a question), there are fewer steps in the EBP process (see Display 4–1). Formulation of a PICOT question in EBP is a similar process to the research question outlined in the steps of the research process, especially in its specificity (see Display 4–2).

Although the EBP steps outlined by Melnyk and Fineout-Overholt (2014) end with evaluation and dissemination, it is generally recognized that the final steps in the research process also apply to EBP. Most EBP research requires human subjects' approval, and dissemination of findings is very important in order to advance the science of nursing and provide effective outcomes for our clients. These steps will be examined in more detail.

Obtain Institutional Review Board or Human Subjects Committee Approval

Whenever research is to be conducted that involves human subjects, prior approval must be gained from either an IRB or an HSC. This can be true for research studies or when measuring client outcomes elicited from EBP-implemented changes in nursing interventions (unless, perhaps, this is a QI effort that affects all clients equally and involves only one setting). The reason for this approval is to safeguard the rights of prospective study participants. Each health department should have a committee or a gatekeeper, such as the health officer, who understands the federal guidelines for protecting subjects involved in research studies.

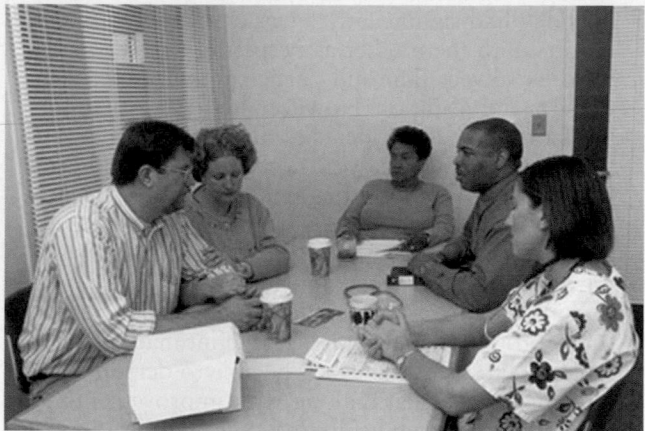

The purpose of an IRB is to protect the rights of human subjects and ensure compliance with federal laws.

Sadly, one of the most egregious examples of exploitation of human subjects was a study carried out by the U.S. Public Health Service. The Tuskegee study, begun in 1932 and ended in 1972, sought to learn more about syphilis and to justify treatment services for blacks in Alabama (Centers for Disease Control and Prevention [CDC], 2013). The 399 men with syphilis who participated in the study had agreed to be examined and treated. However, they were misled about the exact purpose of the study and were not given all of the facts; therefore, they were unable to truly give informed consent. Even after penicillin became the drug of choice for treatment of syphilis in 1947, the researchers failed to offer this treatment to the infected participants. Later, a nurse historian found evidence that research on syphilis was also funded by the Public Health Service and conducted in Guatemala. However, these participants were purposely infected with syphilis, causing even greater outrage and a formal apology from President Barack Obama to Guatemalan President Alvaro Colom (Reverby, 2011). Because of earlier Nazi atrocities, the Nuremberg Code and the Declaration of Helsinki were adopted by the world scientific community and then revised in 1975 as a means of ensuring ethical research practices; the President's Council on Bioethics was established in 2001 after President Clinton apologized on behalf of the nation to the Tuskegee participants and their families in 1997 (Blais & Hayes, 2015; CDC, 2013). See Evidence-Based Practice: Ethics in Action.

The following ethical principles are widely viewed as basic protections for research participants (U.S. Department of Health & Human Services [USDHHS], n.d.a). Freedom from harm or exploitation encompasses several aspects. First, no research can be done that may inflict permanent or serious harm. Second, the research study must be stopped if it becomes evident that harm may come to participants. Debriefing, or allowing participants to ask questions of the researcher at the conclusion of the study, as a means of protecting them from any unseen psychological harm, is also a component.

There should be some identified benefits from participation in the research study, and any costs or risks should be clearly outlined, so that participants can more easily determine the cost–benefit ratio (referred to as *full disclosure*). Subjects should also be told that they are able to withdraw from the study at any time without prejudice or penalty (known as *self-determination*). Consent forms should include full disclosure of the nature of the study, the time and commitment required of subjects, the researcher's contact information, and a pledge of confidentiality (or *assurance of privacy*).

Vulnerable subjects, as determined by federal guidelines, include children, mentally or emotionally disabled people, physically disabled people, institutionalized people (e.g., prisoners), pregnant women, and the terminally ill. Special care must be taken to ensure protection of vulnerable subjects. Once approval has been obtained from the proper entities, data collection can begin (USDHHS, n.d.b).

Collect and Analyze Data

The value of the data collected in any research study or EBP project depends largely on the care taken when measuring the concepts of concern, or variables. The specific tool used to measure the variables in a study, often a questionnaire or interview guide, is called an **instrument**. The accuracy of the instrument used and the appropriateness of the choice of instruments can clearly influence the results. For instance, Spielberger's State-Trait Anxiety Inventory is a well-researched questionnaire used in studying anxiety levels in adults. It has been shown to accurately measure state anxiety and the more stable tendency toward anxious personality—*trait anxiety*. Because of this evidence, one could infer that more accurate measurements of anxiety could be found using this instrument than a researcher-developed questionnaire that has never been tested for validity and reliability.

Validity and Reliability

Two tests are used to evaluate instrument accuracy: validity and reliability. **Validity** is the assurance that an instrument measures the variables it is supposed to measure. If a written questionnaire is being used in the study, the questions included would be evaluated to make certain that they are appropriate to the subject (content validity) and that the variable of interest is actually being measured (construct validity).

Reliability refers to how consistently an instrument measures a given research variable within a particular population. Test–retest reliability ensures that similar results are obtained using the same instrument with the same population at two separate testing times. If similar results are obtained on two separate occasions, the test can be considered reliable.

Statistical tests and measurements are often used to analyze subjects' responses to questionnaires to evaluate internal consistency. A questionnaire is internally consistent to the extent that all of its subparts measure the same characteristic. Cronbach's alpha (a) is often cited as a measure of internal consistency and is reported as a correlation coefficient, so that the closer the value is to +1.0, the greater the degree of internal consistency. Results higher than 0.7 are generally regarded as desirable.

EVIDENCE-BASED PRACTICE
Ethics in Action

Today, safeguards are in place to ensure that studies are stopped when either potential harm or insufficient benefit are noted. In April 2011, a drug trial examining daily use of an antiretroviral medication as a means of pre–HIV exposure prophylaxis was found to be ineffective in preventing HIV infection. No difference in rates of infection was noted for women taking the medication and another group taking a placebo, even though an earlier drug study with men showed some promise in HIV prevention (AllAfrica, 2011). In an earlier drug trial, a major international study of a drug-conserving protocol for AIDS medication was stopped because those who were in the on-again, off-again group got sicker than those taking continuous medication therapy (Associated Press, 2006). More than 5,000 HIV patients in 33 countries participated in this study, which was halted by the National Institutes of Health. This large-scale study was initiated after several smaller studies had suggested a possible benefit from the on-and-off medication strategy. It was hoped that this strategy of only taking medications when immune cell levels dropped would not only cut costs, it would decrease medication side effects for patients. What researchers found was that this episodic strategy actually increased side effects related to the heart, liver, and kidney. Researchers say that the results are difficult to explain, but because of patient safety, it was best to stop the clinical trial.

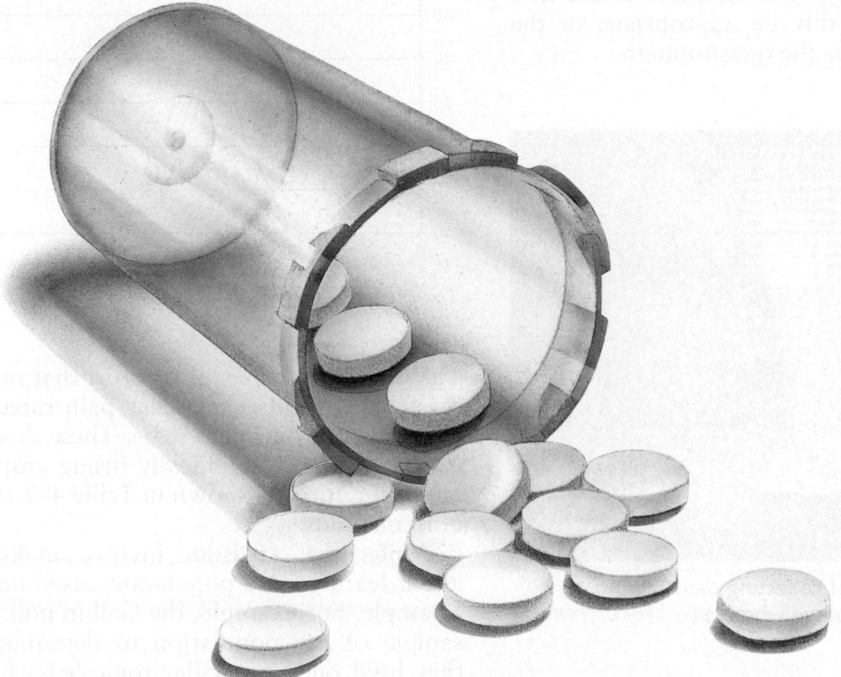

Drug safety was also questioned in a study of Avandia, a drug used by some people with type 2 diabetes. In the summer of 2010, the Food and Drug Administration (FDA) ordered researchers to stop enrolling new participants in a trial of this drug because of heart risks and to notify the more than 1,300 participants already in the study of these risks (Wilson, 2010). In fall of 2010, they significantly restricted access to this drug, and in spring 2011, cardiovascular risk warnings were added to the label and the drug could only now be given to patients enrolled in a special FDA program (FDA, 2011).

What ethical principles are involved? Is there an ethical dilemma? Consider the rights of a few versus the rights of many. Apply Iserson's (1999) three tests (under heading Decision-Making Frameworks).

Within the area of community health nursing research, instruments appropriate to the measurement of nursing concepts may not be available. Researchers may use questionnaires that have been designed and tested by other investigators, or they may begin the tedious task of developing their own. Both approaches to measuring the variables of interest are acceptable; however, using available instruments of known reliability and validity saves considerable time (Melnyk & Fibneout-Overholt, 2014).

Methods of Collecting Data

A variety of methods can be used to collect data, including self-report (subjects report their own experience verbally or in written form), observation (investigators observe subjects and document their observations), physiologic assessment (investigators use measures of physical evidence, such as blood pressure or impaired mobility), and document analysis (investigators review and analyze written materials, such as health records). For example, using these four methods, investigators examining the stress level of the caregiver when a family member chooses to die at home might do the following:

1. Design or use an existing written questionnaire or interview schedule (self-report).
2. Outline a schema, such as a list of potential stress-induced behaviors, for observing caregivers as they function in the home (observation).
3. Measure various physiologic indicators of stress, such as hypertension, insomnia, or poor diet (physiologic assessment).
4. Ask caregivers to keep a diary of their activities and feelings for 2 weeks, and analyze the diaries for evidence of stress (document analysis).

In most instances, the nature of the data to be collected dictates the best method of collection. One or more methods may be appropriate, given the topic of concern. In the example mentioned, a combination of the first three methods would probably be appropriate, or the diary could be substituted for the questionnaire.

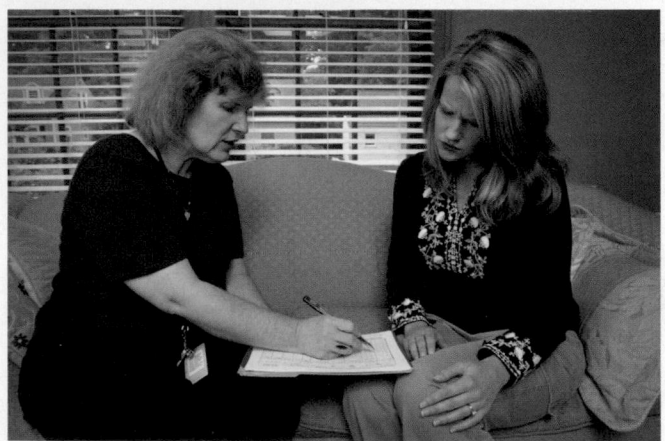

Surveys are common methods of collecting data. (Photo courtesy of CDC Public Health Image Library.)

Methods of Analyzing Data

Once collected, data must be analyzed so that a meaningful interpretation can be made. Statistical procedures reduce great amounts of information to smaller chunks that can be easily interpreted. When deciding on an appropriate statistical procedure, it is helpful to consider the two major categories of statistical analysis: descriptive and inferential statistics.

Descriptive statistics portray the data collected in quantitative or mathematical terms. Commonly used descriptive statistical methods include calculating the average number (or *mean*) of a particular set of occurrences and calculating *standard deviations* (how much each score on the average deviates from the mean) and percentages. For example, an investigator analyzing data collected from 50 clients with chronic pain might find their mean pain score to be 4.96 (on a scale from 0 [no pain] to 10 [worst pain]), with a standard deviation of 0.83. These descriptive statistics suggest that clients are grouped around the middle of the pain scale and differ very little in the amount of pain they experience.

Table 4–1	Pain Ratings	
Value	**Frequency**	**Percent (%)**
3.00	1	2.0
4.00	11	22.0
5.00	30	60.0
6.00	6	12.0
7.00	1	2.0
8.00	1	2.0
Mean 4.96	Standard deviation 0.83	

The investigator may also report that more than 95% of the female clients experience pain rated between 4 and 6 on the 10-point pain scale. These descriptive statistics can be reported graphically (using graphs or charts) or in written form as shown in Table 4–1 for an example of both methods.

Inferential statistics involve making assumptions about features of a population based on observations of a sample. For example, the Gallup poll, which surveys a sample of the population to determine what opinion they hold on a particular topic (e.g., favorite presidential candidate), uses inferential statistics to estimate the proportion of the total population that favors a particular candidate (McKenzie, Neiger, & Thackeray, 2012). The potential for **generalizability**, the ability to apply the research results to other similar populations, has great value to health professionals. It allows researchers to test their hypotheses on smaller groups before instituting widespread changes in methods, programs, and even national health policies.

Inferential statistics are also used to test hypotheses in research; they provide information about the likelihood that an observed difference between two or more groups could have happened just by chance or might be the result of some intervention or manipulation. These statistical procedures provide a determination of the extent to which changes or differences between sets of data are attributable to chance fluctuations and estimate the confidence with which one can make generalizations about the data.

It is appropriate to use both descriptive and inferential statistics to analyze the data from a study. For example, in a study designed to examine the effects of prenatal education on the health status of pregnant women, investigators might use inferential statistics to find a significant difference in health status between the group who experienced the educational program (experimental group) and the group who did not (control group). The investigators might also use descriptive statistics to report the percentage of women from the experimental group who attended all classes and the means and standard deviations for the women's health status scores.

Interpret Results

The explanation of the findings of a study flows from the previously formulated research plan. The findings need to be a logical conclusion, based upon the building blocks of the literature review, conceptual framework, research question, and methodology (Polit & Beck, 2014). You can't jump to a conclusion for which you have not laid a foundation. Findings need to make sense, to be reasonable and logical. When findings support the directions developed in the research plan, their interpretation is relatively straightforward. For example, a group of community health nurse investigators might design a study to determine the effect of parenting classes on the self-esteem of single welfare mothers between 21 and 35 years of age. They could use Coopersmith's (1967) ideas on self-esteem as their conceptual model, hypothesize that self-esteem will improve as a result of the classes, and design an experiment to test their idea. If self-esteem does, in fact, increase, their finding flows logically from their framework.

If the findings do not support the hypothesis of the study, investigators question various aspects of the research to develop an explanation. In this instance, a number of questions could be posed. Coopersmith posited that self-esteem would relate to feelings of success in a given endeavor. Can that position be inaccurate? Could the parenting classes have been ineffective? Perhaps they did not enhance feelings of success. Could the intervention have been too weak to show a statistical difference (not enough sessions)? Were there problems with the methodology used? Were there too few subjects or intervening, confounding factors that affected the results? All of these questions and more should be considered in an attempt to explain the results.

If the study is descriptive in nature (i.e., one that was designed to describe particular characteristics of a population), the direction of the findings is not a concern. A detailed, accurate report of the results and their implications alone is appropriate. Given either an experimental or a descriptive design, the importance of accuracy cannot be overemphasized. Leaps of faith when reporting the results of a study are not appropriate unless labeled as such. For example, one could not conclude from the study on parenting classes that these classes develop expert parenting skills, given that parenting skills were not assessed.

A valuable contribution can be made to the advancement of nursing knowledge when investigators use their results to make suggestions for future research. The investigators' knowledge of a particular area and their experience in conducting a specific study give them an excellent background for identifying future research possibilities.

As in EBP, results should be disseminated through publication, presentation, or other means.

IMPACT OF RESEARCH ON COMMUNITY HEALTH AND NURSING PRACTICE

Research has the potential to have a significant impact on community health nursing in three ways, by affecting public policy and the community's health, the effectiveness of community health nursing practice, and the status and influence of nursing as a profession. Community health nurses have been involved in research addressing all three of these dimensions.

Public Policy and Community Health

Research, with policy implications for addressing the health needs of aggregates, has been conducted on numerous topics. Many studies done by nurses and others have examined issues related to prevention, lifestyle change, quality of life, and health needs of specific at-risk populations (see Evidence-Based Practice: A Change of Position).

Often, both quantitative and qualitative methods are useful when conducting **health policy evaluation** studies to determine whether existing health services are appropriate and accessible, as well as effective. Researchers at the University of California Los Angeles (UCLA) Center for Health Policy Research found that older adults in rural California had higher rates of obesity/overweight, food insecurity, and lower rates of physical activity than their urban or suburban counterparts (Durazo et al., 2011). Utilizing data from the California Health Interview Survey, they noted that these conditions are risk factors for diabetes, heart disease, and repeated falls. Barriers to transportation and health care access, along with financial constraints and social and physical isolation, make this a complex issue that should be addressed on local, state, and national levels. They recommended policies to improve access to healthy food and adequate numbers of health care providers, as well as access to Internet and transportation, as a means of addressing the disparities. PHNs can use this type of research to advocate for resources, apply for grant funding, and negotiate collaborative agreements.

The results of health policy studies can influence public policy, the quality of services, and, in turn, the public's health: This is the conclusion of a Robert Wood Johnson initiative targeting smoking behaviors (Giovino et al., 2009). Examining the history of this paradigm shift in the United States provides a powerful example of the use of research in changing health policies and promoting population health. This change began in a few states and has spread, to varying degrees, across all 50 states. As an example, several studies conducted by a researcher at the University of Miami led to further policy changes regarding cigarette smoking. One study examined the projected health benefits and cost savings of raising the legal age for smoking in the United States to 21 (Ahmad, 2005a). Using a computer simulation model, the researcher concluded that changing the policy would net total savings of $212 billion in the United States and reduce the prevalence of cigarette smoking substantially. A similar study,

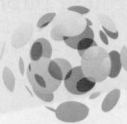

EVIDENCE-BASED PRACTICE

A Change of Position

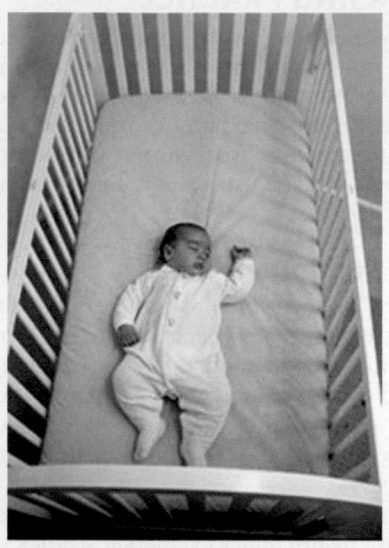

A good number of mothers today place their infants in a supine position—on their backs—to sleep. However, for most of us writing this textbook, the opposite was true—we were placed as sleeping infants in the prone position, on their stomachs. For generations, mothers were told that babies would be at risk of aspiration if they were put to sleep on their backs. Why did this change? In the late 1980s, research indicated that prone positioning of infants was related to greater incidences of SIDS, according to a group at the National Institute of Child Health and Human Development (NIH) who conducted an epidemiologic study examining SIDS risk factors (Hoffman, Damus, Hillman, & Krongrad, 1988). In the early 1990s, an expert panel from the same institute and the American Academy of Pediatrics concluded that infant sleeping positioning was an important factor in prevention of SIDS, and a recommendation was made for parents to place their infants on their backs when sleeping. The *Back to Sleep* campaign began in 1994 (National Institutes of Health, 2010). Since then, the incidence of SIDS has continued to drop steadily in the United States—from 130.3 deaths in 1990 to 39.7 deaths per 100,000 live births in 2013. Despite this decrease, there is still an ethnic difference in incidence with American Indians having a rate of 213.3 deaths compared to 53.8 deaths for Hispanics (CDC, 2015). More recent research has focused on an increased risk with parental use of alcohol (Phillips, Brewer, & Wadensweiler, 2010), possible deficits in serotonin and tryptophan hydroxylase causing increased risk for SIDS (Duncan et al., 2010), and an abnormality in the hippocampal area of the brain that helps control body temperature, heart rate, and breathing (Trachtenberg, Haas, & Krous, 2012). Current recommendations from the American Academy of Pediatrics (2011) include continuing the *Back to Sleep* campaign and advising parents to always:

- Place their sleeping infants in a supine position (not on side or stomach)
- Use a firm sleeping surface (no pillows or quilts under the baby)
- Keep soft objects (e.g., stuffed animals) and loose bedding (e.g., extra quilts, positioners/wedges, bumper pads, or loose bedding) out of baby's crib
- Not smoke during pregnancy and avoid baby's exposure to secondhand smoke
- Not share the bed with baby—put baby in a separate crib or bassinet with parents in the same room
- Offer a pacifier at sleep time throughout the 1st year of life (it has been shown to reduce the risk of SIDS)
- Avoid overheating (keep room temperature comfortable for lightly clothed adults—do not overbundle babies or cover their heads)
- Encourage "tummy time" to aid in development and reduce incidence of positional plagiocephaly (uneven, flat head)
- Avoid the use of apnea monitors (not shown to be effective) and other commercial devices marketed as effective in reducing SIDS cases (not sufficient proof of efficacy)

AAP also recommends that infants get all recommended vaccinations and that mothers breast-feed babies. Do your community health clients put their babies to sleep on their backs? If not, how can you convince them that it is beneficial?

looking only at the state of California, found that raising the legal smoking age to 21 would yield an 82% drop in prevalence in teen smoking and would save $24 billion over 50 years' time (Ahmad, 2005b). Taxes are another disincentive for smokers. California raised excise taxes on cigarettes in 1999, but Ahmad (2005c) used another computer simulation to reveal that an additional "20% tax-induced cigarette price increase would reduce smoking prevalence from 17% to 11.6% ... and reduce smoking-related medical costs by $188 billion" (p. 276). Raising cigarette taxes again would both decrease the number of smokers and increase the tax revenue that could be used

to further reduce smoking in California. However, other effective methods of reducing cigarette smoking exist. Levy et al. (2005) noted that smoking prevalence declined between 1997 and 2003, and, although most of the change could be explained by price increases, researchers also found that clean air laws, widespread media campaigns, and more easily accessible smoking cessation interventions also played a part. They encouraged lawmakers to continue with tax increases and to strengthen clean air laws that ban smoking in public places. In a Minnesota study, smoke-free workplaces were found to be more effective than free nicotine replacement therapy

(Ong & Glantz, 2005). Other researchers have found that antismoking advertising focusing on the addictive nature of cigarettes and the dangers of environmental tobacco smoke to children increased the chances of quitting among adult smokers who have children living in their homes (Netermeyer, Andrews, & Burton, 2005). Consistent and wide-ranging antismoking media campaigns that emphasize social unacceptability and easier access to smoking cessation classes were also emphasized to policy makers (Alamar & Glantz, 2006). A study by nursing researchers found that culturally specific smoking cessation outreach approaches were helpful in motivating rural smokers living in the southeastern United States (Butler et al., 2014).

Another group of nursing researchers examined the use of smokeless tobacco, both alone and in conjunction with cigarette use among blue-collar workers in a national survey of drug use and health (Noonan & Duffy, 2014). Almost 10% of survey respondents currently used smokeless tobacco, and just over 5% of them used it exclusively. The remainder used both forms of tobacco. They examined the factors that were also related to sole use of smokeless tobacco and found that current reported binge drinking, use of marijuana, marital status, age, gender, and race/ethnicity were common, along with type of blue-collar job. For those who used both smokeless tobacco and cigarettes, similar factors were also discovered, but illicit drug use and cigar smoking, rather than use of marijuana, were discovered. Workplace cessation programs were recommended for this population.

Community Health Nursing Practice

A primary purpose for conducting community health research is to gain new knowledge that will improve health services and promote the public's health. Consequently, most nursing research has implications for nursing practice. Many studies focus on a specific health need or at-risk population and then suggest nursing actions to be taken based on study findings. An example is a study examining HIV health education strategies and community outreach to rural Hispanic populations living along the U.S.–Mexico border. Hernandez, Mata, Provencio Vasquez, and Martinez (2014) assessed needs of rural health clinics for linguistically and culturally suitable health education materials. The goal was to integrate education, screening, and referral during routine clinic appointments in order to better address HIV and sexually transmitted infections in this vulnerable and often underserved population. Researchers felt that this addressed health equity and translated local research findings that would improve services and practice. DeGuzman and Kulbok (2012) offer a framework for nurses interested in studying the built population and its impact on vulnerable populations. The framework added to Florence Nightingale's original work on environment and health, and adapted frameworks dealing with social determinants of health and environmental health promotion to better fit with public health nursing research. They encouraged PHNs to conduct research in this area to "gain valuable insight into the pathways linking built environment to health of vulnerable populations" (p. 341), as more evidence is necessary to advocate for policy changes and improve the health of populations. Individual-level measures are not thought to be as effective as population-based approaches in improving the health of a nation (Abbot, 2015). Other issues that can be individual or population-based include obesity, physical activity, vaccinations, and communicable diseases.

Nursing's Professional Status and Influence

The third way in which research has a significant impact on community health nursing is in its potential to enhance nursing's status and influence. As community health nursing research sheds light on the critical health needs of at-risk populations, exposes deficiencies in the health care system, demonstrates more efficient and cost-effective methods for delivering services, and documents the effectiveness of nursing interventions, the profession will gain a stronger voice and have a greater impact on health policy and programs. After all, PHNs have always been advocates for their clients and promoted policies that improved health.

A recent example of CBPR assessed tribal youth physical activity and programming among an American Indian tribe of 1,000 people (Perry & Hoffman, 2010). **Community-based participatory research (CBPR)** is defined as research done in communities in which those persons affected by the condition or issue of interest and other key community stakeholders have an opportunity to participate fully in each phase of the research study—from conception to design and during execution, analysis, and interpretation, as well as formulation of conclusions and communication of results, they actively and equally share in decision-making power (Kulbok, Thatcher, Park, & Meszaros, 2012; NIH, n.d.; Perry & Hoffman, 2010). These community health nurse researchers recognized the inherent mistrust of university researchers among tribal communities and spent considerable time establishing relationships and discussing ideas with tribal members. Because this research involved children and adolescents, they engaged the Tribal Youth Council, as well as the adult Tribal Council, and established a Community Advisory Board to help them design their study. This board met an average of twice monthly for 8 months. They produced a data-sharing agreement that specified the type of data and how it would be collected, along with how to protect confidentiality of the data and who would have access to the data (Perry & Hoffman, 2010). They also collaborated on development of a questionnaire to collect information on favorite and least favorite exercise, motivators and barriers to exercise, and some demographic questions. They also designed two focus groups (one with 8- to 11-year-olds and another with 15- to 18-year-olds) to determine types and amounts of daily physical activity, as well as preferences and ideas to promote physical activity among the youth. The goal of the research project was to determine tribal youths' current patterns of behavior patterns, beliefs, and preferences related to physical activity. Results showed that youth "differentiated exercise and sports" and had different barriers and motivators for each (p. 111). They saw exercise as "work" that could improve mood and health and stabilize their weight, along with improving strength and conditioning. None of the tribal youth met the national recommendations for physical activity (60 minutes of moderate to vigorous physical activity daily), and they were less active, on average, than youth in national studies. They reported spending 50% of their day in "sedentary activities" (p. 111) and cited motivators for physical activity to be coaches, friends, team, and school. Barriers were deemed to be lack of time, lack of programs, and school and/or work. The results were presented to the tribe, and much discussion ensued. The tribe began boys' and girls' basketball groups and planned for additional baseball and wrestling teams. They are exploring other alternatives to promote physical activity (e.g., family days to teach traditional games, building walking trails) and felt that they had ownership of this research and their destiny. The researchers respected "tribal knowledge, traditions, and beliefs"—a theme of CBPR and of public health nursing—while helping to provide effective solutions to potential health problems.

Strong documentation supports the effectiveness of community health nursing interventions. Nurses in the community setting must provide empirical proof of their worth as professionals while serving the needs of their clients. This kind of information must be made visible if it is to influence legislators, planners, administrators, and other decision-makers in health care (Hinshaw & Grady, 2011). As visibility increases, nursing's status and influence will increase.

THE COMMUNITY HEALTH NURSE'S ROLE IN RESEARCH

Community health nursing has a focus on health promotion and disease prevention and providing services across the lifespan where people live, work, and learn. PHNs also focus on the development of community capacity building for health, and work with partnerships, coalitions, and policy makers to promote a healthier environment. Community health nurses have two important responsibilities with respect to research in community health: to apply research findings to practice (EBP) and to conduct or participate in nursing research. Because research results provide essential information for improving health policy and the delivery of health services, community health nurses must be knowledgeable consumers of research. That is, they need to be able to critically examine research reports and apply study findings to improve the public's health.

Community health nurses have many opportunities to apply the results of other investigators' research and systematic reviews, but a necessary prerequisite is to be informed about research findings. As an essential part of their role, community health nurses must read the journals focusing on public health and community health nursing. Subscribing to some of these journals enables nurses to make a regular review of research an ongoing part of their professional practice. Nursing agencies and employment sites in community health can encourage nurses to become more knowledgeable about research findings by subscribing to journals and circulating them among staff, by holding seminars to discuss recent research results, and by promoting nurses' application of research findings in their practice.

Although the amount of health nursing research is expanding, and its quality is improving, many more community health nurses need to conduct research and participate in EBP. An increasing number of nurses have developed skill in research through advanced preparation, and they are conducting investigations related to aggregate health needs. Other community health nurses work collaboratively with trained investigators on a variety of research projects affecting community health. Whether initiated by the nurse or involving the nurse as a team member, these projects are an opportunity to influence the types of research questions that are addressed and the ways in which the research is carried out, factors that ultimately affect the community's health (Kulbok et al., 2012).

VALUES AND ETHICS IN COMMUNITY HEALTH NURSING

Whereas the research process leads to EBP and expands nursing theory, there are other ways to develop knowledge in nursing. According to the classic treatise by Carper (1978), there is an art to nursing, which comes from our aesthetic sensibilities. Our personal history and experiences inform our practice, as well as our values and beliefs about what it means to be a good nurse. These values and beliefs support your own decisions about the right course of action to take, how to be just and fair in dealing with others, and what outcomes you deem to be right. Every profession has ethical codes that guide decision-making and provide a framework for thinking about practice issues that have a moral dimension. In this chapter, we consider the philosophical background for nursing ethics and discuss some of the recent issues that you may encounter in your community health nursing experiences that will stimulate your thinking about how you define your own philosophy of nursing.

For well over a decade, nurses have ranked highest in a Gallup poll for perceived honesty and ethical standards, beating out the clergy, physicians, and police officers (Gallup, 2016). Clearly, the public has a favorable impression of nursing as a profession that can be trusted. Nursing has had an ethical code for practice since 1910, when Gettner published "The Nightingale Pledge." This evolved into the current "Code of Ethics for Nurses," as the American Nurses Association (ANA) has updated the code to reflect current issues and ideologies. The latest revision was approved in 2015.

The Code of Ethics for Nurses is based on respect for persons. Respect for the dignity and value of each individual encompasses not only our patients but also our colleagues, our workplaces, and society at large. It also includes a mandate to respect the values and beliefs of each individual nurse. Because our personal experiences, our education, and our cultural and social values shape our beliefs, we have an obligation to think about those values that shape our practice. Having a greater awareness of our personal beliefs is a process called values clarification. This is an essential first step in a discussion of ethics, so that we have established moral beliefs, against which ethical dilemmas can be evaluated. As EBP is the result of the rigorous application of scientific method, our philosophy of nursing is based on clarity about our ethical code of practice, and a logical system for moral reasoning so

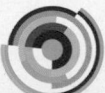
CODE OF ETHICS FOR NURSES—PROVISIONS, APPROVED AS OF JANUARY 6, 2015

The nurse, in all professional relationships, practices with compassion and respect for the inherent dignity, worth, and uniqueness of every individual, unrestricted by considerations of social or economic status, personal attributes, or the nature of their health problems.

1. The nurse respects the unique attributes of every person, practices with compassion and respect for each person's self-worth and dignity.

2. "The nurse's primary commitment is to the patient, whether an individual, family, group, community, or population" (p. v).

3. The nurse promotes, advocates for, and strives to protect the health, safety, and rights of the patient.

4. The nurse is responsible and accountable for individual nursing practice and determines actions consistent with the nurse's obligation to provide optimum patient care, with a focus on health promotion.

5. The nurse owes the same duties to self as to others, including the responsibility to preserve integrity and safety, to "maintain competence, and to continue personal and professional growth" (p. v).

6. The nurse is a key member of the team in maintaining and improving ethical environments for both patient care and the work of nursing in the provision of safe and quality care.

7. The nurse plays a leadership role in advancement of the profession through contributions to practice, education, administration, and knowledge development and most importantly the development of health policy and nursing policy.

8. The nurse works together with "other health professionals and the public" to protect and promote human rights and diminish health disparity and improve health diplomacy in the community and globally (p. v).

9. The profession of nursing, as represented by associations and their members, is responsible for articulating nursing values, for maintaining the reliability and integrity of the nursing profession and its practice, and for shaping social policy.

Adapted from American Nurses Association (ANA). (2015). *Code of ethics for nurses with interpretive statements.* Silver Spring, MD: Author.

that we are able to practice with integrity and within the context of social justice (ANA, 2015).

For the nurse in community health, the focus is on providing care for populations within our community of concern. This is a potential source for ethical conflict, when the needs of the individual must be evaluated in light of the needs of the larger group. There are social, political, and economic issues that must be separated out from the ethical concerns (ANA, 2010). Consider the following situations:

- Imagine, for example, that you are providing health care to a population of migrant farm workers whose housing lacks adequate toilets, bathing facilities, heating, and equipment for cooking and refrigerating food. You recognize that this is a valid health and safety issue. However, when you report the situation to your supervisor, you are told to ignore the conditions because the wineries that employ the workers contribute heavily to a high-profile clinic for all low-income children in your area. What would you do?

- What if you were working in a homeless shelter and were told to evict someone who would not agree to take a tuberculin skin test? You agree that residents should comply with this demand, but would you hesitate to implement the eviction if the resident were elderly or the teenage mother of a newborn?

Within the United States, many marginalized people are failed by the public health care system or may go without any health care at all. At the same time, affluent individuals enjoy a plethora of health care options, including preventive screenings and health promotion classes. For instance, seven surgical operations are the average for an American over their lifetime, and each year, approximately 5 million people will be admitted to an ICU in this country (Gawande, 2010; 2012). Community health nurses often are confronted by this disparity when making ethical decisions about client care. Social justice, human rights, and equality are hallmarks of public health nursing ethics (see more in Chapters 13, 25, and 29).

In addition to these dilemmas, progress in the United States often is linked to the exploitation of people in less-developed countries, and this contributes to widening disparities in health, wealth, and human rights. Distributive justice, or the fair allocation of goods and services, comes into play (discussed later in this chapter and in Chapter 29). Failure to respond to such global challenges only leads to greater poverty and deprivation, continuing conflict, escalating migration, and the spread of infectious disease, all further adding to our ethical dilemmas.

Advances in technology also contribute to ethical dilemmas. For example, electronic health records make client information readily accessible, thus raising issues of confidentiality, clients' rights, issues of empowerment, and informed consent (Vezyridis & Timmons, 2015). Sensitive information is now frequently stored electronically and may be accessed through unethical means (Widup, Bassett, Hylender, Rudis, & Spitler, 2015). Technology also forces nurses to confront the issues of genetic testing and stem cell research, as well as assisted suicide and euthanasia (Katz, 2015). Further ethical questions arise regarding organ, tissue, and limb transplants and the decisions about who is to receive them, as well as what happens to tissues removed during biopsy or surgery (Ertin, Harmanci, Mahmutoglu, & Basagaoglu, 2010). See Display 4–4. Ethical issues in nursing practice have been

---

DISPLAY 4–4 IMMORTAL CELLS, ETHICAL DILEMMA

How would you feel if tissues or cells taken from you during surgery or a routine biopsy were subsequently used in health research without your knowledge or permission (or remuneration)? That happened to Henrietta Lacks, a black woman from Baltimore, whose cells (known as HeLa cells) were the first immortal human cells and used in the development of the field of virology. HeLa cells were tested in the first space missions to determine zero gravity's effects and were vital to the development polio and hepatitis B vaccines, as well as chemotherapy, in vitro fertilization, cloning, and gene mapping (Skloot, 2011). These cells, taken from a biopsy of her cervix a few months before she died of cervical cancer in 1951, were useful in the development of medications for leukemia, herpes, hemophilia, and influenza. They have been used in innumerable studies around the world, to test the effects of massive radiation (e.g., nuclear blasts), hormones, vitamins, steroids, TB, salmonella, and hemorrhagic fever. HeLa cells were also instrumental in many historic scientific discoveries (e.g., cigarettes caused lung cancer, how cancer cells grew differently from normal cells, how HIV infected cells) and continue to be used today in scientific research. Although this happened in the 1950s, today, it is still often considered legal for a researcher to use tissues removed from your body for scientific research without your consent. It has been considered by law to be "abandoned waste" and may be used for gain without the knowledge, consent, or reimbursement to the donor.

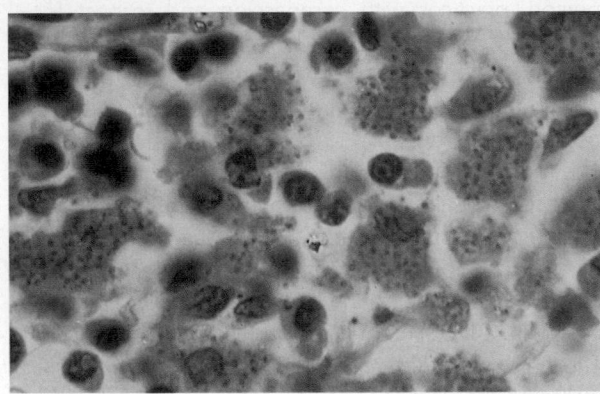

From Skloot, R. (2011). The immortal life of Henrietta Lacks. New York, NY: Random House/Broadway Books.

---

described as a "moving picture," with challenges, values, and obligations continually being questioned (Izumi, Nagae, Sakurai, & Inamura, 2012).

Underlying every issue and influencing every ethical and professional decision are *values*. Ethics and values are inextricably intertwined in professional decision-making, because values are the criteria by which decisions are made.

VALUES

What are values? A **value** is something that is perceived as desirable or a personally held abstract belief about the worth and truth associated with behaviors, thoughts, or objects (Guido, 2013). A value motivates people to behave in certain ways that are personally or socially preferable. Values are usually derived from societal norms, as well as from family and/or religious beliefs. We develop our value system as a result of our experiences with others (e.g., family, peers, schools, churches, jobs). As seen in Chapter 5, a group's culture often is defined by its members' common or shared values.

STANDARDS FOR BEHAVIOR

In general, values function as standards that guide actions and behavior in daily situations or act as a code of conduct for living one's life. Once internalized by an individual, a value, such as honesty, becomes a criterion for that individual's personal conduct. Values may function as criteria for developing and maintaining attitudes toward objects and situations or for justifying a person's own actions and attitudes. Values also may be the standard by which people pass moral judgments on themselves and others (Guido, 2013).

Values have a long-term function in giving expression to human needs. Values motivate people in their work setting, in their personal lives, and in dealing with their health, as well as with the larger society. In addition, values are used as standards to guide presentation of the self to others, to ascertain personal morality and competency, and to persuade and influence others by indicating which beliefs, attitudes, and actions of others are worth trying to reinforce or change. As a practitioner, values act as a compass to direct the nurse when working with clients.

QUALITIES OF VALUES

The nature of values can be described according to five qualities: endurance, hierarchical arrangement, prescriptive–proscriptive belief, reference, and preference.

Endurance

Values remain relatively stable over time, persisting to provide continuity to personal and social existence. Enduring religious beliefs, for example, offer stability to many people. This is not to say that values are completely stable over time; values do change throughout a person's life. Certainly, the values of children are different from adults. Moral development generally follows a prescribed path, according to Lawrence Kohlberg (Colby & Kohlberg, 1987) and Carol Gilligan (1982), researchers studying changes in moral behavior and judgment from childhood to adulthood. Yet social existence in the community requires standards within the individual as well as an agreement about standards among groups of individuals (Pereira, 2015). As Kluckhohn (1951, p. 400) once pointed out, without values, "the functioning of the social system could not continue to achieve group goals; individuals … could not feel within themselves a requisite measure of order and unified purpose." A group's culture provides such a set of enduring values. By adding an element of collective purpose in social life, values most often guarantee endurance and stability in social existence.

Hierarchical System

Isolated values usually are organized into a hierarchical system in which certain values have more weight or importance than others. For instance, in a team sport such as baseball, values regarding individual performance, batting and running records, speed, and throwing and catching all fall into a hierarchy, with the values of team and winning being at the top. As an individual confronts social situations throughout life, isolated values learned in early childhood come into competition with other values, requiring a weighing of one value against another. Concern for others' welfare, for instance, competes with self-interest. Through experience and maturation, the individual integrates values learned in different contexts into systems in which each value is ordered relative to other values (Harris, 2011; Iacobucci, Daly Luindell, & Griffin, 2012).

Prescriptive–Proscriptive Beliefs

Rokeach (1973) described values as a subcategory of beliefs. He argues that some beliefs are *descriptive* or capable of being true or false (e.g., the chair on which I am sitting will hold me up). Other beliefs are *evaluative*, involving judgments of good and bad (e.g., that was an excellent lecture). Still other beliefs are *prescriptive–proscriptive*, determining whether an action is desirable or undesirable (e.g., this music is too loud, those baseball fans shouldn't yell when the pitcher is winding up). Values, Rokeach says, are prescriptive–proscriptive beliefs. They are concerned with desirable behavior or "what ought to be." For example, parents' values about child behavior determine how they choose to discipline their children, using corporal punishment, a time-out, or a laissez-faire attitude where behavior is largely ignored. Some parents believe that their 2-year-old child has the capacity to control his bladder, and when the child wets his pants, he is being "rebellious" and should be punished. Values have cognitive, affective, and behavioral components. According to Rokeach, to have a value, it is important to know the correct way to behave or the correct end state for which to strive (cognitive component); to feel emotional about it—to be affectively for or against it (affective component); and to take action based on it (behavioral component). More recent research has further delineated moral regulation within the framework of avoidance versus approach motivation (Else-Quest, Higgins, Allison, & Morton, 2012; Sheikh & Janoff-Bulman, 2010). For example if you used duty as a basis for action, these would be proscriptive moral emotions. Duty is a consequential emotion, where you would think about concrete negative consequences to an action. For

example, what would happen if you did not study well for an exam in nursing school? Prescriptive moral emotions might focus more abstractly and in a positive manner on what ought to be done; these might inspire you to study so that you can be a "crackerjack" nurse at the bedside. Think about which beliefs or values (prescriptive/proscriptive) inspire you to do well in nursing school (Cornwall & Higgins, 2015).

Reference

Values also have a reference quality. That is, they may refer to end states of existence called **terminal values**, such as spiritual salvation, peace of mind, or world peace, or they may refer to modes of conduct called **instrumental values**, such as confidentiality, keeping promises, and honesty. The latter can have a moral focus or a nonmoral focus, and these values may conflict (Husted, Scotto, Husted, & Wolf, 2015).

For example, a nurse may experience a conflict between two moral values, such as whether to act honestly (tell a client about a fatal diagnosis) or to act respectfully (honor the family's request not to tell the client). Similarly, the nurse may experience conflict between two nonmoral values, such as whether to plan logically (design a traditional group intervention for mental health clients) or to plan creatively (design an innovative field experience). The nurse also may experience conflict between a nonmoral value and a moral value, such as whether to act efficiently or to act fairly when establishing priorities for funding among community health programs. Ethical reasoning in nursing develops over time, as novice nurses are exposed to various situations. Students and novice nurses struggle to apply ethics, even when exposed to theoretical underpinnings. Although nurses may inherently have great moral courage, its use is limited because of lack of confidence in ethical decision-making in practice (Iacobucci et al., 2012; Laabs, 2012; Murray, 2010).

Adults generally possess only a few—perhaps no more than 20—terminal values, such as peace of mind or achievement. These are influenced by complex physiologic and social factors. The needs for security, love, self-esteem, and self-actualization, proposed by Maslow (1969), are believed to be the greatest influences on terminal values. Although an individual may have only a few terminal values, the same person may possess as many as 50 to 75 instrumental values. Any single instrumental value, or several instrumental values combined, also may help to determine terminal values. For example, the instrumental values of acceptance, taking it easy, living 1 day at a time, and not being concerned about the future can shape the terminal value of peace of mind, whereas the instrumental values of hard work, driving oneself to compete, and not letting anyone get in the way can influence the terminal value of achievement. Figure 4–2 illustrates the influence of instrumental values and human needs on the development of terminal values.

Preference

A value may show preference for one mode of behavior over another, such as exercise over inactivity, or it may show a preference for one end state over another, such as physical fitness and leanness over sedentary lifestyle and

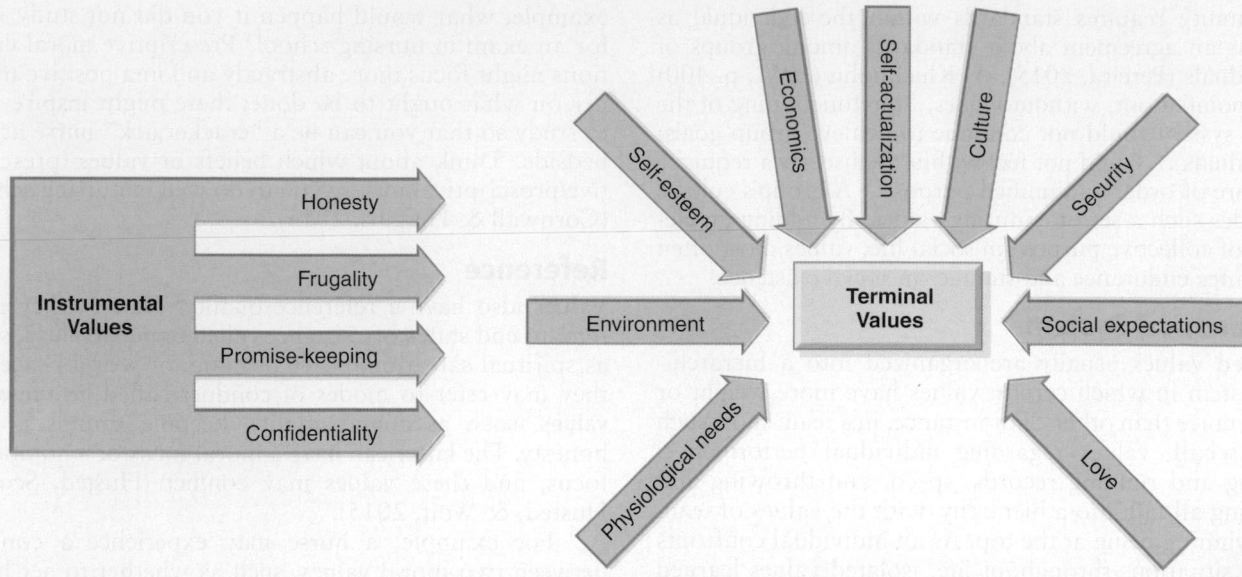

FIGURE 4–2 Factors influencing terminal values.

obesity. The preferred end state, or mode of behavior, is located higher in the personal value hierarchy.

VALUE SYSTEMS

Value systems generally are considered organizations of beliefs that are of relative importance in guiding individual behavior (Harris, 2011; Rokeach, 1973; Weiner, McConnell, Latella, & Ludi, 2013). Instead of being guided by single or isolated values, however, behavior at any point in time (or over a period of time) is influenced by multiple or changing clusters of values. Therefore, it is important to understand how values are integrated into a person's total belief system, how values assume a place in a hierarchy of values, and how this hierarchical system changes over time.

Hierarchical System of Values

Learned values are integrated into an organized system of values, and each value has an ordered priority with respect to other values (Harris, 2011; Rokeach, 1973; Wiener et al., 2013). For example, a person may place a higher value on physical comfort than on exercising. This system of ordered priority is stable enough to reflect the continuity of someone's personality and behavior within culture and society, yet it is sufficiently flexible to allow a reordering of value priorities in response to changes in the environment or social setting (e.g., society's emphasis on physical fitness and youth) or changes based on personal experiences (e.g., diagnosis of type 2 diabetes). Behavioral change would be regarded as the visible response to a reordering of values within an individual's hierarchical value system.

Conflict Between Values in a System

Nurses often enter patient and community situations that activate several values in their system of beliefs. Because not all of the activated values are compatible with one another, conflict between values occurs. This conflict between values is a part of the decision-making process,

and resolving these value conflicts is crucial to making good decisions. Community health nurses face such conflicts of values when caring for patients whose determinants of health create a situation where we must decide how to use of scarce resources for care (Blacksher, 2015). This can be a struggle when patients want the freedom to choose how to live their life but don't want to suffer either. One example is how the smoker with COPD wants home health visits but refuses to quit smoking. Even within a single community agency, nurses may find that they prioritize client service or programming values differently.

Some values seem to consistently triumph over others, persisting as stronger directives for individual behavior; an example is the value placed on high achievement in the United States. Providing quality health care for all without sacrificing the basic rights of a few is an ongoing ethical struggle for most people (Sorrell, 2012). Other values lose their positions of importance in a value hierarchy (e.g., resuscitation of all hospital patients vs. Do Not Resuscitate orders) (Fagerlin et al., 2013). It is this changing arrangement of values in a hierarchical system that determines, in part, how conflicts are resolved and how decisions are made. In this way, people's value systems function as a learned organization of principles and rules that help them to choose among alternative courses of action to reach decisions.

VALUES CLARIFICATION

One way to understand the influence and prioritize values in your own behavior, as well as in that of community health clients, is to use various values clarification techniques in decision-making. **Values clarification** is a process that helps to identify the personal and professional values that guide your actions, by prompting you to examine what you believe about the worth, truth, or beauty of any object, thought, or behavior and where this belief ranks compared with your other values. Because individuals are largely unaware of the motives underlying their choices, values clarification is important for understanding and shaping the kind of decisions people make. Only by understanding your values and their hierarchy can you ascertain whether your choices are the result of rational thinking or of external influences, such as cultural or social conditioning. Values clarification by itself does not yield a set of rules for future decision-making and does not indicate the rightness or wrongness of alternative actions. It does, however, help to guarantee that any course of action chosen by people is consistent and in accordance with their beliefs and values (Abhyankar, Bekker, Summers, & Velikova, 2011).

Process of Valuing

Before values clarification can take place, it must be understood how the process of valuing occurs in individuals. In 1977, Uustal listed the following seven steps, which remain useful today:

1. Choose the value freely and individually.
2. Choose the value from among alternatives.
3. Carefully consider the consequences of the choice.
4. Cherish or prize the value—feel good about the choice.
5. Publicly affirm the chosen value.
6. Incorporate the value into behavior, so that it becomes a standard or a pattern of behavior.
7. Consciously use the value in decision-making.

These steps provide specific actions for the discovery and identification of people's values. They also assist the decision-making process by explicating the process of valuing itself. For example, some people may choose to value honesty in a presidential candidate. They may choose this over other values, such as knowledge of foreign affairs or public speaking ability, because, when considering the consequences, they want a leader who will deliver on promises made and who will continue to be the person represented to the public during the campaign. They prize this value of honesty, affirm it publicly, and consciously use it as a standard when deciding on whom to vote into office or to reject.

Values Clarification Strategies

In 1978, Uustal offered several values clarification strategies that are ultimately useful to the decision-making process in community health nursing practice today. Strategy 1 is a way for nurses to come to know themselves and their values better (Fig. 4–3). Strategy 2 assists in discovering value patterns and the priority of values within personal value systems (Fig. 4–4). Strategy 3 can be used to examine personal responses to selected issues in nursing practice. Each response helps to establish priorities of values by asking the nurse to choose among the alternatives presented or to indicate degree of agreement or disagreement (Fig. 4–5). Other values clarification strategies are included in the critical thinking activities at the end of this chapter to assist in understanding personal ordering of values and when considering directions for change. These strategies also help the nurse to assist community health clients to become clearer about their own values.

All of these strategies can be used to analyze and understand how values are meaningful to people and ultimately influence their choices and behavior. Clarification

of a person's values is the first step in the decision-making process, and it affects the ability of people to make ethical decisions. Values clarification also promotes understanding and respect for values held by others, such as community health clients and other health care providers. As pointed out by Uustal (1977, p. 10), "Nurses cannot hope to give optimal, sensitive care to any patient without first understanding their own opinions, attitudes,

---

Name Tag

Take a piece of paper and write your name in the middle of it. In each of the four corners, write your responses to these four questions:

1. What two things would you like your colleagues to say about you?
2. What single most important thing do you do (or would you like to do) to make your nurse–client relationships positive ones?
3. What do you do on a daily basis that indicates you value your health?
4. What are the three values you believe in most strongly?

In the space around your name, write at least six adjectives that you feel best describe who you are.

Take a closer look at your responses to the questions and to the ways in which you described yourself. What values are reflected in your answers?

FIGURE 4–3 Values clarification strategy 1.

Patterns

Which of the following words describe you? Draw a circle around the seven words that best describe you as an individual. Underline the seven words that most accurately describe you as a professional person. (You may circle and underline the same word.)

ambitious   reserved   assertive   opinionated

concerned   generous   independent

easily hurt   outgoing   reliable   indifferent

capable   self-controlled   fun-loving

suspicious   solitary   likable   dependent

intellectual   argumentative   dynamic   unpredictable

compromising   thoughtful   affectionate   obedient

logical   imaginative   self-disciplined

moody   easily led   helpful   slow to relate

Reflect on the following questions:

1. What values are reflected in the patterns you have chosen?
2. What is the relationship between these patterns and your personal values?
3. What patterns indicate inconsistencies in attitudes or behavior?
4. What patterns do you think a nurse should cultivate?

FIGURE 4–4 Values clarification strategy 2.

Forced Choice Ranking

How do you order the following alternatives by priority? (There is no correct set of priorities.) What values emerge in response to each question?

1. With whom on a nursing team would you become most angry? The nurse who
   _____ never completes assignments.
   _____ rarely helps other team members.
   _____ projects his or her feelings on clients.

2. If you had a serious health problem, you would rather
   _____ not be told.
   _____ be told directly.
   _____ find out by accident.

3. You are made happiest in your work when you use
   _____ your technical skills in caring for adults with complex needs.
   _____ your ability to compile data and arrive at a nursing diagnosis.
   _____ your ability to communicate easily and skillfully with clients.

4. It would be most difficult for you to
   _____ listen to and counsel a dying person.
   _____ advise a pregnant adolescent.
   _____ handle a situation of obvious child abuse.

FIGURE 4–5 Values clarification strategy 3.

---

and values." This values clarification process provides a backdrop for next exploring the role of values in ethical decision-making. Values clarification has also proven helpful with clients. A recent study in patient choice of anticoagulant showed how this method could assist with clarity in drug choice (Palacio, Kirolos, & Tamariz, 2015). Focused values clarification exercises, as part of a package of decision aids (e.g., pamphlets, videos), for patients making treatment or screening decisions were found to improve knowledge of options/risks/benefits and promote decision-making in choosing the best anticoagulant for the patient's lifestyle and preferences.

ETHICS

Values are central to any consideration of ethics or ethical decision-making. Yet, it is not always obvious at first what constitutes an ethical problem in health care or in the practice of community health nursing. Most nurses easily recognize the moral crisis in some kinds of decisions—for example, whether to let seriously deformed newborn infants die, whether to terminate pregnancies resulting from rape, or whether to provide universal health care coverage. However, other, less obvious moral dilemmas often found in the routine practice of community health nursing are not always considered to be ethical in nature.

What is **ethics** and what is *ethical*? The *Merriam Webster Online Dictionary (2015)* defines **ethics** as "the principles of conduct governing a group" (para. 1). Ethics may also be viewed as a set of moral principles or a theory or system of moral values. Ethics are often idealized as "what ought to be." **Ethical decision-making**, then, means making a choice that is consistent with a moral code or

that can be justified from an ethical perspective. Of necessity, the decision-maker must exercise moral judgment. Remember that the term **moral** refers to conforming to a standard that is right and good. Community health nurses become "moral agents" by making decisions that have direct and indirect consequences for the welfare of themselves and others. **Bioethics** refers to using ethical principles and methods of decision-making in questions involving biologic, medical, or health care issues all while keeping the centrality of the patient to practice in the face of contemporary systems issues in care (Burkhardt, & Nathaniel, 2014). The next section examines how a PHN makes these moral decisions.

Public Health Ethics

Protection and promotion of health are at the core of public health nursing. Ethical principles are further clarified in this specialty area. Public health ethics is defined as "a systematic process to clarify, prioritize and justify possible courses of public health action based on ethical principles, values and beliefs of stakeholders, and scientific and other information" (CDC, 2016, para. 1). Specific ethical principles apply to public health in general (e.g., advocacy for healthy communities and equitable distribution of limited resources; balance between individual rights and the collective good) and public health nursing specifically (e.g., professional ethics). Preventing disease or harm, respecting individual rights, and encouraging community input are common values, as well as empowerment of the disenfranchised and equal access to resources. Promoting health, protecting confidentiality (except where justified), and collaborating or partnering with other community agencies are viewed as universal practices. Other principles include respecting diverse values/beliefs and working effectively with different cultural groups to enhance the social and physical environment while employing competent public health professionals. Public health is most often concerned distribution of resources and shaping behavior and thoughts, which may include resources such as clean water and constraints, such as quarantine. We need to keep in mind the responsibility of the world to global justice when implementing public health programs and policy (Jennings, 2015). Without care in global justice, there may be an uneasy balance between individual and public interests and rights.

A framework is applied in public health ethics inquiry. Three core functions of this inquiry include

1. Identifying and clarifying the ethical dilemma
2. Analyzing it in terms of alternative courses of action and their consequences
3. Resolving the dilemma by deciding which course of action best incorporates and balances the guiding principles and values (CDC, 2016, para. 5)

Identifying Ethical Situations

Ethics involves making evaluative judgments. To be ethically responsible in the practice of community health nursing, it is important to develop the ability to recognize evaluative judgments as they are made and implemented in nursing practice. Nurses must be able to distinguish between evaluative and nonevaluative judgments. Evaluative statements involve judgments of value, rights, duties, and responsibilities. Examples are "Parents should never strike their children" and "It is the duty of every citizen to vote." Among the words to watch for are verbs such as *want, desire, refer, should,* or *ought* and nouns such as *benefit, harm, duty, responsibility, right,* or *obligation.*

Sometimes, the evaluations are expressed in terms that are not direct expressions of evaluations but clearly are functioning as value judgments. Winland-Brown et al. (2015) provide useful clinical applications of the ANA code of ethics and refer to the obligations or duties of nurses to both patient and self (see "Code of Ethics for Nurses: Provisions"). Another important step is to distinguish between moral and nonmoral evaluations. **Moral evaluations** refer to judgments that conform to standards of what is right and good. Moral evaluations assess human actions, institutions, or character traits rather than inanimate objects, such as parks or architectural structures. They are prescriptive–proscriptive beliefs having certain characteristics separating them from other evaluations such as aesthetic judgments, personal preferences, or matters of taste. Moral evaluations also have distinctive characteristics (Brambilla & Leach, 2014):

- Morality and sociability impact social judgment. We want to be able to anticipate others' actions that could lead to benefit or harm or their skill and ability.
- Values possess universality or reflect a standpoint that applies to everyone. They are evaluations that everyone in principle ought to be able to make and understand, even if some individuals, in fact, do not.
- Moral evaluations avoid giving a special place to a person's own welfare. They have a focus that keeps others in view, or at least considers one's own welfare on a par with that of others.

Moral evaluations, like "parents should take care of their children," meet these criteria. A nonmoral evaluation, like "Mrs. X has five children," does not evoke a moral judgment of Mrs. X, but only an assessment of her family composition.

Resolving Moral Conflicts and Ethical Dilemmas

When judgments involve moral values, conflicts are inevitable. In clinical practice, the nurse may be faced with moral conflicts, such as the choice between preserving the welfare of one set of clients over that of others. For example, the nurse may have to choose whether to keep a promise of confidentiality to persons who are infected by HIV when these individuals continue to have unprotected sex with unknowing partners. Nurses may have to choose between protecting the interests of colleagues or the interests of the employing institution by reporting a nurse who makes phone visits rather than home visits, so that she can spend more time shopping online from work. They may have to decide whether to serve future clients by striking for better conditions or to serve present clients by refusing to strike. Often, nurses' values are at odds with their employers' values and procedures. The moral values of a nurse may conflict with the policies and practices of a particular bureaucracy, as nurses are taught that their clients (individuals, families, aggregates) are their focus of concern (Wright & Brajtman, 2011). Each decision involves a potential conflict between moral values and is called an **ethical dilemma**. An ethical dilemma occurs when morals conflict with one another, causing the nurse to face a choice with equally attractive or equally undesirable alternatives (Burkhardt & Nathaniel, 2014). If you are faced with two or more values of equal importance that will lead to different actions, then you are dealing with an ethical dilemma. It can create a decision-making problem, even in ordinary nursing situations.

Decision-Making Frameworks

To resolve ethical dilemmas or the conflict between moral values in community health nursing practice, and to provide morally accountable nursing service, several frameworks for ethical decision-making have been proposed. Among these frameworks, three key steps are considered as fundamental to choosing alternative courses of action that reflect moral reasoning: separate questions of fact from questions of value, identify both clients' and nurse's value systems, and consider ethical principles and concepts (see Fig. 4–6).

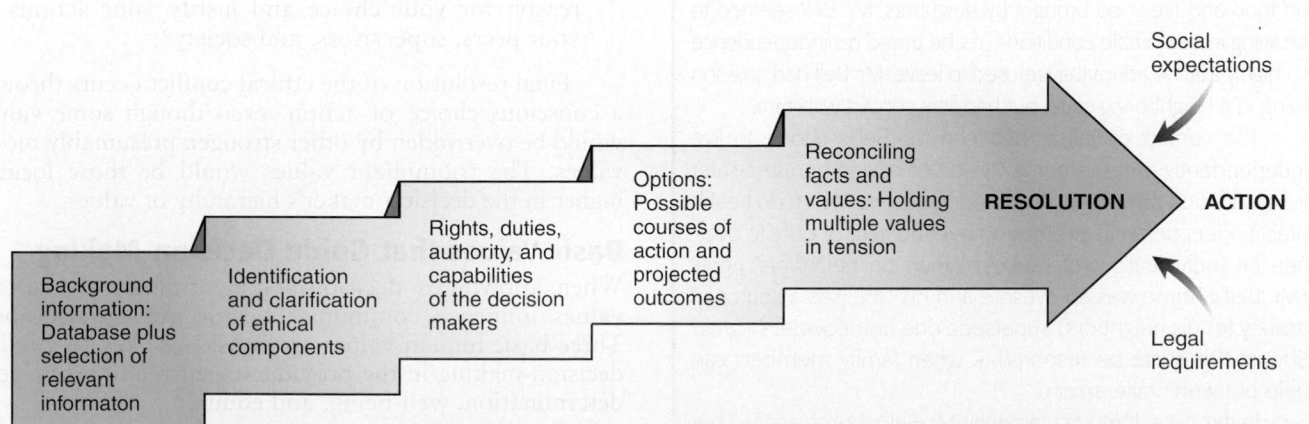

FIGURE 4–6 An ethical decision-making framework. Although legal requirements or social expectations may sway a decision one way or another, they are extrinsic to the ethical analysis and should not be confused with right and wrong. What is legal and what is expected are not necessarily right and wrong.

The identification of clients' values and those of other persons involved in conflict situations is an important part of ethical decision-making. In the example given in From the Case Files I, what are Mr. Bell's values? What are the values of neighbors who are concerned about him, but feel that they can no longer care for him? What are the nurse's values? What are the values of the nurse's employer? What are society's values?

An ethical decision-making framework referred to as the DECIDE model is initially useful in determining the problem and reviewing options. What is missing from this model is the patients' preference, a vital component (Park, 2012). For public health, patients' preference may be replaced with the harm versus benefit argument. The DECIDE model It includes the following steps:

D—*Define the problem (or problems)*. What are the key facts of the situation? Who is involved?

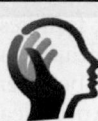

From the Case Files **I**

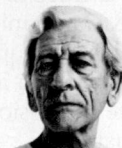

Mr. Bell

Community health nurses encounter value differences every day, and value differences, in turn, create ethical problems. Consider, for example, the dilemma faced by one nurse in Seattle on her first home visit to an elderly man, Mr. Bell, referred by concerned neighbors. This 82-year-old gentleman was homebound and living alone with severe arthritis under steadily deteriorating conditions. Overgrown shrubs and vines covered the yard and house, making access impossible except through the back door. A wood burning stove in the kitchen was the sole source of heat. The kitchen, along with a corner of the dining room, constituted Mr. Bell's living quarters. The remainder of the once-lovely three-bedroom home, including the bathroom, was layered with dust, unused. His bed was a cot in the dining room; his toilet, a 2-pound coffee can sitting under the cot. Unbathed, unshaven, and existing on food and firewood brought by neighbors, Mr. Bell seemed to be living in deplorable conditions. Yet he prized his independence so highly that he adamantly refused to leave. Mr. Bell had one son living in a neighboring state, but had little contact with him.

The conflict of values between Mr. Bell's choice to live independently and the nurse's value of having him in a safer living situation raises several ethical questions. When do health practitioners or family members have the right or duty to override an individual's preferences? When do neighbors' rights (Mr. Bell's home was an eyesore and his care was a source of anxiety for his neighbors) supersede one homeowner's rights? Should the nurse be responsible when family members can help but won't take action?

In this case, the nurse entering Mr. Bell's home applied her values of respect for the individual and his right to autonomy even at the risk of public safety. Not until he fell and broke a hip did he reluctantly agree to be moved into a nursing home.

What are their rights and duties and your rights and duties?

E—*Ethical review*. What ethical principles have a bearing on the situation, and which principle or principles should be given priority in making a decision?

C—*Consider the options*. What options do you have in the situation? What alternative courses of action exist? What help, means, and methods do you need to use?

I—*Investigate outcomes*. Given each available option, what consequences are likely to follow from each course of action open to you? Which is the most ethical thing to do?

D—*Decide on action*. Having chosen the best available option, determine a specific action plan, set clear objectives, and then act decisively and effectively.

E—*Evaluate results*. Having initiated a course of action, assess how things progress, and when concluded, evaluate carefully whether or not you achieved your goals.

Other frameworks can be used. The framework for ethical decision-making shown in Display 4–5 helps to organize thoughts and acts as a guide through the decision-making process. The steps help to determine a course of action, with heavy responsibility at the evaluation level: here the outcomes need to be judged and decisions repeated or rejected in future situations. Figure 4–6 summarizes several views in the field on ethical decision-making. This framework advocates keeping multiple values in tension before resolution of conflict and action on the part of the nurse. It suggests that value conflict is not capable of resolution until all possible alternative actions have been explored. Three tests may be helpful in your decision-making process (Edwards & Robey, 2010; Iserson, 1999):

● Impartiality test—Would you be willing to have this done to you? The "golden rule."
● Universalizability test—If every nurse in similar circumstances did the same as you, would you be comfortable with that "universal rule"?
● Interpersonal justifiability test—Can you state a reason for your choice and justify your actions to your peers, supervisors, and society?

Final resolution of the ethical conflict occurs through a conscious choice of action, even though some values would be overridden by other stronger, presumably moral values. The triumphant values would be those located higher in the decision-maker's hierarchy of values.

Basic Values that Guide Decision-Making

When applying a decision-making framework, certain values influence community health nursing decisions. Three basic human values are considered key to guiding decision-making in the provider–client relationship: self-determination, well-being, and equity.

Self-Determination

The value of **self-determination** or individual autonomy is a person's exercise of the capacity to shape and pursue personal plans for life. Self-determination is instrumentally

---

DISPLAY 4–5 A FRAMEWORK FOR ETHICAL DECISION-MAKING

Clarify the ethical dilemma: Whose problem is it? Who should make the decision? Who is affected by the decision? What ethical principles are related to the problem?

Gather additional data: Have as much information about the situation as possible. Be up to date on any legal cases related to the ethical question.

Identify options: Brainstorm with others to identify as many alternatives as possible. The more options identified, the more likely it is that an acceptable solution will be found.

Make a decision: Choose from the options identified and determine the most acceptable option, the one more feasible than others.

Act: Carry out the decision. It may be necessary to collaborate with others to implement the decision and identify options.

Evaluate: After acting on a decision, evaluate its impact. Was the best course of action chosen? Would an alternative have been better? Why? What went right and what went wrong? Why?

---

valued because self-judgment about a person's goals and choices is conducive to an individual's sense of well-being. Informed consent derives from self-determination. When one respects self-determination, it is based on the belief that better outcomes will result when autonomy is held in high regard. The outcomes that could be maximized by respecting self-determination or autonomy include enhanced self-concept, enhanced health-promoting behaviors, and enhanced quality of care. Self-determination is a major value in the United States, but does not receive the same emphasis in all societies or ethnic groups (Owens & Cribb, 2013; Soenens & Vansteenkiste, 2010).

In health care contexts, the desire for self-determination has been of such high ethical importance in U.S. society that it overrides practitioner determinations in many situations. Client empowerment is an approach that differs from the paternalistic approach to health care in which decisions are made for, rather than with, the client; instead, it enables patients and professionals to work in partnership (Cawley & McNamara, 2011). Many physicians and other health providers, including community health nurses, fail to recognize the high value attributed to self-determination by many consumers or the differences in views of self-determination among ethnic groups. The freedom of our patients must be respected and integrated into the matrix of health care decisions in any encounter or program (Risjord, 2014).

The conflict between provider and consumer may be broader. When self-determination deteriorates into self-interest, it poses a major roadblock to equitable health care. **Self-interest** is the fulfillment of one's own desires, without regard for the greater good. Consumers mostly have to fend for themselves when they encounter the world of for-profit health care, just as they do in other commercial markets, where "buyers beware" is the standard. This is well discussed in litigation against for-profit nursing homes as it looks at the impact of poor staffing on care, numerous citations, but no action taken in defense of the patients in the home (Harrington, Stockton, & Hooper, 2014).

When providing health care, self-determination and taking personal responsibility for health care decisions should be nurtured. This includes informing clients of options and the reasoning behind all recommendations. Yet self-determination and personal autonomy at times

are impermissible or even impossible. For example, society must impose restrictions on unacceptable client choices, such as child abuse and other abusive behaviors, or situations in which clients are not competent to exercise self-determination, as is true for certain levels of mental illness or dementia. There are two situations in which self-determination should be restricted: when some objectives of individuals are contrary to the public interest or the interests of others in society (e.g., endangering others with a communicable disease) and when a person's decision-making is so defective or mistaken that the decision fails to promote the person's own values or goals. When a person cannot fully comprehend the options, the consequences of actions related to the options, and the true costs and benefits, he may not have adequate capacity for making health care decisions. In these situations, self-determination is justifiably overridden on the basis of the promotion of one's own well-being or the well-being of others—another important value in health care decision-making (Kelly, 2013; Soenens & Vansteenkisrte, 2010).

Well-being

Well-being is a state of positive health. Although all therapeutic interventions by health care professionals are intended to improve clients' health and promote well-being, well-intended interventions sometimes fall short if they are in conflict with clients' preferences and needs. Determining what constitutes health for people and how their well-being can be promoted often requires knowledge of clients' subjective preferences. It is generally recognized that clients may be inclined to pursue different directions in treatment procedures based on individual goals, values, and interests. Community health nurses, who are committed not only to helping clients but also to respecting their wishes and avoiding harming them, must understand each client group's needs and develop reasonable alternatives for service from which clients may choose (see From the Case Files II). In addition, when individuals are not capable of making a choice, the nurse or other surrogate decision-maker is obliged to make health care decisions that promote the value of well-being. This may mean that the alternatives presented by the nurse for choice are only the alternatives that will promote well-being. With shared decision-making, the nurse seeks not only to understand

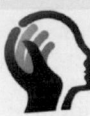

From The **Case Files** II

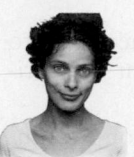

Andrea Vargas, PHN: A Family Living in Poverty

Contrasting value systems may be seen in many community health practice settings. Andrea Vargas, a community health nurse, experienced such a contrast on her first home visit to a family living in poverty. Referred by a school nurse for the children's recurring problems with head lice and staphylococcal infections, the family was living in a converted outbuilding on the outskirts of town. Although basically clean and orderly, nonetheless the living conditions were cramped, inadequate, and unsafe. Three hammocks were strung, stacked one upon the other, across the far corner of the room to accommodate the three younger children (out of a total of six). The older two children slept on the couch and the floor, while the baby slept with the single mother in the small bed. There was an old gas stove for cooking, and it was currently being used to heat the room, as the wall heater did not work. The mother did not know why it was no longer working. She seemed "stuck"—unable to muster the effort to talk with the landlord about the lack of a working heater. Even though using a gas stove to heat the room was dangerous (because of carbon monoxide), it seemed to her to be the easiest way to deal with the problem. Andrea knew that landlords were sometimes slow to respond to the needs of low-income renters and she saw this as unjust. The mother's main pleasure in life was watching soap operas on television, and Andrea felt that the mother seemed disinterested in trying to improve her circumstances. The nurse interpreted the situation through the framework of her own value system, in which health and safety were priorities, and justice was an instrumental value. Yet the mother, who might have shared those values in the past, appeared to prize pleasurable diversion, perhaps as a way to cope with her situation. In this instance, it is possible that environmental influences reordered the family's value system priorities. Rather than imposing her own values, Andrea chose to determine the priorities of the family, assess their needs, and begin where they were. Will she have a greater chance at success by doing this?

clients' needs and develop reasonable alternatives to meet those needs but also to present the alternatives in a way that enables clients to choose those they prefer. Well-being and self-determination are two values that are intricately related when providing community health nursing services (Jormfeldt, 2014; Rath & Harter, 2010).

Equity

The third value that is important to decision-making in health care contexts is the value of **equity** or justice, which means being treated equally or fairly. The principle of equity implies that it is unjust (or inequitable) to treat people the same if they are, in significant respects, unalike. In other words, different people have different needs in health care, but all must be served equally and adequately (Maiese, 2013). Equity generally means that all individuals should have the same access to health care according to benefit or needs (see Levels of Prevention Pyramid). However, effectively applying this value is often a complex enterprise and fraught with difficulties (McLeod, Blakelu, Kvizhinadze, & Harris, 2014).

The major problem with this definition of equity is, of course, that it assumes that an adequate level of health care can be economically available to all citizens. In times of limited technical, human, and financial resources, however, it may be impossible to fully respect the value of equity (Hussein, 2010; Karadag & Hakan, 2012). Choices must be made and resources allotted, while the value obligations of professional practice create conflicts of values that seem impossible to resolve. Many of these conflicts are reflected in current health care reform efforts that focus on access to services, quality of services, and ways to control rising costs. We also have many new genomics issues with access to care paramount in equity decisions (Rogowski, Grosse, Schmidtke, & Marckmann, 2014). The following list represents some of the most pressing aggregate health problems related to inequities in the distribution of and access to health and illness care facing patients worldwide.

- *Too many women go without preventive care.* The overall rate of infant mortality (all infant deaths before 1 year of age) is 5.1 per 1,000 in the United States, which is good news, as it is lower than previous rates. Although rates for infant mortality remain high, rates have declined among African Americans over the last few years, from 12.9 to 11.3 per 1,000 in the United States (Kaiser Family Foundation [KFF], 2015a). Native Hawaiian and other Pacific Islanders and Native American infant mortality rates have also declined—but all infant mortality rates among people of color are higher than those for White, non-Hispanic, and Hispanic Americans (5.1). Forty-nine percent of pregnancies in the United States during 2001 were unintended—among White and Hispanic females, 40% and 54%, respectively, were reported as unintended. But among African American females, 69% report unintended pregnancies. Poverty is strongly related to difficulty in accessing family planning services (Snow, Laski, & Mutumba, 2015) as are health care system factors (e.g., access), provider-related factors (e.g., similar culture), and patient preferences (Dehlendorf, Rodrigue, Levy, Borrero, & Steinauer, 2010).

- *Immunization rates for children entering kindergarten are an example of how public health works.* In most states, exemption rates are low, with Idaho having the highest exemption rates (CDC, 2015). Compliance with scheduled vaccines is high. Less than 1% of children between 19 and 35 months are unvaccinated. According to the CDC, "consistent, high coverage rates are needed to provide community immunity (herd immunity) and protect children from disease outbreaks like measles" (CDC, 2015, para. 7). Childhood immunization rate disparities have been dramatically reduced through multiple interventions and a strong infrastructure of vaccine services (Walker,

LEVELS OF PREVENTION PYRAMID

SITUATION: Provide distributive justice for battered women and children by changing a proposed state law that would eliminate funding for shelters for battered women and children to a law that preserves resources for this population.

GOAL: Using the three levels of prevention, negative health conditions are avoided or promptly diagnosed and treated, and the fullest possible potential is restored.

TERTIARY PREVENTION

Rehabilitation	Primary Prevention	
	Health Promotion and Education	*Health Protection*
If unable to stop the proposed law: • Seek volunteer services to fill the gaps in funding paid employees. • Seek donations to support existing shelter buildings.	• Educate the public regarding the need for lost/limited services using various forms of media and/or venues.	• Seek private resources or grants to fund shelters. • Propose a new bill to match private funding for shelters at the next legislative session.

SECONDARY PREVENTION

Early Diagnosis	Prompt Treatment
• Recognition that the proposed bill is going to pass	• Advocate for amendments to the proposed bill to preserve limited funding for shelters.

PRIMARY PREVENTION

Health Promotion and Education	Health Protection
• Advocacy • Active lobbying against the bill • Garnering community support in favor of the revised bill	• Community understand the impact of the potential loss • Put a "human face" on the problem

Smith, & Kolasa, 2014). The many interventions and programs implemented during this period, including Vaccines for Children (VFC), have built a successful infrastructure for vaccination services.

- *Vast disparities in immunization rates exist* for adults along racial and ethnic lines, as well as poverty level. Even with a number of health care encounters and socioeconomic factors controlled for in a study comparing non-Hispanic White and non-Hispanic Black influenza vaccination rates, the rate for Blacks was only 70% that of Whites (Liu, 2011).
- *The uninsured are likely to go without physician care.* Differences in access to expensive, discretionary procedures emerge according to health insurance status, race, and ethnicity, as well as other sociodemographic factors. The Affordable Care Act has helped to improve the numbers of previously uninsured in America from a high of 32 million without insurance, to current levels of 9 million people uninsured. Those who remain uninsured are the working poor. Over half of those without health insurance live at 200% below the poverty level White non-Hispanic Americans remain more likely to be insured than people of color (Kaiser Family Foundation, 2015b).
- *Environmental hazards threaten global health.* Global trade, travel, and changing social and cultural patterns make the population vulnerable to diseases that are endemic to other parts of the world, as well as to previously unknown diseases. The Ebola outbreak highlighted the need for better preparation for pandemics (DeMoro, 2014). Pollution of air, water, and soil to support industry contributes to pathogen mutations and threatens public health. Specific geological exposures to pathogens can also affect health, such as long-term arsenic exposure (Wardrop & LeBlond, 2015).
- *Equity is tied to social justice* (see below) and can be a difficult concept to truly grasp because we have difficulty understanding how our own privilege creates equity and, therefore, cannot see how those who lack what we have live in a socially *unjust world*. People are socialized to see the world through the eyes of their own experience. Once we can break that cycle of socialization and "unpack" how race, gender, income, education, age, and sexual identity influence equity and social justice, we then become allies to those who lack privilege. True equity occurs when we first understand our own privilege. Social justice happens when those who are seen as "other" are treated to the same equity as the historically privileged (Adams et al., 2013). See Display 4–6, Society and Individual Responsibility in Health Care.

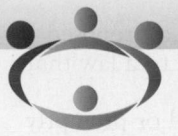

DISPLAY 4-6 SOCIETY AND INDIVIDUAL RESPONSIBILITY IN HEALTH CARE

To promote the achievement of equity, self-determination, and clients' well-being, certain conclusions drawn from the literature can enhance community health nursing practice (Badzek, Henaghan, & Turner, 2013; Blacksher, 2014; Holt & Convey, 2012). *Society has an ethical obligation to ensure equitable access to health care for all.* This obligation is centered on the special importance of health care and is derived from its role in relieving suffering, preventing premature death, restoring functioning, increasing opportunity, providing information about an individual's condition, and giving evidence of mutual empathy and compassion.

1. *The societal obligation is balanced by individual obligations.* Individuals ought to pay a fair share of the cost of their own health care and take reasonable steps to provide for such care when they can do so without excessive burdens.
2. *Equitable access to health care requires that all citizens can secure an adequate level of care without excessive burdens.* Equitable access also means that the burdens borne by individuals in obtaining adequate care ought not to be excessive or to fall disproportionately on particular individuals. Communities need to be empowered to address distribution problems.
3. *When equity occurs through the operation of private forces, there is no need for government involvement.*

However, the ultimate responsibility for ensuring that society's obligation is met—through a combination of public and private sector arrangements—rests with the federal government.

4. *The cost of achieving equitable access to health care ought to be shared fairly.* The cost of securing health care for those who are unable to pay ought to be spread equitably at the national level and should not fall more heavily on the shoulders of particular practitioners, institutions, or residents of different localities.
5. *Efforts to contain rising health care costs are important but should not focus on limiting the attainment of equitable access for the least-served portion of the public.* Measures designed to contain health care costs that exacerbate existing inequities or impede the achievement of equity are unacceptable from a moral standpoint. Aggregates in the community should be involved in planning and problem solving to increase the distribution of resources where those resources are most needed.

Badzek, L., Henaghan, M., & Turner, M. (2013). Ethical, legal, and social issues in the translation of genomics into health care. *Journal of Nursing Scholarship, 45*(1), 15–24.

Blacksher, E. (2014). *Public health ethics.* Retrieved from https://depts.washington.edu/bioethx/topics/public.html

Holt, J., & Convey, H. (2012). Ethical practice in nursing care. *Nursing Standard, 27*(13), 51–56.

Ethical Decision-Making in Community Health Nursing

The key values of self-determination, well-being, and equity influence nursing practice in many ways. The value of self-determination has implications for how community health nurses regard the following:

- The choices of clients
- Privacy
- Informed consent
- Diminished capacity for self-determination

The value of well-being has implications for how community health nurses seek to:

- Prevent harm and provide benefits to client populations
- Determine effectiveness of nursing services
- Weigh costs of services against real client benefits

The value of equity has implications for community health nursing in terms of its priorities for:

- Distributing health goods (macro allocation issues)
- Deciding which populations will obtain available health goods and services (microallocation issues)

Decisions based on one value means that this value often will conflict with other values. For example, deciding primarily on the basis of client well-being may conflict with deciding on the basis of self-determination or equity. How community health nurses balance these values may even conflict with their own personal values or the professional values of nursing as a whole. In these situations, values clarification techniques used with an ethical decision-making process may assist in producing decisions that promote the greatest well-being for clients without substantially reducing their self-determination or ignoring equity.

Ethical Principles

Based in utilitarianism and deontology, seven fundamental ethical principles provide guidance in making decisions regarding clients' care: respect, autonomy, beneficence, nonmaleficence, justice, veracity, and fidelity (Guido, 2013).

Respect

The principle of **respect** refers to treating people as unique, equal, and responsible moral agents. This principle emphasizes one's importance as a member of the community and of the health services team. To apply this principle in decision-making is to acknowledge community clients as valued participants in shaping their own and the community's health outcomes. It includes treating them as equals on the health team and holding them, as well as their views, in high regard (Guido, 2013).

Autonomy

The principle of **autonomy** means freedom of choice and the exercise of people's rights. Individualism and self-determination are dominant values underlying this principle (William Glasser Institute, 2010). As nurses apply this principle in community health, they promote individuals' and groups' rights to and involvement in decision-making. This is true, however, only so long as those decisions enhance these individuals' and groups' well-being and do not harm the well-being of others. When applying this principle, nurses should make certain that clients are fully informed and that the decisions are made deliberately, with careful consideration of the consequences (see From the Case Files III).

Beneficence

The ethical principle of **beneficence** means doing good or benefiting others. It is the promotion of good or taking action to ensure positive outcomes on behalf of clients (Burkhardt & Nathaniel, 2014). In community health, the nurse applies the principle of beneficence by making decisions that actively promote community clients' stated interests and their view of well-being (Husted et al., 2015). Examples might encompass the development of a seniors' health program that ensures equal access to all in the community who are in need, and the support of programs to encourage preschool immunizations.

Nonmaleficence

The principle of **nonmaleficence** means avoiding or preventing harm to others as a consequence of a person's own choices and actions (Burkhardt & Nathaniel, 2014).

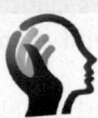

From the **Case Files** III

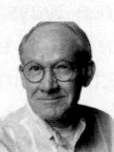

Tom Hardy, PHN: An Elderly Client Gives Up

Tom Hardy, PHN, has been assigned to monitor Mr. Jack, an elderly man who was diagnosed with TB (positive skin test, positive sputum and x-ray). Mr. Jack's wife unexpectedly died recently, and he is depressed and wants to "join her." He is not eating or sleeping much. He refuses to take TB medications, or his eight other medications for heart disease, thyroid insufficiency, type 2 diabetes, glaucoma, high cholesterol and triglycerides, and hypertension. He has consistently refused any of Tom's suggestions or assistance. He does not want to see a mental health counselor, and Tom wonders if he should continue to make home visits. He has a busy caseload and needs to focus on the most pressing cases. Mr. Jack's children feel that his depression and refusal of medications are a "temporary condition" in response to his wife's death and have asked for Tom's assistance in keeping their father healthy. Why is this an ethical dilemma? What are the ethical principles involved? What does Mr. Jack value? What are his children's values? What are Tom's values? Prioritize your values. What are the possible actions you could take?

This involves taking steps to avoid negative consequences. Community health nurses can apply this ethical principle in decision-making by actions such as encouraging physicians to prescribe drugs with the fewest side effects, promoting legislation to protect the environment from pollutants emitted from gasoline even if it raises prices, and lobbying for lower speed limits or gun controls to save lives.

Justice

The principle of **justice** refers to treating people fairly (Guido, 2013). It means the fair distribution of both benefits and costs among society's members. Examples might include equal access to health care, equitable distribution of services to rural as well as urban populations, not limiting the amount or quality of services because of income level, and fair distribution of resources—all of these draw on the principle of justice.

Within this principle are three different views on allocation, or what constitutes the meaning of "fair" distribution. One, **distributive justice**, says that benefits should be given first to the disadvantaged or those who need them most (see Levels of Prevention Pyramid). Decisions based on this view particularly help the needy, although it may mean withholding goods from others who may also be deserving, but less in need (e.g., food stamps). The second view, **egalitarian justice**, promotes decisions based on equal distribution of benefits to everyone, regardless of need (e.g., Medicare). The third, **restorative justice**, determines that benefits should go primarily to those who have been wronged by prior injustice, such as victims of crime or racial discrimination. Programs are in place to compensate victims for their injury or families for their loss—a beginning step to "restore justice." Another example includes the funds that were set up by several agencies, corporations, and groups to assist the families of the victims of the September 11, 2001, terrorist attacks. The principle of justice seeks to promote equity, a value that was discussed in the previous section.

Social justice refers to the fair and equitable distribution of wealth, economic opportunity, and access to privileges in society and is tied to human rights (Adams et al., 2013). The National Association of Social Workers (2011) describes social justice as the "view that everyone deserves equal economic, political and social rights and responsibilities." See Chapter 25 for more on social justice.

Veracity

The principle of **veracity** refers to telling the truth. Community clients deserve to be given accurate information in a timely manner. To withhold information or not tell the truth can be self-serving to the nurse or other health care providers and hurtful, as well as disrespectful, to clients. Truth-telling involves treating clients as equals, and it expands the opportunity for greater client involvement, as well as provides needed information for decision-making (Husted et al., 2015).

Fidelity

The final ethical principle, **fidelity**, means keeping promises. People deserve to count on commitments being met. This principle involves the issues of trust and trustworthiness (Brambilla, Rusconi, Sacchi, & Cherubini, 2011; Guido, 2013). Nurses who follow through on what they have said earn their clients' respect and trust. In turn, this influences the quality of the nurse's relationship with clients, who then are more likely to share information, which leads to improved decisions and better health. Conversely, when a promise (e.g., a commitment to institute child care during health classes) is not kept, community members may lose faith and interest in participation.

Ethical Standards and Guidelines

As the number and complexity of ethical decisions in community health increase, so too does the need for ethical standards and guidelines to help nurses make the best choices possible. The ANA's *Code for Nurses with Interpretive Statements* (2015) provides a helpful guide. Some health care organizations and community agencies, using the ANA code or a similar document, have developed their own specific standards and guidelines. For instance, the Public Healthy Leadership Society's veteran text, *Principles of the Ethical Practice of Public Health* (2002), guides both institutions and individual practitioners as they serve the public. More recently, the Association of State and Territorial Directors of Nursing (ASTDN, n.d.), a public health nursing organization, published a text on how to incorporate ethical principles into local health department processes and provide guidelines for the PHN role in eliminating health inequalities.

More health care organizations are using ethics committees or ethics rounds to deal with ethical aspects of client services (Guido, 2013). These committees are common in the acute care setting and in senior and long-term care settings, and they often focus on such issues as caregiving dilemmas involving practitioner negligence or poor client outcomes and the related health care decisions. In long-term care and home care settings, such a committee may consider conflicts in client care issues that involve family members. However, these committees also function in a variety of community health care settings. In public health agencies, cases of clients with complicated communicable disease diagnoses and health care provider concerns are discussed as they relate to policy, protocols, and the health and safety of the broader population.

S U M M A R Y

Implementation of EBP enables community health nurses to promote health and prevent illness among at-risk populations and to design and evaluate community-based interventions. EBP is essential to ensuring economical and effective interventions for our clients. Systematic reviews can provide direction for those who have developed a "burning clinical question." Finding accurate, complete information and critically appraising it is vital (see Evidence-Based Practice: Hand washing).

Research is defined as the systematic collection and analysis of data related to a particular problem or phenomenon. *EBP* is characterized as the use of best evidence, along with the nurse's clinical judgment and knowledge of patient's wishes, in making decisions about nursing practice and client outcomes. It encompasses the steps outlined in Display 4–1.

Systematic reviews are summaries of evidence usually compiled and analyzed by expert panels on a specific problem of interest, using predetermined criteria.

Research has a significant impact on community health and nursing practice in three ways. It provides new knowledge that helps to shape health policy, improve service delivery, and promote the public's health. It contributes to nursing knowledge and the improvement of nursing practice. And it offers the potential to enhance nursing's status and influence through documentation of the effectiveness of nursing interventions and broader recognition of nursing's contributions to health services.

Nurses must become responsible consumers of research, keeping abreast of new knowledge and applying it in practice. Nurses must learn to evaluate evidence critically, assessing the validity and applicability to their own practice. Nurses should search for current evidence and discuss EBP initiatives with colleagues and supervisors. More community health nurses must also conduct EBP implementation studies of their own or collaborate with other community health professionals in doing clinical research. A commitment to the use and conduct of research will move the nursing profession forward and enhance its influence on the health of at-risk populations.

Values and ethical principles strongly influence community health nursing practice and ethical decision-making. *Values* are lasting beliefs that are important to individuals, groups, and cultures. A value system organizes these beliefs into a hierarchy of relative importance that motivates and guides human behavior. Values function as standards for behavior, as criteria for attitudes, and as standards for moral judgments, and they give expression to human needs. The nature of values can be understood by examining their qualities of endurance, their hierarchical arrangement, and their function as prescriptive–proscriptive beliefs and by examining them in terms of reference and preference.

The nurse often is faced with decisions that affect client's values and involve conflicting moral values and ethical dilemmas. Understanding what personal values are and how they affect behavior assists

EVIDENCE-BASED PRACTICE
Hand washing

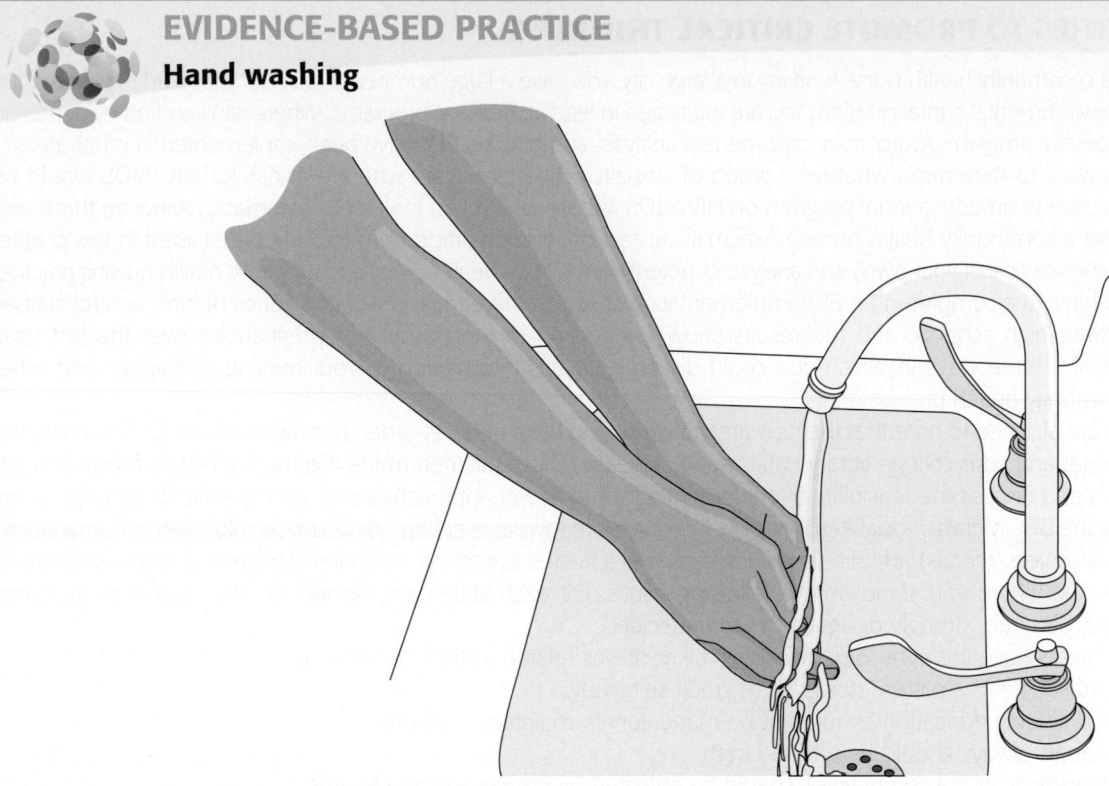

As nurses, we are taught the importance of hand washing. In nursing school, we are educated to wash our hands before and after patient care—it is often drilled into us. But, when you work in the community, you do not always have ready access to soap and water. Many PHNs choose to carry small bottles of hand sanitizer as a practical alternative to hand washing. Community-based research has confirmed the effectiveness of waterless alcohol-based hand sanitizers for new mothers living in areas without adequate water supplies and for reducing microbes on the soiled hands of farmworkers harvesting produce in the fields (deAceituno et al., 2015; Pickering, Boehm, Mwanjali, & Davis, 2010). It is also important to educate our patients, both at home and in acute care environments, about the importance of hand washing. Use of waterless wash and traditional hand washing are both effective (Sunni, Kennedy, Davis, Thompson, & Jones, 2014). Where would you go to find a systematic or integrative review of this subject? How would you go about presenting this information at a staff meeting to stimulate changes in policies and procedures?

the nurse in making ethical evaluations and addressing ethical conflicts in practice. Various strategies can guide the nurse in making these decisions; one example is values clarification, which clarifies what values are important. Several frameworks for ethical decision-making that include the identification and clarification of values impinging on the making of ethical decisions were discussed in this chapter.

Three key human values influence client health and nurse decision-making: the right to make decisions regarding a person's health (self-determination), the right to health and well-being, and the right to equal access and quality of health care. At times, these values are affected by the value of self-interest on the part of another person or a system. Seven fundamental principles guide community health nurses in making ethical decisions: respect, autonomy, beneficence, nonmaleficence, justice, veracity, and fidelity.

This chapter discusses current research as it relates to and impacts community health nursing practice. The steps of EBP are emphasized. The chapter includes information on constructing a clinical question and incorporating client considerations and clinical guidelines, as well as helpful resources for finding and analyzing research studies. Ethics and values are also examined, as they relate to both research and community health nursing practice. This chapter explores the nature and function of values and value systems, the role of values and value systems in ethical decision-making, the central values related to health care choices and their potential conflicts, and the implications of values and ethics for community health nursing decision-making and practice.

ACTIVITIES TO PROMOTE **CRITICAL THINKING**

1. As a community health nurse working in a large city, you have a large number of children with lead poisoning due to environmental contamination. You are interested in lead abatement programs. Where can you find evidence on successful programs/outcomes, cost–benefit analysis, and policies that have been implemented in other areas?

2. You want to determine whether a group of sexually active teenagers who are at risk for HIV/AIDS would be receptive to an educational program on HIV/AIDS. Where would you look for a systematic review on this topic?

3. Select a community health nursing systematic review or research article from the references listed in this chapter (or choose one of your own) and analyze its potential impact on health policy and on public health nursing practice.

4. You have just completed an EBP implementation study on the effectiveness of a series of birth control classes in three high schools, and the results show a reduction in the number of pregnancies over the last year. Describe three ways in which you could disseminate this information to your nursing colleagues and other community health professionals.

5. You are alarmed to note that the new area to which you have been assigned has high rates of TB. Searching the Internet and your college library databases to research this topic, determine the most effective forms of treatment and discuss the feasibility of implementing some newer approaches with your specific target population.

6. Take the BBC Morals–Social Responsibility Questionnaire (available at http://www.bbc.co.uk/science/humanbody/mind/surveys/morals) and discuss your results with a trusted classmate. How similar were your responses? Why?

7. Describe where you stand on the following issues. For each statement, decide whether you strongly agree, agree, disagree, strongly disagree, or are undecided:
   a. Clients have the right to participate in all decisions related to their health care.
   b. Nurses need a system designed to credit self-study.
   c. Continuing education should not be mandatory to maintain licensure.
   d. Clients always should be told the truth.
   e. Standards of nursing practice should be enforced by state examining boards.
   f. Nurses should be required to take relicensure examinations every 5 years.
   g. Clients should be allowed to read their health record on request.
   h. Abortion on demand should be an option available to every woman.
   i. Critically ill newborns should be allowed to die.
   j. Laws should guarantee desired health care for each person in this country.
   k. Organ donorship should be automatic unless a waiver to refuse has been signed.

8. In a grid similar to the one shown, write a statement of belief in the space provided and examine it in relation to the seven steps of the process of valuing. Areas of confusion and conflict in nursing practice that should be examined are peer review, accountability, confidentiality, euthanasia, licensure, clients' rights, organ donation, abortion, informed consent, and terminating treatment. To the right of your statements, check the appropriate boxes to indicate when your beliefs reflect one or more of the seven steps in the valuing process. Is your belief a value according to the valuing process?

9. Rank in order the following 12 potential nursing actions, using "1" to indicate the most important choice in a client–community health nurse relationship and "12" to indicate the least important choice:

Statement	Freely chosen	Alternatives	Consequences	Cherished	Affirmed	Incorporated	Employed
	1	2	3	4	5	6	7

_____ Touching clients
_____ Empathetically listening to clients

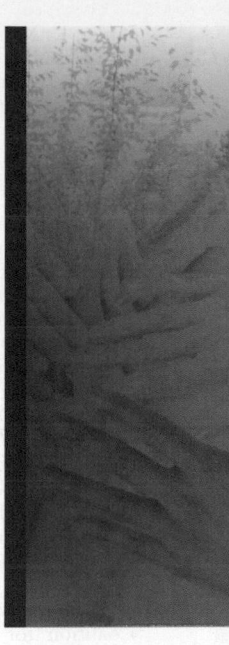

_____ Disclosing yourself to clients

_____ Becoming emotionally involved with clients

_____ Teaching clients

_____ Being honest in answering clients' questions

_____ Seeing that clients conform to professionals' advice

_____ Helping to decrease clients' anxiety

_____ Making sure that clients are involved in decision-making

_____ Following legal mandates regarding health practices

_____ Remaining "professional" with clients

_____ (Add an alternative of your own)

Examine your ordering of these options. What values can be identified based on your responses in this exercise? How do these values emerge in your behavior?

10. Request to attend one or two sessions of an ethics committee meeting of a community health agency or a local acute care hospital. Observe and make notes on (a) what values are evident in the discussion, (b) what ethical principles are used, (c) what decision-making framework is used, and (d) what you would have liked to contribute if you had been a member of the committee.

REFERENCES

Abbot, L. S. (2015). Evaluation of nursing interventions designed to impact knowledge, behaviors, and health outcomes for rural African-Americans: An integrative review. *Public Health Nursing, 32*(5), 408–420.

Abhyankar, P., Bekker, H., Summers, B., & Velikova, G. (2011). Why values elicitation techniques enable people to make informed decisions about cancer trial participation. *Health Expectations, 14*(Suppl 1), 20–32.

Adams, M., Blumenfeld, W., Castañeda, C., Hackman, H., Peters, M., & Zúñiga, X. (2013). *Readings for diversity and social justice* (3rd ed.). New York, NY: Routledge.

Ahmad, S. (2005a). Closing the youth access gap: The projected health benefits and cost savings of a national policy to raise the legal smoking age to 21 in the United States. *Health Policy, 75*(1), 74–84.

Ahmad, S. (2005b). The cost-effectiveness of raising the legal smoking age in California. *Medical Decision Making, 25*(3), 330–340.

Ahmad, S. (2005c). Increasing excise taxes on cigarettes in California: A dynamic simulation of health and economic impacts. *Preventive Medicine, 41*(1), 276–283.

Alamar, B., & Glantz, S. A. (2006). Effect of increased social unacceptability of cigarette smoking on reduction in cigarette consumption. *American Journal of Public Health, 96*(8), 1359–1363.

Albrecht, S., Kelly-Thomas, K., Osborne, J. W., & Ogbagaber, S. (2011). The SUCCESS program for smoking cessation for pregnant women. *Journal of Obstetric, Gynecologic, & Neonatal Nursing, 40*(5), 520–531.

AllAfrica. (2011, April 18). *Africa: Prevention drug trial disappoints.* Retrieved from http://allafrica.com/stories/201104190163.html

American Academy of Pediatrics (AAP). (2011). *AAP expands guidelines for infant sleep safety and SIDS risk reduction.* Retrieved from https://www.aap.org/en-us/about-the-aap/aap-press-room/pages/aap-expands-guidelines-for-infant-sleep-safety-and-sids-risk-reduction.aspx

American Nurses Association (ANA). (2010). *Nursing's social policy statement the essence of the profession.* Washington, DC: Author.

American Nurses Association (ANA). (2015). *Code for nurses with interpretive statements.* Washington, DC: Author.

Associated Press. (2006). *U.S. halts enrollment in major AIDS drug study.* Retrieved from http//www.msnbc.msn.com/id/10907973/print/1/displaymode/1098/

Association of State and Territorial Directors of Nursing (ASTDN). (n.d.). The public health nurse's role in achieving health equity: Eliminating inequalities in health. Position Paper. Author. Retrieved from http://www.astdn.org/downloadablefiles/ASTDN-health-equity-11-08.pdf

Association of Women's Health, Obstetric, and Neonatal Nurses (AWHONN). (2014). *Women's health and perinatal nursing care quality draft measures specifications.* Retrieved from https://www.awhonn.org/awhonn/content.do?name=02_PracticeResources%2F02_perinatalqualitymeasures.htm

Backonja, U., Royer, J. R., & Lauver, D. R. (2014). Young women's reasons to seek sexually transmitted infection screening. *Public Health Nursing, 31*(5), 395–404.

Badzek, L., Henaghan, M., & Turner, M. (2013). Ethical, legal, and social issues in the translation of genomics into health care. *Journal of Nursing Scholarship, 45*(1), 15–24.

Baker, D., Dang, M., Ly, M., & Diaz, R. (2010). Perception of barriers to immunization among parents of Hmong origin in California. *American Journal of Public Health, 100*(5), 839–845.

Barlow, J., Smailagic, N., Bennett, C., Huband, N., Jones, H., & Coren, E. (2011). Individual and group parenting for improving psychosocial outcomes for teenage parents and their children. *Campbell Systematic Reviews.* Retrieved from http://www.campbellcollaboration.org/library.php

Black, A. T., Baineaves, L. G., Garossino, C., Puyat, J. H., & Qian, H. (2015). Promoting evidence-based practice through a research training program for point-of-care clinicians. *Journal of Nursing Administration, 45*(1), 14–20.

Blacksher, E. (2014). *Public health ethics.* Retrieved from https://depts.washington.edu/bioethx/topics/public.html

Blacksher, E. (2015). *Public health ethics. Ethics in medicine.* Retrieved from https://depts.washington.edu/bioethx/topics/public.html

Blais, K. K., & Hayes, J. S. (2015). *Professional nursing practice: Concepts and perspectives* (7th ed.). Upper Saddle River, NJ: Pearson Prentice Hall.

Bradley, E. H., Curry, L., Horwitz, L. I., Sipsma, H., Wang, Y., Walsh, M. N., … Krumholz, H. M. (2013). Hospital strategies associated with 30-day readmission rates for patients with heart failure. *Circulation: Cardiovascular Quality and Outcomes, 6*, 444–450.

Brambilla, M., & Leach, C. (2014). On the importance of being moral: The distinctive role of morality in social judgment. *Social Cognition, 32*(4), 397–408.

Brambilla, M., Rusconi, P., Sacchi, S., & Cherubini, P. (2011). Looking for honesty: the primary role of morality (vs. sociability and competence) in information gathering. *European Journal of Social Psychology, 41*, 135–143.

Bryant, K., Haynes, T., Kim Yeary, K. H., Greer-Williams, N., & Hartwig, N. (2014). A rural African American faith community's solutions to depression disparities. *Public Health Nursing, 31*(3), 262–271.

Burkhardt, M., & Nathaniel, A., (2014). *Ethics & issues in contemporary nursing* (4th ed.). Stamford, CT: Cengage Learning.

Butler, K. M., Rayens, M. K., Adkins, S., Record, R., Langley, R., ..., Hahn, E.J. (2014). Culturally-specific smoking cessation outreach in a rural community. *Public Health Nursing, 31*(1), 44–54.

Canadian Nurse-Family Partnership Network. (2010). Implementing the NFP in Canada. *Canadian NFP Network,* 1(3), 1–2.

Carper, B. A. (1978). Fundamental patterns of knowing in nursing. *Advances in Nursing Science, 1*(1), 13–23.

Cawley, T., & McNamara, P. M. (2011). Public health nurse perceptions of empowerment and advocacy in child health surveillance in West Ireland. *Public Health Nursing, 28*(2), 1–9.

Centers for Disease Control and Prevention (CDC). (2013). *The Tuskegee timeline.* Retrieved from http://www.cdc.gov/tuskegee/timeline.htm

Centers for Disease Control and Prevention (CDC). (2015). *Sudden unexpected infant death and sudden infant death syndrome.* Retrieved from http://www.cdc.gov/sids/data.htm

Centers for Disease Control and Prevention (CDC). (2016). *Public health ethics.* Retrieved from http://www.cdc.gov/od/science/integrity/phethics/

Chaiyachati, K. H., Ogbuoji, O., Price, M., Suthar, A., & Barnighausen, T. (2014). Interventions to improve adherence to antiretroviral therapy: A rapid systematic review. *AIDS, 28*(Suppl 2), s187–s204.

Chassin, M., Loeb, J., Schmaltz, S., & Wachter, R. (2010). Accountability measures: Using measurement to promote quality improvement. *New England Journal of Medicine, 363*(7), 683–688.

Coalition for Evidence-Based Policy. (2015). *Social programs that work: Nurse-Family Partnership—top tier.* Retrieved from http://evidencebasedprograms.org/1366-2/nurse-family-partnership

Colby, A., & Kohlberg, L. (1987). The measurement of moral judgment: Theoretical foundations and research validation (Vol. 1). New York, NY: Cambridge University Press.

Conner, B. (2014). Differentiating research, evidence-based practice, and quality improvement. *American Nurse Today, 9*(6). Retrieved from http://www.americannursetoday.com/differentiating-research-evidence-based-practice-and-quality-improvement/

Coopersmith, S. (1967). *The antecedents of self-esteem.* San Francisco, CA: Freeman & Company.

Cornwall, J., & Higgins, T. (2015). Approach and avoidance in moral psychology: Evidence for three distinct motivational levels. *Personality & Individual Differences, 86,* 139–149.

Quad Council. (2011). *Quad Council competencies for public health nurses.* Retrieved from http://www.achne.org/files/quad%20council/quadcouncilcompetenciesforpublichealthnurses.pdf

Davis, M. V., Mahanna, E., Joly, B., Zelek, M., ..., Riley, W., Verma, P., & Fisher, J. S. (2014). Creating quality improvement culture in public health agencies. *American Journal of Public Health, 104*(1), e98–e104.

deAceituno, A. F., Bartz, F. E., Hodge, D. W., Shumaker, D. J., Grubb, J. E., Arbogast, J. W., ..., Leon, J. S. (2015). Ability of hand hygiene interventions using alcohol-based hand sanitizers and soap to reduce microbial load on farmworker hands soiled during harvest. *Journal of Food Protection, 78*(11), 2024–2032.

DeGuzman, P. B., & Kolbok, P. A. (2012). Changing health outcomes of vulnerable populations through nursing's influence on neighborhood built environment: A framework for nursing research. *Journal of Nursing Scholarship, 44*(4), 341–348.

Dehlendorf, C., Rodriguez, M., Levy, K., Borrero, S., & Steinauer, J. (2010). Disparities in family planning. *American Journal of Obstetrics and Gynecology, 202*(3), 214–220.

DeMoro, R. (2014). In it together. *National Nurse, 110*(5), 13–27.

Doren, D., Haynes, R., Kushniruk, A., Straus, S., Grimshaw, J., Hall, L., ..., Jedras, D. (2010). Supporting evidence-based practice for nurses through informational technologies. *Worldviews on Evidence-Based Practice, 7*(1), 4–15.

Douglas, M. R., Mallonee, S., & Istre, G. R. (1999). Estimating the proportion of homes with functioning smoke alarms: A comparison of telephone survey and household survey results. *American Journal of Public Health, 89*(7), 1112–1114.

Duncan, J. R., Paterson, D. S., Hoffman, J. M., Mokler, D. J., Borenstein, N. S., Belliveau, R. A., et al. (2010). Brainstem serotonergic deficiency in sudden infant death syndrome. *Journal of the American Medical Association, 303*(5), 430–437.

Durazo E., Jones, M., Wallace, S., Van Arsdale, J., Aydin, M., & Stewart, C. (2011, June). The health status and unique health challenges of rural older adults in California. *Health Policy Brief.* Retrieved from http://www.healthpolicy.ucla.edu/pubs/files/ruralolderadultspb.pdf

Eckenrode, J., Ganzel, B., Henderson, C., Smith, E., Olds, D. L., Powers, J., et al. (2000). Preventing child abuse and neglect with a program of nurse home visitation: The limiting effects of domestic violence. *Journal of the American Medical Association, 284*(11), 1385–1391.

Eckenrode, J., Zielinski, D., Smith, E., Marcynyszyn, L., Henderson, C., Kitzman, H., et al. (2001). Child maltreatment and the early onset of problem behaviors: Can a program of nurse home visitation break the link? *Developmental Psychopathology, 13*(4), 873–890.

Eckenrode, J., Campa, M., Luckey, D., Henderson, C., Cole, R., Kitzman, H., et al. (2010). Long-term effects of prenatal and infancy nurse home visitation on the life course of youths. *Archives of Pediatrics and Adolescent Medicine, 164*(1), 9–15.

Edwards, K. A., & Robey, T. (2010). Preparing for the unexpected: Teaching ER ethics. *Virtual Mentor, 12*(6), 455–458.

Else-Quest, N. M., Higgins, A., Allison, C., & Morton, L. C. (2012). Gender differences in self-conscious emotional experience: A meta-analysis. *Psychological Bulletin, 138*(5), 947–981.

Ertin, H., Harmanci, A., Mahmutoglu, F., & Basagaoglu, I. (2010). Nurse-focused ethical solutions to problems in organ transplantation. *Nursing Ethics, 17*(6), 705–714.

Fagerlin, A., et al. (2013). Clarifying values: An updated review. *BMC Medical Informatics & Decision Making, Supplement, 2*(13), S8.

Ferng, Y. H., Wong-McLoughlin, J., Barrett, A., Currie, L., & Larson, E. (2011). Barriers to mask wearing for influenza-like illnesses among urban Hispanic households. *Public Health Nursing, 28*(1), 13–23.

Fleming, R. (2011). Use of school nurse services among poor ethnic minority students in the urban Pacific Northwest. *Public Health Nursing, 28*(4), 308–316.

Food and Drug Administration (FDA). (2010, September 23). FDA significantly restricts access to the diabetes drug Avandia. *FDA News Release.* Retrieved from http://www.fda.gov/newsevents/newsroom/pressannouncements/ucm226975.htm

Food and Drug Administration (FDA). (2011, May 18). Avandia: REMS—risk of cardiovascular events. *FDA News Release.* Retrieved from http://www.fda.gov/Safety/MedWatch/SafetyInformation/SafetyAlertsforHumanMedicalProducts/ucm226994.htm

Gallup. (2016). *Honesty/ethics in professions.* Retrieved from http://www.gallup.com/poll/1654/honesty-ethics-professions.aspx

Gawande, A. (2010). *The checklist manifesto: How to get things right.* New York, NY: Metropolitan Books.

Gawande, A. (2012, August 13). Annals of health care: Big med. *The New Yorker.* Retrieved from http://www.newyorker.com/magazine/2012/08/13/big-med

Gilligan, C. (1982). *In a different voice.* Cambridge, MA: Harvard University Press.

Giovino, G. A., Chaloupka, F. J., Hartman, A. M., Gerlach Joyce, K., Chriqui, J., Orleans, C. T., et al. (2009). *Cigarette smoking prevalence and policies in the 50 states: An era of change—The Robert Wood Johnson Foundation impact Teen Tobacco Chart Book.* Buffalo, NY: State University of New York.

Glavin, K., Smith, L., Sorum, R., & Ellefsen, B. (2010). Supportive counseling by public health nurses for women with postpartum depression. *Journal of Advanced Nursing, 66*(6), 1317–1327.

Grant, H. S., Stuhlmacher, A., & Bonte-Eley, S. (2012). Overcoming barriers to research utilization and evidence-based practice among staff nurses. *Journal of Nurses in Staff Development, 28*(4), 163–165.

Guido, G. W. (2013). *Legal and ethical issues in nursing* (6th ed.). Upper Saddle River, NJ: Pearson-Prentice Hall.

Harrington, C., Stockton, J., & Hooper, S. (2014). The effects of regulation and litigation on a large for-profit nursing home chain. *Journal of Health Politics, Policy & Law, 39*(4), 781–809.

Harris, S. (2011). *The moral landscape: How science can determine moral values.* New York, NY: Free Press.

Hernandez, K., Mata, H., Provencio Vasquez, E., & Martinez, J. (2014). Community outreach along the U.S.-Mexico border: Developing HIV health education strategies to engage rural populations. *Online Journal of Rural Nursing & Health Care, 14*(1), 3–17.

Hinshaw, A. S., & Grady, P. A. (Eds.). (2011). *Shaping health policy through nursing research.* New York, NY: Springer.

Hoffman, H., Damus, K., Hillman, L., & Krongrad, E. (1988). Risk factors for SIDS. Results of the National Institute of Child Health and Human Development SIDS Cooperative Epidemiological Study. *Annals of the New York Academy of Sciences, 533,* 13–30.

Hogan, C. (2014). Socioeconomic factors affecting infant sleep-related deaths in St. Louis. *Public Health Nursing, 31*(1), 10–18.

Holt, J., & Convey, H. (2012). Ethical practice in nursing care. *Nursing Standard*, 27(13), 51–56.

Hussein, G. M. A. (2010). When ethics survive where people do not. *Public Health Ethics* 3(10), 72–77.

Husted, G., Scott, C., Husted, J., & Wolf, K. (2015). *Bioethical decision making in nursing* (5th ed.). New York, NY: Springer.

Iacobucci, T. A., Daly, B. J., Lindell, D., & Griffin, M. Q. (2012). Professional values, self-esteem, and ethical confidence of baccalaureate nursing students. *Nursing Ethics*, 20(4), 479–490.

Institute of Medicine (IOM). (2000). *To err is human: Building a safer health care system*. Washington, DC: National Academies Press.

Institute of Medicine (IOM). (2001). *Crossing the quality chasm: A new health system for the 21st century*. Washington, DC: National Academies Press.

Institute of Medicine. (2003). *Priority areas for national action: Transforming health care quality*. Washington, DC: National Academies Press.

Institute of Medicine. (2011). *The future of nursing: Leading change, advancing health*. Washington, DC: National Academies Press.

Institute of Medicine. (2014). *Strategies for scaling effective family-focused preventive interventions to promote children's cognitive, affective, and behavioral health. Workshop Summary*. Washington, DC: The National Academies Press.

Isaacs, J. B. (2007). *Cost-effective investments in children*. Washington, DC: The Brookings Institution.

Isaacs, J. B. (2008). *Impacts of early childhood programs: Nurse home visiting*. Washington, DC: The Brookings Institution.

Iserson, K. V. (1999). Ethical issues in emergency medicine. *Emergency Medicine Clinics of North America, 17*(2), 283–306.

Izumi, S., Nagae, H., Sakurai, C., & Inamura, K. (2012). Defining end-of-life care from perspectives of nursing ethics. *Nursing Ethics*, 19(5), 608–618.

Jennings, B. (2015). Relational liberty revisited: Membership, solidarity and public health ethics of place. *Public Health Ethics*, 8(1), 7–17.

Jianzhong, Z., Ma, Y., & Weihua, L. (2014). Strategies for communicating contraceptive effectiveness. *Public Health Nursing*, 31(5), 438–440.

Jormfeldt, H. (2014). Perspectives on health and well-being in nursing. *International Journal on Qualitative Studies on Health and Well-Being, 9*. doi: 10.3402/qhw.v9.23026.

Joyce, B., O'Brien, K., Belew-LaDue, B., Dorjee, T. K. & Smith, C. M. (2015). Revealing the voices of public health nurses by exploring their lived experiences. *Public Health Nursing, 32*(2), 151–160.

Kaiser Family Foundation. (2015a). *Infant mortality rate (deaths per 1,000 live births) by race/ethnicity*. Retrieved from http://kff.org/other/state-indicator/infant-mortality-rate-by-race-ethnicity/

Kaiser Family Foundation. (2015b). *Key facts about the uninsured population*. Retrieved from http://kff.org/uninsured/Karadag, C. O., & Hakan, A. K. (2012). Ethical dilemmas in disaster medicine. *Iranian Red Crescent Medical Journal, 14*(10), 602–612.

Katz, A. (2015, April 2). Cancer genetics: Genetic counseling, ethical issues, and the nurse's role. *Oncology Nurses Society*. Retrieved from http://congress.ons.org/cancer-genetics-genetic-counseling-ethical-issues-and-the-nurses-role/

Kavanagh, K. T., Cimiotti, J. P., Abusalem, S., & Coty, M. B. (2012). Moving healthcare quality forward with nursing-sensitive value-based purchasing. *Journal of Nursing Scholarship, 44*(4), 385–395.

Kelly, C. (2013). *Essentials of nursing leadership and management* (3rd ed.). Clifton Park, NY: Delmar Cengage Learning.

Kitzman, H., Olds, D., Henderson, C., Hanks, C., Cole, R., Arcoleo, K. J., et al. (2010). Enduring effects of prenatal and infancy home visiting by nurses on children. *Archives of Pediatrics and Adolescent Medicine, 164*(5), 412–418.

Kitzman, H., Olds, D., Henderson, C., Hanks, C., Cole, R., Tatelbaum, R, et al. (1997). Effect or prenatal and infancy home visitation by nurses on pregnancy outcomes, childhood injuries, and repeated childbearing: A randomized controlled trial. *Journal of the American Medical Association, 278*(8), 644–652.

Kluckhohn, C. (1951). Values and value-orientations in the theory of action: An exploration in definition and classification. In T. Parsons, & E. A. Shils (Eds.), *Toward a general theory of action* (pp. 388–433). Cambridge, MA: Harvard University Press.

Kobayashi, K., Fukushima, M., Kitaoka, H., Shimizu, Y., & Shimanouchi, S. (2014). The influence of public health nurses in facilitating a healthy family life for families with abused and neglected children by providing care. *Internal Medicine Journal, 22*(1), 6–11.

Kronstadt, J., Beitsch, L.M., & Bender, K. (2015). Marshaling the evidence: The prioritized public health accreditation research agenda. *American Journal of Public Health, 105*(S2), s153–s158.

Kulbok, P. A., Thatcher, E., Park, E., & Meszaros, P. S. (2012). Evolving public health nursing roles: Focus on community participatory health promotion and prevention. *Online Journal of Issues in Nursing, 17*(2), 1. doi: 10.3912/OJIN.Vol17No02Man01.

Laabs, C. (2012). Confidence and knowledge regarding ethics among advanced practice nurses. *Nursing Education Perspectives, 33*(1), 10–14.

Lai, D., Ding, Q., Bodson, J., Warner, E. L., & Kepka, D. (2016). Factors associated with increased HPV vaccine use in rural-frontier U.S. states. *Public Health Nursing, 33*(4), 283–294.

Larsen, R., & Reif, L. (2011). Effectiveness of cultural immersion and culture classes for enhancing nursing students' transcultural self-efficacy. *Journal of Nursing Education, 14*, 1–5.

LeBlanc, E., Zakher, B., Daeges, M., Pappas, M., & Chou, R. (2015). Screening for vitamin D deficiency: a systematic review for the U.S. Preventive Task Force. *Annals of Internal Medicine, 162*(2), 109–122.

Lee, M. C., Johnson, K. L., Newhouse, R. P., & Warren, J. I. (2013a). Evidence-based practice process quality assessment: EPQA guidelines. *Worldviews on Evidence-Based Nursing, 10*(3), 140–149.

Lee, R. H., Weber, T., & Colon-Emeric, C. (2013b). Comparison of cost-effectiveness of vitamin D screening with that of universal supplementation in preventing falls in community-dwelling older adults. *Journal of the American Geriatric Society (JAGS), 61*(5), 707–714.

Levy, D., Nikolayev, I., & Mumford, E. (2005). Recent trends in smoking and the role of public policies: Results from the SimSmoke tobacco control policy simulation model. *Addiction, 100*(10), 1526–1536.

Lindson, N., Aveyard, P., & Hughes, J. (2010). Reduction versus abrupt cessation in smokers who want to quit. *Cochrane Database of Systematic Reviews, 3*, CD008033.

Liu, R. (2011, February 8). Startling racial disparities in vaccination persist. *Doctors for America*. Retrieved from http://www.drsforamerica.org/blog/startling-racial-disparities-in-vaccination-persist

MacDonald, S. E., Newburn-Book, C. V., Allen, M., & Reutter, L. (2012). Embracing the population health framework in nursing research. *Nursing Inquiry, 20*(1), 30–41.

Maiese, M. (2013). *Principles of justice and fairness: Beyond intractability*. Retrieved from http://www.beyondintractability.org/essay/principles-of-justice

Martin, C. T., Keswick, J. L., Crayton, D., & LeVeck, P. (2012). Perceptions of self-esteem in a welfare-to-wellness-to-work program. *Public Health Nursing, 29*(1), 19–26.

Maslow, A. (1969). *Toward a psychology of being* (2nd ed.). New York, NY: Van Nostrand.

McHugh, M. D. (2010). Hospital nurse staffing and public health emergency preparedness: Implications for policy. *Public Health Nursing*, 27(5), 442–449.

McKenzie, J. F., Neiger, B., & Thackeray, R. (2012). *Planning, implementing and evaluating health promotion programs: A primer* (6th ed.). San Francisco, CA: Benjamin Cummings.

McLeod, M., Blakely, T., Kvizhinadze, G., & Harris, R. (2014). Why equal treatment is not always equitable: the impact of existing ethnic health inequalities in cost-effectiveness modeling. *Population Health Metrics, 12*, 2–20.

Mejdoubi, J., van den Haijkant, C. M., Struijf, E., van Leerdam, F., Heymans, M. W., Hirasing, R. A., & Crijnen, A. M. (2011). Addressing risk factors for child abuse among high-risk pregnant women: Design of a randomized controlled trial of the Nurse-Family Partnership in Dutch preventive health care. *BMC Public Health, 11*, 823.

Mejdoubi, J., van den Haijkant, C. M., van Leerdam, F., Heymans, M. W., Crijnen, A. M., & Hirasing, R. A. (2015). The effect of VoorZorg, the Dutch nurse-family partnership, on child maltreatment and development: A randomized controlled trial. *PLOS ONE, 10*(4), e0120182. doi: 10.371/journal.pone.0120182.

Mejdoubi, J., van den Haijkant, C. M., van Leerdam, F., Heymans, M. W., Hirasing, R. A., & Crijnen, A. M. (2013). Effect of nurse home visits vs. usual care on reducing intimate partner violence in young high-risk pregnant women: A randomized controlled trial. *PLOS ONE, 8*(10), e78185.

Melnyk, B., & Fibneout-Overholt, E. (2014). *Evidence-based practice in nursing and healthcare: A guide to best practice* (3rd ed.). Philadelphia, PA: Lippincott Williams & Wilkins.

Melnyk, B., Gallagher-Ford, L., Long, L. E., & Fineout-Overholt, M. (2014). The establishment of evidence-based practice competencies for practicing registered nurses and advanced practice nurses in real-world clinical settings: Proficiencies to improve healthcare quality, reliability, patient outcomes, and cost. *Worldviews on Evidence-Based Nursing, 11*(1), 5–15.

Merriam Webster Online Dictionary. (2015). *Ethics*. Retrieved from http://www.merriam-webster.com/dictionary/ethics

Miller, T. R. (2012, September). *Nurse-Family Partnership home visitation: Costs, outcomes, and return on investment. Executive Summary*. Beltsville, MD: H.B.S.A., Inc.

Murray, J. (2010). Moral courage in healthcare: Acting ethically even in the presence of risk. *Online Journal of Nursing Education, 15*(3), 2.

National Association of Social Workers. (2011). *Social justice*. Retrieved from http://www.socialworkers.org/pressroom/features/issue/peace.asp

National Institutes of Health. (2012). *Back to Sleep public education campaign*. Retrieved from https://www.nichd.nih.gov/sids/

National Institutes of Health. (n.d.a). *Ten landmark nursing research studies*. Retrieved from https://www.ninr.nih.gov/sites/www.ninr.nih.gov/files/10-landmark-nursing-research-studies.pdf

National Institutes of Health. (n.d.b). *Community-based participatory research*. Offices of Behavioral and Social Sciences Research. Retrieved from https://obssr.od.nih.gov/scientific_areas/methodology/community_based_participatory_research/

Naylor, M. D., Aiken, L. H., Kurtzman, E. T., Olds, D. M., & Hirschman, K. B. (2011). The care span: The importance of transitional care in achieving health reform. *Health Affairs, 30*(4), 746–754.

Netermeyer, R., Andrews, J. C., & Burton, S. (2005). Effects of anti-smoking advertising-based beliefs on adult smokers' consideration of quitting. *American Journal of Public Health, 95*(6), 1062–1066.

Neuman, B., & Fawcett, J. (2011). *The Neuman systems model* (5th ed.). Boston, MA: Pearson.

Nightingale, F. (1859/1992). *Notes on nursing: What it is, and what it is not [Commemorative ed.]*. Philadelphia, PA: Lippincott.

Noonan, D., & Duffy, S.A. (2014). Factors associated with smokeless tobacco use and dual use among blue-collar workers. *Public Health Nursing, 31*(1), 19–27.

Nurse-Family Partnership (NFP). (2011a). *Locations*. Retrieved from http://www.nursefamilypartnership.org/locations

Nurse-Family Partnership (NFP). (2011b). *Proven effective through extensive research*. Retrieved from http://www.nursefamilypartnership.org/proven-results

Nurse-Family Partnership (NFP). (2011c). *Evidence-based policy and program impact*. Retrieved from http://www.nursefamilypartnership.org/assets/PDF/Fact-sheets/NFP_Evidence-Based-2014pdf.aspx

Nurse-Family Partnership (NFP). (2015, April 15). *US Congress extends funding for the bipartisan-supported federal home visiting program*. Retrieved from http://www.nursefamilypartnership.org/NFP/media/Press-Release/NFP_Congress_MIECHV.pdf?ext=.pdf

Nurse–Family Partnership (NFP). (2010). *Evidentiary foundations of Nurse-Family Partnership*. Retrieved from http://www.nursefamilypartnership.org/assets/PDF/Policy/NFP_Evidentiary_Standards

O'Leary, D. F., & Mhaolrunaigh, S. N. (2012). Information-seeking behaviour of nurses: Where is information sought and what processes are followed? *Journal of Advanced Nursing, 68*(2), 379–390.

Olds, D. (2010). The nurse-family partnership. In R. Haskins, & W. S. Barnett (Eds.). *Investing in young children: New directions in federal preschool and early childhood policy*. Washington, DC: Brookings Institution.

Olds, D., Donelan-McCall, N., O'Brien, R., MacMillan, H., Jack, S., Jenkins, T., …, Beeber, L. (2013). Improving the nurse-family partnership in community practice. *Pediatrics, 132*(S110), s110–s117.

Olds, D., Eckenrode, J., Henderson, C., Kitzman, H., Powers, J., Cole, R., et al. (1997). Long-term effects of home visitation on maternal life course and child abuse and neglect: Fifteen-year follow-up of a randomized trial. *Journal of the American Medical Association, 278*(8), 637–643.

Olds, D. L., Holmberg, J. R., Donelan-McCall, N., Luckey, D. W., Knudtson, M. D., & Robinson, J. (2014a). Effects of home visits by paraprofessionals and by nurses on children: Follow-up of a randomized trial at ages 6 and 9 years. *JAMA Pediatrics, 168*(2), 114–121.

Olds, D. L., Kitzman, H., Cole, R., Hanks, C., Arcoleo, K., Anson, E., et al. (2010). Enduring effects of prenatal and infancy home visiting by nurses on maternal life course and government spending. *Archives of Pediatrics & Adolescent Medicine, 164*(5), 419–424.

Olds, D. L., Kitzman, H., Knudtson, M. D., Andson, E., Smith, J. A., & Cole, R. (2014b). Effect of home visiting by nurses on maternal and child mortality results of a 2-decade follow-up of a randomized clinical trial. *JAMA Pediatrics, 168*(9), 800–806.

Olds, D., Robinson, J., Pettitt, L., Luckey, D., Holmberg, J., Ng, R. K., et al. (2004). Effects of home visits by paraprofessionals and by nurses: Age 4 follow-up results of a randomized trial. *Pediatrics, 114*(6), 1560–1568.

Olson Keller, L., & Strohschein, S. (2011a, June 1). Show me the evidence: Evidence-based public health nursing practice. *Webinar Handouts*. Retrieved from http://publichealthnurses.org/images/uploads/Webinar_I_Slides_Updated.pdf

Olson Keller, L., & Strohschein, S. (2011b, June 15). Innovations in translating evidence into practice. *Webinar Handouts*. Retrieved from http://publichealthnurses.org/images/uploads/Web_II_Handout_(1).pdf

Ong, M., & Glantz, S. A. (2005). Free nicotine replacement therapy programs vs. implementing smoke-free workplaces: A cost-effectiveness comparison. *American Journal of Public Health, 95*(1), 969–975.

Owens, J., & Cribb, A. (2013). Beyond choice and individualism: Understanding autonomy for public health ethics. *Public Health Ethics, 6*(3), 262–271.

Palacio, A., Kirolos, I., & Tamariz, L. (2015). Patient values and preferences when choosing anticoagulants. *Patient Preference and Adherence, 9*, 133–138.

Park, E. (2012). An integrated ethical decision making model for nurses. *Nursing ethics, 19*(1), 139–159.

Park, Y. H., & Han, H. R. (2010). Nurses' perceptions and experiences at daycare for elderly with stroke. *Journal of Nursing Scholarship, 42*(3), 262–269.

Pereira, G. (2015). What do we need to be part of dialogue? From Discursive Ethics to Critical Social Justice, *Critical Horizons, 16*(3), 280–298.

Perry, C., & Hoffman, B. (2010). Assessing tribal youth physical activity and programming using a community-based participatory research approach. *Public Health Nursing, 27*(2), 104–114.

Phillips, D, Brewer, K., & Wadensweiler, P. (2010). Alcohol as a risk factor for sudden infant death syndrome (SIDS). *Addiction, 106*(3), 516–525.

Pickering, C. E. Z., & Phillips, L. R. (2014). Development of a causal model for elder mistreatment. *Public Health Nursing, 31*(4), 363–372.

Pickering, A., Boehm, A., Mwanjali, M., & Davis, J. (2010). Efficacy of waterless hand hygiene compared with handwashing with soap: A field study in Dar es Salaam, Tanzania. *American Journal of Tropical Medicine, 82*(2), 270–278.

Polit, D., & Beck, C. T. (2012). *Nursing research: Generating and assessing evidence for nursing practice* (9th ed.). Philadelphia, PA: Lippincott Williams & Wilkins.

Polit, D., & Beck, C. T. (2014). *Essentials of nursing research: Appraising evidence for nursing practice* (8th ed.). Philadelphia, PA: Lippincott Williams & Wilkins.

Porter, E., Matsuda, S., & Lindbloom, E. (2010). Intentions of older homebound women to reduce the risk of falling again. *Journal of Nursing Scholarship, 42*(1), 101–109.

Porter-O'Grady, T. (2010). A new age for practice: Creating the framework for evidence. In K. Malloch, & T. Porter-O'Grady (Eds.), *Introduction to evidence-based practice in nursing and health care* (2nd ed., pp. 1–30). Sudbury, MA: Jones & Bartlett Publishers.

Raffo, J., Meghea, C., Zhu, Q., & Roman, L. A. (2010). Psychological and physical abuse among pregnant women in a Medicaid-sponsored prenatal program. *Public Health Nursing, 27*(5), 385–398.

Rath, T., & Harter, J. (2010). *Wellbeing: the five essential elements*. New York, NY: Gallup Press.

Rebar, C., Gersch, C., Macnee, C., & McCabe, S. (2014). *Understanding nursing research: Using research in evidence-based practice* (4th ed.). Philadelphia, PA: Lippincott Williams & Wilkins.

Renault, K., Norgaard, K., Secher N. J., Andreasen, K. R., Baldur-Felskov, B., & Nilas, L. (2012). Physical activity during pregnancy in normal-weight and obese women: Compliance using pedometer assessment. *Journal of Obstetrics & Gynecology, 32*, 430–433.

Reverby, S. M. (2011). "Normal exposure" and inoculation syphilis: a PHS "Tuskegee" doctor in Guatemala. *The Journal of Policy History, 23*(1), 6–28.

Risjord, M. (2014). Nursing and human freedom. Nursing *Philosophy,15*(1), 35–45.

Rogowski, W., Grosse, S., Schmidtke, J., Marckmann, G. (2014). Criteria for fairly allocating scarce health-care resources to genetic tests: Which matter most? *European Journal of Human Genetics, 22*(1), 25–31.

Rokeach, M. (1973). *The nature of human values*. New York, NY: Free Press.

Schaffer, M. A., & Mbibi, N. (2014). Public health nurse mentorship of pregnant and parenting adolescents. *Public Health Nursing, 31*(5), 428–437.

Schaffer, M. A., Goodhue, A., Stennes, K., & Lanigan, C. (2012). Evaluation of a public health nurse visiting program for pregnant and parenting teens. *Public Health Nursing, 29*(3), 218–231.

Schmit, S., Schott, L., Pavetti, L., & Matthews, H. (2015, February 9). Effective, evidence-based home visiting programs in every state at risk if Congress does not extend funding. *Center on Budget and Policy Priorities.* Retrieved from http://www.cbpp.org/research/effective-evidence-based-home-visiting-programs-in-every-state-at-risk-if-congress-does-not

Sharps, P., Campbell, J., Baty, M., Walker, K., & Bair-Merritt, M. (2008). Current evidence on perinatal home visiting and intimate partner violence. *Journal of Obstetrical, Gynecological, & Neonatal Nursing, 37*(4), 480–490.

Sheikh, S., & Janoff-Bulman, R. (2010). The "shoulds" and "should nots" of moral emotions: A self-regulatory perspective on shame and guilt. *Journal of Personality & Social Psychology, 36*(2), 213–224.

Sierau, S., Dahne, V., Brand, T., Kurtz, V., von Klitzing, K., & Jungmann, T. (2016). Effects of home visitation on maternal competencies, family environment, and child development: A randomized controlled trial. *Prevention Science, 17*(1):40–51.

Snow, R., Laski, L., & Mutumba, M. (2015). Sexual and reproductive health: Progress and outstanding needs. *Global Public Health, 10*(2), 149–173.

Soenens, B., & Vansteenkiste, M. (2010). A theoretical upgrade of the concept of parental psychological control: Proposing new insights on the basis of self-determination theory. *Developmental Review, 30,* 74–99.

Sorrell, J. (2012). Ethics: The Patient protection and affordable care act: Ethical perspectives in 21st century health care. *Online Journal of Issues in Nursing, 18*(1). Retrieved from http://www.nursingworld.org/MainMenuCategories/ANAMarketplace/ANAPeriodicals/OJIN/Columns/Ethics/Patient-Protection-and-Affordable-Care-Act-Ethical-Perspectives.html

Speck, B., & Looney, S. (2006). Self-reported physical activity validated by pedometer: A pilot study. *Public Health Nursing, 23*(1), 88–94.

Stauffer, B. D., Fullerton, C., Fleming, N., Ogola, G., Herrin, J., Stafford, P. M., & Ballard, D. J. (2011). Effectiveness and cost of a transitional care program for heart failure: A prospective study with concurrent controls. *Archives of Internal Medicine, 171*(14), 1238–1243.

Stausmire, J. M. (2014). Quality improvement of research: Deciding which road to take. *Critical Care Nurse, 34*(6), 58–63.

Stevens, K. R. (2013). The impact of evidence-based practice in nursing and the next big idea. *The Online Journal of Issues in Nursing, 18*(2), 4.

Sunni, B., Kennedy, B., Davis, S., Thompson, H., & Jones, J. (2014). Assessing patient awareness of hand hygiene. *Nursing, 45*(5), 27–30.

Sweet, L. L., Polivka, B. J., Chaudry, R. V., & Bouton, P. (2014). The impact of an urban home-based intervention program on asthma outcomes in children. *Public Health Nursing, 31*(3), 243–252.

Terabe, Y., Harada, A., Tokuda, H., Okuizumi, H., Nagaya, M., & Shimokata, H. (2012). Vitamin D deficiency in elderly women in nursing homes: Investigation with consideration of decreased activation function from the kidneys. *Journal of the American Geriatrics Society (JAGS), 60*(2), 251–255.

The Cochrane Collaboration. (2015). *Our name.* Retrieved from http://www.cochrane.org/about-us/our-name

Thomas, C. W., Corso, L., Monroe, J. A. (2015). The value of the "system" in public health services and systems research. *American Journal of Public Health, 105*(s2), s147–s149.

Thompson, M., Tiwari, A., Moe, E., & Buckley, D. I. (2012). *A framework to facilitate the use of systematic reviews and meta-analysis in the design of primary research studies.* Rockville, MD: Agency for Healthcare Research & Quality.

Trachtenberg, F. L., Haas, E. A., Kinney, H. C., Stanley, C., & Krous, H. F. (2012). Risk factor changes for sudden infant death syndrome after initiation of Back-to-Sleep campaign. *Pediatrics, 129*(4), 630–638.

U.S. Congress. (2010, January 5). *H.R. 3590 The Patient Protection an Affordable Care Act.* Retrieved from http://frwebgate.access.gpo.gov/cgi-bin/getdoc.cgi?dbname=111_cong_bills&docid=f:h3590enr.txt.pdf

U.S. Department of Health and Human Services (USDHHS). (2011a). *Home visiting evidence of effectiveness: Implementing NFP.* Retrieved from http://homvee.acf.hhs.gov/Implementation/3/Nurse-Family-Partnership-NFP—Program-Model-Overview/14

U.S. Department of Health and Human Services (USDHHS). (2011b). *Home visiting evidence of effectiveness: Nurse Family Partnership (NFP) in brief.* Retrieved from http://homvee.acf.hhs.gov/Model/1/Nurse-Famiy-Partnership-NFP--In-Brief/14

U.S. Department of Health and Human Services (USDHHS). (n.d.a). *The Belmont report: Ethical principles and guidelines for the protection of human subjects of research.* Retrieved from http://www.hhs.gov/ohrp/policy/belmont.html

U.S. Department of Health and Human Services (USDHHS). (n.d.b). Informed consent FAQs. Retrieved from http://answers.hhs.gov/ohrp/categories/1566

Uustal, D. B. (1977). The use of values clarification in nursing practice. *Journal of Continuing Education in Nursing, 8,* 8–13.

Uustal, D. B. (1978). Values clarification in nursing. *American Journal of Nursing, 78,* 2058–2063.

Vezyridis, P., & Timmons, S. (2015). On the adoption of personal health records: Some problematic issues for patient empowerment. *Ethics and Information Technology, 17*(2), 113–124.

Walker, A., Smith, P. & Kolasa, M. (2014). Reduction of racial/ethnic disparities in vaccination coverage, 1995–2011. *MMWR Surveillance Summaries, 63*(1), 7–12.

Wardrop, N., & LeBlond, J. (2015). Assessing correlations between geological hazards and health outcomes: Addressing complexity in medical geology. *Environment International, 84,* 90–93.

Weekes, C. V., Haas, B. K., & Gosselin, K. P. (2014). Expectations and self-efficacy of African American parents who discuss sexuality with their adolescent sons: An intervention study. *Public Health Nursing, 31*(3), 253–261.

Whittemore, R., Rosenberg, A., Gilmore, L., Withey, M., & Breault, A. (2014). Implementation of a diabetes prevention program in public housing communities. *Public Health Nursing, 31*(4), 317–326.

Widup, S., Bassett, G., Rudis, B., & Spitler, M. (2015). *2015 protected health information data breach report.* Retrieved from http://www.verizonenterprise.com/resources/reports/rp_2015-protected-health-information-data-breach-report_en_xg.pdf

Wiener, L., McConnell, D. G., Latella, L., & Ludi, E. (2013). Cultural and religious considerations in pediatric palliative care. *Palliative & Supportive Care, 11*(1), 47–67.

Wilfond, B. S. (2013). Quality improvement ethics: Lessons from the SUPPORT study. *American Journal of Bioethics, 13*(12), 14–19.

William Glasser Institute. (2010). *Choice theory.* Retrieved from http://www.wglasser.com/index.php?option=com_content&task=view&id=12&Itemid=27

Wilson, D. (2010, July 21). Glaxo ordered to end drug trial enrollment. *The New York Times.* Retrieved from http://www.nytimes.com/2010/07/22/business/22avandia.html

Winland-Brown, J., Lachman, V. D., & Swanson, E. O. (2015). The new 'Code of Ethics for Nurses with Interpretive Statements' 2015: Practical clinical application, part I. *Medsurg Nursing, 24*(4), 269–271.

Wright, D., & Brajtman, S. (2011). Relational and embodied knowing: Nursing ethics within the interprofessional team. *Nursing Ethics, 18*(1), 20–30.

Yang, Z., Scott, C. A., Mao, C., Tang, J., & Farmer, A. J. (2013). Resistance exercise versus aerobic exercise for type 2 diabetes: A systematic review and meta-analysis. *Sports Medicine.* doi: 10.1007/s40279-013-0128-8.

Young, C., & Skorga, P. (2011). Reduction versus abrupt cessation in smokers who want to quit: A review summary. *Public Health Nursing, 28*(1), 54–56.

Transcultural Nursing in the Community

"People everywhere share common biological and psychological needs, and the function of all cultures is to fulfill such needs; the nature of the culture is determined by its function."

—Bronislaw Malinowski (1884–1942), Cultural Anthropologist

"Looking from far and above, from our high places of safety in the developed civilization, it is easy to see all the crudity and irrelevance of magic. But without its power and guidance early man could not have mastered his practical difficulties as he has done, nor could man have advanced to the higher stages of civilization."

—Horace Miner (1912–1993), Anthropologist

KEY TERMS

Complementary therapies
Cultural assessment
Cultural diversity
Cultural relativism
Cultural self-awareness
Cultural sensitivity
Culture

Culture shock
Dominant values
Enculturation
Ethnic group
Ethnicity
Ethnocentrism
Ethnorelativism

Folk medicine
Home remedies
Integrated health care
Microculture
Minority group
Norms
Race

Subcultures
Tacit
Transcultural nursing
Value

LEARNING OBJECTIVES

Upon mastery of this chapter, you should be able to:

- Define and explain the concept of culture.
- Discuss the meaning of cultural diversity and its significance for community health nursing.
- Describe the meaning and effects of ethnocentrism on community health nursing practice.
- Identify five characteristics shared by all cultures.
- Contrast the health-related values, beliefs, and practices of selected culturally diverse populations with those of the dominant U.S. culture.
- Conduct a cultural assessment.
- Apply principles of transcultural nursing in community health nursing practice.

American society values individuality, and we are a country of immigrants. Many different cultural groups and races built this nation. For example, pilgrims came here hundreds of years ago, to seek freedom to practice their religious beliefs. It took a powerful independent resolve to pioneer the West in the 1800s. Partly because of this pioneer spirit, people from all nations have sought to live in America. Some came of their own free will for adventure and opportunity. Others saw this land as a refuge from political, religious, or economic strife. Still others were brought here against their will. Consequently, we have not become the ideal *melting pot* once described, but, rather, an amalgamation of people who have different values, ideals, and behaviors.

Americans have many differences, but we also have much in common. In the Western culture, there is joy in seeing children grow and develop in unique ways. An individual's creative achievements are applauded. There is also respect for one another's personal preferences about food, dress, or personal beliefs. The right to be oneself—and thereby to be different from others—is even protected by state and federal laws.

Although individuality is a cherished American value, there are limits to the range of differences most Americans find acceptable. People whose behavior falls outside the acceptable range may be labeled as misfits. For example, the U.S. culture approves of moderate social drinking, but not alcoholism. The beliefs and sanctions of the dominant or majority culture are called **dominant values**. In the United States, the majority culture is made up largely of non-Hispanic Whites, whose dominant values include the work ethic, thrift, success, independence, initiative, privacy, cleanliness, youthfulness, attractive appearance, and a focus on the future. However, in some regions and states, non-Hispanic Whites are not the majority. For example, in California, only 40% of the population is non-Hispanic White (California Pan-Ethnic Health Network, 2015). Between 2010 and 2050, the proportion of the population identified as White is projected to continue to fall below other ethnicities (U.S. Census Bureau, n.d.a.).

Dominant values reflect the cultural power differentials that exist in this country in that powerful groups "invoke structure in their own interests while the less powerful are more constrained" (Roscigno, 2012, para. 8). The powerful exert control over political, economic, and social structures that influence all members of society. Many years ago, this country put laws into place prohibiting discrimination on the basis of "race, color, religion, national origin, and sex," as well as qualified disabled persons (U.S. Equal Employment Opportunity Commission, n.d., para. 1). But, Alexander (2012, p. *x*) sees a new "racial caste system alive and well in the age of colorblindness" as evidenced by the high proportion of incarcerations among nondominant groups, especially Blacks. Schrecker and Bambra (2015) argue that political decisions affect the health of populations, specifically those that began with deregulation, private sector growth, and reductions in government spending in this country and others, have led to increased rates in poverty, inequality, obesity, and other health problems tied to the social determinants of health. (See Chapters 13 and 25 for more on social determinants of health.)

Given this awareness, dominant values are important to consider in the practice of community health nursing because they can shape people's thoughts and behaviors. Why are some client behaviors acceptable to health professionals and others not? Why do nurses have such difficulty persuading certain clients to accept new ways of thinking and acting? Explanations can be found by examining the concept of culture, especially its influence on health and on community health nursing practice. For example, an emphasis on the need for milk in the diet may reflect cultural blindness, considering the number of people from diverse ethnic groups who are lactose intolerant, and food allergies appear to go undiagnosed in minority children (Taylor-Black & Wang, 2012). Regardless of their own cultural backgrounds, nurses are socialized throughout the educational process; the biomedical model is frequently the framework, and dominant social values are often involuntarily reinforced.

THE MEANING OF CULTURE

Culture refers to the beliefs, values, and behavior that are shared by members of a society and provide a template or "road map" for living. Culture tells people what is acceptable or unacceptable in a given situation. Culture dictates what to do, say, or believe. Culture is learned. As children grow up, they learn from their parents and others around them how to interpret the world. In turn, these assimilated beliefs and values prescribe desired behavior. We think of this as learned behavior, but can culture actually impact your neurobiology? For more on this see What Do You Think?

Generally, anthropologists describe culture as systems of beliefs, values, and norms of behavior found in all societies. This is more than simply custom or ritual; it is a way of organizing and thinking about life. It gives people a sense of security about their behavior; without having to consciously think about it, they know how to act. Culture also provides the underlying values and beliefs on which people's behavior is based. For example, culture determines the value placed on achievement, independence, work, and leisure. It forms the basis for the definitions of male and female roles. It influences a person's response to authority figures, dictates religious beliefs and practices, and shapes child-rearing. Giger (2017) describes culture as a patterned response of

What do *you* think?

CAN CULTURE AFFECT YOUR NEUROBIOLOGY?

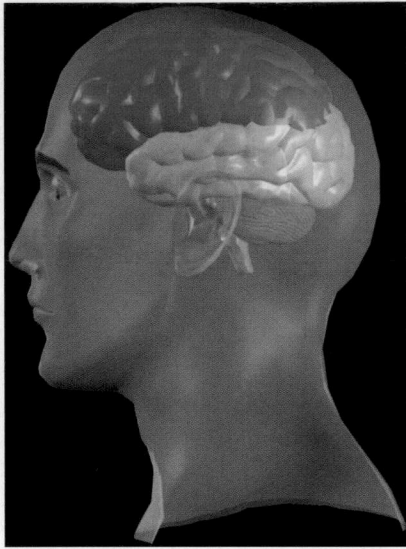

The neuroscience of culture is an emerging area of research. Studies that link cognitive neuroscience with cultural and social psychology include those examining "emotion, perspective-taking, memory, object perception, attention, language, and the self" (Rule, Freeman, & Ambady, 2013, p. 3). For instance, researchers studied brain activity through the use of functional magnetic resonance imaging (fMRI) while both young and elderly American and East Asian participants were shown a series of images depicting various objects on different backgrounds. For both cultures, the younger subjects demonstrated similar brain activity. But a marked contrast was noted between the older subjects, with the neural responses of those only from the East Asian culture showing minimal activity to changes of single objects while the Americans' activity in the lateral occipital complex was continually active (Burton, 2007). Americans were more focused on the individual objects as new ones were introduced, but the East Asians maintained focus on the background information and not on new individual objects, according to earlier research. The explanation for this is that Asian culture is "less individual-oriented than Western culture" and more interdependent (p. 6). Even with Westernization, they feel that these differences demonstrate that "culture is sculpting the brain at the level of perception"—evidence that culture can impact us on a biological level (p. 6).

A later study by Ng, Han, Mao, and Lai (2010) used similar methods to examine neural representation of self and significant others among a sample of "Westernized bicultural Chinese" (p. 83). While undergoing fMRI imaging, participants were asked to make trait judgments regarding self, mother, or an unidentified individual. Either Western or Chinese culture priming was used before the testing. Those with Western priming demonstrated an increased differentiation of self from either mother or unidentified individual, but Chinese priming subjects showed less differentiation. The results of a quantitative meta-analysis of 35 fMRI studies "suggest that cultural differences in social and nonsocial processes are mediated by distinct neural networks" (Han & Ma, 2014, p. 293). The differences between Western and East Asian study participant neural activity emphasized the individual versus other-oriented cultures.

Korn et al. (2014, para. 1) used the board game, *Monopoly*, to test "cultural influences on social conformity, positivity biases, and self-related neural activity" in two groups of participants (one of German and the other of Chinese origin). Each participant played a timed game with three other people from the same cultural background, and all of them were asked to rate the other three players on 40 negative and 40 positive adjectives (using a 4-point Likert scale). The means were shared with each participant before a second timed game began, and participants were tested to determine how much influence this feedback had in their own personality ratings before and after the feedback. Greater conformity to social feedback was found among the Chinese participants and less among the Germans. Also, all participants processed the feedback from others in a way that was biased toward the positive, or changed behavior based on more pleasant feedback, and cultural groups showed no differences. Germans had greater self-related changes in prefrontal activity during the feedback-processing period when compared to Chinese; the researchers noted that this real-life interaction by way of a board game added to the knowledge of cultural diversity.

Functional MRI was used to examine the neurobiological basis of shame and guilt (Michl et al., 2014). One study examined German participants, and compared results with a previous study using Japanese participants. Both groups demonstrated similar areas of brain activity for both shame and guilt states; however, the similarity did not extend to gender, as there was a difference for women experiencing guilt. Women showed neural activity in the temporal regions, but men had additional activity in the frontal and occipital areas of the brain, as well as the amygdala. Could this be due to culturally different gender roles?

Burton, K. W. (2007). Cultural experience affects perception. *Brain Work: The Neuroscience Newsletter, 17*(5), 6.

Han, S., & Ma, Y. (2014). Cultural differences in human brain activity: A quantitative meta-analysis. *NeuroImage, 99*, 293–300.

Korn, C. W., Fan, Y., Zhang, K., Wang, C., Han, S., & Heekeren, H. R. (2014). Cultural influences on social feedback processing of character traits. *Frontiers in Human Neuroscience, 8*, 192. Retrieved from http://www.ncbi.nlm.nih.gov/pmc/articles/PMC3983486/

Michl, P., Meindl, T., Meister, F., Born, C., Engel, R. R., Reiser, M., Hennig-Fast, K (2014). Neurobiological underpinnings of shame and guilt: A pilot fMRI study. *Social Cognitive and Affective Neuroscience, 9*(2), 150–157.

Ng, S. H., Han, S., Mao, L., & Lai, J. C. (2010). Dynamic bicultural brains: fMRI study of their flexible neural representation of self and significant others in response to culture primes. *Asian Journal of Social Psychology, 13*, 83–91.

Rule, N. O., Freeman, J. B., & Ambady, N. (2013). Culture in social neuroscience: A review. *Social Neuroscience, 8*(1), 3–10.

behavior that develops from the impact of social and religious structures in a community. This develops over time from infancy through old age and can be apparent in a community's intellectual and artistic achievements.

Every community and social or ethnic group has its own culture. Furthermore, all of the individual members believe and act based on what they have learned within that specific culture. As anthropologist Edward Hall (1959) said over a half-century ago, culture controls our lives. Even the smallest elements of everyday living are influenced by culture. For instance, culture determines the proper distance to stand from another person while talking with him or her. A comfortable talking distance for Americans is at least 2.5 feet, whereas Latin Americans prefer a shorter distance for dialogue, often only 18 inches. Culture also influences one's perception of time. In the non-Hispanic White American culture, when someone makes an appointment, it is expected that the other person will be on time, or not more than a few minutes late; to keep a person waiting (or to be kept waiting) for 45 minutes or more is considered insulting. Yet other cultural groups, including Native Americans and Hispanics, have a much more flexible response to time. Their members feel that time is much more elastic, and if someone is kept waiting, it is not considered a thoughtless act. So, as you can see, culture is the knowledge people use to design their own actions and, in turn, to interpret others' behavior (Spradley, McCurdy, & Shandy, 2015).

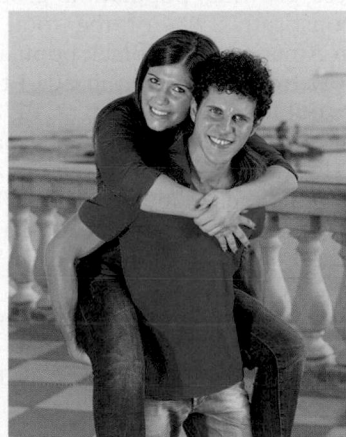

Culture influences rules about the appropriateness of public displays of affection.

Cultural Diversity

Race refers to biologically designated groups of people whose distinguishing features, such as skin color, are inherited; examples include Asian, Black, and White, although the term race is more of a social construct because humans are one species. An **ethnic group** is an assemblage of people who have common origins and a shared culture and identity; they may share a common geographic origin, race, language, religion, traditions, values, and food preferences (Spector, 2013). When a variety of racial or ethnic groups join a common, larger population, cultural diversity becomes more apparent and more easily distinguished. **Cultural diversity**, also called *cultural plurality*, means that a variety of cultural patterns coexist within a designated geographic area. Cultural diversity

occurs not only between countries or continents but also within many countries, including the United States (Spector, 2013). However, the term *culture*, used alone, has no single definition. We have defined it for use in this book at the beginning of this section. Others have described culture as meaning the total, socially inherited characteristics of a group, comprising everything that one generation can tell, convey, or hand down to the next generation.

Cultural diversity in the United States began when Native Americans were challenged by early foreign settlements. Early settlers came primarily from European countries through the 1800s, peaking in numbers just after the turn of the 20th century, with almost 9 million immigrants admitted in the first decade. During much of that time, especially during the late 1600s through the early 1800s, Africans were enslaved and brought to the United States against their will, mostly to southern states, where they were sold to plantation owners as property in order to labor on large plantations and farms. Slavery and cultural oppression has had profound effects for many generations (Klein, 2012). Immigration stayed high during the early 1900s, and then dropped sharply from 1930 to 1950. Immigration from non-European regions, such as Asia and South America, then steadily increased. The total number of immigrants from all countries in the 1990s actually exceeded the number who arrived during the first decade of the 1900s, when immigration was formerly at its peak (Table 5–1).

Currently, the foreign-born population is believed to be a difficult group to count, and that increases the likelihood of coverage error for this population. English language ability, literacy skills, understanding of the census, residential attachment, and legal status are all factors

Table 5–1	Immigrants to the United States, 1901–2013
Decade	**Number of Immigrants**
1901–1910	8,795,386
1911–1920	5,735,611
1921–1930	4,107,209
1931–1940	528,431
1941–1950	1,035,039
1951–1960	2,515,479
1961–1970	3,322,677
1971–1980	4,493,314
1981–1990	7,338,062
1991–2000	9,095,417
2001–2013	2,052,593

From Baker, B., & Rytina, N. (2014). U.S. lawful permanent residents 2013. *Department of Homeland Security Annual Flow Report.* Retrieved from https://www.dhs.gov/sites/default/files/publications/ois_lpr_pe_2013_0.pdf

Table 5–2 Persons Obtaining Legal Permanent Resident Status by Region of Birth, 2013

Origin	Number
All countries	1,130,818
Africa	98,304
Asia	400,348
Europe	86,556
North America	315,660
Oceania	5,277
South America	80,945

From Baker, B., & Rytina, N. (2014). U.S. lawful permanent residents 2013. *Department of Homeland Security Annual Flow Report.* Retrieved from https://www.dhs.gov/sites/default/files/publications/ois_lpr_pe_2013_0.pdf

that contribute to coverage error in censuses and surveys (Jensen, Bhaskar, & Scopilliti, 2015). More accurate counts come from the immigrants seeking naturalization, becoming United States citizens. As shown in Table 5–2, immigrants come from all regions of the world, in greater numbers from some areas than others (Monger & Yankay, 2014).

Although the numbers of legal immigrants have dropped, illegal immigration continues to be a controversial topic in this country, especially after the tragedy of 9/11. Plans to end the flow of illegal immigrants from Mexico included building a 700-mile fence along the border, and legislation that more stiffly penalized employers of undocumented workers. In the late 20th and early years of the 21st century, the numbers of migrants losing their lives while crossing illegally into this country rose dramatically, from 87 in 1999 to 417 in 2009. That number only includes the known deaths, and does not include those who may have died and whose bodies were not found (Sacchetti, 2014). While social justice is an important issue in public health nursing, what is often not considered in the national debate over this issue is the economic desperation that drives people to put themselves in such jeopardy. The issue of social justice is discussed more in Chapters 13 and 29.

The United States is changing to a majority–minority nation (Table 5–3). A recent census projection report states that by 2044, more than 50% of Americans will belong to a minority group, or one other than non-Hispanic White. In some states, especially those bordering Mexico and some industrialized states in the eastern part of the country, the most current information reveals that this change already has occurred or will occur much sooner than 2044 (Colby & Ortman, 2015). See Display 5–1.

The fastest growing group is projected to be those people reporting two or more races, growing from 8 million in 2014 to 26 million in 2060. This would increase from 2.5% of the total U.S. population in 2014 to 6.2% by 2060. The second fastest growing group is projected to be Asians, growing from 5.4% of the total population in 2014 to 9.3% of the total population in 2060 (Colby & Ortman, 2015)

Hispanics surpassed the African American population as the largest minority group in the United States in 2010 and in the 2014 census, constituted 17.4% of the population with 55 million people (Office of Minority Health, 2015). This population group is expected to increase to 119 million in 2060. Although this is only the third fastest growing population group, they are expected to constitute 29% of the total population. Among African Americans, the Black population alone is expected to grow from 42 million in 2014 to 60 million in 2060. This would place the group at 14% of the U.S. population, well below the percent of Hispanics (Colby & Ortman, 2015). Asian–Pacific Islanders are expected to more than double their numbers, to 9.3% of the U.S. population; the American Indian and Alaska Native population is expected to be stable at or near 1% (Colby & Ortman, 2015).

Immigration patterns are strongly influenced by immigration laws established since the 1800s. The Immigration Reform and Control Act of 1986 (Public

Table 5–3 U.S. Population by Race and Hispanic/Latino Origin, Census 2000 and 2010 Estimate

Race and Hispanic/Latino Origin	Census 2000, Population	Percent of Population	Census 2010, Population	Percent of Population	Percent Change, 2000–2010
Total Population	**281,421,906**	**100.0%**	**308,745,538**	**100.0%**	**+9.7%**
White	211,460,626	75.1	196,817,552	63.7	−5.7
Black or African American	34,658,190	12.3	37,685,848	12.2	+12.3
American Indian and Alaska Native	2,475,956	0.9	2,247,098	0.7	−18.4
Asian	10,242,998	3.6	14,465,124	4.7	−43.3
Native Hawaiian and other Pacific Islander	398,835	0.1	481,576	0.15	+35.4
Hispanic or Latino	35,305,818	12.5	50,477,594	16.3	+43.0

From Humes, K. R., Jones, N. A., & Ramirez, R. R. (2011, March). *Overview of race and Hispanic origin: 2010.* Retrieved from http://www.census.gov/prod/cen2010/briefs/c2010br-02.pdf

DISPLAY 5–1   HISPANIC POPULATION TREND IN THE UNITED STATES

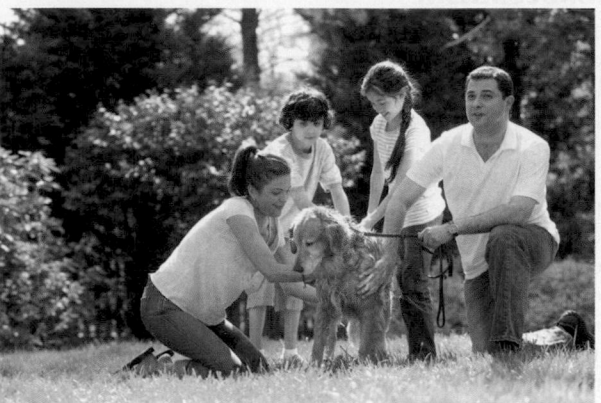

In 2013, a record number of 41.3 million (or 13.1%) of the population were foreign born. Of the total immigrant population in the United States, 25.8% are from Mexico, 25.8% from Asia, 24% from Latin America and only 14.2% from Europe and Canada. The face of immigration has shifted, from Europe and Canada sending the largest proportion in the 1960s to the current larger influx from Mexico, Asia, and Latin America. The mean age of immigrants also differs by region of origin; the median age for those from Europe and Canada is 52 years, whereas Mexican immigrants have a median age of 39 years. Children of immigrants who are born in the

United States, considered second-generation Americans, constitute 11.7% of our U.S. population. The level of education of immigrants has risen steadily since the 1960s, with the most dramatic gains among those from Asia, Europe, and the Middle East. The unauthorized immigrant population has grown rapidly over the past three decades, hitting a peak at 12.2 million. It had since dropped to 11.2 million and continues to remain fairly steady at about 4% of the population. Unauthorized Mexican immigrants fell from a 6.9 million peak in 2007 to 5.9 million in 2012. It estimated that about one fourth of the foreign-born population in the United States are unauthorized immigrants; the vast majority are in the United States legally, and 41.8% are naturalized citizens (Pew Research Center, 2015).

A common political talking point is the number of infants born in the United States to unauthorized immigrants. This number has declined to 295,000 in 2013 from a high of 370,000 in 2006–2007. The 14th Amendment of the Constitution automatically grants the right to citizenship to anyone born within the United States Currently, there are approximately 4.5 million U.S.-born children under age 18 living with parents who are unauthorized immigrants. Also, these immigrants are now more likely to be long-term U.S. residents than in the past (Pew Research Center, 2015).

From Pew Research Center. (2015). *Hispanic trends*. Retrieved from http://www.pewhispanic.org

---

Law 99-603) and the Immigration Act of 1990 (Public Law 101-649) set new limits on the number of immigrants admitted. These laws set annual numerical ceilings on certain immigrant groups while authorizing increases for highly skilled workers or family members of aliens who have recently achieved legal status. After the terrorist attacks on September 11, 2001, U.S. President George Bush suspended all immigration for 2 months. Suspicion about people from Middle Eastern countries permeated the nation—worsening the social climate for immigrants. More currently, political upheaval and war have sent refugees and migrants from the Middle East, South Asia, and Africa are flooding into Europe. Almost one half million migrants crossed boundaries in Europe during just the first 9 months of 2015, many seeking asylum from Syria's civil war (Park, 2015). As countries, including the United States, wrestle with the social and political issues, there is no coordinated effort to quickly find placements for the continual stream of people. The social climate in the U.S and many other countries is characterized by ambivalence about whether immigrants should be accepted and ambiguity about their status. The newcomers find an environment that is both welcoming and hostile. On the one hand, they may find tolerance of diversity in the United States—demonstrated by interest in ethnic food, cultural celebrations, and sensitivity to employees from different backgrounds. On the other

hand, a backlash is demonstrated by a rise in hate crimes, national and local policies that limit services to undocumented immigrants, restriction in English as a Second Language (ESL) and bilingual education, and limits to potential class action suits challenging practices of the U.S. Citizenship and Immigration Services and Department of Homeland Security.

Although broad cultural values are shared by most large national societies, those societies contain smaller cultural groups—called subcultures. **Subcultures** are relatively large aggregates of people within a society who share separate distinguishing characteristics, such as **ethnicity** (e.g., African American, Hispanic American), occupation (e.g., farmers, physicians), religion (e.g., Catholics, Muslims), geographic area (e.g., New Englanders, Southerners), age (e.g., the elderly, school-age children), gender (e.g., women, men), or sexual preference (e.g., gay, lesbian). Within these subcultures are even smaller groups that anthropologists call **microcultures**. Microcultures have been described as collections of knowledge that is unique or characteristic of specific subgroups within a larger culture. People belonging to a microculture usually share much of what they know with others in the community as they hold a special cultural knowledge that is unique to the subgroup (Spradley et al., 2015). Examples of microcultures can range from a group of Hmong immigrants from Southeast Asia adopting selected aspects of U.S. culture to a third-generation

Norwegian American community whose members share unique foods, dress, and values.

The members of each subculture and microculture retain some of the characteristics of the society from which they came or in which their ancestors lived, as noted by the eminent anthropologist Margaret Mead (1960). Some of their beliefs and practices—such as the food they eat, the language they speak at home, the way they celebrate holidays, or their ideas about sickness and healing—remain an important part of their everyday life. American Indian or Native American groups have retained some aspects of their traditional cultures. Mexican Americans, Irish Americans, Swedish Americans, Italian Americans, African Americans, Puerto Rican Americans, Chinese Americans, Japanese Americans, Vietnamese Americans, and many other ethnic groups have their own microcultures.

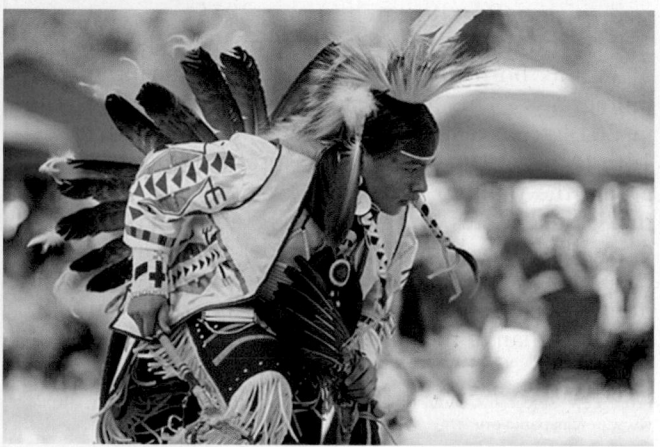

Native American groups retain some aspects of their traditional culture. (Photo courtesy USA.gov)

Furthermore, certain customs, values, and ideas are unique to the poor, the rich, the middle class, women, men, youth, or the elderly. Many deviant groups, such as narcotics abusers, transient alcoholics, gangs, criminals, and terrorist groups, have developed their own microcultures. Regional microcultures, such as that of the White and Black Appalachian people living in the hills and hollows of Kentucky or West Virginia, also have distinctive ways of defining the world and coping with life. Other microcultures, such as those of rural migrant farm workers or urban homeless families, acquire their own sets of beliefs and patterns for dealing with their environments.

Many religious groups have their own microcultures. Even occupational and professional groups, such as nurses or attorneys, develop their own special languages, beliefs, and perspectives.

Ethnocentrism

There is a difference between a healthy cultural or ethnic identification and ethnocentrism. Anthropologists generally note that **ethnocentrism** is an expression of the belief that one's culture of origin is the best approach to life. It is a reflection of judgment on the beliefs and practices of others using our native culture as a reference point (Spradley et al., 2015). It causes people to believe that their way of doing things is right and to judge others' methods as inferior, ignorant, or irrational. Ethnocentrism blocks effective communication by creating biases and misconceptions about human behavior. In turn, this can cause serious damage to interpersonal relationships and interfere with the effectiveness of nursing interventions (McFarland & Wehbe-Alamah, 2015).

People can experience a developmental progression along a continuum from ethnocentrism, feeling one's own culture is best, to **ethnorelativism**—seeing all behavior in a cultural context (Blair & Jansen, 2015). Some people may stop progressing and remain stagnated at one step, and others may move backward on the continuum. The left side of the continuum represents the most extreme reaction to intercultural differences: refusal or denial. On the right side is the characterization of people who show the most sensitivity to intercultural differences: incorporation (Fig. 5–1).

CHARACTERISTICS OF CULTURE

In their study of culture, anthropologists and sociologists have made significant contributions to the field of community health. Their findings shed light on why and how culture influences behavior. Five characteristics shared by all cultures are especially pertinent to nursing's efforts to improve community health: culture is learned, it is integrated, it is shared, it is tacit, and it is dynamic.

Culture Is Learned

Patterns of cultural behavior are acquired, not inherited. Rather than being genetically determined, the way people dress, what they eat, and how they talk are all learned. Spradley et al. (2015) described that when born, we do not have culture and lack a system of beliefs, knowledge and patterns of behavior. In the family and community environment throughout our lives, we are part

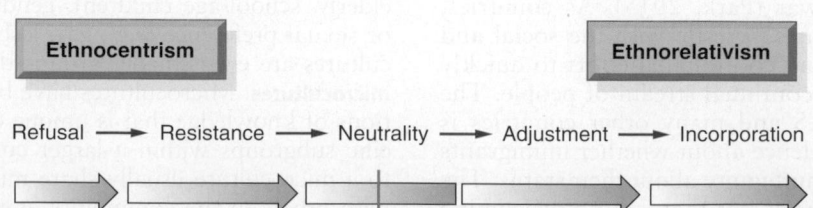

FIGURE 5–1 Cross-cultural sensitivity continuum. Being extremely ethnocentric (**left of midpoint**) and totally ethnorelative (**far right**) are reflected in the diagram. The steps toward ethnorelativism begin at the most ethnocentric view, with refusal and resistance. Neutrality is midpoint, and adjustment and incorporation bring the person to an ethnorelative perspective.

of a general system of learning in our home culture. For example, laughing and smiling are general human responses, but we learn from our culture when to laugh, when to smile, what is considered humorous. All humans can cry, but when we cry and how we cry is tied to our cultural practices.

Each person learns about culture through socialization with the family or significant group, a process called **enculturation**. As a child grows up in a given society, he or she acquires certain attitudes, beliefs, and values and learns how to behave in ways appropriate to that group's definition of the female or male role; by doing so, children are learning about their culture (Spector, 2013; Spradley et al., 2015).

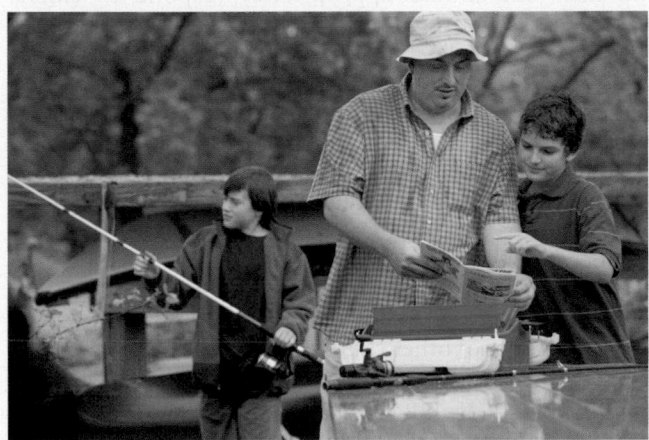

Family socialization helps acculturate children to acquire shared values and attitudes. (Photo courtesy of CDC Photo Image Library.)

Although culture is learned, the process and results of that learning are different for each person. Each individual has a unique personality and experiences life in a singular way; these factors influence the acquisition of culture. Families, social classes, and other groups within a society differ from one another, and this sociocultural variation has important implications (Andrews & Boyle, 2016). Because culture is learned, parts of it can be relearned. People might change certain cultural elements or adopt new behaviors or values. Some individuals and groups are more willing and able than others to try new ways and thereby influence change.

Culture is Integrated

Rather than being merely an assortment of various customs and traits, a culture is a functional, integrated whole. As in any system, all parts of a culture are interrelated and interdependent. The various components of a culture, such as its social mores or religious beliefs, perform separate functions but come into relative harmony with each other to form an operating and cohesive whole. In other words, to understand culture, single traits should not be described independently. Each part must be viewed in terms of its relationship to other parts and to the whole.

A person's culture is an integrated web of ideas and practices. For example, a nurse may promote the need for consuming three balanced meals a day, a practice tied to the beliefs that good nutrition leads to good health and that prevention is better than cure. These cultural beliefs, in turn, are related to the nurse's values about health. Health, the nurse believes, is essential for maximum energy output and productivity at work. Productivity is important because it enables people to reach goals. These values are linked to social or religious beliefs about hard work and taboos against laziness. Through such connections, these ideas and beliefs about nutrition, health, economics, religion, and family are all interrelated and work to motivate behavior.

For example, parents who are Jehovah's Witnesses may refuse a blood transfusion for their child. Their actions might seem irrational or ignorant to those who do not understand the parents' religious beliefs. However, the couple's choice represents behavior consistent with their cultural values and standards. The single behavior of refusing blood transfusions, when viewed in context, is seen to be part of a larger religious belief system and a basic component of the parents' culture. Even mothers' expectations for their children's development can vary between cultures (Damon, Borstein, & Leventhal, 2015)—something to keep in mind when we use developmental screening tools.

In some cultural groups (e.g., Muslims), modesty for women may make it uncomfortable and perhaps traumatic to be examined by a person of the opposite sex (Lovering, 2012). Asking certain Native American groups to comply with rigid appointment scheduling requires them to reframe their concept of time. It also violates their values of patience and pride (Spector, 2013). Before nurses attempt to change a person's or group's behavior, they need to ask how that change will affect the people involved through its influence on other parts of their culture. Extra time and patience or different strategies may be needed if change still is indicated. Nurses often may find, however, that their own practice system can be modified to preserve clients' cultural values.

Culture Is Shared

Culture is the product of aggregate behavior, not individual habit. Certainly, individuals practice a culture, but customs are phenomena shared by all members of the group. More than 40 years ago, anthropologist George Murdock explained (1972, p. 258):

> Culture does not depend on individuals. An ordinary habit dies with its possessor, but a group habit lives on in the survivors and is transmitted from generation to generation. Moreover, the individual is not a free agent with respect to culture. He is born and reared in a certain cultural environment, which impinges on him at every moment of his life. From earliest childhood his behavior is conditioned by the habits of those around him. He has no choice but to conform to the folkways current in his group.

A culture's values are among its most important elements (see Chapter 4). A **value** is a notion or idea designating relative worth or desirability. For example, some cultures place value on honesty, loyalty, and faithfulness more than other traits. Also, there may be strong values against lying, stealing, and cheating—behaviors to avoid. Each culture classifies phenomena into good and bad, desirable and undesirable, right and wrong. When people respond in favor of or against some practice, they are reflecting their culture's values about that practice. One person may eagerly anticipate eating a steak for dinner; another, who believes that eating meat is sacrilegious or unhealthful, experiences revulsion at the idea of steak for a meal. Some American subcultures think that loud, vocal expressions are a necessary way to deal with pain; others value silence and stoicism. Some have high regard for speed and efficiency, whereas others prefer patience and thoughtfulness. Either way, values serve a purpose. Shared values give people in a specific culture stability and security and provide a standard for behavior. From these values, members know what to believe and how to act (Andrews & Boyle, 2016). The normative criteria by which people justify their decisions are based on values that are more deeply rooted than behaviors and, consequently, more difficult to change.

Knowing that culture is shared helps us to better understand human behavior. For example, a community health nurse tried unsuccessfully to persuade a mother to limit the amount of catnip tea she fed her infant. The infant was pacified with the tea and was not consuming a sufficient amount of infant formula, thus putting him at risk for nutritional deficiencies and developmental problems. The nurse discovered that the mother was acting in the tradition of her rural subculture, which held that catnip promoted good health as it acts as an antispasmodic, perhaps causing relaxation and resulting in a more contented infant with fewer symptoms of colic (Spector, 2013). The fact that all of the other mothers in her small rural community also used catnip with their babies proved a powerful deterrent to the change suggested by the nurse. Other members of the same culture frequently influence health behaviors. It is difficult for one person to eliminate a cultural practice, especially if reinforced by so many other members of the group. Group acceptance and a sense of membership usually depend on conforming to these shared cultural practices (Spradley et al., 2015).

Community health nurses may need to focus on an entire group's health behavior to affect individual practices. In the example described, the pattern of consuming large amounts of catnip tea was modified after the nurse worked with the entire rural community. She began with a well-recognized cultural strategy: working through formal or informal leaders. She contacted the oldest woman in the community and discussed the cultural practice. The elder shared the group's beliefs that catnip tea is vital to the well-being of infants for the first 6 months. When the nurse explained her concerns about low formula intake and low weight gain, the community leader clarified that only 1 or 2 ounces of the tea a day was needed. The nurse and the community leader shared this information among the women, and, as a result, the mothers gradually reduced the amount of tea they gave their infants. Consequently, the clients' infants drank more formula and gained weight. A cultural tradition was retained while the health of the infants improved. The community health nurse could then use this new information and other supportive information from the community leader to improve the health of more infants (Spector, 2013).

Culture Is Generally Tacit

Culture provides a guide for human interaction that is **tacit**—that is, mostly unexpressed and at the unconscious level. Members of a cultural group, without the need for discussion, know how to act and what to expect from one another. Culture provides an implicit set of cues for behavior, not a written set of rules. Spradley et al., (2015) explained that culture often lies below a conscious level because it is such a regular and pervasive part of the daily environment. It is like a memory bank in which knowledge is stored for recall when the situation requires it, but this recall process is mostly unconscious. Culture teaches the proper tone of voice to use for each occasion. It prescribes how close to stand when talking with someone and how one should appropriately respond to elders. Individuals learn to make responses that are appropriate to their gender, role, and status. They know what is right and wrong. As an example, one study's researchers found that children's storybooks authored by Native Americans portrayed humans as more connected to nature than did those by non-Native authors (Dehghani et al., 2013). All of these attitudes and behaviors become so ingrained—so tacit—that they are seldom, if ever, discussed.

Because culture is mostly tacit, realizing which of one's own behaviors may be offensive to people from other groups is difficult. It also is difficult to know the meaning and significance of other cultural practices. In some groups, such as American Indians or Islamic women, silence is valued and expected, but may make others uncomfortable. Offering food to a guest in many cultures is not merely a social gesture but an important symbol of hospitality and acceptance; to refuse it, for any reason, may be an insult and a rejection. Touching or calling someone by their first name may be viewed as a demonstration of caring by some groups, but is seen as disrespectful and offensive by others. Even how one trusts others in a group context is affected by cultural influences, and communities with multiple ethnic groups may not exhibit social cohesiveness (van der Meer & Tolsma, 2014). Consequently, community health nurses have a twofold task in developing cultural sensitivity: not only must we try to learn clients' cultures, but we also must try to make our own culture less tacit and more explicit. We must be more aware of our own biases and preconceived values and beliefs. Nurses bring both their professional and personal cultural history to the workplace, often developing unique values not shared with others who are not in the profession (Blais & Hayes, 2015). Cross-cultural tension can be resolved through conscious efforts to develop awareness, patience, and acceptance of cultural differences (Display 5–2).

Culture is Dynamic

Every culture undergoes change; none is entirely static. Within every cultural group, some individuals generate innovations. More important, some members see advantages in doing things differently and are willing to adopt new practices. Each culture is an amalgamation of ideas, values, and practices from a variety of sources. This process depends on the extent of exposure to other groups. Nonetheless, every culture is in a dynamic state of adding or deleting components. Functional aspects are retained; less functional ones are eliminated.

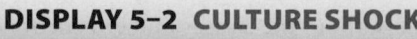

DISPLAY 5–2 CULTURE SHOCK

An increasing number of immigrants and refugees from many different countries have been assimilated into American culture in recent years. Although they quickly adapt in many respects, such as learning the language and seeking housing and employment, they continue to operate within the framework of their own cultural beliefs and behaviors. The conflict between their culture and American culture often causes **culture shock**. This has been termed as a state of anxiety that may result from cross-cultural misunderstanding; people in culture shock may experience difficulty interacting with others in the new environment (Spradley et al., 2015). Immigrants and refugees find themselves in a strange setting with people who act in unfamiliar ways. Speaking their own language in their homes and retaining values and familiar practices all help to promote some sense of security in the new environment.

The same is true for nurses and others working in unfamiliar countries. No longer are the small but important cues available that orient a stranger to appropriate behavior. Instead, a person in a different culture may feel isolated and anxious and even become dysfunctional or ill. Immersion in the culture over time and learning the new culture are the major remedies. As adjustment occurs, old beliefs and practices that are still functional in the new setting can be retained, but others that are not functional must be replaced.

When this adaptation does not occur, the cultural group may face serious difficulty. For example, Hmong teenagers from Southeast Asian refugee families in the United States are among the first generation to be raised in America. Their parents had high hopes for them to restore honor and pride to a displaced people, but the teens struggle to balance their American lifestyle with Hmong traditions. The stresses they feel as a result of the generational and cultural gaps between themselves and their parents are often overwhelming. Hmong community leaders, community health workers, school districts, law enforcement, and Hmong families have joined together to develop interventions to address these issues (see Perspectives: Voices From the Community). Recent prospective research indicates that ethnic identity is positively associated with self-esteem among Asian American adolescents, including Hmong community members (Gertner, Kiang, & Supple, 2014).

Another example of problematic cultural adaptation is the case of the "one child rule" in China. In an effort to contain population growth, in 1979, China began limiting married couples to having only one child. For several years, the government strictly enforced this policy, with few exceptions. Because male offspring are more highly valued than female in the Chinese culture, there was a significant increase in the ratio of male to female births. Couples who had a female infant might choose to place the baby in an orphanage and make her available for adoption, and, although they are considered illegal, it is thought that a large number of sex-selective abortions occur. The goal of the government's policy was to change the Chinese culture from large-to small-family preference, and recent surveys indicate that this appears to be taking place. However, there are unplanned consequences of this cultural shift; inadvertently improving gender equality in education of children (Lee, 2012). Another interesting finding is that mothers having only one child show a higher probability of being overweight (Wu & Li, 2012). In 2013, the government had relaxed the one-child policy for those spouses who were only children; however, only about 12% of eligible couples had applied to have a second child by May of 2015. In late 2015, the Chinese government announced its plans to permit married couples to

PERSPECTIVES
VOICES FROM THE COMMUNITY

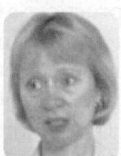

"The European immigrants who emerged from the Ford Motor Company melting pot came to the United States because they hoped to assimilate into mainstream American society. The Hmong came to the United States for the same reason they had left China in the 19th century: because they were trying to resist assimilation. What the Hmong wanted here [in the United States] was to be left alone to be Hmong: clustered in all-Hmong enclaves, protected from government interference, self-sufficient, and agrarian (p. 183)."

—Fadiman, A. (1998). *The spirit catches you and you fall down: A Hmong child, her American doctors, and the collision of two cultures.* New York, NY: Farrar Straus & Giroux.

"You are talking about parents who are medieval, coming to a country that is hundreds of years ahead of theirs. They're trying to catch up, but it's hard."

—Mymee (college instructor)

"There is much research that shows people who stand in the middle of two cultures are really at risk of depression and anxiety."

—Valerie (psychologist)

"The kids are constantly living between two cultures. At some point, they may give up."

—Leng (psychologist, Southeast Asian adult services center)

"I think it's a topic that nobody wants to talk about. It's hard for me to say if the Hmong community is ready to deal with it."

—Xong (social worker, Hmong suicide task force)

"We parents think we know only one way to raise our kids. We ignore that these children are living in America and are espousing everything that is American, good and bad."

—Andy (Hmong parent)

Adapted from Ellis, A. D. (2002, August 11). Hmong Teens: Lost in America [special report]. *The Fresno Bee,* 1–12.

now have two children. A government commission noted that this would help to reduce economic pressures from an aging population, and would also eventually lead to a larger labor supply. When asked about plans for more children, many Chinese citizens expressed an indifferent attitude. Many were concerned about the cost of an additional child, as well as the greater parenting burden, but were glad to see this change (Buckley, 2015).

Community health nurses must remember the dynamic nature of culture for several reasons. First, cultures and subcultures do change over time. Patience and persistence are key attributes to cultivate when working toward improving health behaviors. Second, cultures change as their members see greater advantages in adopting "new ways." Discussions of these advantages need to be conducted in a language understood by members and in the context of their own cultural value system. This is an important reason for nurses to develop an understanding of their clients' culture and to deliver culturally competent care (Andrews & Boyle, 2016; McFarland & Wehbe-Alamah, 2015). Third, it is important to remember that, within a culture, change may occur because of certain key individuals who are receptive to new ideas and are able to influence their peers. These key persons can adapt the change process, so that "new" practices are culturally consistent and fit with group values. Tapping into this resource becomes imperative for successful change. Finally, the health care culture is dynamic, too. Westerners are just beginning to appreciate the validity of many non-Western health care practices such as acupuncture, meditation, and the use of various therapeutic herbs and spices (e.g., turmeric, fenugreek). We can learn much from our clients and their cultures (Grandbois & Sanders, 2012; Spector, 2013) (see Perspectives: Voices From the Community).

ETHNOCULTURAL HEALTH CARE PRACTICES

Throughout history, people have relied on natural elements to treat various maladies that family, clan, tribe, or community members experience. Knowledge of culturally recognized practices or substances, such as berries, plants, barks, or rituals and incantations usually becomes the responsibility of one person in the community. This revered community leader is known as a medicine man/woman, healer, or shaman (Spector, 2013). As time passes, this person teaches the skills of recognizing and treating ailments or performing rituals to an apprentice, thereby continuing the healing knowledge and traditions.

In the following sections, we discuss how various geographic or ethnocultural groups view health care, including the biomedical, magicoreligious, and holistic views. You may encounter many distinctive ways that your clients manage their health and illness, so we will discuss selected folk medicines and home remedies, such as herbs, over-the-counter (OTC) drugs, and patent medications. In addition to these forms of treatments, there are complementary or alternative therapies (e.g., folk remedies) and various self-care practices. This section concludes with the community health nurse's role and responsibilities to provide culturally competent care in relation to caring for, respecting, teaching, and treating clients from different cultures.

The World Community

Beliefs about the causes and effects of illness, health practices, and health-seeking behaviors are all influenced by a person's, a group's, or a community's perception of what causes illness and injury and what actions can best treat or cure the health problem. The three major views in the world community are biomedical, magicoreligious, and holistic health beliefs (Spector, 2013).

Biomedical View

Western societies in general have a biomedical view of health and illness. The biomedical view relies on scientific principles and sees diseases and injuries as life events controlled by physical and biochemical processes that can be manipulated through medication, surgery, and other treatments. Examples of this view include the following beliefs:

- Elements, such as bacteria, fungi, or viruses, are causes of illness.
- Lack of certain elements, such as an adequate diet, calcium, or iron, causes other health problems, such as malnutrition, osteoporosis, or anemia.
- An accepted treatment for many physical ailments is to remove diseased organs, or to treat injuries from falls or accidents.

People living in countries where Western medicine is practiced believe that theirs is the best and, perhaps the only way, to deal with illness or injury. The dominant values presume that science is value free and not constructed by the social norms of the cultural group. The same is true, however, where Western medicine is not practiced and the social norms of the cultural group support the healing practices of that group (McFarland & Wehbe-Alamah, 2015; Spector, 2013). Many people, including community health nurses, are not open to other ways of looking at a person's wellness capabilities. As a result, clients may not receive culturally competent care from their caregivers. To be effective with clients, community health nurses must be knowledgeable and accepting of others' cultural practices.

Magicoreligious View

Magicoreligious themes of health and illness, which focus on the control of health and illness by supernatural forces, are prominent in some cultural groups. Diseases occur as a result of "committing sins" or "going against God's will." Good health is a gift from God, and illness is a form of punishment that affords an opportunity to be forgiven and to realign oneself with God. Prayer to God or other religious figures is used to cope with illness, seek intervention for healing, and ask for forgiveness and entrance into heaven, if death be God's will.

Some cultures mix traditional folk beliefs with organized religious practices and participate in forms of magic or voodoo. In cultures that have such beliefs, a hex or spell can be placed on another person through the use of incantations, elixirs, or an object resembling the person. For some, illness results from a look or a touch from another person considered to have special powers or intent to harm (McFarland & Wehbe-Alamah, 2015; Spector, 2013). Later in this chapter, we discuss some specific health beliefs and practices common to cultural groups in North America.

Religious beliefs, an individual's spirituality, and how these factors interface with feelings of wellness and specific healing practices are personal and important to clients and cannot be separated from their culture. This makes it imperative for community health nurses to be familiar with folk beliefs commonly seen in their practice. Only then can culturally competent nursing care be provided.

Holistic View

Holistic health believers come from many different cultural groups and generally view the world as being in harmonious balance. If the principles guiding natural laws to maintain order are disturbed, an imbalance in the forces of nature is created, resulting in chaos and disease. For an individual to be healthy, all facets of the individual's nature—physical, mental, emotional, and spiritual—must be in balance.

Some cultural groups believe that all things in creation or the universe have a spirit and therefore are considered equal in value, purpose, and contribution (Grandbois & Sanders, 2012). Individuals have universal connectedness and are viewed as holistic beings. Persons are extensions of and integrated with family, community, tribe, and the universe. For example, a pregnant woman and her fetus are seen as integrally related and affecting each other. While physically they are part of a family, they are also two individual spirits in the process of becoming one.

Folk Medicine and Home Remedies

Many of us remember our mothers giving us hot herbal tea with lemon, or slathering on ointments and piling on blankets to lessen the effects of a mild illness. Many folk medicines and home remedies came about as a means of providing health care to family members when no medical care was available or deemed affordable.

Folk medicine is a body of preserved treatment practices that has been handed down verbally from generation to generation. It exists today as the first line of treatment for many individuals. Some clients may never plan to seek Western medical treatment but may share with you, the community health nurse, a practice they are using to treat a family member. Your response and actions may mean the difference between health and illness or injury. Some maternal–child health practices from the U.S. rural Midwest or South that may be encountered in community health nursing practice include the following (Andrews & Boyle, 2016; Spector, 2013):

- Not reaching above your head if you are pregnant, because doing so will cause the umbilical cord to strangle the baby
- Pregnant women eating handfuls of clay, dirt, or cornstarch
- Taping coins over a newborn's umbilical area to prevent hernias
- Giving catnip tea to infants because it saves their lives
- Holding a baby upside down by the heel to "wake up the liver"
- Not letting a cat in a room with a sleeping baby, because the cat will "suck the life" out of the baby

Home remedies are individualized caregiving practices that are passed down within families. Even individuals who routinely seek the guidance of a health care practitioner for diagnosis and treatment may try home remedies before seeking professional advice. Each of us has a set of home remedies our parents used on us that we are likely to use on our own children before or instead of calling the pediatrician. Examples include using baking soda paste on a bee sting, ice on a "cold sore," or cranberry juice to prevent a urinary tract infection.

Herbalism

Textbooks have been written on the many uses of medicinal herbs (Barrett, 2015; Gardner & McGuffin, 2013; Pizzorno, Murray, & Joiner-Bey, 2016). The use of some herbs has waxed and waned in favor. Some continue to be much touted, whereas others have been designated as dangerous and to be avoided (Gardner & McGuffin, 2013; Medline Plus, 2015). Increasingly, the public is using herbal preparations in the form of self-selected OTC products for therapeutic or preventive purposes.

In an increasingly multicultural society, the source, form, and identity of many herbs, roots, barks, and liquid preparations become impossible for most community health nurses to distinguish. The most astute among us may be familiar with herbs used by one cultural group, whereas herbs used by another escape us. A book with pictures and descriptions, botanical form, purported indications and uses, and implications for nursing management is an important tool to keep handy when interacting with clients (Barrett, 2015). Basic safety questions that community health nurses should answer about an herb when teaching or interacting with families include the following:

- Is the herb contraindicated with prescription medications the client is taking?
- Is the herb harmful? Does it have negative side effects?
- Is the client relying on the herb, without positive health changes, while neglecting to get effective treatment from a health care practitioner?

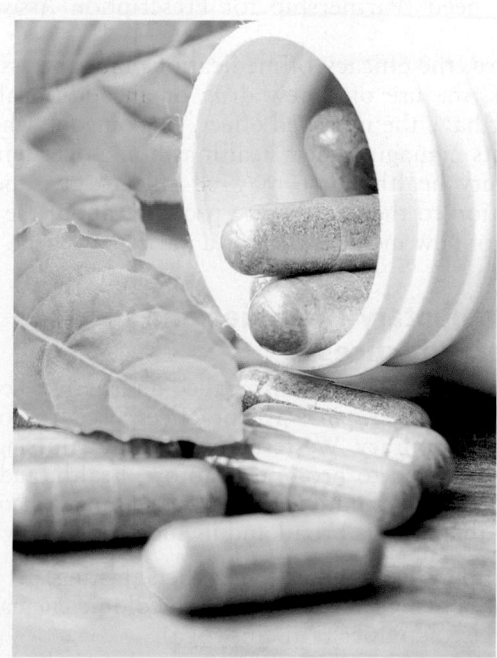

Herbal remedies are increasingly in popularity.

Herbs are not regulated as drugs and are not risk free. Dosages are not standardized and are left to the individual. Quality of the product may be suspect. For these reasons, herbs must be used only in moderation and with caution, preferably with guidance by a health care practitioner.

Prescription and Over-the-Counter Drugs

The cautions mentioned about herbs can also apply to prescription and OTC preparations. First, they are not risk free. In this country, prescription drugs are reviewed and tested by the U.S. Food and Drug Administration's (FDA's) Center for Drug Evaluation and Research (CDER), and OTC drugs go through a somewhat less-rigorous process through the CDER's Division of OTC Drug Products. Many OTC drugs were once available only by prescription, and remain powerful medicines. All drugs can have major side effects, may be contraindicated in people with certain conditions, and may not be safe to use in combination with certain other drugs. Medication instruction and review is an important part of the community health nurse's role on home visits, especially with elderly clients (see Chapter 24).

Second, some new prescription medications are so expensive that clients cannot afford to take them as prescribed. Often, older, less expensive, and more frequently used drugs work as well as the newer, more expensive ones, which are heavily marketed by drug companies to health care practitioners and consumers. If you encounter clients who are unable to pay for drugs, you may need to advocate for them with health care providers to prescribe a less expensive medication or change to the generic form of the same drug, usually sold at a fraction of the cost. Some health care practitioners have samples of drugs available and may be able to use them for medically indigent clients. Many pharmaceutical companies now have low-cost prescription assistance programs for those in need (Partnership for Prescription Assistance, 2015).

Third, the efficacy of medications must be assessed. At times, the use of a new drug or an additional drug does not have the intended effect. As someone who sees the clients managing their health at home over time, the community health nurse may be able to give the best information to the health care provider about the effectiveness of new medications for a particular client.

Complementary Therapies and Self-Care Practices

Complementary therapies (also called alternative medicine or alternative therapies) are practices used to complement contemporary Western medical and nursing care and are designed to promote comfort, health, and well-being (Snyder & Lindquist, 2014). The range of complementary therapies is broad and includes the following:

- Therapies (cancer diets, juice diets, fasting)
- Treatments (coffee enemas, high colonic enemas)
- Exercise activities (t'ai-chi, yoga)
- Exposure (aromatherapy, music therapy, light therapy)
- Manipulation (acupuncture, acupressure, reflexology)

Most cultural groups engage in some form of complementary therapy, either alone or in conjunction with Western medicine. **Integrated health care** is defined as the combination of complementary therapies with biomedical or Western health care (Snyder, Lindquist, & Tracy, 2014). Complementary therapies have become so commonplace today that many states are developing policies and guidelines for their use.

Consumers need to be well informed regarding the efficacy and safety of complementary therapies and how they can be true complements to other treatment modalities. The community health nurse should be aware of the variety of therapies available and how to get information for clients while remaining objective and supportive of the client's choices. At times, if a therapy contradicts the recommendations of the client's health care practitioner, the nurse may be in a position to provide the pros and cons of continuing the complementary therapy. On the other hand, the nurse may be able to suggest therapy forms that would complement Western medicine for the client, such as music therapy to promote relaxation and reduce stress or biofeedback for chronic pain management.

Self-care activities include complementary therapies, medications, and spiritual and cultural practices. They are uniquely individual for each person, as well as among different cultural groups. Chapter 19 includes a Self-Care Assessment Guide that may be helpful in assessing the self-care practices of families.

Role of the Community Health Nurse

When working with different cultural groups in the area of health care practices, the community health nurse can be an effective advocate for the client. First, however, the nurse must be prepared to speak knowledgeably about health care practices and choices. The nurse also must be able to assess the client or family adequately, so as to know what belief system motivates their choices. Finally, the nurse must be prepared to teach clients about the limits and benefits of cultural health care practices. The community health nurse should always individualize assessment and caregiving for the client within her culture and should not generalize about the client based on cultural group norms.

Preparation of the Community Health Nurse

To be effective when working with clients in the area of cultural health care and spirituality, the nurse must be prepared. Many ways exist for you to increase your cultural awareness and promote sensitivity to the differences among people from ethnocultural groups different from your own. You can acquire information from peers who are from the same cultural group as your clients; attend workshops or conferences on chosen cultural topics; read books on ethnocultural health care practices, herbalism, or complementary therapies; talk with clients about their views and practices and learn from them; keep an open mind and be curious about various practices; or attend community cultural events, such as Native American pow-wows, ethnic food events held in some cities, or Cinco de Mayo celebrations. There are textbooks, novels, and articles about cultures in the community in which one practices. For example, the classic book *The Spirit Catches*

You and You Fall Down (Fadiman, 1998) describes a Hmong child, her American doctors, and the collision of two cultures. Universities offer courses in transcultural nursing, ethnic studies courses or programs, and cultural events that can be valuable. The experience of public health nurse Karin Urso, who worked with people from many different countries and cultures, illustrates the benefits of being open-minded (see From the Case Files I).

Assessment

When beginning to work with a group or family, it is important for you to become as familiar with them as possible. In addition to a family assessment or an individual health assessment, you can enhance your aggregate care by doing an ethnocultural or self-care assessment. Such an assessment reveals information about day-to-day living, cultural/spiritual influences, traditional/cultural health care choices and practices, and cultural taboos. Often this type of information is most useful as you work with clients on a regular basis. Useful tools include the two cultural assessment reviews at the end of this chapter and the self-care assessment tool in Chapter 19.

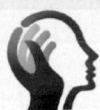

From the **Case Files** I

Learning About Other Cultures

I was always interested in learning about other countries and cultures. But, I didn't realize that an overseas assignment would teach me so much about myself in addition to other cultures and ways of living. The lessons were sometimes difficult, but always rewarding. I knew that my expectations would not always be met and, yet it did surprise me how different the experience was from what I had imagined it would be. My job assignment, location, and team members changed frequently. Flexibility, comfort with ambiguity, a sense of humor, a deeper reliance upon my faith, patience, when results were not forthcoming, trust in others, and the ability to cross multiple cultures with some degree of ease were all skills that I developed over time. Most important to being successful at my job was to maintain the attitude of a "learner," not a "solver of problems" or the person "with all the answers." I made friends with people from all over the world who graciously accepted me into their lives, thus enriching mine. I learned that we all are different, but that every behavior has a reasonable explanation when you take the time to listen with your heart as well as with your ears. I found that I actually preferred other ways of doing and being while still maintaining those parts of my identity that were valuable to me. When I returned home, I found that my newly developed skills were still necessary—as I had changed and had to adjust to reentry into my home culture!

Karin Urso, PHN

Teaching

As you are aware from your studies and preparation, teaching is the most important role in nursing, both in acute care settings and in the home. When working with families as a community health nurse, teaching takes a good deal of your time, because health care education is vitally important to communities, groups, and families. However, teaching that is undertaken in ways that are incomplete, culturally inappropriate, or inadequate may be frustrating and even harmful to your clients. Becoming ethnoculturally focused and prepared to teach from the client's view of the world will start you in the right direction. The suggestions in Display 5–3 offer ideas for providing culturally competent care. Chapter 11 on health promotion and education will help prepare you as well.

SELECTED CULTURAL COMMUNITIES

An examination of the meaning and nature of culture clearly underscores the need to recognize cultural differences and to understand clients in the context of their cultural backgrounds. Practically speaking, how can knowledge of cultural diversity be integrated into everyday community health nursing practice? What are the diverse cultural communities served by community health nurses? What are their differences? Do they share some features?

To provide insights and answers to these questions, this section describes 5 cultural communities, out of the more than 100 different ethnic groups living in the United States. Three are dominant in the United States; the other two represent populations native to North America and people from a Middle Eastern culture, an expanding group in the United States. These brief descriptions should not to be considered as a stand-alone guide to cultural competence; each culture is complex and unique, deserving of a more comprehensive study than is possible within the scope of this chapter. Many good references are available for nurses on cultural diversity (see References and Selected Readings).

Four of the groups highlighted represent those identified in *Healthy People 2020* (U.S. Department of Health and Human Services [U.S. DHHS], 2015). The fifth group, Arab populations, is presented because of the significant media attention people of the Middle East have received in recent years. *Healthy People 2010* (U.S. DHHS, 2015) described significant disparities among members of some of the five groups highlighted here. Several of the disparities are given in Table 5–4. *Healthy People 2020* objectives expand on the work done through *Healthy People 2010*.

Native American Indians, Aleut, and Eskimo Communities

Native American Indians and Alaska Natives (Eskimo communities residing in Alaska), the first known settlers of this continent, form a large cluster of tribal groups whose members are descendants of the original Native Americans who inhabited this country before White Europeans settled here. The earliest European explorers

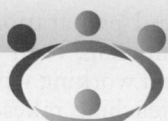

DISPLAY 5–3 DEVELOPING CULTURAL COMPETENCE

First: Know that culture is dynamic.
It is a continuous and cumulative process.
It is learned and shared by people.
People exhibit cultural behaviors and values.
Culture is creative and meaningful to our lives.
It is symbolically represented through language and interaction.
Culture guides us in our thinking, feeling, and acting.

Second: Become aware of culture in yourself.
Thought processes that occur within you also occur within others but may take on a different shape or meaning.
Cultural values and biases are interpreted internally.
Cultural values are not always obvious because they are shared socially with those you meet on a daily basis and are perceived through your senses.

Third: Become aware of culture in others, especially among client groups you serve.
This is best represented by the belief that there are many cultural ways that are correct, each in its own location and context.
It is essential to build respect for cultural differences and appreciation for cultural similarities.
Develop the ability to work within others' cultural context, free from ethnocentric judgments.

were the Vikings (circa 1010 AD). Various other Europeans followed in the 16th century (Spector, 2013). Native Americans, Aleuts, and Eskimos have adopted many European American values and practices, yet they preserve many aspects of their own culture.

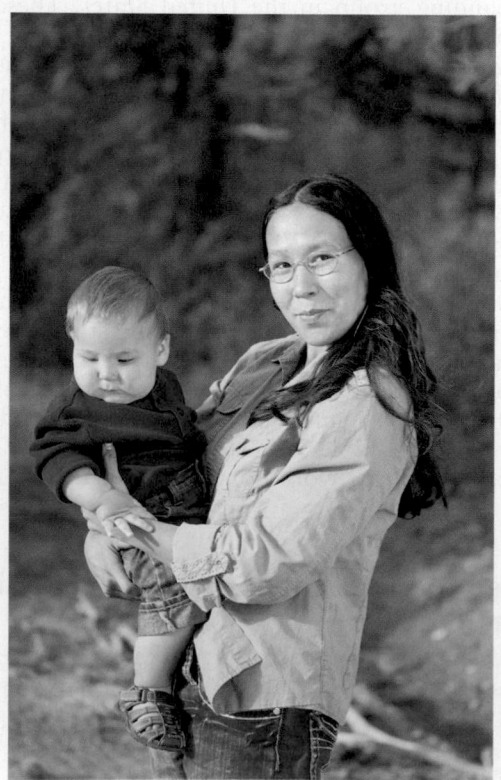

Native American mother and child.

Population Characteristics and Culture

Native Americans and Alaska Natives are a diverse group made up of different tribes and 562 federally recognized nations that speak approximately 250 languages. Eskimos, Aleuts, and Native Americans living in Alaska are known as Alaska Natives; those living in other states are known as Native Americans or American Indians. In this chapter, the term *Native American* is used to encompass all facets of this diverse group of people. Many people in this group identify with more than one race or ethnicity. In the 2010 census, an estimated 6.5 million people identified at least "part" Native American, whereas 4.0 million self-identified only as Native American or Alaska Native (Colby & Ortman, 2015). These people proudly identify themselves as being Native American, unlike in the past, when to claim Native American blood carried a social stigma. In addition to societal changes in the acceptance of Native Americans, financial incentives exist for many Americans who are recognized tribal members. Roughly 224 of the tribal governments receive revenue from gambling casinos—roughly half of all tribes have casinos in 28 states (Tribal Court Clearinghouse, n.d.). In 1988, when Congress passed the Indian Gaming Regulatory Act, casinos owned by Native Americans made $212 million; by 2015, a total of 486 gaming operations grossed $28.5 billion (National Indian Gaming Council, 2015). Some, but not all, tribes pay per capita payments to tribal members (Tribal Court Clearinghouse, n.d.).

Even though the poverty rate fell for Native Americans overall, it is over twice the U.S. average (Office of Minority Health, 2015), and unemployment is nearly three times the national rate—making Native Americans among the nation's poorest groups (Native

Table 5-4 *Healthy People 2020*, Selected Objectives and Disparities

Healthy People 2020 Goals	Baseline Progress: Most Current Values (2012–2013)						
	Total	White	American Indian/A.N.	Hispanic/Latino	Black	Asian	Native Hawaiian
AHS-1.1 Increase proportion of persons with medical insurance 100% of population	83.5%	83.7%	70.6%	69.3%	81.1%	85.8%	89.3%
PA-2.4 Increase proportion of adults engaged in physical activity (aerobic and muscle strengthening) 20.1% of population	18.2%	23.5%	23.8%	15.1%	20.0%	17.5%	—
NWS-9 Reduce proportion of adults who are obese 30.5% of population	33.9%	36.4%	—	42.6	48.4%	—	—
NWS-10.4 Reduce the proportion of 2- to 19-year-olds who are obese 14.5%	16.1%	14.0%	—	21.8%	22.1%	—	—
AH-5.1 Increase the proportion of students who graduate from high school in 4 y 87%	79%	87%	78%	75%	71%	—	—
SA-14.3 Decrease the proportion of adults binge drinking in past 30 d 24.4%	27.1%	28.1%	28.3%	28.6%	23.6%	14.4%	28.7%
TU-1.1 Decrease proportion of adults who are current cigarette smokers 12.0%	20.6%	20.2%	21.5%	11.7%	18.0%	9.4%	27.8%
MICH-1.3 Decrease infant mortality rate 6/1,000	6.7	10.4	7.6	5.0	11.1	4.1	4.1
MICH-9.1 Decrease percentage of infants born preterm 11.4% of live births	12.7%	10.2%	13.1%	11.3%	16.3%	10.2%	10.2%
FP-7.1 Increase the proportion of sexually active females (15–44) receiving reproductive health services in past 12 mo 86.5%	78.6%	76.1%	—	77.5%	84.8%	—	—
HIV-13 Increase proportion of those 13 y and over aware of their HIV infection 90.0% living w/ HIV	80.9%	89.8%	81.1%	85.3%	86.4%	79.4%	76.9%
MHMD-1 Decrease the rate for suicide 10.2/100,000	11.3	15.9	11.7	—	5.6%	—	—

From U.S. Department of Health and Human Services. (2016). Healthy People 2020: LHI topics. *Selected Topics & Objectives with Racial/Ethnic Disparities Reported.* Retrieved from https://www.healthypeople.gov/2020/leading-health-indicators/2020-LHI-Topics

American Rights Fund, n.d.). Although gaming and other ventures have improved access to health, education, and employment for most Native Americans, access still falls behind that of other U.S. citizens.

The population of Native Americans and Alaska Natives is primarily concentrated in 26 states in the United States, including Alaska and the Aleutian Islands (Spector, 2013). Many live on reservations and in rural areas; however, more than half live in urban counties and have greater difficulty accessing the health care available to them through Indian Health Service, a federal program providing comprehensive health care to Native Americans (Office of Minority Health, 2015). The largest numbers live in Oklahoma, Arizona, California, New Mexico, North Carolina, and Alaska, as a result of forced westward migration (Spector, 2013). By 2050, the U.S. Census Bureau estimates about 4.5 million Native Americans will live in the United States, nearly double the number in 2000 (Colby & Ortman, 2015). Some of this increase can be attributed to official recognition of persons who can provide information linking them to a tribe or nation; if they are accepted, they can then declare themselves to be Native Americans.

Each tribe or nation has its own distinct language, beliefs, customs, and rituals. The community health nurse cannot assume that knowledge of one group can be generalized to others. Knowledge of various Native American cultures (Display 5–4) can assist nurses working with members of a specific tribe. For many Native American groups, large, extended family networks reinforce cultural standards and expectations and provide emotional support and practical assistance.

Health Problems

Health problems among Native Americans tend to be both chronic and socially related. One third of Native Americans live in abject poverty and experience the afflictions associated with poor living conditions, including malnutrition, tuberculosis (TB), and high maternal and infant death rates (Office of Minority Health, 2015;

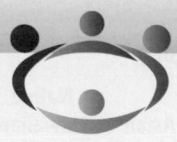

DISPLAY 5–4 SIMILARITIES AMONG NATIVE AMERICAN CULTURES

All of creation/universe has Spirit and is considered equal in value.

Everything is considered alive with energy and importance.

People have universal connectedness.

Harmony is a way of life based on cooperation and sharing.

Dignity of the individual, family, and community is valued.

Respect for advancing age is valued; elders are leaders.

There is present-time orientation, grounded in what is happening at the moment.

Symbolic arts and crafts are valued.

A strong sense of identity fosters resilience.

Generosity, harmony, and sharing are valued.

Religion is integrated into everyday life.

Herbal medicines and traditional healing practices are used.

Rituals and ceremonies are valued.

Silence is used as a way to practice presence and strength.

Thoughtful speech and patience are valued.

Cultural resilience is important when confronting stereotypes.

Adapted from Grandbois, D. M., & Sanders, G. F. (2012). Resilience and stereotyping the experiences of Native American elders. *Journal of Transcultural Nursing, 23*(4), 389–396; Spector, R. E. (2013). *Cultural diversity in health and illness* (8th ed.). Upper Saddle River, NJ: Pearson Education.

Spector, 2013). The highest-ranking health problems in children include a postneonatal mortality rate double that of White infants (due largely to sudden infant death syndrome [SIDS], injuries, and congenital anomalies); overweight, obesity, and Type 2 diabetes; and morbidity and mortality as a result of unintentional and intentional injuries, often motor vehicle injuries (Office of Minority Health, 2015). For adults, diabetes, TB, and obesity all rank higher among Native Americans than in the general population. Deaths from TB (5 times higher), alcoholism (5 times higher), diabetes (almost 2 times higher), unintentional injuries (1.5 times higher), and suicide and homicide (combined, 1.6 times higher) are higher for Native Americans than other Americans (Office of Minority Health, 2015). Mortality from heart disease and cardiovascular disease is slightly higher than the general U.S. population (269.4 per 100,000 deaths compared with 267 per 100,000 deaths; Office of Minority Health, 2015). Poor sanitation, crowded housing, and low immunization levels contribute to the prevalence of a variety of communicable diseases.

Alcoholism is the major health problem of Native Americans. Both traditional/cultural and medical explanations exist for the disproportionate number of alcohol-related health problems in Native Americans. Tribal medicine men have attributed the problems of alcoholism to losing the community's loss of chance to make choices, and advocate for people to gain a sense of cultural identification in order to minimize or eliminate alcoholism (Spector, 2013). Medically, it appears that Native Americans have a much lower tolerance for alcohol and therefore demonstrate the effects of alcohol with lower amounts consumed. When individuals are under the influence of alcohol, other health and safety problems occur. Instances of domestic violence, child abuse and neglect, traffic injuries and deaths, and homicides are more frequent because of alcohol abuse. Along with these high rates of injuries and deaths, alcohol's destructive effects on the unborn lead to a high incidence of fetal alcohol syndrome (FAS) and fetal alcohol effects (FAE). Substance abuse is also prevalent among those living on reservations, and increasingly among youth using alcohol, tobacco, and other drugs (U.S. Substance Abuse & Mental Health Services Administration [U.S. SAMHSA], 2014).

Health Beliefs and Practices

Native Americans as a group prefer traditional healing practices and folk medicine to Western medicine. Most Native Americans today still seek out a medicine man or rely on traditional remedies before going to a health clinic. Many of their beliefs about health and illness have common traditional roots, regardless of tribe or location. Health and dietary practices are closely tied to cultural and religious beliefs. Beliefs about health reflect living in total harmony with nature. Cultural resilience has been identified as an important component of well-being in this cultural group (Grandbois & Sanders, 2012). The Earth is considered a living organism that should be treated with respect, as should the body (Spector, 2013). Native Americans practice purification rituals such as immersion in water and the use of sweat lodges to maintain their harmony with nature and to cleanse the body and spirit. The basis of therapy lies in nature, with herbal teas, charms, and fetishes used as preventive and curative measures (Gardner & McGuffin, 2013; McGaa, 2011). Depending upon location, tribes use available plants or herbs to treat illnesses. For instance, those in the West often used sage (or sagebrush) tea for sore eyes, stomachache, or the pain of childbirth.

Because of decades of racism and government paternalism, many Native Americans feel oppressed and dehumanized and carry considerable resentment and lack of trust toward Whites. As a result, many maintain a degree of separateness from overall American culture. Nurses must overcome these barriers through patience, acceptance, and respect for their clients' culture, as illustrated in the case study of the community health nurse, Sandra

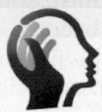

From the *Case* Files II

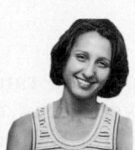

Sandra's New Clients

As she drove down the dirt road and parked her car next to the community hall, Sandra Josten felt apprehensive. The previous public health nurse had alerted her about the difficulty of working with these Native American people: "This tribe is lazy and unappreciative. You can't get anywhere with them." Only through the urging of Mrs. Brown, an Indian community aid, had a group of the women reluctantly agreed to meet with the new nurse. They would see what she had to say.

Sandra's steps echoed hollowly as she walked across the wooden floor of the large room to the far corner where a group of women sat silently in a circle. Only their eyes turned; their faces remained impassive. Mrs. Brown rose slowly, greeted the nurse, and introduced her to the group. Swallowing her fear, Sandra smiled. She told them of her background and explained that she had not worked with Indian people before. There was a long silence. No one spoke. Sandra continued, "I'd like to help you if I can, maybe with problems about care of your children when they are sick or questions about how to keep them healthy, but I don't know what you need or want." Silence fell again. She would like to learn from them, she repeated. Would they help her? Again, Sandra felt an uncomfortable silence.

Then one woman began to speak. Quietly, but with deep feeling, she described several bad experiences with the previous nurse and the county social worker. Then others spoke up: "They tell us what we should do. They don't listen. They say our way is not good." Seeing Sandra's interest and concern, the women continued. One of their main concerns was their children's health. Another was the high incidence of accidents and injuries on the reservation. They wanted to learn how to give first aid. Other concerns were expressed. The group agreed that Sandra could help them by teaching a first-aid class.

In the weeks that followed, Sandra taught several classes on first aid and emergency care. She then began a series of sessions on child health. Each time, she asked the women to choose a topic or problem for discussion and then elicited from them their accustomed ways of dealing with each problem; for example, how they handled toilet training or taught their children to eat solid foods. Her goal was to learn as much as she could about their culture and to incorporate that information into her teaching, which preserved as many of their practices as possible. Sandra also visited informally with the women in their homes and at community gatherings.

She learned about their way of life, their history, and their values. For example, patience was highly valued. It was important to be able to wait patiently, even if a scheduled meeting was delayed as much as 2 hours. It also was important for others to speak, which explained the Indian women's comfort with silences during a conversation. Other values influenced their way of life. Courage, pride, generosity, and honesty all were important determinants of behavior. These also were values by which they judged Sandra and other professionals. Sandra's honesty in keeping her promises enabled the women to trust her. Her generosity in giving her time, helping them occasionally with some household task, and arranging for childcare during classes won their respect.

The women came to accept her, and Sandra was invited to eat with them and share in tribal get-togethers. The women criticized and advised her on acceptable ways to speak and act. Her openness and patience to learn and her respect for them as a people had paved the way to improving their health. At first, Sandra felt that her progress was slow, but this slowness was an advantage. She had built a solid foundation of cross-cultural trust, and in the months that followed she saw many changes in her clients' health practices.

Josten, and her new client from a Native American community (see From the Case Files II).

Blacks or African Americans

Some of the ancestors of Black Americans, or African Americans, originally came to this continent as free settlers as early as 1619, but most of the approximately 4 million who followed came as slaves in the 17th and 18th centuries, mostly from the west coast of Africa (Klein, 2012). Most Black Americans alive today were born in the United States; some, however, are immigrants from African countries. Other Black Americans come from the West Indies, the Dominican Republic, Haiti, and Jamaica, often to escape poverty or political persecution (Spector, 2013)

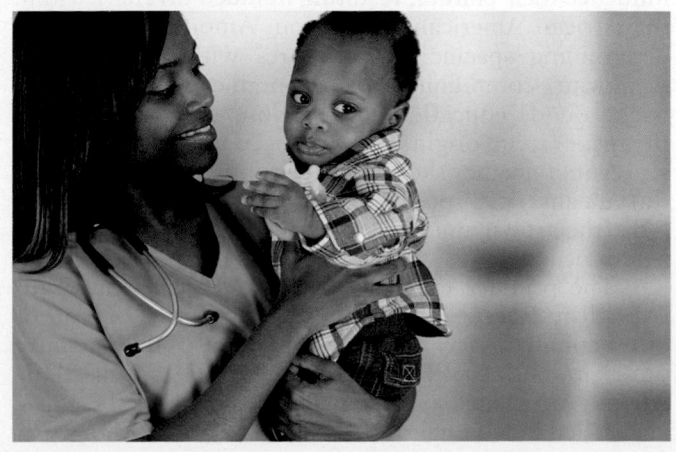

Population Characteristics and Culture

The U.S. Census Bureau estimated that African Americans numbered 45 million and constituted approximately 13.2% of the U.S. population in 2014. By 2060, the projected black population of the United States (including those of more than one race) is estimated to reach 74.5 million. Based on these projections, by that time, blacks would constitute 17.9% of the United States' total population (U.S. Census Bureau, n.d.a.) One third of the African American population is younger than 18 years of age. Slightly more than 8% of African Americans are older than 65 years, and most of them are women; in comparison, 13% of the total population is older than 65 years. Some 58% of Black children live with their mothers only, compared with 21% of White children (Office of Minority Health, 2015).

Despite improvements in the legal and social climate for African Americans, great disparities exist between them and White Americans (Office of Minority Health, 2015). In 2012, the average family income for African Americans was $33,762 and $56,565 for White families. More than 28% of African Americans live in poverty, compared with 1% of Whites. Although African Americans make up only 13.5% of the population, more than 50% of prison inmates are Black.

Educational and employment disparities also exist. Unemployment among African Americans is 10.3, compared with 4.8% for Whites (Office of Minority Health, 2015). Among people aged 25 years and older, 83% of Blacks and 92% of Whites have a high school education (Office of Minority Health, 2015). More than half of those African Americans with less than a high school education are not in the workforce, compared with 36% of Whites with a similar education. African American women acquire more educational training than their Black male counterparts do, but their earnings are lower than those of the men, as is also the case with White and Hispanic women compared with men in those groups. In a recent study of racial discrimination in the labor market for recent college graduates, the authors report finding strong evidence of differential treatment by race (Nunley, Pugh, Romero, & Seals, 2014).

Like Native Americans and Asian Americans, African Americans do not constitute a single culture; rather, this group forms a heterogeneous community. As with other large ethnic and racial groups, many factors influence their culture, resulting in much diversity within the African American population. Among the variables determining specific microcultures within the African American community are economic level, religious background, education, occupation, social class identity, geographic origin, and residence in an integrated or segregated neighborhood. For community health nurses, this means that specific groups of African Americans have their own unique values, character, lifestyle, and health needs.

The primary language of most African Americans is English. Recent Black immigrants from Caribbean or other countries may retain the language of their country of origin, but usually learn to use English as well. Many African Americans speak nonstandard dialects of English, also called Black English or African American Vernacular English. These dialects evolved from *pidgin* English spoken during the era of slavery, and they have become a dynamic and meaningful language of their own. For some African Americans, this dialect symbolizes racial pride and identity—it can also be used to differentiate them from the mainstream culture (Spector, 2013).

Health Problems

African Americans have much higher mortality rates than do White Americans, with a life expectancy of 75.1 years (Arias, 2014). Life expectancy for Whites in 2010 was 78.7 years (Arias, 2014). The number for African Americans is the same as the life expectancy of Whites in 1980, revealing a 30-year lag for the Black population compared with the White population and demonstrates the inequality in mortality and life expectancy, an outcome of health care, economic, and educational disparity.

Stress and discrimination, poverty, lack of education, high rates of teen pregnancy, inadequate housing, and inadequate insurance for health care are among the risk factors influencing the health of this population. Female-headed households, single-parent births (most frequently among teenagers), and a limited presence of male role models have exacerbated family vulnerability. This situation is improving with a reported reduction of female-headed households with children under the age of 18 decreasing from 56% in 1985 to 52% in 2014 (U.S. Census Bureau, n.d.b.).

The major health problems for Blacks include cardiovascular disease and stroke, cancer, diabetes mellitus, cirrhosis, a high infant mortality rate (twice that of Whites), homicide, accidents, and malnutrition (Display 5–5). Leading causes of death for African Americans are heart disease, cancer, and stroke. As noted, infant death rates are higher in Blacks than in other groups (11.1 per 1,000 live births), leading many health departments to focus on services for African American pregnant women (Office of Minority Health, 2015). Mortality rates for communicable diseases, including acquired immunodeficiency syndrome (AIDS), also are higher for Blacks than for Whites. The incidence of TB in this population is rising, with many cases being diagnosed in conjunction with AIDS (see Chapters 8 and 26). Other infectious and parasitic diseases are three to six times more prevalent among African Americans than among Whites (Office of Minority Health, 2015). Hypertension is a real concern in this population; 40.5% of men and 44.3% of women over the age of 20 report having hypertension. In the same age group, 70% of men and 80% of women are reported as overweight (Office of Minority Health, 2015). In two health-related areas, Blacks demonstrate a lower incidence than do Whites: suicide is 50% less prevalent among Blacks, and the rate of chronic obstructive pulmonary disease (COPD) is 20% to 30% less. All other leading causes of death are higher for Black populations, much of which can be attributed to lifestyle and poverty factors (Office of Minority Health, 2015). However, some genetic studies have shown significant differences between African Americans and Whites in those genes associated with hypertension and cardiovascular disease (Non, Gravlee, & Mulligan, 2012).

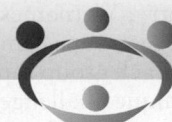

DISPLAY 5–5 EXAMPLES OF CULTURAL PHENOMENA AFFECTING HEALTH CARE AMONG BLACK OR AFRICAN AMERICANS

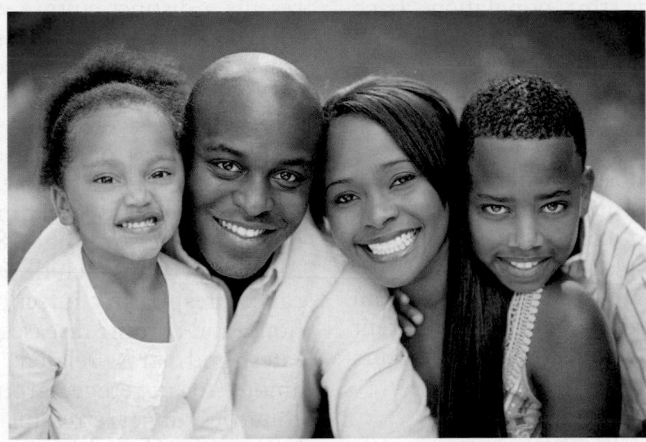

Nations of Origin	Many West African countries (as slaves) West Indian Islands The Dominican Republic, Haiti, Jamaica
Environmental Control	Traditional health and illness beliefs may continue to be observed by "traditional" people
Biological Variations	Sickle cell anemia, hypertension, cancer of the esophagus, stomach cancer, coccidioidomycosis, lactose intolerance
Social Organization	Family: many single-parent households headed by females Large, extended family networks Strong church affiliations within the community Community social organizations
Communication	National languages Dialect: Pidgin French, Spanish, Creole
Spatial Distancing	Close personal space
Time Orientation	Present over future

Adapted from Spector, R. E. (2013). *Cultural diversity in health and illness* (8th ed.). Upper Saddle River, NJ: Pearson Education.

Blacks may have specific skin problems (e.g., keloids, melasma). In addition, sickle cell anemia and sickle cell trait occurs in Blacks, an inherited genetic trait thought to have originated in Africa as a defense against malaria (Spector, 2013).

Health Beliefs and Practices

Although African Americans have assimilated into the more dominant non-Hispanic White American culture in the United States, some retain aspects of their ancestors' traditional values and practices. Some, for example, hold traditional African beliefs about health being a sign of harmony with nature and illness being evidence of disharmony. Evil spirits, the punishment of God, or a hex placed on the person might account for this disharmony. Healers treat body, mind, and spirit. Prayer, laying on of hands, magic or other rituals, special diets, wearing of preventive charms or copper bracelets, ointments, and other folk remedies sometimes are practiced (Spector, 2013). African Americans have a high degree of religious involvement; 80% consider themselves to be either very or fairly religious. Higher levels of active religious participation are associated on average with less illness and better health (Lumpkins, Greiner, Daley, Mabachi, & Neuhaus, 2013). Church attendance for African Americans is significantly associated with positive health care practices, including mental health conditions such as depression and substance abuse (Hankerson & Weissman, 2012), as well as decreased pain in sickle cell anemia (Cotton, Grossoehme, & McCrady, 2012). Such an effect is even stronger for the chronically ill and uninsured subgroups. This is an important consideration when public health nurses plan programs targeting this population. Each African American community has its own set of health beliefs and practices that must be determined by the community health nurse before any interventions are planned.

Asian Americans

A third cultural cluster is composed of immigrants and refugees from various Pacific Rim countries, such as China, Korea, Japan, Thailand, Laos, the Philippines, Vietnam, and Cambodia (Display 5–6). Some Asian Americans have been transplanted fairly recently from their native countries and cultures to an entirely different culture, whereas others may have lived here many years or were born in the United States.

Population Characteristics and Culture

In the 2010 census, more than 16.7 million Asians and Pacific Islanders were living in the United States, representing 5.5% of the total population (Jensen et al., 2015).

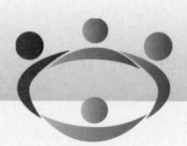

DISPLAY 5–6 ASIAN–PACIFIC POPULATIONS

Asian refers to:	Pacific Islander refers to:
Chinese	Polynesian
Filipino	Hawaiian
Japanese	Samoan
Asian Indian	Tongan
Korean	Micronesian
Vietnamese	Guamanian
Laotian	Melanesian
Thai	Fijian
Cambodian	Tahitian
Pakistan	Marshallese
Indonesian	Trilese
Hmong	
Mein	
Lahu	

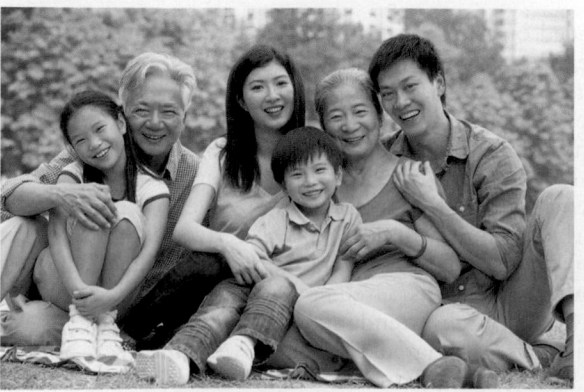

The largest groups were Chinese and Filipinos, with more than 1.5 million persons from each country; Vietnamese numbered a close second. Other fairly large groups came from Korea, India, Laos, and Cambodia. Each group represents a distinct culture with its own unique challenges for community health nurses, as illustrated in the case study of the Kim family (see From the Case Files III).

Health Problems

Leading causes of death among Asians include cancer, heart disease, and stroke (Office of Minority Health, 2015). Smoking is lower in this group (18% of males and 6% of females over age 18 smoke). Health problems for Asian Americans include malnutrition, TB, mental illness, cancer, respiratory infections, arthritis, parasitic infestations, and chronic diseases associated with aging. Suicide rates and stress-related illness are particularly high among Asian refugee groups who have had to flee their countries under stressful conditions and among teens born in the United States to Asian immigrants; many of these children have difficulty living between two cultures (Kim, Sangalang, & Kihl, 2012). However, Asians can view mental illness as shameful, and the stigma attached to it prompts them to express the mental illness as a disturbed bodily function or to hide it as long as possible (Kim et al., 2012; Spector, 2013).

Health Beliefs and Practices

Asian health beliefs vary among subcultures. Many Asians believe in the Chinese concepts of *yin* (cold) and *yang* (hot), which do not refer to temperature but to the opposing forces of the universe regulating normal flow of energy. A balance of yin and yang results in *qi* (pronounced *chee*), which is the desired state of harmony. Illness results when an imbalance occurs in these forces. If the imbalance is an excess of yin, then "cold" foods, such as vegetables and fruits, are avoided, and "hot" foods, such as rice, chicken, eggs, and pork, are offered. Some Asians view Western medicines as "hot" and Eastern folk medicines and herbal treatments as "cold," which explains why some groups practice both for balance. The Vietnamese have a similar hot-and-cold belief, but call it *am* and *dong*. Other Asian groups, such as the Filipinos, view illness as an act of God and pray for healing, reflecting their strong religious beliefs as Catholics or Muslims. The Khmer of Cambodia believe that illness reflects a deviation from moral standards, and the Hmong consider illness to be a visitation by spirits (Paniaguia 2014; Spector, 2013).

Many Asian groups have traditional healers, who, depending on the culture, may include acupuncturists, herbalists, herb pharmacists, spirit and magic experts, or a shaman. Most Asian cultures also exercise traditional self-care practices, including herbal medicines and poultices, types of acupuncture, and massage (Andrews & Boyle, 2016; Spector, 2013). Southeast Asians also practice dermabrasive techniques of coining, cupping, pinching, rubbing, and burning. These methods are used to relieve symptoms such as headache, sore throat, cough, fever, and diarrhea by bringing toxins to the skin surface or compensating for heat lost. Because these techniques leave a bruise-like lesion on the skin, they can be mistaken for physical abuse (Chirali, 2014). Each client requires

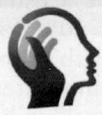

From the Case Files III

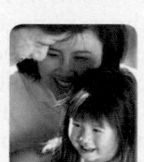

The Kim Family

Armed with enthusiasm and pamphlets on pregnancy and prenatal diet, Paula Morrow, the community health nurse, began home visits to the Kim family. Paula's initial plan was to discuss pregnancy and fetal development, teach diet, and prepare the mother for delivery. Mr. Kim, a graduate student, was present to interpret, because Mrs. Kim spoke little English. Their two children, ages 1 and 3 years, played happily on the kitchen floor. The family offered tea to the nurse and listened politely as she explained her reasons for coming and asked, "How can I be most helpful to you? What would you like from my visits?"

The Kims were grateful for this approach. Hesitant at first, they hinted at Mrs. Kim's fears of American doctors and hospitals; her first two children had been born in Korea. None of the family had any experience with Western medicine. They shared some concerns about adjustment to living in the United States. It was difficult to shop in American food stores with their overwhelming variety of foods, many of which the Kims found unfamiliar. Mrs. Kim, who had come from a family whose servants prepared the food, was an inexperienced cook. Servants also had cared for the children, and her role had been that of an aristocrat in hand-tailored silk gowns.

Listening carefully, Paula began to realize the striking differences between her own culture and that of her clients. Her care plans changed. In subsequent visits, she determined to learn about Korean culture and base her nursing intervention on that knowledge. She learned about their traditional ways of raising children, the traditional male and female roles, and practices related to pregnancy and lactation. She respected their value of "saving face" and attempted never to offend their pride or dignity. As time went on, her interest and respect for their way of life won their trust. She inquired about their cultural practices before attempting any intervention. As a result, the Kims were receptive to her suggestions. Whenever possible, Paula adapted her teaching and suggestions to comply with the Kims' culture. For example, appropriate changes were made to Mrs. Kim's diet plan to incorporate her food preferences and cultural eating patterns. Because she was not accustomed to drinking milk, she increased her calcium intake by learning to prepare custards (which disguised the milk flavor) and by eating more portions of leafy, green vegetables. After 5 months, a strong, positive relationship had been established between this family and the nurse. Mrs. Kim delivered a healthy baby girl and looked forward to continued supportive visits from the community health nurse.

Whereas each Asian culture is distinct in language, values, and customs, many Asians share some general traits. Traditional Asian families tend to be patriarchal (the father is the head of the household) and patrilineal (the genealogy is carried through the male line). Male members are valued over female members, and elders are respected. The male role generally is that of provider, whereas the female role is that of homemaker. Traditional Asians value achievement because it brings honor to the family name. Saving face or preserving dignity and family pride is important. Cooperation is valued over competition (McFarland & Wehbe-Alamah, 2015; Spector, 2013).

---

a careful **cultural assessment** (a detailed data-gathering about the client's cultural practices) before nursing action is implemented.

Hispanic Americans

A fourth cultural cluster constitutes groups who are of Hispanic or Latino origin and have immigrated to the United States, some many generations ago. More than half come from Mexico, followed by Puerto Rico, Cuba, the Dominican Republic, and Central and South America (Colby & Ortman, 2015; Spector, 2013). Those with Mexican and Central American backgrounds generally are referred to as Latinos. Depending on the region of the country, socioeconomic status, immigration or citizenship status, or age, members of this large minority group refer to themselves as Mexican American, Spanish American, Chicano, Latin American, Latin, Latino, or Mexican (Colby & Ortman, 2015; Spector, 2013). In this chapter, for convenience, the term *Hispanic* is used to encompass this entire diverse population.

The subgroups of Hispanics vary by their patterns of geographic distribution in the United States. Of the almost 55 million Hispanics in the United States, Mexicans are the largest percentage at 64.3%. Central and South Americans constitute almost 15%, and Puerto Ricans make up 9.4% and Cubans 3.7% of the Hispanic population. The states with the largest Hispanic populations include California (14.5 million), Texas (10 million), New York (3.5 million), Florida (4.5 million), and Illinois (2.1 million). The Hispanic population is young, with 33.2% under the age of 18, compared to 19.7% non-Hispanic Whites (Office of Minority Health, 2015).

Population Characteristics and Culture

With 55 million self-identifying Hispanics, this population is the largest ethnic group in the United States. People identifying Hispanic origin are predicted to number more than 119 million by 2060 (U.S. Census Bureau, n.d.a.).

The Hispanic population uses Spanish as its common and primary language; nonetheless, its diverse cultural and linguistic backgrounds account for diversity in dialects. Currently about 74% of the Hispanic population in the United States speaks Spanish at home (Office of Minority Health, 2015). Compared to Whites, Hispanics have lower achievement of a high school diploma (92% vs. 64%). In 2012, 25.4% of Hispanics, compared with 11% of Whites, lived at the poverty level (Office of Minority Health, 2015). Of particular note to public health nurses, Hispanics have the highest uninsured rates of any racial/ethnic group, with 19.9% not covered by any health insurance. Although this coverage rate has improved within the past 5 years, it continues to far exceed the rate for Non-Hispanic Whites at 7.6%, African Americans at 11.8%, and Asians at 9.3% (Smith & Medalia, 2015).

Hispanic people value extended, cohesive families. Families have generally been patriarchal, with male members perceived as superior and female members seen as a family-bonding life force. These traditional family structures are changing because of migration, urbanization, women in the workforce, and social movements. Spousal roles are becoming more egalitarian (Andrews & Boyle, 2016; Spector, 2013). However, vestiges of the *macho* man and the self-sacrificing woman still are evident in Hispanic culture and continue to shape behavior (see From the Case Files IV).

Health Problems

Leading causes of death for the Hispanic population include heart disease, cancer, unintentional injuries (accidents), stroke, and diabetes. A large number of this population is uninsured and does not have a usual source of health care—31% for adults, almost 10% for children (Office of Minority Health, 2015). Health problems among the Hispanic population are complicated by experiences in their countries of origin, as well as by socioeconomic and lifestyle factors in this country. TB is high in this group, especially among those younger than 35 years of age. Hypertension, diabetes, and obesity are major concerns. Obesity is higher in Hispanics than Whites, and asthma, COPD, suicide, and liver disease also significantly impact Hispanics. Other problems include infectious diseases, particularly AIDS and pneumonia, parasitic infections, malnutrition, gastroenteritis, alcohol and drug abuse, unintentional injuries, and violence. Frequently, the most important health issues for Hispanics are related to the fact that the population is young and has a high birth rate at 97.7 per 1,000 births (Office of Minority Health, 2015). The rate of low-birth-weight infants is lower in Hispanics overall but higher among Puerto Ricans, for whom low birth weight occurs twice as often as in Non-Hispanic Whites. Puerto Ricans also experience disproportionate levels of asthma, infant mortality, and HIV/AIDS. Mexicans have higher rates of diabetes; they are 1.2 times more likely than Whites to be diagnosed with diabetes. Mexican women are 1.2 times more likely to be overweight or obese than White women

---

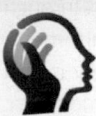 ## From the **Case Files** IV

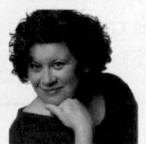 ### Maria Juarez

Maria Juarez, a 53-year-old Mexican American widow, was referred to a public health nursing agency by a clinic. Her married daughter reported that Mrs. Juarez was having severe and prolonged vaginal bleeding and needed medical attention. The daughter had made several appointments for her mother at the clinic, but Mrs. Juarez had refused at the last minute to keep any of them.

After two broken home visit appointments, the community health nurse made a drop-in call and found Mrs. Juarez at home. The nurse was greeted courteously and invited to have a seat. After introductions, the nurse explained that she and the others were only trying to help. Mrs. Juarez had caused a lot of unnecessary concern to everyone by not cooperating, she scolded in a friendly tone. Mrs. Juarez quickly apologized and explained that she had felt fine on the days of her broken appointments and saw no need "to bother" anyone. Questioned about her vaginal bleeding, Mrs. Juarez was evasive. "It's nothing," she said. "It comes and goes like always, only maybe a little more." She listened politely, nodding in agreement as the nurse explained the need for her to see a physician. Her promise to come to the clinic the next day, however, was not kept. The staff labeled Mrs. Juarez as unreliable and uncooperative.

Mrs. Juarez had been brought up in traditional Mexican American culture that taught her to be submissive and interested primarily in the welfare of her husband and children. She had learned long ago to ignore her own needs and found it difficult to identify any personal wants. Her major concern was to avoid causing trouble for others. To have a medical problem, then, was a difficult adjustment. The pain and bleeding had caused her great apprehension. Many Mexican Americans have a particular dread of sickness and especially hospitalization. Furthermore, Mrs. Juarez's culture had taught her the value of modesty. "Female problems" were not discussed openly. This cultural orientation meant that the sickness threatened her modesty and created intense embarrassment. Conforming to Mexican American cultural values, she had first turned to her family for support. Often, only under dire circumstances do members of this ethnic/cultural group seek help from others; to do so means sacrificing pride and dignity. Mrs. Juarez agreed to go to the clinic because refusal would have been disrespectful, but her fear of physicians and her reluctance to discuss such a sensitive problem kept her from going. Mrs. Juarez was being asked to take action that violated several deeply felt cultural values. Her behavior was far from unreliable and uncooperative. With no opportunity to discuss and resolve the conflicts, she had no other choice.

(Office of Minority Health, 2015). Posttraumatic stress disorder is a major problem among refugees from Central and South America who have experienced war and physical and emotional torture.

Health Beliefs and Practices

Religion plays an important part in Hispanic culture. For most Hispanics, Catholicism is the dominant religion (e.g., 95% of Mexican Americans are Catholic), but religious beliefs often consist of a blend of Catholicism and pre-Columbian Indian beliefs and ideology, along with magicoreligious practices. Hispanics believe in submission to the will of God and that illness may be a form of *castigo*, or punishment for sins. They cope with illness through prayers and faith that God will heal them. Their religion also determines the rituals used in healing; for example, *solito*, a condition of depression in women similar to a midlife crisis seen in the American culture, is treated by having the patient lie on the floor while her body is stroked by the *curandero* (native healer) until the depression passes. Latino culture includes beliefs that witchcraft (*brujeria*) and the evil eye (*mal de ojo*) are supernatural causes of illness that cannot be treated by "Anglo" or Western medicine. *Empacho*, a stomachache

in children that occurs after a traumatic event, is treated by the *curandero* with herbal mixtures made into teas. After tender loving care and a bowel movement, the child is considered healed (Table 5–5). As with Asians, Hispanics use "hot" and "cold" categories of foods to influence their diet during illness. Many Hispanics tend to be present-oriented, and consequently are not as concerned as the mainstream culture about keeping to time schedules or preparing for the future (Giger, 2017; McFarland & Wehbe-Alamah, 2015; Spector, 2013).

Arab Populations and Muslims

The final cultural community selected for this discussion is made up of groups of people who come from Arabic countries, especially those who espouse the Muslim religion. By comparison with the groups previously mentioned, the number of people from Arabic countries in the United States is small, but because of the terrorist attacks of September 11, 2001 and ongoing terrorism, as well as the wars in the Middle East, increasing racial and religious animosity has been directed toward people from this part of the world and against those who bear physical resemblance to members of these groups. This unwarranted ostracism has led to mental anguish and distress

Table 5–5	Hispanic Health Beliefs and Folk Diseases
Belief Name	**Explanation/Treatment**
Ataque	Severe expression of shock, anxiety, or sadness characterized by screaming, falling to the ground, thrashing about, hyperventilation, violence, mutism, and uncommunicative behavior. Is a culturally appropriate reaction to shocking or unexpected news that ends spontaneously.
Bilis	Vomiting, diarrhea, headaches, dizziness, nightmares, loss of appetite, and the inability to urinate brought on by livid rage and revenge fantasies. Believed to come from bile pouring into the bloodstream in response to strong emotions and the person "boiling over."
Bilong (hex)	Any illness may result from this; proper diagnosis and treatment requires consulting with a *santero* or *santera* (priest or priestess).
Caide de mollera	A condition thought to cause a fallen or sunken anterior fontanelle, crying, failure to nurse, sunken eyes, and vomiting in infants. Popular home remedies include holding the child upside down over a pan of water, applying a poultice to the depressed area of the head, or inserting a finger in the child's mouth and pushing up on the palate. (Note: According to Western medicine, these symptoms are indicative of dehydration and can be life threatening. The community health nurse role is imperative—to promoting hydration and definitive health care.)
Empacho	Lack of appetite, stomachache, diarrhea, and vomiting caused by poorly digested food. Food forms into a ball and clings to the stomach, causing pain and cramping. Treated by strongly massaging the stomach, gently pinching and rubbing the spine, drinking a purgative tea (*estafiate*), or by administering *azarcon* or *greta*, medicines that have been implicated, in some cases, in lead poisoning. (Note: The community health nurse must assess family for the use of these "medicines" and initiate appropriate follow-up.)
Fatigue	Asthma-like symptoms treated with Western health care practices, including oxygen and medications.
Mal de ojo	A sudden and unexplained illness including vomiting, fever, crying, and restlessness in a well child (most vulnerable) or adult. Brought on by an admiring or covetous look from a person with an "evil eye." It can be prevented if the person with the "evil eye" touches the child when admiring him or her if the child wears a special charm. Treated by a spiritualistic sweeping of the body with eggs, lemons, and bay leaves accompanied by prayer.
Pasmo	Paralysis-like symptoms in the face and limbs treated by massage.
Susto	Anorexia, insomnia, weakness, hallucinations, and various painful sensations brought on by traumatic situations such as witnessing a death. Treatment includes relaxation, herb tea, and prayer.

Adapted from Spector, R. E. (2013). *Cultural diversity in health and illness* (8th ed.). Upper Saddle River, NJ: Pearson Education.

in Arab and Muslim communities (Giger, 2017). Factual information about these groups of people should dispel myths and alleviate fear.

About 4 million people of Arab descent live in the United States. For U.S. census purposes, Arabs are listed as White, and this may include those from Lebanon and Palestine, as well as Algerians, Moroccans, and Egyptians. (U.S. Census Bureau, 2011). Arab Americans have done very well economically, with many having college degrees, owning homes, and being employed as professionals or managers, with the accompanying incomes. Many Arab-Americans immigrants practice Islam and have expressed feeling misunderstood since the terrorist attacks on Washington, DC and New York in 2001 (Nimer, 2013).

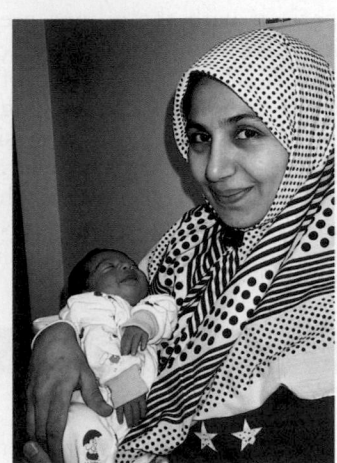

A large percentage of Arabs own their own homes, are college graduates, and work as professionals, for example, in business, medicine, nursing, and education.

A common language (Arabic) and background unite them, yet only 18% of Muslims (followers of Islam) reside in Middle Eastern countries. Arabs are largely Christian or Muslim, although some Arabs may be Jews or Druze (Arab American Institute [AAI], 2015). Christian Arabs first began immigrating to the United States in the late 19th and early 20th centuries (mostly from Syria and Lebanon), but during the middle of the 20th century, Muslim Arabs began to emigrate in greater numbers (commonly from Palestine, Egypt, Iraq, and Yemen). Islam is the fastest-growing global religion, with more than 1 billion followers worldwide. The Council on American–Islamic Relations (CAIR, 2015) reports that there are 6 to 7 million Muslims living in the United States. Most Muslims live in China, India, and South Asia (CAIR, 2015). The tenets of Islam are interpreted more liberally in some nations and more strictly in others, but all practicing Muslims adhere to the five tenets of Islam in some fashion (Table 5–6).

Population Characteristics and Culture

An Arab is generally defined as someone from 1 of the 22 Arab countries who speaks an Arabic dialect and shares the values and beliefs of an Arab culture (AAI, 2015). Arab Americans can trace their ancestry to the North African countries of Morocco, Tunisia, Algeria, Libya, Sudan, and Egypt, as well as the Western Asian countries of Lebanon, Palestine, Syria, Jordan, Bahrain, Qatar, Oman, Saudi Arabia, Kuwait, the United Arab Emirates, and Yemen. Iran is sometimes listed in this group, although Iranians generally consider themselves to be Persian, not Arab AAI, 2015. Assyrian/Chaldean/Syriac and sub-Saharan (Somalian and Sudanese) groups are also noted as Arab. In general, the beliefs and practices of people from such disparate and distant countries cannot be encompassed into one culture. Despite the fact that some of these countries are highly Westernized, enjoy natural resources such as crude oil and the riches that may follow, and are more liberal in following traditional cultural practices, others do not.

Arabs are mostly divided into two distinct religious groups: Muslims and Christians. Arabs generally value Western medicine, trust American health care workers, and do not generally postpone seeking medical care (Lovering, 2012). Several practices, however, are unfamiliar to most Americans. Many Arabic women stay at home and are not in the workforce. Families impose stricter rules for girls than for boys. After menarche, teenage girls may not socialize with boys. The adolescent female also begins to cover her

Table 5–6	The Five Pillars (Tenets) of Islam
1. Faith	Declaration of faith (*shahada*) that there is no God but Allah and that Mohammad is the messenger of Allah
2. Prayer	Obligatory prayers five times a day at dawn, noon, mid-afternoon, sunset, and when night falls (called *salat*) link the worshipper to God. Prayers are led by a learned man who knows the Quran, as there is no hierarchical authority in Islam (like a minister or priest).
3. Almsgiving	This is like tithing and is a very important principle as all wealth is thought to belong to God. It is called *zakat*, and each Muslim is expected to pay 2.5% of his or her wealth annually for the benefit of others in need.
4. The Fast	To abstain from food, drink, and sexual intercourse during daytime (from dawn to sunset) throughout the 9th lunar month (Ramadan). It is a means of self-purification and spirituality. The sick, elderly, or pregnant/nursing women may be permitted to break the fast.
5. The Pilgrimage	The pilgrimage to Makkah (Mecca, or the Hajj) once in a lifetime for those who are physically and financially able to do so. About 2 million people go to Makkah every year (located in Saudi Arabia).

Khan Academy. (2016). *The five pillars of Islam.* Retrieved from https://www.khanacademy.org/humanities/art-islam/beginners-guide-islamic/a/the-five-pillars-of-islam

head and perhaps wears a *hajab*, which takes the form of a modest dress and veil designed to diminish attractiveness and appeal to the opposite sex. Some Arab groups take this mode of dress to extremes, not even allowing a woman's eyes to show out of the *hajab*. Modesty is one of the core values for Arabs; it is expressed by both genders, although more evidently by females (Lovering, 2012; Padela, Gunter, Killawi, & Heisler, 2012).

Within the Arabic population, strict sexual taboos and social practices exist. All sexual contacts outside the marital bond are considered illegal. Those known to have been involved in such activities can be socially rejected, or in some countries even put to death. The stigma of lost honor can continue with their families for generations to come. Another social practice, at times mistakenly related to the Islamic religion, is the practice of female genital mutilation. This is practiced in a few of the Arabic countries on the African continent and has spread to southern Egypt, but it is rare or nonexistent in other Arabic countries. This practice may include the removal of a young woman's labia, clitoris, or both, and it sometimes includes closing the vaginal opening by suturing. Such mutilation can result in prolonged labor and obstetric lacerations, along with urinary and fecal fistula (Berg & Underland, 2013).

Health Problems

Health problems among Middle Easterners are most frequently lifestyle related. These include poor nutritional practices, resulting in obesity, especially among women; smoking among men; and lack of physical exercise (Padela et al., 2012). In some rural areas, especially in Saudi Arabia, men and women chew tobacco, and an increase of oral cancers is seen. Major public health concerns for most Arabs are related to motor vehicle accidents, maternal–child health, TB, malaria, trachoma, typhus, hepatitis, typhoid fever, dysentery, and parasitic infection (Giger, 2017).

Most social restrictions are directed toward women and can affect their health. As mentioned earlier in this chapter, pregnancy can be complicated by genital mutilation, with infections and difficult deliveries. Childbearing continues up until menopause. There is often a desire to have more sons than daughters, and this may result in very large families and closely spaced pregnancies—often without the benefit of family planning. It is often debated whether birth control methods are sanctioned by Islam or not, but Akbar (2015) states that Muslims can reason for themselves, and notes that family planning is not forbidden by the beliefs of Islam. Abortion and infanticide are not accepted, however.

Health Beliefs and Practices

Traditional medicine is practiced in spite of the growth of Western medical services in some of the richer Arab nations. Traditional health care practices are much more common in the poorer Middle Eastern countries and in rural areas of all Arabic countries.

Muslims believe in predestination—that life is determined beforehand—and they attribute the occurrence of disease to the will of Allah. However, this does not prevent people from seeking medical treatment. Islamic law prohibits the use of illicit drugs, which include alcohol.

Users of such substances are liable to trial, and those convicted of smuggling substances into an Arab country can be sentenced to death in some cases. *Sharaf*, or honor, is an important concept in Arab American beliefs, and drug addiction, mental illness, or unwed pregnancy of a family member brings shame to the entire family (Padela et al., 2012). Conversely, when a member does something good or is recognized for an achievement, that honor is reflected on the family as a whole.

Cleanliness is paramount and ritualistic, especially before prayers and after sexual intercourse. The bodies of both genders are kept free of axillary and pubic hair. The left hand is used for cleaning the genitals and the right one is reserved for eating, hand shaking, and other hygienic activities. Muslims fast during Ramadan from sunrise to sunset, and this can include abstinence from all things (including medications or intravenous fluids). Illness can be an exception to this rule, but public health nurses should consult with a family elder or Muslim leader to encourage the client to continue with any necessary treatments. Also, Muslims pray several times daily, facing toward Mecca. Home visits should be planned so that prayers are not interrupted (Padela et al., 2012).

When caring for Arabs in clinics or at home, a nurse of the same sex as the client should be assigned. It is important to note that only women may discuss many topics (e.g., menstruation, family planning, pregnancy, and childbirth), and men are not included in these discussions.

Additional guidelines for nurses working with all immigrant groups include the following:

- Make no assumptions about a client's understanding of health care issues.
- Permit more time for interviewing; allow time to evaluate beliefs and provide appropriate interventions.
- Provide educational programs to correct any misconceptions about health issues; this can occur in clinics, mosques, schools, or homes.
- Provide an appropriate interpreter to improve communication with immigrants who do not speak English well.

TRANSCULTURAL COMMUNITY HEALTH NURSING PRINCIPLES

Culture profoundly influences thinking and behavior and has an enormous impact on the effectiveness of health care. Just as physical and psychological factors determine clients' needs and attitudes toward health and illness, so too can culture. Kark emphasized over 30 years ago that "culture is perhaps the most relevant social determinant of community health" (1974, p. 149). Culture determines how people rear their children, react to pain, cope with stress, deal with death, respond to health practitioners, and value the past, present, and future. Culture also influences diet and eating practices. Partly because of culturally derived preferences, dietary practices can be very difficult to change (McFarland & Wehbe-Alamah, 2015; Spector, 2013).

Despite its importance, the client's culture often is misunderstood or ignored in the delivery of health care (McFarland & Wehbe-Alamah, 2015). With the growth in non-White populations, it is essential that nurses, physicians and other professional health care providers are ready to interact with cultural diversity in their health care team members and in their clients (Andrews & Boyle, 2016). Especially in public health, the nurse must avoid ethnocentric attitudes and must attempt to understand and bridge cultural differences when working with others. It is important to develop knowledge and skill in serving multicultural clients and an ability to place clients' responses to experiences within the context of their lives, or else risk ineffectiveness in the face of a limited understanding and interpretation of client experience.

Overcoming ethnocentrism requires a concerted effort on the nurse's part to see the world through the eyes of clients. It means being willing to examine one's own culture carefully and to become aware that alternative viewpoints are possible. It also consists of attempting to understand the meaning other people derive from their culture and appreciating their culture as important and useful to them (Campinha-Bacote, 2011). Ignoring consideration of clients' different cultural origins often has negative results, as illustrated in From the Case Files IV discussion about Maria Juarez.

Culture is a universal experience. Each person is part of some group, and that group helps to shape the values, beliefs, and behaviors that make up their culture. In addition, every cultural group is different from all others. Even within fairly homogeneous cultural groups, subcultures and microcultures have their own distinctive characteristics. Further differences, based on such factors as socioeconomic status, social class, age, or degree of acculturation, can be found within microcultures. These latter differences, called *intraethnic variations*, only underscore the range of culturally diverse clients served by community health nurses.

Given such diversity, community health nurses face a considerable challenge in providing service to cross-cultural groups. This kind of practice, known as **transcultural nursing**, means providing culturally sensitive nursing service to people of an ethnic or racial background different from the nurse's (Andrews & Boyle, 2016; McFarland & Wehbe-Alamah, 2015). Community health nurses in transcultural practice with client groups can be guided by several principles: develop cultural self-awareness, cultivate cultural sensitivity, assess the client group's culture, show respect and patience while learning about other cultures, and examine culturally derived health practices.

Develop Cultural Self-Awareness

The first principle of transcultural nursing focuses on the nurse's own culture. Self-awareness is crucial for the nurse working with people from other cultures (Andrews & Boyle, 2016; McFarland & Wehbe-Alamah, 2015). Nurses must remember that their culture often is sharply different from the culture of their clients. **Cultural self-awareness** means recognizing the values, beliefs, and practices that make up one's own culture. It also means becoming sensitive to the impact of one's culturally based responses. The community health nurse who assisted Mrs. Juarez in the fourth Case File discussion probably thought that she was being friendly, efficient, and helpful. In terms of her own culture, this nurse's behavior was intended to reassure clients and meet their needs.

Unaware of the negative consequences of her behavior, the nurse caused damage rather than met needs.

To gain skill in understanding their own culturally based behavior, nurses can complete a cultural self-assessment by analyzing their own:

- Influences related to racial background
- Verbal and nonverbal communication patterns
- Values and **norms** (expected cultural practices or behaviors)
- Beliefs and practices

Start with a detailed list of values, beliefs, and practices relative to each point. Next, enlist one or more close friends to call attention to selected behaviors, to bring them to a more conscious level. Videotaping practice interviews with colleagues and actual interviews with selected clients creates further awareness of the nurse's unconscious, culturally based responses. Finally, ask selected clients to critique nursing actions in light of the clients' own culture. Feedback from clients' perspectives can reveal many of the nurse's own cultural responses.

Because culture is mostly tacit, as discussed earlier, it takes conscious effort and hard work to bring the nurse's own cultural biases or influence to the surface. Doing so, however, rewards the nurse with a more effective understanding of self and enhanced ability to provide culturally relevant service to clients (Andrews & Boyle, 2016; Spector, 2013).

Cultivate Cultural Sensitivity

The second transcultural nursing principle seeks to expand the nurse's awareness of the significance of culture on behavior. Nurses' beliefs and ways of doing things frequently conflict with those of their clients. A first step toward bridging cultural barriers is to recognize those differences and develop cultural sensitivity. **Cultural sensitivity** requires recognizing that culturally based values, beliefs, and practices influence people's health and lifestyles and need to be considered in plans for service (Campinha-Bacote, 2011; McFarland & Wehbe-Alamah, 2015). Mrs. Juarez's values and health practices sharply contrasted with those of the clinic's staff. Failure to recognize these differences led to a breakdown in communication and ineffective care. Once differences in culture are recognized, it is important to accept and appreciate them. A nurse's ways are valid for the nurse; clients' ways work for them. The nurse visiting the Kim family in the third case file discussion avoided the dangerous ethnocentric trap of assuming that her way was best, and she consequently developed a fruitful relationship with her clients.

As a part of developing cultural sensitivity, nurses need to try to understand clients' points of view. They need to stand in their clients' shoes and try to see the world through their eyes. By listening, observing, and gradually learning other cultures, the nurse must add a further step of choosing to avoid ethnocentrism. Otherwise, the nurse's view of a different culture will remain distorted and perhaps prejudiced (Andrews & Boyle, 2016; McFarland & Wehbe-Alamah, 2015). The ability to show interest, concern, and compassion enabled one nurse to win the trust and respect of the Native American women in the second case file example and told the Kims that their nurse cared about them. These nurses attempted to understand the feelings and ideas of their clients; in this way, they established a trusting relationship and opened the door to the possibility of their clients' adopting healthier behaviors

Assess the Client Group's Culture

A third transcultural nursing principle emphasizes the need to learn clients' cultures. All clients' actions, like one's own, are based on underlying culturally learned beliefs, values, and ideas (Andrews & Boyle, 2016; Spector, 2013). Mrs. Kim did not like milk because her culture had taught her that it was distasteful and she believed many Asians are lactose intolerant (Reicks et al., 2012). The Native American women's response to waiting or keeping someone else waiting was influenced by their valuing patience. There usually is some culturally based reason that causes clients to engage in (or avoid) certain actions. Instead of making assumptions or judging clients' behavior, the nurse first must learn about the culture that guides that behavior. During a cultural assessment (Giger, 2017), the nurse obtains health-related information about the values, beliefs, and practices of a designated cultural group. Learning the culture of the client first is critical to effective nursing practice. The Transcultural Assessment Model (Giger, 2017) proposes six interrelated factors for assessing differences between people in cultural groups (Fig. 5–2). Understanding these phenomena is a first step toward

appreciating the diversity that exists among people from different cultural backgrounds. Interviewing members of a subcultural group can provide valuable data to enhance understanding (Andrews & Boyle, 2016).

To fully understand a group's culture, it should be studied in depth. Immersion in a given culture is needed to better understand the patterns and teachings that shape individual behavior. The concept of diversity can be generally understood, but each individual group should be appreciated within its own cultural and historical context.

Practically speaking, however, it is not possible to study in depth all of the cultural groups that the nurse encounters. Instead, the nurse can conduct a cultural assessment by questioning key informants, observing the cultural group, and reading additional information in the literature. The data can be grouped into six categories:

1. *Ethnic or racial background*: Where did the client group originate, and how does that influence their status and identity?
2. *Language and communication patterns*: What is the preferred language spoken, and what are the group's culturally based communication patterns?
3. *Cultural values and norms*: What are the client group's values, beliefs, and standards regarding such things as family roles and functions, education, child-rearing, work and leisure, aging, death and dying, and rites of passage?
4. *Biocultural factors*: Are there physical or genetic traits unique to this cultural group that predispose them to certain conditions or illnesses?
5. *Religious beliefs and practices*: What are the group's religious beliefs, and how do they influence life events, roles, health, and illness?
6. *Health beliefs and practices*: What are the group's beliefs and practices regarding prevention, causes, and treatment of illnesses?

The cultural assessment guide presented in Table 5–7 gives suggestions for more detailed data collection.

Many cultural assessment guides can be found throughout the nursing literature. Nonetheless, a thorough cultural assessment may be too time-consuming and costly. Instead, the two-phase assessment process is proposed, as outlined in Table 5–8. Categories to explore in the assessment include values, beliefs, customs, and social structure components. Two methods that have proved highly effective for in-depth study of cultural groups are ethnographic interviewing and participant observation. Spradley (1979, 1980) provides classic descriptions of these methods.

Show Respect and Patience While Learning About Other Cultures

The fourth transcultural nursing principle emphasizes key behaviors for the nurse to practice during the cultural learning process. Respect is the first behavior, and it is shown in many ways. When Sandra Josten involved the Native American women in decisions and gave them choices, she was showing respect. When the nurse gave positive recognition to the importance of the Kims' culture, she was showing respect. Attentive listening is a way to show respect and to learn about a client's culture.

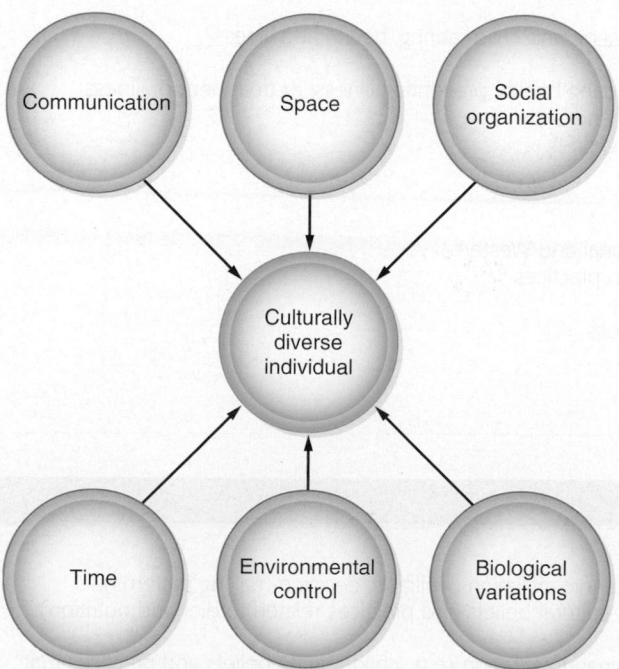

FIGURE 5–2 Components of the Giger and Davidhizar Transcultural Assessment Model showing the culturally diverse individual through communication, space, social organization, time, environmental control, and biologic variations. (Adapted from Giger, J. M. (2017). Culturally competent care: Emphasis on understanding the people of Afghanistan, Afghan Americans, and Islamic culture and religion. *International Nursing Review*, 49(2), 79–86, with permission.)

Table 5–7   Cultural Assessment Guide

Category	Sample Data
Ethnic/racial background	Countries of origin Mostly native born or U.S. born? Reasons for emigrating if applicable Racial/ethnic identity Experience with racism or racial discrimination?
Language and communication patterns	Languages of origin Languages spoken in the home Preferred language for communication How verbal communication patterns are affected by age, sex, other? Preferences for use of interpreters Nonverbal communication patterns (e.g., eye contact, touching)
Cultural values and norms	Group beliefs and standards for male and female roles and functions Standards for modesty and sexuality Family/extended family structures and functions Values regarding work, leisure, success, time Values regarding education and occupation Norms for child-rearing and socialization Norms for social networks and supports Values regarding aging and treatment of elders Values regarding authority Norms for dress and appearance
Biocultural factors	Group genetic predisposition to health conditions (e.g., hypertension, anemia) Socioculturally associated illnesses (e.g., AIDS, alcoholism) Group attitudes toward body parts and functions Group vulnerability or resistance to health threats? Folk illnesses common to group? Group physical/genetic differences (e.g., bone mass, height, weight, longevity)
Religious beliefs and practices	Religious beliefs affecting roles, childbearing and child-rearing, health and illness? Recognized religious healers? Religious beliefs and practices for promoting health, preventing illness, or treatment of illness Beliefs and rituals regarding conception and birth Beliefs and rituals regarding death, dying, grief
Health beliefs and practices	Beliefs regarding causes of illness Beliefs regarding treatment of illness Beliefs regarding use of healers (traditional and Western) Health promotion and illness prevention practices Folk medicine practices Beliefs regarding mental health and illness Dietary, herbal, and other folk cures Food beliefs, preparation, consumption Experience with Western medicine

Table 5–8   Two-Phased Cultural Assessment Process

Phase I—Data Collection

Stage 1	Assess values, beliefs, and customs (e.g., ethnic affiliations, religion, decision-making patterns).
Stage 2	Collect problem-specific cultural data (e.g., cultural beliefs and practices related to diet and nutrition).
Stage 3	Make nursing diagnoses. Determine cultural factors influencing nursing intervention (e.g., child-rearing beliefs and practices that might affect nurse teaching toilet training or child discipline).

Phase II—Data Organization

Step 1	Compare cultural data with: Standards of client's own culture (e.g., client's diet compared with cultural norms) Standards of the nurse's culture Standards of the health facility providing service.
Step 2	Determine incongruities in above standards.
Step 3	Seek to modify one or more systems (client's, nurse's, or the facility's) to achieve maximum congruity.

Within the United States, people of minority groups particularly need respect (Renzaho, Romios, Crock, & Sønderlund, 2013). At times, for groups with limited English skills and a community health nurse who is not bilingual, an interpreter who can assist with communication becomes a necessity (Display 5–7).

A **minority group** is part of a population that differs from the majority and often receives different and unequal treatment. Their ways contrast with those of the dominant culture. It is difficult for them to retain pride in their lifestyles, or in themselves, when the majority culture suggests that they are inferior (McFarland & Wehbe-Alamah, 2015; Spector, 2013). This message may be only implied or even unintentional, as was the case for Mrs. Juarez in From the Case Files IV. The clinic's routine and the manner of the staff were not intended to show disrespect. They did, nevertheless, and Mrs. Juarez was intimidated and was unable to receive the help that she needed. Everyone needs respect to enhance pride, dignity, and self-esteem; it is an important contributor to good mental health. Showing respect also is an important means for breaking down barriers in cross-cultural communication. For community health nurses, culturally relevant care means practicing cultural relativism. **Cultural relativism** is recognizing and respecting alternative viewpoints and understanding values, beliefs, and practices within their cultural context.

In addition to respect, patience is essential. It takes time to build trust and effect cultural change. It can be difficult to establish the nurse–client relationship when it involves two different cultures. Trust must be won, and winning it may take weeks, months, or years. Time must be allowed for both nurse and clients to learn how to communicate with one another, to test one another's trustworthiness, and to learn about one another. Change in behavior (learned aspects of the culture) occurs gradually. Some aspects of both the nurse's and the clients' cultures can, and probably will, change. The Kims' nurse, Paula Morrow, for example, modified some of her usual practices and adapted them to the Kims' culture and needs. They, in turn, began to assume some American practices and values. However, the process took several months. Time, respect, and patience help to break down cultural barriers (Campinha-Bacote, 2011).

Examine Culturally Derived Health Practices

The final transcultural nursing principle involves scrutiny of the client group's cultural practices, as they affect the group's health status. Once the community health nurse has assessed the culture of the client group, cultural practices affecting the health of the client group need to be

---

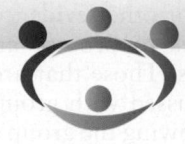

DISPLAY 5–7 INTERPRETER GUIDELINES

1. Unless the community health nurse is thoroughly effective and fluent in the client's language, an interpreter should be used.

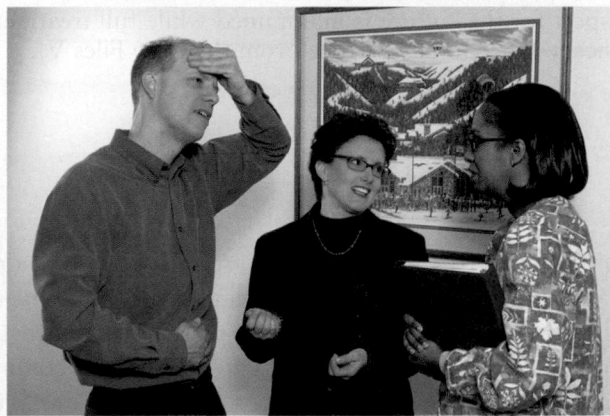

Hearing-impaired client helped by interpreter using sign language.

2. Become familiar with your interpreters. Meet with them on a regular basis, because they provide both a window and a mirror when dealing with clients.

3. The interpreter must maintain confidentiality and can divulge nothing without the full approval of the client and community health nurse.

4. Evaluate the interpreter's style, approach to clients, and ability to develop a relationship of trust and respect. Try to match the interpreter to the client.

5. Maintain eye contact with and address the client, not the interpreter. Remember that clients may understand what is being said (to some degree) even if they don't feel comfortable speaking English.

6. Be patient. Careful interpretation often requires that the interpreter use long, explanatory phrases. Confirm the client's understanding and agreement to promote improved care.

7. Interpreters must interpret everything that is said by all of the people in the interaction but should inform the community health nurse if the content might be perceived as offensive, insensitive, or harmful to the dignity and well-being of the client.

8. When appropriate, encourage interpreters to explain cultural differences to the client and to yourself.

9. Interpretation conveys the content and spirit of what is said, with nothing omitted or added.

10. Volunteer interpreters receive no fee. Employed interpreters usually receive their fee or salary from the hiring agency. They should not accept money or favors from clients or the community health nurse. A sincere "thank you" is the most appropriate gratuity.

From Massachusetts General Hospital. (2015). *Working with an interpreter.* Retrieved from http://www2.massgeneral.org/interpreters/working.asp

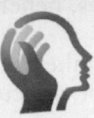

From the Case Files V

The Importance of Cultural Sensitivity

In Australia, well-intentioned government officials, including representatives of the health ministry, identified problems related to substandard housing among a particular aggregate of aboriginal people. To assist this community, the officials spent a great deal of time, energy, and finances planning and building homes for the Aborigines. The homes were small but modern and offered many of the conveniences that officials believed would improve the quality of life for the community.

The Aborigines were appreciative of the group's efforts and moved into their new homes. Before long, however, officials realized that one by one the community members were moving back to their "substandard" housing. When asked about their lack of appreciation for the improved lifestyle, the group informed the officials that their watering hole was their lifeline

and that the houses were not only uncomfortable to them but were too far from their watering hole. Soon, all of the aboriginal families had returned to living on the land, and the homes were part of a veritable ghost town in the middle of nowhere.

Questions

- Was the aboriginal community truly "poor," as the officials seemed to think?
- Discuss your perception of the following issues: Cultural imposition, cultural poverty, dignity and spirit.
- If you were part of an international health team assigned to return to the community to try again to improve their quality of life, what steps would you take to ensure that previous mistakes are not repeated?

examined. Are these behaviors preserving and enhancing the group's health, or are they harmful to their health? Some traditional practices, such as customary diet, birth rituals, and certain folk remedies, may promote both physical and psychological health. These can be considered healthful. Other practices may be neither harmful nor particularly health promoting but are useful in preserving the culture, security, and sense of identity of a particular ethnic group. And some traditional practices may be directly harmful to health. Examples include using herbal poultices to treat an infected wound or "burning" the abdomen to compensate for heat loss associated with diarrhea (Gardner & McGuffin, 2013; McFarland & Wehbe-Alamah, 2015).

Cultural assessment and aggregate health assessment must go hand in hand. If the group is experiencing a high incidence of low-birth-weight babies, pregnancy complications, skin infections, mental illness, or other evidence of health problems, these can be clues to prompt an examination of cultural health practices. Those that are clearly damaging to health can be discussed with group leaders and healers. In this situation, knowing the group's cultural norms for authority and decision-making can be helpful. Often, a cultural practice can be continued or modified while combined with Western medicine, so that respect for the culture is maintained while full treatment efficacy is accomplished (see From the Case Files V).

SUMMARY

Community health clients belong to a variety of cultural groups. A culture is a design for living; it provides a set of norms and values that offer stability and security for members of a society and plays a major role in motivating behaviors. Cultural differences exist, and values of the dominant culture can result in power differentials that can affect the population health. The increase in and great variety of cultural groups reinforce the need for community health nurses to understand and appreciate cultural diversity. Ethnocentrism is the bias that a person's own culture is best and others are wrong or inferior. It can create serious barriers to effective nursing care. Understanding cultural diversity and being sensitive to the values and behaviors of cultural groups often is the key to effective community health intervention.

Culture has five characteristics: it is learned from others; it is an integrated system of customs and traits; it is shared; it is tacit; and it is dynamic. Every culture preserves its integrity by deleting nonfunctional practices and acquiring new components that better serve the group. To gain acceptance, nurses must strive to introduce improved health practices that are presented in a manner consistent with clients' cultural values.

Five transcultural nursing principles, drawn from an understanding of the concept of culture, can guide community health nursing practice: (1) develop cultural self-awareness, (2) cultivate cultural sensitivity, (3) assess the client group's culture, (4) show respect and patience while learning other cultures, and (5) examine culturally derived health practices.

ACTIVITIES TO PROMOTE **CRITICAL THINKING**

1. Based on your own cultural background, how would you feel and what behaviors would you exhibit if you were:
   a. A client sitting in a clinic waiting room in a foreign country whose language you did not know?
   b. Part of a nutrition class being told to eat foods you had never heard about before?
   c. Visited in your home by a nurse who told you to discipline your child in a way that contradicted everything you had been raised to believe about parenting?

2. Describe three tacit cultural rules that govern your own behavior. How might these affect your interactions with clients from another culture?

3. What does the term *ethnocentrism* mean to you? Have you ever experienced someone else being ethnocentric in their attitude toward you? If so, describe that experience. Using the Cross-Cultural Sensitivity Continuum (see Fig. 5–1), explore where your own attitudes are on the continuum toward several of the cultural groups with which you regularly come in contact or from which you know people well.

4. Imagine that you are a PHN assigned to work with a Mexican American migrant population. What are the steps that you would take to gather the appropriate information to provide culturally relevant nursing service? What sources might provide that information?

5. A Hmong father who severely beat his 12-year-old son with a belt, leaving cuts and bruises, is charged with child abuse. "If I can't discipline my son, how can he be a good child?" said the father. What nursing responses would show respect for this cultural group's norms and values and yet be constructive in resolving the cultural conflict?

6. Find Web sites that elaborate on transcultural nursing and cross-cultural health care concerns. What is most surprising or interesting to you? What information is most helpful to you in your nursing practice (in the acute care setting or public health nursing)?

7. Interprofessional communication techniques among diverse health care disciplines are imperative to effective caregiving. How comfortable are you with knowing the linguistic style, practice, and research backgrounds of social workers, pharmacists, physical therapists, educators, psychologists, and others? Seek out a colleague from a different interprofessional discipline and discuss developing a "shared language."

8. Sample exam questions for material in this chapter:
   a. A new nurse in the health department comments that the elderly Vietnamese woman was "stupid" because she could not tell the nurse how long she had been coughing up blood. What is the best response you can give to the nurse?
      1. "Some Asians are long-time smokers and the hemoptysis is probably from smoking."
      2. "That patient may be afraid of TB and not want to tell you. Try asking her a different way."
      3. "That patient does not look like she understands English, and I doubt it is blood; it is probably food."
      4. "Tell her to come back in 3 weeks, when the Vietnamese interpreter is here."
   b. Your caseload includes a Columbian refugee family who witnessed the torture of their neighbors before coming to this country. The mother reports through an interpreter that her 11-year-old son is misbehaving in school, does not sleep through the night, and has lost interest in games he used to enjoy. What is your best response?
      1. In America, boys this age focus on their peers, and often develop interests outside their family. This is normal behavior.
      2. It sounds like he is disobedient. You should set behavioral rules and be strict with him.
      3. He is probably tired. You should go to our clinic doctor to get sleeping medication for him.
      4. His behavior may be related to things he saw years ago. We have a doctor at the clinic that might be able to help with that.

Key for Sample Exam Questions
   a. The correct response is (2). In the response, the nurse uses clinical knowledge about potential health problems in the ethnic group. The nurse suggests that the new employee use patience to achieve effective communication with the patient.
   b. The correct response is (4). In the response, the nurse is using clinical knowledge about this population and mental or physical health problems for which they may be at high risk. The nurse is addressing the mother's concerns with a referral to rule out a posttraumatic stress condition.

REFERENCES

Akbar, K. F. (2015). *Family planning and Islam: A review.* Retrieved from http://muslimcanada.org/family.pdf

Alexander, M. (2012). *The new Jim Crow: Mass incarceration in the age of colorblindness.* New York, NY: The New Press.

Andrews, M., & Boyle, J. (2016). *Transcultural concepts in nursing care* (8th ed.). Philadelphia, PA: Wolters Kluwer, Lippincott Williams & Wilkins.

Arab American Institute [AAI]. (2015). *Demographics.* Retrieved September 20, 2015 from http://www.aaiusa.org/demographics

Arias, E. (2014). United States life tables, 2010. *National Vital Statistics Report 63(7). U.S. Department of Health and Human Services.* Retrieved from http://www.cdc.gov/nchs/data/nvsr/nvsr63/nvsr63_07.pdf

Barrett, M. (Ed.). (2015). *Handbook of clinically tested herbal remedies* (Vols. 1 & 2). New York, NY: Routledge, Taylor & Francis Group.

Berg, R., & Underland, V. (2013). The obstetric consequences of female genital mutilation/cutting: a systematic review and meta-analysis. *Obstetrics and Gynecology International.* doi: 10.1155/2013/496564.

Blair, K., & Jansen, M. (Eds.). (2015). *Advanced practice nursing: Core concepts for professional role development* (5th ed.). New York, NY: Springer Publishing Company.

Blais, K. K., & Hayes, J. S. (2015). *Professional nursing practice: Concepts and perspectives* (7th ed.). Upper Saddle River, NJ: Prentice Hall.

Buckley, C. (2015, October 29). China ends one-child policy, allowing families two children. *The New York Times.* Retrieved from http://www.nytimes.com/2015/10/30/world/asia/china-end-one-child-policy.html?_r=0

California Pan-Ethnic Health Network. (2015). *Mapping the landscape of opportunity.* Retrieved from http://www.healthycity.org/group/cpehn_landscape

Campinha-Bacote, J. (2011). Delivering patient-centered care in the midst of a cultural conflict: the role of cultural competence. *Online Journal of Issues in Nursing, 16(2).* Retrieved from http://www.nursingworld.org/MainMenuCategories/ANAMarketplace/ANAPeriodicals/OJIN/TableofContents/Vol-16-2011/No2-May-2011/Delivering-Patient-Centered-Care-in-the-Midst-of-a-Cultural-Conflict.html

Chirali, I. (2014). *Traditional Chinese medicine cupping therapy* (3rd ed.). St. Louis, MO: Elsevier.

Colby, S., & Ortman, J. (2015). Projections of the size and composition of the United States population, 2014 to 2060. *United States Census Bureau, Current Population Reports.* Retrieved from http://www.census.gov/content/dam/Census/library/publications/2015/demo/p25-1143.pdf

Cotton, S., Grossoehme, D., & McGrady, M. (2012). Religious coping and the use of prayer in children with sickle cell disease. *Pediatric Blood & Cancer, 58(2),* 244–249.

Council on American-Islamic Relations (CAIR). (2015). *About Islam & American Muslims.* Retrieved from http://www.cair.com/publications/about-islam.html

Damon, W., Borstein, M., & Leventhal, T. (Eds.). (2015). *Handbook of child psychology: Child psychology in practice, vol. 4* (7th ed.). New York, NY: John Wiley & Sons.

Dehghani, M., Bang, M., Medin, D., Marin, A., Leddon, L., & Waxman, S. (2013). Epistemologies in the text of children's books: Native- and non-Native-authored books. *International Journal of Science Education, 35(13),* 2133–2151.

Fadiman, A. (1998). *The spirit catches you and you fall down.* New York, NY: Farrar, Straus, & Giroux.

Gardner, Z., & McGuffin, M. (Eds.). (2013). *Botanical safety handbook* (2nd ed.). Boca Raton, FL: Taylor & Francis Group, LLC.

Gertner, M., Kiang, L., & Supple, A. (2014). Prospective links between ethnic socialization, ethnic and American identity, and wellbeing among Asian American adolescents. *Journal of Youth and Adolescence, 43(10),* 1715–1727.

Giger, J. N. (2017). *Transcultural nursing* (7th ed.). St. Louis, MO: Elsevier.

Grandbois, D. M., & Sanders, G. F. (2012). Resilience and stereotyping: the experiences of Native American elders. *Journal of Transcultural Nursing, 23(4),* 389–396.

Hall, E. T. (1959). *The silent language.* Garden City, NY: Doubleday.

Hankerson, S., & Weissman, M. (2012). Church-based health programs for mental disorders among African Americans: A review. *Psychiatric Services, 63(3),* 243–249.

Jensen, E., Bhaskar, R., & Scopilliti, M. (2015). Demographic analysis 2010: Estimates of coverage of the foreign-born population in the American Community Survey. *Population Division, U.S. Census Bureau, Working Paper No. 103.* Retrieved from http://www.census.gov/content/dam/Census/library/working-papers/2015/demo/POP-twps0103.pdf

Kim, B., Sangalang, C., & Kihl, T. (2012). Effects of acculturation and social network support on depression among elderly Korean immigrants. *Aging and Mental Health, 16(6),* 787–794.

Klein, H. (2012). *A population history of the United States* (2nd ed.). New York, NY: Cambridge University Press.

Lee, M. (2012). The one-child policy and gender equality in education in China: Evidence from household data. *Journal of Family and Economic Issues, 33(1),* 41–52.

Lovering, S. (2012). The Crescent of Care: A nursing model to guide the care of Arab Muslim patients. *Diversity and Equality in Health and Care, 9,* 171–178.

Lumpkins, C., Greiner, K., Daley, C., Mabachi, N., & Neuhaus, K. (2013). Promoting healthy behavior from the pulpit: Clergy share their perspectives on effective health communication in the African American church. *Journal of Religion and Health, 52,* 1093–1107.

McFarland, M., & Wehbe-Alamah, H. (2015). *Culture, care, diversity, and universality: A theory of nursing* (3rd ed.). Boston, MA: Jones & Bartlett Publishers.

McGaa, E. (2011). *Mother earth spirituality: Native American paths to healing ourselves and our world.* New York, NY: HarperCollins e-books.

Mead, M. (1960). Cultural contexts of nursing problems. In F. C. MacGregor (Ed.), *Social science in nursing* (pp. 74–88). New York, NY: Wiley.

Medline Plus. (2015). *Herbal medicine.* Retrieved from https://vsearch.nlm.nih.gov/vivisimo/cgi-bin/query-meta?v%3Aproject= medlineplus&v%3Asources=medlineplus-undle&query=Herbal+medicine

Monger, R., & Yankay, J. (2014). U.S. lawful permanent residents 2013. *Department of Homeland Security Annual Flow Report. U.S. Department of Homeland Security, Office of Immigration Statistics.* Retrieved from http://www.dhs.gov/sites/default/files/publications/ois_lpr_fr_2013.pdf

Murdock, G. (1972). The science of culture. In M. Freilich (Ed.), *The meaning of culture: A reader in cultural anthropology* (pp. 252–266). Lexington, MA: Xerox College Publishing.

National Indian Gaming Council (NIGC). (2015). *NIGC fact sheet: Facts at a glance.* Retrieved from http://www.nigc.gov/images/uploads/Fact%20Sheet%20August%202015.pdf

Native American Rights Fund. (n.d.). *Dispelling the myths about Indian gaming.* Retrieved from http://www.narf.org/pubs/misc/gaming.html

Nimer, M. (2013). *The North American Muslim resource guide.* New York, NY: Routledge Taylor & Francis.

Non, A., Gravlee, C., & Mulligan, C. (2012). Education, genetic ancestry, and blood pressure in African Americans and Whites. *American Journal of Public Health, 102(8),* 1559–1565.

Nunley, J., Pugh, A., Romero, N., & Seals, A. (2014). *An examination of racial discrimination in the labor market for recent college graduates: Estimates from the field.* Retrieved from http://cla.auburn.edu/econwp/Archives/2014/2014-06.pdf

Office of Minority Health. (2015). *Minority population profiles.* Retrieved from http://www.minorityhealth.hhs.gov/omh/browse.aspx?lvl=3&lvlid=64

Padela, A., Gunter, K., Killawi, A., & Heisler, M. (2012). Religious values and healthcare accommodations: Voices from the American Muslim community. *Journal of General Internal Medicine, 7(6),* 708–715.

Paniaguia, F. (2014). *Assessing and treating culturally diverse clients.* Thousand Oaks, CA: Sage Publications, Inc.

Park, J. (2015, September 23). Europe's migration crisis. *Council on Foreign Relations.* Retrieved from http://www.cfr.org/migration/europes-migration-crisis/p32874

Partnership for Prescription Assistance. (2015). *Prescription assistance programs.* Retrieved from www.pparx.org/

Pizzorno, J., Murray, M., & Joiner-Bey, H. (2016). *The clinician's handbook of natural medicine* (3rd ed.). St. Louis, MO: Elsevier.

Reicks, M., Degeneffe, D., Ghosh, K., Bruhn, C., Goddell, S., Gunther, C., Zaghloul, S (2012). Parent calcium-rich food practices/perceptions are associated with calcium intake among parents and their early adolescent children. *Public Health Nutrition, 15*(2), 331–340.

Renzaho, A., Romios, P., Crock, C. & Sønderlund, A. (2013). The effectiveness of cultural competence programs in ethnic minority patient-centered health care—a systematic review of the literature. *International Journal for Quality in Health Care, 25*(3), 261–269.

Roscigno, V. J. (2012, November 7). *Power, sociologically speaking.* Retrieved from https://thesocietypages.org/specials/power/

Sacchetti, M. (2014, July 26). *The unforgotten. Boston Globe.* Retrieved from https://www.bostonglobe.com/metro/2014/07/26/students-make-efforts-identify-immigrants-buried-unmarked-graves-near-southwest-border/4iDqnsqHzu9m8N6pPZXffI/story.html

Schrecker, T., & Bambra, C. (2015). *How politics makes us sick: Neoliberal epidemics.* Hampshire, UK: Palgrave Macmillan.

Smith, J., & Medalia, C. (2015). *Health insurance coverage in the United States: 2014. U.S. Census Bureau, Current Population Reports, P60-253.* Washington, DC: U.S. Government Printing Office.

Snyder, M., Lindquist, R., & Tracy, M. (Eds.). (2014). *Complementary and alternative therapies in nursing* (7th ed.). New York, NY: Springer Publishing Company.

Spector, R. E. (2013). *Cultural diversity in health and illness* (8th ed.). Upper Saddle River, NJ: Pearson Education.

Spradley, J. P. (1979). *The ethnographic interview.* New York, NY: Holt.

Spradley, J. P. (1980). *Participant observation.* New York, NY: Holt.

Spradley, J., McCurdy, D., & Shandy, D. (2015). *Conformity and conflict: Readings in cultural anthropology* (15th ed.). New York, NY: Pearson.

Taylor-Black, S., & Wang, J. (2012). The prevalence and characteristics of food allergy in urban minority children. *Annals of Allergy, Asthma, and Immunology, 109*(6), 431–437.

Tribal Court Clearinghouse. (n.d.). *Native gaming resources.* Retrieved from http://www.tribal-institute.org/lists/gaming.htm

U. S. Equal Employment Opportunity Commission. (n.d.). *Laws enforced by EEOC.* Retrieved from http://www.eeoc.gov/laws/statutes/

U.S. Census Bureau. (2011). *The White population.* Retrieved from http://www.census.gov/prod/cen2010/briefs/c200br-05.pdf

U.S. Census Bureau. (n.d.a). *National population summary tables, 2014.* Retrieved from http://www.census.gov/population/projections/data/national/2014/summarytables.html

U.S. Census Bureau. (n.d.b). *Families and living arrangements.* Retrieved from http://www.census.gov/hhes/families/data/families.html

U.S. Department of Health and Human Services (USDHHS) Office of Disease Prevention and Health Promotion. (2015). *Healthy People 2020.* Retrieved from http://www.healthypeople.gov/

U.S. Substance Abuse & Mental Health Services Administration (U.S. SAMHSA). (2014). *Results from the 2014 national survey on drug use and health: National findings.* Retrieved from http://www.samhsa.gov/data/sites/default/files/NSDUH-FRR1-2014/NSDUH-FRR1-2014.pdf

van der Meer, T., & Tolsma, J. (2014). Ethnic diversity and its effects on social cohesion. *Annual Review of Sociology, 40,* 459–478.

Wu, X., & Li, L. (2012). Family size and maternal health: evidence from the One-Child policy in China. *Journal of Population Economics, 25*(4), 1341–1364.

thePoint: Everything You Need to Make the Grade!

thePoint®   Visit http://thePoint.lww.com/Rector9e
for selected readings, study aids for all learning styles, and more!

PUBLIC HEALTH ESSENTIALS FOR COMMUNITY HEALTH NURSING

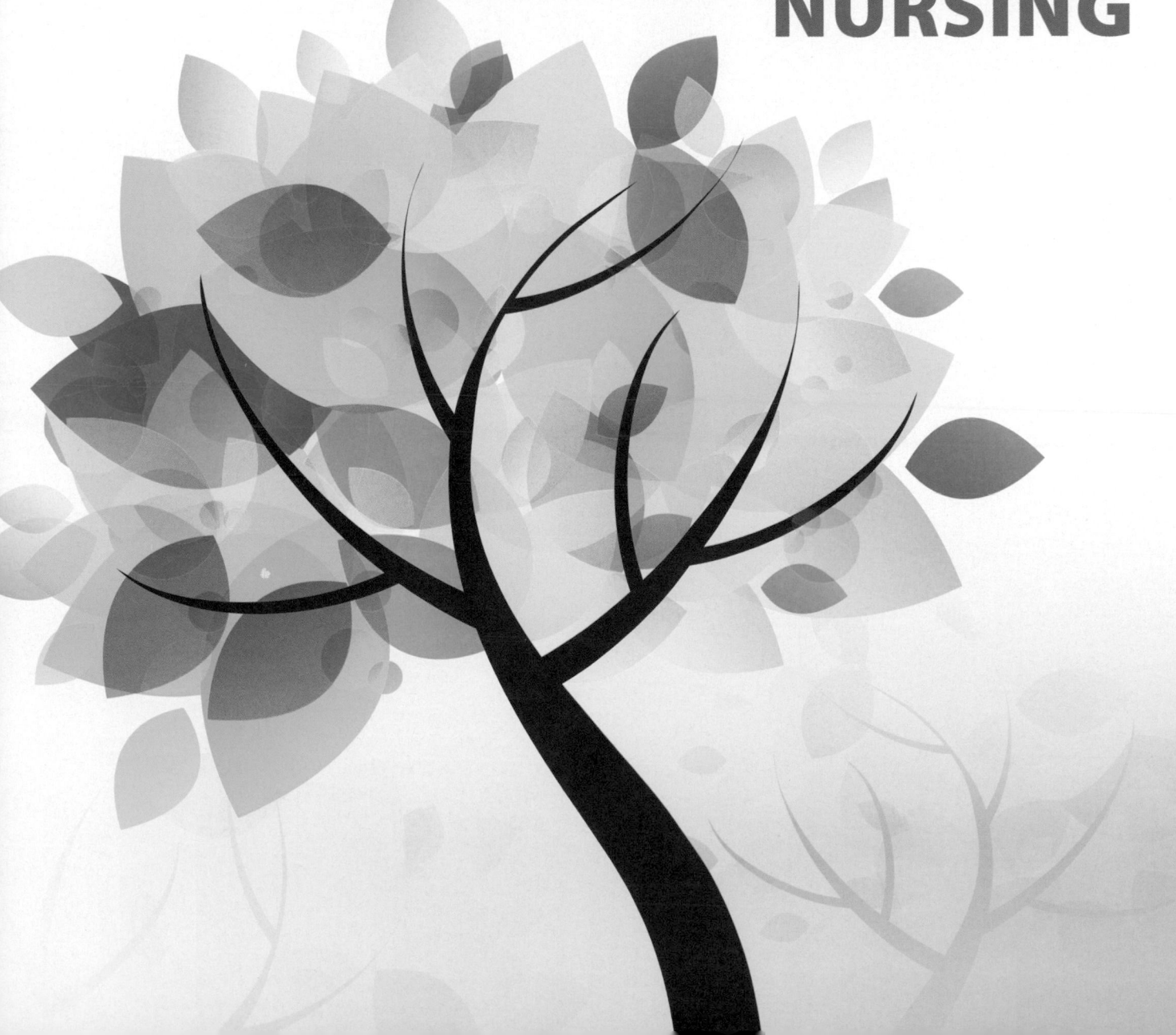

Structure and Economics of Community Health Services

"Healthcare is vital to all of us some of the time, but public health is vital to all of us all of the time."

—*C. Everett Koop,* Former U.S. Surgeon General

"There are 10^{11} stars in the galaxy. That used to be a huge number. But it's only a hundred billion. It's less than the national deficit! We used to call them astronomical numbers. Now we should call them economical numbers."

—*Richard Feynman* (1918–1988)

KEY TERMS

Adverse selection
Assessment
Assurance
Capitation
Capitation rates
Competition
Consumer-driven/high-
  deductible health plan
Core public health functions
Cost sharing
Cost shifting
Demand
Diagnosis-related groups
  (DRGs)
Economics

Fee-for-service (FFS)
Gross domestic product
  (GDP)
Health care economics
Health maintenance
  organization (HMO)
Health savings account
  (HSA)
High-deductible health plan
  (HDHP)
Macroeconomic theory
Managed care organizations
  (MCOs)
Managed competition
Medicaid

Medical home
Medicare
Microeconomic theory
Moral hazard
Nongovernmental
  organizations (NGOs)
Official health agencies
Point-of-service (POS) plan
Policy development
Predictive modeling
Preferred provider
  organization (PPO)
Proprietary health services
Prospective payment
Public Health Service (PHS)

Quarantine
Rationing
Regulation
Retrospective payment
Sanitation
Shattuck Report
Single-payer system
Supply
Third-party payments
Underinsured
Uninsured
Universal coverage
Voluntary health agencies

LEARNING OBJECTIVES

Upon mastery of this chapter, you should be able to:

- Trace historic events and philosophical developments leading to today's health services delivery systems.
- Outline the current organizational structure of the public health care system.
- Examine the three core functions of public health as they apply to health services delivery.
- Differentiate between the functions of public versus private sector health care agencies.
- Examine the public health services provided by selected international health organizations.
- Explain the influence of selected legislative acts in the United States on shaping current health services policy and practice.

- Explore how the structure and functions of community health services affect community health nursing practice.
- Define the concept of health care economics.
- Describe three sources of health care financing.
- Compare and contrast retrospective and prospective health care payment systems.
- Analyze the trends and issues influencing health care economics and community health services delivery.
- Explain the causes and effects of health care rationing.
- List the pros and cons of managed competition as opposed to a single-payer system.
- Discuss health care reform and its potential impact on community health nursing.
- Explain the philosophical implications of health care financing patterns on community health nursing's mission and values.

Nurses preparing for population-based practice need to be familiar with how the health care delivery system is organized and operates, because it is through this system that we are able to offer community health services (see Chapter 3). This system forms an organizing framework for the design and implementation of programs aimed at improving the health of communities and vulnerable groups. It is within this system or framework that community health nurses labor, realize the opportunity to shape future health services, and develop innovative and more effective means of improving community health.

Nurses concerned with the delivery of needed community health services also must understand how those services are financed. In an era when health care costs are rising while resources are limited and providers are competing for scarce dollars, nurses must be well informed about the issues related to health care financing and about ways to obtain funding to address identified health needs in the community. The structure and economics of community health care are intertwined. **Health care economics** is a specialized field of economics that describes and analyzes the production, distribution, and consumption of goods and services, as well as a variety of related problems such as finance, labor, and taxation (Estes, Chapman, Dodd, Hollister, & Harrington, 2013). The goal of health care economics, much like that of public health, is to overcome scarcity by making good choices while providing essential services.

Service delivery systems directed at restoring or promoting the public's health have evolved over centuries. The structure, function, and financing of health care systems have changed dramatically during that time in response to evolving societal needs and demands, scientific advancements, more effective methods of service delivery, new technologies, and varying approaches to resource acquisition and allocation (Knickman & Kovner, 2015). Although progress has been made toward a healthier global society, many problems remain, particularly those of controlling health care costs, assuring equitable distribution and effectiveness of health services, and assuring the quality of and access to those services (Pan American Health Organization, 2016; U.S. Department of Health & Human Services [USDHHS], 2016b).

This chapter examines the current structure and functions of community health services in the United States and reviews historical and legislative events that influenced the planning for and the delivery of those services. It also provides an overview of health care economics and the ever-changing landscape of financial incentives and disincentives for enhancing the public's health.

HISTORICAL INFLUENCES ON HEALTH CARE

Despite centuries of change, some personal and community hygiene and health care practices have continued from the beginning of time. Many primitive tribes engaged in sanitary practices such as burial of excreta, removal of the dead, and isolation of members with certain illnesses. Treatment of the sick has always included using a variety of therapeutic agents administered by a "healer."

Whether health care practices were based on superstition, derived from survival needs, or primarily tied to religious beliefs is unknown. Nonetheless, records show that in India, Egypt, and the Middle East, as early as 3000 BCE, people were building drainage systems, using toilets and systems for water flushing, and practicing personal cleanliness (Rosen, 2015). The Hebrew hygienic code, described in the Bible in Leviticus circa 1500 BCE, probably was the first written code in the world and was the prototype for personal and community sanitation. It emphasized bodily cleanliness, protection against the spread of contagious diseases, isolation of "lepers," disinfection of dwellings after illness, sanitation of campsites, disposal of excreta and refuse, protection of water and food supplies, and maternal hygiene (Erwin & Brownson, 2017; Rosen, 2015). Even more advanced were the Athenians, circa 1000 to 400 BCE, who emphasized personal hygiene, diet, and exercise in addition to a sanitary environment, albeit for the benefit of the wealthy. Their successors, the Romans, added more community health measures, such as laws regulating environmental sanitation and nuisances and construction of paved streets, aqueducts, and a subsurface drainage system. In the Americas, the Inca people (from about 1100 CE to 1550 CE) included cities with clean water supplies and extensive sewage systems (Rosen, 2015).

The Middle Ages (from about 500 to 1500 CE) were distinguished by a public health change in Europe. People gathered in cities for protection, but the cities were unable to meet the needs of the growing population (Rosen, 2015). Farm animals were kept near crowded housing, sanitation systems were nonexistent, streets were not paved, and food and water supplies were insufficient. Contrary to popular belief, bathing was important in the Middle Ages (Polack & Kania, 2015). The ability to bathe, however, was likely limited for the lowest classes of society. These living conditions (overcrowding, poor nutrition, and a lack of hygiene) were ideal for the spread of disease.

Increased trade between Europe and Asia, military conquests, and Christian crusades to the Middle East brought diseases to European cities (Rosen, 2015). Bubonic plague, known as the Black Death, was the most devastating of the epidemics, reportedly killing more than 60 million people in the mid-1300s. Fear of the Black Death caused Venice to ban entry of infected ships and travelers—a form of quarantine. **Quarantine** is a period of enforced isolation of persons exposed to a communicable disease during the incubation period of the disease, to prevent its spread should infection occur. The first known official quarantine measure was instituted in 1377, at the Port of Ragusa (now Dubrovnik, Croatia), where all travelers from plague areas were required to wait 30 days and to be free of disease before entry. This waiting period was then extended to 40 days, leading to the term quarantine.

For many years, people thought that diseases came from magical or religious sources. Because having a clean body was thought to reflect a "clean" (i.e., sin-free) soul, the inability to bathe regularly became associated with an image of the poor as morally corrupt (Polack & Kania, 2015). To some extent, the association between disease and behavior still exists today. Despite knowing the cause of disease, stigma regarding conditions such as leprosy and tuberculosis (TB) still exists, and some regard sexually transmitted diseases (STDs) and HIV/AIDS as punishment for immoral conduct (Erwin & Brownson, 2017).

During the 16th and 17th centuries, diseases were categorized and described in more detail (Rosen, 2015). Towns and cities continued to use quarantine to protect their populations from epidemics. Concern with sailors' health, followed by miners' health, led to early occupational health interventions. This was followed by new efforts at reform during the Enlightenment period, influenced by a growing emphasis on human dignity, human rights, and the search for scientific truth (Erwin & Brownson, 2017). Despite these improvements, serious problems persisted and new ones developed (Lindemann, 2010). Industrialization, masses of people moving to cities, and low regard for human life all contributed to deplorable living and working conditions. Hundreds of children who were poor died in England's abusive, yet socially approved, workhouses and apprentice system.

As early as the 16th century, London was one of the largest cities in the world, with the population tripling by the end of the 17th century (Cockayne, 2007). By the mid-18th century, noise from carriages and carts, animals, and vendors created a "hideous din" (Cockayne, 2007, p. 107). Air pollution from burning coal and wood for fuel caused Londoners to cough and spit. People "rarely washed their bodies and lived in the constant sight and smell of human feces and human urine" (Cockayne, 2007, p. 60). Householders dumped their refuse from windows or doors into the streets. Rivers and water supplies were seriously contaminated (Lindemann, 2010). Diseases, including cholera, typhus, typhoid, smallpox, and TB, took a tremendous toll on human life.

Around the turn of the 19th century, England's leaders became increasingly concerned about social and sanitary reform (Richardson, 1887). The term **sanitation** refers to the promotion of hygiene and prevention of disease by maintenance of health-enhancing (sanitary) conditions. The first sanitary legislation, passed in 1837, established vaccination stations in London. One of the most notable reformers, Edwin Chadwick, the father of modern public health, published his *Report on an Inquiry into the Sanitary Conditions of the Laboring Population of Great Britain* in 1842. His efforts resulted in passage of the English Public Health Act and establishment of a General Board of Health for England in 1848, as reported by Lewis (1952) more than a century later.

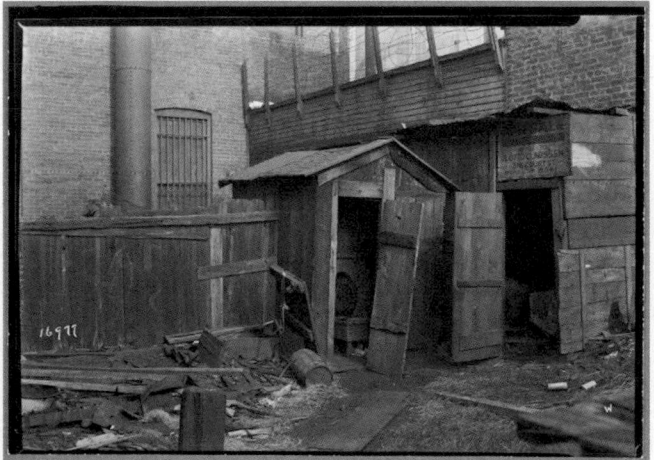

Dilapidated outhouse and debris behind old tenement building in New York City (around 1930).

John Snow, a London physician, investigated several cholera outbreaks in London neighborhoods (Rosen, 2015). In 1854, he was able to connect addresses of cholera deaths to a particular water source. Thus, Snow is considered one of the founders of epidemiology. His conclusions eventually led to changes in the practice of sewage dumping into the Thames River, thus improving London's morbidity and mortality from cholera (see Chapter 7). His 1855 work, *On the Mode of Communication of Cholera*, was a landmark public health contribution. Conditions improved, and scientific study advanced in England and, concurrently, in France, Germany, Scandinavia, and other European countries. England, however, set the pace for application of research, particularly with reference to public health measures, through steadily improved legislation. British laws subsequently became the pattern for sanitary ordinances in the United States.

PUBLIC HEALTH CARE SYSTEM DEVELOPMENT IN THE UNITED STATES

The current U.S. public health care system was long in developing (Trust for America's Health [TFAH], 2013). Most health-related services in the United States were initially reactive, responding to the pressure of immediate needs and uncoordinated from one locality to another. Over time, events and insights contributed to a gradually improving system of programs and services, along with recognition that the health of individuals was affected by the health of the wider community. (Table 6–1 highlights some of these changes.) Our current public health system is not really a single entity, but more of a loosely affiliated network of federal, state, and local health agencies that have been chronically underfunded.

Precursors to a Health Care System

Early health care in the American colonies consisted of private practice, with occasional (but infrequent) governmental action for the public good (Erwin & Brownson, 2017). Action usually was in the form of isolated local responses to specific dangers or nuisances, such as the 1647 regulation to prevent pollution of Boston Harbor or the 1701 Massachusetts law requiring ship quarantine and isolation of smallpox patients. New York City,

Table 6–1   Changes in Health Status and Health Care Services

Turn of the 20th Century	Turn of the 21st Century
Morbidity and Mortality	
THEN	NOW
High communicable disease and mortality	High chronic disease morbidity and mortality
Little prevention	Old and new sexually transmitted diseases
Infrequent cure	Resurgence of TB
Life span of 47 y	Life span of 76 y
High infant mortality	Significant infant mortality
High maternal mortality	High teenage pregnancy
Alcohol abuse	Multiple substance abuse
Many undiagnosed and untreated conditions	New strains of multidrug-resistant diseases, long-term chronic illnesses, and disability
Causes of many diseases unknown	Increased emphasis on personal responsibility (e.g., smoking, overweight)
Access to Health Care	
Access primarily for those who could pay a fee	Access for those with health insurance
No health insurance	Insurance with co-payments; costs shifting from employers to employees; health care reform
Public health clinics for people who were poor and underserved	Free health clinics for uninsured (especially children)
Limited treatments available	Multitude of treatments with regular new advances
Health Care Delivery System	
Extended hospital stays	Short-term, acute care hospitalizations
Discharge on recovery	Recovery occurs at home or in a transitional setting.
Extended maternal and newborn hospitalization	Short-stay maternal and newborn care
Many home deliveries with lay assistance	Few home deliveries with skilled assistance
Handwritten charts and notes	Electronic records, bar-coded medication
Home care through not-for-profit agencies	Home care through not-for-profit and proprietary agencies
PHN begun in health departments	Shifting PHN role in health departments
Health departments provide personal care	Health department's personal care services now part of managed care systems
	Public health departments partner with health care systems to share data and offer expertise in population health

Adapted from American Public Health Association. (2015). *Healthy outlook: Public health resources for systems transformation*. Retrieved from https://www.apha.org/~/media/files/pdf/topics/aca/tranformation/healthyoutlookcomplete.ashx; Erickson, G. P. (1996). To pauperize or empower: Public health nursing at the turn of the 20th and 21st centuries. *Public Health Nursing*, 13(3), 163–169; Frist, W. H. (2005). Healthcare in the 21st century. *New England Journal of Medicine*, 352, 267–272.

in the late 1700s, formed a public health committee to monitor water quality, sewer construction, marsh drainage, and burial of the dead. Physicians in the early 19th century had few tools at their disposal and could do little to change the course of illness. They made house calls, as most quality care was given in the home, not in hospitals (Cutler, 2005). The U.S. Constitution, adopted in 1789, made no direct reference to public health, nor did the federal government take an active stance on health matters. It was the responsibility of each sovereign state to manage its own health affairs. The first federal intervention for health problems was the Marine Hospital Service Act of 1798 (Rosen, 2015). It subsidized medical and hospital care for sick and injured merchant seamen, with the first marine hospital being located in Boston.

When Europeans came to the Americas, a scourge of epidemics, especially smallpox, cholera, typhoid, and typhus, caused deaths among the colonists but decimated the Native American population (Woodward, 1932). Extensive travel between colonies made local control of quarantine efforts ineffective. In 1837, Congress finally instituted the national port quarantine system, which was regulated and enforced by the Marine Hospital Service. Epidemics were quickly

checked, causing society to recognize the benefits of uniform central government policy. However, improvements in public health and sanitation on a state and local level competed with other needs, such as police and fire protection (Greene, 2001; Lee, Teutsch, Thacker, & St. Louis, 2010). See Table 6–2 for examples of this.

Calls for Sanitary Reforms

The **Shattuck Report** (1850), a landmark document in the United States, made a tremendous impact on sanitary progress. Lemuel Shattuck, a physician and legislator, chaired a legislative committee that studied health and sanitary problems in the Commonwealth of Massachusetts. In 1850, he produced the *Report of the Sanitary Commission of Massachusetts*, describing the public health concepts and methods that form the basis for current public health practice. Shattuck advocated the establishment of state and local boards of health, environmental sanitation, collection and use of vital statistics, systematic study of diseases, control of food and drugs, urban planning, establishment of nurses' training schools (there were none before this time), and preventive medicine.

Table 6–2 Societal Events and Situations Affecting Health Care Needs

Turn of the 20th Century	Turn of the 21st Century
Societal and Population Shifts	
THEN	NOW
Industrial society focusing on production	Postindustrial, service and information oriented
Rural to urban	Urban to suburban
Limited violence	Rampant violence and terrorism
Wide gaps between rich and poor	Widening gaps between rich and poor
Growing philanthropy	Declining support for charitable health care
Intense immigration from eastern Europe	Moderate immigration—Africa, Europe, Asia
Environment	
Overcrowded, unsanitary housing	Deteriorating inner-city neighborhoods
Unsafe workplaces, lack of worker safeguards	Environmental hazards in some workplaces
Rampant child labor	Homelessness
Poor public sanitation	Good public sanitation
Multiple health risks	Increasing environmental and behavioral risks
Skill Changes and Employment	
Farm to factory	Factory to service and information
Low wages	Improved but stagnant wages, limited benefits
Dramatic disparity in wages between men and women	Slowly resolving disparity in male/female wage differences
Not enough jobs	Downsizing, layoffs, corporate streamlining, failing companies
People Living in Poverty	
Women and children	Women, children, and the aged
Immigrants—European	Immigrants—Hispanic, Caribbean, Middle Eastern, and Asian
Migration—south to north	Seasonal migration of farm workers

Adapted from American Public Health Association. (2015). *Healthy outlook: Public health resources for systems transformation.* Retrieved from https://www.apha.org/~/media/files/pdf/topics/aca/tranformation/healthyoutlookcomplete.ashx; Erickson, G. P. (1996). To pauperize or empower: Public health nursing at the turn of the 20th and 21st centuries. *Public Health Nursing, 13*(3), 163–169; Frist, W. H. (2005). Healthcare in the 21st century. *New England Journal of Medicine, 352,* 267–272.

A similar report by John Griscom on conditions of workers who remained poor in New York City, published in 1845, concluded that illness, premature death, and poverty were directly related and were not the result of immoral or intemperate behaviors, as many public officials advocated. He recommended sanitary reform as did others, among them Barton, Jarvis, and Snow (Duffy, 1990). Almost 25 years passed before these recommendations were fully appreciated and implemented.

Recent Calls to Action

In 1988, the Institute of Medicine (IOM) published *The Future of Public Health*, highlighting the state of disarray in our current public health system and calling for improvements in the public health infrastructure—largely focusing on governmental responsibilities. In 2002, the IOM issued a new publication, *The Future of the Public's Health in the 21st Century*. This report called for expanding the responsibilities of the public health system beyond governmental agencies to include private and nongovernmental entities. The report outlined how partnerships could be formed with communities, businesses, the media, universities, and other components of the health care delivery system to expand the reach of public health and achieve the *Healthy People 2010* goals (IOM, 2002). Other needed changes included a spotlight on multiple determinants of health, a strong population focus, transdisciplinary utilization of evidence-based practice, better communication, and systems of accountability. The IOM again reported on the state of the U.S. public health system in 2012 with *For the Public's Health: Investing in a Healthier Future*. This report noted the need for additional focus on population-based prevention, rather than on clinical care, if the United States is to improve health outcomes. It also called for federal spending on public health to be doubled and that minimum public health services and costs should be determined. Public health departments are positioned to collaborate with community partners and solve existing health problems, but they do not receive enough funding to fulfill their mission. In the report, the IOM calls for stable, long-term financing of public health services. The IOM (2013) publication, *U.S. Health in International Perspective: Shorter Lives, Poorer Health*, provides a timely investigation of the misconceptions that persist about the performance and quality of our health care system.

About 75% of health care spending goes toward preventable conditions such as cardiovascular disease, diabetes, cancer, lung diseases, injuries, STDs, and vaccine preventable diseases, yet <5% of health care spending goes into prevention and public health (Mays, 2013). More research is needed to demonstrate the effects of public health services on population statistics for diabetes, tobacco use, vaccination rates, food safety, nutrition/physical activity, environmental health, and HIV/STD prevention (Mays, 2013). Sir Michael Marmot, a British professor of public health, researches the "social gradient" of health and life expectancy (Boseley, 2010, para. 3). He estimates that if all of their population had a college education, about 200,000 people over the age of 30 would not experience premature deaths; that equates to a 40% drop. Those premature deaths represent lost productivity and diminished tax revenues, so it benefits the entire population to help prevent these inequalities (see Chapter 25).

Official Health Agencies

The beginnings of an organized health care system in the United States came in the form of **official health agencies,** later called public health agencies. These were publicly funded and operated by state or local governments with a goal of providing population-based health services. Development occurred initially at the local level. Many cities established local boards of health in the late 1700s and early to middle 1800s. Among the earliest were those in Baltimore, Maryland (1798); Charleston, South Carolina (1815); and Philadelphia, Pennsylvania (1818). As their efforts expanded from handling public "nuisances" to dealing with epidemics and complex public health problems, local health boards recognized that full-time staffs were needed, and thus, health departments were formed. Louisiana was first in 1855; Massachusetts followed in 1869.

Again at the national level, the Marine Hospital Service gained a broader function, becoming the Public Health and Marine Hospital Service in 1902. Congress gave it a more clearly defined organizational structure and specific functions for its director, the Surgeon General. In 1912, it was renamed the U.S. Public Health Service (PHS) (USDHHS, 2016a).

Rapidly expanding through World War I and the Great Depression, the PHS strengthened its research activity through the National Institutes of Health (NIH, founded in 1912), added demonstration projects, and initiated greater cooperation with the states. Responding to increasingly complex needs, the NIH added programs significant to public health, such as the Children's Bureau (1912); the National Leprosarium at Carville, Louisiana (1917); examination of arriving aliens (1917); the Division of Venereal Diseases (1918); the Food and Drug Administration [FDA] (1927); and the Narcotics Division (1929), which later became the Division of Mental Hygiene. Title VI of the 1935 Social Security Act promoted stronger federal support of state and local public health services, including health workforce training (USDHHS, 2014a).

As health, welfare, and educational services proliferated, the need for consolidation prompted the creation of the Federal Security Agency in 1939. In 1953, the agency was enlarged and renamed the Department of Health, Education, and Welfare (DHEW), under President Eisenhower. In 1979, education was made a separate cabinet-level department, and the DHEW was renamed the U.S. Department of Health & Human Services (USDHHS, 2015). Other significant events include the establishment during World War II of the Communicable Disease Center in Atlanta, currently known as the Centers for Disease Control and Prevention (CDC), and the development after World War II of the National Office of Vital Statistics, now called the National Center for Health Statistics (NCHS) (CDC, 2015b).

Voluntary Health Agencies

The private sector responded first to health problems in the United States and continues to complement and supplement the government's role in providing health services. By the late 1800s, **voluntary health agencies** (sometimes called private agencies or **nongovernmental organizations [NGOs]**) began to emerge. They were privately funded and operated to address specific health needs. The first of these was the Anti-Tuberculosis Society of Philadelphia, which was formed in 1892 to educate the public and the government about TB, then causing 10% of all deaths. Other agencies followed: the National Society to Prevent Blindness was formed in 1908, the Mental Health Association in 1909, the American Cancer Society in 1913, the National Easter Seal Society for Crippled Children and Adults in 1921, and the Planned Parenthood Federation of America, also in 1921. In the late 1800s, organized charities such as the Red Cross, previously denounced for promoting dependent poverty, began to be recognized for their contributions to health and welfare. Philanthropy, too, became prominent with the establishment of the Rockefeller Foundation in 1913, followed by the Carnegie-Mellon, Kellogg, and Robert Wood Johnson Foundations (National Philanthropic Trust, 2016).

Health-Related Professional Associations

Many health-related professional associations have influenced the quality and type of community health services delivery. Among these, the National Organization for Public Health Nursing, from 1912 to 1952, significantly influenced early preparation for and the quality of public health nursing services (Abrams, 2004). The American Public Health Association (APHA), founded in 1872, maintains a prominent role in the dissemination of public health information, influence on health policy, and advocacy for the nation's health. Other nursing and community health organizations that have promoted quality efforts in community health include the Association of Public Health Nurses (APHN) (formerly the Association of State and Territorial Directors of Nursing), the Association of State and Territorial Health Officers (ASTHO), the National League for Nursing (NLN), the American Nurses Association (ANA), and the Association for Community Health Nursing Educators (ACHNE), among others (APHN, n.d.; Levin et al., 2008).

HEALTH ORGANIZATIONS IN THE UNITED STATES

Over the years, responsibility for meeting community health needs has shifted between private groups and governing institutions, each offering different viewpoints and benefits. Only within the last century have they gradually begun to work together to create a loosely structured system of health care (Rosen, 2015).

Turnock (2016) and others have noted the growing interdependence of the public and private sectors, and this partnership was encouraged by the IOM (2002). How does that system work today? What are its strengths and weaknesses? To answer these questions, its structure must first be examined. Structure is important because it becomes the operational base for assessment, diagnosis, planning, implementation, and evaluation of services—and it provides a framework for intersystem and intrasystem communication and coordination. Health services occur at four levels: local, state, national, and

international. Like ever-widening concentric circles, these levels encompass broader populations. The organization of health services at each level can generally be classified as one of two types: public or private sector.

Public Sector Health Services

Government health agencies, the tax-supported arm of the public health effort, perform a vital function in community health practice. With their jurisdiction and types of service dictated by law, they coordinate and administer activities that often can be carried out only by group or community-wide action (e.g., proper sewage disposal, provision of sanitary water systems, or regulation of toxic wastes). Many community health activities require an authoritative legal backing to ensure enforcement—another useful function of public health agencies—in areas such as environmental pollution, highway safety practices, communicable disease control, and proper, safe handling of food. Official public health agencies provide important record-keeping services, including the collection and monitoring of vital statistics. They also conduct research, provide consultation, and sometimes financially support other community health efforts.

Core Public Health Functions

Public health agencies perform a wide variety of activities, but all can be grouped under one of three **core public health functions** (CDC, 2015a; IOM, 1988). These are assessment, policy development, and assurance (Table 6–3). As discussed in Chapters 1 and 3, public health nurses (PHNs) practice as partners with other public health professionals within these core functions.

Table 6–3 Core Public Health Functions Applied to Populations and People at Risk
Population-Wide Services
Assessment
• Health status monitoring and disease surveillance
Public Policy
• Leadership, policy, planning, and administration
Assurance
• Investigation and control of diseases and injuries
• Protection of environment, workplaces, housing, food, and water
• Laboratory services to support disease control and environmental protection
• Health education and information
• Community mobilization for health-related issues
• Targeted outreach and linkage to personal services
• Health services quality assurance and accountability
• Training and education of public health professionals
Personal Services and Home Visits for People at Risk
• Primary care for underserved and those people not served through health care system
• Treatment services for targeted conditions
• Clinical preventive services
• Payments for personal services delivered by others

Assessment refers to measuring and monitoring the health status and needs of a designated community or population. As a core function, it is a continuous process of collecting data and disseminating information about health, diseases, injuries, air and water quality, food safety, and available resources. This function helps to identify trends in morbidity, mortality, and causative factors. It identifies available health resources, unmet needs, and community perceptions about health issues. This is commonly done through community needs assessments (CDC, 2015a).

Policy development is the formation of a guide for action that determines present and future decisions affecting the public's health (CDC, 2015a). As a core public health function, good public policy development builds on data from the assessment function and incorporates community values and citizen input. It provides leadership and administration for the development of sound health policy and planning. This can include local ordinances, as well as statewide initiatives (e.g., water safety, clean indoor air, alcohol regulation, etc.).

Assurance is the process of translating established policies into services (CDC, 2015a). This function ensures that population-based services are provided, whether by public health agencies or private sources. It also monitors the quality of and access to those services. Training for employees, to assure current knowledge, is another assurance function.

The roles of public health agencies vary by level, with each level carrying out the core functions in different ways to form a partnership in protecting the public's health (Turnock, 2015). International health agencies focus on issues of global concern, setting policy, developing standards, and monitoring health conditions and programs. At the national level, government health agencies engage in similar functions aimed at regional or nationwide concerns.

The federal level provides funds (e.g., through the Medicaid program, block grants, categorical grants) and develops policy (e.g., air pollution policy, occupational safety) but depends on the states to implement them. Agencies at the federal level also develop facilities and programs for special groups, such as Native Americans, migrant workers, inmates of federal prisons, and military personnel and veterans, whose health care is not the direct responsibility of any one state or locality (Erwin & Brownson, 2017; Turnock, 2015; U.S. Environmental Protection Agency, 2015). At the federal level, public health responsibilities include

- Assuring the capacity of all levels of government to provide essential public health services
- Acting when health threats span many states, regions, or the whole country
- Acting where the solution may be beyond the jurisdiction of individual states
- Acting to assist states when they do not have the expertise or resources to mount an effective response in a public health emergency (e.g., natural disaster, bioterrorism, emerging disease, etc.)
- Facilitating the formulation of public health goals in collaboration with state and local governments and other relevant stakeholders (e.g., *Healthy People 2020*)

- Acting transparently and accountably for public health investments
- Disseminating innovation and best practices from state and local public health (TFAH, 2006, p. 7)

State government health agencies function fairly autonomously while working within federal guidelines. They assess, develop, and monitor statewide health needs and services. Historically, they have been responsible for communicable disease control, vital statistics, laboratory services, environmental sanitation and hygiene, health education, and maternal–child health, with the addition of categorical programs (e.g., heart disease, migrant health) in the 1950s (Erwin & Brownson, 2017). In the 1980s, block grants became the primary way to provide federal funding for state actions. While block grants gave states more flexibility to provide targeted services, they were also seen as a way to decrease overall federal support of public health services (Dilger & Boyd, 2014).

At the local level, a city government health agency, a county agency, or a combination of both assess, plan, and serve the health needs of that locality. Most local health departments (LHDs) are under county jurisdiction, with only a small percentage of cities (usually large cities) having LHDs. Some are city–county agencies or special districts, and most LHDs report to either local government councils or boards of health (Erwin & Brownson, 2017). In some states, LHDs also report to state public health agencies. In about 30% of states, LHDs are operated by the state health agency, which provides services locally, without city or county oversight (Turnock, 2016).

Unlike private organizations that tend to have a specific focus, government health agencies exist to accomplish a broad goal of protecting and promoting the health of the total population under their jurisdiction. Such a task requires a wide range of services and the combined talents of many types of professional disciplines. Among them are nurses, physicians, health educators, sanitarians, epidemiologists, statisticians, engineers, administrators, accountants, computer programmers, planners, sociologists, nutritionists, laboratory technicians, chemists, physicists, veterinarians, dentists, pharmacists, demographers, and meteorologists. Furthermore, public health agencies must function not only on an interdisciplinary basis but also on an interorganizational basis. Other government services (e.g., education) can meet their goals fairly autonomously, but public health cannot accomplish its important objectives without the collaboration of many agencies and organizations, both public and private (Turnock, 2015). To manage the HIV/AIDS epidemic, for example, public health agencies, educational institutions, welfare agencies, mental health programs, home care services, Medicaid, and private groups, among others, have been called upon to collaborate.

Many different government agencies contribute to the health of a community. Most obvious are the local and state health departments, which provide a variety of direct and indirect health services, including community health nursing. Other tax-supported agencies that sponsor health care or health-related services include welfare departments, departments of public works, public schools and hospitals, police departments, county agricultural services, and local housing authorities.

Local Public Health Agencies

At the grassroots level, government health agencies vary considerably in structure and function from one locality to the next. This partly results from variations in local needs and the size and resources of the community. For example, a rural community served by a county or state health department may have needs and services that differ widely from those of a densely populated urban community (see Chapter 29). Differing health care standards and regulations, as well as the type and stipulations of funding sources, also contribute to variations in the structure and function of health agencies. Nonetheless, each local governmental health agency shares some commonly held responsibilities, functions, and structural features.

The primary responsibilities of the LHD are to assess the local population's health status and needs, determine how well those needs are being met, and take action toward satisfying unmet needs (Erwin & Brownson, 2017). Specifically, local government health agencies should fulfill these core functions as follows:

- Monitor local health needs and the resources for addressing them
- Develop policy and provide leadership in advocating equitable distribution of resources and services, both public and private
- Evaluate availability, accessibility, and quality of health services for all members of the community
- Keep the community informed about how to access public health services

The local health agency represents a critical level of health services' provision because of its closeness to the ultimate recipients—health care consumers. In a classic study by Barry, Centra, Pratt, and Giordano in 1998, a survey of LHDs revealed the top three expenditure categories were enforcing laws and regulations; informing, educating, and empowering people; and ensuring the provision of care. A systematic review of the literature by Hyde and Shortell (2012) included four studies that examined local public health expenditures. The authors found that expenditures were largely focused on providing services to individual patients and clients, with little spending on population-level programs.

The structure of the LHD varies in complexity with the setting. Rural and small urban agencies need a simple organization, whereas large metropolitan agencies require more complex structures to support the greater diversity and quantity of work.

Where a board of health exists, it holds the legal responsibility for the health of its citizens. About 70% of LHDs work with a board of health, and they are more commonly found with smaller populations (National Association of County and City Health Officials [NACCHO], 2014). An elected official may appoint board of health members (e.g., a mayor if the board of health serves a city or a board of supervisors if it serves a county), or voters may elect board of health members. In turn, the board of health often hires a health officer; about 65% do so (NACCHO, 2014). The health officer directs health department activities and usually has specialty training in public health (22%), nursing (32%), or medicine (12%). Most LHDs employ registered nurses (96%) and environmental health workers (85%). Other public health workers, such as nutritionists, health educators, statisticians, epidemiologists, social workers, mental health workers, physical therapists, veterinarians, or public health dentists, may be added as needs and resources dictate. The number of staff at LHDs can range from 5 to nearly 500, depending upon the size of the agency and population served (NACCHO, 2014). Figure 6–1 depicts the organization of one LHD serving a population of approximately 300,000.

Revenues to support LHDs come from various sources. A small amount of money comes directly from the federal government, specifically between 2% and 7%, depending on LHD size (NACCHO, 2014). Additional federal funds are provided to LHDs via state health departments. These are known as federal "pass-through" dollars and are generally intended for federal programs delivered at the local level, such as family planning, HIV/AIDS services, or nutrition programs. Approximately 16% of LHD finances come from this source. State funds represent 21% of LHD budgets, and local sources constitute 26% (NACCHO, 2014). In the *2013 Profile of Local Health Departments*, NACCHO (2014) found that local sources made up 30% of LHD budgets. This increase in the percent of the budget coming from local sources reflects cuts in state funding; state health department budgets were cut in 48 states between 2008 and 2013 (TFAH, 2015). About 14% of LDH funds are reimbursement for clinical services, mostly from Medicaid (NACCHO, 2014). According to Turnock (2016), fees, reimbursements, and additional miscellaneous sources, such as state laboratory revenues and food supply supplements, make up the remaining portion of the budget (between 11% and 18%). Cuts in federal, state, and local spending for public health services have led to job cuts across the United States (TFAH, 2015). In 2011, more than half of LHDs reported that they decreased or eliminated at least one type of service.

State Public Health Agencies

State-level government health agencies also vary in structure and in how they carry out the core functions. Each state, as a sovereign government, establishes its own health department, which in turn determines its goals, actions, and administrative structure. In 42% of states and territories (eight U.S. territories have health departments), the health department is part of a larger, umbrella agency (ASTHO, 2014). Other services in the umbrella agency may include public assistance, substance abuse services, and Medicaid reimbursement.

The state health department is responsible for providing leadership in and monitoring of comprehensive public health needs and services in the state. Most state health departments provide training or technical assistance to LHDs; common topics are disease prevention, tobacco, and disaster preparedness (ASTHO, 2014). State health agencies may also provide some direct services, particularly for populations served by small LHDs, such as HIV counseling and partner notification. A new role for state health agencies is state-level health insurance exchanges, developed under the Patient Protection and Affordable Care Act (ACA); a total of 20 health departments participated in implementing the exchange in the 28 states that did so.

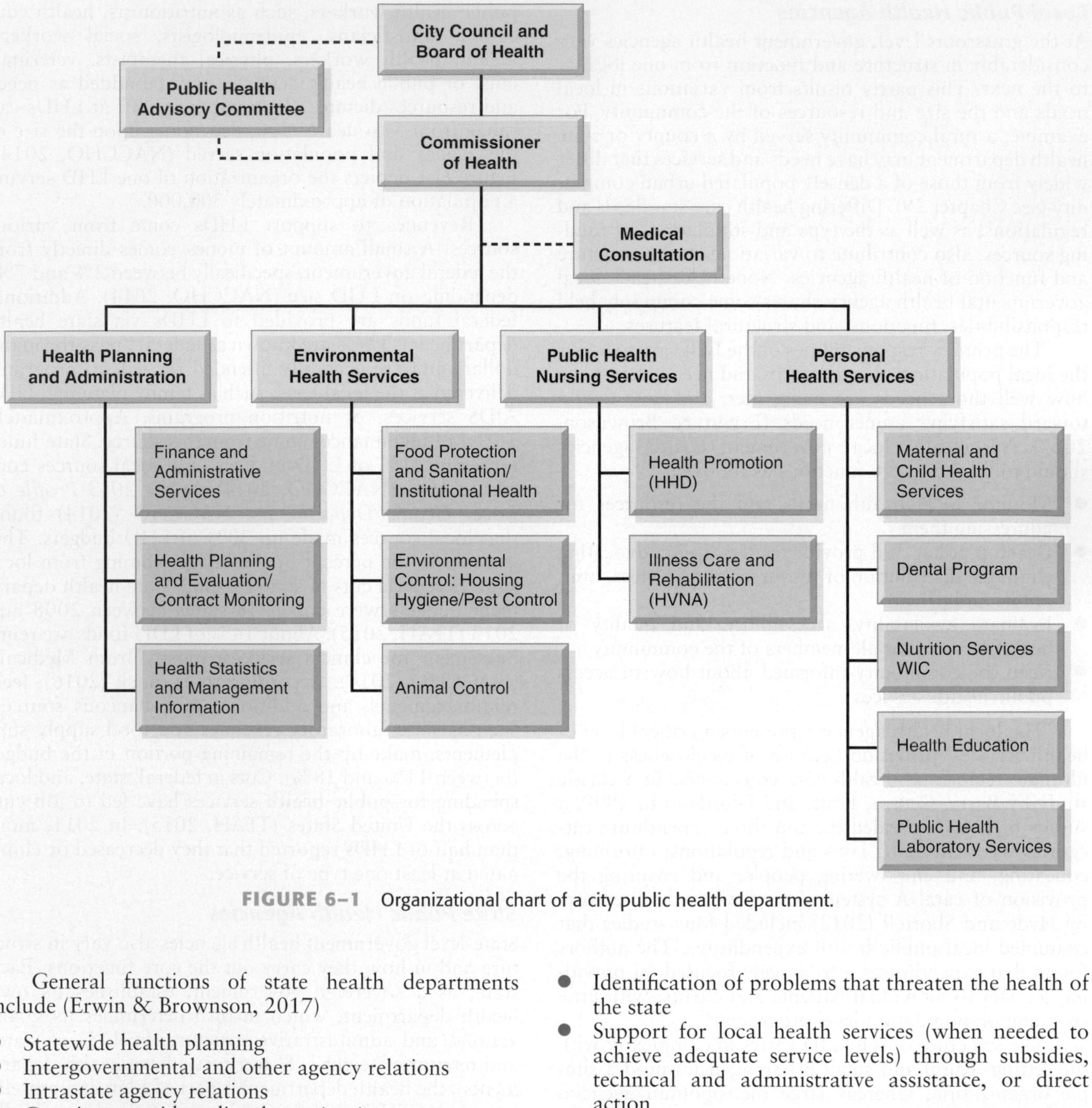

FIGURE 6–1   Organizational chart of a city public health department.

General functions of state health departments include (Erwin & Brownson, 2017)

- Statewide health planning
- Intergovernmental and other agency relations
- Intrastate agency relations
- Certain statewide policy determinations
- Standards setting
- Health regulatory functions

Specifically, the IOM (1988) described the role of state government related to health. Summarized, it includes

- A statewide method of collecting and analyzing data to assess health needs
- Adequate statutory base for state health activities
- Statewide health objectives (holding localities accountable where power for implementation has been delegated)
- Statewide development and maintenance of essential personal, educational, and environmental health services

- Identification of problems that threaten the health of the state
- Support for local health services (when needed to achieve adequate service levels) through subsidies, technical and administrative assistance, or direct action

State public health agencies face a challenge in addressing the health-related issues confronting them. Health care reform, uninsured and underinsured populations (those who are unable to pay for all or some medical services), long-term care, HIV/AIDS, emerging infectious diseases, and chronic disease are among the problems faced by most states. Clearly, state health departments must collaborate closely with other agencies, such as social services, education, public works, and the housing bureau, and the legislature, to effectively solve such problems. Thus, the solution of state health problems and delivery of health services requires the functioning of an interdependent network of organizations, many of which are not traditional health agencies. Fragmentation of public health roles and functions among different state agencies poses problems for coordinating the core public health functions at this level (Turnock, 2016).

Budgetary sources for a state health department include state-generated funds, federal grants and contracts, and fees and reimbursements. A large source of federal monies to the states comes through the U.S. Department of Agriculture (USDA), which supports the Women, Infants, and Children (WIC) program, a supplemental nutrition program that targets women who are pregnant or breast-feeding, infants, and children up to age 5 (see Chapter 21 for information about WIC). State health agencies often provide grant opportunities for LHDs (either from state funds or through federal grant monies awarded to states). Funding for state public health agencies comes mostly from federal funds (53% of revenue), with less than one quarter (24%) from general state funds (ASTHO, 2014). Other sources of funding are targeted state funds (10%), fees and fines (4%), and miscellaneous sources (9%).

Because the federal government provides the largest portion of state health agency funds, cuts in federal spending for public health have direct consequences for states. Federal funding for key public health agencies, such as the USDA, the CDC, the Health Resources and Services Administration (HRSA), has been reduced in recent years (TFAH, 2015). The USDA provided more than 50% of the federal money given to state health departments in 2011 (ASTHO, 2014). The CDC and HRSA provide most of their budgets to state health agencies, LHDs, and other public or private organizations (TFAH, 2015). In addition, the amount of spending is not distributed equally among the states. Federal funding spent on prevention in 2015 ranged from approximately $15 in Indiana to just over $50 in Alaska. The Milbank Memorial Fund, National Association of State Budget Officers, and Reforming States Group (2005), in the most recent information available, note that <1.7% of all state expenditures go toward population health (e.g., health promotion and chronic disease control). Most state public health expenditures in 2012 dealt with improving consumer health (27%), WIC programs (26%), and infectious (10%) or chronic disease (5%) control (ASTHO, 2014). Environmental health, disaster preparation and response, and quality of health services are also common public health expenditure categories.

Each of the 50 state health departments in the United States has a unique structure. Some are strongly centralized organizations, whereas others are decentralized. In most states, the appointed director or executive of the agency reports to a state board of health or directly to the governor. Some states have advisory boards that make health policy recommendations and review departmental activities. Organizational structures vary from state to state, but there are usually several divisions or bureaus under the director. Those divisions most commonly found in state health department organizational structures are disease prevention and control, community health services, maternal and child health, health systems and technical services, laboratory services, environmental health, and a state center for health statistics. Figure 6–2 shows the organizational chart of one state health department. Significant variation occurs in the types of programs managed by state health agencies. In 2013, 100% of state health departments reported

primary administrative responsibility for emergency preparedness, and nearly all reported administrative responsibility for maternal–child health services (98%) and vital statistics (98%) (ASTHO, 2014). Many state public health agencies regulate health care facilities and deal with food safety and some environmental health issues, especially in areas not covered by an LHD.

National Public Health Agencies

At the national level, public health organization can be clustered into four groups of government agencies:

- The **Public Health Service (PHS)**
- The U.S. Department of Health & Human Services (USDHHS)
- Federal departments that oversee areas that impact health, such as the Departments of Labor, Education, Agriculture, and Transportation, among others
- Federal agencies that focus on international health concerns, such as the U.S. Agency for International Development (AID) and the Office of International Health Affairs, which is part of the Department of State (Turnock, 2015)

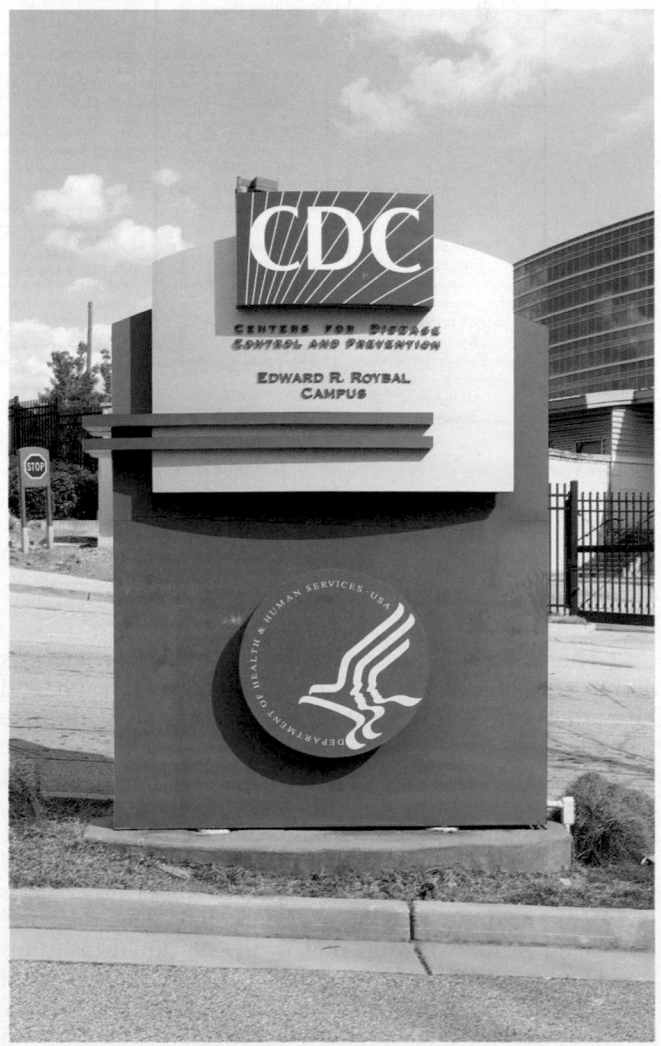

The Centers for Disease Control and Prevention (CDC) headquarters is located in Atlanta, Georgia.

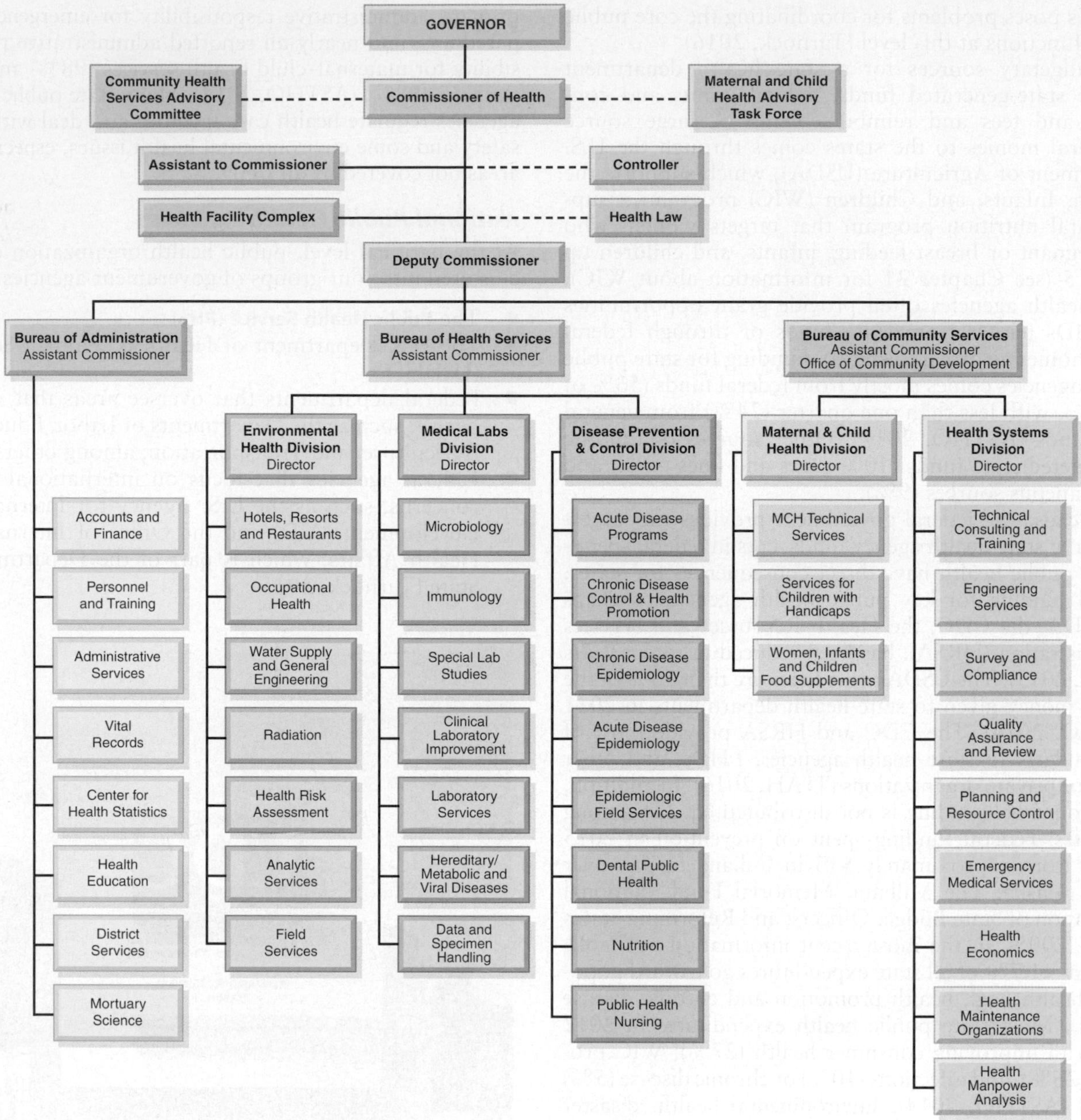

GOVERNOR

Community Health Services Advisory Committee - - - - - **Commissioner of Health** - - - - - Maternal and Child Health Advisory Task Force

Assistant to Commissioner - - - - - - - Controller

Health Facility Complex - - - - - - - Health Law

Deputy Commissioner

Bureau of Administration
Assistant Commissioner

Bureau of Health Services
Assistant Commissioner

Bureau of Community Services
Assistant Commissioner
Office of Community Development

Bureau of Administration
- Accounts and Finance
- Personnel and Training
- Administrative Services
- Vital Records
- Center for Health Statistics
- Health Education
- District Services
- Mortuary Science

Environmental Health Division
Director
- Hotels, Resorts and Restaurants
- Occupational Health
- Water Supply and General Engineering
- Radiation
- Health Risk Assessment
- Analytic Services
- Field Services

Medical Labs Division
Director
- Microbiology
- Immunology
- Special Lab Studies
- Clinical Laboratory Improvement
- Laboratory Services
- Hereditary/Metabolic and Viral Diseases
- Data and Specimen Handling

Disease Prevention & Control Division
Director
- Acute Disease Programs
- Chronic Disease Control & Health Promotion
- Chronic Disease Epidemiology
- Acute Disease Epidemiology
- Epidemiologic Field Services
- Dental Public Health
- Nutrition
- Public Health Nursing

Maternal & Child Health Division
Director
- MCH Technical Services
- Services for Children with Handicaps
- Women, Infants and Children Food Supplements

Health Systems Division
Director
- Technical Consulting and Training
- Engineering Services
- Survey and Compliance
- Quality Assurance and Review
- Planning and Resource Control
- Emergency Medical Services
- Health Economics
- Health Maintenance Organizations
- Health Manpower Analysis

FIGURE 6–2 Organizational chart of a state public health department.

The PHS is concerned with broad health interests across the United States. The Secretary of Health and Human Services (a cabinet-level position) has ultimate responsibility for the PHS. The PHS consists of the Office of Public Health and Science (headed by the Assistant Secretary for Health), the Office of the Surgeon General, and 10 regional offices across the country. The PHS has 11 functional branches: the Administration for Children and Families, the Centers for Medicare and Medicaid Services (CMS), the Administration on Aging, the CDC, the Food and Drug Administration (FDA), the National Institutes for Health (NIH), the Substance Abuse and Mental Health Services Administration (SAMHSA), the Agency for Healthcare Research and Quality (HRSA), the Indian Health Service, and the Agency for Toxic Substances and Disease Registry (ATSDR). One of its major functions through these 11 branches is the administration of grants and contracts with other government agencies, private organizations, and individuals. In some instances, the PHS provides hospital, clinical, and other types of health services, for example, for Native Americans and Eskimos through the Indian Health Service. Through the CDC and the NIH, it provides epidemiologic surveillance and numerous research programs. The FDA monitors the safety and usefulness of various food and drug products, as well as cosmetics, toys, and flammable fabrics (USDHHS, 2015). Much of the PHS is staffed by the Commissioned Core, which consists of over 6,700 uniformed health professionals (see Chapter 30 for more on the PHS Commissioned Corps).

Through its staff offices, the PHS offers other services. It has responsibility for the formation, planning, and evaluation of health policy; health promotion; health services management; health research and statistics; intergovernmental affairs; legislation; population affairs; and international health. It provides financial assistance to the states through grants-in-aid—monies raised by Congress through taxes for specific purposes. It also offers consultation through national advisory health councils and special advisory committees made up of lay experts. The PHS maintains 10 regional offices to make its services more readily available to the states. These offices are located in Boston, New York City, Philadelphia, Atlanta, Chicago, Dallas, Kansas City, Denver, San Francisco, and Seattle.

The second group of federal agencies concerned with public health is organized under the USDHHS. Assistant secretaries manage offices for Health, Administration, Financial Resources, Planning and Evaluation, Preparedness and Response, Legislation, and Public Affairs. Within the USDHHS, clusters of federal agencies deal with the needs of particular population groups, such as older adults (Administration on Aging), children (Administration for Children and Families), and Native Americans/Alaska Natives (Bureau of Indian Affairs), and government health insurance programs (USDHHS, 2015). Figure 6–3 is the organizational chart for USDHHS.

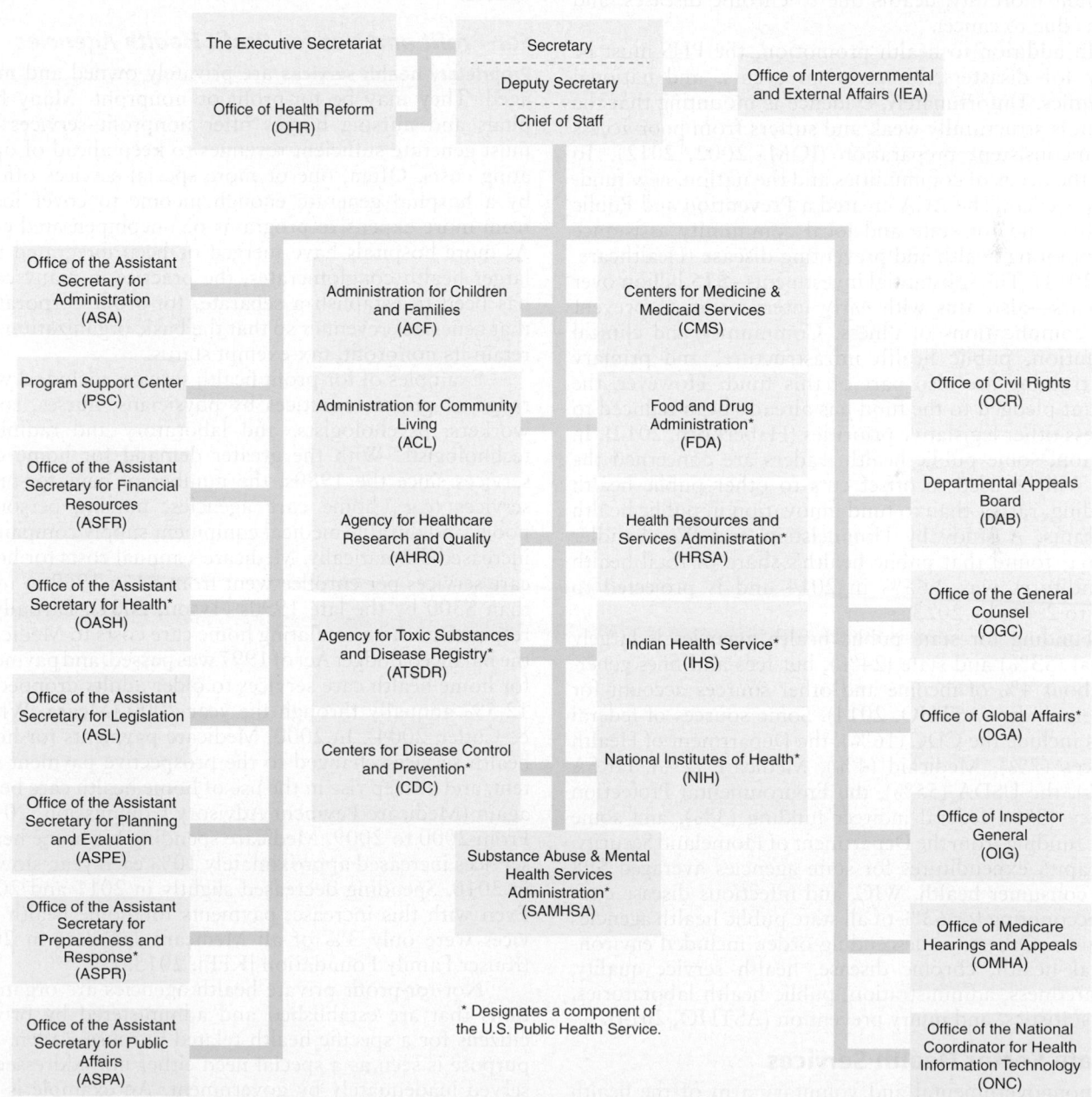

FIGURE 6–3 Department of Health and Human Services Organizational Chart, February 2016. (From U.S. Department of Health & Human Services. (2016). *HHS organizational chart.* Content created by Assistant Secretary for Public Affairs. Last reviewed February, 1, 2016. Retrieved from http://www.hhs.gov/sites/default/files/hhs-org-chart.gif)

Budgets and Funding for Public Health

U.S. government public health spending represented 2.6% of the total health spending in 2014 (CMS, 2015a). The per capita annual health expenditure in 2014 was $9,523 (CMS, n.d.b). Combining national, state, and local spending, public health funding in 2013 was 10% lower than prerecession levels in 2009 (TFAH, 2015). Yet, an IOM report in 2012 recommended an increase in public health spending to twice the amount spent in 2009 (APHA, 2012). This disproportionate funding for public health continues despite evidence that public health spending results in a significant return on investment. Mays and Smith (2011) found that each 10% increase in local public health spending resulted in reductions in infant mortality, deaths due to chronic diseases, and deaths due to cancer.

In addition to health promotion, the PHS must be ready for disasters, bioterrorism events, and national epidemics. Unfortunately, evidence is mounting that the system is structurally weak and suffers from poor access and inconsistent preparation (IOM, 2002, 2012). To meet the needs of communities and the nation, new funding is needed. The ACA created a Prevention and Public Health Fund for state and local community assistance in promoting health and preventing disease (Healthcare. gov, 2011). The substantial investment—$15 billion over 10 years—also aids with early intervention to prevent later complications of illness. Community and clinical prevention, public health infrastructure, and primary care training are also part of this fund. However, the amount pledged to the fund has already been reduced to address other legislative priorities (Haberkorn, 2012). In addition, some public health leaders are concerned the fund will be used to offset cuts to other public health spending, rather than to fund innovation in public health programs. A study by Himmelstein and Woolhandler (2016a) found that public health's share of total health expenditures was 2.65% in 2014 and is projected to drop to 2.4% by 2023.

Funding for state public health agencies is largely federal (53%) and state (24%), but fees and fines generate about 4% of income and other sources account for the remainder (ASTHO, 2014). Some sources of federal funds include the CDC (16%), the Department of Health Services (7%), Medicaid (4%), Medicare (2%), HRSA (10%), the USDA (55%), the Environmental Protection Agency (3%), federal indirect funding (3%), and some grant funding from the Department of Homeland Security. Per capita expenditures for state agencies averaged $98 with consumer health, WIC, and infectious disease control accounting for 63% of all state public health agencies expenses. Others, in descending order, included environmental health, chronic disease, health service quality, preparedness, administration, public health laboratories, vital statistics, and injury prevention (ASTHO, 2014).

Private Sector Health Services

The nongovernmental and voluntary arm of the health care delivery system includes many types of services. Privately owned, nonprofit health agencies (most hospitals and social agencies) make up one large group. Privately owned (proprietary), for-profit agencies are another.

Private professional health care practice, composed largely of physicians in solo or group practice, forms a third group. These make up the non–tax-supported, nongovernmental dimension of community health care.

Private health services are complementary and supplementary to government health agencies. They often meet the needs of special groups, such as those with cancer or heart disease; they offer an avenue for private enterprise or philanthropy; they are less constrained than are government agencies in developing innovations in health care; and they have been spurred to development, in part, by impatience or dissatisfaction with government programs (Erwin & Brownson, 2017). Their financial support comes from voluntary contributions, bequests, or fees.

For-Profit and Not-for-Profit Health Agencies

Proprietary health services are privately owned and managed. They may be for-profit or nonprofit. Many hospitals and nursing homes offer nonprofit services but must generate sufficient revenues to keep ahead of operating costs. Often, one or more special services offered by a hospital generate enough income to cover losses from more expensive programs or uncompensated care. As more hospitals have merged or been integrated into larger health conglomerates, the practice in many cases has been to establish a separate, for-profit corporation that generates revenues so that the basic organization can retain its nonprofit, tax-exempt status.

Examples of for-profit health services include a wide range of private practices by physicians, nurses, social workers, psychologists, and laboratory and radiology technologists. With the greater demand for home care services since the 1980s, the number of new, for-profit services (e.g., home care agencies, nursing personnel pools, and durable medical equipment supply companies) increased dramatically. Medicare's annual costs for home care services per enrollee went from $4 in 1969 to more than $300 by the late 1990s (Tyson, 2001). Partially in response to these escalating home care costs to Medicare, the Balanced Budget Act of 1997 was passed, and payments for home health care services to older adults dropped by 12.5% annually through the year 2000 (Meara, White, & Cutler, 2004). In 2000, Medicare payments for home health services changed to the prospective payment system, and a steep rise in the use of home health care began again (Medicare Payment Advisory Commission, 2014). From 2000 to 2009, Medicare spending for home health services increased approximately 10% each year, slowing in 2010. Spending decreased slightly in 2011 and 2012. Even with this increase, payments for home health services were only 3% of all Medicare spending in 2014 (Kaiser Family Foundation [KFF], 2015a).

Not-for-profit private health agencies are organizations that are established and administered by private citizens for a specific health-related purpose. Often, this purpose is seen as a special need either not addressed or served inadequately by government. An example is visiting nurse associations, which were formed to provide care for the sick in their homes. The contribution of the private, not-for-profit health agency then becomes complementary to public health services.

Three types of private, not-for-profit health agencies have specialized interests. Some, such as the American Cancer Society and the American Diabetes Association, focus on specific diseases. Others, such as the National Society for Autistic Children, Planned Parenthood Federation of America, and the National Council on Aging, focus on the needs of special populations. A third group, including agencies such as the American Heart Association and the National Kidney Foundation, is concerned with diseases of specific organs. All of these agencies are funded through private contributions. TFAH is a nonpartisan, nonprofit organization sponsored by foundation and individual support is focused on disease prevention and protection of individuals and communities.

Another group of private, not-for-profit agencies affecting health and health care includes the many foundations that support health programs, research, and professional education. Examples include the W.K. Kellogg Foundation, the Pew Charitable Trusts, the Robert Wood Johnson Foundation, and the Bill and Melinda Gates Foundation. Some agencies, such as the United Way, exist to fund other voluntary efforts.

Professional associations that work to improve the public's health through the promotion of standards, research, information, and programs constitute the third group of agencies. Examples are the American Public Health Association (APHA), Association of Public Health Nurses (APHN), Association of State and Territorial Health Officials (ASTHO), National Association of County and City Health Officials (NACCHO), National League for Nursing (NLN), American Nurses Association (ANA), Association of Community Health Nursing Educators (ACHNE), and the American Medical Association (AMA). These organizations are funded primarily through membership dues, bequests, and contributions.

Functions of Private Sector Health Agencies

The general functions of private sector health agencies may include (Stallworthy, Boahene, Ohiri, Pamba, & Knezovich, 2014)

- Detecting unmet needs or exploring better methods for meeting needs already identified
- Piloting or subsidizing demonstration projects
- Promoting public knowledge
- Assisting official agencies with innovative programs not otherwise possible
- Evaluating official programs and assuming a public advocacy role
- Promoting health legislation and policies
- Planning and coordinating to promote collaboration among voluntary services and between voluntary and official agencies
- Developing well-balanced community health programs that seek to make services relevant and comprehensive

Both public and private agencies are needed to maintain a viable public health system (Turnock, 2015, 2016). Future functions of both private and public sectors most likely will remain much the same. However, the structure of the organizations within both sectors is changing dramatically and will continue to do so as **managed care organizations (MCOs)** blur the lines between private and public sectors. The blurring of the private and public health care sectors has opened the doors to emerging creative health care services.

INTERNATIONAL HEALTH ORGANIZATIONS

The health of countries around the world cannot be ignored. Besides important humanitarian and moral concerns, there are pragmatic reasons for addressing health issues at the international level. Today, health—along with politics and economics—has become a global issue. Health care among most of the world's population continues to be based on traditional (non-Western) medicine. At the same time, technology is revolutionizing health practices via distance education, training, and telemedicine. Health care information technology has the potential to empower all nations, rich and poor, to enhance the health of their citizens, and many governments and private organizations collect data on a daily basis (Luna, Mayan, Garcia, Almerares, & Househ, 2014). To use all of these data, however, information systems need to be interconnected. Currently, data within one nation, let alone between nations, are generally fragmented. In addition, many countries lack the infrastructure needed to analyze the volume of data available.

It may not seem possible that the health of a resident of a country 9,000 miles away can affect that of a student from the United States or vice versa; however, when boarding an international flight for a school holiday, the student will likely be seated among people from many nations. Despite close scrutiny of airline passengers for passports, visas, customs regulations, weapons, and drugs, how can anyone know whether any passenger sitting near the student has an airborne communicable disease that is resistant to known antibiotics? (See From the Case Files I.)

International cooperation in health dates back to early concerns for epidemics. In 1851, representatives from 12 countries met in Paris for the First International Sanitary Conference. They later established a more permanent organization, the Office International d'Hygiène Publique, in 1907. Epidemics in the Western Hemisphere also prompted representatives from 21 American republics to meet for the First International Sanitary Conference in Mexico City in 1902. In that same year, the International Sanitary Bureau was formed and, later, renamed the Pan American Sanitary Bureau. It is now called the Pan American Health Organization (PAHO) (World Health Organization [WHO], n.d.). See Chapter 16 for more on global health.

World Health Organization

The WHO, an agency of the United Nations, was developed to direct and coordinate the promotion of health worldwide. It was formed after World War II, in 1948, and assumed the functions of the League of Nation's health organization. The PAHO remained separate but

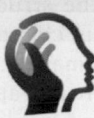

From the Case Files I

Medication-Resistant Tuberculosis, an International Problem

In 2007, the Centers for Disease Control and Prevention (CDC) ordered federal isolation (or quarantine)—something it hadn't done since 1963—for a 31-year-old Atlanta lawyer diagnosed with tuberculosis (TB). In his initial examination, Andrew Speaker says he was told he had TB but wasn't contagious or a danger to anyone else and was not forbidden to fly to Greece and Europe for his wedding and honeymoon; he was reportedly told by county health officials that they preferred that he didn't fly (Ogilvie, 2007; Ruger, 2010). The CDC contends that they instructed him not to travel abroad, but he ignored them (Kvinta, 2011). While he and his new wife were honeymooning, lab test results revealed that he had an extensively drug-resistant (XDR) strain of TB, and the CDC warned him not to take a commercial flight home but to turn himself over to Italian health authorities so that he could be isolated (Kvinta, 2011). However, he and his wife disregarded this admonition, flying back to Canada on Czech Air and then "sneaking" across the border to the United States. He was quarantined a day later and then sent to National Jewish Medical and Research Center in Denver, Colorado—a hospital with a long history of TB research and treatment. Several months later, new tests showed that his sputum samples were positive for multidrug-resistant (MDR) TB, with no signs of the XDR TB first noted on bronchoscopy samples. MDR TB is less resistant to antituberculosis medications and requires less intensive treatment than does XDR TB (Prasad, 2012). Mr. Speaker later had surgery to remove the infected lung and was subsequently diagnosed as noncontagious. At the time of the incident, the CDC recommended that fellow travelers on Mr. Speaker's transatlantic flights have TB tests to determine if they contracted the disease. This incident brought TB to the forefront and reinforced the concept of the world as a global community. It also highlighted international public health law and the need for countries to work together to protect the health of all citizens. Mr. Speaker filed suit against the CDC in 2009, claiming his privacy was invaded, but the U.S. District Court subsequently dismissed the lawsuit. In 2010, the U.S. Court of Appeals ruled that his lawsuit could go forward, but in 2012, his lawsuit was dismissed again because Speaker was not able to provide evidence to support his claim of a specific CDC employee releasing his name to the press (Chrysler, 2012).

In 2013, there were about 100 cases of multidrug-resistant TB (MDR TB) in the United States, and about 480,000 worldwide; treatment only works in about 10% of cases. Annually, over 1.5 million people around the world die from TB (Weber, 2015). Prompt diagnosis and treatment are essential to prevent these drug-resistant forms of TB (Chang & Yew, 2013). In 2010, the average cost of treatment for TB was $17,000; for MDR TB, it was $260,000; for XDR TB, the treatment cost jumps to $554,000. In 2015, a woman from India with XDR TB flew to the United States and visited three states before she saw a physician for treatment of her illness. Hundreds of people could have been exposed to this frightening strain of TB, and it was theorized that she might have come to the United States because of the better chance of successful treatment available here (Weber, 2015). The CDC has a surveillance system that monitors epidemics around the world, and the World Health Organization has regulations in place to encourage its member nations to report and respond to various diseases of international concern (Ruger, 2010).

Chang, K. C., & Yew, W. W. (2013). Management of difficult multidrug-resistant tuberculosis and extensively drug-resistant tuberculosis: Update 2012. Respirology, 18(1), 8–21.

Chrysler, D. (2012, March 22). Andrew Speaker vs. CDC: Speaker's lawsuit dismissed...again. Retrieved from https://www.networkforphl.org/the_network_blog/2012/03/22/95/andrew_speaker_vs_cdc_speakers_lawsuit_dismissed_again/

Kvinta, B. (2011). Quarantine powers, biodefense, and Andrew Speaker. Journal of Biosecurity, Biosafety, and Biodefense Law, 1(1), article 5.

Ogilvie, M. (2007, July 13). TB-infected man sued by plane passengers. Toronto Star. Retrieved from http://www.thestar.com/article/235524

Prasad, R. (2012). Multidrug and extensively drug-resistant tuberculosis management: Evidences and controversies. Lung India, 29(2), 154–159.

Ruger, J. P. (2010). Control of extensively drug-resistant (XDR-TB): A root cause analysis. Global Health Governance, 3(2), 1–20.

Weber, L. (2015, December 10). This disease could kill 75 million people by 2050. Retrieved from http://www.huffingtonpost.com/entry/tuberculosis-mdr-tb-treatment_us_56211f2be4b06462a13bc8fd

became the WHO regional office for the Americas. The WHO began with 61 member nations, one of which was the United States. There are currently 194 member nations (WHO, 2016a). The mission of the WHO is to serve as the one directing and coordinating authority on international health. From its inception, it has influenced international thinking with its classic definition of health as "a state of complete physical, mental, and social wellbeing and not merely the absence of disease or infirmity" (WHO, 2016b, para. 1). The primary function of the WHO is to help countries improve their health status and services by assisting them to help themselves and each other. To accomplish this, it provides member countries with technical services, information from epidemiology and statistics reports, advisory and consulting services, and demonstration teams.

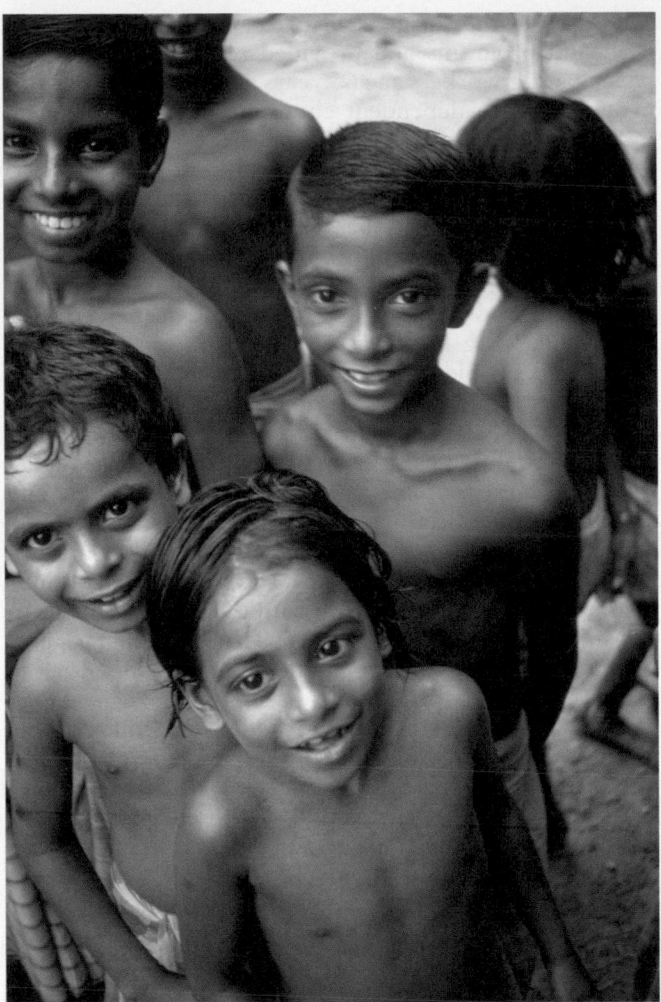

The WHO helps countries improve health services and the health of their citizens, such as these Bangladeshi children examined during a smallpox search.

For 20 years, the WHO focused on achieving the Millennium Development Goals (MDGs), which stated that, by the year 2000, no individual in any country would have a level of health below an acceptable minimum (WHO, 1998). Progress was made, but not all goals were entirely met. Member nations then renewed goals for 2015 to "combat poverty, hunger, disease, illiteracy, environmental degradation, and discrimination against women" (WHO, 2015a para. 3). Currently, the MDGs are transitioning to a set of 17 Sustainable Development Goals (SDGs) (WHO, 2015b, 2016c). The SDGs, "comprise a broad range of economic, social and environmental objectives, and offer the prospect of more peaceful and inclusive societies" (p. 3). The SDGs build on the MDGs, which focused on population targets for health. The SDGs focus on equity and building a strong health infrastructure in all nations.

Headquartered in Geneva, Switzerland, the WHO has six regional offices (WHO, 2016d). The Regional Office for the Americas is located in Washington, DC. The other regional offices are in Copenhagen, Denmark (Europe); Cairo, Egypt (Eastern Mediterranean); Brazzaville, Congo (Africa); New Delhi, India (Southeast Asia); and Manila, Philippines (Western Pacific). Funding comes from member countries and from the United Nations. The WHO holds an annual World Health Assembly to discuss international health policies and programs. The organization publishes several periodicals of interest to the global community, which are available by subscription for a fee and in partial text through WHO's Web site (www.who.int/publications/en/) and include the following:

> *Bulletin of the World Health Organization*—monthly
> *WHO Drug Information*—quarterly
> *Weekly Epidemiological Record*—weekly
> *Pan American Journal of Public Health*—monthly

Pan American Health Organization

The PAHO, the central coordinating organization for public health in the Western Hemisphere, is the oldest continuously functioning international health organization in the world (PAHO, 2016). Its budget comes from assessments contributed by member states, augmented by funds from WHO, the United Nations, and other sources, including private donations.

As the World Health Organization's regional office for the Americas, PAHO disseminates epidemiologic information, provides technical assistance, finances fellowships, and promotes cooperative research and professional education (PAHO, 2016). Conferences convened by PAHO provide an opportunity for delegates from member nations to discuss issues of concern and plan strategies for addressing health needs. The most widely read journal published by PAHO is the *Pan American Journal of Public Health*, an open-access journal, published monthly (PAHO, 2016).

United Nations International Children's Emergency Fund

Organized in 1946, the United Nations Children's Fund, now called the United Nations International Children's Emergency Fund (UNICEF), was established initially as a temporary emergency program to assist the children of war-torn countries (UNICEF, 2016). That focus has broadened, and UNICEF is now a permanent agency for promoting child and maternal health and welfare globally, through a variety of programs and activities, including provision of food and supplies to underdeveloped countries, immunization programs in cooperation with the WHO, disease control (especially HIV/AIDS), creating protective environments for children, and the education of girls.

U.S. Agency for International Development

The USAID (2016) is the "lead U.S. Government agency that works to end extreme global poverty and enable resilient, democratic societies to realize their potential" (para. 1). USAID was formed in 1961 under the John F. Kennedy administration and lists goals of improving the health, education, and well-being of the populations of developing countries. Its initial focus was on technical and monetary assistance, changing to an agenda that addressed basic human needs in the 1970s.

USAID invests in methods to improve the lives of millions of men, women, and children by

- Investing in agricultural productivity so countries can feed their people
- Combating maternal and child mortality and deadly diseases like HIV, malaria, and tuberculosis
- Providing lifesaving assistance in the wake of disasters
- Promoting democracy, human rights, and good governance around the world
- Fostering private sector development and sustainable economic growth
- Helping communities adapt to a changing environment
- Elevating the role of women and girls throughout all our work (USAID, 2016, para. 3)

Other International Health Organizations

Many other organizations deal with health concerns at the international level. The United Nations Educational, Scientific, and Cultural Organization (UNESCO) goal is to assist people in forming peaceful and inclusive societies (UNESCO, 2016). UNESCO promotes sports, social integration, health, and education without regard to geographical borders or social classes. The World Bank addresses health problems through funding and technical assistance. The Food and Agriculture Organization (2016) works to achieve food security by ending hunger and malnutrition, eliminating poverty, and improving economic and social progress. It also promotes sustainable management of resources used to grow food (land, water, air, etc.). *Medecins Sans Frontieres*, or Doctors Without Borders (n.d.), is an international, neutral organization that sends emergency medical assistance to people in need because of war, epidemics, disasters, or denial of health care. Founded in France in 1971 by 13 doctors and journalists, it initially had 300 volunteer workers, including doctors, nurses, and other staff. MSF now has 30,000 employees around the world. The group was awarded the Nobel Peace Prize in 1999, in recognition of the humanitarian work of their medical staff. MSF has taken care of more than 100 million people in 80 countries. Doctors Without Borders is also known for speaking out—telling the world what they have seen and criticizing those who interfere with their impartial medical mission.

SIGNIFICANT LEGISLATION

During the past century in the United States, an ever-widening sense of responsibility for health in the public sector led to passage of an increasing amount of health-related legislation. Some acts are of particular significance to the financing and delivery of community health services (see list on thePoint). Early health-related legislation focused on particular population groups: merchant seamen (1798), Native Americans (1920), and mothers and infants (1921). During the Great Depression, the U.S. government enacted the first significant legislation that affected the health and well-being of a wide range of citizens (Rosen, 2015).

In 1935, the Social Security Act ensured greater public health programs and provided retirement income to participating workers age 65 years and older. The act also included aid to dependent children and unemployment insurance (Social Security Administration [SSA], n.d.). Later legislation provided federal support for expansion of hospitals; care for individuals with mental retardation; research and support for heart disease, cancer, and stroke; and training for health care personnel.

The landmark Medicare and Medicaid legislation in 1965 moved the federal government deeper into the role of financing health care, especially for many older adults and people living in poverty, who, prior to this time, either could not get services or had to rely on charity care (CMS, 2011). Health care legislation in the 1980s sought to contain health care spending, ensure the quality of health care, promote national health objectives, and facilitate data collection and research (see Display 6–1). More recent laws have protected the confidentiality of health records and made it easier for workers to continue insurance coverage after being laid off. As described earlier in this chapter, the ACA is the most recent legislation to impact health care financing in the United States (Knickman & Kovner, 2015).

President Bill Clinton made an unsuccessful attempt at universal health care during his first term in office. In 1997, the State Children's Health Insurance Program (SCHIP) was created to expand coverage to uninsured children at no or low cost, and this coverage was extended in 2009 under President Barak Obama (CMS, n.d.a). The ACA requires states to maintain the SCHIP through 2019. The Medicare Modernization Act of 2003, signed into law by President George W. Bush, added prescription drug benefits and disease screening to Medicare and promoted Health Savings Accounts (HSAs). President Barak Obama signed the ACA into law in 2010. The ACA enacted several health insurance reforms, which have made "healthcare more affordable, accessible and of a higher quality, for families, seniors, businesses, and taxpayers alike" (USDHHS, 2014a, para. 1).

Development of the Current Health Care System

In 1900, a total of 20% of infants died before they reached the age of 10, and life expectancy was about 47 years. Infectious diseases and poor sanitation and nutrition contributed to the poor outcomes. Physicians were not well trained, and the AMA had only 8,000 members (Public Broadcasting System, n.d.). Hospital infection rates were high, and most care was given in the home—and then only to those who could afford to pay for it or those who received charity care. (See From the Case Files II.)

As the public health system acted to improve water supplies, sanitation, and personal hygiene, the incidence of infectious disease began to diminish. Antibiotics, first widely available during World War II, and better-trained physicians began to change the health care system in the 1950s—although medical and surgical care was not at all

(*Text continues on page 185*)

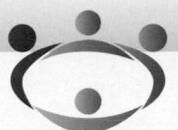

DISPLAY 6-1 DATA COLLECTION SYSTEMS

The National Center for Health Statistics Data Collection Systems

Some collection systems of the NCHS are ongoing annual systems, and others are conducted periodically. There are two major types of data systems: those based on populations (these data are collected by personal interview and examination) and those based on records, with data collected from vital and medical records.

National Health Interview Survey

The National Health Interview Survey is a continuous nationwide survey of illness and disability. It is the main source of data on the health of the U.S. population (nonmilitary, noninstitutionalized). This survey, which monitors the health of the nation, has been conducted since 1957.

National Health and Nutrition Examination Survey

The National Health and Nutrition Examination Survey (NHANES) provides physical, physiologic, and biochemical data related to nutrition of national population samples. Conducted for over 40 years, NHANES provided data that led to the development of pediatric growth charts, vitamin fortification of grains and cereals, and phasing out of lead-based gasoline. It also provided information about the link between cholesterol and heart disease and information on smoking, bone density, obesity, and changes in diet over time.

National Health Care Surveys

The National Health Care Surveys are a series of surveys of providers that yields clear information about health care services, patients, organizations, and providers.

National Ambulatory Medical Care Survey: Gathers data from nonfederal, office-based physicians giving direct patient care

National Hospital Ambulatory Medical Care Survey: Gathers data from physicians on ambulatory services by specialty and target population

National Hospital Care Survey: A new survey describing patterns of care delivery in hospitals and freestanding ambulatory surgery centers

National Hospital Discharge Survey: Provides annual data on such things as length of stay, diagnosis, procedures performed, and patient use patterns

National Survey of Ambulatory Surgery: Data on use and services given in hospital emergency and outpatient departments

National Home and Hospice Care Survey: Administrators and staff are personally interviewed to retrieve information about patients and discharges.

National Home Health Aide Survey: Information on home health aides employed by home health agencies and/or hospice

National Nursing Home Survey: Collects data about nursing home services, staff, and residents regarding need, level of care, costs, and use patterns

National Employer Health Insurance Survey: Provides estimates on employer-sponsored health insurance, the types of plans provided, and detailed information about the plans

National Nursing Assistant Survey: Information on nursing assistants employed by nursing homes.

National Survey of Residential Care Facilities: Information from a national sample of residential care facilities.

National Vital Statistics System

The National Vital Statistics System is the oldest survey and best example of public health intergovernmental data sharing. Vital statistics registries around the country provide uniform data to the national system on the following categories: births, marriages, divorces, deaths, and fetal deaths. Specific data are available through the following systems:

- Birth data
- Mortality data
- Fetal death data
- Linked birth/infant deaths
- National Mortality Followback Survey
- National Maternal and Infant Health Survey

National Survey of Family Growth

The National Survey of Family Growth assembles information on marriage and divorce, pregnancy, use of contraception, family life, infertility, and women's and men's health. The data are used to plan health programs and services.

National Immunization Survey

The National Immunization Survey is a list-assisted random digit–dialing survey employed to gather information on vaccination coverage rates for children between the ages of 19 and 35 months. A mailed survey follows the telephone call, and this produces timely estimates of the rates of recommended vaccine doses.

The Longitudinal Studies of Aging

The Longitudinal Studies of Aging are done as a collaboration between the NCHS and the National Institute on Aging. These studies measure changes in functional status, living arrangements, health, and the utilization of health services for persons aged 70 and above. They involve two cohorts of U.S. citizens moving through old age and the oldest ages.

State and Local Area Integrated Telephone Survey

The State and Local Area Integrated Telephone Survey collects in-depth data needed at the state and local levels to meet the needs of program planners, policymakers, and government agencies. Some of the topics researched include access to care, utilization of services, health insurance coverage, perceived health status, and measurement of child well-being. The same random digit–dialing method employed by NIS is utilized on a regional basis.

From National Center for Health Statistics. (2016). *Surveys and data collection systems.* Retrieved from http://www.cdc.gov/nchs/surveys.htm

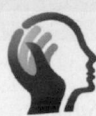

From the **Case Files** **II**

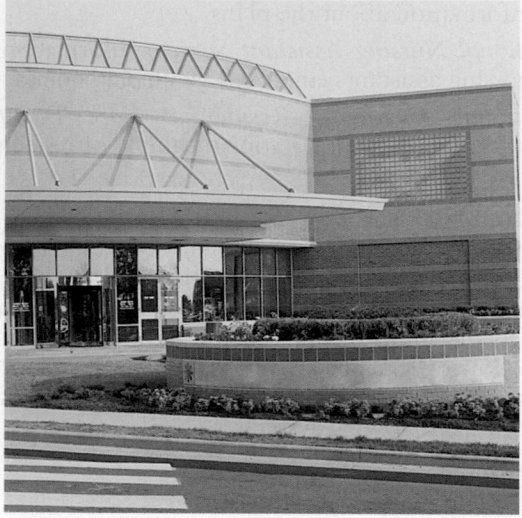

Hospital Care: Comparisons Between the 20th and 21st Centuries

In the 1890s, riots occurred in Milwaukee when a child suspected of having smallpox was ordered by a public health official to be taken by ambulance to a local hospital for isolation. One of the child's siblings had already died of smallpox in the same hospital, and his family did not want the second child to risk death at the same institution especially while upper- and middle-class children were quarantined in their own homes (not sent to isolation hospitals). A crowd of 3,000 or more people, carrying clubs, kept the ambulance attendants at bay. Why was there such concern about hospitalizing a sick child? When this occurred, hospitals were rife with infection, and doctors could do little to halt its spread. Also, the inequity of how smallpox cases were handled stirred feelings of injustice and discrimination (Cutler, 2005; Solnit, 2009).

In the early 21st century, are hospitals any safer? Almost half a million Americans die each year from preventable hospital errors—making this the third leading cause of death (Leapfrog Group, 2015). According to the (CDC, 2016), a total of 721,800 hospital-associated infections were reported in 2011. The Society of Actuaries projected the cost of medical errors in 2008 to be almost $20 billion (2010). Andel, Davidow, Hollander, and Moreno (2012) estimate an even higher number—$1 trillion annually—when they apply quality-adjusted life years (QALYs) to deaths from medical errors. With repeated calls for safety and quality improvement in our health care system, would you think that today's hospitals must be safer?

Can you be assured of good care when you or your loved one enters a hospital? In the case of a busy trauma center located in South Los Angeles, you might have reason for concern. Martin Luther King/Drew Medical Center was created after the

1965 Watts Riot, with a history of providing stellar neonatal care (95% of babies under 2 pounds survive) and excellent training for trauma surgeons—one fourth of U.S. military surgeons have trained there (Associated Press, 2004). But numerous problems began to be reported in the early 1970s; employees were inebriated on the job, and some stole medications from the pharmacy and sold them on the street. There were numerous cases of gross medical malpractice at a time when only one physician in a 5-year period was formally disciplined by the hospital (Kuypers & Gellert, 2012). The hospital came to be known as "killer King" (para. 28) because of the numerous deaths, unsanitary conditions, and employee absenteeism or working under the influence of drugs or alcohol. Nurses would leave the units with patients needing care, took meal breaks without authorization, or left their shifts early; they also turned off monitors. In one case, a toddler on a ventilator suffered "profound mental retardation" after his nurse left the floor for an early dinner and his ventilator tubing was dislodged (Kuypers & Gellert, 2012, para. 34). An AIDS patient's monitors were turned off and the nurse falsified the patient records showing that she checked on him, but the patient died at 5 PM with no one in attendance. Emergency room and orthopedic units had to close because of staff not reporting for duty. Medication errors were made, and patients were instructed by nurses to sign waivers, releasing them from any disciplinary actions. The hospital hired a convicted child abuser as a physician assistant, as well as hiring hospital staff who were unlicensed and dropped or failed out of medical school. They failed to discipline physicians who administered lethal doses of medications, performed incorrect surgeries, grossly misdiagnosed patients, and delayed deliveries that resulted in babies' deaths or mental retardation (Kuypers & Gellert, 2012). Other mistakes included infusing a woman with HIV-infected blood, causing her to contract the disease, and slicing the throat of a teenaged shooting victim (Karlamangla, 2015).

Numerous incidents of patients in the ER going untreated and unnoticed were reported. A patient died in the ER after waiting 22 hours to be treated. The patient had a gangrenous leg, a pneumothorax, and was in kidney failure. Inpatient care was often no better, though, as a 46-year-old man admitted for meningitis was given chemotherapy medication for 4 days. Even after the pharmacy error was noted, nurses continued to give medications in error (at least 40 incidents). The patient subsequently lost vision in one eye. In 2007, a 43-year-old woman was admitted to the now-named Martin Luther King/Harbor Medical Center three times in 3 days complaining of intense stomach pain. Her diagnosis was listed as gallstones and she was prescribed pain medication and released each time. After the third discharge, she remained on the hospital grounds and was eventually taken to the ER by police, who were notified of a woman screaming for help. According to the police officers,

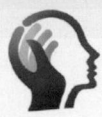

From the Case Files II (Continued)

the ER triage nurse refused to help the woman, and she lay on the floor in severe pain for almost an hour. She "spit up a dark-colored substance, which her boyfriend said was blood" and security cameras showed a janitor mopping around her as she lay in agony on the floor (Rosenblatt, 2007, p. 11).

By fall 2007, after the federal government withdrew $200 million in annual funding, the hospital closed its doors (Ornstein, Weber, & Leonard, 2007). An urgent care center/outpatient clinic remained open. However, the community voiced concern over the closure. One study found "increased delays in access to care for needed medical services after the closure of Martin Luther King, Jr. Hospital" in a survey of older minority adults in South Los Angeles (Walker et al., 2011, p. 356). The Los Angeles County Board of Supervisors voted to reopen the hospital, with staffing by University of California physicians, and provided $50 million in start-up funding (CBS Los Angeles, 2011). In 2015, the new $250 million 131-bed King/Drew Medical Center opened its doors as the community celebrated. A mental health facility, outpatient center, and urgent care are also part of the new medical campus (Jennings, 2015). The new hospital

uses a team approach to patient care, with a nurse managing each team. Care coordinators work with every patient, not just those who are high-risk, and nurses do patient rounds with physicians every morning. Administrators reported careful vetting of physicians and have new technology such as beds that provide patient weights and other diagnostics that are digitally transmitted EHRs (Karlamangla, 2015). Will these improvements override the past problems and reputation? Time will tell.

What is different about these two scenarios is the reaction of the public. In the 1890s case, it was an angry mob trying to keep a child out of harm's way by not allowing ambulance personnel to take him to the hospital. In this century, it was the federal and local government who moved to close what was deemed an unsafe facility. Some in the community were happy to see the closure, especially those who lost loved ones to what they feel was substandard care. But many others were sad to see a much-needed neighborhood medical center close—its ER saw almost 50,000 patients in 2006—and they worked with county supervisors to build the new facility and encourage a culture of patient safety (CBS Los Angeles, 2011; Karlamangla, 2015).

Andel, C., Davidow, S. L., Hollander, M., & Moreno, D. A. (2012). The economics of health care quality and medical errors. Journal of Health Care Finance, 39(1), 39–50.

Associated Press. (2004). Crisis threatens landmark medical center: Five top administrators have been fired for ignoring problems. Retrieved from http://www.msnbc.msn.com/id/4780341/

CBS Los Angeles. (2011, March 8). L.A. County OKs $50M for new King-Harbor Hospital. Retrieved from http://losangeles.cbslocal.com/2011/03/08/la-county-to-spend-50m-on-new-king-harbor-hospital/

Centers for Disease Control and Prevention (CDC). (2016). HAI data and statistics. Retrieved from http://www.cdc.gov/hai/surveillance/

Jennings, A. (2015, July 7). Community celebrates opening of Martin Luther King hospital. Retrieved from http://www.latimes.com/local/california/la-me-0708-king-drew-20150708-story.html

Karlamangla, S. (2015, September 22). How the new King hospital hopes to put its "Killer King" image 'far behind'. Retrieved from http://www.latimes.com/local/california/la-me-mlk-care-20150922-story.html

Kuypers, J. A., & Gellert, A. (2012). The story of King/Drew Hospital: Guilt and deferred purification. Journal of the Kenneth Burke Society, 8(1). Retrieved from http://kbjournal.org/kuypers_gellert_king_drew_hospital

Ornstein, C., Weber, T., & Leonard, J. (2007, August 11). King-Harbor fails final check, will close soon. Los Angeles Times. Retrieved from http://pqasb.pqarchiver.com/latimes/results.html?st=advanced&QryTxt=&type=current&sortby=RELEVANCE&datetype=0&frommonth=01&fromday=01&fromyear=1985&tomonth=10&today=20&toyear=2011&By=&Title=King-Harbor+fails+final+check&at_curr=ALL&Sect=ALL

Rosenblatt, S. (2007, November 6). Family seeks $45 million in King-Harbor death; Edith Rodriguez died after writhing in pain on the hospital floor as employees ignored her. Los Angeles Times. Retrieved from http://pqasb.pqarchiver.com/latimes/access/1377858201.html?FMT=ABS&FMTS=ABS:FT&type=current&date=Nov+6%2C+2007&author=Susannah+Rosenblatt&pub=Los+Angeles+Times&edition=&startpage=B.6&desc=Family+seeks+%2445+million+in+King-Harbor+death%3B+Edith+Rodriguez+died+after+writhing+in+pain+on+the+hospital+floor+as+employees+ignored+her.+A+lawsuit+accuses+L.A.+County+of+negligence

Society of Actuaries. (2010). The economic measurement of medical errors. Retrieved from https://www.soa.org/Research/Research-Projects/Health/research-econ-measurement.aspx

Solnit, R. (2009). A paradise built in hell: The extraordinary communities that arise in disaster. New York, NY: Penguin Group.

Walker, K., Leng, M., Liang, L., Forge, N., Morales, L., Jones, L., & Brown, A. (2011). Increased patient delays in care after the closure of Martin Luther King hospital: Implications for monitoring health system changes. Ethnicity Disease, 21(3), 356–360.

sophisticated by today's standards. (See From the Case Files III.)

Since the 1950s, U.S. citizens have come to expect longer lives made possible by medications and treatments that can cure or control a wide variety of diseases. At the same time, expanding technology and services provide a

dizzying array of choices to health care consumers. These advances have come at a price, however. Health spending in 2013 was estimated at 17.4% of the U.S. **gross domestic product (GDP)**—the total amount of goods and services produced within a year (Keehan et al., 2015). To put that in perspective, health spending in 1960 was only

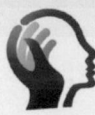

From the Case Files III

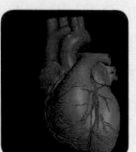

Care for Cardiovascular Patients

In developed countries, the most common cause of mortality is cardiovascular disease (CVD). In 2015, one third of worldwide deaths can be attributed to CVD. Although these statistics are daunting, it is important to note that in the 1940s, 50% of all U.S. deaths were due to CVD. Little was known about the causes of heart disease and stroke. Many people died from what most thought simply was the result of "old age." It wasn't until the Framingham Heart Study began in 1948 that the epidemiology of CVD was studied; this was the first longitudinal study of any kind in the United States. Initial findings were not reported until 1957, when a 400% greater incidence of coronary heart disease was noted in patients with blood pressures of ≥160/95 mm Hg (Mahmood, Levy, Vasan, & Wang, 2014). Later, stroke was also noted as a consequence of hypertension. A common rule of thumb for physicians of that time was to add the person's age (e.g., 60) to the baseline of 100 (totaling 160), as a "permissible" systolic blood pressure (p. 2003). In 1969, the Offspring Cohort was recruited and the study continued to gather data. In 1971, results were reported that demonstrated elevated systolic blood pressure as a predictor for heart failure and stroke. Control of hypertension was not formally incorporated into practice guidelines until 1977. Over the next decade or two, the focus widened to include prevention of CVD and not just treatment of those who already had developed it.

But this was not the case in 1932, when Franklin Delano Roosevelt ran for President and made his medical records public, including a blood pressure reading of 140/100 mm Hg. By the time of the WWII Normandy invasion in 1944, his blood pressure had risen to 186/108 mm Hg, and he was seen by one of a small number of cardiac specialists who noted that he had signs of slight cyanosis. He diagnosed him with "hypertension, hypertensive heart disease, and cardiac failure" but could only offer him digitalis to relieve some symptoms (p. 2001). His blood pressure rose to 240/130 mm Hg within a couple of months, and by the Yalta Conference with Churchill and Stalin in 1945, he appeared to be very ill. He died 2 months later "from cerebral hemorrhage with a blood pressure of 300/190 mm Hg" (p. 2001).

In 1950, the role that hypertension and high cholesterol levels played in heart disease was still unclear. Only when someone presented with chest pain were they then monitored for blood pressure and cholesterol control. Doctors frequently recommended that their patients cut down on salt consumption and lose weight. They were also counseled to reduce their schedules and "rest around midday," as there were essentially no effective medications to treat these two problems (Cutler, 2005, p. 50; Jaquish, 2007). Cardiac patients were treated with absolute bed rest for a minimum of 6 weeks, morphine for pain, and oxygen. That was the state-of-the-art regimen prescribed for President Eisenhower after his heart attack in 1955 (Gilbert, 2008; Jaquish, 2007).

It was not until the Framingham Heart Study confirmed that hypertension leads to CVD, and oral antidiuretic medications were used to control it. In the 1950s and 1960s, epidemiologist Ancel Keys' research revealed that high cholesterol intake was also associated with CVD (Jaquish, 2007).

Today, bed rest is known to promote blood clots and is ineffective in treating myocardial infarctions (MIs). Quick, intensive therapy is the standard. Aspirin, heparin, beta (β)-blockers, and thrombolytic medications help to prevent and reduce blood clots, reduce the workload on the heart, and dissolve tiny clots in cardiac vessels (Zafari et al., 2016). Nitrates are given to reduce pain and the heart's workload. Other commonly administered medications include β-blockers, calcium channel blockers, antiplatelet medications, and continued anticoagulant therapies. Cardiac catheterization permits physicians to visualize arterial blockages. Percutaneous angioplasty to open the blocked arteries or coronary artery bypass graft (CABG) surgery is now routine; stents may also be used. Well-trained emergency medical service personnel and specialized cardiac intensive care units with highly expert nurses are found in most communities. Cardiopulmonary resuscitation (CPR) is promoted and automated external defibrillators (AEDs), now commonly placed in schools, shopping malls, government buildings, and other common spaces, have saved the lives of many victims of heart disease (Zafari et al., 2016). Because of all of these advances in the last 50 years, post-MI death rates have dropped by 75%. Antihypertensive and cholesterol-lowering medications, along with healthier lifestyles that include no smoking, regular exercise, and diets low in sodium and saturated fats, have also reduced the rates of hypertension and hyperlipidemia. Compared to 1950 rates, the age-adjusted mortality rate for CVD dropped 60% by the year 1996 (CDC, 1999). The rate of CVD death dropped 60% between 1997 and 2006 for adults without diabetes (American Heart Association, 2015).

With all of these advances over the past half-century plus, it is reasonable to expect increased health care costs. In return, more lives have been saved and extended. But, how much can we afford to pay for future improvements in health care? How many more new advances lie ahead? And, what will we receive in return for our investment?

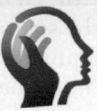

From the Case Files III *(Continued)*

American Heart Association. (2015). Heart disease and stroke statistics—2015 update. Retrieved from http://circ.ahajournals.org/content/early/2014/12/18/CIR.0000000000000152.full.pdf

Centers for Disease Control and Prevention (CDC). (1999). Achievements in public health, 1900–1999: Decline in deaths from heart disease and stroke—United States, 1900-1999. Morbidity & Mortality Weekly Report (MMWR), 48(30), 649–656.

Cutler, D. M. (2005). Your money or your life: Strong medicine for America's health care system. New York, NY: Oxford University Press.

Gilbert, R. E. (2008). Eisenhower's 1955 heart attack: Medical treatment, political effects, and the "behind the scenes" leadership style. Politics and the Life Sciences, 27(1), 2–21.

Jaquish, C. E. (2007). The Framingham Heart Study: On its way to becoming the gold standard for cardiovascular genetic epidemiology? BMC Medical Genetics, 8, 63.

Mahmood, S. S., Levy, D., Vasan, R. S., & Wang, T. J. (2014). The Framingham Heart Study and the epidemiology of cardiovascular diseases: A historical perspective. Lancet, 383(9921), 999–1008.

Zafari, A. M., Abdou, M. H., Talavera, F., Yang, E. H., Garas, S. M., & Jeroudi, A. M. (2016). Myocardial infarction treatment & management. Retrieved from http://emedicine.medscape.com/article/155919-treatment

at 5.0% (Catlin & Cowan, 2015). Keehan et al. (2015) predicts that health care spending will increase to 19.6% of U.S. GDP in 2024—meaning that almost one fifth of all goods and services produced in the United States will go toward health care. Total spending on health care services was $3.1 trillion in 2014 and is predicted to grow to more than $5 trillion in 2024. Viewed as a separate economy, the U.S. health care system would be the fifth largest economy in the world (Blumenthal & Osborn, 2013). Clearly, to gain a deeper understanding of this phenomenon, some basic economic concepts must be examined.

THE ECONOMICS OF HEALTH CARE

Economics is defined as the science of making decisions regarding scarce resources. It is concerned with the "production, distribution, and consumption of services" (Rambur, 2015, p. 8). Economics permeates our social structure—it affects and is affected by policies. Consequently, health is closely tied to economic growth

and development, in that a healthy population is necessary for adequate national productivity. Ample evidence exists for a health–income gradient, as personal income (specifically poverty) is linked to health status, and is especially critical for children between the ages of 6 and 12 (Fletcher & Wolfe, 2012; deChesnay & Anderson, 2012).

Health economics can be better understood by examining the two basic theories underlying the science of economics: microeconomics and macroeconomics. In addition, concepts of health care payment must be understood.

Microeconomics

Microeconomic theory is concerned with supply and demand. **Supply** is the quantity of goods or services that providers are willing to sell at a particular price. **Demand** denotes the consumer's willingness to purchase goods or services at a specified price (Estes et al., 2013). In our free-market–driven economy, supply and demand is a key concept. Economists using microeconomic theory study the supply of goods and services: how we, as consumers, allocate and distribute our resources, and how those marketing goods and services compete. They further study how allocation and distribution affect consumer demand for these goods and services. The concepts of supply and demand are influenced by each other and, in turn, affect prices. In a simplified example, an increase in, or oversupply of, certain products usually leads to less overall consumption (decreased demand) and, usually, lowered prices. The opposite also is true. Limited availability of desired products means that supply does not meet demand, and prices usually increase. An example is the price of a gallon of gasoline. When demand for oil is high and supply begins to dwindle, the prices go up. When demand drops and supplies become more plentiful, prices go down to attract more purchasers. This occurs as long as there are no monopolies to artificially control prices, or only a few choices for goods and services that inhibit competition.

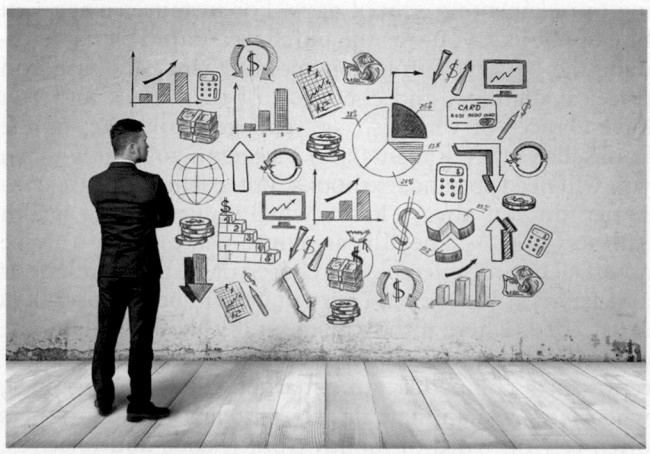

Health care economics can seem very complicated.

In health care, demand-side policies are enacted to reduce demand for health care (e.g., raising insurance deductibles and co-payments), and supply-side policies restrict the supply of resources (e.g., denial of coverage for specific services, utilization of preferred providers who practice within boundaries set by insurance companies) (Estes et al., 2013). Under the ACA, some traditional demand-side policies were removed to improve access to care. For example, preventive services must now be offered without deductibles or co-payments and insurance companies are limited in their ability to deny coverage for preexisting conditions (Healthcare.gov, 2015).

Microeconomic theory is useful for understanding price determination, resource allocation, consumer income, and spending distribution at the level of individuals and organizations (Estes et al., 2013). Microeconomic theory comes into play when health care competition increases, because the success of the supply-and-demand concept depends upon a competitive market. Issues such as cost containment, competition between providers, accessibility of services, quality, and need for accountability continue as targets of major concern in the 21st century. Several ACA provisions address these issues as well (Healthcare.gov, 2015). The law established the Center for Medicare and Medicaid Innovation, which will test ways to improve quality and efficiency of care. In addition, payments to hospitals and physicians will increase or decrease based on the quality of care provided, and all hospitals must publicly report several indicators of quality. Evaluation of how these provisions affect the supply and demand for health services is ongoing.

Macroeconomics

Macroeconomic theory is concerned with the broad variables that affect the status of the economy as a whole. Economists using macroeconomics study factors influencing aggregate demand and supply. In other words, it deals with production, consumption, investment, international trade, inflation, and unemployment on an aggregate level (Rice University, 2016). The focus is on the larger view of economic stability and growth. Macroeconomic theory is useful for providing a global or aggregate perspective of the variables affecting the total economic picture (Estes et al., 2013). Macroeconomic theory has been useful in providing a large-scale perspective on health care financing and led to various proposals for national health plans, health care rationing, competition, and managed care. For instance, when the United States compares overall health spending with countries across the world, it becomes clear that we spend a large percentage of our GDP on health care—more than any other country—and we often have worse indicators of health than do countries who spend much less, for example, lower life expectancy and higher infant mortality rates (Squires & Anderson, 2015). A report from the National Research Council and Institute of Medicine (NRC & IOM, 2013) cites a growing body of evidence that "Americans live shorter lives and experience more injuries and illnesses that people in other high-income countries" indicating a "U.S. health disadvantage" (p. 1) (see A Nursing Professor's Perspectives)

A recent review of 13 high-income countries found that U.S. spending on health care (17.4% of GDP in 2013) was about 50% more than in France (11.6% of GDP; the second highest amount) and nearly double the spending in the United Kingdom (8.8% of GDP) (Squires & Anderson, 2015). At the same time, the United States had the lowest life expectancy, the highest infant mortality rate (nearly twice as high), and the highest prevalence of chronic disease. Possible reasons for the high spending in the United States include high rates of obesity, higher costs for prescription drugs and physician services, and frequent use of expensive technology (Squires & Anderson, 2015). High rates of adverse events (e.g., medication errors, receiving incorrect test results) are another indicator of the poor quality of care received despite high payments. Adverse events are also one reason for high health costs; estimates of preventable hospital costs in the United States range from $16 billion to $18 billion annually (Corrigan, Wakeam, Gandhi, & Leape, 2015). Recent interventions to improve hospital safety are beginning to show promise. The Agency for Health Research and Quality (2015) found a 17% decrease in hospital-acquired conditions from 2010 to 2013, saving approximately $12 billion in health care costs. Whereas those of us with adequate health insurance report good access to services and cutting-edge care from well-trained health care professionals, many of our fellow citizens experience significant barriers to care and a fragmented, poorly staffed health care system. See Figure 6–4 for a comparison of U.S. health care expenditure and health status indicators with eight other countries.

The economics of health care encompasses both microeconomics and macroeconomics and an intricate and complex set of interacting variables. Health care economics is concerned with supply and demand: Are available resources sufficient to meet the demand for use by consumers? Are the resources expended achieving the desired outcomes? When health care resources are scarce or insufficient to address all needs (e.g., for programs and services for at-risk populations), how should they be applied? Should there be a move toward national health insurance (NHI) to improve our nation's health because a healthy population promotes productivity and a more robust economy?

Supply and Demand in Health Care Economics

We learned about supply-and-demand economics during our elementary school days. For instance, when you buy textbooks, you—as the purchaser—are able to determine the best value for your money (generally based on price, availability, and condition of the book), and you have choices of vendors (e.g., college bookstore, online bookseller, other students). As a student, you know when you will need specific textbooks, but as a health care consumer, do you always know when you will need health care services? As a health care consumer, can you truly be an efficient and effective purchaser of health care goods and services? How does a patient determine what services are needed, where to buy them, and how to evaluate the quality of the goods and services? Does health care truly represent a competitive free market, then? For instance, when purchasing a new flat-screen television, consumers often rely on word of mouth from friends and relatives, advice from experts, past experiences with brands,

A NURSING PROFESSOR'S PERSPECTIVE
STRUCTURE AND EVALUATION OF CUBAN VERSUS THE UNITED STATES HEALTH CARE SYSTEMS

Despite being the closest island neighbor to the United States, Cuba could not be any more different compared to the U.S. related to cultural foundations. The political differences alone provide juxtaposition when surveying the two countries. Cuba is quite an intriguing country. Despite a lack of economic resources, Cuba enjoys health outcomes that meet and surpass many of those when compared to the United States. As a nurse involved in public health, it is always important to consider the structure of health care systems and how they shape health outcomes. Because Cuba presents a unique structure, evaluating the two countries and their health systems could prove to be a useful tool in identifying tools and interventions to improve health. The prevailing sentiment about Cuba since as long as I could remember was that Cuba was an impoverished, communist country, and the thought of the United States is that it was the land of opportunity. When I had the chance to visit Cuba, I had the thought that it would be just that, a stark, poor contrast between the United States. However, I was struck by the health interventions I observed. When I drive around the United States, I see children and young families in parks, but in Cuba, older adults were enjoying group exercise classes. In the United States, I see older adults in retirement homes and communities, but in Cuba, I learned that older adults are supported through community-based older adult activity programs designed to engage and support their mental and physical needs. I was able to tour the Cuban equivalent of a U.S. multispecialty health care group, but the Cuba equivalent is 100% government funded and based in the community. This novelty is known as the policlinico and consisted of several nurses and physicians, physical and occupational therapy, Reiki, massage therapy, and a dental clinic. This was in one location, and the patients were able to move from one area of the clinic to the other without waiting for their appointment to be scheduled. In the United States, childhood immunizations are delivered in vaccine clinics and at the provider's office, but in Cuba, I saw vaccines being delivered door to door. Besides costly concierge physicians, I have not seen physicians in the United States visit patients in their home, but I walked around the community with a physician and a nurse that were able to meet children on the street and see that they were developing appropriately. The structure

of the Cuban health care system is centered on the policlinico. This model was focused on preventative health care, and this differs from what we see in the United States where the health care model is really focused on caring for those that are ill. I was able to see how physicians and nurses are educated in Cuba, and this model allows for greater access and output of physicians. One school, funded by the Cuban government, supported the medical education of students from African, Central American, South American, and even students from the United States. This program provided the necessary medical education for the students to return to their home country and work to improve health and health outcomes. Although the United States has many medical schools and accepts students from across the globe, an entire school similar to the Latin American School of Medicine, where medical education is provided to foreigners free of charge, is unknown. Perhaps the most intriguing finding while visiting Cuba was learning of their initiatives to enhance maternal–child health. It was explained to me that many years ago, the Cuban government noticed that maternal–child health outcomes were extremely poor, and they worked toward creating systems to improve these outcomes. One of these interventions is called a maternity home. Maternity homes are places that high-risk pregnant women can live until they deliver their baby. The homes are residential and provide nutrition, medical, nursing, and social services care for the woman and her family. The goal of the maternity home is to provide a homelike environment where women can deliver full-term, healthy babies. In the United States, high-risk pregnant ladies are on home bed rest and must journey to the clinic for their obstetrics appointments or are hospitalized. Although there are distinct structural differences between the two countries and their health outcomes, there are opportunities to compare the two structures and identify how culturally appropriate the interventions are comparing the U.S. approach to the Cuban approach and vice versa. Visiting Cuba was eye opening to cultural, political, and health approaches, and it provided food for thought as the United States strives to improve health for our citizens.

Colleen Marzilli, PhD, DNP, RN-BC, CCM, APHN-BC, CNE
Nursing Professor

customer ratings on Web sites, and rating services like *Consumer Reports*. Also, we most often plan in advance for large purchases, like newer and bigger televisions, saving a little money each month to keep within our budget.

With health care, this is seldom the case; health care is typically unpredictable and often difficult to research (Ubel, 2014). Even with the growth of health information (and, often, misinformation) available on the Internet, physicians are still the system's main gatekeepers, and patients must trust that these care providers have the competence to appropriately diagnose and treat them, as well as coordinate necessary resources to provide quality health care. Further, they must trust that physicians will

put patients' interests before their own (i.e., give them accurate information about risks and benefits and not induce them to have expensive procedures to enrich the provider). Now, enter health insurance companies and managed care into the mix—each agency likely pays a different price for the same service. Hence, health care purchases are not easily understood. In a free-market system, competition is an important factor, but is competition truly possible with employer-based health insurance that limits the choice of plans and providers?

In 1963, economist Kenneth Arrow wrote an influential article about health care economics detailing the lack of information in the medical marketplace (reprinted as Arrow,

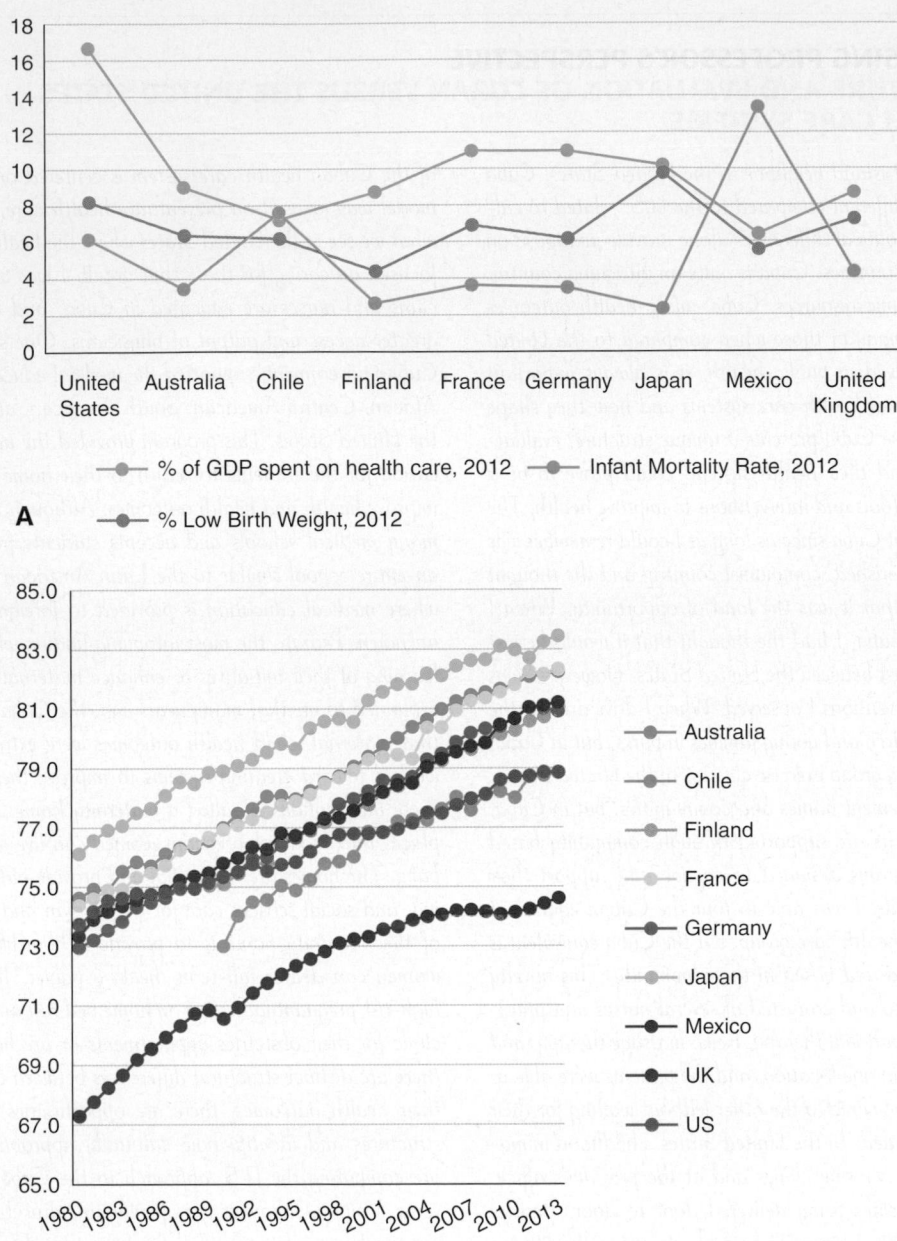

FIGURE 6–4   A: Comparison of United States with eight other countries on selected health status indicators and percentage of gross domestic product (GDP) spent on health. **B:** Comparison of United States with eight other countries on life expectancy rates from 1980 to 2013. (From Organization of Economic Cooperation & Development (OECD). (2016). *Health statistics, selected OECD countries.* Retrieved from http://stats.oecd.org/Index.aspx?DataSetCode=SHA)

2004; also cited in Krugman, 2009, 2011). The main points of the article noted that risk and uncertainty prohibit a true market economy in health care because consumers:

- Do not know when or if they will become ill—but they know they will need and want medical treatment, thus the demand for health insurance
- Do not know what services will be needed and what works best for their condition—thus the need for physicians
- Do not know about the quality of health care good and services—thus the need for government regulation (e.g., licensing, certification) and malpractice lawsuits

- Have an asymmetric level of information, compared to the insurer, about the likely demand for health care services, resulting in **adverse selection** (e.g., high-risk patients are denied insurance or care) and market failure (e.g., inefficiencies and lack of appropriate competition)—although this is less severe in large group insurance plans that spread out the risk

Thus, a fundamental problem of the health care economy is the difficulty of any one person or organization (e.g., patient, physician, health plan, government) to act as an effective consumer of health care goods and services (Ubel, 2014). One area of health care, however, that has been thought to more closely follow the free-market supply-and-demand model is with cosmetic procedures, especially laser eye surgery (Herrick, 2013). Between 1992 and 2011, while the costs of health care increased approximately 118%, the cost of cosmetic surgeries increased only 30%—despite increases in demand and quality. The price of conventional LASIK eye surgery decreased about 25% between 1999 and 2011, whereas the price of newer, better quality laser eye surgeries in 2011 was nearly the same as the LASIK price in 1999. Report of a 30% decrease in LASIK procedures during the 2007–2009 recession and decreased Google queries for LASIK between 2007 and 2011 indicate that market forces have an impact on this procedure (Kuo, 2011; Stein, Childers, Nan, & Mian, 2013. FDA (2014) studies, first reported in 2008, indicated that 45% of patients developed visual symptoms following LASIK surgery (e.g., halos, dry eye, glare, starbursts). This new information was also thought to influence decreased Internet searches (Stein et al., 2013). Leonhardt (2014) argued that much of the slowdown in the growth of health care costs was due to economic trends (e.g., recession) rather than effects of the ACA. The LASIK evidence seems to echo that. These examples indicate that consumers influence the price of a service when they can accurately compare cost, quality, and services from different providers. It should be noted, however, that cosmetic and laser eye surgery are elective procedures, and this makes comparison between these procedures and other health care costs more complicated.

Health Insurance Concepts

Conventional economic theories posit that people pay small premiums monthly to offset the risk of large medical bills should they become seriously ill. This represents an *indemnity policy* (much like car or homeowners' insurance) and this is the type of health insurance first offered in the United States. In the past, patients could choose any doctor or hospital and submit the providers' bills to the insurance company for payment. **Moral hazard** is the term used by economists to explain how health insurance changes the behavior of people, resulting in more risk-taking and wasteful actions. They liken it to fire insurance without a deductible, noting that a person may be less careful about clearing brush from a house or may even resort to arson if it costs the owner nothing to have the home replaced. If a person has health insurance, many economists hypothesize, they are less likely to take good care of themselves, and if they don't pay for their health care (through premiums, co-payments, and deductibles), they are more likely to overuse it, although empirical evidence of this is sparse (Dranove, 2008; Nickitas, Middaugh, & Aries, 2016). In other words, economists theorize that insurance has a paradoxical effect and may lead to wasteful or risk-taking behaviors. In this scenario, patients will demand expensive health care, even if it provides only the smallest benefit. The concept of moral hazard is the reason behind larger deductibles and co-payments—it is an effort to control wasteful or excessive use of health care resources.

A newer supposition states that consumers purchase health insurance not to avoid risk but to earn a claim for additional income (i.e., insurance paying for medical care) when they become ill and that co-payments and managed care actually work against the system by reducing the amount of income transferred to ill persons or limiting their access to needed services. Think about what would happen if you or your loved one were to suddenly need an expensive heart surgery or lengthy cancer treatment—without health insurance. You would want health insurance to protect against this possibility—to be able to pay medical bills without losing your assets (e.g., home, belongings). Houle and Keene (2014) found that individuals experiencing a decrease in health were almost three times as likely to default on a mortgage compared to those who did not report such a change. Having health insurance decreased the risk slightly. This substantiates the claim of a genuine risk of financial disaster when confronted with a serious medical emergency or long-term illness and helps explain why some economists argue that a focus on moral hazard in the insurance industry has actually worked against reducing health care costs (Stone, 2011). Another reason that moral hazard doesn't accurately apply to health insurance is that its effects may not be as predictable as in other instances of indemnity (Ubel, 2015). The case can surely be made that even those with unlimited insurance coverage don't just "check into the hospital because it's free" as noted in a classic article by Gladwell (2005, para. 11). Most people do not seek infinite numbers of mammograms, colonoscopies, or other invasive procedures or surgeries, for example.

Cost sharing, which includes co-payments and deductibles, divides the cost of health care services between insurance companies and patients. Insurance companies use cost sharing to prevent overuse of health services. The amount of a co-payment or deductible may change for some types of care, such as a visit to the ED. In a systematic review of the literature, Kiil and Houlberg (2014) found some evidence that cost sharing reduces the use of prescription medication, primary care and specialty office visits, and ambulatory care, possibly lowering overall health care costs. At the same time, is it possible that individuals are attempting to avoid higher costs by not following through on medical appointments or medication? Also, the effect of cost sharing on use of services is not equal. Individuals with low incomes decrease their use of medications and services more than do others. The ACA limits cost sharing for people with low or moderate incomes, in plans offered by employers and plans purchased through the marketplace (Healthcare.gov, 2015).

For some people, the cost-sharing component of their health insurance is so high that they are considered **underinsured**. They fall into one or more of three categories: (1) medical expenses totaling more than 10% of their yearly income, (2) annual income 200% of federal poverty level (FPL) with medical expenses >5% of yearly income, and (3) health insurance deductibles ≥5% of their annual income (Collins, Rasmussen, Beutel, & Doty, 2015). Prior to the ACA, about half of those underinsured and 58% of those without insurance reported problems paying for medical bills, being contacted by a collection agency about unpaid medical bills, and having to pay off medical bills over time (Schoen, Doty, Robertson, & Collins, 2011). They often exhausted their savings, ran up credit card debt, or else delayed necessary medical care to avoid going into debt. Woolhandler and Himmelstein (2013, p. 1122) reported that high deductibles for the privately insured "increased the risk of dying by 21%" among sicker, low-income patients but didn't cause problems for healthier, more affluent patients. Those gaining access through ACA-expanded Medicaid plans (projected to reach about 40%) will be "woefully uninsured" as many states have "reduced benefits, cut provider payments, and narrowed provider networks" (p. 1123). Even those with private insurance Bronze plans (minimum coverage allowed by ACA) will only have 60% of medical costs covered. This goes up to 70% for Silver plans; Gold plans, like most employment-based policies, will cover about 80% of medical costs. It is important to remember that people who have insurance, whether they have always had insurance or gained coverage through the ACA, may continue to have very high out-of-pocket costs for their income level and are essentially underinsured. Efficiency (or net benefit to consumers) of plans may need to include regulation of premiums (Glazer & McGuire, 2011) (see What Do You Think?).

Employer-Sponsored Health Insurance

Employer-sponsored health insurance is the leading source of coverage for nonelderly U.S. citizens. Historically, employers became the leading source of coverage because of three policy decisions in the 1940s

and 1950s. First, during World War II, wage controls did not apply to health insurance, so employers used health insurance to lure workers from their competitors. Later, the U.S. government determined that health insurance could be part of collective bargaining. Finally, in 1954, the IRS exempted health insurance premiums paid by employers from federal income tax (Rook, 2015). In a 2015 annual survey, 57% of companies offered health insurance to their workers, unchanged from the previous year but considerably lower than the high of 69% in 2010 (KFF & Health Research and Educational Trust [HRET], 2015). However, only 79% of those workers are eligible for health coverage because of minimum work hours or mandatory waiting periods. Seventy-nine percent of those eligible participate in health insurance. Because not all employers offer health insurance, only about 56% of workers in the United States are covered by employer-sponsored health plans. Many small businesses do not offer employee health insurance because of the high costs.

In 2015, the average cost of group health insurance was $17,545 for a family policy and $6,251 for an individual (KFF & HRET, 2015). These figures are 4% higher than 2014 costs (wages increased <2% from 2014 to 2015). The cost for family coverage increased 61% from 2005 to 2015, and employee contributions for family coverage increased 83%. The average worker contributed about 28% of the premium for family coverage, and 16% for individual coverage in 2015. See Figure 6–5 for trends in health insurance premium costs as compared to wages and overall inflation.

The percent of employers offering health insurance decreased prior to the ACA but has not significantly decreased since implementation of its reforms (KFF & HRET, 2015). Employers are continuing to pass along some of the higher costs of health insurance to employees in the form of higher employee premiums, deductibles, co-payments, and stricter enrollment requirements. Workers having insurance that includes an annual deductible have increased from 55% in 2006 to 70% in 2010 to 81% in 2015 (KFF & HRET, 2015). Similarly, the percentage of covered workers enrolled in employer health plans with a deductible of $1,000 or more for single coverage increased from 10% in 2006 to 27% in 2010 to 46% in 2015.

Those people whose employers do not offer health insurance coverage or who are self-employed can purchase nongroup health insurance. However, premiums are greater than the worker's share of employer group coverage. The ACA has made purchasing a nongroup policy easier and subsidizes the premiums for eligible people. Even in states that did not expand Medicaid, a greater number of people with lower incomes purchased insurance on the federal marketplace (Sommers, Blendon, & Orav, 2016). Variations in costs were an issue prior to the ACA; one large-scale survey found that annual premiums for family coverage ranged from $2,325 to $9,201 and individual coverage varied (depending upon age) from $1,163 and $2,325 (KFF, 2008). Variation in costs has not been eliminated with the ACA, but the variation is geographical; specifically, costs vary by location, not within one location (Gabel et al., 2016). Premiums for benchmark plans increased 6% nationally from 2015

What do *you* think?

If you make 399% over the poverty level in annual income ($45,900 in 2013) and are eligible for ACA premium subsidies, you are expected to pay about $4,361 for individual Bronze insurance premiums and about $4,167 in co-payments and additional deductibles. But, if you earn 401% over the poverty level ($46,100), subsidies are no longer provided and your premium would then be $10,585 annually, with capped out-of-pocket costs estimated at $6,250.

Do you think the higher cost sharing will ultimately reduce health care expenditures? International research has shown this method is generally not effective at controlling costs (Woolhandler & Himmelstein, 2013). Canada outlawed deductibles and co-payments in 1981 and has experienced slower growth in spending and more rapid improvements in health. They highlight that single-payer systems reduce administrative costs and Canada has demonstrated that costs can be controlled through other measures (e.g., negotiated physician fee schedules, global hospital budgeting). Scotland, with health costs half those of the United States, views patients as "owners of their healthcare system, not its customers" (p. 1123).

What do you think the United States should do to control costs and improve health?

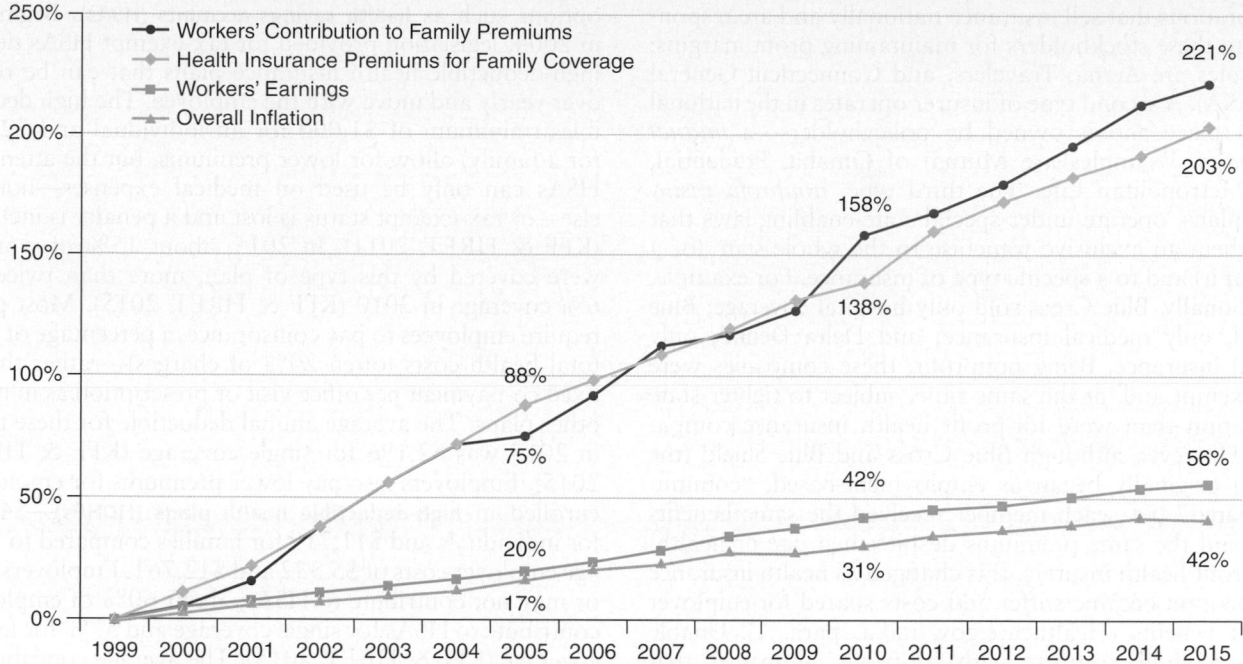

FIGURE 6–5 Increases in average annual premiums for health insurance, worker contributions, and earnings, 1999–2015. (From Kaiser Family Foundation & Health Research & Educational Trust. (2015). *Employer health benefits survey 2015*. Retrieved from http://files.kff. org/attachment/report-2015-employer-health-benefits-survey)

to 2016 but increased by 10% or more in 21 states and decreased in seven states and the District of Columbia. In addition, premiums increased more in suburban and rural areas than in urban areas.

The cost of health insurance is a deterrent for many people. Prior to the ACA, only 4% to 11% of those at the lower income levels purchased nongroup health coverage (Bernard, Banthin, & Encinosa, 2009). Although coverage levels generally increase as income rises, only 25% of those earning 10 times the poverty level purchased health insurance. As of 2015, 32.3 million nonelderly people in the United States were uninsured (Garfield, Damico, Cox, Claxton, & Levitt, 2016). More than 25% of these individuals are likely eligible for coverage by Medicaid or CHIP. Another 22% could receive subsidies to purchase a nongroup plan from the marketplace. Approximately 42% are not eligible for any of the insurance options available under the ACA, as 15% are undocumented immigrants, 15% have an employer who offers an insurance plan, and 12% have an income too high to qualify for tax credits. The remaining people (about 10%) fall into a "coverage gap" because their state did not expand Medicaid. A survey by the KFF in December of 2014 found that many people who remained uninsured were not aware of the financial assistance available under the ACA (Garfield & Young, 2015). Some were incorrectly told that they were not eligible for assistance.

Further understanding of health economics and its impact on community health and community health nursing can be obtained by examining methods of health care finance, trends and issues influencing health care economics, and the effects of finance patterns on community health practice.

SOURCES OF HEALTH CARE FINANCING: PUBLIC AND PRIVATE

Financing of health care significantly affects community health and public health nursing practice. It influences the type and quality of services offered, as well as the ways in which those services are used. Sources of payment may be grouped into three categories: third-party payments, direct consumer payment, and private or philanthropic support.

Third-Party Payments

Third-party payments are monetary reimbursements made to providers of health care by someone other than the consumer who received the care. The organizations that administer these funds are called *third-party payers* because they are a third party, or external, to the consumer–provider relationship. Included in this category are four types of payment sources: private insurance companies, independent or self-insured health plans, government health programs, and claims payment agents (Estes et al., 2013).

Private Insurance Companies

Private insurance companies currently pay the majority of U.S. health care expenditures for those under age 65. Payments from private companies make up approximately 20% of total health care spending (CMS, 2015b). They market and underwrite policies aimed at decreasing consumer risk of economic loss because of a need to use health services. There are three types of private insurers. First are commercial stock companies that sell health insurance, usually as a sideline. They are private, stockholder-owned corporations that sell insurance nationally and are responsible to these stockholders for maintaining profit margins; examples are Aetna, Travelers, and Connecticut General (CIGNA). A second type of insurer operates in the national marketplace and is owned by policyholders—a *mutual company*. Examples are Mutual of Omaha, Prudential, and Metropolitan Life. The third type, *nonprofit insurance* plans, operate under special state-enabling laws that give them an exclusive franchise to the whole state (or a part of it) and to a specific type of insurance. For example, traditionally, Blue Cross sold only hospital coverage; Blue Shield, only medical insurance; and Delta Dental, only dental insurance. Being nonprofit, these companies were tax exempt and, at the same time, subject to tighter state regulation than were for-profit health insurance companies. However, although Blue Cross and Blue Shield (the Blues) originally began as employment-based, "community-rated" (i.e., each member received the same benefits and paid the same premiums despite their age or health) nonprofit health insurers, this changed as health insurance competition became stiffer and costs soared for employer health benefits (Healthcare.gov, n.d.a, para. 1). Unable to successfully compete with for-profit companies that employed traditional underwriting practices (i.e., charging more to those at higher risk), the Blues sought for-profit status so that some of their franchises could be publicly traded (i.e., sell stocks and raise capital). They often used this extra money to merge and expand market share and began adopting business strategies used by other for-profit companies. In 2004, two of these for-profit arms, Wellpoint and Anthem, merged to become the largest health insurer in the United States. The Blues nonprofit arms became virtually indistinguishable as profits moved to the forefront, and in 2015, California ordered that the tax-exempt status of Blue Shield of California be revoked and that the company be ordered file tax returns back to 2013 because of increasing profits ($3.19 to $4.18 billion from 2009 to 2014) and $13.6 billion in revenue reported in 2014 (Terhune, 2015; Varney, 2010). Many insurance plans, including the Blues, sought "double-digit rate increases" to defray added costs of additional insured patients under ACA (Rappleye, 2015, para. 14). Today, about one third of Americans are covered by a health plan offered by the Blues (Blue Cross Blue Shield, 2016). Maintaining profits for stockholders means that insurance companies must control the *medical loss ratio*, or the money paid for health services. If they can reduce the amount paid for health care services, then profits are increased and the stock is more attractive to potential buyers. Four common ways that were used to reduce the medical loss ratio included (1) reduce covered services, (2) raise deductibles and co-payments, (3) exclude people with preexisting conditions, and (4) targeted marketing to young, healthy populations. Previously, insurers also resorted to *rescission* of coverage—or canceling coverage for failure to disclose a preexisting condition (often unrelated to the person's current health care problem) or some other means of disqualifying coverage after large medical claims have been filed (Healthcare.gov, n.d.b; Nelson, 2009). However, the ACA made this practice illegal, except in cases of consumer misrepresentation or fraud.

A recent trend in private insurance is the move to **consumer-driven/high-deductible health plans** with savings options such as **health savings accounts (HSAs)**. Beginning in 2004, legislation provided for tax-exempt HSAs tied to high-deductible health insurance plans that can be rolled over yearly and move with the employee. The high deductibles (minimum of $1,000 for an individual and $2,000 for a family) allow for lower premiums, but the attendant HSAs can only be used on medical expenses—nothing else—or tax-exempt status is lost and a penalty is incurred (KFF & HRET, 2011). In 2015, about 15% of workers were covered by this type of plan, more than twice the 6% coverage in 2010 (KFF & HRET, 2015). Most plans require employees to pay coinsurance, a percentage of their total health costs (often 20% of charges)—rather than a fixed co-payment per office visit or prescription as in many other plans. The average annual deductible for these plans in 2015 was $2,196 for single coverage (KFF & HRET, 2015). Employers also pay lower premiums for employees enrolled in **high-deductible health plans (HDHPs)**—$4,539 for individuals and $11,719 for families compared to average employer costs of $5,332 and $12,761. Employers may or may not contribute to HSAs; about 60% of employers contribute to HSAs for single coverage and 57% for family coverage (KFF & HRET, 2015). The average contribution is $568 for individuals and $991 for families.

Most workers with employer-sponsored health insurance also have prescription drug coverage (more than 99%), with some cost sharing, such as co-payment or coinsurance (KFF & HRET, 2015). Only 12% are in plans that pay 100% of prescription drug costs after a deductible is met. Often, co-payments are based on tiered systems, for example, $10 co-payment for less expensive drugs in the first tier and $25 for slightly more expensive drugs in the second tier. These co-payments can affect medication adherence. A meta-analysis of studies of people with public insurance found that those with co-payments for prescriptions had 11% higher odds for nonadherence (Sinnott, Buckley, O'Riordan, Bradley, & Whelton, 2013). A systematic review of the literature concluded that lower (or no) co-payments for medications not only improved adherence and patient outcomes but also decreased the use of other health care services (Kesselheim et al., 2015).

Independent or Self-Insured Health Plans

Independent or self-insured health plans underwrite the remaining private health insurance in the United States. These plans have been offered through a limited number of organizations, such as large businesses, unions, school districts, consumer cooperatives, and medical groups. Employers with self-insured plans take on all or a major part of the risk for health care costs of their employees. These plans may be self-administered or utilize third-party claims administrators. Minimum premium plans are another form of self-insurance for which employers pay medical costs up to an agreed-upon limit, and insurers assume responsibility for the excess claims (Bureau of Labor Statistics, n.d.). Sixty-three percent of employees receiving work-related insurance benefits were part of self-insured plans in 2015 (KFF & HRET, 2015). The ACA encourages self-insured employers to limit the overall value of their plans (Claxton & Levitt, 2015). This will result in employees having lower-cost health insurance options, which are not taxed, and (theoretically) higher wages, which are taxed.

Government Health Programs

Government health programs currently make up the largest source of third-party reimbursement in the United States. Payments from federal sources increased to 28% in 2014, from 26% in 2013 (CMS, 2015a). This increase is primarily due to the Medicaid expansion under the ACA, which is 100% funded by the federal government until 2017 (Healthcare.gov, 2015). State and local government spending was 17% of health care spending. As a whole, the proportion of government funding of health care in the United States is less than that of 34 other developed countries (Organization for Economic Cooperation & Development [OECD], 2015). In 2013, 48% of health care spending was estimated to be paid by public sources in the United States, compared with the Netherlands at 87%, United Kingdom at 83%, France at 79%, Japan at 83%, Canada at 70%, and Mexico at 51%. Whereas the percent of public money in the United States is low compared to other countries, overall public spending in the United States in 2013 was $4,197 per capita, more than any other country except Norway and the Netherlands (Squires & Anderson, 2015).

The U.S. government's four major health insurance programs are Medicare, Medicaid, the Federal Employees Health Benefits Plan, and the Civilian Health and Medical Program of the Uniformed Services. The largest programs are Medicare and Medicaid. In addition to payments from Medicare and Medicaid, the U.S. government reimburses safety-net hospitals and other entities involved in care of the uninsured. The Centers for Medicare and Medicaid (CMS, 2015b) anticipates spending $6.4 billion for uncompensated care in fiscal year 2016—exemplifying just some of the costs to taxpayers.

Medicare and Social Security Disability Insurance

Medicare, known as Title XVIII of the Social Security Act Amendments of 1965, has provided mandatory federal health insurance since July 1, 1966, for adults aged 65 years and older who have paid into the Social Security system (CMS, 2015a). It also covers certain people with disabilities (regardless of age). Medicare is administered by the CMS (formerly the Healthcare Financing Administration) of the USDHHS. In 2014, Medicare covered more than 55 million people. The majority of recipients are age 65 or older (46.3 million), and Medicare paid health care costs of $618.7 billion. In 2015, 15% of total federal spending was for Medicare (KFF, 2016). Financing of Medicare is through general tax revenues (41%), payroll taxes (38%), premiums from beneficiaries (13%), and other sources. Out-of-pocket spending for Medicare beneficiaries was $5,368 in 2011, almost equally divided between medical/long-term care and premiums. About 85% of beneficiaries were over the age of 65; the remaining beneficiaries qualified for Medicare 24 months after they became eligible for Social Security Disability Insurance. These recipients are younger than age 65 and permanently disabled or chronically ill, including those with end-stage renal disease (added in 1973). Most enrollees are between the ages of 65 and 84, 16% are under age 65 (and qualify for Medicare because of a permanent disability), and 13% are age 85 and older. The Medicare population is projected to grow to 81 million by 2030, more than twice the number of recipients in 2000 (see Fig. 6–6).

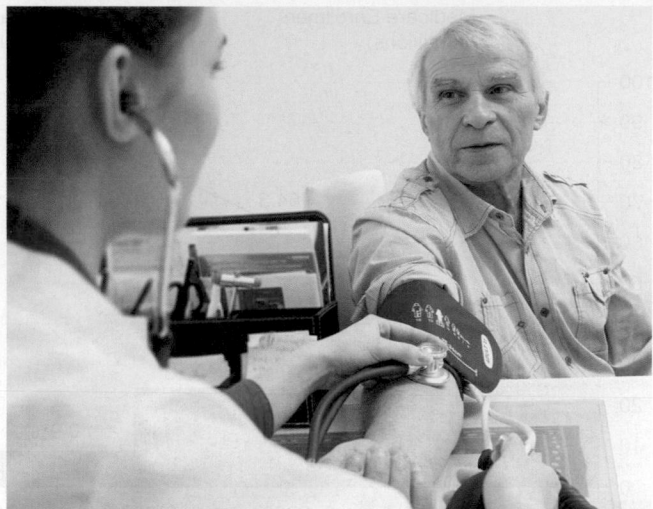

Medicare plays an important part in protecting the health of Americans.

Part A of Medicare, the hospital insurance program, covers inpatient hospitals, limited-skilled nursing facilities, home health, and hospice services to participants eligible for Social Security Disability Income (Cubanski et al., 2015). The 2015 deductible per episode (not annual) for Part A is $1,260, and some coinsurance costs apply. Part A is primarily financed through trust funds derived from employment payroll taxes. A total tax of 2.9% of employee wages is split between the employer and employee. These payroll taxes, along with interest earned on trust fund investments, provide the income for this program. In 2013, the payroll tax for employees was increased from 1.45% to 2.35% for individuals making more than $200,000.

Part B of Medicare, the supplementary and voluntary medical insurance program, primarily covers physician services but also covers home health care for beneficiaries not covered under Part A (Cubanski et al., 2015). The 2015 annual deductible was $147 and recipients pay 20% for services once the deductible is met. No out-of-pocket charges are applied for annual wellness visits or preventive services that are rated "A" or "B" by the U.S. Preventive Services Task Force (USPSTF). Part B is funded through general revenue and enrollee monthly premiums ($146.90 in 2015). For couples earning over $170,000 annually, premiums can range from $146.90 to $335.70; very few Medicare recipients pay the higher-income premiums.

Part C Medicare plans, also called Medicare Advantage, are private plans generously subsidized by the federal government (Cubanski et al., 2015). Part C plans are not supplemental to Part A and Part B—they take the place of Part A and Part B. Some may also cover vision, dental, and prescriptions. Most people enrolled in Part C pay the Part B premium and may also pay an additional amount to the private company. Part C plans must limit out-of-pocket expenses annually; the cap was $6,700 in 2015. This limit is only applied to Part C plans; Part A and Part B plans do not have a limit. Also unlike traditional Medicare, Part C plans use provider networks, which limit the choice of physicians or hospitals. They are regional, which may be problematic for seniors who want to spend winters in Florida and summers in Montana, for instance. There were

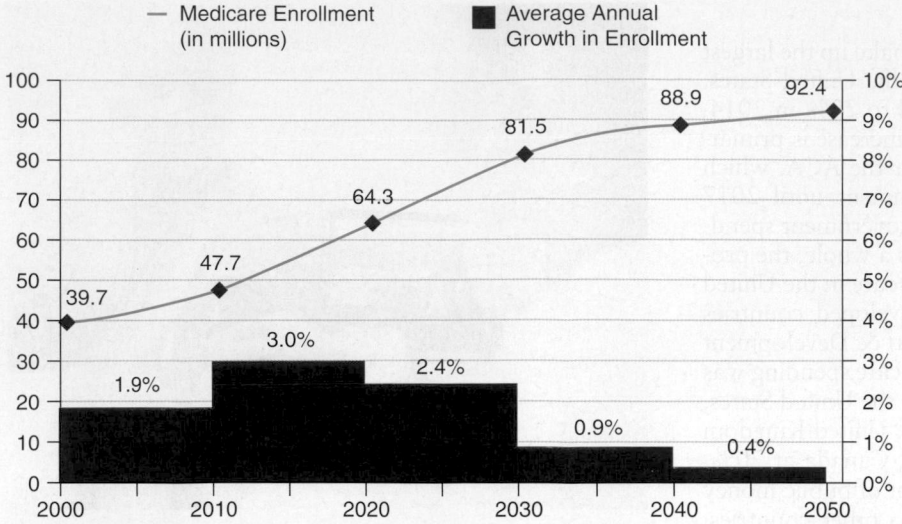

FIGURE 6–6 Projected change in Medicare enrollment, 2000–2050: Depicting growth in beneficiaries and decline in ratio of workers. (From Kaiser Family Foundation. (2015). *Fact sheet: Medicare spending and financing*. Retrieved from http://kff.org/medicare/fact-sheet/medicare-spending-and-financing-fact-sheet/. This information was reprinted with permission from the Henry J. Kaiser Family Foundation. The Kaiser Family Foundation, based in Menlo Park, California, is a nonprofit, private operating foundation focusing on the major health care issues facing the nation and is not associated with Kaiser Permanente or Kaiser Industries.)

approximately 18 Medicare Advantage plans available in each region in 2015; each is required to provide all benefits covered under Part A and Part B, but many offer additional services, including prescription drug coverage. Seniors can change their Part C plan during open enrollment periods or revert back to traditional Medicare Part A and Part B. In 2015, 15.7 million Medicare participants had Part C plans, nearly three times the number in 2003. Other types of Medicare plans include Medicare Medical Savings Account (MSA) plans, Medicare cost plans, Programs of All-Inclusive Care for the Elderly (PACE), and Medication Therapy Management (MTM) program; these are not available in all areas (Medicare.gov, n.d.a).

Forty-five percent of Medicare beneficiaries have supplemental coverage through a private company or employer retiree health insurance plans—known as *Medigap* coverage—added to Medicare Part A and Part B (Cubanski et al., 2015). Medigap coverage helps enrollees pay for out-of-pocket expenses. This supplemental coverage cannot be combined with Part C plans, because they already have a limit on enrollee cost sharing. People with Medigap coverage through their employers' retiree health plan generally pay lower premiums than people with coverage through a private company do. With rising costs of health care coverage, companies are increasing premium costs for retirees, offering new options, such as Medicare Advantage to replace traditional health plans, or paying only a set amount for health coverage and leaving retirees to purchase their own insurance.

Part D, the prescription benefit plan added through the Medicare Prescription Drug Improvement and Modernization Act of 2003, became available to seniors in 2006 (Cubanski et al., 2015). Offered by private companies (but supported by government funds), Part D plans can be combined either with Part A/Part B or with a Medicare Advantage plan (Part C) that does not cover prescriptions. Part D is primarily financed through general revenue and participant premiums. Seniors can change plans during open enrollment periods, and plans vary in coverage. Beneficiaries must review what prescriptions and what pharmacies each plan will cover when selecting a Part D plan. Each region has, on average, 30

plans available. Part D plans cost (on average) around $26 per month in 2006 and about $39 per month in 2015 (Cubanski et al., 2015). The premiums for these plans vary by location and plan chosen. For instance, one can find a premium as low as $12.60 in New Mexico and one as high as $171.50 in Florida. Because of the high costs of Part D plans, people with incomes up to 150% of the FPL and limited assets (e.g., a home, a car) are eligible for low-income subsidies that pay for all or part of the Part D premium. Similar to Part B, enrollees with higher incomes (more than $85,000 for an individual) pay an additional fee as part of their Part D premium.

All part D plans must offer at least the standard benefit set by the U.S. government (Cubanski et al., 2015). In 2015, Part D beneficiaries pay a deductible of $320 and then pay 25% of prescription costs until total drug costs (costs paid by the plan and by the enrollee) reach $2,960. This is followed by a coverage gap, often called the "doughnut hole"; this ends when total drug costs reach the catastrophic coverage limit of $7,062 (~$4,700 in out-of-pocket spending). During the coverage gap, enrollees pay 45% of brand-name drug costs, and 65% of generic drug costs. Many enrollees have plans that provide some additional coverage during the gap period. Medicare is gradually phasing in subsidies in the coverage gap for brand-name drugs and generic drugs, reducing the beneficiary coinsurance rate from 100% in 2010 to 25% in 2020. This is called closing the gap, and ACA provisions over time will close the doughnut hole (Rice et al., 2014).

Briesacher et al. (2010) published a study of household spending on prescription drugs prior to Part D implementation. Medicare enrollees and their families spent a large portion of their income on housing, food, transportation, and personal care expenses, with little left over for medication expenses. Enrollees took, on average, four to five medications per week, leading to decisions to not adhere to medication instructions because they could not pay for them. Part D only partially alleviated this situation. A follow-up study by Naci et al. (2014) indicated that more Medicare beneficiaries could afford their prescription medications in the first three years after Part D implementation. After that, the recession led to economic hardships for many people, and the number of enrollees reporting that they did not take a medication because of its cost increased during the 2009 to 2011 time period. Part D does not benefit all racial and ethnic groups equally. Recipients from minority groups often have more difficulty obtaining a Part D plan and do not receive adequate assistance from plan administrators (Haviland et al., 2012). When the "doughnut hole" closes in 2020, some enrollees may still have difficulty purchasing brand-name drugs (Sacks, Burgess, Cabral, Pizer, & McDonnell, 2013). Finally, most beneficiaries do not choose the least expensive plan relevant to their health care needs (Zhou & Zhang, 2012).

The majority of Medicare beneficiaries participate in both Part A and Part B, often with supplemental private insurance, or they choose a Medicare Advantage plan (Part C). Less than 14% relied solely on Medicare coverage in 2010 (Cubanski et al., 2015). Some Medicare beneficiaries, especially those in need of long-term care, will also be enrolled in Medicaid. Although Medicare is generally viewed as a helpful program, there are concerns related to continued funding with an older population.

Average total Medicare expenditures grew from $5,080 per person in 1991 to $7,310 in 2001 and $11,728 in 2014 (Congressional Budget Office, 2005, 2009; Keehan et al., 2015). Overall, spending per beneficiary increased at a rate of 7.0% between 2000 and 2010, compared to 1.0% between 2010 and 2014 (KFF, 2015c). The rate of growth is projected to be 4.1% annually from 2014 to 2024. Medicare spending, like most health care spending, is skewed in that 10% of beneficiaries are responsible for nearly 60% of total spending, representing $61,722 per capita (Cubanski et al., 2015). A study by Hellander, Himmelstein, and Woolhandler (2013) estimated that Medicare had overpaid private insurers (e.g., Medicare Advantage plans) $282.6 billion since 1985 and called for an end to privatization of Medicare. **Capitation rates** for Medicare Advantage plans are being reduced under provisions of the ACA, with a financial incentive for plans with higher-quality scores; those scoring poorly face penalties (Rice et al., 2014). Medicare home health costs have increased and quality has diminished, as the majority of home health agencies providing care for Medicare patients are now for-profit. Higher per-patient costs were demonstrated ($4,827 vs. $4,075), as these agencies had higher profits and administrative costs (Cabin, Himmelstein, Siman, & Woolhandler, 2014). An analysis of acute care costs for Medicare patients found that 10% of patients were responsible for more than 70% of total spending (Joynt, Gawande, Orav, & Jha, 2013). An interesting footnote involves unauthorized immigrants paying into the Medicare Trust Fund; this was estimated at between $2.2 and $3.8 billion more annually than what was withdrawn between 2000 and 2011 for a $35.1 billion surplus (Zallman et al., 2016). For more information on Medicare trends and concerns about its solvency, see Chapter 24.

Medicaid

Medicaid, known as Title XIX of the Social Security Amendments Act of 1965, provides medical assistance for children, pregnant women, parents with dependent children, seniors, and people with severe disabilities (Paradise, 2015; Paradise, Lyons, & Roland, 2015). Medicaid is an optional program for states, but all states currently participate. Over time, the scope of Medicaid increased, and states opting to provide Medicaid were required to implement each increase—or lose their federal Medicaid funding. Medicaid covered more than 71 million people in 2015, an increase of nearly 13 million since 2013, largely due to the Medicaid expansion under the ACA (CMS, 2015b). Spending for Medicaid was $495.8 billion. Because Medicaid covers so many people, many of whom have complex health needs, it is a large component of health care spending in the United States (Paradise et al., 2015). Medicaid covers 37% all children and 77% of children living below poverty level. It covers 20% of all Medicare beneficiaries and 64% of enrollees living in nursing homes. However, Medicaid only covers 35% of adults living below poverty level. Prior to the ACA, childless adults without disabilities were not eligible for Medicaid. Under the ACA, Medicaid was expanded to all nonelderly adults with incomes up to 138% of the FPL, $16,250 for an individual in 2015. Other changes made through the ACA were to extend Medicaid coverage for children in foster care until age 26 (equal to the requirement that private plans allow dependent children to remain on a parent's plan until that age). States also needed to make the Medicaid application process easier.

The ACA initially required all states to expand Medicaid. This was legally challenged by several states, leading to a Supreme Court case called *National Federation of Independent Business v. Sebelius* (KFF, 2012). On the last day of the 2011–2012 term, the court released their ruling: The Medicaid expansion was unconstitutional because it was highly coercive. Although states participating in Medicaid had been required to comply with all of its provisions, the Supreme Court ruling stated that this increase was too sudden and the penalty of withholding all existing Medicaid funds for noncompliance was too high. Thus, the Medicaid expansion became optional for states. Currently, 24 states have not expanded Medicaid coverage under the ACA, and Dickman, Himelstein, McCormick, and Woolhandler (2015) estimate that this led to 7.74 million people remaining uninsured. They project that there will be between 7,076 and 16, 945 more deaths resulting from this action, compared to states that opted in. And this will also result in 441,260 fewer Pap smears along with 420,273 diabetics unable to receive medications.

Medicaid spending is important to the U.S. health care system overall, paying $1 of every $6 of personal health spending (Paradise et al., 2015). The largest portion of Medicaid spending goes toward people with disabilities (42%) and older adults (21%). This group is only 24% of Medicaid enrollees. Nearly 10 million people are eligible for both Medicaid and Medicare, 14% of Medicaid enrollees. This small group uses 40% of all Medicaid spending. In addition to these high-cost groups, Medicaid finances

- 25% of all behavioral health care
- Nearly half of all births
- 50% of all long-term care expenses
- 35% of safety-net hospitals' income
- 40% of health center income

Medicaid is jointly funded between federal and state governments to assist the states in providing adequate medical care to eligible persons (Paradise et al., 2015). The federal government matches state Medicaid spending, and this is the largest source of federal funding for states. The federal government pays a portion of the costs, called the Federal Medical Assistance Percentage (FMAP). Historically, the FMAP is around 50%, but it is higher in poorer states; it can reach as high as 76%. The average FMAP, for all states, is 57%. The federal government will pay 100% of the expenses for care provided to people enrolled in Medicaid because of the ACA expansion through 2016, and 90% of these expenses after 2016. These rules, and other increased federal payments for specific groups, will raise the average FMAP to 64% (through 2016) and 62% (after 2016).

The funding model for Medicaid has benefits and problems. There isn't a limit on federal spending, so as states expand their Medicaid programs, more federal funding flows to states (Paradise et al., 2015). This allows Medicaid to expand during epidemics, natural or man-made disasters, or short economic downturns. At the same time, when the economy contracts, as in the recent recession, many more people become eligible for Medicaid at a time when state and federal funds are decreasing.

The states have some discretion in determining which population groups their Medicaid programs cover and the financial criteria for Medicaid eligibility, as well as the scope of services, rate of payment, and how the program will be administered, so long as they meet the minimum requirements set by the federal government (Paradise et al., 2015).

Medicaid mandatory services include the following (CMS, n.d.b):

- Outpatient and inpatient hospital services
- Early childhood screenings and well-child checkups (to age 21)
- Physician and nurse practitioner/certified nurse midwife services
- Lab and x-ray services
- Family planning services
- Tobacco cessation counseling for pregnant women
- Home health care and nursing home services for those over age 21 (including rehabilitation centers)
- Federally qualified health center and rural health clinic services
- Transportation to medical care

As with Medicare, Medicaid programs moved to a managed care concept, following mandates within the Balanced Budget Act of 1997, to attempt to restrain costs (Paradise et al., 2015). In 2015, more than half of Medicaid beneficiaries have managed care programs; in some states, a managed care plan is required. Medicaid beneficiaries are economically disadvantaged, frequently reside in medically underserved areas, and often have more complex health and social needs than other adults with higher incomes do. They often must choose between multiple plans, yet few providers, and may need to drive long distances to see specialists. Some managed care plans lack sufficient oversight, leading to fragmented services and poor health outcomes.

Medicaid is also a source of innovation in health care (Paradise et al., 2015). States implemented medical homes, care coordination, integration of physical and mental health care, and other "new" services earlier than private health plans. The flexibility built into the federal requirements for Medicaid, Medicaid rule waivers to test ideas, and the new Innovation Center in CMS (part of the ACA) allow states to develop new models of health care delivery.

Patient advocates (e.g., physicians, nurses, community leaders) often express concerns that many managed care plans (or state administrators) are more focused on keeping their costs down than on improving patient care. The system has wide variability in cost-effectiveness and quality (Paradise et al., 2015). Ensuring access and quality of care in a managed care environment will require fiscally solvent plans, established provider networks, education of providers and beneficiaries about managed care, and awareness of the unique needs of the Medicaid population. A key factor to Medicaid's future success is reimbursements to providers, both the amount of payments and administrative delays. Medicaid has historically reimbursed providers at a lower rate than Medicare and other insurance programs and may require significant effort to file for reimbursement. States may also take a long time to make the reimbursement payment. These issues create burdens for clinics and private physician offices, leading to a lack of provider participation—and a lack of access to care for enrollees.

Despite these issues, Medicaid provides societal benefits. Medicaid coverage is associated with reduced rates of infant mortality and low-birth-weight infants (Paradise et al., 2015). In addition, providing coverage to children early in life leads to higher educational achievement, higher income, and decreased use of public programs. Medicaid coverage led to an increase in health-related quality of life and happiness in an Oregon study (Baicker et al., 2013). Medicaid enrollees were also less likely to report financial strain due to health care costs and more likely to have a usual place of care. Although there are access and quality problems with Medicaid, one large study examining differences between an uninsured population and those with Medicaid found that similar patients with Medicaid were more likely to see a physician at least once annually; among low-income populations with high blood pressure, those with Medicaid had greater awareness and control of hypertension (Christopher et al., 2016). This did not extend, however, to those with high cholesterol or with diabetes.

Children's Health Insurance Plan

Enacted as part of the Balanced Budget Act in 1997, the Children's Health Insurance Plan (CHIP) provides health coverage to uninsured children under age 19 for families caught in the gap between Medicaid and affordable health insurance (CMS, n.d.b). In 2013, the program covered 8.1 million children, spending more than $13 billion (Pew Charitable Trusts, 2014). CHIP decreased the rate of uninsured children from 15% in 1997 to 9% in 2012. All 50 states participate, but eligibility guidelines and covered services vary (CMS, n.d.b). The ACA extended funding for the program through 2015, and, after contentious debate, Congress passed a bill to reauthorize spending through 2017 (Kardish, 2015). The federal portion of CHIP spending increased with the ACA as well, to a state average of 93% of costs (Pew Charitable Trusts, 2014). The program is authorized, including currently eligibility guidelines, through 2019. However, congress will have to reauthorize funding after 2017.

Other Government Programs

In addition to third-party reimbursement, the government offers some direct health services to selected populations, including Native Americans, military personnel, veterans, merchant marines, and federal employees. Government support, largely through grants administered through the CDC, provides immunizations and well-child care, as well as prenatal care and other programs at the state and local level.

Payment Concepts in Health Care

Reimbursement for health care services generally has been accomplished through one of two approaches: retrospective or prospective payment. Conceptually, these approaches are polar opposites. It is helpful to understand their differences and their meaning for the financing and delivery of health services, past and present.

Retrospective Payment

A traditional form of reimbursement for any kind of service, including health care, is **retrospective payment**, which is reimbursement for a service after it has been rendered (Rambur, 2015). A fee may be established in advance. However, payment of that fee occurs after the fact, or retrospectively. This is known as the **fee-for-service (FFS)** approach.

In health care, limited accountability in the use of retrospective payment has created several problems (Estes et al., 2013). With third-party payers (e.g., insurance companies, the government) serving as intermediaries, neither consumers nor providers of health services were accountable for containing costs. Many physicians were unaware of the cost of tests and therefore did not hesitate to order repeated testing (Agrawal, Taitsman, & Cassel, 2013). Patients and providers alike often insisted on expensive tests and treatments, believing these to be the best option for patient care (Estes et al., 2013). As more advanced technology and new medications became available, costs increased. Third-party reimbursement also increased, along with other factors, to create an inflationary spiral of escalating costs.

A further problem associated with the FFS concept was its tendency to encourage sickness care rather than wellness services. Physicians and other providers were rewarded financially for treating illness and for providing additional tests and services. There were few incentives for prevention or health promotion in an industry that reaped its revenues from keeping hospital beds full and caring for the sick and injured. Although retrospective payment worked well in other industries, from a cost-containment as well as a public health perspective, it was problematic in health care.

Prospective Payment

Prospective reimbursement, although not a new concept, was implemented for inpatient Medicare services in 1983, in response to the health care system's desperate need for cost containment (Rambur, 2015). It has since influenced the Medicaid program, as well as private health insurers. The prospective payment form of reimbursement has virtually eliminated the retrospective payment system (Estes et al., 2013; Nickitas et al., 2016). **Prospective payment** is a payment method based on rates derived from predictions of annual service costs that are set in advance of service delivery. Providers receive payment for services according to these fixed rates, set in advance. Payments may be in the form of premiums paid before receipt of service or in response to fixed-rate (not cost) charges. To correct unlimited reimbursement patterns and counteract disincentives to contain costs, prospective payment involves four classic steps (Dowling, 1979; Longest, 2016):

1. An external authority is empowered (by statute, market power, or voluntary compliance by providers) to set provider charges, third-party payment rates, or both.
2. Rates are set in advance of the prospective year during which they will apply and are considered fixed for the year (except for major, uncontrollable occurrences). The provider accepts the assignment of fees.
3. Patients, third-party payers, or both pay the prospective rates rather than the costs incurred by providers during the year (or charges adjusted to cover these costs).
4. Providers are at risk for losses or surpluses.

The concept of prepayment, or consumers paying in advance of health care, has existed for many years. As far back as 1933, prepaid medical groups were advocated to reduce costs and make services more accessible (Rambur, 2015). Examples of early plans were the Group Health Association of Washington, DC, the Health Insurance Plan of Greater New York City, and the Kaiser Plan (Knickman & Kovner, 2015; National Council on Disability, 2013). The success of these plans helped to influence the growth of the Health Maintenance Organization (HMO), a type of managed care discussed later in this chapter.

Prospective payment imposes constraints on spending and provides incentives for cutting costs. The federal government, as mentioned earlier, enacted a prospective payment plan (The Social Security Amendments Act of 1983; see Landmark Healthcare Legislation). The plan is a billing classification system known as **diagnosis-related groups (DRGs)**. The system is based on about 500 diagnosis and procedure groups. It provides fixed Medicare reimbursement to hospitals based on weighted formulas. Flat rates of payment are based on average national costs for a specific group, adjusted annually, with some regional variations accounting for higher wages and other costs (Longest, 2016; Rambur, 2015). This system was enacted to curb Medicare spending in hospitals and to extend the program's solvency period. The regulatory approach of DRGs changed Medicare hospital reimbursement from a cost-based retrospective payment system, in which a hospital was paid its costs, to a fixed-price prospective payment system. It was designed to create incentives for hospitals to be more efficient in delivering services.

Indeed, the prospective payment system reduced Medicare's rate of increase in inpatient hospital spending and increased hospital productivity (Clifton, 2009; Rambur, 2015). Thought to reduce hospital stays and unnecessary admissions, the system however led to DRG creep or "upcoding" (i.e., classifying patients into more lucrative categories) and patient dumping (i.e., transferring patients whose reimbursement is expected to be lower than actual costs of services) in an effort to counteract the losses in revenue to hospitals that spend more on Medicare patients than they are reimbursed (Angeles & Park, 2009, para. 3). It also led to fierce competition among providers and mounting concern about quality of care—in hospitals, ambulatory settings, and home care. Kinney (2013) notes that the three major concerns faced by Medicare (and the ACA) are "cost and volume inflation, quality assurance, and fraud and abuse" (p. 253). Whereas cost inflation was addressed by DRGs, quality was addressed in October 2008, when Medicare began withholding payments to hospitals for preventable errors in an effort to provide an incentive to prevent avoidable mistakes and improve patient care. The 10 preventable errors (often called "never events") included

1. Foreign objects retained after surgery
2. Air embolism
3. Incompatible blood transfusions
4. Stage III and IV pressure ulcers
5. Injuries sustained because of falls and trauma
6. Some types of poor glycemic control (e.g., diabetic ketoacidosis, hypoglycemic coma)
7. Catheter-associated urinary tract infections
8. Vascular catheter-associated infections
9. Surgical site infections
10. Deep vein thrombosis (DVT)/pulmonary emboli following a total knee or hip replacement (CMS, 2008, p. 2)

These changes were instituted at the request of Congress, and initially, many hospitals complained that their payments would be substantially reduced, especially for frail, complicated patients. However, even though Medicare did not pay for an initial pressure ulcer, for instance, the resulting medication-resistant staph infection or sepsis resulting from that bed sore was covered. In January 2009, CMS ceased all payments for cases involving wrong surgical procedures and surgery on the wrong patient or on the wrong body part. The days of paying physicians providing substandard care resulting in subsequent procedures, hospitalizations, and thus greater income have ended. The policy successfully reduced Medicare payments in fiscal years 2009 and 2010, saving $44 million (CMS, 2012). New quality reporting requirements were added, and policies for Hospital Value-Based Purchasing and hospital readmission rate reductions (CMS, 2012, 2013). The National Quality Forum (n.d.) has developed a lengthier list of serious reportable events (see Table 6–4).

"Never events" are medical errors or adverse events that should not happen and are largely preventable (Agency for Healthcare Research & Quality, 2014, para. 1). An expanded list of 24 never events for hospitals—serious incidents that could have been prevented—was approved for nonpayment by Medicaid beginning in July 2012 for all states (in 2011, about 21 states had already begun nonpayment). The ACA changes this system from evaluating payments on a case-by-case basis to evaluating payments based on the rate of "never events." The goal was to reduce serious medical errors and preventable infections that should reduce costs and improve patient care. Some physician groups objected to this, as they noted that some complications are "not entirely preventable"

Table 6–4   National Quality Forum List of Serious Reportable Events

Category	Events
1. Surgical or Invasive Events	Wrong surgery; surgery to wrong patient/site; retained foreign object; postop death
2. Product or Device Events	Serious injury or death from contaminated medications or devices (or devices used not as intended) or air embolism while in health care setting
3. Patient Protection Events	Inappropriate release/discharge (to unauthorized person if incapacitated); injury or death after patient disappearance; patient self-harm or suicide while in health care setting
4. Case Management Events	Serious injury or death because of unsafe administration of blood/products, "irretrievable loss of an irreplaceable biological specimen" (para. 19), medication error, not giving information or following up on x-rays, lab, or pathology results, during low-risk labor/delivery, or after a fall in health care setting. Also, stage III, IV, or not staged pressure ulcers after admission. Errors in artificial insemination (wrong egg/sperm)
5. Environmental Events	Serious injury or death to either patient or staff because of electric shock or burns during patient care; incidents with contaminated or wrong gas (or no gas available); serious injury or death with use of bedrails or restraints while in health care setting
6. Radiologic Events	Serious injury or death to either patient or staff related to metallic object in MRI areas
7. Potential Criminal Events	Care ordered/provided by someone impersonating a licensed health care professional; patient abduction; assault or sexual abuse of staff or patient in or on grounds of health care setting (and serious injury or death resulting from assault/abuse)

Source: National Quality Forum. (n.d.). *List of Serious Reportable Events (SREs)*. Retrieved from http://www.qualityforum.org/Topics/SREs/List_of_SREs.aspx

(Galewitz, 2011, para. 6). Patients have benefitted from increased attention to the quality of care (KFF, 2015b). The number of hospital-acquired conditions decreased from 2010 to 2013, and 30-day hospital readmission rates decreased for Medicare enrollees from 2007 to 2013 (USDHHS, 2014b). Plans to expand nonpayment to other settings have yet to be implemented. Rather, the ACA includes incentive payments to primary care providers who meet quality goals. Debate continues about nonpayment outside of hospital settings and about which conditions should be included in the list of never events (see What Do You Think?).

Private insurers also moved to nonpayment for medical errors and never events, although the list of conditions varies by company (Sorensen, Jarrett, Tant, Bernard, & McCall, 2014). In 2009, Milstein reported that preventable complications within 90 days after inpatient surgery costs an average of between $11,797 and $19,480 for private insurers whose enrollees develop metabolic problems, pressure ulcers, or infections. In 2015, the average hospital costs for patients with inpatient surgery complications was calculated to be 119% higher (or $19,626) than for those without complications, and the average third-party reimbursement was 105% higher (or $18,497) for those patients with surgical complications. For hospitals, the profit margin dropped from 5.8% to 0.1% for those patients with complications (Healy, Mullard, Campbell, & Dimick, 2016).

A more vigorous version of prospective payment is **capitation**. As noted before, capitation refers to a fixed fee per person that is paid to an MCO for a specified package of services. Fees remain in effect until renegotiated, regardless of the number of services provided. Because profit margins are very tight, utilization, quality, and costs are carefully monitored (Nickitas et al., 2016).

The prospective payment concept has proved useful from a public health perspective. Prepaid services create incentives for providers to keep their enrollees healthy, thus reducing provider costs. A potential, indirect benefit from fixed rates and reduced costs is that more of the health care dollar is available to spend on prevention programs.

Claims Payment Agents

Claims payment agents administer the process for government third-party payments. That is, the government contracts with private fiscal agents to handle the claims payment process and function as an intermediary between them and the health care provider. More than 80% of the government's third-party payments have been handled by these private contractors, who sometimes are known as fiscal intermediaries (when processing Medicare hospital claims), carriers (when dealing with insurance under Medicare), or fiscal agents (as applied to Medicaid programs). As an example, Blue Cross and Blue Shield, in addition to being a private insurance company, has also acted as a claims payment agent for Medicare since its inception (Blue Cross Blue Shield, 2016).

Direct Consumer Reimbursement or Out-of-Pocket Payment

Another source of health care financing comes from direct fees paid by consumers. This refers to individual out-of-pocket payments made for several different reasons, such as payments made by individuals who have no insurance coverage (fees must be paid directly for health and medical services) or payments for limited coverage, insurance caps, and exclusions (services for which the consumer must bear the entire expense). For example, some individuals carry only major medical insurance and must pay directly for physician office visits, prescriptions, eyeglasses, and dental care. In other instances, the insurance contract may include a deductible amount that must be paid by the insured before reimbursement begins (e.g., $500 for individuals or $1,500 for a family). The contract may be established on a coinsurance basis, which determines a percentage to be paid by the insurer and the rest by the individual (e.g., 80/20 plans mean that individuals pay 20% of costs after deductibles are met). Or the individual may pay the remainder of a health service bill after the insurer has paid a previously agreed-on fixed amount, such as a fixed fee (known as a coverage cap) for a particular service (labor and delivery, knee surgery, etc.). In 2015, 11% of people between 19 and 64 years of age with private health insurance had high out-of-pocket costs, such as 10% or more of income or 7% or more if low income (Collins, Gunja, Doty, & Beutel, 2015).

Another important factor for those paying directly for their health care expenses is **cost shifting**. This practice of charging different prices to different consumers most often affects those without health insurance who are paying out-of-pocket for care (Coughlin, Holahan, Caswell, & McGrath, 2014). As health insurance plans or large companies contract with hospitals and physicians for services, they purchase these services at a reduced cost. Those without this "buying power" pay full price. For example, a $500 radiology procedure may be discounted to $225 for an insurance plan, but an individual paying out-of-pocket will pay the full price. This also can occur with government-sponsored plans. When

---

What do *you* think?

What if you were to hire a glass company to replace a broken windshield in your car, and while completing the repair, they accidentally broke off your rear view mirror. Would you expect them to pay for that mistake? Or would you just absorb the cost yourself? In the past, we the taxpayers have been paying Medicare payments to hospitals and physicians who have made serious errors that have led to adverse events, spiraling costs, and resulted in poor patient outcomes. Congress and others feel that this is unfair and have enacted legislation to stop paying for these types of errors or preventable events. Do you think this is fair? Can these conditions always be prevented? Are there extenuating circumstances that should be taken into account? Are there benefits to patients and taxpayers from holding health care providers accountable for errors and poor care?

Medicare payment changes to hospitals were instituted with the Balanced Budget Act of 1997, cost shifting to private patients in order to cover their losses became more difficult for those hospitals with large Medicare patient loads and more financial distress. Smaller hospitals with higher market power and a lower proportion of Medicare patients were found to be able to shift up to 37% of their cuts to private patients in a 2010 study by Wu. Other studies have found that cost shifting is uncommon (Frakt, 2011) and that lower Medicare payments actually resulted in lower costs for other payers (White, 2013). A review of research on hospital cost shifting concluded that evidence for cost shifting shows that if it does occur, it generally is not substantial (Robert Wood Johnson Foundation, 2011).

Private and Philanthropic Support

Private or philanthropic support, a third funding source, contributes both directly and indirectly to health care financing. Many private agencies fund programs, underwrite research, and provide benefits for people who otherwise would go without services. Charitable donations to nonprofit health care institutions, after a drop of 11% in 2009 compared to 2008, increased 7% in 2011 compared to 2010 (PRNewswire, 2013; Shinkman, 2010). Contributions were stable in 2012, with more than $8.9 billion raised. On average, 8% to 10% of hospital budgets come from charitable giving (Jones, 2012). Nearly one third of donations were major gifts from individuals or groups and 24.1% of donations came from businesses or foundations (PRNewswire, 2013). In addition, volunteerism, the efforts of numerous individuals and organizations that donate their time and services (e.g., hospital guild members), provides tremendous cost savings to health care institutions. It also enables many individuals to receive services, such as home-delivered meals or transportation to health care facilities, at no charge.

Philanthropic financing of health care has significantly decreased in the last two decades. Free medical clinics, beginning in the 1960s, have provided services to those without other sources of health care. They have helped many people but have also helped health care professionals by providing another place for research as well as a venue for teaching students outside the acute care setting. These clinics often rely on volunteer clinicians in addition to students. In 2010, free clinics in the United States served more than 1.8 million individuals (Swan & Foley, 2016).

Clinicians have historically provided uncompensated (charity) care to individuals outside of free clinics as well. The amount of charity care is decreasing, however. Much of this trend is explained by the increase in individuals covered by Medicaid (Sabik & Gandhi, 2013). Expanded insurance coverage due to the ACA has changed the amount of charity care provided by hospitals, too. Hospitals in the United States provide about $50 billion in charity care each year (DeLeire, Joynt, & McDonald, 2014). In 2014, because of increased insurance coverage under the ACA, hospitals saved an estimated $5.7 billion in charity care costs; nearly 75% of these savings are in states that expanded Medicaid.

TRENDS AND ISSUES INFLUENCING HEALTH CARE ECONOMICS

The High Cost of Health in the United States

The United States per person costs for health care in 2013 was over $9,255 (KFF, 2014), paid through a combination of public tax money, individual and corporate contributions to insurance plans, and other sources. In 2012, our costs were 42% higher than the second highest country, Norway. Not only do we pay almost twice the per capita expenditure of Canada and Germany and almost three times that of Japan and Italy, but also we have had one of the largest increases in health care spending since 1980. As noted earlier, health spending in 2013 was estimated at 17.4% of the U.S. GDP, whereas the United Kingdom spent only 8.8% of their GDP (KFF, 2014). U.S. tax-funded health care expenditures encompassed 64.3% of 2013 total health spending, and it is projected to rise to roughly two thirds by 2024. Private employer spending constituted 18.5% of health spending in 2001 but is projected to drop to 14.5% by 2024. Increased government share of spending on health care is largely due to the aging population and ACA spending on subsidies and Medicaid expansion (Himmelstein & Woolhandler, 2016b).

In 2010, the World Health Organization's *World Health Report* focused on health financing. The report notes that the composition of services needed to achieve good health for all people varies in different countries or regions. However, a strong health system requires accountability and oversight. The report estimates that between 20% and 40% of health care spending is the result of inefficiency and waste. The goal of universal coverage for health needs could be partially met by improving efficiency and using resources more effectively. It notes that, around the world, the high cost of medical care and lack of sufficient coverage causes "150 million people (to) suffer financial catastrophe annually while 100 million are pushed below the poverty line" (p. 8).

In a global comparison of health care costs totaling over $6.5 trillion, the WHO (2012) found that the United States had the highest total per person annual expenditure ($8,362), compared to global per person annual spending of only $948. An earlier WHO (2000) study found that the U.S. health care system was the "most expensive … in the world" largely because of high administrative costs (estimated then to range between 19.3% and 24.1%), the system of complex multiple payers, and the rising costs of prescription medications and advanced medical technology (p. 2). They also noted the shift from nonprofit to for-profit hospitals and the aging population as causative factors, along with the high proportion of people without insurance and the high cost of their untreated illnesses. WHO (2011) has outlined key components of well functioning health care systems, indicating some of the areas that are problematic for the U.S. system. A comparison study of hospital administrative costs among eight developed nations revealed that these costs made up over 25% of the U.S. total hospital expenditures. These costs in England were 15.5%, and in Canada and Scotland about 12%. The researchers projected cost saving of over $150 billion in 2011 if our levels had been as low as Canada's (Himmelstein, Jun, et al., 2014). Another study examined the billing and insurance-related administrative costs of our fragmented system and noted that by moving to a more simplified system of financing health care, the United States could save over $350 billion a year, or almost 15% of total health care spending (Jiwani, Himmelstein, Woolhandler, & Kahn, 2014). The average physician is reported to spend almost 17% of their workweek in administrative duties, and this is rising with the increased use of electronic health records (EHRs) (Woolhandler & Himmelstein, 2014).

Why does health care cost so much? Explanations include the following:

- Medical malpractice costs and physicians' perceived need to practice *defensive medicine* by ordering excessive tests and x-rays. A landmark study found that this increased health care spending by 2.4% in 2008 (Mello, Chandra, Gawande, & Studdert, 2010). Defensive medicine is not evidence based and may even harm healthy patients (Hoffman & Kanzaria, 2014).
- An aging population and the greater prevalence of chronic disease (Knickman & Kovner, 2015; Shi & Singh, 2014).
- Advances in and the spread of medical technology; patient demand for cutting-edge technology and physician responsiveness both contribute to this problem (Chandra & Skinner, 2011; Hayden, 2014; Hoffman & Kanzaria, 2014). In 2009, Callahan reported economists' projections about the use of newer technologies leading to 40% to 50% of annual health care cost increases.
- Rapidly rising prescription drug costs (Cox, Kamal, Jankiewicz, Rousseau, 2016).
- High costs of insurance administration: The amount of private health insurance companies in the United States leads to higher costs compared to countries with a government-run insurance system (Mathauer & Nicolle, 2011).
- Ineffective, inappropriate, and inadequate health care leading to increased morbidity and mortality and costs; a "highly fragmented" health care system, large number of uninsured population, and restricted primary care and public health resources (IOM, 2001, 2013, p. 4).
- Those who have lived most of their lives without insurance have higher costs when they enroll in Medicare (Joynt et al., 2013). This would likely decrease if new beneficiaries were covered by insurance throughout their lives, and costs of uncompensated care would also decrease with universal coverage.

Many U.S. citizens believe that their health care system provides the most advanced medical care, which makes up for other deficits in the U.S. health care system. In fact, as noted above, use of the most advanced medical technology and medications is one cause of high health care costs in the United States. What does the U.S. health care system deliver for the price paid? The Commonwealth Fund (2015) studied the health systems in seven countries: Australia, Canada, Germany, the Netherlands, New Zealand, the United Kingdom, and the United States.

The U.S. health system ranked last or near last on access, efficiency, and equity. The WHO (2000) noted at the start of the 21st century that the United States was found to be "the only country in the developed world, except for South Africa, that does not provide healthcare for all of its citizens" (p. 3). In the United States, the patchwork quilt of private and public insurance—mostly tied to either employment or low-income status—makes it difficult for many people to get the care they need. The researchers noted that those without health insurance are "sicker and die younger than people with health insurance" (p. 4). Although the ACA has expanded health insurance coverage to many, there are still uninsured individuals in the United States. In 2012, 47 million Americans under age 65 were uninsured, but that number is expected to drop to 31 million by 2020 as a result of the ACA (Rice et al., 2014).

The news is not all bad; the United States ranked fifth overall in timeliness of care compared to other OECD countries in 2013 (Davis, Stremikis, Squires, & Schoen, 2014). People in the United States report low wait times for elective surgery despite having fewer acute care hospital beds compared to other countries (Mossialos, Wenzl, Osborn, & Sarnak, 2016). This might be because in the United States focus is on decreasing hospital stays, so space is available to bring in more new patients. In addition, the United States performs more ambulatory surgical procedures than other countries do (Mossialos et al., 2016). However, less than half (48%) of U.S. citizens can get a physician appointment on the same day; only Canada is lower at 41%. In Germany and New Zealand, more than 70% of people can be seen the same day they call for an appointment. Another good outcome is that the United States ranked first in 2000 among all WHO countries on *responsiveness*—a construct relating to how respectfully clients are treated. However, as noted in Chapters 5 and 25, for many racial and ethnic minorities, this is not the case.

The United States leads other countries in cancer screening and survival (Ho & Preston, 2010; NRC & IOM, 2013) and heart disease management, or control of cholesterol and blood pressure. Lower rates of mortality due to stroke and lower smoking rates, as well as higher household average income, also characterize positive comparisons; also, recent immigrants have better health than those of us who are native born (NRC & IOM, 2013). At the same time, the U.S. health care system scores very low in other areas, including medical errors (Ho & Preston, 2010). U.S. citizens do not have longer, healthier lives overall when compared to other high-income countries (NRC & IOM, 2013). The United States ranked 34th for overall life expectancy in 2011 and 31st in healthy life expectancy (the average number of healthy years expected in a population) in 2007 when compared to other WHO nations (Bezruchka, 2012).

In recent years, debate about the ACA has focused public attention on many issues with the U.S. health care system. In a study of OECD countries, only 25% of people in the United States reported that they felt the U.S. health care system worked well, compared with 40% in France (the next lowest) and 63% in the United Kingdom (Mossialos et al., 2016). Conversely, 27% of people in the United States reported that the U.S. system needed to be thrown out and rebuilt, compared with 12% in Norway, the second highest country.

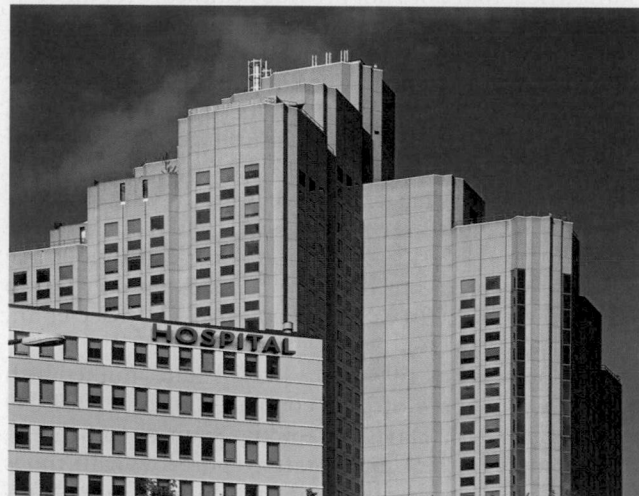

U.S. hospitals are increasingly using electronic health records (EHRs).

The U.S. health care system is changing. Promising improvements include an increase in the percentage of physicians (83%) and hospitals (76%) using EHRs according to Mossialos et al. (2016). Using an incentive program, the federal government will continue to push health care providers to increase the use and functions of EHRs. The use of EHRs permits examination of not just cost, but also operational and clinical performance, and a greater "emphasis on population-based patient care management" (Bodycombe, 2013, para. 2). **Predictive modeling**, using statistics from EHRs, can be used to determine high-risk patients and move them into interventions to more efficiently address their health care needs. It is also used to help address readmissions and control complications and costs. It will also be helpful in monitoring pain medication misuse and developing more complex health risk assessment data (Bodycombe, 2013). We encounter the use of some type of predictive modeling on an everyday basis. Google, Facebook, and others use analyses such as this to determine which ads or articles you may see when you login to Web sites. The use of statistics is improving health care in many ways.

To measure and monitor health care quality, the Commonwealth Fund developed a scoring method that compares actual performance to achievable performance (McCarthy, How, Fryer, Radley, & Schoen, 2011). Comparing data from the 2011 scorecard to those reported in 2008, control of hypertension improved from 31% to 50% (although the benchmark rate is 75%). Cigarette smoking decreased from 21% to 17%, and pressure sores among short-stay nursing home residents dropped from 19% to 14%. Access to care and health insurance and the rising costs of care and insurance are growing concerns. The infant mortality rate in the United States is over 35% higher than the best state-level

rates. These best state rates are two times higher than rates in many other industrialized nations. Childhood obesity and care for minorities and low-income populations are also troubling. Although the United States has made some progress, the goal of safe, effective, and high-quality health care remains unreached.

In order to reach benchmark performance levels of leading nations, states, or regions, the U.S. health care system would have to improve performance by 40% or more (McCarthy et al., 2011). If this were done, the following outcomes are possible:

- 91,000 fewer annual premature deaths from causes "amenable to health care"—this is twice the number of people dying in motor vehicle accidents (p. 15)
- 38 million more adults with access to a primary care provider
- 66 million more adults getting all recommended preventive care
- Savings of $1.6 to $3.1 billion in annual medical costs by improving control of hypertension and diabetes (reducing disease complications)
- Medicare savings of $12 billion annually by reducing hospital readmissions
- Savings of $55 billion by reducing health insurance administrative costs to the average of other countries with private–public insurance systems

Mossialos et al. (2016) reported health care comparisons across OECD countries and found that the United States ranked last on *amenable mortality levels* (deaths prior to age 75 that may be prevented through effective, timely health care). Other U.S. indicators included

- Among the lowest nations in the percentage of adults who smoke daily
- The highest percentage of adults who are obese
- A breast cancer 5-year survival rate among the three highest nations
- Childhood (measles) vaccination rates below average, but above-average flu vaccination rates for adults age 65 or older.
- The highest percentage of adults who were unable to access health care because of costs

Controlling Costs

The ACA has introduced many strategies to control the rise of health care costs, including increased funding for primary prevention strategies. A focus on primary prevention demands a paradigm shift in thinking about the practice and delivery of health care (see Chapter 1). It is one that fits more closely with the mission of public health. It expects that citizens are involved in their health care, are knowledgeable about their health status, can manage self-care practices, and can modify lifestyle behaviors to promote wellness. This creates a rich environment for community health nurses to collaborate with primary care practitioners and other health care professionals to control health care costs while providing quality care focusing on primary prevention. Our focus on illness and not health promotion or prevention has proven costly. Prevention should be at the forefront of a new era in health care. Trust for America's Health

(TFAH) (2016) has developed 10 Top Priorities for a National Prevention Strategy:

1. Promoting Disease Prevention
2. Combating the Obesity Epidemic
3. Preventing Tobacco Use/Exposure
4. Preventing/Controlling Infectious Diseases
5. Preparing for Potential Health Emergencies/Bioterrorism Attacks
6. Recognizing the Relationship Between Health and U.S. Economic Competitiveness
7. Safeguarding the Nation's Food Supply
8. Planning for Changing Health Care Needs of Seniors
9. Improving the Health of Low-Income/Minority Communities
10. Reducing Environmental Threats (para. 4)

Access to Health Services: The Uninsured and Underinsured

Many services, preventive or illness focused, are not available to a large portion of our population. The U.S. Census Bureau (2010) reported that 50.7 million people (16.7% of the population) were **uninsured** in 2009. This was the first year to show an actual drop in the number of people with health insurance since tracking of these data first occurred in 1987. By 2014, the number of people who were uninsured decreased to 33 million or 10.4% of the population (U.S. Census Bureau, 2015).

The rate of those lacking health insurance varies by age group (U.S. Census Bureau, 2015). Of those age 65 or older, 1.4% report being uninsured, compared to 6.2% of children under the age of 19 and 14.3% of adults age 19 to 64. The uninsured rate is higher for children in poverty (8.6%) compared to children not in poverty (5.6%) and higher for Hispanics (19.9%), African Americans (11.8%), and Asians (9.3%) compared to non-Hispanic Whites (7.6%). Even after the Medicaid expansion under the ACA, variation in insurance coverage continues from state to state. Massachusetts has had the lowest uninsured rate for several years, which decreased slightly in 2014 to 3.3%. Texas has the highest uninsured rate (19.1%). Kentucky's rate decreased the most between 2013 and 2014, from 14.3% to 8.5%.

As described earlier, a significant portion of the population with insurance coverage is still considered underinsured. Difficulty paying the out-of-pocket costs creates the same lack of health care services experienced by the uninsured. For example, 46% of underinsured and 63% of uninsured reported that they did not see a doctor when they were ill, did not fill a prescription, or went without a recommended medical treatment or test (Schoen et al., 2011). This compared with only 28% of those who had adequate health care coverage. The ACA has helped increase the number of people who are insured; approximately 9 million fewer Americans were uninsured in 2014 than in 2013 (KFF, 2015b). But it has not completely resolved the problem of an underinsured population. In 2014, the Commonwealth Fund's Biennial Health Insurance Survey found that 23% of nonelderly adults with yearlong health insurance were underinsured, and this number was not significantly different compared to the survey's findings in 2010 and 2012

(Collins, Rasmussen, Beutel, et al., 2015). In addition, many underinsured have no dental or vision coverage, and few prescription drug benefits, yet still experience higher deductibles compared to insurance plans with these services.

Even those with Medicaid and Medicare can be underinsured. In 2013, more than 25% of Medicaid recipients and 65% of Medicare enrollees were underinsured (Magge, Cabral, Kazis, & Sommers, 2013). Although Medicaid recipients were less likely to be underinsured than were adults with private insurance, the Medicaid expansion in 2014 would not necessarily provide access to new enrollees with low income. A particularly vulnerable group is adults age 50 to 64 (Smolka, Multack, & Figueiredo, 2012). Although 85% of people in this age group were insured in 2012, 75% of those insured rely on employer-sponsored plans. Workers with low and midlevel incomes often experience gaps in insurance coverage due to unstable job situations. Many employers do not offer health insurance to their employees, and a large number of the uninsured are employees of these companies (or their dependents). Finally, self-employed individuals may find it difficult to pay the high costs of insurance premiums without the benefit of group rates. Consequently, many of the self-employed can access health services only by purchasing expensive individual insurance policies with high deductibles and coinsurance or by making expensive out-of-pocket payments. Self-employed individuals are able to access insurance through ACA, but 48% of uninsured adults in 2014 stated that they did not have health insurance because of high costs (KFF, 2015a). There are subsidies available to offset insurance costs for those individuals below 400% of the poverty line (Collins, Gunja, Rasmussen, Beutel, & Doty, 2015).

Another issue related to access is where people receive care. Historically, they first saw their family physician when a new health concern arose. Prior to the ACA, a study found that 42% of visits for new health problems were made to a regular primary care physician whereas an average of 37% were made to the ED. Using the ED for a new, nonurgent health problem occurs for several reasons, including convenience, negative perceptions of non-ED sources of care, and the legal requirement that the ED provide care for everyone without regard for ability to pay (Uscher-Pines, Pines, Kellermann, Gillen, & Mehrotra, 2013). A study in Massachusetts indicated increased ED use after that state's health care reform implementation, occurring years before the ACA (Hosseini & Weinberg, 2014). In addition to increased cost, visits to the ED are a missed opportunity to establish a relationship with a primary care provider (Uscher-Pines et al., 2013). People who lack insurance or who are underinsured may experience more duplicate testing and poor chronic disease management, due to the lack of a **medical home** (seeing the same health care provider for regular care). While Medicaid patients often use the ED, the numbers of people with private insurance using EDs is increasing rapidly. From 1995 to 2008, 60% of the increased ED use was due to privately insured individuals; only 9% was due to the uninsured (Cunningham, 2011).

Medical Bankruptcies

A wide variety of medical issues can lead to financial insecurity and bankruptcy. If you don't have health insurance and you undergo emergency surgery for appendicitis, it may take a great effort to pay off your medical debt (or you may turn to high-interest credit cards). Even if you have health insurance, long-term cancer treatments will likely mean large out-of-pocket costs—and your inability to work may lead to further financial problems. Many people with significant financial stressors, such as medical debt, may not file for bankruptcy, because of either lack of financial resources for legal fees or other reasons. Middle-income groups are more likely to file bankruptcy, whereas lower-income groups are more often found to suffer from late payments that affect their credit scores and their subsequent ability to purchase a home or apply for credit (McCloud & Dwyer, 2011). Bankruptcy filings rose significantly from 1980 to 2004—as much as 360% (Himmelstein, Warren, Thorne, & Woolhandler, 2005; Cammarosano, 2015). Filings decreased drastically in 2007 and then began to rise again through 2011 (Cammarosano, 2015). In 2015, personal bankruptcy filings were nearly as low as they were in 2008. Medical debt is thought to be a major contributor to personal bankruptcy filings. In a classic study, Himmelstein, Thorne, Warren, and Woolhandler (2009) reported that 62% of bankruptcy filings were associated with medical expenses in a five-state study. This number has been widely cited—in academic journals, in the media, and in political speeches. A later study found that medical bankruptcies in Massachusetts increased by over 33% and in 2009, and 89% of the bankruptcy debtors and their families reported having health insurance whereas about 25% had recently had insurance coverage lapses. The bankruptcy rate increase in the state was lower than the national statistics (Himmelstein, Thorne, & Woolhandler, 2011). However, a national study using more recent data (2005–2013) found that medical bankruptcies accounted for about 18% to 25% of all bankruptcies (Austin, 2014). Although this estimate is much lower than 62%, Austin (2014) did find that medical debt was the single largest cause of personal bankruptcy. In a survey of Canadian bankruptcy filers, over 40% reported loss of income due to personal injury or illness-related work absences, and over 8% reported the income loss due to caregiving duties. Less than 7% had medical bills that totaled over $5,000 in the past two years. With Canada's socialized health system, researchers concluded that some bankruptcies occur because of work-related income losses rather than medical costs (Himmelstein, Woolhandler, Sarra, & Guyatt, 2014c).

Medical debt that doesn't lead to bankruptcy is still problematic. Cutshaw, Woolhandler, Himmelstein, and Robertson (2016) studied medical causes and consequences of home foreclosures in Arizona and found that about 10% of those affected were uninsured, but 28% reported a coverage gap within the previous 2 years. Medical debt or other medical causes were cited by 57%, and 54% stated that they incurred new debt in an effort to pay medical bills (10% had mortgaged homes). About 57% reported having a chronic condition, and over 50% had either delayed or missed medical visits. Five months after the first data collection, 33% reported that they could not afford food, and 63% had new medical debts. A few respondents were homeless. Kalousova and Burgard (2013) found that people with medical debt were more likely to delay or miss needed medical care than people with other types of debt. Although medically related bankruptcies have dropped slightly, approximately 60% of bankruptcy filings are still due to medical debt, and the high-deductible insurance plans can strain family budgets. It is estimated that 10 million U.S. adults, having full health insurance coverage year-round, will struggle to pay off medical debts that they incur in 2013 (Mangan, 2013). This is further evidence that the underinsured, along with those individuals without health insurance, are in danger of financial disaster when confronted with a serious medical emergency or long-term illness.

Managed Care

The term managed care became popular in the late 1980s. It refers to systems that contract to coordinate medical care for specific groups in order to promote provider efficiency and control costs. Although the term *managed care* is relatively new, the concept has been practiced for many years through various models of alternative health care delivery. Managed care is a cost-control strategy used in both public and private sectors of health care. Care is *managed* by regulating the use of services and levels of provider payment. This approach includes using HMOs and PPOs. HMOs represent 14% of employer-sponsored group insurance and PPOs enroll about 52% of workers (KFF, 2015c).

In contrast to FFS models, managed care plans operate on a prospective payment basis and control costs by managing utilization and provider payments. The managed care model encourages the provision of services within fixed budgets, thus avoiding cost escalation. Because costs are tight, preventive services are generally encouraged, so that more expensive tertiary care costs can be avoided if possible.

Health Maintenance Organizations

Health maintenance organizations (HMOs) are systems in which participants prepay a fixed monthly premium to receive comprehensive health services delivered by a defined network of providers. A traditional HMO offers both health insurance and health care services (Corlette, Volk, Berenson, & Feder, 2014). HMOs typically cover a large group of individuals, generating a large amount of premium revenues, and strictly control use of services. Consumers and providers have often resisted the strenuous cost-containment policies of many HMOs, because of the limits placed on health care decisions. However, employers are often drawn to HMO alternatives to traditional FFS plans as a potential cost-saving method. But 2015 costs for employee health coverage are similar for HMO, PPO, and point-of-service (POS) plans (KFF, 2015c). Also, industry projections for HMO premium rates and cost increases vary little from other types of plans, ranging from 5.8% to 6.2%; for PPOs, the range is from 5.4% to 7.8%; and for consumer-driven/high-deductible health plans, it is about 7.9% (Managed Care Online [MCOL], 2015).

HMOs are the oldest model of managed care. Several HMOs have existed for decades (e.g., Kaiser

Permanente), but many have developed more recently. HMO enrollees were told that they could benefit from lower-cost premiums, reduced cost sharing, and fewer administrative costs. From 1930 to 1965, the HMO movement, supported initially by the private sector, gradually gained federal backing. Group plans were included as a part of Medicare and Medicaid legislation. The skyrocketing employer health insurance costs of the 1980s and 1990s encouraged many companies to move from traditional insurance and FFS to HMOs. The number of HMO enrollees peaked in 1999 to 2000 but encompassed nearly 75 million in 2014 (MCOL, 2015). Currently, there are numerous HMOs with a variety of configurations. The unique set of properties of HMOs includes the following:

- A contract between the HMO and the beneficiaries (or their representative), the enrolled population.
- Absorption of prospective risk by the HMO.
- A regular (usually monthly) premium to cover specified (typically comprehensive) benefits paid by each enrollee of the HMO. Few additional charges are levied, because the payment mechanism is not FFS.
- An integrated delivery system with provider incentives for efficiency. The HMO contracts with professional providers to deliver the services due the enrollees, and the basis for reimbursing those providers varies among HMOs (Estes et al., 2013).

Official encouragement, government subsidies, and the pressures for cost control spurred the growth of HMOs. Some HMOs follow the traditional model, employing health professionals (e.g., physicians, nurses), building their own hospital and clinic facilities, and serving only their own enrollees. Other HMOs provide some services while contracting for the rest. HMOs have penetrated Medicare (29%) and Medicaid (67%) markets, as well as nearly all commercial insurance markets (MCOL, 2015). They have historically been viewed as a positive alternative delivery system because of their potential for conserving costs, which results from their emphasis on prevention, health promotion, and ambulatory care, and with a corresponding reduction in hospital and medical care utilization. However, there are questions as to whether the cost savings result partly from favorable selection of enrollees. Quality concerns also have been raised about the dangers of underserving enrollees in order to stay within payment limits (Sultz & Young, 2014). Scanlon, Swaminathan, Chernew, and Lee (2006) examined longitudinal data and found that HMO competition was related to consumer satisfaction surveys, but not necessarily to better quality of care for chronic conditions. Later research verified that increased HMO competition did not lead to improved HMO quality (Scanlon, Swaminathan, Lee, & Chernew, 2008). A study examining Medicare Advantage plans, which have a managed care model, with traditional FFS Medicare noted increased cost and little evidence for improved management of outpatient chronic conditions (Nicholas, 2009). Archer (2011) observes that the costs of private plans have increased more rapidly than Medicare, often driven by little true competition; lower administrative costs for Medicare also contribute to the cost differences.

A large-scale, longitudinal study of 11 quality indicators found that Medicaid-managed care enrollees received lower-quality care than managed care commercial plan enrollees (Landon et al., 2007). The Medicare Rights Center (2010) reported that almost half of Medicare private plan disenrollment is due to problems with provider access and marketing abuse or misinformation. Problems related to coverage for medical services and transfer problems affected almost 40% of patients. As mentioned earlier, Medicare overpayments to private plans have been estimated to be in excess of $282.6 billion since 1985 (Hellander et al., 2013). A Cochrane review (Scott et al., 2011) found inconclusive evidence for the impact of financial incentives to primary care physicians on the quality of health care provided.

These concerns about HMOs and managed care in general have not gone unanswered. The Health Insurance Portability and Accountability Act (HIPAA) and the Newborns' and Mothers' Health Protection Act are both significant pieces of legislation from 1996 addressing health care concerns among the nation's citizens. HIPAA, in addition to protecting the privacy of health information, strengthened rules protecting continued health care coverage when people changed jobs. Protection for newborns and mothers became necessary when many insurance companies covered a hospital stay for labor and delivery for 24 hours—for some, this meant 24 hours from admission, and infants and mother left the hospital in potentially unstable postdelivery conditions. Newborns would go home when younger than one day of age, in some cases so soon after birth that body temperature was not stabilized and the ability to suck and take breast milk or formula was not established. The Newborns' and Mothers' Health Protection Act eliminated these "drive-through deliveries," ensuring that mothers and newborns would have the right to remain in the acute care setting for at least 48 hours, covered by their insurance plan (see Landmark Healthcare Legislation). In response to concerns from managed care clients, the government developed a patient bill of rights stipulating the patient's right to timely emergency services, respect and nondiscrimination, as well as participation in treatment decisions and a more consumer-friendly appeals process.

Preferred Provider Organizations

A **preferred provider organization (PPO)** is another model of managed or coordinated care that developed earlier than the HMO (Knickman & Kovner, 2015). A PPO is a network of physicians, hospitals, and other health-related services that contract with a third-party payer organization to provide comprehensive health services to subscribers on a fixed FFS basis. Because of contractual fixed costs, employing organizations that subscribe can offer medical services to their employees at discounted rates. In PPOs, consumer choice exists. Enrollees have a choice among providers within the plan and contracted providers out of the plan. The PPOs practice utilization review and often use formal standards for selecting providers.

PPOs did not exist in their present form until after 1980. Enrollment in PPOs grew from about 10 plans in 1981 to more than 700 plans in the 1990s (Dranove, 2008). The number of people enrolled in PPOs also increased, from an estimated 10.4% of individuals with private insurance in 1988 to 40% by the late 1990s, with the numbers leveling off as the decade came to a close. As consumers became more frustrated with limits imposed by HMOs, they began to move toward PPOs that provide more choices. In 2014, 152.8 million people were enrolled in a PPO, more than twice the number in HMOs (MCOL, 2015). In 2015, PPOs were the most common form of health insurance offered by employers—with 72% of workers able to choose this type of policy (KFF, 2015c). Early use of PPOs appeared to promote cost savings, but the long-range cost-effectiveness of this model has yet to be fully proven. PPOs have been criticized in the past for their lack of vigorous case management—more often found in HMOs—and some larger plans have moved toward this model, especially in the case of chronic diseases, such as hypertension and diabetes, or with palliative care (Kogut, Johnson, Higgins, & Quilliam, 2012). The ACA encourages comprehensive case management of chronic disease as one way to decrease hospitalizations and the cost of care. New methods of determining cost-effectiveness are being utilized to determine the realistic impact of population interventions (Arbel & Greenberg, 2016).

Point-of-Service Plans

A variation on the just-mentioned plans is the **point-of-service (POS) plan**, which permits more freedom of choice than a standard HMO or PPO. Enrollees choose a primary physician from within the plan (POS) who monitors

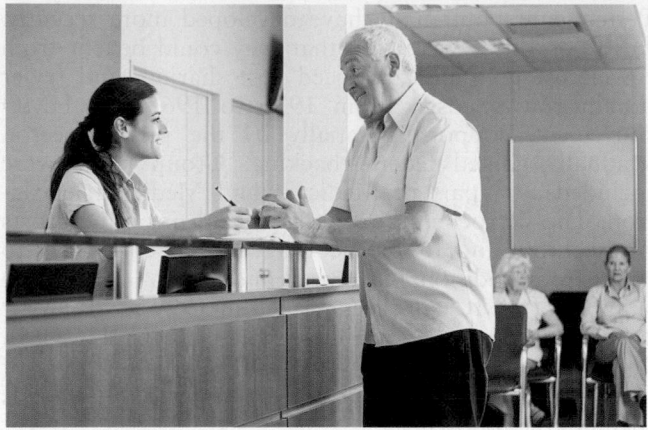

Primary health care providers are chosen by patients of POS, PPO, and HMO plans.

their care and makes outside referrals when necessary. At an extra cost, enrollees can go outside the HMO or PPO network of contracted providers unless their primary physician has made a specific referral (Small Business Majority, 2012). It is a hybrid or combination of an HMO and PPO. In 2015, about 10% of employees were enrolled in POS plans (KFF, 2015c). See Figure 6–7 for a look at the trend in types of health plan coverage among those employees who are covered by their employers.

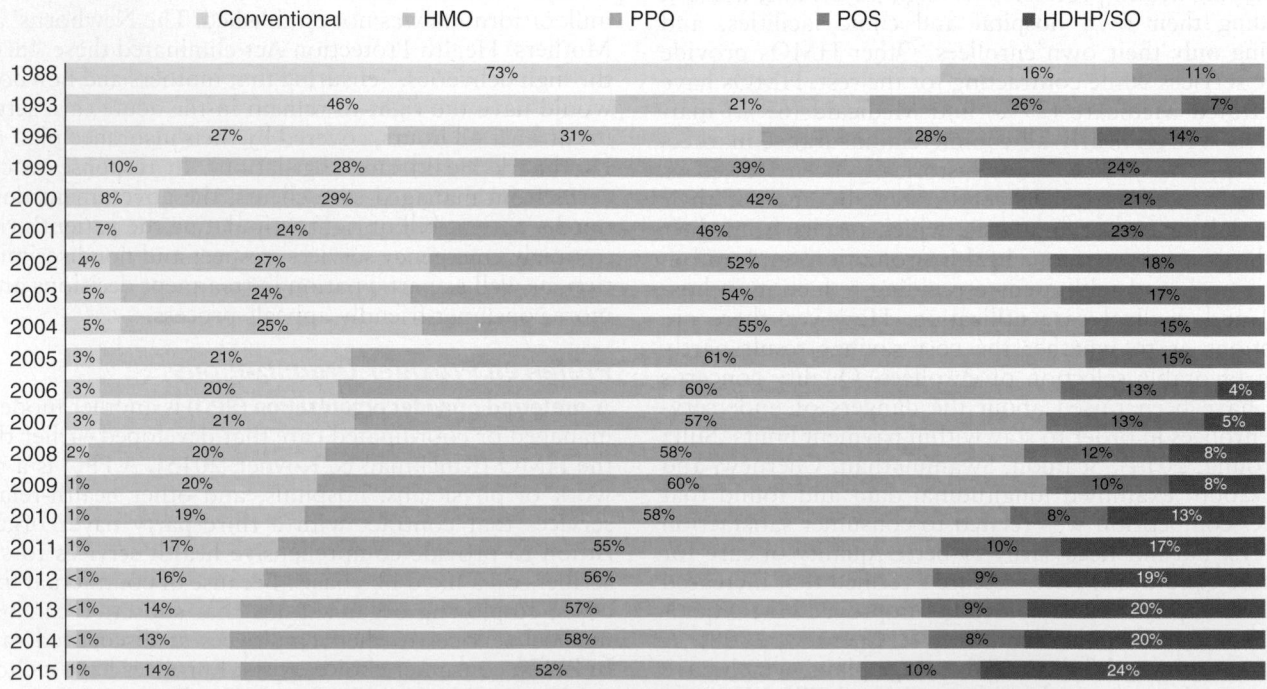

Year	Conventional	HMO	PPO	POS	HDHP/SO
1988	73%			16%	11%
1993	46%		21%	26%	7%
1996	27%		31%	28%	14%
1999	10%	28%	39%	24%	
2000	8%	29%	42%	21%	
2001	7%	24%	46%	23%	
2002	4%	27%	52%	18%	
2003	5%	24%	54%	17%	
2004	5%	25%	55%	15%	
2005	3%	21%	61%	15%	
2006	3%	20%	60%	13%	4%
2007	3%	21%	57%	13%	5%
2008	2%	20%	58%	12%	8%
2009	1%	20%	60%	10%	8%
2010	1%	19%	58%	8%	13%
2011	1%	17%	55%	10%	17%
2012	<1%	16%	56%	9%	19%
2013	<1%	14%	57%	9%	20%
2014	<1%	13%	58%	8%	20%
2015	1%	14%	52%	10%	24%

FIGURE 6–7 Distribution of health plan enrollment among covered workers, by type of plan, 1988–2015. (From Kaiser Family Foundation & Health Research & Educational Trust. (2015). *Employer health benefits survey 2015*. Retrieved from http://files.kff.org/attachment/report-2015-employer-health-benefits-survey. This information was reprinted with permission from the Henry J. Kaiser Family Foundation. The Kaiser Family Foundation, based in Menlo Park, California, is a nonprofit, private operating foundation focusing on the major health care issues facing the nation and is not associated with Kaiser Permanente or Kaiser Industries.)

Health Care Rationing

Health care in the United States is allocated based on price and the willingness and ability of patients to pay. In other words, patients are entitled to purchase a share of the medical services that they value. Social justice, in contrast, emphasizes the well-being of the community over the individual. Under this view, health care is regarded as a social good (as opposed to an economic good) that should be collectively financed and available to everyone regardless of ability to pay (Hoffman, 2013). The United States rations chiefly by price and the ability to pay (Hughes, 2011).

The concept of **rationing** in health care refers to limiting the provision of health care services. Rationing may occur according to a social justice or market justice model (Bowser, 2015). Rationing implies that resources are fixed or limited and, therefore, cannot meet every need. Scheunemann and White (2011, p. 1625) state "need is limitless and resources are not," thus there is a certain inevitability of rationing. Rationing in the United States today is more likely to be described with words such as quality, value, or evidence-based care (Ubel, 2015). The use of these words separates the need to distribute limited resources from the "emotional and historical baggage" attached to the word rationing (p. 15).

When rationing is based on social justice principles, it is a rational, fair and equal distribution of resources according to a clinical need or potential for effectiveness and is not based on income or where one lives. In this way, rationing focuses on the needs of the population more than the individual (Bowser, 2015). Rationing may occur by restricting people's choices, by denying access to services, or by limiting the supply of services or personnel. It may be overt, as in the oft-cited case of the United Kingdom, or more covert, as practiced by some health plans. When rationing is based on market justice principles, limited resources are distributed based on the ability to pay (Bowser, 2015). This has been the main model of rationing in the United States, as we have rationed by income, as access to health care has been based on ability to pay (Hughes, 2011).

Rationing may jeopardize the well-being of groups of individuals (Bowser, 2015). With limited resources for health services delivery, the government, insurers, and providers of health care services make rationing decisions to contain costs (Rosoff, 2014). This has included strict eligibility levels or monitoring the use of resources to ensure the most equitable distribution. In the past, private insurers engaged in rationing by excluding enrollees who are at greatest risk for health problems—and, thus, higher expenditures (Rosoff, 2014). This practice is no longer allowed under the rules of the ACA.

Advances in knowledge and technical capabilities through research and technology compound rationing decisions. When several individuals need an organ transplant and only one organ is available, what criteria should be used to select the recipient? Now that it is commonly accepted that certain lifestyle behaviors, such as smoking and alcohol consumption, or driving without restraints, create health risks, should people who engage in these activities pay a higher price for health care or be excluded from certain services? Should a younger person needing specialized surgery take priority over an older person needing similar care? There are no easy answers. Individual providers, insurance companies, governments, and consumers have struggled with these difficult ideas for years. With health care costs, the problems are even more complex. As health care spending rose, calls for rationing often intensified (Kelly & Cronin, 2011). Total health care spending was projected to rise to 25% of GDP by 2020, and 37% by 2050; it could even reach 49% by 2082 unless something were to be done, and this was a considerable impetus for health care reform (Rosoff, 2014). The spending for Medicare and Medicaid has grown rapidly. Over the last 30 years, Medicare spending has grown 2.4% per year faster than the GDP, and a 2009 predictive study by Friedman found that it could account for 31% of GDP in 2082 if no adjustments were made. Societal and medical advances have increased life expectancy and improved national welfare, but as spending continued to consume more and more of the GDP, more people have questioned if the costs outweighed the benefits. This may lead to limiting access to high-cost, low-benefit health procedures, such as expensive MRIs for rare conditions or conditions with no effective treatments or cures. Already, the organ allocation system controls or rations who gets an organ and when they get it; it is illegal to purchase an organ. Other types of rationing include congressional budget decisions; for instance, what proportion of the total budget goes to the Department of Defense versus agencies dealing with health and human services or medical research. When it comes to rationing, Americans need to realize that some rationing must occur or we will face financial destruction, but our society is not accepting of the idea of rationing because of our individualistic value orientation and because we are often easily influenced by those having financial interests in opposing this discussion (Rosoff, 2014).

Oregon began an overt system of rationing in 1994. The state approached the problem pragmatically and openly. In an effort to reach universal coverage, Medicaid was expanded to cover all state residents with incomes below the FPL, and then health care services rationing was planned in order to pay for the increased public coverage. Community meetings were held, and over 1,000 citizens spoke out. Thirteen health-related values, under three headings, (1) value to society, (2) value to individuals at risk, and (3) essential to basic health care, were put forward. An original list of 709 medical services was decided upon. The state envisioned a plan for legislative determination of a cutoff point, depending on yearly budget allocations; the list changed yearly, and in 1995, 581 out of 745 procedures were covered (Perry & Hotze, 2011). In 1999, Oregon's Medicaid program covered 574 of 743 conditions, but in the early part of the 2000s, an economic downturn prevented further expansion of the Oregon Health Plan (OHP). Cuts were made and co-pays instituted that eventually led to unmet health care needs. In the year between 2002 and 2003, enrollment dropped more than 50%, and by 2007, it was down by 75% to 77% (Perry & Hotze, 2011). In 2007, the prioritized list became the basis of the essential benefits package and was divided into tiers. Lower-priority items had higher cost sharing, and higher-priority items (e.g., tobacco and substance abuse, obesity), although prevalent among the low-income population, did not focus on personal responsibility and risk behaviors or the individual's response to treatment. Faguet (2013) concluded that Oregon's health rationing plan was ineffective, as no real systematic rationing took place and coverage was actually more broad than the previous Medicaid plan, especially for dental and mental health services. Although more individuals were covered under the plan—only 11% were uninsured versus national rate of 16%—only minimal Medicaid savings were realized. The plan was underfunded, so cigarette taxes were increased and Medicaid clients were moved into managed care plans. Also, it was difficult for legislators were influenced by political influence of pressure groups and those seeking to game the rankings for their own benefit (Faguet, 2013). With the passage of ACA, Oregon has established Patient-Centered Primary Care Homes and regional Coordinated Care Organizations or networks of physicians, mental health and dental providers working under a capitated budget to provide coordinated and comprehensive services to OHP members. Financial incentives are offered for those patients needing chemical dependency, mental health, and chronic illness care (Howard, Bernell, Yoon, Luck, & Ranit, 2015). (See What Do You Think?)

Competition and Regulation

Often, competition and regulation in health economics have been viewed as antagonistic and incompatible concepts. **Competition** means a contest between rival health care organizations for resources and clients. **Regulation** refers to mandated procedures and practices affecting health services delivery that are enforced by law. In a society in which long-held values of freedom of choice and individualism reign supreme, competition provides opportunities for entrepreneurial endeavor, free enterprise, and scientific advancement. Yet, to promote the public good, oversee equitable distribution of health services, and foster community-wide participation, regulation also serves an important role.

Health care incorporates four major kinds of regulation (Longest, 2016; Sultz & Young, 2014):

- Laws
- Regulations
- Programs
- Policies

Laws that regulate health care include any legislation that governs financing or delivery of health services, such as legislation regulating Medicare reimbursement to

---

What do *you* think?

Put yourself in the place of Manny Alvarez, a 23-year-old college student. He has a particularly devastating form of cancer—a very rare form of sarcoma. His physician has worked diligently to find a chemotherapy that looks promising against his specific tumor cells, but it is not approved for his cancer. It is only FDA approved to treat leukemia. In order to find this drug, tumor specimens were taken from his knee and femur and tested against 200 other potential medications. He had tried a drug offered through an NIH clinical trial, but it was completely ineffective against his tumor. The leukemia drug killed his cancer cells in lab tests, but his insurance company, Blue Cross Blue Shield of Florida, has declined his claim for treatment. The reason given was because this was "not established as a standard of therapy" for his type of sarcoma. But the cost of the medication is at least $300,000 (Katz, 2015, para. 4).

What would you do? If Manny does not receive treatment, he will die. Is there a moral duty to give him the medication? The pharmaceutical company should be paid for their product, but where will Manny and his family get the money for his treatment? Is there an obligation for the insurance company to provide the treatment? Or, should they wait until more clear evidence of effectiveness is available? This is a very rare form of sarcoma, and no insurance company has unlimited resources. Also, there is no federal standard that offers "clear criteria for differentiating valid from invalid

requests," so insurers follow their own rulebooks (Katz, 2015, para. 7).

Do you think we should have some type of federal standard that governs the rights of insurers to deny coverage or care?

Katz (2015) suggests that nonstandard care should be covered if a qualified physician documents a "desperate need for treatment," and there evidence that supports "potential efficacy" for a specific treatment (para. 8). Because of our collective fear of the word *rationing*, we do not engage in discussions about what should and should not be covered, and our health care system often engages in heroic, but misguided, measures in some very futile scenarios, especially with very ill patients near the end of their lives. If we chose not to ration health care, then Manny would receive treatment; but insurance companies could become financially insolvent. If we "choose to rational rationally," Manny could receive care depending upon the standards set. However, if we "ration irrationally," care will most often be denied to Manny and still provided in cases of "misguided futility" (para. 15).

Do you think we should have a debate about how we divide up our health care resources? Is rationing a dirty word, or something we need to examine as a society?

Katz, D. (2015, June 12). *The irrational rationing of health care*. Retrieved from http://www.huffingtonpost.com/david-katz-md/the-irrational-rationing-_b_7565580.html

hospitals. Regulations guide and clarify implementation; they are issued under the authority of law and are part of most federal health care programs. Examples include regulations governing project grants such as HMO development; formula grants, such as those provided under the Hill–Burton Act; and entitlements, such as Medicare and Medicaid. Regulatory programs are created from legislative enactments and are designed to accomplish specific goals, such as accreditation and licensing rules for hospitals, public health agencies, and other health service providers. Regulatory policies have a broader focus and involve decisions that shape the health care system by channeling the flow of resources into it and setting limits on key players' actions. Examples of regulatory policies are found by reviewing state or federal budget proposals for funding programs, such as health manpower training, research, and technology development (Kingdon, 2011; Longest, 2016). See Chapter 13.

From the 1950s through the 1970s, the federal government assumed an increasing role in regulating health services (Sultz & Young, 2014). First, federal subsidy of health care costs increased, and there was greater federal control of state programs. Health services became regionalized and more comprehensive. Federal appropriations supported operational as well as capital and planning costs. Health research and the training of health professionals gained greater federal support. Group medical practice multiplied as a cost-saving measure. More than 60% of the population was covered by some form of prepaid health insurance, largely because of the effects of Medicare and Medicaid. Interagency health planning cooperation increased, and health program evaluation improved. Neighborhood health centers, community mental health centers, and other programs were developed to improve health care access for everyone. Although costs rose, the period was one of relative economic stability that emphasized quality of care, with the federal government assuming a major role in regulating the planning, use, and reimbursement of health care services.

In the early 1980s, government cost-control measures were greatly diminished as the Reagan era ushered in deregulation in many areas of debate (Sultz & Young, 2014). The passage of the Omnibus Budget Reconciliation Act caused dramatic changes affecting health care. The federal government, having failed to contain rising health care costs, shifted responsibility for the public's health and welfare back to state and local governments. Large amounts of federal funding for health research, health manpower training, and public health programs were withdrawn. Continued escalation of health care costs prompted a concentrated effort among public and private providers alike to find cost-containment measures. From all this grew the competition-versus-regulation debate.

The 1990s were characterized by numerous hospital mergers and nonprofit to for-profit status. The Clinton health plan failed to gain support and many hospitals downsized and reduced the number of nurses on staff. Managed care became more popular as a means of reducing employer premiums in the early 1990s, but by the late 1990s, as they restricted benefits, fears were raised about MCOs withholding necessary care and a consumer

"backlash" resulted (RAND Health, 2010). Many states and the federal government enacted benefit laws between 1990 and 2002, in response to these concerns. We are still feeling the results of these changes, and one of the most obvious consequences deals with competition in health care.

Competition, its proponents say, offers wider consumer choice and positive incentives for cost containment and enhanced efficiency (Sultz & Young, 2014); that is, consumers are free to select among various health plans on the basis of cost, quality, and range of services. Competing providers must develop efficient production and distribution methods to stay in business, and consumers are more likely to use only necessary services, because of the required cost sharing that is part of the competition model. One downside is fragmentation of services, lack of coordination, and subsequent waste. Integrated delivery systems, such as Kaiser Permanente's fully integrated system or more loosely organized public–private partnerships, could lead to improved quality, outcomes, and reduced costs (Enthoven, 2009b; Mate & Compton-Phillips, 2014; Reich, Rapold, & Flatscher-Thöni, 2012).

Examples of competition have been very evident as more health plans, including HMOs and PPOs, vied with traditional insurance plans for subscribers: Currently, only one percent of workers are covered by their employers through a conventional insurance plan (KFF, 2015c). However, costs have not dropped substantially. Many hospitals, too, compete aggressively for patients. Some hospitals now advertise maternity care depicting a new mother and father having a candlelight dinner in the hospital with their newborn infant in the bassinet beside them. Some surgical centers advance the "hotel guest" concept, with beautifully appointed rooms, including meals and lodging for a guest. Some research has shown that a greater concentration of hospital markets can lead to higher prices, although prices can be lower when health plan market concentration is also high (Melnick, Shen, & Wu, 2011).

Although it may appear that competition offers the best service for the least cost, regulation advocates have for almost 20 years argued that there are at least four problems associated with the competition model: (1) consumers often do not make proper health care choices because of limited knowledge of health services; (2) competition may discriminate against enrolling certain consumers, especially high-risk, high-cost patients, thus excluding those who may need services the most; (3) the competition model may not encourage enough teaching and research—expensive elements of our present system; and (4) quality may be sacrificed to keep costs down.

Regulation advocates conclude that standardization and controls are needed to guarantee quality and equal access. Our capitalist system can be driven by profits, and the profit motive in health care can lead to excesses and higher costs for taxpayers and patients. The five largest health insurance companies posted $3.3 billion in profits between just the months of April and June 2011; however, nonprofit health insurer Blue Cross/Blue Shield of Illinois paid their CEO $16 million in 2012, and the Mayo Clinic's CEO made $2 million (Ubel, 2014). Leaders in the field have concluded that both competition and regulation are needed (Longest, 2016; Sultz & Young, 2014). With foresight, McNerney (1980) wrote, "It is rapidly becoming apparent that what we need is a proper balance between competition and regulation with more effective links [and] regulation [should be] used as a force to keep the market honest" (p. 1091).

HEALTH CARE REFORM

HMOs and PPOs have become accepted methods of delivering health care in the United States in the past 30 years. Over several generations, other methods have been considered, yet not passed by legislation and adopted as law. Health care reform became a reality in 2010, with the passage of the ACA. It is helpful to look at earlier attempts and thought processes that moved us toward this reality. Managed competition and universal coverage, as well as single-payer systems, have been part of the discussion in health care reform (Squires & Anderson, 2015).

Two plans worth further review are managed competition and universal coverage, with and without a single-payer system. The benefits and drawbacks of each are important to discuss here.

Managed Competition

The idea of managed competition, as a health care delivery method, was born from the controversy regarding competition versus regulation and was driven by the need for health care reform. **Managed competition**, it was hoped, would combine with market competition to achieve cost savings with government regulation to achieve expanded coverage. This idea, whose origin is credited to cconomist Alain C. Enthoven of Stanford University, has played a major part in debates on health care reform. It sought to address the two fundamental issues driving reform: cost containment and universal access to health care (Enthoven, 2009a).

Managed competition has been viewed as a market-based solution that places accountability for resolving the health care crisis with the insurance industry and with consumers. Insurers would be required to accept all applicants, without excluding those at more risk. At the same time, the insurers must control costs. Consumers would choose among competing health insurance plans, paying above fixed amounts paid by their employers to receive the best value. But for true competition, employers must offer real choices and a wide variety of plans. To do this, Enthoven and colleagues envisioned "regional insurance exchanges" that select health plans, manage risk selection, and establish equity rules, for example, those plans with sicker participants would be subsidized by plans with younger, healthier participants (Arrow et al., 2009, p. 493).

Another concept of managed competition is consumer choice, and consumers must be able to access information, so that they can make responsible choices and feel that they have purchased something of value for their money (Vaiana, 2011). Other common features of managed competition proposals include regulations that prevent screening out of high-risk enrollees, penalties for companies that try to achieve better risk pools, community ratings to prevent companies from setting rates by risk pool, and guaranteed coverage for all who apply. Another

critical component involves management; some standardization must be established among benefit packages and an effort must be made to dismantle health care monopolies that endeavor to gain uneven market power—in other words, a more level playing field (Enthoven and Wynand, 2007; Mikkers & Ryan, 2014). There is also recognition that the transition period can be lengthy.

Proponents of managed competition cite many advantages. Managed competition would encourage insurance companies to compete on price and quality of services to attract enrollees. It would also offer consumers tax incentives to purchase the lowest-cost plans that meet minimum benefit requirements. Managed competition, although market driven, would be highly regulated to ensure quality and access. Cost-effectiveness and quality/outcomes information must be made available to consumers, although currently this information is not always easy to find or to decipher. Providers have not widely accepted systems of ranking on measures of quality. According to its proponents, managed competition, as a reform concept, would have the potential for reducing expenditures and improving access to health care coverage and is being used successfully in other countries (Enthoven & Wynand, 2007; van Ginneken, Schäfer, & Kroneman, 2011).

Duijmelinck and van de Ven (2016) summarize the lessons to be learned from the U.S. experience with managed care: Health care providers are often the most critical toward this change, consumers will accept some loss of provider choice if lower premiums are provided, information should be provided to consumers about quality of in network and out of network providers, and quality indicators and national guidelines help promote acceptance of managed care. This highlights some of the problems and potential benefits regarding managed competition. Can market forces really work in the health care market? Similar models, such as HMOs and the Federal Employee Health Benefits Program, have failed to reign in ever-increasing health care costs (Sultz & Young, 2014).

Another major criticism of managed competition is its potential failure to provide equitable and universal coverage. It is possible that large employers would benefit financially under managed competition, but small businesses would find the cost burden heavy, and many individuals, such as the self-employed, could remain uninsured. A basic benefits package, critics argue, must address the special concerns affecting groups such as women and older adults, including coverage for long-term care, home care, mental health, dental care, and prescribed drugs. Competition among providers would be inefficient in rural areas, where there are fewer provider choices, such as county nursing agencies and isolated small-town hospitals scattered over great distances (Rice et al., 2014).

Universal Coverage and a Single-Payer System

A different approach to health care reform emphasizes universal health insurance coverage, often through a stronger role played by government. Some proponents of this system of health care promote a **single-payer system** that would replace the health insurance companies in the United States with a single, public sector insurer that would entitle all citizens to **universal coverage** (everyone would have health insurance of some type, ensuring better access to care). Efforts to accomplish this approach have been evident for many years.

Since the time of Teddy Roosevelt in 1912, NHI has been debated while its proponents have sought comprehensive health care protection, in particular, for the aged, children, and the needy. Presidents Roosevelt (both Theodore and Franklin), Truman, Nixon, Carter, and Clinton have all lobbied for some form of NHI or universal health coverage, and Senator Edward Kennedy was also a long-time supporter (Kingdon, 2011). Growing concern over the cost and accessibility of health services in the 1960s and again in the mid-1970s led to a renewed focus on NHI as a solution by which health insurance coverage could be provided for all citizens through a single-payer system or a mix of public and private insurers. Numerous attempts to pass some form of NHI resulted in piecemeal legislation that added various benefits for Social Security recipients. The Kerr–Mills bill (1960) set a precedent of public financing for older adults who were medically needy but not receiving public assistance. Medicare (1965) was the first compulsory NHI program in the United States. By 2001, it reached some 40 million people—only 16% of the total U.S. population.

Most other developed countries offer some type of NHI or attempt to provide universal health coverage to their citizens. Other countries believe that health care is a fundamental right, and provide it as a social service, unlike the United States, which tends to view it as a commodity that is only available based on one's ability to pay (IOM, 2013; Quadagno, 2010). The APHA (2010) has long been an advocate of universal health care, including a single-payer system, and they strongly endorsed passage of the ACA health care reform legislation.

Although many agree that insuring all U.S. citizens will improve overall national health and performance, the concept of a government-sponsored, single-payer system is controversial, as many think that this equates to socialized medicine; however, a single-payer system is more consistent with Medicare where the single payer is the government, but the care is provided by various private entities (physicians, nurse practitioners, hospitals, clinics). A socialized system is more like the Veterans Administration where care and payment are both provided by the government (Rovner, 2016). Even though polls have often revealed that people were dissatisfied with the health care system before health care reform (ACA), they generally reported being satisfied with their own arrangements for health care—and they were uncomfortable with the idea of a government-controlled health plan. A 2016 Kaiser Health Tracking poll revealed that 36% of people want to "build on the existing law" to make it more affordable and accessible to greater numbers of citizens, and 24% would like to see universal coverage guaranteed to all through a single government health plan (McCanne, 2016, para. 1). However, 16% would like to completely do away with the ACA, and 13% would like its replacement to be a Republican-sponsored plan. A 2013 survey of 1,151 adults making ED visits in Massachusetts found that the majority would prefer NHI over the health care reform instituted there 7 years earlier. This was true across demographic groups, although the majority of respondents were non-White and low income. NHI garnered high levels of support among those who were not satisfied with their current health plans, those who couldn't buy medications because of the high cost, and those who reported delaying medical care (between 81.2% and 87.3%). Saluja et al. (2016) concluded that this level of support indicated that the ACA does not completely meet the needs of underserved individuals.

The "Medicare-for-all" plan promoted by Senator Bernie Sanders is favorable to 53% of Democrats. Semantics is important, as 49% of those polled viewed socialized medicine as negative, but only 38% found guaranteed universal coverage to have a negative connotation (McCanne, 2016). Logic indicated that single-payer plans could provide cost savings from reduced overhead and administrative costs. But other questions remained, such as: What is the best way to provide universal coverage? Should health insurance still be linked to employment? How can the expense be funded? Should citizens become more responsible for their health outcomes? How can quality be ensured and costs managed? (See Table 6–5).

In testimony to Congress, experts from the Commonwealth Fund and other groups encouraged the design of a universal health care system that meets four criteria: improves access to care, has the potential to slow cost increases and improve efficiency, improves equity in the system, and has the potential to improve health care quality (Collins, 2007; Collins et al., 2007; Kingdon, 2011). Some politicians proposed expanding Medicare, Medicaid, and the CHIP programs or focusing more on prevention and individual responsibility. Other groups supported a system of tax credits, employer and individual taxes, and a more transparent evaluation of costs and quality. Aspects of each of these ideas are included in the ACA (see Perspectives: Health Care Reform).

Some states initiated legislation to extend coverage to uninsured residents. Massachusetts required all residents above a set income level to get insurance coverage from their employer or purchase it individually; adults earning up to 150% of FPL and children of parents earning up to 300% of FPL are fully subsidized by the state. Results are mixed; more people are insured, but costs have not been curbed. Before this legislation, about 94% of residents were insured; currently, 98% of residents (and 99.8% of children) are covered. The percentage of private employers providing employee health insurance rose from 70% to 77%, and companies with more than 11 full-time employees are expected to contribute to health insurance or face penalties. Increased costs to the state in the 2010 budget were only 1%, but a cost shift burden from employers to individuals is problematic. Medical bankruptcies rose by over 33% between 2007 and 2009 but are currently lower in Massachusetts than in other states (Falla, n.d.). Although most residents are supportive of the law, and 88% of physicians in a recent survey stated it improved care or didn't affect the quality of care, per capita health care spending is projected to be almost twice the current rate by 2020 for this precursor to the ACA (Khan, 2011). Primary care providers are also stretched thin with additional patients seeking physician gatekeepers, and safety-net hospitals have also been shortchanged as funds have

Table 6-5 **Health Care System Comparisons: Australia, Canada, France, Germany, Japan, Sweden, and United States, 2014**

Country	Type of Coverage Model	HC % of GDP	Average Annual Growth Rate	Per Capita Out-of-Pocket	Practicing MDs/1,000 People	Average MD Visits/Capita	Number Hospital Beds Per Capita	MRI Machines/ Million People	MRI Exams/ 1,000 People	MD Use of EHRs	Obesity	Life Expectancy at Birth
Australia	NHI	9.1%	2.4%	$731	3.31	6.9	3.40	15.0	26.0	92%	28.3%	79.27
Canada	NHI	10.9%	2.4%	$690	2.48	7.9	1.72	8.8	53.7	56%	25.4%	78.35
France	Bismarck	11.6%	1.4%	$320	3.08	6.7	3.39	8.7	82.0	67%	14.5%	77.41
Germany	Bismarck	10.3%	2.0%	$627	3.96	9.7	5.38	n/a	n/a	82%	n/a	77.11
Japan	Bismarck	10.3%	3.5%	$483	2.29	13.0	7.94	46.9	n/a	n/a	3.6%	79.20
Sweden	Beveridge	9.6%	1.9%	$678	3.92	n/a	1.95	n/a	n/a	88%	11.8%	77.92
United States	Private/public no universal coverage	16.9%	2.4%	$1,045	2.46	4.0	2.56	34.5	104.8	69%	35.3%	75.64

From Mossialos, E., Wenzl, M., Osborn, R., & Anderson, C. (Eds.). (2015, January). *2014 International profiles of health care systems: Australia, Canada, Denmark, England, France, Germany, Italy, Japan, The Netherlands, New Zealand, Norway, Singapore, Sweden Switzerland, and the United States.* Retrieved from http://www.commonwealthfund.org/~/media/files/publications/fund-report/2015/jan/1802_mossialos_intl_profiles_2014_v7.pdf Institute of Medicine (IOM). (2013). *U.S. health in international perspective: Shorter lives, poorer health.* Washington, DC: National Academies Press.

The Patient Protection and Affordable Care Act (ACA) was signed into law by President Barak Obama on March 23, 2010. Provisions included expanded coverage of dependent children on parents' health insurance until age 26, and care for screenings/preventive services, along with a prohibition on canceling policies for those who become ill. However, many provisions of the act did not become fully implemented until 2014, and others are still in the process of being fully implemented (Gaynor, 2013; Rice et al., 2014). Key provisions of the ACA include the following:

Private Insurance Coverage Expansion

- An individual mandate requires health insurance (private or public) for every American and documented immigrant. Those choosing not to get health insurance are subject to an annual financial penalty of $695 for an individual and $2,085 for a family (or 2.5% of income) by the 2016 deadline. The penalties will be recovered from federal income tax refunds. Subsidies, offered on a sliding scale, help uninsured families and individuals purchase private insurance through health insurance exchanges.
- Health insurance exchanges may be accessed online (state or federal) and must offer the same minimum benefit packages (i.e., ambulatory and emergency services, hospitalization, maternity/neonatal care, pediatric care, mental health/substance abuse services including behavioral health counseling, prescription drugs, rehabilitation services/devices, laboratory, and preventive/wellness services along with management of chronic diseases). Preexisting conditions may no longer be a consideration (Rice et al., 2014).
- Insurance premiums can vary only by age, by geographical location, and, in some cases, by smoking status. Insurers may not set annual or lifetime policy limits, and they must return 80% of premiums either to the policyholders or provide them additional health benefits. However, Day, Himmelstein, Broder, and Woolhandler (2015) found that the medical loss ratio (or overhead spending) for private insurers had not substantially changed during a 3-year period before the ACA and a 3-year period after ACA.

Changes in Medicaid and Medicare

- Medicaid coverage was extended to those making 138% of the federal poverty level.
  - Federal government pays 100% of the expansion cost to states at first, and then, the amount drops to 90% by 2020 (ANA, 2014).
  - The Supreme Court ruled that states had the right to determine if they wanted to participate in the Medicaid expansion, and, by 2016, 31 states (and the District of Columbia) chose to do so.
- Medicare now offers preventive services without co-payments, and the prescription drug coverage gap (doughnut hole) will eventually be closed.
  - Capitation rates for Medicare Advantage plans will be reduced, and bonuses will be given to plans that reach high-quality scores; penalties will be incurred for those with low-quality scores.
  - Independent Payment Advisory Board will make cost-containment recommendations if fee-for-services expenses growth more than 1% more than the GDP. Congress may override the recommendations (Rice et al., 2014).

Changes for Employers

- Large employers (100 employees) must offer health insurance by 2015. Those with 50 to 99 employees must offer health insurance by 2016. Monthly penalties can range from $2,160 to $3,240 divided by 12 months per employee who either was not provided health insurance or was provided insurance that did not meet minimum requirements (KFF, 2015a). Some tax credits are offered to small employers who offer coverage. The Cadillac Tax for expensive health plans will go into effect by 2020 (Himmelstein, Ariely, & Woolhandler, 2014; Woolhandler & Himmelstein, 2016).

Changes for Health Care Providers

- Scholarships/loans offered to primary care physicians who are willing to work in underserved areas (Rice et al., 2014). Grant funding for nursing education, and other nursing workforce grants, was expanded (ANA, 2014).
- Providers are encouraged to become part of Accountable Care Organizations (ACOs), or voluntary groups/networks of hospitals, home health agencies, pharmacies, physicians, and other health care providers that offer "coordinated, high-quality care" to patients without duplication of services or medical errors (CMS, 2015b, para. 1). The Medicare Shared Savings Program also encourages ACOs but provides no specific instructions about their structure (Brill, 2015).
  - Since 2011, 744 ACOs have formed and about 6 million Medicare patients are part of an ACO. Incentives are given for keeping patients healthy, controlling costs, and providing quality care. A hope for ACOs is that burgeoning costs for care of our aging population will be controlled. Some large private insurers have created ACOs. They seem similar to HMOs, but patients are not required to remain within the ACO and may see providers outside that network (Gold, 2015).
  - ACOs much meet four quality standards—patient/caregiver experiences, patient safety/care coordination, preventive health services, and chronic disease populations (Rice et al., 2014).
  - Some are concerned that the integrated systems created by ACOs may lead to a monopoly when it comes to raising costs or that providers will be pressured to control costs at the expense of quality because of financial incentives offered (Rice et al., 2014). The Federal Trade Commission monitors health care enforcement and mergers (Brill, 2015). Research has demonstrated that financial rewards have caused problems with motivation and performance in health care settings (Himmelstein, Ariely, et al., 2014). Physician governance is needed to avoid this, but medical education must also include more content on processes of care delivery and managing costs (Dranove, 2014).

Changes for Consumers

- Individuals and families with incomes of $200,000 and $250,000, respectively, will begin to pay higher taxes on investment and unearned income in 2013.
  - They will also pay higher payroll taxes that will be used to finance Medicare (Rice et al., 2014).

Some economists and researchers feel that the ACA is a move in the right direction but does not go far enough and may actually end up causing problems because of narrow markets and high premiums and deductibles. Many encourage a single-payer system of national health plan to reduce administrative costs and better control rising health care costs (Dranove, 2012; Gaffney, Woolhandler, & Himmelstein, 2016; Gaynor, 2013).

been diverted to help pay for the costs of health care reform (Norbash, Hindson, & Heineke, 2012).

With the lack of quality health outcomes in the United States, as described above, even if everyone received health insurance, how could quality be assured? Some believe that the overall performance of the health care system should improve as everyone gains access to care. However, a system that provides incentives to *both* providers and patients to use services efficiently and effectively produces the best results (Bouffard, 2015; Collins, 2007; Collins et al., 2007). Providing information to consumers is another component of quality assurance, and this is sorely lacking. But information is becoming more readily available. For instance, since 2000, the Leapfrog Group (n.d.) has promoted *transparency* through surveys of standard measurements and practices to enable comparisons and reimbursement incentives to encourage quality and efficiency. Scores for local hospitals can be reviewed at the Leapfrog Web site (http://www.leapfroggroup.org/compare-hospitals). The quality of insurance plans, measured by the Health Plan Employer Data and Information Set (HEDIS), includes information on patient satisfaction, data on risk factor control, and procedures such as prescribing β-blockers after heart attacks and is monitored by the National Committee for Quality Assurance (NCQA). Nursing students are aware of the Quality and Safety Education for Nurses (QSEN) project that provides a basis for continuous quality improvement and health care safety (Case Western Reserve University, 2014). Other systems of quality measurement, like health outcomes, the process of care, and adherence to standardized guidelines, are still required. The ACA requires hospitals, providers, and insurance plans to include quality ratings on their Web sites, increasing transparency (Dash, Corlette, & Thomas, 2014).

Health Care Reform: Making the Change

The cry for health care reform is not new. In a classic study, Perkins examined the work of the 1927 to 1932 Committee on the Costs of Medical Care. More than 75 years ago, the committee defined *costs* as the major problem and *business models of organization* as the major solution (Perkins, 1998).

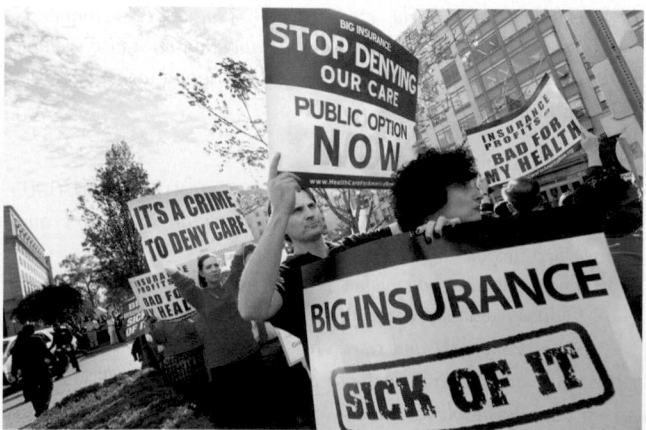

Health care reform advocates march in Washington, DC.

A standard set of benefits, set by law and enjoyed by the entire population, regardless of age, health, income, and employment status, is an important health care reform element. Many countries have successfully implemented such a package under a plan called a *statutory model*. Various versions of this model have worked well in Austria, France, Belgium, Japan, Germany, Israel, Poland, the Netherlands, and Switzerland. In this model, health insurance falls under the rubric of social security and is funded through government-mandated payroll premiums or taxes. Payment is made to private sector health insurers, from a fund called a *sickness fund* in some countries (IOM, 2013). Individuals select among nationwide plans and choose their doctor and hospital and can switch plans when desired. This statutory model eliminates the need for separate programs such as Medicaid and Medicare. It also provides uniform and comprehensive benefits (Estes et al., 2013). See Display 6–2 for a description of four models of health care and a comparison of health systems in five developed countries.

Other issues include making the system more accountable, eliminating adverse risk selection, and providing informed choices to consumers. Furthermore, health reform must focus on the central question: Is there coverage for the promotion of health and prevention of illness or simply payment for the diagnosis and treatment of those who are already ill? Research has shown that public health interventions have been found to be consistently more cost-effective than medical services, yet past health reform has often paid minimal attention to this critical issue (Shroufi et al., 2013; Tanner, 2015). In addition, our frequent emphasis on medical care cost containment does not take into account the social determinants of health that need to be addressed outside the health care system. PHNs can play an influential role in emphasizing health promotion services as being central to future health reform efforts through political involvement and policy development.

Designers of health reform have faced a difficult challenge in reconciling these conflicting views. As a result, elements of both models have been used to shape an improved system. Recent health care reform includes an incremental plan that allows for a flexible transition and opportunities for states to experiment with approaches. With the successful passage of HR 3590 (Public Law [PL] 111–148), *The Patient Protection and Affordable Care Act*, on March 23, 2010, and the March 25 passage of HR 4872 (PL 111–152), *Health Care and Education Affordability Reconciliation Act of 2010*, amending HR 3590, the long journey toward health care system reform crossed a threshold. Both pieces of legislation are referred to as the *Affordable Care Act* (ACA). Although by no means a grand vision for change with its incremental implementation, it has been called "among the most consequential pieces of social policy passed since the Great Society" of Lyndon Johnson in the 1960s (Klein, 2011, para 5).

Beginning in 2010, dependent coverage for adult children was extended to age 26, and prohibition on lifetime limits on coverage and preexisting conditions for children, along with tax credits to small employers (25 employees or less) providing health insurance began, among other things. In 2011, grants were awarded to states to investigate current tort litigations, and to small employers to establish wellness programs, as well as implementation of 50% discounts on Medicare Part D brand-name prescriptions from pharmaceutical

DISPLAY 6-2 MODELS OF HEALTH CARE AND HOW FIVE OTHER COUNTRIES PROVIDE HEALTH CARE

According to Reid (2010), there are four models of health care:

1. *Bismarck Model*—This is named after the Prussian Chancellor, Otto von Bismarck, who proposed this model as part of the 19th century unification of Germany. Private insurance (funded by employers and employee payroll deductions) and private health care providers characterize this system. Many hospitals are also private, and everyone is covered. There are over 200 funds that pay for services, but there are strict controls on medical fees and services to keep costs down. Belgium, Germany, Japan, and Switzerland have this type of health care system.

2. *Beveridge Model*—This is inspired by the British social reformer, William Beveridge, who envisioned a system of health care both financed and provided by the government through taxes. Like using the public library, services are not billed but are provided as a public service. Hospitals, clinics, and physicians are part of the governmental system, but some private physicians are paid fees by the government. The government is the single payer in this system, and this is how costs are controlled. It has been called socialized medicine, but that is actually more representative of the U.S. Veterans Administration system. This type of health care system is found in Great Britain, Hong Kong, Italy, Span, and many Scandinavian countries.

3. *National Health Insurance Model*—This is considered to be a hybrid of the Beveridge and Bismarck models. The government pays for services from private health care providers through an insurance system paid for by taxpayers. This is considered universal health care, and savings are achieved through lower administrative, marketing, and underwriting costs. Better prices are negotiated, and covered services are sometimes limited or patient wait times may be increased. Canada's health care system uses this model, and Australia, South Korea, and Taiwan have variations of this model.

4. *Out-of-Pocket Model*—This system is found in less developed countries where the rich can afford health care services and the poor cannot afford care (about 160 of the world's 200 countries). In rural areas of Africa or South American, for instance, "hundreds of millions of people go their whole lives without ever seeing a doctor " (p. 19). The government has no system of care or type of plan to cover citizens. Examples include Cambodia, Egypt, and India where 73% to 91% of health care costs are paid out-of-pocket by patients.

Reid (2010) notes that the United States has some components of each of these models. The Bismarck Model can be found among American workers with employer-sponsored health insurance. The Beveridge Model applies to those Americans who are military personnel and veterans, as well as Native Americans using the Indian Health Service. Medicare recipients participate in a plan very similar to the National Health Insurance Model, as there are low administrative costs and almost universal involvement. For those Americans who still remain uninsured after ACA, they rely on care in emergency departments or charity clinics or are required to pay out of pocket for their care.

Germany
Percentage of GDP spent on health care: 10.7%
Average family premium: $750 per month (depending on income)
Co-payments: 10 euros ($15) every 3 months; some patients exempt

- German Statutory Health Insurance began in 1883. Germans buy insurance from private, nonprofit sickness funds. Fund manager pay is based on enrollment, and there is competition for members as well as negotiations with physicians for competitive pricing.
- Single-payment system. Physician salaries are two-thirds U.S. salaries, but medical school is free and malpractice insurance costs are much lower.
- Choice of physician (can see specialists first), hospital, long-term care facility and medication and dental.
- The richest 10% can opt out and purchase for-profit insurance that pays physicians higher fees (so they may see patients sooner); Germans living in poverty receive public assistance in paying sickness fund premiums.

Great Britain (United Kingdom)
Percentage of GDP spent on health care: 8.3%
Average family premium: Tax-funded, no additional cost
Co-payments: None for most services; some dental and vision co-pays; 5% for prescriptions (exempt for older adults and children)

- National Health Service (NHS) since World War II (funded from general revenues). This is considered "socialized medicine" as the government both pays for and provides health care services. Hospital physicians are paid salaries from taxes, and family physicians' salaries are based on the numbers of patients seen. A few specialists work outside the NHS, seeing private-paying patients.
- Low administrative costs and no claims to review or bills to collect. Family physicians provide medical homes and make referrals to specialists. They are paid bonuses for keeping their patients well and focusing on prevention. Well-designed system, but chronically underfunded
- Tax-based, free at point of service (covers ambulatory care, hospital, medications, long-term care, vision)

(continued)

DISPLAY 6–2 MODELS OF HEALTH CARE AND HOW FIVE OTHER COUNTRIES PROVIDE HEALTH CARE (*Continued*)

- Choice of physician; generally short waiting times for appointments, but longer waiting lists for elective referrals to specialists. Government reforms are making care more competitive and providing wider choices. Hospitals now compete for NHS funds and patients can choose where they want treatment for many procedures.

Japan

Percentage of GDP spent on health care: 8%
Average family premium: $280 per month, with employers paying over 50% of this
Co-payments: Procedures (30%), but total amount paid per month is capped per income level

- Japan utilizes a "social insurance" system, and all citizens are mandated to have health insurance (through employers or from nonprofit, community-based plans). Public assistance is given to those unable to afford insurance. Physicians and most hospitals are in the private (not public) sector, and most health insurance is private.
- There are no gatekeepers, as in the UK system, and Japanese may go to any specialist as often as they wish without first seeing a family physician. The Ministry of Health negotiates with physicians on pricing every 2 years.
- Japan, perhaps partially because of diet and lifestyle, has excellent health statistics (e.g., life expectancy).
- Because there is no gatekeeper, there is no incentive for patients to have a medical home. Because they have been successful in cost containment, 50% of hospitals now have budget losses.

Switzerland

Percentage of GDP spent on health care: 11.6%
Average monthly family premium: $750 paid by patients, with government assistance for people who are poor
Co-payments: 10% of the cost of services ($420 per year cap)

- Switzerland employs "social insurance," which began with a national referendum in 1994. At that time, 95% of their population was insured, but all citizens are now required to have health insurance. They have universal coverage, despite being a capitalistic society with large pharmaceutical and insurance industries.
- Insurance companies are forbidden from making a profit on basic care and cannot "cherry-pick" enrollees. They do make profits on supplemental insurance.

- Insurers negotiate with providers (e.g., hospitals, physicians), but the government sets prescription prices. Some, but not all, plans require physician gatekeepers; others give discounts to patients who use medical homes.
- The Swiss have the second most expensive system (still much less spent than the United States), and prices of medications are higher than in other euro countries. (Some Swiss drug companies are said to make 33% of their profits in the U.S. market.)

Taiwan

Percentage GDP spent on health care: 6.3%
Average family premium: $650 per year for a family of 4
Co-payments: Prescriptions (20% of cost, up to $6.50); outpatient care ($7); dental and traditional Chinese medicine ($1.80); many exemptions apply (e.g., preventive services, major diseases, childbirth, care for veterans/children/those living in poverty)

- In 1995, Taiwan adopted the "National Insurance Model." Insurance is mandatory for all citizens, and there is one, government-run health insurer. Employers and workers split premiums, and other citizens pay flat rates for insurance (with government assistance). Care for veterans and people who are poor is subsidized by the government. This system is similar to Canada and Medicare in the United States.
- Health insurance was extended to 40% of the uninsured population, and health care spending was actually decreased. Any physician can be seen without a referral, and smart cards are used to store medical history and for billing purposes. Public health officials are also assisted in monitoring standards, and Taiwan's administrative costs are the lowest in the world.
- Taiwan does not bring in enough money to cover all medical care provided. The parliament must approve insurance premium increases, and it has only done this once since 1995.

How do you think these systems compare with the U.S. health care system between 1965 and 2009? How do they compare with health care reform (ACA)? Which one of Reid's models, or combination of models, do you think would be most effective in the United States?

Adapted from Frontline. (2010). *Sick around the world: Five capitalist democracies & how they do it*. Retrieved from http://www.pbs.org/wgbh/pages/frontline/sickaroundtheworld/countries/
Reid, T. R. (2010). *The healing of America: A quest for better, cheaper, and fairer health care*. New York, NY: Penguin Books.

manufacturers. An Innovation Center within CMS was created, and a national quality improvement strategy developed. Small businesses have been allowed to keep insurance plans in effect—"grandfathering"—and about

72% of those with 100 or fewer workers have done so (KFF, 2012). In 2012, the Medicare Independence at Home Demonstration program was created and other cost-cutting measures came into effect, along with enhanced collection and reporting of data. Adoption of a single set of operating rules for verification of eligibility and claims status, enrollment, premium payments, and referrals began in 2013, as did increased Medicaid payments to primary care providers.

More dramatic reforms occurred the following year, including the creation of an essential health benefits package and permission for states to have an option to create a Basic Health Plan for uninsured residents making between 133% and 200% of the FPL. As of 2014, all U.S. citizens and legal residents are now required to have health coverage, with a phased-in penalty for those not covered. Employers with 50 or more employees who do not offer health coverage will be assessed a fine of $2,000 per full-time employee (first 30 excluded). Employers with more than 200 employees must automatically enroll all employees into health insurance plans. American Health Benefit Exchanges and Small Business Health Options Program Exchanges have been created, and deductibles for health plans in small group markets have limits of $2,000 for individuals and $4,000 for families. Waiting periods for full coverage is limited to 90 days. After 2015, states could form health care choice compacts and allow insurers to sell policies in any state in the compact after January 2016. Additional Medicare payment reductions for hospital-acquired infections began in 2015, and an excise tax on employers who offer "Cadillac health plans" (i.e., 40% on values >$10,200 for individuals and $27,500 for families) are scheduled for 2020 and are considered by some economic researchers to harm middle-class families making between 2009 incomes of $38,550 to $100,000 but will not affect the wealthy (Himmelstein, Ariely, et al., 2014). For a summary of the ACA, see http://kff.org/health-reform/fact-sheet/summary-of-the-affordable-care-act/.

The ACA has been described as "consumer-friendly" because applicants in each state will be screened for all available health subsidy programs and enrolled through a standardized process. Coordination and seamless transition between programs is the goal. Uniform income rules and forms, along with streamlined enrollment, will make administrative functions simpler and less costly. Paperless verification is required through secure Web portals, where information can be securely exchanged. The goal is to help individuals better understand their choices, as well as access and maintain health coverage. Families were able to apply online, but early on, it became clear that many needed assistance. Coordination between insurance exchanges, Medicaid, and CHIP provides for better coverage (Rosenbaum & Riley, 2012). Also, exchanges have the power to remove insurers who abuse the system or provide inadequate service.

Rapidly rising health care costs cannot be reined in overnight. Projections by 2030, with health care reform, are expected to be only 0.5% lower than they would have been without reform. But the federal budget deficit is projected to be $100 billion less after the first decade of ACA and $1 trillion less in the decade beyond 2020. Total health care expenditures could even end up $600 billion less in the first decade. There is flexibility and a focus on quality improvement that should help restrain unnecessary growth in health care costs. In controlling costs, new fraud and abuse measures in both Medicare and Medicaid are being instituted, and administrative savings should occur with standardization and electronic records (Orszag & Emanuel, 2010; RAND Health, 2011). An Independent Advisory Board (comprising experts and stakeholders) is assisting in controlling Medicare costs and has the power to make changes in the system without waiting for Congress to act (Klein, 2011). As Medicare's costs per capita exceed a prescribed threshold (general inflation plus 1% after 2018), this advisory board is empowered to develop and propose new policies for reducing inflationary costs that will be implemented by USDHHS, unless Congress enacts legislation resulting in similar cost savings (Orszag & Emanuel, 2010). The Patient-Centered Outcomes Research Institute will provide additional information on effectiveness of treatments and interventions, and the Innovation Center at CMS will develop, evaluate, and test new programs and policies that reduce cost and enhance care for Medicaid and Medicare patients. Improved value and quality outcomes are the proposed benefits of these three innovations (Orszag & Emanuel, 2010). ACA also increases incentives for change that will improve patient care and outcomes (e.g., hospital readmissions, hospital-acquired infections) and improve coordination of care (e.g., bundled payments to MDs and hospitals for patients with chronic illnesses, accountable care organizations, medical homes). These changes in the delivery of health care, as well as cost-control reforms suggested by economists, health policy experts, and physicians, are hoped to achieve cost reductions while providing expanded health insurance coverage (Orszag & Emanuel, 2010; RAND Health, 2011). Others note that lower payment increases to physicians seeing Medicare patients and reductions for insurers participating in Medicare, along with the increased Medicare tax on higher-income earners, will save the system money but will be largely offset by expenditures in Medicaid expansion, small business and exchange credits, and other expenses (Klein, 2011). Only time will tell; if the reform is dynamic and flexible, as touted, perhaps we can stay a step ahead of costs.

Not everyone is convinced that health care reform is a good idea. Republican legislators have continued to threaten repeal but have failed to provide a viable alternative solution. As of January 2012, 19 states have passed legislation that opposes at least some elements of the ACA, and 45 states had filed over 200 measures either proposing alternative policies or opposing elements of health reform. Several lawsuits over the "individual mandate" (penalty for not purchasing health insurance) have been field. In June, 2012, the Supreme Court ruled that that the ACA individual mandate was constitutional and constituted a tax, as those who do not obtain health insurance coverage are required to pay a penalty ("shared responsibility payment") to be collected by the IRS (p. 2). At the same time, it found the Medicaid expansion "unconstitutionally coercive of states" and ruled that the Secretary of Health and Human Services could not enforce this provision by withholding more than expansion Medicaid funding to states that choose to opt out of the Medicaid expansion outlined in the ACA (Musumeci, 2012, para. 1). See Perspectives: Why Did the Obama Administration Succeed With Health Care Reform?

PERSPECTIVES
WHY DID THE OBAMA ADMINISTRATION SUCCEED WITH HEALTH CARE REFORM WHEN OTHERS DID NOT?

President Bill Clinton had tried, unsuccessfully, to pass health care reform legislation during his time in office. Many other presidents had also tried this, beginning with Theodore Roosevelt, and including Truman, Nixon, and Carter. President Franklin D. Roosevelt's Social Security program and President Lyndon B. Johnson's reforms leading to Medicare and Medicaid coverage were large policy leaps, but access was not afforded all Americans.

Kingdon (2011) explains that the enormous size of the American health care system (about one sixth of our total economy), with many stakeholders (patients/consumers, health care providers, hospitals and clinics, pharmaceutical/managed care and insurance companies), makes change difficult. There are also many special interest groups among the stakeholders, as well as business interests, labor unions, and professional organizations, that control powerful lobbying interests in the nation's capital and across the country.

Also, our governmental system (separation of powers, legislative rules) makes it difficult to pass significant legislative changes — like health care reform — unless there is overwhelming support behind it. Americans also are not fond of higher taxes or big government programs, and most of them (about 85%) already had employer-sponsored or government health insurance. So, how was it possible to make policy changes despite these seemingly high odds? Kingdon (2011, p. 241) divides it into problems, policies, and the political stream leading to the "open window" permitting policy changes in health care reform (see Chapter 13 for more on Kingdon's Model).

Problems:
- Rising costs of health care, health insurance, and coverage gaps
- Rising long-term national debt and concerns over entitlement programs (e.g., Medicaid, Medicare, Social Security)
- Several academic studies/economic reports on our inefficient health care system
- Aging population and "baby boomer" increases in retirements
- Great Recession and loss of 700,000 jobs, along with employer-sponsored insurance for many
- Globalization revealed America's economic disadvantage compared to countries with national health plans (labor unions and businesses ultimately both agreed on need for changes)

These problems existed, to a lesser degree, during President Clinton's term. However, they became much more pressing issues during President Obama's first years in office.

Policies:
- It is important to forge a "consensus on policy options before a window opens" (p. 236).
  - Because health policy experts held markedly different views on how to solve the problem of health care reform during President Clinton's term, this was difficult to achieve. His wife, Hillary Clinton, led a task force on reform, but meetings were held in private and consensus was difficult to achieve. The final plan was "unfamiliar and untested" (p. 236) and was shot down by insurance companies, professional associations, and business interests.
- Policy experts had achieved some agreement by the time President Obama was elected and common views on the individual mandate, leaving private health insurance intact and expanding access to government insurance, were widely supported. Also, Congress was given the responsibility of drafting the legislation. This was not a "top-down" approach but allowed for conversation and consensus building in committees, as well as fostering public discussion.
- A similar approach was already in place in Massachusetts, which gave coverage to most residents of the state and was generally popular, despite some problems.

Political Stream:
- Health care had been a topic of debate during the 2008 election, with both Democratic candidates (Obama and Clinton) discussing it.
- Democrats now had a majority in the Senate and had enough votes so that they could prevent the opposition's filibuster. They also had a majority in the House. This was also the case when President Clinton was first elected, but not enough Senators to prevent a filibuster.
- Since President Clinton's attempt at reform, many of the interest groups involved had formed coalitions and were more open to reform. Members of President Obama's administration immediately began to meet with them and broker a "good deal" (p. 240).
  - Drug companies discounted prices for Medicare and gave up other income, and physicians, hospitals, AARP, and other groups also found common ground. Insurance companies had to give up their cost savings by using preexisting conditions to exclude individuals and lifetime caps on coverage; in return, they received new customers because of the individual mandate. Others that had opposed the Clinton reform were now neutral.
- The "strategic decision" (p. 240) to have Congress, not the administration, draft the health care reform bill helped build consensus — this was a lesson learned from the Clinton attempt at reform with an administration task force and bill that did not involve assistance from Congress in its development.
  - Some downside to this stance included a variety of bills that had to be melded into one final bill in order to be passed by both houses of Congress. At times, the Congress needed a nudge to keep things moving along, and this made it difficult for the administration that had promised a hands-off approach.
  - Some congressional opponents veered off course with wild claims of "death panels" and other off-the-wall misrepresentations.

With all of the pieces in place for President Obama, he moved quickly, before the "open window" closed. Despite attempts to repeal the legislation and several court challenges, the Patient Protection and Affordable Care Act was signed into law March 23, 2010. The U.S. Supreme Court upheld the majority of its provisions on June 28, 2012.

What are your views on this legislation and why? Did it go too far, or not far enough?

EFFECTS OF HEALTH ECONOMICS ON COMMUNITY HEALTH PRACTICE

Health economics has significantly affected community health and community health practice by advancing disincentives for efficient use of resources, incentives for illness care, and conflicts with public health values.

Disincentives for Efficient Use of Resources

All of the system structures that directly or indirectly promote cost escalation and prevent cost containment contribute to disincentives for efficient use of resources. For example, retrospective financial reimbursement, with its lack of setting limits, encourages spending on nonessential tests and treatments and drives up costs. Tax-deductible employer contributions for health care coverage and nontaxable employee health benefits encourage unnecessary use of services and result in cost increases. Some economists propose limiting or doing away with employer-sponsored health insurance tax deductions (Dranove, 2012). Lack of cost sharing by consumers and of financial risk for decisions made by providers may create further disincentives to keep costs down (Knickman & Kovner, 2015).

Public health has been affected in several ways. Abuse of resources in some parts of the system leads to depletion in other areas. The trend of diminished federal and state allocations has had profound effects on community and public health programs, and severe budget cuts have affected even basic public health services. The ACA has forced public health agencies to reexamine their traditional programs and seek new avenues for the provision of services, along with new revenue sources, and new collaborative health care partners (Hester et al., 2015). Public health agencies may need to consider working with other providers in Accountable Care Organizations and providing their expertise in community assessment and design of population-based interventions.

Incentives for Illness Care

The traditional U.S. health care system tends to promote illness, because health care providers have primarily been rewarded for treating problems, not for preventing them. Hospitals derive more income when their beds are full of sick or injured people. Health insurance plans compete, not by lowering costs or increasing quality but by avoiding the sick and seeking healthy enrollees—leaving many without access to necessary health care (IOM, 2013; Rambur, 2015).

The bulk of most reimbursable health services centers on treating illness or disability in hospitals, nursing homes, and ambulatory care facilities, using physicians or skilled nursing care in the home (home health services)—situations in which the individual must play the role of patient. Our disease-focused system of health care has been a basic problem, but, with ACA, that focus is moving more toward preventive services and cost-effective, quality care (IOM, 2013). Most preventive care is woefully inadequate and largely overlooked by both practitioners and patients alike: Remember, about half of all U.S. adults receive recommended health screening tests annually (Shires et al., 2012); health promotion nursing activities, such as comprehensive prenatal, maternal, and infant care; health education; childhood immunizations; and home services to enable older adults to live independently have not always been consistently covered by most insurers but are now generally covered through the ACA (Rice et al., 2014).

A system that has historically financially supported illness care affects public health practice in several ways. The number and severity of health problems in a community increase when individuals postpone care because they cannot afford visits to the doctor or clinic. Also, it has been more difficult in the past to encourage community clients to assume responsibility for their own health and to engage in self-care, prevention, and active health promotion. Furthermore, such illness-oriented incentives have created a basic societal valuing of illness care that, conversely, devalues wellness care. Health promotion and disease prevention efforts now need to be emphasized. In communities where a greater proportion of community health practice is spent in the treatment of disorders and rehabilitation, resources for prevention and health promotion need to be developed (Hester et al., 2015).

Prepayment methods and the growth of managed care have been positive moves in the direction of a more wellness-oriented financial incentive structure. An HMO has the incentive to offer preventive and health-promoting services, such as early detection and treatment of symptoms, regular physical examinations, and health teaching, because the HMO loses money when it must pay out for expensive tertiary care. With health care reform, there is a change in focus as newer *accountable health care organizations* proliferate, and a variety of innovative, evidence-based programs, such as the YMCA's Diabetes Prevention Program, become more widely available. In this yearlong, group-based program, trained lifestyle coaches promote physical activity and healthy eating with prediabetic individuals. Over 30 different health plans now include this program in their coverage, as it has shown that participants lost 5% to 7% of body weight and their chance of developing diabetes greatly decreased (Frist & Rivlin, 2015).

Managed Care and Public Health Values

Initially, MCOs focused on event-driven cost avoidance. Strategies included decreasing inpatient days, decreasing specialty physician use, using physician extenders, and implementing provider discounting. This evolved into a second stage, in which the principal objective was to control resource intensity and improve the delivery process. Strategies used to meet this objective included capitation of specialist costs, controls on units of service, patient-focused redesign, clinical pathways, and total quality management. But emphasis is shifting to a focus on health promotion and population health. Community assessments are an important part of this approach, so that high-risk groups can be identified and provided early interventions. Case management of individuals with chronic illness is also a focus.

Community health assessments could become standard quality tools for not only public health interventions but also health care in general (Feldman, Hile, & Weinberg, 2011). The ACA requires hospitals to conduct regular community assessments, and many have partnered with LHDs to do so (NACCHO, 2014). Community assessments establish the baseline health status of a community and measure changes in the health of the community over time. Community health assessments must include source information that is both primary (health status assessment surveys, focus groups, and satisfaction surveys) and secondary (data collected by public health agencies and state agencies, such as birth rates, mortality rates, and incidence of communicable diseases in the community). Health care reform legislation includes a requirement for community needs assessment every three years for state-licensed, tax-exempt health organizations such as hospitals and imposes a $50,000 annual penalty if this is not done. Prioritization of health needs and a description of community resources are to be included, as in input from those with expertise in public health (Adams, 2011). See Chapter 15 for more on Community Assessment.

Improving the health status of a community mandates that health care agencies be actively involved in accurately assessing the community's health status and the major issues facing the community. This involves health teaching and health promotion, as well as developing community action plans to promote collaboration and focus on early intervention and treatment (Brownson, Baker, Leet, Gillespie, & True, 2011). Are these not the proposals that public health advocates have been making for more than a century?

Competition in health care is a reality with which public health practice must cope. Although competition offers several benefits, it poses some dilemmas for community health that may be difficult to resolve. Values underlying the competition model can be in direct conflict with several basic public health values (Erwin & Brownson, 2017). With the new focus on coordination and collaboration in health care reform, this emphasis on competition may be diminished.

Public health is committed to serving all persons in need, regardless of ability to pay. Traditionally, the competition model has focused on individuals and has been oriented to the present. Public health is concerned with aggregates and is future oriented, emphasizing prevention. Competition establishes relatively fixed limits for service, whereas public health must remain flexible if it is to respond to the health needs of the entire population. These dramatic differences are beginning to blur and, out of necessity, will continue to be less adversarial and more collegial. By shifting their focus to public health as a systems outcome, health care insurers can create several positive changes, including a safe environment, wholesome nutrition, healthy lifestyle, adequate education, sufficient income, meaningful spirituality, challenging work, recreation, and functional families (Brownson et al., 2011). As more people are covered by ACA, public health department clinics may scale down or chose to "claim reimbursement from private and public insurance" (Bovbjerg, Ormand, & Waidman, 2011, p. 1). Public health needs to embrace EHRs, big data, and research that validate interventions and services; we also need to get better at communicating our value in promoting the nation's health (Bovbjerg et al., 2011).

Over time, a greater number and variety of services have been offered through public health agencies. An early nurse-directed diabetes management program at a county public health clinic in Los Angeles County reflects the potential benefits of public health services for clients of MCOs and other private health care plans. PHNs were able to significantly reduce the numbers of urgent care and ED visits, along with hospitalizations, for diabetic patients from a minority population (Davidson, Ansari, & Karlan, 2007). Another example is the University of Pittsburgh Medical Center Health Plan program utilizing certified diabetes educators as "hub resources to a network of diverse care management services" (Siminerio, DePasquale, Johnson, & Thearle, 2015, p. 71). Through the use of patient-centered medical homes, ongoing staff training and support, and teaching and collaboration with community members (e.g., nursing homes, mobile clinics, coaches/ community education programs), mean A1C reductions were noted in high-risk patients and staff reported greater confidence in their ability to work with diabetic patients. Working together, better health can be achieved for large numbers of patients.

IMPLICATIONS FOR COMMUNITY HEALTH NURSING

The structure and functions of the health care delivery system, as well as particular legislative acts, have had a significant impact on community health nursing. PHNs have had to adapt to a constantly changing system. They have developed innovative modes of service delivery, such as community-based nursing centers for health education, counseling, and screening of low-income populations. They have learned to practice in a variety of settings extending beyond homes, worksites, schools, churches, clinics, and voluntary agencies. They have acquired skills in teamwork, leadership, and political activism. They have recognized the importance of outcomes research to document the value of nursing interventions with at-risk populations (Kulbok, Thatcher, Park, & Meszaros, 2012). As with public health agencies, PHNs will need to become adept at EHRs. The benefits include the use of a common language, a better connection between nursing assessment and interventions, as well as meaningful use of data to recognize trends, patterns, and quality indicators. PHNs in the state of Washington began using a Web-based EHR coordinated with the Omaha System to "extract meaningful data and measure outcomes" (Plemmons, Lipton, Fong, & Acosta, 2012). This enabled them to show administrators that services and resources were being used appropriately and effectively. PHNs were also able to use the data to better guide their practice, strategic planning, and in policy development. Data collected through this program include source of referral, demographic information, initial patient assessment (knowledge, behavior, status ratings for problems identified), and any changes noted on subsequent visits. Increased patient referral, outreach, data collection, and nurse performance, along with improved patient care, have been noted by PHNs. Community nurses should recognize the benefits accrued with the use of EHRs and promote their use. See Chapter 10 for more on EHRs.

At the national, state, and local level, community health nursing has important ties to both private and public health agencies. When serving in the public sector, nurses often provide consultation, serve on boards, volunteer their services, or collaborate with private sector health organizations to ensure quality and access of care to the broader community. Examples include joint efforts to promote certain types of health legislation and collaboration to produce and disseminate health education materials targeting specific populations (Bowman et al., 2012; Evans, 2013). Sometimes, public health nursing services operate within a single organization that combines public and private sector organization and funding. An example is the Metropolitan Visiting Nurse Association of Minneapolis, Minnesota, which is a combined public–private agency supported by taxes and voluntary funds (MVNA, 2014).

Community health nurses also have many opportunities to serve in international health. Some work with the WHO, PAHO, or other agencies to assist in direct care projects such as famine relief, immunization efforts, or nutritional screening and education programs (see Chapter 16). Other nurses serve as health planners, assist with policy development, conduct collaborative needs assessment projects and research efforts, or engage in program development (Kulbok et al., 2012).

SUMMARY

Many factors and events have influenced the current structure, function, and financing of community health services. Understanding this background gives the community health nurse a stronger base for planning for the health of the population under her care.

Historically, health care has progressed unevenly, marked by numerous influences. Primitive practices of early centuries were replaced with more advanced sanitary measures by the Greeks and Romans. The Middle Ages saw a serious health decline in Europe, with raging epidemics leading to extensive 19th-century reform efforts in England and, later, in the United States.

Organized health care in the United States developed slowly. Public health problems, such as the need for isolation of persons with communicable diseases and control of environmental pollution, prompted the gradual development of official interventions. For example, quarantines to control the spread of communicable disease were imposed in the late 1700s. Sanitary reform was pursued more vigorously during the 1800s. Local and then state health departments were formed starting in the late 1700s. By the early 1900s, the federal government had assumed a more active role in public health, with a proliferation of health, education, and welfare services.

For years, efforts to address community health needs have been made by public agencies and private individuals. These two arms of service were not well coordinated in the past. Only gradually and recently have they begun to work together to form an emerging health care system.

The public arm of health services includes all government, tax-supported health agencies and occurs at four levels: local, state, national, and international. Each level deals with the health needs of the population encompassed within its boundaries. Each level has a different structure and set of functions. Public health services include three core public health functions: assessment, policy development, and assurance.

Private health services are the unofficial arm of the community health system. They include voluntary nonprofit agencies as well as privately owned (proprietary) and for-profit agencies. Their financial support comes from voluntary contributions, bequests, or fees. Private health organizations often supplement and complement the work of official agencies.

The delivery and financing of community health services have been significantly affected by various legislative acts. These acts have prompted such innovations as health insurance and assistance for people who are poor, elderly, or disabled; money to train health personnel and conduct health research; standards for health planning and delivery; health protection for workers on the job; and the financing of health services.

Health care economics studies the production, distribution, and consumption of health care goods and services to maximize the use of scarce resources to benefit the most people. This science underlies the financing of the health care system. It is influenced by microeconomics as well as macroeconomics.

Health care is funded through public and private sources, which fall into three categories: third-party payers, direct consumer payment, and private support. Health care services have been reimbursed either retrospectively, typical of FFS plans, or prospectively, typical of most preferred provider organizations (PPOs) or managed care plans.

Several trends and issues have influenced community health care financing and delivery and are important in understanding health care economics and helping to improve community health. They include cost control, financial access, managed care, health care rationing, competition and regulation, managed competition, universal coverage, a single-payer system, and health care reform.

The changing nature of health care financing has adversely affected community health and its practice two ways: (1) because the health care system traditionally has reimbursed only for treatment of people who are ill or disabled, with no reward for health promotion and prevention efforts, it has promoted incentives to focus only on illness care; and (2) the competition model, which has long driven up health care costs and eliminated many from being able to afford health care services, has generated a conflict with the basic public health values of health promotion and disease prevention for all persons. Health care reform has reduced the number of uninsured Americans, but access for many people is still difficult. Some health policy experts feel that reform did not go far enough, and that waste still exists. The United States remains the only industrialized nation without some type of universal health coverage. We also rank significantly lower than most other developed countries on health indicators, such as infant mortality and life expectancy, and we spend the highest percentage of GDP on health care.

PHNs can lead the effort in making health care more accessible to all citizens and encourage policies and practices that promote health, rather than reward illness. The ability to utilize data provided through EHRs can be helpful to PHNs in developing programs and interventions. PHNs can serve in many capacities and in private or government settings, including work with international health organizations.

ACTIVITIES TO PROMOTE **CRITICAL THINKING**

1. If possible, interview someone at your local health department. How do the services offered compare with those listed in this chapter? How do PHNs in this agency incorporate the core public health functions?
2. Look up your state health department's Web site. Compare its functions with the core public health functions described in this chapter. Identify areas where improvement may be needed.
3. If possible, conduct an interview on-site or by telephone with someone at a private health agency, voluntary agency, or community-based NGO. Compare the agency's functions with those listed in this chapter for private health agencies. Describe how this agency works collaboratively with public health agencies and other community organizations. What is the role of the nurse in this agency? How does the role compare to PHNs in the local public health agency?
4. Look up various international health agencies online. Explore Web sites that discuss current international health care issues. What topics are of current concern? For example, are new epidemics or emerging strains of a virus being highlighted? What could (or should) a community health nurse in your local community do with this information?
5. With your classmates, debate the pros and cons of a strong federal role in health care provision, as opposed to decentralized (state and local) control.
6. Interview two consumers about their perception of the problems and strengths of our health care system. What are their thoughts and feelings about health care reform (the Affordable Care Act [ACA] enacted in 2010)? Select people who represent distinctly different age groups and life situations, such as a single 25-year-old mother of three children making minimum wage and a 75-year-old widower.
7. Form two teams and debate the advantages and disadvantages of managed competition as opposed to mandatory universal coverage. What are the advantages and disadvantages of a single-payer system? Is further health care reform feasible in the United States? What is the most efficient way of ensuring universal coverage, as evidenced by other countries?
8. Locate recent articles and legislation on health care reform, strengths and weakness of the public health system, and the uninsured population. What are the most common themes on each issue? What most surprised you about your results?
9. Talk with your classmates and other students at your college or university about their access to health care and if they have some type of health insurance. Does your campus have a student health center? What services are offered there? What are the average costs to students?

REFERENCES

Abrams, S. E. (2004). From function to competency in public health nursing, 1931 to 2003. *Public Health Nursing, 21*(5), 507–510.

Adams, A. (2011, August 4). *Guidance issued on community health needs assessments for exempt hospitals.* Retrieved from http://www.healthcarereforminsights.com/2011/08/04/guidance-issued-on-community-health-needs-assessments-for-exempt-hospitals/

Agency for Healthcare Research & Quality. (2014). *Patient safety primer: Never events.* Retrieved from https://psnet.ahrq.gov/primers/primer/3/never-events

Agency for Health Research and Quality. (2015, April). Health care-associated infections. Retrieved from https://psnet.ahrq.gov/primers/primer/7/health-care-associated-infections

American Nurses Association (ANA). (2014, June 18). *Healthcare transformation: The Affordable Care Act and more.* Retrieved from http://nursingworld.org/MainMenuCategories/Policy-Advocacy/HealthSystemReform/AffordableCareAct.pdf

American Public Health Association (APHA). (2010, March 15). *APHA strongly supports congressional efforts to finalize comprehensive health reform this week.* Retrieved from http://www.apha.org/about/news/pressreleases/2010/healtHREForm3_15.htm

American Public Health Association (APHA). (2012, June). *The Prevention and Public Health Fund: A critical investment in our nation's physical and fiscal health.* Washington, DC: Author. Retrieved from https://www.apha.org/~/media/files/pdf/factsheets/apha_prevfundbrief_june2012.ashx

Angeles, J., & Park, E. (2009, September 13). *"Upcoding" problem exacerbates overpayments to Medicare Advantage plans.* Retrieved from http://www.cbpp.org/research/upcoding-problem-exacerbates-overpayments-to-medicare-advantage-plans

Agrawal, S., Taitsman, J., & Cassel, C. (2013). Educating physicians about responsible management of finite resources. *Journal of the American Medical Association, 309,* 1115–1116. doi: 10.1001/jama.2013.1013.

Arbel, R., & Greenberg, D. (2016). Rethinking cost-effectiveness in the era of zero healthcare spending growth. *International Journal for Equity in Health, 15,* 33. doi: 10.1186/s12939-016-0326-8.

Archer, D. (2011, September 20). *Medicare is more efficient than private insurance.* Retrieved from http://healthaffairs.org/blog/2011/09/20/medicare-is-more-efficient-than-private-insurance/

Arrow, K. (2004). Uncertainty and the welfare economics of medical care. *Bulletin of the World Health Organization, 82*(2), 141–149. Retrieved from http://www.who.int/bulletin/volume/82/2/PHCBP.pdf

Arrow, K., Auerbach, A., Bertko, J., Brownlee, S., Casalino, J., Cooper, F. J., ... van de Ven, W. P. (2009). Toward a 21st-century health care system: Recommendations for health care reform. *Annals of Internal Medicine, 150*(7), 493–495.

Association of Public Health Nurses (APHN). (n.d.). *APHN's history.* Retrieved from http://www.phnurse.org/APHNs-Story

Association of State and Territorial Health Officials (ASTHO). (2014). *ASTHO profile of state public health, volume three.* Washington, DC: Author. Retrieved from http://www.astho.org/Profile/Volume-Three/

Austin, D. A. (2014). Medical debt as a cause of consumer bankruptcy. *Maine Law Review, 67,* 1–23.

Baicker, K., Taubman, S. L., Allen, H. L., Bernstein, M., Gruber, J. H., Newhouse, J. P., ... Finkelstein, A. N. (2013). The Oregon experiment: Effects of Medicaid on clinical outcomes. *New England Journal of Medicine, 368,* 1713–1722. doi: 10.1056/NEJMsa1212321.

Barry, M. A., Centra, L., Pratt, D., & Gioradano, L. (1998). *Where do the dollars go? Measuring local public health expenditures.* Washington, DC: National Association of County and City Health Officials.

Bernard, D., Banthin, J., & Encinosa, W. (2009). Wealth, income, and the affordability of health insurance. *Health Affairs, 28*(3), 887–896.

Bezruchka, S. (2012). The hurrier I go the behinder I get: The deteriorating international ranking of US health status. *Public Health, 33,* 157. doi: 10.1146/annurev-publhealth-031811-124649.

Blue Cross Blue Shield. (2016). *Blue facts: Healthcare coverage designed for your community, accessible across the country.* Retrieved from http://www.bcbs.com/healthcare-news/press-center/blue-facts.html

Blumenthal, D., & Osborn, R. (2013, April 30). *In pursuit of better care at lower costs: The value of cross-national learning.* Retrieved from http://www.commonwealthfund.org/publications/blog/2013/apr/the-value-of-cross-national-learning

Bodycombe, D. (2013, February). *More data in health care will enable predictive modeling advances.* Retrieved from http://www.managedcaremag.com/archives/2013/2/more-data-health-care-will-enable-predictive-modeling-advances

Boseley, S. (2010, October 28). *Public health advances "could prevent 200,000 premature deaths a year."* Retrieved from http://www.theguardian.com/politics/2010/oct/28/michael-marmot-health-prospects-report

Bowman, S., Unwin, N., Critchley, J., Capewell, S., Husseini, A., Maziak, W., ... Ahmad, B. (2012). Use of evidence to support healthy public policy: A policy effectiveness-feasibility loop. *Bulletin of the World Health Organization,* Article ID BLT.12.104968. Retrieved from http://www.who.int/bulletin/online_first/12-104968.pdf

Bowser, R. (2015). Race and rationing. *Health Matrix, 25,* 87.

Bovbjerg, R. R., Ormand, B. A., & Waidman, T. A. (2011). *What directions for public health under the Affordable Care Act?* Retrieved from http://www.nhchc.org/wp-content/uploads/2011/09/Urban-public-health-ACA-Nov-2011.pdf

Briesacher, B. A., Ross-Degnan, D., Wagner, A., Fouayzi, H., Zhang, F., Gurwitz, J., ... Soumerai, S. B. (2010). Out-of-pocket burden of health care spending and the adequacy of the Medicare Part D low-income subsidy. *Medical Care, 48*(6), 503–509.

Brill, J. (2015, January 26). Competition in the health care markets. *Health Affairs Blog.* Retrieved from http://healthaffairs.org/blog/2015/01/26/competition-in-health-care-markets/

Bouffard, K. (2015, April 6). Blue Cross incentives save $50 million in health care costs. *The Detroit News.* Retrieved from http://www.detroitnews.com/story/business/2015/04/06/blue-cross-incentives/25392361/

Brownson, R. C., Baker, E., Leet, T., Gillespie, K., & True, W. (2011). *Evidence-based public health* (2nd ed.). New York, NY: Oxford University Press.

Bureau of Labor Statistics. (n.d.). *Definitions of health insurance terms.* Retrieved from http://www.bls.gov/ncs/ebs/sp/healthterms.pdf

Cabin, W., Himmelstein, D. U., Siman, M. L., & Woolhandler, S. (2014). For-profit Medicare home health agencies' costs appear higher and quality appears lower compared to nonprofit agencies. *Health Affairs, 33*(8), 1460–1465.

Callahan, D. (2009). *Taming the beloved beast: How medical technology costs are destroying our health care system.* Princeton, NJ: Princeton University Press.

Cammarosano, L. (2015, May 31). *Bankruptcy in America.* Retrieved from https://smaulgld.com/bankruptcy-in-america/

Case Western Reserve University. (2014). *QSEN.* Retrieved from http://qsen.org/about-qsen/

Catlin, C. A., & Howard, A. (2015, November 19). *History of health spending in the United States: 1960–2013.* Retrieved from https://www.cms.gov/Research-Statistics-Data-and-Systems/Statistics-Trends-and-Reports/NationalHealthExpendData/Downloads/HistoricalNHEPaper.pdf

Cauchi, R. (2012, January 27). *State legislation and actions challenging certain health reforms, 2011–2012.* Retrieved from http://www.ncsl.org/issues-research/health/state-laws-and-actions-challenging-aca.aspx

Centers for Disease Control and Prevention (CDC). (2015a). *Core functions of public health and how they relate to the 10 essential services.* Retrieved from http://www.cdc.gov/nceh/ehs/ephli/core_ess.htm

Centers for Disease Control and Prevention (CDC). (2015b). *National Center for Health Statistics: Celebrating 50 years.* Retrieved from http://www.cdc.gov/nchs/about/50th_anniversary.htm

Centers for Disease Control and Prevention (CDC). (2016). *HAI data and statistics.* Retrieved from http://www.cdc.gov/hai/surveillance/

Centers for Medicare and Medicaid Services (CMS). (n.d.a). *The nation's health dollar ($2.5 trillion) calendar year 2009: Where it went.* Retrieved from https://www.cms.gov/nationalhealthexpend-data/downloads/PieChartSourcesExpenditures2009.pdf

Centers for Medicare and Medicaid Services (CMS). (n.d.b). *National health expenditures 2009 highlights.* Retrieved from https://www.cms.gov/nationalhealthexpenddata/downloads/highlights.pdf

Centers for Medicare and Medicaid Services (CMS). (2008). *Never events: SMDL #08-004.* Retrieved from https://downloads.cms.gov/cmsgov/archived-downloads/SMDL/downloads/smd073108.pdf

Centers for Medicare and Medicaid Services (CMS). (2011). *History overview.* Retrieved from https://www.cms.gov/history/

Centers for Medicare and Medicaid Services. (2012). *CMS report to Congress: Assessing the feasibility of extending the hospital acquired conditions (HAC) IPPS payment policy to Non-IPPS settings.* Retrieved from https://innovation.cms.gov/Files/x/Hosp AcquiredConditionsRTC.pdf

Centers for Medicare and Medicaid Services (CMS). (2013). Medicare program; hospital inpatient prospective payment systems for acute care hospitals and the long-term care hospital prospective payment system and fiscal year 2014 rates; quality reporting requirements for specific providers; hospital conditions of participation; payment policies related to patient status. Final rules. *Federal Register, 78*(160), 50495–51040.

Centers for Medicare and Medicaid Services (CMS). (2015a). *National health expenditures 2014 highlights.* Retrieved from https://www.cms.gov/research-statistics-data-and-systems/statistics-trends-and-reports/nationalhealthexpenddata/downloads/highlights.pdf

Centers for Medicare and Medicaid Services (CMS). (2015b). *National health expenditures: Nominal dollars, real dollars, price indexes, and annual percent change: Selected calendar years 1980–2014.* Retrieved from https://www.cms.gov/Research-Statistics-Data-and-Systems/Statistics-Trends-and-Reports/NationalHealthExpendData/NationalHealthAccountsHistorical.html

Chandra, A., & Skinner, J. S. (2011). Technology growth and expenditure growth in health care (Working Paper No. 16953, Summary). *National Bureau of Economic Research: Bulletin on Aging and Health, 2*, 1–2.

Christopher, A. S., McCormick, D., Woolhandler, S., Himmelstein, D. U., Bor, D. H., & Wilper, A. P. (2016). Access to care and chronic disease outcomes among Medicaid-insured persons versus the uninsured. *American Journal of Public Health, 106*(1), 63–69.

Claxton, G., & Levitt, L. (2015, August 25). *How many employers could be affected by the Cadillac tax plan? Kaiser Family Foundation.* Retrieved from http://kff.org/health-costs/issue-brief/how-many-employers-could-be-affected-by-the-cadillac-plan-tax/

Clifton, G. L. (2009). *Flatlined: Resuscitating American medicine.* New Brunswick, NJ: Rutgers University Press.

Cockayne, E. (2007). *Hubbub, filth, noise and stench in England 1600–1770.* New Haven, CT: Yale University Press.

Collins, S. (2007). *Congressional testimony: Universal health insurance: Why it is essential to a high performing health system and why design matters.* Retrieved from http://www.commonwealthfund.org/Publications/Testimonies/2007/Nov/Congressional-Testimony–Widening-Gaps-in-Health-Insurance-Coverage-in-the-United-States–The-Need-f.aspx

Collins, S. R., Gunja, M., Rasmussen, P. W., Beutel, S., & Doty, M. M. (2015a). *Are marketplace plans affordable? Consumer perspectives from the Commonwealth Fund Affordable Care Act tracking survey, March-May 2015.* Retrieved from http://www.commonwealthfund.org/publications/issue-briefs/2015/sep/are-marketplace-plans-affordable

Collins, S. R., Gunja, M., Doty, M. M., & Beutel, S. (2015b). *How high is America's health care cost burden? Findings from the Commonwealth Fund health care affordability tracking survey, July–August 2015.* Retrieved from http://www.commonwealthfund.org/publications/issue-briefs/2015/nov/how-high-health-care-burden

Collins, S. R., Rasmussen, P. W., Beutel, S., & Doty, M. M. (2015c, May 20). *The problem of underinsurance and how rising deductibles will make it worse: Findings from the Commonwealth fund biennial health insurance survey, 2014.* Retrieved from http://www.commonwealthfund.org/publications/issue-briefs/2015/may/problem-of-underinsurance

Collins, S. R., Schoen, C., Davis, K., Gauthier, A. K., & Schoenbaum, S. C. (2007, October). *A roadmap to health insurance for all: Principles for reform.* Retrieved from http://www.commonwealthfund.org/usr_doc/Collins_roadmaphltinsforall_1066.pdf?section=4039

Commonwealth Fund. (2015). *U.S. health system ranks last among eleven countries on measures of access, equity, quality, efficiency, and healthy lives.* Retrieved from http://www.commonwealthfund.org/publications/press-releases/2014/jun/us-health-system-ranks-last

Congressional Budget Office. (2005, May). *High-cost Medicare beneficiaries.* Retrieved from http://www.cbo.gov/ftpdocs/63xx/doc6332/05-03-MediSpending.pdf

Congressional Budget Office. (2009). *The long-term outlook for Medicare, Medicaid, and total health care spending.* Retrieved from http://www.cbo.gov/ftpdocs/102xx/doc10297/Chapter2.5.1.shtml#1091397

Corlette, S., Volk, J., Berenson, R., & Feder, J. (2014). *Narrow provider networks in new health plans: Balancing affordability with access to quality care.* Retrieved from http://www.urban.org/health.policy/url.cfm

Corrigan, J. M., Wakeam, E., Gandhi, T. K., & Leape, L. L. (2015). On the safe side: The move to value-based payment models could mean improvements in patient safety. *Healthcare Financial Management, 69*(8), 94–97.

Cox, C., Kamal, R., Jankiewicz, A., & Rousseau, D. (2016). Recent trends in prescription drug costs. *Journal of the American Medical Association, 315*, 1326–1326. doi: 10.1001/jama.2016.2646.

Coughlin, T. A., Holahan, J., Caswell, K., & McGrath, M. (2014). *Uncompensated care for the uninsured in 2013: A detailed examination.* Retrieved from http://kff.org/report-section/uncompensated-care-for-the-uninsured-in-2013-a-detailed-examination-introduction/

Cubanski, J., Lyons, B., Neuman, T., Snyder, L., Jankiewicz, A., & Rousseau, D. (2015). Medicaid and Medicare trends and challenges. *Journal of the American Medical Association, 314*, 329–329. doi: 10.1001/jama.2015.8130.

Cunningham, P. (2011, May 11). *Nonurgent use of hospital emergency departments.* Retrieved from http://hschange.org/CONTENT/1204/1204.pdf

Cutler, D. M. (2005). *Your money or your life: Strong medicine for America's health care system.* New York, NY: Oxford University Press.

Cutshaw, C. A., Woolhandler, S., Himmelstein, D. U., & Robertson, C. (2016). Medical causes and consequences of home foreclosures. *International Journal of Health Services, 45*(1), 36–47.

Davidson, M., Ansari, A., & Karlan, V. (2007). Effect of a nurse-directed diabetes disease management program on urgent care/emergency room visits and hospitalizations in a minority population. *Diabetes Care, 30*(2), 224–227.

Davidson, M. B., Blanco-Castellanos, M., & Duran, P. (2010). Integrating nurse-directed diabetes management into a primary care setting. *American Journal of Managed Care, 16*(9), 652–656.

Davis, K., Stremikis, K., Squires, D., & Schoen, C. (2014). *Mirror, mirror on the wall: How the performance of the US healthcare system compares internationally.* Retrieved from http://www.resbr.net.br/wp-content/uploads/historico/Espelhoespelhomeu.pdf

Dash, S. J., Corlette, S., & Thomas, A. (2014, July). *Implementing the Affordable Care Act: State action on quality improvement in state-based marketplaces.* Retrieved from http://www.commonwealthfund.org/~/media/files/publications/issuebrief/2014/jul/1763_dash_implementing_aca_state_action_quality_improvement_rb_v2.pdf

Day, B., Himmelstein, D., Broder, M., & Woolhandler, S. (2015). The Affordable Care Act and medical loss ratios: No impact first three years. *International Journal of Health Services, 45*(1), 127–131.

deChesnay, M., & Anderson, B. A. (2012). *Caring for the vulnerable: Perspectives in nursing theory, practice, and research* (3rd ed.). Burlington, MA: Jones & Bartlett Learning.

DeLeire, T., Joynt, K., & McDonald, R. (2014). *Impact of insurance expansion on hospital uncompensated care costs in 2014.* Retrieved from https://aspe.hhs.gov/pdf-report/impact-insurance-expansion-hospital-uncompensated-care-costs-2014

Dickman, S. L., Himmelstein, D. U., McCormick, D., & Woolhandler, S. (2015). Health and financial consequences of 24 states' decision to opt out of Medicaid expansion. *International Journal of Health Services, 45*(1), 133–142.

Dilger, R. J., & Boyd, E. (2014, July 15). *Block grants: Perspectives and controversies.* Congressional Research Service. Retrieved from https://www.fas.org/sgp/crs/misc/R40486.pdf

Doctors Without Borders. (n.d.). *About us: History and principles.* Retrieved from http://www.doctorswithoutborders.org/aboutus/?ref=main-menu

Dowling, W. L. (1979). Prospective rate setting: Concept and practice. *Topics in Health Care Financing, 3*(2), 35–42.

Dranove, D. (2008). *Code red: An economist explains how to revive the healthcare system without destroying it.* Princeton, NJ: Princeton University Press.

Dranove, D. (2012). Recommendations for improving the health system: Academics speak out. *Health Management, Policy and Innovation, 1*(1), 44–59.

Dranove, D. (2014, July 12). *In ACO era, physicians will still play a leading—but changing role.* Retrieved from http://www.modernhealthcare.com/article/20140712/magazine/307129979

Drevdahl, D. (2002). Social justice or market justice? The paradoxes of public health partnerships with managed care. *Public Health Nursing, 19*(3), 161–169.

Duffy, J. (1990). *The sanitarians: A history of American public health.* Urbana, IL: University of Illinois Press.

Duijmelinck, D., & van de Ven, W. (2016). What can Europe learn from the managed care backlash in the United States? *Health Policy, 120*(5), 509–518.

Enthoven, A. C. (2009a). *Building a health marketplace that works.* Retrieved from http://healthaffairs.org/blog/2009/07/31/building-a-health-marketplace-that-works/

Enthoven, A. C. (2009b). Integrated delivery systems: The cure for fragmentation. *American Journal of Managed Care, 15,* s284–s290.

Enthoven, A. C., & Wynand, P. M. (2007). Going Dutch: Managed-competition health insurance in the Netherlands. *New England Journal of Medicine, 357,* 2421–2423.

Erwin, P. C., & Brownson, R. C. (Eds.). (2017). *Scutchfield and Keck's Principles of public health practice* (4th ed.). Boston, MA: Cengage Learning.

Estes, C. L., Chapman, S. A., Dodd, C., Hollister, B., & Harrington, C. (2013). *Health policy: Crisis and reform* (6th ed.). Sudbury, MA: Jones & Bartlett Publishers.

Evans, K. A. (2013, June 9). *Health policy: What's your role?* Retrieved from http://nurse-practitioners-and-physician-assistants.advanceweb.com/Columns/Role-Growth/Health-Policy-Whats-Your-Role.aspx

Faguet, G. B. (2013). *The Affordable Care Act: A missed opportunity, a better way forward.* New York, NY: Algora Publishing.

Falla, R. (n.d.). *Massachusetts State Senate research internship report: The state of our current health care system.* Retrieved from http://iop.harvard.edu/sites/default/files_new/Programs/MA_HealthPolicyPaper.pdf

Feldman, M., Hile, S., & Weinberg, G. (2011). A community needs assessment to inform HIV and substance abuse prevention services for Black and Latino young men who have sex with men in New York City. *Journal of Gay Lesbian Social Services, 23*(4), 465–506.

Fletcher, J., & Wolfe, B. L. (2012). *Increasing our understanding of the health-income gradient in children.* Retrieved from http://www.nber.org/papers/w18639.pdf

Food and Agriculture Organization. (2016). *About FAO.* Retrieved from http://www.fao.org/about/en/

Food and Drug Administration (FDA). (2014). *LASIK Quality of Life Collaboration Project.* Retrieved from http://www.fda.gov/MedicalDevices/ProductsandMedicalProcedures/SurgeryandLifeSupport/LASIK/ucm190291.htm

Frakt, A. B. (2011). How much do hospitals cost shift? A review of the evidence. *Milbank Quarterly, 89,* 90–130. doi: 10.1111/j.1468-0009.2011.00621.x.

Frist, B., & Rivlin, A. (2015, May 28). The power of prevention: U.S. health care reform should focus on prevention efforts to cut skyrocketing costs. *U.S. News & World Report.* Retrieved from http://www.usnews.com/opinion/blogs/policy-dose/2015/05/28/focus-on-prevention-to-cut-us-health-care-costs

Gabel, J. R., Whitmore, H., Call, A., Green, M., Oran, R., & Stromberg, S. (2016, January 28). *Modest changes in 2016 health insurance marketplace premiums and insurer participation.* Retrieved from http://www.commonwealthfund.org/publications/blog/2016/jan/2016-health-insurance-marketplace-premiums

Gaffney, A., Woolhandler, S., & Himmelstein, D. (2016). Moving forward from the Affordable Care Act to a single-payer system. *American Journal of Public Health, 106*(6), 987–988.

Galewitz, P. (2011, June 1). Medicaid to stop paying for hospital mistakes. *Kaiser Health News.* Retrieved from http://www.kaiserhealthnews.org/Stories/2011/June/01/medicaid-hospital-medical-error-payment-short-take.aspx

Garfield, R., Damico, A., Cox, C., Claxton, G., & Levitt, R. (2016). *New estimates of eligibility for ACA coverage among the uninsured.* Retrieved from http://kff.org/health-reform/issue-brief/new-estimates-of-eligibility-for-aca-coverage-among-the-uninsured/

Garfield, R., & Young, K. (2015). *Adults who remained uninsured at the end of 2014.* Retrieved from http://kff.org/health-reform/issue-brief/adults-who-remained-uninsured-at-the-end-of-2014/

Gaynor, M. (2013, August 9). *Beyond the Affordable Care Act: A framework for getting health care reform right.* Retrieved from http://thehealthcareblog.com/blog/2013/08/09/beyond-the-affordable-care-act-a-framework-for-getting-health-care-reform-right/

Gladwell, M. (2005, August 29). The moral-hazard myth. *The New Yorker.* Retrieved from http://www.newyorker.com/archive/2005/08/29/050829fa_fact

Glazer, J., & McGuire, T. G. (2011). Gold and silver health plans: Accommodating demand heterogeneity in managed competition. *Journal of Health Economics, 30*(5), 1011–1019.

Gold, J. (2015, September 14). *Accountable Care Organizations, explained.* Retrieved from http://khn.org/news/aco-accountable-care-organization-faq/

Greene, V. W. (2001). Personal hygiene and life expectancy improvements since 1850: Historic and epidemiologic associations. *American Journal of Infection Control, 29*(4), 203–206.

Haberkorn, J. (2012, February 23). *The prevention and public health fund.* Retrieved from http://www.healthaffairs.org/healthpolicybriefs/brief.php?brief_id=63

Haviland, A. M., Elliott, M. N., Weech-Maldonado, R., Hambarsoomian, K., Orr, N., & Hays, R. D. (2012). Racial/ethnic disparities in Medicare Part D experiences. *Medical Care, 50*(Suppl.), s40–s47.

Hayden, T. P. (2014). Using the medical loss ratio to incentivize the adoption of innovative medical technology. *Vanderbilt Journal of Entertainment & Technology Law, 17,* 239–265.

Healthcare.gov. (n.d.a). *Glossary: Community rating.* Retrieved from https://www.healthcare.gov/glossary/community-rating/

Healthcare.gov. (n.d.b). *Glossary: Recession.* Retrieved from https://www.healthcare.gov/glossary/rescission/

Healthcare.gov. (2011). *Key features of the Affordable Care Act, by year.* Retrieved from http://www.healthcare.gov/law/timeline/full.html

Healthcare.gov. (2015, August 13). *About the law.* Retrieved from http://www.hhs.gov/healthcare/facts-and-features/key-features-of-aca/index.html

Healy, M. A., Mullard, A. J., Campbell, D. A., & Dimick, J. B. (2016, May 11). *Hospital and payer costs associated with surgical complications.* Retrieved from http://archsurg.jamanetwork.com/article.aspx?articleid=2519879

Hellander, I., Himmelstein, D. U., & Woolhandler, S. (2013). Medicare overpayments to private plans, 1985–2012: Shifting seniors to private plans has already cost Medicare $282.6 billion. *International Journal of Health Services, 43*(2), 305–319.

Herrick, D. M. (2013, May). *The market for medical care should work like cosmetic surgery.* Retrieved from http://www.ncpa.org/pdfs/st349.pdf

Hester, J., Auerbach, J., Choucair, B., Heishman, H., Kuehnert, P., & Monroe, J. (2015, June). New directions in public health services and systems research. Retrieved from http://www.academyhealth.org/files/phsr/PHSSR%20Paper%202015_FINAL.pdf

Himmelstein, D., Ariely, D., & Woolhandler, S. (2014a). Pay-for-performance: Toxic to quality? Insights from behavioral economics. *International Journal of Health Services, 44*(2), 203–214.

Himmelstein, D., Jun, M., Busse, R., Chevreul, K., Geissler, A., Jeurissen, P., … Woolhandler, S. (2014b). A comparison of hospital administrative costs in eight nations: US costs exceed all others by far. *Health Affairs, 33*(9), 1586–1594.

Himmelstein, D. U., Woolhandler, S., Sarra, J., & Guyatt, G. (2014c). Health issues and health care expenses in Canadian bankruptcies and insolvencies. *International Journal of Health Services, 44*(1), 7–23.

Himmelstein, D. A., Thorne, D., Warren, E., & Woolhandler, S. (2009). Bankruptcy in the US, 2007: Results of a national study. *American Journal of Medicine, 122*(8), 741–746.

Himmelstein, D., Thorne, D., & Woolhandler, S. (2011). Medical bankruptcy in Massachusetts: Has health reform made a difference? *American Journal of Medicine, 124*(3), 224–228.

Himmelstein, D., Warren, E., Thorne, D., & Woolhandler, S. (2005). Market Watch: Illness and injury as contributors to bankruptcy. *Health Affairs.* doi: 10.1377/hlthaff.w5.63.

Himmelstein, D., & Woolhandler, S. (2016a). Public health's falling share of US health spending. *American Journal of Public Health, 106*(1), 56–57.

Himmelstein, D., & Woolhandler, S. (2016b). The current and projected taxpayer shares of US health costs. *American Journal of Public Health, 106*(3), 449–452.

Ho, J. Y., & Preston, S. H. (2010). US mortality in an international context: Age variations. *Population and Development Review, 36,* 749–773. doi: 10.1111/j.1728-4457.2010.00356.x.

Hoffman, B. (2013, January 18). *Health care rationing is nothing new (excerpt).* Retrieved from http://www.scientificamerican.com/article/health-care-rationing-is/

Hoffman, J. R., & Kanzaria, H. K. (2014). Intolerance of error and culture of blame drive medical excess. *British Medical Journal, 349*, g5702. doi: 10.1136/bmj.g5702.

Hosseini, N., & Weinberg, S. (2014). The effect of the Massachusetts healthcare reform on emergency department use. *World Medical & Health Policy, 6*, 9–21. doi: 10.1002/wmh3.77.

Houle, J. N., & Keene, D. E. (2014). Getting sick and falling behind: Health and the risk of mortgage default and home foreclosure. *Journal of Epidemiology and Community Health, 69*, 382–387. doi: 10.1136/jech-2014-204637.

Howard, S. W., Bernell, S. L., Yoon, J., Luck, J., & Ranit, C. M. (2015). Oregon's experiment in health care delivery and payment reform: Coordinated care organizations replacing managed care. *Journal of Health Politics, Policy, and Law, 40*(1), 246–255.

Hughes, C. (2011, December 8). *Rationing of healthcare in America*. Retrieved from http://www.drsforamerica.org/blog/rationing-of-healthcare-in-america

Hyde, J., & Shortell, S. M. (2012). The structure and organization of local and state public health agencies in the U. S. *American Journal of Preventive Medicine, 42*(5 Suppl. 1), s29–s41.

Institute of Medicine (IOM). (1988). *The future of public health.* Washington, DC: National Academies Press.

Institute of Medicine (IOM). (2001). *Crossing the quality chasm: A new health system for the 21st century.* Washington, DC: National Academies Press.

Institute of Medicine (IOM). (2002). *The future of the public's health in the 21st century.* Washington, DC: National Academies Press.

Institute of Medicine (IOM). (2012). *For the public's health: Investing in a healthier future.* Washington, DC: National Academies Press.

Institute of Medicine (IOM). (2013). *U. S. health in international perspective: Shorter lives, poorer health.* Washington, DC: National Academies Press.

Jiwani, A., Himmelstein, D., Woolhandler, S., & Kahn, J. G. (2014). Billing and insurance-related administrative costs in United States' health care: Synthesis of micro-costing evidence. *BMC Health Services Research, 14*, 556.

Jones, L. (2012). *Millions from millions*. Retrieved from http://www.philanthropyroundtable.org/topic/excellence_in_philanthropy/millions_from_millions

Joynt, K. E., Gawande, A. A., Orav, E. J., & Jha, A. K. (2013). Contribution of preventable acute care spending to total spending for high-cost Medicare patients. *Journal of the American Medical Association, 309*, 2572–2578. doi: 10.1001/jama.2013.7103.

Kaiser Family Foundation (KFF). (2008). *How non-group health coverage varies with income.* Retrieved from http://www.kff.org/insurance/upload/7737.pdf

Kaiser Family Foundation (KFF). (2012, January). *Explaining health care reform: How will the Affordable Care Act affect small businesses and their employees?* Retrieved from http://www.kff.org/healthHREForm/upload/8275.pdf

Kaiser Family Foundation (KFF). (2014, April). *Healthcare spending in the United States and selected OECD countries.* Retrieved from http://www.kff.org/insurance/snapshot/OECD042111.cfm

Kaiser Family Foundation (KFF). (2015a). *Employer responsibility under the Affordable Care Act.* Retrieved from http://kff.org/infographic/employer-responsibility-under-the-affordable-care-act/

Kaiser Family Foundation (KFF). (2015b). *Key facts about the uninsured population.* Retrieved from http://kff.org/uninsured/fact-sheet/key-facts-about-the-uninsured-population/

Kaiser Family Foundation (KFF). (2015c). *The facts on Medicare spending and financing [Fact Sheet].* Retrieved from http://kff.org/medicare/fact-sheet/medicare-spending-and-financing-fact-sheet/

Kaiser Family Foundation (KFF). (2016, April 1). *An overview of Medicare.* Retrieved from http://kff.org/medicare/issue-brief/an-overview-of-medicare/

Kaiser Family Foundation (KFF) & Health Research and Educational Trust (HRET). (2011). *Employer health benefits 2011 annual survey.* Retrieved from http://ehbs.kff.org/pdf/2011/8225.pdf

Kaiser Family Foundation (KFF) & Health Research and Educational Trust (HRET). (2015). *Employer health benefits 2015 annual survey.* Retrieved from http://files.kff.org/attachment/report-2015-employer-health-benefits-survey

Kalousova, L. & Burgard, S. A. (2013). Debt and foregone medical care. *Journal of Health and Social Behavior, 54*, 203–219. doi: 10.1177/0022146513483772.

Kardish, C. (2015, April 21). Children's health insurance is safe now, but uncertainty awaits. *Governing the states and localities.* Retrieved from http://www.governing.com/topics/health-human-services/gov-childrens-health-insurance-uncertain-future.html

Keehan, S. P., Cuckler, G. A., Sisko, A. M., Madison, A. J., Smith, S. D., Stone, D. A., … Lizonitz, J. M. (2015). National health expenditure projections, 2014–24: Spending growth faster than recent trends. *Health Affairs, 34*, 1407–1417. doi: 10.1377/hlthaff.2015.0600.

Kelly, A. M., & Cronin, P. (2011). Rationing and health care reform: Not a question of if, but when. *Journal of the American College of Radiology, 8*(12), 830–837.

Kesselheim, A. S., Huybrechts, K. F., Choudry, N. K., Fulchino, L. A., Isaman, D. L., Kowal, M. K., & Brennan, T. A. (2015). Prescription drug insurance coverage and patient health outcomes: A systematic review. *American Journal of Public Health, 105*(2), e17–e30.

Khan, H. (2011, May 12). *Has Mitt Romney's Massachusetts health care law worked?* Retrieved from http://abcnews.go.com/blogs/politics/2011/05/has-mitt-romneys-massachusetts-health-care-law-worked/

Kiil, A., & Houlberg, K. (2014). How does copayment for health care services affect demand, health and redistribution? A systematic review of the empirical evidence from 1990 to 2011. *European Journal of Health Economics, 15*, 813–828. doi: 10.1007/s10198-013-0526-8.

Kingdon, J. W. (2011). *Agendas, alternatives and public policies* (2nd ed.). Boston, MA: Pearson/Longman.

Kinney, E. D. (2013). The Affordable Care Act and the Medicare program: The engines of true health reform. *Yale Journal of Health Policy, Law & Ethics, 13*(2), 253–325.

Klein, E. (2011, January 11). The Affordable Care Act in one table. *The Washington Post.* Retrieved from http://voices.washingtonpost.com/ezra-klein/2011/01/the_affordable_care_act_in_one.html

Knickman, J. R. & Kovner, A. R. (Eds.). (2015). *Jonas & Kovner's health care delivery in the United States* (11th ed.). New York, NY: Springer Publishing Company.

Kogut, S. J., Johnson, S., Higgins, T., & Quilliam, B. (2012). Evaluation of a program to improve diabetes care through intensified care management of activities and diabetes medication copayment reduction. *Journal of Managed Care Pharmacy, 18*(4), 297–310.

Krugman, P. (2009, July 25). Why markets can't cure healthcare. *The New York Times.* Retrieved from http://krugman.blogs.nytimes.com/2009/07/25/why-markets-cant-cure-healthcare/

Krugman, P. (2011, September 16). Free to die. *The New York Times*, A29.

Kulbok, P. A., Thatcher, E., Park, E., & Meszaros, P. S. (2012). Evolving public health nursing roles: Focus on community participatory health promotion and prevention. *Online Journal of Issues in Nursing, 17*(2), Manuscript 1. doi: 10.3912/OJIN.Vol17No02Man01.

Kuo, I. C. (2011). Trends in refractive surgery at an academic center, 2007–2009. *BMC Opthalmology, 11*, 11. Retrieved from http://bmcophthalmol.biomedcentral.com/articles/10.1186/1471-2415-11-11

Landon, B., Schneider, E., Normand, S., Scholle, S., Pawlson, L. G., & Epstein A. M. (2007). Quality of care in Medicaid managed care and commercial health plans. *Journal of the American Medical Association, 298*(14), 1674–1681.

Leapfrog Group. (n.d.). *Leapfrog accomplishments.* Retrieved from http://www.leapfroggroup.org/media/file/Leapfrog_Accomplishments_3-07.pdf

Lee, L., Teutsch, S., Thacker, S., & St. Louis, M. (Eds.). (2010). *Principles and practice of public health surveillance* (3rd ed.). New York, NY: Oxford University Press.

Leonhardt, D. (2014, December 5). The health-cost slowdown isn't just about the economy. The New York Times. Retrieved from http://pnhp.org/blog/2014/12/23/health-care-inflation-slowdown-is-due-to-the-economy-not-aca-reforms/

Levin, P., Cary, A., Kulbok, P., Leffers, J., Molle, M., & Polivka, B. (2008). Graduate education for advanced practice public health nursing: At the crossroads. *Public Health Nursing, 25*(2), 176–193.

Lewis, R. A. (1952). *Edwin Chadwick and the public health movement, 1832–1854.* New York, NY: Longman's.

Lindemann, M. (2010). *Medicine and society in early modern Europe* (2nd ed.). New York, NY: Cambridge University Press.

Longest, B. B. (2016). *Health policymaking in the United States* (6th ed.). Chicago, IL: Health Administration Press.

Luna, D. R., Mayan, J. C., García, M. J., Almerares, A. A., & Househ, M. (2014). Challenges and potential solutions for big data implementations in developing countries. *IMIA Yearbook of Medical Informatics, 9*, 36–41. doi: 10.15265/IY-2014-0012.

Magge, H., Cabral, H. J., Kazis, L. E., & Sommers, B. D. (2013). Prevalence and predictors of underinsurance among low-income adults. *Journal of General Internal Medicine, 28*, 1136–1142. doi: 10.1007/s11606-013-2354-z.

Managed Care Online (MCOL). (2015). *National managed care enrollment, 2014*. Retrieved from http://www.mcol.com/current_enrollment

Mangan, D. (2013, June 25). Medical bills are the biggest cause of US bankruptcies: Study. Retrieved from http://www.cnbc.com/id/100840148

Mate, K. S., & Compton-Phillips, A. L. (2014, December 15). The antidote to fragmented health care. *Harvard Business Review*. Retrieved from https://hbr.org/2014/12/the-antidote-to-fragmented-health-care

Mathauer, I., & Nicolle, E. (2011). A global overview of health insurance administrative costs: What are the reasons for variations found? *Health Policy, 102*, 235–246. doi: 10.1016/j.healthpol.2011.07.009.

Mays, G. P. (2013, March 6). *Building the science of public health delivery: Advances in public health services and systems research*. Retrieved from http://uknowledge.uky.edu/cgi/viewcontent.cgi?article=1032&context=hsm_present

Mays, G. P., & Smith, S. A. (2011). Evidence links increases in public health spending to declines in preventable deaths. *Health Affairs, 30*, 1585–1593. doi: 10.1377/hlthaff.2011.0196.

McCanne, D. (2016, February 25). *Lessons from Kaiser poll on single payer*. Retrieved from http://pnhp.org/blog/2016/02/25/lessons-from-kaiser-poll-on-single-payer/

McCarthy, D., How, S. K. H., Fryer, A., Radley, D., & Schoen, C. (2011). *Why not the best? Results from the national scorecard on U.S. health system performance, 2011*. Retrieved from http://www.commonwealthfund.org/publications/fund-reports/2011/oct/why-not-the-best-2011

McCloud, L., & Dwyer, R. (2011). The fragile American: Hardship and financial troubles in the 21st century. *Sociological Quarterly, 52*(1), 13–35.

McNerney, W. J. (1980). Control of health care costs in the 1980s. *New England Journal of Medicine, 303*, 1088–1095.

Meara, E., White, C., & Cutler, D. (2004). Trends in medical spending by age, 1963–2000. *Health Affairs, 23*(4), 176–183.

Medicare.gov. (n.d.a). *About Medicare health plans*. Retrieved from https://www.medicare.gov/sign-up-change-plans/medicare-health-plans/medicare-health-plans.html

Medicare Rights Center. (2010, Summer). *Why consumers disenroll from Medicare private health plans*. Retrieved from http://www.medicarerights.org/pdf/Why-Consumers-Disenroll-from-MA.pdf

Mello, M., Chandra, A., Gawande, A., & Studdert, D. (2010). National costs of the medical liability system. *Health Affairs, 29*(9), 1569–1577.

Melnick, G. A., Shen, Y., & Wu, V. Y. (2011). The increased concentration of health plan markets can benefit consumers through lower hospital prices. *Health Affairs, 30*(9), 1728–1733.

Metropolitan Visiting Nurse Association of Minneapolis, Minnesota (MVNA). (2014). *About MVNA*. Retrieved from http://www.mvna.org

Mikkers, M., & Ryan, P. (2014). "Managed competition" for Ireland? The single versus multiple payer debate. *BMC Health Services Research, 14*, 442.

Milbank Memorial Fund, National Association of State Budget Officers, & Reforming States Group. (2005). *2002–2003 state health care expenditure report*. Retrieved from http://www.milbank.org/reports/05NASBO/NASBO2005.pdf

Mossialos, E., Wenzl, M., Osborn, R., & Sarnak, D. (2016). *2015 international profiles of health care systems*. Retrieved from http://www.commonwealthfund.org/~/media/files/publications/fund-report/2016/jan/1857_mossialos_intl_profiles_2015_v7.pdf

Musumeci, M. (2012, July). *A guide to the Supreme Court's Affordable Care Act decision. Focus on healthcare reform*. Menlo Park, CA: Kaiser Family Foundation.

Naci, H., Soumerai, S. B., Ross-Degnan, D., Zhang, F., Briesascher, B. A., Gurwitz, J. H., & Madden, J. M. (2014). Medication affordability gains following Medicare Part D are eroding among elderly with multiple chronic conditions. *Health Affairs, 33*(8), 1435–1443.

National Association of County and City Health Officials (NACCHO). (2014). *2013 National profile of local health departments*. Retrieved from http://archived.naccho.org/topics/infrastructure/profile/upload/2013-national-profile-of-local-health-departments-report.pdf

National Council on Disability. (2013). *Medicare managed care for people with disabilities: Appendix B. A brief history of managed care*. Retrieved from https://www.ncd.gov/publications/2013/20130315/20130513_AppendixB

National Philanthropic Trust. (2016). *Giving in the 1900s*. Retrieved from http://www.nptrust.org/history-of-giving/timeline/1900s/

National Quality Forum. (n.d.). *List of serious reportable events (SREs)*. Retrieved from http://www.qualityforum.org/Topics/SREs/List_of_SREs.aspx

National Research Council & Institute of Medicine. (2013). *Shorter lives, poorer health: US health in international perspective*. Washington, DC: National Academies Press.

Nelson, D. I. (2009). *A short history of major changes in the U.S. health care system since 1994; costs, coverage and quality*. Retrieved from http://lwvsfc.org/files/healthcare.history_of_changes.pdf

Nicholas, L. H. (2009). *Medicare advantage? The effects of managed care on quality of care*. Retrieved from http://www.psc.isr.umich.edu/pubs/pdf/rr09-672.pdf

Nickitas, D. M., Middaugh, D. J., & Aries, N. (Eds.). (2016). *Policy and politics for nurses and other health professionals* (2nd ed.). Burlington, MA: Jones & Bartlett Publishers.

Norbash, A., Hindson, D., & Heineke, J. (2012). The accountable health care act of Massachusetts: Mixed results for an experiment in universal health care coverage. *Journal of the American College of Radiologists, 9*(10), 734–739.

Organization for Economic Cooperation & Development (OECD). (2015). *Country note: How does health spending in the United States compare?* Retrieved from http://www.oecd.org/united-states/Country-Note-UNITED%20STATES-OECD-Health-Statistics-2015.pdf

Orszag, P. R., & Emanuel, E. J. (2010). Health care reform and cost control. *New England Journal of Medicine, 363*, 601–603.

Pan American Health Organization (PAHO). (2016). *About the Pan American Health Organization (PAHO): Who we are*. Retrieved from http://www.paho.org/hq/index.php?option=com_content&view=article&id=91%3Aabout-paho&Itemid=220&lang=en

Paradise, J. (2015, March 9). *Medicaid moving forward*. Retrieved from http://kff.org/health-reform/issue-brief/medicaid-moving-forward/

Paradise, J., Lyons, B., & Rowland, D. (2015, May 6). *Medicaid at 50*. Retrieved from http://kff.org/medicaid/report/medicaid-at-50/

Public Broadcasting System. (n.d.). *Healthcare crisis: Healthcare timeline*. Retrieved from http://www.pbs.org/healthcarecrisis/history.htm

Perry, P. A., & Hotze, T. (2011). Oregon's experiment with prioritizing public health care services. *Virtual Mentor, 13*, 4, 241–247.

Perkins, B. B. (1998). Economic organization of medicine and the Committee on the Costs of Medical Care. *American Journal of Public Health, 88*(11), 1721–1726.

Pew Charitable Trusts. (2014). *The Children's Health Insurance Program: A 50-state examination of CHIP spending and enrollment*. Retrieved from http://www.pewtrusts.org/~/media/assets/2014/10/childrens_health_insurance_program_report.pdf

Plemmons, S., Lipton, B., Fong, Y., & Acosta, N. (2012). Measurable outcomes from standardized nursing documentation in an electronic health record. *AINA Caring, 2nd quarter*, 4–8.

Polack, G., & Kania, K. (2015). *The middle ages unlocked: A guide to life in medieval England, 1050-1300*. Gloucestershire, UK: Amberley Publishing

PRNewswire. (2013). *Philanthropic giving to nonprofit hospitals and health care systems held steady in fiscal 2012, AHP reports*. Retrieved from http://www.prnewswire.com/news-releases/philanthropic-giving-to-nonprofit-hospitals-and-health-care-systems-held-steady-in-fiscal-2012-ahp-reports-224057501.html

Quadagno, J. (2010). Institutions, interest groups, and ideology: An agenda for the sociology of health care reform. *Journal of Health and Social Behavior, 51*(2), 125–136.

Rambur, B. (2015). *Health care finance, economics, and policy for nurses: A foundational guide*. New York, NY: Springer Publishing.

RAND Health. (2010). *Managed care backlash: Did consumers vote with their feet?* Retrieved from http://www.rand.org/content/dam/rand/pubs/research_briefs/2005/RAND_RB9121.pdf

RAND Health. (2011). *How will health care reform affect costs and coverage?* Retrieved from http://www.rand.org/content/dam/rand/pubs/research_briefs/2011/RAND_RB9589.pdf

Rappleye, E. (2015, June 10). *25 things to know about Blue Cross Blue Shield*. Retrieved from http://www.beckershospitalreview.com/payer-issues/25-things-to-know-about-blue-cross-blue-shield.html

Reich, O., Rapold, R., & Flatscher-Thöni, M. (2012). An empirical investigation of the efficiency effects of integrated care models in Switzerland. *International Journal of Integrated Care, 12*, e2.

Rice, T., Unruh, L. Y., Rosenau, P., Barnes, A. J., Saltman, R. B., & van Ginneken, E. (2014). Challenges facing the United States of America in implementing universal coverage. *Bulletin of the World Health Organization, 92*, 894–902.

Rice University. (2016). *How the AD/AS model incorporates growth, unemployment, and inflation.* Retrieved from http://cnx.org/contents/zJqU35Tm@5/How-the-ADAS-Model-Incorporate

Richardson, B. W. (1887). *The health of nations: A review of the works of Edwin Chadwick* (Vol. 2). London, UK: Longmans, Green.

Robert Wood Johnson Foundation. (2011, May). *Findings brief: A review of the evidence on hospital cost shifting.* Retrieved from https://www.academyhealth.org/files/HCFO/HCFOBriefMay2011FINAL.pdf

Rook, D. (2015, August 17). *How we got to now: A brief history of employer-sponsored healthcare.* Retrieved from http://www.griffinbenefits.com/employeebenefitsblog/history-of-employer-sponsored-healthcare

Rosen, G. (2015). *A history of public health* (rev. expanded ed.). Baltimore, MD: Johns Hopkins University Press.

Rosenbaum, S., & Riley, T. (2012, January). *Building a relationship between Medicaid, the exchange and the individual insurance market.* Retrieved from http://www.nasi.org/sites/default/files/research/Building_A_Relationship_Between_Medicaid:the_Exchange_and_the_Individual_Insuranc

Rosoff, P. M. (2014). *Rationing is not a four-letter word: Setting limits on healthcare.* Cambridge, MA: The MIT Press.

Rovner, J. (2016, January 22). *Debate sharpens over single-payer health care, but what is it exactly?* Retrieved from http://www.npr.org/sections/health-shots/2016/01/22/463976098/debate-sharpens-over-single-payer-health-care-but-what-is-it-exactly

Sabik, L. M., & Gandhi, S. O. (2013). Impact of changes in Medicaid coverage on physician provision of safety net care. *Medical Care, 51*, 978–984. doi: 10.1097/MLR.0b013e3182a50305.

Sacks, N. C., Burgess, J. F., Cabral, H. J., Pizer, S. D., & McDonnell, M. E. (2013). Cost sharing and decreased branded oral anti-diabetic medication adherence among elderly Part D Medicare beneficiaries. *Journal of General Internal Medicine, 28*(7), 876–885.

Saluja, S., Zallman, L., Nardin, R., Bor, D., Woolhandler, S., Himmelstein, D. U., & McCormick, D. (2016). Support for national health insurance seven years into Massachusetts healthcare reform: Views of populations targeted by the reform. *International Journal of Health Services, 46*(1), 185–200.

Scanlon, D., Swaminathan, S., Chernew, M., & Lee, W. (2006). Market and plan characteristics related to HMO quality and improvement. *Medical Care Research & Review, 63*(6 Suppl.), 56–89.

Scanlon, D., Swaminathan, S., Lee, W., & Chernew, M. (2008). Does competition improve health care quality? *Health Services Research, 43*(6), 1931–1951.

Schoen, C., Doty, M., Robertson, R., & Collins, S. (2011). Affordable Care Act reforms could reduce the number of underinsured US adults by 70 percent. *Health Affairs, 30*(9), 1762–1771.

Scheunemann, L. P., & White, D. B. (2011). The ethics and reality of rationing medicine. *Chest, 140*(6), 1625–1632.

Scott, A., Sivey, P., Ouakrim, A., Willenberg, L., Naccarella, L., Furler, J., & Young, D. (2011, September 7). The effect of financial incentives on the quality of health care provided by primary care physicians. *Cochrane Database Systematic Review, 9*, CD008451.

Shattuck, L. (1850). *Report of the Sanitary Commission of Massachusetts.* Cambridge, MA: Harvard University Press.

Shi, L., & Singh, D. A. (2014). *Delivering health care in America: A systems approach* (6th ed.). Burlington, MA: Jones & Bartlett Learning.

Shinkman, R. (2010, September 28). *Healthcare philanthropy plummets.* Retrieved from http://www.fiercehealthfinance.com/story/healthcare-philanthropy-takes-big-dip/2010-09-28

Shires, D., Stange, K., Divine, G., Ratliff, S., Vashi, R., Tai-Seale, M., & Lafata, J. E. (2012). Prioritization of evidence-based preventive health services during periodic health examinations. *American Journal of Preventive Medicine, 42*(2), 164–173.

Shroufi, A., Chowdhury, R., Anchala, R., Stevens, S., Blanco, P., Han, T., ... Franco, O. H. (2013). Cost effective interventions for the prevention of cardiovascular disease in low and middle income countries: A systematic review. *BMC Public Health, 13*, 285. Retrieved from http://bmcpublichealth.biomedcentral.com/articles/10.1186/1471-2458-13-285

Siminerio, L. M., DePasquale, K., Johnson, P., & Thearle, M. (2015). An insurer-based diabetes educator-community partnership: Leveraging Education and Diabetes Support (LEADS). *Clinical Diabetes, 33*(2), 70–72.

Sinnott, S. J., Buckley, C., O'Riordan, D., Bradley, C., & Whelton, H. (2013). The effect of copayments for prescriptions on adherence to prescription medicines in publicly insured populations: A systematic review and meta-analysis. *PLoS One, 8*(5):e64914. doi: 10.1371/journal.pone.0064914.

Small Business Majority. (2012). *Reference guide: Coverage types. Point-of-service plan (POS).* Retrieved from http://healthcoverage-guide.org/reference-guide/coverage-types/point-of-service-plan-pos/

Smolka, G., Multack, M. & Figueiredo, C. (2012, February). *Health coverage among 50- to 64-year olds. AARP Public Policy Institute.* Retrieved from http://www.aarp.org/content/dam/aarp/research/public_policy_institute/health/Health-Insurance-Coverage-for-50-64-year-olds-insight-AARP-ppi-health.pdf

Social Security Administration (SSA). (n.d.). *Historical background and development of Social Security.* Retrieved from http://www.ssa.gov/history/briefhistory3.html

Sommers, B. D., Blendon, R. J., & Orav, E. J. (2016). Both the 'private option' and traditional Medicaid expansions improved access to care for low-income adults. *Health Affairs, 35*, 96–105. doi: 10.1377/hlthaff.2015.0917.

Sorensen, A., Jarrett, N., Tant, E., Bernard, S., & McCall, N. (2014). HAC-POA policy effects on hospitals, other payers, and patients. *Medicare & Medicaid Research Review, 4*(3), e1–e13. doi: 10.5600/mmrr.004.03.a07.

Squires, D., & Anderson, C. (2015). *U.S. health care from a global perspective: Spending, use of services, prices, and health in 13 countries.* Retrieved from http://www.commonwealthfund.org/publications/issue-briefs/2015/oct/us-health-care-from-a-global-perspective

Stallworthy, G., Boahene, K., Ohiri, K., Pamba, A., & Knezovich, J. (2014). Roundtable discussion: What is the future role of the private sector in health? *Globalization and Health, 10*, 55. Retrieved from https://globalizationandhealth.biomedcentral.com/articles/10.1186/1744-8603-10-55

Stein, J. D., Childrs, D. M., Nan, B., & Mian, S. I. (2013). Gauging interest of the general public in laser-assisted in situ keratomileusis (LASIK) eye surgery. *Cornea, 32*(7), 1015–1018.

Stone, D. (2011). Moral hazard. *Journal of Health Politics, Policy and Law, 36*, 887–896. doi: 10.1215/03616878-1407676.

Sultz, H. A., & Young, K. A. (2014). *Health care USA: Understanding its organization and delivery* (8th ed.). Burlington, MA: Jones & Bartlett Learning.

Swan, G. A., & Foley, K. L. (2016). The perceived impact of the Patient Protection and Affordable Care Act on North Carolina's free clinics. *North Carolina Medical Journal, 77*, 23–29. doi: 10.18043/ncm.77.1.23.

Tanner, J. (2015, December 9). *Reducing maternal and child mortality—What does the evidence show?* Retrieved from https://ieg.worldbankgroup.org/blog/reducing-maternal-and-child-mortality-what-does-evidence-show

Terhune, C. (2015, March 18). *With billions in the bank, Blue Shield of California loses its state tax-exempt status.* Retrieved from http://www.latimes.com/business/la-fi-blue-shield-california-20150318-story.html

Trust for America's Health (TFAH). (2006). *Public health leadership initiative: An action plan for healthy people in healthy communities in the 21st century.* Retrieved from http://healthyamericans.org/policy/files/ActionPlan.pdf

Trust for America's Health (TFAH). (2013). *Investing in America's health: A state-by-state look at public health funding and key health facts.* Washington, DC: Author.

Trust for America's Health (TFAH). (2015). *Investing in America's health: A state-by-state look at public health funding and key health facts, 2015.* Retrieved from http://healthyamericans.org/assets/files/TFAH-2015-InvestInAmericaRpt-FINAL.pdf

Trust for America's Health (TFAH). (2016). *Ten top priorities for prevention.* Retrieved from http://healthyamericans.org/pages/?id=126

Turnock, B. J. (2015). *Public health: What it is and how it works* (6th ed.). Sudbury, MA: Jones & Bartlett Learning.

Turnock, B. J. (2016). *Essentials of public health* (3rd ed.). Sudbury, MA: Jones & Bartlett Learning.

Tyson, L. D. (2001). Healing Medicare. In E. C. Hein (Ed.), *Nursing issues in the 21st century: Perspectives from the literature* (pp. 459–468). Philadelphia, PA: Lippincott Williams & Wilkins.

Ubel, P. (2014, February 12). *Is the profit motive ruining American healthcare?* Retrieved from http://www.forbes.com/sites/peterubel/2014/02/12/is-the-profit-motive-ruining-american-healthcare/#542f6e2ca0ce

Ubel, P.A. (2015). Why it's not time for health care rationing. *Hastings Center Report, 45*(2), 15–19. doi: 10.1002/hast.427.

United Nations Educational, Scientific, & Cultural Organization (UNESCO). (2016). *Bureau of strategic planning.* Retrieved from http://www.unesco.org/new/en/bureau-of-strategic-planning/resources/medium-term-strategy-c4/

United Nations International Children's Emergency Fund (UNICEF). (2016). *Frequently asked questions: What is UNICEF?* Retrieved from https://www.unicefusa.org/about/faq

U.S. Agency for International Development (USAID). (2016). *What we do.* Retrieved from http://www.usaid.gov/what-we-do

U.S. Census Bureau. (2010, September 16). *Income, poverty and health insurance coverage in the United States: Summary of key findings.* Retrieved from http://www.census.gov/newsroom/releases/archives/income_wealth/cb10-144.html

U.S. Census Bureau. (2015). *Comparison of the prevalence of uninsured persons from the National Health Interview Survey and the Current Population Survey: January–April 2014.* Retrieved from https://www.cdc.gov/nchs/data/nhis/health_insurance/NCHS_CPS_Comparison092014.pdf

U.S. Department of Health & Human Services (USDHHS). (2014a). *Historical highlights.* Retrieved from http://www.hhs.gov/about/hhshist.html

U.S. Department of Health & Human Services (USDHHS). (2014b). *New HHS data shows major strides made in patient safety, leading to improved care and savings.* Retrieved from https://innovation.cms.gov/Files/reports/patient-safety-results.pdf

U.S. Department of Health & Human Services (USDHHS). (2015). *HHS Agencies & Offices.* Retrieved from http://www.hhs.gov/about/agencies/hhs-agencies-and-offices/index.html

U.S. Department of Health & Human Services (USDHHS). (2016a). *U.S. Department of Health and Human Services Organizational Chart.* Retrieved from http://www.hhs.gov/about/orgchart/

U.S. Department of Health & Human Services (USDHHS). (2016b). *About Healthy People.* Retrieved from http://www.healthypeople.gov/2020/about/default.aspx

U.S. Environmental Protection Agency. (2015). *Summary of the Occupational Safety and Health Act (1970).* Retrieved from http://www.epa.gov/laws-regulations/summary-occupational-safety-and-health-act

Uscher-Pines, L., Pines, J., Kellermann, A., Gillen, E., & Mehrotra, A. (2013). Deciding to visit the emergency department for non-urgent conditions: A systematic review of the literature. *American Journal of Managed Care, 19*, 47–59.

Vaiana, M. E. (2011). *How does growth in health care costs affect the American family?* Retrieved from http://www.rand.org/pubs/research_briefs/RB9605/index1.html

Van Ginneken, E., Schäfer, W., & Kroneman, M. (2011). Managed competition in the Netherlands: An example for others? *Eurohealth, 16*(4), 23–26.

Varney, S. (2010, March 18). *Did Blue Cross' mission stray when plans became for-profit?* Retrieved from http://www.npr.org/templates/story/story.php?storyId=124807720

White, C. (2013). Contrary to cost-shift theory, lower Medicare hospital payment rates for inpatient care lead to lower private payment rates. *Health Affairs, 32*, 935-943. doi: 10.1377/hlthaff.2012.0332.

Woodward, S. B. (1932). The story of smallpox in Massachusetts. *New England Journal of Medicine, 206*, 1181.

Woolhandler, D., & Himmelstein, D. U. (2013). Life or debt: Underinsurance in America. *Journal of General Internal Medicine, 28*(9), 1122–1124.

Woolhandler, D., & Himmelstein, D. U. (2014). Administrative work consumes one-sixth of U.S. physicians' working hours and lowers their career satisfaction. *International Journal of Health Services, 44*(4), 635–642.

Woolhandler, D., & Himmelstein, D. U. (2016). The "Cadillac Tax" on health benefits in the United States will hit the middle class hardest: Refuting the myth that health benefit tax subsidies are regressive. *International Journal of Health Services, 46*(2), 325–330.

World Health Organization (WHO). (n.d.). *History of WHO and international cooperation in public health.* Retrieved from https://apps.who.int/aboutwho/en/history.htm

World Health Organization (WHO). (1998). *Health for all policy for the twenty-first century (Resolution WHA51.7).* Geneva, Switzerland: Author.

World Health Organization (WHO). (2000). *The world health report 2000. Health systems: Improving performance.* Retrieved from http://www.who.int/whr/2000/en/index.html

World Health Organization (WHO). (2011). *Key components of a well functioning health care system.* Retrieved from http://www.who.int/healthsystems/EN_HSSkeycomponents.pdf

World Health Organization (WHO). (2012). *Spending on health: A global overview.* Retrieved from http://www.who.int/mediacentre/factsheets/fs319/en/

World Health Organization (WHO). (2015a). *Media centre: Millennium development goals.* Retrieved from http://www.who.int/entity/mediacentre/factsheets/fs290/en/index.html

World Health Organization (WHO). (2015b). *World health statistics, 2015.* Retrieved from http://www.who.int/gho/publications/world_health_statistics/en/

World Health Organization (WHO). (2016a). *Countries.* Retrieved from http://www.who.int/countries/en/

World Health Organization (WHO). (2016b). *Health.* Retrieved from http://www.who.int/trade/glossary/story046/en/

World Health Organization (WHO). (2016c). *Sustainable development goals.* Retrieved from http://www.who.int/topics/sustainable-development-goals/en/

World Health Organization (WHO). (2016d). *WHO—Its people and offices.* Retrieved from http://www.who.int/about/structure/en/index.html

Wu, V. (2010). Hospital cost shifting revisited: New evidence from the balanced budget act of 1997. *International Journal of Health Care Finance and Economics, 10*(1), 61–83.

Zallman, L., Wilson, F. A., Stimpson, J. P., Bearse, A., Arsenault, L., Dube, B., … Woolhandler, S. (2016). Unauthorized immigrants prolong the life of Medicare's Trust Fund. *Journal of General Internal Medicine, 31*(1), 122–127.

Zhou, C., & Zhang, Y. (2012). The vast majority of Medicare Part D beneficiaries still don't choose the cheapest plans that meet their medication needs. *Health Affairs, 31*(10), 2259–2265.

thePoint: Everything You Need to Make the Grade!

thePoint® Visit http://thePoint.lww.com/Rector9e
for selected readings, study aids for all learning styles, and more!

CHAPTER 7

Epidemiology in Community Health Care

"Let me tell you the secret that has led me to my goal. My strength lies solely in my tenacity."

—*Louis Pasteur*

KEY TERMS

Agent
Bushmeat
Causal matrix
Causality
Chain of causation
Ebola virus disease
Endemic

Environment
Epidemic
Epidemiology
Global health patterns
Host
Immune-privileged
Immunity

Incidence
Morbidity rate
Mortality rate
Natural history
Nosology
Pandemic
Prevalence

Reservoir
Risk
Vector
Web of causation

LEARNING OBJECTIVES

Upon mastery of this chapter, you should be able to:

- Explore the historical roots of epidemiology.
- Explain the host, agent, and environment model.
- Describe theories of causality in health and illness.
- Explain a *web of causation* matrix that assists you with recognizing multicausal factors in disease or injury occurrences.
- Define immunity and compare passive immunity, active immunity, cross-immunity, and herd immunity.
- Explain how epidemiologists determine populations at risk.
- Identify the four stages of a disease or health condition.
- List the major sources of epidemiologic information.
- Distinguish between incidence and prevalence in health and illness states.
- Use epidemiologic methods to describe an aggregate's health.
- Discuss the types of epidemiologic studies that are useful for researching aggregate health.
- Use the seven-step research process when conducting an epidemiologic study.

Epidemiology is a "discipline that describes, quantifies, and postulates causal mechanisms for diseases in populations, and develops methods for the control of diseases" (Friis & Sellers, 2014, p. 8). Epidemiology examines determinants and distribution of diseases, disabilities, morbidity, and mortality, as well as health. It is a specialized form of scientific research that can provide health care workers, including community health nurses, with a body of knowledge on which to base their practice and methods for studying new and existing problems. The term is derived from the Greek words *epi* (upon), *demos* (the people), and *logos* (knowledge); the knowledge or study of what happens to people. Epidemiologists ask such questions as the following:

- What is the occurrence of health and disease in a population?
- Has there been an increase or decrease in a health state over the years?
- Does one geographic area have a higher frequency of disease than another?
- What characteristics of people with a particular condition distinguish them from those without the condition?
- What factors need to be present to cause disease or injury?
- Is one treatment or program more effective than another in changing the health of affected people?
- Why do some people recover from a disease and others do not?

Epidemiology is the scientific discipline that studies the "distribution and determinants of health-related states or events in specified populations, and the application of this study to the control of health problems" (U.S. Department of Health and Human Services [USDHHS], 2012, pp. 1–2). It is data driven and relies on an unbiased and systematic approach to collecting and analyzing and interpreting data. It draws on methods from other areas, such as biostatistics and informatics. It also includes principles from the biologic, social, and economic and behavioral sciences.

Epidemiology offers community health nurses a specific methodology for assessing the health of aggregates. Furthermore, it provides a frame of reference for investigating and improving clinical practice in any setting. For example, if a PHN goal is to lower the incidence of sexually transmitted diseases/infections (STDs/STIs) in a given community, such a prevention plan requires information about population groups. How many STD cases have been reported in this community over the past year? What is the expected number of STD cases (the morbidity rate)? Which members of the community are at highest risk of contracting STDs? To be effective, any program of screening, treatment, or health promotion regarding STDs must be based on this kind of information about population groups. Whether the community health nurse's goals are to improve a population's nutrition, control the spread of human immunodeficiency virus (HIV), deal with health problems created by a flood, protect and promote the health of battered women, or reduce the number of automobile crash injuries and fatalities at a specific intersection, epidemiologic data are essential.

HISTORICAL ROOTS OF EPIDEMIOLOGY

Most of the early contributions to epidemiology were made by physicians who sought the cause of disease through methodical observation and conducting experiments to test their theories of new treatment methodologies. The work of these physicians formed the basic concepts that served as a foundation for the science of epidemiology.

Early Physician–Epidemiologists

The roots of epidemiology can be traced to Hippocrates (460 to 375 BCE), a Greek physician who is sometimes referred to as the first epidemiologist. Hippocrates tried to explain disease occurrences from a rational, rather than a supernatural, viewpoint. His essay, *On Airs, Waters, and Places*, suggested that environmental and host factors (e.g., lifestyle behaviors) might influence disease development (USDHHS, 2012). Basic epidemiologic concepts introduced by Hippocrates included observations of how diseases spread and affect populations. He looked at diseases in relation to time and season, place, environmental conditions and disease control. His main contribution to epidemiology is the emphasis on epidemiologic observation.

Thomas Sydenham (1624 to 1689) advanced strong empirical approaches to medicine and close observations of disease. He developed a classification of fevers that plagued London in the 1660s and 1670s. He advocated for exercise, fresh air, and a healthy diet as treatments and remedies that were not in vogue among other physicians at the time (Merrill, 2013).

James Lind (1716 to 1794) identified the effect of diet on disease based on clinical observations and experimental design. He identified that the spread of scurvy among British naval seamen was effectively addressed by eating oranges and limes. This practice gave rise to the use of the term "limeys" for British seamen (Merrill, 2013).

Edward Jenner (1749 to 1823) invented a vaccination for smallpox based on observations and experiments by Benjamin Jesty, a farmer/dairyman. Jesty noticed that his dairymaids never got smallpox, but did develop cowpox from the cows they milked. He theorized that by getting cowpox, dairymaids were protected from developing smallpox. Jenner applied this theory in developing the smallpox vaccine (Merrill, 2013).

Ignaz Semmelweis (1818 to 1865) was the clinical director of the Viennese Maternity Hospital in the mid-1800s when many women died from childbed (puerperal) fever shortly after giving birth. This is an infection of female reproductive tract that often begins at the uterine wall. Through careful clinical observation, retrospective study, and the collection and analysis of maternal death data, he concluded that it wasn't the actual labor that was the cause, but bacterial contamination during the doctors' pelvic examinations immediately after performing autopsies of infected and decaying bodies without first washing their hands. Semmelweis instituted the use of chlorinated lime in hand washing between patient examinations. As a result, maternal deaths plummeted to 1.3% in 1848 from a high of 12.1% in 1842 (Merrill, 2013).

John Snow's (1813 to 1858) approaches, concepts, and methods used to identify the cause of cholera in 1800s London were his greatest contributions to the field of epidemiology. He conducted a descriptive epidemiologic investigation of a cholera outbreak in London's Soho district, and an analytic epidemiologic investigation of a cholera epidemic by comparing death rates of those getting their water from either the Lambeth Water Company or the Southward and Vauxhall Water Company. His spot (or dot) mapping of cholera cases, which plotted where cholera deaths were occurring, helped to characterize when the epidemic started, peaked, and subsided. The removal of the handle from the Broad Street pump (so people could not get water from that public water pump) was the control measure that finally stopped the epidemic. Because of Snow's many contributions to epidemiology, he became known as the Father of Epidemiology (Merrill, 2013) (see Figs. 7–1 and 7–2).

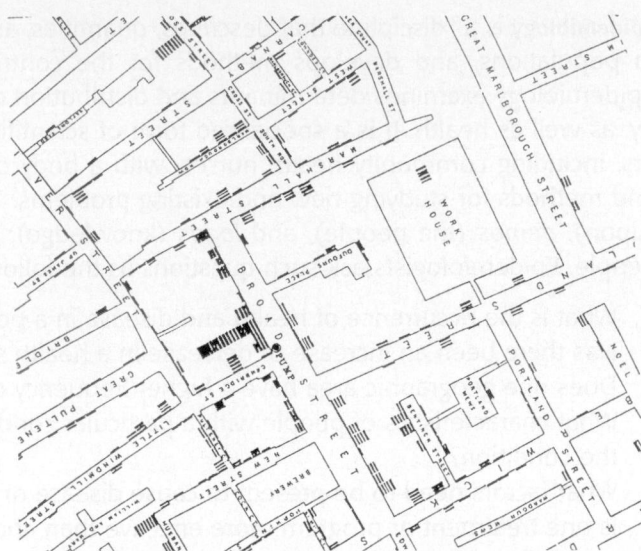

FIGURE 7–2 Spot map. (*Source*: http://www.cdc.gov/ophss/csels/dsepd/ss1978/lesson1/section2.html; Snow, J. (1936). *Snow on cholera*. London, UK: Humphrey Milford/Oxford University Press.)

Florence Nightingale: Nurse Epidemiologist

Nursing's epidemiologic roots can be traced to Florence Nightingale (1820 to 1910). Wanting to make nursing a respectable profession, Nightingale advocated training in science, strict discipline, attention to cleanliness, and the development of empathy for patients. She also established a nursing school at London's St. Thomas Hospital, and is commonly referred to as "The Lady with the Lamp" for nursing soldiers throughout the night during the Crimean War (Florence Nightingale Museum, n.d.).

Her detailed records, morbidity (sickness) statistics, and careful description of the health conditions among the soldiers fighting in the Crimean War represent one of the first systematic descriptive studies of the distribution and patterns of disease in a population. She used wedge-shaped graphs that were shaded and colored to illustrate preventable deaths of the hospitalized Crimean soldiers, compared with hospitalized soldiers in England at the time. The sophisticated level of detail in her studies heralded her as the first nurse researcher. She conducted an exhaustive study of the health of the British Army and published several reports about her findings that resulted in creating changes in hygiene and overall treatment of patients. Her monitoring of disease mortality rates was used to improve sanitary methods in hospitals that led to decreased death rates. Nightingale used applied statistical methods for displaying data, and introduced a new way for improving medical and surgical practices. During her lifetime, Queen Victoria recognized Nightingale's contributions to nursing and epidemiology; she was awarded the highest civilian medal, the Order of Merit, and was the first woman to receive it (Merrill, 2013; Florence Nightingale Museum, n.d.). Florence Nightingale learned to "use statistics as evidence" to gain the attention of politicians and powerful people in her quest for hospital and public health reforms, and she was aided in that effort by William Farr (Schiotz, 2015, p. 3).

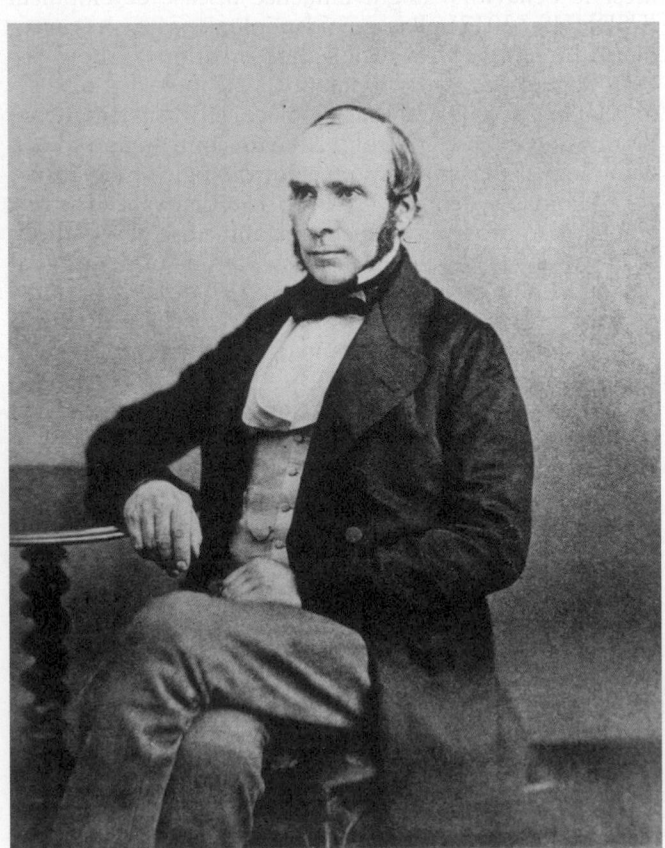

FIGURE 7–1 John Snow.

William Farr

William Farr (1807 to 1883) served as the Compiler of Abstracts in the Office of the Registrar General for England and Wales. He created the first national vital statistics system. He also began compiling vital statistics data on an annual basis, which included analyses of causes of death and assessments of mortality by occupation. To support his work, he developed a **nosology** (classification of diseases) from which today's International Classification of Diseases (ICD) developed. His collaborative work with contemporaries helped to advance the value of epidemiology for controlling diseases. His epidemiologic investigations into the spread of cholera supported John Snow's efforts to control its spread. He collaborated with Florence Nightingale in her British Army studies, publicizing the value of vital statistics. He supported Greenhow's systematic studies in occupational epidemiology and Seaton's analyses of the efficacy of smallpox vaccinations. This work later formed the scientific basis for English public health policy that lasted for over 50 years. By careful analysis of mortality data and disease patterns among different geographical areas, he "called attention to the connection between socioeconomic class and disease" (Lilienfeld, 2007; Schiotz, 2015, p. 5).

Eras in the Evolution of Modern Epidemiology

Modern epidemiology can be described as having four distinct eras, each based on causal thinking, sanitary statistics, infectious-disease epidemiology, and chronic-disease epidemiology. In light of new research, the eco-epidemiology era is emerging.

Early causal thinking was dominated by the *miasma theory*, which had its origins in the work of the Hippocratic School and was formally developed in the early 1700s. This theory held that a substance called *miasma* was composed of malodorous and poisonous particles generated by the decomposition of organic matter and was the cause of disease. Prevention based on this theory attempted to eliminate the sources of the miasma or polluted vapors. Despite the faulty reasoning, this type of prevention had positive consequences because it made people aware that decaying organic matter can be a source of infectious diseases. This theory dominated until the first half of the 19th century (Schiotz, 2015).

Similarly, the pioneering work of John Snow in identifying the source of cholera in England in the mid-1800s was based on a faulty assumption that the climate was involved. Even so, he was able to trace the source of the infectious agent to the water supply and brought public attention to the link between sanitary conditions and disease. We owe much to these individuals; that they didn't understand the exact mechanisms in disease causation does not lessen their pioneering work in applied epidemiology.

The era of infectious-disease epidemiology was dominated by the *contagion theory* of disease, which developed during the mid-18th century. Prompted by the development of increasingly sophisticated microscopes, this theory attempted to identify the microorganisms that cause diseases as a first step in prevention. It inspired various theories of immunity, and even prompted some initial attempts at vaccination against smallpox. Additionally, once an agent had been identified, measures were taken to contain its spread. Fumigating ships to kill rats, protecting wharf buildings and human habitations from rats, and removing rat food supplies from easy access were all measures taken to protect the public by further preventing the spread of plague bacilli. Based on the work of Louis Pasteur, Jakob Henle, and Robert Koch (see Koch's Postulates Display 7–1), the contagion theory was refined and became best known as the *germ theory of disease* that was predominant from the late 19th century through the first half of the 20th century (McKenzie, Pinger, & Kotecki, 2012).

In the era of infectious-disease epidemiology, scientists viewed disease in terms of a simple cause-and-effect relationship. Finding a single cause (e.g., plague bacilli) and attacking it (e.g., eliminating rats) seemed to be the solution for preventing many diseases. In the case of bubonic plague, this approach appeared to be quite effective. However, scientific research eventually revealed that disease causation was much more complex than first suspected. For example, although most members of a group might be exposed to the plague, many did not contract it.

With bubonic plague, as with many other infectious diseases, host characteristics can determine both the spread of the disease and its individual impact. Not everyone in a population is at equal risk; it is now known that untreated bubonic plague has a case fatality rate of 40% to 70%, meaning that about half of those who contract the disease and are not treated will eventually die. Furthermore, the agent and course of transmission can be quite complex. Although a flea carries the bacilli from rats to humans in bubonic plague, many infectious diseases spread directly from one human being to another. Finally, the environment must be considered as part of the

---

DISPLAY 7–1 KOCH'S POSTULATES

1. The microorganism must be observed in every case of the disease.
2. It must be isolated and grown in pure culture.
3. The pure culture must, when inoculated into a susceptible animal, reproduce the disease.

4. The microorganism must be observed in, and recovered from, the experimentally diseased animal.

King, L. S. (1952). Dr. Koch's postulates. *Journal of Historical Medicine, 350–361.* As cited in Friis, R. H., & Sellers, T. A. (2014). *Epidemiology for public health practice* (5th ed., p. 38). Burlington, MA: Jones and Bartlett Learning.

cause of disease. Evidence suggests that the plague originated in the high plains of Asia and spread to other parts of the world (Centers for Disease Control & Prevention [CDC], 2014). However, questions remain as to whether the bacillus spread from rats to ground squirrels or had always been part of the squirrels' ecology.

After World War II, the causative agents of major infectious diseases were identified, methods of prevention were recognized, and antibiotics were added to the arsenal to fight communicable diseases. The focus then became understanding and controlling the new chronic disease epidemics, ushering in the era of chronic disease epidemiology. Researchers completed case–control and cohort studies, to be discussed more fully later, that linked the causative factors of cholesterol levels and smoking with coronary heart disease (CHD) and associated smoking with lung cancer. Today, the major causes of mortality in the United States are noninfectious diseases. In 2012, the top two leading causes of death, heart disease and cancer, accounted for 46.5% of all deaths. Chronic lower respiratory diseases (3rd), cerebrovascular diseases (4th) and unintentional injuries (5th) accounted for 15.7% of all deaths in 2012. Alzheimer's disease (6th), diabetes mellitus (7th), influenza and pneumonia (8th), kidney disease (9th), and suicide (10th) together accounted for 11.6% of deaths in 2012 (Heron, 2015). As you can see, infectious agents are not to blame for most of today's major health problems. See more in Chapters 23 and 24.

We are entering a new era of *eco-epidemiology*, distinguished by transforming global health patterns and technological advances. **Global health patterns**, the route, form, and virulence in which diseases appear in countries around the world, with consideration of environmental, ecologic, human, technologic, and political factors, are in transformation. With this, new and emerging infections are now a concern, as is the spread of medication-resistant diseases. See more in Chapters 8, 9, and 16. The West Nile virus, sudden acute respiratory syndrome (SARS), influenza A (H1N1), multidrug-resistant tuberculosis (MDR TB), HIV, and Ebola virus disease (EVD) illustrate this transformation. In most cases, causative organisms and critical risk factors are known, yet diseases occur, spread, and suddenly appear in countries or regions previously free of them (Bain & Awah, 2014). We know which social behaviors need to change, but we are at a loss about how to create a climate of permanent change, even when entire populations are at stake. For example, we know how to prevent the transmission of HIV, yet thousands of new cases are reported each year. How can preventive practices be promoted among populations at risk for communicable diseases? The same situation is true for many current chronic diseases. For instance, how many nurses smoke? Do you exercise as often as you know you should? Do you know your cholesterol level, and eat appropriate foods accordingly? Do you regularly use sunscreen? What are we missing to effectively change social behaviors?

Developments in technology drive research, primarily in biology and biomedical techniques and in information system capabilities. For example, genetic influence in some cases of insulin-dependent diabetes is linked to human leukocyte antigens (HLAs) and particular combinations of this gene variant can predict risk of Type 1 diabetes, whereas other combinations either cause no problems or may be protective (National Institute of Diabetes and Digestive and Kidney Diseases, 2014). HIV, tuberculosis, and other infections can be tracked from person to person through identifying the molecular specificity of the organisms. BRCA1 and BRCA2 genes have been found to cause about one-quarter of hereditary breast cancers and up to 10% of all breast cancers, as well as 15% of ovarian cancers, and genetic screening tests are used to screen for these genes (National Cancer Institute, 2015).

On a broader scale, using new technology, we are now able to track the geographic distribution of disease and correlate those data with other important health risks. For instance, using these geocoding systems, overweight and obesity in children can be correlated with other factors, such as after-school recreation opportunities, distribution of fast food restaurants, farmer's markets, or socioeconomic status. (See Chapter 10 for more on technology in public health). The possibilities of learning through technology have just begun in this current epidemiologic era. Table 7–1 summarizes the four eras in the evolution of modern epidemiology.

Epidemics

An **epidemic** refers to a disease occurrence that clearly exceeds the normal or expected frequency in a community or region. In past centuries, epidemics of cholera, bubonic plague, and smallpox swept through community after community, killing thousands of people, changing the community structure, and altering the lifestyle of masses of people. When an epidemic, such as the bubonic plague (also called pneumonic plague or the Black Death) or HIV/AIDS, is worldwide in distribution, it is known as a **pandemic**.

Epidemic and pandemic diseases clearly prompted the development of epidemiology as a science. Epidemiology became a distinct branch of medical science through its concern with massive waves of infectious diseases. While epidemiology provides public health with the tools to investigate disease outbreaks, it also provides strategies for controlling disease to prevent future outbreaks. Despite hundreds of years of experience with disease outbreaks, new diseases arise all the time, challenging us to come up with new methods. Eradication would be ideal, but sometimes it may take a long time, or it may not happen at all. Read about smallpox eradication in Chapter 16.

Historically, as the threat of the great epidemic diseases declined, epidemiologists began to focus on other infectious diseases, such as diphtheria, infant diarrhea, typhoid, tuberculosis and syphilis. They also studied diseases linked to occupations, such as scurvy among sailors and scrotal cancer among chimney sweeps. In recent years, epidemiologists turned to the study of major causes of death and disability, such as cancer, cardiovascular disorders, AIDS, violence, mental illness, accidents, arthritis, and congenital defects (Remington & Brownson, 2011).

Ebola Virus Disease: A 21st Century Disease Epidemic

As of December 2, 2015, the Centers for Disease Control and Prevention (CDC) reported a total of 11,864 laboratory confirmed cases of Ebola in Guinea, Sierra Leone,

Table 7–1   Eras in the Evolution of Modern Epidemiology

Era	Paradigm	Analytic Approach	Prevention Approach
Sanitary statistics (1800–1850)	Miasma: poisoning from foul emanations	Clustering of morbidity and mortality	Drainage, sewage, sanitation
Infectious disease epidemiology (1850–1950)	Germ theory: single agent related to specific disease	Laboratory isolation and culture from disease sites and experimental transmission/reproduction of lesions	Interrupt transmission (vaccines, isolation, and antibiotics)
Chronic disease epidemiology (1950–2000)	Exposure related to outcome	Risk ratio of exposure to outcome at individual level in populations	Control risk factors by modifying lifestyle (diet), agent (guns), or environment (pollution)
Eco-epidemiology (emerging)	Relations within and between localized structures organized in a hierarchy of levels	Analysis of determinants and outcomes at different levels of organization using new information systems and biomedical techniques	Apply both information and biomedical technology to find leverage at efficacious levels

Adapted from Susser, M., & Susser, E. (1996a). Choosing a future for epidemiology: I. Eras and paradigms. *American Journal of Public Health, 86*(5), 668–673; Susser, M., & Susser, E. (1996b). Choosing a future for epidemiology: II. From black box to Chinese boxes and eco-epidemiology. *American Journal of Public Health, 86*(5), 674–677.

and Liberia, with a total of 8,764 deaths (73.9%) since the Ebola epidemic started in March 2014 (CDC, 2015a). The most recent death occurred in November 2015, when an outbreak occurred after Liberia was declared disease free for 2 months. According to the World Health Organization (WHO), Liberia has recorded more than 4,800 deaths during the worst and largest Ebola outbreak in history (Paye-Layleh, 2015). Two imported cases, including one death, and instances of locally acquired cases in two nurses were reported in the United States (CDC, 2015b). See Chapter 8 (Fig. 7–3).

Ebola virus disease (EVD) is a viral hemorrhagic fever (VHF) that is characterized by fever, diarrhea, and unexplained bleeding (bruising, petechiae, bloody stools, mucosal hemorrhage) and is definitively diagnosed at reference laboratories that have advanced biocontainment capability, such as the CDC. Early clinical diagnosis minimizes potential nosocomial spread. Antiviral therapy is useful, with intensive supportive care, and those infected must be cared for under strict contact precautions, including hand hygiene, double gloves, gowns, shoe and leg coverings, and face shield or goggles. Airborne precautions should be instituted, and at minimum, a fit-tested, HEPA filter–equipped respirator (e.g., N-95 mask) and a battery-powered, air-purifying respirator (PAPR), or a positive pressure-supplied air respirator, should by worn by personnel sharing an enclosed space within 6 feet of a VHF patient (CDC, 2015c).

VHFs are a diverse group of illnesses caused by RNA viruses. The four viral families are *Arenaviridae, Bunyaviridae, Filoviridae, and Flaviviridae*. The *Filoviridae* family includes the Ebola and Marburg viruses. There are five species of the Ebola virus (Zaire, Sudan, Bundibugyo, Reston, Ivory Coast—now known as Taï Forest). The Reston virus has not caused disease in humans. The first recognized EVD outbreak caused by the Zaire and Sudan species occurred in 1976, and an outbreak of 316 cases from a single index case occurred in Zaire in 1995. Subsequent outbreaks from the Zaire virus (*Zaire ebolavirus*) and

Sudan virus (*Sudan ebolavirus*) occurred in Gabon, Ivory Coast, Uganda, Democratic Republic of Congo (DRC) (former Zaire), and Sudan, with the last reported Ebola-Zaire epidemic in the DRC reported in 2007. The Reston virus (*Reston ebolavirus*) was isolated from monkeys in 1989, and caused outbreaks in nonhuman primate facilities. Although the Reston virus (*Reston ebolavirus*) is not recognized as a human pathogen, exposed animal handlers did seroconvert without manifesting clinical disease. In 2008, humans also seroconverted without clinical disease when exposed to pigs infected with Ebola-Reston in the Philippines. At that time a scientist also contracted the Taï Forest virus (*Taï Forest ebolavirus*) after working with postmortem tissues, became ill, but fully recovered. The Bundibugyo virus (*Bundibugyo ebolavirus*) was responsible for a 2007 outbreak in Uganda, and recent data implicated bats as the likely reservoir, but initial mode of spread to humans and the ecology of these diseases remain unclear. Scientists do not know why it occurs intermittently (CDC, 2015c; United States Army Medical Research Institute of Infectious Diseases, 2011) (Fig. 7–4).

Studies have found, however, that the Ebola virus lives in fruit bats and can infect humans through contact with bodily secretions (e.g., blood and sweat). Once people are infected, they can pass the virus to other humans through direct exposure to bodily fluids (Kahn, 2015). In a Guinea village in 2014, an EVD outbreak in which a toddler had died was blamed on a bat-filled tree. Children would catch and play with the bats. Before any definitive testing of the bats could be done, the tree was burned down and the villagers ate all the bats (Geggel, 2014). Investigations into the 2014 outbreak have uncovered the eating of bushmeat as a potential mode of transmission. **Bushmeat** is any animal killed for food (including bats). Because Africans often have no alternative, they frequently eat bushmeat. People hunt gorillas, chimpanzees, and other animals that may have been infected eating the droppings from bats that have been identified as an Ebola **vector,** or carrier (Cooney, 2014).

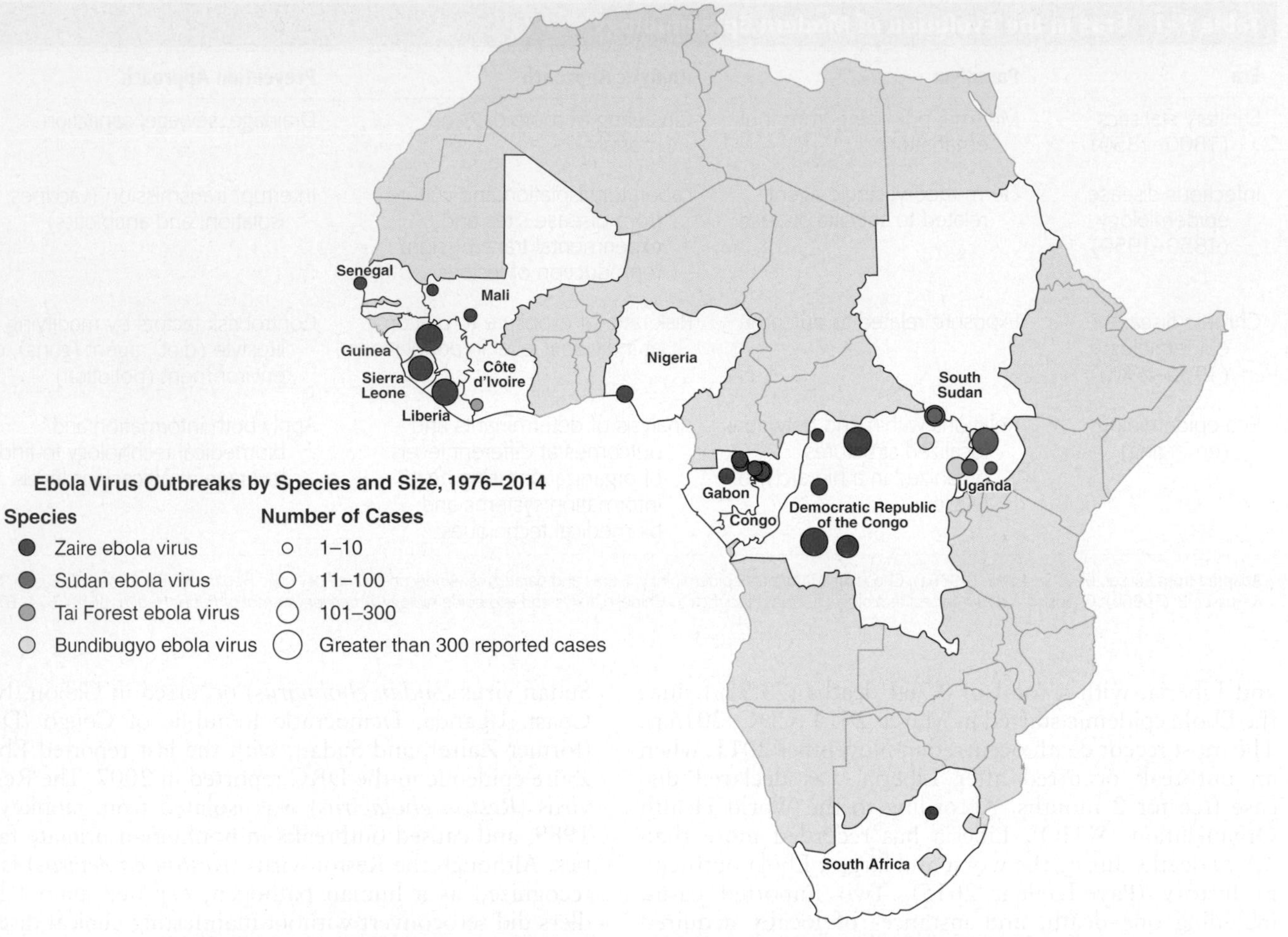

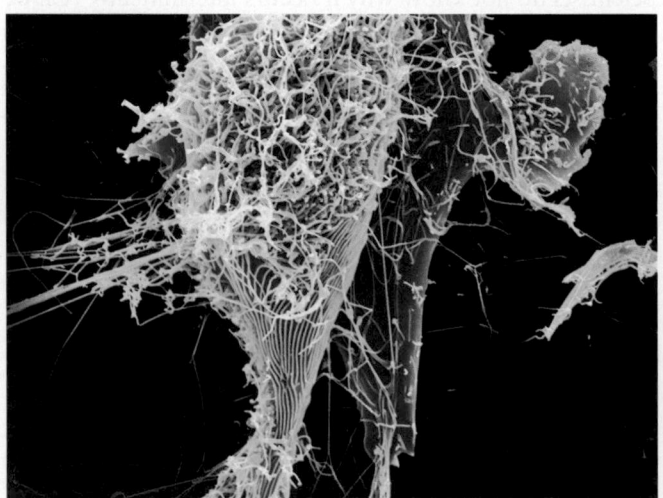

Ebola Virus Outbreaks by Species and Size, 1976–2014

Species	Number of Cases
● Zaire ebola virus	○ 1–10
● Sudan ebola virus	○ 11–100
● Tai Forest ebola virus	○ 101–300
● Bundibugyo ebola virus	○ Greater than 300 reported cases

FIGURE 7–3 Cases of Ebola virus disease in Africa, 1976 to 2015. (*Source*: http://www.cdc.gov/vhf/ebola/outbreaks/history/distributionmap.html#modalIdString_CDCImage_0)

Of greater concern was the *New England Journal of Medicine* report that there was now molecular evidence that EVD can be sexually transmitted. While the Ebola virus is detectable in the bloodstream only during acute illness, the virus may persist in the body within

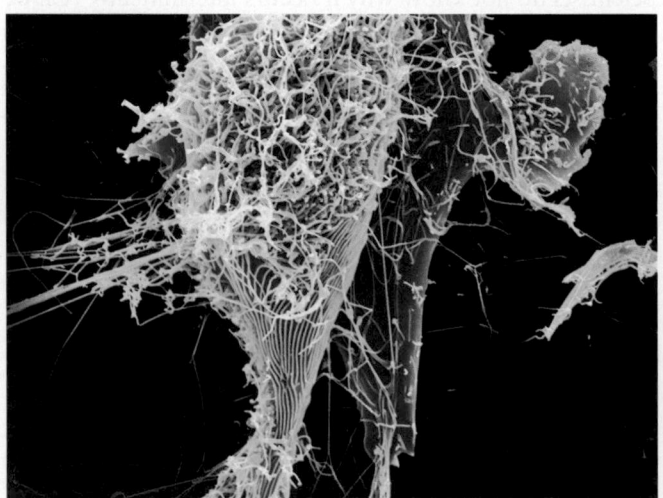

FIGURE 7–4 Ebola virus (string-like Ebola virus was peeling off an infected cell). (*Source*: http://images.nigms.nih.gov/index.cfm?event=viewDetail&imageID=3619)

immune-privileged sites (e.g., eye, testes; where inflammatory immune response does not occur following exposure to an antigen). Ebola RNA has been detected in breast milk up to 15 days, in vaginal secretions up to 33 days, in ocular aqueous humor up to 98 days, and in semen up to 101 days after disease onset. Specifically, with semen, the Ebola virus has been cultured from samples 40, 61, and 82 days after disease onset when the virus has been cleared from the blood (Mate et al., 2015).

This long-term persistence of the virus in the semen of survivors provides opportunities for sexually transmitting the disease even when the outbreak may be deemed officially over. In this report, the WHO and the CDC advised survivors of EVD to abstain from sexual intercourse or to use condoms for at least 3 months after the onset of EVD (Mate et al., 2015). However, the CDC has since advised that condoms should be worn correctly and consistently every time until further information becomes known (Christie et al., 2015; Rettner, 2015).

Furthermore, WHO's criteria of a 42-day cut-off period for declaring a country "Ebola free" (after the last confirmed case tests negative for the virus) has been questioned. In the November 2015 Liberia outbreak, individuals have tested positive for Ebola antibodies while testing negative for the virus, suggesting the possibility of human-to-human transmission from previously undocumented or mildly symptomatic cases. Recent reports that the virus can linger in semen (Deen et al., 2015), breast milk, and the eye for as long as 9 months after survivors recover, and the differing behaviors of the different Ebola strains have caused the WHO to add a 90-day high-surveillance phase to those countries passing the 42-day cut-off period. Additionally, animal-to-human transmission in **endemic** areas (where disease is most frequently found), such as Sierra Leone, Liberia, and Guinea, cannot be adequately addressed because of "an animal reservoir of unknown origin," thus making it impossible to eradicate the disease in those areas (Thomas, 2015a, para. 5).

While the overall case fatality rate is high for EVD (52%), it can vary by geographic location (e.g., 42% for Sierra Leone, 66% for Guinea) (WHO, 2014a). Survivors from the 2014 outbreak are starting to report serious sequelae. About half of EVD survivors report what is now referred to as the "post-Ebola syndrome." Reports include blurred vision, retro-orbital pain, hearing loss, sleep disturbances, neurological abnormalities, memory loss, arthralgias (joint pain), confusion, difficulty swallowing, and chronic health problems. These health issues can persist for more than 2 years. The most severe involve the eyes where viral genome or infectious virus have been found, causing pressure, uveitis (inflammation), and even blindness. The virus has not been found in tears, reducing the potential for infecting others (Mackay, 2015).

EVD is a prime example of how epidemiology can help characterize an infectious disease so it can be controlled to prevent its spread. Knowing that EVD can be sexually transmitted has led the CDC to advise EVD survivors to use condoms indefinitely in order to prevent this mode of transmission. Another mode of transmission, such as the eating of bushmeat, however, is not so easy to address. This will probably require a broader approach with public health education and culturally sensitive strategies to assist this population in finding alternative food sources.

Furthermore, there is much more to learn about Ebola before it can be eradicated.

Periodic outbreaks in which previous known modes of transmission no longer apply have left researchers puzzled, questioning their expertise (Beaubien, 2015). Genomic sequencing of the Ebola virus has revealed a high mutation rate without changing the characteristics of the virus itself. This technology has been useful in matching new viral infections to earlier ones, but has not been sufficient to help eradicate the disease (Thomas, 2015b). However, as we learn more about the virus, control measures can be implemented. For example, WHO has issued a protocol for the safe management of dead bodies and burial of those who have died from suspected or confirmed EVD (WHO, 2014b).

CONCEPTS BASIC TO EPIDEMIOLOGY

The science of epidemiology draws on certain basic concepts and principles to analyze and understand patterns of occurrence among aggregate health conditions.

Host, Agent, and Environment Model

Through their early study of infectious diseases, epidemiologists began to consider disease states generally in terms of the *epidemiologic triad*, or the *host, agent, and*

environment model. Interactions among these three elements explained infectious and other disease patterns.

Host

The **host** is a susceptible human or animal who harbors and nourishes a disease-causing agent. Many physical, psychological, and lifestyle factors influence the host's susceptibility and response to an agent. Physical factors include age, sex, race, and genetic influences on the host's vulnerability or resistance. Psychological factors, such as outlook and response to stress, can strongly influence host susceptibility. Lifestyle factors also play a major role. Diet, exercise, sleep patterns, and healthy or unhealthy habits all contribute to either increased or decreased vulnerability to the disease-causing agent (Fletcher & Fletcher, 2012).

The concept of resistance is important for public health nursing practice. People sometimes have an ability to resist pathogens. This is called *inherent resistance.* Typically, these people have inherited or acquired characteristics, such as the various factors mentioned earlier, that make them less vulnerable. People who maintain a healthful lifestyle may not contract influenza even if exposed to the flu virus. Resistance can be promoted through preventive interventions that support a healthful lifestyle.

For example, Walker et al. (2011) demonstrated that participants ($n = 7,867$) taking multivitamins with folic acid during the early second trimester were 63% less likely to have preeclampsia. In another study, folic acid supplementation and higher dietary folate intake during pregnancy were found to reduce the risk of preeclampsia (Wang et al., 2015). If confirmed by additional studies, multivitamin use with folic acid could be recommended as a preventive measure for preeclampsia. The American Academy of Pediatrics (AAP, 2015) and the U.S. Public Health Service already recommend that women capable of becoming pregnant take 400 µg of folic acid each day to prevent neural tube defects such as spina bifida. Further study may reveal other benefits from the use of folic acid during pregnancy.

Agent

An **agent** is a factor that causes or contributes to a health problem or condition. Causative agents can be factors that are present (e.g., bacteria that cause tuberculosis, rocks on a mountain road that contribute to an automobile crash) or factors that are lacking (e.g., a low serum iron level that causes anemia or the lack of seat belt use that contributes to the extent of injury during an automobile crash) (Fig. 7–5).

Agents vary considerably and include five types: biologic, chemical, nutrient, physical, and psychological. Biologic agents include bacteria, viruses, fungi, protozoa, worms, and insects. Some biologic agents are infectious, such as Influenza virus or HIV. Chemical agents may be in the form of liquids, solids, gases, dusts, or fumes. Examples are poisonous sprays used on garden pests and industrial chemical wastes. The degree of toxicity of the chemical agent influences its impact on health. Nutrient agents include essential dietary components that can produce illness conditions if they are deficient or are taken in excess. For example, a deficiency of niacin can cause pellagra, and too much vitamin A can be toxic. Physical agents

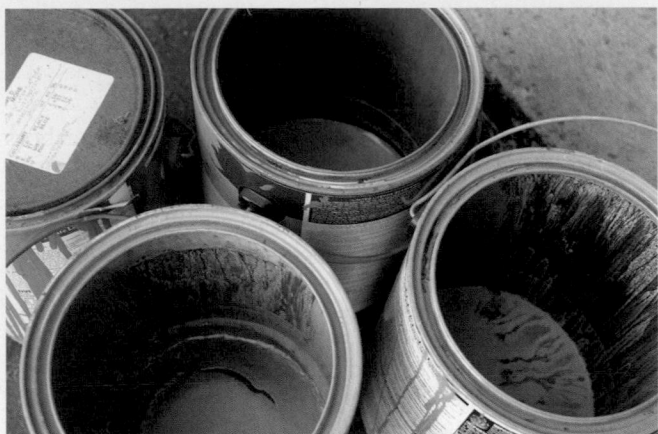

FIGURE 7–5 Old paint cans may be a source of lead and other toxins.

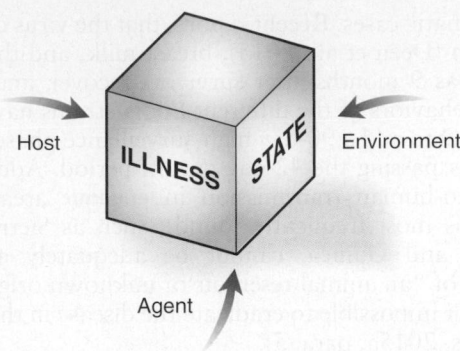

FIGURE 7–6 Epidemiologic triad. Epidemiologists study the causal agent, the susceptible host, and environmental factors that contribute to an illness, an injury, or a wellness state. Intervention may focus on any of these three to prevent the spread of illness or to improve health in a population.

include anything mechanical (e.g., chainsaw, automobile), material (e.g., rock slide), atmospheric (e.g., ultraviolet radiation), geologic (e.g., earthquake), or genetically transmitted that causes injury to humans. The shape, size, and force of physical agents influence the degree of harm to the host. Psychological agents are events that produce stress leading to health problems (e.g., war, terrorism).

Agents may also be classified as infectious or noninfectious. Infectious agents cause communicable diseases, such as AIDS or tuberculosis—that is, the disease can be spread from one person to another. Certain characteristics of infectious agents are important for community health nurses to understand. Extent of *exposure* to the agent, the agent's *pathogenicity* (capacity to cause disease in the host), its *infectivity* (capacity to enter the host and multiply), its *virulence* (severity of disease), *toxigenicity* (capacity to produce a toxin or poison), *resistance* (ability of the agent to survive environmental conditions), *antigenicity* (ability to induce an antibody response in the host), and its structure and chemical composition all influence the effect of the agent on the host (Friis & Sellers, 2014). Chapter 8 examines the subject of communicable disease in greater depth. Noninfectious agents have similar characteristics in that their relative abilities to harm the host vary with type of agent and intensity and duration of exposure (Fletcher & Fletcher, 2012).

Environment

The **environment** refers to all the external factors surrounding the host that might influence vulnerability or resistance. The physical environment includes factors such as geography, climate and weather, safety of buildings, water and food supply, and presence of animals, plants, insects, and microorganisms that have the capacity to serve as reservoirs (storage sites for disease-causing agents) or vectors (carriers) for transmitting disease. The psychosocial environment refers to social, cultural, economic, and psychological influences and conditions that affect health, such as access to health care, cultural health practices, poverty, and work stressors, which can all contribute to disease or health (Fletcher & Fletcher, 2012).

Host, agent, and environment interact to cause a disease or health condition. For example, the agent responsible for

Lyme disease is the spirochete *Borrelia burgdorferi*; humans of all ages are susceptible hosts, along with dogs, cattle, and horses. Ticks (a vector) that feed on wild rodents and deer transfer the spirochete to human hosts after feeding on them for several hours. Environmental factors, such as working or playing in tick-infested areas, influence host vulnerability. The host, agent, and environment model, shown in Figure 7–6, offered plan for intervention for the epidemiologists who first studied Lyme disease in 1982. As soon as the agent was identified, measures could be taken to keep the spirochete from infecting human hosts, such as wearing protective clothing or tick repellent in tick-infested areas and promptly removing the attached ticks (Heymann, 2014).

In another example, the West Nile virus, which was widespread in Africa and the Middle East, arrived in the United States in 1999 and began to spread. The first reported cases were in New York, where 45 people were infected. In that year, the region experienced a total of 59 hospitalized cases of West Nile disease, resulting in seven deaths (Sejvar, 2003). By 2006, West Nile virus had been reported in 43 states and the District of Columbia, with a total of 4,269 cases and 177 deaths. In 2011, there were 690 confirmed cases and 43 deaths in the United States. As of January 2012, only Alaska, Hawaii, and Oregon had no confirmed presence of the virus in humans, birds, animals, or mosquitoes (CDC, 2015f). The infected mosquitoes (vector) pass the virus on to birds, humans, or horses through bites. Many dead birds in an area may mean that the virus is circulating between the bird and mosquito populations and should be reported. In humans and animals with intact immune systems, the virus is usually destroyed in the bloodstream. If the virus survives in the body, it can infect membranes around the spinal cord and brain and cause encephalitis. Those at highest risk are the elderly, children, and people with impaired immune systems (CDC, 2015f).

Prevention of West Nile virus infections includes avoiding mosquito bites by applying insect repellent containing N,N-diethyl-meta-toluamide (DEET) when outdoors; wearing long-sleeved clothing and long pants treated with DEET-containing repellents; staying indoors at dawn, at dusk, and in the early evening; eliminating standing water sources where mosquitoes lay their eggs; reporting dead birds; and ensuring that an organized mosquito control program exists in the area (CDC, 2015f). Using the model in Figure 7–6, can you categorize each of these six recommendations by their target (host, agent, or environment)?

Causality

Causality refers to the relationship between a cause and its effect. A purpose of epidemiologic study has been to discover causal relationships, in order to understand why conditions develop, and to offer effective prevention and protection (Fletcher & Fletcher, 2012). As scientific knowledge of health and disease has expanded, epidemiology has changed its view of causality. The following section discusses some of those changes in thinking that began in the 1960s and is being continually refined.

Chain of Causation

As the scientific community's thinking about disease causation and the tripartite model (host–agent–environment) grew more complex, epidemiologists began to use the idea of a **chain of causation** (Fig. 7–7). The chain begins by identifying the **reservoir** (i.e., where the causal agent can live and multiply). With plague, that reservoir may be other humans, rats, squirrels, and a few other animals. With malaria, infected humans are the major reservoir for the parasitic agents, although certain nonhuman primates also act as reservoirs (Heymann, 2014). Next, the agent must have a portal of exit from the reservoir, as well as some mode of transmission. For example, the bite of an *Anopheles* mosquito provides a portal of exit for the malaria parasites, which spend part of their life cycle in the mosquito's body; the mosquito in this case is the mode of transmission. The next link in the chain of causation is the agent itself. Malaria, for example, actually consists of four distinct diseases caused by four kinds of microscopic protozoa (Heymann, 2014). The next link is the portal of entry. In the case of malaria, the mosquito

bite provides a portal of exit as well as a portal of entry into the human host.

The box surrounding the chain of causation in Figure 7–6 represents the environment, which can have a profound influence at almost any point along the chain. Consider the impact of environmental factors on the 1934-to-1935 malaria epidemic in Sri Lanka (an island country in the Indian Ocean off southern India). Historically, malaria occurred frequently in the dry northern area, where sparse vegetation allowed pools of water to be exposed to the sun, providing excellent breeding grounds for the *Anopheles* mosquito. In contrast, the more populous southwestern area usually had heavy monsoon rains and was relatively free from malaria. In 1934, however, a severe drought changed this environment drastically; throughout Sri Lanka, rivers almost dried up, leaving stagnant pools of water for mosquito breeding. Widespread crop failure caused the population to become badly undernourished, which added to conditions that would foster a malaria epidemic. The epidemic occurred in October 1934, affecting 2 to 3 million people and causing 80,000 deaths. The environment must certainly be seen as a major part of this causal chain (Karunaweera, Galappaththy, & Wirth, 2014). See Chapter 9.

Causation in Noninfectious Disease

With the availability of vaccines and antibiotics to thwart most infectious diseases in the United States and the developed world, attention shifted to the causes of noninfectious diseases such as cancer and diabetes. A new causal paradigm was clearly needed. The linear thinking embodied in models such as the *chain of causation* was insufficient in understanding the causes of these emerging health threats. Beginning in the 1950s, there was a growing interest in the role smoking played in the development of lung cancer. In 1964, the publication of *Smoking and Health: Report of the Advisory Committee to the Surgeon General of the Public Health Service* concluded that smoking caused lung and laryngeal cancer in men (U.S. Public Health Service,

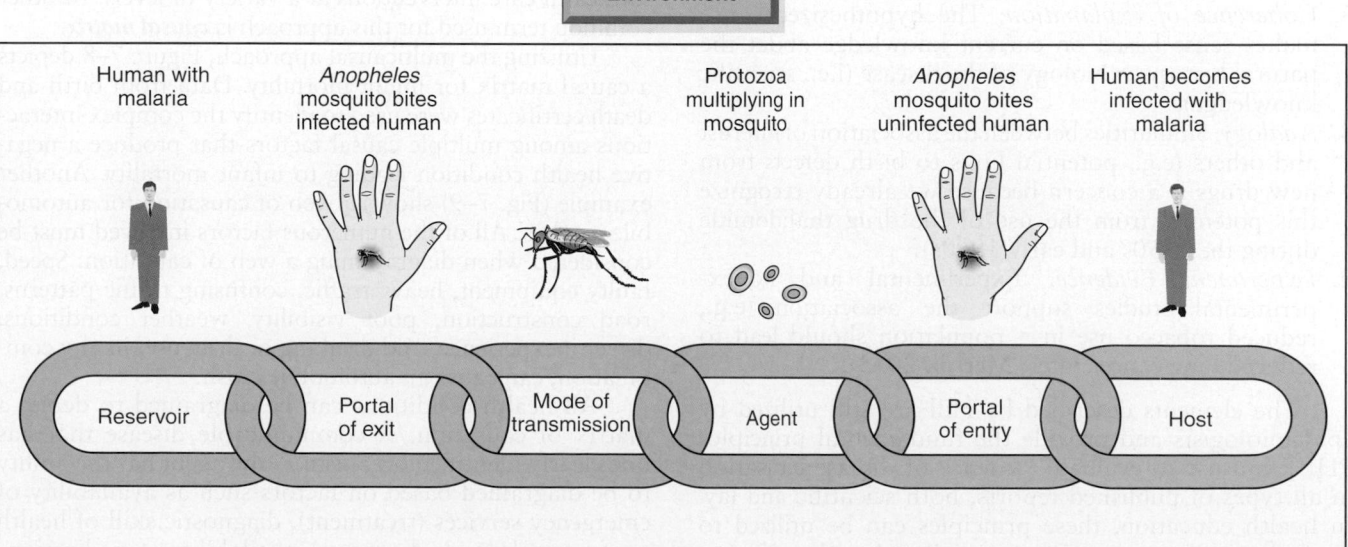

FIGURE 7–7 Chain of causation.

1964). Fifty years later, the Surgeon General released *The Health Consequences of Smoking—50 Years of Progress: A Report of the Surgeon General, 2014*. Additional findings further implicate smoking, such as causing liver and colon cancer, diabetes mellitus and rheumatoid arthritis, as well as general adverse health effects from inflammation and impairment of immune function. The report further states that those exposed to secondhand smoke were at increased risk of stroke, and that smoking increases a smoker's risk of dying from cancer and other diseases (USDHHS, 2014).

In 1856, John Stuart Mill formed three methods of hypothesis formulation for determining disease etiology. These methods include method of difference, method of agreement, and method of concomitant variation. In 1965, Sir Austin Bradford Hill proposed expanding on Mill's postulates about causality by developing nine criteria to evaluate the relationship between environmental exposure and potential health outcomes. The criteria can be used with infectious disease as well as noninfectious disease. These elements are summarized below:

1. *Strength of association*: This refers to the ratio of disease rates in those with and without the suspected causal factor. A strong association would be noted if rates of disease are much higher in the group with the factor than in the group without it.
2. *Consistency of association*: An association is demonstrated in varying types of studies among diverse study groups (i.e., replication).
3. *Specificity*: A cause leads to one effect (not always the case in noninfectious diseases).
4. *Temporality*: Exposure to the suspected factor must precede the onset of disease (i.e., time order or time sequence).
5. *Biological gradient*: This relationship is demonstrated if, with increasing levels of exposure to the factor, there is a corresponding increase in occurrence of the disease (i.e., dose–response relationship).
6. *Biological Plausibility*: The hypothesized cause makes sense based on current biologic or social models (i.e., it is possible).
7. *Coherence of explanation*: The hypothesized cause makes sense based on current knowledge about the natural history or biology of the disease (i.e., scientific knowledge).
8. *Analogy*: Similarities between the association of interest and others (e.g., potential links to birth defects from new drugs is a concern because we already recognize this potential from the use of the drug thalidomide during the 1950s and early 1960s).
9. *Experiment Evidence*: Experimental and nonexperimental studies support the association (e.g., reduced tobacco use in a population should lead to reduced lung cancer rates; Merrill, 2013).

The elements described by Hill are still utilized by epidemiologists and provide the fundamental principles PHNs can use to evaluate evidence of disease causation in all types of published reports, both scientific and lay. In health education, these principles can be utilized to teach disease causation risk, especially when the evidence is not yet complete. For instance, a pregnant teen asks a nurse if she should drink diet soda while she is pregnant. The nurse can share with her that the evidence to date supports the safety of artificial sweeteners for most adults (experiment), but that it is probably not wise to drink diet soda while pregnant. When she asks why (because there isn't any reported risk), the nurse can respond that any chemical has the potential to cause harm (plausibility and analogy), and the effects on a growing fetus (biologic gradient) are often unknown until decades later (temporality and experiment).

Multiple Causations

As health care professionals began to understand the complexity of many of the infectious and noninfectious disease threats, they came to realize that causation was never completely straightforward. Even with long-recognized contagious diseases like cholera, the organism was only part of the equation. Factors such as availability of clean water, the number of trained nurses and doctors, the overall nutrition of the population, and even political upheaval could influence the spread of disease and the number who ultimately died. Causation was beginning to be viewed as multifactorial. Fortunately, with recognition of the complexity of each health threat, came multiple opportunities to find solutions. The following section discusses the complexity of causal factors on health outcomes and implications for reduced morbidity and mortality.

Web of Causation

In the 1960s, the concept of multiple causation emerged to explain the existence of health and illness states and to provide guiding principles for epidemiologic practice. A causal paradigm that gained attention was referred to as the **web of causation**. The implication was that intervention (or breaking of the web at any point nearest to the disease) could profoundly impact the development of that disease (Fletcher & Fletcher, 2012; Merrill, 2013). This was a significant shift in thinking about disease and health, positing that the combination of multiple factors was the deciding factor in the development of poor outcomes. This refinement in causal thinking also provided opportunities for health care interventions at a variety of levels. Another common term used for this approach is ***causal matrix***.

Utilizing the multicausal approach, Figure 7–8 depicts a causal matrix for infant mortality. Data from birth and death certificates were used to identify the complex interactions among multiple causal factors that produce a negative health condition leading to infant mortality. Another example (Fig. 7–9) shows a web of causation for automobile crashes. All of the numerous factors involved must be considered when diagramming a web of causation. Speed, faulty equipment, heavy traffic, confusing traffic patterns, road construction, poor visibility, weather conditions, driver inexperience, and drinking or drug use, in any combination, can cause an automobile crash.

All health conditions can be diagramed to depict a matrix of causation. A communicable disease that has one clearly identified organism as the agent has the ability to be diagramed based on factors such as availability of emergency services (treatment), diagnostic skill of health professionals (early diagnosis), availability of medications and vaccines to treat the disease (reduced morbidity), and

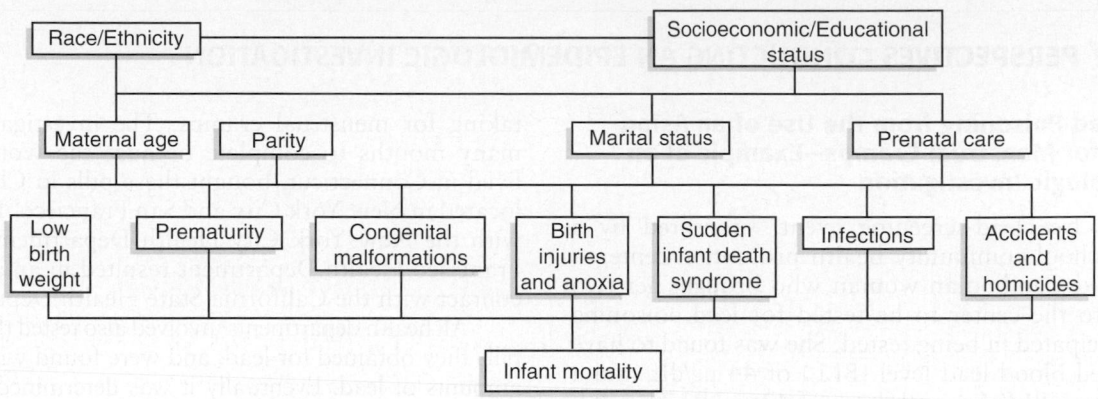

FIGURE 7–8 Web of causation for infant mortality.

community communication networks (public awareness). Any of these factors could greatly influence the progression of disease within the community.

Association is a concept that is helpful in determining multiple causalities. Events are said to be associated if they appear together more often than would be the case by chance alone (see Perspectives). Such events may include risk factors or other characteristics affecting disease or health states. Examples are the frequent association of cigarette smoking with lung cancer, obesity with heart disease, and severe prematurity with infant mortality. The study of associated factors suggests possible causality and points for intervention. Contemporary epidemiologists continue to explore new and more comprehensive ways of viewing health and illness. The associations among lifestyle, behavior, environment, and stress of all kinds and the ways in which they affect health states are gaining importance in epidemiology (Fletcher & Fletcher, 2012).

In the host, agent, and environment model, a shifting emphasis of investigation over time may be noted. Early epidemiologists worked to identify and manage the causative agent; the focus of concern was the disease state.

The emphasis then shifted to the host: Who was susceptible? What characteristics led to susceptibility? Through immunization and health promotion, efforts were made to improve host resistance. Increasingly, however, public health workers came to realize the limitations imposed on individual control of health. Even individuals who are in the best of health cannot withstand toxic agents in the workplace—for example, nuclear wastes in the atmosphere from power plant accidents—or other debilitating conditions created by modern society. More and more, public health professionals are studying the environment and looking for methods to change conditions that contribute to illness. See Chapter 9.

Immunity

Immunity refers to a host's ability to resist a particular infectious disease–causing agent. This occurs when the body forms antibodies and lymphocytes that react with the foreign antigenic molecules and render them harmless (Fletcher & Fletcher, 2012). For public health nursing, this concept has significance in determining which individuals and groups are protected against disease and

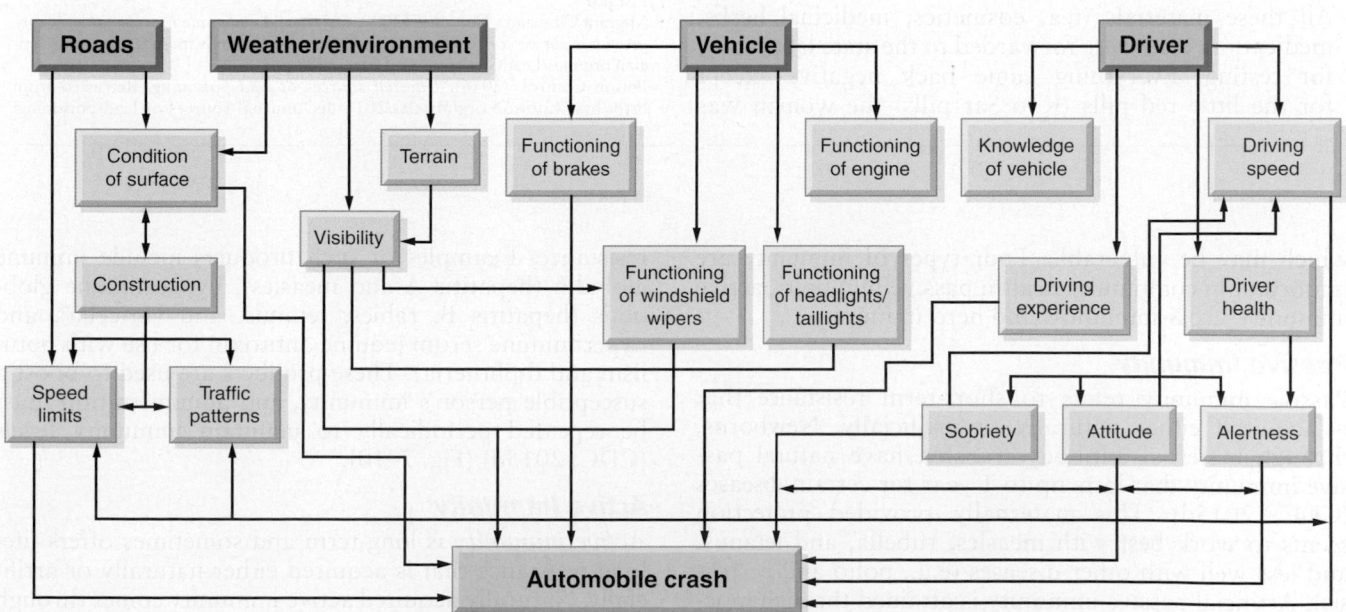

FIGURE 7–9 Web of causation for automobile crashes.

 **PERSPECTIVES** CONDUCTING AN EPIDEMIOLOGIC INVESTIGATION

Adult Lead Poisoning from the Use of an Asian Remedy for Menstrual Cramps—Example of an Epidemiologic Investigation

During a free lead-screening event, sponsored by a nursing school community health promotion center, a 33-year-old Cambodian woman who brought her two children to the center to be tested for lead poisoning also participated in being tested. She was found to have an elevated blood lead level (BLL) of 44 µg/dL, and a confirmatory BLL 1 month later of 42 µg/dL. The children and her husband were found to have normal BLLs. This woman was referred by the director of the health promotion center for follow-up to the Connecticut Department of Public Health.

As the Connecticut Adult Blood Lead Surveillance Program's Adult Lead Registry and Case Management Coordinator, I was responsible for compiling and analyzing BLL data from Connecticut laboratories performing these tests, and to follow up on any reports of elevated lead levels, such as this woman who was identified through a community screening event sponsored by a nursing school.

Although ideally there should be no lead in the blood, levels below 10 µg/dL are considered normal (because of ambient exposures), and any value above 10 µg/dL was considered abnormal and required follow-up regarding the cause. The Connecticut Adult Lead Poisoning Program is funded by the CDC's Adult Blood Lead Epidemiology and Surveillance Program (ABLES), with a primary interest in studying and reducing occupational exposure to lead. In this particular case, occupational exposure was ruled out (she was not working), but an epidemiological investigation was still conducted to identify the source of lead exposure.

The woman was requested to send in any possible causes of lead exposure to the state health department. All these materials (tea, cosmetics, medicinal herbs, medication, etc.) were forwarded to the state laboratory for testing. Everything came back negative except for the little red pills (Koo Sar pills) the woman was taking for menstrual cramps. The investigation took many months to complete because the woman, who lived in Connecticut, bought these pills in Chinatowns located in New York City and San Francisco. Follow-up with the New York City Health Department and San Francisco Health Department resulted in an additional contact with the California State Health Department.

All health departments involved also tested the Koo Sar pills they obtained for lead, and were found with varying amounts of lead. Eventually it was determined that lead was not a listed ingredient of these pills but a contaminant during the manufacturing process. The investigation was reported in an issue of the CDC's *Morbidity and Mortality Weekly Report*. This report led to a greater awareness among public health professionals, health care providers, and environmental workers of the potential for lead poisoning from herbal remedies.

–BC Jung, MPH, RN, MCHES

For more information please see
Centers for Disease Control and Prevention. (1999). Adult Lead Poisoning from an Asian Remedy for Menstrual Cramps—Connecticut, 1997. *Morbidity and Mortality Weekly Report, 48*(20), 27–29. Retrieved from http://www.cdc.gov/mmwr/preview/mmwrhtml/00056277.htm

Chen, A. (2015, August 3). *Toxic lead contaminates some traditional Ayurvedic medicines.* Retrieved from http://www.npr.org/sections/health-shots/2015/07/31/428016419/toxic-lead-contaminates-some-traditional-ayurvedic-medicines

City of New York, Department of Health and Mental Hygiene. (n.d.). *Imported herbal medicine products known to contain lead, mercury, or arsenic.* Retrieved from http://www.nyc.gov/html/doh/downloads/pdf/lead/lead-herbalmed.pdf

Food & Drug Administration (FDA). (2015). *Guidance for the industry: The safety of imported traditional pottery intended for use with food.* Retrieved from http://www.fda.gov/food/guidanceregulation/guidancedocumentsregulatoryinformation/ucm214740.htm

Food & Drug Administration (FDA). (2015). *Lipstick & lead: Questions & answers.* Retrieved from http://www.fda.gov/Cosmetics/ProductsIngredients/Products/ucm137224.htm

Los Angeles County Childhood Lead Poisoning Prevention Program. (2009). *Traditional remedies and other products reported to contain lead.* Retrieved from http://www.lapublichealth.org/lead/reports/Home%20Remedies%20List.pdf

Migrant Clinician's Network. (2009, October). *Lead guidelines for primary care providers caring for migrant children.* Retrieved from http://www.migrantclinician.org/files/LeadGuidelinesChildren_2009.pdf

Poison Control. (2016). *Unusual sources of lead poisoning.* Retrieved from http://www.poison.org/articles/2011-dec/unusual-sources-of-lead-poisoning

which may be vulnerable. Four types of immunity are important in community health: passive immunity, active immunity, cross-immunity, and herd immunity.

Passive Immunity

Passive immunity refers to short-term resistance that is acquired either naturally or artificially. Newborns, through maternal antibody transfer, have natural passive immunity that lasts up to 1 year for certain diseases (CDC, 2015d). This maternally provided protection seems to work best with measles, rubella, and tetanus, and less well with other diseases (e.g., polio and pertussis). Artificial passive immunity is attained through inoculation with antibody products to provide temporary resistance. Examples of such products include immune globulin (hepatitis A and measles), hyperimmune globulins (hepatitis B, rabies, tetanus, and varicella), and hyperimmune serum (equine antitoxin for use with botulism and diphtheria). These products are used to boost a susceptible person's immunity, and administration must be repeated periodically to maintain immunity levels (CDC, 2015d) (Fig. 7–10).

Active Immunity

Active immunity is long-term and sometimes offers lifelong resistance that is acquired either naturally or artificially. Naturally acquired active immunity comes through host infection. That is, a person who contracts a disease

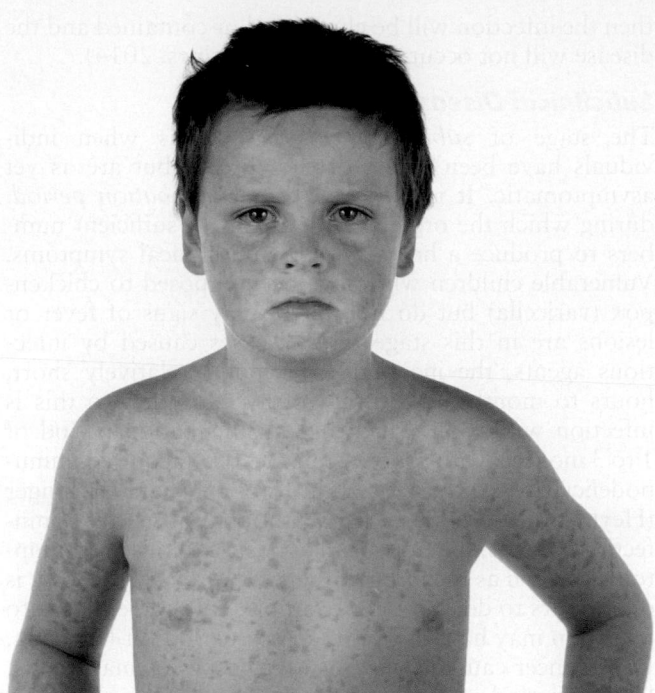

FIGURE 7–10 Child with red, watery eyes and a rash.

often develops long-lasting antibodies that provide immunity against future exposures. Artificially acquired active immunity is attained through vaccine inoculation. Such vaccines are prepared from killed (inactivated) or live attenuated (weakened) organisms administered to artificially produce or increase immunity to a particular disease (CDC, 2015d). The concept of active immunity underlies public health immunization programs that have successfully kept polio, diphtheria, smallpox, and other major diseases under control worldwide.

Cross-Immunity

Cross-immunity refers to a situation in which a person's immunity to one agent provides immunity to a related agent as well. The immunity can be either passive or active. Sometimes, infection with one disease, such as cowpox, gives immunity to a related disease, such as smallpox. The concept of cross-immunity has also been useful in the development and administration of vaccines. Inoculation with a vaccine made from one disease-causing organism can provide immunity to a related disease-causing organism. Field trials in Uganda and Papua, New Guinea and a study in India in the 1990s examined the administration of *bacille Calmette-Guérin* (BCG) vaccine, which is used to prevent tuberculosis, to people who had been exposed to Hansen's disease (leprosy). The vaccine against *Mycobacterium tuberculosis* appeared to provide these individuals with a degree of cross-immunity to the related infectious agent, *Mycobacterium leprae*, and prevented their contracting disease (Heymann, 2014).

Herd Immunity

Herd immunity describes the immunity level that is present in a population group. A population with low herd immunity is one with few immune members; consequently, it is more susceptible to a particular disease. Nonimmune

people are more likely to contract the disease and spread it throughout the group, placing the entire population at greater risk. Conversely, a population with high herd immunity is one in which the immune people in the group outnumber the susceptible people; consequently, the incidence of a particular disease is reduced (Merrill, 2013; Willingham & Helft, 2014). The level of herd immunity may vary with diseases. For instance, a level of community immunity of between 83% and 85% may be necessary for rubella, but for diphtheria a level of 85% may be effective (Merrill, 2013; Willingham & Helft, 2014). Mandatory preschool immunizations and required travel vaccinations are applications of the herd immunity concept. A figure in Chapter 8 provides a depiction of herd immunity.

Risk

To determine the chances that a disease or health problem will occur, epidemiologists are concerned with **risk**, or the probability that a disease or other unfavorable health condition will develop. For any given group of people, the risk of developing a health problem is directly influenced by their biology, environment, lifestyle, and system of health care (McKenzie et al., 2012). A person's inherited health capacity, the environment lived in, the person's lifestyle choices, and the quality and accessibility of the health care system either negatively or positively affect health, thereby increasing or decreasing the likelihood that a health problem will occur. Negative influences are called *risk factors*. For example, low-birth-weight babies (biology, environment, and system of health care) tend to be at greater risk for health problems, as are people who smoke cigarettes, have diets high in cholesterol, and are sedentary (lifestyle). The degree of risk is directly linked to susceptibility or vulnerability to a given health problem.

Epidemiologists study populations at risk. A *population at risk* is a collection of people among whom a health problem has the possibility of developing because certain influencing factors are present (e.g., exposure to HIV) or absent (e.g., lack of childhood immunizations, lack of specific vitamins in the diet), or because there are modifiable risk factors present (e.g., cardiovascular disease). A population at risk has a greater probability of developing a given health problem than other groups do. Epidemiologists measure this difference using the *relative risk ratio*, which statistically compares the disease occurrence in the population at risk with the occurrence of the same disease in people without that risk factor.

$$\text{Relative risk ratio} = \frac{\text{Incidence in exposed group}}{\text{Incidence rate in unexposed group}}$$

If the risk of acquiring the disease is the same regardless of exposure to the risk factor studied, the ratio will be 1:1, and the relative risk will be 1.0. A relative risk >1.0 indicates that those with the risk factor have a greater likelihood of acquiring the disease than do those without it; for instance, a relative risk of 2.54 means that the exposed group is 2.54 times more likely to acquire the disease than the unexposed group. This statistic may be used, for example, to compare the incidence of heart disease among smokers (smoking is a risk factor) with the incidence among nonsmokers, assuming that all other factors are the same. The relative risk ratio assists in determining the most effective points for community health intervention in regard to particular health problems. It also provides a more easily understood method for explaining the risk of certain behaviors in the development of illness or injury to the public (Gordis, 2014).

Natural History of a Disease or Health Condition

Any disease or health condition follows a progression known as its **natural history;** this refers to events that occur before its development, during its course, and during its conclusion. This process involves the interactions among a susceptible host, the causative agent, and the environment. The natural progression of a disease occurs in four stages as they affect a population—susceptibility, preclinical (subclinical) disease, clinical disease, and resolution (Fig. 7–11). The last stage, resolution, includes recovery, disability, or death (Gerstman, 2013).

Susceptibility Stage

The first stage is *susceptibility*. During this state, the disease is not present and individuals have not been exposed. However, host and environmental factors could very likely influence people's susceptibility to a causative agent and lead to development of the disease. Infection occurs when a pathogen invades body cells and reproduces. Usually, infection leads to an immune response. If the immune system's response is effective,

then the infection will be eliminated or contained and the disease will not occur (History of Vaccines, 2014).

Subclinical Disease Stage

The stage of *subclinical disease* begins when individuals have been exposed to a disease but are as yet asymptomatic. It is followed by an *incubation period*, during which the organism multiplies to sufficient numbers to produce a host reaction and clinical symptoms. Vulnerable children who have been exposed to chickenpox (varicella) but do not yet display signs of fever or lesions are in this stage. For diseases caused by infectious agents, the incubation period is relatively short, hours to months. One noteworthy exception to this is infection with HIV, which has an incubation period of 1 to 3 months, with progression to AIDS (acquired immunodeficiency syndrome) from 1 to 15 years or longer (Heymann, 2014). In other conditions caused by noninfectious agents, the time from exposure to onset of symptoms, known as the *induction period* or *latency period*, is often years to decades. For example, children exposed to radiation may have a 5-year latency period for leukemia. Lung cancer caused by exposure to asbestos may have a latency period of up to 40 years between exposure and detection of the disease.

Clinical Disease Stage

During the *clinical disease stage*, signs and symptoms of the disease or condition develop. In the early phase of this period, the signs may be evident only through laboratory test findings, such as tubercular lesions on radiographs or

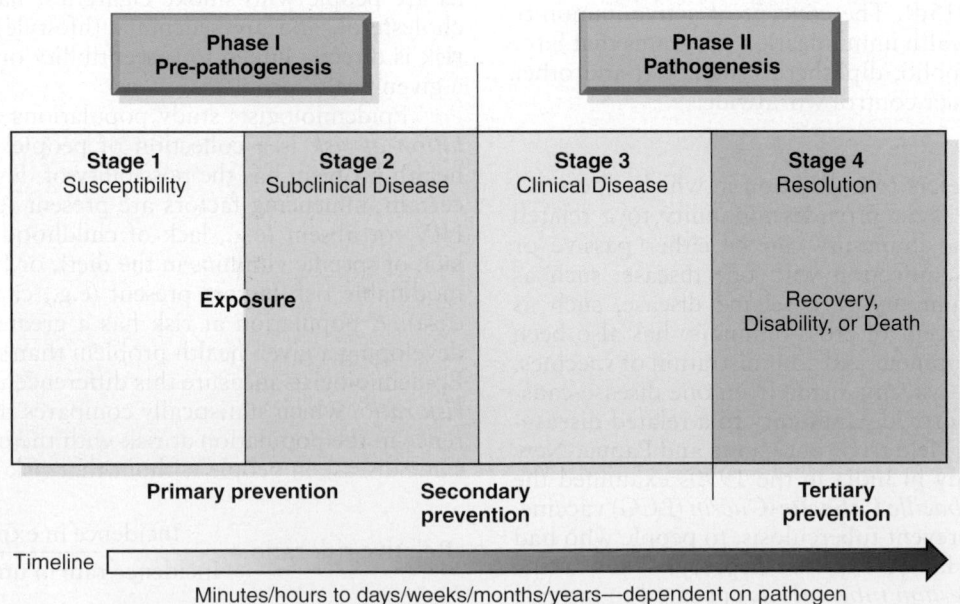

Stage 1—Host and environment factors influence population's vulnerability
Stage 2—Invasion by causative agent; people are asymptomatic
Stage 3—Disease or condition evident in population
Stage 4—Disease or condition concludes in renewed health, disability, or death

FIGURE 7–11 Natural history stages of a disease. (Adapted from Gerstman, B. B. (2013). *Epidemiology kept simple: An introduction to traditional and modern epidemiology* (3rd ed.). Hoboken, NJ: John Wiley & Sons Ltd.)

premalignant cervical changes evident on Papanicolaou (Pap) smears. Later in this stage, acute symptoms are clearly visible, as in the case of widespread enterocolitis in a salmonellosis (food poisoning) outbreak. In this early clinical stage or early discernible lesions stage, evidence of the disease or condition is present and diagnosis occurs (Heymann, 2014).

Resolution Stage

In the *resolution stage,* the disease or health condition causes sufficient anatomic or functional changes to produce recognizable signs and symptoms. Disease severity may vary from mild to severe. The disease may conclude with a return to health, a residual or chronic form of the disease with some disabling limitations, or death. This can also be called the *advanced disease stage,* because the disease or condition has completed its course (Gerstman, 2013).

Community health nurses can intervene at any point during these four stages to delay, arrest, or prevent the progression of the disease or condition. Primary, secondary, and tertiary prevention can be applied to each of the stages (see Levels of Prevention Pyramid).

Epidemiology of Wellness

The public health science of epidemiology has traditionally studied the occurrence of disease and health problems. Because of their devastating effect on the health of populations, infectious diseases such as plague, cholera, and AIDS, as well as chronic illnesses such as heart disease or cancer, and fatal or debilitating injuries all require a continued epidemiologic focus. Nonetheless, the need to examine the epidemiology of wellness grows increasingly urgent, for if we continually examine and uncover new health promotion practices and encourage them, we can focus on wellness at the ideal primary level of prevention. See Chapter 11 on health promotion.

Epidemiology has moved from concentrating only on illness to examining how host, agent, and environment are involved in wellness at various levels. In response to an escalating need for improved methods of health planning and health policy analysis, epidemiology has developed more holistic models of health (Kiefer, 2015). These evolving epidemiologic models are organized around four attributes that influence health: (1) the physical, social, and psychological environment; (2) lifestyle with

---

LEVELS OF PREVENTION PYRAMID

SITUATION: Apply the levels of prevention during the four stages of the natural history of a disease to eradicate or reduce risk factors (examples of possible conditions provided).

GOAL: Using the three levels of prevention negative health conditions are avoided, or promptly diagnosed and treated, and the fullest possible potential is restored.

TERTIARY PREVENTION

Rehabilitation	Primary Prevention	
	Health Promotion and Education	*Health Protection*
• Reduce the extent and severity of a health problem to minimize disability • Restore or preserve function	• Training for employment—homeless population • Group treatment and rehabilitation—adolescent drug users • Food, shelter, rest/sleep, exercise	• Health services • Immunizations as needed

SECONDARY PREVENTION

Early Diagnosis	Prompt Treatment
The third stage in the natural history of disease, the early pathogenesis or onset stage: • Screening programs—breast and testicular cancer, vision and hearing loss, hypertension, tuberculosis, diabetes	• Initiate prompt treatment • Arrest progression • Prevent associated disability

PRIMARY PREVENTION

Health Promotion & Education	Health Protection
May include • Nutrition counseling—diabetes • Sex education—pregnancy • Smoking cessation—lung cancer	May include • Improved housing and sanitation—waterborne diseases • Immunizations—communicable diseases • Removal of environmental hazards—accidents

its self-created risks; (3) human biology and genetic influences; and (4) the system of health care organization. In the United States, *Healthy People 2020* (USDHHS, 2015) and greater recognition of the importance and cost-effectiveness of illness prevention and health promotion are driving new efforts to develop policy and research initiatives that can improve the public's health (see Display 7–2). There is also growing recognition of the collective impact of social determinants of health on health outcomes and conditions, not merely their individual role. Social determinants of health are "conditions in the environments in which people are born, live, play, worship, and age that affect a wide range of health, functioning, and quality of life outcomes and risks" (CDC, 2015e). Population disparities result when these social determinants disproportionately impact individuals owing to race/ethnicity, socioeconomic status, gender, age, disability status, sexual orientation, and geographic location (USDHHS, 2015, para. 6). See Chapters 15 and 25 for more on this.

Wellness models that at first focused on individual behavior now include approaches that encompass aggregates. A variety of wellness models can be found for groups of seniors (see Chapter 24), in occupational health settings (see Chapter 31), at innovative schools where wellness programs for children and teens are initiated (see Chapter 22), and throughout the services provided for beginning and growing families (see Chapter 21). Programs designed for aggregates focus on a wellness approach to growth and development. Examples include programs for pregnant teens and for infant and child development (e.g., Healthy Start, Head Start) that are funded by state and federal monies. Societal changes, such as the aging population, the technological revolution, the global economy, environmental threats, health care reform with its focus on prevention, and the health and

---

DISPLAY 7–2 *HEALTHY PEOPLE 2020*

Epidemiological Focus Objectives

Data and Information Systems

PHI-7—Increase the proportion of population-based *Healthy People 2020* objectives for which national data are available for all major population groups

PHI-7.1—Increase the proportion of population-based *Healthy People 2020* objectives for which national data are available by race and ethnicity

PHI-7.2—Increase the proportion of population-based *Healthy People 2020* objectives for which national data are available by sex

PHI-7.3—Increase the proportion of population-based *Healthy People 2020* objectives for which national data are available by socioeconomic status

PHI-8—Increase the proportion of *Healthy People 2020* objectives that are tracked regularly at the national level

PHI-8.1—Increase the proportion of *Healthy People 2020* objectives that have at least one data point

PHI-8.2—Increase the proportion of *Healthy People 2020* objectives that have at least two data points

PHI-8.3—Increase the proportion of *Healthy People 2020* objectives that are tracked at least every 3 years

PHI-9—(Developmental) Increase the proportion of *Healthy People 2020* objectives for which national data are released within 1 year of the end of data collection

PHI-10—Increase the number of States that record vital events using the latest U.S. standard certificates and report

PHI-10.1—Increase the number of States that record vital events using the latest U.S. standard certificate of birth

PHI-10.2—Increase the number of States that record vital events using the latest U.S. standard certificate of death

PHI-10.3—Increase the number of States that record vital events using the latest U.S. standard report of fetal death

Public Health Organizations

PHI-11—Increase the proportion of Tribal and State public health agencies that provide or assure comprehensive laboratory services to support essential public health services

PHI-12—Increase the proportion of public health laboratory systems (including State, Tribal, and local) that perform at a high level of quality in support of the 10 Essential Public Health Services

PHI-13—Increase the proportion of Tribal, State, and local public health agencies that provide or assure comprehensive epidemiology services to support essential public health services

PHI-14—Increase the proportion of State and local public health jurisdictions that conduct a public health system assessment using national performance standards

PHI-15—Increase the proportion of Tribal, State, and local public health agencies that have developed a health improvement plan and increase the proportion of local health jurisdictions that have a health improvement plan linked with their State plan

PHI-16—Increase the proportion of Tribal, State, and local public health agencies that have implemented an agency-wide quality improvement process

PHI-17—Increase the number or proportion of Tribal, State and local public health agencies that are accredited

From U.S. Department of Health and Human Services. (2016). *Healthy People 2020: Public health infrastructure*. Retrieved from http://www.healthypeople.gov/2020/topics-objectives/topic/public-health-infrastructure/objectives?topicId=35

wellness movements, are driving these new approaches. See Chapter 12.

The four stages of the natural history of disease can apply to an understanding of any health condition, including wellness states. In stage one, *susceptibility*, people can become amenable to healthier practices and improved health system organization. In stage two, *subclinical*, a community can learn about these health-promoting behaviors. Stage three, *clinical disease stage*, could be a period of trying out the beneficial policies and activities, and stage four, *resolution*, could encompass full adoption and a higher level of well-being for the community. This approach has important implications for preventive and health-promotion practices in community health nursing.

Community health nursing can play a primary role in the investigation and identification of factors that not only prevent illness but also promote health. This means sharpening skills in epidemiologic research to uncover the factors that contribute to a full measure of healthful living. The time for an epidemiology of wellness has come.

Causal Relationships

One of the main challenges to epidemiology is to identify causal relationships in disease and health conditions among populations. As was previously suggested, the assessment of causality in human health is difficult at best; no single study is adequate to establish causality. Causal inference is based on consistent results obtained from many studies. Frequently, the accumulation of evidence begins with a clinical observation or an educated guess that a certain factor may be causally related to a health problem (Gordis, 2014).

A *cross-sectional study* (which explores a health condition's relation to other variables in a specified population at a specific point in time) can show that the factor and the problem coexist. For example, one classic study compared the incidence of gonorrhea in a 55-block area in urban New Orleans with a "broken window index," which measured housing quality, abandoned cars, graffiti, trash, and public school deterioration (Cohen et al., 2000). Broken windows theory is a symbol of lack of social control in neighborhoods and has been used to predict crime and social isolation (Aiyer, Zimmerman, Morrel-Samuels, & Reischl, 2015). The broken window index predicted the variance for gonorrhea rates more accurately than did a poverty index measuring income, unemployment, and low education.

A *retrospective study* (which looks backward in time to find a causal relationship) allows a fairly quick assessment of whether an association exists. Such studies use existing data that have been recorded for reasons other than research, and are generally less expensive and labor intensive. One disadvantage is that the data may not be collected with a research outcome in mind. An example of a short-term retrospective cohort study occurred with an outbreak of *Giardia* among members of a golfing club in Massachusetts. Cases had already begun to diminish before the health department became involved. They examined the facilities and found both an adult pool and a kiddie pool at the golfing club; best guess was that a child in could have contaminated the kiddie pool with *Giardia*-shedding stool. They questioned adults by asking if they spent any time in the kiddie pool, and this gave them the number of people exposed to the kiddie pool, along with the number of them who developed *Giardia*, versus the ones exposed to the adult pool and the number of them who developed *Giardia*. There were 9 additional cases per 100 people for those who used the kiddie pool than those who did not, and they calculated the risk ratio as 3.27 (Boston University School of Public Health, 2015).

A *prospective study* (which looks forward in time to find a causal relationship) is crucial to ensure that the presumed causal factor actually precedes the onset of the health problem. The prospective approach is concerned with current information and provides a direct measure of the variables in question. For example, in the Nurses' Health Study (Channing Laboratory, 2013) many prospective analyses of numerous risk factors that impact health were performed. Studies have found the following:

Alcohol: One or more drinks a day increases the risk of breast cancer; two or more drinks a day increase the risk of colon cancer; high consumption increases the risk of hip fracture.

Diet: Higher intake of red meat increases the risk of premenopausal breast cancer and colon cancer. Mediterranean-type diets reduce risk of incident CHD and stroke. Refined carbohydrates and trans fats increase the risk of CHD. Higher vegetable intake (green leafy vegetables) reduces the risk of cognitive impairment.

Obesity: Increases the risk of breast cancer among postmenopausal women (postmenopause weight loss reduces the risk). A positive relationship was found between weight (BMI) and the risk of CHD and stroke. Weight gain after age 18 increases the risk of stroke and CHD; it also increases the risk of colon cancer, cataracts and age-related macular degeneration (AMD). It is protective against hip fracture owing to extra hip padding.

Oral Contraceptive Use: Current use increased the risk of breast cancer and CHD, and reduced the risk of colon cancer, hip fracture, and high-tension glaucoma, as well as "wet" AMD.

Physical Activity: >3 hours per week of physical activity reduces the risk of breast cancer, CHD, and stroke (walking), as well as colon cancer and risk of hip fracture (walking). Moderate physical activity reduces the risk of cognitive impairment.

Postmenopausal Hormones: With more than 5 years of estrogen plus progestins taken, the risk of breast cancer is increased. It is also increased with more than 10 years of estrogen alone. Current use increases the risk of stroke and reduces the risk of CHD among recently menopausal women. Reduced risk of colon cancer and of hip fracture and high-tension glaucoma and "wet" AMD was found for current users.

Smoking: Has a strong positive association with CHD and stroke, and the risk can be reduced within 2 to 4 years of smoking cessation. Smoking increases the risk of colon cancer, hip fracture, and cataracts, along with "wet" AMD.

Other factors: Family history of breast cancer, high breast density, high circulating hormone levels, and shift work all increased the risk of breast cancer. Snoring is associated with a modest but significant increased risk of CHD and stroke. Diabetes, as well as rotating night shifts, increased the risk of hip fracture, as well as the risk of glaucoma and cataracts. Type 2 diabetes and higher insulin levels in women without diabetes increases the risk of cognitive impairment. Positive family history and African heritage increases the risk of glaucoma (Channing Laboratory, 2013).

Studies such as these provide a mechanism to evaluate a variety of factors that precede the development of disease and then assess issues of association and ultimately causation.

Finally, if ethically possible, an *experimental study* (in which the investigator controls or changes factors suspected of causing the condition and observes results) is used to confirm the associations obtained from observational studies (in which the investigator merely observes data or people without controlling or changing any factors). It often requires many years to accumulate enough evidence to suggest a causal relationship. An example of this may be manufacturing plants that agree to participate in CHD prevention. One plant gets the intervention—education and screening for CHD—and the other serves as a control with no intervention given. Years later, the incidence of CHD is measured and the numbers for the two groups are compared to determine if the intervention may have made a difference (BMJ Publishing Group, 2015).

Epidemiologically, a causal relationship may be said to exist if two major conditions are met: (a) the factor of interest (causal agent) is shown to increase the probability of occurrence of the disease or condition as observed in many studies in different populations, and (b) evidence suggests that a reduction in the factor decreases the frequency of the given disease. The synthesis of data begins by selecting as many of the various types of epidemiologic studies of the problem as possible. After those studies that are not methodologically sound are discarded, the studies are reviewed. The better the data meet the criteria outlined by Hill (discussed earlier), the more likely it is that the factor of interest is one of several causes of the disease (strength of association, consistency, specificity, time sequence, biologic gradient, plausibility, coherence, experiment, and analogy).

The goal of any epidemiologic investigation is to identify causal mechanisms that meet Hill's nine criteria for disease causation and to develop measures for preventing illness and promoting health (Gordis, 2014). The PHN may need to gather new data for this type of investigation, but pertinent existing data should be thoroughly examined first. This type of information can be obtained from a variety of sources, which are discussed in the next section.

SOURCES OF INFORMATION FOR EPIDEMIOLOGIC STUDY

Epidemiologic investigators may draw data from any of three major sources: existing data, informal investigations, and scientific studies. The public health nurse will find all three sources useful in efforts to improve the health of aggregates. See Chapter 15 on community assessment for more on sources of data.

Existing Data

A variety of information is available nationally, by state, and by section (e.g., county, region, census tract, metropolitan statistical area [MSA]). This information includes vital statistics, census data, and morbidity statistics on certain communicable or infectious diseases. Local health departments often can provide these data on request. Public health nurses seeking information on communities may find local health system agencies helpful. These agencies collect health information for groups of counties within states and interact with health planning authorities at the state level. They have access to many types of information and can give advice on specific problems. One newer source of data is social media. (See Population-Focus on Epidemiology and Social Media.)

Vital Statistics

Vital statistics refers to the information gathered from ongoing registration of births, deaths, adoptions, divorces, and marriages. Certification of births, deaths, and fetal deaths are the most useful vital statistics in epidemiologic studies. The community health nurse can obtain blank copies of a state's birth and death certificates to become familiar with the information contained in each (Displays 7–3 and 7–4). Much more information is recorded on the death certificate than the fact and cause of death on the death. Birth certificates also can provide helpful information (e.g., weight of the infant, amount of prenatal care received by the mother), which can be used to identify high-risk mothers and infants.

Sources for vital statistical information include state Web sites, local and state health departments, city halls, and county halls of records (see list of Internet resources on *thePoint*). Statistics regarding general aggregate morbidity and mortality for specific states are available from the Centers for Disease Control and Prevention (CDC) at the national level (National Center for Health Statistics [NCHS]). State statistics are obtained from state health departments, and county information (specific cities or census tracts) can be obtained from either the state or the county health department.

Census Data

Data from population censuses taken every 10 years in many countries are the main source of population statistics. This information can be a valuable assessment tool for the PHN who is taking part in health planning for aggregates. Population statistics can be analyzed by age, sex, race, ethnic background, type of occupation, income gradient, marital status, educational level, or other standards, such as housing quality. Analysis of population statistics can provide the community health nurse with a better understanding of the community and help identify specific areas that may warrant further epidemiologic investigation. Data from the 2010 Census can be found on the U.S. Census Bureau Web site, and is an easily accessed source of population-level data.

POPULATION-FOCUS ON EPIDEMIOLOGY AND SOCIAL MEDIA

Most of us use some form of social media daily. But, did you know that epidemiologists and PHNs have used Twitter and Yelp in food-borne illness investigations? Traditionally, most investigations begin with either a physician report to the local health department or a self-report called in by someone who became ill after eating out at a restaurant or a food truck. But, two large progressive health departments found ways to utilize social media to assist them in these epidemiological investigations.

In Chicago, the health department and civic partners established a Web site, FoodBorne Chicago (https://www.foodbornechicago.org), to more quickly identify and respond to complaints on Twitter about possible signs and symptoms of food-borne illness. An algorithm was used to identify tweets that would later be reviewed by staff members (e.g., diarrhea, vomiting, stomach cramps after ingesting food prepared outside homes). Replies to identified tweets were made by staff members, inviting Twitter users to report the illness and giving them the Web site link. Submitted forms from the Web site went to the city's 311 system. Over a 10-month period, 270 tweets complained of symptoms related to food-borne illness, and 3% noted visits to the emergency room or a physician as a result. Web site complaints totaled 193, but the number of those originating from Twitter could not be identified. Almost 9% of these sought medical care. All of the complaints identified a total of 179 restaurants, and 133 locations had unannounced health inspection visits. This represented 6.9% of all food establishment health inspections due to complaints during that time. Almost 92% of the 133 inspections led to at least one violation; this is similar to rates of the other inspections during the study period. However, 20.3% of the inspections prompted by the study had a minimum of one critical violation (high-risk or immediate hazard) versus 16.4% for the other inspections. A total of 21 restaurants were closed after failing FoodBorne Chicago inspections, and 33 with critical violations corrected them and were cleared on later inspections. Thirty tweets were linked directly to a "corresponding complaint" by clicking on "reply tweet" to fill in the form (p. 684). FoodBorne Chicago has made their open-source software available on GitHub, and is working with both New York City and Boston on adapting their program for use in these cities.

Harris, J. K., Mansour, R., Choucair, B., Olson, J., Nissin, C., & Bhatt, J. (2014). Health department use of social media to identify foodborne illness: Chicago, Illinois, 2013–2014. Morbidity and Mortality Weekly Report, 63(32), 681–685.

In New York City, health department staff noticed patron reports of illness after eating at the same restaurant they were investigating for a recent gastrointestinal disease outbreak; most of these had not been reported to the health department. Thinking that this might be a reliable source for population-based investigation into food-borne illnesses, the New York City Department of Health and Mental Hygiene worked with Yelp to use data mining software to download weekly data that met the following criteria: (a) symptoms occurred after a meal, (b) symptoms occurred within 4 weeks of the posted review, and (c) two or more people became ill (or one person with symptoms of severe neurologic illness). Of about 294,000 reviews, 468 were identified as possibly meeting the criteria for a recent illness, after an epidemiologist specializing in food-borne illness reviewed 893 potential postings. Messages were sent through Yelp that the reviewers contact the health department for a telephone interview. Ultimately, 27 out of 129 accepted the request, and 3 outbreaks causing 16 illnesses were discovered. The food in question included shrimp and lobster cannelloni, a house salad, and macaroni and cheese spring rolls from three different restaurants. These establishments were inspected, and multiple violations were found. Although the city has a 311 service for reporting nonemergencies to city agencies, most reviewers who were informed of this service did not know about it (78%). The 311 system identifies outbreaks in about 1% of reported cases, whereas the Yelp reviews netted 3% in this pilot project. Daily review feeds are now being provided by Yelp, and the health department is investigating links to other review sites and multiple complaints to a particular restaurant in an effort to get better data and resolve violations more quickly.

Harrison, C., Jorder, M., Stern, H., Stravinsky, F., Reddy, V., Hanson, H., ... Balter, S. (2014). Using online reviews by restaurant patrons to identify unreported cases of foodborne illness: New York City, 2012–2013. Morbidity and Mortality Weekly Report, 63(20), 441–446.

Reportable Diseases

Each state has developed laws or regulations that require health organizations and practitioners to report to their local health authority cases of certain communicable and infectious diseases that can be spread through the community (Heymann, 2014). This reporting enables the health department to take the most appropriate and efficient action, for instance, in the case of food-borne illnesses. All states require that diseases subject to international quarantine regulations be reported immediately. However, many of these diseases (e.g., plague, cholera, yellow fever, polio) are virtually unknown now in developed countries (WHO, 2015). Health care professionals have not had experience identifying another reportable disease, smallpox, because no cases have been reported since 1977 (CDC, 2007; Scheibner, 2012). In 1980, the World Health Organization (WHO) declared the global eradication of smallpox after more than 10 years of international effort. (Chapter 17 discusses the concern over the use of smallpox as a bioterrorism threat.)

The World Health Organization (2007) has numerous other diseases under surveillance (e.g., tuberculosis,

(*Text continues on page 255*)

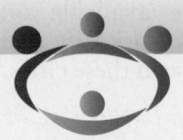

DISPLAY 7–3 STANDARD BIRTH CERTIFICATE

U.S. STANDARD CERTIFICATE OF LIVE BIRTH

LOCAL FILE NO.

BIRTH NUMBER:

CHILD

1. CHILD'S NAME (First, Middle, Last, Suffix)	2. TIME OF BIRTH (24 hr)	3. SEX	4. DATE OF BIRTH (Mo/Day/Yr)

5. FACILITY NAME (If not institution, give street and number)	6. CITY, TOWN, OR LOCATION OF BIRTH	7. COUNTY OF BIRTH

MOTHER

8a. MOTHER'S CURRENT LEGAL NAME (First, Middle, Last, Suffix)	8b. DATE OF BIRTH (Mo/Day/Yr)

8c. MOTHER'S NAME PRIOR TO FIRST MARRIAGE (First, Middle, Last, Suffix)	8d. BIRTHPLACE (State, Territory, or Foreign Country)

9a. RESIDENCE OF MOTHER-STATE	9b. COUNTY	9c. CITY, TOWN, OR LOCATION

9d. STREET AND NUMBER	9e. APT. NO.	9f. ZIP CODE	9g. INSIDE CITY LIMITS? ☐ Yes ☐ No

FATHER

10a. FATHER'S CURRENT LEGAL NAME (First, Middle, Last, Suffix)	10b. DATE OF BIRTH (Mo/Day/Yr)	10c. BIRTHPLACE (State, Territory, or Foreign Country)

CERTIFIER

11. CERTIFIER'S NAME: _____ TITLE: ☐ MD ☐ DO ☐ HOSPITAL ADMIN. ☐ CNM/CM ☐ OTHER MIDWIFE ☐ OTHER (Specify)_____	12. DATE CERTIFIED ___ / ___ / ___ MM DD YYYY	13. DATE FILED BY REGISTRAR ___ / ___ / ___ MM DD YYYY

INFORMATION FOR ADMINISTRATIVE USE

MOTHER

14. MOTHER'S MAILING ADDRESS: ☐ Same as residence, or: State:	City, Town, or Location:	
Street & Number:	Apartment No.:	Zip Code:

15. MOTHER MARRIED? (At birth, conception, or any time between) ☐ Yes ☐ No IF NO, HAS PATERNITY ACKNOWLEDGEMENT BEEN SIGNED IN THE HOSPITAL? ☐ Yes ☐ No	16. SOCIAL SECURITY NUMBER REQUESTED FOR CHILD? ☐ Yes ☐ No	17. FACILITY ID. (NPI)

18. MOTHER'S SOCIAL SECURITY NUMBER:	19. FATHER'S SOCIAL SECURITY NUMBER:

INFORMATION FOR MEDICAL AND HEALTH PURPOSES ONLY

MOTHER

20. MOTHER'S EDUCATION (Check the box that best describes the highest degree or level of school completed at the time of delivery) ☐ 8th grade or less ☐ 9th - 12th grade, no diploma ☐ High school graduate or GED completed ☐ Some college credit but no degree ☐ Associate degree (e.g., AA, AS) ☐ Bachelor's degree (e.g., BA, AB, BS) ☐ Master's degree (e.g., MA, MS, MEng, MEd, MSW, MBA) ☐ Doctorate (e.g., PhD, EdD) or Professional degree (e.g., MD, DDS, DVM, LLB, JD)	21. MOTHER OF HISPANIC ORIGIN? (Check the box that best describes whether the mother is Spanish/Hispanic/Latina. Check the "No" box if mother is not Spanish/Hispanic/Latina) ☐ No, not Spanish/Hispanic/Latina ☐ Yes, Mexican, Mexican American, Chicana ☐ Yes, Puerto Rican ☐ Yes, Cuban ☐ Yes, other Spanish/Hispanic/Latina (Specify)_____	22. MOTHER'S RACE (Check one or more races to indicate what the mother considers herself to be) ☐ White ☐ Black or African American ☐ American Indian or Alaska Native (Name of the enrolled or principal tribe)_____ ☐ Asian Indian ☐ Chinese ☐ Filipino ☐ Japanese ☐ Korean ☐ Vietnamese ☐ Other Asian (Specify)_____ ☐ Native Hawaiian ☐ Guamanian or Chamorro ☐ Samoan ☐ Other Pacific Islander (Specify)_____ ☐ Other (Specify)_____

FATHER

23. FATHER'S EDUCATION (Check the box that best describes the highest degree or level of school completed at the time of delivery) ☐ 8th grade or less ☐ 9th - 12th grade, no diploma ☐ High school graduate or GED completed ☐ Some college credit but no degree ☐ Associate degree (e.g., AA, AS) ☐ Bachelor's degree (e.g., BA, AB, BS) ☐ Master's degree (e.g., MA, MS, MEng, MEd, MSW, MBA) ☐ Doctorate (e.g., PhD, EdD) or Professional degree (e.g., MD, DDS, DVM, LLB, JD)	24. FATHER OF HISPANIC ORIGIN? (Check the box that best describes whether the father is Spanish/Hispanic/Latino. Check the "No" box if father is not Spanish/Hispanic/Latino) ☐ No, not Spanish/Hispanic/Latino ☐ Yes, Mexican, Mexican American, Chicano ☐ Yes, Puerto Rican ☐ Yes, Cuban ☐ Yes, other Spanish/Hispanic/Latino (Specify)_____	25. FATHER'S RACE (Check one or more races to indicate what the father considers himself to be) ☐ White ☐ Black or African American ☐ American Indian or Alaska Native (Name of the enrolled or principal tribe)_____ ☐ Asian Indian ☐ Chinese ☐ Filipino ☐ Japanese ☐ Korean ☐ Vietnamese ☐ Other Asian (Specify)_____ ☐ Native Hawaiian ☐ Guamanian or Chamorro ☐ Samoan ☐ Other Pacific Islander (Specify)_____ ☐ Other (Specify)_____

Mother's Name   _Mother's Medical Record No._

26. PLACE WHERE BIRTH OCCURRED (Check one) ☐ Hospital ☐ Freestanding birthing center ☐ Home Birth: Planned to deliver at home? ☐ Yes ☐ No ☐ Clinic/Doctor's office ☐ Other (Specify)_____	27. ATTENDANT'S NAME, TITLE, AND NPI NAME: _____ NPI:_____ TITLE: ☐ MD ☐ DO ☐ CNM/CM ☐ OTHER MIDWIFE ☐ OTHER (Specify)_____	28. MOTHER TRANSFERRED FOR MATERNAL MEDICAL OR FETAL INDICATIONS FOR DELIVERY? ☐ Yes ☐ No IF YES, ENTER NAME OF FACILITY MOTHER TRANSFERRED FROM: _____

REV. 11/2003

MOTHER

29a. DATE OF FIRST PRENATAL CARE VISIT	29b. DATE OF LAST PRENATAL CARE VISIT	30. TOTAL NUMBER OF PRENATAL VISITS FOR THIS PREGNANCY
____/____/_____ MM DD YYYY ☐ No Prenatal Care	____/____/_____ MM DD YYYY	_____ (If none, enter ʌ0".)

31. MOTHER'S HEIGHT _____ (feet/inches)	32. MOTHER'S PREPREGNANCY WEIGHT _____ (pounds)	33. MOTHER'S WEIGHT AT DELIVERY _____ (pounds)	34. DID MOTHER GET WIC FOOD FOR HERSELF DURING THIS PREGNANCY? ☐ Yes ☐ No

35. NUMBER OF PREVIOUS LIVE BIRTHS (Do not include this child)	36. NUMBER OF OTHER PREGNANCY OUTCOMES (spontaneous or induced losses or ectopic pregnancies)	37. CIGARETTE SMOKING BEFORE AND DURING PREGNANCY For each time period, enter either the number of cigarettes or the number of packs of cigarettes smoked. IF NONE, ENTER ʌ0".	38. PRINCIPAL SOURCE OF PAYMENT FOR THIS DELIVERY

35a. Now Living	35b. Now Dead	36a. Other Outcomes	Average number of cigarettes or packs of cigarettes smoked per day.		☐ Private Insurance ☐ Medicaid ☐ Self-pay ☐ Other (Specify) _____
Number _____ ☐ None	Number _____ ☐ None	Number _____ ☐ None	# of cigarettes / # of packs		

Three Months Before Pregnancy _____ OR _____
First Three Months of Pregnancy _____ OR _____
Second Three Months of Pregnancy _____ OR _____
Third Trimester of Pregnancy _____ OR _____

35c. DATE OF LAST LIVE BIRTH ____/_____ MM YYYY	36b. DATE OF LAST OTHER PREGNANCY OUTCOME ____/_____ MM YYYY	39. DATE LAST NORMAL MENSES BEGAN ____/____/_____ MM DD YYYY	40. MOTHER'S MEDICAL RECORD NUMBER

MEDICAL AND HEALTH INFORMATION

41. RISK FACTORS IN THIS PREGNANCY (Check all that apply)

Diabetes
☐ Prepregnancy (Diagnosis prior to this pregnancy)
☐ Gestational (Diagnosis in this pregnancy)

Hypertension
☐ Prepregnancy (Chronic)
☐ Gestational (PIH, preeclampsia)
☐ Eclampsia

☐ Previous preterm birth

☐ Other previous poor pregnancy outcome (Includes perinatal death, small-for-gestational age/intrauterine growth restricted birth)

☐ Pregnancy resulted from infertility treatment-If yes, check all that apply:
  ☐ Fertility-enhancing drugs, Artificial insemination or Intrauterine insemination
  ☐ Assisted reproductive technology (e.g., in vitro fertilization (IVF), gamete intrafallopian transfer (GIFT))

☐ Mother had a previous cesarean delivery If yes, how many _____
☐ None of the above

42. INFECTIONS PRESENT AND/OR TREATED DURING THIS PREGNANCY (Check all that apply)

☐ Gonorrhea
☐ Syphilis
☐ Chlamydia
☐ Hepatitis B
☐ Hepatitis C
☐ None of the above

43. OBSTETRIC PROCEDURES (Check all that apply)

☐ Cervical cerclage
☐ Tocolysis

External cephalic version:
☐ Successful
☐ Failed

☐ None of the above

44. ONSET OF LABOR (Check all that apply)

☐ Premature Rupture of the Membranes (prolonged, ∃12 hrs.)
☐ Precipitous Labor (<3 hrs.)
☐ Prolonged Labor (∃ 20 hrs.)
☐ None of the above

45. CHARACTERISTICS OF LABOR AND DELIVERY (Check all that apply)

☐ Induction of labor
☐ Augmentation of labor
☐ Non-vertex presentation
☐ Steroids (glucocorticoids) for fetal lung maturation received by the mother prior to delivery
☐ Antibiotics received by the mother during labor
☐ Clinical chorioamnionitis diagnosed during labor or maternal temperature ≥38°C (100.4°F)
☐ Moderate/heavy meconium staining of the amniotic fluid
☐ Fetal intolerance of labor such that one or more of the following actions was taken: in-utero resuscitative measures, further fetal assessment, or operative delivery
☐ Epidural or spinal anesthesia during labor
☐ None of the above

46. METHOD OF DELIVERY

A. Was delivery with forceps attempted but unsuccessful?
  ☐ Yes ☐ No

B. Was delivery with vacuum extraction attempted but unsuccessful?
  ☐ Yes ☐ No

C. Fetal presentation at birth
  ☐ Cephalic
  ☐ Breech
  ☐ Other

D. Final route and method of delivery (Check one)
  ☐ Vaginal/Spontaneous
  ☐ Vaginal/Forceps
  ☐ Vaginal/Vacuum
  ☐ Cesarean
  If cesarean, was a trial of labor attempted?
  ☐ Yes
  ☐ No

47. MATERNAL MORBIDITY (Check all that apply) (Complications associated with labor and delivery)

☐ Maternal transfusion
☐ Third or fourth degree perineal laceration
☐ Ruptured uterus
☐ Unplanned hysterectomy
☐ Admission to intensive care unit
☐ Unplanned operating room procedure following delivery
☐ None of the above

NEWBORN INFORMATION

NEWBORN

Mother's Name   Mother's Medical Record No.

48. NEWBORN MEDICAL RECORD NUMBER

49. BIRTHWEIGHT (grams preferred, specify unit)
9 grams   9 lb/oz

50. OBSTETRIC ESTIMATE OF GESTATION:
_____ (completed weeks)

51. APGAR SCORE:
Score at 5 minutes: _____
If 5 minute score is less than 6,
Score at 10 minutes: _____

52. PLURALITY - Single, Twin, Triplet, etc.
(Specify) _____

53. IF NOT SINGLE BIRTH - Born First, Second, Third, etc. (Specify) _____

54. ABNORMAL CONDITIONS OF THE NEWBORN (Check all that apply)

☐ Assisted ventilation required immediately following delivery
☐ Assisted ventilation required for more than six hours
☐ NICU admission
☐ Newborn given surfactant replacement therapy
☐ Antibiotics received by the newborn for suspected neonatal sepsis
☐ Seizure or serious neurologic dysfunction
☐ Significant birth injury (skeletal fracture(s), peripheral nerve injury, and/or soft tissue/solid organ hemorrhage which requires intervention)
9 None of the above

55. CONGENITAL ANOMALIES OF THE NEWBORN (Check all that apply)

☐ Anencephaly
☐ Meningomyelocele/Spina bifida
☐ Cyanotic congenital heart disease
☐ Congenital diaphragmatic hernia
☐ Omphalocele
☐ Gastroschisis
☐ Limb reduction defect (excluding congenital amputation and dwarfing syndromes)
☐ Cleft Lip with or without Cleft Palate
☐ Cleft Palate alone
☐ Down Syndrome
  ☐ Karyotype confirmed
  ☐ Karyotype pending
☐ Suspected chromosomal disorder
  ☐ Karyotype confirmed
  ☐ Karyotype pending
☐ Hypospadias
☐ None of the anomalies listed above

56. WAS INFANT TRANSFERRED WITHIN 24 HOURS OF DELIVERY? 9 Yes 9 No IF YES, NAME OF FACILITY INFANT TRANSFERRED TO: _____	57. IS INFANT LIVING AT TIME OF REPORT? ☐ Yes ☐ No ☐ Infant transferred, status unknown	58. IS THE INFANT BEING BREASTFED AT DISCHARGE? ☐ Yes ☐ No

Rev. 11/2003
NOTE: This recommended standard birth certificate is the result of an extensive evaluation process. Information on the process and resulting recommendations as well as plans for future activities is available on the Internet at: http://www.cdc.gov/nchs/vital_certs_rev.htm.

Retrieved from http://www.cdc.gov/nchs/data/dvs/birth11-03final-acc.pdf

DISPLAY 7–4　STANDARD DEATH CERTIFICATE

U.S. STANDARD
CERTIFICATE OF DEATH

LOCAL FILE NUMBER   STATE FILE NUMBER

TYPE/PRINT IN PERMANENT BLACK INK FOR INSTRUCTIONS SEE OTHER SIDE AND HANDBOOK

DECEDENT

1. DECEDENT'S NAME (First, Middle, Last)

2. SEX

3. DATE OF DEATH (Month, Day, Year)

4. SOCIAL SECURITY NUMBER

5a. AGE—Last Birthday (Years)

5b. UNDER 1 YEAR — Months | Days

5c. UNDER 1 DAY — Hours | Minutes

6. DATE OF BIRTH (Month, Day, Year)

7. BIRTHPLACE (City and State or Foreign Country)

8. WAS DECEDENT EVER IN U.S. ARMED FORCES? (Yes or no)

9a. PLACE OF DEATH (Check only one; see instructions on other side)
HOSPITAL: ☐ Inpatient ☐ ER/Outpatient ☐ DOA
OTHER: ☐ Nursing Home ☐ Residence ☐ Other (Specify)

9b. FACILITY NAME (If not institution, give street and number)

9c. CITY, TOWN, OR LOCATION OF DEATH

9d. COUNTY OF DEATH

10. MARITAL STATUS—Married, Never Married, Widowed, Divorced (Specify)

11. SURVIVING SPOUSE (If wife, give maiden name)

12a. DECEDENT'S USUAL OCCUPATION (Give kind of work done during most of working life. Do not use retired.)

12b. KIND OF BUSINESS/INDUSTRY

13a. RESIDENCE—STATE

13b. COUNTY

13c. CITY, TOWN, OR LOCATION

13d. STREET AND NUMBER

13e. INSIDE CITY LIMITS? (Yes or no)

13f. ZIP CODE

14. WAS DECEDENT OF HISPANIC ORIGIN? (Specify No or Yes—If yes, specify Cuban, Mexican, Puerto Rican, etc.) ☐ No ☐ Yes Specify:

15. RACE—American Indian, Black, White, etc. (Specify)

16. DECEDENT'S EDUCATION (Specify only highest grade completed)
Elementary/Secondary (0-12) | College (1-4 or 5+)

PARENTS

17. FATHER'S NAME (First, Middle, Last)

18. MOTHER'S NAME (First, Middle, Maiden Surname)

INFORMANT

19a. INFORMANT'S NAME (Type/Print)

19b. MAILING ADDRESS (Street and Number or Rural Route Number, City or Town, State, Zip Code)

DISPOSITION

20a. METHOD OF DISPOSITION
☐ Burial ☐ Cremation ☐ Removal from State
☐ Donation ☐ Other (Specify) _____

20b. PLACE OF DISPOSITION (Name of cemetery, crematory, or other place)

20c. LOCATION—City or Town, State

21a. SIGNATURE OF FUNERAL SERVICE LICENSEE OR PERSON ACTING AS SUCH

21b. LICENSE NUMBER (of Licensee)

22. NAME AND ADDRESS OF FACILITY

PRONOUNCING PHYSICIAN ONLY

ITEMS 24-26 MUST BE COMPLETED BY PERSON WHO PRONOUNCES DEATH

Complete items 23a-c only when certifying physician is not available at time of death to certify cause of death.

23a. To the best of my knowledge, death occurred at the time, date, and place stated.
Signature and Title ▶

23b. LICENSE NUMBER

23c. DATE SIGNED (Month, Day, Year)

24. TIME OF DEATH　M

25. DATE PRONOUNCED DEAD (Month, Day, Year)

26. WAS CASE REFERRED TO MEDICAL EXAMINER/CORONER? (Yes or no)

CAUSE OF DEATH

SEE INSTRUCTIONS ON OTHER SIDE

27. PART I. Enter the diseases, injuries, or complications that caused the death. Do not enter the mode of dying, such as cardiac or respiratory arrest, shock, or heart failure. List only one cause on each line.

IMMEDIATE CAUSE (Final disease or condition resulting in death) ▶
a. _____
DUE TO (OR AS A CONSEQUENCE OF):

Sequentially list conditions, if any, leading to immediate cause. Enter UNDERLYING CAUSE (Disease or injury that initiated events resulting in death) LAST
b. _____
DUE TO (OR AS A CONSEQUENCE OF):
c. _____
DUE TO (OR AS A CONSEQUENCE OF):
d. _____

Approximate Interval Between Onset and Death

PART II. Other significant conditions contributing to death but not resulting in the underlying cause given in Part I.

28a. WAS AN AUTOPSY PERFORMED? (Yes or no)

28b. WERE AUTOPSY FINDINGS AVAILABLE PRIOR TO COMPLETION OF CAUSE OF DEATH? (Yes or no)

29. MANNER OF DEATH
☐ Natural ☐ Pending Investigation
☐ Accident
☐ Suicide ☐ Could not be Determined
☐ Homicide

30a. DATE OF INJURY (Month, Day, Year)

30b. TIME OF INJURY　M

30c. INJURY AT WORK? (Yes or no)

30d. DESCRIBE HOW INJURY OCCURRED

30e. PLACE OF INJURY—At home, farm, street, factory, office building, etc. (Specify)

30f. LOCATION (Street and Number or Rural Route Number, City or Town, State)

CERTIFIER

SEE DEFINITION ON OTHER SIDE

31a. CERTIFIER (Check only one)

☐ CERTIFYING PHYSICIAN (Physician certifying cause of death when another physician has pronounced death and completed Item 23)
To the best of my knowledge, death occurred due to the cause(s) and manner as stated.

☐ PRONOUNCING AND CERTIFYING PHYSICIAN (Physician both pronouncing death and certifying to cause of death)
To the best of my knowledge, death occurred at the time, date, and place, and due to the cause(s) and manner as stated.

☐ MEDICAL EXAMINER/CORONER
On the basis of examination and/or investigation, in my opinion, death occurred at the time, date, and place, and due to the cause(s) and manner as stated.

31b. SIGNATURE AND TITLE OF CERTIFIER

31c. LICENSE NUMBER

31d. DATE SIGNED (Month, Day, Year)

32. NAME AND ADDRESS OF PERSON WHO COMPLETED CAUSE OF DEATH (ITEM 27) (Type/Print)

REGISTRAR

33. REGISTRAR'S SIGNATURE

34. DATE FILED (Month, Day, Year)

NAME OF DECEDENT: For use by physician or institution

SEE INSTRUCTIONS ON OTHER SIDE

DEPARTMENT OF HEALTH AND HUMAN SERVICES – PUBLIC HEALTH SERVICE – NATIONAL CENTER FOR HEALTH STATISTICS – 1989 REVISION

SEE DEFINITION ON OTHER SIDE

PHS-T-003

Retrieved from http://www.cdc.gov/nchs/data/dvs/death11-03final-acc.pdf

malaria, viral influenza), and these must also be reported. The World Health Organization's *International Health Regulations* (2nd ed.), published in 2005, remains in effect. Review efforts are under way to determine whether or not these regulations need updating. A review committee is set to finalize its work in Geneva in May 2016. If it is determined that updating is needed, it will take several years to complete a revised document (Hofmann, T. D., *personal communication*, November 24, 2015).

Other reportable diseases (numbering between 20 and 40 in each state) are usually classified according to the speed with which the health department should be notified. Some should be reported by phone or e-mail, others weekly by regular mail. They vary in potential severity from varicella (chickenpox) to rabies and include AIDS, encephalitis, measles, meningitis, pertussis (whooping cough), syphilis, and toxic shock syndrome (MedlinePlus, 2013). Community health nurses should obtain the list of reportable diseases from their local or state health department office. Following up on occurrences of these diseases is a task frequently assigned to public health nurses working for local health departments. Chapter 8 includes an example of a Confidential Morbidity Report (CMR) used to report and track communicable diseases at the local, regional, and national levels.

Disease Registries

Some areas or states have disease registries or rosters for conditions with major public health impact. Tuberculosis and rheumatic fever registries were more common when these diseases occurred more frequently. Cancer registries provide useful incidence, prevalence, and survival data, and assist the community health nurse in monitoring cancer patterns within a community. Community health nurses can access these registries through state health department Web sites.

At the federal level, the Agency for Toxic Substances and Disease Registry (ATSDR, 2014) maintains four registries of major public concern: the World Trade Center Health Registry (comprehensive and confidential health survey of those directly exposed to fallout and debris on September 11, 2001), the National Amyotrophic Lateral Sclerosis (ALS) Registry (population-based registry to assist scientists in the study of this disease), the Katrina and Rita Exposures Registry (KARE; monitors people who lived in trailers provided by federal agencies after hurricanes Katrina and Rita), and the Rapid Response Registry (collects and shares information with state, local, and federal public health and disaster response agencies regarding exposures or potential exposures to harmful substances during catastrophic events).

Also at the federal level, the Surveillance, Epidemiology, and End Results (SEER) Program of the National Cancer Institute collects and publishes cancer incidence and survival data from population-based cancer registries that cover a portion of the U.S. population (National Cancer Institute, n.d.).

Surveillance Systems

The Centers for Disease Control and Prevention (CDC) maintains various surveillance systems to monitor diseases so it can develop and evaluate control strategies. The data from its two most popular systems are used by public health entities to determine which populations are most affected, and to evaluate the effectiveness of interventions to address disease entities, many of which are chronic in nature.

The Behavioral Risk Factor Surveillance System (BRFSS) conducts an ongoing state-based telephone survey of the civilian, noninstitutional adult population. The survey ascertains the prevalence of high-risk behaviors, such as excessive alcohol consumption, cigarette smoking, physical inactivity and lack of preventive health care, such as screening for cancer. Results are published on a periodic basis in the Mortality and Morbidity Weekly Report (MMWR)'s CDC Surveillance Summaries, and are available online at http://www.cdc.gov/brfss/

The Youth Risk Behavior Surveillance System (YRBSS) monitors six categories of priority health-risk behaviors in young adults, as well as the prevalence of obesity and asthma with the use of the national Youth Risk Behavior Survey (YRBS). The survey is conducted every 2 years with 9th to 12th grade students in public and private schools. The survey includes questions about unintentional injuries and violence, tobacco use, alcohol and other drug use, sexual behaviors that contribute to unintended pregnancy and STDs, unhealthy dietary behaviors, and physical inactivity. Results are available online at http://www.cdc.gov/healthyyouth/data/yrbs/index.htm (McKenzie et al., 2012).

Environmental Monitoring

State governments, through health departments or other agencies, now monitor health hazards found in the environment. Pesticides, industrial wastes, radioactive or nuclear materials, chemical additives in foods, and medicinal drugs have joined the list of pollutants (see Chapter 9 for a detailed discussion). Concerned community members and leaders view these as risk factors that affect health at both community and individual levels. Public health nurses can also obtain data from federal agencies such as the Food and Drug Administration (FDA), the Consumer Product Safety Commission, the Environmental Protection Agency (EPA), and, as previously mentioned, the ATSDR.

National Center for Health Statistics Health Surveys

The National Center for Health Statistics (NCHS) furnishes valuable health prevalence data from surveys of Americans. Published data are also frequently available for regions. Examples are as follows:

- The National Health Interview Survey (formerly known as National Health Survey) was established by Congress in 1956, and provides a continual source of information about the health status and needs of the entire nation. The National Health Interview Survey includes interviews from approximately 43,000 households each year and provides information about the health status and needs of the entire country (NCHS, 2015a).
- The National Nursing Home Survey primarily samples institutional records of hospitals and nursing homes; it provides information on those who are using these services, along with diagnoses and other characteristics (NCHS, 2015b).

- The National Health and Nutrition Examination Survey (NHANES) reports physical measurements on smaller samples of the population and augments the information provided by interviews. It also provides prevalence information on injuries, diseases, and disabilities that appear frequently in the population (NCHS, 2015b).
- The National Survey of Family Growth (NSFG) focuses on fertility and family planning as well as other aspects of family health (NCHS, 2015b).

Other studies investigate vital statistics events and characteristics of ambulatory patients in physicians' community practices. Each of these nationally sponsored efforts suggest ways in which community health nurses can examine health problems or concerns affecting their communities (see From the Case Files). Interviews, physical examinations of subsets of community members, and surveillance of institutions, clinics, and private physicians' practices can be carried out locally after needs are identified and funds made available. Other sources may be found in data kept routinely, but not centrally, on the health problems of workers in local industries or the health problems of schoolchildren; a key issue for many community health nurses. Existing epidemiologic data can be used to plan parent education programs, health promotion among students, and almost any other type of service.

Centers for Disease Control and Prevention Reports

The CDC issues the *Mortality and Morbidity Weekly Report (MMWR)*. This publication presents weekly summaries of disease and death data trends for the nation. It includes reports on outbreaks or occurrences of diseases in specific regions of the country and international trends in disease occurrences that may affect the U.S. population. Most health departments subscribe to this publication, which provides important information both for epidemiologists and PHNs. It is also available free online from the CDC at http://www.cdc.gov/mmwr/index.html

The CDC also provides administrative, research, and technical support for the Community Preventive Services Task Force, which maintains the "Guide to Community Preventive Services" Web site. This Web site houses the official collection of all the CPSTF findings and the systematic reviews upon which they are based. It is offered as a free resource to help public health nurses and other public health professionals choose programs and policies to improve health and prevent disease within the communities with whom they work (Community Preventive Services Task Force, 2015).

For example, before a public health education program is developed to address a community health problem, program planners can access the Web site to review programs that have already been developed to address a similar issue and have been evaluated for program effectiveness. Such a literature review can form a more scientific foundation for developing new programs that may address a similar problem but with a different target population. This can reduce trial and error efforts that may not be cost-effective, given the limited funding that may be available for program development. Currently available topics include "Adolescent Health, Alcohol—Excessive Consumption, Asthma, Birth Defects, Cancer, Cardiovascular Disease, Diabetes, Emergency Preparedness, Health Communication, Health Equity, HIV/AIDS, STDs/STIs, Pregnancy, Mental Health, Motor Vehicle Injury, Nutrition, Obesity, Oral Health, Physical Activity, Social Environment, Tobacco, Vaccination, and Violence and Worksite" (Community Preventive Services Task Force, 2015, para. 1).

Informal Observational Studies

A second information source in epidemiologic study is informal observation and description. Almost any client group encountered by the community health nurse can trigger such a study. If, for example, the nurse encounters an abused child at a clinic, a study of the clinic's records to screen for additional possible instances of child abuse and neglect could lead to more case finding. If several cases of diabetes come to the attention of a nurse serving on a Navajo reservation, a widespread problem might come to light through informal inquiries about the incidence and age at onset of the disease among this Native American population. Informal observational study often raises questions and suggests hypotheses that form the basis for designing larger-scale epidemiologic investigations.

Scientific Studies

The third source of information used in epidemiologic inquiry involves carefully designed scientific studies. The nursing profession has recognized the need to develop a systematic body of knowledge upon which to base nursing practice. Systematic research is becoming an accepted part of the community health nurse's role. Findings from

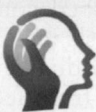

From the Case Files I

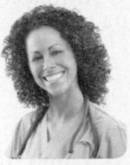

Public health nurses working for a local or county health department will find themselves more involved with program planning than direct patient care. Many times they will be asked to help develop a health education program based on what is affecting the community the most. Many times the health department is limited by budgetary constraints or the reporting requirements of grant funders.

Let's say your health department has been given the opportunity to apply for funding from three sponsoring organizations. The choices are to develop public health education programs about alcohol consumption, smoking cessation, and community HIV testing. In an upcoming department meeting you are asked to make a case for and against for applying for the funding of each of these programs.

In preparing for this presentation, what specific types of data would you recommend to the department? What would be the sources of this data? Are those sources from local, state, or national resources? How could *Healthy People 2020* help frame this presentation?

epidemiologic studies conducted by or involving nurses are appearing more frequently in the literature. The Cochrane Database of Systematic Reviews (CDSR) is the most popular resource for systematic reviews in health care and includes a section on public health. Its Web site is searchable by topic or Cochrane Review Group. Additionally, the Web site includes reviews, methods studies, technology assessments, and economic evaluations (Wiley Online Library, 2015). Systematic reviews can routinely be found in many professional journals and the aforementioned Community Guide. Systematic studies, as well as informal studies and existing epidemiologic data, can provide the community health nurse with valuable information that can be used to positively affect aggregate health.

METHODS IN THE EPIDEMIOLOGIC INVESTIGATIVE PROCESS

The goals of epidemiologic investigation are to identify the causal mechanisms of health and illness states and to develop measures for preventing illness and promoting health. Epidemiologists employ an investigative process that involves a sequence of three approaches that build on one another: descriptive, analytic, and experimental studies. All three approaches have relevance for community health nursing (see Chapter 4 for a more detailed description).

Descriptive Epidemiology

Descriptive epidemiology includes investigations that seek to observe and describe patterns of health-related conditions that occur naturally in a population. For example, a community health nurse might seek to learn how many children in a school district have been immunized for measles, how many home births occur each year in the county, how many cases of STDs have occurred in the city in the past month, or how many automobile crashes have occurred near the community high school. At this stage in the epidemiologic investigation, the researcher seeks to establish the occurrence of a problem. Data from descriptive studies suggest hypotheses for further testing. Descriptive studies almost always involve some form of broad-based quantification and statistical analysis (Gordis, 2014). An example of a descriptive epidemiological study looked at work organization, physical and mental health, and quality of life among a population of Hispanic female farm workers in North Carolina (Arcury, Grzywacz, Chen, Mora, & Quandt, 2014). This cross-sectional study surveyed 319 female farm workers over a 2-year period, and found that heavier job demands (e.g., increased psychological demands, heavier loads, awkward posture) were correlated with higher depressive and musculoskeletal symptoms. When workers had little job control or were lower skilled, these symptoms were higher. If there was a safety climate and greater support from supervisors, fewer depressive symptoms were found. Chapter 29 has more on migrant health.

Counts

The simplest measure of description is a count. For example, an epidemiologic study to assess the impact of the routine 2-dose varicella vaccination program on death due to the disease used the National Vital Statistics System data for 2008–2011, the first years of the routine 2-dose varicella vaccination program, and characteristics of varicella deaths reported to CDC during 1996–2013, using the 2008–2011 Mortality Multiple Cause-of-Death records. Calculated rates were used to compare the prevaccine and mature 1-dose varicella vaccination program eras. Findings include an 87% reduction from the prevaccine years, with an annual average age-adjusted mortality rate for varicella as the underlying cause to be 0.05 per million population during 2008–2011. Varicella deaths among persons aged <20 years declined by 99% in 2008–2011 when compared with prevaccine years, and a 70% decline when compared to 2005–2007. Of the 83 deaths reported to the CDC, 24 (29%) were among those who were immunocompromised. Authors concluded that the vaccine program significantly reduced varicella disease burden (Leung, Bialek, & Marin, 2015).

Obtaining a count of this type always depends on the definition of what is being counted and when it was counted. This particular count, for example, utilizes a large database that takes time to be made public and therefore may not provide a current picture of actual deaths. Use of this type of data should always consider the time delay involved. If a community health nurse needs more current information within a specific community or state, hospital records or death certificates may be another source. However, before making use of any statistics, whether from official state offices, the Census Bureau, or a health agency, it is necessary to determine what the information represents.

Rates

Rates are statistical measures expressing the proportion of people with a given health problem among a population at risk. The total number of people in the group serves as the denominator for various types of rates. To express a count as a proportion, or rate, the population to be studied must first be identified. For instance, total West Nile virus fatalities in the United States for 2011 were 43 out of 690 confirmed infections (CDC, 2015f). If those deaths are considered in relation to the total number of cases in the country, there will be one rate; if, however, those fatalities are considered in relation to the total population, there will be a quite different rate. It is important when reviewing rates that you understand which measures are being compared.

In epidemiology, the population represents the universe of people defined as the objects of a study. Because it is often difficult, if not impossible, to study an entire population, most epidemiologic studies draw a sample to represent that group. Sometimes, it is important to seek a random sample (in which everyone in the population has an equal chance of selection for study and choice is made without bias). At other times, a sample of convenience (in which study subjects are selected because of their availability) is sufficient. In many small epidemiologic studies, it may be possible to study almost every person in the population, eliminating the need for a sample. Several rates have wide use in epidemiology (Gordis, 2014). Those most important for the public health nurse to understand are the prevalence rate, the period prevalence rate, and the incidence rate.

Prevalence

Prevalence refers to all of the people with a particular health condition existing in a given population at a given point in time. The *prevalence rate* describes a situation at a specific point in time (McKenzie et al., 2012). If a nurse discovers 50 cases of measles in an elementary school, that is a simple count. When this number is divided by the total number of students in the school, the result is the prevalence of measles. For instance, if the school has 500 students, the prevalence of measles on that day would be 10% (50 measles/500 population).

$$\text{Prevalence rate} = \frac{\text{Number of persons with a characteristic}}{\text{Total number in population}}$$

The prevalence rate over a defined period of time is called a *period prevalence rate*:

$$\text{Period prevalence rate} = \frac{\text{Number of persons with a characteristic during a period of time}}{\text{Total number in population}}$$

Incidence

Not everyone in a population is at risk for developing a disease, incurring an injury, or having some other health-related characteristic. The *incidence rate* recognizes this fact. **Incidence** refers to all new cases of a disease or health condition appearing during a given time. Incidence rate describes a proportion in which the numerator is all new cases appearing during a given period of time and the denominator is the population at risk during the same period (Gordis, 2014). For example, some childhood diseases give lifelong immunity. The school children having had such diseases would be removed from the total number of children at risk in the school population. Three weeks after the start of a measles epidemic in a school, the incidence rate describes the number of cases of measles appearing during that period in terms of the number of persons at risk:

$$\frac{200}{1,000} \text{ or } \frac{200 \text{ new cases}}{1,000 \text{ persons at risk}}$$

The health literature is not always consistent in the use of the term *incidence;* sometimes, this word is used synonymously with *prevalence rates,* and the reader must take this into consideration.

$$\text{Incidence rate} = \frac{\text{Number of persons developing a disease}}{\text{Total number at risk per unit of time}}$$

Another rate that describes incidence is the attack rate. An *attack rate* describes the proportion of a group or population that develops a disease among all those exposed to a particular risk. This term is used frequently in investigations of outbreaks of infectious diseases such as influenza. If the attack rate changes, it may suggest an alteration in the population's immune status or that the disease-causing organism is present in a more or less virulent strain (Gordis, 2014).

Computing Rates

To make comparisons between populations, epidemiologists often use a common base population in computing rates. For example, instead of merely saying that the rate of an illness is 13% in one city and 25% in another, the comparison is made per 100,000 people in the population. This population base can vary for different purposes from 100 to 100,000. To describe the **morbidity rate**, which is the relative incidence of disease in a population, the ratio of the number of sick individuals to the total population is determined. The **mortality rate** refers to the relative death rate, or the sum of deaths in a given population at a given time (Gordis, 2014). Display 7–5 includes formulas for computing rates commonly used in community health.

The goal of descriptive studies is to identify the patterns of occurrence of any health-related condition. They can be *retrospective* (identify cases and controls, then go back to review existing data) or *prospective* (identify groups and exposure factors, and then follow them forward in time). In a descriptive study of child abuse, for example, the investigator would note the age, gender, race or ethnic group, and physical and emotional conditions of the children affected. In addition, data would be collected that described the economic status and occupation of parents, the location and setting of abusive behavior, and the time and season of the year when abuse occurred. In the retrospective study on reported varicella deaths, the investigators described the age, sex, ethnic background, and birthplace of victims and other information. Describing facets of these deaths provides information for further study and suggests avenues for intervention or prevention.

Analytic Epidemiology

A second type of investigation, *analytic epidemiology,* goes beyond simple description or observation and seeks to identify associations between a particular human disease or health problem and its possible causes. Analytic studies tend to be more specific than descriptive studies in their focus. They test hypotheses or seek to answer specific questions and can be retrospective or prospective in design (Merrill, 2013). Analytic studies fall into three types: prevalence studies, case–control studies, and cohort studies.

Prevalence Studies

When examining prevalence, it is helpful to remember that the health condition may be new or may have affected some people for many years. A *prevalence study* describes patterns of occurrence, as in the study of varicella-related deaths. It may examine causal factors, but a prevalence study always looks at factors from the same point in time and in the same population. Hypothesized causal factors are based on inferences from a single examination and most likely need further testing for validation (Fletcher & Fletcher, 2012; Merrill, 2013).

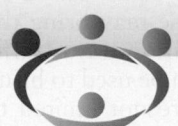

DISPLAY 7–5 COMMON EPIDEMIOLOGIC RATES

General Mortality Rates

Crude Mortality Rate =

$$\frac{\text{Number of Reported Deaths During 1 Year}}{\begin{array}{c}\text{Estimated Population as of July 1}\\\text{of Same Year}\end{array}} \times 100{,}000$$

Cause - Specific Mortality Rate =

$$\frac{\begin{array}{c}\text{Number of Deaths From a Stand}\\\text{Cause During 1 Year}\end{array}}{\begin{array}{c}\text{Estimated Population as of}\\\text{July 1 of Same Year}\end{array}} \times 100{,}000$$

Case Fatality Rate =

$$\frac{\text{Number of Deaths From a Particular Disease}}{\text{Total Number With the Same Disease}} \times 100$$

Proportional Mortality Ratio =

$$\frac{\begin{array}{c}\text{Number of Deaths From a Specific}\\\text{Cause Within a Given Time Period}\end{array}}{\text{Total Deaths in the Same Time Period}} \times 100$$

Age - Specific Mortality Rate =

$$\frac{\begin{array}{c}\text{Number of Persons in a Specific}\\\text{Age Group Dying During 1 Year}\end{array}}{\begin{array}{c}\text{Estimated Population of the Specific Age}\\\text{Group as of July 1 of Same Year}\end{array}} \times 100{,}000$$

Specific Rates for Maternal and Infant Populations

Crude Birth Rate =

$$\frac{\text{Number of Live Births During 1 Year}}{\text{Estimated Population as of July of Same Year}} \times 1{,}000$$

General Fertility Rate =

$$\frac{\text{Number of Live Births During 1 Year}}{\begin{array}{c}\text{Number of Females Aged 15 \quad 44 as}\\\text{of July of Same Year}\end{array}} \times 1{,}000$$

Maternal Mortality Rate =

$$\frac{\begin{array}{c}\text{Number of Deaths From}\\\text{Purepeal Causes During 1 Year}\end{array}}{\begin{array}{c}\text{Number of Live Births}\\\text{During Same Year}\end{array}} \times 100{,}000$$

Infant Mortality Rate =

$$\frac{\begin{array}{c}\text{Number of Deaths Under}\\\text{1 Year of Age for Given Year}\end{array}}{\begin{array}{c}\text{Number of Live Births Reported}\\\text{for Same Year}\end{array}} \times 1{,}000$$

Perinatal Mortality Rate =

$$\frac{\begin{array}{c}\text{Number of Fetal Deaths Plus Infant}\\\text{Deaths Under 7 Days of Age During 1 Year}\end{array}}{\begin{array}{c}\text{Number of Live Births Plus}\\\text{Fetal Deaths During Same Year}\end{array}} \times 1{,}000$$

Case–Control Studies

A *case–control study* compares people who have a health or illness condition (number of cases with the condition) with those who lack this condition (controls). These studies begin with the cases and look back over time (retrospectively) for presence or absence of the suspected causal factor in both cases and controls (Merrill, 2013). In a case–control study, researchers explored if exposure to endocrine-disrupting chemicals and carcinogens in occupational environments increases breast cancer risk. Comparison was made between 1,005 breast cancer cases referred by a regional cancer center and 1,146 randomly selected community controls. The study found that across all sectors, women in jobs with potentially high exposures to endocrine disruptors and carcinogens had an elevated breast cancer risk (OR = 1.42 for 10 years of exposure direction). The risk varied by occupational environment, and premenopausal breast cancer risk was highest for automotive plastics (OR = 4.76) and food canning (OR = 5.70) (Brophy et al., 2012).

Cohort Studies

A *cohort* is a group of people who share a common experience in a specific time period. Examples are a group of the elderly or the employees of an industry. In epidemiology, a cohort of people often becomes a focus of study. Cohort studies, rather than measuring the relationship of variables in existing conditions, study the development of a condition over time. A cohort study begins by selecting a group of people who display certain defined characteristics before the onset of the condition being investigated (Gordis, 2014). In studying a disease, the cohort might include individuals who are initially free of the disease but were known to have been exposed to a particular factor. They would be observed over time to evaluate which variables were associated with the development or nondevelopment of the disease. These types of studies are often utilized with environmental hazard exposures, as with the Health Registry and the National Toxic Substance Incidents Program discussed earlier (ATSDR, 2014). These sources of data provide the capability to conduct a cohort study on postexposure disease development and enable those affected to access the most current information on their exposure risks.

In 1993, the Women's Health Study, a 10-year national longitudinal, experimental, cohort study involving nearly 40,000 female health professionals was initiated (National Institutes of Health, 2012). Sponsored by the National Heart, Lung, and Blood Institute and the National Cancer Institute, it consisted of a randomized trial evaluating the benefits and risks of low-dose aspirin and vitamin E in the prevention of cancer and cardiovascular disease. Depending on the random assignment of the women, participants took 100 mg of aspirin or placebo and 600 IU of vitamin E or placebo every other day. This was a double-blind study: neither the participants nor the researchers knew which subjects were taking the study drugs or placebos. The study was funded through 2009 to provide observational follow-up of study participants. The study findings were that women over age 65 might benefit from low-dose aspirin to prevent strokes. The aspirin regimen was not effective in preventing a first heart attack or death from cardiovascular causes. With respect to cardiovascular health and vitamin E, there was no demonstrated benefit or risk.

In practice, the various types of studies just discussed are frequently mixed. A case–control study may include description and analysis with a retrospective focus; a cohort study may be conducted prospectively or retrospectively. The Women's Health Study is an example of a case–control study, a cohort study, and an experimental study. Flexibility is essential to allow the investigator as much freedom as possible in choosing the most useful methodology.

Experimental Epidemiology

Experimental epidemiology follows and builds on information gathered from descriptive and analytic approaches. In an experimental study, the investigator actually controls or changes the factors suspected of causing the health condition under study and then observes what happens to the health state (Merrill, 2013). In human populations, experimental studies should focus on disease prevention or health promotion rather than testing the causes of disease, which is done primarily on animals.

Experimental studies are carried out under carefully controlled conditions, and must be approved by an Institutional Review Board (IRB). The investigator exposes an experimental group to some factor thought to cause disease, improve health, prevent disease, or influence health in some way (as in the Women's Health Study). Simultaneously, the investigator observes a control group that is similar in characteristics to the experimental group but without the exposure factor. See Chapter 4 for more on experimental research studies.

The public health nurse should be alert for opportunities to conduct experimental studies in the course of working with groups. A study need not be elaborate to provide important data for future nursing practice. For example, a community health nurse can provide focused instruction to 20 new mothers encouraging them to breast-feed and then compare the health of their infants with infants of 20 mothers in the same service area who use formula.

A nurse can look at the number of automobile crashes at an intersection having a traffic light compared with a similar intersection that has stop signs. Based on the results of the investigation, the nurse may bring the information to the city council and petition for a traffic light at the intersection. Study results can be used to bring about change in the community and are not limited to communicable or chronic diseases. Improving community safety is also an essential outcome.

An expanding area of experimental epidemiology involves the use of computers to simulate epidemics. With mathematical models, it is possible to determine the probabilities of various aspects of disease occurrence (Honner, 2014; Yang et al., 2015). This approach is making an increased contribution to epidemiologists' knowledge of etiology and prevention.

Occasionally, an experiment occurs naturally, thus affording the researcher a chance to make important discoveries. John Snow discovered such a "natural experiment" in London in 1854 (as discussed earlier in the chapter). In his seminal study of an epidemic of cholera, he observed one group that contracted the disease and another that did not. Closer inspection revealed that the major difference between these groups was their water supply. See Chapter 9 for an example from Flint, Michigan's lead-contaminated water.

A *community trial* is a type of experimental study done at the community level. Geographic communities are assigned to intervention (experimental) or nonintervention (control) groups and compared to determine whether the intervention produces a positive change in the community (Merrill, 2013). Community trials can be extremely expensive and are not undertaken unless there is substantial evidence that the intervention will make a difference at the aggregate level. There are times when these community trials occur spontaneously, and it is important for the community health nurse to recognize these opportunities. For instance, one community public health department institutes an aggressive campaign to educate health care workers on the signs of elder abuse. Selecting a similar community where that level of training is not available, the community health nurse can then compare the rates of elder abuse reporting between these two communities. If you were conducting this research, what outcome would you expect in the community with the enhanced training? Where could you obtain this information? Think about what other measures you might also want to compare between these two communities.

CONDUCTING EPIDEMIOLOGIC RESEARCH

The community health nurse who engages in an epidemiologic investigation becomes a kind of detective. First, there is a problem to solve, a puzzle to unravel, or a question to answer. The nurse begins to search for basic information, for clues that might help answer the question. Information is never self-explanatory, and, like a detective, the nurse must analyze and interpret every additional clue. Slowly, there is a narrowing of possible suspects until the causes of a particular disease, the consequences of a prevention plan, or the results of treatment are identified. On the basis of this investigation, the nurse can draw further conclusions and make new applications to improve health services.

As discussed previously, epidemiologic studies are a form of research. The steps outlined here are similar to those discussed in Chapter 4. Epidemiologic research involves seven steps. Everything from an informal study in the course of nursing practice to the most comprehensive epidemiologic research project can be undertaken with these steps: (1) identify the problem, (2) review the literature, (3) design the study, (4) collect the data, (5) analyze the findings, (6) develop conclusions and applications, and (7) disseminate the findings.

Although research in the PHN role is covered in Chapter 4, the analysis of one epidemiologic study reinforces the integration of research in the nurse's role.

Identify the Problem

Community health nurses are constantly confronted with threats to the health and well-being of the community. Almost daily, questions are raised, puzzles presented, and problems identified. Pregnant women who smoke or use cocaine threaten the health of their unborn children: What can be done to reduce this behavior? Rape is increasing: What can be done to prevent such violence or to bring aid to victims? Children are injured and die from bicycle accidents: Why do these occur and how can they be prevented? Many farm workers have been killed or injured in farm equipment accidents: What can be done to prevent them? Any threat to the health of a group offers fertile ground for epidemiologic investigation. One example is study conducted by public health nurses in an effort to address the disproportionate burden of asthma among low-income and African American children (Sweet, Polivka, Chaudry, & Bouton, 2014). The purpose of the study was to improve asthma symptoms by attempting to control indoor triggers (Fig. 7–12).

Review the Literature

Sometimes, after identifying a problem, health professionals rush to take immediate action without reviewing solutions that have been tried previously. Every epidemiologic investigation should begin with a review of the literature. Even discovering that little research has been done on the problem can be valuable information. A good source for conducting a literature review is the

Community Guide Web site (see Internet resources on *thePoint*). Conversely, if many studies have already been conducted in the area, this information can help narrow the study to areas that have not previously been investigated or allow researchers to replicate earlier studies to confirm findings in a different setting. One of the most valuable sources in the literature is the systematic review, which evaluates research studies done on specific topics. Sweet et al. (2014), in preparing for their interventional study with families of children with asthma, examined factors that may lead to asthma disparities, home-based intervention studies, and the role of nurses in interventional studies on asthma. They found that adverse home environments, with pest infestations, poor ventilation, dampness and mold, smoking in the home, and exposure to dust mite allergens, increased the likelihood of children developing asthma. They also noted that home-based interventions had generally shown promise in helping to relieve asthma symptoms, as well as emergency room visits and hospitalizations. Interventions provided by nurses were not common, as most of them involved community health workers.

Design the Study

The first step in designing a study is to formulate one or more specific questions to answer or hypotheses to test. Sometimes, the question or hypothesis emerges from the review of the literature; it also may be developed through the researcher's own analysis and hunches. It is a good idea to write out one or more hypotheses to test or questions to answer.

The next step is to plan what study type (descriptive, analytic, or experimental) or combination of study types, best suits the goals of the research and how the study will be conducted. Will the data be collected retrospectively from existing records, or will new data be collected? Who will conduct interviews? What kinds of data will be needed to measure the outcomes of intervention?

The purpose of the Sweet et al. (2014, p. 244) study was to evaluate an intervention designed for "low-income families of children with asthma in an urban setting." Further, they wanted to determine both short-term and long-term impact on asthma severity, if caregivers' quality of life was impacted, and household activities that were asthma triggers, along with families' use of asthma management techniques. This was a large study: 115 participants with pre- and posttest data, conduced over a 3-year period. After referral from various community sources (MDs, school nurses, children's hospitals), a registered sanitarian determined safety hazards and asthma triggers per a home assessment. Such things as smoking, pets, pests, mold, ventilation, presence of clutter, and overall cleanliness were reported. Then, a PHN made a home visit (sometimes along with a health educator) and "provided comprehensive education" on how to control asthma triggers in the home and mediate asthma symptoms (p. 245). An action plan was discussed with the families; bedding supplies, a HEPA vacuum cleaner, cleaning supplies, and safety supplies were provided, along with pest control information and supplies. If needed, assistance with structural problems was provided by a community agency (e.g., repairing bathroom vents, removing

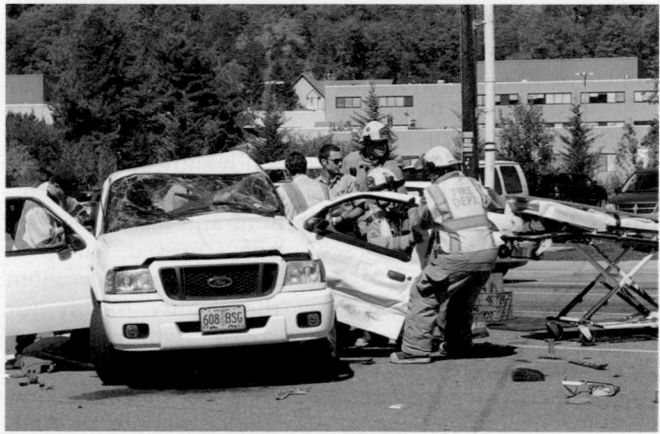

FIGURE 7–12 Firefighters extricating victims of an automobile crash.

mold). One or two additional home visits were made over the next 2 to 4 weeks, as well as 1 to 2 phone calls.

Collect the Data

The PHN then needs to begin to gather data from available sources that are pertinent to the research topic. For example, demographic data are available online from the U.S. Census Web site, and health-related data are available from the National Center for Health Statistics. Geographic-based behavioral risk factor data are available from the Behavior Risk Factor Surveillance System Web site. Geographic information systems (GIS) data are available from the CDC, the U.S. Geological Survey, and the Environmental Protection Agency, as well as state and local agencies and nongovernmental organizations (Sheldon Margen Public Health Library, 2014). Data about a particular community may be available from the state, county, or local health departments, upon request.

Once you have gathered whatever you can from available sources, you then may have to develop data collecting tools to gather additional information. The Community Guide Web site may provide ideas about how to collect data for a particular purpose (e.g., assessment, evaluation, pilot testing), and what works and doesn't work. Development of data collection tools should start with why the data are being collected and what data are needed at the end of the study. This will help determine what kinds of data collection are most suited (e.g., mail surveys, telephone surveys, online surveys, face-to face surveys, focus groups, etc.) in order to gather the data.

There are many freely available data collection tools online. The most popular in use today is SurveyMonkey (https://www.surveymonkey.com/). It is free to use for gathering survey data from small populations (e.g., 10 questions, 100 responses), with limited online analysis. More ongoing data gathering for larger populations requires a paid subscription. As with any data collection tool, pros and cons to the method used needs to be considered. For example, disadvantages with the use of Internet surveys include biased respondent demographics, inability to probe, and poor response rates (DJS Research Ltd., 2014).

In the asthma intervention study, pretest and posttest evaluations were done. The sanitarian verbally administered the baseline survey at the initial home assessment, and a PHN did the posttest survey 6 months later by phone. Assessment tools had been developed in previous studies conducted by some of the researchers (Polivka, Chaudry, Crawford, Bouton, & Sweet, 2011) to record the child's age, race/ethnicity, and the caregiver's education, employment status, and relationship to the child (e.g., mother, father, grandmother). Short-term indicators were chosen (i.e., asthma episodes within prior 2 weeks, number of days with no asthma symptoms or waking at night, number of days quick-relief asthma medication was used, and number of days that asthma limited the child's activity). Hospitalizations, emergency room visits, school days missed, and days of work missed by caregiver were chosen as long-term indicators. A survey that assessed the caregiver's quality of life was used. Asthma-related trigger activities that could be controlled within the home were assessed (e.g., smoking, using bathroom vents to reduce moisture, use of cleaning products without fragrances). Also, asthma management activities, like the use of a spacer with inhalers and the adherence to an asthma action plan, were assessed (Sweet et al., 2014).

Analyze the Findings

In most epidemiologic studies, data analysis consists of summarizing the findings, computing rates and ratios, and displaying the findings in tables and graphs. At this stage, the data are used to address the original question or test the original hypothesis. Was the hypothesis supported or not supported by the data? Summarized data can also generate more questions or indicate areas that warrant further investigation.

Develop Conclusions and Applications

Stating conclusions is an outcome of analysis and interpretation. The investigators summarize the results and their meaning for the purpose of making this information useful to other health services providers. Many times, research has direct practical application for improving health services, continuing or discontinuing services, or conducting future research. It is also important to describe mistakes made and lessons learned about study design and other aspects of the research and to propose further areas of study, to assist future investigators.

Returning to the asthma intervention study, Sweet et al. (2014) used descriptive statistics to analyze their data. They compared pre- and posttest results on the key outcomes (e.g., asthma severity, asthma triggers in the home, asthma management activities, caregiver quality of life). They used statistical tests to determine the significance of their findings.

Disseminate the Findings

Finally, research findings should be shared. The audience for the reporting of findings should be considered during the development of the study to ensure that the concerns and questions of the audience will be addressed by the study. Of course, if the study is being sponsored, then the purpose for the study is clear, making the dissemination of the findings easier. Sponsorship, however, can affect how the findings are perceived. In medical research, financial conflicts of interest (e.g., pharmaceutical-funded studies) can negatively impact the value of the findings (Johnston, 2015). Nevertheless, information gained from epidemiologic studies must be disseminated throughout the professional community to strengthen the knowledge base for improved practice and to promote future research.

A research article was written and submitted to a public health nursing journal and accepted for publication (Sweet et al., 2014). Results of this study showed significant reductions in "asthma symptom days, nighttime awakenings, days with activity limitation, and albuterol use" (p. 243). The number of school days missed, caregiver work days missed, and the number of emergency room visits was significantly lower; the quality of life for caregivers was significantly improved. Asthma triggers were reduced, and this home-based intervention was deemed successful in meeting the goals and objectives outlined for this population. Because the researchers disseminated this research by writing a journal article, you and your clients benefit from their hard work and knowledge.

SUMMARY

Epidemiology is the study of the distribution and determinants of health, health conditions, and disease in human population groups. It shares with public health nursing the common focus of the health of populations. It is a specialized form of scientific research that can provide public health professionals with a body of knowledge on which to base their practice and methods for studying new and existing problems. To understand epidemiology, one must first understand some basic epidemiologic concepts: the host, agent, and environment model; causality; immunity; the natural history of disease or health conditions; risk; and prevention strategies.

Community health nurses can use three sources of information when conducting epidemiologic investigations: existing epidemiologic data, informal investigations, and carefully designed scientific studies.

Epidemiology employs three investigative approaches: descriptive studies, analytic studies, and experimental studies. Although studies can be either retrospective or prospective, some merely describe existing conditions (descriptive studies), whereas others seek to explain causes (analytic studies). Experimental studies seek to confirm causal relationships identified in descriptive and analytic studies. Analytic studies can be of three types: prevalence, case–control, or cohort. In practice, all these types of studies often become combined in various ways. They also make use of quantitative concepts such as count, prevalence rate, incidence rate, mortality rate, and various types of morbidity (sickness) rates.

Epidemiologic research includes seven steps: (1) identifying the problem, which is usually a threat to the population's health, (2) reviewing the literature to determine what other studies have found, (3) carefully designing the study, (4) collecting the data, (5) analyzing the findings, (6) developing conclusions and applications, and (7) disseminating the findings.

Thinking epidemiologically can significantly enhance community health nursing practice. Epidemiology provides both the body of knowledge—information on the distribution and determinants of health conditions—and methods for investigating health problems and evaluating services.

ACTIVITIES TO PROMOTE **CRITICAL THINKING**

1. Identify an aggregate-level health problem in your community. Using the host, agent, and environment model, explains who the host is, what the causative agents are, and what environmental factors have promoted or delayed the development of the problem. When needed, consider vector control programs that may be needed or enhanced.
2. Select an aggregate health (wellness) condition, such as preschoolers' normal growth and development or elders' healthy aging, and list all the causal factors that might contribute to this healthy state. Now, plot these schematically in a diagram to show the web of causation model for this condition.
3. Using the same health condition that you selected in the previous exercise, describe the natural history of this condition, outlining its four stages. Identify three preventive nursing interventions, one for each level of prevention that could apply to this condition.
4. Select an article that reports an epidemiologic study from a recent nursing or public health journal, and record your responses to the following questions:
   - What prompted the study, and what was its purpose?
   - Was it descriptive, analytic, or experimental research?
   - Was the study design retrospective or prospective?
   - Why did the investigators choose this design?
   - What existing sources of epidemiologic data did this study use? List all sources specifically, such as *Morbidity and Mortality Weekly Report* or incomes by household in census data.
   - What were the study findings? Identify the population group that will benefit from this research.
5. Interview one or more practicing public health nurses in your community, and identify an aggregate-level problem that needs epidemiologic investigation. Propose a rough draft study design to research this problem.
6. Search for local or national news regarding a new disease threat (e.g., Zika virus), an example of a food-borne illness outbreak (e.g., bacterial contamination of produce), or another example requiring epidemiological investigation. Work with a small group of classmates to develop a hypothetical case investigation and a potential epidemiological plan for action. Are there specific environmental factors that should be considered? If possible, watch for the resolution of the issue (e.g., conclusions of the investigation, public health recommendations).

REFERENCES

Agency for Toxic Substances and Disease Registry (ATSDR). (2014). *Exposure and health registries*. Retrieved from http://www.atsdr.cdc.gov/publications_health_registries.html

Aiyer, S. M., Zimmerman, M. A., Morrel-Samuels, S., & Reischl, T. M. (2015). From broken windows to busy streets: A community empowerment perspective. *Health Education & Behavior, 42*(2), 137–147.

American Academy of Pediatrics (AAP). (2015). *Where we stand: Folic acid*. Retrieved from http://www.healthychildren.org/English/ages-stages/prenatal/pages/Where-We-Stand-Folic-Acid.aspx

Arcury, T., Grzywacz, J., Chen, H., Mora, D., & Quandt, S. (2014). Work organization and health among immigrant women: Latina manual workers in North Carolina. *American Journal of Public Health, 104*(12), 2445–2452.

Bain, L. E., & Awah, P. K. (2014). Eco-epidemiology: Challenges and opportunities for tomorrow's epidemiologists. *Pan African Medical Journal, 17*, 317. doi: 10.11604/pamj.2014.17.317.4080.

Beaubien, J. (2015). *Puzzling ebola deaths shows how little we know about the virus*. Retrieved from http://www.npr.org/sections/goatsandsoda/2015/11/24/457277942/puzzling-ebola-death-shows-how-little-we-know-about-the-virus

BMJ Publishing Group. (2015). *Epidemiology for the uninitiated*. Retrieved from http://www.bmj.com/about-bmj/resources-readers/publications/epidemiology-uninitiated/1-what-epidemiology

Boston University School of Public Health. (2015). *Prospective versus retrospective cohort studies*. Retrieved from http://sphweb.bumc.bu.edu/otlt/MPH-Modules/EP/EP713_CohortStudies/EP713_CohortStudies2.html

Brophy, J. T., Keith, M. M., Watterson, A., Park, R., Gilbertson, M., Maticka-Tyndale, E., ... Luginaah, I. (2012). Breast cancer risk in relation to occupations with exposure to carcinogens and endocrine disruptors: A Canadian case-control study. *Environmental Health, 11*, 87. doi: 10.1186/1476-069X-11-87.

Centers for Disease Control and Prevention (CDC). (2007). *Smallpox fact sheet: Smallpox disease overview*. Retrieved from http://emergency.cdc.gov/agent/smallpox/overview/disease-facts.asp

Centers for Disease Control and Prevention (CDC). (2014). *Plague: History*. Retrieved from http://www.cdc.gov/plague/history/

Centers for Disease Control and Prevention (CDC). (2015a). *2014 Ebola outbreak in West Africa—Case counts*. Retrieved from http://www.cdc.gov/vhf/ebola/outbreaks/2014-west-africa/case-counts.html

Centers for Disease Control and Prevention (CDC). (2015b). *Ebola (Ebola virus disease)*. Retrieved from http://www.cdc.gov/vhf/Ebola/

Centers for Disease Control and Prevention (CDC). (2015c). *Ebola virus disease (EVD) information for clinicians in U.S. healthcare settings*. Retrieved from http://www.cdc.gov/vhf/ebola/healthcare-us/preparing/clinicians.html

Centers for Disease Control and Prevention (CDC). (2015d). *Epidemiology and prevention of vaccine preventable diseases: The pink book, course textbook* (13th ed.). Retrieved from http://www.cdc.gov/vaccines/pubs/pinkbook/index.html

Centers for Disease Control and Prevention (CDC). (2015e). *Social determinants of health: Know what affects health*. Retrieved from http://www.cdc.gov/socialdeterminants/

Centers for Disease Control and Prevention (CDC). (2015f). *West Nile virus: Statistics, surveillance, and control archive*. Retrieved from http://www.cdc.gov/westnile/index.html

Channing Laboratory. (2013). *The nurses' health studies: Our story*. Retrieved from http://www.nhs3.org/index.php/our-story

Christie, A., Davies-Wayne, G. J., Cordier-Lasalle, T., Blackley, D. J., Laney, A. S., Williams, D. E., ... De Cock, K. M. (2015). Possible sexual transmission of Ebola virus—Liberia, 2015. *Morbidity and Mortality Weekly Report, 64*(17), 479–481. Retrieved from http://www.cdc.gov/mmwr/preview/mmwrhtml/mm6417a6.htm

Cohen, D., Spear, S., Scribner, R., Kissinger, P., Mason, K., & Wildgen, J. (2000). "Broken windows" and the risk of gonorrhea. *American Journal of Public Health, 90*, 230–236. Retrieved from http://www.ncbi.nlm.nih.gov/pmc/articles/PMC1446134/pdf/10667184.pdf

Community Preventive Services Task Force. (2015). *What is the community guide?* Retrieved from http://www.thecommunityguide.org/index.html

Cooney, D. (2014). *Ebola and bushmeat in Africa: Q & A with leading researcher*. Retrieved from http://blog.cifor.org/23924/Ebola-and-bushmeat-in-africa-qa-with-leading-researcher#.VER09_ldWSo

Deen, G. F., Knust, B., Broutet, N., Sesay, F. R., Formenty, P., Ross, C., ... Sahr, F. (2015). Ebola RNA persistence in semen of Ebola virus disease survivors—Preliminary report. *New England Journal of Medicine*. doi: 10.1056/NEJMoa1511410.

DJS Research Ltd. (2014). *What are the pros and cons of data collection methods?* Retrieved from http://www.marketresearchworld.net/index.php?option=com_content&task=view&id=2118&Itemid=78

Fletcher, R., & Fletcher, S. W. (2012). *Clinical epidemiology: The essentials* (5th ed.). Philadelphia, PA: Lippincott Williams & Wilkins.

Florence Nightingale Museum. (n.d.). *Biography*. Retrieved from http://www.florence-nightingale.co.uk/the-collection/biography.html

Friis, R. H., & Sellers, T. A. (2014). *Epidemiology for public health practice* (5th ed.). Burlington, MA: Jones and Bartlett Learning.

Geggel, L. (2014). *Bat-filled tree may have been source of current Ebola outbreak*. Retrieved from http://www.livescience.com/49286-ebola-bats-transmission.html

Gerstman, B. B. (2013). *Epidemiology kept simple: An introduction to traditional and modern epidemiology* (3rd ed.). Hoboken, NJ: John Wiley & Sons, Ltd.

Gordis, L. (2014). *Epidemiology* (5th ed.). Philadelphia, PA: Saunders.

Heymann, D. L. (Ed.). (2014). *Control of communicable diseases manual* (20th ed.). Washington, DC: American Public Health Association.

Heron, M. (2015). Deaths: Leading causes for 2012. *National Vital Statistics Reports, 64*(10). Retrieved from http://www.cdc.gov/nchs/data/nvsr/nvsr60/nvsr60_04.pdf http://www.cdc.gov/nchs/data/nvsr/nvsr64/nvsr64_10.pdf

History of Vaccines. (2014). *The human immune system and infectious disease*. Retrieved from http://www.historyofvaccines.org/content/articles/human-immune-system-and-infectious-disease

Honner, P. (2014). *Exponential outbreaks: The mathematics of epidemics*. Retrieved from http://learning.blogs.nytimes.com/2014/11/05/exponential-outbreaks-the-mathematics-of-epidemics/?_r=0

Johnston, J. (2015). *Conflict of interest in biomedical research*. Retrieved from http://www.thehastingscenter.org/Publications/BriefingBook/Detail.aspx?id=2156

Karunaweera, N. D., Galappaththy, G. N. L., & Wirth, D. F. (2014). On the road to eliminate malaria in Sri Lanka: Lessons from history, challenges, gaps in knowledge and research needs. *Malaria Journal, 13*, 59. doi: 10.1186/1475-2875-13-59.

Kahn, R. (2015). *Ebola: Where are we now?* Retrieved from http://www.redbrick.me/tech/ebola-where-are-we-now/

Kiefer, D. (2015). *What is holistic medicine?* Retrieved from http://www.webmd.com/balance/guide/what-is-holistic-medicine

Leung, J., Bialek, S. R., & Marin, M. (2015). Trends in varicella mortality in the United States: Data from vital statistics and the national surveillance system. *Human Vaccines and Immunotherapeutics, 11*(3), 662–668. Retrieved from http://www.tandfonline.com/doi/abs/10.1080/21645515.2015.1008880?src=recsys&

Lilienfeld, D. E. (2007). Celebration: William Farr (1807–1883)—An appreciation on the 200th anniversary of his birth. *International Journal of Epidemiology, 36*(5), 985–987. doi: 10.1093/ije/dym132.

Mackay, I. M. (2015, August 6). *Post-Ebola syndrome or just chronic Ebola virus disease ... ?* Retrieved from http://virology-downunder.blogspot.com/2015/08/post-ebola-syndrome-or-just-chronic.html

Mate, S. E., Kugelman, J. R., Nyenswah, T. G., Ladner, J. T., Wiley, M. R., Cordier-Lassalle, T., ... Palacios, G. (2015). Molecular evidence of sexual transmission of Ebola virus. *New England Journal of Medicine*. doi: 10.1056/NEJMoa1509773.

McKenzie, J. F., Pinger, R. R., & Kotecki, J. E. (2012). *An introduction to community health* (7th ed.). Sudbury, MA: Jones & Bartlett Learning.

MedlinePlus. (2013). *Reportable diseases*. Retrieved from https://www.nlm.nih.gov/medlineplus/ency/article/001929.htm

Merrill, R. M. (2013). *Introduction to epidemiology* (6th ed.). Sudbury, MA: Jones & Bartlett Learning.

National Cancer Institute. (n.d.). *About the SEER registries*. Retrieved from http://seer.cancer.gov/registries/index.html

National Cancer Institute. (2015). *BRCA1 and BRCA2: Cancer risk and genetic testing*. Retrieved from http://www.cancer.gov/about-cancer/causes-prevention/genetics/brca-fact-sheet#q1

National Center for Health Statistics (NCHS). (2015). *National Health Interview Survey. About NHIS*. Retrieved from http://www.cdc.gov/nchs/nhis.htm

National Center for Health Statistics (NCHS). (2015). *Surveys and data collection systems.* Retrieved from http://www.cdc.gov/nchs/

National Institute of Diabetes and Digestive and Kidney Diseases. (2014). *Causes of diabetes.* Retrieved from http://www.niddk.nih.gov/health-information/health-topics/Diabetes/causes-diabetes/Pages/index.aspx

National Institutes of Health. (2012). *Women's health study.* Retrieved from http://clinicaltrials.gov/ct2/show/record/NCT00000479

Paye-layleh, J. (2015, November 23). US officials headed to Liberia to help determine cause of latest Ebola cases, official says. *U.S. News and World Report.* Retrieved from http://www.usnews.com/news/world/articles/2015/11/23/liberia-seeks-us-help-to-determine-cause-of-new-Ebola-cases

Polivka, B. J., Chaudry, R. V., Crawford, J., Bouton, P., & Sweet, L. (2011). Impact of an urban healthy homes intervention. *Journal of Environmental Health, 73*(9), 16–20.

Remington, P. L. & Brownson, R. C. (2011). Fifty years of progress in chronic disease epidemiology and control. *Morbidity and Mortality Weekly, 60*(4), 70–77.

Rettner, R. (2015, May 1). *Ebola survivors should use condoms indefinitely, CDC says.* Retrieved from http://www.livescience.com/50700-ebola-transmission-sex.html

Scheibner, V. (2012, April 2). *Smallpox was considered eradicated, yet still infects humans today.* Retrieved from http://www.vaccinationcouncil.org/2012/04/02/smallpox-declared-eradicated-while-still-alive-and-well-by-viera-scheibner-phd/

Schiotz, A. (2015). Medical statistics and epidemiology: The early history. *Norwegian Journal of Epidemiology, 25*(1–2), 3–9.

Sejvar, J. J. (2003). West Nile Virus: An historical overview. *Ochsner Journals, 5*(3), 6–10. Retrieved from http://www.ncbi.nlm.nih.gov/pmc/articles/PMC3111838/

Sheldon Margen Public Health Library. (2014). *Public health GIS resources.* Retrieved from http://www.lib.berkeley.edu/PUBL/gis.html

Sweet, L. L., Polivka, B. J., Chlaudry, R. V., & Bouton, P. (2014). The impact of an urban home-based intervention program on asthma outcomes in children. *Public Health Nursing, 31*(30), 243–252.

Thomas, K. (2015). *Liberia resurgence: The changing meaning of Ebola-free.* Retrieved from http://www.eboladeeply.org/articles/2015/11/8515/liberia-resurgence-changing-meaning-ebola-free/

Thomas, K. (2015). *The long read. Unlocking Ebola's secrets.* Retrieved from http://www.eboladeeply.org/articles/2015/07/8082/long-read-unlocking-ebolas-secrets-part/

United States Army Medical Research Institute of Infectious Diseases. (2011, September). *Medical management of biological casualties handbook* (7th ed.). Retrieved from http://www.usamriid.army.mil/education/bluebookpdf/USAMRIID%20BlueBook%207th%20Edition%20-%20Sep%202011.pdf

U.S. Department of Health and Human Services (USDHHS). (2012). *Principles of epidemiology in public health practice: An introduction to applied epidemiology and biostatistics* (3rd ed.). Retrieved from http://www.cdc.gov/ophss/csels/dsepd/SS1978/SS1978.pdf

U.S. Department of Health and Human Services (USDHHS). (2014). *The health consequences of smoking—50 years of progress: A report of the Surgeon General.* Retrieved from http://www.surgeongeneral.gov/library/reports/50-years-of-progress/

U.S. Department of Health and Human Services (USDHHS). (2015). *Healthy people 2020: Public health infrastructure.* Retrieved from http://www.healthypeople.gov/2020/topics-objectives/topic/public-health-infrastructure/objectives?topicId=35

U.S. Public Health Service. (1964). *Smoking and health: Report of the Advisory Committee to the Surgeon General of the Public Health Service.* Washington, DC: Author. Retrieved from http://profiles.nlm.nih.gov/ps/retrieve/Narrative/NN/p-nid/60/p-docs/true

Walker, M. C., Finkelstein, S. A., Rennicks White, R., Shachkina, S., Smith, G. N., Wen, S. W., & Rodger, M. (2011). The Ottawa and Kingston (OaK) birth cohort: Development and achievements. *Journal of Obstetrics and Gynaecology Canada, 33,* 1124–1133.

Wang, Y., Zhao, N., Qiu, J., He, J., Zhou, M., Cui, H., ... Zhang, Y. (2015). Folic acid supplementation and dietary folate intake, and risk of preeclampsia. *European Journal of Clinical Nutrition, 69*(10), 1145–1150. doi: 10.1038/ejcn.2014.295.

Wiley Online Library. (2015). *Cochrane database of systematic reviews.* Retrieved from http://www.cochranelibrary.com/cochrane-database-of-systematic-reviews/index.html

Willingham, E. & Helft, L. (2014, September 5). *What is herd immunity?* Retrieved from http://www.pbs.org/wgbh/nova/body/herd-immunity.html

World Health Organization (WHO). (2014a). *Ebola virus disease update—West Africa.* Retrieved from http://www.who.int/csr/don/2014_08_28_ebola/en/

World Health Organization (WHO). (2014b). *How to conduct safe and dignified burial of a patient who has died from suspected or confirmed Ebola virus disease.* Retrieved from http://www.who.int/csr/resources/publications/ebola/safe-burial-protocol/en/

World Health Organization (WHO). (2015). *International health regulations 2005.* Retrieved from http://www.who.int/ihr/en/

Yang, W., Zhang, W., Kargbo, D., Yang, R., Chen, Y., Chen, Z., ... Shaman, J. (2015). Transmission network of the 2014-2015 Ebola epidemic in Sierra Leone. *Journal of the Royal Society Interface, 12*(112). doi: 10.1098/rsif.2015.0536.

SELECTED READINGS

American Academy of Pediatrics. (2012). *Red Book online: Vaccine status table.* Retrieved from http://redbook.solutions.aap.org/vaccine-status.aspx?gbosid=167073

Anderson, C. T., & McFarlane, J. (2010). *Community as partner: Theory and practice in nursing* (6th ed.). Philadelphia, PA: Lippincott Williams & Wilkins.

Centers for Disease Control and Prevention. (2012, May 18). *Historical evolution of epidemiology.* Retrieved from http://www.cdc.gov/ophss/csels/dsepd/ss1978/lesson1/section2.html

Ford, E. S., Zhao, G., Tsai, J., & Li, C. (2011). Low-risk lifestyle behaviors and all-cause mortality: Findings from the National Health and Nutrition Examination Survey III Mortality Study. *American Journal of Public Health, 101,* 1922–1929. doi: 10.2105/ajph.2001.300167.

Gonzalez-Guarda, R. M., Florom-Smith, A. L., & Thomas, T. (2011). A syndemic model of substance abuse, intimate partner violence, HIV infection, and mental health among Hispanics. *Public Health Nursing, 28,* 366–378. doi: 10.1111/j.1525-1446.2010.00928.x.

Vollman, A. (2011). *Canadian community as partner: Theory & multidisciplinary practice* (3rd ed.). Philadelphia, PA: Lippincott Williams & Wilkins.

World Health Organization. (2008). *International health regulations (2005;* 2nd ed.). Geneva, Switzerland: World Health Organization. Retrieved from http://www.who.int/ihr/publications/9789241596664/en/

World Health Organization. (2014). *International Health Regulations (IHR) fact sheet.* Retrieved from http://www.euro.who.int/__data/assets/pdf_file/0004/268438/IHR-Fact-Sheet_December-2014.pdf

INTERNET RESOURCES

Association for Professionals in Infection Control and Epidemiology, Inc.: http://www.apic.org

Centers for Disease Control and Prevention Behavioral Risk Factor Surveillance System: http://www.cdc.gov/brfss

Centers for Disease Control and Prevention Youth Risk Behavior Surveillance System: http://www.cdc.gov/healthyyouth/data/yrbs/index.htm

Centers for Disease Control and Prevention—Epidemiological Case Studies: http://www.cdc.gov/epicasestudies/

Centers for Disease Control and Prevention: http://www.cdc.gov/

Certification Board of Infection Control and Epidemiology, Inc.: http://www.cbic.org

Cochrane: http://www.cochrane.org/

Cochrane Library: http://www.cochranelibrary.com/

Community Preventive Services Task Force. (2011) Community Guide Task Force Findings: 1/1/1997–8/1/2011: http://www.thecommunityguide.org/about/ConclusionReport100311.pdf

Environmental Protection Agency: http://www.epa.gov

Healthy People 2020, Search the Data: http://www.healthypeople.gov/2020/data-search/Search-the-Data

Immunization Action Coalition: http://www.immunize.org

March of Dimes (Perinatal Statistics): http://www.marchofdimes.com/peristats/Peristats.aspx

National Cancer Institute (Surveillance Epidemiology and End Results [SEER]—cancer statistics): http://seer.cancer.gov/

National Health Statistics: http://www.health.gov

Nurses' Health Study: http://www.channing.harvard.edu/nhs/

Safety and Health Statistics: http://www.bls.gov/iif/

UCLA Center for Health Policy Research (University of California, Los Angeles): http://www.healthpolicy.ucla.edu/

UIC School of Public Health (Public Health Games): http://www.publichealthgames.com/

University of Pittsburgh: A Brief Introduction to Epidemiology Lecture Series: http://www.pitt.edu/~super1/courses/epi3.htm

United Nations International Children's Fund (UNICEF; statistics): http://www.unicef.org/statistics/

U.S. Bureau of Census: http://www.census.gov/

Women's Health Initiative—National Heart, Lung, and Blood Institute (NHLBI): http://www.nhlbi.nih.gov/whi/

World Health Organization (statistics): http://www.who.int/gho/publications/world_health_statistics/en/

thePoint: Everything You Need to Make the Grade!

thePoint® Visit http://thePoint.lww.com/Rector9e for selected readings, study aids for all learning styles, and more!

Communicable Disease Control

"The diseases of the present have little to do with the diseases of the past, save that we die of them".

Agnes Repplier (1855–1950), Essayist and Biographer

"There are only two things a child will share willingly; communicable disease and its mother's age".

Benjamin Spock (1903–1998), Pediatrician and Author

KEY TERMS

Active immunity	Fomites	Isolation	Screening
Antigenic shift	Herd immunity	Novel	Surveillance
Cocooning	Immunization	Passive immunity	Vaccine
Communicable disease	Incubation period	Quarantine	Vector
Direct transmission	Indirect transmission	Reservoir	
Disease control	Infectious	Ring vaccination	

LEARNING OBJECTIVES

Upon mastery of this chapter, you should be able to:

- Discuss the nurse's role in communicable disease control.
- Describe the three modes of transmission for communicable diseases.
- Identify major communicable diseases in the United States.
- Explain the strategies used for the three levels of prevention in communicable disease control.
- Explain the significance of immunization as a communicable disease control measure.
- Delineate the major concerns of parents who choose not to vaccinate their children.
- Describe major issues that affect the control and elimination of tuberculosis (TB).
- Discuss specific ways to prevent sexually transmitted diseases, including HIV/AIDS.
- Discuss the consequences of biologic terrorism with weapons such as anthrax and smallpox.
- Discuss ethical issues affecting communicable disease and infection control.

Communicable diseases pose a major threat to public health and are of significant concern to community/public health nurses. A **communicable disease** is caused by an **infectious** agent, such as a virus or bacteria, and can be transmitted from one source to another. Transmission to a susceptible host can occur directly either from person to person or animal to human, or transmission may occur indirectly through a **reservoir** such as contaminated water (Centers for Disease Control and Prevention [CDC], 2014e; Heymann, 2015). Some noncommunicable diseases can also be caused by infectious agents, such as tetanus, but cannot be transmitted from one source to another (CDC, 2014e). Jurisdictional laws and regulations define the infectious and noninfectious diseases to be reported to local, state, and territorial public health departments (CDC, 2015q). The National Notifiable Diseases Surveillance System allows sharing of notifiable disease information nationally and between jurisdictions for surveillance, control, and prevention purposes (CDC, 2015q).

Knowledge of communicable diseases is fundamental to the practice of community/public health nursing because these diseases typically spread through communities of people. Understanding the basic concepts of communicable disease control, as well as the numerous surrounding issues, helps a public health nurse work effectively to prevent and control communicable disease in populations and groups. It also helps nurses teach important and effective preventive measures to community members, advocate for those affected, and protect the well-being of uninfected persons (including health care workers and nurses themselves).

In the last century, numerous changes occurred in the lives of people both nationally and globally related to issues of public health. Communicable disease control is recognized as one of the 10 great public health achievements of the 20th century (CDC, 2013c, 2013e). In the early 1900s, the top three causes of death were pneumonia, tuberculosis (TB), and diarrheal or enteric diseases. Then, control measures including improved sanitation and hygiene, vaccinations, and use of antibiotics and other antimicrobials, along with improved surveillance systems, have all contributed to a significant reduction of infant and child mortality and a nearly 30-year increase in life expectancy overall (National Institute on Aging, 2015). During the first decade of the 21st century, new vaccines reduced the number of serious illness and death due to pneumococcal infection and reduced rotavirus-related hospitalizations among children. Deaths related to other vaccine-preventable diseases (VPDs), including hepatitis A, hepatitis B, and varicella, were also reduced during this 10-year time period (Hinman, Orenstein, & Schuchat, 2011). In addition, improved public health infrastructure and changes in prevention strategies resulted in a 30% reduction in TB and a 58% reduction in bloodstream infections related to central lines. Improved testing has allowed more people with human immunodeficiency virus (HIV)/ acquired immune deficiency syndrome (AIDS) to be identified and receive lifesaving treatment earlier. Rabies control efforts have resulted in the elimination of canine rabies in the United States (CDC, 2011a). The Centers for Disease Control and Prevention is charged to protect Americans against threats of disease, both in the United States and abroad (CDC, 2014k).

But, new challenges in communicable disease control have emerged:

- New and reemerging communicable diseases that threaten the health of populations around the world. Examples include a pandemic of H1N1 influenza in 2009–2010 resulting in over 12,000 deaths in the United States, an outbreak of Ebola in West Africa in 2014 resulting in over 11,000 deaths, and an emergence in 2015–2016 of the Zika virus in the Americas, which, at the time of this writing, was suspected of causing microcephaly in babies born to women who contracted the mosquito-borne illness during pregnancy, as well as West Nile virus and corona viruses such as MERS and SARS (CDC, 2014c, 2016c, 2016f; Heymann, 2015).
- Threat of vector-borne pathogens such as Rift Valley fever and dengue fever emerging in the United States as a result of changes in climate (CDC, 2014d).
- Development of antibiotic-resistant strains of bacteria around the world that threaten the public's health as well as pose significant occupational health risk for health workers. Examples include multi- and/or extreme drug-resistant TB (MDRTB, XDRTB), HIV/ AIDS, malaria, and methicillin-resistant Staphylococcus aureus, or MRSA (WHO, 2016c, 2016i).
- The threat of bioterrorism, which involves the use of biologic agents with the intent to cause harm (Heymann, 2015). An example of this is the deliberate delivery of anthrax spores through the U.S. mail in 2001. See Chapter 17 for more on emerging infections and bioterrorism.

This chapter provides information to help you better understand communicable diseases in communities and around the globe. It describes ways to plan and implement appropriate prevention interventions, including immunization of children and adults, environmental interventions, community education, screening programs, and disease investigation and case/contact finding. Ethical issues of communicable disease control are also discussed. A list of communicable disease information sources useful to you, the community/public health nurse, is also provided.

BASIC CONCEPTS REGARDING COMMUNICABLE DISEASES

Communicable diseases have challenged health care providers for centuries. Exposure to infectious agents can occur out in the community or within health care settings (Heymann, 2015). The threat of these diseases has led to the development of important nursing and medical preventive measures, such as infection control measures including hand washing, use of personal protective equipment, safe handling of contaminated sharp equipment, and appropriate disposal of potentially infectious materials, to community sanitation and the development of vaccines and use of antimicrobial medications (Heymann, 2015).

Evolution of Communicable Disease Control

Although communicable diseases are no longer the leading cause of death in the world, they continue to pose a serious threat. Three of the top 15 causes of death continue to be infectious illnesses. These are HIV, diarrheal diseases, and TB (WHO, 2014). In 2012, 1.5 million people died from HIV/AIDS and another 1.5 million people died from diarrheal illnesses (WHO, 2014). Over 900,000 people died of TB in that same time period (WHO, 2014).

Bubonic plague, caused by *Yersinia pestis*, is one example of how communicable diseases have changed the course of history. The first documented pandemic plague occurred in 541 AD. The next 200 years saw over 25 million deaths due to plague (CDC, 2015t). In 1334, the great plague pandemic, known as "Black Death," killed 60% of the European population. Now, this deadly disease can be controlled through early identification and treatment with antibiotics. *Y. pestis* has been used as a weapon during wars over the centuries. Weaponization of *Y. pestis* remains a threat today (CDC, 2015t).

Historically, as countries became industrialized, increased productivity, trade, and economic growth also brought on the four D's of disruption, deprivation, disease, and death. Industrialization brings large numbers of people close together in condensed living conditions. Trade brings populations together, exposing them to infectious agents they had not previously seen. These conditions, combined with poor sanitation leading to contaminated water supplies and infestation of disease-carrying insects or rodents, have all contributed to devastating epidemics in the past and continue to pose a threat today in developing countries. Planning for built environments that support health and safety is critical for mitigating the risk for disease outbreaks in developing urban regions (Neiderud, 2015).

Control of infectious disease began when microorganisms were identified as the source of these illnesses. In the 20th century, public health measures began to be implemented, resulting in significant achievements in the control of infectious diseases. These interventions included improvements in sanitation and hygiene, animal and pest control, vaccination, and infectious disease detection through testing, monitoring, and treatment with antimicrobials (Rosner, 2010).

Not until the 1700s and 1800s were the causative organisms for various infectious diseases recognized through the assistance of increasingly sophisticated microscopes. With these discoveries came early attempts to create ways to prevent the spread of such organisms, either by decreasing their power or by eliminating them. Pasteurization of milk was invented, and efforts to eliminate rats from ships and food storage areas began. These measures commenced a global effort to eliminate communicable diseases (Schlipköter & Flahault, 2010).

In 1945, as the United Nations (UN) was being formed, they identified a need for a global health program. By 1948, the World Health Organization (WHO, 2016f) came into existence. The WHO continues to be a very active part of the UN. They provide multifaceted services such as promoting health across the lifespan by working toward improving health systems; addressing communicable and noncommunicable diseases; working on emergency preparedness, surveillance, and response; and providing corporate services through their 150 offices around the world (WHO, 2016a). See more on global health in Chapter 16.

Also mentioned in Chapter 6 is the Centers for Disease Control and Prevention (CDC), which is a branch of the U.S. Department of Health and Human Services (USDHHS). Originally tasked with the elimination of malaria in war areas, it has evolved over the years into a health promotion and disease prevention agency. It is recognized globally for its partnerships in disease surveillance, research, data collection, and analysis, as well as for responding nationally and globally with peer agencies to disease outbreaks (CDC, 2012b). Smallpox, caused by the *variola* virus, is a classic example of a communicable disease control success story. The *variola* virus had been associated with devastating epidemics throughout the centuries. Smallpox became endemic in Europe in the 18th century and was responsible for 300 to 500 million deaths worldwide during the 20th century (Thèves, Biagini, & Crubezy, 2014). Smallpox first responded to a crude vaccine that was developed in the 18th century. The vaccine was studied and perfected and used globally for decades. A major worldwide eradication campaign began in 1967, under the direction of the WHO (Heymann, 2015). The last naturally acquired case of smallpox in the world occurred in Somalia in 1977, and WHO certified global eradication 2 years later (Heymann, 2015). In 1980, the World Health Assembly declared the eradication of smallpox and made a call to cease smallpox vaccinations around the globe (WHO, 2016b). Outside of a small accidental laboratory-related outbreak in 1978, there have been no cases of smallpox since that time (Heymann, 2015).

Despite strides in controlling major disease outbreaks, the threat of biologic warfare using smallpox, anthrax, plague, or other disease organisms raises concerns about how to prepare for the future (Heymann, 2015). The Global Health Security Agenda, an international partnership among nearly 50 participating nations, began in 2014. The goal of this program is to make the world safe and secure from biological threats by bringing nations together to address this issue and making security a top priority among global leaders (Global Health

Security Agenda, 2015). Strategies include prevention, detection, and response (Globalhealth.gov, n.d.). This collaborative includes partnerships among both governmental and nongovernmental stakeholders. The U.S. commitments to this agenda include participation from U.S. Department of Health and Human Services, U.S. Department of Defense, U.S. Department of Agriculture, and U.S. Department of International Development (Globalhealth.gov, n.d.). Partnerships are with the governments of neighboring Canada and Mexico, as well as almost 50 other countries around the world.

Surveillance is key to security from biological threats. Health care service providers and laboratories are required to submit reportable information to the local health department. Local health jurisdictions can voluntarily send this information to the CDC National Notifiable Diseases Surveillance System (NNDSS). This system includes an electronic means of sharing surveillance information in place in all 50 states and the District of Columbia, allowing them to send case notifications to NNDSS quickly and securely (CDC, 2015r). The United States, South Africa, and Thailand have led the Global Health Security Agenda (GHSA) in working toward development of a laboratory surveillance system that would allow laboratories across each nation to detect harmful pathogens, both known and new threats, safely and accurately (CDC, 2014f).

Community Health Nurse's Role: Process of Investigating Reportable Communicable Diseases

Diseases in humans are reported to the local health authority (Heymann, 2015) (Fig. 8–1). Each state has a State Health Department, but not all states have local level sites like a county health department. Some of the state and/or local health departments utilize a combination of nurses, epidemiologists, and communicable disease investigators. The CDC and WHO provide guidance documents that assist state public health agencies to develop investigation policies and procedures for the local level investigator to use. The local investigation process must meet the

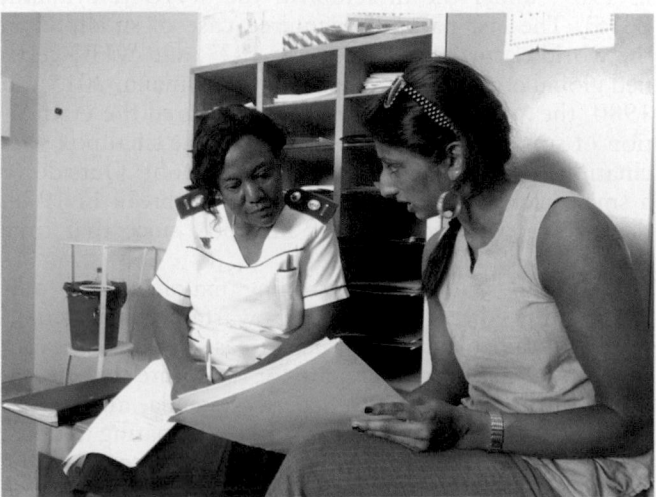

FIGURE 8-1 PHN interviews a health center nurse during TB/HIV investigation.

requirements of the state and federal reporting laws that derive from state, federal, and global health regulations. Individual states utilize the national notifiable infectious disease list as the guidance for developing the state's reportable diseases and may add to this list as they choose, reflecting the types of conditions that are unique to a state or region of the United States (CDC, 2012b). State health departments commonly specify two other circumstances that must be reported: any outbreak or unusually high incidence of any disease and any occurrence of an unusual disease of public health importance (CDC, 2015r). A core function of the CDC is to provide support to any local, tribal, territorial, or state health department to prepare or respond to any health threat (CDC, 2014i). This support comprises information, training, and staff, tools so that local health departments can respond promptly (CDC, 2014i). The CDC is also available to each individual citizen via mail, phone, or the Internet. You can reach them at:

Centers for Disease Control and Prevention
1600 Clifton Rd., Atlanta, Georgia 30333
800-CDC-INFO (800-232-4636); TTY: (888) 232-6348, 24 hours/every day E-mail: cdcinfo@ cdc.gov

The local health department/agency is the initial point of notification of a communicable disease investigation. If a person is identified in one jurisdiction but had been exposed in another, the health agency receiving the report should notify the health agency where the exposure occurred so an investigation can be conducted in the originating region (Heymann, 2015). In most states, reporting known or suspected cases of a reportable disease is generally considered to be an obligation of:

- Physicians, dentists, nurses, and other health professionals
- Medical examiners
- Administrators of hospitals, clinics, nursing homes, schools, and nurseries

Some states also require or request reporting from:

- Laboratory directors
- Any individual who knows of or suspects the existence of a reportable disease

Each state has a disease report form; California uses a form titled *Confidential Morbidity Report*. Display 8–1 is an example of a reporting form. Each local health department or agency will investigate a specific disease using a protocol set by the local, state, or federal public health official. Reportable diseases must be reported to the state health department. Notifiable diseases are voluntarily reported by the state to the CDC (CDC, 2015j). The list of notifiable conditions is updated annually.

Disease investigation requires a systematic approach. The nurse may be assigned to work on individual cases of a disease or several cases that make up a cluster or outbreak. Whether it is a single case of illness in a small town or a multijurisdictional outbreak, similar investigation steps are followed. The investigation will require surveillance to identify additional people who might be infected, determining the possible source of the infection and the means of transmission, identifying others who are at risk so screening

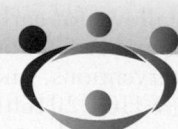

DISPLAY 8-1 CONFIDENTIAL MORBIDITY REPORT

CONFIDENTIAL MORBIDITY REPORT

NOTE: For STD, Hepatitis, or TB, complete appropriate section below. Special reporting requirements and reportable diseases on back.

DISEASE BEING REPORTED: _____

Patient's Last Name

Social Security Number
___ - ___ - ___

Ethnicity (✓ one)
- ☐ Hispanic/Latino
- ☐ Non-Hispanic/Non-Latino

First Name/Middle Name (or initial)

Birth Date
Month Day Year

Age

Race (✓ one)
- ☐ African-American/Black
- ☐ Asian/Pacific Islander (✓ one):

☐ Asian-Indian	☐ Japanese
☐ Cambodian	☐ Korean
☐ Chinese	☐ Laotian
☐ Filipino	☐ Samoan
☐ Guamanian	☐ Vietnamese
☐ Hawaiian	
☐ Other:_____	

Address: Number, Street

Apt./Unit Number

City/Town

State

ZIP Code

- ☐ Native American/Alaskan Native
- ☐ White: _____
- ☐ Other: _____

Area Code **Home Telephone**
___ - ___ - ___

Gender M F

Pregnant? Y N Unk

Estimated Delivery Date
Month Day Year

Area Code **Work Telephone**
___ - ___ - ___

Patient's Occupation/Setting
- ☐ Food service ☐ Day care ☐ Correctional facility
- ☐ Health care ☐ School ☐ Other _____

DATE OF ONSET
Month Day Year

Reporting Health Care Provider

REPORT TO

DATE DIAGNOSED
Month Day Year

Reporting Health Care Facility

Address

City   **State**   **ZIP Code**

DATE OF DEATH
Month Day Year

Telephone Number
( )

Fax
( )

Submitted by

Date Submitted
(Month/Day/Year)

(Obtain additional forms from your local health department.)

SEXUALLY TRANSMITTED DISEASES (STD)

Syphilis
- ☐ Primary (lesion present)
- ☐ Secondary
- ☐ Early latent < 1 year
- ☐ Latent (unknown duration)
- ☐ **Neurosyphilis**

- ☐ Late latent > 1 year
- ☐ Late (tertiary)
- ☐ Congenital

Syphilis Test Results
- ☐ RPR   Titer:_____
- ☐ VDRL   Titer:_____
- ☐ FTA/MHA: ☐ Pos ☐ Neg
- ☐ CSF-VDRL: ☐ Pos ☐ Neg
- ☐ Other:_____

Gonorrhea
- ☐ Urethral/Cervical
- ☐ PID
- ☐ Other: _____

Chlamydia
- ☐ Urethral/Cervical
- ☐ PID
- ☐ Other: _____

- ☐ **PID (Unknown Etiology)**
- ☐ **Chancroid**
- ☐ **Non-Gonococcal Urethritis**

STD TREATMENT INFORMATION
- ☐ Treated (Drugs, Dosage, Route):

_____
_____

Date Treatment Initiated
Month Day Year

- ☐ Untreated
  - ☐ Will treat
  - ☐ Unable to contact patient
  - ☐ Refused treatment
  - ☐ Referred to: _____

VIRAL HEPATITIS

		Pos	Neg	Pend	Not Done
☐ **Hep A**	anti-HAV IgM	☐	☐	☐	☐
☐ **Hep B**	HBsAg	☐	☐	☐	☐
☐ **Acute**	anti-HBc	☐	☐	☐	☐
☐ **Chronic**	anti-HBc IgM	☐	☐	☐	☐
	anti-HBs	☐	☐	☐	☐
☐ **Hep C**	anti-HCV	☐	☐	☐	☐
☐ **Acute**	PCR-HCV	☐	☐	☐	☐
☐ **Chronic**					
☐ **Hep D (Delta)**	anti-Delta	☐	☐	☐	☐
☐ **Other:**_____		☐	☐	☐	☐

Suspected Exposure Type
- ☐ Blood transfusion
- ☐ Other needle exposure
- ☐ Sexual contact
- ☐ Household contact
- ☐ Child care
- ☐ Other:_____

TUBERCULOSIS (TB)

Status
- ☐ **Active Disease**
  - ☐ Confirmed
  - ☐ Suspected
- ☐ **Infected, No Disease**
  - ☐ Convertor
  - ☐ Reactor

Site(s)
- ☐ Pulmonary
- ☐ Extra-Pulmonary
- ☐ Both

Mantoux TB Skin Test
Month Day Year

Date Performed

☐ Pending

Results:_____ mm ☐ Not Done

Chest X-Ray Month Day Year

Date Performed

- ☐ Normal ☐ Pending ☐ Not done
- ☐ Cavitary ☐ Abnormal/Noncavitary

Bacteriology
Month Day Year

Date Specimen Collected

Source _____

Smear: ☐ Pos ☐ Neg ☐ Pending ☐ Not done
Culture: ☐ Pos ☐ Neg ☐ Pending ☐ Not done

Other test(s) _____

TB TREATMENT INFORMATION
- ☐ **Current Treatment**
  - ☐ INH ☐ RIF ☐ PZA
  - ☐ EMB ☐ Other:_____

Month Day Year

Date Treatment Initiated

- ☐ **Untreated**
  - ☐ Will treat
  - ☐ Unable to contact patient
  - ☐ Refused treatment
  - ☐ Referred to:_____

REMARKS

PM 110 (8/05) (Edited 9/05)

and prevention measures can be implemented, preventing further transmission, and monitoring the response to these interventions (Heymann, 2015). In the event of an outbreak, the response should also include confirmation of the outbreak, establishment of a task force to serve as the command-and-control center of the response, communication with the public, managing care for those who are ill, and conducting an outbreak investigation (Heymann, 2015).

Prior to contacting an individual for an interview:

- Review the information received from the mandated reporter for completeness.
- Clarify that the disease is suspect or lab confirmed. Some infections can be reported if they meet a set of clinical criteria or are part of a larger outbreak and a case definition has been defined.
- Review the case definition. A case is the individual who either has a laboratory-confirmed reportable disease or meets the clinical definition in an investigation.
- Review the disease information—reservoir, incubation period, infectious period, symptoms, and treatment. Also, know the methods of control. Be prepared to provide education to the client while also conducting the investigation.
- Many diseases have specific questionnaires that are useful when interviewing the client. Review the questionnaire prior to contacting the client so you understand the intent of the investigation and know the questions you will ask the client to answer. This will allow you to focus on the investigation and can help set the client at ease.
- If no questionnaire exists, you may have to write a narrative report including the information related to onset of illness, symptoms, medical evaluation, treatment if received, recovery state, and individuals the person has been in contact with depending upon the nature of the disease.
- Display 8–2 provides an example of a generic disease investigation form.

Conducting the interview:

- Maintaining a neutral and nonjudgmental attitude during the interview process will elicit information more readily, especially when discussing an STD, for example.
- The interview may be by telephone or in person. The way an interview is pursued depends upon the department protocol and/or disease being addressed.
- Introduce yourself and explain the purpose of the confidential nature of the interview.
- Eliciting what the individual knows about the disease may give the nurse an idea of the individual's knowledge base and what education or reeducation to provide.
- Gathering the information by using a disease-specific questionnaire may lead to a possible source of the disease, or to additional infected contacts.
- The nurse will contact individuals identified as possibly infected by the identified case. By pursuing contacts, the possibility of outbreak status may appear.

Surveillance of communicable diseases is the next step. The WHO defined **surveillance** as the ongoing, systematic, collection, analysis, and interpretation of health data (WHO, 2016h). Surveillance allows for early identification of public health emergencies and evaluation of the effectiveness of public health interventions, and is used to help inform policy changes (WHO, 2016h). Contact tracing can identify additional people who are also affected (Heymann, 2015). Information obtained by the nurse during the interview is sent from the local investigation to the next higher level of government for analysis and interpretation. If an outbreak is occurring, it may be from the next level of government that assistance is garnered (Heymann, 2015). Next is disease control. **Disease control** measures are determined by the characteristics specific to the disease. Public health nurses must understand the characteristics of the infectious agent so that appropriate control measures can be implemented. Prompt, appropriate action could minimize or even prevent an outbreak. Control measures may include testing, counseling, education, environmental modifications such as draining standing water, vaccination, treatment, or prophylaxis as appropriate (Heymann, 2015).

Effective surveillance and control can lead to *elimination* and *eradication* of a disease in many cases. The 1989–1992 International Task Force for Disease Eradication defined the terms of disease elimination and eradication. Elimination is the stopping of a disease in a defined geographical region, whereas eradication is the extinction of a naturally occurring disease (Carter Center, 2016). Eradication eliminates the need for further control measures (Carter Center, 2016). An example of elimination is that there are no natural cases of polio in the Americas. An example of eradication of a disease is smallpox. See Chapter 16 for more on global eradication of infectious diseases.

Modes of Transmission

Transmission of a communicable disease describes how disease is passed from person to person or from another source to a person. Transmission can occur by direct or indirect methods (Heymann, 2015).

Direct Transmission

Direct transmission occurs by immediate transfer of infectious agents from a reservoir to a new susceptible host. This can be through either direct contact or droplet spread. Direct contact with the source could include touching, biting, kissing, or sexual intercourse—that is, contact with oral secretions, blood, or other potentially infectious fluid, such as the drainage from a skin lesion. Coughing or sneezing secretions into the face of a susceptible individual can transmit respiratory infections, such as measles or pertussis, by way of droplet spread. Close proximity of <1 m is required, like sharing the space in a car or small room, to transmit an organism from one person to another (Heymann, 2015) (see Fig. 8–2).

Airborne Transmission

Airborne transmission occurs through droplet nuclei—the small residues that result from evaporation of fluid from droplets emitted by an infected host. Sneezing and coughing are common examples of airborne transmission. Because of the small size and weight of droplet

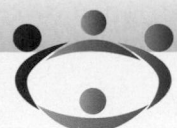

DISPLAY 8-2 SAMPLE GENERIC DISEASE INVESTIGATION FORM

SAMPLE GENERIC DISEASE INVESTIGATION FORM

Name: _____ DOB/age: _____

Address: _____

Telephone(s): _____

Race/ethnicity: _____ Occupation: _____ Gender: _____

Risk Factors

Recent travel outside U.S.?_____ Outside of the County? _____

    If yes, location(s) & date(s) _____

Was client born in U.S.?_____

    If no, country of birth _____ Year arrived in U.S. _____

In 10 days prior to this illness, has individual participated in the following activities? If yes, please explain.

    Attended a social gathering _____

    Was food served? If yes, list foods consumed _____

    Eaten at restaurants, including fast-food restaurants _____

    _____

    Eaten rare/raw animal products, home-canned /unusual foods _____

    _____

    Visited a day care or medical facility _____

    Had visitors in his/her home? _____ Were any of them ill? _____

        If yes, sex and dates of illness _____

    Drunk water from/or swam/bathed in pools, lakes, hot tubs, etc. _____

        If yes, where and when: _____

    What is usual source of drinking water? _____

    Does client have contact with domestic or wild animals? _____

    Were any animals sick? If so, date of contact _____

  I. Comments:

(continued)

DISPLAY 8-2 SAMPLE GENERIC DISEASE INVESTIGATION FORM (*Continued*)

Clinical Information

Date/time of onset: _____   Duration of symptoms: _____

Symptoms: (check all that apply)

☐ Fever _____

☐ Chills   ☐ Nausea   ☐ Vomiting   ☐ Abdominal Cramps

☐ Diarrhea   ☐ Headache   ☐ Neck Stiffness   ☐ Cough

☐ Runny Nose   ☐ Shortness of Breath

Others: _____

_____

_____

Did client see health care provider? _____

    If yes, name of provider, phone and date seen _____

    What was diagnosis? _____

    Was any lab work ordered? _____

    If yes: Test: _____   Results _____

             Test: _____   Results _____

             Test: _____   Results _____

    Was any medication prescribed? _____

Was client hospitalized? _____   Where _____

What was outcome? _____

Does client have any chronic illnesses?   List _____

What medications does client normally take? _____

Does client use any home remedies? _____

Allergies to foods or medications _____

Recent immunizations _____

Is client aware of anyone else with similar symptoms? _____

    If yes, please give identifying information _____

Females: Are you pregnant? _____   If yes, EDC _____

Is there any other information you think may be important for us to know regarding this Illness?

_____

_____

Initial telephone contact by _____   Phone: _____   Date: _____

Person conducting the interview: _____   Phone: _____   Date: _____

California Public Health Nursing Disaster Handbook   IV-5
Second Edition 2008

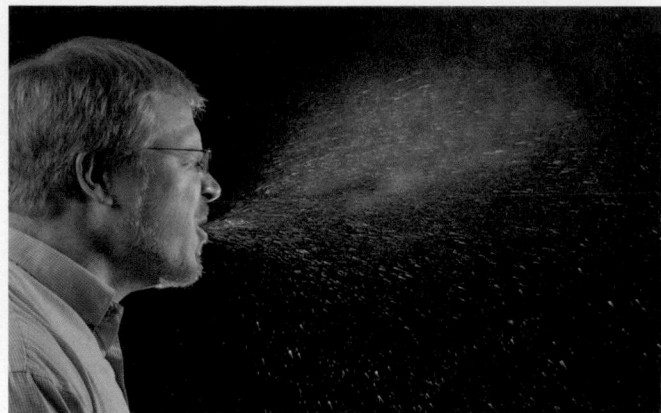

FIGURE 8–2 Sneeze in progress—revealing the plume of droplets expelled in a large cone-shaped array. (From Centers for Disease Control and Prevention. Public Health Image Library. Photo Image ID #11161—James Gathany.)

nuclei, they can remain suspended in the air for long periods before they are inhaled into the respiratory system of a host. Small particles of dust from soil containing fungus spores may cling to clothing, bedding, or floors. The spores may become separated from dry soil by the wind and then be inhaled by the host (Heymann, 2015).

Indirect Transmission

Indirect transmission occurs when the infectious agent is transported within contaminated inanimate materials called **fomites**, including toys, sharp objects, tissues, or even water or food. This type of indirect transmission is also referred to as *vehicle-borne transmission*. The infectious agent may or may not need to multiply while in the inanimate material (Heymann, 2015). Chapter 9 describes both the government's role and the nurse's role in helping to prevent food and water contamination by infectious agents (Heymann, 2015). Another way infectious disease can be transmitted indirectly is by insects. Insects may carry disease on their feet or expel it through their digestive tract. This mechanical transmission does not require the infectious organism to multiply. Insects can also transmit disease when the infectious agent has propagated within the insect (Heymann, 2015). This requires an incubation period for the infectious agent to be passed to the host. Examples of this cycle are malaria that is transmitted by mosquitoes or Lyme disease transmitted by ticks. These modes of transmission that involve insects or animals are called vector-borne transmission (Heymann, 2015).

Vector Transmission

When transmission occurs through a **vector** (i.e., a nonhuman carrier such as an animal or insect), it is known as vector-borne transmission. Vector-borne diseases are a major public health concern (CDC, 2014a). Transmission can be through a bite of the insect (e.g., mosquito) or animal (e.g., rat) or exposure to the infected animal's body fluids, such as the urine from the Hantavirus-infected rodent (Heymann, 2015). Insects such as mosquitoes, fleas, and ticks are responsible for transmission of malaria, plague, and Lyme disease. Rabies and Hantavirus are examples of vector-borne illnesses passed to humans from animals.

Of all the infectious diseases, vector-borne illnesses are the most complex to prevent and control (CDC, 2014a). Control strategies directed toward vector-borne diseases typically involve community education and environmental measures to hinder the vector from reaching the host.

Control strategies may include the following:

- Reduce the population of insects.
- Eradicate rodents that carry diseases, such as rats.
- Use of mechanical or chemical barriers to protect from exposure to vectors, such as mosquitoes or ticks—for example, sprays or mesh bed nets.
- Public education about preventive and protective measures, including avoiding vector habitats, and how to respond when exposed to a vector to prevent disease from developing.

Food- and Water-Related Illness

Food- or water-related illness can be caused by bacteria, viruses, or parasites, such as *Salmonella*, *Shigella*, *Escherichia coli* 0157, listeriosis, and *Campylobacter*, the protozoan agent *Giardia*, and the viral agent hepatitis A (Heymann, 2015). Toxins released in response to bacteria in the intestines can also result in severe illness. Ingestion of the pathogenic organism sets in motion the events of a food- or water-related intestinal illness or even death. The contamination can occur at the source (e.g., contamination by animal waste being introduced into the food or water chain) or through unsanitary food handling or practices. This fecal–oral route results in the ingestion of fecal material. Food storage at improper temperatures can also create an environment allowing microorganisms to grow.

Most commonly, exposure to contaminated food or water results in symptoms related to gastrointestinal function, including diarrhea, nausea, vomiting, stomach cramps, and bloating. Fever may accompany these infections as well. Onset of symptoms may occur within a few hours after exposure or not until days or even weeks later, depending on the microorganism. This time interval between exposure and onset of symptoms is called the **incubation period**.

Microorganism contamination of food resulting in human illness occurs as a result of either infection or intoxication. Infection is related to a pathogen that occurs through ingestion of food contaminated with adequate doses of *Salmonella*, *Shigella*, *E. coli*, or other pathogens. The cycle begins when the infectious agent multiplies and grows in the food medium. The agent subsequently invades the host after ingestion of the food. Then infection occurs—which is the entry and development or multiplication of an infectious agent in the body. Infection is usually accompanied by an immune response, such as the production of antibodies with or without clinical manifestation. The infectious organism produces illness by direct irritation of the normal gastrointestinal mucosa. By contrast, intoxication is caused by the production of toxins as a by-product of the normal bacterial life cycle. This commonly occurs when cooked food is left standing at room temperature. Or it can occur when the bacteria is living on the skin of a food preparer who inadvertently inoculates the food. It is ingestion of the toxin, rather than the microbe itself, that produces the illness (Heymann, 2015). One well-recognized example is the neurotoxin botulinum that is produced by the bacteria *Clostridium botulinum*.

The distinction between infection and intoxication is relevant for a number of reasons. Toxins may be difficult to isolate and identify, particularly in the absence of the bacteria; some suspected food-borne illnesses go unidentified for this reason. Although the bacteria may be killed after heating of foodstuffs before consumption, some bacteria-produced toxins are stable at normal cooking temperatures, so that food cannot be rendered safe even though it has been thoroughly cooked. Bacteria established in the human gastrointestinal system may require medical treatment to be eradicated. In contrast, individuals with food intoxication typically require supportive care while in the process of ridding themselves of the toxin (Heymann, 2015).

Food- and water-related outbreaks can impact large numbers of people. Such outbreaks serve to remind all community health practitioners of the continuing need to teach and observe the most basic methods for preventing food and water contamination. Display 8–3 summarizes correct methods for maintaining the safety and cleanliness of food.

The most important aspect of food- or water-related diseases for nurses in community health is to recognize that outbreaks of illness affecting large numbers of people can occur, despite well-recognized standards for decontamination of water supplies and safe commercial food preparation. The public health nurse may notice they have received similar reports of illness that requires looking for a common source. This may necessitate a higher level of investigatory assistance, such as the state health department (CDC, 2011b). Outbreaks may not be detectable by local surveillance means alone because of the mobility of individuals or the routine transportation of foods from one state or country to the other. It may not be identified as an outbreak until the various reports of illness and laboratory reports from affected communities (or in one if it is a local outbreak) are processed and forwarded to a public health laboratory, and then onto the state public health laboratory. It is at this point that the sentinel surveillance system is triggered. Some states have local county public health laboratories that may make the identification of

---

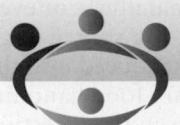

DISPLAY 8–3   CORRECT METHODS FOR PRESERVING THE SAFETY AND CLEANLINESS OF FOOD

Before handling food:
- Wash hands and all food preparation surfaces and utensils thoroughly with soap and water.

When preparing food:
- Wash foods that are to be eaten raw and uncooked thoroughly in clean water. This includes foods that are to be peeled that grow on the ground or come in contact with soil.
- Cook all meat products thoroughly.
- Do not allow cooked meats to come in contact with dishes, utensils, or containers used when the foods were raw and uncooked.

When storing leftover foods:
- Cool cooked foods quickly; store under refrigeration in clean, covered containers.

When reheating leftover foods:
- Heat foods thoroughly. Bacteria contaminating food grow and multiply in a temperature range between 39°F and 140°F.

Adapted from U.S. Department of Agriculture. (n.d.). *Kitchen companion: Your food safe handbook*. Retrieved from http://www.fsis.usda.gov/wps/wcm/connect/6c55c954-20a8-46fd-b617-ecffb4449062/Kitchen_Companion_Single.pdf?MOD=AJPERES

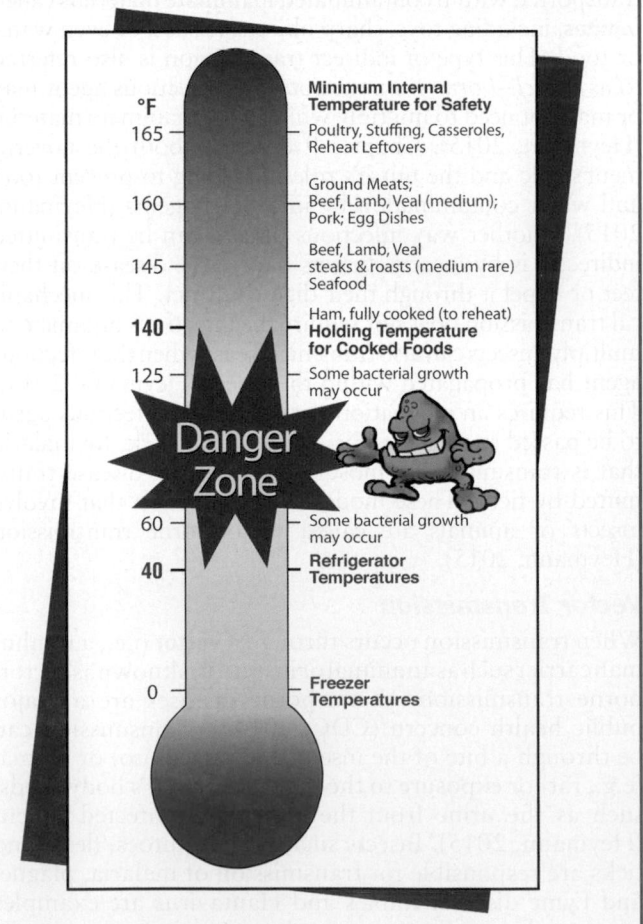

organism clusters. Unfortunately, many states or regions rely primarily on the state public health laboratory for organism identification, which has the potential for delays (CDC, 2011b).

The CDC has a system of surveillance called PulseNet, a program designed to identify organisms that may come from a same source, allowing outbreaks to be identified and sources to be eliminated (CDC, 2013a). This program uses laboratory testing to connect food-borne illness cases. Currently, 87 laboratories participate in this program with at least one lab in each state. Testing is conducted to match ill people in different states using pulsed-field gel electrophoresis to identify the DNA fingerprinting of the various organisms. A cumulative database of over 0.5 million bacterial isolates are stored in the system (CDC, 2013a). When a common source is identified, the food regulatory agency can work with the facility to clean up the problem or close the facility down.

An example of one PulseNet success story occurred in 2014 when this system identified a rare fingerprint of *Salmonella* Newport in specimens from ill patients. This prompted multiple health departments to initiate an investigation. Chia powder was determined to be the common source. Chia powder was being used in people's smoothie drinks. Public health investigators included questions about Chia powder in their questionnaires and identified additional cases in the United States and in Canada. The product was pulled from shelves, eliminating the source from the food supply (CDC, 2014b).

MAJOR COMMUNICABLE DISEASES IN THE UNITED STATES

Community health nurses encounter any number of communicable diseases in their practice. Many are reportable, but some are not—although they are just as transmittable to others as the reportable infections. As mentioned previously, each state department of health has the capacity to determine which diseases will be reportable based upon the federal reportable disease list. These diseases are frequently diagnosed and treated in the community care setting rather than the hospital. The following sections discuss some of the more common communicable diseases, but the list is not inclusive of all that are reportable. Diseases are presented in groups by similarity, rather than by virulence or prevalence.

Influenza (Seasonal or Novel) and Pandemic Preparedness

Influenza (flu) is identified as an acute communicable viral disease of the respiratory tract. Symptoms include fever, headache, myalgia, prostration, coryza, sore throat, and cough. The influenza virus undergoes minor genetic mutations from year to year, and these changes are referred to as antigenic drift. Periodically, the influenza A virus will transform drastically, which is referred to as **antigenic shift**. Most people around the world would not have antibodies to protect them from this **novel** (new) strain, thus making a large percentage of the population susceptible, leading to a pandemic (Heymann, 2015). Influenza A virus causes the most severe and widespread disease (pandemics); influenza B causes milder disease outbreaks;

and influenza C is connected with only sporadic cases of milder respiratory disease. Influenza is usually seasonal in nature but may be found year round if testing is done. Each year, a vaccine is developed to prepare for the upcoming flu season. The strains used in the vaccine is based on the influenza strains identified through the WHO's ongoing surveillance as those currently circulating around the globe (Heymann, 2015).

Influenza derives its importance from the rapidity with which epidemics evolve, the widespread morbidity, and the seriousness of complications, specifically pneumonias (Heymann, 2015). Influenza, an Italian word that means *influence of the cold*, has been recognized since 412 BC and was first described by Hippocrates (Heymann, 2015). It existed throughout the early centuries, and about 30 probable pandemics have been documented in the past 400 years. Three have occurred in the 20th century—in 1918, 1957, and 1968. The 1918 "Spanish flu" pandemic was the most devastating, with 20% to 40% of the world population affected and an estimated death toll of 50 million worldwide; in the United States, roughly 675,000 died (Flu.gov, n.d.). This novel influenza strain spread easily from person to person, resulting in devastating morbidity and mortality rates around the globe. The most recent influenza pandemic occurred in 2009 when the novel strain, H1N1, emerged. Estimates of infection rates range between 43 million and 89 million people, and between 8,800 and 18,300 deaths worldwide are attributed to the flu (Flu.gov, n.d.).

Influenza infections occur primarily in the winter months, affecting individuals in all age groups and causing thousands of deaths and hospitalizations annually in the United States alone. Children have the highest rates of infection, but individuals aged 65 years and older, children younger than 2 years of age, pregnant women, and those with certain medical conditions have the highest rates of serious morbidity, hospitalization, and mortality. Older adults account for more than 90% of the deaths related to influenza and pneumonia (Heymann, 2015).

Community health nurses play a major role in primary prevention. Universal **immunization** is recommended for *all people 6 months of age and older*. In the elderly, immunization may be less effective in preventing illness but can still be of importance because it may reduce the severity of disease. With immunization, the incidence of complications and death among the elderly is reduced. Children younger than 6 months cannot receive the vaccine, so they need to be protected by immunization of the individuals surrounding them. It is important that community/public health nurses promote immunization of those who may suffer the poorest of outcomes and their caretakers:

- Health care workers and personal care providers
- Children younger than 5, but especially children younger than 2 years old
- Adults 65 years of age and older
- Pregnant women
- Individuals with asthma
- Those with chronic disease of any system of the body (neurologic, cardiac, pulmonary, hematologic, renal, hepatic, immune, or metabolic, endocrine, and anyone on long-term medication for an illness)

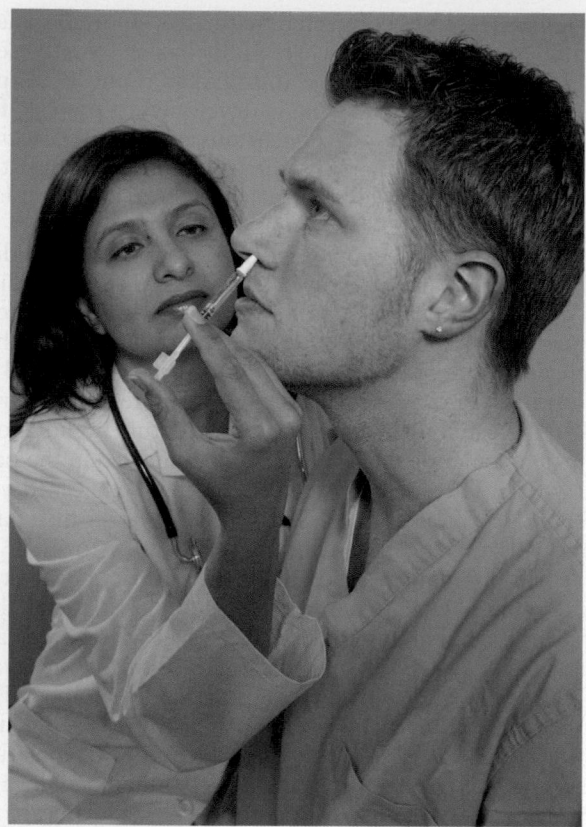

FIGURE 8–3 Administration of nasal spray flu vaccine. (From Centers for Disease Control and Prevention. Public Health Image Library. Photo Image ID #11864—James Gathany.)

The injectable influenza vaccine is inactivated. The nasally inhaled version is a live attenuated vaccine and is licensed for use in people ages 2 to 49 years (Heymann, 2015; see Fig. 8–3). The vaccine should be given every year *before* influenza is expected in the community. The season can begin as early as October, so vaccinating in September may be indicated, but usually it begins by the end of October in most of the United States. For those living or traveling outside the United States, timing of the immunization should be based on the seasonal patterns of influenza in the area to which they are traveling (Heymann, 2015). Influenza immunization clinics are frequently planned and organized by or with the local public health agency, with the injections usually administered by community/public health nurses.

Influenza pandemics occur when a flu subtype has not circulated previously (novel strain) or has reemerged in a population that has never been exposed (CDC, 2015h). The 2009 H1N1 pandemic provides an example of the emergency response to a pandemic event. On April 15, 2009, the first case of H1N1 strain influenza was diagnosed in the United States. Ongoing cases of this novel strain were being reported across the United States and around the world into the summer of 2010. There was a rapid response by the WHO and the CDC in investigating, typing the strain, and initiating the production of a vaccine. Production of a vaccine began by April 21 and on April 26, the federal government declared a public health emergency (Flu.gov, n.d.). Within 6 months,

a monovalent (single-strain) vaccine was available to the public. Eighty million doses were administered during that first season, which minimized the impact of this pandemic event (Flu.gov, n.d.).

The WHO's Global Influenza Surveillance and Response System (GISRS) is an integrated surveillance system that maintains constant vigilance for new influenza viruses. It monitors the evolution of influenza viruses; provides recommendations about diagnostic testing, vaccine development, antiviral susceptibility, and assessment of vulnerable populations; and alerts when a virus is identified to have potential for creating a pandemic (WHO, 2016e). This program began in 1952 and now involves 143 institutions from 113 WHO member states.

FluNet is an Internet-based tool for worldwide influenza surveillance. This program allows for the electronic submission of influenza data from participating global laboratories. Real-time data can be accessed through this resource. As new data arrive and are verified, the maps and tables are revised to give users an up-to-date overview of the influenza situation. Data are provided remotely through the GISRS, the WHO regional databases, and other designated laboratories. Only designated users can submit data, but the results—graphics, maps, and tables of influenza activity on a global scale—are available to the general public. FluNet has expedited the sharing of information on influenza patterns and virus strains and is becoming an essential tool in preparing for and preventing influenza pandemics. Collaborating Influenza Surveillance Centers have created a task force of influenza experts to develop a plan for the global management and control of influenza pandemics. These influenza experts and world public health leaders work diligently to prevent another influenza pandemic similar to the devastating outbreak of 1918 (WHO, 2016d). See more on global disease surveillance in Chapter 16.

Pneumonia

Pneumonia is a pulmonary infection that causes inflammation of the lobes of the lungs, bronchial tree, or interstitial space. It is an important cause of death among the elderly and infants. There are a number of infectious agents that can cause pneumonia. In the United States, the most common bacterial cause of pneumonia is *Streptococcus pneumoniae* (pneumococcus), and the most common viral causes are influenza, parainfluenza, and respiratory syncytial viruses. Symptoms of pneumonia include sudden onset with a shaking chill, fever, pleural pain, dyspnea, a productive cough of "rusty" sputum, and tachypnea. The onset is less abrupt in elderly individuals who may present with fever, shortness of breath, and altered mental status. In infants and young children, fever, vomiting, and convulsions may be the initial symptoms. The diagnosis may need to be confirmed by radiographic studies (Heymann, 2015).

Community-acquired pneumonia is a significant cause of morbidity and mortality. The incidence of pneumonia is highest in winter. An increased incidence of pneumonia often accompanies epidemics of influenza. In the United States and Europe, morbidity rates range between 30 cases per 100,000 adults and 100 cases per 100,000. Incidences are higher among people living in poverty or who have poor nutrition. Case fatality rates of pneumococcal pneumonia range from 5% to 35% and are 10% for children living in developing countries. Children under the age of 6 months who live in developing countries have a 60% fatality rate. Globally, pneumonia kills more than one and a half million children younger than 5 years of age each year. This is greater than the number of deaths from any other infectious disease, such as AIDS, malaria, or TB (Heymann, 2015). Hospital admissions and mortality related to pneumonia are far more common among people older than age 65; the mortality rate is approximately 50%. Although this is not a reportable infectious disease, it can nevertheless have a great impact upon the community (Heymann, 2015).

Pneumonia can be spread by several means (e.g., droplets, direct oral contact, fomites that are defined as any inanimate objects freshly soiled with respiratory discharges). People most susceptible to pneumonia are infants, the elderly, and people with a history of chronic diseases, a compromised immune system, or any condition affecting the anatomic or physiologic integrity of the lower respiratory tract. Malnutrition and smoking also increase risk (Heymann, 2015).

Two vaccines are available to help protect against pneumonia. The pneumococcal protein–polysaccharide conjugate vaccine protects against 10 or 13 of the most common pneumonia serotypes and is included as part of the routine vaccination schedule for infants. The 23-valent pneumococcal polysaccharide vaccine (PPV23) is available for high-risk groups, ages 2 years old and up. High-risk groups include those with chronic diseases, those with immunosuppressing health conditions, or those who are asplenic. Reimmunization is recommended only for high-risk children or adults over 65 years who received their first vaccine before age 65 and at least 5 years has passed since the previous vaccine. The vaccine is not effective in children younger than 2 years of age and is not recommended for the healthy population between the ages of 2 and 65 years. For these people, education about preventing pneumonia is a major part of the community/public health nurse's role (Heymann, 2015).

Hepatitis

Of the five viral hepatitis infections that constitute serious liver disease, the three most commonly reported types are hepatitis A, B, and C. Infection with hepatitis is an ongoing global epidemic. Substantial progress is being made in the elimination of hepatitis viruses through the primary prevention practices of education and immunization with hepatitis A and B vaccines.

Hepatitis A

Hepatitis A is caused by infection with the hepatitis A virus (HAV). It occurs worldwide and is sporadic and epidemic, with cyclic recurrences affecting children and young adults most frequently. Case rates are highest in areas with poor sanitation. This includes Central and South America, the Caribbean, Mexico, Asia (except Japan), Africa, and southern and eastern Europe (Heymann, 2015). The disease is transmitted from person to person by the fecal–oral route with an incubation period of 28 days; however, onset of illness

can range between 15 and 50 days after exposure to the virus. Hepatitis A is characterized by the abrupt onset of symptoms including fever, malaise, anorexia, nausea, and abdominal discomfort, followed by jaundice in more severe cases. Children may be asymptomatic. Mild illnesses last 1 to 2 weeks; more severe cases last 1 month or longer. It is generally a self-limited disease that does not result in chronic infection or chronic liver disease. Recovery from HAV usually confers immunity for the individual. Hepatitis A is identified by the presence of immunoglobulin M antibodies against HAV in the serum of acutely or recently ill individuals. Upon diagnosis, providers are mandated to report hepatitis A to the local health agency (Heymann, 2015). Sensitive occupations include food handlers and health care personnel because of the risk of transmission to others in the course of their work (CDC, 2015s).

In areas of the world where environmental sanitation conditions are poor, endemic infection may exist and cause infection at an early age. In this setting, the majority of adults have immunity due to previous exposure. In industrialized countries, cases will tend to occur in the older population rather than children, in households of the infected, and among travelers returning from countries where the disease is endemic. At times, common-source outbreaks are related to contaminated water, food contaminated by infected food handlers, raw or undercooked shellfish harvested from contaminated water, or contaminated produce. Outbreaks of hepatitis A may warrant mass vaccination outreach with the hepatitis A vaccine or immunoglobulin (Heymann, 2015).

An inactivated hepatitis A vaccine has been available for use since 1995 (CDC, 2015s). Administered in a two-dose series, these vaccines induce protective antibody levels in virtually all who are immunized. Ninety-five percent of immunized adults develop immunity after the first dose and nearly 100% seroconvert after the second dose (CDC, 2015s). This has been a boon to eliminating this disease as a public health problem in the United States. The vaccine is recommended as a routine vaccine for children and, as of 2005, was made available to children older than 12 months. Community/public health nurses play an important role in the prevention and control of this disease. Offering hepatitis A vaccine to travelers, conducting case investigations, providing education, and identifying potential sources and exposed contacts that need referral or assistance in obtaining postexposure prophylaxis and vaccination are vital to preventing and controlling this disease (CDC, 2015s).

Hepatitis B

Hepatitis B is a serious disease. The hepatitis B virus (HBV) is often a lifelong infection and may cause cirrhosis (scarring) of the liver, liver cancer, liver failure, and death. In a very few cases, the infection will resolve, conferring immunity (Heymann, 2015). This is a blood and body fluid pathogen; common transmission patterns are parenteral, sexual, and perinatal transmission from mother to newborn (CDC, 2015s).

Hepatitis B is a global problem. Approximately 2 billion people have evidence of resolved or current HBV infection, and 240 million people are chronic carriers of the virus. Approximately 600,000 people die each year because of hepatitis B infection. Rates are highest in China, Southeast Asia, most of Africa, most of the Pacific Islands, parts of the Middle East, and in the Amazon basin (CDC, 2015s). In countries where hepatitis B has the highest endemic rates, the primary cause of infection is from mother to fetus (Heymann, 2015). The chance of a child developing a chronic HBV infection is 90% if infected at birth, 20% to 50% if infected between 1 and 5 years of age, and only 1% to 10% if infected after the age of 5 years (Heymann, 2015). Symptoms of HBV range from unnoticeable to fulminating and include anorexia, vague abdominal discomfort in the right upper quadrant, nausea and vomiting, light or gray-colored stools, dark urine, arthralgia, arthritis, and rash, often progressing to jaundice (CDC, 2015s). Infants rarely present with symptoms, and <10% of children and only 30% to 50% of adults present with jaundice. The diagnosis is confirmed by the presence of specific antigens to HBV in serum (Heymann, 2015).

Immunization is the most effective way of preventing HBV transmission. The hepatitis B vaccine has been available in the United States since 1981. Since then, rates of HBV infection in the United States have declined by 75% (CDC, 2015s). Almost all infections would be prevented if hepatitis B vaccines were administered to all newborns and infants (Heymann, 2015). After receiving the recommended three doses of vaccine, 95% of infants and children develop immunity whereas only 90% of adults become immune. By age 65 years, only 75% become immune (CDC, 2015s). Infants born to HBV carrier mothers are at an extremely high risk for developing hepatitis B. Hepatitis B vaccination and one dose of hepatitis B immunoglobulin within 24 hours of birth, and completing the three-dose series at one to 2 months and at 6 month of age, is 85% to 95% effective (CDC, 2015s). Community/public health nurses have an important role in the prevention and control of hepatitis B. Most importantly, this role includes teaching that encourages immunization compliance, particularly following up on immunization of infants born to mothers with chronic HBV status, and consistent adherence to universal precautions, especially for people in high-risk lifestyles or occupations.

Hepatitis C

Hepatitis C (HCV) causes a complex infection of the liver and is one of the leading known causes of liver disease in the United States. Seventy-five percent to 85% of people with acute HCV develop chronic disease (Heymann, 2015). It is a common cause of cirrhosis and hepatocellular carcinoma, as well as liver transplantation. It is believed that 3.5 million people in the United States, and 130 to 170 million people worldwide, are infected with HCV (CDC, 2015n; Heymann, 2015). Most HCV infections result from the sharing of contaminated needles or other equipment used for injecting drugs.

Symptoms are similar to those of hepatitis A and B and may be unrecognizably mild or people can present with fulminating symptoms. Only 20% to 30% of people develop symptoms (Heymann, 2015). Many infected people are unaware that they are infected because of lack of symptoms (CDC, 2015n). Diagnosis depends on the detection of antibody to HCV. Testing does not distinguish between acute and chronic disease (Heymann, 2015). Testing is recommended for those individuals at greater risk for HCV infection. These include:

- People born between 1945 and 1965.
- People who inject drugs, including those who injected once or a few times in the past and do not consider themselves drug users.
- Individuals who received transfusions or organ transplants before 1992 and recipients of blood from a positive donor.
- People with selected medical conditions, including recipients of clotting factors before 1987, people undergoing chronic hemodialysis, and those with persistently elevated alanine aminotransferase levels.
- People diagnosed with HIV/AIDS.
- People with symptoms of liver disease.
- Those exposed to HCV-positive sources, such as through needle sticks, sharps, or mucosal exposures.
- Children born to HCV-positive mothers; testing should be done after child is 18 months old to avoid detecting mother's antibodies (CDC, 2015n).

There is currently no vaccine for HCV. The public health nurse's role is primarily supportive, encouraging testing for people who identified as having HCV infection risk factors and referring individuals for care and treatment and to support/educational groups. As with HBV, teaching adherence to universal precautions in the home is important as well (CDC, 2015n). Public health nurses can also educate at-risk populations about risk reduction behaviors (Heymann, 2015).

HIV/AIDS

The *Human Immunodeficiency Virus (HIV)* is a retrovirus that attacks the body's immune system. HIV is contracted through exposure to blood and body fluids from an infected person by a susceptible person. Transmission can occur during unprotected sex, sharing of contaminated needles, and placental transmission from mother to fetus and may also be transmitted through blood or blood components. Two types have been identified: type 1 (HIV-1) and type 2 (HIV-2). These viruses are relatively distinct serologically and geographically, but they have similar epidemiologic characteristics. The pathogenicity of HIV-2 appears to be less than that of HIV-1, and antibodies can be detected in <1 month after exposure whereas onset of AIDS symptoms may take 1 to 15 years (Heymann, 2015). The age at the time of infection has been found to influence the time frame of AIDS symptoms onset, with older people having a more rapid onset than those who acquire the virus at a younger age (Heymann, 2015).

This disease was first recognized in the early 1980s and the retrovirus was identified in 1983. At that time, no treatment existed. Without effective treatment, HIV is highly fatal (Heymann, 2015). An HIV-infected individual may remain symptom free for long periods, but viral replication is active during all stages of infection. The virus destroys the hosts T cells, making it difficult to fight other infections. Opportunistic infections and cancers appear. At this point, the disease has progressed to AIDS (CDC, 2015o). Although there is no cure for HIV/AIDS,

HIV infection is now treated with antiretroviral medications and is viewed by many to be a chronic, manageable disease process, especially in the developed world (Heymann, 2015). HIV continues to devastate populations of people who do not have access to life-extending medical care and medications. Seventy-one percent of those affected by AIDS are living in sub-Sahara Africa. The Caribbean countries of Haiti and the Dominican Republic are other areas heavily impacted by this epidemic (Heymann, 2015). Estimates indicate that in 2013, 35 million people were living with HIV/AIDS worldwide; there were 2.1 million new cases and 1.5 million AIDS-related deaths (Heymann, 2015).

Acquired Immune Deficiency Syndrome (AIDS) is a severe, life-threatening condition, representing the late clinical stage of infection with HIV, in which there is progressive damage to the immune and other organ systems—particularly the central nervous system. AIDS has been delayed or deferred in many individuals by the use of medications during the HIV stage of the spectrum. AIDS reporting is obligatory in most countries (Heymann, 2015).

Public health nurse interventions may include education about risk reduction behaviors for those who are at risk but not yet infected. For those who are infected, public health nurses can provide education about treatment, noting that with early initiation of appropriate treatment, a person with HIV can expect to live almost as long as an uninfected person. Nurses can also play a role in promoting good health for those who are infected, helping them access care, and advising them on how to prevent transmitting the virus to others (CDC, 2015o).

Tuberculosis

TB is a disease primarily of the lungs and larynx, caused by the *Mycobacterium tuberculosis* (MTB) complex, *M. africanum*, *M. tuberculosis*, and *M. canettii*. These are all Gram-positive bacilli. TB can also infect other parts of the body; it is then referred to as *extrapulmonary TB* (outside of the lungs). Extrapulmonary TB occurs in approximately 15% to 30% of all active cases (Heymann, 2015). TB has two stages: latent infection, which is noninfectious to others, and active disease, which is highly infectious to others. The person with latent infection has become infected with the bacilli but has not yet developed active disease. A person with active disease has symptoms of TB. Symptoms of TB include a prolonged cough, fatigue, loss of appetite, weight loss, and night sweats. The cough may begin as a dry cough but then progresses to purulent sputum. The development of hemoptysis indicates progressed disease. A chest x-ray may reveal pulmonary infiltrates or cavitation in the upper lobes. Fibrotic changes and reduced lung volume may indicate advanced disease (Heymann, 2015).

TB is airborne and is spread by droplet nuclei, sprayed from the mouth by coughing, sneezing, laughing, yelling, singing, or any way in which air is expelled vigorously from the lungs through the mouth. A person can be infectious as long as they have viable TB bacilli in their sputum (Heymann, 2015). Infection occurs after inhaling the bacilli exhaled by a person with active TB. Communicability depends upon the duration of the exposure with the infected person as well as the proximity or closeness and ventilation within the space where the exposure occurred. The incubation time for TB is approximately 10 to 12 weeks (Heymann, 2015). Exposure to TB does not lead to actual disease in all cases. A latent period may persist for many years before the infected person develops disease and becomes infectious, if ever.

Most individuals exposed to people with TB do not become infected. Of those who do, all but about 5% to 10% will remain disease free. The remaining 90% harbor the organism in a latent stage; although they are not infectious, these individuals represent a persistent pool of potential cases in a population. The likelihood of being among the 10% who develop clinical infectious disease is variable, depending on the initial dose of infection and certain other risk factors (Heymann, 2015). Groups at increased risk include children younger than 3 years of age, adolescents and young adults, the aged, the immunosuppressed, and those who are early in their infection (<2 years). Health factors can contribute to the development of active TB. Poor nutrition, health status, and chronic illness like diabetes can inhibit the immune system's ability to prevent TB activation from the latent TB dormant state (Heymann, 2015). Figure 8–4 shows the geographic distribution of TB in the United States.

Once almost eradicated, TB has reemerged as a serious public health problem. Nearly one third of the world's population is infected with latent TB (Heymann, 2015; WHO, 2016e). There were a total of 8.6 million cases of active TB in 2013 (CDC, 2015o). Over 95% of all cases of TB are occurring is developing countries with the highest rates found in sub-Sahara Africa (Heymann, 2015). In 2014, over 9,420 new TB cases were reported in the United States, representing a rate of 2.96 cases per 100,000 people. This rate was 2.2% lower than in 2013. Rates continue to drop since 1953, when national reporting was instituted; however, this drop is the smallest decline in rate in the past decade (CDC, 2015u). This illness continues to be a significant health threat in many parts of the world. There are sharply disparate rates among foreign-born and racial/ethnic minority populations. In the United States, 66% of the reported TB cases in 2014 were among foreign-born individuals. The rate of foreign-born TB cases in the United States was 13 times greater than the rate among those born in the United States (CDC, 2015o). Rates per 100,000 people were highest among Asian (17.8 cases) and Native Hawaiian and other Pacific Islanders (16.9 cases), whereas the White population had the lowest rates (0.6 cases). Rates among African Americans, Alaska Natives, and Hispanics/Latinos were 5.0 cases for all three groups (CDC, 2015o).

The WHO characterizes global TB burden into three categories: TB rates, multiresistant TB and TB with HIV coinfection. Fourteen countries fell into all three of the high-burden categories; they are Angola, China, Democratic Republic of Congo, Ethiopia, India, Indonesia, Kenya, Mozambique, Myanmar, Nigeria, Papua New Guinea, South Africa, Thailand, and Zimbabwe (WHO, 2016i).

HIV infection contributes dramatically to the development of active TB. People with HIV/AIDS can develop active TB within weeks after exposure to the mycobacterium, and the disease progresses much faster than in those with a normal, competent immune system. The risk of developing active TB increases from the 10% lifetime

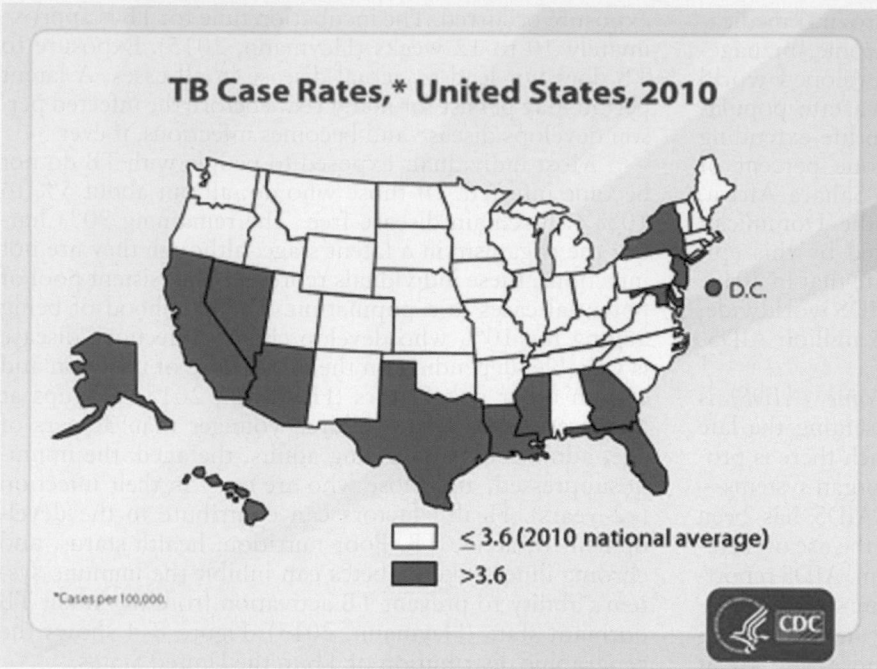

TB Case Rates,* United States, 2010

□ ≤ 3.6 (2010 national average)
■ >3.6

*Cases per 100,000.

FIGURE 8–4 Reported TB cases in the United States, 1982–2014, and TB case rates by state. (From Centers for Disease Control and Prevention (CDC). (2014). *Trends in tuberculosis, 2014.* Retrieved from http://www.cdc.gov/tb/publications/factsheets/statistics/tbtrends-2014.pdf)

risk for the general population to 15% each year, if they are not receiving antiretroviral treatment (Heymann, 2015). It is critical to rule out active disease before treating a person with HIV/AIDS for latent TB infection to also reduce the risk of developing drug-resistant TB (CDC, 2011f; Heymann, 2015).

Screening

TB infection can be detected by screening through either a skin test or blood testing. The tests can only be used to identify a person who has been infected at some point; they do not differentiate between latent and active disease.

Tuberculin skin test (TST): The Mantoux TST can detect if a person is infected with *M. tuberculosis* 2 to 8 weeks after infection (CDC, 2014g). Using the Mantoux technique, the nurse injects 0.1 mL of 5 TU purified protein

derivative (PPD) solution through the intradermal route. The reading must be conducted within 48 to 72 hours after the test had been administered. Interpretation of the results is based on measurement of induration and recorded in millimeters. Induration is described as the raised, hard area (redness is not considered part of the reaction). Results are considered positive based on various factors (CDC, 2014g). See Figure 8–5A and B for information on the correct administration, reading, and interpretation of TB skin tests.

Special considerations: Nurses should not administer the TST to individuals who report a previous positive TST. The BCG vaccine, used in TB-endemic countries to protect infants and young children from life-threatening TB illness, may cause a reaction to the TST. The effect of BCG often wanes over time; however, repeated TST may

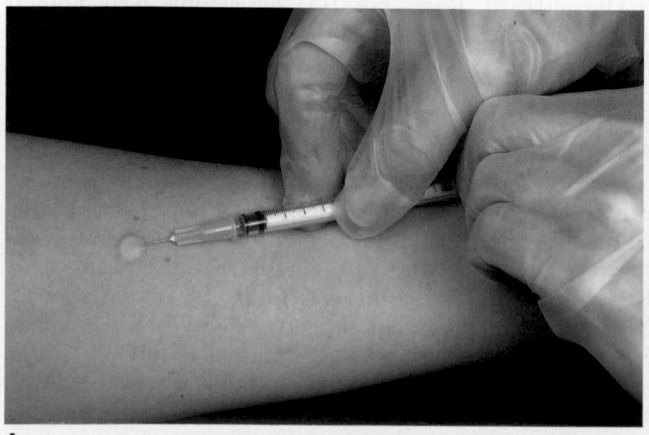
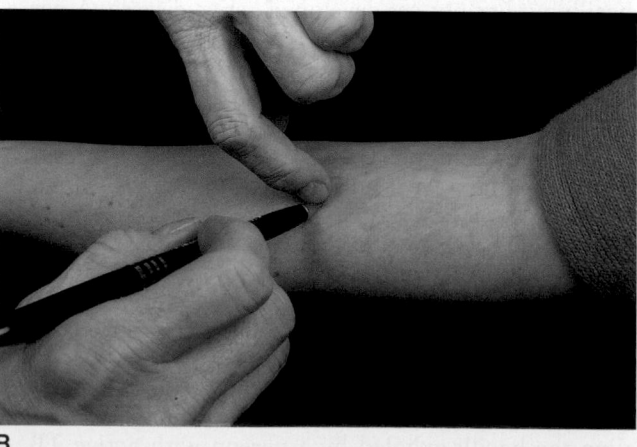

A　　　　　　　　　　　　　　B

FIGURE 8–5　A and B: Mantoux tuberculin skin test. (From Centers for Disease Control and Prevention (CDC) (2013). *Tuberculosis: 2012 surveillance slides.* Retrieved from http://www.cdc.gov/tb/statistics/surv/surv2012/slides/surv24.htm)

Table 8–1 Classification of the Tuberculin Skin Test Reaction

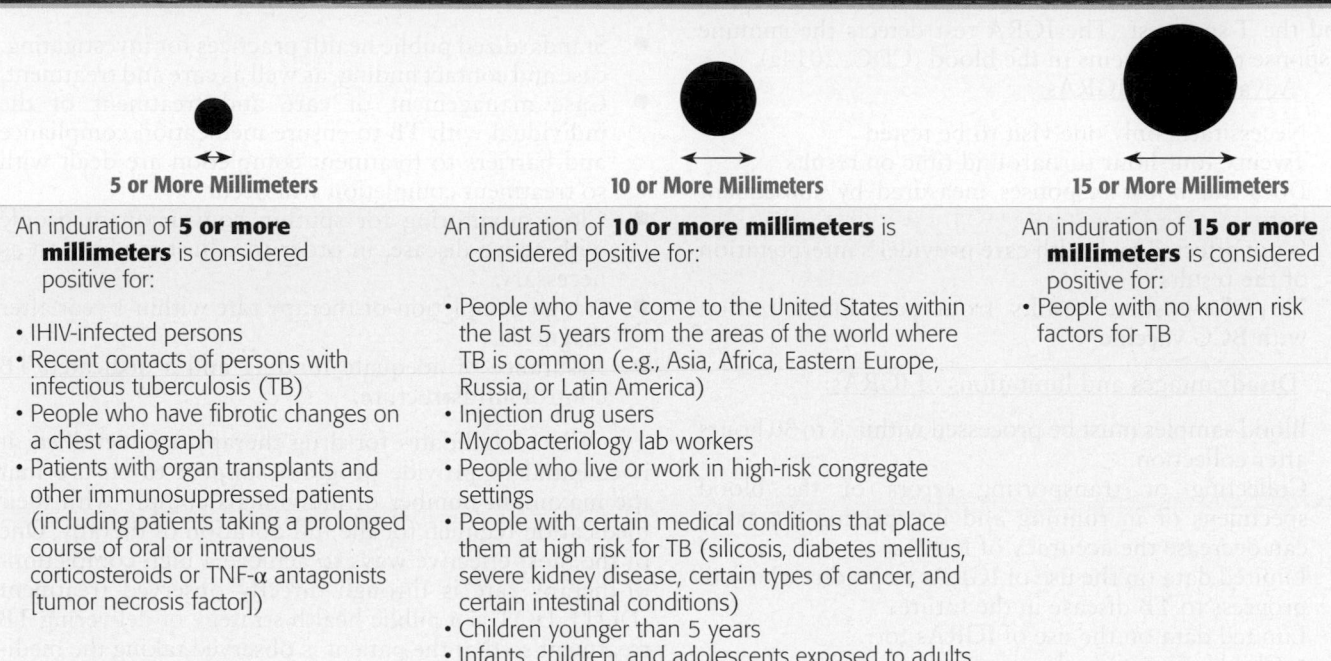

5 or More Millimeters	10 or More Millimeters	15 or More Millimeters
An induration of **5 or more millimeters** is considered positive for: • IHIV-infected persons • Recent contacts of persons with infectious tuberculosis (TB) • People who have fibrotic changes on a chest radiograph • Patients with organ transplants and other immunosuppressed patients (including patients taking a prolonged course of oral or intravenous corticosteroids or TNF-α antagonists [tumor necrosis factor])	An induration of **10 or more millimeters** is considered positive for: • People who have come to the United States within the last 5 years from the areas of the world where TB is common (e.g., Asia, Africa, Eastern Europe, Russia, or Latin America) • Injection drug users • Mycobacteriology lab workers • People who live or work in high-risk congregate settings • People with certain medical conditions that place them at high risk for TB (silicosis, diabetes mellitus, severe kidney disease, certain types of cancer, and certain intestinal conditions) • Children younger than 5 years • Infants, children, and adolescents exposed to adults in high-risk categories	An induration of **15 or more millimeters** is considered positive for: • People with no known risk factors for TB

From Centers for Disease Control and Prevention. (2013). *Core curriculum on tuberculosis: What the clinician should know (6th ed.). Table 3.2 interpreting the TST reaction.* Retrieved from http://www.cdc.gov/tb/education/corecurr/pdf/chapter3.pdf

boost the reactivity in a BCG-vaccinated person. The results should be interpreted based on risk stratification regardless of BCG history. Two-step TST testing may help to identify an infected person who might otherwise not be detected owing to a waning immune response because too much time had lapsed since a previous TST. The two-step approach allows the immune system to wake up and respond using a booster effect (CDC, 2014g). See Table 8–1 with instructions on reading TB skin tests and Table 8–2 for TB classification system.

Table 8–2 Classification System for Tuberculosis (TB)

Class	Type	Description
0	No TB exposure **Not** infected	• No history of TB exposure and no evidence of *M. tuberculosis* infection or disease • Negative reaction to tuberculin skin test (TST) or interferon gamma release assay (IGRA)
1	TB exposure No evidence of infection	• History of exposure to *M. tuberculosis* • Negative reaction to TST or IGRA (given at least 8 to 10 weeks after exposure)
2	TB infection No TB disease	• Positive reaction to TST or IGRA • Negative bacteriological studies (smear and cultures) • No bacteriological or radiographic evidence of active TB disease
3	TB clinically active	• Positive culture for *M. tuberculosis* • Positive reaction to TST or IGRA, plus clinical, bacteriological, or radiographic evidence of current active TB
4	Previous TB disease (**not** clinically active)	• May have past medical history of TB disease • Abnormal but stable radiographic findings • Positive reaction to the TST or IGRA • Negative bacteriologic studies (smear and cultures) • No clinical or radiographic evidence of current active TB disease
5	TB suspected	Signs and symptoms of active TB disease, but medical evaluation **not** complete

From Centers for Disease Control and Prevention. (2013). *Core curriculum on tuberculosis: What the clinician should know (6th ed.). Table 2.8 TB classification system.* Retrieved from http://www.cdc.gov/tb/education/corecurr/pdf/chapter2.pdf

Interferon gamma release assays (IGRAs): There are two IGRA tests, the QuantiFERON test (QFT) and the T-spot test. The IGRA test detects the immune response to TB proteins in the blood (CDC, 2014g).

Advantages of IGRAs:

- Necessitates only one visit to be tested
- Twenty-four-hour turnaround time on results
- Does not boost responses measured by subsequent tests
- Is not affected by health care provider's interpretation of the results
- No false-positive results from past immunization with BCG vaccine

Disadvantages and limitations of IGRAs:

- Blood samples must be processed within 8 to 30 hours after collection.
- Collecting or transporting errors of the blood specimens or in running and interpreting the assay can decrease the accuracy of IGRAs.
- Limited data on the use of IGRAs to predict who will progress to TB disease in the future.
- Limited data on the use of IGRAs for:
  - Children younger than 5 years of age
  - Persons who had been recently exposed to *M. tuberculosis*
  - Immunocompromised persons
  - People requiring serial testing
- Tests may be expensive.

IGRAs are preferred for people who are not likely to return for reading of TST and people who have a history of receiving BCG vaccine. The TST is preferred for children under the age of five (CDC, 2014g).

Diagnosis of Active TB

Diagnosis of suspected active TB disease is initially based on the presence of acid-fast bacilli (AFB) in the sputum. Confirmation is determined by culture that reveals MTB. The culture test also provides information about drug susceptibility that informs the decisions for treatment (Heymann, 2015). A full examination should also be conducted, including obtaining a chest radiograph and reviewing the person's history of risk factors and symptoms.

Prevention and Intervention

The public health nurse can apply all three levels of prevention when working with TB clients. According to the CDC Division of TB Elimination (DTBE) (CDC, 2011d), a well-functioning TB control program must focus resources on those at risk for TB exposure and treating latent TB and active TB. Isoniazid therapy for individuals who are infected with TB but have no evidence of active disease has been shown to be highly effective in preventing progression to infectiousness and clinical symptoms. Isoniazid (also known as INH) is a key component of the treatment for active disease (CDC, 2016d; Heymann, 2015).

Risk factors for active TB can be poor health (HIV/AIDS, chronic disease), lack of access to health care, poverty, malnutrition, and fear of deportation (nonresident status). Prevention and rapid treatment of infection can help prevent active TB and the possible emergence of drug-resistant TB. The functional aspect of the program should ideally strive for:

- Standardized public health practices for investigating, case and contact finding, as well as care and treatment.
- Case management of care and treatment of the individual with TB to ensure medication compliance and barriers to treatment completion are dealt with so treatment completion will occur.
- Close monitoring for sputum conversion in people with active disease, in order to adjust medication as necessary.
- A high completion-of-therapy rate within 1 year after diagnosis.
- Assurance of adequate funding and a dedicated TB control infrastructure.

When candidates for drug therapy are identified, it is essential to provide program support to ensure that the maximum number of individuals comply with their medication regimen for the full duration of therapy. One of the most effective ways to achieve a high completion-of-therapy rate is through directly observed treatment (DOT). DOT is a public health strategy of delivering TB treatment so that the patient is observed taking the medications each day. The benefits of DOT include timely completion of treatment, prevention of drug resistance, and preventing further transmission (California Department of Public Health [CDPH], 2014). In endemic countries, such as Africa, directly observed treatment short course (DOTS) is used. This strategy assures treatment success because the client takes the medication in the presence of a health care worker. The DOT(s) strategy has been demonstrated to work when it is implemented universally with all active TB patients within the county, and it is supported by the CDC and in turn by state and local health departments. It is not mandatory, but health officers may use the laws surrounding TB prevention and public protection to institute policy and statute to mandate its use. By using DOT(s) with the client with active TB, there is a reduction in ongoing potential sources of infection in the community (CDC, 2016d; Moonan et al., 2011).

The DOT approach is obviously labor-intensive, but according to the WHO, it has made a difference in fighting the spread of this disease. The more difficult clients are those who do not realize their personal or social responsibility for health and those who do not have the resources to focus on health when there are other stressors or diversions in their life. For these reasons, clients such as alcohol and drug abusers, transient homeless people, and people stressed by socioeconomic problems may become the source for new cases of TB. DOT therapy ensures that clients take a daily or intermittent dose of prescribed medication, locating them wherever they may be—in neighborhood bars, sleeping on the sidewalk, in a homeless shelter, or in a drug rehabilitation center. Most health departments and TB control programs have a percentage of their clients receiving DOT therapy, with licensed staff or community health workers assigned to administer the TB drug regimen. These outreach workers and sometimes public health nurses meet the people where they are, school, shelter, church, bar, or job, wherever it supports adherence to the mediation regimen. These ancillary staff members are often former program participants, trained and supervised by professional health workers. A program like DOTS needs sustained political commitment, with the governments of nations recognizing the long-term benefits of providing the resources and staff necessary to ensure its proper implementation (CDC, 2011d, 2016d; Moonan et al., 2011).

Multidrug-Resistant Tuberculosis

Epidemiologists and communicable disease specialists cite a number of factors that contribute to the development and spread of TB strains resistant to one or more of the standard arsenal of TB drugs. Strains now exist that are resistant to almost all of the standard anti-TB drugs. According to the WHO, one in four persons contracting XDRTB dies rapidly, within months from the disease. Chief among the factors contributing to drug resistance seems to be the political and social response to declining rates of TB over past decades, which has resulted in funding cuts for surveillance, treatment, and research and a premature sense that TB was defeated. Figure 8–6 demonstrates the disproportionate prevalence of MDRTB in foreign-born persons. On an individual case basis, the most common means by which resistant organisms are acquired is by noncompliance with therapy for the full, recommended period. As previously mentioned, the DOTS intervention can help those with TB successfully treat and cure the disease (Moonan et al., 2011; WHO, 2016g). Figure 8–6 compares MDRTB rates among people born in the United States and those born in other countries now living in the United States.

Clients with HIV and TB

HIV infection is associated with an increased possibility of developing primary TB after exposure to a source. The person living with coinfection of latent TB infection and HIV infection has a 50% higher risk of developing active TB than the immunocompetent individual (Heymann, 2015).

People with HIV infection and TB infection should be counseled thoroughly about the benefit of preventive treatment and possibility of TB activation without treatment. For HIV-infected people, preventive therapy usually consists of isoniazid daily for up to 1 year (the usual regimen for preventive therapy is 6 to 9 months). These clients must be monitored closely for effectiveness of the preventive therapy and for tolerance to isoniazid. This drug has the capacity to develop adverse reactions or negative side effects. Isoniazid can cause hepatitis or damage the liver; close monitoring and regular follow-up are necessary to detect early symptoms such as nausea, vomiting, abdominal pain, fatigue, and dark urine signifying bleeding. Any combination of these symptoms is sufficient to initiate liver function tests (Heymann, 2015).

The HIV-positive client may not have the ability to react to a skin test for TB because of a weakened immune system. Therefore, other methods to determine TB status are employed. If it is determined that TB disease is present, HIV-infected clients should begin a regimen of drugs according to the accepted national and global medication schedule used in their country. The client should be closely monitored for response to treatment; if they do not seem to be responding, they should be reevaluated. Drug sensitivity is key to correct and successful treatment.

TB Case Management

Community health nurses have a responsibility to individuals who are HIV infected and also infected with TB, to experience a successful TB treatment regimen. As previously mentioned, a component of a successful TB program is case management of care and treatment, which includes monitoring for adherence to treatment,

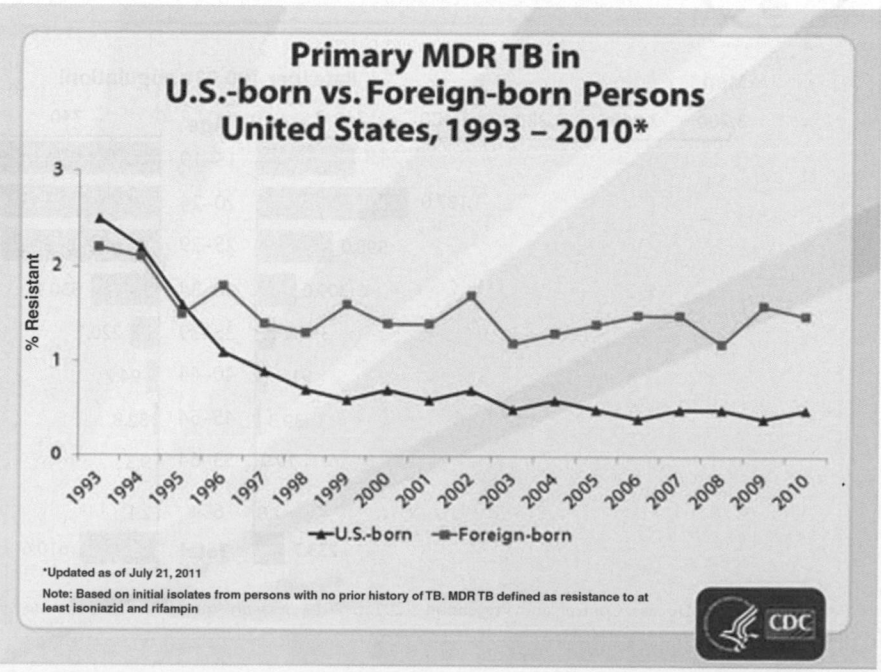

FIGURE 8–6 Multidrug-resistant TB patterns: comparison of U.S.-born and foreign-born persons, 1993–2012. (From Centers for Disease Control and Prevention (CDC). (2013). *Tuberculosis: 2012 surveillance slides*. Retrieved from http://www.cdc.gov/tb/statistics/surv/surv2012/slides/surv24.htm)

administering medications (either directly through DOT or through DOT supervision by ancillary staff), interviewing the individual for signs and symptoms of adverse reactions, collecting lab specimens in a timely manner and monitoring for culture conversion, monitoring for overall health and well-being, educating, and making referrals (CDC, 2011f).

Sexually Transmitted Infections

Chlamydia

Chlamydia trachomatis (CT) infections are the most commonly reported notifiable STD in the United States (CDC, 2015i). In 2014, more than 1,440,000 cases of *Chlamydia* were reported in the United States; however, estimates of actual numbers of infection indicate that there may be 2.86 million actual cases each year. The numbers are likely underrepresented because of the lack of symptoms in most cases. Only 10% of men and 5% to 30% of women with confirmed *Chlamydia* reported having symptoms. This illness is transmitted through sexual contact and through maternal transmission to their newborn (CDC, 2015i). *Chlamydia* is a public health concern because while it remains a "silent" disease for those who are asymptomatic, serious complications can impact women. These complications include pelvic inflammatory disease (PID), fallopian tube issues including ectopic pregnancy and infertility, and chronic pain in the pelvis (CDC, 2015i). Infection during pregnancy can lead to preterm delivery or complications for the newborn including conjunctivitis or pneumonia (CDC, 2015i).

This infection affects young people as the majority of new cases are among people between the ages of 15 and 24.

Estimates are that 1 in 20 young women in the United States are infected with CT (CDC, 2015i). Disparities exist, resulting in infection rates among Black individuals that are 6.7 times higher than the rates of White individuals.

Screening programs have been extremely effective in reducing the overall *Chlamydia* burden and reducing rates of PID in women (CDC, 2015d). The use of the highly sensitive nucleic acid amplification (NAAT) urine tests is easy and more acceptable to most individuals who may be symptomatic or asymptomatic (CDC, 2015d). As a result of increased screening efforts in many settings outside of the medical office, reported rates of *Chlamydia* continue to increase, especially in women aged 15 to 24 years (Display 8–4).

The current CDC (2015i) guidelines for screening recommendations are as follows:

- Yearly screening of all women who are sexually active and 24 years old or younger.
- Women older than 24 years old who have a new sexual partner or multiple partners or whose partner has been diagnosed with an STD.
- Screen all pregnant women at their first obstetrical visit.
- Routine screening of men is not generally recommended; however, screening should be considered among men who have sex with men in settings with high rates of CT infection.

Recommended antibiotics for treatment of *Chlamydia* include azithromycin, doxycycline, levofloxacin, or ofloxacin. Erythromycin may cause gastrointestinal side effects resulting in nonadherence to the treatment regimen (CDC, 2015d). Barriers exist to successful prevention, diagnosis,

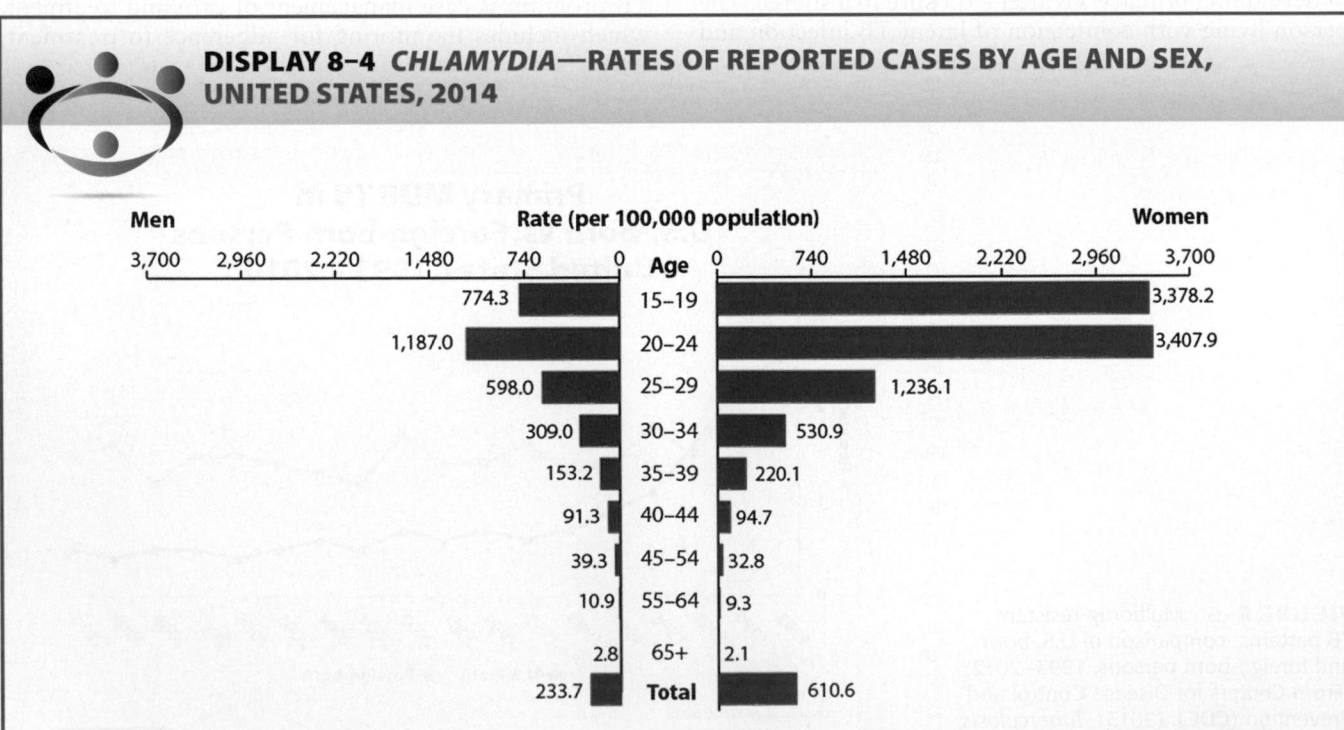

DISPLAY 8-4 *CHLAMYDIA*—RATES OF REPORTED CASES BY AGE AND SEX, UNITED STATES, 2014

Men	Age	Women
774.3	15–19	3,378.2
1,187.0	20–24	3,407.9
598.0	25–29	1,236.1
309.0	30–34	530.9
153.2	35–39	220.1
91.3	40–44	94.7
39.3	45–54	32.8
10.9	55–64	9.3
2.8	65+	2.1
233.7	Total	610.6

Rate (per 100,000 population)

From Centers for Disease Control and Prevention. (2015). *2014 Sexually transmitted diseases surveillance*. Retrieved from http://www.cdc.gov/std/stats14/figures/5.htm

and treatment of *Chlamydia*. Stigma surrounding seeking care, access to affordable care, and completion of extended antibiotic treatment may keep individuals from getting care and treatment. Using a one-dose treatment is far more acceptable than two to three times a day for 7 days treatment plan (CDC, 2011e).

Treating partners disrupts the transmission of disease by preventing reinfection to the person who had received treatment as well as preventing infection of other partners (CDC, 2015d). Some health departments use the Internet to anonymously notify partners of possible exposure to an STD (CDC, 2015e). Another strategy is to use patient-delivered partner treatment or expedited partner treatment (EPT). This entails the giving of either a prescription or medication to the infected patients to, in turn, give to their sex partner. This intervention has been shown to be more effective than encouraging the patient to notify the partner(s) to seek testing and treatment. Each state may have its own legal requirements related to this treatment option; the nurse needs to review and understand their states' law (CDC, 2015e). Another aspect to this method of treatment is to provide very specific written instructions that include self-administration of the medication, warnings about pregnancy and allergic reactions, when to seek medical care, and how to prevent reinfection (CDC, 2015e). However, for men who have sex with men, this practice is not as customary, as there may be other coinfection issues needing evaluation and treatment, such as HIB infection (CDC, 2015e). To minimize the risk for reinfection, clients should be instructed to abstain from sexual intercourse until all of their sex partners have been treated and advised to use condoms as a continued STD prevention method. Testing for cure of infection depends upon the type of antibiotic used and if the person is pregnant or not (CDC, 2015d).

Gonorrhea

The causative agent of gonorrhea (GC) is the gonococcus bacteria—*Neisseria gonorrhoeae*. GC is the second most commonly reported notifiable disease in the United States with 350,062 cases reported in 2014 (CDC, 2015a). Rates had been decreasing with a historic low of 98.1 cases per 100,000 people in 2009; however, since then, there has been an uptick of reported GC cases. In 2014, rate was 110.7 per 100,000. Ninety-three percent of cases were among people 15 to 44 years old. Compared to the rate of reported GC among Whites, the rate was 10.6 times higher in Blacks, 4.2 times higher in American Indian/Alaska Natives, 2.7 times higher in Native Hawaiians and other Pacific Islanders, and 1.9 times higher in Hispanics. Between 2010 and 2014, rates of reported GC infection among men had increased whereas rates among women had decreased. This increase may be due to either increased transmission or increased testing among men (CDC, 2015a).

Gonorrhea commonly manifests in men as a purulent drainage from the penis, accompanied by painful urination within 2 to 7 days after an infecting exposure. Women infected with GC are often asymptomatic or the symptoms such as vaginal discharge or bleeding after intercourse may be so mild as to go unnoticed (Heymann, 2015). Progression of untreated GC in women can lead to serious reproductive system involvement including PID, infertility, or ectopic pregnancy. Disseminated gonococcal infection presents with a petechial or pustular lesions and requires hospitalization for treatment. These patients should be evaluated for complications such as endocarditis and meningitis. Screening criteria are similar to those of *Chlamydia*; refer back to previous section on *Chlamydia* (Heymann, 2015).

Antimicrobial resistance is a great concern when treating GC. In 2007, treatment recommendations switched from the use of fluoroquinolone to cephalosporin because of an emergence of a fluoroquinolone-resistant strain of *N. gonorrhoeae* (CDC, 2015f). Then in 2010, concerns over emerging resistant GC prompted the CDC to recommend dual therapy, combining cephalosporin with azithromycin or doxycycline. Resistance to cefixime, a third-generation cephalosporin, appeared in Asia, Europe, South Africa, and Canada, causing further changes in dual treatment guidelines advising the exclusive use of ceftriaxone and azithromycin (CDC, 2015f). GC can be transmitted to neonates during delivery and presents 2 to 5 days after delivery. This can result in ophthalmia neonatorum and sepsis. Most states have a law that requires a prophylactic agent be given to all infants after delivery to prevent ophthalmia neonatorum. Infants born to mothers infected with GC who had not received treatment are at high risk for infection. Treatment during pregnancy is the best way to prevent GC infection in the newborn (CDC, 2015f).

Sex partners need to be referred to a medical provider for testing and treatment, but if this is not possible, EPT can be used. This is not the preferred partner treatment course for men who have sex with other men owing to concerns of coexisting STD infection including HIV (CDC, 2015f). Once again, it is best to refer to your state's regulations surrounding this method of treatment.

Syphilis

Syphilis is a sexually transmitted infection caused by the spirochete, *Treponema pallidum*. This disease is characterized by three distinct stages. Approximately 3 weeks after exposure, a primary lesion called a *chancre* characteristically appears as a painless ulcer at the site of the spirochete entry point. This first stage is considered primary syphilis. After 4 to 6 weeks, the chancre heals without treatment and is replaced by the development of a more generalized secondary macular-to-papulosquamous skin eruption, classically appearing on the soles of the feet, palms of the hands, and trunk. This rash is often accompanied by fever, sore throat, lymphadenopathy and fatigue. This stage is secondary syphilis. These secondary manifestations can resolve spontaneously within weeks or may persist up to 12 months. During the primary and secondary stages, the spirochete invades the central nervous system. If untreated, a latent period follows, which may last from weeks to years. One third of those infected who do not receive treatment progress to tertiary syphilis. These latent stages are referred to as latent, late latent, and tertiary or neurosyphilis. In the early latent stage, recurring lesions may appear. The third stage is associated with severe systemic involvement, disability, and abnormalities in the cerebral spinal fluid, deafness, meningitis, cranial nerve palsy, or even death (Heymann, 2015).

Transmission of syphilis occurs when a person is exposed to the spirochetes through direct contact with the lesions that are present during the primary or secondary stages of the disease. Syphilis can be transmitted from an infected mother to the fetus during pregnancy. Congenital syphilis can result in fetal death, premature birth, death of the newborn, or a variety of complications including failure to thrive, anemia, lesions, and CNS symptoms. Infection can also occur through blood transfusions if the donor was in the early stages at the time of the donation (Heymann, 2015).

The incidence of syphilis had been declining, with the lowest rates in 2000 and 2001 at 2.1 cases per 100,000 reported, but the number of cases increased to 6.3 cases per 100,000 in 2014. Increased incidence has been seen among men, especially impacting the population of men who have sex with men. The highest rates of syphilis in 2014 were among both men (31.1 cases per 100,000) and women (4.5 cases per 100,000) between the ages of 25 and 29. Rates of congenital syphilis also increase between 2013 and 2014 (CDC, 2015c).

Penicillin is the treatment of choice for syphilis. Patients should be instructed to avoid sexual contact until the treatment is completed and the lesions have resolved; contacts should also receive treatment. For patients with primary syphilis, contacts are defined as sexual partners within the 3 months prior to onset of symptoms; for secondary syphilis, this time period should extend to 6 months prior to onset of symptoms and for those with tertiary syphilis, 1 year for early latent and long-term partners for those diagnosed in the late latent stage. If an infant is diagnosed with congenital syphilis, all immediate family members should be treated (Heymann, 2015). Anyone diagnosed with syphilis should also be evaluated for other STDs.

Genital Herpes

Genital herpes is an STD caused by the herpes simplex viruses type 1 (HSV-1) and type 2 (HSV-2) and is one of the most common STDs in the United States. Most genital herpes infections are caused by HSV-2; however, rates of HSV-1 genital herpes are increasing among college students. Most people with HSV-2 remain undiagnosed because of the symptoms being mild causing the person to not recognize a need to seek medical care (CDC, 2015b). When the infection first occurs, symptoms are systematic and may include fever and malaise, and bilateral lesions appear on the cervix or external genitalia in women or the external genitalia in men. The anus or rectum can be affected in those who engage in anal intercourse. These lesions may last 2 to 3 weeks (Heymann, 2015). The infection can remain in the body indefinitely. Subsequent outbreaks can present in areas beyond the initial exposure site. These lesions are usually unilateral, less severe, and less frequent and resolve more quickly than the primary lesion (Heymann, 2015). HSV can be diagnosed through isolation of the virus, DNA detection through polymerase chain reaction (PCR) testing, or through tests that detect HSV antigens. Viral isolates can be typed to determine whether the infection is due to HSV-1 or HSV-2 (Heymann, 2015).

There is no cure for HSV; however, antiviral medications can prevent or reduce the duration of an outbreak and can reduce the risk of transmission to uninfected sexual partners (CDC, 2015l). If a pregnant woman becomes infected late in the pregnancy, delivery by cesarean section is often advised to reduce the risk of transmission to the neonate. Women who have a history of HSV is <1%, and a cesarean section is only advised if an active lesion is present at the time of delivery. Antiviral therapy can be given to the pregnant woman at 36 weeks gestation to suppress the virus to help reduce the need for a cesarean section birth (Heymann, 2015).

Viral Warts

Condyloma acuminata, verruca vulgaris, papilloma venereum, and the common wart are all forms of a viral disease caused by the *human papillomavirus* (HPV) and manifested by a variety of lesions found on the skin or mucous membranes (Heymann, 2015). Lesions found on the throat or respiratory tract are referred to as recurrent, respiratory papillomatosis. Those found in and around the genital region are condyloma acuminata, otherwise known as genital warts (Heymann, 2015). HPV is transmitted through direct contact, through contact with fomites, or from an infected mother to her neonate during vaginal birth. Genital warts are sexually transmitted via skin-to-skin contact. The incubation period is usually 2 to 3 months (Heymann, 2015).

More than 120 HPV types have been identified and at least 40 of these types of the virus are sexually transmitted. Whereas most infections with HPV are asymptomatic and self-limiting, some can persist and progress to cancer of the oropharynx, anus, cervix, vulva, vagina, or penis (CDC, 2015l). HPV is the most common STD. Each year, 14 million people are infected with HPV, mostly teenagers and young adults, and approximately 17,600 women and 7,300 men are diagnosed with HPV-related cancer. Cervical cancer is the most common HPV cancer among women, affecting approximately 11,000 women annually; 4,400 of them die each year. Oropharyngeal cancer is the most common HPV cancer among men, striking approximately 7,200 men each year (CDC, 2015p). Sexually active individuals are at risk for contracting any one or several of the types of genital warts that exist. Because few produce the actual bumpy, visual signs of warts and some produce no notable symptoms, many cases go undiagnosed. This asymptomatic state leads to ongoing transmission between or among sexual partners (CDC, 2015g). Cervical screenings, such as the Papanicolaou (Pap) smear, are recommended for women between the ages of 21 and 65 (CDC, 2015l). If cervical changes are seen, colposcopy and biopsy may be necessary (Heymann, 2015).

Treatment may include curettage, trichloroacetic acid, cryotherapy with liquid nitrogen, or surgical debunking for larger lesions. Patient-applied treatment may include immunomodulator creams or ointments, but topical treatments may not be appropriate for pregnant women (Heymann, 2015).

Three vaccines are available for the prevention of HPV infection. These vaccines are available to both female and males, and recommendation for administration is between the ages of 11 and 12. They can be given after that age if a person had not been previously vaccinated. Females can receive any of the vaccines; however, males must only receive the quadrivalent or 9-valent HPV vaccine. It is preferable that the vaccine be given prior to onset of sexual activity (CDC, 2015p). Condom use is also recommended to prevent transmission of HPV; however, condoms may not give full protection (CDC, 2015p) (see Chapter 22).

Sexually Transmitted Disease Prevention and Control

Human history has been shaped by disease, and all historical events played a part in creating the preconditions for epidemics. Of all the communicable diseases, perhaps none are as closely interrelated with human activities and attitudes as STDs. Many have occurred in epidemic proportions; most have existed for centuries.

The public health nurse needs to be concerned with the fact that minority populations, as well as women and children, suffer an inordinate STD burden (USDHHS, 2016). The medically underserved, particularly the poor and marginalized, as well as ethnic and racial minorities shoulder a disproportionate share of this problem. And this disparity in health burden is due to social conditions that affect minorities. These include inability to pay for needs services, distrust of the health care system, and fear of discrimination from health care providers (CDC, 2014j). It is important for PHNs to consider the root causes of inequities so that they may be exposed and addressed. Racism has had a long-lasting impact on health in the United States for over 300 years. Nurses need to realize the basic human need to feel accepted. They need to expose the health consequences of chronic stress caused by inequality based on skin color and be involved in intervening in this process (Penman-Aguilar, Harrison, & Dean, 2013). Access to health care is only one part of the equation. Where one lives also has a great impact on their overall health as neighborhoods with appropriate housing, adequate amenities and minimal crime have higher trajectories than do poorer neighborhoods where crime is rampant and resources are limited (Penman-Aguilar et al., 2013). Public health efforts need to be monitored to measure the impact that public health interventions, programs, and policies have on the problem. Personal stories and consistent messages help persuade the public and the policymakers to demand change, for example, by telling a compelling story. The communities need to be included as equal partners with health departments in order to work together and address the health issues they face. Community health nurses can think outside of the box to identify participants that these partnerships may include (Penman-Aguilar et al., 2013) (see Chapters 5 and 25).

As noted earlier in this chapter, women also have higher risk of serious complications from STDs. These include PID, sterility, ectopic pregnancy, and cancer associated with HPV. Children can also be affected by exposure to maternal STDs, resulting in fetal and infant death, birth defects, blindness, and mental retardation. Undiagnosed and untreated STDs result in over 24,000 women becoming infertile each year in the United States. Factors associated with this increased risk are asymptomatic STDs resulting in underdiagnosis or undertreatment, along with gender disparities and age disparities, with young adults having the highest rates of STDs (USDHHS, 2016). Nurses need to be involved in accomplishing the *Healthy People 2020* goal of promoting healthy sexual behaviors, strengthening capacities within communities, and increasing access to quality services (USDHHS, 2016) (see Chapter 21).

Infectious Diseases of Bioterrorism

The deliberate release of biological agents into society with the intent to cause harm is a real risk. Release could come in the form of an overt or a covert event (Heymann, 2015). An overt event would be one in which the public or the authorities are made aware of the threat prior to the release. Such an announcement could result in hysteria and overwhelm the public health system (Heymann, 2015). A covert attack is never announced, but there might be an unusual increase in the number of cases of a respiratory illness or a food-borne illness. Multiple agencies across the nation and around the world need to work together for preparation, surveillance, and response to such a threat (Heymann, 2015). Public health nurses are in a position that allows them to allay fears, provide the public with correct information, and help people in the decision-making process to consider immunization in the event of a possible terrorist attack. A variety of disease-causing organisms may be weaponized. However, anthrax and smallpox, two biological agents that have a history of being used as terrorist weapons, will be discussed here.

Anthrax

Shortly after the terrorist attacks of September 11, 2001, the U.S. population was further terrorized by a deliberate release of anthrax agent into the postal service system. Several people who handled or delivered the infected mail inhaled and touched anthrax spores that had been concealed in envelopes. As a result, 22 people were infected and five died, and 32,000 were identified as potentially exposed and were treated with antibiotics as a precaution (Heymann, 2015).

Anthrax spores are found in nature in the digestive tracks of herbivores and can be found in the soil. Infection in humans is sporadic in most developed countries (Heymann, 2015). There are infrequent and sporadic human infections in most industrialized countries. It is an occupational hazard among workers who process animal hides, hair, bone and bone products, and wool in some countries, leading to it being referred to as *woolsorter disease* and *ragpicker disease* (Heymann, 2015).

In humans, anthrax is an acute bacterial disease that affects mainly the skin or respiratory tract. The two main forms—cutaneous anthrax and inhalation anthrax—account for most human anthrax cases. The case fatality rate for cutaneous anthrax is 5% to 20%. The skin becomes itchy where exposed; a lesion becomes papular and then vesicular. In 2 to 6 days, a depressed black eschar, surrounded by extensive edema, develops. The infection may spread to the lymph system and cause septicemia. With inhalation anthrax, the initial symptoms are mild and may include fever, mild cough, chest pain, and malaise. The disease can then progress to respiratory distress, fever, and shock. There is an 85% fatality rate with inhalational anthrax; however, antimicrobial therapy and supportive therapy could reduce this rate (Heymann, 2015).

The causative organism *Bacillus anthracis* is a Gram-positive, encapsulated, spore-forming agent found in livestock and wildlife as the main reservoirs. The incubation period for cutaneous infection is 5 to 7 days, but for inhalational anthrax, it can vary between 1 and 45 days (Heymann, 2015). Person to person transmission is rare, but articles and soil contaminated with spores may remain infective for decades, and so, these items must be appropriately disposed (Heymann, 2015).

A vaccine that protects against cutaneous and inhalational anthrax exists. This vaccine is generally used only for those laboratory scientists handling specimens and some veterinarians who may have work-related exposure risk (Heymann, 2015).

Smallpox

The variola virus causes smallpox and is transmitted from person to person. Initial infection begins with a febrile prodromal period that includes a fever of 104°F, malaise, headache, abdominal pain, and vomiting (Fig. 8–7). This would be followed by the eruption of a deep-seated rash that transitions from macular to papular, and then, lesions become vesicles and pustules. Eventually, these scab over and fall off approximately 3 to 4 weeks after onset (Heymann, 2015). It was passed from person to person through respiratory droplets or skin inoculation. It is most easily spread by droplet during the first week after the rash has developed (Heymann, 2015).

Smallpox is a disease from our history books. A global eradication campaign had pushed smallpox into extinction. The last known naturally occurring case of smallpox was in Somalia in 1977. Smallpox was declared globally eradicated in May of 1980. Officially, the smallpox virus presently exists at only two places: the CDC in Atlanta and the State Research Centre of Virology and Biotechnology in Koltsovo, Novosibirsk Region, Russian Federation. These samples remain available in the unlikely case of reemergence of smallpox disease (Heymann, 2015).

A vaccine made from the vaccinia virus exists. The vaccinia virus, or also known as cowpox, is a similar organism that confers protection to smallpox. In 1798, Edward Jenner was able to demonstrate that the vaccinia virus could be used to protect people from smallpox (WHO, 2016b). Smallpox vaccination has risks. It is not a benign vaccine, and some experts allege that the morbidity associated with the vaccine has been understated. Serious complications include eye infection or blindness if the vaccinated person has the vaccine virus on the hand and touches the eye, severe rash leading to scarring or even death, encephalitis, or preterm birth or fetal demise if the virus becomes transmitted to a fetus during pregnancy (CDC, n.d.). One to two deaths per 1 million recipients of the vaccine can be expected, and 52 per 1 million may experience a life-threatening reaction (CDC, n.d.; Heymann, 2015). Less severe but more common side effects include the formation of satellite lesions, regional lymphadenopathy, fever, headache, nausea, muscle aches, fatigue, and chills. In addition, the vaccine is contraindicated for those who are immunosuppressed, those with eczema, and for pregnant women (Heymann, 2015) (Fig. 8–8).

Routine immunization against smallpox is no longer recommended for the general public because, at this point in time, the risk of harm from the vaccine is considered to be greater than the risk of contracting the disease. Laboratory workers who work in high-risk areas may still obtain the vaccine (Heymann, 2015).

The response plan for smallpox exposure may utilize the previously successful **ring vaccination** strategy—containing an outbreak by rapidly isolating and vaccinating people who have had close, face-to-face contact with the victim. This method refers to a ring of people around the exposed or ill person. Contacts would be monitored daily for fever and isolated if a fever develops (Heymann, 2015).

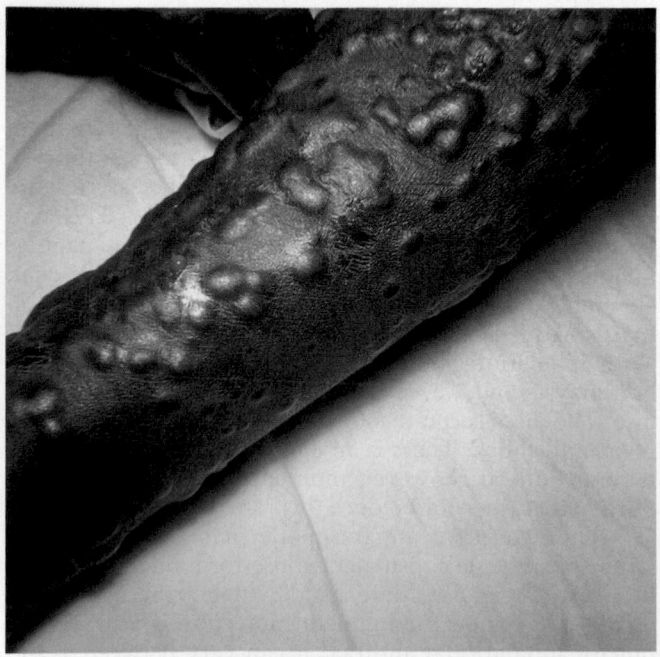

FIGURE 8–7 No longer commonly seen, the maculopapular rash of smallpox is very distinct.

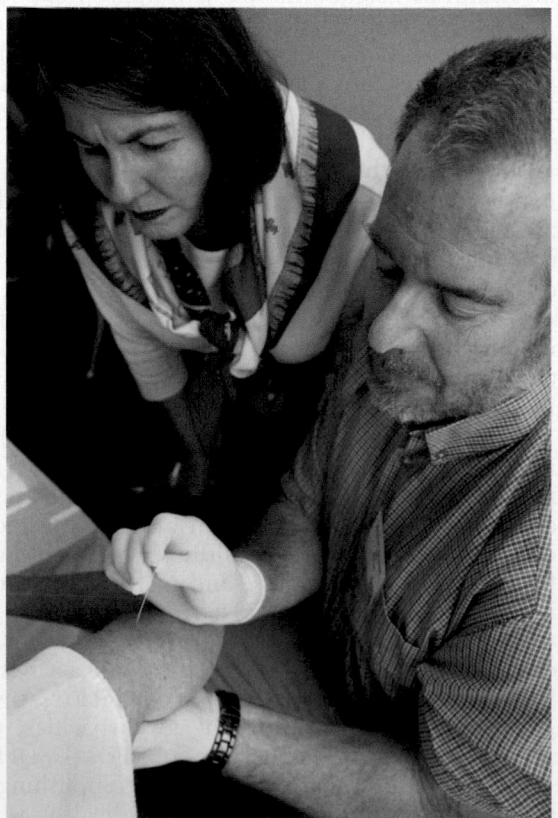

FIGURE 8–8 Smallpox inoculation of public health worker. (From Centers for Disease Control and Prevention. Public Health Image Library. Photo Image ID #2825—James Gathany.)

PRIMARY PREVENTION

In the context of communicable disease control, two approaches are useful in achieving primary prevention: (a) immunizations and (b) education using mass media with targeted health messages to aggregates.

Education

Health education in primary prevention is directed both at helping individuals understand their risk and at promoting healthy behaviors. Chapter 11 deals more extensively with the concepts of learning theory and the variety of health education approaches and materials available to community/public health nurses today.

Targeting Meaningful Health Messages to Aggregates

To effectively deliver a health promotion and disease prevention message, the message must reach the target (at-risk) population (Fig. 8–9). This requires correct identification of the target populations and characteristics specific to this audience in terms of educational level, salience of the issue, involvement of the target audience with the issue, and access of the target audience to the media channels used. Cultural issues affect people's interpretation of messages and must be considered in the presentation of a disease-prevention message to ethnic and racial minority groups. A target market is defined as a group of people with the same needs, interests, and behaviors. Public health practitioners can use marketing strategies to reach out to target populations (CDC, 2011c). Marketing is based on the principles of exchange, paying a price for goods or services. The price may be money, effort, or time. The goods are the outcomes, such as good health.

To adapt health messages to specific population subgroups, include the following:

1. Develop educational materials from the community perspective, reflecting respect for community values and traditions, relevance to community needs and interests, and participation of the community in the preparation and use of the materials.

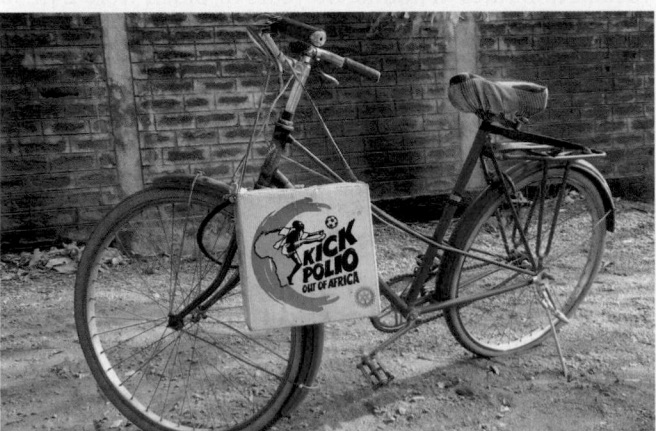

FIGURE 8–9 A targeted health message in Africa: Stop Transmission of Polio (STOP) campaign volunteer's bicycle equipped with a vaccine-carrying satchel with the message "Kick Polio out of Africa."

2. Materials must be related to the delivery of health services that are available, accessible, and acceptable to the target population.
3. All materials must be pretested and have demonstrated attractiveness, comprehension, acceptability, ownership, and persuasiveness.
4. Materials must have a readability level for the intended audience.

Ways to Communicate

Social media, made up of tools such as Facebook and Twitter, offers the ability to engage a large number of participants in an interactive, collaborative, and synchronous manner (Heldman, Schindelar, & Weaver, 2013). Practitioners can reach populations where they might not easily arrange to meet face-to-face. Social media allows people from diverse populations to meet. It also makes sharing of information easier; however, nurses need to take steps in order to ensure that patients' privacy is maintained. This approach can also be integrated with other public health communication strategies. Unfortunately, public health organizations are not utilizing social media engagement to its full potential (Heldman et al., 2013). Nurses can explore ways that social media can be used to augment current public health communication approaches. Chapters 10 and 12 have more information on social marketing and using technology to reach various populations.

Immunization

The extended life expectancy that has been enjoyed during the 20th century was largely due to the expansion of immunization programs that are provided to families. Immunizations are a cost-effective public health intervention that offers a high return on investment. Examples of the benefits gained through immunization programs include saving 33,000 lives and preventing $14 million in lost income from disease while also saving $9.9 billion in health care costs and $33.4 billion in indirect costs (USDHHS, 2014). Immunization and control of infectious diseases remain a national focus through *Healthy People 2020* (USDHHS, 2014). Table 8–3 highlights select objectives related to immunization and infectious diseases.

Challenges still exist. Over 42,000 adults and 300 children die each year from VPDs. Pockets of communities with low vaccination rates among the children exist across the country. In addition, new and emerging diseases may develop to which a vaccine might not yet be developed (USDHHS, 2014).

The Advisory Committee on Immunization Practices (ACIP) reviews the schedule for administration of vaccines for various populations and age groups. The ACIP consists of 15 experts in the field of VPD. The Secretary of the USDHHS chooses the members of this group; it functions to guide and advise on immunization practices (CDC, 2013b). The ACIP provides vaccine recommendations based on research and scientific data related to vaccine safety and efficacy for adult and child vaccines. Recommendations include age when vaccines should be given, dosage, number of doses, time intervals between doses, and precautions and contraindications (CDC, 2013b). They also make recommendations during times of disease outbreaks and vaccine shortages. An example is an outbreak of pertussis (whooping cough) in 2012. More than 14,000 people had

Table 8–3 *Healthy People 2020*

Immunization and Infectious Diseases: Select Objectives

IID-1	Reduce, eliminate, or maintain elimination of cases of vaccine-preventable diseases
IID-5	Reduce outpatient visits for ear infections where antibiotics were prescribed to young children
IID-6	Reduce outpatient visits where antibiotics were prescribed for the sole diagnosis of the common cold.
IID-7	Achieve and maintain effective vaccination coverage levels for universally recommended vaccines among young children
IID-11	Increase routine vaccination coverage levels for adolescents
IID-14	Increase the percentage of adults who are vaccinated against zoster (shingles)
IID-17	Increase the percentage of providers who have had vaccination coverage levels among children in their practice population measured within the past year
IID-18	Increase the percentage of children under age 6 whose immunization records are in fully operational, population-based immunization information systems (IIS)
IID-22	Increase the number of public health laboratories monitoring influenza virus resistance to antiviral agents
IID-24	Reduce chronic hepatitis B virus (HBV) infections in infants and young children (perinatal infections)
IID-27	Increase the percentage of persons aware they have a hepatitis C infection
IID-28	(Developmental) Increase the percentage of persons who have been tested for HBV within minority communities experiencing health disparities

From U.S. Department of Health and Human Services. Office of Disease Prevention and Health Promotion. (2016). *Healthy People 2020 topics & objectives: Immunization and infectious diseases objectives*. Retrieved from http://www.healthypeople.gov/2020/topics-objectives/topic/immunization-and-infectious-diseases/objectives

become infected and 14 babies died of pertussis. Given that young infants cannot receive the first dose of pertussis until they are 2 months old and their immunity would still be developing as they receive subsequent doses, ACIP made recommendations that people who would be near infants get a pertussis immunization so they would be protected and reduce the risk of exposing the infant to the disease until the infant would be old enough to receive the series and develop immunity (CDC, 2013b).

The majority of American society has accepted immunizations as a part of overall health care. However, there are some who challenge the notion of immunizing their children for many reasons. Some oppose government mandates and the sheer number of vaccinations, and others want to veer from the recommended spacing schedule for alternative immunization spacing and will eventually complete the childhood series. Although the ACIP may set the recommendations for immunizations, there are no laws mandating a child be immunized. There are varying laws in each state that may allow for exempting immunizations for various reasons, religion, philosophy, or medical. Not all states accept all of these reasons. The public health nurse should look to their state's immunization agency for the accepted exemption criteria (Immunization Action Coalition, 2013). This subject is further discussed under the section Barriers to Immunization Coverage.

In 1993, the CDC initiated the first National Immunization Survey, and in April of 1994, the first national data set obtained. This data set analyzed the immunization rates of children. Currently, there are data collection surveys for children, adolescents, and adult immunization rates. In 2013, 83% of children represented in the survey who were 19 to 35 months of age had received four doses of DPT, DT, or DTaP vaccine; 93% had received three doses of polio vaccine; 92%

had received one dose of MMR; 82% had received the primary series and a booster of *Haemophilus influenza* type b (HIB); 91% had received three doses of hepatitis B; 91% had received 1 dose of varicella vaccine; and 82% had received four doses of Pneumococcal conjugate vaccine (CDC, 2015k). In the teen population, ages 13 to 17 years, vaccination rates of HPV were low with 60% of the girls and 40% of the boys having been vaccinated (CDC, 2015v). HPV vaccine rates were higher in Hispanic girls than in White girls and higher among girls living in poverty than those living at or above the poverty line. In adults, HPV rates were 63.9% in adult women ages 19 to 26, whereas the HPV vaccination rate in male adults was 5.9% in the male adults in the same age category. Rates of Tdap vaccination in women under the age of 60 years old were 24.2%, and herpes zoster vaccination rates in adults, 60 years or older, were 24.2% (Williams et al., 2015).

Health care providers, public health nurses, and school nurses are in positions to review records, educate families, and provide opportunities for a child to obtain immunizations. Nurses need to realize the effect that negative information available on the Internet and in the media can have on parents' decisions about immunization for their children. In an effort to determine the type of information parents may find on the Internet, one group of researchers conducted Google searches using negative, neutral, and positive search terms related to vaccinations. When negative search terms were used, 37.5% of the recommendations on Web sites retrieved were against vaccination, and 12.5% on those with neutral search terms (Ruiz & Bell, 2014). Researchers noted that if parents are seeking information on the Internet about vaccination risks, they are likely to discover more Web sites perpetuating negative myths and recommending against childhood vaccination. Even though a Cochrane systematic review of a small number of randomized control trials that involved face-to-face education for parents about childhood vaccination had inconclusive results, reviewers noted that talking to parents during health care visits was most likely helpful (Kaufman et al., 2013). It is important for nurses to take the time during their busy workday to talk with parents about their children's immunizations (Donovan & Bedford, 2013; Kestenbaum & Feemster, 2015). Nurses need to listen carefully to the parents' concerns, express empathy, answer their questions, and provide evidence-based information from reputable sources. Parents appreciate nurses who spend time with them and respectfully listen, even if the nurse does not agree with the parents' beliefs.

One common question a parent may have is "Are the vaccines safe?" Nurses can provide information about the safety trials that the vaccines undergo prior to release to the public. They can also advise parents of possible side effects and how to care for the child if side effects do arise. Another concern expressed by the parent is "I'm worried about giving so much at one time; how does that affect my child's immune system?" Nurses can assure parents that the small dose in the vaccine is not nearly as much as children are exposed to in everyday life (Donovan & Bedford, 2013; Dube et al., 2013). Parents may believe that the diseases no longer exist and so vaccination is not needed. Although incidences of diseases have declined, other than polio, they still exist in the natural setting. These diseases can easily resurface and many of them can be life threatening. Parents may also ask why their child should get vaccines at such a young age. Nurses need to explain that to decline giving the immunization at the time they are eligible, the visit becomes a lost opportunity. Their unvaccinated child will not be protected and will be vulnerable until they have completed the series (Donovan & Bedford, 2013). One last question parents commonly ask is if the preservatives or additives will harm their baby. The nurse could explain why the preservative is added to the vaccine. Public health nurses should be aware of any state law prohibiting the administration of a vaccine that contains thimerosal to a newborn. See From the Case Files.

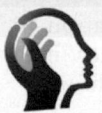 ## From the Case Files

Perspectives, PHN: Personal Belief Exemption and Immunization

A whooping cough (pertussis) outbreak occurred in a small rural community. Whooping cough is a VPD. It is highly contagious and can have devastating outcomes in the very young and very old. In this community, the population is not very ethnically diverse, but it is philosophically diverse. Many community members are against vaccinating their children. The outbreak of pertussis occurred in a small charter school, where the majority of the children were unvaccinated for reasons of parental personal belief objections. Personal belief exemption to vaccination is an option for a family. Unfortunately, with a large unvaccinated population, as in this school, the spark of a contagious, vaccine-preventable infection can spread rapidly. This is what happened in this school, with 22 cases of pertussis among children and family members. The school had to be closed a week early for winter break to help halt continued disease spread. Three waves of illness occurred in this school from November to April.

One might think the entire problem rests with the group of individuals who will not vaccinate their children, but this is not what was discovered upon investigation. The issue of personal belief exemption was discussed among public health nurses and school nurses in this community. The issue was discussed with parents and teachers at the charter school. The two highlights from our discussions were that parents signed the exemption either out of true conviction or out of frustration that the school was hounding them to get their child vaccinated. For whatever reason, some parents just cannot seem to make the time to get the necessary immunizations completed. These parents can be the high-risk families who keep a school nurse busy. It was discovered that in some of the schools with high-risk families, the personal belief exemption was signed in order to keep staff from pestering them.

So, to which group do you extend your efforts as a public health nurse? The answer is both. The parents who will not vaccinate their children will not be convinced otherwise. Parents who chose the easy way out may need more assistance. The county's immunization coordinator, the community's immunization coalition, and the school nurses determined that the school secretaries were the point of entrance to school registration. It was discovered that these individuals needed an in-service on how to properly offer the exemption to a family and what information parents would need to make an informed decision before signing the exemption.

The immunization coordinator developed an education tool that explained to the parents their responsibility to the community at large if their child were to become ill with a vaccine-preventable illness. The document covered points such as the family having a medical plan with their physician, learning how to care for and isolate the child, working with a public health nurse, and so on (see Display 8–5). The school secretaries were asked to give this document to parents who were interested in the exemption, as well as community resource information for families who may not have access to affordable immunizations.

The parents at the charter school were very accepting of the information on what to do for an ill child, and the school secretaries expressed relief regarding dealing with parents who may want to exempt out for convenience rather than conviction.

Karen, PHN

DISPLAY 8–5 WHAT PARENTS SHOULD KNOW WHEN SIGNING A PERSONAL BELIEFS AFFIDAVIT EXEMPTION OF IMMUNIZATION

1. Measles, mumps, rubella, chicken pox, pertussis, diphtheria, polio, *Haemophilus influenza* type b, hepatitis A, and hepatitis B are infectious to others and are avoidable through immunization.

2. Please educate yourself to the symptoms and possible complications that can arise from a vaccine-preventable disease (VPD). Information for parents about these diseases may be found at the National Immunization Program site http://www.cdc.gov/nip/or by calling *Insert Local County Public Health Department Name & Phone Number*.

3. These diseases have many symptoms that require close monitoring and care so that complications are minimized. It is essential to have a plan of care, coordinated with your health care provider, to act upon the mildest to most severe symptoms of the disease.

4. The school or school nurse is responsible for maintaining a list of the school children who have parent-signed exemption to immunization for medical, religious, or personal belief. This list allows the school nurse to quickly identify any child who is at risk of exposure to a VPD.

5. An unimmunized child will be excluded from school by the County Health Officer when a VPD is identified in the school. The ill child will also be excluded from school.

6. When a child is excluded from school, it is the responsibility of the parent or guardian to keep the child isolated* from the public at large to prevent spread of infection to the community.

7. VPDs are considered **reportable communicable diseases** under the Health and Safety Codes of California. If your child contracts one of these diseases, a public health nurse will contact you. Be prepared to provide information about the illness to the investigator. **This information is confidential**.

8. The parent or guardian is also at risk of contracting any of these diseases when exposed to an ill child. If unimmunized, the parent or guardian may also be considered exposed and incubating the disease, because this may continue the cycle of infection to others. This in turn requires that the parent or guardian remain in isolation from the community through the incubation period.

9. The child who is exposed to the disease may be offered preventive medication or immunization to prevent the disease from occurring—either may keep the child from being excluded from school.

_____   _____

Parent signature   Date

*The isolation time frame is determined by the county health officer. Isolation means that the exposed or ill child cannot leave home except for medical care. No social gatherings!

Vaccine-Preventable Diseases

VPDs, such as hepatitis A and B, *H. influenza* type b, measles, polio, diphtheria, pertussis, influenza, and chickenpox, are a few examples of diseases that can be prevented through immunization. Immunization causes the body to become immune to an infectious agent. The immunity allows the body to tolerate the presence of material that is foreign, such as a virus or bacteria. The immune system develops a defense against the invading infectious agent or antigen. Vaccination initiates this process (Hamborsky, Kroger, & Wolfe, 2015). Immunity may be either passive or active. **Passive immunity** is short-term resistance to a specific disease-causing organism; it may be acquired naturally (as with newborns through maternal antibody transfer) or artificially through inoculation with pooled human antibody (e.g., immunoglobulin) that gives temporary protection. **Active immunity** is long-term (sometimes lifelong) resistance to a specific disease-causing organism; it also can be acquired naturally or artificially. Naturally acquired active immunity occurs when a person contracts a disease, whereas artificial immunity occurs when a person receives an inoculation of an antigen through a vaccine. Both prompt an immune response that stimulates the development of long-lasting antibodies that provide immunity against future exposure to that antigen (Hamborsky et al., 2015).

A **vaccine** is a preparation made from either a live organism or an inactivated form of the organism. Live attenuated vaccines are made from weakened wild virus organisms that are able to replicate but generally not make the person ill. It only takes a small amount to initiate an immune response, and the organisms must replicate to be effective. Inactivated vaccines are made from a viral organism that has been inactivated by heat or chemicals. These vaccines cannot replicate in the recipient (Hamborsky et al., 2015). The more similar the vaccine is to the actual agent, the better the immune response to the vaccine. Currently, measles, mumps, rubella, vaccinia, yellow fever, rotavirus, and intranasal influenza are all live attenuated vaccines (Hamborsky et al., 2015).

Because of the success of immunization strategies, few practicing nurses in the United States today have treated clients with tetanus or diphtheria, or even measles, although some may have cared for clients with residual polio disabilities. However, VPDs still exist in force in the developing world, and outbreaks occur in the United States in groups of nonimmunized or susceptible populations. Some people may be medically exempt from immunization, and others may decline immunization for religious or personal reasons. Some states are tightening the use of these exemptions in an effort to prevent disease outbreaks. For instance, California now requires that all children attending school or daycare be fully immunized, unless a physician deems that they are exempt owing to medical reasons. This was spurred by an outbreak of measles at Disneyland, lobbying efforts from professional health care organizations, and concern over the continuing abuse of personal exemptions (Crawford, 2015).

Schedule of Recommended Immunizations

A schedule for the administration of childhood vaccinations, based on recommendations by the ACIP, the American Academy of Pediatrics (AAP), the American Academy of Family Physicians, and the CDC, is published annually (Table 8–4). The CDC also provides "catch-up" schedules for children not receiving their first immunizations at birth, according to the standard schedule. Current recommendations call for a child to receive 10 different vaccines or toxoids (many in combination form and all requiring more than one dose) in six or seven visits to a health care provider between birth and school entry, with boosters in the preteen to early teen years (Hamborsky et al., 2015).

Factors influencing the recommended age at which vaccines are administered include the age-specific risks of the disease, the age-specific risks of complications, the ability of persons of a given age to produce an adequate and lasting immune response, and the potential for interference with the immune response acquired from passively transferred maternal antibodies. In general, vaccines are recommended for the youngest age group at risk whose members are known to develop an acceptable antibody response to vaccination (Hamborsky et al., 2015).

Revisions in recommendations for vaccine administration may be revised in certain circumstances. For example, it is now recommended that infants receive hepatitis B vaccine at birth, whether or not their mothers have a positive or negative response to the hepatitis B surface antigen. This approach will catch any infant born to mothers who lack prenatal testing or who may live in households with individuals with unknown hepatitis B status (Heymann, 2015).

Herd Immunity

Herd immunity, or community immunity, is central to understanding immunization as a means of protecting community health. As described in Chapter 7, *herd immunity* is the immunity level present in a particular group or community of people. If few immune persons exist within a community (i.e., if herd immunity is low), then the spread of disease is more likely (see Fig. 8–10). However, if there

---

Table 8–4 Recommended Immunization Schedules, Ages 0 to 18 (2016)

These recommendations must be read with the footnotes that follow. For those who fall behind or start late, provide catch-up vaccination at the earliest opportunity as indicated by the green bars in Figure 1. To determine minimum intervals between doses, see the catch-up schedule (Figure 2). School entry and adolescent vaccine age groups are shaded.

Vaccine	Birth	1 mo	2 mos	4 mos	6 mos	9 mos	12 mos	15 mos	18 mos	19–23 mos	2-3 yrs	4-6 yrs	7-10 yrs	11-12 yrs	13–15 yrs	16–18 yrs
Hepatitis B[1] (HepB)	1st dose	←— 2nd dose —→			←———————— 3rd dose ————————→											
Rotavirus[2] (RV) RV1 (2-dose series); RV5 (3-dose series)			1st dose	2nd dose	See footnote 2											
Diphtheria, tetanus, & acellular pertussis[3] (DTaP: <7 yrs)			1st dose	2nd dose	3rd dose		←———— 4th dose ————→					5th dose				
Haemophilus influenzae type b[4] (Hib)			1st dose	2nd dose	See footnote 4		3rd or 4th dose, See footnote 4									
Pneumococcal conjugate[5] (PCV13)			1st dose	2nd dose	3rd dose		←———— 4th dose ————→									
Inactivated poliovirus[6] (IPV: <18 yrs)			1st dose	2nd dose	←———————— 3rd dose ————————→							4th dose				
Influenza[7] (IIV; LAIV)					Annual vaccination (IIV only) 1 or 2 doses						Annual vaccination (LAIV or IIV) 1 or 2 doses		Annual vaccination (LAIV or IIV) 1 dose only			
Measles, mumps, rubella[8] (MMR)					See footnote 8		←— 1st dose —→					2nd dose				
Varicella[9] (VAR)							←— 1st dose —→					2nd dose				
Hepatitis A[10] (HepA)							←———— 2-dose series, See footnote 10 ————→									
Meningococcal[11] (Hib-MenCY ≥ 6 weeks; MenACWY-D ≥9 mos; MenACWY-CRM ≥ 2 mos)					See footnote 11									1st dose		Booster
Tetanus, diphtheria, & acellular pertussis[12] (Tdap: ≥7 yrs)														(Tdap)		
Human papillomavirus[13] (2vHPV: females only; 4vHPV, 9vHPV: males and females)														(3-dose series)		
Meningococcal B[11]															See footnote 11	
Pneumococcal polysaccharide[5] (PPSV23)												See footnote 5				

Range of recommended ages for all children | Range of recommended ages for catch-up immunization | Range of recommended ages for certain high-risk groups | Range of recommended ages for non-high-risk groups that may receive vaccine, subject to individual clinical decision making | No recommendation

This schedule includes recommendations in effect as of January 1, 2016. Any dose not administered at the recommended age should be administered at a subsequent visit, when indicated and feasible. The use of a combination vaccine generally is preferred over separate injections of its equivalent component vaccines. Vaccination providers should consult the relevant Advisory Committee on Immunization Practices (ACIP) statement for detailed recommendations, available online at http://www.cdc.gov/vaccines/hcp/acip-recs/index.html. Clinically significant adverse events that follow vaccination should be reported to the Vaccine Adverse Event Reporting System (VAERS) online (http://www.vaers.hhs.gov) or by telephone (800-822-7967). Suspected cases of vaccine-preventable diseases should be reported to the state or local health department. Additional information, including precautions and contraindications for vaccination, is available from CDC online (http://www.cdc.gov/vaccines/recs/vac-admin/contraindications.htm) or by telephone (800-CDC-INFO [800-232-4636]).

This schedule is approved by the Advisory Committee on Immunization Practices (http://www.cdc.gov/vaccines/acip), the American Academy of Pediatrics (http://www.aap.org), the American Academy of Family Physicians (http://www.aafp.org), and the American College of Obstetricians and Gynecologists (http://www.acog.org).

From U.S. Department of Health & Human Services (USDHHS). (2016). *Recommended immunizations schedules for persons aged 0 through 18 years, United States, 2016.* Retrieved from http://www.cdc.gov/vaccines/schedules/downloads/child/0-18yrs-child-combined-schedule.pdf

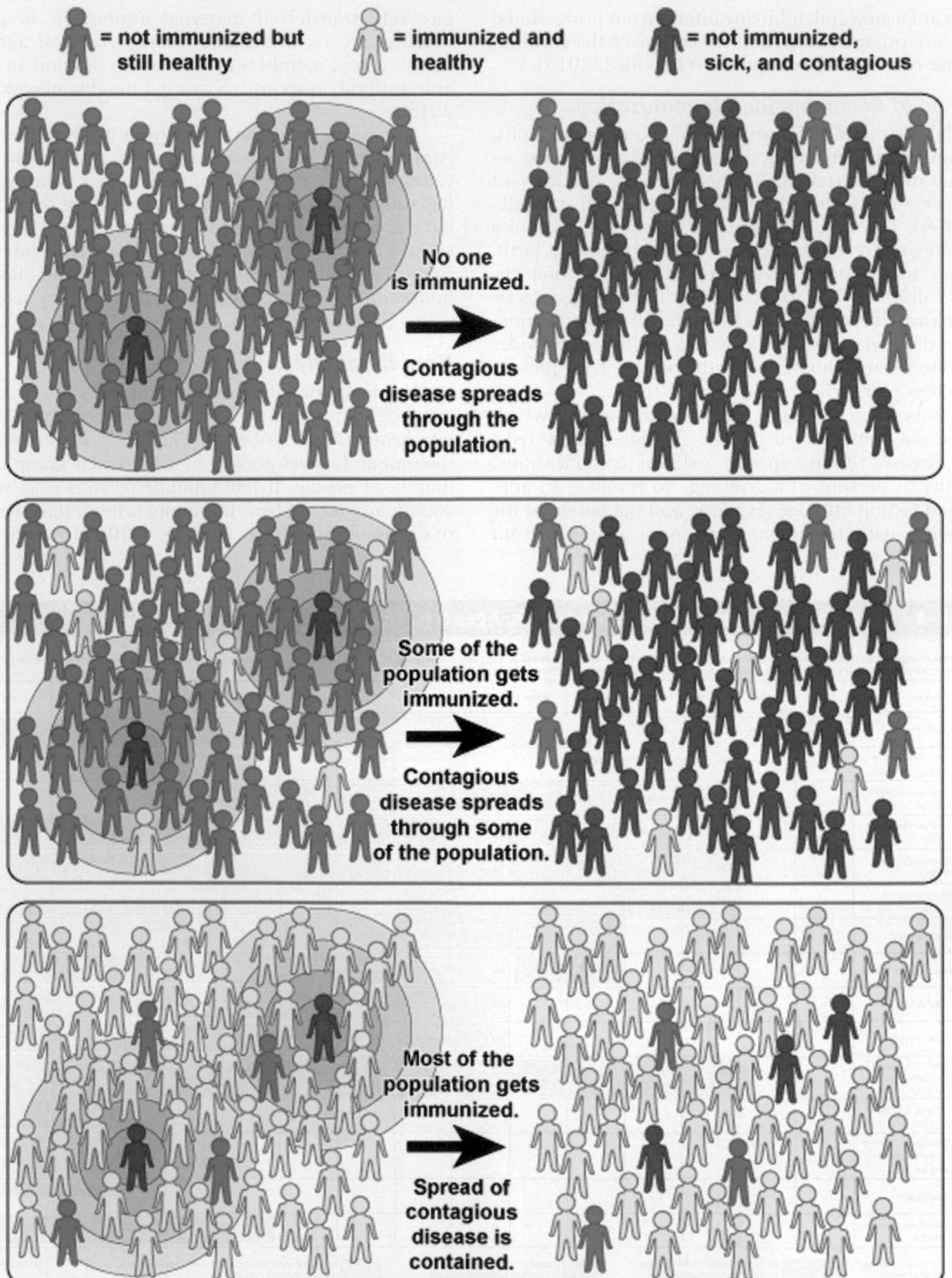

FIGURE 8–10 Community immunity/herd immunity. (From National Institute of Allergies and Infectious Diseases (NIAID). Retrieved from https://www.niaid.nih.gov/topics/pages/communityimmunity.aspx)

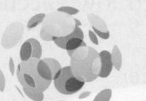

EVIDENCE-BASED PRACTICE

"Cocooning" to Protect Unvaccinated Infants

Over the past years, a practice known as **cocooning** has gained increased attention as a means to prevent communicable diseases, such as influenza and pertussis, in unvaccinated and incompletely vaccinated individuals. It can be thought of as a form of herd immunity within a small group of people such as a family or childcare setting. Infants and children who are at high risk for infection, but not old enough or have other health conditions that prevent them from being immunized, are the target groups for protection. The goal is to immunize (especially for influenza or pertussis) close family and friends or frequent contacts to reduce the risk of exposing the vulnerable person to these diseases (CDC, 2015m).

The PHN has an opportunity to evaluate the emerging research related to the cocoon approach and determine if their community could benefit from this strategy in reducing VPD outbreaks and poor outcomes for the infant at risk. A number of questions must be addressed in considering whether cocooning is a viable option in a community:

Does this approach actually reduce infections in the target population and where is the evidence?
What is the risk to the household members being vaccinated?
What is the cost of this program?
Are there unintended consequences from this approach, such as delayed immunizations in the target population?

Innovations are an important source of improved health-promoting practices and should not be discouraged, but as always, solid research evidence is vital. With limited health care dollars, efforts must target the most cost-effective and proven methods possible. Only time and research will show whether cocooning can be an effective tool in the public health arsenal.

---

are more individuals in the community who are immunized (i.e., if herd immunity is high), this helps minimize the chance that an unvaccinated person will become ill (Heymann, 2015). See Evidence-Based Practice.

Assessing Immunization Status of the Community

Immunization rates still need to be improved. Nurses need to work to ensure that all those who need vaccines are receiving them. Laws have been implemented requiring students to receive vaccines prior to entering school. Community/public health nurses need to assess their community to identify the barriers to receiving the immunizations. These may include transportation issues, financial constraints, or perhaps personal belief barriers such as religion or culture. It may even be that the health care provider is not promoting vaccination according the ACIP schedule. This section will review approaches to address vaccine hesitancy. This hesitancy can lead to reemerging VPDs (Kestenbaum & Feemster, 2015).

It is important to recognize that all clients who refuse vaccination are not all the same. They may have very different concerns. Clients who choose to be unvaccinated or undervaccinated can lead to public health concerns. Antivaccination movement began in the 1950s in response to the smallpox vaccine. There was a belief that the government was impeding on their individual liberties. The subsequent drop in vaccination rates resulted in an increase in smallpox cases in the next two decades. The movement began to emerge again in the early 1990s when the Internet provided a means for disseminating information and groups of concerned parents began pressuring states to expand exception laws; it continues today (Domachowske & Suryadevara, 2013; Ruiz & Bell, 2014).

Although complete refusal to obtain any vaccines is not common, vaccine hesitancy, the intention to delay or avoid vaccines administration as recommended by the ACIP guidelines, is seen quite often. Parents may decide to hesitate or refuse for a variety of reasons. Some parents may be concerned that their child is receiving too many vaccines at one visit, or they may believe that the risk for VPDs is no longer valid, and, in some cases, they may be obtaining their information from noncredible sources. Others may be hesitant for religious reasons. Antivaccinators may feel strongly about vaccination as their personal choice, whereas others may challenge the scientific evidence supporting vaccination (Domachowske & Suryadevara, 2013; Dubé et al., 2013; Kestenbaum & Feemster, 2015).

Nurses and other health care providers should engage families who are hesitant about vaccines in open conversation. This may be a challenging task when a parent is confrontational with the health provider or perhaps even attempting to change the mind of the health care provider. Some who seemed adamant about refusing the vaccine may even decide to accept the vaccine after an honest discussion because they felt that they were heard and their questions were answered.

One approach is called "ASK" (Acknowledging, Steering, and Knowing). The first step is to acknowledge the parents' concerns and then steer the conversation to provide answers and knowing the facts. Another strategy is called "CASE" (Corroborate, About, Science, Explain). Acknowledge the concerns and have a respectful conversation with the parent. Then, be sure the parent is aware of how the health care provider is knowledgeable on the topic (tell them about yourself and your level of expertise). Third is to refer to the scientific evidence, and the final step is to explain and advise, following the

ACIP guidelines (Domachowske & Suryadevara, 2013). These may be time-consuming but the effort may pay off if a parent is able to accept the vaccine for their child.

Offering vaccines at home visiting and WIC offices has also been found to be effective. Another strategy is to work with providers. The AFIX (Assessment, Feedback, Incentives, and Exchange) is designed to help providers recognize the problem. This is accomplished by assessing the current immunization rates within the office to show the provider an accurate picture of their rates. The CDC has computer programming to assist with this process. The next stage is to provide feedback to the provider about their progress in increasing their vaccination rates. This needs to be conveyed in a nonjudgmental way, but it is useful because it helps guide where to go for the next steps. Incentives help to motivate the provider to make the needed changes. The final phase is exchange of information where they can share with other providers about what worked for them (Hamborsky et al., 2015).

Planning and Implementing an Immunization Campaign

Immunization campaigns targeting specific subgroups can be effective if they include the following: (a) community assessment for the target group(s) and (b) assessment of and planning for the needs of the target group(s), such as transportation, need for language interpreters, provision of child care, or dealing with high illiteracy rates. Successful outreach efforts are motivated by the desire to reach the target population, even if specific or unusual accommodations must be made. Clinics can be scheduled and held at times and places specifically intended to make the service more accessible and convenient to the target group. Materials in multilingual form can be obtained through the state's immunization agency or the CDC. The CDC and state immunization agencies have campaigns throughout the year for the public health nurse to participate in and provide to the public. Tool kits with the materials and tips for planning and implementing are available through the state immunization agency (Hamborsky et al., 2015). Display 8–6 outlines an example of the necessary steps and considerations for administering an immunization campaign in a community setting.

Adult Immunization

Many people assume that vaccinations are for children only. Well-advertised influenza vaccination campaigns in recent years have, to some extent, helped to correct this notion.

Adults face risk for becoming infected with a VPD if they are unimmunized or underimmunized. Some of the immunizations that wane, meaning that the protection disappears over time, are tetanus, pertussis, influenza, and pneumococcal. Other vaccines are specific for adults, such as the varicella zoster, otherwise known as the shingles vaccine. The CDC (2016a) provides an adult immunization schedule of recommendations. See Chapter 23 for adult vaccination schedule and adult screenings.

Substantial numbers of VPDs still occur among adults despite the availability of safe and effective vaccines (Appel, 2011). Community health nurses should be aware of factors that may contribute to low vaccination levels among adults:

1. Cost and reimbursement can be a barrier.
2. Insufficient tracking methods for adults as compared to those in place for children.
3. Although statutory requirements exist for vaccination of children, no such requirements exist for all adults.
4. Health care providers may not be current with the adult-recommended immunizations or not consider vaccination at the time of the visit, leading to missed opportunities to vaccinate.
5. Comprehensive vaccination programs have not been established in settings where healthy adults congregate (e.g., the workplace, senior centers).
6. Clients and providers may fear adverse effects after vaccination.

Pertussis is a disease that adults can acquire and pass onto infants, children, and other vulnerable individuals. Because of recent pertussis epidemics, adults are strongly encouraged to receive a dose of Tdap (CDC, 2016b; Domachowske & Suryadevara, 2013).

Shingles is the later version of dormant chickenpox. Shingles appear along the dermatomes, are painful, and can be debilitating (Domachowske & Suryadevara, 2013). The varicella–zoster (shingles) vaccine has been available to adults 60 years or older since 2006 and is protective for shingles. The vaccine is licensed for adults 50 years or older; however, the ACIP recommends not making it available to anyone under 60 owing to limited availability of the vaccine and the low incidence of shingles in that age category (Domachowske & Suryadevara, 2013).

Adults may require immunizations to prevent infection in the event of an occupational exposure to blood, blood products, or other potentially contaminated body fluids. The Occupational Safety and Health Administration (OSHA) has established the requirements for hepatitis B immunization for those whose professions may put them at risk (OSHA, 2011).

All persons should also receive a tetanus vaccine every 10 years unless they experience sharp object injury. If such a wound is sustained, the individual should receive a booster of a tetanus toxoid–containing vaccine on the day of the injury only if more than 5 years has elapsed since the last tetanus toxoid–containing dose (Heymann, 2015).

Other reasons for promoting adult vaccination include pneumococcal vaccine for adults over the age of 65 (or for those who smoke or have a history of high-risk conditions, such as heart disease, diabetes, or chronic respiratory diseases), international travel (possibly requiring vaccines specific to the destination), or suspected failure of earlier vaccines to produce lasting immunity (Domachowske & Suryadevara, 2013).

International Travelers, Immigrants, and Refugees

As Americans interact more and more with their neighbors in other parts of the world, the incidence of Americans with tropical or imported diseases also rises (Fig. 8–11). Within about 36 hours of boarding an airplane, any destination in the world can be reached. An average flight can equal the incubation period of some infectious diseases,

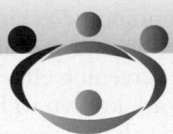

DISPLAY 8-6 ADMINISTRATIVE ASPECTS OF IMMUNIZATION CAMPAIGNS

Study the Target Community
- Assess disease incidence and level of immunization coverage.
- Identify the target group.
- Assess conditions in the community: Is the target group scattered or localized?
- Assess level of community involvement and awareness of the problem.
- Identify means of communicating with target group: through the media or through leaders or other.
- Consider political and social structure of the community. Identify important leaders.
- Identify sites for immunization clinics that are appropriate, accessible, and available.

Plan the Immunization Campaign
- Review budget for immunization services.
- Determine goals for clinic performance or outcome measures.
- Communicate with target group to notify them of need and promote involvement and participation.
- Estimate needs for vaccines and supplies and obtain them. Plan care of vaccines before, during, and after clinic.
- Develop team coordination among staff.
- Plan clinic logistics: Available supply of needed materials, medical waste disposal, anaphylaxis supplies, records and means of clinic registration, staffing, floor plan for traffic control, and efficient management of crowds.
- Prepare staff with information regarding objectives for clinic, criteria for who shall not be immunized,

and mechanisms for referral of clients with other health needs.

Publicity
- Inform target group of date, location, and times of immunization clinic.
- Provide information on reasons for and benefits of (and contraindications to) immunization.
- Encourage parents to bring existing immunization records to clinic.
- Provide contact information for those with questions or inquiries.

Immunization Clinic
- Registration system and records (for parent and clinic) ready.
- Registrar or assistant(s) ready to assist parents not familiar with language of paperwork.
- Parent education: informed consent, reporting of adverse reactions, and date next vaccine due.
- System for call back, follow-up.
- System for dealing with other health issues and/or adverse events.

Evaluation of Campaign
- Assess numbers of immunizations given in relation to goals.
- Assess suitability of approach in identification of target group, selection of sites, means of communication with group, availability of resources, and so forth.
- Invite parental as well as community and staff feedback.
- Evaluate results in relation to expenditures.

---

and before the onset of symptoms are realized, microbial agents could be spread around the globe.

Travelers can take steps to protect themselves prior to embarking on their journey to new and exotic places. Information is available on the CDC Travelers Health

Web site so that potential travelers can stay healthy while on their trip and remain healthy upon their return (CDC, 2016e). Travelers can also make an appointment for a consultation with a tropical medicine or travel clinic to prepare for their international travel. At a minimum, all international travelers should take steps to be adequately immunized as required by international health practices. These steps include being immunized with the recommended vaccines for the particular area of the world, having the necessary chemical prophylaxis on hand (i.e., antimalarial medications as prescribed), and being knowledgeable about food and water hygiene precautions as well as basic first aid for the care of simple injuries (CDC, 2016e). Every year, countless travelers who neglect to take the recommended travel vaccines or medications end up with generally preventable illnesses, which can cost them time, money, and their health (CDC, 2015w).

Refugees and international travelers who arrive in the United States may be unfamiliar with U.S. health systems, health precautions, and practices. Refugees and immigrants must follow prescribed guidelines including extensive health screening mandated by U.S. immigration

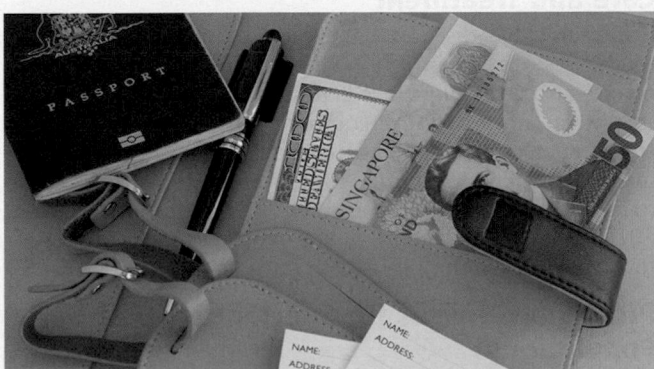

FIGURE 8-11 Careful planning is needed when traveling internationally.

laws, immunizations and treatment, as appropriate (CDC, 2013d). More than ever before, community health nurses have professional contact with these new Americans, whether close to their time of arrival or later, in schools, immunization clinics, or other locations. Visitors from other countries may also require the assistance of other community health professionals. For this reason, public health nurses are encouraged to develop and maintain a global perspective on communicable diseases. See Chapter 16 for more information on global health.

SECONDARY PREVENTION

Two approaches to secondary prevention of communicable disease are possible: (a) screening and (b) disease case and contact investigation and notification (previously discussed).

Screening

The term **screening** is used in community health and disease prevention to describe programs that provide disease-testing opportunities to detect disease in groups of asymptomatic, apparently healthy individuals. Common screening measures can include prenatal hepatitis B, urine *Chlamydia* and GC, and Mantoux TSTs for TB infection. For HIV, several screening tests are available—including oral fluid testing, rapid fingerstick, or the more sensitive screening enzyme immunoassay. The HIV screening tests must be confirmed by a supplemental test such as the Western blot or an immunofluorescence assay when positive results arise (Heymann, 2015). The public health nurse must follow the five C's when conducting HIV/AIDS screening: consent, confidentiality, and counseling, correct results, and connect to care. Screening is a secondary prevention method because asymptomatic cases can be discovered and provided with prompt early treatment. Pregnant women can also be identified and treated to prevent infection to the neonate (Heymann, 2015)

It is important to remember that the screening test itself is not diagnostic but rather a method to identify those persons with positive or suspicious test findings that then require further medical evaluation or treatment. Public health nurse working with clients in a screening setting must be prepared to clearly and correctly explain to individuals that screening tests are not definitive and that positive findings require subsequent investigation before diagnostic conclusions can be drawn.

Criteria for Screening Tests

Some important criteria are used in deciding whether to carry out a screening intervention in a community. They include validity and reliability and predictive value and yield.

Validity and Reliability

The screening test must be valid and reliable. *Validity* refers to the test's ability to accurately identify those with the disease. *Reliability* refers to the test's ability to give consistent results when administered on different occasions by different technicians.

Predictive Value and Yield

The *predictive value* of a screening test is important for determining whether the screening intervention is justified. *Yield* refers to the number of positive results found per number tested. The predictive value and the yield of screening tests become important in planning screening programs for communicable disease detection and prevention because they can help planners locate screening efforts in areas or within population groups that are known to be at high risk for the disease. The predictive value of screening tests increases as the prevalence of the disease increases. For example, a screening test for TB among refugees would have a greater predictive value and yield than would TB screening in the population at large, owing to a higher endemicity of TB in many countries outside of the United States.

Epidemiologic criteria for screening interventions for the detection of health problems include the following:

- Is the disease an important public health problem?
- Is there a valid and reliable test?
- Is there an effective and tolerable treatment that favorably influences the early stages of the disease?
- After a positive screening result, are facilities for diagnosis and treatment available and accessible?
- Is there a recognizable early asymptomatic or latent stage in the disease?
- Do clear guidelines for referral and treatment exist?
- Is the total cost of the screening justifiable compared with the costs of treating the disease if left undiscovered?
- Is the screening test itself acceptable?
- Will screening be ongoing?

The ethics or values represented by these statements include a clear and unwavering respect for the dignity and worth of individuals across racial, gender, religious, sexual, tribal, ethnic, and geographic lines. They include a commitment to ensuring that resources are allocated to areas where they will have the most benefit in preventing disease and premature death. Socioeconomically disadvantaged persons are often at greatest risk for disease, yet they are the least likely to receive screening services because of financial barriers, including lack of health insurance coverage for preventive care (CDC, 2011d, 2012c). See Chapter 7 for more on epidemiology.

TERTIARY PREVENTION

The approaches to tertiary prevention of communicable disease include care and treatment of the infected person, isolation and quarantine of the infected person, and safe handling and control of infectious wastes.

Care and Treatment

Communicable diseases have care and treatment specific to the disease. As mentioned previously, with respect to investigation, the nurse needs to understand the disease, the treatment and follow-up requirements, and the educational component to discuss with the infected person. There are many information resources for the community health nurse to utilize, such as the CDC and state agency resources (CDC, 2012a). The public health agency may have policies and protocols for the community health nurse to utilize as well.

Providing Services for Special High-Risk Populations

The Lesbian, Gay, Bisexual, and Transgender (LGBT) community bears a disproportionate burden of sexually transmitted diseases, particularly among men. Sixty-three percent of the new HIV infections in 2010 were among men who have sex with men. In addition, gay and bisexual men represent 75% of the cases of primary and secondary syphilis. Whereas men are generally at a lower risk for cancer due to HPV, men who have anal sex are 17 times more at risk for anal cancer (CDC, 2014h). Primary prevention measures can include vaccination and use of condoms. Secondary prevention includes screening for HIV and other STDs. Tertiary care involves treating the infection. Fear of bias in provider offices presents a barrier to accessing screening and treatment services. Public health nurses can educate providers about the need to be culturally sensitive to members of the LGBT community and to incorporate LGBT-friendly practices such as nongender questions on patient history forms and nongender bathrooms (CDC, 2014h). This is an example of how nurses can collaborate with health care team members to provide patient-centered care resulting in improved outcomes and reduced harm among a vulnerable population (Case Western Reserve University, 2014).

Isolation and Quarantine

Communicable disease control includes two methods for keeping infected persons and noninfected persons apart to prevent the spread of a disease (Fig. 8–12). **Isolation** refers to separation of the infected persons (or animals) from others for the period of communicability to limit the transmission of the infectious agent to susceptible persons. **Quarantine** refers to restrictions placed on healthy contacts of an infectious case for the duration of the incubation period to prevent disease transmission if infection should develop (Heymann, 2015).

Safe Handling and Control of Infectious Wastes

The control of infection in community health also relies upon the proper disposal of contaminated wastes. The CDC and the OSHA support and encourage *universal precautions* that stress that health care workers think of all blood and body fluids and materials that they may come in contact with as potentially infectious (OSHA, 2011). Although universal precaution observance is primarily considered while the nurse is giving hands-on treatment or care to a patient, keeping these principles in mind while making community health visits in the primary and secondary setting is paramount to the safety of both the client and the nurse (Heymann, 2015).

Universal precautions include the following:

- Hand washing after contact with the client or with potentially contaminated articles and before care of other clients
- Bagging and discarding articles contaminated with infectious material into an appropriate labeled container before it is sent for decontamination
- Use of proper personal protective equipment while dealing with an individual in isolation. This isolation is based on the mode of transmission of the specific disease, which may include strict isolation, contact isolation, respiratory isolation, TB isolation (AFB isolation), enteric precautions, or drainage/secretion precautions.

Infectious waste is waste capable of producing an infectious disease. The agency notes that for waste to be infectious, it must contain pathogens with sufficient virulence and quantity so that exposure to the waste by a susceptible host could result in an infectious disease. Requirements for medical waste disposal are for waste to be segregated into categories of:

- Used and unused sharps
- Cultures and stocks of infectious agents
- Human blood and blood products
- Human pathologic, isolation, and animal waste

Although incineration has long been recognized as an efficient method for disposing safely of sharps and other contaminated medical waste, fewer incinerators are available now because of increasing regulation of emissions and particularly those regulations related to burning chemical wastes (Heymann, 2015; OSHA, 2011).

Four key elements of an infectious waste management program are applicable to community practice:

1. Health professionals must be able to correctly distinguish waste that poses a significant infection hazard from other biomedical waste that poses no greater risk than general municipal waste, and such infectious waste must be clearly defined.
2. The waste management program must have administrative support and authority to institute practice guidelines and provide the containers and other resources needed for safe disposal of infectious wastes.
3. Handling of the infectious wastes must be minimized. Containers should be rigid, leak resistant, and impervious to moisture; they should have sufficient strength to prevent rupture or tearing under normal conditions; and they should be sealed to prevent leakage. Containers for sharps must also be puncture resistant.
4. An enforcement or evaluation mechanism must be in place to ensure that the goal of reducing the potential for exposure to infectious waste in the community is met.

USING THE NURSING PROCESS FOR COMMUNICABLE DISEASE CONTROL

As mentioned in Chapters 4 and 7, the nursing process has steps similar to the research process and the epidemiologic process when approaching any health problem or condition. Therefore, using the nursing process to achieve

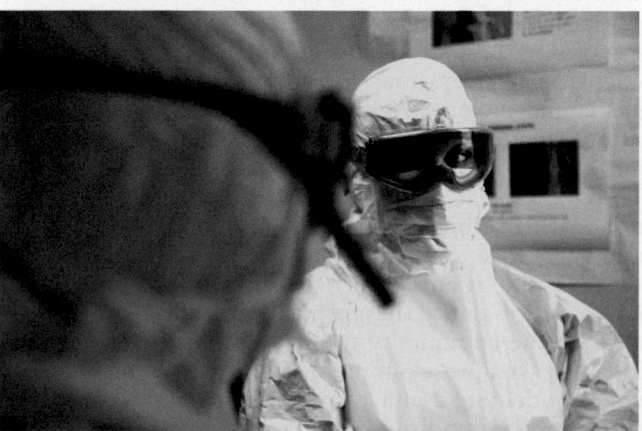

FIGURE 8–12   Personal protective equipment (PPE) used in a mock Ebola treatment unit. Exposed skin is to be avoided, as it presents an opportunity for possible infection.

communicable disease control should be an important and natural process for community health nurses.

Assessment

The first step of the nursing process—assessment—aligns itself with case identification and case finding in communicable disease control. The community health nurse must use all assessment skills and tools available during contact with clients, so as not to overlook the possibility of a communicable disease. Assessment must be comprehensive, producing physical, social, and environmental data. There is no place for assumption. At times, a nurse can become lulled into the usual patterns of inquiry, and this oversight may prove fatal to the client. An example follows:

"Baby Josephine is irritable," says the mother. "Well, babies sometimes are," says the nurse. "How are you feeding her? Show me how you hold her. Does she sleep well? Try rocking her in the rocking chair before bedtime. And burp her more frequently. I'll check back with you in 2 weeks." Did the nurse record the baby's temperature, look at her for a rash, compare present weight with last weight, ask about bowel habits or vomiting, inquire about illnesses in the family, check on breast-feeding technique or watch while the mother demonstrated formula preparation, inspect the family's water source, ask about other foods the baby is eating, and so forth?

Broader inquiry into such a simple statement from the mother in this example may lead to the discovery of a life-threatening, undiagnosed communicable disease.

Assessment in the broader sense with respect to communicable disease control relates to the surveillance for disease. As mentioned previously, communicable diseases are reportable and the public health nurse may be the first to notice a trend in a rise in a particular disease rate.

Diagnosis

This may include identification of the problems associated with the specific communicable disease for the individual (e.g., pain, need for isolation, risk for further infection), the family (e.g., family support systems/stressors, strains of caregiving, preventing spread of infection to others), and the community (e.g., prevention of spread of infection in schools, workplaces, other social settings). Diagnosis of a specific communicable disease may be made through laboratory confirmation, but nursing diagnosis will extend beyond that and include physical, emotional, social, and care needs of the individual, family, and community.

Planning

The planning step in the nursing process involves different activities, depending on whether the intervention is for an individual, family, group, or entire community. At the individual level, the nurse may assist a client or family to obtain an immunization or definitive treatment. Or the nurse may assist the client through education about self-care related to disease symptoms that provide relief and in reducing the chance of transmitting the disease to others in the family or community. With groups and communities, planning interventions include the collaboration with community members and/or organizations. Whether a teen immunization campaign is proposed or a flu shot day is planned for senior citizens, there are location, staff, and supplies to prepare, which may include

writing grants, establishing contracts, and training and orienting staff, before implementation can begin.

Implementation

During the implementation step, the nurse actually takes the action that was identified as necessary during assessment and planning. In the implementation step, the nurse may actually deliver the service or may supervise other staff or volunteers, as with a large immunization event. Implementing plans with small groups or families may involve arranging for transportation, so that several people can get to the immunization site or can be seen by a primary care provider. It may include gathering clinical specimens for laboratory analysis from a family recovering from a *Salmonella* infection. Education on primary prevention to prevent future infections is an essential part of the implementation phase. Agency record keeping, state-required contact investigation, and reports to the next level of government oversight of a communicable disease are essential in this phase.

Evaluation

Evaluation is an essential step in the nursing process with all services community health nurses provide. When dealing with communicable diseases, it is most important to determine whether actions have achieved the established goals. Have the outcomes been accomplished? Are all family members immunized? Are all family members free of the disease? Do families know how to prevent the diseases recurring? What needs to be done now to keep the community safe from communicable diseases? Are there funding issues, programs nearing completion that need support, or growth of services needed that can be addressed before a critical need occurs? These are examples of questions that need answers during evaluation. The community health nurse who is concerned with the health and safety of the community applies the steps of the nursing process to reach healthy community goals.

LEGAL AND ETHICAL ISSUES IN COMMUNICABLE DISEASE CONTROL

The threats presented by communicable diseases can bring public safety and ethical considerations to a crossroad. Public health interventions to protect the public often overlap individual rights (Phua, 2013). The communitarianism concept of what is good for the whole is good for the parts might be applied to public health practice. Considerations for ethical public health practice should include overall benefit to society, collective action, communitarianism, fairness in distribution of burden, harm principle, and paternalism, liberty-limiting continua, social justice/fairness, and global justice. In addition, ethical issues of autonomy, beneficence, nonmaleficence, and justice also need to be taken into consideration (Phua, 2013). Community/public health nurses must balance these ethical principles while working with the community to control the spread of infectious diseases. An example of this conflict might occur while conducting contact investigation for an STD. The nurse must be mindful to conduct the investigation while maintaining confidentiality of the index case. Another example is mandating immunizations resulting in exclusion of unvaccinated children from a school setting

(Phua, 2013). Public health practitioners walk a fine line to protect the rights of the individual while also protecting the health and safety of the community.

Enforced Compliance

Legally, the responsibilities of public health officials in communicable disease control include the police power to enforce compliance with treatment or restrict the activity of infectious people to protect the welfare of others (CDPH, 2013). Regulations that enforce compliance with disease prevention strategies are a justifiable restriction if the measures proposed are demonstrably effective and grounded in ethical principles (CDPH, 2013). Due process protects individuals from government intrusion, particularly ensuring that fundamental fairness has been implemented in situations requiring imprisonment (CDPH, 2013).

Confidentiality, Privacy, and Discrimination

The health officer has the duty to provide communicable disease control, examine the patient, and take steps to prevent the spread of the disease to others (CDPH, 2013).

To carry out communicable disease interventions, client needs for confidentiality and privacy must be ensured. The Health Insurance Portability and Accountability Act (HIPAA) Privacy Rules, last revised in 2003, note that reports must be made to public health in order to protect the public's health. These rules allow for disclosure of only that information needed to protect the public. Information may also be disclosed to a person at risk of contracting an illness, without disclosing identifying information about the source. Only the minimum amount of information to allow the person to obtain the necessary care can be disclosed (USDHHS, n.d.).

Human society has a long-standing aversion to infectious diseases. Ostracism, which in the past included people with leprosy and other contagious conditions, has shifted to discrimination against people with TB or AIDS, for example. People are protected from discrimination under the Americans with Disability Act but not with respect to posing a public health treat, such as with the contagious state of TB (U.S. Equal Employment Opportunity Commission, 2011).

SUMMARY

Communicable diseases pose a major threat to the public's health and have done so since the beginning of humankind. In today's world, such diseases are transmitted globally as the result of mobile populations, increased urbanization, and international travel. Communicable diseases can be transmitted through direct contact from one person to another or indirectly through contaminated objects (air, water, food) or a vector (animal or insect). Communicable diseases affect all types of people and have worldwide significance.

Ideally, prevention of communicable diseases is accomplished through primary prevention methods such as utilizing mass media education campaigns, one-on-one education, and immunization. Knowledge of VPDs, the schedule of vaccinations, a community's immunization status, herd immunity, barriers to immunization coverage, planning and implementing immunization campaigns, adult immunizations, and the immunization needs of international travelers, immigrants, and refugees has been discussed. Health care workers need to practice universal precaution and the safe handling of infectious wastes to maintain worksite safety.

Secondary prevention activities of screening and disease investigation are steps taken when primary prevention activities have failed. Tertiary prevention is needed to ensure additional people are not infected and those who are ill receive care and treatment. Ongoing disease transmission can be interrupted through treatment, isolation, or quarantine.

Becoming familiar with the major communicable diseases affecting our nation is essential baseline information for community health nurses. TB, resurging since the 1980s, may be one of the biggest public health problems in the new millennium. Nurses must be aware of the populations at risk, how the disease is prevented, and the use of appropriate interventions during diagnosis and treatment. Issues compounding the control of TB are twofold: increasing infections with MDR strains, and the increasing number of people with TB and HIV/AIDS, making diagnosis and treatment more complicated.

A second major disease, HIV/AIDS, was first identified in the 1980s. With the success of antiviral drugs, HIV/AIDS is becoming a chronic disease for clients in industrialized nations, with an average life expectancy of 10 to 15 years after diagnosis. Africa is deeply affected by the massive numbers of women and children who are HIV positive, without access to the life-prolonging drugs available to people in developed nations.

STDs threaten the health and lives of millions of citizens. At greater risk are the sexually active, non-monogamous. Control of STDs can be accomplished through effective screening, treatment, contact investigation, and aggressive public education. Several common STDs were discussed, including GC, syphilis, *Chlamydia*, genital herpes, and viral warts.

Hepatitis is more common than HIV and can lead to life-threatening events, such as cirrhosis and liver cancer. Yet, these diseases do not garner the attention they need. Most of the public is unaware of the types of hepatitis, prevention, transmission, and treatment. Vaccines for two of the forms (hepatitis A and hepatitis B) are available.

Influenza and pneumonia are "old" diseases that cause increased morbidity. These diseases cause the most morbidity and mortality in the frailest citizens—the immune compromised, very young, and the very old—although vaccines are available to prevent them.

Smallpox (an eradicated disease) and anthrax have been identified as potential bioterrorism weapons. The community/public health nurse has several areas of responsibility in regard to bioterrorism. First, the nurse must know the signs and symptoms of potential infectious diseases used as weapons. Also, the nurse has a responsibility to the community to allay fears about bioterrorism and to provide information about prevention.

Community/public health nurses use the nursing process in their important role with regard to all populations at risk for communicable diseases. Nurses concerned with communicable disease control must recognize who is at risk, where the potential reservoirs and sources of infectious disease agents are located, what environmental factors promote their spread, and what are the characteristics and vulnerability of community members and groups. Community health nurses must work collaboratively with other public health professionals to establish immunization and education campaigns, work to improve community communicable disease control policies, and develop a broad range of services for at-risk community members.

Ethical issues in communicable disease control include enforced compliance, the justifiability of screening, preservation of confidentiality and privacy, and the avoidance of discrimination against infected people.

ACTIVITIES TO PROMOTE **CRITICAL THINKING**

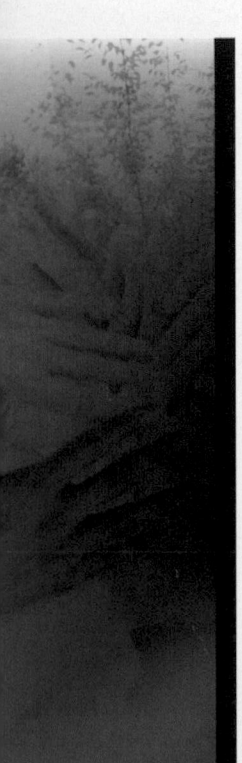

1. Interview a professional in your local or state health department who works in communicable disease control. Determine (a) how he conducts communicable disease surveillance, (b) what diseases must be reported in your state, and (c) which communicable diseases are posing the greatest threat to the health of your state's citizens. Compare this information to national statistics.

2. Compare a recent issue of *Mortality and Morbidity Weekly Report* with the same issue published 5 years earlier, in terms of cases of specific notifiable diseases in the United States. Which diseases appear to be increasing? Decreasing? Select one disease and read at least one recent publication on this subject to determine the reasons for its rise or decline.

3. Through your local health department or county office of education, determine the percentage of preschool children that are immunized in your city or county. Is this a safe level of herd immunity? Propose some recommendations for preserving or raising this level.

4. Select one high-risk population discussed in this chapter, and list the factors that make this group vulnerable to communicable disease. Use at least one other published source to enhance your understanding. Propose one nursing intervention (such as a specific screening or educational program) and outline how it might be best accomplished.

5. Interview a professional who works in STD services or with the HIV-infected population. Determine what methods he or she uses for contact investigation. How does this health care worker preserve privacy and confidentiality? What measures have proved most effective in reaching contacts? How do they evaluate the success of their program?

6. Access the CDC Web site (http://www.cdc.gov) and browse the site to learn about its various services. Are there special travelers' warnings in certain countries at this time? What are some of the CDC's current concerns regarding communicable diseases? Select a communicable disease and identify the number of cases presently reported. Return to the same Web site 1 month later. Has the incidence of the disease increased or decreased?

REFERENCES

Appel, A. (2011). Improving adult immunization rates: Overcoming barriers. *American Family Physician, 8*(9), 977–978. Retrieved from http://www.aafp.org/afp/2011/1101/p977.pdf

California Department of Public Health (CDPH). (2013). *Health officer practice guide for communicable disease control in California.* Retrieved from https://www.cdph.ca.gov/programs/dcdc/Documents/Health-Officer-Practice-Guide-DCDC.pdf

California Department of Public Health (CDPH). (2014). *Information for physicians regarding directly observed therapy (DO) for active tuberculosis (TB).* Retrieved from https://www.cdph.ca.gov/programs/tb/Documents/TBCB-PMD-DOT.pdf

Carter Center. (2016). *International task force for disease eradication: Terms defined.* Retrieved from http://www.cartercenter.org/health/itfde/program_definition.html

Case Western Reserve University. (2014). *QSEN.* Retrieved from http://qsen.org/about-qsen/

CDC. (2011). *Detecting a possible outbreak.* Retrieved from http://www.cdc.gov/outbreaknet/investigations/detection.html

Centers for Disease Control and Prevention. (n.d.). *Smallpox vaccination and adverse events training module.* Retrieved from http://www.bt.cdc.gov/training/smallpoxvaccine/reactions/adverse.html

Centers for Disease Control and Prevention (CDC). (2011a). *Advisory Committee on Immunization Practices (ACIP). General recommendations on immunization.* Retrieved from http://www.cdc.gov/vaccines/pubs/ACIP-list.htm

Centers for Disease Control and Prevention (CDC). (2011b). *Gateway to health communication and social marketing practice: Health marketing basics.* Retrieved from http://www.cdc.gov/healthcommunication/toolstemplates/basics.html

Centers for Disease Control and Prevention (CDC). (2011c). *Menu of suggested provisions for state tuberculosis prevention and control laws/C. treatment/1. Case management, treatment guidelines, and required treatment.* Retrieved from http://www.cdc.gov/tb/programs/laws/menu/treatment.htm

Centers for Disease Control and Prevention (CDC). (2011d). *Sexually transmitted diseases (STDs): 2010 STD treatment guidelines.* Retrieved from http://www.cdc.gov/std/treatment/2010/default.htm

Centers for Disease Control and Prevention (CDC). (2011e). *TB guidelines: Tuberculosis infection control and prevention.* Retrieved from http:www.cdc/gov/tb/topic/infectioncontrol/default.htm

Centers for Disease Control and Prevention (CDC). (2012a). *CDC organization.* Retrieved from http://www.cdc.gov/about/organization/cio.htm

Centers for Disease Control and Prevention (CDC). (2012b). *Epidemiology and prevention of vaccine preventable diseases: The Pink Book* (12th ed.). Washington, DC: Public Health Foundation.

Centers for Disease Control and Prevention (CDC). (2012c). *TB and HIV co-infection.* Retrieved from http://www.cdc.gov/tb/topic/TBHIVcoinfection/default.htm

Centers for Disease Control and Prevention (CDC). (2013a). *About PulseNet.* Retrieved from http://www.cdc.gov/pulsenet/about/faq.html

Centers for Disease Control and Prevention (CDC). (2013b). *The advisory committee on immunization practices (ACIP).* Retrieved from http://www.cdc.gov/vaccines/hcp/conversations/downloads/vacsafe-acip-color-office.pdf

Centers for Disease Control and Prevention (CDC). (2013c). *Ten great public health achievements in the 20th century.* Retrieved from http://www.cdc.gov/about/history/tengpha.htm

Centers for Disease Control and Prevention (CDC). (2013d). *Immigrant and refugee health.* Retrieved from http://www.cdc.gov/immigrantrefugeehealth/

Centers for Disease Control and Prevention (CDC). (2013e). Ten great public health achievements, 1990–1999: Control of infectious diseases. *Morbidity and Mortality Weekly Report, 48*(29), 621–629.

Centers for Disease Control and Prevention (CDC). (2014a). *About the division of vector-borne diseases.* Retrieved from http://www.cdc.gov/ncezid/dvbd/about.html

Centers for Disease Control and Prevention (CDC). (2014b). *Asking the right questions quickly from the beginning.* Retrieved from http://www.cdc.gov/foodcore/successes/questions-from-beginning.html

Centers for Disease Control and Prevention (CDC). (2014c). *CDC estimates of 2009 H1N1 influenza cases, hospitalizations and deaths in the United States.* Retrieved from http://www.cdc.gov/h1n1flu/estimates_2009_h1n1.htm

Centers for Disease Control and Prevention (CDC). (2014d). *Climate and health: Diseases carried by vectors.* Retrieved from http://www.cdc.gov/climateandhealth/effects/vectors.htm

Centers for Disease Control and Prevention (CDC). (2014e). *Emergency preparedness and response.* Retrieved from http://emergency.cdc.gov/preparedness/quarantine/

Centers for Disease Control and Prevention (CDC). (2014f). *Global health security agenda: GHSA national laboratory system action package (GHSA action package detect 1).* Retrieved from http://www.cdc.gov/globalhealth/security/actionpackages/national_laboratory.htm

Centers for Disease Control and Prevention (CDC). (2014g). *Latent tuberculosis infection: A guide for primary health care providers.* Retrieved from www.cdc.gov/tb/publications/ltbi/default.htm

Centers for Disease Control and Prevention (CDC). (2014h). *Lesbian, gay, bi-sexual and transgender health.* Retrieved from http://www.cdc.gov/lgbthealth/

Centers for Disease Control and Prevention (CDC). (2014i). *State, tribal, local, and territorial support.* Retrieved from http://m.cdc.gov/about/report/2014/docs/state-tribal-local-territorial-support.pdf

Centers for Disease Control and Prevention (CDC). (2014j). *STD health equity.* Retrieved from http://www.cdc.gov/std/health-disparities/

Centers for Disease Control and Prevention (CDC). (2014k). *Vision, mission, core values, and pledge.* Retrieved from http://www.cdc.gov/about/organization/mission.htm

Centers for Disease Control and Prevention (CDC). (2015a). *2014 sexually transmitted disease surveillance: Gonorrhea.* Retrieved from http://www.cdc.gov/std/stats14/gonorrhea.htm

Centers for Disease Control and Prevention (CDC). (2015b). *2014 sexually transmitted disease surveillance: Other sexually transmitted diseases.* Retrieved from http://www.cdc.gov/std/stats14/other.htm#herpes

Centers for Disease Control and Prevention (CDC). (2015c). *2014 sexually transmitted diseases guidelines: Syphilis.* Retrieved from http://www.cdc.gov/std/stats14/syphilis.htm

Centers for Disease Control and Prevention (CDC). (2015d). *2015 Sexually transmitted diseases treatment Guidelines: Chlamydial infections.* Retrieved from http://www.cdc.gov/std/tg2015/chlamydia.htm

Centers for Disease Control and Prevention (CDC). (2015e). *2015 Sexually transmitted diseases treatment guidelines: Clinical treatment guidance.* Retrieved from http://www.cdc.gov/std/tg2015/clinical.htm#partner

Centers for Disease Control and Prevention (CDC). (2015f). *2015 sexually transmitted diseases treatment guidelines: Gonococcal infections.* Retrieved from http://www.cdc.gov/std/tg2015/gonorrhea.htm

Centers for Disease Control and Prevention (CDC). (2015g). *2015 sexually transmitted diseases guidelines: Human papillomavirus (HPV) infection.* Retrieved from http://www.cdc.gov/std/tg2015/hpv.htm

Centers for Disease Control and Prevention (CDC). (2015h). *CDC resources for pandemic flu.* Retrieved from http://www.cdc.gov/flu/pandemic-resources/

Centers for Disease Control and Prevention (CDC). (2015i). *Chlamydia: CDC fact sheet (detailed).* Retrieved from www.cdc.gov/std/chlamydia/stdfact-chlamydia-detailed.htm

Centers for Disease Control and Prevention (CDC). (2015j). *Data collection and reporting.* Retrieved from http://wwwn.cdc.gov/nndss/data-collection.html

Centers for Disease Control and Prevention (CDC). (2015k). *FastStats: Immunization.* Retrieved from http://www.cdc.gov/nchs/fastats/immunize.htm

Centers for Disease Control and Prevention (CDC). (2015l). *Genital herpes: Genital herpes treatment and care.* Retrieved from http://www.cdc.gov/std/Herpes/treatment.htm

Centers for Disease Control and Prevention (CDC). (2015m). *Get the whooping cough vaccine while you are pregnant.* Retrieved from http://www.cdc.gov/pertussis/pregnant/mom/get-vaccinated.html

Centers for Disease Control and Prevention (CDC). (2015n). *Hepatitis C FAQ for health professionals.* Retrieved from www.cdc.gov/hepatitis/hcv/hcvfaq.html#section1

Centers for Disease Control and Prevention (CDC). (2015o). *HIV basics.* Retrieved from www.cdc.gov/hiv/basics/index.hml

Centers for Disease Control and Prevention (CDC). (2015p). *HPV vaccine information for clinicians.* Retrieved from http://www.cdc.gov/hpv/hcp/need-to-know.pdf

Centers for Disease Control and Prevention (CDC). (2015q). *National notifiable diseases surveillance system.* Retrieved from http://wwwn.cdc.gov/nndss/

Centers for Disease Control and Prevention (CDC). (2015r). *National notifiable disease surveillance system: NEDSS/NBS.* Retrieved from http://wwwn.cdc.gov/nndss/nedss.html

Centers for Disease Control and Prevention (CDC). (2015s). *The pink book.* Retrieved from www.cdc.gov/vaccines/pbs/pinkbook/index.html

Centers for Disease Control and Prevention (CDC). (2015t). *Plague: History.* Retrieved from http://www.cdc.gov/plague/history/

Centers for Disease Control and Prevention (CDC). (2015u). *TB data and statistics.* Retrieved from www.cdc.gov/tb/statistics/

Centers for Disease Control and Prevention (CDC). (2015v). *Teen vaccination coverage: 2014 national immunization survey-teen (NIS-Teen).* Retrieved from http://www.cdc.gov/vaccines/who/teens/vaccination-coverage.html

Centers for Disease Control and Prevention (CDC). (2015w). *Traveler's health: Yellow book homepage.* Retrieved from http://wwwnc.cdc.gov/travel/page/yellowbook-home-2014

Centers for Disease Control and Prevention (CDC). (2016a). *Adult immunization schedule.* Retrieved from http://www.cdc.gov/vaccines/schedules/hcp/adult.html

Centers for Disease Control and Prevention (CDC). (2016b). *Help protect babies from whooping cough.* Retrieved from http://www.cdc.gov/features/pertussis/

Centers for Disease Control and Prevention (CDC). (2016c). *Nationally notifiable infectious conditions, United States 2016.* Retrieved from http://wwwn.cdc.gov/nndss/conditions/notifiable/2016/

Centers for Disease Control and Prevention (CDC). (2016d). *Tuberculosis (TB).* Retrieved from http://www.cdc.gov/tb/

Centers for Disease Control and Prevention (CDC). (2016e). *Vaccines. Medicines. Advice.* Retrieved from http://wwwnc.cdc.gov/travel

Centers for Disease Control and Prevention (CDC). (2016f). *Zika virus.* Retrieved from http://www.cdc.gov/zika/

Crawford, C. (2015, July 6). *California mandates vaccines for children in school, daycare.* Retrieved from http://www.aafp.org/news/health-of-the-public/20150706califvaccines.html

Domachowske, J. B., & Suryadevara, M. (2013). Practical approaches to vaccine hesitancy issues in the United States: 2013. *Human Vaccines & Immunotherapeutics, 9*(12), 2654–2657.

Donovan, H., & Bedford, H. (2013). Talking with parents about immunization. *Primary Health Care, 23*(4), 16–20.

Dubé, E., Laberge, C., Guay, M., Bramadat, P., Roy, R., & Bettinger, J. (2013). Vaccine hesitancy: An overview. *Human Vaccines & Immunotherapeutics, 9*(8), 1763–1773.

Flu.gov. (n.d.). *Pandemic flu history.* Retrieved from www.flu.gov/pandemic/history

Global Health Security Agenda. (2015). *About.* Retrieved from https://ghsagenda.org/about.html

Globalhealth.gov. (n.d.). *U.S. commitment to the Global Health Security Agenda: Toward a world safe and secure from infectious disease threats.* Retrieved from http://www.globalhealth.gov/global-health-topics/global-health-security/GHS%20US%20Commitments%20Factsheet_a.pdf

Hamborsky, J., Kroger, A., & Wolfe, C. (Eds.). (2015). *Epidemiology and prevention of vaccine-preventable diseases* (13th ed.). Retrieved from http://www.cdc.gov/vaccines/pubs/pinkbook/index.html

Heldman, A. B., Schindelar, J., & Weaver, J. B. (2013). Social media engagement and public health communications: Implications for public health organizations being truly "social." *Public Health Reviews, 35*(1). Retrieved from http://www.publichealthreviews.eu/upload/pdf_files/13/00_Heldman.pdf

Heymann, D. L. (Ed.). (2015). *Control of communicable diseases manual* (20th ed.). Washington, DC: American Public Health Association.

Hinman, A. R., Orenstein, W. A., & Schuchat, A. (2011). *Vaccine-preventable diseases, immunizations, and* MMWR—1961–2011. *Morbidity and Mortality Weekly Report, 60*(4), 49–57.

Immunization Action Coalition. (2013). *State information.* Retrieved from http://www.immunize.org/laws/

Kaufman, J., Synnot, A., Ryan, R., Hill, S., Horey, D., Willis, N., ... Robinson, P. (2013). Face to face interventions for informing or educating parents about early childhood vaccines. *Cochrane Database of Systematic Reviews, 5,* CD010038. doi: 10.1002/14651858.CD010038.pub2.

Kestenbaum, L. A., & Feemster, K. A. (2015). Identifying and addressing vaccine hesitancy. *Pediatric Annals, 44*(4), e71–e75.

Moonan, P. K., Quitugua, T. N., Pogoda, J. M., Woo, G., Drewyer, G., Sahbazian, B., ... Weis, S. W. (2011). Does directly observed therapy (DOT) reduce drug resistant tuberculosis? *BioMed Central, 11,* 19. Retrieved from http://www.ncbi.nlm.nih.gov/pmc/articles/PMC3032680/?tool=pubmed

National Institute on Aging. (2015). *Living longer.* Retrieved from https://www.nia.nih.gov/research/publication/global-health-and-aging/living-longer

Neiderud, C. (2015). How urbanization affects the epidemiology of emerging infectious diseases. *Infection Ecology & Epidemiology, 5,* 27060. doi: 10.3402/lee.v5.27060.

Occupational Safety and Health Administration (OSHA). (2011). *OSHA fact sheet: Bloodborne pathogens standard.* Retrieved from https://www.osha.gov/OshDoc/data_BloodborneFacts/bbfact01.pdf

Penman-Aguilar, A., Harrison, K. M., & Dean, H. D. (2013). Identifying the root causes of health inequities: Reflections on the 2011 National Center for HIV/AIDS, viral hepatitis, STD, and TB prevention health equity symposium. *Public Health Reports, 3*(128), 29–32. Retrieved from http://www.publichealthreports.org/issueopen.cfm?articleID=3045

Phua, K. (2013). Ethical dilemmas in protecting individual rights versus public protection in the case of infectious diseases. *Infectious Diseases: Research and Treatment, 6,* 1–5. doi: 10.4137/IDRT.S11205.

Rosner, D. (2010). Public health in the early 20th century. *Public Health Reports, 125*(Suppl. 3), 37–47.

Ruiz, J. B., & Bell, R. A. (2014). Understanding vaccination resistance: Vaccine search term selection bias and the valence of retrieved information. *Vaccine, 32*(44), 5776–5780.

Schlipköter, U., & Flahault, A. (2010). Communicable diseases: Achievements and challenges for public health. *Public Health Reviews, 32*(1), 90–119.

Thèves, C., Biagini, P., & Crubezy, E. (2014). The rediscovery of smallpox. *Clinical Microbiology and Infection, 20*(3), 210–218. doi: 10.1111/1469.12536.

U.S. Department of Health and Human Services (USDHHS). (n.d.). *Health information privacy: Public health.* Retrieved from http://www.hhs.gov/hipaa/for-professionals/special-topics/public-health/index.html

U.S. Department of Health and Human Services Agency (USDHHS). (2014). *Healthy People: Immunizations and infectious diseases.* Retrieved from http://www.healthypeople.gov/2020/topics-objectives/topic/immunization-and-infectious-diseases

U.S. Department of Health and Human Services Agency (USDHHS). (2016). *Healthy People: Sexually transmitted diseases.* Retrieved from http://www.healthypeople.gov/2020/topics-objectives/topic/sexually-transmitted-diseases

U.S. Equal Employment Opportunity Commission. (2011). *Questions and answers about the association provision of the Americans with Disabilities Act.* Retrieved from http://www.eeoc.gov/facts/association_ada.html

Williams, W. W., Lu, P., O'Halloran, A., Bridges, C. B., Kim, D. K., Pilishvili, T., ... Markowitz, L. E. (2015). Vaccination coverage among adults, excluding influenza vaccination—United States, 2013. *Morbidity and Mortality Weekly Report, 64*(4), 95–102. Retrieved from http://www.cdc.gov/mmwr/preview/mmwrhtml/mm6404a6.htm

World Health Organization (WHO). (2014). *The top 10 causes of death.* Retrieved from http://www.who.int/mediacentre/factsheets/fs310/en/#

World Health Organization (WHO). (2016a). *About WHO: What we do.* Retrieved from http://www.who.int/about/what-we-do/en/

World Health Organization (WHO). (2016b). *Biologicals: Smallpox.* Retrieved http://www.who.int/biologicals/vaccines/smallpox/en/

World Health Organization (WHO). (2016c). *Disease specific drug resistance.* Retrieved from http://www.who.int/drugresistance/diseases/en/

World Health Organization (WHO). (2016d). *FluNet.* Retrieved from www.who.int/influenza/gisrs_laboratory/flunet/en/

World Health Organization (WHO). (2016e). *Global influenza surveillance and response system (GISRS)*. Retrieved from www.who.int/influenza/gisrs_laboraory/en/

World Health Organization (WHO). (2016f). *History of WHO*. Retrieved from http://www.who.int/about/history/en/

World Health Organization (WHO). (2016g). *Multidrug-resistant tuberculosis (MDR-TB)*. Retrieved from http://www.who.int/tb/challenges/mdr/en/

World Health Organization (WHO). (2016h). *Public health surveillance*. Retrieved from http://www.who.int/topics/public_health_surveillance/en/

World Health Organization (WHO). (2016i). Use of high burden country lists for TB by WHO in the post-2015 era: Summary. Retrieved from www.who.int/entity/tb/publications/global_report/high_tb_burdencountrylists2016-2020summary.pdf

thePoint: Everything You Need to Make the Grade!

thePoint® Visit http://thePoint.lww.com/Rector9e for selected readings, study aids for all learning styles, and more!

Environmental Health and Safety

"When we try to pick out anything by itself, we find it hitched to everything else in the Universe."

John Muir (1838–1914), Naturalist

KEY TERMS

Bioaccumulation
Biomonitoring
Brownfields
Built environment
Climate change
Ecology

Ecomedicine
Endocrine disrupting
  chemicals (EDCs)
Environmental epidemiology
Environmental justice
Epigenetics

Exposure pathway
Health disparities
Integrated pest management
  (IPM)
Precautionary principle
Risk assessment

Risk management
Social determinants of
  health
Superfund
Sustainability
Toxicology

LEARNING OBJECTIVES

Upon mastery of this chapter, you should be able to:

- Apply the ecological perspective to human and environmental relationships.
- Discuss concepts of prevention and upstream approaches to health impact and environmental health.
- Discuss guiding documents for public health nursing.
- Discuss how the core functions of public health can be applied to public health nursing.
- Relate the effect of environmental hazards to human health.
- Describe how nurses can collaborate with other professionals, government agencies, and communities to reduce environmental threats to health.

The World Health Organization (WHO, 2015c, para. 1) defines health as "a complete state of physical, mental, and social wellbeing" and environment, as it relates to health, as "all the physical, chemical, and biological factors external to a person, and all the related behaviors" (WHO, 2015a, para. 1). The ability to live in a healthy environment increases not only the number of years of a healthy life but also one's quality of life. In nursing, the concern for the environment dates back to Florence Nightingale who reminds us in her *Notes on Nursing: What It Is and What It Is Not* (1860/1969) that health is dependent upon clean air, clean water, safe food, noise, and light. Increasingly, a number of environmental factors have been recognized as detrimental to health including exposures to hazardous materials in air, water, food, and soil, the rise in development and use of synthetic chemicals not well tested for safety, the adverse effects of natural and man-made disasters, and, more recently, the built environment. The most recent version of Healthy People, *Healthy People 2020*, uses the WHO definition of environmental health and explains that this includes not only the study of the direct pathological effects of various chemical, physical, and biological agents but also the effects on health of the social and broader environment, including urban development, housing, industry, transportation, and agriculture (United States Department of Health and Human Services [USDHHS], 2015b).

ENVIRONMENTAL HEALTH AND NURSING

Nurses are charged to incorporate knowledge of the environment into their nursing practice. Historically, public health and occupational health nurses (OHNs) have been leaders in this effort through their work in homes, in communities, and with governmental organizations. Despite this history, there is a need for increased nursing knowledge, environmental health assessment, engaging with community members to address environmental health issues and policy, and advocacy efforts among public health nurses (PHNs). During the past two decades in particular, several documents challenge nurses to advance their environmental health nursing knowledge and skills. In 1995, the Institute of Medicine report, *Nursing Health and the Environment* (Pope, Snyder, & Mood, 1995), addressed nursing education, practice, and research. The Agency for Toxic Substances and Disease Registry (ATSDR) launched their "Nursing and the Environment" initiative. Public health nursing led the profession with the publication of the *Environmental Principles for Public Health Nursing* in 2005 (see Table 9–1). The American Nurses Association (ANA) produced the *ANA's Principles of Environmental Health for Nursing Practice and Implementation Strategies* in 2007 (see Table 9–2). And most recently, in 2015, the ANA, in *Nursing: Scope and Standards of Practice*, built upon a new standard first introduced in 2010—Standard 17 Environmental Health (see Display 9–1). These guiding documents and initiatives call for all nurses to incorporate environmental health into all areas of nursing practice.

Brief History of Occupational/Environmental Health Movement in Nursing

Since the time of Florence Nightingale, nurses have considered the environment of the home, hospital, or community as a factor for health and illness. However, the specific role of nurses in occupational and environmental health first occurred in the workplace. Nurses who worked with hazardous exposures in the workplace were often called industrial nurses. Now those who work in industry are called OHNs where they both assess worker's health status and work to ensure worker safety and prevent adverse health effects from hazards in the workplace. With specific education and training in toxicology, epidemiology, workplace hazards, regulations, and prevention strategies, OHNs can be certified through the American Board of Occupational Health Nurses (see Chapter 31). Public health has included environmental health as a central aspect of health promotion and disease prevention. More recently, the nursing profession has responded to the call of nurses to establish environmental health competencies for nursing practice.

In 1995, the Institute of Medicine released the report of their meeting on *Nursing, Health, and the Environment* (Pope et al., 1995) that called for nurses to become more knowledgeable about the scientific principles of the relationship between health and environment, to advance their assessment and referral skills for environmental hazards, to advocate for patients and communities, to reduce adverse health effects, and to understand policy and legislation related to environmental health. More specifically, the report called for nurses to recognize pathways of exposure, prevention and control strategies, and the importance of research to develop sound and effective interventions. Interventions would include education and appropriate risk communication (Pope et al., 1995).

From 1995 until 2008, in response to this pivotal report, many schools and colleges increased their capacity to include environmental health into the nursing curriculum. In addition, nurses in practice incorporated environmental health into practice and were instrumental in making significant change in practice settings to reduce hazardous exposures to both health professionals and patients. Nursing research to address nursing interventions for environmental health increased, and nurses became involved in a number of policy and advocacy efforts.

In December 2008, 50 nurse leaders representing a range of nursing organizations including the American Public Health Association (APHA) Public Health Nursing Section, the Association of Community Health Nursing Educators (ACHNE), the Association of Public Health

---

Table 9–1 Guiding Documents: Environmental Health Principles for Public Health Nursing

Environmental Health Principles for Public Health Nursing

1. Safe and sustainable environments are essential conditions for the public's health.

2. Environmental health is integral to the role and responsibilities of all PHNs.

3. All PHNs should possess environmental health knowledge and skills.

4. Environmental health decisions should be grounded in sound science.

5. The precautionary principle is a fundamental tenet for all environmental health endeavors.

6. Environmental justice is a right of all populations.

7. Public awareness and community involvement are essential in environmental health decision-making.

8. Communities have a right to relevant and timely information for decisions on environmental health.

9. Environmental health approaches should respect diverse values, beliefs, cultures, and circumstances.

10. Collaboration is essential to effectively protecting the health of all people from environmental harm.

11. Environmental health advocacy must be rooted in scientific integrity, honesty, respect for all persons, and social justice.

12. Environmental health research addressing the effectiveness and public health impact of nursing interventions should be conducted and disseminated (p. 5).

From American Public Health Association, Public Health Nursing Section. (2005). *Environmental health principles & recommendations for public health nursing.* Washington, DC: Author, with permission.

Table 9–2 ANA's Principles of Environmental Health for Nursing Practice

All nurses are to be aware of the principles of environmental health for nursing. We are to integrate these principles into our practice, education, and research.

1. Knowledge of environmental health concepts is essential to nursing practice (p. 17).

2. The precautionary principle guides nurses in their practice to use products and practices that do not harm human health or the environment and to take preventive action in the fact of uncertainty (p. 18).

3. Nurses have a right to work in an environment that is safe and healthy (p. 20).

4. Healthy environments are sustained through multidisciplinary collaboration (p. 22).

5. Choice of materials, products, technology, and practices in the environment that impact nursing practice are based on the best available evidence (p. 23).

6. Approaches to promoting a healthy environment reflect a respect for the diverse values, beliefs, cultures, and circumstances of patients and their families (p. 24).

7. Nurses participate in assessing the quality of the environment in which they practice and live (p. 25).

8. Nurses, other health care workers, patients, and communities have the right to know relevant and timely information about the potentially harmful products, chemicals, pollutants, and hazards to which they are exposed (p. 27).

9. Nurses participate in research of best practices that promote a safe and healthy environment (p. 29).

10. Nurses must be supported in advocating for and implementing environmental health principles in nursing practice (p. 30).

From American Nurses Association (ANA). (2010). *ANA's principles of environmental health for nursing practice with implementation strategies* (2nd ed.). Silver Spring, MD: Author, with permission.

DISPLAY 9–1 AMERICAN NURSES ASSOCIATION, PUBLIC HEALTH NURSING: SCOPE AND STANDARDS OF PRACTICE

Standard 16. Environmental Health

"The registered nurse practices in an environmentally safe and healthy manner" (p. 62).

The Registered Nurse

1. Has knowledge of current environmental health issues and strategies
2. Promotes a safe and healthy workplace and professional practice environment for populations, for communities, and for individual clients
3. Assesses the environment in the practice setting to identify health risk factors (e.g., chemical, biological, physical)
4. Promotes the safe, cautious, and proper use/disposal of products in the community setting
5. Communicates information about both environmental health risks and strategies to reduce exposure to peers, families, consumers of health care, and the wider community
6. Applies the precautionary principle and current research to ascertain if a practice, policy, or product is a threat to human health or the environment
7. Works with others to promote "healthy communities" (p. 62)
8. Works toward promoting "sustainable environmental health policies and conditions" through partnerships with other professionals and agencies
9. Critically appraises media coverage of issues/incidents relating to environmental health
10. Serves as an advocate for implementing principles of environmental health in public health and nursing practice

Adapted from American Nurses Association (ANA). (2013). *Public health nursing: Scope and standards of practice* (2nd ed.). Silver Spring, MD: Author.

Nurses (APHN), and ANA met to develop an agenda for environmental health nursing. The organization, Alliance of Nurses for Healthy Environments (ANHE), was formed to advance nursing knowledge of environmental health and engage nurses in collaboration to advance environmental health nursing (ANHE, 2015a). Four workgroups were formed: education, research, practice, and advocacy/policy. Since that time, a number of initiatives have placed environmental health at the forefront for nursing education and practice. The ANHE Education Workgroup developed competencies for nursing practice in 2009 (Leffers, McDermott-Levy, Smith, & Sattler, 2014). Working collaboratively with the ANA, Standard 16: Environmental Health was included in the second edition of *Nursing: Scope and Standards of Practice* (ANA, 2010) and revised for the 2015 edition (ANA, 2015b). Since the publication of the 2010 Standard 16: Environmental Health, all nurses must incorporate environmental health principles into nursing practice. In addition to the success of the development of competencies and standards, the nurses who work with ANHE have advanced their advocacy and policy voice, prepared research priorities for environmental health nursing, and held conferences and workshops for nursing practice, education, and advocacy efforts (ANHE, 2015b). Although PHNs have been at the forefront of environmental health nursing, the new competencies provide guidance for all types of nursing practice and can be applied in many community and acute care settings.

Guiding Documents

In addition to the previously mentioned *Environmental Health Principles for Public Health Nursing* (APHA, 2005), the *ANA Principles of Environmental Health for Nursing Practice* (ANA, 2007), and the *Scope and Standards of Nursing Practice* (ANA, 2010; ANA, 2015b), nurses are guided by other public health documents. These include the federal guidelines from the surgeon general report on Healthy People and the core functions of public health (Centers for Disease Control and Prevention [CDC], 2015b).

Healthy People 2020 Initiatives

In 1979, the surgeon general released a report, *Healthy People: The Surgeon General's Report on Health Promotion and Disease Prevention,* to set goals for improving health for the nation. In 1990, the Healthy People initiative set specific objectives to reduce disease, promote health, and improve healthy years of life. The revisions in 2000, 2010, and most recently for *Healthy People 2020* continue this focus upon targets for health improvement. This document provides guidance for nurses to identify targets for health and is used for many public health nursing interventions. The *Healthy People 2020* framework offers specific goals and objectives for environmental health. The overall goal is to "promote health for all through a healthy environment" (USDHHS, 2015b, para. 1). The most recent release of the *Healthy People 2020* Environmental Health objectives focuses in six areas that include

- Outdoor air quality
- Surface and groundwater quality
- Toxic substances and hazardous wastes
- Homes and communities
- Infrastructure and surveillance
- Global environmental health (para. 3)

A number of health conditions are linked to poor air quality such as respiratory disease, cardiovascular disease, and cancer. Toxins found in water have been linked to neurological problems, endocrine disruption, and cancer. Although not all mechanisms for disease from toxic exposures are fully understood or studied, various hazardous chemicals have been linked to birth defects, neurological problems, endocrine disruption, and cancer (USDHHS, 2015a). See Display 9–2 for a full listing of the *Healthy People 2020* Environmental Health objectives.

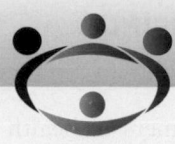

DISPLAY 9–2 *HEALTHY PEOPLE 2020* **OBJECTIVES FOR ENVIRONMENTAL HEALTH TOPIC AREAS**

Goal: Promote health for all through a healthy environment.

Topic and Number Objective

Outdoor Air Quality

EH-1   Reduce the number of days the air quality index (AQI) exceeds 100, weighted by population and AQI.

EH-2   Increase use of alternative modes of transportation for work.

EH-3   Reduce air toxic emissions to decrease the risk of adverse health effects caused by airborne toxics.

Water Quality

EH-4   Increase the proportion of persons served by community water systems who receive a supply of drinking water that meets the regulations of the Safe Drinking Water Act (SDWA).

EH-5   Reduce waterborne disease outbreaks arising from water intended for drinking among persons served by community water systems.

EH-6   Reduce per capita domestic water withdrawals with respect to use and conservation.

EH-7   Increase the proportion of days that beaches are open and safe for swimming.

Toxics and Waste

EH-8   Reduce blood lead levels in children

EH-9   Minimize the risks to human health and the environment posed by hazardous sites.

EH-10   Reduce pesticide exposures that result in visits to a health care facility.

EH-11   Reduce the amount of toxic pollutants released into the environment.

EH-12   Increase recycling of municipal solid waste.

Healthy Homes and Healthy Communities

EH-13   Reduce indoor allergen levels

EH-14   Increase the proportion of homes with an operating radon mitigation system for persons living in homes at risk for radon exposure.

EH-15   Increase the percentage of new single-family homes (SFH) constructed with radon-reducing features, especially in high-radon-potential areas.

EH-16   Increase the proportion of the Nation's elementary, middle, and high schools that have official school policies and engage in practices that promote a healthy and safe physical school environment.

EH-17   (Developmental) Increase the proportion of persons living in pre-1978 housing that has been tested for the presence of lead-based paint or related hazards.

EH-18   Reduce the number of U.S. homes that are found to have lead-based paint or related hazards.

EH-19   Reduce the proportion of occupied housing units that have moderate or severe physical problems.

Infrastructure and Surveillance

EH-20   Reduce exposure to selected environmental chemicals in the population, as measured by blood and urine concentrations of the substances or their metabolites.

EH-21   Improve quality, utility, awareness, and use of existing information systems for environmental health.

EH-22   Increase the number of states, territories, tribes, and the District of Columbia that monitor diseases or conditions that can be caused by exposure to environmental hazards EH-23.

EH-23   Reduce the number of new schools sited within 500 ft of an interstate or federal or state highway.

Global Environmental Health

EH-24   Reduce the global burden of disease due to poor water quality, sanitation, and insufficient hygiene.

Source: U.S. Department of Health and Human Services. (2016). *Healthy People 2020: Environmental health.* Retrieved from http://www.healthypeople.gov/2020/topics-objectives/topic/environmental-health/objectives

Importance of Environmental Health for Nursing

Nurses are essential to improve environmental health through nursing education, research, and practice. The ANHE offers reasons why nurses are important to environmental health that include the role of nurses in promoting healing and safe environments for people. Nurses work with diverse populations in homes, workplaces, and communities and are the largest population of health care providers in the United States with almost 3 million registered nurses. In addition, nurses are in one of the most trusted professions, are able to communicate complex information to their patients and communities, and interact with many other health care organizations and in policy setting roles (Smith, 2015).

CONCEPTS AND FRAMEWORKS FOR ENVIRONMENTAL HEALTH

Ecology

Ecology can be defined as the study of the interactions and relationships between living organisms and their environments. Ecosystems are dynamic communities of plant, animal, and microorganisms as well as the nonliving environments in which they live. No organism, including humans, can live removed from their ecosystem or other species. Ecosystems help regulate water, gases, waste recycling, nutrient cycling, pollination, infectious disease, climate, and biology as well as provide recreational and cultural opportunities for human use (Frumkin, 2010; Wright & Boorse, 2013). The scientific study of ecosystems provides the science to understand the synergistic relationship between humans and the environment and why knowledge of environmental health is so important for nurses. The term **ecomedicine** refers to the adverse human impact upon the environment that, in turn, creates new patterns of disease and poverty (Science and Environmental Health Network [SEHN], 2015a). Specific threats to the environment for human health are discussed using a sustainability perspective.

PHNs find that the science of ecology has been applied to social ecological perspectives that identify not only the physical environment but also the social and cultural factors that exist for populations. In public health, the ecological model of population health is used to illustrate that determinants of health (biological, behavioral, and environmental) interact to affect health (Friis, 2012). In addition, the *Healthy People 2020* approach emphasizes the need to include social, cultural, and environmental conditions into assessments for health determinants. Health behaviors occur within various levels of the ecological model and must be considered to clearly identify the most effective interventions for health promotion (USDHHS, 2015a). See Figure 9–1: Ecological Model of Public Health.

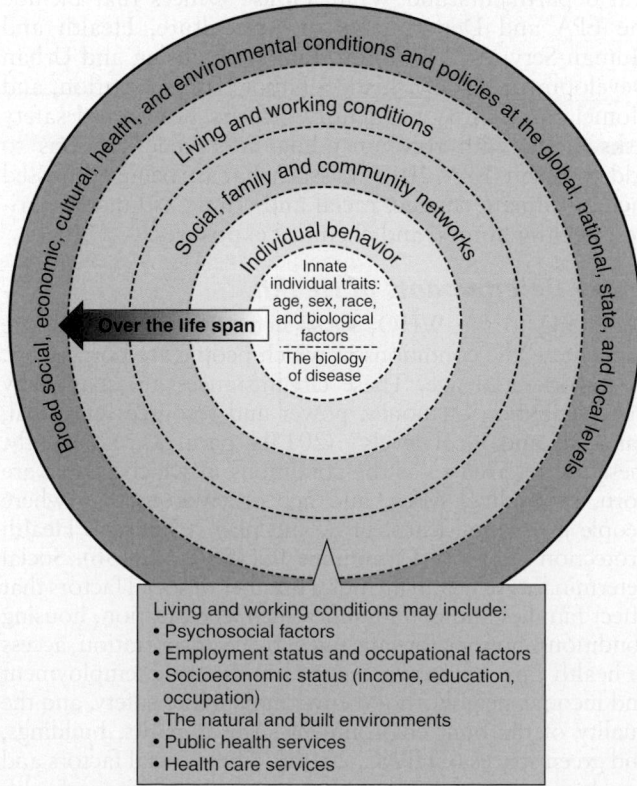

APPROACH AND RATIONALE

A guide to thinking about the determinants of population health

Broad social, economic, cultural, health, and environmental conditions and policies at the global, national, state, and local levels

Living and working conditions

Social, family and community networks

Individual behavior

Innate individual traits: age, sex, race, and biological factors

The biology of disease

Over the life span

Living and working conditions may include:
• Psychosocial factors
• Employment status and occupational factors
• Socioeconomic status (income, education, occupation)
• The natural and built environments
• Public health services
• Health care services

FIGURE 9–1 Ecological model for public health.

Sustainability

Sustainability is based upon the principle that human beings and the natural environment must coexist harmoniously for human survival (U.S. Environmental Protection Agency [EPA], 2015p). When the concept of sustainability is applied to human systems, it is evident that the public must protect the environment and promote healthy characteristics in the population and communities in which they live. Currently, much of human/environment interactions are not sustainable in that energy use exceeds supply and pollutants are changing the natural landscape of plant and animal life and threatening both human life and ecosystems. Solutions to improve sustainability for humans and the environment include strategies that are socially desirable, economically feasible, and ecologically viable (Wright & Boorse, 2013). One example of how increased human demands for energy impact sustainability is the increased use of fossil fuels for home heating and cooling. The increased use of coal, for example, increases air pollution from the toxic emissions released in coal-fired power plants that are often referred to as greenhouse gases and that contribute to climate change. Current estimates indicate that the global need for oil has exceeded available resources that are not sustainable. Further in this chapter, you will learn about the work of nurses to address the health risks associated with hydraulic fracturing. This, too, is a concern for sustainability that impacts human health. Concerns about the depletion of natural resources, disruption of nutrient cycles, widening economic disparities between the rich and poor, and climate change are key issues addressed in the EPA's *Framework for Sustainability Indicators at EPA* (2015l).

Sustainability is an important concept in relationship to nursing and health. The U.S. health care industry is a $2.5 trillion enterprise that contributes to 8% of all greenhouse gases and 7% of all carbon dioxide emissions. Hospitals generate as much as 5 million tons of solid waste annually; much of that includes hazardous materials. Nurses were instrumental in the formation of Health Care Without Harm, a leading organization that promotes environmentally responsible health care (Health Care Without Harm, 2015a). The ANA (2015a) has long supported efforts to address medical and pharmaceutical waste. For example, Denise Choiniere, MS, RN, launched the sustainability effort at the University of Maryland Medical Center (UMMC) in 2007 and now serves as the UMMC Director of Materials Management and Sustainability; Beth Schenk, PhD, MHI, RN, serves as the Nurse Scientist and Sustainability Coordinator with Providence Health Services St. Patrick Hospital in Montana. Director Choiniere, who was employed as a cardiac care nurse at the hospital, led efforts to begin a Green Team and build the sustainability program. The UMMC has won numerous awards for their efforts to move toward sustainability in environmentally preferred purchasing, safer chemicals, use of green cleaners, farmers' market and sustainable food options, green commuting, waste reduction, energy conservation, and building design (Boone, 2012). In Dr. Schenk's role with her shared appointment at Washington State University, she seeks to advance environmental stewardship in health care and promote research for sustainability (Washington State University, 2015). Efforts are ongoing to advance nursing knowledge for sustainability in health care (Butterfield et al., 2014; Woeber, 2013).

While these examples highlight the work of two nurse leaders for large health care systems, nurses who work in community settings must comply with best practices for waste disposal as well as greening their practice environments. Pharmaceutical waste is a serious concern for nurses who work in home and school settings. This topic is more fully addressed in the section about water contaminants.

Upstream Focus

Many PHNs incorporate an "upstream" focus into their work with populations. That approach emerged from the seminal publication by John McKinley in 1979, *A Case for Focusing Upstream*, which identifies root causes of disease and manufacturers of illness. It considers socioeconomic factors and also the environmental origins of disease and health problems. To illustrate this, he uses examples in the food and tobacco industries (McKinley, 1979). PHNs work in prevention and health promotion areas, but an upstream approach moves our thinking to those factors that are at the institutional and system level rather than looking solely at healthy lifestyle issues: in other words, "upstream" from the identified problem or issue. For example, a program to improve heart health in a community using a lifestyle approach would promote healthy diets, increased physical activity, and smoking cessation. An upstream focus looks at the social factors such as secondhand smoke in public places, unhealthy food choices available in schools and other public places, and how the built environment promotes or impedes safe outdoor physical activity. Two related concepts for environmental health nursing are health disparities and the social determinants of health. This focus for public health and environmental health nursing was introduced in a classic article by Butterfield (2002) who reminds the nursing profession that nurses, particularly PHNs, with a presence in worksites, homes, schools, and other community settings can serve to reduce risks. PHNs are often the "sentinels of surveillance" (Butterfield, 2002, p. 33) who detect unusual illness patterns and respond to environmental emergencies in work and community settings. With emphasis upon data estimates that as much as 33% of disease occurrence is attributable to environmental exposures, and that the prevalence of environmentally linked health problems such as asthma, neurological problems, certain cancers, and birth defects are all on the rise, a case can be made for why nurses must use an upstream framework to assess, monitor, educate, advocate, and create policies to reduce environmental health risks. Butterfield (2002) identifies three specific opportunities for nurses to impact these health threats: (1) by nursing presence in hospitals, clinicians worksites, schools, and home settings, (2) because nurses have skills to translate technical information into messages that nonhealth professionals can understand, and (3) because nurses have skills to promote health at both the individual and community level. Strategic actions that can be considered as part of an upstream framework are to include the following components:

- Use of an environmental health history in nursing assessments in order to create better tracking of environmental exposures
- Embedding of environmental health information into nursing practice settings
- Increases in educational efforts to inform individuals and families of environmental health hazards

- Knowledge of information
- Engaging in environmental health research in order to advance our understanding of etiology and prevention
- Advocating for individuals and groups who are at specific risks

By using an upstream approach, PHNs can impact the prevalence of disease by intervening where the root causes exist (Butterfield, 2002).

Health Disparities

Health disparities are a serious concern for overall health in the United States and globally. As noted in the discussion of upstream approaches to health, environmental factors are basic determinants of health and well-being. However, great inequities occur between the environments of people with higher incomes and those of low-income communities, people of color, and tribal populations. Complex relationships exist between genes and environment that are related to social determinants of health (National Institute of Environmental Health Sciences [NIEHS], 2015a). Disparities that may be directly correlated with environmental exposures include rates of asthma among children, elevated blood lead levels (EBLLs), cancers that are linked to environmental exposures, and lung diseases among adults. Disproportionate exposures to pesticides, toxic chemicals in the workplace, poor indoor air quality in schools, and lead in housing have all been linked to the social determinants of health. At the federal level, the U.S. government responds to this important concern for health disparities related to children's health through the President's Task Force for Environmental Health and Safety Risks to Children. This interagency effort includes 17 federal departments and White House Offices that include the EPA and Departments of Agriculture, Health and Human Services, Education, Energy, Housing and Urban Development (HUD), Justice, Labor, Transportation, and Homeland Security to identify priority health and safety risks along with recommending interagency actions to address them (EPA, 2015v). Issues that are being addressed include climate change, racial and ethnic asthma disparities, healthy homes, and chemical exposures.

Social Determinants of Health

According to the WHO, **social determinants of health** are defined as "the conditions in which people are born, grow, live, work, and age. These circumstances are shaped by the distribution of money, power and resources at global, national, and local levels" (2015b, para. 1). Frequently, these are referred to as the conditions in which people are born, grow, live, work, and age or environments where people live, labor, learn, pray, and play (Children's Health Protection Advisory Committee [CHPAC], 2013b). Social determinants of health include a number of social factors that affect families and communities such as education, housing conditions, options for safe and active transportation, access to health care services, access to healthy food, employment and income, neighborhood environment and safety, and the quality of the built environment such as parks, buildings, and green spaces (CHPAC, 2013a). These social factors and nonchemical stressors contribute to the inequities in health outcomes, burden of disease, and quality of life.

Environmental Justice

Closely related to social determinants of health is the issue of environmental justice. The EPA defines **environmental justice** as "the fair treatment and meaningful involvement of all people regardless of race, color, national origin, or income with respect to the development, implementation, and enforcement of environmental laws, regulations, and policies" (EPA, 2015i, para. 1). The key difference between social determinants and environmental justice is that the former addresses social factors that contribute to health disparities, whereas environmental justice is responsive to the inequities in the distribution of environmental hazards and exposure risks. The federal government took action to address environmental injustice though President Clinton's Executive Order 12898 in 1994 (EPA, 2015i). In communities across the United States, people of color, low income, and tribal communities bear a higher burden of exposures to environmental risks where they live (Bullard, Johnson, & Torres, 2011). Communities throughout the United States exhibit examples of environmental injustice where racial and ethnic minorities living in low-income communities are disproportionately affected by toxic exposures (Arnold, 2014; EPA, 2015j; Lougheed, 2014). Children are at particular risk in such disadvantaged communities where they have cumulative risk from exposures in homes, schools, and neighborhoods. Developmental and behavioral factors make children more vulnerable to environmental contaminants, and they have little control over where they live, what they eat, or the socioeconomic factors of their lives. Poor and minority children, who are more likely to live in neighborhoods with incinerators, industrial plants, toxic waste sites, and poor quality housing, show higher rates of asthma, learning disabilities, and EBLLs than do nonminority children and those who come from more affluent families (Leffers et al., 2016). A variety of factors contribute to environmental health disparities; those living in affected areas experience challenges related to physical infrastructure, vulnerability/susceptibility, proximity to sources or environmental hazards, unique exposure pathways, multiple cumulative environmental burdens, chronic psychosocial stress, and diminished capacity to participate in decision-making (Bullard, 2005; Nweke et al., 2011). Communities are able to promote healthier environments through a multifaceted approach to community development, community organizing, and community empowerment by working with advocacy groups, networking, and educational programming (Whitehead, 2015).

Nurses who work in communities observe the impact of health disparities with those people living in poverty or of minority status bearing the greatest health burdens. Through community-based participatory research, partnering with local organizations and collaborating with community members, nurses can build relationships with community members that strengthen their voice to address the environmental risks they face. PHNs' skills in building relationships with community members, working collaboratively with community partners, and advocating for change through governmental programs make them important contributors to environmental justice work (Leffers et al., 2016).

The Partnership for Sustainable Communities is an alliance of three federal agencies, the EPA, the Department of Transportation (DOT), and HUD. Reference to this initiative is made in several places in this chapter. An important feature of this program is that by taking a broad approach across housing, transportation, and aspects of the built environment, the federal government is able to promote health and address environmental justice concerns (EPA, 2015h; Partnership for Sustainable Communities, 2015). See Displays 9–3 and 9–4 for further sources of environmental health information.

DISPLAY 9–3 ENVIRONMENTAL HEALTH REGULATORY AGENCIES

EPA

This federal agency was established in December 1970 for the purpose of standard setting, monitoring, and enforcement of environmental protection in order to work for a cleaner and healthier environment for America. The agency works to ensure that Americans are protected from risks to health in their homes, schools, and workplaces. The agency relies on the best scientific evidence to promote the development of policies to protect the environment and health and enforces federal laws to protect human health.
http://www.epa.gov/aboutepa/history/publications/print/origins.html

FDA

The Food and Drug Administration (FDA or USFDA) is an agency of the USDHHS that regulates food safety, dietary supplements, prescription and over-the-counter pharmaceuticals, cosmetics, biopharmaceuticals, blood transfusions, and tobacco products.

CPSC

The U.S. Consumer Product Safety Commission (CPSC) was created in 1972 as an agency of the U.S. government to protect the public from risks of injury or death from consumer products. Commonly reported products are cribs, toys, household chemicals, and power tools but include any commercially traded product. As an independent agency, the CPSC does not report to any other agency of the U.S. government.
http://www.cpsc.gov/about/about.html

OSHA

The Occupational Safety and Health Administration (OSHA) was created in 1970 as a regulatory federal agency of the United States to assure safe working conditions. OSHA sets and enforces standards for health and safety in work environments.
http://www.osha.gov/

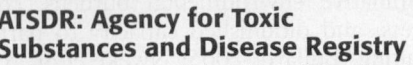

DISPLAY 9–4 ENVIRONMENTAL HEALTH RESOURCES

ATSDR: Agency for Toxic Substances and Disease Registry

ATSDR is a federal public health agency of the USDHHS and division of the CDC. Using science, ATSDR serves the public to take responsive public health actions, by providing information to prevent harmful exposures and diseases. http://www.atsdr.cdc.gov/

ANHE: Alliance of Nurses for Healthy Environments

ANHE is an organization for nurses and health care providers to promote health through knowledge, networking, and action. Their envirn.org Web site and Environmental Health textbook serve as an active learning environment for learning essential environmental health information from experts and connecting with others. Through workgroups that focus upon education, research, practice, and policy/advocacy, nurses can increase their capacity for environmental health nursing. http://envirn.org/

CDC: Centers for Disease Control and Prevention

The overall mission of the CDC "is to collaborate to create the expertise, information, and tools that people and communities need to protect their health—through health promotion, prevention of disease, injury and disability, and preparedness for new health threats" (http://www.cdc.gov/about/organization/mission.htm). In the area of environmental health, they include topics related to air quality, air pollution, biomonitoring, children's health, climate and health, environmental health sciences, rodent control, sun protection, and water. Additionally, they address specific risks such as asbestos, carbon monoxide, lead, mold, natural disasters, radiation, smoking and tobacco use, and wildfires. http://www.cdc.gov/Environmental/

NLM: National Library of Medicine

The United States Library of Medicine is the worlds' largest medical library. Their Web site offers a large number of resources useful for nurses to learn about environmental health.

> TOXNET is a large set of databases on environmental health, toxicology, hazardous chemicals, and toxic releases. It also includes a household products database.

TOXMAP is an environmental health e-map that allows the user to explore toxic chemical releases and hazardous waste sites from the EPA's Toxics Release Inventory (TRI) and the Superfund National Priorities List (NPL).

TOX TOWN is an interactive site that includes a variety of settings from town, to city, to farm, to port to U.S. border lands. In each setting, the user is able to view nontechnical descriptions of chemicals, how the environment affects human health, and other Internet resources on topics useful to the user. The color, graphics animation, and sounds make it an effective strategy to each adolescent, educators, and the general public about environmental exposures.

NIEHS: National Institute of Environmental Health Sciences

The NIEHS is a part of the National Institutes of Health (NIH), which is an institute of the Department of Health and Human Services (DHHS). The mission is to understand how the environment influences health. To accomplish this, NIEHS focuses upon research, global health, and research training. http://www.niehs.nih.gov/

NIOSH: National Institute for Occupational Safety and Health

The National Institute for Occupational Safety and Health (or NIOSH) is a U.S. federal agency that is responsible for both conducting research and translating knowledge into recommendations for the prevention of work-related injury and illness. Created in 1970 in response to the Occupational Safety and Health Act, 1970, NIOSH was established to help ensure safe and healthful working conditions. http://www.cdc.gov/NIOSH/

OSHA: Occupational Safety and Health Administration

The OSHA was created in 1970 as a regulatory federal agency of the United States to assure safe working conditions. OSHA sets and enforces standards for health and safety in work environments. http://www.osha.gov/

Precautionary Principle

The **precautionary principle** states that in the absence of clear data that indicate the safety of an action, chemical, or material that poses a threat to human health, it should not be used. The origin of the precautionary principle is from Germany, and it was used as early as 1970 to restrict the impact of potentially toxic air emissions.

In the United States, the adoption of this perspective that was used in Europe grew during the 1990s and culminated in 1998, when an interdisciplinary team met in Wisconsin at the Wingspread Center to address the environment and human health. The *Wingspread Statement on the Precautionary Principle* is rooted in precaution, scientific uncertainty, and human rights. The Wingspread

Statement posits that based upon the release and use of toxic substances, the failure of environmental regulations to adequately protect human health, and evidence that supports adverse human health effects from environmental exposures, implementation of the precautionary principle is necessary. The principle states, "When an activity raises threats of harm to human health or the environment, precautionary measures should be taken if some cause and effect relationships are not fully established scientifically. In this content the proponent of an activity, rather than the public, should bear the burden of proof" (SEHN, 2015b, para. 2).

The precautionary principle has been applied to public health and its core functions. First, the core function of *assessment* includes two essential services: (1) monitoring health status and (2) the diagnosis and investigation of health hazards in the community. Environmental health surveillance is supported by this principle. Most certainly, the role of risk assessment that is central to environmental health meets the concern for evidence to determine the safety of activities that can pose environmental threats to health. *Policy development* addresses the guidance from the precautionary principle through the essential services that inform and educate the public, mobilize the community to address health issues, and develop policies to address those issues. The precautionary principle engages scientists to analyze and develop policies in order to ensure health based upon sound evidence. The core function of *assurance* requires that policies be enforced. The principle charges that, instead of a focus upon remediation, those activities that could be harmful should not be undertaken (Chaudry, 2008). The application of the precautionary principle to public health nursing can be noted in the *Environmental Health Principles and Recommendations for Public Health Nursing*, where principle 5 states that the precautionary principle is a "fundamental tenet for all environmental health endeavors" (APHA, 2005, p. 5). Chaudry (2008) reports that the precautionary principle is relevant for public health nursing interventions that include surveillance, community organizing, and advocacy and must be incorporated into nursing practice. Stokowski (2014) emphasizes that nurses should be "environmental health stewards" (para. 1).

Specific Vulnerabilities

Various groups are at more risk during specific periods of physical development, through comorbid health issues, or from issues related to where they live, work, or attend school. Exposures for pregnant women create a number of risks to both mother and fetus and can produce lifelong or intergenerational adverse outcomes. Some of these effects include fetal loss, low birth weight infants, menstrual abnormalities, recurrent miscarriage, malformations of the reproductive system, reduced fertility, hormonal changes, intrauterine growth restriction, altered semen quality, and alterations in onset of puberty (Chalupka & Chalupka, 2010; Chan, Chalupka, & Barrett, 2015; Leffers, 2015).

Infants and children are at risk for a number of reasons related to their stage of physical development, behavioral factors, and specific environments such as neonatal intensive care units (NICUs), schools, and homes. Children's exposures begin in utero when many pollutants reach the developing fetus. Although breast-feeding is the best source of nutrition for infants, many chemicals, such as polychlorinated biphenyls (PCBs), dichlorodiphenyltrichloroethane (DDT), dioxin, and benzene, have been identified in breast milk. The stage of physical development of the respiratory, neurological, and excretory systems can all lead to increased risk of exposure and decreased ability to metabolize toxins. Childhood behaviors such as hand-to-mouth exploration, crawling and playing on or near the ground, and use of toys all contribute to specific vulnerability to hazards. Toxic materials on floors or in soil where children play and playthings (e.g., pressure-treated wood, toys, and paints) can all increase risk for childhood exposures. Exposures to lead, mercury, and PCBs increase the risk for developmental disabilities. Studies suggest that the rise in attention deficit hyperactivity disorder (ADHD), as well as antisocial and aggressive behavior diagnoses, can be attributed to the harmful effects of neurotoxic agents in the environment (Kalkbrenner, Schmidt & Penlesky, 2014; Landrigan & Goldman, 2011).

Prenatal Exposure to EDCs and Effect on Future Generations

Evidence indicates that many chronic diseases arise from complex interactions between the environment and the genes (Fig. 9–2). **Epigenetics** is the field of study that examines the gene–environment interaction to study the processes where genes are expressed differently as a result of environmental influences (EPA, 2015k). **Endocrine disrupting chemicals** (EDCs) mimic or block natural hormones in the human body and are linked to changes in genes inherited by offspring (Engel & Wolff, 2013; English, Healy, Jagais, & Sly, 2015). One example of epigenetic change was the use of DES (diethylstilbestrol) to treat women at risk of miscarriage. Female offspring of mothers who took DES showed increased rates of vaginal adenocarcinoma. This type of cancer is now linked to the estrogen taken by their mothers during pregnancy (Malahingahiah et al., 2015). In addition, a long-term follow-up study of 4,653 women who were exposed to DES in utero (comparison group of 1,927

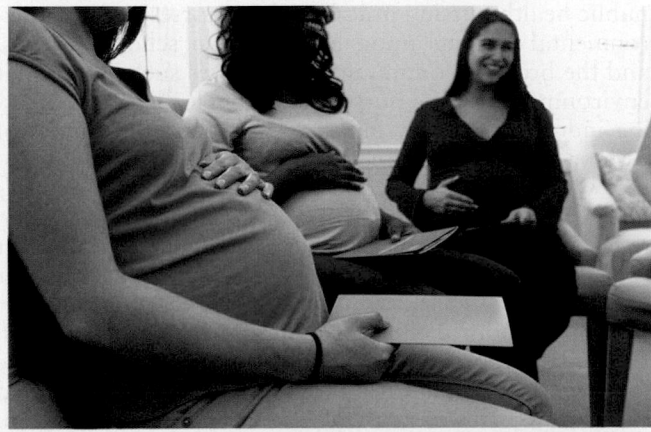

FIGURE 9–2 Pregnant women should avoid exposure to EDCs.

women not exposed) found that those women exposed to DES while in utero were 1.42 to 3.77 times more likely to suffer from reproductive problems such as infertility, spontaneous abortion, preterm delivery, loss of second-trimester pregnancy, ectopic pregnancy, preeclampsia, stillbirth, gynecological conditions such as early menopause, grade 2 or higher cervical intraepithelial neoplasia, and breast cancer at 40 years of age or older (Hoover et al., 2011). Experts argue that the genetic changes that result from epigenetic processes because of developmental exposure to environmental stressors create negative effects on the health of future generations and contribute to rising rates of neurological conditions, alterations in reproductive organ development, and cancer (Grandjean et al., 2015).

CORE FUNCTIONS OF PUBLIC HEALTH

In 1988, the Institute of Medicine convened to address what they called "the disarray of public health" and developed the mission, role of government in fulfilling this mission, and specific responsibilities for level of government. This resulted in the core functions of public health and the 10 essential services. The core functions, assessment, policy development, and assurance, will be applied to the important aspects of environmental health for public health nursing. Assessment includes the investigation of health hazards, surveillance of health issues such as disease or injury, examining causes, and assessing needs. Policy development relies upon science for decision-making and educates people to create community involvement in order to develop polices. Assurance is a function that seeks innovative solutions to health issues, guarantees necessary services are provided, and provides oversight to policy implementation (Institute of Medicine, 1988, p. 19). See Chapter 3.

PHNs fulfill these functions but extend them by their strong emphasis upon education for health promotion, disease prevention, as well as advocacy by integrating nursing knowledge and practice into these functions. In addition, PHNs work collaboratively with others in the community to promote health for the people they serve. This chapter will review essential environmental health information for PHNs using the core functions as an organizational framework.

Some of the most commonly recognized areas of public health nursing practice where nurses address environmental impacts upon health are in schools, homes, and the broader community, with issues such as the built environment. School nurses have been leaders in addressing indoor air quality in schools particularly as rates of asthma in children rise (EPA, 2015cc). Many collaborate with the U.S. EPA and their *IAQ Tools for Schools* program (EPA, 2015n). More recently, in response to the Federal Insecticide, Fungicide, and Rodenticide Act (FIFRA), school nurses are serving as advocates for **integrated pest management (IPM)** programs for pest prevention without increasing exposure to harmful toxins. PHNs have been part of the Healthy Homes Initiative (HHI). Occupational health nurses (OHNs) have served to educate, enforce safety standards, monitor health, and advocate for workers' health. At the community

level, PHNs are involved with efforts to reduce pediatric obesity by participation in efforts to improve the built environment through safe walking paths, advocating for safe parks and recreational areas, and in reducing exposure to pesticides in playgrounds (Gilden, 2011).

Assessment

The breadth of environmental health information available exceeds the scope of this chapter. Our discussion is organized around the settings where people live, work, and go to school, the routes of exposure, the types of hazards, and the health effects of environmental toxins. In particular for nurses in the community, it is important to identify priority concerns for the locations where people spend the majority of their time (home, work, school) to better prepare health promotion and disease prevention interventions. To help the learner, we begin with some common types of exposures and the resultant adverse health effects. Later in the chapter, we will discuss the settings and common exposures there. While community assessment and epidemiology are essential skills for public health nursing, the ability to perform critical assessments for environmental health requires background in the environmental health sciences.

Sciences for Environmental Health

Environmental health sciences include environmental epidemiology, toxicology, risk assessment, and risk management. In Chapter 7, you have learned about the principles of epidemiology. *Environmental epidemiology* is a particular branch of epidemiology that focuses upon environmental exposures and the risks that contribute to adverse health effects such as cancer, developmental disabilities, neurological problems, reproductive health issues, or death. Environmental epidemiology seeks to understand the specific vulnerabilities of population groups, to understand how toxic exposures adversely affect health, and to contribute to public health policies that address risk and risk management (National Cancer Institute, 2015).

Toxicology is the "study of how the body processes the toxicants to which it is exposed and of the ultimate effects of these toxicants in the body" (Maxwell, 2014, p. 18). Toxicants are those substances that are harmful and made by humans or result from human activities, in contrast to toxins that are naturally produced. By studying the physical properties of chemicals, scientists are able to examine the toxicity of chemicals as manifested by enzyme inhibition, cytotoxicity, inflammation, necrosis, immune hypersensitivity or immune suppression, neoplasia, and mutagenic reactions. These processes should be familiar to nurses as they parallel the effects and adverse effects of pharmacotherapeutic chemicals. Chemicals are classified as alcohols, solvents, heavy metals, oxidants, and acids and may be found as industrial wastes, agricultural chemicals, waterborne toxicants, air pollutants, or food additives. Factors such as dose level and timing can make a difference in efficacy or toxicity of a drug; dose and timing can also affect the toxicity of chemicals. Toxicity is affected by factors such as gender, age, lifestyle, diet, genetics, and disease states. Further, **exposure pathways**, or the route by which a chemical enters

LEVELS OF PREVENTION PYRAMID

SITUATION: *Healthy People 2020* Pesticides Exposures

TERTIARY PREVENTION

Rehabilitation	Primary Prevention
Call Poison Control Center at 1-800-222-1222 HAZMAT teams Disaster preparedness	Health Education: Educate employers and workers about the Material Safety Data Sheets to understand hazardous chemicals Health Protection: Advocate for safe use of pesticides and prepare for emergencies

SECONDARY PREVENTION

Early Diagnosis	Prompt Treatment
Recognition of early signs or pesticide poisoning. Laboratory screening for pesticide toxicity (blood or urine samples)	Poisoning signs can be seen, for example, vomiting, sweating, or pinpoint pupils. Symptoms are any functional changes in normal condition that can be described by the victim of poisoning and may include nausea, headache, weakness, dizziness, and others. National Pesticide Information Center http://npic.orst.edu/ingred/index.html

PRIMARY PREVENTION

Health Promotion and Education	Health Protection
Educate community members to reduce exposures to pesticides in their homes and outdoor areas. Educate employers and workers about the Safety Data Sheets to understand hazardous chemicals.	Advocate for community level policy to restrict exposures to hazardous chemicals in pesticides in public places and use IPM for schools and playgrounds Advocate for safe use of pesticides and prepare for emergencies

the body, can affect toxicity, absorption, and metabolism. For example, children have less well-developed metabolic processes and are less able to detoxify chemical exposures. Likewise, older adults have reduced defense mechanisms in their lungs, skin, and other systems that make them more prone to adverse health effects (Leffers, 2015). Nurses can learn more about toxicology through the National Library of Medicine (2011) TOXNET site available at http://toxnet.nlm.nih.gov/.

It is important to understand that although health care screening does not test for most hazardous chemicals, some studies highlight the importance of biomonitoring. **Biomonitoring** refers to body burden of toxic chemicals or, more precisely, the "standard for assessing people's exposure to toxic substances as well as for responding to serious environmental public health problems" (CDC, 2015d, para. 1). Nurses can learn more about the CDC National Biomonitoring Program on the CDC Web site (CDC, 2015e).

Risk assessment is a process that uses scientific information by identifying and evaluating adverse events to aid in judgments about hazards in the environment. The process uses hazard identification, the dose response assessment, and exposure assessment to characterize risk. As scientists identify health risks from epidemiology and toxicology, government agencies must determine how to regulate hazards. For example, the EPA uses risk assessments to "characterize the nature and magnitude of health risks to humans (e.g. residents, workers, recreational visitors) and ecological receptors (e.g. birds, fish, wildlife) from chemical contaminants and other stressors that may be present in the environment" (EPA, 2015d). **Risk management** requires that judgments be made about the significance of those risks (Frumkin, 2010; Maxwell, 2014).

Public Health Nursing Assessments

In public health nursing practice, nurses routinely complete a variety of assessments for individuals, families, groups, and communities. There are a number of assessment tools available to help guide both PHNs and the people they serve in order to assess environmental health risks.

What do *you* think?

How many chemicals do you come in contact with on a daily basis? Of particular interest to nurses is the study conducted by Physicians for Social Responsibility (PSR) and titled *Hazardous Chemicals in Health Care: Snapshot of Chemicals in Doctors and Nurses*. This study involved the testing of 20 American doctors and nurses from a variety of practice settings for six chemicals or chemical groups totaling 62 chemicals. Each participant was found to have at least 24 hazardous chemicals in their bodies. This study is significant not only to health care workers but also to their patients who are exposed to the same health care environments and chemicals (PSR, 2015). In addition, the Environmental Working Group (EWG) (2012) video, *10 Americans*, referenced in the "How safe is your home and hospital?" exercise at the end of this chapter is a compelling argument for body burden and the importance of biomonitoring. Blood draws from a random sample of 10 Americans showed that they had 287 chemicals in their bloodstream representing exposures from waste products, commonly used chemicals in the home, as well as more than 200 chemicals and pesticides that were banned more than 30 years ago (EWG, 2012).

Environmental Working Group. (2015). *10 Americans (video)*. Retrieved from http://www.ewg.org/news/videos/10-americans
Physicians for Social Responsibility. (2015). Hazardous chemicals in health care: Snapshots of chemicals in doctors and nurses. Retrieved from http://www.psr.org/assets/pdfs/hazardous-chemicals-in-health-care.pdf

Individual Assessments

At the individual level, individuals should complete a personal environmental health exposure assessment. Ideally, this should be part of every health visit, workplace assessment, or other health history. Though humans share some characteristics for environmental exposures, their individual risks from work, home, school, and recreation all contribute to their overall risk. The ATSDR provides continuing education credits for learning about a variety of environmental risks and how to take an exposure history. This is available at their Web site (http://www.atsdr.cdc.gov/csem/conteduc.html). In addition, they created an environmental exposure history card using the mnemonic "I PREPARE" to aid nurses and other health professionals in adding environmental health exposure questions to patient assessment. This tool that is both brief and easy to remember can be incorporated into any health assessment easily. Pocket-sized guides are available for order on the ATSDR Web site (see Table 9–3).

While completing an individual assessment, it is important to consider those exposures specific to the workplace, school, or neighborhood. Workplace exposures are often addressed by OHNs and include not only physical hazards such as injuries from machinery, burns, falls, and crushing injuries but also hazardous exposure to toxic chemicals, particulate matter in the form of dust, VOCs and aerosols, heavy metals, and other chemicals that can contribute to poor indoor air quality (EPA, 2015o). See Chapter 31.

School nurses often address children's and adults' exposures in school settings, but it is very important for PHNs to identify potential risks in order to educate parents about environmental hazards in the school setting. Similar to the workplace, many schools have issues of poor indoor air quality with the increased use of synthetics in building materials and reduced access to outdoor air. Neighborhood exposures affect individual health, but are discussed in the community assessment section of this chapter. Specifically important to assess for hazards among school-aged children are the routes taken to school and playgrounds. See Chapter 30.

Home Assessments

PHNs generally conduct home assessments when making a visit to a client's home for case finding, follow-up, screening, or other public health services. Home assessments often involve looking for safety hazards in the home, but do not always include potential hazardous environmental toxic exposures. Families can be exposed to a number of serious environmental toxins in their own homes. Allison Del Bene Davis, PhD, RN created a *Home Environmental Health and Safety Assessment Tool* at the University of Maryland Environmental Health Education Center that is easy to use and addresses key exposure topics (Davis, 2007). These are grouped in areas such as the home itself, source of heat, gas appliances, source of water and lead pipes, fire safety, and carbon monoxide detector. This is available at http://envirn.org/pg/file/read/4387/home-environmental-health-amp-safety-assessment-tool. The EWG (2015) offers a *Healthy Home Checklist* available on their Web site, and the National Center for Healthy Housing (2015) published their checklist as well. In addition, PHNs must assess the home for environmental tobacco smoke, possibility of asbestos in the home, lead paint, and other hazardous materials. PHNs should ensure that the family has their home tested for radon (EPA, 2015x, 2015w). Likewise, family members should be reminded to safely dispose of their mercury thermometers and any other devices containing mercury. Cleaning products, paints, varnishes, strippers and other home remodeling materials, gardening fertilizers and pesticides, pest management insecticides and other materials, air fresheners, and presence of mold and moisture can all be sources of exposure in the home and land around the home (Butterfield, Hill, Postma, Butterfield, & Odom-Maryon, 2011). Pets can bring pesticides applied to lawns and gardens into the home, and adults and children can carry pesticides into the home on their shoes (see Chapter 29). Finally, a home assessment should address nearby environmental hazards or potential sources of hazards such as coal-fired power plants, farms, industries, **brownfields** (properties where pollutants, contaminants, or hazardous substances may be present), toxic waste sites, highways, and contaminated waterways (EPA, 2015f). Frequently, these hazards

Table 9-3   Environmental Health Assessment "I PREPARE"

Mnemonic Cue	Examples of Questions
I Investigate potential exposures	Have you ever felt sick after coming in contact with a chemical, pesticide, or other substance? Do you have any symptoms that improve when you are away from your usual location (e.g., home or work)?
P Present work	Are you exposed to solvents, dusts, fumes, radiation, loud noise, pesticides, or other chemicals? Do you know where to find Safety Data Sheets on chemicals that you work with? Do you wear personal protective equipment? Are work clothes worn home? Do coworkers have similar health problems?
R Residence	When was your residence built? What type of heating do you have? Have you recently remodeled your home? What chemicals are stored on your property? Where does your drinking water come from?
E Environmental concerns	Are there environmental concerns in your neighborhood (i.e., air, water, soil)? What types of industries or farms are near your home? Do you live near a hazardous waste site or landfill?
P Past work	What are your past work experiences? What is the longest job held? Have you ever been in the military, worked on a farm, or done volunteer or seasonal work?
A Activities	In what type of activities and hobbies do you and your family engage in? Do you burn, solder, or melt any products? Do you garden, fish, or hunt? Do you eat what you catch or grow? Do you use pesticides? Do you engage in any alternative healing or cultural practices?
R Referrals and resources	Use these key referrals and resources: Agency for Toxic Substances and Disease Registry www.atsdr.cdc.gov Association of Occupational and Environmental Clinics www.aoec.org Environmental Protection Agency www.epa.gov Safety Data Sheets https://www.osha.gov/Publications/HazComm_QuickCard_SafetyData.html Occupational Safety and Health Administration www.osha.gov Local Health Department, Environmental Agency, Poison Control Center
E Educate	Are materials available to educate the patient? Are alternatives available to minimize the risk of exposure? Have prevention strategies been discussed? What is the plan for follow-up?

From Agency for Toxic Substances and Disease Registry. (n.d.). *Environmental exposure history*. Retrieved from http://www.atsdr.cdc.gov/asbestos/site-kit/docs/IPrepareCard.pdf

are visible in the neighborhood, but often, there are hidden routes of exposure from contaminated groundwater, ambient air, and contaminated soil. See Table 9–4 for Common Hazards in the Home Setting.

Community Assessments

A comprehensive community health assessment considers environmental factors in a number of ways. In Chapter 15 of this book, community health assessment is introduced with a focus on aspects of the community that promote health or provide risks to health. Environment refers to more than the natural environment but also includes the **built environment**, that is, all structures (homes, schools, workplaces, and business areas), roadways, and parks or recreational areas. It includes waste disposal areas and changes in land use for agriculture and other purposes. The impact of the built environment includes both indoor and outdoor physical environments, which in turn affect social environments where people live, work, and engage with others (Lopez, 2012).

Table 9–4   Common Hazards in the Home Setting

Hazard	Source	Exposure Pathway	Risk Groups	Health Effects
Asbestos	Asbestos is a fiber that has been used for insulation and as a fire retardant Used in shipbuilding and other occupational exposures to metal work	Inhalation	Children of metal workers Home residents	Lung cancer (mesothelioma) and lung disease
Arsenic	Used in pressure-treated wood, was formerly used in industrial sites, can be present in soil and water	Drinking water Inhalation from indoor or outdoor air	Children playing in playgrounds with pressure-treated wood, those with contaminated water supply	High levels are lethal. Exposure can cause decreased red and white blood cells
Carbon monoxide	Colorless and odorless gas that is a by-product of combustion from home heating sources as well as automobiles housed in attached garage	Inhalation	Persons with respiratory and cardiovascular disease	Unconsciousness and death due to hypoxia
Environmental tobacco smoke	Cigarette smoking	Inhalation	Those people in area where smoking occurs in indoor space/home	Lung disease; lung cancer; cardiovascular problems
Formaldehyde	Carpeting, particle board, glues, adhesives used in home construction, or decorating Also some personal care products	Inhalation		Cancer
Lead	Paint used prior to 1978; leaded gasoline prior to ban in 1970s; ceramics, pottery, pipes, soil; some alternative medical therapies	Ingestion from dust in home or soil	Children	Nervous system
Mold	Normal growth of fungi in and outside of home Can produce VOCs	Spores travel in the air Inhalation	Those people most sensitive to molds	Respiratory symptoms
Pests	Mites, cockroaches	Inhalation, physical contact with droppings	Children and those with asthma	Exacerbation of asthma
Pesticides	Used in homes and outside lawns and gardens to protect plants from pests, home from insects	Indoor or outdoor air; inhalation Dermal absorption	Children All people exposed	Specific types of pesticides have been linked to neurological problems, others to cancer, and many as EDCs.
Radon	Naturally occurring radioactive gas	Seeps into homes through cracks in foundation of home; inhalation	Residents of home	Lung damage particularly lung cancer
Solvents such as paint thinners, varnishes, and resins (ethers)	Dry cleaning, home improvements	Inhalation Percutaneous absorption	Home residents	Neurological problems renal, liver, and reproductive effects
Personal care products	Shampoo, soaps, cosmetics	Percutaneous	Individuals using them, children, adolescents	Varied EDCs, cancer, and neurological effects
Volatile organic compounds (VOCs)	Alcohols, ketones, and esters that are present in thousands of products such as paint thinners, cleaning supplies, pesticides, building materials, office equipment, copiers, printers, glues, adhesives	Inhalation	Those exposed in indoor settings	Eye, nose, and throat irritation; headaches; kidney damage; and central nervous system disorders

Community assessment is central to public health nursing practice and to the core functions of public health. For environmental health, it is imperative that nurses incorporate key assessment data into the overall assessment in order to identify community risks from environmental sources. Typically, a *windshield* or walking survey is very useful for observation of environmental hazards (see Chapter 15). By incorporating knowledge of likely hazards in the community, the PHNs can identify many possible toxins simply by observation while traveling in the community. Various tools have been developed to assist nurses in their work. Though most community assessment tools address environment, it is important that PHNs also consider specific threats for areas more broadly assessed. For air quality, nurses should look for visible sources of air pollution from smokestacks, identify exhaust from various vehicles, and learn of significant industries, power sources, and incinerators in the community. To better understand water quality, PHNs must identify the source of drinking water as public or private, understand water treatment and quality, recognize evidence of pollution and whether there are fish alerts for local waterways, examine stagnant water and possible vectors, and identify issues related to sewer function and possible overflow and contamination as well as likelihood of floods and other water emergencies. Land use is another area for possible exposures. Nurses must assess not only the current land use but also how the land was formerly used. **Superfund** refers to funding made possible by the Comprehensive Environmental Response, Compensation, and Liability Act of 1980 to address those contaminated areas of the United States that needed to be remediated; the EPA administers the funding. Well-known examples are Love Canal in New York State and Times Beach, Missouri. Nurses must be aware of such sites in their communities that are listed on the National Priorities List and can be located by searching on the EPA Web site (EPA, 2015ee). Brownfield sites refer to real "property, the expansion, redevelopment, or reuse of which may be complicated by the presence or potential presence of a hazardous substance, pollutant, or contaminant" (EPA, 2015g, para. 2). These sites may remain undeveloped in communities but can also be redeveloped for public or private use. Playgrounds and schools that have been built upon former brownfield sites alarm community residents who often express concerns for the safety of their children. The EPA Brownfields Program seeks to ensure that the hazards are removed prior to redevelopment. The EPA also promotes the successful redevelopment of sites such as the redevelopment of a former petroleum storage terminal used from 1922 until 1977 into the Festival Pier in Pawtucket, RI. The former brownfield was dismantled and the land donated to the city where it sat unused and contaminated. In the spring of 2015, the Rhode Island Department of Environmental Management completed cleanup activities, removing contaminated soil and capping the entire property. Redevelopment of the area included planting of trees to remediate the groundwater and creating recreational areas for picnics, fishing, boat ramps, and viewing area for the annual Dragon Boat Races (EPA, 2015dd). This example is not unique, but one of thousands of instances of urban and rural communities nationwide that address the risks in their community and have a voice to advocate for the citizens of their localities.

Built Environment

The built environment refers to all aspects of our human environment that are not naturally occurring and includes not only the physical structures (e.g., dams, roadways, buildings) but also the features that contribute to social cohesiveness or disruption (Fig. 9–3). For the last decade, environmental health experts have called for a shift from a focus on disease causation that can result from a lack of discipline and poor lifestyle choices, to a focus that examines how the built environment contributes to health (Jackson, 2012; Srinivasan, O'Fallon, & Dearry, 2003). Evidence suggests that many physical and mental health problems are related to the built environment, such as asthma, cardiovascular disease, lung conditions, obesity, and cancer. Efforts to conduct research that demonstrates the positive effect of well-designed communities with safe walking and biking paths, environmentally safe public transportation, public spaces to encourage social interaction, and accessible green spaces for recreation will provide evidence to help increase efforts for improving the built environment for better health. Neighborhoods must be designed to encourage social interaction such as parks with shady areas that encourage people to congregate, ponds and trees that also help our ecological environment, and safe walkways and bikeways for access (Jackson, 2012).

PHNs also must assess the quality of the housing stock. Buildings that were constructed prior to 1978 are likely to have lead-based paint. Homes or buildings constructed between 1930 and 1950 are likely to have asbestos in the insulation as well as in the hot water and steam pipes (U.S. Consumer Product Safety Commission, n.d.). The overall condition of the community indicates sanitation factors, safe waste disposal, and contamination sources in the community. The location of schools, playgrounds, and public transportation and access to green spaces should be part of the community assessment. Examination of the overall community environment provides community health nurses with essential information about how the residents can use the environment to maintain health or how the residents are more likely to

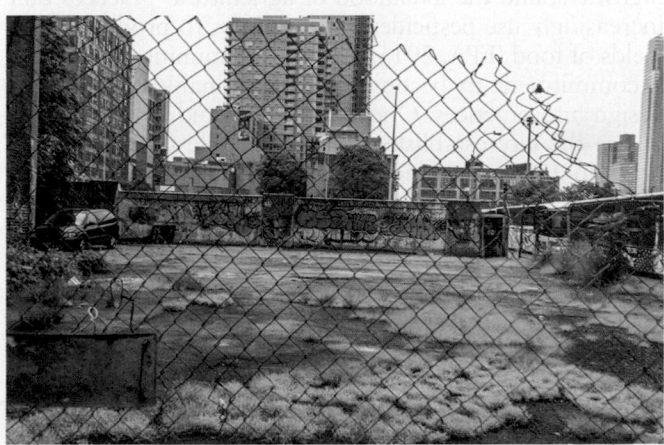

FIGURE 9–3 Neighborhoods, or the built environment, can contribute to population health or illness.

PERSPECTIVES—A STUDENT VIEWPOINT OF COMMUNITY HEALTH NURSING, ENVIRONMENTAL HEALTH

I am a senior nursing student who works as a collegiate aide in the hospital while I complete my nursing program. This semester I am learning about environmental health in my public health nursing course. We learned about the work of nurses to improve health care environments. I recalled a story my mother told me about when she was a nursing student and worked as a student aide years ago. She had been exposed to a cleaning product used on the floors that had been left in the hallway and overturned onto the stairway where she walked to her unit. She had a severe skin reaction to the cleaning product and had to visit employee health. This really got me thinking about all the chemicals used in the hospital where I work. I decided to see if my hospital had a Green Team and if nurses were involved with it. Once I began my quest, I found that indeed my hospital had a Green Team and was hard at work to improve purchasing in order to reduce harmful exposures and increase the use of safer products for hospital use, as well as efforts to reduce medical waste. I decided to learn more about products and looked first at the

USDHHS Household Products Database http://householdproducts.nlm.nih.gov/ to learn more about the types of exposures that I and my patients might have in the hospital setting. I looked at the personal care products, the cleaners, pesticides, and maintenance products and thought how many are used regularly in the hospital. Because there were no nurses on the Green Team, I contacted the Green Team, and they invited me to come to one of their meetings. From the team members, I learned about two organizations, Practice Greenhealth (https://practicegreenhealth.org/) and Health Care Without Harm (https://noharm.org/) that both work to improve health care settings to be safer and more sustainable. As a student, I was thrilled to be part of the work and have now invited members of the unit where I work to join in as well. Though I have not decided what area of nursing might be my future professional focus, I know that I will include environmental health in my work!

Anna, senior nursing student

be at risk for adverse health outcomes. See Perspectives: A Student Viewpoint of Community Health Nursing, Environmental Health.

Sustainable Communities

Community assessments can provide evidence that a community is striving to be sustainable in practices to promote health for community members and to protect the natural environment. The President's Council in 1993 defined sustainable communities as "healthy communities where natural and historic resources are preserved, jobs are available, sprawl is contained, neighborhoods are secure, education is lifelong, transportation and health care are accessible, and all citizens have opportunities to improve the quality of their lives" (Clinton, n.d., para. 8). This definition uses examples that are often considered causes of unsustainable practices such as urban sprawl that increases automobile use, use of highways, and the likelihood of agricultural practices that increasingly use pesticides and products to produce larger yields of food (EPA, 2015j). Many communities have made a commitment to become more sustainable in their city design and practices. One example is Oakland, California where the city established a "Sustainable Oakland" program in 1997. Oakland had suffered from poor land use planning that created many sources for toxic exposures, noted by high rates of asthma and other environmentally related health problems (Jackson, 2012). Their goal is to provide city residents opportunities to live safe, happy, and healthy lives through sustainable development. They focus upon buildings, energy, climate, housing, land use, transportation, waste, natural resources, health, safety, education, and economic prosperity. The city has been recognized as a bicycle-friendly city, a top ten city by the National Resource Defense Council, a top ten sustainable city, and recognition for solar efforts, storm management, and climate protection. Recent activities include the Energy

and Climate Action Plan and the Sustainable Oakland 2013 to 2014 Report (City of Oakland, California, 2015). See Population Focus.

Climate Change

Climate issues are a great concern for health. In the community assessment, the nurse can note the presence of animal and insect vectors that can transmit disease. With **climate change**, there have been changes in the distribution of infection due to global warming. For example, locally transmitted malaria has been reported in Florida, Georgia, and Texas. Scientists track these changes and note that health professionals must be aware of the changing patterns of disease transmission from warming trends. In addition, there will likely be risks related to food and water quality and availability, heat stress for those most vulnerable, increased air pollution, and severe weather-related events. Vulnerable populations such as infants, children, and older adults must be protected from the impacts of climate change (U.S. Global Change Research Program, 2015). Severe weather events such as flooding, droughts, hurricanes, and tornados require emergency preparedness and disaster response from the public health sector. Specifically, PHNs must be prepared for surge events with skills such as the ability to (1) be personally prepared, (2) comprehend state and local disaster plans, (3) conduct a rapid needs assessment, (4) investigate outbreaks, (5) perform public health triages, (6) communicate risk effectively, (7) participate effectively in mass dispensing interventions, and (8) respond post event to the debriefing and public health impact of the event (Polivka et al., 2008).

Nurses are working to disseminate timely and accurate information for nursing practice through resources and collaboration with national organizations. All nurses

POPULATION-FOCUS
ON SUSTAINABLE COMMUNITIES

In public health nursing, the focus on community or population is often used synonymously. In contrast to clinical experiences early in undergraduate nursing education, the community/public health nursing curriculum uses a population approach to assessment and planning (Callen et al., 2013). Most nursing theories focus upon individual or families as the focus of nursing care. Fawcett and Ellenbacker (2015) propose a conceptual model for population health and nursing practice. They define a population focus as "life span wellness and disease experiences of aggregate groups of people residing in local, state, national or international geographic regions or those population with common characteristics." (p. 290). Conceptual model elements include upstream factors, socioeconomic environment, physical environment, population factors, genetic factors, behavioral factors, physiological factors, resilience, health state, health care system factors, providers, organizations and institutions, hospitals, inpatient and outpatient clinics, community health centers, home health care agencies, payers, policies, nursing activities, population-based nursing practice processes, culturally appropriate wellness, promotion, restoration and maintenance, culturally appropriate disease prevention, population health outcomes, population-level wellness, population-level functional status, population-level life expectancy, population-level mortality, and population-level quality of life. The upstream factors look at social

determinants of health; socioeconomic factors such as income, education, and employment; and physical environment factors such as atmosphere, air, pollutants, weather, housing, radiation, and the built environment. These upstream factors help nurses to understand the broad population-level factors that impact communities. Like root cause analysis, a systems approach used by hospital staff to analyze adverse events, analysis of upstream factors helps to determine underlying problems. Current emphasis upon sustainable communities by agencies such as the EPA include indicators such as land use, walkability, access to recreational areas, crime rates, access to healthy food options, brownfield remediation, transportation, bicycle accessibility, and housing. Bridgeport, Connecticut, set goals to become Green 2020 with grant funding from three federal agencies: the EPA, DOT, and Housing and Human Development. The video available at https://www.sustainablecommunities.gov/video/bridgeport-connecticut helps us learn how sustainable communities can promote health and address population health.

Callen, B., Smith, C., Joyce, B., Lutz, J., Brown-Schott, N., & Block, D. (2013). Teaching/learning strategies for the essentials of baccalaureate nursing education for entry-level community/public health nursing. *Public Health Nursing,* 30(6), 537–547.
Fawcett, J. & Ellenbacker, C. H. (2015). A proposed conceptual model of nursing and population health. Nursing Outlook, 63(3), 288–298.

must understand the implications of climate change upon health. The ANHE offers information about the work of Laura Anderko, PhD, RN; Stephanie Chalupka, EdD, RN, PHCNS-BC, FAAOHN; and Brenda M. Afzal, MS, RN, all nurses with public health expertise that collaborated with the Catholic Health Association (ANHE, 2015c). With funding from the U.S. Climate Action Network, nurses also developed a set of modules to address clean air and climate available on the ANHE Web site (ANHE, 2015a). This includes an opportunity for continuing education credit based upon a workbook and three video modules. In addition, the U.S. Global Change Research Program releases the full report, *Impacts of Climate Change on Human Health in the U.S.: A Scientific Assessment,* for the public in early 2016.

Land Use

Topics that must be considered to address land use for a community health assessment include zoning regulations and enforcement, industries and their toxic releases, types of transportation with an emphasis upon sidewalks, bikeways, public transportation, recreational space including green space, what fertilizers or pesticides are applied to the fields, safe play areas for children, and information regarding a tree ordinance to promote health environments (EPA, 2015j). School locations should be examined for accessibility by foot or bicycle, surrounding area,

and the use of pesticides on school fields. The community should be assessed for commercial lots, their safety and use, and vacant lots or unused property. Specific commercial businesses such as gas stations, auto repair shops, and dry cleaners are often sources of toxic exposures. If the community has agricultural areas, these must be assessed for irritation practices, use of pesticides, runoff, and land use practices. In addition, waste can be a source of environmental hazards so PHNs must assess the presence of landfills or municipal waste incinerators, medical waste incinerators, and municipal trash collection or presence of dumpsters throughout the community.

Recent evidence suggests that land use and transportation patterns and plans can influence the health of the community. The design of a city, community, or neighborhood affects physical activity, automobile dependence, ability of those of older age and those with physical disabilities to navigate the community, and opportunities for children to walk to school. Community design also highlights concerns for environmental justice when those who live in areas of low accessibility and high exposure to pollution are more likely to be of minority status or living in poverty. Researchers call for further research that will include walking as an indicator of community health; measuring physical activity levels and contributory factors; examining the public health consequences of public safety design choices; determining the types and determinants of travel to school; examining the influence of community design on risk of injury; explaining the influence of community design on emissions of overall and specific pollutants; measuring physical activity, mobility, and social integration in persons with disabilities; characterizing social equity and health outcomes in relation to community design; and examining the influence of physical setting characteristics on mental health. For example, zoning codes that require minimum requirements for parking areas per housing unit but do not require sidewalks promote dependence upon automobile travel that increases air emissions and poor air quality, possible water contamination from auto exhaust, risk of injury, or death and reduce opportunities for safe areas for physical activity (Dannenberg et al., 2003; Jackson, 2012; Lopez, 2012).

Types of Toxic Exposures

Air

Air quality is a major variable in the health of populations. Those geographic areas that suffer poor air quality demonstrate higher rates of disease and adverse health effects. As we have discussed, climate change contributes to air pollution and adversely affects health. Ambient air, the air humans breathe, can be affected by a number of air pollutants. Air pollution is composed of a number of materials such as aerosols, criteria air pollutants (carbon monoxide, lead, ground-level ozone, nitrogen dioxide, sulfur dioxide, particulate matter), volatile organic compounds (VOCs), hydrofluorocarbons, as well as radon and other gases that contain toxins harmful to health. In response to the Clean Air Act of 1970, air quality is monitored by the EPA. The public is informed of air quality through the AQI that is often reported in media sources on a daily basis. The AQI measures the criteria air pollutants in communities to see if they exceed the national air quality standard set by the EPA. The EPA publishes a *Plain English Guide to the Clean Air Act* available on their Web site for the public to learn more about air quality (EPA, 2015u, 2015ff).

Reports from the EPA monitoring of air pollution indicate that from 1990 to 2010, the overall levels of the six major pollutants measured by the federal government (carbon monoxide, ozone, sulfur dioxide, nitrogen dioxide, lead, and particulate matter) declined by a high of 83% for lead and a low of 17% for ozone because of cleaner cars, industries, and consumer products. However, millions of people live in areas that exceeded the national ambient air quality standard (NAAQS) set by the EPA (2012b). Additionally, as discussed earlier, climate can adversely affect outdoor air quality.

The outdoor and indoor air humans breathe can be affected by a variety of factors. Ambient air, or that air that is composed of gases such as nitrogen, oxygen, argon, carbon dioxide, hydrogen, neon, helium, and other gases, is part of the atmosphere. It also contains moisture and particulate matter. The amount of hazardous matter that is contained in ambient air is the reason that the Clean Air Act of 1970 was created. In an effort to inform citizens about the air quality in their own community, the EPA created the AQI as seen in Table 9–5. The AQI is a tool to report daily air quality in communities. It is calculated for four of the six criteria air pollutants (ground-level ozone, particle pollution, carbon monoxide, and sulfur dioxide) with an emphasis upon how these affect health. On their Web site, they provide a

Table 9–5 Air Quality Index

AQI Value	Level of Health Concern	Color
When AQI is in this range…	Air quality conditions are….	As symbolized by this color
0–50	Good	Green
51–100	Moderate	Yellow
101–150	Unhealthy for sensitive groups	Orange
151–200	Unhealthy	Red
201–300	Very unhealthy	Purple
301–500	Hazardous	Maroon

AIRNow. (2016). *Air Quality Index (AQI)—A guide to air quality and your health*. Retrieved from http://www.airnow.gov/index.cfm?action=aqi_brochure.index
Each category corresponds to a different level of health concern. The six levels of health concern and what they mean are:
- "Good" AQI is 0–50. Air quality is considered satisfactory, and air pollution poses little or no risk.
- "Moderate" AQI is 51–100. Air quality is acceptable; however, for some pollutants, there may be a moderate health concern for a very small number of people. For example, people who are unusually sensitive to ozone may experience respiratory symptoms.
- "Unhealthy for sensitive groups" AQI is 101–150. Although general public is not likely to be affected at this AQI range, people with lung disease, older adults, and children are at a greater risk from exposure to ozone, whereas persons with heart and lung disease, older adults, and children are at greater risk from the presence of particles in the air.
- "Unhealthy" AQI is 151–200. Everyone may begin to experience some adverse health effects, and members of the sensitive groups may experience more serious effects.
- "Very unhealthy" AQI is 201–300. This would trigger a health alert signifying that everyone may experience more serious health effects.
- "Hazardous" AQI >300. This would trigger a health warning of emergency conditions. The entire population is more likely to be affected.

Environmental Protection Agency. (2016). *Air quality index (AQI) basics*. Retrieved from http://www.airnow.gov/index.cfm?action=aqibasics.aqi

guide for citizens to understand the importance of monitoring the ambient air, what the six criteria air pollutants are and how they affect health, and efforts to monitor air quality to provide public health advisories (EPA, 2015c). See Table 9–5: Air Quality Index.

PHNs must understand the adverse effects of ambient air pollution in order to assess, monitor, and advocate for those most vulnerable that includes children, people with lung disease, older adults, and even healthy individuals who are active outdoors. Health effects include irritation of the respiratory system with inflammation of the cell lining. This makes the lungs more susceptible to infection. Air pollution can also exacerbate asthma and cause chronic lung disease, reduced lung function, and permanent lung damage. In addition, air pollution causes increased risk of cardiac disease, in particular acute myocardial infarctions and arrhythmias (EPA, 2015c). Indoor air quality is particularly important for home, school, and workplace assessments. During advisories when the ambient AQI is high and people are asked to remain inside, humans are exposed to those pollutants that commonly affect indoor air. Air pollution in homes occurs from exposure to heating or combustion sources such as oil, coal, kerosene or wood, radon gas, secondhand smoke from cigarettes, building materials and furniture that contains pressed wood products, carpeting and adhesives that emit VOCs, asbestos in insulation, cleaning products, paints, varnishes, and paint removers, personal care products, and other sources used around the home such as pesticides. Mild health effects might be headaches and nausea; the more serious health effects include damage

to the liver, kidneys, and central nervous system, as well as cancer. In addition, molds, dust, and known asthma triggers in the home can not only exacerbate the asthma symptoms but also cause irritation to those with heart and lung conditions. Air quality in school buildings is very important for staff, teachers, and students. More than 56 million children and adults spend up to 6 to 8 hours in elementary and secondary school each day. In particular, children are at increased risk for a variety of reasons. Young children are more likely to spend time on or near the floor where toxins are likely to settle; they use more hand-to-mouth behavior, and they take in more air per size than adults. Although exposures can be the same as in the home, those who attend or work in schools are in the same air environment for 6 to 8 hours or more where they are exposed to the toxins for long periods of time (EPA, 2015bb). Nurses who work in the school setting can access information through the EPA Web site to aid in assessments and interventions in order to improve air quality in schools. A comprehensive guide to healthier school environments is available on their Web site (EPA, 2012c). In addition, the EPA offers guidance for healthy buildings that includes information on design, construction, renovation, cleaning, and maintenance as well as efficiency improvement advice (EPA, 2015o). See Evidence-Based Practice.

Water

The human body is composed of upward of 50% to 60% water. So too, water is necessary for human survival. In public health, the concern is for safe water consumption;

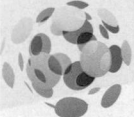

EVIDENCE-BASED PRACTICE
Local and Global Issues

What Must PHNs Know About Climate Change?

The Obama Administration, the EPA, and the APHA all call for the public health community and for health care providers to play a critical role in addressing issues of health protection and climate solutions. An important role for community and PHNs is that of disaster preparedness (also see Chapter 17 for more information on this important topic). The report, Climate Change and Health: Is There a Role for the Health Care Sector?, provides important information to help nurses learn about health risks from climate change (Anderko, Chalupka & Afzal, 2012). Because climate change has increased the number of climate events globally, such as hurricanes, flooding, forest fires, and severe storms, we witness an increase in not only in the number disasters but other health impacts as well. These impacts include poor birth outcomes, malnutrition, water quality and disease, vector-borne diseases, respiratory diseases, and psychological impacts. Certain vulnerable populations such as infants, children, and older adults are at higher risk for adverse health outcomes as well at those living in poverty. This is a global health issue for all nurses.

Polivka, Chaudry, and Crawford (2012) concur that this is an important role for nurses, in particular PHNs. To address this, they surveyed 786 practicing PHNs (with a response rate of $n = 176$) to identify their knowledge and attitudes regarding climate change. The majority of the sample identified air quality–related illnesses, flooding-related displacement, vector-borne diseases, and mental health conditions as health impacts of climate change, but they did not identify food and water impacts. However, the respondents did acknowledge a role for PHNs to address the health impacts of climate change for the populations they serve. The evidence indicates that all nurses and in particular PHNs across the globe must have the knowledge and skills to address health impacts of climate change in their practice.

Anderko, L., Chalupka, S., & Afzal, B. M. (2012). *Climate change and health: Is there a role for the health care sector?* Washington, DC: Catholic Health Association.
Polivka, B., Chaudry, R., & Crawford, J. (2012). Public health nurses knowledge and attitudes regarding climate change. *Environmental Health Perspectives, 120*(3), 321–325.

EVIDENCE-BASED PRACTICE

Indoor Air Quality in Schools

School environments can influence child health. This has been demonstrated in research studies. For example, environmental triggers have been shown to worsen asthma symptoms in children. The Louisiana Asthma Management and Prevention Program initiated an Asthma-Friendly Schools project that addressed improvement in the school environment, along with individualized asthma action plans and school policy changes in order to improve asthma outcomes in 70 public schools. After the changes to improve indoor air quality (and reduce asthma triggers), institution of policy changes that permitted students to carry asthma medication with them, and the improved adherence to asthma action plans, researchers noted that asthma-related symptoms and problems were improved (Nuss et al., 2016).

Traffic-related air pollution has been associated with adverse health effects, including decreased cognitive development in schoolchildren attending schools in close proximity to high-traffic areas (Sunyer et al., 2015). Canadian researchers wanted to know if changes in the timing of outdoor air intake might reduce the concentration levels of traffic-related pollutants in schools. They changed the ventilation timing so that it did not move air into schools during periods of rush hour traffic and studied it over a 2-month period in four school buildings. They noted statistically significant reductions in most pollutant concentrations with this intervention and recommended timing changes for outdoor air intake ventilation, especially for schools near high-traffic areas or major roadways (MacNeil et al., 2015).

MacNeil, M., Dobbin, N., St-Jean, M., Wallace, L., Marro, L., ... Wheeler, A. J. (2015). Can changing the timing of outdoor air intake reduce indoor concentrations of traffic-related pollutants in schools? *Indoor Air.* doi: 10.1111/ina.12252

Nuss, H. J., Hester, L. L., Perry, M. A., Stewart-Briley, C., Reagon, V. M., & Collins, P. (2016). Applying the social ecological model to creating asthma-friendly schools in Louisiana. *Journal of School Health, 86*(3), 225–232.

Sunyer, J., Esnaola, M., Alvarez-Pederol, M., Forns, J., Rivas, I., Lopez-Vicente, M., ... Querol, X. (2015). Association between traffic-related air pollution in schools and cognitive development in primary school children: A prospective cohort study. *PLoS Medicine, 12*(3), e1001792.

safe lakes, rivers, and streams for recreation; and safe waterways to support animal and plant life necessary for transport of nutrients and ecology of the environment. Globally, the availability of clean water is becoming a very serious threat to human survival. Globally, 748 million people lack access to safe water, and in 2012, approximately 2.5 million did not have access to an improved sanitation facility creating threats to safe water (United Nations, 2015). Poverty is linked with lack of access to clean water and sanitation globally (Fig. 9–4). Reports identify the lack of safe drinking water as the leading cause of hunger, disease, and poverty worldwide (Global Water, 2015).

Water in the environment is available in two forms: surface water and groundwater. Lakes, rivers, and streams are examples of surface water, as is the surface run off from rainfall. Groundwater is found in underground aquifers that run beneath the surface of the earth. Both are sources of contamination or pollution. Drinking water is available from both surface and groundwater. Surface water sources include lakes, streams, and municipal reservoirs for water use. Underground sources include aquifers that run beneath the ground level and are reached via wells and springs. Many municipalities use reservoirs and other surface sources for their water supply, whereas in many areas, people must rely upon wells to provide their source of water. Safe drinking water is essential for human health. Public water systems provide water for community members through pipes for human consumption. More than 90% of Americans are

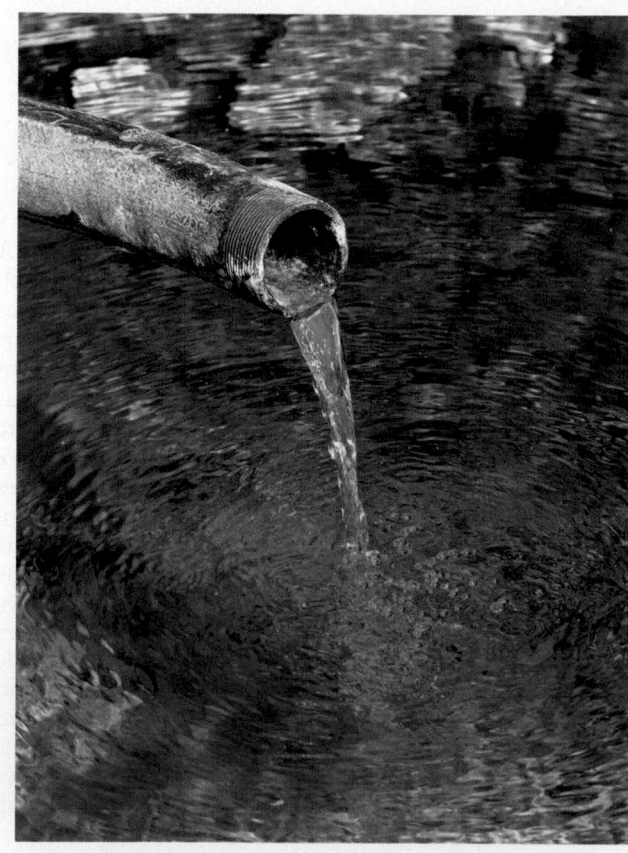

FIGURE 9–4 Clean water is vital to life and health.

served by public water systems. Public water systems are monitored and regulated through the EPA. These regulations require that public water suppliers protect consumers from microorganisms that are harmful to health. The EPA does not regulate private sources of water from private wells, and individual users must be responsible for monitoring their own wells. As a result, those using

private wells are likely to have fecal contamination or microorganisms in their water as well as a number of toxic agents that are linked to bladder, kidney, and liver cancers (Friis, 2012). See From the Case Files I: Flint, Michigan.

Water can become contaminated from a number of sources, including both point and nonpoint sources. Point

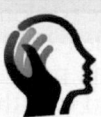

From the Case Files I

Flint, Michigan

The public health of citizens in Flint, Michigan, was compromised when the city changed its water supply in April 2014 from Lake Huron water supplied by Detroit to the Flint River, in a temporary attempt to save money while waiting for a new pipeline to be built to Lake Huron. Flint was once a booming automotive manufacturing area and the site of early labor strikes and conflicts. Now, the plants are closed and jobs are scarce. Since 1980, 77% of jobs from manufacturing were lost and currently 42% of Flint children live in poverty compared to 16.2% for the state and 14.8% for the nation. It has some of the highest levels of violent crime, preterm birth/infant mortality, domestic violence, and illicit drug use in the state, as well as some of the poorest health outcomes (Hanna-Attisha, LaChance, Sadler, & Schnepp, 2016). It is also marred by the effects of largely unrestrained industrial pollution from the industries that dominated the area for 80 years, as "huge amounts of lead and other toxins were pumped into the air, water, streams, and ground" (Rosner, 2016).

After the water supply switch, residents noted concerns with the taste, odor, and color of the water in their homes. Flint's water system was old (with estimates of 10% to 80% of it with lead plumbing), and the city has struggled to maintain basic services in the face of declining tax revenues and high unemployment. By August 2015, researchers had found high levels of lead in the Flint water supply, noting that the water was likely corroding the plumbing lines (Edwards, 2015). In October 2015, the Flint water supply was switched back to Detroit water from Lake Huron, but by then, 80 Legionnaires disease cases (and 10 deaths) were noted. Investigators are examining the possible relationship of corroding pipes and the potential growth and spread of the Legionella bacteria (Keuhn, 2016). In January 2016, President Obama declared federal emergency status to help resolve the water issues.

In the meantime, researchers from Flint's Hurley Children's Hospital conducted a spatial analysis of risk and pre–/post–water system change blood lead levels for over 700 Flint children tested in their facility. They found statistically significant changes in EBLL in blood collected between the months of January to September 2014, compared to blood drawn from January to September 2015. Before the water system change, 2.4% of Flint children had EBLL, but after the change, the

proportion increased to 4.9%; those children living in outside Flint with no change in water source had no significant changes and low levels of lead in both samples. There were also statistically significant changes noted on demographic data, with higher proportions of African American children and greater levels of socioeconomic disadvantages. The "preexisting disparity in lead poisoning" broadened for those children living in Flint, especially for those with high levels of lead in their home water supply (Hanna-Attisha et al., 2016).

PHNs and others are concerned about the current situation, as well as the long-term consequences of lead exposure for the citizens of Flint, Michigan. Given the recent findings of the potential for multigenerational epigenetic changes in grandchildren linked to lead exposure in pregnant women, this environmental exposure has exponential potential for harm (Sen et al., 2015).

What is the role of the public health nurse in addressing this issue?

Which primary, secondary, and tertiary interventions could be applied?

What are the ethical issues involved in this case?

Can you identify issues related to environmental justice in this case?

Edwards, M. (2015, September 8). Our sampling of 252 homes demonstrates a high lead in water risk: Flint should be failing to meet the EPA Lead and Copper Rule. Retrieved from http://flintwaterstudy.org/2015/09/our-sampling-of-252-homes-demonstrates-a-high-lead-in-water-risk-flint-should-be-failing-to-meet-the-epa-lead-and-copper-rule/

Hanna-Attisha, M., LaChance, J., Sadler, R. C., & Schnepp, A. C. (2016). Elevated blood lead levels in children associated with the Flint drinking water crisis: A spatial analysis of risk and public health response. American Journal of Public Health, 106(2), 283–290.

Keuhn, B. M. (2016). Pediatrician sees long road ahead for Flint after lead poisoning crisis. JAMA, 315(10), 967–969.

Rosner, D. (2016). Flint, Michigan: A century of environmental injustice. American Journal of Public Health, 106(2), 200–201.

Sen, A., Heredia, N., Senut, M. C., Land, S., Hollocher, K., Lu, X., … Ruden, D. M. (2015). Multigenerational epigenetic inheritance in humans: DNA methylation changes associated with maternal exposure to lead can be transmitted to the grandchildren. Scientific Reports, 5, 14466.

sources are those that can be traced to one source, such as a wastewater facility release into municipal water or discharge from an industrial site. Nonpoint sources are runoff from agricultural areas, gasoline stations, and other contaminants carried by rain and waterways. Some common water contaminants are microbial (frequently cryptosporidium and giardia), and to rid public water systems of microorganisms, disinfection processes are used. These disinfectants that are chlorine based produce disinfection by-products that can also be hazardous to health. Additionally, other inorganic (such as nitrogen derivatives, arsenic, lead, fluoride, cadmium, and mercury) and organic chemicals (commonly organophosphates, phthalates), as well as radionuclides, are frequent contaminants (EPA, 2015b, 2015h, 2015aa). More recently, there is a global concern about pharmaceutical waste contaminants in water. In a landmark study by the U.S. Geological Survey (2015a) in 1999 to 2000, chemicals such as medications for humans and animals, natural and synthetic hormones, metabolites, pesticides, insecticides, plasticizers, and fire retardants were found in 80% of the streams sampled (Health Care Without Harm, 2015b; U.S. Geological Survey, 2015b). Not only are pharmaceuticals used by humans, excreted in their urine, and discarded into locations where they can reach water supplies but also animals are fed hormones and antibiotics in animal feeding operations that also leach into water supplies (Hribar, 2010; Snyder, Westeroff, Yoon, & Sedlak, 2003). PHNs must be aware of this source of water contamination that puts vulnerable population groups such as the growing fetus, infants and children,

older adults, and those with compromised immunity at great risk (Marcoux & Vogenburg, 2015). Organizations such as Health Care Without Harm seek to address the pharmaceutical waste issue through measures that address production, use, discharge, and disposal, treatment in wastewater facilities, and collection of unused medications (Health Care Without Harm, 2015b).

Finally, a risk to community water supplies occurs in the communities where hydraulic fracturing (fracking) occurs. Methane, benzene, and other chemicals have been found in the groundwater in communities where fracking takes place (McDermott-Levy, Katkins, & Sattler, 2013). This can occur either from the actual fracturing process or from the pits used to store fluid waste. See From the Case Files: Fracking.

Food

Food quality and safety is essential to human health. Food quality refers to the relative nutritional value, cost, and variety of food available. The CDC estimates that each year more than 3,000 people die from food-borne illness and one in six Americans become ill from food consumption (CDC, 2015a). PHNs frequently work closely with environmental sanitarians in state and local health departments who routinely monitor food establishments for their safety in order to prevent exposure to microbial agents that cause food-borne illness (CDC, 2015c). Environmental issues that affect food quality extend beyond the microbial exposures and include the availability of adequate nutritious food, chemical exposures

---

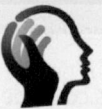 *From the* **Case Files** **II**

Fracking

Scenario

Pleasantville is a small community in rural northeastern Pennsylvania where the local citizens have become concerned about their drinking water as a result of hydraulic fracturing (fracking) activities. In your work in the local community hospital, you have noted more patients with skin rashes and complaints of gastric distress. Fracking, as the hydraulic fracturing process is commonly referred to, is a process to extract natural gas from deep underground for public use. This process has the potential to contaminate air and water from chemical sources such as methane, benzene, and other hydrocarbons and pose health risks to community members as well as those workers involved in extraction operations. In 2012, the ANA passed a resolution, "Nurses' Role in Recognizing, Educating, and Advocating for Healthy Energy Choices," that states nurses must be knowledgeable about the health risks involved with fossil fuel energy. It is important not only for nurses who work in the community but also for all nurses in regions where there are fracking operations, to include appraisal of exposure risk to air or water from drilling

operations into their patient assessments (McDermott-Levy, Katkins, & Sattler, 2013). Because the local community shows great trust for nurses and seeks advice from nurses in hospitals, schools, and community settings, it is important for all nurses to understand and provide education for community members about this health concern.

Questions

1. How might you learn more about hydraulic fracturing and the associated health risks?
2. Describe the role of the nurse working in communities where hydraulic fracturing occurs.
3. Read the article by McDermott-Levy et al. (2013) from the American Journal of Nursing and identify 3 implications for nursing practice.
4. How might you identify issues related to environmental justice in this scenario?

McDermott-Levy, R., Katkins, N., & Sattler, B. (2013). Fracking, the environment, and health: New energy practices may threaten public health. American Journal of Nursing, 133(6), 45–51.

through food additives and from agrichemicals and antibiotics, contaminated food from diseased animals, and improper food handling. Pesticides are ubiquitous in the environment and are transmitted to humans through foods (EPA, 2015b). Fresh fruits and vegetables must be thoroughly washed to remove pesticide residue. In addition, antibiotics fed to animals in animal feeding operations are transmitted through this food (EPA, 2015t).

Risks occur at all points from food production to food consumption. For example, agrichemicals such as chemical fertilizers and pesticides are applied in the production of fruits and vegetables, while hormones and antibiotics are often fed to animals in animal feeding operations. Pesticides have been found in foods, particularly in strawberries, blueberries, and apples (Chiu et al., 2015; Gilden, Huffing, & Sattler, 2010). After production, many foods are processed for market. Food additives such as dyes and flavors provide the color and often improve flavor of foods. Leavening and thickening agents improve consistency, while preservatives keep food from spoiling on the shelf. Many of these additives can be harmful to health with examples being linked to cancer and endocrine disruption. Recently, there is a concern about genetically modified foods being marketed. These concerns not only address the safety of the food for human consumption but also raise questions about the ecological impact and sustainability. Although the U.S. Department of Agriculture sets policy for practices such as this, many organizations call for a more thorough examination of the consequences of this practice (EPA, 2015z; Whitney, Maltby, & Carr, 2004). In addition, food is often irradiated to kill microorganisms. Although many experts cite the safety of this process that can reduce the risk of microbial contamination, there can be concern about the use of radiation in any form for the workers and local community members (CDC, 2015c). After production, food is stored, transported, and prepared for sale in markets. At each phase of this food cycle, there are risks from improper food handling, refrigeration, or time in transit that affect the quality and safety of the food.

Microbial outbreaks are common from a variety of bacteria (shigella, salmonella, campylobacter, *E. coli*) and parasites (*Cryptosporidium parvum*, amoeba) (CDC, 2015c). Although the public often hears about these outbreaks through the media, they may not be as aware of the risks from chemical contaminants. The USFDA is charged with the responsibility to ensure the safety of food produced, shipped, imported, and sold in the United States. This includes the monitoring of not only microbial toxins but also chemicals such as lead and cadmium, pesticides, food additives, and packaging (EPA, 2015e; FDA, 2015b). Although the FDA operates to insure that the genetically modified foods meet the same safety standards as other foods, the technology used to modify or engineer new food varieties from plant and animal breeding techniques is expanding rapidly (FDA, 2015a).

Vulnerable Groups

PHNs must also be aware of the increased vulnerability of certain groups. For example, pregnant women are likely to transmit their exposure to chemicals, pesticides, and toxins to the unborn fetus, children are more susceptible to hazards from food because of their immature gastrointestinal systems and increased food intake per size compared to adults, and those with altered immunity due to cancer, diabetes, and other health conditions are more likely to be affected by food exposures.

In addition, the effect of climate change upon weather extremes (droughts, foods, and storms), changes in rainfall and water supply for soil, and the ecology of microbial growth will have negative impacts upon the food supply. Extreme weather events increase the likelihood of chemical contaminants and pesticide exposures from runoff that occurs with flooding. Agriculture and fisheries industries are sensitive to specific climate conditions related to changes in temperature and levels of CO_2 in the atmosphere. Globally, these changes can also affect human health. Scientists report the risks for waterborne and food-borne pathogens in drinking water, seafood, and fresh produce from climate variability and the potential for ecological changes that can affect watershed and drainage (EPA, 2015a).

Exposure to waterborne and food-borne pathogens can occur via drinking water (associated with fecal contamination), seafood (due to natural microbial hazards, toxins, or wastewater disposal), or fresh produce (irrigated or processed with contaminated water). Weather influences the transport and dissemination of these microbial agents via rainfall and runoff and the survival and/or growth through such factors as temperature. Federal and state laws and regulatory programs protect much of the U.S. population from waterborne disease; however, if climate variability increases, current and future deficiencies in areas such as watershed protection, infrastructure, and storm drainage systems will probably increase the risk of contamination events. Knowledge about transport processes and the fate of microbial pollutants associated with rainfall and snowmelt is key to predicting risks from a change in weather variability (Cann, Thomas, Salmon, Wyn-Jones, & Kay, 2013; Smith et al., 2015).

Toxic Waste

WASTE MANAGEMENT. Individuals, families, schools, governmental agencies, health care facilities, and industries all create waste that must be managed to minimize environmental impact and to protect human health. The EPA reports that in 2012, Americans generated about 251 million tons of trash, a rate higher than all other countries. However, Americans also recycled and composted 87 million tons of these waste products. In response to efforts nationwide to reduce, reuse, and recycle, the average amount of waste per person sent to landfills has decreased during the last 50 years and the percent of municipal solid waste generated and sent to landfills decreased from a high of 89% in 1980 to <54% in 2012 (EPA, 2015r). As landfills enlarge, many municipalities have chosen to incinerate municipal waste. Waste incineration produces particulate air pollution and releases toxins into areas where they affect water and food sources.

More problematic for human health are the hazardous wastes that are produced. These wastes include solvent wastes, dioxins, and wastes from electroplating and other metal finishing operations, wastes from oil refineries, organic chemicals, pesticides, explosives, lead processing materials, and wood preservatives. Communities may be burdened with many brownfield sites, as well as those listed on the National Priorities List of hazardous sites as Superfund sites (EPA, 2015ee). Humans are exposed to these chemicals if they are aerosolized into the ambient air, leach into groundwater or wells, and reach the soil where children play or crops are produced. What is particularly dangerous for human exposure is the fact that most community members are unaware of the hazards in their communities.

TOXIC WASTE AND COMMUNITIES. Many nurses have become aware of communities affected by toxic waste through films such as *A Civil Action* and *Erin Brockovich*. Both films highlighted real community stories where community residents were exposed to hazards through the water they drank from public water systems. In the first movie, released in 1998, residents of Woburn, Massachusetts, were exposed to trichloroethylene (TCE) through contamination of the town's water supply. The hazardous chemical leached from buried storage at the site of a former tannery and affected residents of the community; it was later identified as the source of a leukemia cluster in the community. The latter film, released in 2000, depicted the true story of Erin Brockovich, who worked for an attorney that brought suit against Pacific Gas and Electric for the contamination of the residential water supply with hexavalent chromium used to prevent rust in the machinery at the plant near Hinkley, California. Hexavalent chromium is a known carcinogen. The suit represented more than 1,000 people affected by the release of hexavalent chromium in their water (Penningroth, 2010). Residents still have concerns about residual pollution in their community (Esquivel, 2015).

Nurses should be knowledgeable about the toxic hazards in their own communities and those where the patients and families they care for reside. Through the EPA Superfund Web site (EPA, 2015ee), nurses can assist community members in learning about Superfund sites that impact their communities. Further, on the EPA Brownfields Web site, nurses and community members can learn about *Brownfields Near You* (EPA, 2015f).

Radiation

Humans are exposed to radiation in a variety of forms. Risks and forms of radiation are generally categorized as ionizing and nonionizing radiation. Ionization refers to the process where the atomic particle (ion) breaks away from the nucleus of the atom. Ionizing radiation occurs in natural forms as radon gas and cosmic radiation from the atmosphere. Radon is a leading cause of death from lung cancer. As an odorless gas, it can seep into the foundation of homes from the ground and expose home residents to the radiation effects. Nonionizing radiation refers to radiation from sources such as infrared, microwave, and radio wave radiation (EPA, 2015m, 2015o, 2015w). Nurses should be sure that community members are educated about the risks of radon and carbon monoxide. Personal radon and carbon monoxide detector kits are available at hardware and home improvement stores for use in homes, and their use can save lives as well as prevent disease exposure. Community members can access the EPA's *A Citizen's Guide to Radon: The Guide to Protecting Yourself and Your Family from Radon* from the their Web site (EPA, 2012a). Interactive maps for radon zones in the United States are also available from the EPA (2015hh).

Policy Development

Community health nurses, once informed about the risks to health through environmental exposures, participate in the other core functions of public health for environmental health nursing. Policy development is the core function that addresses the need for legislation to protect human health but also the opportunities for nurses to engage communities to address their own health and create policy specific to their needs (CDC, 2015b).

Nurses must be a catalyst for change in order to protect community members from hazards in the environment. To advocate for change, PHNs must be informed about the hazards in the community, existing legislation that protects people in the community, and governmental and nongovernmental groups in communities that can be partners in the efforts to protect health (Benton, 2012; Gilden, 2003). To advance nursing knowledge in Michigan, *The Nurse and the Environment: Tools for Action (NETFA)* program was developed to increase nurse's knowledge of environmental risks and promote advocacy for change (Ortner, 2004). High school students have participated in a curriculum designed by Stanford University faculty members focusing on upstream issues affecting population health and the need for advocacy in dealing with environmental issues (Curran, Ned, & Winkleby, 2014).

Nurses can begin their advocacy work by writing letters to their legislators to support strengthening laws as the Toxic Substances Control Act (TSCA) or the Federal Insecticide, Fungicide, and Rodenticide Act (FIFRA). Recommendations to reform TSCA include roles for nurses to lobby their legislators but to also inform community members about the need for reform (Denison, 2009; Farquhar, 2014; Sattler, 2011). Additionally, letters to local newspapers and periodicals can remind community members of safe practices in the home and personal use of chemicals. Nurses can present testimony at public forums or hearings (Waddell, Audette, DeLong, & Brostoff, 2016). As knowledgeable and trusted members of the community, PHNs help to educate and empower community members; nurses in many other settings are also realizing the benefits of population-based advocacy (Benton, 2012; Christopher, Duhl, Rosati, & Sheehan, 2015; Snell, 2015; Waddell et al., 2016).

PHNs can organize public educational programs in schools and agencies in their community to inform the public about local hazards in their homes, schools, and communities and to learn about resources to help reduce their exposures (EPA, 2015y). In order to facilitate community involvement in environmental health issues, nurses can help build coalitions in the community to partner with other organizations to promote healthy communities. PHNs serve on local and national committees and boards to advocate for change. Examples of agencies where nurses play an advocacy role are the Children's Environmental Health Network, the EPA

Children's Health Protection Advisory Committee, Just Green Partnership, local and country environmental groups, state nurses association environmental affairs committees, EPA Pesticide Committee, and Health Care Without Harm, to name just a few. Nurses engaged in environmental health research can share the findings of successful environmental health nursing interventions to promote policy change (Snell, 2015).

In order for nurses to function effectively as advocates for safer environments, it is essential to be aware of important legislation for environmental health. To learn more about important legislation for environmental protection, see Display 9–5 for a list of laws enacted in the United States. Nurses can also use the *EnviRN* Web site to follow current advocacy efforts in nursing practice (ANHE, 2015b). An example where nurses participated in important advocacy work was the People's Climate March in September 2014, where many nurses marched to support action to address climate change. Nurses joined the Safer Chemicals, Safer Families Stroller Brigade in 2013, where nurses across the United States took action to promote healthier environments by calling attention to the Safe Chemicals Act (S.696) of 2013. This legislation would improve the regulation of chemical toxins that are currently regulated under the Toxic Chemicals Safety Act (TSCA) of 1976. The limitation of TSCA is that more than 60,000 of the 80,000 chemicals in use today are not tested for safety because of the fact that their safety was "grandfathered" in 1976 (ANHE, 2015a). See Display 9–5.

Assurance

The regulatory function for policy ensures that appropriate services are provided. This public health function demands that PHNs must incorporate environmental health principles into practice (ANA, 2015b; Polivka & Wills, 2014). For example, a nurse can educate families to reduce their risks from environmental hazards in the home, an OHN will ensure that safety regulations are followed in the work settings, or a school nurse can ensure that indoor air quality is monitored for the school setting. Assurance guarantees that policy and regulatory functions are followed through the provision of essential services. Nurses are vital to assuring that essential services are provided in the community. The following examples illustrate how community nurses fulfill the assurance function.

Home

People spend large amounts of time in their homes where environmental hazards contribute to serious adverse health effects and death. To assure that all nurses have essential information about environmental risks to health in home settings, competencies for nursing education include home assessment strategies (ANHE, 2015d; Leffers et al., 2015). Nurses who work with families and in communities participate in research programs and collaborative projects that can impact home environments. To address some of the health issues, particularly for children, the U.S. Department of Housing and Urban Development (USHUD) created the HHI to protect children and their families from health and safety hazards in their homes (Ashley, 2015; USHUD, 2015b).

The program targets multiple childhood diseases and injuries in the home by using a comprehensive approach. Some of the environmental health concerns addressed by the HHI are lead, carbon monoxide, pesticides, radon, mold, home safety, and asthma. In Ohio, PHNs collaborated with other professionals (program manager, health educator, sanitarians, community outreach worker) through a Healthy Homes Program Grant to perform housing control assessments, education, and interventions in housing units. The interventions included home visits and education, and they were found to reduce asthma symptoms, schools days missed, work days missed, and the number of emergency room visits for asthma events (Polivka, Chaudry, Crawford, Bouton, & Sweet, 2011). A Healthy Homes program headed by PHNs in Baltimore, Maryland, focused upon home assessments for environmental health risks (lead, asthma triggers, carbon monoxide, pesticide use, environmental tobacco smoke, and source of heating in the home). Other components of the program were educational sessions to review home environmental health risks and a targeted hazard reduction intervention (USHUD, 2015a, 2015b). In Lowell, Massachusetts, PHNs were involved in a Healthy Homes grant to improve training and education among community and faith-based organizations to develop culturally appropriate home assessments and educational tools for a culturally diverse population in the community (USHUD, 2015a, 2015b, 2015c). See QSEN: Focus on Quality.

Severe Weather Events

A second area for nurses to assure that essential services are provided to community members is in response to severe weather events (Figs. 9–5 and 9–6). Although studies indicate that nurses are involved in disaster response, results indicate that nurses are not always prepared for their role in emergency response (Baack & Alfred, 2013; Usher et al., 2015; Yan, Turale, Stone, & Turini, 2015). In 2015, extreme weather events caused damage and destruction across the United States. During 2015, severe blizzards in the north began in January with Winter Storm Juno, followed by almost 900 confirmed tornados such as the devastation centered in Moore, Oklahoma, in March. More tornados occurred during the spring and summer, causing damage in many areas of the country. Serious flooding of the Mississippi and Missouri Rivers, among others, caused serious damage from Washington State to areas of the south in Texas and South Carolina. Extreme heat and drought contributed to wildfires that destroyed almost 10 million acres of land in California, Oregon, Washington, Idaho, Montana, Wyoming, and Texas. Serious earthquakes occurred in Nepal, Chile, and Afghanistan. Although the United States did not experience severe earthquakes in 2015, during the past decade, notable earthquakes occurred in Alaska, Arkansas, California, Colorado, Oklahoma, Oregon, and Virginia (U.S. Geological Survey, 2015a). Although none were as serious as those reported in other parts of the world, the loss of power from earthquakes and hurricanes put many people at risk from natural disasters. See Perspectives: Hurricane Katrina Stories From a Survivor and a Rescuer.

While Chapter 17 discusses disasters and the role for public health, there are some specific issues related

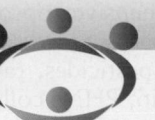

DISPLAY 9–5 IMPORTANT ENVIRONMENTAL PROTECTION LEGISLATION

Clean Air Act 1972

The Clean Air Act (CAA) was established in 1972 to exact controls on air quality through regulation of both stationary (industrial) sources and mobile sources. Through this act, the National Air Quality Standards were created, and the EPA was created and assumed the regulatory responsibility for monitoring these standards. Although this legislation has been amended at various times since 1970, it continues to be the major source of control for air pollution.

Occupational Safety and Health Act (OSHA) 1970

In 1970, Congress passed the Occupational and Safety Health Act to protect workers and promote workplace safety. This act served to protect workers in their place of employment from hazards to their safety and health. This act is regulated through the OSHA and is supported by the work of the NIOSH. It is designed to protect workers from exposure to toxic chemicals, heat or cold stress, and mechanical dangers in the workplace, unsafe noise levels, or unsanitary conditions.

FIFRA 1972

Congress passed an early version of the FIFRA in 1947. Through this act, EPA regulates pesticides through the registration process of chemical manufacturing and enforcement of compliance with banned or unregistered pesticides.

Safe Drinking Water Act 1974

Congress passed the Safe Drinking Water Act (SDWA) in 1974 to protect health by ensuring that water quality of the public water supply would comply with water quality standards. This act is regulated by the EPA to oversee that state and local water supplies meet standards. This act has been amended since 1974 and threats to safe water are reviewed regularly. Primary contaminant sources include human and animal waste, pesticides, hazardous chemicals, and some naturally occurring hazards that get into the water supply.

Toxic Substances Control Act 1976

The TSCA passed in 1976 addresses the production, use, and disposal of specific chemicals, but various materials such as food, drugs, pesticides, cosmetics, and personal care products are excluded.

Clean Water Act 1977

The Clean Water Act (CWA) provides basic structure for regulating discharges of pollutants into the waters of the United States as well as regulating quality standards for surface waters. Wastewater standards are set and regulated to control hazardous contamination of water.

Comprehensive Environmental Response, Compensation, and Liability Act (Superfund) 1980

Superfund is the name given to the environmental program established to address abandoned hazardous waste sites. The Comprehensive Environmental Response, Compensation, and Liability Act (CERCLA), commonly referred to as Superfund, is a program created to fund remediation of hazardous waste sites. CERCLA was created in response to the discovery of toxic waste dumps in the 1970s. By taxing the petroleum and chemical industries, the funds were provided for the cleanup of the most damaging toxic waste sites.

Emergency Planning and Community Right to Know Act 1986

This act is often referred to as "Community Right to Know." This legislation helps communities to ensure environmental safety from hazardous chemicals. Through state and local planning, communities establish emergency planning committees. This act enables the pubic to gain access to information to increase their knowledge of chemicals in individual locations, their uses, and how they are released into the environment.

Federal Actions to Address Environmental Justice in Minority Populations and Low-Income Populations Executive Order 12898 of 1994

Executive Order 12898 focuses attention to the human and environmental health effects of actions upon minority and low-income populations to achieve environmental protection for all. This legislation was developed because of the disproportionate exposures to environmental toxins experienced by people of color, tribal populations, and low-income populations.

FIFRA Amended, 1996

FIFRA was established to provide regulation of pesticides for distribution and use in the United States. In order to register a pesticide, it is necessary to provide evidence that there will not be adverse effects upon the environment, including humans. EPA's Office of Pesticide Programs regulates the use of pesticides.

Protection of Children from Environmental Health Risks and Safety Risks Executive Order 13045 of 1997

As a result of this executive order, the EPA established the Office of Children's Health Protection to ensure that toxic exposures do not adversely affect children. Because of various physical, developmental, behavioral, and social factors, children are more vulnerable to environmental threats in the environment.

Adapted from National Resource Defense Council. (n.d.). *U. S. environmental laws & treaties.* Retrieved from http://www.nrdc.org/reference/laws.asp

QSEN—Focus on Quality: Teamwork and Collaboration

Definition: Function effectively within nursing and inter professional teams, fostering open communication, mutual respect, and shared decision-making to achieve quality patient care.

Knowledge

Recognize contributions of other individuals and groups in helping patient/family achieve health goals.

Analyze differences in communication style preferences among patients and families, nurses, and other members of the health team.

Skills

• Demonstrate awareness of own strengths and limitations as a team member.

• Act with integrity, consistency, and respect for differing views.

• Clarify roles and accountabilities under conditions or potential overlap in team member functioning.

• Integrate the contributions of others who play a role in helping patient/family achieve health goals.

• Communicate with team members, adapting own style of community to the needs of the team and situation.

• Participate in designing systems that support effective teamwork.

Attitudes

Respect the centrality of the patient/family as core members of any health care team.

Value the influence of system solutions in achieving effective team functioning.

Nurses work with patients, families, and populations. Thus far in your nursing education, you have worked primarily with individuals and family members. In the community setting, you now extend your perspective to the care of groups (aggregates) and populations. How do the QSEN competencies apply to aggregates such as persons who are immigrants to this country, or to population groups such as children and the disabled in your community?

Nurses are now expected to shift from solely an individual focus for patient care to systems thinking. Dolansky and Moore (2013) explain that the key to safety in nursing is systems thinking. The QSEN competencies must not be solely for the care of the individual and families but in the work to improve overall health care quality and safety. One area of the QSEN competencies for teamwork and collaboration, and this is particularly important in dealing with environmental health hazards. PHNs may be the first provider to notice a problem with a client, but other professionals must become involved in order to fully resolve most issues. For example, a PHN working in a small, rural community made a home visit to check on a 4-year-old needing a referral to a pediatric cardiologist for a congenital heart defect. In locating the residence, she found that the family was living in a small, stand-alone one-car garage that had been made into a one-room apartment. It was a cold, early December morning, and the family welcomed her inside; she noted the homemade decorations strung across the wall with the phrase, "Happy Birthday, Baby Jesus." The mother, father, 4-year-old, and a newborn baby were huddled together and dressed in coats and sweaters because the outdated wall heater was not working and in need of repair. They generated a small amount of heat by turning on the gas oven and leaving the door open. When asked about having their landlady fix the heater, they responded that they had requested this, but she refused to do it. Because they were undocumented farm workers, the landlady knew that they would not report this to anyone (e.g., the county housing inspectors or the health department environmental health specialists). What risks does this pose to the family, and especially the children? If you were this PHN, how would you begin to address the problem? How would you collaborate to resolve this problem? Who would you seek out as a team member? How can you best respect the family, their feelings, and their difficult position? (If you report the landlady, she may retaliate against the family and evict them.)

The PHN needs to work closely with environmental health professionals in the public health departments, social workers, physicians, community agencies, charities, and others in order to provide safe and quality care for the community clients he serves.

Dolansky, M. A. & Moore, S. M. (2013). Quality and safety education for nurses (QSEN): The key is systems thinking. *The Online Journal of Issues in Nursing*, *18*(3), 1. doi: 10.3912/OJIN.Vol18No3Man01.

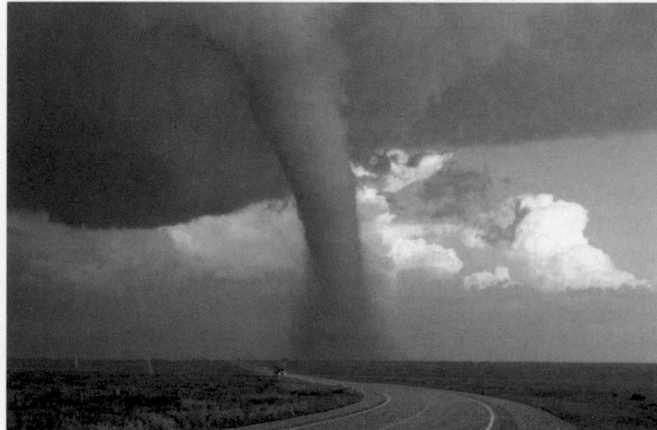

FIGURE 9–5 Severe weather, like tornadoes, can have a serious impact on the environment and population health.

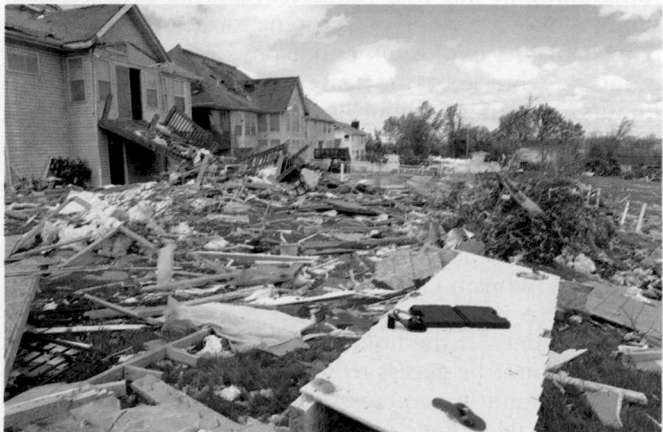

FIGURE 9–6 Severe weather, like tornadoes, can have a serious impact on the environment and population health.

PERSPECTIVES HURRICANE KATRINA STORIES FROM A SURVIVOR AND A RESCUER

I lived in New Orleans during Hurricane Katrina. It was a horrible time for me and for my young children. I called 911 and told them "I am in the attic of my house with my 4 kids. The water is touching my feet now, and none of us can swim. I have a 4-week-old baby." The person on the other end of the phone told me to put my baby in a box, and to put that box on a high beam in the attic. They couldn't promise that someone would come soon to rescue us; I wanted someone to come right away and help us get to safety. I finally realized that no one was coming. I sent my oldest son out an attic window and onto the roof. A man we didn't know finally came by in his boat. He had been searching for other people who were stranded, and he helped us get to a shelter. I was sad that our house and all of our possessions were lost, but I was so relieved that we were together and finally on safe ground.

Tisha, hurricane survivor

No amount of preparation or disaster drills can actually train you for the real thing. After Katrina hit, the power was out and the streets were flooded. I had been called in to work when we knew the storm was going to be a bad one and told that I would be there for a "few days." I had to leave my family and my home without knowing what might happen while I was gone. I work for New Orleans EMS, and we were in bad shape; underfunded and underequipped; we had no capacity for the surge that hit us. For a time, I tended to evacuees in the Super Dome. Then I shifted to assisting with the helicopter rescues of patients at a flooded hospital. After that, it was another 36 hours at the Super Dome, helping to get those evacuees on buses to take them out of the city and to safer shelter. At that point, the 911 dispatchers were completely exhausted from nonstop calls, and some of us gave them a break and took over the phones. Those calls were haunting. Most of the time, we could do nothing. One elderly woman was desperate because her husband depended on oxygen and she couldn't change the tank. Another woman cried because her baby was no longer breathing and she needed paramedics. There was no way to get help to them. A week after the flooding began, we rode the streets, trying to find people who had called 911 and whose cases were backlogged. Some of them we found and helped; others were dead. Bodies of a few of the dead were washing onto streets and freeway on-ramps. No one could rush to pick them up, because we were focusing on those still living. Some of my coworkers lost their homes and were left only with the clothes on their backs. Others lost pets, and some had to find their family members who were forced to leave the area suddenly and were unable to make contact with them. The stress from these horrible weeks took a toll, as some of our coworkers later developed various cancers and many suffered from PTSD. This experience sent many of us into private practice or out of the state, but for those of us who stayed in public service, it has reinforced our commitment to never let this happen again.

Anonymous, EMS Worker

Adapted from Sternberg, S. (2015, August 28). Battle scarred: The personal stories of the Katrina rescuers. Retrieved from http://www.usnews.com/news/articles/2015/08/28/battle-scarred-the-personal-stories-of-the-katrina-rescuers

to environmental risks that occur after severe weather events and are important for community health nurses. These include power outages, safe water and food supply, wastewater, mold, and toxic exposures. For example, when there is a power outage, many families depend upon generators to supply electricity. These can be a source of carbon monoxide poisoning if not effectively functioning or not well ventilated. During cold weather, families may use wood or kerosene for heat that can pose danger of fire, explosion, and asphyxiation from carbon monoxide, but kerosene heaters can also emit other pollutants including carbon dioxide, nitrogen dioxide, and sulfur dioxide. In particular, pregnant women, asthmatics, individuals with cardiovascular disease, older adults, and young children are at particular risk from these toxic emissions. Nurses must inform community members of safety in the home when using alternate sources of heat or power (Wisconsin Department of Health Services, 2015). If a home is without power, there is a risk for food storage and safety. If the home has a well and water pump, there may not be access to water during the power outage. Community members should be informed of issues related to safe storage of food and the need to dispose of improperly refrigerated foods.

Homes that have septic systems may find that they have overflowed if there is any flooding from a severe storm. It is important to understand when it is safe to return to well or septic system use after ground-level flooding. Floods also pose a problem to residents who have water enter their homes. Standing water can cause mold and mildew, possibly harm home furnaces, pose a risk of fire, and release toxins into the water and air. Small children and older adults are at more risk of environmental exposures during and after a natural disaster and the public health nurse must address not only emergency planning but also safe remediation strategies to avoid toxic exposures among community members (EPA, 2015s).

Food Safety in the Community

Another area where nurses can assure health and safety for environmental health risks is for food safety. Although you learned about health risks from food, it is necessary to be able to advise individuals and families about this important information. PHNs participate in efforts to ensure food safety through the prevention of food-borne illness. A great resource for families and community members is the Partnership for Food Safety Education (2015) that promotes safe food handling and education for both children and adults. However, as discussed earlier, food can also be a source of hazardous chemicals both from pesticides and fertilizers used and also from other chemicals found in soil, packaging, and cookware (EPA, 2015t). Nurses can be a resource to ensure that community members learn about the specific risks, particularly in their own localities, and identify ways to decrease their risk. The EPA produces a booklet entitled *Citizen's Guide to Pesticides and Pesticide Safety* that is available from their Web site (EPA, 2015t). The booklet is written to help nonprofessionals understand pesticides. Although it is not directly focused upon pesticides in food, it helps community members understand the hazards present in pesticides and strategies to reduce their use and to ensure safety when using pesticides. The Pesticide Action Network (2011) uses data from the USDA Pesticide Program to identify commonly applied pesticides for many foods. Consumers can consult their Web site to be informed of foods that pose the most serious threats to health, particularly for the most vulnerable groups (Fig. 9–7).

One specific area where nurses have been involved in education, advocacy, and policy efforts is with fish advisories. The EPA National listing of Fish Advisories reports almost 5,000 fish advisories representing 42% of the nation's lake acreage and 36% of the nation's total river miles (EPA, 2015a). Advisories warn consumers of contaminants (mercury, PCBs, chlordane, dioxins, and DDT). These contaminants persist in the environment, particularly in river and lake sediments where fish consume them from bottom-feeding organisms. **Bioaccumulation** refers to the process where toxins accumulate in greater concentration in an organism than the rate of elimination. Toxins can accumulate from direct exposure or from eating contaminated food products. Through biomagnifications, the toxins present at lower levels of the food chain are in greater concentration in those species further up the chain. Therefore, humans who eat contaminated fish are exposed to toxins at all levels across the food chain. Public health nurse and Georgetown University faculty member, Dr. Laura Anderko, has been involved with fish advisories for many years (2015). In collaboration with the EPA, she prepared the educational set of four modules on this topic: *Fish Facts for Health Professionals: Methylmercury Exposure, Fish Consumption, and Health Risks/Benefits.* This is available through the Web site (www.fish-facts.org).

Nurses who work with community agencies can use collaborative strategies to ensure that the population served is protected from environmental hazards, learns how to advocate for a safer community, and identifies appropriate sources of information. The Right to Know legislation and use of Safety Data Sheets provide some assurance and can be helpful in teaching our clients how to better protect themselves as well. PHNs can direct community members to consult the EPA Web site to learn about their right to know. To locate local information, nurses and community members can visit the EPA Web site at www.epa.gov. One link connects to "your own community" and leads to *MyEnvironment* where consumers can learn more about the risks for one's own community, how to address specific pollution, and ensure safe drinking water. Nurses can teach their community partners how to access a consumer confidence report. Every public water system is required to provide information to consumers that identify any detected contaminants or factors that affect the water quality for those customers that they serve. Common contamination is microbial or from chemicals in fertilizers, and other contaminants, such as lead and arsenic, may also be present. This responsibility to provide the public with information about public water systems is mandated through the SDWA enacted in 1974 that established standards for safe drinking water. Individuals can access information from their own water supplier or can visit the EPA Web site (EPA, 2015q). In addition, PHNs can access for themselves and their community partners the EPA resource, *Water on Tap: What you Need to Know,* that is available in English, Chinese, and Spanish through the EPA Web site. This guide discusses not only the safety of public water systems but what individuals using well water can do to ensure the safety of their drinking water. Ways to conserve water use are addressed, as well as the various types of treatment devices such as filters that can be used at the point of entry or point of use for the water in one's home (EPA, 2015gg).

Global Environmental Health

Nurses must engage in strategies to protect human health in their communities through the core functions of public health: assessment, policy development, and assurance. To effectively do this, nurses must think globally in order to be effective locally. This means that considering global conditions of climate change and the effect upon human health is an important beginning (NIEHS, 2015b). However, broadening our perspectives to consider foods imported from countries around the world, toys made in other countries and used in the United States, and the manufacture of products in locations where the regulations for safety are not as stringent

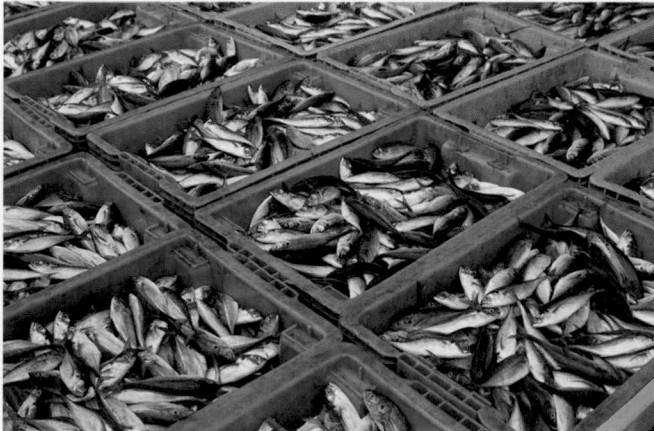

FIGURE 9–7 Fish market: How contaminated is the fish you eat? (Reprinted with permission from Institute of Medicine. (2003). *The future of the public's health in the 21st century.* Washington, DC: National Academies Press. Adapted from Dahlgren, G. & Whitehead, M. (1991). *Policies and strategies to promote social equity in health.* Stockholm (Mimeo): Institute for Future Studies.)

(or in some cases more stringent) as in the United States assists nurses in efforts to address environmental health knowledge and advocacy. Nurses who endorse "green nursing" by promoting more ecological and environmentally safe practices in their workplace are making an impact upon global environmental health. The United Nations Millennium Development Goals (MDGs) for 2015 (that are being updated as the Sustainability Development Goals) addressed a number of health issues that relate to the environment. See Chapter 16 on Global Health. McDermott-Levy, Leffers, and Huffling (2014) examine each of the eight MDGs from an environmental health perspective in order to illustrate the broad range of global environmental health issues. Some of the issues included concerns about nutrition, pesticide use, effects of climate change on agriculture, and impact of sanitation upon nutrition in relation to MDG 1: Eradicate extreme poverty and hunger. MDG 2: Achieving universal primary education is threatened by the fact that in most low-income countries, women, particularly young girls, spend long hours fetching water for home use. The lack of safe drinking water is a serious global health concern. Likewise, household energy use is a concern to women who bear the responsibility for food preparation and shelter for their children. This threatens the goals of gender equality and maternal health. With MDG 6: Combating HIV/AIDS, malaria, and other diseases, there are environmental health implications from the effects of climate change and vector-borne disease, as well as the use of pesticides for these vectors.

Although it is now illegal in most countries to dump waste into the ocean or to ship waste to less developed countries that have less stringent laws to protect their citizens from toxins, large quantities of toxic industrial waste, medical waste, toxic ash from incinerators, as well as the growing issue of e-waste from computers and other electronic products have found their way to ocean waters and poorer countries. In order to fully promote the health of populations, nurses must take personal action to reduce their use of products (particularly those with toxic chemicals), reuse as much as possible, and recycle (in safe processes) to decrease their personal environmental footprint. Nurses must also incorporate the environmental health knowledge and skills mandated by the ANA *Scope and Standards of Nursing Practice* into their nursing practice (ANA, 2015b).

SUMMARY

Environmental health is a discipline encompassing all of the elements of the environment that influence the health and well-being of its inhabitants. PHNs need to monitor and determine causal links between people and their environment with a concern as to how they may promote the health and well-being of both. An ecologic perspective of environmental health is essential for nurses to understand the human–environment relationship and how the health of one affects the health of the other. Prevention and strategic or long-range concerns are also important in considering environmental health, because what is done today may affect the health of future generations. Examples such as DES use in pregnancy and the effects on the children of those women are cautionary tales of the unintended consequences of toxic substances, even when used for beneficial purposes. The precautionary principle reminds us that absence of proof that an action, chemical, or material poses a threat to individuals and the environment is not proof of its safety.

Use of an "upstream" approach challenges the public health nurse to understand the social determinants of health and address system level factors that are at the root of health problems rather than looking solely at healthy lifestyle issues. The disproportionate impact of environmental hazards on low-income populations and people of color argue for the use of environmental justice to remedy those situations. The built environment can both negatively and positively influence the health of a community. Efforts made to promote sustainability, community cohesiveness, and healthy lifestyles can and are being successfully implemented across the county.

Both public and private sectors are involved in regulating, monitoring, and preventing environmental health problems. Health professionals, especially PHNs, and the general public should be aware of reliable sources of information so that best evidence can inform decisions. Utilizing the core functions for public health, the public health nurse recognizes the key role of assessment, assurance, and policy development to influence change in the health of individuals, families, communities, and the environment. The public health nurse should be a leader of the team of health professionals who promote and protect the reciprocal relationship between the environment and the public's health.

ACTIVITIES TO PROMOTE **CRITICAL THINKING**

Understanding Body Burden by Examining the Risks to Health From Personal Care Products

Many people lack awareness of their exposures to harmful chemicals in the environment. Children and adolescents are most vulnerable to exposures from personal care products because of their developmental stage. To gain a better understanding of common risks to health from commonly used personal care products, you will use the resources of the EWG.

1. Begin by watching the EWG video *10 Americans*. There is an 8-minute version available on YouTube. Then consider one specific area where humans are exposed to toxic chemicals: personal care products. Consider more than just cosmetics, and consider also soaps, toothpaste, and other products used several times a day for personal care.
2. Visit the EWG Web site http://www.ewg.org/. Select their *Skin Deep* database of commonly used products. Search for those you use frequently and identify the risks posed to your personal health.
3. Next, select a population group in the community that might be at risk (e.g., neonates, adolescents, elderly) and consider how you might educate that group about their body burden or exposures.

Environmental Protection Agency Activity

As a nursing student, it is important for you to know about common community hazards in order to educate the community members. Visit the EPA *My Environment* site and enter your home zip code or that of the community where you work. The link for this Web site is http://www.epa.gov/myenvironment/. There you will find headings for *MyAir, MyWater, MyHealth, MyEnergy, MyLand, MyEnvironmentReports*, and *MyCommunity*.

1. Look through these headings to identify the hazards in your community. What is the air quality? Are there particular industries, power plants, or high areas for auto emissions that affect health? What about water quality? How might you advise community members to learn about their water quality? Are there significant toxic waste sites? What types of exposures are there in the community?
2. Can you identify possible risks from climate change and severe weather events? What might be ways to ensure emergency preparedness for those most at risk?
3. Using the framework of this chapter and the core public health functions, select a strategy for each area: assessment, policy development, and assurance that is most appropriate for your community.

Air Quality Activity

Have you heard alerts on TV or radio, or seen Internet reports about unhealthy air quality? Do you know what toxic substances are in your community's air? How do these impact you and sensitive groups such as children and older adults? You can find out by examining the EPA's My Environment and AirNow Web sites (http://www.airnow.gov/). Other helpful sites may be found through the CDC, the EPA, and local air resources boards or agencies. Go on a computer scavenger hunt and see what you can find:

- Look around your city or neighborhood. What are the most common environmental hazards? Visit the EPA "My Environment" site. Look at the AQI and air facilities on the map on this site. Be sure to read about radon too. How might these impact the air you breathe? Find the AirNow Web site and enter your zip code. For your city or area, which three companies have the highest amounts of emissions? Are there any VOCs, metals, or polycyclic aromatic hydrocarbons listed for the top company?
- If you were an OHN, what safety measures would you want in place to respond to accidental exposures to these chemicals? What could you do for emergency first aid until assistance arrives?
- If you were a school nurse, what would be your concerns for the children's exposures to air pollution?
- If you were a home care nurse, what would be your concerns for the elderly patients you care for?

ACTIVITY TO PROMOTE **CRITICAL THINKING II**

How Safe Is Your Home and Hospital? Personal Care and Cleaning Products Activity

Most nursing students can relate to the number of chemicals that are used in hospital settings. Begin this exercise by visiting the ToxTown site http://toxtown.nlm.nih.gov/flash/city/flash.php and click on the hospital you see in the city view. Consider the types of exposures there. As you read in our student perspective from Anna, there are many chemicals used in homes and hospitals that carry environmental exposure risks. Many of these are personal care products or cleaning products. To gain a better understanding of common risks to health from commonly used personal care products you will use resources from the EWG and the DHHS Household Products Database.

1. Begin by watching the EWG (2012) video 10 Americans. There is a version available on YouTube at this link https://www.youtube.com/watch?v=0-kc3AIM_LU. Then consider one specific area where humans are exposed to toxic chemicals: personal care products. This includes not only cosmetics but also soaps, toothpaste, and other products used several times a day for personal care.

2. Visit the EWG Web site http://www.ewg.org/. Select their Skin Deep database of commonly used products. Search for those you use frequently and identify the risks posed to your personal health and that of your patients.

3. Visit the DHHS Web site for the Household Products Database http://householdproducts.nlm.nih.gov/index.htm and examine other common products.

4. Finally consider a population group in the community that might be at risk when hospitalized (neonates, adolescents, older adults) and consider how you might educate that group about their exposures.

ACTIVITY TO PROMOTE **CRITICAL THINKING III**

Environmental Protection Agency Activity

As a nursing student, it is important for you to know about common community hazards in order to educate community members. Visit the EPA's MyEnvironment Web site and enter you home zip code or that of the community where you work. The link for this site is http://www3.epa.gov/enviro/myenviro/. There you will find headings for MyMaps, MyAir, MyWater, MyEnergy, MyHealth, MyClimate, MyLand, MyEnvironmentReports, and MyCommunity.

1. Look through these headings to identify the hazards in your community. What is the air quality? Are there particular industries, power plants, or high areas for auto emissions that affect health? What about water quality? Are there significant toxic waste sites? What types of exposures are there in the community?

2. Can you identify possible risks from climate change and severe weather events? What might be ways to assure emergency preparedness for those most at risk?

3. Using the framework for this chapter, the core public health functions, select a strategy that is most appropriate for your community for each area: assessment, policy development, and assurance.

REFERENCES

Alliance of Nurses for Healthy Environments (ANHE). (2015a). *Advancing clean air, climate & health: Opportunities for nurses.* Retrieved from http://envirn.org/pg/pages/view/82102/advancing-clean-air-climate-amp-health-opportunities-for-nurses

Alliance of Nurses for Healthy Environments (ANHE). (2015b). *Alliance of nurses for healthy environments.* Retrieved from http://envirn.org/pg/groups/world/?tag=anhe

Alliance of Nurses for Healthy Environments (ANHE). (2015c). *Climate change and health: Is there a role for the health care sector?* Retrieved from http://envirn.org/pg/file/read/78711/climate-change-and-health-is-there-a-role-for-the-health-care-sector

Alliance of Nurses for Healthy Environments (ANHE). (2015d). *Community/public health nursing. Environmental health curriculum recommendations. E-Text.* Retrieved from http://envirn.org/pg/pages/view/38244/communitypublic-health-nursing-populationcommunity-focused-nursing

American Nurses Association (ANA). (2007). *ANA's principles of environmental health for nursing practice with implementation strategies.* Silver Spring, MD: Author.

American Nurses Association (ANA). (2010). *Nursing: Scope and standards of practice* (2nd ed.). Silver Spring, MD: Author.

American Nurses Association (ANA). (2015a). *Medical waste.* Retrieved from http://www.nursingworld.org/MainMenuCategories/WorkplaceSafety/Healthy-Work-Environment/Environmental-Health/Issues/Facility/MedicalWaste

American Nurses Association (ANA). (2015b). *Nursing: Scope and standards of practice* (3rd ed.). Silver Spring, MD: Author.

American Public Health Association (APHA). (2005). *Environmental health principles for public health nursing.* Retrieved from http://www.apha.org/membergroups/newsletters/sectionnewsletters/public_nur/winter06/default.htm#{D58E85AF-5B7D-4549-A5B3-EC45B9B1216B

Anderko, L. (2015). *Fish facts for health professionals: Methylmercury exposure, fish consumption, and health risks/benefits.* Retrieved from http://www.fish-facts.org/fishfactsworkbook.pdf

Arnold, C. (2014). Once upon a mine: The legacy of uranium on the Navajo nation. *Environmental Health Perspectives, 122*(2), A44–A49. Retrieved from http://ehp.niehs.nih.gov/wp-content/uploads/122/12/ehp.122-A324.alt.pdf

Anderko, L., Chalupka, S., & Afzal, B. M. (2012). *Climate change and health: Is there a role for the health care sector?* Washington, DC: Catholic Health Association.

Ashley, P. J. (2015). HUD's healthy homes program: Progress and future directions. *Journal of Environmental Health, 78*(2), 50–53.

Baack, S., & Alfred, D. (2013). Nurses' preparedness and perceived competence in managing disasters. *Journal of Nursing Scholarship, 45*(3), 281–287.

Benton, D. (2012). Advocating globally to shape policy and strengthen nursing's influence. *The Online Journal of Issues in Nursing, 17*(1), 5. Retrieved from http://www.nursingworld.org/MainMenuCategories/ANAMarketplace/ANAPeriodicals/OJIN/TableofContents/Vol-17-2012/No1-Jan-2012/Advocating-Globally-to-Shape-.html

Boone, T. (2012). *Creating a culture of sustainability: Leadership, coordination and performance management decisions in healthcare.* Retrieved from http://noharm.org/lib/downloads/other/Creating_a_Culture_of_Sustainability.pdf

Bullard, R. D. (2005). *The quest for environmental justice: Human rights and the politics of prevention.* San Francisco, CA: Sierra Club.

Bullard, R. D., Johnson, G. S., & Torres, A. O. (2011). *Environmental health and racial equity in the United States: Building environmentally just, sustainable and livable communities.* Washington, DC: American Public Health Association.

Butterfield, P. G. (2002). Upstream reflections on environmental health: An abbreviated history and framework for action. *Advances in Nursing Science, 25*(1), 32–49.

Butterfield, P. G., Hill, W., Postma, J., Butterfield, P. W., & Odom-Maryon, T. (2011). Effectiveness of a household environmental health intervention delivered by rural public health nurses. *American Journal of Public Health, 101*(S1), S262–S270.

Butterfield, P., Schenk, E., Eide, P., Hahn, L., Postma, J., Fitzgerald, C., & O'Neal, G. (2014). Implementing AACN's recommendations for environmental sustainability in colleges of nursing: From concept to impact. *Journal of Professional Nursing, 30*(3), 196–202.

Callen, B., Smith, C., Joyce, B., Lutz, J., Brown-Schott, N., & Block, D. (2013). Teaching/learning strategies for the essentials of baccalaureate nursing education for entry-level community/public health nursing. *Public Health Nursing, 30*(6), 537–547.

Centers for Disease Control and Prevention (CDC). (2015a). *CDC and food safety.* Retrieved from http://www.cdc.gov/foodsafety/cdc-and-food-safety.html

Centers for Disease Control and Prevention (CDC). (2015b). *Environmental health services: Core functions of public health and how they relate to the 10 essential services.* Retrieved from http://www.cdc.gov/nceh/ehs/ephli/core_ess.htm

Centers for Disease Control and Prevention (CDC). (2015c). *Foodborne germs and illnesses.* Retrieved from http://www.cdc.gov/foodsafety/foodborne-germs.html

Centers for Disease Control and Prevention (CDC). (2015d). *Irradiation of food.* Retrieved from http://www.cdc.gov/nczved/divisions/dfbmd/diseases/irradiation_food/

Centers for Disease Control and Prevention (CDC). (2015e). *National biomonitoring program.* Retrieved from http://www.cdc.gov/biomonitoring/about.html

Chalupka, S., & Chalupka, A. N. (2010). The impact of environmental and occupational exposures on reproductive health. *Journal of Obstetric, Gynecologic, and Neonatal Nursing, 39*, 84–102. doi: 10.1111/j.1552-6909.2009.01091.x.

Chan, L. M., Chalupka, S. M., & Barrett, R. (2015). Female college student awareness of exposures to environmental toxins in personal care products and their effect on preconception health. *Workplace Health & Safety, 63*(2), 64–70.

Chaudry, R. V. (2008). The precautionary principle, public health, and public health nursing. *Public Health Nursing, 25*(3), 261–268.

Children's Health Protection Advisory Committee (CHPAC). (2013). *Letter to administrator Gina McCarthy.* Retrieved from http://www2.epa.gov/sites/production/files/201405/documents/chpac-sdh-letter-nov-2013-final.pdf

Children's Health Protection Advisory Committee (CHPAC). (2013). *Social determinants of health letter to administrator McCarthy: Appendix A the importance of social determinants of health for children.* Retrieved from http://www2.epa.gov/sites/production/files/2014-05/documents/chpac-sdh-appendices-final.pdf

Chiu, Y. H., Afeiche, M. C., Gzskins, A. J., Williams, P. L., Petrozza, J. C., Tanrikut, C., … Chavarro, J. E. (2015). Fruit and vegetable intake and its relation to semen quality among men from a fertility clinic. *Human Reproduction, 30*(6), 1342–1351.

Christopher, A., Duhl, J., Rosati, R., & Sheehan, K. (2015). Advocacy for vulnerable patients: How grassroots organizations can influence health care policy. *American Journal of Nursing, 115*(3), 66–69.

City of Oakland, California. (2015). *Sustainable Oakland.* Retrieved from http://www2.oaklandnet.com/Government/o/PWA/o/FE/s/SO/index.htm

Clinton, W. J. (n.d.). *National goals toward sustainable development.* Retrieved from http://clinton5.nara.gov/PCSD/Publications/TF_Reports/amer-chap1.html

Curran, N., Ned, J., & Winkleby, M. (2014). Engaging students in community health: A public health advocacy curriculum. *Health Promotion Practice, 15*(2), 2271–289.

Dannenberg, A. L., Jackson, R. J., Frumkin, H., Schieber, R. A., Pratt, M., Kochtitzky, C., & Tilson, H. H. (2003). The impact of community design and land-use choices on public health: A research agenda. *American Journal of Public Health, 93*(9), 1500–1508.

Davis, A. (2007). Home environmental health risks. *OJIN: The Online Journal of Issues in Nursing, 12*(4), 4. Retrieved from http://www.nursingworld.org/MainMenuCategories/ANAMarketplace/ANAPeriodicals/OJIN/TableofContents/Volume122007/No2May07/HomeEnvironmentalHealthRisks.html

Denison, R. A. (2009). *Ten essential elements in TSCA reform.* Washington, DC: Environmental Law Institute. Retrieved from http://www.edf.org/sites/default/files/9279_Denison_10_Elements_TSCA_Reform_0.pdf

Dolansky, M. A. & Moore, S. M. (2013). Quality and safety education for nurses (QSEN): The key is systems thinking. *The Online Journal of Issues in Nursing, 18*(3), 1. doi: 10.3912/OJIN.Vol18No3Man01.

Edwards, M. (2015, September 8). *Our sampling of 252 homes demonstrates a high lead in water risk: Flint should be failing to meet the EPA Lead and Copper Rule.* Retrieved from http://flintwaterstudy.org/2015/09/our-sampling-of-252-homes-demonstrates-a-high-lead-in-water-risk-flint-should-be-failing-to-meet-the-epa-lead-and-copper-rule/

Engel, S. M., & Wolff, M. S. (2013). Causal inference considerations for endocrine disruptor research in children's health. *Annual Review of Public Health, 34*, 139–158. doi: 10.1146/annurev-publhealth-031811-124556.

English, K., Healy, B., Jagais, P., & Sly, P. D. (2015). Assessing exposure of young children to common endocrine disrupting chemicals in the home environment: A review and commentary of the questionnaire approach. *Reviews on Environmental Health, 30*(1), 25–49.

Environmental Working Group (EWG). (2012). *10 Americans.* Retrieved from http://www.ewg.org/news/videos/10-americans

Environmental Working Group (EWG). (2015). *Healthy home tips.* Retrieved from http://www.ewg.org/research/healthy-home-tips/tip-14-your-healthy-home-checklist

Esquivel, P. (2015, April 12). 15 years after 'Erin Brockovich', town still fearful of polluted water. *Los Angeles Times.* Retrieved from http://www.latimes.com/local/california/la-me-hinkley-20150413-story.html

Farquhar, D. (2014). Chemical quandary: Chemicals are essential to our way of life, but who's ensuring their safe use? *State Legislatures Magazine, 40*(10), 32–34.

Fawcett, J. & Ellenbacker, C. H. (2015). A proposed conceptual model of nursing and population health. *Nursing Outlook, 63*(3), 288–298.

Cann, K. F., Thomas, D. R., Salmon, R. L., Wyn-Jones, A. P., & Kay, D. (2013). Extreme water-related weather events and waterborne disease. *Epidemiology and Infection, 141*, 671–686. doi: 10.1017/s0950268812001653.

Friis, R. H. (2012). *Essentials of environmental health* (2nd ed.). Sudbury, MA: Jones and Bartlett.

Frumkin, H. (2010). *Environmental health: From global to local.* San Francisco, CA: John Wiley.

Gilden, R. C. (2003). Community involvement at hazardous waste sites: A review of policies from a nursing perspective. *Policy, Politics, and Nursing Practice, 4*, 29–35. doi: 10.1177/1527154402239452.

Gilden, R. (2011, November). Potential health effects related to pesticide use on athletic fields. *Presented at the American Public Health Association Meeting, Washington, DC.*

Gilden, R., Huffing, K., & Sattler, B. (2010). Pesticides and health risks. *Journal of Obstetrical, Gynecological, and Neonatal Nursing, 39*, 103–110.

Global Water. (2015). *Why water.* Retrieved from http://globalwater.org/whywater.htm

Grandjean, P., Barouki, R., Bellinger, D. C., Castelevn, L., Chadiwck, L. H., Cordier, S., … Paige, L. B. (2015). Life-long implications of developmental exposure to environmental stressors: New perspectives. *Endocrinology, 156*(10), 3408–3415. doi: 10.1210/EN.2015-1350.

Hanna-Attisha, M., LaChance, J., Sadler, R. C., & Schnepp, A. C. (2016). Elevated blood lead levels in children associated with the Flint drinking water crisis: A spatial analysis of risk and public health response. *American Journal of Public Health, 106*(2), 283–290.

Health Care Without Harm. (2015a). *Leading the global movement for environmentally responsible healthcare.* Retrieved from https://noharm.org/

Health Care Without Harm. (2015b). *Pharmaceutical pollution.* Retrieved from https://noharm-europe.org/content/europe/pharmaceutical-pollution-faqs

Hoover, R. N., Hyer, M., Pfeiffer, R. M., Adam, E., Bond, B., Cheville, A. L., … Troisi, R. (2011). Adverse health outcomes in women exposed in utero to diethylstilbestrol. *New England Journal of Medicine, 365*(14), 1304–1314.

Hribar, C. (2010). *Understanding concentrated animal feeding operations and their impact on communities.* Bowling Green, OH: National Association of Local Boards of Health.

Institute of Medicine. (1988). *Future of public health.* Washington, DC: National Academy Press.

Jackson, R. L. (2012). *Designing healthy communities.* San Francisco, CA: Jossey-Bass.

Kalkbrenner, A. E., Schmidt, R. J., & Penlesky, A. C. (2014). Environmental chemical exposures and autism spectrum disorders: A review of epidemiological evidence. *Current Problems in Pediatric Adolescent Health Care, 10*, 277–318. Retrieved from http://www.ncbi.nlm.nih.gov/pubmed/25199954

Keuhn, B. M. (2016). Pediatrician sees long road ahead for Flint after lead poisoning crisis. *Journal of American Medical Association, 315*(10), 967–969.

Landrigan, P. J., & Goldman, L. R. (2011). Children's vulnerability to toxic chemicals: A challenge and opportunity to strengthen health and environmental policy. *Health Affairs, 30*(5), 842–850.

Leffers, J. (2015). *Vulnerable populations. EnviRN essentials.* Retrieved from http://envirn.org/pg/groups/16/vulnerable-populations/

Leffers, J., McDermott-Levy, R., Smith, C., & Sattler, B. (2014). Nursing education's response to the 1995 Institute of Medicine report: Nursing Health and the Environment. *Nursing Forum, 49*(4), 214–224.

Leffers, J., Smith, C. M., Huffling, K., McDermott-Levy, R., & Sattler, B. (Eds.). (2016). *Environmental Health in Nursing.* Mt. Rainier, MD: Alliance of Nurses for Healthy Environments.

Leffers, J., Smith, C., McDermott-Levy, R., Resick, L. K., Hanson, M. J., Jorsan, L. C., ... Huffling, K. (2015). Developing curriculum recommendations for environmental health nursing. *Nurse Educator, 40*(3), 139–143.

Lopez, R. (2012). *The built environment and public health.* San Francisco, CA: Jossey-Bass.

Lougheed, T. (2014). Arising from the ashes: Environmental health in Detroit. *Environmental Health Perspectives. 122*(12), A324–A331. Retrieved from http://ehp.niehs.nih.gov/wp-content/uploads/122/12/ehp.122-A324.alt.pdf

MacNeil, M., Dobbin, N., St-Jean, M., Wallace, L., Marro, L., ... Wheeler, A. J. (2015). Can changing the timing of outdoor air intake reduce indoor concentrations of traffic-related pollutants in schools? *Indoor Air.* doi: 10.1111/ina.12252.

Malahingaiah, S., Hart, J. E., Wise, L. A., Terry, K. L., Boynton-Jarret, R. & Missmer, S. A. (2015). Prenatal diethylstilbestrol exposure and risk of uterine leiomyomata in Nurses' Health Study II. *American Journal of Epidemiology, 179*(2), 186–191.

Marcoux, R. M., & Vogenberg, F. R. (2015). Hazardous waste compliance in community settings. *Pharmacy & Therapeutics, 40*(2), 115–118.

Maxwell, N. I. (2014). *Understanding environmental health: How we live in the world* (2nd ed.). Sudbury, MA: Jones & Bartlett.

McDermott-Levy, R., Katkins, N., & Sattler, B. (2013). Fracking, the environment, and health: New energy practices may threaten public health. *American Journal of Nursing, 133*(6), 45–51.

McDermott-Levy, R., Leffers, J., & Huffling, K. (2014). Global earth caring through the millennium development goals and beyond. *International Journal for Human Caring, 18*(2), 9–17.

McKinley, J. (1979, June). *A case for focusing upstream: The political economy of illness.* Proceedings of the American Heart Association Conference: Applying Behavioral Science to Cardiovascular Risk, Seattle, WA.

National Cancer Institute. (2015). *Environmental epidemiology.* Retrieved from http://epi.grants.cancer.gov/environmental/

National Center for Healthy Housing. (2015). *Healthy homes checklist.* Retrieved from http://www.nchh.org/Portals/0/Contents/Healthy_Housing_Checklist.pdf

National Institute of Environmental Health Sciences (NIEHS). (2015a). *Environmental health disparities and environmental justice.* Retrieved from http://www.niehs.nih.gov/research/supported/dert/programs/justice/

National Institute of Environmental Health Sciences (NIEHS). (2015b). *Health impacts of climate change.* Retrieved from http://www.niehs.nih.gov/research/programs/geh/climatechange/health_impacts/index.cfm

National Library of Medicine. (2011). *TOXNET.* Retrieved from http://toxnet.nln.nih.gov/

Nightingale, F. (1969). *Notes on nursing: What it is and what it is not.* New York, NY: Dover Publications, Inc. (Original work published 1860)

Nuss, H. J., Hester, L. L., Perry, M. A., Stewart-Briley, C., Reagon, V. M., & Collins, P. (2016). Applying the social ecological model to creating asthma-friendly schools in Louisiana. *Journal of School Health, 86*(3), 225–232.

Nweke, O. C., Payne-Sturges, D., Garcia, L., Lee, C., Zenick, H., Grevatt, P., ... Dankwa-Mullan, I. (2011). Symposium on integrating the science of environmental justice into decision-making at the Environmental Protection Agency. *American Journal of Public Health, 101*(s1), S19–S26.

Ortner, P. M. (2004). The nurse as change agent: An approach to environmental health advocacy training. *Policy Politics and Nursing Practice, 5*(2), 125–130.

Partnership for Food Safety Education. (2015). *Food safety.* Retrieved from http://www.fightbac.org/

Partnership for Sustainable Communities. (2015). *Indicators.* Retrieved from https://www.sustainablecommunities.gov/indicators/discover

Penningroth, S. (2010). *Toxic chemical risk: Science and society.* Boca Raton, FL: CRC Press.

Pesticide Action Network. (2011). *What's on my food?* Retrieved from http://whatsinmyfood.org/index.jsp

Physicians for Social Responsibility (PSR). (2015). *Hazardous chemicals in health care: Snapshot of chemicals in doctors and nurses.* Retrieved from http://www.psr.org/resources/hazardous-chemicals-in-health.html

Polivka, B., & Wills, C. (2014). Student nurses' risk perceptions of home environmental hazards. *Public Health Nursing, 31*(4), 298–308.

Polivka, B., Chaudry, R., & Crawford, J. (2012). Public health nurses knowledge and attitudes regarding climate change. *Environmental Health Perspectives, 120*(3), 321–325.

Polivka, B. J., Chaudry, R. V., Crawford, J., Bouton, P., & Sweet, L. (2011). Impact of an urban healthy homes intervention. *Journal of Environmental Health, 73*(9), 16–20.

Polivka, B. J., Stanley, S. A., Gordon, D., Taulbee, K., Kieffer, G., & McCorkle, S. M. (2008). Public health nursing competencies for public health surge events. *Public Health Nursing, 25*(2), 159–165.

Pope, A. M., Snyder, M. A., & Mood, L. H. (1995). *Nursing, health and the environment: Strengthening the relationship to improve the public's health.* Washington, DC: National Academy Press.

Rosner, D. (2016). Flint, Michigan: A century of environmental injustice. *American Journal of Public Health, 106*(2), 200–201.

Sattler, B. (2011). Chemical policy reform—nurses must say 'yes'. *Alabama Nurse, 38*(20), 18.

Science and Environmental Health Network (SEHN). (2015a). *Ecological medicine.* Retrieved from http://www.sehn.org/emandeh.html

Science and Environmental Health Network (SEHN). (2015b). *Precautionary principle.* Retrieved from http://www.sehn.org/precaution.html

Sen, A., Heredia, N., Senut, M. C., Land, S., Hollocher, K., Lu, X., ... Ruden, D. M. (2015). Multigenerational epigenetic inheritance in humans: DNA methylation changes associated with maternal exposure to lead can be transmitted to the grandchildren. *Scientific Reports, 5*, 14466.

Smith, C. (2015). *Why nursing and environmental health?* Retrieved from http://envirn.org/pg/pages/view/1785/why-nursing-and-environmental-health

Smith, B. A., Ruthman, T., Sparling, E., Auld, H., Comer, N., Young, I., ...Fazil, A. (2015). A risk-modeling framework to evaluate the impacts of climate change and adaptation on food and water safety. *Food Research International, 68*, 78–85.

Snell, D. (2015). Leading the way: Implementing a domestic violence assessment pilot project by public health nurses. *Nursing Leadership, 28*(1), 65–72.

Snyder, S. A., Westerhoff, P., Yoon, Y., & Sedlak, D. L. (2003). Pharmaceuticals, personal care products, and endocrine disruptors in water: Implications for the water industry. *Environmental Engineering Science, 20*(5), 449–469.

Srinivasan, S., O'Fallon, L. R., & Dearry, A. (2003). Creating healthy communities, healthy homes, healthy people: Initiating a research agenda on the built environment and public health. *American Journal of Public Health, 93*(9), 1446–1450.

Stokowski, L. A. (2014). *Nurses: Are you environmental health stewards?* Medscape: Nursing Perspectives. Retrieved from http://www.medscape.com/viewarticle/829068_3

Sunyer, J., Esnaola, M., Alvarez-Pederol, M., Forns, J., Rivas, I., Lopez-Vicente, M., ... Querol, X. (2015). Association between traffic-related air pollution in schools and cognitive development in primary school children: A prospective cohort study. *PLoS Medicine, 12*(3), e1001792.

U.S. Consumer Product Safety Commission. (n.d.). *Asbestos in the home*. Retrieved from http://www.cpsc.gov/safety-education/safety-guides/home/asbestos-in-the-home/

U.S. Department of Health and Human Services (USDHHS). (2015a). *Healthy people 2020*. Retrieved from http://www.healthypeople.gov/2020/about/default.aspx

U.S. Department of Health and Human Services (USDHHS). (2015b). *Healthy people 2020 environmental health objectives*. Retrieved from http://www.healthypeople.gov/2020/topics-objectives/topic/environmental-health

U.S. Department of Housing and Urban Development (USHUD). (2015a). *Healthy homes demonstration grant program*. Retrieved from http://portal.hud.gov/hudportal/HUD?src=/program_offices/healthy_homes/hhi/hhd

U.S. Department of Housing and Urban Development (USHUD). (2015b). *Healthy homes program. Abstracts by region*. Retrieved from http://portal.hud.gov/hudportal/HUD?src=/program_offices/healthy_homes/hhi/hhabstracts

U.S. Department of Housing and Urban Development (USHUD). (2015c). *Healthy homes program*. Retrieved from http://portal.hud.gov/hudportal/HUD?src=/program_offices/healthy_homes/hhi

U.S. Environmental Protection Agency (EPA). (2012a). *A citizen's guide to radon: The guide to protecting yourself and your family from radon*. Retrieved from http://www2.epa.gov/sites/production/files/2015-05/documents/citizensguide.pdf

U.S. Environmental Protection Agency (EPA). (2012b). *Our nation's air: Status and trends through 2010*. Retrieved from http://www3.epa.gov/airtrends/2011/report/fullreport.pdf

U.S. Environmental Protection Agency (EPA). (2012c). *Sensible steps to healthier school environments*. Retrieved from http://www2.epa.gov/sites/production/files/2014-05/documents/sensible_steps.pdf

U.S. Environmental Protection Agency (EPA). (2015a). *Advisories and technical resources for fish and shellfish consumption*. Retrieved from http://www2.epa.gov/fish-tech

U.S. Environmental Protection Agency (EPA). (2015b). *Agriculture and food supply*. Retrieved from http://www3.epa.gov/climatechange/impacts/agriculture.html

U.S. Environmental Protection Agency (EPA). (2015c). *Air quality*. Retrieved from http://www.epa.gov/airquality/peg_caa/

U.S. Environmental Protection Agency (EPA). (2015d). *About risk assessment*. Retrieved from http://www2.epa.gov/risk/about-risk-assessment#whatisrisk

U.S. Environmental Protection Agency (EPA). (2015e). *Assessing human health risk from pesticides*. Retrieved from http://www2.epa.gov/pesticide-science-and-assessing-pesticide-risks/assessing-human-health-risk-pesticides

U.S. Environmental Protection Agency (EPA). (2015f). *Brownfields*. Retrieved from http://www2.epa.gov/brownfields

U.S. Environmental Protection Agency (EPA). (2015g). *Brownfields overview and definition*. Retrieved from http://www2.epa.gov/brownfields/brownfield-overview-and-definition

U.S. Environmental Protection Agency (EPA). (2015h). *Drinking water contaminants*. Retrieved from http://water.epa.gov/drink/contaminants/index.cfm

U.S. Environmental Protection Agency (EPA). (2015i). *Environmental justice*. Retrieved from http://www.epa.gov/environmentaljustice/

U.S. Environmental Protection Agency (EPA). (2015j). *Environmental justice equals healthy, sustainable, and equitable communities*. Retrieved from http://www3.epa.gov/environmentaljustice/sustainability/index.html

U.S. Environmental Protection Agency (EPA). (2015k). *EPA workshop on epigenetics and cumulative risk assessment*. Retrieved from http://cfpub.epa.gov/ncea/risk/recordisplay.cfm?deid=308271&CFID=51323330&CFTOKEN=62079592

U.S. Environmental Protection Agency (EPA). (2015l). *Framework for sustainability indicators at EPA*. Retrieved from http://www2.epa.gov/sites/production/files/2014-10/documents/framework-for-sustainability-indicators-at-epa.pdf

U.S. Environmental Protection Agency (EPA). (2015m). *Health risks of radon*. Retrieved from http://www2.epa.gov/radon/health-risk-radon

U.S. Environmental Protection Agency (EPA). (2015n). *IAQ tools for schools action kit*. Retrieved from http://www2.epa.gov/iaq-schools/indoor-air-quality-tools-schools-action-kit

U.S. Environmental Protection Agency (EPA). (2015o). *Indoor air quality*. Retrieved from http://www2.epa.gov/indoor-air-quality-iaq

U.S. Environmental Protection Agency (EPA). (2015p). *Learn about sustainability*. Retrieved from http://www2.epa.gov/sustainability/learn-about-sustainability#what

U.S. Environmental Protection Agency (EPA). (2015q). *Local drinking water information*. Retrieved from http://water.epa.gov/drink/local/

U.S. Environmental Protection Agency (EPA). (2015r). *Municipal solid waste (MSW) generation, recycling and disposal in the United States: Facts and figures 2012*. Retrieved from http://www3.epa.gov/epawaste/nonhaz/municipal/pubs/2012_msw_fs.pdf

U.S. Environmental Protection Agency (EPA). (2015s). *Natural disasters and weather emergencies*. Retrieved from http://www2.epa.gov/natural-disasters

U.S. Environmental Protection Agency (EPA). (2015t). *Pesticides and food: What you and your family need to know*. Retrieved from http://www2.epa.gov/safepestcontrol

U.S. Environmental Protection Agency (EPA). (2015u). *Plain English guide to the Clean Air Act*. Retrieved from http://www2.epa.gov/clean-air-act-overview/plain-english-guide-clean-air-act

U.S. Environmental Protection Agency (EPA). (2015v). *President's task force for environmental health and safety risks to children*. Retrieved from http://www2.epa.gov/children/presidents-task-force-environmental-health-and-safety-risks-children

U.S. Environmental Protection Agency (EPA). (2015w). *Radiation protection*. Retrieved from http://epa.gov/radiation/understand/ionize_nonionize.html#nonionizing

U.S. Environmental Protection Agency (EPA). (2015x). *Radon*. Retrieved from http://www2.epa.gov/radon

U.S. Environmental Protection Agency (EPA). (2015y). *Resources in your community*. Retrieved from http://epa.gov/epahome/community.htm

U.S. Environmental Protection Agency (EPA). (2015z). *Risk management research: Genetically modified foods*. Retrieved from http://www.epa.gov/nrmrl/news/052010/news052010.html

U.S. Environmental Protection Agency (EPA). (2015aa). *Safe Drinking Water Act*. Retrieved from http://water.epa.gov/lawsregs/rulesregs/sdwa/

U.S. Environmental Protection Agency (EPA). (2015bb). *Schools*. Retrieved from http://www.epa.gov/schools/

U.S. Environmental Protection Agency (EPA). (2015cc). *Schools: Healthy buildings*. Retrieved from http://www2.epa.gov/schools-healthy-buildings

U.S. Environmental Protection Agency (EPA). (2015dd). *State and tribal response program highlights*. Retrieved from http://www2.epa.gov/sites/production/files/2015-09/documents/state_tribal_program_highlights_apr_may_june_2015_508.pdf

U.S. Environmental Protection Agency (EPA). (2015ee). *Superfund*. Retrieved from http://www2.epa.gov/superfund

U.S. Environmental Protection Agency (EPA). (2015ff). *Urban air*. Retrieved from http://www.epa.gov/airquality/urbanair/

U.S. Environmental Protection Agency (EPA). (2015gg). *Water on tap*. Retrieved from http://water.epa.gov/drink/guide/

U.S. Environmental Protection Agency (EPA). (2015hh). *Radon*. Retrieved from http://www2.epa.gov/radon/find-information-about-local-radon-zones-and-radon-programs#radonmap

U.S. Food and Drug Administration (FDA). (2015a). *Consumer info about food from genetically engineered plants*. Retrieved from http://www.fda.gov/food/foodscienceresearch/geplants/ucm461805.htm

U.S. Food and Drug Administration (FDA). (2015b). *Food safety*. Retrieved from http://www.fda.gov/

U.S. Geological Survey. (2015a). *Significant earthquakes*. Retrieved from http://earthquake.usgs.gov/earthquakes/eqinthenews/

U.S. Geological Survey. (2015b). *Water quality data for pharmaceuticals, hormones and other organic wastewater contaminants in streams, 1999–2000*. Retrieved from http://toxics.usgs.gov/pubs/OFR-02-94/index.html

U.S. Global Change Research Program. (2015). *Climate change impacts the U.S. southeast*. Retrieved from http://www.globalchange.gov/

United Nations. (2015). *Water for a sustainable world: United Nations world water development report 2015*. Retrieved from http://unesdoc.unesco.org/images/0023/002318/231823E.pdf

Usher, K., Mills, J., West, C., Casella, E., Dorji, P., Guo, A., ... Woods, C. (2015). Cross-sectional survey of the nurses across the Asia-Pacific region. *Nursing & Health Sciences, 17*(4), 434–443.

Waddell, A., Audette, K., DeLong, A., & Brostoff, M. (2016). A hospital-based interdisciplinary model for increasing nurses' engagement in legislative advocacy. *Policy, Politics, & Nursing Practice, 17*(1), 15–23.

Washington State University. (2015). *College of Nursing faculty*. Retrieved from http://directory.nursing.wsu.edu/default.aspx?id=1876

Whitehead, L. (2015). The road towards environmental justice from a multifaceted lens. *Journal of Environmental Health*, 77(6), 106–108.

Whitney, S. L., Maltby, H. J. & Carr, J. M. (2004). "This food may contain…": What nurses need to know about genetically engineered foods. *Nursing Outlook*, 52, 262–266.

Wisconsin Department of Health Services. (2015). *Portable generator hazards*. Retrieved from https://www.dhs.wisconsin.gov/air/generators.htm

Woeber, K. (2013). A sustainability framework to guide community assessment and problem solving. *Nurse Educator, 38*(3), 89–91.

World Health Organization (WHO). (2015a). *Environmental health*. Retrieved from http://www.who.int/topics/environmental_health/en/

World Health Organization (WHO). (2015b). *Social determinants of health*. Retrieved from http://www.who.int/social_determinants/sdh_definition/en/

World Health Organization (WHO). (2015c). *WHO definition of health*. New York, NY: World Health Organization. (Original work published 1948). Retrieved from https://apps.who.int/aboutwho/en/definition.html

Wright, R. T., & Boorse, D. F. (2013). *Environmental science: Toward a sustainable future* (12th ed.). Upper Saddle River, NY: Pearson.

Yan, Y. E., Turale, S., Stone, T., & Petrini, M. (2015). Nursing skills, knowledge, and attitudes required in earthquake relief: implications for nursing education. *International Nursing Review, 62*, 351–359.

thePoint: Everything You Need to Make the Grade!

thePoint® Visit http://thePoint.lww.com/Rector9e for selected readings, study aids for all learning styles, and more!

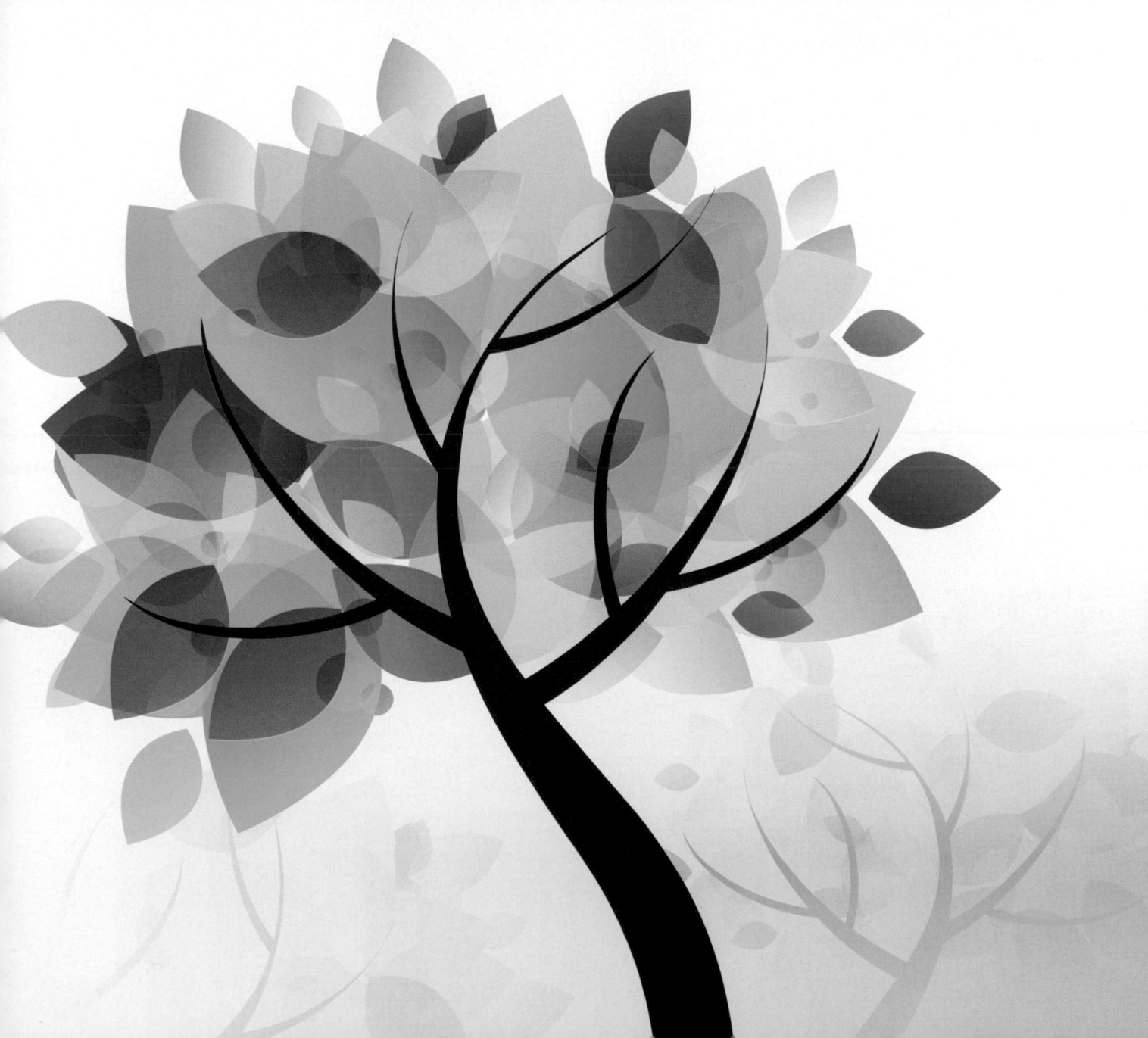

COMMUNITY HEALTH
NURSING TOOLBOX

Communication and Collaboration in the 21st Century: Informatics and Health Technology in Community Health Nursing

"Think like a wise man but communicate in the language of the people."

—**William Butler Yeats** (1865–1939)

"Technology gives us power, but it does not and cannot tell us how to use that power. Thanks to technology, we can instantly communicate across the world, but it still doesn't help us know what to say."

—**Jonathan Sacks** (1948–), British Rabbi and Philosopher

KEY TERMS

Active listening
Asset-based community
    development
Big data
Brainstorming
Channel
Communication
Community-based
    participatory research

Contracting
Critical pathway
Decoding
Electronic health records
Empathy
Encoding
Feedback loop
Formal contracting
Group process

Health literacy
Informal contracting
Integrative strategies
Interactive strategies
Message
Mobile health (mHealth)
Multimedia
Multivoting
Nominal group technique

Nonverbal messages
Nursing informatics
Paraphrasing
Receiver
Sender
Telehealth
Verbal messages

LEARNING OBJECTIVES

Upon mastery of this chapter, you should be able to:

- Identify the seven basic parts of the communication process.
- Describe five barriers to effective communication in community health nursing and how to deal with them.
- Summarize the key issues related to health literacy.
- Explain the stages of group process.
- Describe five characteristics of collaboration in community health.

- Discuss the value of contracting to both clients and public health nurses.
- Design a contract useful in community health nursing.
- Debate the pros and the cons of using electronic health records (EHRs).
- Describe the unique features of big data and areas of public health where it is most helpful.
- Explain the three main trends in mHealth and give a public health-related example of each.
- Identify a current example of the combination of data and GIS applications in public health.

Communication, collaboration, and contracting are primary tools for community health nurses. They form the basis for effective relationships that contribute both to the prevention of illness and to the protection and promotion of population health. Because of its relationship to health promotion and disease prevention and management, health literacy is a concept that is important to health care providers, especially those in public settings. For the nurse accustomed to communicating one-on-one with clients, communicating with community groups, along with a wide range of professionals and lay community workers, requires new skills. Group work is a key component of community health nursing, and effective application of group process skills will facilitate work with both task and support groups. Unlike ordinary social relationships, collaborative relationships are based on a team approach with shared responsibilities and mutual participation in establishing and carrying out goals. Effective professional collaboration can improve health outcomes and foster organizational commitment. The concept of contracting can further assist the collaborative process. Clients and health care professionals enter into a working agreement, or contract, tailored to address specific client needs.

Leveraging the power of health technology is one of the ways we can improve health for vulnerable and minority communities. The implementation and evaluation of technology innovations will help to address public health concerns. Health technology serves as a powerful equalizer for improving health education and access to care among vulnerable and minority populations by reaching people where they are and in whatever environment they live. This chapter examines these tools and discusses their integration into community health nursing practice.

COMMUNICATION IN COMMUNITY HEALTH NURSING

The importance of communication is often taken for granted because people spend most of their waking hours communicating through speaking, listening, reading, or writing. Yet, the quality of people's communication has far-reaching effects. In nursing, lack of effective communication can lead to misunderstanding, poor performance, interpersonal conflict, ineffective program development, medical mistakes, and many other undesirable outcomes. Therefore, to be successful nurses, we must use both our clinical skills and good communication skills (Arnold & Boggs, 2016).

Effective communication is vital to all areas of nursing but is considered to be a fundamental core competency needed in public health nursing practice. The Quad Council PHN Competencies (Swider, Krothe, Reyes, & Cravetz, 2013) includes communication

skills as one of the eight essential core competencies. Communicating effectively, soliciting input from others, and listening to others in a nonjudgmental way are a few of the necessary skills highlighted in that document. Nurses working in community health must be skilled in effective communication to be able to maintain relationships with individual clients, family members and aggregate populations, members of the health care team, and community partners. Good communication skills will enable public health nurses to provide quality health care and health education; advocate effectively for clients, families, and populations; initiate public health policy; and implement programs designed to meet the needs of clients (Vertino, 2014). Ineffective communication is one of the major causes of preventable adverse events in acute care settings (James, 2013). In community health nursing, effective individual and group communication can improve patient outcomes, enhance professional collaboration, and foster organizational commitment.

Communication provides a two-way flow of information that nourishes professional–client and professional–professional relationships. It also establishes the base of information on which health planning decisions are made and programs developed. For communication to take place, clients and professionals need to send and receive messages. As participants in the communication process, community health nurses play both roles: sender and receiver. The nurse working with a group of abused women must learn to "read" the messages these women send. Similarly, as a member of a health planning team, the nurse must be able to elicit ideas as well as contribute to the planning process by speaking and acting in ways that promote information sharing.

Communication serves several functions in community health nursing. It provides information for decision making at all levels of community health. From the choice of goals for a small client support group to health policy affecting a population at risk, decisions are enhanced through effective communication. Communication functions as a motivator by clarifying information, so that consensus is reached and the people involved can move forward with commitment to shared goals. Effective communication facilitates the expression of feelings and promotes closer working relationships. It also controls behavior by providing clear expectations and boundaries for group member actions.

The Communication Process

Communication in its simplest form is the sending and receiving of a **message**, a process by which one assigns and conveys meaning in an attempt to create shared understanding. This process incorporates the conventional aspects of communication—sender, receiver, message, channel, feedback, the **encoding**, and the **decoding** of the messages (Tonn, 2012). This seven-step process is described in Figure 10–1.

It is often suggested that the message is the most important aspect of communication because without the message, there can be no communication. However, for effective communication to occur, we must take a closer look at the seven steps of the communication process. First, the **sender** must effectively encode the message for the receiver. To transmit the message, the sender must decide which specific signals or codes, such as language, words, gestures, and body language, to use. The degree of the sender's success in encoding a message is influenced by the sender's communication skills, knowledge about the topic, attitudes, and feelings related to the message.

The **channel** is the medium through which the sender conveys the message. The channel may be a written, spoken, or nonverbal expression, and communication channels may be formal, such as a written grant proposal, or informal, such as a face-to-face verbal statement. Other examples include e-mail messages, a written report to provide information, a written care plan, or a facial expression indicating confusion. Once the sender has conveyed a message through a channel, the **receiver** must translate (decode) the message into an understandable form. The receiver's ability to decode the message is influenced

by knowledge of the topic, skills in reading and listening, and attitudes, beliefs, and sociocultural values.

Although communication has been exchanged, this does not mean that the exchange is meaningful. All communication involves perception and expectation. We interpret messages based upon prior experiences with either the sender/receiver or with others who have influenced our lives. The final part of the communication process, the **feedback loop**, allows both the sender and the receiver to check on the success of the transference of meaning and to renegotiate the message to allow for clarity and better understanding. Effective communication is seen only when the message sent is received and interpreted by the receiver as intended (Borkowski, 2016).

Communication Barriers and Strategies to Overcome Them

Community health nurses should be aware of the barriers that block effective communication. Display 10–1 lists barriers that nurses working in community health may encounter.

Overcoming barriers to effective communication requires development of sound communication skills that include sending skills, receiving skills, and interpersonal skills.

Sending Skills

Sending skills enable nurses to transmit messages effectively. Through these skills, nurses convey information to clients and other persons. Two important considerations influence the clarity and effectiveness of message sending. First, the extent of the nurse's self-awareness affects communication. Does the nurse feel anxious, angry, tired, impatient, or concerned? Does the nurse find certain individuals irritating or offensive? What motives and interests prompt the communication? Second, the nurse's awareness of the receiver influences the sending of messages. What do clients or the professionals with whom the nurse is interacting want or need? Is the message suited to their cultural background and level of understanding? Does the message have significance for them? How are receivers responding as the nurse sends the message?

Two main channels are used to send messages: nonverbal and verbal. **Nonverbal messages**, those conveyed without words, constitute a large portion of the messages transmitted in normal communication. Nonverbal statements may enhance or discredit what someone says verbally and, thus, are even more important than the spoken words (Phutela, 2015). People send messages

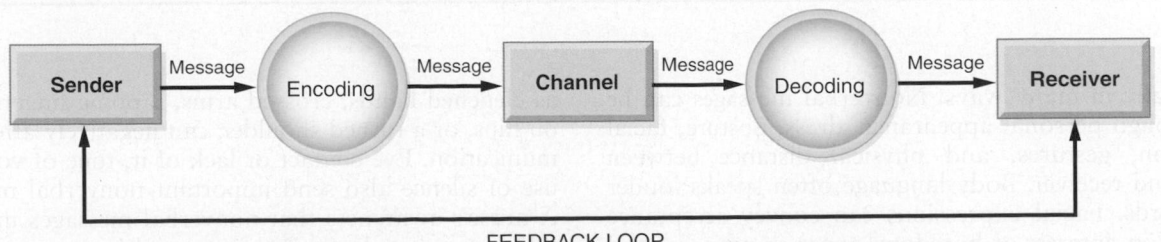

FEEDBACK LOOP

FIGURE 10–1 The communication process (the feedback loop).

DISPLAY 10–1 BARRIERS TO EFFECTIVE COMMUNICATION IN COMMUNITY HEALTH NURSING

Selective Perception

Receivers in the communication process interpret a message through their own perceptions, which are influenced by their own experience, interests, values, motivations, and expectations. They project this perceptual screen onto the communication process as they decode a message, leading to possible distortion or misinterpretation of the meaning from the sender's original intent. Nurses can overcome this barrier by using the feedback loop to ask clients or others involved to voice their understanding of the message. This provides an opportunity for clarification and correction of misunderstandings, which is an essential step in the communication process and helps to prevent miscommunication that can lead to mistakes.

Filtering

Filtering is described as manipulation of information by the sender in order to make it seem more favorable to the receiver. To gain favor with receivers, senders sometimes say what they believe receivers want to hear rather than the whole truth (Tuhovsky, 2015).

Clients sometimes use filtering during a needs assessment process, giving only partial or distorted information because they think this is what health professionals want to hear. Filtering can also affect PHNs. Cole (1990), in a classic work, notes that we have "filters" through which we view others—often influenced by culture, ethnicity, and socioeconomic class or even gender—and these can lead to miscommunication. Cole's premise is that people from different backgrounds actually view the world differently, thus confounding communication and leading to prejudice and stereotyping. PHNs should consider the communication style and preferences of the people with whom they come in contact and avoid stereotyping (Tuhovsky, 2015). Another intent of filtering is to slant information. Prepared minutes from a meeting or a department's quarterly report can emphasize some points and omit or de-emphasize others, giving (sometimes unintentionally) false impressions that influence decision making.

Emotional Influence

How a person feels at the time a message is sent or received influences the meaning. Senders can distort messages, and receivers can interpret messages incorrectly when emotions cloud their perception. Emotions can interfere with rational and objective reasoning, thus blocking communication. Nurses need to be aware of their own emotions as they send messages. To avoid misunderstandings, they also need to ascertain the emotional status of clients or health professionals with whom they are communicating. For example, it is important for PHNs to remain calm and unruffled when dealing with families in crisis. Family communication may be angry, blaming, and confrontational because of a child's serious health crisis, for instance. A PHN who responds with frustration, defensiveness, or anger only heightens the family's emotional reactions. A calm, firm, reassuring presence can go far in diffusing the situation and promoting clearer and more constructive communication. It is always helpful to be aware of the receiver's emotional status and help the receiver to identify it. You may say, "I sense that you are feeling upset about Joey's diagnosis. Are there any questions I can answer for you? How can I be helpful?"

Language Barriers

People interpret the meaning of words differently, depending on many variables, such as age, education, cultural background, and primary spoken language. An adolescent understands the terms dope and bad to mean that something is good or desirable, whereas an 80-year-old woman might understand the terms to mean drugs or marijuana and unacceptable or unpleasant, respectively. In the community health, nurses work with a wide range of clients and professionals whose disparate ages, education levels, and cultural backgrounds lead to different communication patterns.

Language of Nursing

The context of health care provides nurses with a unique vocabulary that may not be understood by clients, family, and community members. The use of scientific terminology or jargon by some health professionals can be confusing. For example, the terms critical pathways or case management approach may have little meaning to a community group. PHNs should be able to adjust their communication styles as appropriate; for instance, communication techniques would be different when educating a new mother on proper breast-feeding techniques than when discussing community health needs with the director of a community health department (Tuhovsky, 2015).

nonverbally in many ways. Nonverbal messages can be sent through personal appearance, dress, posture, facial expression, gestures, and physical distance between sender and receiver. Body language often speaks louder than words. Facial expressions can convey acceptance or rejection, interest or boredom, anger or patience, and fear or confidence. Gestures and bodily movements, such as clenched hands, crossed arms, tapping fingers, hands on hips, or a turned shoulder, can negatively affect communication. Eye contact or lack of it, tone of voice, and use of silence also send important nonverbal messages. A nurse's awareness that nonverbal messages may have different cultural meanings or social interpretations can save considerable misunderstanding.

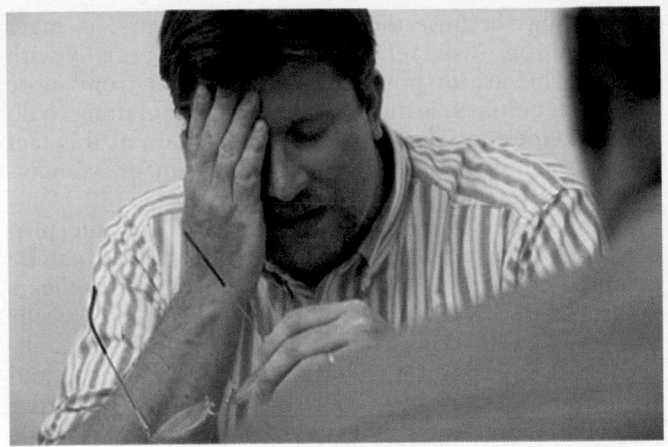

Verbal messages are communicated ideas, attitudes, and feelings transmitted by speaking or writing. Effective sending skills depend on asking for feedback to make certain that receivers have understood the verbal message's intent. Nurses cannot always assume clients or other professionals completely understand the exact intent of their words. Communication is more effective if speakers avoid using jargon that is unfamiliar to clients. Like all occupations, nursing has its own vocabulary, or jargon, which may not be understood by clients and may make them feel inferior.

The basic rules for effective sending can be summarized in this manner:

1. Keep the message honest and uncomplicated.
2. Use as few words as possible to state it.
3. Ask for reactions (feedback) to make certain that the message is understood.

Receiving Skills

Receiving skills are as important to communication as sending skills. They involve not only listening to what people say but also observing their behavior and nonverbal cues. They enable nurses to receive accurate and complete messages. Effective receiving skills require attending to nonverbal as well as verbal messages and seeking feedback to understand their meaning.

If members of a seniors' exercise class agree to certain exercises but do not participate in them, they are sending a message. What message is their behavior sending? Were the proposed exercises too difficult? Did they misunderstand the nurse's instructions about how to perform the exercises? Are they resisting in other areas of the program? The nurse's role is to clarify the intent of the message through effective communication skills.

An essential skill needed for receiving messages is **active listening** or reflective listening, which is considered to be the most useful and important listening skill. Active listening is the skill of assuming responsibility for and striving to understand the feelings and thoughts in a sender's message, thus giving importance to the person speaking (Karp, 2015). Understanding the message from the sender's perspective demands careful attention, which arises from a genuine interest in what the speaker has to say. Active listeners demonstrate their interest, often by remaining quiet when appropriate, sitting forward

with arms relaxed, sustaining eye contact, nodding the head, and asking occasional questions for clarification (Heslip, 2015; Wolf, 2015). The content and feeling of the sender's message may be overwhelming at times, and the receiver can become preoccupied with formulating a response rather than listening actively so it is important to tune out distractions. Sometimes, it is helpful to let the speaker's words mentally repeat as your client speaks. At times, **paraphrasing**, or repeating back to the sender what the receiver heard, is helpful in clarifying the sender's meaning (Harmon, 2016). Summarizing your perceptions at the end of a home visit, for instance, helps to ensure that the client's communication has been accurately interpreted.

Active listening helps to communicate acceptance and increase trust, especially when the listener is empathetic and nonjudgmental. However, often we listen to our own personal beliefs and values when clients are speaking, and we make judgments about their messages. A critical response to the client's message by the nurse cuts off communication. Many nurses note that "a curtain drops"—a visible change of expression takes place—when the client *disengages* in response to a nurse's judgmental response. Refraining from making any negative judgments of the message or the way it is delivered will allow clients to be heard and acknowledged, which ultimately increases acceptance of suggestions (Karp, 2015).

Nurses also can listen actively by asking reflective questions that restate what clients or others have said to clarify the received meaning. Reflective questions have a twofold purpose: to show a sincere attempt to understand the sender's message and to demonstrate the importance of the message. An example of a reflective question follows:

Client states: "Quitting smoking is impossible."
The nurse asks: "Do you feel you can't quit smoking?"

By asking reflective questions, the nurse continues to clarify the messages clients send. You can reflect back to clients their:

- Account of the facts
- Thoughts and beliefs
- Feelings and emotions
- Wants, needs, and motivations
- Hopes and expectations

Active listening allows us to more accurately understand another person's viewpoint and helps to bring issues and concerns into the open where they can be more easily resolved. And if a misunderstanding has occurred, active listening will allow community health nurses to address any misunderstanding immediately (Canpolat, Kuzu, Yildirim, & Canpolat, 2015).

Interpersonal Skills

Effective communication in community health nursing also requires interpersonal skills. Three types of interpersonal skills build on sending and receiving skills, but go beyond the mere exchange of messages. They are showing respect, empathizing, and developing trust and rapport.

Showing Respect

Showing respect means conveying the attitude that clients and others have importance, dignity, and worth—a concept basic to nursing practice (Sabatino, Rocco, Stievano, & Alvaro, 2015). Respect can be expressed by treating clients' ideas and comments as valuable and worthy of attention, as well as demonstrating an interest in wanting to understand the situation from the other person's point of view. We show respect by the manner in which we address people—for instance, by using the courtesy titles of "Mr." or "Mrs." until it is determined how the client wants to be addressed. On a more subtle level, the tone of voice the nurse uses can show respect or make people feel inferior and insignificant. Nonverbal cues and active listening can indicate to clients that you are fully engaged and interested in their issues. Clients, community members, and other professionals all need to feel respected if they are to enter fully into the mutual exchange necessary for effective communication and optimal health care.

Empathizing

Empathy is a critical component of the communication process and is essential to the nursing process (Maruca, Díaz, Kuhnly, & Jeffries, 2015). The capacity to empathize communicates a sensitive awareness of another person's feelings, emotional state, and point of view. We show empathy by striving to put ourselves in our client's shoes—by reflecting their feelings and expressing the message in the receiver's language. This action allows us to convey the message, "This is the way it seems to me. Am I understanding that correctly?" The nurse should keep validating the speaker's true feelings to be certain that the message is being interpreted correctly. The nurse should use the same terms and, if possible, the same tone of voice as the other person did. For example, you should assume a serious manner if the speaker seems serious. Effective empathetic responses facilitate the development of mutual trust and a sense of shared understanding (Meyer-Junco, 2015).

Developing Trust and Rapport

Building trust and rapport with clients is usually the first goal for community health nurses, and the strongest tool a community health nurse can use in order to develop a trusting relationship is communication. Effective communication can aid in establishing a trusting relationship that is open, genuine, and demonstrates true concern for their clients (O'Hagan et al., 2014). Clients note that a trusting relationship is developed when the community health nurse shows respect and enhances dignity by being open, accepting, nonjudgmental, and showing empathy (Clancy, Gressnes, & Svensson, 2013). Clients appreciate nurses using a transparent process of communication; this includes being reliable, honest, and admitting when they don't have all of the answers (Elcock, 2014). However, power differences that may exist between the nurse and client may present difficulties in creating a trusting relationship. This is important to understand as clients and others will not express their true feelings if they do not fully trust the nurse (Rutherford, 2014). Many times, clients may say what they think the nurse wants to hear. They may agree to a plan of action simply because they do not want to displease the nurse or they may hide their true feelings because they think that the nurse is eager for a decision. Also, agreeing with others, especially with people who are in powerful positions and from more dominant cultures, is the polite and respectful thing to do in some cultures. The nurse who is unaware of this fact may mistakenly interpret the client's agreement as understanding, thus a "teachable moment" is lost.

Building a trusting relationship is a dynamic process essential in community health nursing. Trust can be nurtured through a consistent relationship with clients (Soares, 2016). Unexpected circumstances can occur and result in breaking your word (and trust) with a client, but it is important to acknowledge that breach and work more carefully to fulfill your obligations in order to rebuild trust (Rodwell & Ellershaw, in press). A trusting relationship can enable our clients to have the necessary strength needed to accomplish important lifestyle changes (see Evidence-Based Practice). Therefore, we need to promote trust in all relationships by:

- Committing to have knowledge and experience of the patient and situation.
- Clarifying expectations, anticipated behaviors, and boundaries of the nurse–client relationship
- Demonstrating consistency
- Being aware of attitudes and behaviors that do not promote trust (Dawson-Rose et al., in press; Kulbok, Thatcher, Park, & Meszaros, 2012)

Factors Influencing Communication

In a helping relationship, it is important for the public health nurse to demonstrate effective communication. Display 10–2 lists key components that assist in promoting a helping relationship.

Effective communication is also strongly influenced by previous experiences and culture of both the nurse and the client. Previous experiences of both sender and receiver influence their perceptions and the meanings they attach to messages. For example, adolescents who are having difficulty with parents' authority may hear the nurse's suggestion to "learn more about sexually transmitted diseases" as an authoritarian command or effort to exert control. Requests for clarification help to verify that messages are being received as intended.

The respective cultures of sender and receiver influence both understanding and acceptance of messages. Communication between health care providers and clients who share the same culture and language background is often complex, but differences in culture, ethnicity, and linguistics pose even greater challenges in establishing a helping relationship (see From the Case Files: Mr. Sanchez Needs an Interpreter).

In community health nursing, nurses often find themselves communicating cross-culturally (sometimes through an interpreter), which requires patience and constant effort to ensure accurate and inoffensive messages. For example, a nervous laugh, appropriate as an outlet in one culture, may appear rude and disrespectful to someone from another culture. Silence, which in Native American cultures indicates patience and thoughtfulness, may be interpreted as weakness or indifference to someone not familiar with these cultural practices. As culture

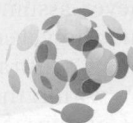

EVIDENCE-BASED PRACTICE
Community Health Nurse–Client Communication

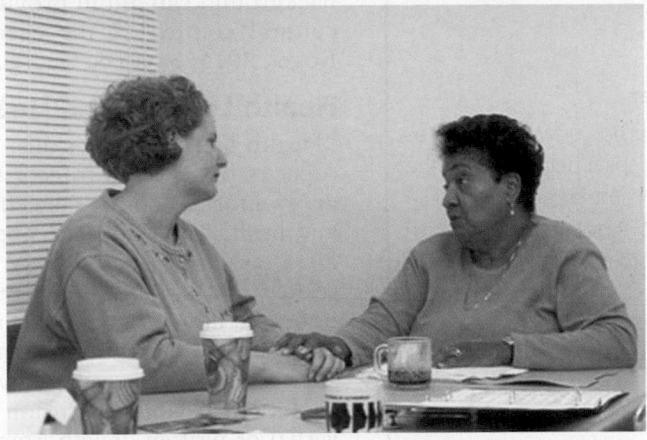

Early research on community health nurse–client communication revealed that this relationship supported self-confidence through the verbal communication patterns of information sharing/advising, negotiating, encouraging, calming, confirming, joking, listening, and silence (Vehvilamen-Julkunen, 1992). Newer research has verified the importance of establishing rapport and trust, understanding our clients, and describes the complex communication skills used by nurses with their clients. A review of studies conducted over a 30-year period revealed that preconditions for trust between nurses and patients exist. These included a level of preexisting trust due to past experiences with nurses and the health care system, the accessibility or availability of the nurse, the technical skill and bedside manner of the nurse, and the nurse's continual presence or service (Dinç & Gastmans, 2013). A trusting relationship was developed over time and was dynamic and changing; it is a reciprocal relationship and the nurse earns continued trust by meeting patient expectations. Characteristics of the nurse that facilitate trust include being honest, sensitive, authentic, respectful, caring, accepting of the patient, encouraging, and being committed to giving good care. Barriers to trust include language barriers (e.g., jargon), not understanding the needs of the patient, being neglectful or not having adequate time or knowledge/skill, and conflicts involving power or time. Murray and McCrone (2015) noted similar findings in their integrative review of studies done over a 15-year period. Trust in health care providers and the system promotes more positive patient outcomes, better management of chronic diseases, and increased use of preventive health care. Mistrust leads to underuse of health care when needed, reduced adherence to treatment regiments, and may result in higher health care costs. The trust relationship is negotiated over time and becomes more stable as the patient feels respected and accepted and values the ethical and moral practice of the nurse. Motivational counseling is a PHN task, and preconditions needed for establishment of a trusting relationship during health counseling involve establishment of trust and rapport. Taking the time to get to know the patient as a person enhances the development of trust. Setting goals and contracting with patients, rather than taking control, supports continued trust. Their conceptual definition of promoting trust is "provider demonstration of interpersonal and technical competence, moral comportment and vigilance to support positive patient outcomes" (Murray & McCrone, 2015, p. 4).

Talk with your instructor and PHNs about these findings. Do they concur? How can you use this information to promote more effective trusting relationships with your clients?

DISPLAY 10–2 CHARACTERISTICS OF A HELPING RELATIONSHIP

In a helping relationship, it is important to promote:

- Openness, genuineness, trustworthiness, and self-awareness (ability to reflect on one's strengths and weaknesses)
- Sensitivity, acceptance, and concern for the client
- Respect for the client as an individual, which includes:

- Encouraging client to take an active role in health care and to be included in all decisions and choices
- Considering ethnic and cultural backgrounds
- Considering family background, beliefs, and values
- Knowledge, self-confidence, creativity, compassion, and empathy
- Ability to problem solve and to confront or direct when necessary (Miller & Rollnick, 2013)

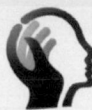

From the Case Files I

Mr. Sanchez Needs an Interpreter

I am a student in community health nursing now, but I work as an extern at our small, local county hospital helping out in the emergency department (ED). A man came in one Saturday a month or so ago with a bad cut to his right hand from a push lawnmower—you know, the kind without a motor. Mr. Sanchez was trying to clean the grass from the blades and cut himself pretty badly. The ED doc asked him if he had received a tetanus shot recently, and he quickly nodded "yes." He spoke a little English, but I could tell that he was having some trouble understanding some of our questions. His friend, who brought him to the ED, did not speak English at all. We couldn't find an interpreter—they are always stretched so thin. None of us spoke Spanish. Anyway, he wasn't given a tetanus booster—we just cleaned his wound, closed it with stitches, bandaged it, and told him to keep it clean. He was given a prescription for an antibiotic medication. It was a busy night, and I didn't think about it much. A few weeks later, Mr. Sanchez was back in the hospital because his wound had gotten infected, and he had used a needle to drain some pus from his hand (he hadn't gotten the prescription filled because he had no insurance and no money due to being off work now because of his injury). Unfortunately, by poking around with the needle, he had provided a perfect, anaerobic place for tetanus to flourish. He now was in the ICU with full-blown tetanus. I have never seen anything like this! He was on a ventilator and had to be "paralyzed," so that we could get air into him. I had only read about opisthotonos—in which the body arches with only feet and head touching the bed because of a tetanic spasm—but now I was seeing it firsthand. This poor man was completely rigid, and we were trying to give him meds to relax him and permit the ventilator to work, but at the same time, we were working to keep his blood pressure from dropping too low from the meds. Mr. Sanchez spent 30 agonizing days in ICU—all because he nodded "yes" to the doc's question about the tetanus booster. With hindsight I think he probably just wanted to get out of the ED and didn't truly understand the question. A $5 tetanus booster could have prevented all of this misery and expense. (He had no insurance and was an undocumented alien, so the county paid the bill.) We should have used an interpreter, should have insisted on it, and should have waited until one was available. They are always in short supply—but I truly understand the importance of a translator now. I have some Spanish-speaking clients in my community health nursing rotation. I do my best to speak with them, and they are usually very welcoming and patient, but when I need to be sure that something is fully understood, I request that an interpreter accompany me on my home visits. I always remember Mr. Sanchez and what can happen when you don't use an interpreter.

Amy, age 24

is dynamic, community health nurses can never assume they know what is typical of another's culture; however, it has been shown that knowledge of someone's cultural background can aid in providing quality care within the cultural context of the client (Crawford, Candlin, & Roger, 2015; Savio & George, 2013). See Chapter 5.

Health Literacy and Health Outcomes

"Health literacy is the skills, knowledge, motivation and capacity of a person to access, understand, appraise and apply information to make effective decision about health and health care and take appropriate action" (Johnson, 2015, p. 21). **Health literacy** includes several tasks that relate to the ability to understand basic medical information, like how to take medicine, follow orders from the provider, access health care, and use health education from print and online sources (Rowlands, Berry, Protheroe, & Rudd, 2015). Comprehension of health information, either verbal or written, is important for clients in maintaining their health and the health of their families. However, many people lack the ability to read, understand, and act on health information presented to them on a regular basis. The *National Action Plan to Improve Health Literacy* addresses these issues and cites research showing that limited health literacy affects people of all races, incomes, ages, and educational levels, with the impact of limited health literacy disproportionately affecting minority and lower socioeconomic groups, and nearly 9 out of 10 adults have difficulty with using the health information that is routinely presented to them (USDHHS, 2010). Clear communication and understanding is important to health care outcomes; the interchange between health care provider and the patient is a vital part of health literacy (Nouri & Rudd, 2015). Cultural belief systems and styles of communication affect comprehension and responses to health information (National Network of Libraries of Medicine, 2013). The level of health literacy among rural heart failure patients has been shown to predict morbidity and mortality rates (Moser et al., 2015). It is important to be able to communicate with health care personnel and to fully comprehend instructions and information. (See Display 10–3 for further explanation.)

Low health literacy has a negative impact on a patient's health status and health outcomes. Research studies show that patients with limited reading skills are:

- Less likely to engage in health screenings and preventive action
- Less likely to have chronic disease under control
- More likely to be hospitalized
- More likely to report being in poor health
- More likely to die

Poor health literacy skills have been associated with poorer health status and increased health care costs and use of EDs as patients with low health literacy levels are less knowledgeable about their health conditions and are less likely to seek preventative care (Jihye, Namhee, & So Young, 2014; Wang et al., 2014). A systematic review of articles assessed health literacy rates for patients seeking care through hospital EDs found that a substantial portion of patients seen in EDs have limited health literacy and that older adults (≥65) with lower health literacy

---

DISPLAY 10-3 HEALTH COMMUNICATION—ONE DISPARITY: LOW-LITERACY CLIENTS

Most poorly educated populations, those with the lowest literacy levels, have the highest mortality and morbidity. Changing demographics suggest that low literacy is an increasing problem among adults over age 65, certain racial and ethnic groups, recent refugee and immigrant populations, low-income populations, people with less than a high school degree or GED, nonnative speakers of English, and those living with chronic mental and/ or physical health conditions (National Network of Libraries of Medicine, 2013; USDHHS, 2010). Yet it has been well documented that most health information pamphlets, brochures, and other materials cannot be read or comprehended by low-literacy adults. Communication with these high-risk groups should be simplified and should include easy-to-read materials.

At the same time, there is the danger of making the communication so simple that the reader feels insulted. Low literacy does not necessarily mean low intelligence. How does the nurse find the right balance?

The goal of communication is to achieve understanding. If clients are to understand health communication—whether the messages are spoken or written—they must be given ample opportunity to provide feedback. Before final printing and distribution, pamphlets and other written health information should be reviewed by members of the intended audience. Proposed users should comment on the readability and acceptability of both text and graphics. With spoken communication, nurses should regularly solicit feedback to make certain that messages are understood.

---

were more likely to use the ED as a primary source for care—leading to increased health care costs (Mantwill & Schulz, 2015). For children, low literacy skills in both the children and their caregivers have been tied to poor health outcomes. A systematic review of parent health literacy found that those parents with low literacy skills had worse health behaviors and had less knowledge about their child's condition and less likely to engage in behaviors to help improve their child's condition, thus leading to worse health outcomes for their children (Morrison, Myrvik, Brousseau, Hoffmann, & Stanley, 2013).

Health literacy is characterized as critical to health promotion and disease prevention; therefore, it is important to recognize that health literacy goes beyond the basic definitions of literacy and can include such things as cultural literacy and computer literacy, as well as scientific, media, and technological literacy (National Network of Libraries of Medicine, 2013; USDHHS, 2010). Vulnerable groups are most affected by low health literacy, and strengthening skills in this area can help address health disparities. For instance, the elderly, recent immigrants, migrants, ethnic minorities, and low levels of education and dominant language proficiency are those most often to be unable to effectively manage their health, gain service access, and understand information presented to them; they are also proportionately more likely to have chronic illnesses such as diabetes, heart disease, and other noncommunicable diseases (Kickbusch, Pelikan, Apfel, & Tsouros, 2013). Recognizing the factors that affect health literacy is important as we strive to improve health literacy because it "builds resilience" and improves the health of individuals and populations (p. 22). An individual who is health literate can

- Understand and complete self-care instructions, including complex daily medical regimens
- Plan and attain necessary lifestyle adjustments to improve their health
- Make positive, informed health-related decisions

- Know when and how to access necessary health care
- Address health issues in their community and society by sharing health-promoting activities with others (p. 23)

The USDHHS developed the National Action Plan to Improve Health Literacy based on the vision and principles that "(1) everyone has the right to health information that helps them make informed decisions and (2) health services are delivered in ways that are understandable and beneficial to health, longevity, and quality of life" (USDHHS, 2010, p. 16) (Display 10–4).

To be sure that these goals are being met, the improvement of health literacy and health communication for our population continues to be a priority in the *Healthy People 2020* goals (Display 10–5).

Health communication not only encompasses the concept of health literacy but also incorporates health messages and campaigns, along with mass media and consumer health issues that are targeted to populations. Population health promotion is best achieved by health communication that uses multiple communication channels to reach individuals, families, and community members. Those mass media communication sources may include TV, radio, newspapers, Web sites, social media sites, smartphones/applications, text messaging, educational pamphlets, health care providers, nutrition, and medication labels. To manage disease and promote health, we must make sure our patients can understand the health information they see, hear, and read from multiple sources (Kickbusch et al., 2013). More information on these topics can be found in Chapter 11.

CONTRACTING IN COMMUNITY HEALTH NURSING

Contracting means negotiating a working agreement between two or more parties in which they come to a shared understanding and mutually consent to the purposes and terms of the transaction. Some kinds

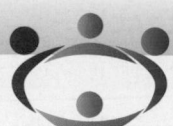

DISPLAY 10-4 THE NATIONAL ACTION PLAN TO IMPROVE HEALTH LITERACY

Vision for the Future
- An engaged and informed public that values health promotion, protection, and preparedness

The vision informing this plan is of a society that

- Provides everyone with access to accurate and accountable health information
- Delivers person-centered health information and services
- Supports lifelong learning and skills to promote good health

This vision depends on achieving the following seven goals:

1. Develop and disseminate health and safety information that is accurate, accessible, and actionable.
2. Promote changes in the health care system that improves health information, communication, informed decision making, and access to health services.
3. Incorporate accurate, standards-based, and developmentally appropriate health and science information and curricula in childcare and education through the university level.
4. Support and expand local efforts to provide adult education, English language instruction, and culturally and linguistically appropriate health information services in the community.
5. Build partnerships, develop guidance, and change policies.
6. Increase basic research and the development, implementation, and evaluation of practices and interventions to improve health literacy.
7. Increase the dissemination and use of evidenced-based health literacy practices and interventions.

From U.S. Department of Health and Human Services: Office of Disease Prevention and Promotion. (2010). *National action plan to improve health literacy*. Retrieved from http://www.health.gov/communication/HLActionPlan/pdf/Health_Literacy_Action_Plan.pdf

of contracts are familiar, such as when a buyer signs a contract agreeing to pay a certain amount over a specified period of time to purchase an automobile. Paying tuition for an education involves a form of contracting. Although no formal document is signed, students agree with an educational institution on a purpose (to obtain a degree), with the terms of the contract being regular tuition payments and regular learning opportunities over a planned period of time. For students in individual university courses, the syllabus is an informal contract. It spells out what is offered, what is expected, and what the outcomes may include. Sometimes, learning contracts are utilized within a course to further clarify roles and responsibilities, and students may "contract" for a

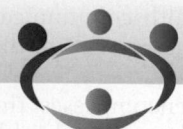

DISPLAY 10-5 HEALTH COMMUNICATION, HEALTH INFORMATION TECHNOLOGY, AND HEALTH LITERACY

Selected *Healthy People 2020* objectives related to health literacy or health communication are listed below:

Health Communication (HC) and Health Information Technology (HIT)

HC/HIT-1: Improve the health literacy of the population.

HC/HIT-2: Increase the proportion of persons who report that their health care providers have satisfactory communication skills.

HC/HIT-3: Increase the proportion of persons who report that their health care providers always involved them in decisions about their health care as much as they wanted.

HC/HIT-4: Increase the proportion of patients whose doctor recommends personalized health information resources to help them manage their health.

HC/HIT-5: Increase the proportion of persons who use electronic personal health management tools.

HC/HIT-6: Increase individuals' access to the Internet.

HC/HIT-7: Increase the proportion of adults who report having friends or family members whom they talk with about their health.

HC/HIT-8: Increase the proportion of quality, health-related Web sites.

HC/HIT-9: Increase the proportion of online health information seekers who report easily accessing health information.

HC/HIT-10: Increase the proportion of medical practices that use electronic health records.

HC/HIT-12: Increase the proportion of crisis and emergency risk messages intended to protect the public's health that demonstrate the use of best practices.

HC/HIT-13: Increase social marketing in health promotion and disease prevention.

U.S. Department of Health and Human Services (USDHHS). (2016). *Healthy People 2020: Health communication and health information technology*. Retrieved from https://www.healthypeople.gov/2020/topics-objectives/topic/health-communication-and-health-information-technology/objectives

grade—agree to do a specific number of assignments in exchange for a predetermined grade.

In contrast to legal contracts, which are written and legally binding, contracts in community health nursing can be either a verbal or written agreement that clients make with themselves, with family members, or with health care practitioners. This agreement commits clients to a set of behaviors, with the goal to improve adherence to a health promotion program or plan. Display 10–6 shows a contract used by community health nurses when counseling clients who desire to stop smoking. Contracts in a collaborative relationship or a nurse–client alliance may be flexible and changing and are based on mutual understanding and trust. The flexibility built into nurse–client contracting makes it a valuable tool for community health nurses.

The same format is followed with clients who are receiving home health care services. The contract that develops from the partnership between client and home health care nurse often is referred to as a **critical pathway**. It consists of the written plans for client care with a timetable. This represents a more formal type of contracting: it is typically a fiscally driven and agency-required tool designed to document standards and quality of care while reducing costs (see Chapters 12 and 32).

Characteristics of Contracting

The concept of contracting, as used in the collaborative relationship, incorporates four distinctive characteristics: partnership and mutuality, commitment, format, and negotiation.

Partnership and Mutuality

All aspects of contracting involve shared participation and agreement between team members; they become partners in the relationship. There is also mutuality to the nurse–client relationship: If we were to document

---

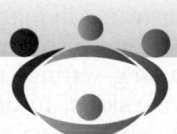 **DISPLAY 10–6 CLIENT SERVICE PLAN WITH CONTRACT**

Madera County Public Health Department
Public Health Nursing: Client Individual Service Plan

Client Name: _Angelica Luz-Smith_   Client's Signature: _____

RN Case Manager: _C. Rector, PHN_   Start Date: _3/1/2017_

Date: 3/1/2017	Client Goal:	Case Manager: Teaching/Counseling/ Referral Case Manager will:	Follow-up/ Reassessment Date: 5/2017
Strengths Identified: Angelica desires to improve the length and quality of life to be healthier to spend time with grandchildren	ANGELICA will decrease to fewer than 10 cigarettes per day within the next 2 months. Contract agreement: Angelica will avoid temptations or situations associated with pleasurable aspects of smoking by:	• Promote positive expectations for success; encourage self-efficacy. • Prepare Angelica for relapse.	Outcome/Evaluation Angelica will be smoking fewer than 10 cigarettes (1/2 pack) per day by 5/2017.
Problems/Risks: Has smoked 1–2 packs per day for 20 years	• Instead of smoking after meals, brush teeth or take a walk. • Limit social activities to where smoking is prohibited. • Find new activities that make smoking difficult such as swimming or bicycle riding. • Identify new activity to spend time on during work breaks (reading, crosswords, etc.). • Avoid alcoholic drinks. • Keep oral substitutes such as carrots, pickles, sugarless gum handy. • Take a yoga class to learn relaxation techniques. Angelica will explore community resources: • American Lung Association Program: Freedom from Smoking • California Smokers' Helpline: 1-800-NO-BUTTS	• Assist in developing timeframe with goal ultimately to be that Angelica will stop smoking completely. • Partner with Angelica for evaluation, feedback, and revision of health plan as needed. • Provide resources for Freedom from Smoking and California Smoker's Helpline.	

Adapted from Gulanik, M., & Myers, J. (2014). *Nursing care plans: Diagnosis, interventions, and outcomes* (8th ed.). Philadelphia, PA: Elsevier/Mosby.

nurse–client collaboration on a continuum, paternalism would be at one extreme and autonomy at the other. Mutuality becomes the midpoint balance or ideal of these two extreme positions (Duiveman & Bonner, 2012). For example, a parenting group of 15 couples requested community health nursing involvement. The group entered into a mutual partnership with the nurse and came to an agreement on what they needed and what the nurse could provide. Together, they developed goals, outlined methods to meet those goals, explored resources to help achieve them, defined the time limits for the contract, and outlined their separate responsibilities. The contract involved reciprocal negotiation and shared evaluation. A partnership with mutuality means that all parties are responsible for setting up and carrying out the terms of the agreement within a dynamic balance.

Commitment

Second, every contract implies a commitment. The involved parties make a decision that binds them to fulfilling the purpose of the contract (Hufford, Williams, Malec, & Cravotta, 2012). In community health collaboration, contracting does not mean making a binding agreement in the legal sense, but it is a pledge of trust and dedication. Accompanying that sense of dedication is a strong motivation to see the contract through to completion. All parties feel responsible for keeping promises; all want to achieve the intended outcomes. When the nurse and the parenting group identified their separate tasks, they committed themselves: "Yes, we will do thus and so."

Format

Format, the third distinctive feature of contracting, involves outlining the specific terms of the relationship. Clients and professionals gain a clear idea of the purpose of the relationship, their respective responsibilities, and the specific limits within which they will work. Expectations are clarified for all parties involved. The format of contracting provides the framework for collaboration. Once the terms of the contract have been spelled out, there is no question about what has to be done, who is to do it, or within what timeframe it is to be accomplished. This format helps to avoid the difficulty of terminating long-term relationships and shifts health care responsibilities from the professionals to the individual or group. At times, having something in writing helps the client "legitimize" the nurse–client interaction.

Negotiation

Finally, contracting always involves negotiation. The nurse and other team members propose certain responsibilities and then ask whether the clients agree. The nurse might ask, "What do you feel you can do to achieve this goal?" A period of give-and-take then occurs in which ideas are discussed and conclusions and consensus are reached—no coercion should be involved. Team members may find over time that terms or goals on which they had agreed need modification. Perhaps clients have assumed more responsibility than they can realistically handle at this time and need to redefine their specific responsibilities. Perhaps the nurse feels a need to involve another professional in the collaborative process. The

importance of effective interpersonal communication between clients and professionals to keep contracts updated is emphasized. Negotiation during contracting allows for changes that facilitate the ultimate achievement of goals. It provides built-in flexibility and encourages ongoing communication among all team members. Negotiation gives contracting a dynamic quality. Also, we need to remember that, although we may be experts in community health nursing and feel that we know best what is needed for our clients, they know more about their life circumstances and how health and illness impact them. Mutual respect and regard are necessary before effective contracting can take place. Duiveman and Bonner (2012) conducted a qualitative study of community health nurses contracting with clients and noted that negotiation was one of three themes that emerged, along with needs assessment and education toward self-care. Negotiation was used to develop the contract and to periodically change it as needed.

Value of Contracting

The value of contracting has been demonstrated in many settings and disciplines. Contracts have been used for many years in psychiatric and other nursing settings to promote client self-respect, problem-solving skills, autonomy, and motivation. Other disciplines, such as social work and counseling, have long used contracting as a tool in helping to enhance realistic planning and emphasize partnership (Hufford et al., 2012). For example, both nurses and social workers can utilize contracting to help a frustrated young mother develop a child safety plan. If a young mother feels that she may hit her child out of anger or frustration, a plan can be developed to identify a family member or friend who can be called in a time of crisis. This process identifies the potential problem and allows the mother to identify a resource that can help her in a time of need—ultimately keeping her baby safe (Kobayashi, Fukushima, Kitaoka, Shimizu, & Shimanouchi, 2015). Dieticians have used contracting to improve patient motivation and compliance with dietary interventions (Desroches et al., 2015). Educational contracts between students and instructors have proven valuable for facilitating learning. Negotiating with students to develop contracts gives them the opportunity to realize that what they want does matter, and it allows them to become more responsible for their own work and more enthusiastic about their education.

Public health nursing has used the concept of contracting for many years, developing partnerships with clients to address issues such as weight loss, exercise, and substance abuse. Without always labeling it contracting, these techniques have been used with clients who, for example, want to lose weight. In this case, the contract involves mutual agreement on certain exercise and eating patterns for clients and teaching and support responsibilities for the nurse. Often, it has a set time limit, such as 6 months, within which to achieve the intended weight loss. For chronically ill older adults, PHNs can help take a complex behavior and break it into manageable steps. For example, the idea of exercise may seem overwhelming to an older adult struggling with chronic health issues; however, contracting to walk at a moderate pace for 30 minutes three times a week may seem feasible. And, success in meeting the contract may aid in stimulating future efforts to increase exercise activities. In each case, a partnership is developed, with agreement about the partnership and the conditions under which it will be carried out. Nurses and clients are, in effect, contracting even though they may see it simply as setting goals with clients, and no written documentation is developed.

As more nurses seek to promote client autonomy and self-care, the wide applicability of contracting within nursing practice is recognized. PHNs may use contracting when implementing health promotion programs. Community health interventions where contracting may be helpful include stopping or reducing substance abuse, changing eating habits, increasing physical activity, improving diabetes care, and addressing depression and medication compliance. Display 10–7 is a simple contract that can be used by community health nurses and other providers when working with families to combat childhood obesity.

Common concepts of contracting in community health nursing:

1. Involves clients in promoting their own health
2. Motivates clients to perform necessary tasks
3. Focuses on clients' unique needs, regardless of aggregate size
4. Increases the possibility of achieving the health goals identified by collaborating team members
5. Enhances all team members' problem-solving skills
6. Fosters client participation in the decision-making process
7. Promotes clients' autonomy and self-esteem as they learn self-care
8. Makes nursing service more efficient and cost-effective (Duiveman & Bonner, 2012)

Contracting can also be done with groups or aggregates and with agencies (e.g., schools, businesses). For instance, a school district may want to contract with a public health agency to provide PHNs and health educators to address pregnancy prevention. The nurse working with the adolescents in the pregnancy prevention program may want to informally contract with them about sharing information gleaned in the small-group teaching exercises with their parents to encourage adolescent–parent communication.

Potential Problems with Contracting

Emphasis on contracting as a method rather than a concept can create problems. If a client has experienced contracts only in a business setting, it is possible to carry the stereotype of a cold, formal arrangement into the nursing practice setting. Some nurses fear that asking clients to negotiate a contract will place clients under stress, impede the development of trust, and negatively influence the relationship. Others have found that some clients prefer to have the nurse make decisions for them and are not ready to enter into any kind of negotiation. These problems in contracting can be overcome by understanding the true conception of contracting. Contracting is not a panacea. Some clients cannot fully participate in a collaborative relationship. Developmentally delayed clients and those with serious mental or cognitive impairments (e.g., mental illness, dementia) may be unable to fully participate in the nurse–client contract. Also, the use of contracting should not be used in place of developing a therapeutic relationship with clients. For example, when working with clients with suicidal ideations, practitioners may use contracting to address suicide prevention—developing a written agreement between the health care provider and the client stating that the client will refrain from suicidal behavior for a specified time period. However, it has been found

---

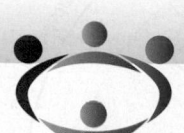

DISPLAY 10–7 RX FOR HEALTHIER LIVING

IDEAS FOR HEALTHIER LIVING

5	Eat at least 5 fruits and vegetables every day.
2	Limit screen time (e.g., TV, video games, computer) to 2 hours or less per day.
1	Get 1 hour or more of physical activity every day.
0	Drink fewer sugar-sweetened drinks. Try water and low-fat milk instead.

MY HEALTHY LIFE STYLE

- Eat ____ fruits and vegetables each day.
- Reduce screen time to ____ minutes per day.
- Get ____ minutes of physical activity each day.
- Reduce number of sugared drinks to ____ per day.

_____ Client's name/Signature

_____ Parent's/Caregiver Signature

_____ Provider's Signature

_____ Date

Adapted from Let's Move: America's move to raise a healthier generation of kids. (n.d.). *Prescribe activity and healthy habits*. Retrieved from http://www.letsmove. gov/prescribe-activity-and-healthy-habits

that formal contracting in suicide prevention is often used in place of a therapeutic alliance and also can weaken an existing therapeutic relationship. Suicide prevention contracting should be done very carefully as it has the potential to produce negative outcomes when used in high-risk patients who are unlikely to be able to give informed consent (Wortzel, Matarazzo, & Homaifar, 2013).

Problems can arise when contracting with aggregates or agencies, as well. In the earlier example of contracting with a school district on pregnancy prevention, the community health nurse may need to take into account the culture of the school, as well as the community in general. If the school is concerned about teen pregnancy, but the community is against "sex education," it may be an unrealistic alliance. The community or agency culture may prevent real progress on this issue.

Principles of Contracting

Contracting applies the basic principles of adult education: self-direction, mutual negotiation, and mutual evaluation. It need not be a formal, written, or complex negotiation; it may be formal or informal, written or verbal, simple or detailed, and signed or unsigned by client and nurse. It should be adapted to the particular client's abilities to assess, plan, implement, and evaluate, which may vary greatly from situation to situation. The tool shown in Display 10–12 seeks input from the client. The client's goals are mutually set, and the goals are spelled out. Initial interventions are dated, as are follow-up and reassessment visits. In addition, there is a place for a continuing assessment of outcomes and for evaluation on future dates. Like all nursing tools, contracting enhances a client's health only if it is adapted to each particular set of client needs and abilities.

Contracting in Steps

Contracting follows a sequence of steps. As a working agreement, it depends on knowing what clients want, agreeing on goals, identifying methods to achieve these goals, knowing the resources that collaborating members bring to the relationship, using appropriate outside resources, setting limits, deciding on responsibilities, and providing for periodic reviews. Each of these tasks requires discussion among members of the contractual group. The tasks are incorporated into the contracting process and can be described in eight phases that follow the nursing process.

Assessment

1. *Explore needs*: Assess clients' health and needs: done by clients, nurse, and other relevant persons.

Nursing Diagnosis/Goal Setting

2. *Establish goals*: Discussion followed by agreement among contracting members on goals and objectives

Plan/Intervention

3. *Explore resources*: Define what each member has to offer (clarify PHN role) and can expect from the others; identify appropriate resources and agencies.
4. *Develop a plan*: Identify methods, activities, and a timeline for achieving the stated goals.
5. *Divide responsibilities*: Negotiate the activities for which each member will be responsible.
6. *Agree on time frame*: Setting limits for the contract in terms of length of time or number of meetings.

Evaluation

7. *Evaluation*: Formative and summative assessments of progress toward goals occur at agreed-on intervals.
8. *Renegotiation or termination*: Agree to modify, renegotiate, or terminate the contract.

As community health nurses use this process to negotiate a contract, they must adapt it to each situation. The sequence of phases may change, and some steps may overlap. Nevertheless, the basic elements remain important considerations for successful contracting (Fig. 10–2).

Levels of Contracting

Community health nurses use contracts at levels ranging from formal to informal. The degree of formality depends on the demands of the situation. To fund a community health program for preventing child abuse, for example, a formal contract in the form of a written grant proposal may be needed. To conduct a wide-scale needs assessment of a homeless population, the services of an epidemiologist and statistician may require a formal contract to clarify roles and expectations, as well as fees. **Formal contracting** involves all parties negotiating a written contract by mutual agreement, signing the agreement, and sometimes having it witnessed or notarized. This level of contract has been used with mental health or substance-abusing clients, where the seriousness of the working agreement and the need to actively involve the client are important aspects of therapy.

Some situations best lend themselves to a modified and less formal use of contracting, in which the nursing plan

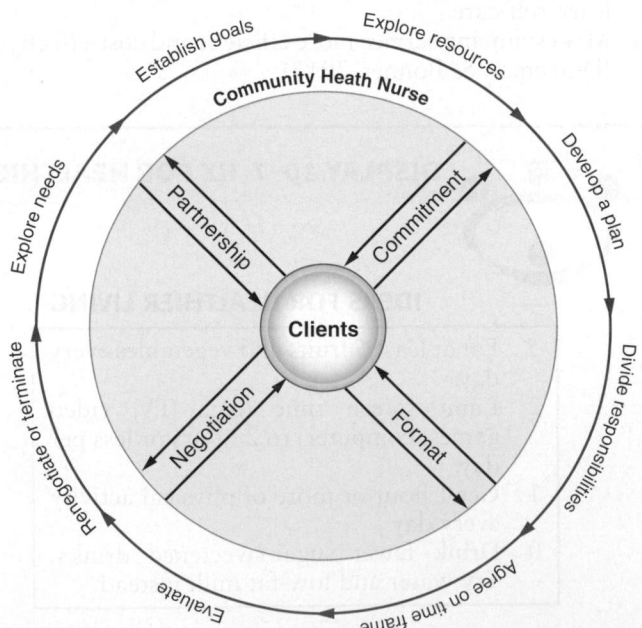

FIGURE 10–2 The concept and process of contracting. Contracting is based on four distinctive features, shown here as spokes that support a wheel. These features form the basis for a reciprocal relationship among clients, nurse, and other persons. This relationship is not static; it is a dynamic process that moves through phases, represented here as the outer rim of the wheel. The process moves forward, focused on meeting clients' needs, and enables the collaborating group to facilitate ultimate achievement of clients' goals.

becomes the written contract. For example, a school nurse forms a support group for pregnant adolescents. The nurse uses modified contracting by discussing with the girls the purpose of the group and the number of sessions needed and obtaining their agreement to attend all sessions.

Informal contracting involves some form of verbal agreement about relatively clear-cut purposes and tasks. A client group may agree to prioritize their list of needs, the nurse may agree to conduct health teaching sessions, the social worker may agree to obtain informational materials, and so on. Sometimes, nurses use contracting informally without realizing it. They conclude a session with clients by agreeing with them about the purpose and time of the next meeting. Conscious use of contracting, however, is a more effective way to provide structure for the relationship and foster client involvement, regardless of the level at which it is applied.

The level of contracting also may change during the development of communication and collaboration. Clients often need education about their options. Initially, they may have difficulty in identifying needs and making choices. The professional team can work to promote clients' self-confidence and help them assume increasing responsibility for their own health. Through these efforts, contracting becomes a consciously recognized part of the relationship, and clients become fully participating partners.

COMMUNICATING WITH GROUPS

An important aspect of communication in community health nursing involves working with groups of people. Community health nurses are regularly involved in committees, task forces, and other work-related groups; they also work with aggregates in small groups—often teaching and facilitating support groups. Group communication patterns can be complex, and interaction requires skill on the nurse's part to elicit feedback from all members and to generate a common understanding among the group's members. Because the relationships among group members can significantly influence the effectiveness of communication, community health nurses need to understand how to organize groups and how groups function and develop over time, as well as techniques for facilitating group support and decision making.

Group Development

Think about the first time you walked into a nursing classroom—you didn't know the teacher or any of the other students in your group. What were your feelings? What did you expect or need the teacher to do? How did your feelings and expectations about the students and teacher change by the end of the term? Changes in "group dynamics" over time are termed **group process**.

In 1977, Tuckman and Jenson were credited with identifying the five most commonly used stages of group development (Display 10–8). The first stage of their model is termed *forming*. In this stage, members feel awkward and hesitant, needing to be reassured and accepted. Members depend on the group leader or facilitator to help them develop mutual trust and give them structure and guidance (Carter & Mossholder, 2015). At this stage, the group leader's task is to help the members become oriented to each other and to the work or purpose at hand.

"Ice-breaker" activities, to introduce members to each other and move past the awkwardness and hesitancy, are often used at the first group meeting. Conflict and sensitive topics, or too much self-disclosure by leaders or group members, are avoided at this stage. Rather, it is important to set ground rules (e.g., no sharing personal information outside of support group) and define the scope of work and timeline for completion. As group interaction is established in the first stage, task roles are the major focus with maintenance roles emerging in later stages (see Task, Maintenance, and Nonfunctional Roles in Group, Display 10–9).

The next stage is called *storming*, which is when the group begins to work together. In this stage, conflict and competition become more common as different agendas, ideas, and approaches begin to compete for attention. However, this period of role ambiguity is necessary to allow group members to identify roles and expectations and get a feel for how the group will work together. The storming stage can be difficult, but an effective group leader can guide group members in problem solving and setting goals. Modeling maintenance roles such as encouraging all group members to participate, asking for a quiet member to share an idea with the group, and summarizing group feelings is helpful in moving group members along in maintenance as well as task roles.

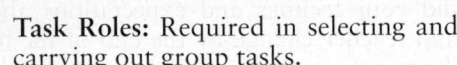

DISPLAY 10–8 STAGES OF GROUP DEVELOPMENT

Forming—Group dependent on facilitator; anxiety high, need safe environment, structure, and avoid too much self-disclosure; agree on guidelines for group work/behavior; orient to task or purpose of group.

Storming—Competition and conflict; need for structure; problem solving; need to draw out quiet members; continue to clarify group task or purpose.

Norming—Group now more cohesive and creative; acknowledge others' contributions; shared leadership; trust increases; work moves along more quickly.

Performing—Not reached by all groups; true interdependence—can work as group, or as individuals, and in subgroups; most productive; least reliant on facilitator.

Adjourning—The termination phase; conclusion of activities and resolution of relationships; formal acknowledgment of group work.

DISPLAY 10–9 TASK, MAINTENANCE, AND NONFUNCTIONAL ROLES IN GROUPS

Task Roles: Required in selecting and carrying out group tasks.

Maintenance Roles: Required in strengthening and maintaining group relationships and activities.

Nonfunctional Roles: Roles that harm the group and its work—often self-oriented behavior.

Task Role Behaviors

Initiating Activity: Proposing solutions; suggesting new ideas, new definitions of the problem, and new approaches to the problem or new organization of material.

Seeking Information: Asking for clarification of suggestions; requesting additional information or facts.

Seeking Opinions: Looking for an expression of feeling about something from members; seeking clarification of values, suggestions, or ideas.

Giving Information: Offering facts or generalizations; relating one's own experiences to the group problem to illustrate a point.

Giving Opinions: Stating an opinion or belief concerning a suggestion or suggestions; particularly concerning its value rather than its factual basis.

Elaborating: Clarifying, giving examples or developing meanings, and trying to envision how a proposal might work if adopted.

Coordinating: Showing relationships among various ideas or suggestions, trying to pull ideas and suggestions together, trying to draw together activities of various subgroups or members.

Summarizing: Pulling together related ideas or suggestions; restating suggestions after the group has discussed them.

Maintenance Role Behaviors

Encouraging: Being friendly, warm, and responsive to others, praising others and their ideas, agreeing with and accepting contributions of others.

Gatekeeping: Trying to make it possible for another member to make a contribution to the group by saying "We haven't heard anything from Jim yet" or suggesting limited talking time for everyone, so that all will have a chance to be heard.

Standard Setting: Expressing standards for the group to use in choosing its content or procedures or in evaluating its decisions; reminding the group to avoid decisions that conflict with group standards.

Following: Going along with decisions of the group, thoughtfully accepting ideas of others, and serving as audience during group discussion.

Expressing Group Feelings: Summarizing what group feeling is sensed to be and describing reactions of the group to ideas or solutions.

Both Task and Maintenance Role Behaviors

Evaluating: Submitting group decisions or accomplishments to compare with group standards and measuring accomplishments against goals.

Diagnosing: Determining sources of difficulties, appropriate steps to take next, and analyzing the main block to progress.

Testing for Consensus: Tentatively asking for group opinions in order to find out whether the group is nearing consensus on a decision and sending up trial balloons to test group opinions.

Mediating: Harmonizing, conciliating differences in points of view, and suggesting compromise solutions.

DISPLAY 10-9 TASK, MAINTENANCE, AND NONFUNCTIONAL ROLES IN GROUPS (*Continued*)

Relieving Tension: Draining off negative feelings by jesting or pouring oil on troubled waters and putting a tense situation in a wider context.

Types of Nonfunctional Behaviors

Being Aggressive: Working for status by criticizing or blaming others, showing hostility toward the group or some individual, and deflating egos or status of others.

Blocking: Interfering with the progress of the group by going off on a tangent, citing personal experiences unrelated to the problem, arguing too much on a point, and rejecting ideas without consideration.

Self-confessing: Using the group as a sounding board and expressing personal, nongroup-oriented feelings or points of view.

Competing: Vying with others to produce the best idea, talk the most, play the most roles, and gain favor with the leader.

Seeking Sympathy: Trying to induce other group members to be sympathetic to one's problems or misfortunes, deploring one's own situation, or disparaging one's own ideas to gain support.

Special Pleading: Introducing or supporting suggestions related to one's own pet concerns or philosophies and lobbying.

Horsing Around: Clowning, joking, mimicking, and disrupting the work of the group.

Seeking Recognition: Attempting to call attention to one's self by loud or excessive talking, extreme ideas, and unusual behavior.

Withdrawal: Acting indifferent or passive, using excessive formality, daydreaming, doodling, whispering to others, and wandering off the subject.

Adapted from Boyd, M. A. (2015). *Psychiatric nursing: Contemporary practice* (6th ed.). Philadelphia, PA: Wolters Kluwer.
Kirst-Ashman, K., & Hull, G. (2011). *Understanding generalist practice* (6th ed.). Belmont, CA: Cengage Learning.

By the time group members begin to show signs of cohesiveness, they have moved on to the *norming* stage, and work begins to progress. Trust and openness are much more apparent, and there is a shared sense of "belonging" to the group. Creativity and shared ideas and opinions characterize this stage. Until this time, most groups function at the task level, but by this stage, maintenance activities are more apparent as members draw others in and constructively share feelings. The leader should continue to role model good maintenance behaviors to move the group along in its work.

The *performing* stage may not occur with all groups; it is characterized by the ability to work as a total group, in subgroups or independently. This stage is considered the most productive, as group members are motivated and able to handle the decision-making process in a competent and autonomous manner. A high level of team satisfaction is seen in this stage as members are now able to work together more smoothly and do not need a lot of direction from the facilitator.

When either work or support groups end, the final stage of development is termed *adjourning*. In adjourning, the emphasis is on wrapping up the project, and this results in a withdrawal from both task and relationship or maintenance activities. Group members often feel happy that they have accomplished their goal but are sad about the loss or disbanding of the group. PHN group leaders can support the group as they prepare to disengage through a closure activity such as a small party or ceremony (Betts & Healy, 2015).

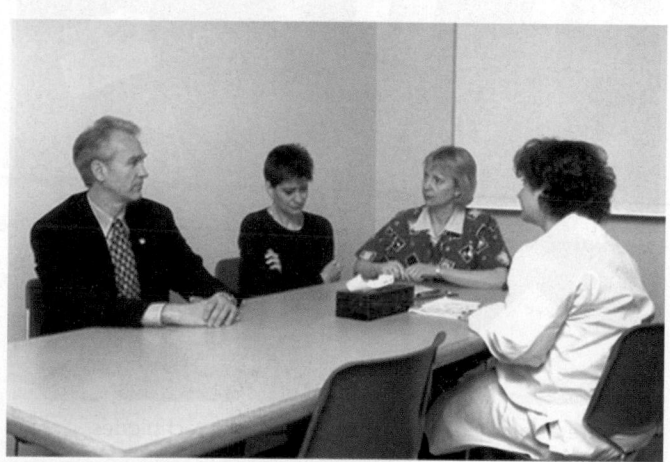

Group Functions in Decision Making

Groups, regardless of size, perform many functions. Four functions of particular relevance to group decision making include:

1. *Group members share information.* In public health nursing, groups often include clients, health professionals, and community members who share their experience and expertise to arrive at solutions and decisions. Something one member says may spur others to think of more creative solutions or share similar problems allowing group members to gain insight and develop trust (Kilpatrick, Lavoie-Tremblay, Ritchie, & Lamothe, 2014).

2. *Groups are heterogeneous and present diverse views* that enrich the number and types of alternatives in the problem-solving process. Group decisions are often better than individual ones because of the diversity of experiences and perspectives. However, group facilitators should promote open, prejudiced-free attitudes within the group to increase the positive benefits of diversity (Kilpatrick et al., 2014).

3. *Groups influence their members, thinking* by broadening their perspectives and presenting new ways of thinking about the issues. This allows group members to gain more insight in understanding the issue at hand (Hare, 2010). This influencing function can improve the quality of group decision making and increase the likelihood of decisions that support positive outcomes (Kilpatrick et al., 2014).

4. *Groups progress toward consensus* or resolution by planning tasks that allow members to discuss a set of alternatives and arrive at solutions to meet established goals. Time pressures and desire for completion help to move this process along (Kilpatrick et al., 2014).

Techniques for Enhancing Group Decision Making

As a member of many decision-making groups in the community, the community health nurse can facilitate the process through certain techniques. Three strategies commonly used in community health settings include brainstorming, multivoting technique, and nominal group technique.

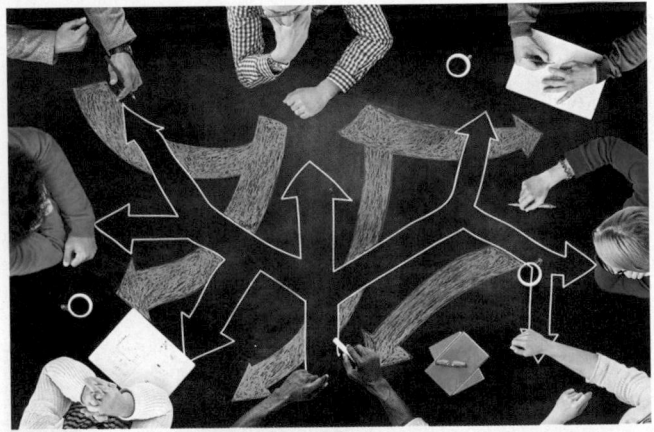

There are a variety of group decision-making techniques.

Brainstorming

Brainstorming is an idea-generating process that encourages group members to freely offer suggestions. When brainstorming, group members are asked to present ideas. They are encouraged to be creative and "think out of the box"; no idea is too bizarre or wild. Furthermore, no criticism or discussion is allowed until all ideas have been exhausted and recorded. This technique is helpful for generating creative possibilities and is most useful in the early stages of decision making. Research has shown that brainstorming is considered to be the most widely used method of generating creative ideas, but is often less effective than nominal group techniques (Gobble, 2014).

Multivoting

Multivoting is a decision-making tool that enables members to prioritize a long list of ideas with minimal discussion and difficulty. Multivoting often follows brainstorming to narrow the list to a few items worthy of immediate attention. All of the ideas are listed on a flip chart and members are allowed to vote on one third of the total number of items. For example, if there are 60 items, members are given 20 stickers to place their "vote" beside their top priorities on the flip chart. Once everyone has voted, the stickers are tallied to arrive at a shorter list of priorities (Minnesota Department of Health, 2016).

Nominal Group Technique

Nominal group technique is a group decision-making method in which group members are asked to not speak to each other but instead are asked to write down their ideas, along with the advantages and disadvantages of the issue being addressed. After everyone has completed the task, the members' ideas are presented to the group, and discussion takes place so that the information can be categorized and prioritized (Baheiraei, Mirghafourvand, Mohammadi, Mohammad-Alizadeh, & Nedjat, 2013). Nominal group technique affords researchers a means of collecting data that are inclusive and respectful of participants' opinions, while allowing both shy and talkative members to join in the discussion.

Other Group Communication Techniques

Not all community health nursing work with groups involves group process and group decision making. Sometimes, community health nurses are asked to speak to groups of concerned citizens at public meetings to raise awareness of an issue (e.g., preparing for disasters) or provide information to parent-teacher groups (e.g., immunization compliance). Often, they are called upon to incorporate group-teaching methods to change behaviors (see Chapter 11 for more on health teaching). Group teaching can be an effective tool for many health care challenges such as for diabetes teaching and education (Aeyoung, De Gagne, Sunah, & Young-Oak, 2015; Kewming, D'Amore, & Mitchell, 2016).

Group or public education and communication occur routinely in public health nursing. However, it is even more critical during disasters and other public health emergencies. Consistent public messages, interagency communication, and providing education and guidance on disaster preparedness are essential communication techniques for the garnering trust and reducing anxieties (Humphreys & Thompson, 2014).

COLLABORATION AND PARTNERSHIPS IN COMMUNITY HEALTH NURSING

Effective interdisciplinary and interprofessional collaboration is essential in the health care system to achieve quality health care and assure successful outcomes (Morgan, Pullon, & McKinlay, 2015). The definition of collaboration implies working together for the greater good; however, a more detailed definition will help facilitate the development of collaboration into practice for community health nurses. In this context, **collaboration** means a purposeful interaction among nurses, clients, other professionals, and community members to develop strategies for improving the health of individuals, families, and communities (Mitchell et al., 2013).

Although collaboration is a complex dynamic process, there are really only two basic features of collaboration: (1) it has a goal, and (2) it involves several parties assisting one another to achieve that goal. The overriding purpose or goal of collaboration in community health practice is to benefit the health of the public. Therefore, many players must work together (e.g., agencies, professionals, clients, lay health workers) to effectively achieve that goal. Partners will be able to meet their goals more effectively if the collaborative process promotes an atmosphere of mutual trust and respect, maintains open and honest communication, and accepts the roles and skills of the participating partners (Mitchell et al., 2013).

Asset-based community development (ABCD) is a methodology that starts with community assets and strengths including local persons, community associations and networks, natural resources, and institutions as a means of working with residents to create sustainable communities. Rather than a needs-focused approach, ABCD starts with identifying the types of skills and resources in the community and then consults with the community members on improvements they would like to make (Nel, 2015). Similarly, **community-based participatory research** (CBPR) involves community members in the entire research process from identifying a topic of importance to the community through implementation and dissemination (Kulbok et al., 2012; Pavlish & Pharris, 2012). See more on CPBR in Chapter 4. Involving stakeholders in planning and implementing programs and research increases their buy-in and the likelihood of success.

Key principles for establishing partnerships and collaboration with communities and interprofessional team members include:

- Think "outside the box" when looking for partners or collaborators.
- Plans are guides toward a goal; stay flexible.
- Partners must be part of the planning; continuously widen the circle of participants.
- When adding new partners, be prepared to replan.
- Maintain different levels of collaboration (different team members have more resources, come in later to the project, or leave the project earlier).
- Use consensus-building techniques that are creative and visual.
- Establish a shared vision; then share the plans and leadership (Bryant, 2014; Nel, 2015; Ng, Fraser, Goding, Paroissien, & Ryan, 2013).

To meet the needs of aggregate populations, public health nursing practice draws on the expertise and assistance of numerous individuals. The list of team members can include health planners, policy makers, epidemiologists, biostatisticians, community citizens, demographers, environmentalists, educators, politicians, housing experts, safety professionals, and industrial hygienists in addition to nurses, physicians, social workers, dieticians, psychologists, physical therapists, dentists, and other professionals involved in health services. All partners should be encouraged and allowed to utilize their skills and knowledge to optimize outcomes (Bryant, 2014; Kulbok et al., 2012).

Depending on the need to be addressed, community health nurses may work with many people on a single project or on multiple endeavors; it is important to remember to involve the most important team players. Therefore, representatives from the identified client population should always be included as key members of the collaborative process. For example, to address the increasing prevalence of childhood obesity and adolescent metabolic syndrome, research is beginning to show promise beyond just family-based programs to involve school-based interventions (IOM, 2012). Therefore, overweight and obese adolescents and their parents should be included in the process of designing and implementing school-based nutritional and physical activity interventions. By including members of the identified population, potential barriers, such as having few healthy food and drink choices at school, lack of consistent opportunities for exercise, and poor understanding about how to maintain weight loss, can be addressed. In a CBPR study about developing weight management lesson plans and audiovisual aids for a school-based health center intervention in New Mexico, researchers sought advice on adolescents' definition of health and motivation for weight loss, as well as how to best provide culturally and developmentally appropriate interventions and aids, along with incorporation of Internet activities and resources so that their program was attractive to a population of largely Hispanic, Black, and American Indian teens. Outcomes after participating in the intervention revealed significant improvement in BMI percentile and waist circumference compared to a control group (Sussman et al., 2013). Another example involves developing a culturally based intervention program to address HIV/AIDS among Latino youth, and the collaborative process including members of the targeted population while also including HIV prevention and treatment providers, HIV case management agencies, funding partners, and community members. By involving the appropriate interdisciplinary members, effective community health programs can be designed and implemented (Salerno, Delaney, Swartwout, & Tsui-Sui, 2015). Chapter 4 has more information on CBPR. Display 10–10 presents a case study illustrating the concept of community collaboration.

In the Levels of Prevention display, the levels of prevention pyramid are utilized to provide a framework of the collaborative process in community health nursing. One of the objectives seen in *Healthy People 2020* is Environmental Health objective HP2020-13: Eliminate elevated blood lead levels in children (U.S. Department of Health and Human Services [USDHHS], 2014). To achieve this objective, community health nurses need to be able to collaborate effectively with community partners in the design and implementation of health programs that address this very significant issue. However, the same nurses may work directly with individuals and families to educate them on the importance of having their children tested for elevated lead blood levels, and once a child is identified with an elevated lead blood level, the nurse may collaborate with individual clients to understand the importance of medical treatment for their child.

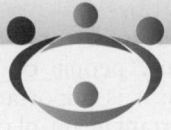

DISPLAY 10–10 COMMUNITY COLLABORATION

Case Study: Community Health Improvement Partnership

Problem #1:

The proportion of people who are uninsured in the United States is problematic. In the state of Florida, 2010 data from the Census Bureau indicates that one in four Floridians under the age of 65 lack health insurance that puts Florida third on the list of states with the highest percentage of uninsured. For the total population, 22.5% were uninsured. This high percentage of uninsured residents in Florida affects all Floridians through higher medical costs, insurance premiums, and taxes. The health insurance crisis in Florida puts all communities at risk. Floridians without health insurance are more likely to be sicker as access to care is late or not at all, thus impacting quality of life greatly. In Sarasota County, Florida, 38% of uninsured residents report that they delayed or did not get needed medical care when sick, with 12% reporting their health care status as fair or poor.

What can a community do to address the number of uninsured individuals in their neighborhoods? In Sarasota County, community leaders believed that a community is only as strong as its weakest member and that finding ways to expand coverage and increase access to affordable care for the uninsured was vital to the health of their entire county. The Community Health Improvement Partnership (CHIP) in Sarasota County brought together a dynamic collaboration of individuals, community leaders, not-for-profit organizations, and hospitals that are dedicated to improving the physical, mental, social, and environmental health of all citizens in Sarasota County. Community Health Action Teams (CHATs), comprising community volunteers and organizational partners, were formed in several areas of the county to focus on improving the health of a specific community. CHATs identified and studied health issues and then took action to tackle priority issues. For example, the North Port CHAT helped bring additional health care and transportation services to its community and also promoted youth activities and efforts to reduce substance abuse.

The Health Provocateur Project is another example of CHIP's initiatives. This initiative convened major stakeholders of the local health care system, including hospital chief executive officers (CEOs) and health department administrators on a quarterly basis to discuss and act on local issues. A team of collaborators from 12 hospitals and health departments created Sarasota Healthcare Access, a model system of care to improve services to the uninsured. Using a large-scale systems approach, the goals of this initiative included:

- Creating a formal system of the exchange of patient health information, data, and information on program/providers services
- Developing a universal referral system
- Utilizing existing capacity of providers to increase the number of residents who are enrolled in primary care and oral health service programs

- Providing case management services for uninsured clients with identified medical conditions to reduce unnecessary emergency room visits and hospital readmissions
- Enhancing access to low-cost medication
- Increasing community awareness of available health care resources for the uninsured

Effective collaboration in Sarasota County has led to the creation of a coordinated system of care that moved Sarasota County one step closer to improving the quality of life for all its residents.

Problem #2:

In 2013, data indicated that obesity were the most pressing challenge, and a new action plan was developed. The main components of that plan included the following:

- Development of a consistent message that promoted healthy weight.
- Applying EBP protocols to assess current weight of individuals.
- Developing a standard template for a healthy weight plan.
- Building capacity to meet the needs of the obese population (prevention, assessment, treatment, follow-up).
- Implementing interventions to improve environments that promoted healthy weight.
- School nurses, school nutrition programs, and parents were engaged to promote healthier eating in schools, and day care providers were also contacted. Worksite wellness collaborative and CHAT teams worked to improve healthy food access in the community.

Once the new assessment processes and healthy weight templates were in place, a pilot program showed early improvements in BMI.

From Ellingstad, K. (2013). *Healthy Sarasota County: Working together to improve community health.* Retrieved from https://www.scgov.net/Sustainability/Sarasota%20Sustainability%20Partnership%20Meeting%20Presen/2013_07%20Healthy%20Sarasota%20-Ellingstad.pdf
Sarasota County Health Department. (2012). *Community health improvement plan.* Retrieved from http://www.floridahealth.gov/provider-and-partner-resources/community-partnerships/floridamapp/state-and-community-reports/sarasota-county/_documents/sarasota-cha.pdf
Sarasota County Health Department. (2011). *Community health improvement partnership.* Retrieved from http://www.sarasotahealth.org/community-programs/chip.htm

Case Study Analysis Questions

Directions: Explore the CHIP Web site (http://www.chip4health.org) to learn more about this initiative and help answer the following questions:

1. What characteristics of collaborative partnerships are evident in this case study? Provide examples.
2. How are community members engaged in the CHIP initiatives? What is the role of CHAT teams in both problems?
3. What barriers to communication would you anticipate in working with CHIP teams?

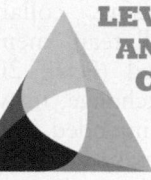 **DISPLAY 10–10 COMMUNITY COLLABORATION** (*Continued*)

4. Provide examples of three task and maintenance roles that the public health nurse can use to facilitate effective communication during CHIP and Health Provocateur Project meetings.

5. Discuss the stages of group development that you would expect the CHAT team to experience. What interventions can the community health nurse employ to help the CHAT move to the performing stage?

6. The hospitals and health departments in the Health Provocateur Project are a mix of government, for-profit, and not-for-profit organizations. What are the benefits and challenges of these entities working together?

7. What barriers to collaboration would you expect in the Health Provocateur Project? In the Obesity Project? What communication interventions could the public health nurse use to address the barriers?

LEVELS OF PREVENTION PYRAMID APPLIED TO CHILDREN'S HEALTH AND THE ENVIRONMENT: COLLABORATIVE OPPORTUNITIES FOR COMMUNITY HEALTH NURSES AT ALL THREE LEVELS OF PREVENTION

SITUATION: High lead blood levels were identified in a community
GOAL: Using the three levels of prevention:

- Programs and policies will be developed to prevent childhood lead poisoning.
- Children will be screened for elevated blood levels.
- Lead-poisoned infants and children will receive appropriate medical care and environmental follow-up.

TERTIARY PREVENTION (REDUCE THE MORBIDITY RELATED TO LEAD EXPOSURE OR POISONING)

Prevent Death and Further Disability	Interventions
• Restore child to healthful state. • Restore the environment to a healthful state.	• Medical treatment as indicated; may include chelation therapy • Removal of child from environment • Aggressive environmental remediation

SECONDARY PREVENTION (MINIMIZE ABSORPTION OF LEAD AND ELIMINATE CHRONIC EXPOSURE)

Early Diagnosis	Prompt Treatment
Surveillance and screening activities for early detection, treatment, and referral for management of environmental lead exposure	Identification of children with elevated blood lead levels Routine maintenance and repair of homes in high-risk communities

PRIMARY PREVENTION (REMOVE LEAD FROM THE ENVIRONMENT SO THAT EXPOSURE CANNOT OCCUR)

Health Promotion and Education	Health Protection
• Identify high-risk areas, populations, and activities associated with housing-based lead exposure. • Use local data and expertise to expand resources and motivate action for primary prevention. • Develop strategies and ensure the creation of lead-safe housing. • Collaborative partnerships in communities to provide educational programs to increase knowledge of lead safety in at-risk populations • Evaluate and redesign current prevention programs to achieve primary prevention while ensuring adequate secondary interventions.	• Use surveillance, demographic, and housing data to identify high-risk geographic areas • Identify high-risk families who could benefit from immediate assessment and services to reduce lead exposure. • Educate community partners on the cost of inaction to the community and affected families; highlight risk disparities. • Incorporate lead hazard screening into home visits by community health nurses. • Assure current programs are meeting the community's needs or readjust priorities.

Adapted from Centers for Disease Control and Prevention (CDC) (2015a).

Culture and Collaborative Services

Culture is a set of shared understandings related to knowledge, attitudes, and behaviors that give meaning to an experience. In public health nursing, clients and providers are often separated by their own distinct set of understandings or culture. Therefore, clients' cultural background, experience in collaboration and partnership building, perspectives, and expressions of need provide important information for the planning and delivery of services (Display 10–11). PHNs, by being aware of one's own culture and the difference between their culture and their clients', will be able to participate in cultural exchanges with clients that will promote stronger alliances, allowing them to develop greater understanding, acceptance, and commitment to more fully use the health programs designed for their benefit (Tucker et al., 2014). See Chapter 5 for more on culture in community health nursing.

Characteristics of Collaborative Partnerships in Community Health Nursing

To explore the meaning of collaboration in the context of community health nursing, this section examines five characteristics that distinguish collaboration from other types of interaction: shared goals, mutual participation, maximized resources, clear responsibilities, and set boundaries.

Shared Goals

First, collaboration in community health nursing is goal directed. The nurse, clients, and others involved in the collaborative effort or partnership recognize specific reasons for entering into the relationship. For example, a lumber company with 150 employees seeks to develop a wellness program. The community health nurse, company employee representatives, a safety expert, an industrial hygienist, a health educator, an exercise therapist, a nutritionist, and a psychologist might work together to develop specific physical and mental health goals. The team enters into the collaborative relationship with broad needs or purposes to be met and specific objectives to accomplish.

Mutual Participation

Second, in community health nursing, collaboration involves mutual participation; all team members contribute and are mutually benefited (Petri, 2010). Collaboration involves a reciprocal exchange, in which individual team players discuss their intended involvement and contribution, and it is important for all members of a team to feel equally valued—no hierarchies should exist (Davis & Travers Gustafson, 2015). The lumber company representatives may outline assessed areas of need, such as back-strengthening exercises to

---

DISPLAY 10–11 CROSS-CULTURAL GUIDELINES

1. Community health nurses should strive to ensure all population members receive care and services that are respectful and sensitive to their client's cultural beliefs and practices.
2. Be aware of your own belief system and values; understand and acknowledge that cultural differences may exist.
3. Develop a basic understanding and knowledge of other cultures, but do not use generalizations about other cultures to stereotype or oversimplify your ideas to another person or group. Remember there are differences within each cultural group that are influenced by individual characteristics and geographical location; therefore, never assume you understand what a person from another culture thinks or feels.
4. Demonstrate a genuine interest in the client's personal circumstances and seek to establish trust. Suspend judgments and respect the opinion of others.
5. Be aware of power imbalances and the effect on communication. Identify members who are accorded higher status and authority in family or group and respect the status hierarchy. Respect gender and age differences.
6. Do not assume that there is only one way (yours) to communicate. Keep working on ways to improve your cross-cultural communication skills. For example, avoid using jargon or slang that may not be understood cross-culturally. Use very clear and simple English.
7. Unspoken communication can be powerful; be aware and use appropriate body language.
8. Practice active listening. Try to put yourself in the other person's shoes, especially when another person's ideas or perceptions are different from your own. Be willing to step outside your comfort zone.
9. Do not assume that just because clients say they understand the information that they really do. Clarify questions and statements. Seek feedback by reframing the question in a different form to ensure understanding.
10. Apologize for cultural mistakes. Admit your own limitations and state willingness to learn from others. Show appreciation for the opportunity to learn from others.
11. Easily understood information and services should be delivered in the preferred language of the population served. Whenever possible, utilize interpreters who are trained in culturally competent care, and if possible, avoid using family members or friends to interpret. Look directly at the client, not the interpreter, when speaking.
12. Practice—we get better at cross-cultural collaboration when we practice it.

Adapted from Eubanks, R. L., McFarland, M. R., Mixer, S. J., Munoz, C., Pacquiao, D. F., & Wenger, A. F. (2010). Chapter 4: Cross-cultural communication. *Journal of Transcultural Nursing, 22*(Suppl 1), 137S–150S.
Rowe, J., & Paterson, J. (2010). Culturally competent communication with refugees. *Home Health Care Management Practice, 22*(5), 334–338.

facilitate lifting and reduce strain. The professionals, including the nurse involved in the collaboration, will offer their own specific ideas and expertise to design the wellness program. In interdisciplinary teams, physicians, nurses, lay community health workers, clients, outside agency personnel, and others must be able to effectively share ideas and frustrations on an equal, reciprocal basis.

Maximized Use of Resources

A third characteristic of collaboration is that it maximizes the use of community assets (Majee, Goodman, Vetter-Smith, & Canfield, 2016). That is, the collaborative partnership is designed to draw on the expertise of those who are most knowledgeable and in the best positions to influence a favorable outcome. If the lumber company team has identified a need for health education materials, the nurse and other members of the collaborating team may explore health education resources through the local health department and within their own professions. In this age of dwindling resources, it is now common for public health agencies to seek additional funding assistance from other agencies to support new community health programs or to provide educational information or interventions. Acute care hospitals and public health agencies may align over common interests (e.g., influenza, diabetes, and other lifestyle diseases). Outside funding agencies, both government and nonprofit, are increasingly looking for proof of effective collaboration and coalition building before approving grant or government funding. Being able to demonstrate fiscal responsibility and evidence-based outcomes will assist community health nurses in sustaining health promotion efforts on a long-term basis, and this may be facilitated by collaborative partnerships.

Clear Responsibilities

Fourth, the collaborating team members work in partnership and assume clearly defined responsibilities. As in a football team, each member in the partnership plays a specific role with related tasks. The nurse may play a case management or group-leadership role, whereas others assume roles appropriate to their areas of expertise. Effective collaboration clearly designates what each member will do to accomplish the identified goals. The nurse, for example, might coordinate the planning effort for the lumber company wellness program and work with the health educator to develop classes on various topics. The psychologist might advise on a chemical dependency program, and the industrial hygienist would provide assistance with safety measures. Each member of the team develops an understanding of individual responsibilities based on realistic and honest expectations. This understanding comes through effective communication. The collaborating partners explore necessary resources, assess their capabilities, and determine their willingness to assume tasks.

Boundaries

Fifth, collaboration in community health practice has set boundaries, with a beginning and an end, that fall within the goals of the partnership. An important part of defining collaboration is determining the conditions under which it occurs and when it will be terminated. The temporal boundaries sometimes are determined by progress toward the goal, sometimes by the number of team member contacts and often by setting a time limit (Browning, Torain, & Patterson, 2016). The collaborating group might target 6 months as a completion date for the lumber company wellness program and establish a timeline with designated activities to reach the goal. Once the purpose for the collaboration has been accomplished, the group as a formal entity can be terminated.

In some settings, the partnership may desire to continue to work on other, mutually agreed upon activities. If so, the process begins again with different goals. Some partnerships are ongoing. For example, a university with a department of nursing might use a neighborhood community center for clinical experiences for their students. The community center has needs that may include health assessments and in-home health teaching among community members, flu shots given at the center for elders without transportation, or health education classes for the adults in an English-as-a-Second-Language (ESL) class or for preschoolers in a Head Start program. The center and the university work in partnership so that, each semester, ongoing services are provided by the nursing students and coordinated by a faculty member or graduate nursing student in collaboration with the community center staff. Each partner wins. The students receive a rich educational experience, and the neighborhood center gets services they would otherwise do without. Within such a model, there are opportunities for students and volunteers. Students from other educational disciplines— social work, theater arts, physical therapy, early elementary education, and other areas—can be integrated into a center that serves people of all ages. Professionals (e.g., dentists, pediatricians) who are willing to volunteer (e.g., one-half or 1 day per week) enhance the services provided, as can lay volunteers, who can read to the children, answer the telephone, or participate in fund raising. When people collaborate and work together in partnership, a great number of possibilities exist.

Fostering Client Participation

This chapter has stressed that communication and collaboration are based on mutual participation. The extent of clients' involvement in that participation varies, however, depending on their readiness and ability to participate (Albarran, Heilemann, & Koniak-Griffin, 2014). The client's level of wellness at the time of the initial professional–client encounter directly influences participation. Some people are not physically or emotionally healthy enough to assume an active role in the relationship. Women recently discharged from the hospital after a mastectomy, for example, have many physical and emotional adjustments with which to cope. Their families, too, must expend additional energies to provide needed support and to cope with the temporary loss of the woman's usual role in the family. They may find it difficult to engage actively in identifying their needs and goals at the start of the collaborative process. The nurse may have to take a stronger initial leadership role; however, the goals of collaboration are not abandoned. Gradually, as the client's wellness level improves or the client's family becomes more involved, the nurse can encourage more active participation. Developmentally disabled clients, or others who are cognitively impaired, may not have the full capacity for true collaboration, but a collaborative team can work together with them in designing an effective plan.

Engaging clients in a collaborative process may be difficult at times. Clients with lower literacy skills or from low-income levels or minority or different cultural backgrounds may need extensive encouragement to actively participate in a collaborative relationship. Sometimes, a client's previous experience with health personnel limits participation in collaboration; clients who were not previously encouraged to participate in decision making by physicians, nurses, or other professionals may follow the pattern of a passive role and may not feel that they can truly collaborate. Unless the nurse persists in efforts to reduce the dependence of clients, the relationship can fall short of therapeutic goals (Dawson-Rose et al., 2016; Kulbok et al., 2012).

The nurse's own view of collaboration also influences the degree of client participation. Nurses who are accustomed to relating to clients in an adult-to-child manner restrict client involvement. If nurses see their position as more informed, and the client's position as one of complete ignorance and need, a paternalistic relationship may develop. All clients have resources on which to build, and the community health nurse should help clients to discover these resources and use them to enhance collaboration and attain health goals.

Structure of Collaborative Relationships

Like group process, collaboration among agencies or groups of people may occur in stages (Display 10–12). During this process, the work of identifying and meeting the client's needs takes place. Because most collaborative and partner relationships are bound by time, the structure involves several phases: (1) a beginning phase when the team relationship is just being established; (2) a middle, working phase; and (3) a termination phase when the relationship or project ends.

The first phase is a period of establishing and defining the team relationship. All of the team members, including clients, are getting to know each other; they seek to establish communication patterns and develop trust. In this phase, they identify the clients'/projects' needs and determine the goals toward which they will work.

The second phase occurs when team members start working together to accomplish desired goals. Their work may include assessment and planning as well as implementation and evaluation. The cycle of the nursing process is repeated as needed during this working phase until goals are satisfactorily accomplished.

The third or termination phase occurs when the need for team members to work together has ended. When team members have grown close in the relationship, termination can be difficult. Termination should never occur abruptly or without participation. It often requires careful advance preparation to make certain that all parties understand when and why it is taking place. Termination helps to ensure a clear-cut end to the collaborative relationship. For example, a nurse, physician, social worker, psychologist, and nutritionist collaborated with a refugee group for almost 1 year. As the group's multiple needs declined, the professionals began to taper off their assistance. Two months before the relationship was ended, termination of the group was discussed. At first, client group members were frightened at the loss of group support, but slowly they took ownership and control, and with their newly acquired skills, they assumed more responsibility for their health needs.

Barriers to Effective Collaboration

Communication barriers and miscommunication can inhibit effective collaboration. This is sometimes caused by misconceptions on the part of team members regarding the professional knowledge and motives of other team members. Stereotypes and the perception of unequal power and authority granted to certain disciplines can sabotage the effectiveness of communication and true collaboration. Apprehension about sharing information with the team, inflexibility and uneasiness with the

---

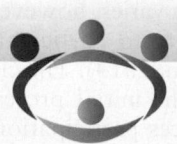

DISPLAY 10–12 STAGES OF COLLABORATION

Competition: Competing backgrounds, ideas, and motivations and a search to find shared values, goals, and ethical principles.

Networking/Communication: Sharing information promotes development of trust and role clarity and reduces miscommunication caused by stereotypical views of other disciplines, professions, or entities.

Cooperation/Coordination: More sharing of resources, less duplication, and formal communication through structure and agreements and more mutual respect.

Coordination/Partnership: Becoming more invested in the success of all partners, better able to manage and share resources, and full support of agencies involved.

Coalition: Shared leadership and decision making; resources benefit all members; sufficient power and authority to work collectively.

Collaboration: Shared mission and vision, open and trusting communication, strong relationships, sense of belonging, and shared accomplishments and goals.

Adapted from Institute of Medicine. (2016). *Collaboration between health care and public health*. Washington, DC: National Academies Press.
Northern Illinois University. (n.d.). *Stages of collaboration*. Retrieved from http://www.niu.edu/rcrportal/collabresearch/stages/stages.html

more fluid boundaries required in collaboration, and a failure to develop a common purpose and goals are all barriers for effective teamwork and collaboration. It is essential that team members share information about their respective disciplines and backgrounds, as well as personal expectations related to collaborative efforts that includes their perspective on what they see as the goal of the process (Shaw, Mitchell, & Del Fabbro, 2015). Organizational or structural factors, such as inadequate time, lack of resources, and lack of agency support are also cited as barriers to effective collaboration (Al Sayah, Szafran, Robertson, Bell, & Williams, 2014).

Conflict is inevitable when dealing with groups of diverse individuals, but how potential anger, resentment, and mistrust are handled is the key to getting beyond conflict (Soares Lopes, Meira Albino, de Menezes, & Muniz Ribeiro, 2015). Open, honest communication must prevail. One strategy to handle conflict is to introduce "carefronting"—described as a method of addressing and resolving conflict by confronting others in a caring, responsible, yet self-asserting manner. This method involves honest communication that sends the message that both parties in the situation should be treated with respect. Using "I" messages ensures that all parties in the conflict matter and that you care enough to negotiate differences so that common goals can be met. It is more fruitful to focus on the issue or problem at hand in a safe environment where all members can voice their opinions openly and not on personal determinations of who is right or wrong (Klinkhamer, 2015).

HEALTH TECHNOLOGY

Health technology/informatics utilizes processes, procedures theories, and concepts from information and computer science, health sciences, and social sciences. Nurses use the tools of information technology (IT) to support delivery of care and improve the health status of all. Health data, information, wisdom, and knowledge can be collected, stored, processed, and communicated. Nurses and other health professionals, administrators, policy and decision makers, as well as consumers, and clients/patients can use IT, hardware, and software (Nelson & Staggers, 2014).

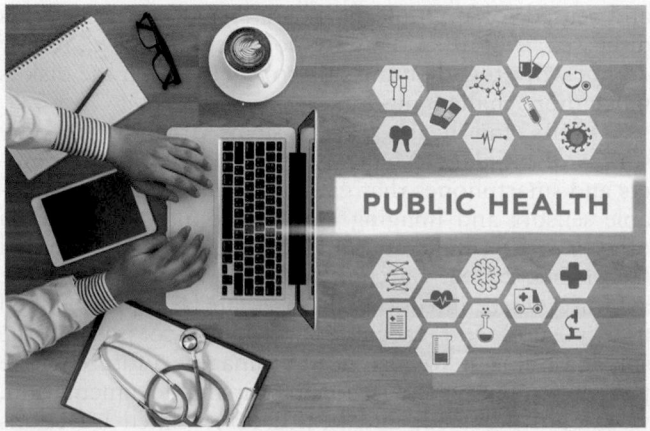

Health technology provides many opportunities for public health nurses to reach clients.

Early Use of Computers in Health Care

The successful application of innovative developments in the computer and information sciences to complex problems in health care promoted the birth of a new distinct specialty, health care informatics. This specialty is usually thought to have begun in the 1950s with the beginning use of computers in health care, as noted in a classic article by Dezelic (2007). Connie Settlemeyer created an example of early **nursing informatics** applications. Connie, while a graduate student at University of Pittsburg in the late 1960s, designed a mainframe-based computer-assisted instruction for teaching nursing students how to chart using a common problem-oriented format. The application was used to teach nursing at the University of Pittsburg throughout the 1970s (Nelson & Staggers, 2014). In the 1960s, El Camino hospital, conveniently located in Silicon Valley, collaborated with Lockheed to install the first computer-aided medical information system, which was known as MIS. Also in the 1960s, Dr. Lawrence Weed at the University of Vermont developed a system to reorganize and automate patient medical records. Weed's work was ultimately the basis for the Mayo health system medical record (Health Technology Review, n.d.). Information systems began to be installed by a number of hospitals to manage inventory and business data. El Camino hospital currently describes itself as a cutting-edge medical technology ecosystem (El Camino Hospital, 2016).

In the 1970s, order entry and results reporting were some of the first hospital information systems. In this decade, computer use was confined to specialty areas such as hemodynamic monitoring in intensive care and procedure areas. Libraries also began the switch to computerized databases, which helped to expand accessibility to medical information. This allowed for access to conference proceedings and journals allowing the knowledge specific to a specialty to become organized and readily available (Health Technology Review, n.d.).

Electronic Health Records Today

Electronic health records (EHRs) are, at their simplest, digital (computerized) versions of patients' paper charts. The contemporary EHR is a complex piece of software with multiple functions and capabilities. It enables a health care provider to record patient progress in free text, place prescription orders, receive decision-support alerts and reminders, order laboratory tests, receive and review results electronically, message patients or fellow providers, and perform a variety of other documentation and clinical tasks. Most nurses practicing today complete charting electronically, either exclusively or at least some of the time. Most U.S. hospitals and health care systems are using a form of EHRs currently. The Centers for Medicare and Medicaid Services (CMS) incentivized hospitals and health care systems to move to EHRs. The American Recovery and Reinvestment Act, signed in 2009 by President Obama, included the Health Information Technology for Economic and Clinical Health Act (HITECH). The CMS were directed through HITECH to motivate eligible providers to begin using EHRs, rather than paper. Financial incentives to health care systems were offered beginning in 2011, and penalties for not using EHRs began in 2015. CMS promoted the adoption of EHRs into three "meaningful use" stages (Duffy, 2015, para. 2). Stage 1 involves data capture and sharing. Stage 2 is about advancing clinical processes, whereas the third stage covers improved outcomes (Duffy, 2015).

By May 2013, about 80% of hospitals were using EHRs (Wu, 2014). The long-term goal of the federal EHR incentive program is to improve the quality and safety of health care. Adoption of EHRs was done with the best intentions in reaction to the mandates, but sometimes without adequate planning and or training. One of the most significant problems encountered is discrete EHR systems within departments in the same hospital or system. Chosen EHR systems may meet the needs of a specific clinical area but may not interact with other EHR systems used in other clinical areas in the same facility. Health care systems may have multiple ways to register patients that do not feed into each other. This leads to frustration on the part of nurses and other clinicians, as well as clients or patients.

One of the most beneficial advantages of using EHRs is the ability to enter data once and reuse them multiple times. This capability reduces redundancy and can reduce errors by providing the history from previous encounters. When an individual is readmitted, the previous data can be reviewed and update with the goal of decreasing charting time and improving continuity of care. Sensmeier (2015) suggests that nurses, as knowledge workers, can use EHR's clinical data to:

- Optimize workflow and support decision making.
- Tell the patient's story.
- Collaborate to foster knowledge translation.
- Leverage analytics to extract actionable knowledge.
- Use sharable, comparable data.
- Build evidence out of nursing practice.

The use of EHRs in public health has followed a slower progression than in hospitals. Reporting (e.g., communicable disease, immunizations) has moved from paper to unidirectional electronic reporting in many areas. Only a few states have capability for bidirectional data exchange between EHRs and immunization monitoring systems. A report of stage 1 implementation noted that 40% of eligible health care providers have submitted data on immunizations to public health agencies. A total of 54% of hospitals have submitted data to immunization registries, and 15% have electronically transferred lab results to public health agencies (Wu, 2014). A program, BioSense 2.0, collects data on ED visits and hospitalizations from multiple sources and works with local and state public health departments to determine the health of local communities (Wu, 2014). Public health agencies may also work with Health Information Exchanges (HIEs) in order to connect with local health care providers, hospitals, pharmacies, and laboratories in sharing health-related information; HIEs have the potential to provide real-time surveillance (e.g., location tracking of high-risk clients during emergencies, syndrome surveillance). Agencies may also find EHRs helpful in areas such as epidemiology, large-scale planning and budgets, and with grant writing (Birkhead, Klompas, & Shah, 2015; Tomines, Readhead, Readhead, & Teutsch, 2013). For example, an agency may search for specific characteristics and target vulnerable populations to best determine more effective planning and targeted interventions (e.g., clients with specific chronic diseases, current smokers). Individuals may also gain access to their own health information, and this is especially helpful in the case of immunization records (Wu, 2014).

Big Data

The McKinsey Global Institute defines **big data** as "datasets whose sizes are beyond the ability of typical database software tools to capture, store, manage and analyze" (Maynika et al., 2011, p. 1). Garcia (2015, p. 53) shared, "broadly speaking, big data refers to a large complex data set that can be analyzed to reveal patterns, trends, and associations, related to human behavior and interactions." The "big" in big data is not solely related to size, but it suggests the use of new statistical tools and the need for massive and/or multiple computers to process the data. Big data today may be considered ordinary or small in the future (Garcia, 2015).

Nurses in all settings add to big data through sharable and comparable documentation in the EHR (Garcia, 2015). The health care industry historically has generated large amounts of data, through record keeping, compliance and regulatory requirements, and patient care. EHRs lead to large amounts of electronic data. With mandatory EHR requirements and the potential to improve the quality of health care delivery meanwhile reducing costs, these massive quantities of data ("big data") can support a wide range of medical and health care functions, including clinical decision support, disease surveillance, and population health management, as well as many others (Raghupathi & Raghupathi, 2014). The use of big data makes it easier to drill down (or view more detailed information), drill up (or see data in an aggregate view), as well as "slicing-and-dicing" (or combining different data variables) than when using more traditional forms of data collection and analysis (Tomines et al., 2013, para. 12).

A goal of EHR documentation is capturing health and care data in structured ways that help build a foundation for accurate, reliable, clinically meaningful measurement across systems and settings of care. Big data are the core of that documentation, all of data entered in EHRs and more. The consistent and reliable use of data elements will allow information to be collected once and reused for multiple purposes (Sensmeier, 2015). As discussed, if EHR systems are not integrated (e.g., if they do not work together and talk to teach other), the task is much more challenging.

EHRs and health care systems are not the only source of big data. Medical data generated by computers and smartphones that gather information from wearable sensors and imaging devices are also included. In other words, a huge amount of data are being gathered (Sensmeier, 2015). Garcia (2015) asks nurses to imagine a future where infectious disease can be rapidly linked to exposures and vaccination patterns to prevent the spread of illness. We also need to imagine a future where patient acuity is calculated from nursing documentation, workloads adjusted, and health care–related infections reduced by the utilization of big data-driven evidence-based protocols.

Mobile Health (mHealth)

The rapid expansion of mobile technology provides an opportunity for nurses and other clinicians to improve health and health care through forms of interactive **mobile health (mHealth)**, referred to as mHealth services. mHealth includes the use of wireless technologies, such as smartphones, tablets, and notebooks for improving health. Mobile technology use in health care is evolving beyond the initial use as direct communication between nurses/clinicians and clients with one-way monitoring. mHealth offers great opportunities for improving global health, safety, and preparedness. The potential of mobile technology's impact on sharing health information and collecting disease/health data is tremendous due to its portability, affordability, and availability; it also has the potential to save billions of dollars in health care costs (Grant, 2013). The potential of mHealth will be further established as patients' experiences with technology and clinical/psychosocial outcomes are evaluated (Park, Howie-Esquivel, Whooley, & Dracup, 2014).

Three current mHealth trends have been identified by the U.S. Department of Health and Human Services (USDHHS, 2014). The trends include mHealth technology that is interactive, integrated, and multimedia. **Interactive strategies** enable "two-way flow of information that engages patients more actively" in their health management. **Integrative strategies** use multiple "self-management applications to share health information between patients and providers through text messages, centralized web-based" tracking and management programs, and mobile monitoring (such as glucose monitoring). **Multimedia** use "games and quizzes" to communicate preventive messages and motivate behavior change (USDHHS, 2014, p. 5).

mHealth is extending health care to underserved areas. Technology puts health care providers in a position to change how health care is delivered, the quality of the patient experience, and the cost of health care. Advantages include management of chronic disease, empowering the elderly and expectant mothers, reminding people to take medication, serving underserved areas, and improving health outcomes and medical system efficiency.

Big differentials exist between developed and developing nations. Africa has lowest rate of mHealth adoption, whereas North America, South America, and Southeast Asia showed the highest adoption levels. A number of countries have initiatives in the pilot stage or have informal activities that are underway. Chronic disease management is the greatest need in many areas. Remote monitoring devices enable individuals with long-term health alterations to manage their illness with clinician consultation (USDHHS, 2014). This keeps them out of doctor's offices for routine care and thereby helps to reduce health care costs. Real-time management is especially important in the case of chronic diseases. More research is required to link mobile technology to health outcomes. See From the Case Files: Monitoring a Cholera Outbreak Using Cell phones.

Mobile Phones

Approximately 91% Americans own a mobile phone, and 64% of those are smartphones (Pew Research Center, 2016). Most people keep mobile phones close by,

---

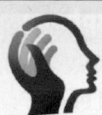

From the **Case Files** II

Monitoring a Cholera Outbreak Using Cell Phones

Cholera outbreaks in the African country of Rawanda sickened hundreds of people over a 2-year period. Nathan Eagle, an engineer and adjunct professor of epidemiology at Harvard University, wondered if tracking the location of individuals using cell phone data might indicate an early sign of an outbreak. For instance, if he tracked 100 individuals within a specific radius and noted that their movements slowed suddenly, it might indicate that there was a new outbreak. He had used mHealth earlier in assisting a small African hospital to prevent shortages of blood by using text messaging to alert the main blood bank early before the blood shortages became an emergency. So, he was familiar with cell phone use in Africa.

For the cholera outbreak, he used the cell phone service providers' call data records to track individuals' movements. When combining that data with public health records, he then had "big data" to use in testing his hypothesis. As luck would have it, as his experiment got started, the roads began to wash out during a flood, and people stopped moving around because they could no longer travel the roadways. However, he still found the data useful because cholera outbreaks often occur approximately 2 weeks following a flood.

Using cell phones in the developing world is a promising approach, as about 90% of the worldwide population has wireless coverage, and around 65% of cell phone subscribers live in areas of the developing world (Harvard University, 2012).

Source: Harvard University. T. H. Chan School of Public Health. (2012). Mobilizing a revolution: How cellphones are transforming public health. Retrieved from http://www.hsph.harvard.edu/news/magazine/mobilizing-a-revolution/

---

and check them several times throughout the day. Konok, Gigler, Bereczky, and Miklósi (2016) reported that people are extremely attached to their mobile phones, and most were kept within arm's reach. Mobile phone use is highest among individuals who use cell phones as their primary methods of communication. Mobile phone technologies offer promising opportunities for nurses working in the community setting (Christofferson, Hamlett-Berry, & Augustson, 2015; Lin et al., 2015).

Nearly two thirds (63%) of cell phone owners now use their phone to go online, according to the Pew Research Center's *Internet & American Life Project* (Duggan & Smith, 2013), and because 91% of all Americans own a cell phone, 57% of all American adults are cell Internet users. This is an 8% increase from the 55% of cell owners who did so at a similar point in 2012, and a twofold increase over the 31% who did so in 2009. See Table 10–1.

Table 10–1	Demographics of Cell and Smartphone Owners, 2014
	Have a Cell Phone
All Adults	90%
Men	93%
Women	88%
Race/Ethnicity	
Hispanic	92%
White and Black	90% each
Age Group	
18–29 years	98%
30–49 years	97%
50–64; 65 and over	88%; 74%
Household Income	
$50,000–$74,999	99%
$75,000 +	98%
$30,000–$49,999	90%
Under $30,000/yr.	84%
Level of Education	
College/some college	93% each
High school or less	87%
Type of Community	
Suburban	92%
Rural and urban	88% each

Adapted from Pew Research Center. (2016). *Cell phone and smartphone ownership demographics*. Retrieved from http://www.pewinternet.org/data-trend/mobile/cell-phone-and-smartphone-ownership-demographics/

Table 10–2	Americans' Cell Phone Activities
81%	Sending or receiving text messages
60%	Use it to access the Internet
52%	Sending or receiving e-mails
50%	Use it to download apps
49%	Use it to get recommendations, directions, or for other location-based services and information
48%	Listening to music
21%	Use it for video calls or chats
8%	Use it to share location or to "check-in"

Adapted from Duggan, M. (2013, September 19). *Cell phone activities* 2013. Retrieved from http://pewinternet.org/Reports/2013/Cell-Activities.aspx

Sixty-seven percent of cell owners find themselves checking their phone for messages, alerts, or calls—even when they don't notice their phone ringing or vibrating. Forty-four percent of cell owners have slept with their phone next to their bed because they wanted to make sure they didn't miss any calls, text messages, or other updates during the night. Twenty nine percent of cell owners describe their cell phone as something they can't imagine doing without (Duggan, 2013). See Table 10–2 for cell phone activities.

Connected health offers the patient the opportunity to feel constantly linked to the health delivery system and offers the system a just-in-time messaging opportunity that can be motivating, educational, and caring. A disadvantage is that mobile or cellular phones are frequently less reliable than landlines, with users citing spotty service, dropped calls, and text messages delayed or lost in cyberspace. To use this network for essential health care communication, improvements are needed (Kvedar, Nesbitt, Kvedar, & Darkins, 2011). Connected health offers the patient the opportunity to feel constantly connected to the health delivery system and offers the system a just-in-time messaging opportunity that can be motivating, educational, and caring (Health Information and Management Systems Society, 2016).

Text messages are the initial, simplest, and most common type of mobile data service and are becoming a vital tool for the delivery of health information and engaging users to improve their health (AHRQ, 2014; CDC, 2015b). Text messaging is a way of connecting quickly with a large population (Nelson, Joos, & Wolf, 2013). Global penetration of mobile text messages approaches 100% worldwide and is a widely recognized communication method in most societies (Kannisto, Koivunen, & Välimäki, 2014). Mobile phones are the most commonly used type of technology globally and have the potential to positively influence health-related behavioral change and self-management of both acute and chronic conditions (Park, Howie-Esquivel, & Dracup, 2014). The use of text messaging has been advocated for people living with HIV as a means of improving health quality and preventing complications (Coomes et al., 2012). Kannisto et al. (2014) conducted a systematic literature review of studies on text message reminders. Although the evidence for text messaging application recommendations is still limited, 77% (46 out of 60) of the studies showed improved outcomes with a text messaging intervention. The outcome measures included adherence to medication or treatment, appointment attendance, appointment nonattendance, and patient satisfaction. Park, Howie-Esquival, and Dracup (2014) conducted a systematic review of text messaging and medication adherence and reported that 62% of studies revealed that text messaging was efficacious in improving medication adherence. Given the widespread use of mobile phone text message reminders among different patient groups, it may have the potential to improve adherence to medication and attendance at clinical appointments globally.

Text messaging is simple, low cost, and ubiquitous. It continues to increase as a form of communication. As noted earlier, mobile phones are often kept close to people, checked several times throughout the day. Cole-Lewis and Kershaw found that people had their phones in the room with them 90% of the time, and 50% of the time they were within arm's reach (2010). Text messaging is considered more private and less intrusive than a phone call. Pictures, video, and text can be sent. Text messaging allows for automatic contact with groups of clients without the sender having send an individual message to each intended recipient. Response may be real time or at the leisure of the recipient. Text messages are less expensive than phone calls and less prone to spam than e-mail. Texts may be stored and revisited, and all languages are supported (Hebda & Czar, 2013). However, health literacy and cultural appropriateness for diverse populations must be considered when using text messages (USDHHS, 2014).

Reminder and educational text messages have the ability to be disseminated widely and broadly, reaching mass number of recipients quickly and inexpensively (Militello, Kelley, & Melnyk, 2012). Tailored, user-friendly interventions delivered by mobile phone may be a better fit with many individuals' lifestyles than traditional treatment and an attractive option for both clinicians and patients or clients. Mobile phones have a broad range of users, diverse functions, and the ability to intercede in "real time." Text messaging can overcome barriers of time and access to reach even high-risk populations (Militello et al., 2012).

Much research in public health has found that it is possible to use text messages to help deliver health-related information and to help people manage disease (e.g., diabetes) and make better health decisions such as smoking less and exercising more. Text message interventions promote healthy lifestyle behaviors, have become widely integrated into routine daily life, and are simple, low cost, and nonlabor intensive. Use of text messaging to deliver information about more sensitive topics, such as sexual health and reducing risky behaviors, seems promising. Opt in features, which allow choice for the recipient, can also be used (Militello et al., 2012).

Text messaging can deliver tailored, convenient, and regular reminders to assist clients with medication regimes as described with cardiac medications (Park, Howie-Esquivel, Chung, & Dracup, 2014) and those with human immunodeficiency virus (Sharma & Agarwal, 2012). For instance, daily text messages including medication reminders and education were sent for 6 weeks to adolescents and adults with atopic dermatitis. Significant improvements were noted in treatment adherence, self-care behaviors, skin severity, and quality of life (Pena-Robichaux, Kvedar, & Watson, 2010). Another study looked at acceptability of text messaging as an intervention with a cohort of African Americans who had uncontrolled hypertension (Buis, Artinian, Schwiebert, Yarandi, & Levy, 2015).

Timely administration of immunizations is a high priority in public health nursing practice. Kharbanda, Stockwell, Fox, and Rickert (2009) found that immunization reminders delivered by text message were preferred over mail or phone reminders. A later study found that parents' choice to enroll in a text message reminder-recall programs effectively promoted on-time receipt of subsequent HPV vaccine doses (Kharbanda et al., 2011). Stockwell et al. (2012) report that text messaging was effective in encouraging a change in behavior that led to higher rates of influenza vaccination.

See examples of text messaging interventions and research in Table 10–3.

Text messages may be used for simple reminders to have blood pressure checked or to notify individuals about an upcoming appointment or to pick up prescriptions (Nelson et al., 2013). Buchholz, Wilbur, Ingram, and Fogg (2013) conducted a systematic review of research studies on adult physical activity and a text messaging intervention. They concluded that a small group of researchers have studied text messaging as a method to promote physical activity, but that those studies show improvement in physical activity outcomes.

Text messaging is used globally to communicate, motivate individuals to engage in healthy or healthier behaviors, deliver public health messages, and alert populations about available resources or disasters. Nurses and other clinicians use of texting may be to assist patients and caregivers with management of chronic conditions and disease prevention. Text messaging provides a venue to deliver information to hard-to-reach populations and the opportunity to have a positive influence on health knowledge, behaviors, and clinical outcomes (USDHHS, 2014). See Display 10–13.

Applications

A mobile software application (app) is a program created for use on such devices as smartphones and tablet computers. Most devices are purchased with several apps as preinstalled software. Additional apps (those that are not preinstalled) are obtained through digital distribution platforms or app stores. In 2008, apps began to be popularized and are operated by mobile operating system owners, including Apple's App Store or iTunes Store, Windows Phone Store, Google Play, and Blackberry World. Some apps are free, and others must be purchased. It is common for a simplified version of an app to be available at no cost, which may entice the user to ultimately purchase the full version. Usually, they are downloaded from the platform to a target device, but sometimes they can be downloaded to laptops or desktop computers (Wikipedia, 2016).

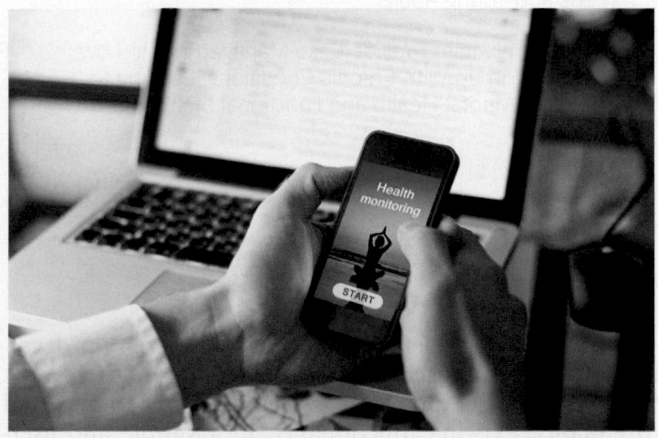

Mobile phone health applications are available to both health care providers and individuals.

Table 10-3 Selected Examples of Text Messaging Interventions and Research

Innovation	Description
Text Messages to Parents Increase Influenza Immunization Rate for Low-Income, Minority Children	A series of automated text messages to predominantly low-income, Latino parents about influenza and the importance of influenza vaccines leads to a small but meaningful increase in the percentage of children vaccinated
Sexual Health Clinics Provide Most Test Results via Text Message, Leading to Faster Diagnosis and Treatment, Greater Capacity to Serve Patients	Sexual health clinics communicate most test results via text message, leading to faster diagnosis and treatment and greater clinic capacity for handling new cases.
Weekly Text Messaging Service Enhances Access to Local Clinics and Accurate Information on Sexual Health for Teens and Young Adults	Weekly text messaging service for teens and young adults enhances access to sexual health information and services and generates positive changes in behavior and knowledge.
Low-Income, Rural HIV/AIDS Patients Receive Regular Text Messages, Leading to Higher Quality of Life and Greater Engagement in Care	Low-income, African American, rural HIV patients receive regular self-written text message reminders that encourage them to regularly access HIV/AIDS primary care, leading to greater retention in care and enhanced quality of life.
Daily Text Messages and Nurse Follow-up Improve Self-Management Behaviors in Patients with Diabetes, Leading to Better Glycemic Control and Lower Costs.	Daily, automated text messages combined with nurse follow-up improved self-management behaviors among patients with diabetes, leading to significant improvements in glycemic control, fewer doctor visits, lower costs, and high patient satisfaction.
Texting Service Enhances Minority Youth Access to HIV/AIDS Information and Testing. A statewide text messaging service provides minority youth and young adults in Illinois with accurate information on HIV/AIDS and connects them to free HIV testing and related services.	A statewide text messaging service provides minority youth and young adults in Illinois with accurate information on HIV/AIDS and connects them to free HIV testing and related services.
Monthly Text Messages Increase Compliance With Recommended Blood Glucose Testing in Medicaid Managed Care Enrollees With Diabetes.	A Medicaid managed care organization uses cell phone text messaging to remind members with type 2 diabetes to get regular blood glucose testing, leading to a significant increase in the percentage of members receiving tests on a regular basis.
Regular Reminders via Text Message Increase Adherence to Medication Regimen, Significantly Reduce Risk of Organ Rejection in Pediatric Liver Transplant Patients	Regular reminders via text message enhance adherence to medication regimens and reduce risk of organ rejection in pediatric liver transplant patients.
Text Messaging Program Increases Awareness and Concern About Sexually Transmitted Diseases Among At-Risk Youth, Particularly African Americans.	SexInfo provided free basic information and referrals for in-person health consultations to at-risk youth in San Francisco via an opt-in text messaging service.
Weekly Text Messaging Service Enhances Access to Local Clinics and Accurate Information on Sexual Health for Teens and Young Adults.	Weekly text messaging service for teens and young adults enhances access to sexual health information and services and generates positive changes in behavior and knowledge.
Public Health Nurses Provide Case Management to Low-Income Women With Chronic Conditions, Leading to Improved Mental Health and Functional Status.	Public health nurses provide case management services to women with one or more chronic conditions who receive Temporary Assistance for Needy Families, leading to enhanced access to mental health services, fewer depressive symptoms, and improved functional status. Nurses used text messaging as necessary to ensure health-related needs were met.

Selected from Agency for Health Care Quality & Research (AHRQ). (n.d.). *Innovations exchange: Search innovations*. Retrieved from https://innovations.ahrq.gov/search/innovations/Text%20Messaging?page=1

Apps may be defined as a software program developed to help the user perform specific tasks (Nelson & Staggers, 2014). Apps are self-contained programs, used to enhance existing functionality, in a simple and user-friendly way. Today's modern smartphones come with powerful web browsers, meaning nearly anything that can be done on a desktop computer can be done with a smartphone's browser. Mobile applications may be a limited version of a larger program and perform limited functions as compared to a more complete Internet-based program, such as is seen in banking. Mobile apps are easily installed and are typically cheaper than those designed

DISPLAY 10–13 TEXT MESSAGING BEST PRACTICES

1. *Keep messages short.* Text messages should be short and concise. The entire message should be <160 characters, including spaces and punctuation and any branding or links to additional information (p. 25).

2. *Make messages engaging.* Write relevant, timely, clear, and actionable messages. Try to begin each message with an interesting fact or question so that users will be more likely to open the text message and read the remainder of the message.

3. *Make content readable.* Content should be at or below an 8th grade reading level.

4. *Use abbreviations sparingly.* Because text messages have a character limit, it is acceptable to use abbreviations, but only use those that are easily understood and don't change the message's meaning.

5. *Limit foreign language characters.* Depending on the mobile carrier, for instance, accented letters do not work well in texts.

6. *Provide access to additional information.* Be sure to include your agency's name in the text so users know who is sending the message and include a way for users to follow up or respond to the message (e.g., URL, phone number, mobile Web site).

7. *Include opt-out options.* Text messages may also include information on how to opt-out of the text message program (p. 25).

8. *Promote your text messaging efforts.* To maximize your reach, create a promotion plan that includes advertising on mobile sites and social media.

9. *Evaluate your efforts.* Evaluation can be accomplished with surveys and metrics reviews (p. 25).

From Centers for Disease Control and Prevention (CDC). (2011). *The health communicator's social media toolkit.* Retrieved from http://www.cdc.gov/socialmedia/tools/guidelines/pdf/socialmediatoolkit_bm.pdf

---

to run on laptop and desktop computers. The portability of the app that allows the user to remain connected is very appealing to both clinicians and patients. Mobile platforms have become more user friendly, computationally powerful, and readily available, leading to the development of mobile apps of increasing complexity to leverage the portability mobile platforms can offer. Many new mobile apps are targeted to assist individuals in their own health and wellness management. Some apps may assist family caregivers. Other mobile apps are targeted to health care providers as tools to improve and facilitate the delivery of patient care (Nelson & Staggers, 2014).

Application developers have noticed the potential of health care apps. Apple had more than 1,500,000 apps on iTunes as of September 2015, with nearly 43,700 identified as health or medical apps. Android features more than 3,300 medical apps. Sixty-nine percent of apps targeted consumers and patients, whereas 31% were developed for use by clinicians. It is unclear if the apps are evidence based, developed without conflicts of interest, and reliable. Health professionals are necessary in app development to peer-review the reliability, usability, and usefulness of the medical apps. Data are not available regarding the number of "real" health care apps, and this presents problem for users. The Institute for Healthcare Informatics (2015) report, *Patient Adoption of mHealth: Use, Evidence and Remaining Barriers to Mainstream Acceptance,* includes a prediction that patient adoption of mHealth apps will move from novelty to mainstream within 5 years (Institute for Healthcare Informatics, 2015). As the use of tablets and smartphones increase, the app market will also expand; one estimate is over 60% by the end of 2017, making it worth $26 billion (Deruy, 2013).

The Food and Drug Administration (FDA) is responsible for the protection of public health by assuring the safety, effectiveness, quality, and security of human and veterinary drugs, vaccines and other biological products, and medical devices (Smith, 2014). The FDA intends to apply regulatory oversight to medical mobile apps and identifies apps as medical devices whose functionality could pose a risk to an individual's safety if the mobile app did not function as intended (FDA, 2015). Some app developers express concern about the FDA's new role in app development. However, it is important to consider that if dangerous errors and disproven apps are allowed to proliferate, distrust could undermine acceptance of other useful products.

Cellular phones are all around, and the number of smart phone users is growing rapidly. Text messaging, the use of applications, and other mHealth interventions can reduce geographic and economic barriers to health information and services. These interventions have the potential to reduce health disparities and leverage a profound effect on health (USDHHS, 2014). mHealth apps are more likely to be used by Hispanics and African Americans than Whites, and this information is not lost on government agencies. For instance, apps that target Type II diabetes and obesity, as well as cancer, among minority populations are being developed to engage hard-to-reach communities (Deruy, 2013).

FastStats

FastStats is an official, free application from the Centers for Disease Control and Prevention's (CDC) National Center for Health Statistics (NCHS). Over 100 public health topics are alphabetically organized and readily available including diseases and conditions, family life, health care and insurance, health status and risk factors, injuries, life stages and populations, and reproductive health. Links provide sources of more data and related Web pages. When the device, phone, tablet, or computer is connected to the Internet, updates occur automatically. Along with getting the most up-to-date health statistics available, the app allows for highlighting, annotating, and bookmarking, as well as sharing of data through social media such as Facebook and Twitter; the mobile app is available through Apple's App Store or for Android phones from Google Play (CDC, 2015b). FastStats homepage and statistics by topics are available at: http://www.cdc.gov/nchs/fastats/

Twitter

Twitter is a micromessaging/microblogging technology and an online social networking service that enables users to send and read short 140-character messages called "tweets." Posts are delineated by a hashtag (#) symbol to organize topics (Nelson & Staggers, 2014). Microblogging began with the advent of Twitter in 2006 and is a method of mass communication. "Followers" or users sign up to follow the microblog. Most microblogs have a setting that requires acceptance of new followers (Nelson et al., 2013). Twitter is real time and designed for mobility (Kvedar et al., 2011). E-registered users can read and post tweets, but those who are unregistered can only read them. Users can post tweets on a smartphone. Twitter is very simple and easy to use and exists somewhere between the worlds of e-mail, blogging, and instant messaging, with the users getting almost immediate responses to tweets. Twitter is extremely popular between individuals looking for means of promotion such as bloggers, online marketers, and entertainers, as it acts as a communication stream that has a continuous flow unlike most other networks. Twitter is one of the top three social media applications, used by 19% of all adults and 23% of online adults in the United States (Duggan, Ellison, Lampe, Lenhart, & Madden, 2015). Access to Twitter is through the Web site interface, text messaging, or mobile device app. Twitter was initially a convenient way to stay in touch with friends and family, but is now emerging as a potentially valuable means of real-time, on-the-go communication of health care information and medical alerts (Liebert, 2009). When an individual tweets or sends a message via Twitter, all of the people who have chosen to follow them will receive it.

Duggan et al. (2015) found that Twitter was used by more men than women and by more young adults (18 to 49 years) than older adults (50 to ≥65 years). Twitter use rates are higher for non-Hispanic Blacks and Hispanics than for non-Hispanic Whites. Nurses/clinicians and health care systems can use Twitter to communicate timely information, both within the medical community and to patients, as well as the general public. Short messages, or "tweets," are delivered to a group of recipients simultaneously, providing an easy and quick method to reach large groups in limited time. There are obvious advantages for sharing time-critical information such as disaster alerts and drug safety warnings, tracking disease outbreaks, or disseminating health care information. Twitter applications can deliver information about clinical trials, for example, or to link brief news alerts from the CDC to reliable Web sites that provide more detailed information (Liebert, 2009).

Professionals are now using Twitter to share informational and web resources. Organizations use Twitter to share news and member updates, and it can be used to share

information among professional conference presenters in real time. Clinicians can "tweet" from the operating room or a disaster site allowing live updates (Hebda & Czar, 2013).

Twitter and texting services both have character limits, so acronyms and shortened forms of the words are used in messages. The character limit of Twitter is 140 characters, whereas the usual character limit of texting is 160 characters. The biggest difference is that Twitter is an Internet-based service and texting is provided through the user's mobile network or cellular phone service. The original intention was that access to Twitter would be via the computer, whereas texting is done using a mobile phone. Twitter has been considered and is described as a social networking program, whereas texting is more of a personalized way of sending messages. In general, texts only go to a single recipient or a small group, whereas tweets on Twitter can be visible to the general public. Individual messages can be sent via Twitter, but it is largely a social networking tool.

Twitter is a free service, whereas texting is a service that usually incurs charges from the mobile companies that provide the services. Both tweet and text contain various characters (e.g., #, &, @, etc.) that allow the messenger to use fewer words. Using characters like # and @ has another function at Twitter where the hash symbol is used to make the tweets more searchable, and @ is used to link another user to the message. The use of these specific functions attached to specific characters is not seen in texting. Unlike some other social media sites, an individual can follow anyone they want on Twitter, even if they don't know them personally (Hebda & Czar, 2013; McGonigle & Mastrian, 2015).

Twitter can be useful to public health agencies and in other health care situations. For instance, it could be used to collect data for epidemiological investigations (e.g., foodborne illness), as a means of tissue recruitment (e.g., organs, blood), for disaster alert and response, as a means of providing FDA drug safety alerts, for Amber alerts, for prescription management, for food and product safety alerts, for community health outreach and policy discussion, and for public safety announcements (Baumann, 2016). A list of 140 health care uses for Twitter can be found at: http://philbaumann.com/140-health-care-uses-for-twitter/

Blogging and Online Support Communities

Blogs or weblogs are web-based chronological journals (Nelson & Staggers, 2014). They are free or low cost and easy to use. Blogs typically include date-stamped, multiple entries in chronological order and are updated frequently. Blogs usually focus on a particular subject or topic. One type of blog, referred to as a simple blog, is a form of online personal diaries. Other blogs relate to group causes such as political or social concerns, and some may ask for contributions. Blogs may contain reflections, commentaries, comments, images, videos, and often hyperlinks to other information of interest to the blogger or that she/he feels will be of interest to their readers. Blogger is the term used for the person who creates and maintains the blog site. The ability for readers to leave comments on a blog post depends on the settings that the blog administrator uses (Nelson et al., 2013).

The popularity or success of a blog is judged by its ability to draw individuals together who are interested in a specialized topic. Many journals, health care systems, nursing and other professional organizations, health care provider networks, and educational institutions create blogs to provide the latest information and promote discussion (Nelson & Staggers, 2014). Many people create personal blogs when faced with an illness or are a family member/support for someone facing health challenges. Participating in the creation of health information through blogging and social networking contributions influences experiences and supports an individual's understanding of their role in health care management and information (DeGroot & Carmack, 2012). Individuals may turn to the Internet to grieve and manage the traumatic experience of loss or to cope with emotional pain after a loss. Personal blogs are often established following the death of a parent, spouse or partner, sibling, close family member, or child. Blogging may serve as an emotional release, therapy, and healing. It can serve as a public way to cope with grief (DeGroot & Carmack, 2012). Some report comfort in sharing information on the Internet, even among those that choose not to share with family or close friends. Individuals or relatives of a person suffering from cancer or other life-changing or threatening disease are affected both physically and psychologically. Canning, Rosenberg, and Yates (2013) found that blogging among family member of cancer patients facilitated everyday life, introduced the relatives to others with similar experiences, assisted in their grief process, and helped to preserve memories.

Advances in medical treatment allow many to survive for long periods of time with diagnoses that previously would have been rapidly fatal. Individuals and families face the physical as well as the social and emotional consequences of chronic pain and extended illness. This creates a new paradigm of medical care for chronic conditions and a need for effective interventions that could provide support throughout the journey of diagnosis, treatment, and management. Many have suggested that expressing emotional or traumatic experiences with the written word through the process of expressive writing may have therapeutic benefit for individuals. Internet-based blogs allow this expression (Ressler, Bradshaw, Gualtieri, & Chui, 2012).

Traditional forms of contact and support groups are limited to certain hours of the day, week, or month. Some face-to-face support groups meet weekly or monthly and may require considerable travel and effort. Telephone help lines may be available only during office hours. Contact and support are available at any hour of the day or night via the Internet. Those with a home computer can access an extraordinary range of resources for private and anonymous communications with others in real time. Individuals who have joined an online support group benefit from venting their feelings and from the support they receive, as well as feeling connected by helping and supporting others (Diefenbeck, Klemm, & Hayes, 2014). Online supportive relationships generally provide a safe environment (Varga & Paulus, 2014). Others' experiences can induce feelings of compassion, and one becomes less self-absorbed and may gain a better perspective (Varga & Paulus, 2014). In a study of online support groups, Mo and Coulson (2014) describe the process of being emotionally empowered when information is exchanged and emotional support is shared, as well as a recognition gained through sharing experiences. Chung (2014) suggests the online support groups simply help people feel better. Ziebland and Wyke (2012, p. 219) stated their study respondents saw this process as important, meaning that you knew you "were not alone" because hearing about other people's experiences gave you a sense of "being supported." Finding a safe place to share can be very empowering.

A study of parents of children with a genetic condition (Schaffer, Kuczynski, & Skinner, 2008) reported most trusted and valued source of information was not clinicians but the other parents in internet communities, whose shared information was combined with a personal stake. As cancer patient Dave de Bronkert (known as e-patient Dave in his popular TED Talk) stated, "Patients know what patients need to know" and are, therefore, the most underused resource in health care. For individuals who have unusual or stigmatizing conditions, who are undergoing atypical treatments, or who are geographically isolated, the online resources may be their best source of support (Mo & Coulson, 2014). The value of first-person accounts, the appeal and memorability of stories, and the need to make contact with peers all strongly suggest that reading and hearing others' accounts of their own experiences of health and illness will remain an important component of health management/care.

PatientsLikeMe, available at: (https://www.patientslikeme.com/), is a great example of a free Internet-based tool for sharing and learning. Individual and clinician accounts are available. Two brothers, Jamie and Ben Heywood, began this site when their brother Stephen was living with amyotrophic lateral sclerosis (ALS). A quote attributed to the brothers is on the home page "Our brother Stephen was living with ALS and we thought, 'there has to be a better way.' There is. By sharing our experiences, we can all contribute new data that can accelerate research and help create better treatments. Our experiences can actually change medicine... for good" (Heywood & Heywood, 2015, para. 4).

Video Games

Half of American adults have played video games, and 10% call themselves gamers. Public attitudes toward video games and the people who play them are complex and often mixed (Duggan, 2015). Video games are typically thought of as entertainment. However, there is a growing interest in video games as a means to facilitate healthy behaviors (Kim, Prestopnik, & Biocca, 2014). Exercise programs based on video game activities (VGA) provide an alternative to motivate and increase adherence to activity and pulmonary rehabilitation programs, especially in the younger population (del Corral, Percegona, Seborga, Rabinovich, & Vilaró, 2014).

A great deal of attention has been given to the negative effects of playing video games, but there can be positive effects of engaging in this activity. Health or training goals can be met using existing commercial games. Tailor-made games may engage patients and make it easier to meet treatment goals. Video games may be used for educational purposes for clinicians. Video games have been used with patients since the 1980s. Tailor-made games for different disease groups are a more recent endeavor and are evaluated in scientific trials (Kim et al., 2014).

Games can serve as a means to engage patients behaviorally in order to improve their health outcomes. Behaviors, often necessary to maintain and improve health, are reinforced. With game play, tension and fears are released in a safe setting, and aversive or shameful aspects of an illness may be managed. The focus of attention on an engaging distraction (the game) may explain how individuals manage aversive symptoms through video game play. An example of distractive use of a game is SnowWorld (see Table 10–4 for description) that is used to distract patients during burn care. The repetitive nature of video game play may promote learning (Kato, 2010; Pauschenwein, Goldgruber, & Sfiri, 2013).

Telehealth

Telehealth is the use of technology to deliver health care, health information, or health education at a distance (National Advisory Committee on Rural Health & Human Services, 2015). The American Academy of Ambulatory Care Nursing's definition of telehealth is:

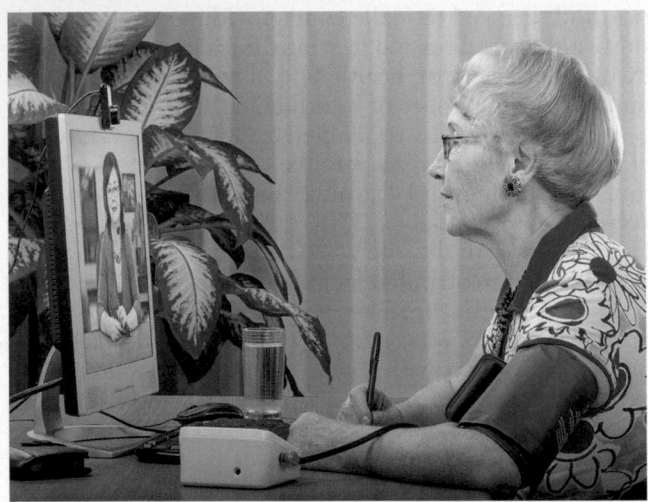

Telehealth gives the public health nurse an opportunity to see and speak with clients located at remote sites, as well as provide education and counseling.

> The delivery, management, and coordination of health services that integrate electronic information and telecommunication technologies to increase access, to improve outcome and contain or reduce costs of health care. Telehealth is an umbrella term used to describe the services delivered across distances by all health professions (Espensen, 2012, p. 42).

Telehealth provides access to care and the ability to export clinical expertise to individuals who require care, regardless or geographic location of the patient or the clinician (Nelson & Staggers, 2014). The boundaries of telehealth are limited only by the technology available, and new applications are being developed and tested every day. Telehealth can be divided into two general types of applications: real-time or synchronous communication

and store-and-forward or asynchronous communication. Real-time communication scenarios include a patient and clinician consulting with a specialist via a live audio/video link or a clinician and a patient in an exam room communicating through an interpreter connected by phone or webcam. Another example is a meeting with a clinician in one location and an individual in another who communicate through Skype. A clinician holding a teleconference with other clinicians about new best practices also could be classified as telehealth. With synchronous or real-time telehealth communication, all members are technologically present at the same time. Asynchronous or store-and-forward applications utilize the transmission of digital images, records or results for a diagnosis, consultation, and information sharing and/or treatment interventions and suggestions. With asynchronous telehealth, members are not technologically present at the same time, but share the same information at the time most convenient to each one (National Advisory Committee on Rural Health & Human Services, 2015). Many online education programs utilize asynchronous methods of instruction.

The American Telemedicine Association (2015) states telehealth has been growing rapidly because it offers four fundamental benefits:

- Improved Access—For over 40 years, telehealth has been used to bring health care services to patients in distant locations.
- Cost Efficiencies—Telehealth has been shown to reduce the cost of health care and increase efficiency through improved management of chronic diseases, shared health professional staffing, reduced travel times, and reduced hospital stays.
- Improved Quality—Studies have consistently shown that the quality of health care services delivered via telehealth is equal to those given in traditional in-person care.
- Patient Demand—Consumers want telehealth that reduces travel time and related stresses for patients/families. Services and/or providers may not be available otherwise (para. 7).

Telehealth applications require IT, but not every use of health-related technology is telehealth. Stand-alone systems like EHRs, discussed earlier, are not typically thought of as a telehealth application. One outstanding value of telehealth is that it can increase contact between an individual patient or a family with the health care system. Additional expertise can be brought to the patient's home or bedside, clinicians can reach out to patients when they are at home, and save travel time and expense for both practitioners and patients. Telehealth shows great potential for advancing preventative medicine and the treatment of chronic conditions (American Telemedicine Association, 2015). The first year of reimbursement for telehealth services delivered outside of care settings occurred in 2015 (Wicklund, 2015).

Geographic Information Systems (GIS)

A geographic information system (GIS) is a computer-based information system designed to capture, store, manipulate, analyze, manage, and present all types of spatial (relating to space) or geographical data. GIS allows

Table 10–4 **Selected Tailor-Made Video Games for Health**		
Name of Game if Specifically Named	**Medical Condition Targeted**	**Game Description**
Snow World	Burn pain	Users travel through an "icy landscape of a canyon, cold river, and waterfall through gently falling snow." Along the way, they can "shoot snowballs at snowmen, penguins, igloos, and robots." This game was "designed specifically to minimize body motion during gameplay to enable wound care (debridement) by nurses." Players control movements and activities by manipulating a fixed joystick (p. 116).
Packy and Marlon, originally made for the Super Nintendo game console system.	Diabetes for children	The game characters are two elephants attending a diabetes summer camp. The goal is to get rid of a "gang of marauding rats" that keep campers from their healthy food and diabetic supplies. To win, players have to "successfully manage their insulin levels and food intake while keeping their characters' glucose levels within an acceptable range" (p. 116).
Bronkie the Bronchiasaurus is a video game on the Super Nintendo Entertainment	Asthma for children	This game takes place in prehistoric times when the world was covered in dust. A fan needed to control the dust has broken. Players help the characters keep their asthma in control by "avoiding triggers such as dust and smoke" while on their quest. Question-and-answer inserts, needing correct responses, are interspersed and must be successfully answered in order to keep going (p. 116).
SpiroGame	Compromised lung function for preschool children	Measures and gives a readout of breathing function for spirometry and is helpful for patients with compromised lung functioning associated with asthma or cystic fibrosis. Spirometry depends highly on patient cooperation and effort during the procedure. Measurement conducted with *SpiroGame* promotes lung functioning in preschool children, inhalation and exhalation, and helps to control their breathing. Children control an animated caterpillar with their breathing. The caterpillar crawls to an apple over a period of 30 seconds as long as the child's breathing reaches predetermined targets. Another mini-game teaches children how to do a breathing test by "moving an animated bee flying from flower to flower" (p. 116).
Nonspecifically titled games that use biofeedback to control gameplay	Bladder and bowel dysfunction Pediatric voiding dysfunction in children	The child's compliance and motivation influence the success of biofeedback. Children are often not interested in dealing with embarrassing topics and may have difficulty staying focused on a biofeedback-training task. When combined with a game interface, interest and motivation in biofeedback are increased. Sensors are placed on the child's perineum to detect pelvic floor muscle activity. "Leads from the sensors connect to a port on the computer in which electrical activity from the sensors is transformed through algorithms to relate to actions in the game" (p. 117). The games included golf, spaceships, baseball, basketball, and a safari adventure. For example, in the golf game, the distance a golf ball traveled was determined by pelvic floor contractions. "In the basketball game, accuracy of shooting a basketball through a hoop was related to the patient's ability to relax the pelvic floor muscles" (p. 117). The games helped improve symptoms and treatment compliance, "even in children young as 4 years old, a group previously thought to be too young for biofeedback muscle training" (p. 117).
Nonspecifically titled games that employee biofeedback to control gameplay	Irritable bowel syndrome in adults	A computer biofeedback game designed for patients with IBS. The game teaches "stress management through deep relaxation exercises" (p. 117). Biofeedback sensors on the patients' fingers measure electrodermal activity (e.g., microchanges in sweat response). Patients control an "animated representation of bowel movement through changes in electrodermal conductivity" detected by biofeedback sensors when the patient engaged in both physical and mental relaxation (p. 117). The patients had more control of the animated gut movement when they were more relaxed.
Re-Mission	Cancer in adolescents and young adults	The goal of the game is to improve treatment, and players control a nanobot named Roxxi, who flies through tumors with chemotherapy and radiation. Roxxi "also combats side effects of treatment such as pain, nausea, infection, and constipation" (p. 117). Animations and direct interactions with environments provide information. Studies revealed greater knowledge, self-efficacy, and treatment compliance.

Kato, P. M. (2010). Video games in health care: Closing the gap. *Review of General Psychology, 14*(2), 113–121.

the user to visualize, question, analyze, and interpret data to understand relationships, patterns, and trends. Spatial or mappable data are integrated with conventional data. GIS can be thought of as a two-dimensional Google earth map. Google earth allows you to zoom in and out and pan around, and GIS additionally allows users to select a feature on the map and, in return, will be provided with any information in the database associated with that feature (University of Mary Washington, 2016). Much of community health is spatially related, so the use of GIS can provide information about demographic, epidemiological, and logistical issues and emerging trends. GIS output is location-based information. GIS can provide:

- Better understanding of a current situation
- Planning/targeting of appropriate interventions
- Monitoring and revision of interventions as needed
- An opportunity for cooperation with other organizations and government departments through a culture of data sharing and working together

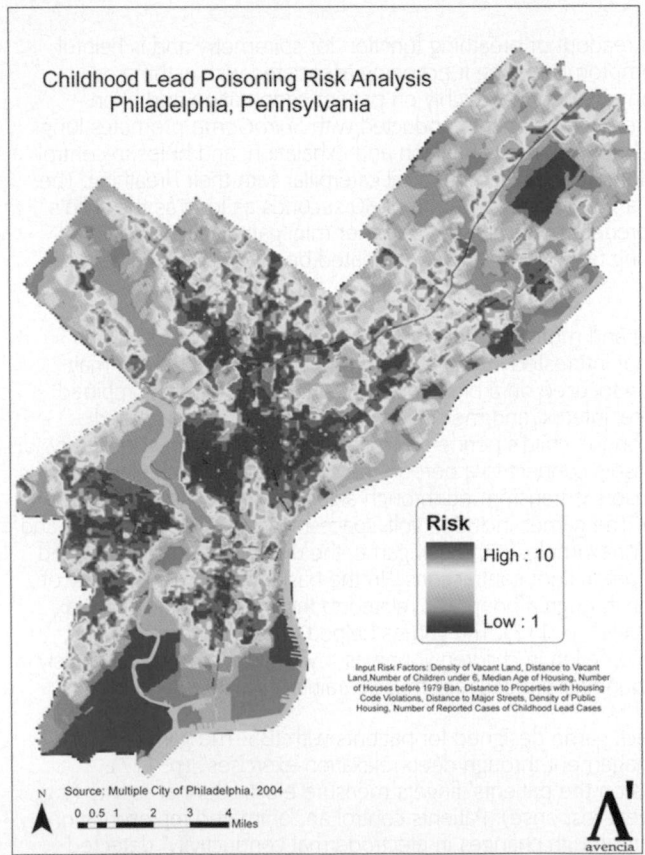

Example of GIS use in a lead poisoning project. (Photo courtesy of USA.gov.)

Sharing, comparing, and integrating data will eliminate silos and result in better outcomes (Detres, Lucio, & Vitucci, 2014; Edward & Biddle, in press; Jones & Ku, 2015).

There is great potential for GIS to inform public health nursing. Nurses can play an important role in demonstrating how various data sources come together to enable informed decisions for populations and

individuals (Kolifarhood, Khorasani-Zavareh, Salarilak, Shoghli, & Khosravi, 2015). It can be helpful in eliminating access barriers and providing policy-based interventions to decrease health inequities (Edward & Biddle, in press). Understanding of GIS may be considered an essential skill for the evolution of nursing practice (Semple et al., 2013). Smartphone and other devices are fitted with GIS technology, and many of us have GIS satellite navigation units in our vehicles or in our pockets. People rely on satellite imagery and digital mapping to get to their destination. These data are often freely available; each time a person asks for directions, the device connects to the satellite network (Mason, 2015).

The tremendous potential of GIS to benefit health care delivery is being realized. Both public and private organizations are developing innovative ways to use GIS, from public health departments and public health policy and research organizations to hospitals, medical centers, and health insurance organizations. Public health uses of GIS include tracking child immunizations, evaluating the spread and clustering of diseases, conducting health policy research, and establishing service areas and districts. Medical information is significantly more useful when combined with knowledge of the environmental factors associated with patients, locations, and conditions (Edward & Biddle, in press; Mason, 2015). A health system utilizing GIS technology will provide a more precise understanding of the links between an individual's health and where they reside, work, and play (Cromley & McLafferty, 2012).

Electronic Health Literacy and the Digital Divide

The rapid development of communication technology affects every aspect of society. Information is instantly available. The rapid proliferation of mobile devices makes information retrieval easier than ever before (Robb & Shellenbarger, 2014). The multitude of electronic health applications (e.g., online health information Web sites, interactive EHRs, health decision support programs, tailored health education programs, health care system portals, mHealth communication programs, advanced telelectronic health applications) hold great promise to increase access to health information, enhance the quality of care, reduce health care errors, increase collaboration, and encourage the adoption of healthy behaviors (Berkowitz & McCarthy, 2013).

Health communication and health information technology competencies are identified as vital skills of an informed consumer and essential for improving population health outcomes and health care quality. The term digital literacy appeared in the literature since the 1990s. A consensus definition may not exist but Nelson et al. (2013, p. 15) define digital literacy as including:

- Competency with digital devices of all types, including cameras, eReaders, smartphones, computers, tablets, video games
- The skills to operate the above devices as well as the knowledge to understand their functionality
- The ability to creatively and critically use these devices to access, manipulate, evaluate, and apply data, information, and wisdom

- The ability to apply basic emotional intelligence in collaborating and communicating with others
- The ethical values and sense of community responsibility to use digital devices for the enjoyment and benefit of society

Electronic health literacy is how people use electronic information and communication to improve health and access health care (Vajaean & Baban, 2015). People with low electronic health literacy represent a vulnerable population who are at risk (Levy, Janke, & Langa, 2015). As mentioned earlier, computer literacy and knowledge of the use of current technologies are part of health literacy. *Healthy People 2020* goals endeavor to increase health literacy skills and acknowledge that these skills may have a significant positive impact on improving health care quality and safety. Potential areas include supporting care, facilitating health care decision making, and building health skills and knowledge (Robb & Shellenbarger, 2014; USDHHS, 2016). Individuals must be able to use technology and navigate through a vast array of information, tools, and sources to acquire and critically analyze the information necessary to make appropriate and informed decisions (Vajaean & Baban, 2015).

Recent technological developments have elevated the importance of assessing how electronic health tools have empowered patients and improved health, especially among the most vulnerable populations. With an awareness of disparities in chronic health outcomes across racial/ethnic and social groups, it is essential that clinicians work to strengthen electronic health skills, particularly in groups that bear a disproportionate burden of disease (Kontos, Blake, Chou, & Prestin, 2014).

> The idea of the "digital divide" refers to the growing gap between the underprivileged members of society, especially the poor, rural, elderly, and handicapped portion of the population who do not have access to computers or the internet; and the wealthy, middle-class, and young Americans living in urban and suburban areas who have access (Stanford University, n.d., para. 2).

Kontos et al. (2014) describe the digital divide through a generational lens; younger generations who have grown up with technology are described as "digital natives" and are more comfortable using technology for everyday needs. Older generations are described as "digital immigrants" and have had to acquire the skills needed to use the Internet; thus they are less comfortable using technology. Technology is continually advancing, and the "digital divide" must be considered when addressing individual and population needs in public health nursing. Those with computers and access to the Internet are gaining skill, knowledge, and power through access to information (Stanford University, n.d.).

Technological literacy cannot be promoted if basic literacy skills are lacking. One in four adults in the United States is illiterate or has limited literacy skill. Adults with low literacy scores may not possess the basic skills required to function successfully within the health care system. Tasks such as reading prescription labels or care instructions, interpreting directions, and managing the health of their family may be daunting (Toronto & Weatherford, 2015). With new and exciting health technology developments comes the daunting responsibility to design interoperable, easy-to-use, engaging, and accessible electronic health applications that communicate the right information needed to guide health care and health promotion for diverse audiences (Kreps & Neuhauser, 2010). There is potential for electronic health technologies to aid in reducing communication inequalities and disparities in health. The need exists to educate at-risk and needy groups (e.g., chronically ill) and design technology in a way that works for them. Addressing these areas may not diminish the digital divide, but it may ameliorate its consequences (Neter & Brainin, 2012).

SUMMARY

Communication and collaboration are important tools for community health nurses to promote aggregate health. Communication involves the transfer and understanding of meaning between individuals (see Display 10–13). The communication process comprises seen parts: a message, a sender, a receiver, encoding, a channel, decoding, and a feedback loop. Barriers to effective communication include selective perception, language barriers, clients filtering out parts of the message, and emotional influence. Core skills essential to effective communication in community health nursing include sending skills, which allow the nurse to transmit messages effectively; receiving skills, which allow the nurse to receive accurate and complete messages; and interpersonal skills, which allow the nurse to interact and respond to the messages from clients. These skills include special techniques of active listening, the ability to show respect regardless of the message (whether positive or negative), the ability to empathize with clients' thoughts and feelings, and the ability to develop trust. Many factors can influence the quality of communication, such as negative previous experience, cultural influence, and relationships among the people involved. The community health nurse must consider all of these factors when trying to foster good communication.

In community health, nurses frequently need to promote communication in groups and in-group decision making. Decisions made by groups have many advantages, including sharing of members' experience and expertise, diversity of opinions, potential for broadening members' perspectives, and a focus on arriving at consensus solutions. Several methods of enhancing group decision making are available, including brainstorming, nominal group technique, and multivoting technique. IT, encompassing all of the computer-generated and other tools created to enhance communication, is changing the form of communication in PHN, as it has in the acute care setting.

Collaboration and partnership building are purposeful interactions among the nurse, clients, community members, and other professionals based on mutual participation and joint effort. It is characterized by shared goals, mutual participation, maximized use of resources, clear responsibilities, and set boundaries. Clients play an important role in the collaborative relationship.

Contracting is a helpful tool in promoting clients' participation, independence, and motivation. It is used at all levels of public health nursing to promote partnership in the collaborative process, to encourage commitment to health goals, and to ensure a format and a means for negotiation among the collaborating parties. Contracts may be formal or informal, written or verbal, and simple or complex. The nurse must know the needs and abilities of clients and must tailor the type of contracting to best suit the client's particular situation. Health technology incorporates large information systems and the use of EHRs. These are common in acute care settings, but are beginning to be used in public health settings. HIEs provide a hub for public health agencies, hospitals, health care providers, and others to share information to improve the health of individuals and populations.

Big data include very large and complex data sets that are analyzed to uncover trends, associations, and patterns. This is very helpful in public health agencies in the areas of disease surveillance, population health management, and immunization trends.

mHealth involves the use of mobile devices (e.g., smartphones, tablets, notebooks) for communication between clients and PHNs. Trends in mHealth include interactive (two-way communication), integrative (patient/provider and tracking systems), and multimedia uses (games/quizzes to promote health). A majority of Americans and people around the world have mobile phones. Text messaging can be useful in promoting health and encouraging immunizations, reminding clients of appointments or the need to pick up prescriptions, as well as encouraging exercise, or diabetes management behaviors, and blood pressure self-checks.

Applications are used for computers, tablets, and smartphones, and more health-related apps are available every year. Because of a lack of regulation, the quality or effectiveness of health apps is not researched. The FDA intends to provide oversight and identify apps that may be detrimental. FastStats is a free app from the CDC that provides information on more than 100 health topics. Twitter is a popular social networking site that has potential public health uses (e.g., disaster alert/response, epidemiological investigations).

Blogging and online support communities have proven to be helpful to those with chronic diseases or others needing emotional support. Those living in rural areas may especially find them useful, as they can connect to a larger group of people for information and support.

Video games are being used for health applications, in addition to their usual entertainment value. Exercise programs, and others that are specifically developed for patients with particular illnesses or conditions (e.g., pulmonary rehabilitation, burn patients), have been found to be beneficial.

Telehealth provides health information or health care to many individuals and groups who may otherwise not be able to access it. It may be done synchronously (in real time) or asynchronously (store-and-forward; accessed when convenient). GIS are mapping programs that can be used along with data to analyze and interpret relationships between a location and a disease or condition (e.g., area of a city and diabetes rates). Both telehealth and GIS have great potential for public health, as access barriers can be eliminated and disease patterns can be more closely studied and addressed. Childhood immunizations can be better tracked, as well as the spread of diseases, and vulnerable groups can be better served.

Electronic health literacy and the digital divide often prevent full use of technology among vulnerable and rural populations. It is important for PHNs to keep these in mind when working with elderly, disabled, poor, and rural clients, for instance, who may need additional assistance, education, and accommodations.

ACTIVITIES TO PROMOTE **CRITICAL THINKING**

1. Practice active listening with a colleague and subsequently analyze the factors that interfered with your total concentration. Identify three actions to take to improve your active listening, and apply them during the next week, keeping a log of your progress.

2. Think of a patient you have worked with who may have low health literacy. What kinds of things can you do to help them better communicate with their physician and other health professionals? Why is good health literacy important not only for the patient as an individual, but for the community and society as a whole?

3. Use nominal group technique with a group of classmates to arrive at a rank ordering of barriers to cross-cultural communication. What did you learn about arriving at a quality decision in the process?

4. Attend an open meeting (e.g., student body council, school board, city council) and watch for task and maintenance roles among the members. Are any members displaying nonfunctional role behaviors? Can you recognize task, maintenance, and nonfunctional role behaviors in some of the student groups in which you participate?

5. Organize a group of classmates to represent a group of clients, professionals, and community members who are collaborating to address the needs of an inner-city homeless population. Analyze how well you integrated the five characteristics of collaboration into your activity.

6. Explain the concept of contracting as it applies to aggregates. Discuss its four distinctive characteristics and the advantages that contracting offers to the community health nurse.

7. Develop a hypothetical contract with a group of elderly widows who need support and outlets to alleviate their loneliness. What other community members and professionals might be helpful as part of a collaborative team to address the widows' needs? How could your collaborative team plan for online support group to meet their needs? Name three benefits to clients who participate in online groups. Discuss any downside or barriers to participation.

8. Search state and local public health agency Web sites (or speak to PHN administrators) about use of electronic health records (EHRs). How common is this practice compared with hospitals in the same locality? Compare and contrast the functionality and use of the EHRs in public health and acute care.

9. Search for state and national examples of the use of big data in assessing public health problems and designing interventions. How are these data more helpful than traditional data? How is this most useful in public health?

10. Consider the various types of technology available (e.g., mHealth, mobile health applications, video games, telehealth, GIS). Which would you find most helpful as you design public health interventions for various age groups and populations (e.g., low-income, Spanish-speaking Latino women needing nutritional information; adolescents needing information on STDs and sexual health; addressing an outbreak of foodborne illness in a large metropolitan area; exercise needs of elderly living in rural areas; a group of young mothers wanting information on normal child development; parents of newly diagnosed children with muscular dystrophy; 10 to 14 year olds with asthma)?

REFERENCES

Aeyoung, S., De Gagne, J. C., Sunah, P., & Young-Oak, K. (2015). The effect of a workshop on a urinary incontinence self-management teaching program for community health nurses. *Journal of Korean Academy of Community Health Nursing, 26*(3), 260–267. doi: 10.12799/jkachn.2015.26.3.260.

Agency for Healthcare Research and Quality. (2014). *AHRQ innovations exchange*. Retrieved from https://innovations.ahrq.gov/search/innovations/TextMessaging

Al Sayah, F., Szafran, O., Robertson, S., Bell, N. R., & Williams, B. (2014). Nursing perspectives on factors influencing interdisciplinary teamwork in the Canadian primary care setting. *Journal of Clinical Nursing, 23*(19/20), 2968–2979. doi: 10.1111/jocn.12547.

Albarran, C. R., Heilemann, M. V., & Koniak-Griffin, D. (2014). Promotoras as facilitators of change: Latinas' perspectives after participating in a lifestyle behaviour intervention program. *Journal of Advanced Nursing, 70*(10), 2303–2313. doi: 10.1111/jan.12383.

American Telemedicine Association. (2015). *What is telemedicine?* Retrieved from http://www.americantelemed.org/about-telemedicine/what-is-telemedicine#.Vo7QiE3QceE

Arnold, E. C., & Boggs, K. U. (2016). *Interpersonal relationships: Professional communication skills for nurses* (7th ed.). St. Louis, MO: Elsevier.

Baheiraei, A., Mirghafourvand, M., Mohammadi, E., Mohammad-Alizadeh C., & Nedjat, S. (2013). Determining appropriate strategies for improving women's health promoting behaviours: Using the nominal group technique. *Eastern Mediterranean Health Journal, 19*(5), 409–416.

Baumann, P. (2016). *140 health care uses for Twitter*. Retrieved from http://philbaumann.com/140-health-care-uses-for-twitter/

Berkowitz, L., & McCarthy, C. (Eds.). (2013). *Innovation with information technologies in healthcare*. London, UK: Springer-Verlag.

Betts, S., & Healy, W. (2015). Having a ball catching on to teamwork: An experiential learning approach to teaching the phases of group development. *Academy of Educational Leadership Journal, 19*(2), 1–9.

Birkhead, G. S., Klompas, M., & Shah, N. R. (2015). Uses of electronic health records for public health surveillance to advance public health. *Annual Review of Public Health, 36*, 345–359.

Borkowski, N. (2016). *Organizational behavior in health care* (3rd ed.). Burlington, MA: Jones and Bartlett.

Browning, H. W., Torain, D. J., & Patterson, T. E. (2016). *Collaborative healthcare leadership: A six-part model for adapting and thriving during a time of transformative change*. Retrieved from http://insights.ccl.org/wp-content/uploads/2015/04/CollaborativeHealthcareLeadership.pdf

Bryant, L. O. (2014). Partnerships and collaborations in promoting health and wellness in minority communities: Lessons learned and future directions. *New Directions for Adult and Continuing Education, 2014*(142), 91–95.

Buchholz, S. W., Wilbur, J., Ingram, D., & Fogg, L. (2013). Physical activity text messaging interventions in adults: A systematic review. *Evidenced-Based Nursing, 10*(3), 163–173.

Buis, L. R., Artinian, N. T., Schwiebert, L., Yarandi, H., & Levy P. D. (2015). Text messaging to improve hypertension medication adherence in African Americans: BPMED intervention development and study protocol. *Journal of Medical Internet Research, 4*(1), e222.

Canning, D., Rosenberg, J. P., & Yates, P. (2013). Therapeutic relationships in specialist palliative care nursing practice. *International Journal of Palliative Nursing, 13*(5), 222–229.

Canpolat, M., Kuzu, S., Yildirim, B., & Canpolat, S. (2015). Active listening strategies of academically successful university students. *Eurasian Journal of Educational Research,* (60), 163–180. doi: 10.14689/ejer.2015.60.10.

Carter, M. Z., & Mossholder, K. W. (2015). Are we on the same page? The performance effects of congruence between supervisor and group trust. *Journal of Applied Psychology, 100*(5), 1349–1363. doi: 10.1037/a0038798.

Centers for Disease Control and Prevention (CDC). (2015a). *CDC's childhood lead poisoning prevention program.* Retrieved from http://www.cdc.gov/nceh/lead/about/program.htm

Centers for Disease Control and Prevention (CDC). (2015b). *The health communicator's social media toolkit.* Retrieved from http://www.cdc.gov/socialmedia/Tools/guidelines/pdf/SocialMediaToolkit_BM.pdf

Christofferson, D. E., Hamlett-Berry, K., & Augustson, E. (2015). Suicide prevention referrals in a mobile health smoking cessation intervention. *American Journal of Public Health, 105*(8), e7–e9.

Chung, J. E. (2014). Social networking in online support groups for health: How online social networking benefits patients. *Journal of Health Communication, 19*(6), 639–659. doi: 10.1080/10810730.2012.757396.

Clancy, A., Gressnes, T., & Svensson, T. (2013). Public health nursing and interprofessional collaboration in Norwegian municipalities: A questionnaire study. *Scandinavian Journal of Caring Sciences, 27*(3), 659–668.

Colc, J. (1990). *Filtering people: Understanding and confronting our prejudice.* Philadelphia, PA: New Society Publishers.

Cole-Lewis, H., & Kershaw, T. (2010). Text messaging as a tool for behavior change in disease prevention and management. *Epidemiologic Reviews, 32*(1), 56–69.

Coomes, C. M., Lewis, M. A., Uhrig, J. D., Furberg, R. D., Harris, J. L., & Bann, C. M. (2012). Beyond reminders: A conceptual framework for using short message service to promote prevention and improve healthcare quality and clinical outcomes for people living with HIV. *AIDS Care, 24*(3), 348–357.

Crawford, T., Candlin, S., & Roger, P. (2015). New perspectives on understanding cultural diversity in nurse–patient communication. *Collegian.* doi: 10.1016/j.colegn.2015.09.00.

Cromley, E. K., & McLafferty, S. L. (2012). *GIS and public health* (2nd ed.). New York, NY: Guilford Press.

Davis, R. A., & Travers Gustafson, D. (2015). Academic-practice partnership in public health nursing: Working with families in a village-based collaboration. *Public Health Nursing, 32*(4), 327–338. doi: 10.1111/phn.12135.

Dawson-Rose, C., Cuca, Y. P., Webel, A. R., Solis Báez, S. S., Holzemer, W. L., Rivero-Méndez, M., … Lindgren, T. (2016). Building trust and relationships between patients and providers: An essential complement to health literacy in HIV care. *Journal of the Association of Nurses in AIDS Care, 27*(5), 574–584.

DeGroot, J. M., & Carmack, H. J. (2012). Blogging as a means of grieving. In T. Dumova & R. Fiordo (Eds.), *Blogging in the global society: Cultural, political and geographical aspects* (pp. 161–178). Hershey, PA: Publisher Information Science Reference.

del Corral, T., Percegona, P., Seborga, M., Rabinovich, R. A., & Vilaró, J. (2014). Physiological response during activity programs using Wii-based video games in patients with cystic fibrosis (CF). *Journal of Cystic Fibrosis, 13*(6), 706–711. doi: http://dx.doi.org/10.1016/j.jcf.2014.05.004.

Deruy, E. (2013, June 3). *Can mobile health apps help more low-income patients?* Retrieved from http://abcnews.go.com/ABC_Univision/News/mobile-apps-healthcare-providers-connect-low-income-patients/story?id=19243999

Desroches, S., Lapointe, A., Deschenes, S., Bissonette-Maheux, V., Gravel, K., Thirsk, J., & Légaré, F. (2015). Dietitians' perspectives on interventions to enhance adherence to dietary advice for chronic diseases in adults. *Canadian Journal of Dietetic Practice and Research, 76*(3), 103–108.

Detres, M., Lucio, R., & Vitucci, J. (2014). GIS as a community engagement tool: Developing a plan to reduce infant mortality risk factors. *Maternal and Child Health Journal, 18*(5), 1049–1055. doi: 10.1007/s10995-013-1337-3.

Dezelic, G. (2007). A short review of medical informatics history. *Acta Informatica Medica, 15*(3), 178–188. Retrieved from http://www.healthtechnologyreview.com/art135_history_of_electronic_medical_records.php

Diefenbeck, C. A., Klemm, P. R., & Hayes, E. R. (2014). Emergence of Yalom's Therapeutic Factors in a peer-led, asynchronous, online support group for family caregivers. *Issues in Mental Health Nursing, 35*(1), 21–32. doi: 10.3109/01612840.2013.836260.

Dinç, L., & Gastmans, C. (2013). Trust in nurse–patient relationships: A literature review. *Nursing Ethics, 20*(5), 501–516.

Duffy, K. (2015, December 21). *Can we make meaningful use our primary barometer to determine EHR success—Part I.* Retrieved from https://www.healthcareguys.com/2015/12/21/37490/

Duggan, M. (2013, September 19). *Cell phone activities* 2013. Retrieved from http://pewinternet.org/Reports/2013/Cell-Activities.aspx

Duggan, M. (2015, December 15). *Gaming and gamers.* Retrieved from http://www.pewinternet.org/files/2015/12/PI_2015-12-15_gaming-and-gamers_FINAL.pdf

Duggan, M., & Smith, A. (2013, September 16). *Cell Internet use 2013: Main findings.* Retrieved from http://www.pewinternet.org/2013/09/16/main-findings-2/

Duggan, M., Ellison N. B., Lampe, C., Lenhart, A., & Madden, M. (2015). *While Facebook remains the most popular site, other platforms see higher rates of growth.* Retrieved from http://www.pewinternet.org/2015/01/09/social-media-update-2014/

Duiveman, T., & Bonner, A. (2012). Negotiating: Experiences of community nurses when contracting with clients. *Contemporary Nurse, 41*(1), 120–125.

Edward, J., & Biddle, D. J. (2016). Using geographic information systems (GIS) to examine barriers to healthcare access for Hispanic and Latino immigrants in the U.S. south. *Journal of Racial & Ethnic Disparities.* doi: 10.1077/s40615-016-0229-9.

El Camino Hospital. (2016). *El Camino Hospital careers.* Retrieved from https://www.elcaminohospital.org/careers

Elcock, K. (2014). Working in partnership: The need for candour and transparency. *British Journal of Nursing, 23*(1), 62.

Espensen, M. (2012). *Telehealth nursing practice essentials.* Pitman, NJ: American Academy of Ambulatory Care Nursing.

Food and Drug Administration (FDA). (2015). *Mobile medical applications.* Retrieved from http://www.fda.gov/MedicalDevices/DigitalHealth/MobileMedicalApplications/default.htm

Garcia, A. L. (2015). How big data can improve health care. *American Nurse Today, 10*(7), 53–55.

Gobble, M. M. (2014). The persistence of brainstorming. *Research-Technology Management, 57*(1), 64–66.

Grant, R. (2013, May 20). *Mobile technology could save billions of dollars on health care costs.* Retrieved from http://venturebeat.com/2013/05/20/mobile-technology-could-save-billions-of-dollars-on-healthcare-costs/

Hare, A. P. (2010). Theories of group development and categories for interaction analysis. *Small Group Research, 41*(1), 106–140.

Harmon, J. (2016). The top 4 communication skills of effective student leaders. *Campus Activities Programming, 48*(7), 30–34.

Health Information and Management Systems Society. (2016). *Connected health survey: Executive summary.* Retrieved from http://www.himss.org/2016-connected-health-survey/executive-summary

Health Technology Review. (n.d.). *History of electronic medical records.* Retrieved from http://www.healthtechnologyreview.com/art135_history_of_electronic_medical_records.php

Hebda, T., & Czar, P. (2013). *Handbook of informatics for nurses and healthcare professionals* (5th ed.). Saddle River, NJ: Pearson.

Heslip, N. (2015). Active listening: An important audit skill. *New Perspectives on Healthcare Risk Management, Control, and Governance, 34*(1), 14–15.

Heywood, J., & Heywood, B. (2015). *PatientsLikeMe.* Retrieved from https://www.patientslikeme.com/

Hufford, B. J., Williams, M. K., Malec, J. F., & Cravotta, D. (2012). Use of behavioural contracting to increase adherence with rehabilitation treatments on an inpatient brain injury unit: A case report. *Brain Injury, 26*(13/14), 1743–1749.

Humphreys, A., & Thompson, C. J. (2014). Branding disaster: Reestablishing trust through the ideological containment of systemic risk anxieties. *Journal of Consumer Research, 41*(4), 877–910. doi: 10.1086/677905.

Institute for Healthcare Informatics. (2015). *Patient adoption of mHealth: Use, evidence and remaining barriers to mainstream acceptance.* Retrieved from http://www.imshealth.com/en/thought-leadership/ims-institute

Institute of Medicine. (2012). *Accelerating progress in obesity prevention: Solving the weight of the nation.* Washington, DC: National Academies Press.

James, J. T. (2013). A new, evidence-based estimate of patient harms associated with hospital care. *Journal of Patient Safety, 9*(3), 122–128.

Jihye, J., Namhee, P., & So Young, S. (2014). The influence of health literacy and diabetes knowledge on diabetes self-care activities in Korean low-income elders with diabetes. *Journal of Korean Academy of Community Health Nursing, 25*(3), 217–224. doi: 10.12799/jkachn.2014.25.3.217.

Johnson, A. (2015). Health literacy: How nurses can make a difference. *Australian Journal of Advanced Nursing, 33*(2), 20–27.

Jones, E. B., & Ku, L. (2015). Sharing a playbook: Integrated care in community health centers in the United States. *American Journal of Public Health, 105*(10), 2028–2034. doi: 10.2105/AJPH.2015.302710.

Kannisto, K. A., Koivunen, M. H., & Välimäki, M. A. (2014). Use of mobile phone text message reminders in health care services: A narrative literature review. *Journal of Medical Internet Research, 16*(10), e222.

Karp, L. (2015). Can empathy be taught? Reflections from a medical student active-listening workshop. *Rhode Island Medical Journal, 98*(6), 14–15.

Kato, P. M. (2010). Video games in health care: Closing the gap. *Review of General Psychology, 14*(2), 113–121.

Kewming, S., D'Amore, A., & Mitchell, E. L. (2016). Conversation maps and diabetes education groups: An evaluation at an Australian rural health service. *Diabetes Spectrum, 29*(1), 32–36. doi: 10.2337/diaspect.29.1.32.

Kharbanda, E. Q., Stockwell, M. S., Fox, H. W., Andres, R., Lara, M., & Rickert, V. I. (2011). Text message reminders to promote human papillomavirus vaccination. *Vaccine, 29*(14), 2537–2531.

Kharbanda, E. Q., Stockwell, M. S., Fox, H. W., & Rickert, V. I. (2009). Text4Health: A qualitative evaluation of parental readiness for text message immunization reminders. *American Journal of Public Health, 99*(12), 2176–2178.

Kickbusch, I., Pelikan, J. M., Apfel, F., & Tsouros, A. D. (2013). *Health literacy: The solid facts.* Retrieved from http://www.euro.who.int/__data/assets/pdf_file/0008/190655/e96854.pdf

Kilpatrick, K., Lavoie-Tremblay, M., Ritchie, J. A., & Lamothe, L. (2014). Advanced practice nursing, health care teams, and perceptions of team effectiveness. *Journal of Trauma Nursing, 21*(6), 291–299. doi: 10.1097/JTN.0000000000000090.

Kim, S., Prestopnik, N., & Biocca, F. (2014). Body in the interactive game: How interface embodiment affects physical activity and health behavior change. *Computers in Human Behavior, 36*, 376–384. doi: 10.1016/j.chb.2014.03.067.

Klinkhamer, F. (2015). School nurse team leaders' experience and management of workplace conflict. *British Journal of School Nursing, 10*(7), 337–347.

Kobayashi, K., Fukushima, M., Kitaoka, H., Shimizu, Y., & Shimanouchi, S. (2015). The influence of public health nurses in facilitating a healthy family life for families with abused and neglected children by providing care. *International Medical Journal, 22*(1), 6–11.

Kolifarhood, G., Khorasani-Zavareh, D., Salarilak, S., Shoghli, A., & Khosravi, N. (2015). Spatial and non-spatial determinants of successful tuberculosis treatment outcomes: An implication of Geographical Information Systems in health policy-making in a developing country. *Journal of Epidemiology and Global Health, 5*, 221–230. doi: 10.1016/j.jegh.2014.11.001.

Konok, V., Gigler, D., Bereczky, B. M., & Miklósi, Á. (2016). Full length article: Humans' attachment to their mobile phones and its relationship with interpersonal attachment style. *Computers in Human Behavior, 61*, 537–547. doi: 10.1016/j.chb.2016.03.062.

Kontos, E., Blake, K. D., Chou, W. Y. S., & Prestin, A. (2014). Predictors of eHealth usage: Insights on the digital divide from the health information national trends survey. *Journal Medical Internet Research, 16*(7), e172. doi: 10.2196/jmir.3117.

Kreps, G. L., & Neuhauser, L. (2010). New directions in eHealth communication: Opportunities and challenges. *Patient Education and Counseling, 78*(3), 329–336.

Kulbok, P. A., Thatcher, E., Park, E., & Meszaros, P. S. (2012). Evolving public health nursing roles: Focus on community participatory health promotion and prevention. *Online Journal of Issues in Nursing, 17*(2), Manuscript 1.

Kvedar, J. C., Nesbitt, T., Kvedar, J. G., & Darkins, A. (2011). E-patient connectivity and the near term future. *Journal of General Internal Medicine, 26*(Suppl 2), 636–638. Retrieved from http://doi.org/10.1007/s11606-011-1763-0

Levy, H., Janke, A., & Langa, K. M. (2015). Health literacy and the digital divide among older Americans. *Journal of General Internal Medicine, 30*(3), 284–289.

Liebert, M. (2009). *Twitter and health care: Can a tweet a day keep the doctor away?* Retrieved from http://www.sciencedaily.com/releases/2009/08/090824141043.htm

Lin, P., Intille, S., Bennett, G., Bosworth, H. B., Corsino, L., Voils, C., … Svetkey, L. P. (2015). Adaptive intervention design in mobile health: Intervention design and development in the Cell Phone Intervention for You trial. *Clinical Trials, 12*(6), 634–645. doi: 10.1177/1740774515597222.

Majee, W., Goodman, L., Vetter-Smith, M., & Canfield, S. (2016). Healthy communities initiative: A preliminary assessment of the University of Missouri-Sedalia health promotion partnership. *Community Development, 47*(1), 91. doi: 10.1080/15575330.2015.1100643.

Mantwill, S., & Schulz, P. J. (2015). Low health literacy associated with higher medication costs in patients with type 2 diabetes mellitus: Evidence from matched survey and health insurance data. *Patient Education and Counseling, 98*, 1625–1630. doi: 10.1016/j.pec.2015.07.006.

Maruca, A. T., Díaz, D. A., Kuhnly, J. E., & Jeffries, P. R. (2015). Enhancing empathy in undergraduate nursing students: An experiential ostomate simulation. *Nursing Education Perspectives, 36*(6), 367–371. doi: 10.5480/15-1578.

Mason, M. (2015). *Geospatial technology: An introduction and overview.* Retrieved from http://www.environmentalscience.org/geospatial-technology

Maynika, J., Chui, M., Brown, B., Bughin, J., Dobbs, R., Roxburgh, C., & Hung Byers, A. (2011). *Big data: The next frontier for innovation, competition, and productivity.* Retrieved from http://www.mckinsey.com/insights/business_technology/big_data_the_next_frontier

McGonigle, D. & Mastrian, K. G. (2015). *Nursing informatics and the foundation of knowledge* (3rd ed.). Burlington, MA: Jones & Bartlett.

Meyer-Junco, L. (2015). Empathy and the new practitioner. *American Journal of Health-System Pharmacy, 72*(23), 2042–2058. doi: 10.2146/ajhp150020.

Militello, L. A., Kelley, S. A., & Melnyk, B. M. (2012). Systematic review of text messaging interventions to promote healthy behaviors in pediatric and adolescent populations: Implications for clinical practice and research. *Worldviews on Evidence-Based Nursing, 9*(2), 66–77.

Miller, W. R., & Rollnick, S. (2013). *Motivational interviewing: Helping people change* (3rd ed.). New York, NY: Guilford Press.

Minnesota Department of Health. (2016). *Multivoting.* Retrieved from http://www.health.state.mn.us/divs/opi/qi/toolbox/nominalgroup.html

Mitchell, R., Paliadelis, P., McNeil, K., Parker, V., Giles, M., Higgins, I., … Ahrens, Y. (2013). Effective interprofessional collaboration in rural contexts: A research protocol. *Journal of Advanced Nursing, 69*(10), 2317–2326. doi: 10.1111/jan.12083.

Mo, P. K., & Coulson, N. S. (2014). Are online support groups always beneficial? A qualitative exploration of the empowering and disempowering processes of participation within HIV/AIDS-related online support groups. *International Journal of Nursing Studies, 51*, 983–993. doi: 10.1016/j.ijnurstu.2013.11.006.

Morgan, S., Pullon, S., & McKinlay, E. (2015). Observation of interprofessional collaborative practice in primary care teams: An integrative literature review. *International Journal of Nursing Studies, 52*(7), 1217–1230. doi: 10.1016/j.ijnurstu.2015.03.008.

Morrison, A. K., Myrvik, M. P., Brousseau, D. C., Hoffmann, R. G., & Stanley, R. M. (2013). The relationship between parent health literacy and pediatric emergency department utilization: A systematic review. *Academic Pediatrics, 13*(5), 421–429.

Moser, D. K., Robinson, S., Biddle, M. J., Pelter, M. M., Nesbitt, T. S., Southard, J., ... Dracup, K. (2015). Clinical investigation: Health literacy predicts morbidity and mortality in rural patients with heart failure. *Journal of Cardiac Failure, 21,* 612–618. doi: 10.1016/j.cardfail.2015.04.004.

Murray, B., & McCrone, S. (2015). An integrative review of promoting trust in the patient-primary care provider relationship. *Journal of Advanced Nursing, 71*(1), 3–23. doi: 10.1111/jan.12502.

National Advisory Committee on Rural Health & Human Services. (2015). *Telehealth in rural America*. Retrieved from http://www.hrsa.gov/advisorycommittees/rural/publications/telehealthmarch2015.pdf

National Network of Libraries of Medicine. (2013). *Health literacy*. Retrieved from https://nnlm.gov/outreach/consumer/hlthlit.html

Nel, H. (2015). An integration of the livelihoods and asset-based community development approaches: A South African case study. *Development Southern Africa, 32*(4), 511–525. doi: 10.1080/0376835X.2015.1039706.

Nelson, R., & Staggers, N. (2014). *Health informatics*. St. Louis, MO: Elsevier Mosby.

Nelson, R., Joos, I., & Wolf, D. M. (2013). *Social media for nurses*. New York, NY: Springer.

Neter, E., & Brainin, E. (2012). eHealth literacy: Extending the digital divide to the realm of health information. *Journal of Medical Internet Research, 14*(1), e19.

Ng, C., Fraser, J., Goding, M., Paroissien, D., & Ryan, B. (2013). Partnerships for community mental health in the Asia-Pacific: Principles and best-practice models across different sectors. *Australasian Psychiatry, 21*(1), 38–45. doi: 10.1177/1039856212465348.

Nouri, S. S., & Rudd, R. E. (2015). Health literacy in the "oral exchange": An important element of patient-provider communication. *Patient Education and Counseling, 98,* 565–571.

O'Hagan, S., Manias, E., Elder, C., Pill, J., Woodward-Kron, R., McNamara, T., ... McColl, G. (2014). What counts as effective communication in nursing? Evidence from nurse educators' and clinicians' feedback on nurse interactions with simulated patients. *Journal of Advanced Nursing, 70*(6), 1344–1355. doi: 10.1111/jan.12296.

Park, L. G., Howie-Esquivel, J., & Dracup, K. (2014). A quantitative systematic review of the efficacy of mobile phone interventions to improve medication adherence. *Journal of Advanced Nursing, 70*(9), 1932–1953.

Park, L. G., Howie-Esquivel, J., Chung, M. L., & Dracup, K. (2014). A text messaging intervention to promote medication adherence for patients with coronary heart disease: A randomized control trial. *Patient Education and Counseling, 94*(2), 261–268.

Pauschenwein, J. J., Goldgruber, E. E., & Sfiri, A. A. (2013). The identification of the potential of game-based learning in vocational education within the context of the project "Play the Learning Game." *International Journal of Emerging Technologies in Learning, 8*(1), 20–23. doi: 10.3991/ijet.v8i1.2359.

Pavlish, C. P., & Pharris, M. D. (2012). *Community-based collaborative action research: A nursing approach*. Sudbury, MA: Jones & Bartlett Learning.

Pena-Robichaux, V., Kvedar, J. C., & Watson, A. J. (2010). Text messages as a reminder aid and educational tool in adults and adolescents with atopic dermatitis: A pilot study. *Dermatology Research and Practice, 2010,* 1–6. doi: 10.1155/2010/894258.

Petri, L. (2010). Concept analysis of interdisciplinary collaboration. *Nursing Forum, 45*(2), 73–82.

Pew Research Center. (2016). *Cell phone and smartphone ownership demographics*. Retrieved from http://www.pewinternet.org/data-trend/mobile/cell-phone-and-smartphone-ownership-demographics/

Phutela, D. (2015). The importance of non-verbal communication. *IUP Journal of Soft Skills, 9*(4), 43–49.

Raghupathi, V., & Raghupathi, W. (2014). Big data analytics in healthcare: Promise and potential. *Health Information Science and Systems, 2*(3). Retrieved from http://www.hissjournal.com/content/2/1/3

Ressler, P. K., Bradshaw, Y., Gualtieri, L., & Chui, K. (2012). Communicating the experience of illness through patient blogs. *Journal of Medical Internet Research, 14*(5), e143. doi: 10.2196/jmir.2002.2012.

Robb, M., & Shellenbarger, T. (2014). Influential factors and perceptions of eHealth literacy among undergraduate college students. *Online Journal of Nursing Informatics, 18*(3). Retrieved from http://www.himss.org/ResourceLibrary/GenResourceDetail.aspx?ItemNumber=33519

Rodwell, J., & Ellershaw, J. (2016). Fulfill promises and avoid breaches to retain satisfied, committed nurses. *Journal of Nursing Scholarship, 48*(4), 406–413.

Rowlands, G., Berry, J., Protheroe, J., & Rudd, R. E. (2015). Building on research evidence to change health literacy policy and practice in England. *Journal of Communication in Healthcare, 8*(1), 22–31.

Rutherford, M. M. (2014). The value of trust to nursing. *Nursing Economics, 32*(6), 283–289.

Sabatino, L., Rocco, G., Stievano, A., & Alvaro, R. (2015). Learning and teaching in clinical practice: Perceptions of Italian student nurses of the concept of professional respect during their clinical practice learning experience. *Nurse Education in Practice, 15,* 314–320. doi: 10.1016/j.nepr.2014.09.002.

Salerno, J., Delaney, K. R., Swartwout, K. D., & Tsui-Sui, A. K. (2015). Improving interdisciplinary professionals' capacity to motivate adolescent behavior change. *Journal for Nurse Practitioners, 11*(6), 626–632. doi: 10.1016/j.nurpra.2015.03.013.

Savio, N., & George, A. (2013). The perceived communication barriers and attitude on communication among staff nurses in caring for patients from culturally and linguistically diverse background. *International Journal of Nursing Education, 5*(1), 141–146. doi: 10.5958/j.0974-9357.5.1.036.

Schaffer, R., Kuczynski, K., & Skinner, D. (2008). Producing genetic knowledge and citizenship through the Internet: Mothers, pediatric genetics, and cybermedicine. *Sociology of Health & Illness, 30*(1), 145–149.

Semple, H., Cudnik, M., Sayre, M., Keseg, D., Warden, C., & Sasson, C. (2013). Identification of high-risk communities for unattended out-of-hospital cardiac arrests using GIS. *Journal of Community Health, 38*(2), 277–284. doi: 10.1007/s10900-012-9611-7.

Sensmeier, J. (2015). Big data and the future of nursing knowledge: How can we use these technologies to improve care quality, optimize outcomes, and reduce healthcare costs? *Nursing Management, 46*(4), 22–27.

Sharma, P., & Agarwal, P. (2012, October). *Mobile phone text messaging for promoting adherence to antiretroviral therapy in patients with HIV infection: RHL commentary. The WHO Reproductive Health Library*. Geneva, Switzerland: World Health Organization.

Shaw, J., Mitchell, C., & Del Fabbro, L. (2015). Group work: Facilitating the learning of international and domestic undergraduate nursing students. *Education for Health: Change in Learning & Practice, 28*(2), 124–129. doi: 10.4103/1357-6283.170123.

Smith, R. (2014). Insights into the FDA regulation of mobile medical apps. *Business2Community*. Retrieved from http://www.business-2community.com/mobile-apps/insights-fda-regulation-mobile-medical-apps-0955123#3uE1IkdRRSQW5gqd.97

Soares, H. (2016). "Touchpoints" by nurses: Impact on maternal representations, child development, quality of mother-infant interaction, and mothers' perception of the quality of relationships with nurses. *Nursing Children and Young People, 28*(4), 51.

Soares Lopes, R., Meira Albino, L. R., de Menezes, H. F., & Muniz Ribeiro, M. C. (2015). Nurse as mediator of conflicts and power relations among the multiprofessional team in surgical center. *Journal of Nursing UFPE, 9*(8), 8825–8830. doi: 10.5205/reuol.7696-67533-1-SP-1.0908201509.

Stanford University. (n.d.). *Digital divide: Overview*. Retrieved from http://cs.stanford.edu/people/eroberts/cs201/projects/digital-divide/start.html

Stockwell, M. S., Kharbanda, E., Martinez, R., Vargas, C. Y., Vawdrey, D. K. & Camargo, S. (2012). Effect of a text messaging intervention on influenza vaccination in an urban, low-income pediatric and adolescent population: A randomized controlled trial. *Journal of the American Medical Association, 7*(16), 1702–1708. doi: 10.1001/jama.2012.502.

Sussman, A. L., Montoya, C., Werder, O., Davis, S., Wallerstein, N., & Kong, A. S. (2013). An adaptive CBPR approach to create weight management materials for a school-based health center intervention. *Journal of Obesity*, Article ID 978482. doi: 10.1155/2013/978482.

Swider, S., Krothe, J., Reyes, D., & Cravetz, M. (2013). The Quad Council practice competencies for public health nursing. *Public Health Nursing, 30*(6), 519–536.

Tomines, A., Readhead, H., Readhead, A., & Teutsch, S. (2013). Applications of electronic health information in public health: Uses, opportunities & barriers. *eGEMS, 1*(2), 1019.

Tonn, V. L. (2012). From meanings, images, and states of mind to structural commonality between communication and poetry and communication competence—A systematic approach to communication study. *Intercultural Communication Studies, 21*(3), 124–137.

Toronto, C., & Weatherford, B. (2015). Health literacy education in health professions schools: An integrative review. *Journal of Nursing Education, 54*(12), 669–676.

Tucker, C. M., Lopez, M. T., Campbell, K., Marsiske, M., Daly, K., Nghiem, K., ... Patel, A. (2014). The effects of a culturally sensitive, empowerment-focused, community-based health promotion program on health outcomes of adults with type 2 diabetes. *Journal of Health Care for the Poor and Underserved, 25*(1), 292–307.

Tuhovsky, I. (2015). *Communication skills: A practical guide to improving your social intelligence, presentation, persuasion and public speaking.* Self-published.

U.S. Department of Health & Human Services (USDHHS). (2014). *Using health text messages to improve consumer health knowledge, behaviors, and outcomes: An environmental scan.* Retrieved from http://www.hrsa.gov/healthit/txt4tots/environmentalscan.pdf

U.S. Department of Health & Human Services (USDHHS). (2016). *2020 Topics and objectives: Health communication and health information technology.* Retrieved from http://www.healthypeople.gov/2020/topicsobjectives2020/overview.aspx?topicId=18

U.S. Department of Health and Human Services: Office of Disease Prevention & Promotion. (2010). *National action plan to improve health literacy.* Retrieved from http://www.health.gov/communication/HLActionPlan/pdf/Health_Literacy_Action_Plan.pdf

University of Mary Washington. (2016). *Geographic information science: What is GIS?* Retrieved from http://cas.umw.edu/gis/what-is-gis/

Vajaean, C. C., & Baban, A. (2015). Emotional and behavioral consequences of online health information-seeking: The role of ehealth literacy. *Cognitie, Creier, Comportament/Cognition, Brain, Behavior, 19*(4), 327–345.

Varga, M. A., & Paulus, T. M. (2014). Grieving online: Newcomers' constructions of grief in an online support group. *Death Studies, 38*(6–10), 443–449.

Vehvilamen-Julkunen, K. (1992). Client-public health nurse relationships in child health care: A grounded theory study. *Journal of Advanced Nursing, 17,* 896–904.

Vertino, K. A. (2014). Effective interpersonal communication: A practical guide to improve your life. *Online Journal of Issues in Nursing, 19*(3), 1.

Wang, K., Chu, N., Lin, S., Chiang, I., Perng, W., & Lai, H. (2014). Examining the causal model linking health literacy to health outcomes of asthma patients. *Journal of Clinical Nursing, 23*(13/14), 2031–2042, 12 p. doi: 10.1111/jocn.12434.

Wicklund, E. (2015). CMS boosts telehealth in 2015 physician pay schedule. *Mhealth News: The Voice of Mobile Care.* Retrieved from http://www.mhealthnews.com/news/cms-boosts-telehealth-2015-physician-pay-schedule

Wikipedia. (2016). *Mobile app.* Retrieved from https://en.wikipedia.org/wiki/Mobile_app

Wolf, J. (2015). You hear, but do you listen? Follow these 6 steps. *HR Specialist, 13*(10), 7.

Wortzel, H. S., Matarazzo, B., & Homaifar, B. (2013). A model for therapeutic risk management of the suicidal patient. *Law and Psychiatry Column, Journal of Psychiatric Practice, 19*(4), 323–326.

Wu, L. (2014, April 29). *Issue brief: Health IT for public health reporting and information systems.* Retrieved from https://www.healthit.gov/sites/default/files/phissuebrief04-24-14.pdf

Ziebland, S., & Wyke, S. (2012). Health and illness in a connected world: How might sharing experiences on the Internet affect people's health? *The Milbank Quarterly, 90*(2), 219–249. http://doi.org/10.1111/j.1468-0009.2012.00662.x

thePoint: Everything You Need to Make the Grade!

the**Point**® Visit http://thePoint.lww.com/Rector9e for selected readings, study aids for all learning styles, and more!

CHAPTER 11

Health Promotion: Achieving Change Through Education

"As I see it, every day you do one of two things: build health or produce disease in yourself."

—*Adelle Davis* (1904–1974), Nutritionist and Author

KEY TERMS

Adult learners
Affective domain
Anticipatory guidance
Change
Cognitive domain

Empiric–rational change
    strategy
Force field analysis
Health promotion
Learning theories

Normative–reeducative
    change strategy
Planned change
Power–coercive change
    strategy
Psychomotor domain

Social determinants of
    health
Social marketing
Stages of change
Transtheoretical Model

LEARNING OBJECTIVES

Upon mastery of this chapter, you should be able to:

- Explain the three stages of change.
- Identify three planned-change strategies.
- Summarize six principles for effecting change in community health.
- Describe the community health nurse's role as educator in promoting health and preventing or postponing morbidity.
- Identify educational activities for the nurse to use that are appropriate for each of the three domains of learning.
- Identify health teaching models for use when planning health education activities.
- Discuss methods of education and social marketing that may be used to improve health promotion with communities and populations.
- Develop teaching plans focusing on primary, secondary, and tertiary levels of prevention for clients of all ages.
- Identify teaching strategies for the community health nurse to use when encountering clients with special learning needs.
- Describe social determinants of health and how each relates to health inequities.

Think of a time when you were so influenced by a teacher that you stopped an unhealthy habit, altered a long-held belief, or embarked on a new endeavor. What precisely was it that motivated the change? Was it simply the content of the teaching, or was it how the teacher presented the content or your involvement in the learning process? What is good teaching, and why is it so important to community health nursing?

Teaching has been a critical part of the community health nurse's role since the origins of the profession, and it frequently is the primary role or function. PHNs develop partnerships with clients to achieve behavior changes that promote, maintain, or restore health. This partnership focuses on self-care—the ability to effectively advocate and manage a person's own health. The rationale for health teaching is to equip people with the knowledge, attitudes, and practices that will allow them to live the fullest possible life for the greatest length of time. The vision of *Healthy People 2020* is for "a society in which all people live long, healthy lives" (U.S. Department of Health and Human Services [USDHHS], 2016a, para. 3). Figure 11–1 depicts a graphic model of *Healthy People 2020*, including overarching goals. This model demonstrates the influence of social determinants of health to the positive health outcomes envisioned in the Healthy People initiative. *Healthy People 2020* objectives for educational, community-based programs, which address the goal of increasing the "quality, availability and effectiveness of educational and community-based programs designed to prevent disease and injury, improve health and enhance the quality of life," are listed in Table 11–1 (USDHHS, 2016b, para.1). These objectives when viewed in the broader context depicted in the model can be used to identify client needs and align educational efforts that will advance this national initiative.

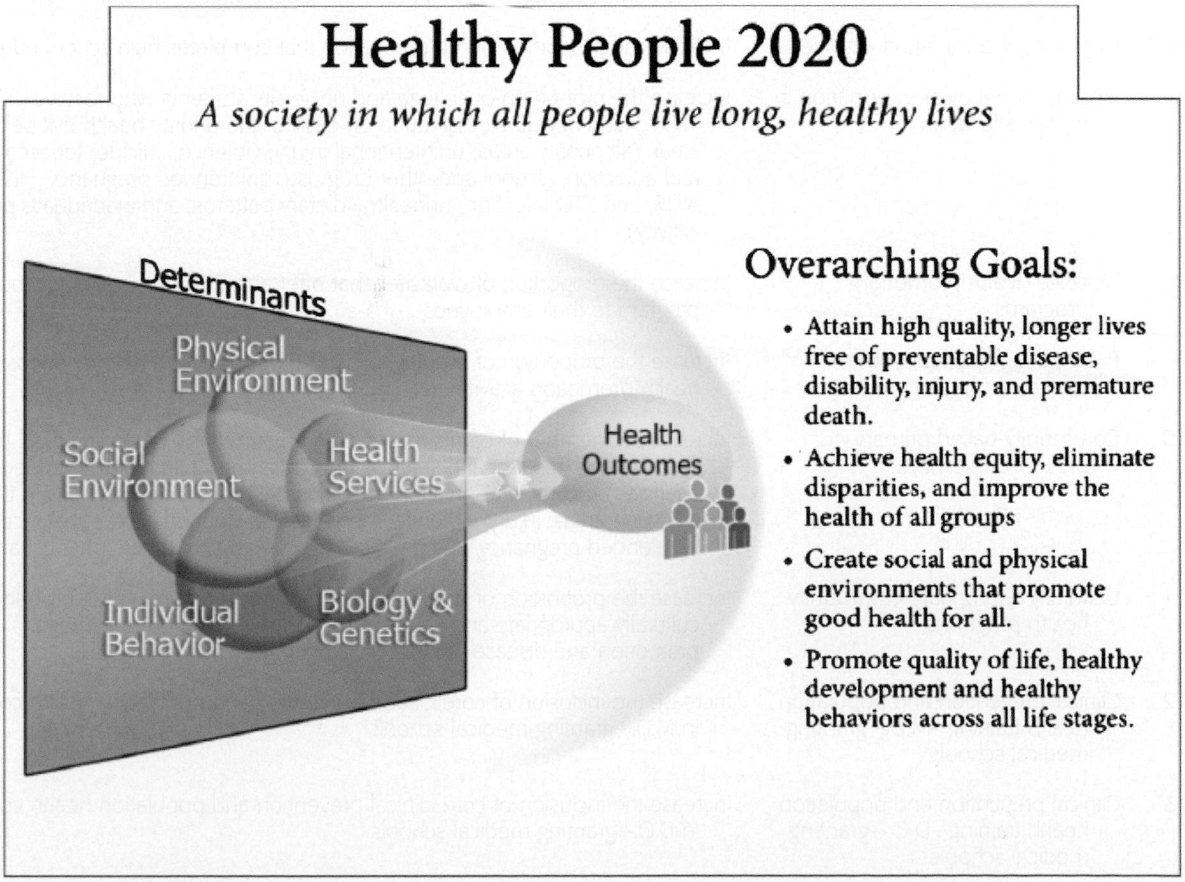

Healthy People 2020

A society in which all people live long, healthy lives

Determinants

Physical Environment

Social Environment

Health Services

Individual Behavior

Biology & Genetics

Health Outcomes

Overarching Goals:

- Attain high quality, longer lives free of preventable disease, disability, injury, and premature death.

- Achieve health equity, eliminate disparities, and improve the health of all groups

- Create social and physical environments that promote good health for all.

- Promote quality of life, healthy development and healthy behaviors across all life stages.

FIGURE 11–1   Health People 2020 framework. (From U.S. Department of Health and Human Services (USDHHS), Office of Disease Prevention and Health Promotion. (n.d.). *Healthy People 2020. Healthy People 2020 Framework: The vision, mission, and goals of Healthy People 2020.* Retrieved from http://www.healthypeople.gov/sites/default/files/HP2020Framework.pdf)

Table 11-1 *Healthy People 2020* **Objectives for Educational and Community-Based Programs**

	Objective	2020 Goal
ECBP-1	Preschool health education	Increase the proportion of preschool Early Head Start and Head Start programs that provide health education to prevent health problems in the following areas: unintentional injury; violence; tobacco use and addiction; alcohol or other drug use; unhealthy dietary patterns; and inadequate physical activity, dental health, and safety
ECBP-2	School health education	Increase the proportion of elementary, middle, and senior high schools that provide comprehensive school health education to prevent health problems in the following areas: unintentional injury; violence; suicide; tobacco use and addiction; alcohol or other drug use; unintended pregnancy, HIV/AIDS, and STD infection; unhealthy dietary patterns; and inadequate physical activity
ECBP-3	School health education standards	Increase the proportion of elementary, middle, and senior high schools that have health education goals or objectives which address the knowledge and skills articulated in the National Health Education Standards (high school, middle, and elementary).
ECBP-4	School health education on personal growth and wellness	Increase the proportion of elementary, middle, and senior high schools that provide school health education to promote personal health and wellness in the following areas: hand washing or hand hygiene, oral health, growth and development, sun safety and skin cancer prevention, benefits of rest and sleep, ways to prevent vision and hearing loss, and the importance of health screenings and checkups
ECBP-5	School nurse-to-student ratio	Increase the proportion of elementary, middle, and senior high schools that have a full-time registered school nurse-to-student ratio of at least 1:750
ECBP-6	High school completion activities	Increase the proportion of the population that completes high school education
ECBP-7v	Health risk behavior information in higher education	Increase the proportion of college and university students who receive information from their institution on each of the priority health risk behavior areas (all priority areas; unintentional injury; violence; suicide; tobacco use and addiction; alcohol and other drug use; unintended pregnancy, HIV/AIDS, and STD infection; unhealthy dietary patterns; and inadequate physical activity)
ECBP-8	Worksite health promotion programs	Increase the proportion of worksites that offer an employee health promotion program to their employees
ECBP-9	Participation in employer-sponsored health promotion	Increase the proportion of employees who participate in employer-sponsored health promotion activities
ECBP-10	Community-based primary prevention services	Increase the number of community-based organizations (including local health departments, tribal health services, nongovernmental organizations, and state agencies) providing population-based primary prevention services in the following areas: injury, violence, mental illness, tobacco use, substance abuse, unintended pregnancy, chronic disease programs, nutrition, physical activity
ECBP-11	Culturally appropriate community health programs	Increase the proportion of local health departments that have established culturally appropriate and linguistically competent community health promotion and disease prevention programs.
ECBP-12	Clinical prevention and population health training—M.D.—granting medical schools	Increase the inclusion of core clinical prevention and population health content in M.D.—granting medical schools
ECBP-13	Clinical prevention and population health training—D.O.—granting medical schools	Increase the inclusion of core clinical prevention and population health content in D.O.—granting medical schools
ECBP-14	Clinical prevention and population health training—undergraduate nursing	Increase the inclusion of core clinical prevention and population health content in undergraduate nursing

Table 11–1 *Healthy People 2020* **Objectives for Educational and Community-Based Programs (*Continued*)**

	Objective	2020 Goal
ECBP-15	Clinical prevention and population health training—nurse practitioner	Increase the inclusion of core clinical prevention and population health content in nurse practitioner training
ECBP-16	Clinical prevention and population health training—physician assistant	Increase the inclusion of core clinical prevention and population health content in physician assistant training
ECBP-17	Clinical prevention and population health training—PharmD—granting colleges and schools of pharmacy	Increase the inclusion of core clinical prevention and population health content in Doctor of Pharmacy (PharmD) granting colleges and schools of pharmacy
ECBP-18	Clinical prevention and population health training—DDS/DDM—granting colleges and schools of Dentistry	Increase the inclusion of core clinical prevention and population health content in Doctor of Dental Surgery and/or Doctor of Dental Medicine granting colleges and schools of Dentistry.
ECBP-19	Clinical prevention and population health training	Increase the proportion of academic institutions with health professions education programs whose prevention curricula include interprofessional educational experiences

From U.S. Department of Health and Human Services (USDHHS). (2016). *Healthy People 2020: Educational and community-based programs.* Retrieved from http://www.healthypeople.gov/2020/topics-objectives/topic/educational-and-community-based-programs/objectives

When the community health nurse identifies a need that is best met through health education, the nurse is faced with a series of questions: What is the overall goal? How can I teach effectively? What content should I cover? What method of presentation will communicate most effectively? What resources can I use as teaching tools? How do I know when the client has grasped the information or mastered the skills? How do I involve the client in the learning process? How do I assist clients with special learning needs? The nurse must understand what makes teaching effective, how teaching skills are acquired, and how mastery is measured. The PHN might also need to consider why some individuals adopt new health practices and others do not, as well as how social determinants influence health outcomes. This chapter addresses these questions and discusses teaching as a basic intervention tool in community health nursing practice. For health education to be effective, awareness of the underlying principles of behavior change is vital. The community health nurse should consider what motivates individuals and groups to adopt new behaviors and what factors may inhibit or prevent that change. By understanding the principles of teaching and behavior change, the community health nurse can work toward the ultimate goal of health promotion for individuals, families, groups, and communities (USDHHS, 2016d).

HEALTH PROMOTION THROUGH CHANGE

Health promotion has been defined as health behaviors that improve well-being and lead to a desire to meet one's human potential (Pender, Murdaugh, & Parsons, 2015). Another term often confused with health promotion is *disease prevention* (or *health protection*), which is "behavior motivated by a desire to actively avoid illness, detect it early, or maintain functioning within the constraints of illness" (Pender et al., 2015, p. 17). These two terms, so often used interchangeably, are clearly both important aspects of health education efforts, yet they imply a decidedly different motivation. For the PHN, both terms relate to practice at the primary level of prevention. The Levels of Prevention Pyramid at the end of this chapter describes educational activities within both of these approaches in relation to primary prevention. For instance, a community health nurse may plan an educational program for community-dwelling older adults to learn about the need for a balanced diet, rich in fruits and vegetables. This would be an example of a health promotion focus, because there is no clear disease or condition at issue. As the nurse continues to work with these individuals, the nurse learns that several clients have had recent falls. Fortunately, none of the falls were serious, yet the nurse recognizes the need to discuss foods that will help reduce bone loss and promote healthy bone growth. To protect the clients' health, the nurse provides information on a variety of foods rich in calcium and explains the need for adequate vitamin D. This effort would be still primary prevention, but with the purpose of health protection.

For the community health nurse, teaching is the primary means to influence health at all levels, primary, secondary, and tertiary. But consider the educational program just described: The PHN has provided a well-developed educational program that was well received by the participants. They listened attentively, took the nurse's well-prepared handouts home, and even promised to add more fruits, vegetables, and calcium-rich foods to their diet. A few weeks later, in another educational program, the nurse learns from the participants that they have not altered their dietary patterns in the slightest. This is an example of how understanding the principles of behavior change may provide guidance to this PHN in planning a more effective program, with a greater chance for success.

The Nature of Change

To be a PHN is to be a health educator with the goal of effecting change in people's behaviors. When nurses suggest that families adopt healthier communication patterns, they are asking them to change. Teaching parenting skills to teenagers is introducing a **change**. Promoting a community's self-determination in choosing a safer environment requires that the individuals involved must change. Therefore, it becomes imperative for community health nurses to understand the nature of change, how people respond to it, and how to effect change for improved community health.

Definitions and Types of Change

Change is "any planned or unplanned alteration of the status quo in an organism, situation, or process," per Lippitt's (1973, p. 37) classic definition. This definition explains that change may occur either by design or by default. Over the years, various theorists have contributed to understanding the nature of change (Burke, 2013). From a systems perspective, change means that things are out of balance or the system's equilibrium is upset (Roussel, Harris, & Thomas, 2016). For instance, when a community is ravaged by floodwaters, its normal functioning is thrown off balance. Adjustments are required; new patterns of behavior become necessary.

Other classic theorists have explained change as the process of adopting an innovation (Spradley & McCurdy, 1994). Something different, such as an organization-wide smoke-free policy, is introduced; change occurs when the innovation is accepted, tried, and integrated into daily practice. Some have explained change in terms of its effect on behavior—change requires adjustment in thinking and behavior, and people's responses to change vary according to their perceptions of it. Change threatens the security that people feel when abiding by established and familiar patterns. It generally requires adopting new roles. Change is disruptive. The way people respond to change depends partly on the type of change required. Others have categorized groups or populations by their willingness to accept innovation and change. Rogers' diffusion of innovation theory helps explain how new ideas or healthy behaviors gain momentum and diffuse (or disperse) throughout a population and are then adopted (Boston University School of Public Health, 2013). People fall into five categories of adopters: (a) innovators who are usually the first to try something new, (b) early adopters who are often opinion leaders that have some awareness of a need for change, (c) early majority who are usually followers (not leaders) who want to examine the evidence before trying out a new behavior, (d) late majority who often are suspicious of change and only adopt a behavior after the majority of the population have done so, and (e) laggards who are very traditional, skeptical, and conservative and represent the most difficult group to convince. For instance, when jogging first gained widespread attention in the early 1970s, only a small number

of people were involved (e.g., innovators). Over time, more people heard about the benefits and wanted to improve their fitness (e.g., early adopters, early majority). Now, regular exercise of some type is considered to be necessary for good health. The change process can be described as sudden or drastic (revolutionary) or gradual over time (evolutionary).

Evolutionary change is change that is gradual and requires adjustment on an incremental basis. It modifies rather than replaces a current way of operating. Some examples of evolutionary change include becoming parents, gradually cutting back on the number of cigarettes smoked each day, and losing weight by eliminating desserts and snacks. Because it is gradual, this kind of change does not require radical shifts in goals or values. For the most part, people resist discarding their own ideas. Accepting another's idea may reduce their self-esteem and is therefore resisted. Gradual change may "ease the pain" that change brings to some individuals. Sometimes, this type of change may be viewed as *reform*.

Revolutionary change, in contrast, is a more rapid, drastic, and threatening type of change that may completely upset the balance of a system (Borwick, 2013). It involves different goals and perhaps radically new patterns of behavior. Sudden unemployment, stopping smoking overnight, losing the town's football team in a plane accident, removing children from abusive parents, or rapidly replacing human workers with computers are examples of revolutionary changes. In each instance, the people affected have little or no advance warning and little or no time to prepare. High levels of emotional, mental, and sometimes physical energy and rapid behavior change are required to adapt to revolutionary change. If the demands are too great, some may experience defense mechanisms such as incapacitation, resistance, or denial of the new situation.

The impact of a proposed change on a system clearly depends on the degree of the change's evolutionary or revolutionary qualities, a factor to be considered in planning for change. Some situations lend themselves better to one kind of change than to another. A community in need of improved facilities for the handicapped (e.g., ramps, wider doors) can introduce this change on an evolutionary, incremental basis, whereas a community that is involved in an unsafe, intolerable, or life-threatening situation, such as a hurricane or serious influenza epidemic, may require revolutionary change.

Two powerful examples of social and public health change occurred during the last decades of the 20th century—dramatic decreases in both motor vehicle crashes and tobacco consumption. These changes did not come about simply through education alone. Rather, "multilevel and multicomponent" approaches were used, and social norms were changed by the use of epidemiology and surveillance as a basis for **social marketing** in bringing the problems to the attention of the American public; with the social influence of individuals, along with supportive legislation and policies, changes in health behaviors occurred (Gielen & Green, 2015, p. 21s). Because of research, surveillance, monitoring of risk factors, and subsequent interventions related to these two problems, more people became aware of the significance of them. Although cigarettes had been proclaimed a health risk in 1964, many people still smoked. It was not until smoking cessation research began to show promise and new over-the-counter treatments and medications became available that more people attempted to stop smoking. In 1992, secondhand smoke was declared to be a carcinogen. Mass media was used to educate the public on the risks and the benefits of quitting; this also began to change public opinion. At the same time, legislation to control the advertising of tobacco products and tighten sales to minors gained momentum. Smoke-free policies were enacted, and higher cigarette taxes made it more difficult for some to smoke. Counseling and education strategies were increasingly empowering individuals and communities to change health behaviors, and multiple attempts at quitting were accepted. Cigarette sales began to drop, and stroke and heart attack death rates quickly improved after smoke-free zones were established. Child asthma admissions to hospitals and premature births also significantly declined within a year after the United States enacted bans on smoking in public places. Researchers point to the synergistic effect of the interventions (Gielen & Green, 2015). Similarly, with environmental (e.g., safer cars, improved roads, better signage) and behavioral changes (e.g., use of seat belts and child safety seats, buying newer/safer vehicles, fewer drunk drivers), motor vehicles crashes drastically dropped. Public information campaigns led by individuals who had been impacted by drunk drivers (e.g., MADD, SADD), along with education and training programs for beverage servers, tougher laws and penalties for drinking and driving, periodic sobriety checkpoints, and campaigns to encourage designated drivers and discourage driving for those who have been drinking led to a change in social norms and reductions in motor vehicle crashes. Because federal highway money was used as an incentive for states to lower the legal limit for drinking and driving, and to move to graduated driver licensing programs for teen drivers, the changes became widespread and more lasting. With the change in public opinion and health behaviors, seat belt use increased from 11% in 1981 to 86% in 2012 and child safety seat use is often cited at 92% to 99%. In this nation that prizes individual rights, public opinion was reframed from "a matter of personal risk to one of imposing risks on others" (Gielen & Green, 2015, p. 24s).

Stages of Change

The phrase **stages of change** refers to the three sequential steps leading to change:

- Unfreezing (when desire for change develops)
- Changing (when new ideas are accepted and tried out)
- Refreezing (when the change is integrated and stabilized in practice)

Kurt Lewin first described these stages in the 1940s and early 1950s, and they have become a cornerstone for understanding the change process (Kaminski, 2011; Lewin, 1947, 1951; Lippitt, Watson, & Westley, 1958).

Unfreezing

The first stage, unfreezing, occurs when a developing need for change causes disequilibrium in the system. A system in disequilibrium is more vulnerable to change. People are motivated to change either intrinsically or by some external force. People have a sense of dissatisfaction; they feel a void that they would like to fill. The unfreezing stage involves initiating the change. Unfreezing may occur spontaneously: A family requests help in solving a problem with alcoholism, a group seeks assistance in adjusting to retirement, and a community desires a solution to noise pollution. However, the nurse as change agent may need to initiate the unfreezing stage by attempting to motivate clients, through education or other strategies, to see the need for change. Rarely do individuals understand the immediate impact of unhealthy decisions and tend to develop poor health habits over time (Koeppl & Robertson, 2015). Being proactive and recognizing the importance that daily choices influence health instead of being reactive to negative health behaviors is essential. The reactive behavior has been termed as "just-in-time" involvement, when clients are motivated to change once illness seems imminent. This concept is discussed further in Chapter 17 in relation to emergency preparedness.

Changing/Moving

The second stage of the change process, changing or moving, occurs when people examine, accept, and try the innovation (Kaminski, 2011). For instance, this is the period when participants in a prenatal class are learning exercises or when elderly clients in a senior citizens' center are discussing and trying ways to make their apartments safe from accidents. During the changing stage, people experience a series of attitude transformations, ranging from early questioning of the innovation's worth to full acceptance and commitment and then to accomplishing the change. The change agent's role during this moving stage is to help clients see the value of the change, encourage them to try it out, and assist them in adopting it.

Refreezing

The third and final stage in the change process, refreezing, occurs when change is established as an accepted and permanent part of the system (Kaminski, 2011). The rest of the system has adapted to it. Because it is no longer viewed as disruptive, threatening, or new, people no longer feel resistant to it. As the change is integrated, the system becomes refrozen and stabilized. It is evident that refreezing has occurred when weight loss clients, for example, are routinely following their diets and losing weight, when senior citizens are using grab bars in their bathrooms and have removed scatter rugs from their homes, or when a community has erected stop signs and established crosswalks at dangerous intersections. Refreezing involves integrating or internalizing the change into the system and then maintaining it. Because a change has been accepted and tried does not guarantee that it will last. Often, there is a tendency for old patterns and habits to return. Consequently, the change agent must take special measures to ensure maintenance of the new behavior (Wills, 2014). A later section discusses ways to stabilize change.

Planned/Managed Change

Leaders in community health nursing have been change agents for decades. They have planned and managed change in a variety of systems. **Planned change** is a purposeful, designed effort to effect improvement in a system with the assistance of a change agent per Spradley's classic definition (1980). Planned change, also known as managed change, is crucial to the development of successful community health nursing programs (Roussel et al., 2016). In fact, the ability to manage and influence change is considered to be an important competency in the field of public health (Reyes, Bekemeier, & Issel, 2014). The following characteristics of planned change are key to its success:

- *The change is purposeful and intentional:* There are specific reasons or goals prompting the change. These goals give the change effort a unifying focus and a specific target. Unplanned change occurs haphazardly, and its outcomes are unpredictable.
- *The change is by design, not by default:* Thorough, systematic planning provides structure for the change process and a map to follow toward a planned destination.
- *Planned change in community health aims at improvement:* That is, it seeks to better the current

situation, to promote a higher level of efficiency, safety, or health enhancement. Planned change aims to facilitate growth and positive improvements. Plans to provide shelter and health care for a homeless population, for example, are designed to improve this group's well-being.

- *Planned change is accomplished through an influencing agent:* The change agent is a catalyst in developing and carrying out the design; the change agent's role is a leadership role, often as an educator.

Planned-Change Process

The planned-change process involves a systematic sequence of activities that follows the nursing process. Following its eight basic steps leads to the successful management of change: (1) recognize symptoms, (2) diagnose need, (3) analyze alternative solutions, (4) select a change, (5) plan the change, (6) implement the change, (7) evaluate the change, and (8) stabilize the change (Spradley, 1980). Figure 11–2 shows how forces acting on a system create a need for change using the planned-change model.

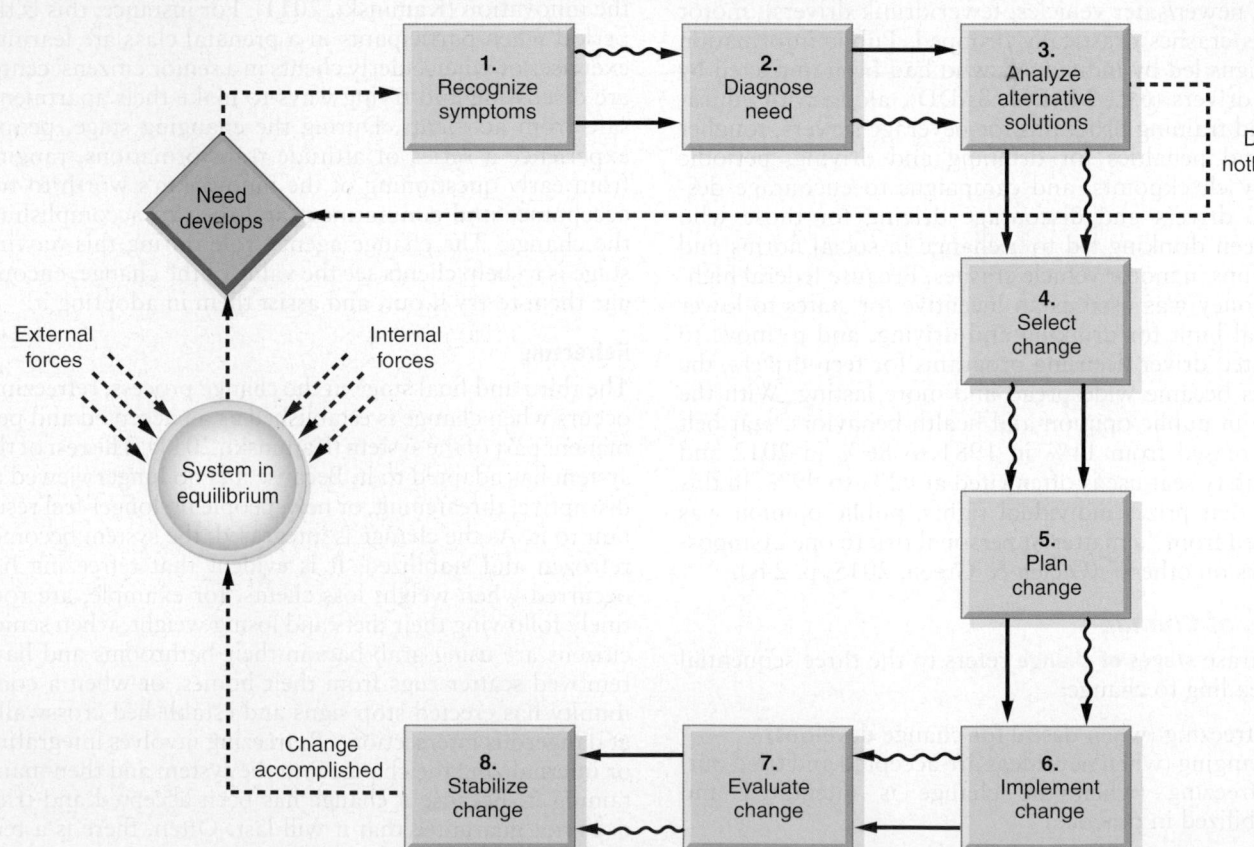

Planned Change Model

FIGURE 11–2 Planned-change model. The planned-change process begins when one recognizes a need. When the change agent fails to respond to a need for change, the need continues and may escalate. Client system (those involved and affected by the change) and change agent must work together throughout the entire planned-change process. Their respective roles vary depending on the situation and the players' abilities, but no planned change is truly effective without utilization of this collaborative relationship. The client system (*wavy arrow*), which may be an entire community, will fluctuate in its involvement with the change process. The change agent (*straight arrow*), as a good leader, analyzes the situation thoroughly, plans carefully, and sets a steady course for effecting the change.

Step 1: Recognize (Assess) Symptoms

The first step in managing change is to recognize and assess the symptoms that indicate a need for change (DiClemente, Salazar, & Crosby, 2013). This step requires gathering and examining the presenting evidence, not diagnosing or jumping ahead to treatment. For instance, assume that a group of clients shows interest in receiving help with parenting skills. The nurse cannot assume that these clients feel inadequate in the parent role, nor can the nurse assume that they lack information about parenting or are having difficulty with their children. The nurse must assess the specific needs to discover that some of the parents have trouble talking to their teenagers, others wonder whether their children's behavior is normal, a few question how strictly they should set limits, and still others are not certain about how to handle discipline. These symptoms are pieces of evidence that will assist diagnosis in the next step. This first step is an assessment phase. Before moving on, however, change agents need to ask themselves what their motives are for pursuing this change. Inappropriate motives on the change agent's part, such as wanting to feel needed, can cloud judgment and interfere with effective management of change.

Step 2: Diagnose Need

Diagnosis involves analyzing the symptoms and reaching a conclusion about what needs changing. First, describe the situation as it is now (the real) and compare it with the way it should be (the ideal). For example, loud arguing and conflict may be normal and functional behavior for an adolescent support group. There is no discrepancy between the real and the ideal and, therefore, no need for change within the group. If, however, a discrepancy exists between the real and the ideal, then a need exists and a change effort is justified (Hersey, Blanchard, & Johnson, 2012). For example, the community health nurse, in talking with a group of parents, hears the following comment: "I'm not sure how much freedom to allow Ashley. She came in late twice last week and I'm not sure how to discipline her." Clearly, the nurse notices a discrepancy between this family's present and ideal situations; so, a need exists.

The next step is to determine the nature and cause of the need (Hersey et al., 2012). Gathering data by questioning clients, checking the literature, or seeking consultation is important for making a more accurate diagnosis. The parents should be questioned in more detail about the difficulties that they are having with their children. The nurse asks questions such as the following: What are your concerns? How do you feel about being parents? What are the most difficult aspects of parenting for you? Have you read any books or used any other resources to help with parenting activities? To whom do you talk about parenting problems? When you have a problem with your children, how do you usually solve it? Secondary data should be obtained by checking the literature to determine the most effective approaches to solving parenting problems or by consulting an expert on family life to get ideas about what this group of parents might need. The parents also should be asked directly what information they desire or need. Conclusions should be drawn about the specific changes needed for these parents. Unless the diagnosis is made accurately, the entire change effort may address the wrong problem. Also, the clients help the nurse to diagnose their problem; the first question the nurse should ask the parents is what it is that they want and need.

These findings should be formulated into a single, diagnostic statement that also includes the problem's cause. After data collection, the nurse discovers that the parents are insecure in their parenting roles, partially because of lack of knowledge about how to carry out parental responsibilities, but primarily because they lack a support system. Most of them live some distance from relatives or no longer maintain close ties with them. The diagnosis for these parents is insecurity in the parenting role resulting from a lack of support and knowledge.

Step 3: Analyze Alternative Solutions

Once the diagnosis and its cause are determined, it is time to identify solutions or alternative directions to follow. Brainstorming is helpful here, and the client system should be involved as much as possible in the process. Reviewing the literature is helpful at this point to suggest solutions tried by others. Make a list of all reasonable, broad alternatives and then analyze them thoroughly to determine the advantages, disadvantages, possible consequences, and risks involved in each (Hersey, Blanchard, & Johnson, 2012). For the parents, general alternatives might be considered, such as family counseling, a support group, or parenting education. Each of these alternatives includes some advantages and disadvantages toward meeting the parents' need for confidence in their roles.

Next, each alternative should be analyzed. For example, the counseling solution could provide insight and awareness into family behavior. It would give family members opportunities to express feelings and gain understanding of how other family members feel. However, it would not provide a frame of reference that the clients could use to compare their own parenting behaviors with other acceptable ones, nor would it provide adult peer support for the parents. The consequences of this alternative most likely would be to promote parents' self-understanding and better family communication. Risks would include the possibility that children, especially teenagers, might not be willing to participate and that parents might not gain self-confidence in their roles. Each alternative should be examined to determine its usefulness and feasibility; again, literature and other resources (e.g., consultants) can be used to determine the best ways to meet the parents' need for change.

Step 4: Select a Change

After all alternatives have been carefully analyzed, the best solution must be selected. The parents favor the idea that the best solution is a parenting support group. The risks involved in the choice of change should be reexamined, such as whether this action might be too costly in terms of time, money, or potential for failure. Ways to reduce these risks might be explored.

To know what the change is aiming to accomplish, a clearly stated goal should be formulated. For this parenting group, the mutually agreed-on goal is to provide a supportive, reinforcing climate while increasing members' parenting skills. "Useful goals should be (1) specific; (2) attainable (doable); and (3) forgiving [less than perfect]" (National Heart Lung and Blood Institute, 2012). For example, setting a goal of walking 30 minutes a day, 5 days a week is more likely to be successful than a goal of walking 5 miles every day because the first goal is specific, doable, and forgiving.

Step 5: Plan the Change

This step is at the heart of planned change, because at this stage, the change agent and client system together prepare the design, or blueprint, that guides the change action. In steps 1 through 4, data are gathered, a diagnosis is made, resources are assessed, and a goal is established—all preparatory actions for planning the change. The plan tells the change agent and the clients how to meet that goal. Preferably, they develop the plan together.

The nurse talks with the parents about ways to meet their goal, considering such possibilities as weekly discussion groups on selected topics, monthly meetings with an informed speaker, or reading books and articles on parenting and holding regular sessions to discuss their application. After analysis and discussion, the group decides to meet one evening a month, rotating the location among members' homes. Group sessions will include a variety of approaches: a speaker will be invited every 2 months, a book or article discussion will be held quarterly, and the remaining meetings will be spent on topics of the group's choice. All sessions will provide opportunities for parents to discuss their concerns or problems. The nurse and the group design this plan around a set of objectives.

The most important activity in planning is to have clear, specific objectives. These should be measurable and, preferably, stated as outcomes. For example, the following objective is measurable and describes an outcome: "By the end of the second session, each parent

in the group will have participated in the discussion at least once." It is helpful to prepare a list of activities to help accomplish each objective and to develop a time plan. It also is important to assess the potential costs in terms of time, money, materials, and the number of people needed, as well as determine the resources available. Then the evaluation plan is designed, and a list of ways to maintain (refreeze) the change is made.

During planning, it is useful to perform a *force field analysis* (Hersey et al., 2012), a technique developed by Kurt Lewin for examining all positive (driving) and negative (restraining) forces that are influencing a change situation. *Force field theory* describes driving forces, which favor change, and restraining forces, which decrease or discourage change. Examples of driving forces include clients' desire to be healthier, to be more productive, or to have a safer environment. Examples of restraining forces include apathy, habits, anxiety or fear of something new, perceived loss of power, low self-esteem, insecurity, and hostility (Roussel et al., 2016). When the strength of the driving forces is equal to the strength of the restraining forces, equilibrium exists. To introduce a change and move the client system to a higher level of health, that balance must be altered. The change agent increases the driving forces, decreases the restraining forces, or both. The change agent uses force field analysis to study both sets of forces and to develop strategies to influence the forces in favor of the change (Fig. 11–3).

The procedure for conducting a force field analysis follows a few simple steps. The change agent may perform the analysis alone but preferably consults with clients and a change-planning resource group such as public health colleagues. Steps for conducting force field analysis include the following (Minnesota Department of Health, n.d.):

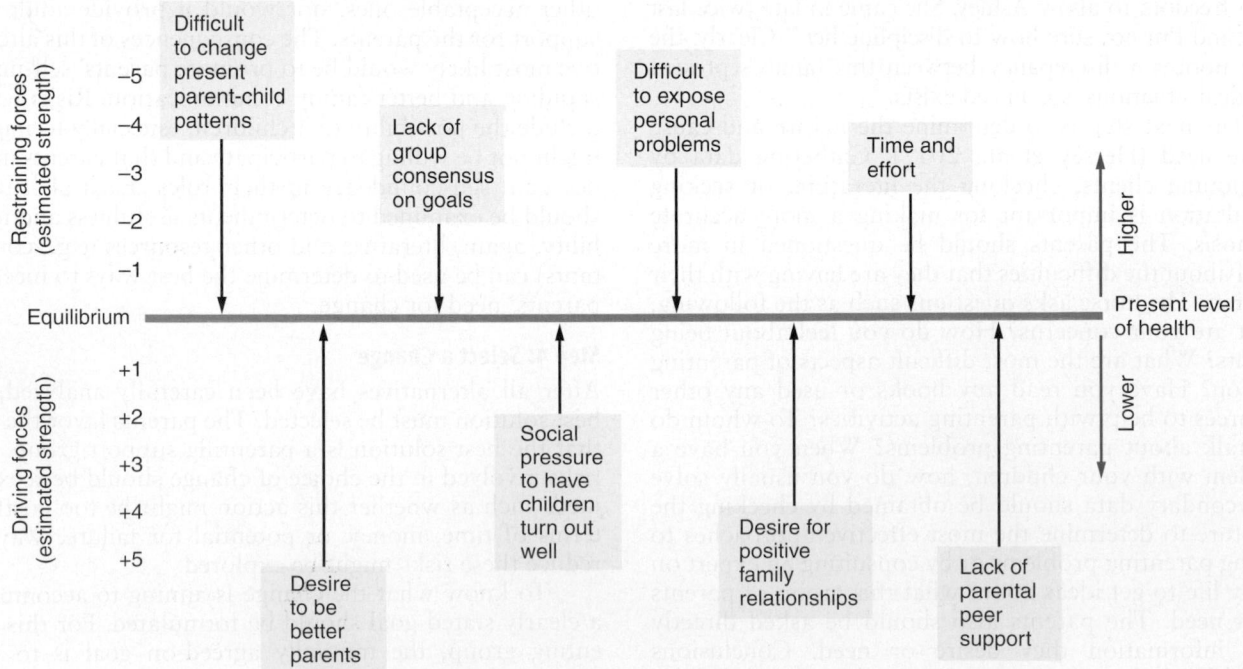

FIGURE 11–3 Analysis of restraining and driving forces.

- Brainstorm to produce a list of all driving and restraining forces. (For the parenting group, one driving force is the parents' desire to be more successful parents; a restraining force might be lack of group agreement on discussion topics.)
- Estimate the strength of each force.
- Plot the forces on a chart such as the one shown in Figure 11–3.
- Note the most important forces, then research and analyze them.
- List and document possible responses or actions that might strengthen each important driving force or weaken each important restraining force.

Finally, as a consideration in planning the change and in analyzing the driving and restraining forces, the change agent studies the social network and interactions within the system involved in the change. The change agent needs to be aware of formal and informal leaders, cliques within larger groups, influential persons, and all other social network influences on the change process. For instance, one nurse attempting to improve the infant-feeding practices among a group of young Southeast Asian mothers failed to consider the strong cultural influence of the infants' grandmothers living nearby. The older women had strong opinions based on long-held cultural traditions about what infants were to eat and how they were to be fed. To ignore their influence could cause the proposed change to fail; involving the grandmothers could be a way of turning their influence into a driving force for the change.

Step 6: Implement the Change

The implementation step involves enacting the change plan. Because the objectives and activities have been clearly defined in previous steps, the change agent and clients know what needs to be done and how to begin the process (Davies, 2011). For example, the parenting group and their nurse/change agent begin group discussions meeting every Tuesday evening at a local school.

At the start of implementation, be certain that all persons concerned clearly understand and are prepared for the change. When working with an aggregate, for example, the nurse may do most of the planning with a few key members. The nurse must be sure that each member who will be affected by the proposed change understands (a) what to expect, (b) the meaning of the change, and (c) what will be required of them in adapting to it. An unprepared client system, especially in a large group or organization, may lead to failure. No matter how well a change effort is planned, people who are unprepared for it may resist it strongly and render it useless.

When implementing change that will affect a large group of people, such as introduction of a mass screening or immunization program, it is helpful to do a *pilot study*. The pilot study is done to test the change on a small scale, iron out problems, and revise the change before implementing it in the larger system. One advantage of a pilot study is that it demonstrates the change to the client system on a small scale, which is less threatening, so that clients are more receptive. It gives people time to adjust their thinking and to discover that the change will not disrupt their lives too much or require drastic adaptations. It is also useful in working out the kinks and making necessary improvements before moving to the larger scale program.

Step 7: Evaluate the Change

The success of step 7 depends on how well the change is planned. Well-written objectives with specific criteria for their measurement make the evaluation step simpler. However, evaluation does not end with saying whether the objectives were met. Each objective requires analysis: Was it met? What evidence (documentation) shows that it was met? Was it accomplished using the best means possible, or would another method have been better? The objective for the parenting group stated that each member should enter into the discussion by the end of the second session. Although the nurse leader could easily evaluate this objective, the objective could have been improved by a more specific description of how this participation would occur. A better method to achieve this objective would have been to suggest that more active group members solicit ideas from those who did not have an opportunity to speak. This would facilitate more group participation, rather than having the nurse educator call on less verbal participants to speak. Finally, considering the evaluation, the change agent makes needed modifications in the change before stabilization.

Step 8: Stabilize the Change

The final step in the planned-change process requires taking measures to reinforce and maintain the change. A well-developed change plan includes a design for stabilization. The change agent actively encourages continued use of the innovation by establishing two-way communication. In this way, future resistance can be overcome, and the client's full commitment to the change can be maintained (Davies, 2011). Stabilization occurs by soliciting reactions from the client system. Do the clients perceive any potential problems? Do they have doubts? Reinforcing the desired behavior and following up on the change as long as necessary will help to ensure its continuation.

Alcoholics Anonymous, for example, stabilizes the change to nondrinking by providing a regular support group that reinforces the nondrinking pattern. The group rewards compliance with praise and replaces drinking with other satisfying experiences, such as social support and acceptance, to keep the alcoholic from returning to the old behavior. In the example of the parenting group, the nurse stabilizes changed behaviors by focusing on the group's increased confidence in their parenting roles and emphasizing the increased success in coping with their children, as group members share their experiences and stories. The group decides to reward successes by giving a "Parent of the Month" award to the member who demonstrates the most growth in parenting skills, and they agree to nominate one member as "Parent of the Year" in the community newspaper contest. After stabilization occurs and the system achieves a new equilibrium, the change agent–client system relationship may no longer be needed.

Applying Planned Change to Larger Aggregates

We have viewed the planned-change process primarily in the context of introducing change to smaller aggregates. Community health nurses also use these eight steps when managing change at organization, population group, community, and larger aggregate levels. For example, a nurse may suspect that there is a widespread lack of confidence among young parents. This hypothesis could be tested through a social media survey to determine parenting needs among the entire community's population of young parents. If symptoms are present (step 1), the nurse, in collaboration with health department personnel or other appropriate professionals, could analyze the symptoms and reach a diagnosis (step 2) that many young parents in the community are lacking in confidence and knowledge of parenting skills. Several approaches to meeting this need could be considered, such as instituting a parenting center in the community with satellite clinics, organizing churches or clubs to sponsor parenting support groups, or working through the community college system to hold workshops and classes on parenting skills (step 3). The most feasible and useful alternative could be selected (step 4), and a parenting program for the community could be planned (step 5) and implemented (step 6). The nurse, with parents and other professionals involved, would then evaluate the outcomes (step 7) and make necessary adjustments in the parenting program before finally stabilizing it (step 8), making certain that this change, undertaken to meet a population group need, remains an established and effectively functioning service (Fig. 11–4).

Change and Health Promotion Within Communities/Populations

Changes in behavior and health promotion can also be directed to even larger audiences—communities and larger populations. Similar approaches can be used, but may be varied depending upon age, most pertinent issues, and how to best reach targeted audiences. For instance, in an effort to address cardiovascular health by encouraging prevention and health promotion, researchers stratified their approaches based upon what they determined were the most beneficial age ranges. They began with 3- to 5-year-olds, and a family-centered educational strategy about hearts

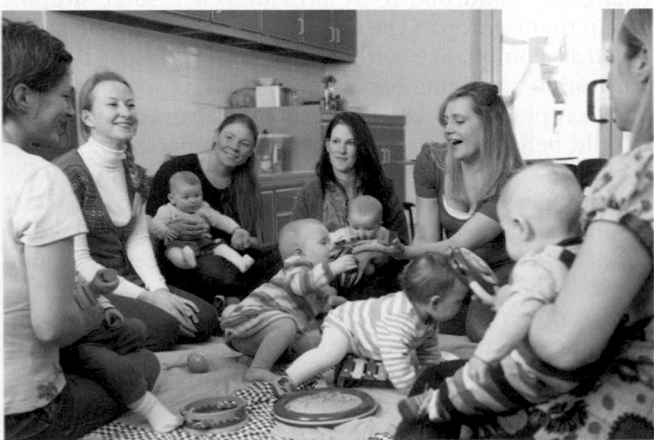

FIGURE 11–4 An aggregate, mothers with infants, at a new mothers' class.

and how to keep them healthy by reducing obesity and other risk factors. Then, between 25 and 50 years of age, the focus changes to education about screening and early detection of potential problems. Over age 50, the approach is directed more toward education about discovering cardiovascular disease and early treatment. In 2015, Mount Sinai Hospital in New York began an educational program for preschoolers and their parents that had been piloted in Spain and Colombia (Science Daily, 2015). This shift to prevention of cardiovascular disease is expected to eventually lead to shorter hospital stays and increased ambulatory care options. A classic systematic review by Jepson, Harris, Platt, and Tannahill (2010) on the effectiveness of interventions used in population health promotion found that workplace or school-based programs, along with mass media efforts, were effective in changing health behaviors.

One model for communicating with populations is CDCynergy Lite, developed by the Centers for Disease Control and Prevention (CDC, n.d.). It involves six phases in developing a social marketing campaign:

1. Problem definition and description (e.g., health problem of concern, who this affects, how you can address it)
2. Problem analysis/market research (e.g., analyze data on problem, target audience's values, behaviors, beliefs, attitudes, and barriers/facilitators to changing behavior)
3. Planning communication/market strategy (e.g., determine target audience, what behaviors that you wish to address, benefits offered [such as better health] with interventions to support change)
4. Program planning/interventions (e.g., methods you will use to influence change [for instance, a Web site to promote better nutrition/physical activity for adolescents], plan, objectives)
5. Program evaluation (e.g., is your program useful, feasible, accurate, ethical)
6. Implementation (e.g., plan for launching program, publicity, threats/opportunities)

This method has been used with many health problems and issues (e.g., arthritis, breast-feeding, drug abuse prevention, smoking cessation, HIV/AIDS, colorectal cancer screening, chronic fatigue syndrome, immunizations, influenza) and is a helpful means of reaching targeted populations (CDC, 2014). See Chapters 10, 12, and 15 for more on health promotion, communication, and use of technology in assessing communities and developing programs for health promotion.

Planned-Change Strategies

Here we focus on the three major change strategies: (1) empiric–rational, (2) normative–reeducative, and (3) power–coercive. In a given situation, the change agent may use one or a combination of these strategies to effect a change (Burke, 2013).

Empiric–Rational Change Strategies

Empiric–rational change strategies are used to effect change based on the assumption that people are rational and, when presented with empiric information, will adopt new practices that appear to be in their best interest

(DiClemente et al., 2013). To use this approach, which is common in community health, new information is offered to people. For instance, most family planning programs use empiric–rational strategies. Clients are given basic information (communication-related strategy) on reproductive anatomy and physiology, and they are told about the benefits of contraception with an explanation of a variety of family planning methods. Health workers hope that once clients have this information, they will adopt some method of family planning. Some clients respond well to this approach, and others do not. The difference lies in client ability and interest in self-help. The nurse/change agent uses empiric–rational strategies with clients who can assume a relatively high degree of responsibility for their own health.

Normative–Reeducative Change Strategies

Normative–reeducative change strategies are used to influence change that not only presents new information but also directly influences people's attitudes and behaviors through persuasion. It is a sociocultural reeducation. This approach assumes that people's attitudes and practices are determined by sociocultural norms and that they need more than presentation of information to change behavior (DiClemente et al., 2013). This approach strengthens client self-understanding, self-control, and commitment to new patterns through direct urging and influence. For example, a health education program that aims to increase safety practices in an industrial setting not only provides safety information, such as posters and warning signs, but also uses persuasive tactics, such as individual rewards for safe practices, division recognition for minimum number of accidents, or discipline for noncompliance. Nurses use normative–reeducative strategies with clients who have a measure of self-care skill but at the same time need external assistance to effect lasting behavioral change. This type of client is often found in teaching, counseling, and therapy situations.

Power–Coercive Change Strategies

Power–coercive change strategies use coercion based on fear to effect change (DiClemente et al., 2013). Change agents may derive power from the law (health regulations, administrative policies), from position (political, social, or managerial), from a group (social, work, or professional), or from personal power (personal charisma, competence, respect of followers). They use this power to coerce change; the result is forced compliance on the part of the client system. Some situations, particularly those that are life threatening, may require power–coercive strategies. In public health practice, power–coercive strategies may be used with people who cannot help themselves or in situations that threaten individuals' safety or the public's health. An example is the stringent enforcement of infection control policies regarding the treatment of contaminated objects such as used needles and the safe disposal of infectious wastes. In another example, if officials find a restaurant to be in violation of health codes, they will either force compliance with the code or close the restaurant. Occasionally, clients cannot exercise responsibility because of temporary or permanent physical or psychological incapacitation; examples may include mentally ill individuals, abusive parents, or developmentally disabled persons. In such cases, the nurse may need to use the power of the law to effect changes that are in clients' best interests. Although power–coercive strategies are appropriate in some situations, they should be used with caution because they can rob people of opportunities to grow in autonomy and capacity for self-care.

Planned-change strategies may be combined; for instance, a normative–reeducative approach might have a power–coercive backup. This combination is evident in programs that educate and persuade groups of people to be immunized against an impending epidemic or to keep their garbage contained to avoid insect and rodent infestation. Behind this normative–reeducative strategy is an implied coercive threat of official disapproval, or worse, if the clients are noncompliant.

The effectiveness of a change strategy varies with each situation and particularly with the degree of client capacity for self-care. The community health nurse as a change agent must adapt strategies to fit each change situation. It is important to remember that not only strategy, culture, and systems change but also the person's perception of the proposed change and how it affects his or her feelings and behaviors toward the change are important.

Principles for Effecting Positive Change

Community health nurses introduce change every day that they practice. Every effort to solve a problem, prevent another problem from occurring, meet a potential community need, or promote people's optimal health requires changes. For these changes to be truly successful, so that desired outcomes are reached, they must be well thought out and managed. The following six principles provide guidelines for effecting positive change: (1) principle of participation, (2) principle of resistance to change, (3) principle of proper timing, (4) principle of interdependence, (5) principle of flexibility, and (6) principle of self-understanding.

Principle of Participation

Persons affected by a proposed change should participate as much as possible in every step of the planned-change process. This involvement is important for several reasons. Collaboration with those who have a vested interest in the change can produce a wealth of ideas and insights that can greatly improve the change plan. Furthermore, such participation can help remove obstacles and reduce resistance. One nurse, for instance, when planning with a school's parent–teacher association for a drug education program, involved students as well as teachers and parents. As a result, the nurse secured this group's support and cooperation, gained many helpful suggestions that had not been previously considered, and discovered that students were more responsive to the program because the change plan was specifically tailored to their needs. Participation ensures a greater likelihood that the change will be accepted and maintained. Participation is the mainstay of community-based participatory research (CBPR), a method of ensuring that community needs are being met and encouraging buy in (see Chapter 4). In cross-cultural or international arenas, community participation is paramount to effective change. For example, a project targeting improved hygiene practices in India involved various community outreach initiatives and partnerships aimed to reduce overall childhood mortality (World Health Organization, 2014). A national examination of CBPR studies involving cancer noted that when interventions were adapted to the local area with integration of cultural wisdom and local investigators were used, mistrust was diminished and cancer disparities were reduced (Simonds, Wallerstein, Duran, & Villegas, 2013).

Principle of Resistance to Change

Because all systems instinctively preserve the status quo, the change agent can expect people to resist change. The homeostatic mechanism operating in any system seeks to maintain equilibrium; change poses a threat to that stability and security. Furthermore, all systems experience inertia, that is, they resist beginning movement. People do not undertake a change until they are convinced of its worth. Resistance may also come from a conflict over goals and methods or from misunderstanding about what the change will mean and require. Involving people in the planned-change process, as discussed in the previous section, is one way to overcome resistance. Another way is establishing and maintaining open lines of communication to make ideas clearly understood and to resolve disagreements quickly. The nurse must prepare clients thoroughly for the change, provide support and patience during the change process, and encourage response and expression of feelings. The world of business can offer great suggestions for PHNs facing resistance from clients and communities. Goulston (2013), a business psychiatrist, offers these words of wisdom, shut up and listen when faced with resistance, and realize that "you never win on the strength of your argument, you win on the strength of your relationship" (para. 20). Building rapport and listening to client/community concerns will engender consensus more quickly than repeated lectures on the why something is needed.

Principle of Proper Timing

Sometimes, a change, even a well-designed and much-needed one, should be postponed because it is not the right time to introduce it. For example, perhaps the client system is experiencing too many other changes to handle the stress of this one. Other projects or activities in which the client system is currently engaged may compete for energy and other resources, depleting the energy and resources needed to make the proposed change successful. For example, in November, some middle-aged women, eager to start a book club that focused on preparing for midlife changes (including menopause, "empty-nest" syndrome, and planning for retirement), had to postpone the project because the holidays were approaching. Shopping, entertaining, and vacations made it impossible to give the kind of time and energy needed to make the book club effective. In hospitals, for instance, major changes to nursing procedures or processes are not usually initiated during flu season when hospitals are overcrowded.

Proper timing is as important to a planned change as well-timed seed planting is to a good harvest. The change idea must be appropriate, the change recipient prepared, the climate right, and the resources available before the change can be fostered to grow into full maturity and usefulness.

Principle of Interdependence

Every system has many subsystems that are intricately related to and interdependent on one another. A change in one part of a system affects its other parts, and a change in one system may affect other systems (Trickett et al., 2011). For example, a county public health nursing agency made a change in its use of home health aides. Because many homebound clients needed more care than the agency staff could provide, the agency contracted with a private home care service for extra home health aides. These paraprofessionals worked in the homes of agency clients, supplementing the care given by agency staff. The private company preferred to supervise its own aides, whereas the county agency had a policy of using community health nurses to supervise aides. The county agency was legally responsible and professionally accountable for the quality of care given to clients. The private company wanted to retain control of its workers. The matter was resolved by contracting with a different private service that would accept the county agency's supervision. The change, however, had affected the roles of nurses and aides within the system, as well as the relationships between the two systems.

This principle of interdependence reminds the nurse that change does not take place in a vacuum. When workers learn new health and safety practices associated with their jobs, their relationships with one another, and their bosses, their overall productivity in the organization may easily be affected. One must anticipate and prepare for the impact of the proposed change on the clients involved, other persons, departments, organizations, or even geographic areas. Also, community interventions should be "ecologically based, multilevel, collaborative approaches to health" and should reflect the complexities of each unique community (Trickett et al., 2011, p. 1410) (Fig. 11–5).

Principle of Flexibility

Unexpected events can occur in every situation. This fifth principle—flexibility—emphasizes two points. First, the nurse needs to be able to adapt to unexpected events and make the most of them. Perseverance and flexibility are

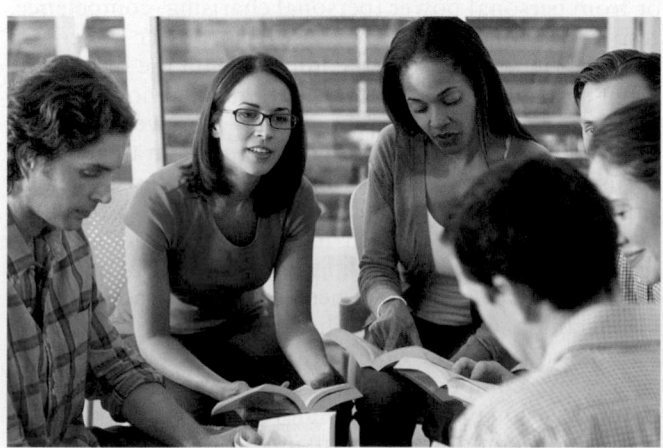

FIGURE 11–5   PHN leading a group.

the marks of a creative change manager (Roussel et al., 2016). One community health nurse had tried unsuccessfully to contact a young mother who was reportedly abusing her 2-year-old son. After several phone calls and visits to an empty house, the nurse finally found the mother and son at home with a neighbor who insisted on staying for the entire visit. At first, the nurse was irritated by the neighbor's presence and viewed it as interfering with the goal of getting to know the mother and child. When the nurse realized that the neighbor's presence offered an opportunity to learn more about the situation through the neighbor's input, the nurse viewed it as an opportunity to influence another client as well. She asked whether the neighbor had children and began to include both women in the discussion, explaining what could be offered in terms of health teaching and support. This nurse was flexible in her approach to this situation.

The second point to remember about flexibility is that a good change planner anticipates possible blocks or problems by preparing strategies and alternative plans. During step 3 of the planned-change process, it is helpful to rank the alternative solutions considered. Then, if the first choice does not work out for some reason, an alternative is ready to be put into action. Flexibility involves a willingness to consider a variety of options and suggestions from many sources, and it is the hallmark of public health professionals, along with curiosity and communication skills (Morris, 2014).

Principle of Self-Understanding

Self-understanding is essential for an effective change agent (Hersey et al., 2012). The community nurse (as change agent) should be able to clearly define his or her role and seek to understand how others define it. It is important to understand your own values and motives in relation to each change that you are asking people to make. Nurses should also understand their own personality traits, so that they can capitalize on or adjust them in order to be more effective change agents. Understanding yourself is crucial to learning to make use of your best qualities and skills in order to effect change (Jerome & Powell, 2016). Change is inevitable. Understanding the principles of planned change can assist the community health nurse in guiding individuals, families, and communities toward achieving the highest level of health.

SOCIAL DETERMINANTS OF HEALTH

Social justice has long been a tenant of our society, dating back to the industrial revolution (Hendrickson, 2015). Social justice, as it relates to health, is an increasing concern primarily because of the growing inequity in the distribution of disease, illness, and wellness across our society. **Social determinants of health** are "conditions in the environments in which people are born, live, learn, work, play, worship, and age that affect a wide range of health, functioning, and quality-of-life outcomes and risks" (USDHHS, 2016c, para. 6). *Healthy People 2020* initiative addresses social determinants of health as a new topic, with the goal of "creating social and physical environments that promote good health for all" (USDHHS, 2016c, para. 1) (Fig. 11–6).

Understanding social determinants of health requires examination of numerous factors, beyond individual

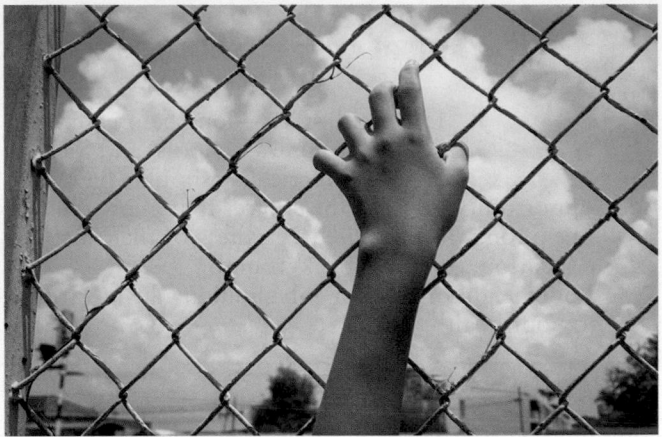

FIGURE 11–6 Social determinants of health, or the environments in which we live and work, affect our health and our quality of life.

behavior, that contribute to our state of health. Factors that influence an individual's ability to maintain good health include social, economic, and physical factors such as access to social and economic opportunities; safe housing; quality education; clean water, food, and air; safe workplaces; equitable social interactions (class, race, and gender); and adequate community resources (USDHHS, 2016c, n.d.). Addressing these factors in a manner that has a positive impact on social, economic, and physical conditions and supports positive health behavior change can improve the health of our communities over time.

"Nursing has a clear mandate to ensure access to health and health-care by providing sensitive empowering care to those experiencing inequities and working to change underlying social conditions that result in and perpetuate health inequities" (Reutter & Kushner, 2012, p. 269). The public health nurse can play a significant role in addressing social determinants of health by first being aware and educated about factors that influence health beyond an individual's choices, looking at root causes of disease.

Secondly, the PHN can incorporate social determinant factors when assessing individuals, families, and communities. One resource for this is the Health Impact Project. This project seeks to advance policies for healthier communities by examining social, economic, and environmental influences, building consensus across community members and other stakeholders, and advocating for health considerations in all policies (Pew Charitable Trusts, 2015).

Finally, community health nurses can educate their client base on the social determinants of health, facilitate community action that supports positive change, and advocate for policies that address the root causes of disease and health inequities (USDHHS, 2016c, 2010e).

The Robert Wood Johnson Foundation conducted research to determine the most effective messages on social determinants of health that are meaningful and understandable to Americans (Robert Wood Johnson Foundation, 2015). The community health nurse educator can use these messages to communicate concepts about social determinants of health to clients and

DISPLAY 11–1   SIX WAYS TO TALK ABOUT SOCIAL DETERMINANTS OF HEALTH

1. Health starts—long before illness—in our homes, schools, and jobs.
2. All Americans should have the opportunity to make the choices that allow them to live a long, healthy life, regardless of their income, education, or ethnic background.
3. Your neighborhood or job shouldn't be hazardous to your health.

4. Your opportunity for health starts long before you need medical care.
5. Health begins where we live, learn, work, and play.
6. The opportunity for health begins in our families, neighborhoods, schools, and jobs (p. 53).

From Robert Wood Johnson Foundation. (2010). A new way to talk about the social determinants of health. Retrieved from http://www.rwjf.org/content/dam/farm/reports/reports/2010/rwjf63023/subassets/rwjf63023_1

communities (see Display 11–1). See Chapters 15, 19, and 25 for additional information.

Facilitating community action is most effective when using participatory action research approaches (Bergold & Thomas, 2012). One such approach is known as the Community Action Model (Fig. 11–7) that seeks to identify actions that are achievable, sustainable, and compels change for the well-being of all. This model builds on

concepts presented in the planned-change process earlier in this chapter. The cyclical five-step process is outlined more fully in Display 11–2. The community health nurse educator can use this model to facilitate community participation and ownership of change that has a positive impact on the community's health. An example of a successful application of the Community Action Model is Pennsylvania's School Nutrition Policy Initiative, targeted

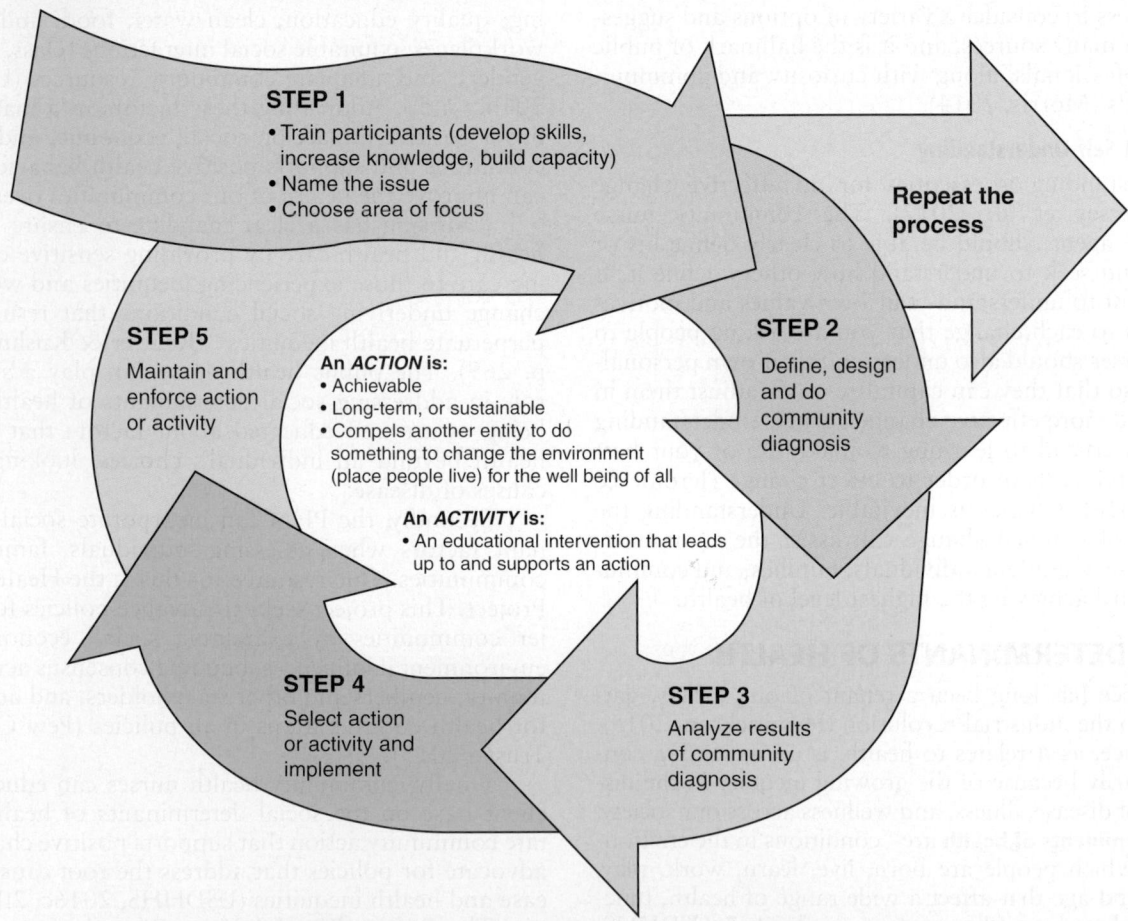

STEP 1
• Train participants (develop skills, increase knowledge, build capacity)
• Name the issue
• Choose area of focus

Repeat the process

STEP 5
Maintain and enforce action or activity

An *ACTION* is:
• Achievable
• Long-term, or sustainable
• Compels another entity to do something to change the environment (place people live) for the well being of all

An *ACTIVITY* is:
• An educational intervention that leads up to and supports an action

STEP 2
Define, design and do community diagnosis

STEP 4
Select action or activity and implement

STEP 3
Analyze results of community diagnosis

FIGURE 11–7 Community action model—creating change by building community capacity. (From Community Health Education Section, San Francisco Department of Public Health. (2002). *Community action training.* Retrieved from http://www.sfdph.org/dph/files/CAMdocs/intro_and_overview/CAMCreatingChangebyBuildingCommunityCapacity.pdf; Brennan Ramirez, L. K., Baker, E. A., & Metzler, M. (2008). *Promoting health equity: A resource to help communities address social determinants of health.* Atlanta, GA: Centers for Disease Control and Prevention.)

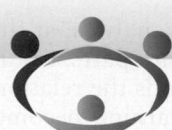

DISPLAY 11–2 FIVE-STEP COMMUNITY ACTION MODEL

Step 1. Skills-based trainings where advocates choose an area of focus

Step 2. Action research where advocates define, design, and do a community diagnosis (action research)

Step 3. Analysis where advocates analyze the result of the diagnosis and prepare findings

Step 4. Organizing where advocates select, plan, and implement an action for change and education to support it

Step 5. Implementing where advocates ensure that the policy outcome is enforced and maintained (p. 360)

From Hofrichter, R., & Bhatia, R. (2010). *Tackling health inequities through public health practice, theory to action* (2nd ed.). New York, NY: Oxford University Press.

---

to combat obesity in 4th to 6th graders. About 48 hours yearly of interactive nutrition lessons are presented in classrooms, and families and local community partners also participate. Incentives are provided to students who choose healthier snacks, and program evaluation found that there was a reduction in overweight incidence by 50%. Overall prevalence rate was decreased for those in the program (10.3%) versus those not participating (25.9%). Other examples incorporate farm-fresh foods into school lunches and snacks or aim to reduce consumption of soda (Healthy Sonoma, 2015).

Policy advocacy is most successful when approached through intersystem collaboration involving key stakeholders as well as beneficiaries of the policies (Reutter & Kushner, 2012). This requires that the community health educator think beyond health and engage with sectors to tackle inequities through policy analysis and advocacy. Advocating for "Health in All Policies" (HiAP) is one approach to addressing multisector policy change as it relates to social determinants of health (World Health Organization, Government of South Australia, 2010). Because many factors outside of health impact health outcomes, it is vital that all policies, regardless of the sector, be viewed from a health lens. Examples of sectors that often have a direct impact on health include agriculture, education, energy, environment, global warming, housing, trade, and transportation, among others (Aspen Institute, 2012). See Chapter 13 for more on policy and advocacy in public health nursing.

CHANGE THROUGH HEALTH EDUCATION

Early in this chapter, you were introduced to one definition of health promotion, with a clear focus on individual and aggregate behavior (Pender et al., 2015). Consider another viewpoint: "the health of populations varies with the interaction of behavior, environment, human biology, social conditions, and community organization" (Green, Ottoson, & Roditis, 2014, p. 478). This definition points out the need for a system-wide approach to promoting healthy behaviors, one that includes education. For the community health nurse, health education is a foundation of practice. Whether the nurse is providing one-on-one education to a new mother about the benefits of breast-feeding, briefing county officials on the need to maintain breast-feeding support centers, or working with community partners and grant funders to develop

a Web-based social marketing campaign to promote breast-feeding among adolescent mothers, educational techniques are being used to promote health in the community. Knowledge of educational theories and teaching methods can assist the nurse to frame these "health messages" for the greatest impact and chance of success.

Teaching is a specialized communication process in which desired behavior changes are achieved. The goal of all teaching is learning. Learning is gaining knowledge, comprehension, or mastery. These can seem like vague terms, and a more concrete definition suggests that *learning* is a process of assimilating new information that promotes a permanent change in behavior. All people have been presented with information that was not interesting, relevant to their needs, or even understandable. In such situations, learning is difficult, if not impossible. The PHN as teacher seeks to convey information in such a way that the client demonstrates a relatively permanent change in behavior. After learning, clients are capable of doing something that they could not do before learning took place. Effective teaching is a cause; learning becomes the effect. To teach effectively, especially in the community where teaching is the focus of care, nurses need to understand the various domains of learning and related learning theories.

DOMAINS OF LEARNING

Learning occurs in several realms or domains: cognitive, affective, and psychomotor. Understanding of the differences among the domains and of the related roles of the nurse provides the background necessary to teach effectively.

Cognitive Domain

The **cognitive domain** of learning involves the mind and thinking processes. When the meaning and relationship of a series of facts is grasped, cognitive learning has occurred. The cognitive domain deals with the recall or recognition of knowledge and the development of intellectual abilities and skills (Bloom, 1956). There are six major levels in the cognitive domain (Miller, Linn, & Gronlund, 2012): knowledge, comprehension, application, analysis, synthesis, and evaluation. To *operationalize* these levels (i.e., put these ideas or concepts into words that can be used), action verbs are used. As the goal of the learning or behavioral objective changes, so do the verbs, indicating the learning to be accomplished within that particular level of the cognitive domain. Notice that the objectives at the beginning of each chapter in this text follow this format, using a variety of verbs to indicate the expected level of learning. A representative sample of behavioral objectives focusing on nutrition and appropriate cognitive-level verbs is included in the discussion of each level.

Knowledge

Knowledge, the lowest level of learning, according to Bloom's taxonomy, involves recall (Miller et al., 2012). If students remember material previously learned, they have acquired knowledge. This level may be used with clients who are unable to understand underlying reasons or rationales, such as young children or people who have had strokes. Stroke clients may need to remember that medication should be taken daily, that regular exercise restores function, and that drinking alcohol should be avoided, although they may not grasp the reasons behind these measures. Five-year-olds may need to identify healthful foods, but may not understand why they are nutritious.

A knowledge-level behavioral objective might be "The client can *recall* the names of six fruits to eat as nutritious snacks." Other knowledge-level verbs include *repeat*, *define*, *list*, and *name*.

Comprehension

The second level of cognitive learning, comprehension, combines remembering with understanding (Miller et al., 2012). Teaching aims at instilling at least a minimal understanding. Nurses want clients to grasp the meaning and to recognize the importance of suggested health behaviors.

An example of a comprehension-level behavioral objective might be, "The pregnant client will *describe* a well-balanced diet during pregnancy." Other appropriate verbs at the comprehension level include *discuss*, *explain*, *identify*, *summarize*, and *report*.

Application

Application is the third level of cognitive learning, in which the learner cannot only understand material but also apply it to new situations (Miller et al., 2012). Application approaches the possibility of self-care when clients use their knowledge to improve their own health. The test of application is a transfer of understanding into practice. Therefore, to encourage application, the nurse can design teaching plans that provide clients with knowledge that they can put into practice. In the home setting, a PHN may suggest that a diabetic client write down glucometer readings to show the nurse at the next visit. A school nurse could ask adolescents in a weight loss group to keep a food and exercise record for a week, draw up a diet plan, and share this plan with the group at the next meeting. In contrast, the construction worker who understands on-the-job hazards, but seldom wears a protective hat in the work area, has yet to transfer knowledge and comprehension into practice or application.

An example of an application-level behavioral objective might be "The client will *practice* eating well-balanced meals at least two times a day." Other verbs at this level include *apply*, *use*, *demonstrate*, *discover*, *prepare*, and *illustrate*.

Analysis

The fourth level of cognitive learning is analysis; at this level, the learner breaks down material into parts, distinguishes between elements, and understands the relationships among the parts. This level of learning becomes a preliminary step toward problem solving. The learner carefully examines all of the variables or elements and their relationships to each other in order to explain the situation (Miller et al., 2012). A family that studies its own communication patterns to identify sources of conflict is using analysis. A mother analyzes when she seeks to determine the cause of an infant's crying. After viewing the total situation, she breaks it down into variables such as hunger, pain, overstimulation, loneliness, type of crying, and intensity of crying. She examines these parts and draws conclusions about their relationships. In health teaching, community health nurses foster clients' analytic skills by (a) demonstrating how to isolate the parts in a situation and (b) encouraging the clients to consider the relationships among the parts and to draw conclusions from their thinking. It is also important to help clients distinguish between facts and what may be inferred.

An analysis-level behavioral objective for senior citizens trying to learn more about low-fat foods might be "The seniors should be able to *distinguish* the fat content in a variety of packaged foods." Other verbs at the analysis level include *differentiate*, *discriminate*, *select*, *contrast*, *debate*, *question*, and *examine*.

Synthesis

Synthesis, the fifth level of cognitive learning, is the ability not only to break down and understand the elements of a situation but also to form elements into a new whole. Synthesis combines all of the earlier levels of cognitive learning to culminate in the production of a unique plan or solution. Clients who achieve learning at this level not only analyze their problems but also find solutions for them (Miller et al., 2012). For example, a community health nurse may assist mental health clients in a therapy group to examine their frequent depression and then to generate their own plan for alleviating it. A young couple that wants to toilet train their 2-year-old child may learn the physiologic and psychological dimensions of toilet training, then begin to analyze their own situation, and develop strategies (their own plan) for working with the child. Nurses facilitate synthesis by assisting and encouraging clients to develop their own solutions with specific plans. After a problem is identified, the client should be asked, "What are some possible causes? Do you see anything that has been overlooked about the problem?" If the client asks for a quick solution, the PHN could encourage synthesis by asking, "What are some possible solutions to this problem that you might carry out?"

An example of a synthesis-level behavioral objective for a client on a sodium-restricted diet might be, "The client will be able to *create* an enjoyable meal using low-sodium foods." Other verbs at this level include *compose*, *compile*, *design*, *formulate*, *create*, *plan*, and *organize*.

Evaluation

The highest level of cognitive learning is evaluation; at this level, the learner judges the usefulness of new material compared with a stated purpose or specific criteria (Miller et al., 2012). Clients can learn to judge their own health behavior by comparing it with standards established by others—such as complete abstinence from smoking, maintenance of normal weight, or exercising three times a week. Alternatively, clients may establish their own criteria. For example, a parent support group might design activities to enhance parent–child communication and then judge their performance by using their desired outcomes as evaluation criteria. When nurses aim for this level of client learning, they have made self-care a concrete objective. Evaluation, because it goes beyond attempts at problem solving, enables the client to judge the adequacy of solutions, to critique lifestyle and health-related behaviors, and to anticipate needed improvements.

An example of a behavioral objective at the evaluation level might be, "The clients in a nutrition class will be able to *appraise* the fat content in one serving of the low-fat dish they brought to share." Other verbs at this level include *judge, compare, contrast, rate, conclude,* and *summarize.*

How to Measure Cognitive Learning

Cognitive learning at any of the levels described can be measured easily in terms of learner behaviors. Nurses know, for instance, that clients have achieved teaching objectives for the application of knowledge if their behavior demonstrates actual use of the information taught. Client roles in cognitive learning range from relatively passive (at the knowledge level) to a more active role (at the evaluation level). Conversely, as clients become more active, the nurse's role becomes less overtly directive. Not all clients need to be brought through all levels of cognitive learning, and not every client needs to reach the evaluation level for each aspect of care. For some clients and situations, comprehension is an adequate and effective level; for others, the nurse should focus on the application level. Table 11–2 illustrates client and nurse behaviors for each cognitive level.

Affective Domain

The **affective domain** involves learning that occurs through emotion, feeling, or *affect*. This kind of learning deals with changes in interest, attitudes, and values (Bloom, 1956; Miller et al., 2012). Here, nurses face the task of trying to influence what their clients may value and feel. Nurses want clients to develop an ability to accept ideas that promote healthier behaviors, even if those ideas conflict with the clients' own values.

Attitudes and values are learned. They develop gradually, as family, peers, experiences, and culture influence the way an individual feels and responds (see Chapter 4). These feelings and responses are the result of imitation and conditioning. In this way, clients acquire their health-related beliefs and practices. Because attitudes and values become part of the person, they are difficult to change unless the nurse is aware of how they develop.

Affective learning occurs on several levels as learners respond with varying degrees of involvement and commitment. At the first level, learners are simply receptive; they are willing to listen, to show awareness, and to be attentive. The nurse aims at acquiring and focusing learners' attention (Miller et al., 2012). This limited goal may be all that clients can achieve during the early stages of the nurse–client relationship. An example of an affective objective at this level might be "The client closely *attends* to the lesson on child development." Other verbs might include *asks, gives, points to,* and *uses.*

At the second level, learners become active participants by responding to the information in some way. Examples are a willingness to read educational material, to participate in discussions, to complete assignments (e.g., keeping a diet record), or to voluntarily seek out more information (Miller et al., 2012). An example of an objective at this level is "The client actively *participates* in group discussions about living with diabetes." Some other verbs indicative of affective learning at this level include *answers, compiles, presents, tells,* and *reports.*

Table 11–2 Cognitive Learning: Case Study in Controlling Diabetes		
Level	**Illustrative Client Behavior**	**Illustrative Nurse Behavior**
Knowledge (recalls, knows)	States that insulin, if taken, will control own diabetes	Provides information
Comprehension (understands)	Describes insulin action and purpose	Explains information
Application (uses learning)	Adjusts insulin dosage daily to maintain proper blood sugar level	Suggests how to use learning
Analysis (examines, explains)	Discusses relationships between insulin, diet, activity, and diabetic control	Demonstrates and encourages analysis
Synthesis (integrates with other learning, generates new ideas)	Develops a plan, incorporating above learning, for controlling own diabetes	Promotes client formulation of own plan
Evaluation (judges according to a standard)	Compares degree of diabetic control (outcomes) with desired control (objectives)	Facilitates evaluation

At the third level, learners attach value to the information. Valuing ranges from simple acceptance through appreciation to commitment (Miller et al., 2012). For example, a PHN taught members of a support group several principles concerning group effectiveness. An explanation of the importance of a democratic group process and ways to improve group skills was given. Members showed acceptance when they acknowledged the importance of these ideas. They showed appreciation of the ideas by starting to practice them. Commitment came when they assumed responsibility for having their group function smoothly. Some verbs for objectives related to valuing are *follows*, *initiates*, *justifies*, *proposes*, *shares*, and *works*.

The final level of affective learning occurs when learners internalize an idea or value. The value system now controls learner behavior. Consistent practice is a crucial test at this level (Miller et al., 2012). Verbs used at this level include *acts*, *performs*, and *verifies*. Clients who know and respect the value of exercise, but only occasionally play tennis or go for a walk, have not internalized this value. Even several weeks of enthusiastic walking are not true evidence of an internalized value. If the walking continues for 6 months, 12 months, or longer, learning may have been internalized.

Affective learning often is difficult to measure and is often attempted through self-report surveys or tools (Miller et al., 2012). This elusiveness may influence PHNs to concentrate their efforts on cognitive learning goals instead. Yet, client attitudes and values have a major effect on the outcome of cognitive learning—which is desired behavioral changes. Therefore, both cognitive and affective domains must be linked when teaching clients about health-related topics; otherwise, results may quickly fade (Hales, 2014).

Attitudes and values can change in the same way that they were first learned, that is, through imitation and conditioning. Role models, particularly individuals from the client's peer group who practice the desired health behaviors, can be a strong influence. Effective health education considers group norms and seeks to influence them (Centers for Disease Control and Prevention [CDC], 2015). Support groups, such as mastectomy or chemical dependency support groups, can have a powerful role model effect. Frequently, clients view nurses as a positive role model; for this reason, nurses should try to demonstrate healthy behaviors. The American Nurses Association (ANA), working with Pfizer, conducted a health risk appraisal study and discovered that RNs found their workplaces stressful, citing instances of incivility, bullying, and physical assaults by patients/families (39% worked in acute care/hospital settings). The majority was overweight, and a cited safety risk was talking on the phone or texting while driving. However, few nurses smoked, and most had access to workplace health promotion or wellness programs (ANA, 2015). They continue to collect data and recognize the importance of a healthy nursing workforce, as well as the example (good or bad) that nurses can set for their clients/patients.

Encouragement is key. Attitudes often change when the PHN provides clients with a satisfying experience during the learning process. The community health nurse who recognizes clients' participation in a group, praises them for completing assignments, or commends them for sticking to diet plans will have more success than the nurse who only criticizes failures. Another point to remember is that clients can develop a close relationship with the PHN during the teaching–learning process. When this occurs, you may want to share a few of your own experiences in managing personal health issues. This can help develop trust and rapport with your clients. Table 11–3 delineates client and nurse behaviors for each level of affective learning.

To influence affective learning requires patience. Values and attitudes seldom change overnight. Remember that other forces continue to reinforce former values. For example, a single young mother may want to pursue an exercise and weight loss plan, but she might not do so because she has several small children and feels that their needs come first. A young man who can verbalize to the nurse the importance of safe sex may be uncomfortable discussing the subject with his partner, thus affecting his compliance with the health teaching plan. Knowledge alone is not usually sufficient to change behaviors. Motivation and attitude are needed.

Psychomotor Domain

The **psychomotor domain** includes visible, demonstrable performance skills that require some kind of neuromuscular coordination (Miller et al., 2012). Clients in the community need to learn skills such as infant bathing, temperature taking, breast or testicular self-examination,

Table 11–3	**Affective Learning: Case Study in Family Planning**	
Level	**Illustrative Client Behavior**	**Illustrative Nurse Behavior**
Receptive (listens, pays attention)	Attentive to family planning instruction	Directs client's attention
Responsive (participates, reacts)	Discusses pros and cons of various methods	Encourages client involvement
Valuing (accepts, appreciates, commits)	Selects a method for use	Respects client's right to decide
Internal consistency (organizes values to fit together)	Understands and accepts responsibility for planning for desired number of children	Brings client into contact with role models
Adoption (incorporates new values into lifestyle)	Consistently practices birth control	Positively reinforces healthy behaviors

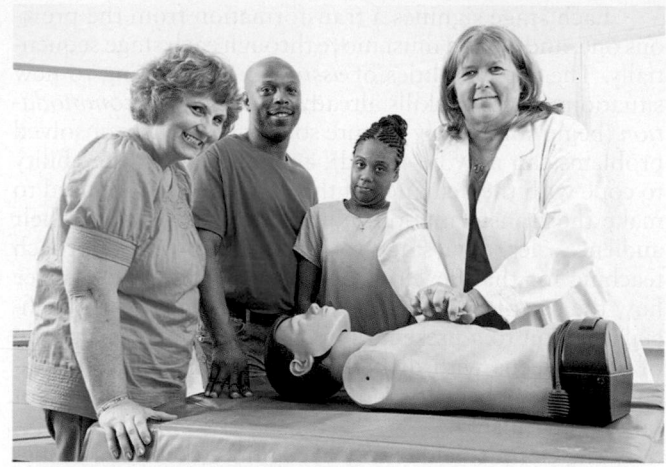

FIGURE 11-8 A community health nurse demonstrates CPR to clients before having them return the demonstration to show that they can put this learning into practice.

prenatal breathing exercises, range-of-motion exercises, catheter irrigation, walking with crutches, and how to change dressings (Fig. 11–8).

For psychomotor learning to take place, three conditions must be met: (1) learners must be capable of the skill, (2) learners must have a sensory image of how to perform the skill, and (3) learners must practice the skill.

PHNs must be certain that the client is physically, intellectually, and emotionally capable of performing the skill. It may be difficult for an elderly diabetic man with tremulous hands and fading vision to give his own insulin injections; it could frustrate and harm him. He may need some assistance or accommodations. Clients' intellectual and emotional capabilities also influence their capacity to learn motor skills. It may be inappropriate to expect persons with significant developmental delays to learn complex skills. The degree of complexity should match the learners' level of functioning. However, educational level should not be equated with intelligence. Many clients have had limited formal schooling, but are able to learn complex skills for themselves or as caregivers after appropriate instruction. Developmental stage is another point to consider in determining whether it is appropriate to teach a particular skill. For example, most children can put on some article of clothing at 2 years of age, but are not ready to learn to fasten buttons until they are past their third birthday.

Learners also must have a sensory image of how to perform the skill through sight, hearing, touch, and sometimes taste or smell. This sensory image is gained by demonstration. To teach clients motor skills effectively, the PHN has to provide them with an adequate sensory image. It is best to demonstrate and explain slowly, one

point at a time, and sometimes repeatedly, until clients understand the proper sequence or combination of actions necessary to carry out the skill.

The third necessary condition for psychomotor learning is practice. After acquiring a sensory image, clients can start to perform the skill. Mastery comes over time as clients repeat the task until it is smooth, coordinated, and unhesitating (Miller et al., 2012). During this process, the PHN should be available to provide guidance and encouragement. In the early stages of practice, you may need to use hands-on guidance to give clients a sense of how the performance should feel. When clients give return demonstrations, you can make suggestions, give encouragement, and thereby maximize the learning. For example, a community health nurse demonstrates passive range-of-motion exercises on a client's wife to show her how the exercises should feel (giving her a sensory image). The wife then learns to perform the exercises on her husband. During practice, feedback from the nurse enables the wife to know whether the skill is being performed correctly. At this guided response stage, objectives may include action verbs such as *fastens*, *manipulates*, *measures*, *organizes*, and *calibrates*.

The psychomotor domain, like the cognitive and affective domains, ranges from simple to complex levels of functioning. It is necessary to exercise judgment in assessing a client's ability to perform a skill. Even clients with limited ability often can move to higher levels once they have mastered simple skills. Nurse behavior that influences psychomotor learning is shown in Table 11–4.

LEARNING THEORIES

A *learning theory* is a systematic and integrated look into the nature of the process whereby people relate to their surroundings in such ways as to enhance their ability to use both themselves and their surroundings more effectively. Each nurse has and uses a particular theory of learning, whether consciously or unconsciously, and that theory, in turn, dictates the way the PHN teaches clients. It is useful to discover what each nurse's learning theory is and how it affects the role of health educator.

Some of the learning theories developed by educational psychologists in the 20th century remain influential. They are grouped into four categories: behavioral, cognitive, social, and humanistic. Additionally, the adult learning theory of Malcolm (Knowles, 1980, 1984, 1989, 1990; Knowles, Holton, & Swanson, 2015) has influenced client teaching. A brief examination of these categories and the specific theories follows.

Behavioral Learning Theories

Behavioral theory (also known as stimulus–response or conditioning theory) approaches the study of learning by focusing on behaviors that can be observed, measured,

Table 11-4 Nurse Behaviors in Psychomotor Learning		
The Nurse	**Provides Sensory Image**	**Encourages Practice**
Determines capability: assesses client's physical, intellectual, and emotional ability	Demonstrates and explains	Uses guidance and positive reinforcement

and changed. Developed early in the 20th century, behavioral theory work is associated primarily with three famous names: Ivan Pavlov (1957), Edward Thorndike (1932, 1969), and B. F. Skinner (1974, 1987). To a behaviorist, learning is a behavioral change—a response to certain stimuli. Therefore, the behavioristic teacher seeks to significantly change learners' behaviors through a series of selected stimuli.

The stimulus–response "bond" theory proposes that, with conditioning, certain causes (stimuli) evoke certain effects (responses). The teacher promotes acquisition of the desired stimulus–response connections so that transfer of learning can occur in another situation having the same stimulus–response elements. You undoubtedly learned about Pavlov's work with stimulus–response and involuntary reflex actions in your psychology classes. Pavlov conditioned a dog to anticipate food by ringing a bell at feeding time. Initially, the dog would salivate as the food was brought to the cage. However, after time, the dog would salivate at hearing the bell, before seeing or smelling the food (Pavlov, 1957).

Two other behavioral theories are conditioning with no reinforcement (Thorndike) and conditioning through reinforcement (Skinner). With the no-reinforcement approach, the focus is on the learner's innate reflexive drives to accomplish the desired response after conditioning (e.g., when the PHN repeatedly emphasizes to a group of pregnant women that their prenatal classes promote a positive delivery experience and healthy newborns). In contrast, the reinforcement theorists use successive, systematic changes in the learner's environment to enhance the probability of desired responses. For example, a school nurse might give rewards (e.g., stickers, activity books) to children who attend each class on safety.

Cognitive Learning Theories

Jean Piaget is the most widely known cognitive theorist. His theory of cognitive development contributed to the theories of Kohlberg (moral development) and Fowler (development of faith). Piaget (1966, 1970) believed that cognitive development is an orderly, sequential, and interactive process in which a variety of new experiences must exist before intellectual abilities can develop. His work with children led him to develop five phases of cognitive development, from birth to 15 years of age (Table 11–5).

Each stage signifies a transformation from the previous one, and a child must move through each stage sequentially. The three abilities of *assimilation* (reacting to new situations by using skills already possessed), *accommodation* (being sufficiently mature so that previously unsolved problems can now be solved), and *adaptation* (the ability to cope with the demands of the environment) are used to make the transformation. Nurses must understand their audience's learning stage to ascertain how to approach teaching for that developmental stage. The nurse can see how the use of puppets with 3-year-olds may be a beneficial addition to a presentation on safety, whereas a group of young teens with diabetes may respond to group discussion on the benefits and consequences of taking or not taking their insulin.

The Gestalt-field family of cognitive theories assumes that people are neither good nor bad—they simply interact with their environment, and their learning is related to perception (Wertheimer, 1945/1959, 1980). A principal assumption of this approach is that every person hears, interprets, and reacts to a variety of situations in a way that is unique to them (Bates, 2016).

The first Gestalt-field theory, called *insight theory*, regards learning as a process in which the learner develops new insights or changes old ones. Learners intuitively and intelligently sense their way through problems. However, the "insight" is useful only if the learner understands its significance. For example, Amy dropped out of high school after the birth of her daughter; after attending a career planning class offered by a community health nurse, she realizes that she has limited job skills and that if she learned more about computer skills, she could get a better job. This learner understood the significance of her insight.

The second theory, *goal–insight*, is similar to the insight theory but goes beyond intuitive hunches to tested insights. Teachers subscribing to this theory promote insightful learning but assist learners in developing higher-quality insights. For example, Amy takes a beginning and then an advanced computer class and is offered a higher-paying job. The community health nurse discusses Amy's successes with her and asks Amy whether she ever thought about going to college. The nurse mentions the added benefits of college-level course work. Amy then reflects on this for a while and begins to think

Table 11–5	Piaget's Five Phases of Cognitive Development	
Age	**Stage**	**Behavior**
Birth to 2 years	Sensorimotor stage	The child moves focus from self to the environment (rituals are important).
2–4 years	Preconceptual stage	Language development is rapid and everything is related to "me."
4–7 years	Intuitive thought stage	Egocentric thinking diminishes, and words are used to express thoughts.
7–11 years	Concrete operations stage	Child can solve concrete problems and recognize others' viewpoints.
11–15 years	Formal operations stage	Child uses rational thinking and can develop ideas from general principles (deductive reasoning) and apply them to future situations.

Adapted from Young, G. (2011). *Development and causality: Neo-Piagetian perspectives.* New York, NY: Springer Publishing.

about completing the requirements to go to community college, because if she had an associate degree she could be promoted to a supervisory position and make more money.

In the third theory, *cognitive-field theory*, the learner is seen as purposive and problem centered. Teachers seek to help learners gain new insights and restructure their lives accordingly. For example, Amy confers with the community health nurse about her choices and has changed her thinking about herself so much that she is planning to get an apartment in a neighborhood that is better for her child and she may continue taking classes "for the fun of it" after she completes her degree in a few months.

Social Learning Theories

The aim of social learning theory is to explain behavior and facilitate learning (Bates, 2016). Bandura (1977, 1986), an important theorist, pointed out that apparent but not real relationships often are dysfunctional and produce undesirable or inappropriate behavior. He described three ways that dysfunctional beliefs develop:

1. In *coincidental association*, outcomes typically are preceded by numerous events, and the client selects the wrong events as predictors of an outcome. For example, Juanita had a negative experience with a man who wore a hearing aid. Afterward, all of her experiences with men who wore hearing aids were negative. She reached the conclusion that all men who wear hearing aids were undesirable. This client's beliefs became a self-fulfilling prophecy.
2. In *inappropriate generalization*, one negative experience provokes negative feelings for future experiences. For example, Dorothy, a senior citizen, had a purse snatched by a teenager and generalized that all teenagers are bad. Three-year-old Ryan accidentally drank some spoiled milk. He generalized that milk tastes bad and now refuses to drink it.
3. In *perceived self-inefficacy*, "Persons who judge themselves as lacking coping capabilities, whether the self-appraisal is objectively warranted or not, will perceive all kinds of dangers in situations and exaggerate their potential harmfulness" (Bandura, 1986, p. 220). For example, an older client, William, tells the community health nurse about two missing Social Security checks, but he refuses to take a bus to the post office. He states that he does not know what to say to the postal clerk and has read about senior citizens getting mugged on buses. He refused to follow up on his lost income.

Social learning theory focuses on the learners, who are influenced by role models, building self-confidence, persuasion, and personal mastery. Self-efficacy can lead to the desired behaviors and outcomes. Juanita may begin to separate her negative experiences with men from their hearing disabilities after attending a class on building self-esteem suggested by the PHN. Through some positive experiences with teenagers organized by the community health nurse working with the senior center, Dorothy may come to learn that not all teenagers are bad. The nurse can suggest to Ryan's mother that she might have Ryan try chocolate milk. She then can slowly reintroduce plain milk. William might find the courage and self-confidence to solve future problems after the PHN introduces him to another gentleman in the apartment complex who feels confident in the neighborhood.

Humanistic Learning Theories

Humanistic theories assume that people possess a natural tendency to learn and that learning flourishes in an encouraging environment. Two of the best-known humanists are Abraham Maslow and Carl Rogers (Bates, 2016). Abraham Maslow developed the classic hierarchy of human needs in the 1940s. It suggests that a person's first needs are physiologic (air, food, water). Once these needs are met, people work to fulfill safety and security needs. Next is the need for love and a sense of belonging; then come self-esteem needs (positive feelings of self-worth). Only after these needs are met do people work toward self-actualization or becoming all that we are meant to be (Maslow, 1970). Maslow's work is often taught in psychology and early nursing courses.

In community health nursing, the clients' needs must be considered when planning health education programs. For example, it would be difficult for a group of young mothers to concentrate on learning about proper infant nutrition if they are worried about their babies crying in the next room or anxious about an abusive partner who doesn't want them to leave the house to participate in activities. Their need to care for their children (need for love and belonging) or for their personal well-being (security and safety) would be greater than the need to learn about future health considerations (self-esteem and self-actualization). Likewise, it is impossible for learning to take place if a room is so warm that the participants are falling asleep (i.e., physiologic needs are not being met).

Carl Rogers developed the client-centered counseling approach that has long been important in psychotherapy. He believed the role of the therapist should be nondirective and accepting, and proposed approaching clients in a warm, positive, and empathetic manner to get in touch with their feelings and thoughts (Bates, 2016). Rogers (1969, 1989) soon applied his beliefs to education, suggesting that the learning environment be learner centered. The outcome of a learner-centered educational environment is that students become more self-directed and guide their own learning. Rogers believed that the learner is the person most capable of deciding how to find the solutions to problems. The client identifies the problem and, given time and space, can find a way through the problem to a solution. The PHN acts as a facilitator in this learning process when, for example, a 55-year-old man wants to quit smoking after a prolonged upper respiratory tract infection that is aggravated by his habit, and comes to a stop-smoking class led by the PHN at the county health department.

Knowles' Adult Learning Theory

In the last 20 to 30 years, a variety of techniques have been developed to help adults learn. One of the main discoveries is that adults as learners are different from children. They do not learn differently, but rather are a different kind of learner (Bates, 2016). Knowles (1984) and Knowles et al. (2015) suggested that there are four characteristics of "**adult learners**", and these characteristics have implications for learning. Adults are self-directed in their learning; they have a lifetime of experience to draw on when learning; their readiness to learn is focused on requirements for their personal and occupational roles; and adults have a problem-centered time perspective, in that the learners have a need to learn so that it can be applied and tried out quickly. Display 11–3 describes the characteristics of adult learners and implications for nurses working with adults in more detail.

CHARACTERISTICS OF EFFECTIVE INSTRUCTORS

There are certain characteristics of teachers that most students (yourself included) will recognize. These can apply to PHNs who do health promotion education. Common characteristics include the following:

- Organization and ability to make things clear—The teacher has clear knowledge of the material; objectives and material are organized, presented in context and in an orderly manner, and explained by using examples, case studies, and a variety of methods to hold the learner's interest.
- Positive, enthusiastic attitude—The instructor is excited about teaching; is welcoming, engaged, positive, and interested in individual students; and also works well with groups. Being respectful, approachable, and responsive are also characteristics

often mentioned by students as helpful. Use of humor and a professional attitude are also cited.
- Good communicator—The teacher listens as well as provides information and gives thorough responses to student questions. Constructive feedback is appreciated, and empowerment approaches are utilized to encourage participation and learning (Goodenough, Galway, Badenhorst, & Kelly, 2013; Singh et al., 2013).

Public health nurses can incorporate these principles by exhibiting thorough preparation for instruction (e.g., well-planned and well-executed presentations), displaying positive and welcoming behaviors with clients (e.g., encouraging participation, showing respect), and listening carefully to clients' questions and comments, as well as encouraging positive social interactions and fostering ability and self-efficacy.

HEALTH TEACHING MODELS

Theories on learning provide a general understanding of how people learn. In addition, various health teaching models specifically focus on explaining individual health experiences, behaviors, and actions. These models fit with the learning theories to give nurses a more accurate picture of the client and the clients' learning needs. Four useful models are described here: the Health Belief Model (HBM), Pender's Health Promotion Model (revised) (HPM), the Transtheoretical or Stages of Change Model, and the PRECEDE and PROCEED models (Fig. 11–9).

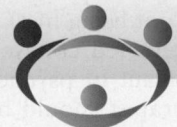

DISPLAY 11–3 CHARACTERISTICS AND IMPLICATIONS FOR KNOWLES' ADULT LEARNING THEORY

Characteristics	Learning Implications
Self-Concept Adult learners are self-directed.	Openness and respect between teacher and learner. The learner plans and carries out own learning activities. Learner evaluates own progress toward self-chosen goals.
Experience Adults have a lifetime of experience and define self in terms of this experience.	Teaching methods focus on experiential activities. Discovering how to learn from experience is key to self-actualization. Mistakes are opportunities for learning.
Readiness to Learn Learning is focused on social and occupational roles.	Experiential learning opportunities focus on requirements for occupational and social roles. Learning peaks when there is a need to know. Adults can best assess own readiness to learn and teachable moments.
Need to Learn Adults have a problem-centered time perspective.	Teaching needs to be problem centered rather than theoretically oriented. Teacher needs to teach what the learners need to learn. Learners need to apply and try out learning quickly.

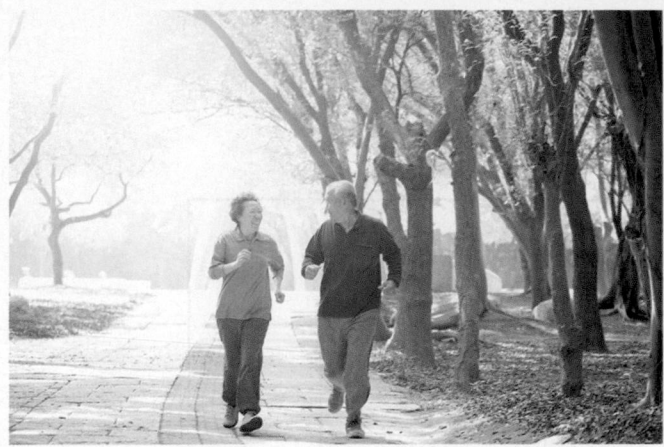

FIGURE 11–9 A goal of health promotion is to encourage clients to develop healthy behaviors.

Health Belief Model

This section and the next describe two closely associated health models. The Health Belief Model (HBM), which was developed by social psychologists and brought to the attention of health care professionals by Rosenstock (1966), has undergone much empiric testing. The HBM is useful for explaining the behaviors and actions taken by people to prevent illness and injury. It postulates that readiness to act on behalf of a person's own health is predicated on the following (Skinner, Tiro, & Champion, 2015):

- Perceived susceptibility to the condition in question
- Perceived seriousness of the condition in question
- Perceived benefits to taking action
- Barriers to taking action
- Cues to action, such as knowledge that someone else has the condition or attention from the media
- Self-efficacy—the ability to take action to achieve the desired outcome

For example, researchers in Iran used the HBM to evaluate an educational program intervention to improve self-management among diabetic patients. The findings revealed improved self-management among those diabetics that participated in the HBM-based education program (Jalilian, Motlagh, Solhi, & Gharibnavaz, 2014). Community health nurses may find the use of the HBM (and variations) to be helpful in assessing the health behaviors and beliefs of culturally diverse populations.

Pender's Health Promotion Model

First published in the 1980s by nurse Nola Pender, the Health Promotion Model (HPM) was envisioned as a framework for exploring health-related behaviors within a nursing and behavioral science context (Pender et al., 2015). Reflecting the growing body of literature relevant to the HPM, Pender revised the model to reflect a number of major theoretical changes. Consistent with the original, the revised model is derived from social cognitive theory and expectancy–value theory. The revised HPM includes three general areas of concern to health-promoting behavior: *Individual characteristics and experiences* are seen to interact with *behavior-specific cognitions and affect*

to influence specific *behavioral outcomes* (Pender et al., 2015). The revised HPM focuses on predicting behaviors that influence health promotion. In addition, the HPM includes the variable of interpersonal influence of others, including family and health professionals.

Being able to predict health promotion behaviors enhances the community health nurse's ability to work with clients. Awareness of their characteristics, experiences, comprehension of their health-related issues, perceived barriers, self-efficacy, support (or lack of it) from significant others, and commitment provides the nurse with a picture that clarifies the client–nurse role and gives direction for action taking. The HPM (Fig. 11–10) is based on the theoretical propositions found in Display 11–4.

Using these propositions, researchers explored clients' health behaviors in many studies conducted in the 1980s, 1990s, and into the 21st century. Examples of research using the model include surveying health-promoting behaviors and predictors of health among Iranian women (Mirghafourvand et al., 2014) and surveying health-promoting lifestyle behaviors among adult survivors of childhood cancer in Israel (Liebergall-Wischnitzer, Buyum, & Ganz, 2015). Research on incorporating anger management training with high-risk soldiers (Asadzandi, Sekarifard, Ebadi, Morovvati Sharif Abad, & Salari, 2015) and surveying health behaviors in pregnant minority women (Kominiarek, 2014) have been completed. And, research using this model has also been done with nurses and nursing students (Belguzar, 2015; Rector, Gilchrist, Camarena, & Cauthen, 2014).

Transtheoretical or Stages of Change Model

Researchers discovered, when working with smokers who wanted to quit smoking, that behavioral change doesn't suddenly happen after an "aha" moment during a health education class, but rather occurs in small increments or stages. This discovery led to a new approach in health promotion programs (Glanz et al., 2015). We have all tried to change a behavior (e.g., consistent dental hygiene, exercising regularly, eating a better diet, being careful to not text while driving), but have we all found immediate success after one attempt? Most people have to work up to making a significant change (e.g., gorge over the holidays and then diet at the start of the new year) and then are often not successful and relapse into old, familiar behaviors. The **Transtheoretical Model** (TTM) recognizes this human frailty and addresses it by anticipating relapses and recognizing them as an opportunity to better plan for how to sustain the needed change in future attempts (Bartholomew et al., 2015; Prochaska, Norcross, & DiClemente, 2007). The model, sometimes called Stages of Change, is not linear but is depicted as a spiral, with plateaus, relapses, and false starts. It can be used with individuals, groups, and populations. The stages include the following (Prochaska, et al., 2007, p. 39):

- Precontemplation—This is usually the normal state of denial or the problem may not be perceived (either don't know about it or don't want to think acknowledge it). Clients may say, "I don't really smoke that many cigarettes, so I don't have to worry about lung cancer or the other health problems."

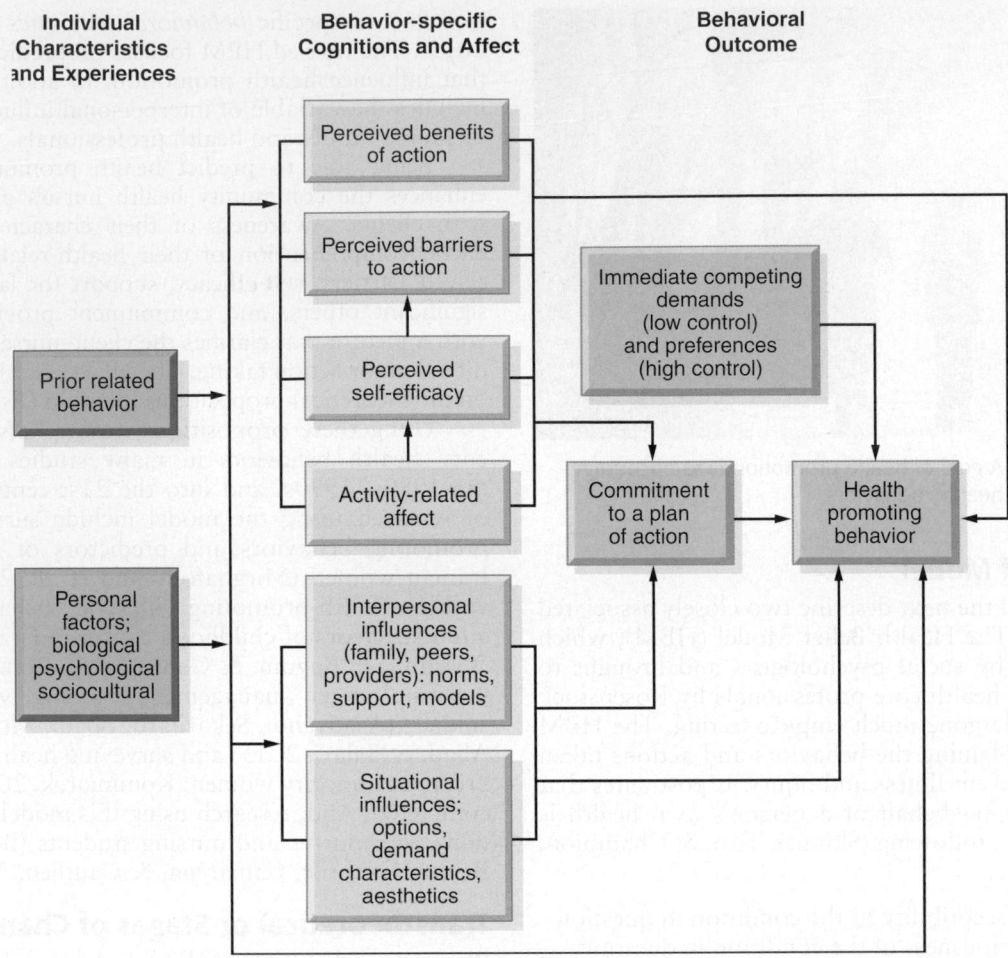

Individual Characteristics and Experiences	Behavior-specific Cognitions and Affect	Behavioral Outcome

FIGURE 11–10   Health promotion model. (From Pender, N. J., Murdaugh, C. L., & Parsons, M. A. (2015). *Health promotion in nursing practice* (7th ed.). Upper Saddle River, NJ: Pearson Education, Inc., with permission.)

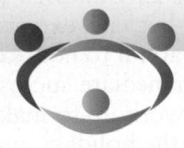

DISPLAY 11–4 THEORETICAL PROPOSITIONS OF THE HEALTH PROMOTION MODEL

1. Inherited and acquired characteristics along with prior behavior influence beliefs, affect, and health-promoting behavior.
2. People engage in behaviors from which they anticipate deriving personally valued benefits.
3. Perceived barriers can constrain action to change behavior and the behavior itself.
4. Perceived self-efficacy to embrace a given behavior increases the likelihood to commit to action and implementing the behavior.
5. Greater perceived self-efficacy results in fewer perceived barriers.
6. Positive affect toward a behavior results in greater perceived self-efficacy, which can result in increased positive affect.
7. When positive affect is associated with a behavior, commitment and action are increased.
8. People are more likely to commit to and participate in health-promoting behaviors when significant others model the behavior, expect it, and provide assistance and support for the behavior.

9. Others—family members, peers, and health care providers—are important sources of influence that can positively or negatively influence commitment to and implementation of health-promoting behavior.
10. Situational influences can positively or negatively influence commitment to and implementation of health-promoting behavior.
11. The greater the commitment to a behavior change, the more likely the change will be maintained over time.
12. Distracting demands over which the person has little control may affect commitment to a behavior change.
13. Commitment to a behavior change is less likely to be maintained when other actions are more attractive and preferred.
14. People can modify the interpersonal and physical environments to create incentives for behavior changes.

Adapted from Pender, N. J., Murdaugh, C. L., & Parsons, M. A. (2015). *Health promotion in nursing practice* (7th ed.). Upper Saddle River, NJ: Pearson Education, Inc.

- Contemplation—At this stage, the client is more realistic and may be more open to discussing the problem of smoking. However, the client may not be able to seriously consider behavior change or feel able to confront the issue. The client may say, "I know I should probably try to quit smoking, but I am really stressed right now and can't think about it."
- Preparation—During this stage, the client is moving away from contemplation toward action. The client may be trying to gather information and may be talking to others about how they quit smoking. They may be concerned that it may take more than one try to accomplish their goal. A client may talk to the physician about medications that are helpful, tell friends and family that he or she is planning to quit smoking, and may even begin to cut back on the number of cigarettes smoked each day.
- Action—This stage is the beginning of the behavioral change. The client sets a date to quit smoking, begins using a nicotine patch or medication, and finds replacement behaviors for smoking (e.g., using breath mints, exercising during usual smoking breaks). The client knows that this attempt may not be successful the first time and should be encouraged to acknowledge and plan for this.
- Maintenance—In this stage, the behavior has been changed. The smoker has stopped smoking, but now needs to be vigilant in avoiding a relapse. The client needs a support system and rewards to encourage maintenance. If the client relapses, the PHN and others can help the client learn from this and begin their preparation and action stages again until longer periods of maintenance are achieved.
- Termination—This occurs when the former behavior is no longer appealing. The smoker no longer has an interest in cigarettes and does not have to exert the constant vigilance needed in the maintenance stage. Prochaska et al. (2007) note that not everyone can truly reach this stage, and therefore, it is not always included in health promotion programs or research.

Researchers have used this model with many topics related to health promotion and prevention (e.g., substance abuse, smoking cessation, weight loss, physical activity). One research study found that this model could help determine which patients had lower adherence scores for antiretroviral medications (ART). Those clients in the action and maintenance stages had significantly higher adherence scores than those in the earlier stages. This was consistent, despite demographic characteristics or HIV risk factors. The researchers determined the stages of change by asking questions on a survey tool, validated by previous research. For those stating yes to the question, "I do not take and right now am not considering taking my ART as directed," they were placed in the precontemplation stage, and those indicating that they were not currently taking ART but were "considering taking my ART as directed" were categorized as being in the contemplation stage. Indicating that they were "planning to start taking my ART as directed" verified that they were in the planning stage, and stating that they "consistently take my ART as directed" showed that they were in the action

stage (Genberg, Lee, Rogers, Wiley, & Wilson, 2013, p. 568). Determining a client's stage and tailoring education and interventions at that level can be helpful.

This model has shown mixed results in other research. A Cochrane systematic review indicated that studies showed "inconclusive evidence" of the model's effectiveness in weight loss and physical activity studies, often because of the need for additional well-designed research and consistent application of the model (Mastellos, Gunn, Felix, Car, & Majeed, 2014, para. 6). Nigg, Geller, Horwath, Wertin, and Dishman (2011) found that the model's strength lies in being able to make individually based interventions relevant to the population level when it comes to physical activity research. Selecting those aggregates that are only beginning to consider starting an exercise program, and targeting specific interventions to them, is an efficient means of addressing this issue. It is also a model that is easy to understand and apply in public health settings, but cross-sectional studies may not be the best application and more longitudinal or trend studies may be needed.

The PRECEDE and PROCEED Models

First published by Green in 1974, the PRECEDE model was developed for educational diagnosis (Glanz et al., 2015). The acronym PRECEDE has been slightly revised from the original to stand for *p*redisposing, *r*einforcing, and *e*nabling *c*onstructs in *e*ducational/ecological *d*iagnosis and *e*valuation (Bartholomew, Markham, Mullen, & Fernandez, 2015; Green & Kreuter, 2005).

The PROCEED model (Green & Kreuter, 1991, 2005) works in tandem with the PRECEDE model as the community health nurse proceeds to plan, implement, and evaluate health education programs. This acronym stands for *p*olicy, *r*egulatory, and *o*rganizational *c*onstructs for *e*ducational and *e*nvironmental *d*evelopment (Bartholomew et al., 2015). The entire PRECEDE–PROCEED model includes eight phases in the formulation and evaluation of health educational programs. The first five of these phases are included in the PRECEDE portion of the model and include (1) social, (2) epidemiologic, and (3) education/ecological assessments, followed by (4) administrative and policy assessment and intervention alignment, and (5) implementation. The PROCEED model is emphasized in the last three phases: (1) process evaluation, (2) impact evaluation, and (3) outcome evaluation.

A hallmark of the PRECEDE–PROCEED model is the emphasis on the desired outcome. The model both begins and ends with *quality of life*, which includes "subjectively defined problems and priorities of individuals and communities" (Green & Kreuter, 2005, p. 11). The emphasis on what the individual or community perceives as the problem, not what the professional believes it to be, is crucial. Outcome evaluation is logically linked back to that same individual or community in assessing achievement of the desired change.

The steps in this model are similar to those of the nursing process. Because of this familiarity, the model has become a useful tool for nurses teaching in the community. The nurse builds on the assessment formulated from the PRECEDE model, determines the best interventions, and

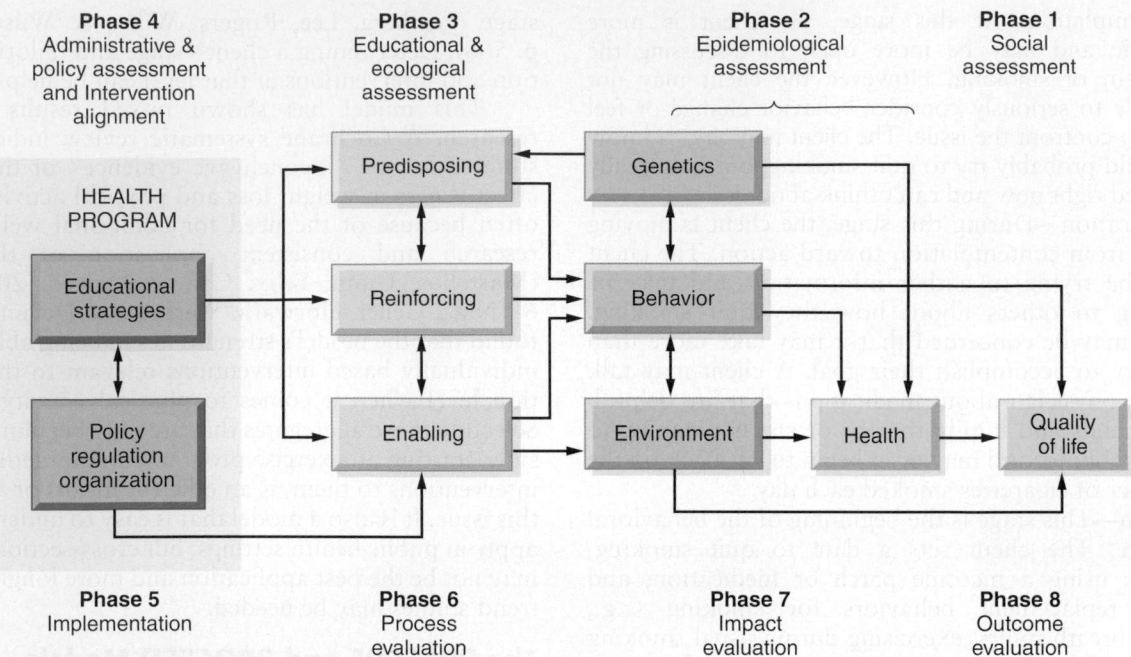

Phase 4
Administrative &
policy assessment
and Intervention
alignment

Phase 3
Educational &
ecological
assessment

Phase 2
Epidemiological
assessment

Phase 1
Social
assessment

HEALTH
PROGRAM

Educational
strategies

Policy
regulation
organization

Predisposing

Reinforcing

Enabling

Genetics

Behavior

Environment

Health

Quality
of life

Phase 5
Implementation

Phase 6
Process
evaluation

Phase 7
Impact
evaluation

Phase 8
Outcome
evaluation

FIGURE 11–11 The PRECEDE–PROCEED model. (From Green, L. W., & Kreuter, M. W. (2005). *Health program planning: An educational and ecological approach* (4th ed., p. 10). New York, NY: McGraw-Hill, with permission.)

then proceeds to evaluate the outcome of those interventions. The emphasis on the perceived needs of the individual or community as the starting point for all community efforts is consistent with public health nursing practice. The model reminds us of the importance of an organized approach to health educational programs, one that begins and ends with the "experts"—the individuals, families, and communities we hope to help through our efforts. The PRECEDE–PROCEED model can be seen in Figure 11–11.

This model has been used to address many public health problems. Over 1,000 examples of published applications of PRECEDE–PROCEED may be found at www.lgreen.net, including studies on health care workers' hand hygiene behaviors, follow-up with multicultural women with abnormal mammograms, implementation of church-based heart health promotion programs for older adults, developing a healthy-eating curriculum for schools, evaluation of a physical activity and nutrition program for senior citizens, and determining health promotion motivators in Asian populations. Other models used in community assessment and intervention may be found in Chapter 15.

TEACHING AT THREE LEVELS OF PREVENTION

PHNs should develop teaching programs that coincide with the level of prevention needed by the client. The three levels of primary, secondary, and tertiary prevention are demonstrated in the Levels of Prevention Pyramid for nurses who teach clients, families, aggregates, or populations.

Ideally, the community health nurse focuses teaching at the primary level. If nurses were able to reach more people at this level, it would help to diminish years of

morbidity and limit subsequent incapacity. Many people experience disabilities that could have been prevented if primary prevention behaviors had been incorporated into their daily activities.

Because the primary level of prevention is not possible in all cases, a significant share of the nurse's time is spent teaching at the secondary or tertiary level. An example is an 88-year-old woman with a fractured hip who has returned home after 3 weeks of physical therapy at a skilled nursing facility. The PHN assesses the client's environment, gait, functional limitations, safety, and adherence to medication and then initiates needed referrals. The teaching focuses on rehabilitation and prevention of a secondary problem that may affect the healing process and the client's health and safety in general.

EFFECTIVE TEACHING

Teaching is an art. It can be performed with such skill and grace that the client becomes part of a well-orchestrated event, with learning as the natural outcome. Instead of relying on prescribed teaching methods, the skillful PHN can make judgments based largely on client qualities, situations, and needs that guide the experience. The desired changes emerge in the course of the interaction rather than at a level conceived before the teaching. Before the community health nurse can reach this level of artistry, there is much to learn about being an effective teacher.

Teaching–Learning Principles

Teaching lies at one end of a continuum. At the other end is learning. Without learning, teaching becomes useless in the same way that communication does not occur unless a message is both sent and received. Both the teacher and the learner have responsibilities on that continuum.

LEVELS OF PREVENTION PYRAMID

SITUATION: Several examples of teaching at three levels of prevention.
GOAL: Using the three levels of prevention, negative health conditions are avoided or promptly diagnosed and treated, and the fullest possible potential is restored.

TERTIARY PREVENTION

Rehabilitation	Primary Prevention	
	Health Promotion and Education	*Health Protection*
• Restore function: a nurse teaches a stroke survivor about home safety, alternative housing options, physical therapy, and retraining opportunities	• Health teaching: a nurse teaches about the importance of diet, rest, and exercise to prevent a secondary health problem	• Maintenance: a nurse observes clients with tuberculosis where they live while taking their oral medication on a daily basis (DOT—Directly Observed Therapy)

SECONDARY PREVENTION

Early Diagnosis	Prompt Treatment
• Screening and case finding: a nurse takes blood pressure measurements from all family members at each home visit and teaches them the importance of maintaining a healthy blood pressure reading	• Treatment: a nurse teaches clients how to navigate through the complexities of the health care delivery system to receive prompt treatment

PRIMARY PREVENTION

Health Promotion and Education	Health Protection
• Health education: a nurse teaches a class on sensible weight control for teenagers	• Immunizations: a nurse teaches about the importance of pneumonia and flu vaccines for seniors, followed by an immunization clinic

Learners must take responsibility for their own learning. Teachers obstruct that process if they assume complete responsibility for bringing about changed behavior. Clients can be directed toward health knowledge, but they will not acquire knowledge unless they have the desire to learn. Davies (2011) lists the factors that influence clients' lifestyle-related health behaviors:

- Attitudes (how someone feels about or values health)
- Beliefs (personal opinions or convictions about health)
- Motivation (incentive or drive for choosing healthy behaviors)
- Intention (a plan for engaging in healthy behaviors)
- Volition (one's own choice or decision to be healthy)
- Planning (developing specific goals and objectives)
- Social support
- Self-monitoring
- Social and material environment (changing one's environment to improve health)

Teaching, then, becomes a matter of facilitating both the desire and the best conditions for satisfying it (Gilbert, Sawyer, & McNeill, 2015). Teaching in community health nursing means to influence, motivate, and act as a catalyst in the learning process. Nurses bring information and learners together and stimulate a reaction that leads to a change (Muma & Lyons, 2012). Nurses facilitate learning when they make it as easy as possible for clients to change. To do this, the PHN needs to understand the basic principles underlying the art and science of the teaching–learning process and the use of appropriate materials to influence learning (Table 11–6).

Client Readiness

The client's readiness to learn influences the PHN's teaching effectiveness. Four facets of client readiness have been identified (Kitchie, 2011, p. 115):

1. Physical readiness, which deals with their ability, task complexity, environment, health status, and gender
2. Emotional readiness, which deals with the state of receptivity to learning (e.g., motivation, anxiety, developmental stage, risk-taking behavior)
3. Experiential readiness, which reflects the learner's past experiences with learning (cultural background, orientation, locus of control, coping mechanisms used)
4. Knowledge readiness, which encompasses the learner's knowledge and understanding (e.g., learning disabilities, learning style, current knowledge base)

Table 11–6   Seven Principles for Maximizing the Teaching–Learning Process

Teaching Principles	Learning Principles
1. Adapt teaching to clients' level of readiness.	1. The learning process makes use of clients' experience and is geared to their level of understanding.
2. Determine clients' perceptions about the subject matter before and during teaching.	2. Clients are given the opportunity to provide frequent feedback on their understanding of the material taught.
3. Create an environment that is conducive to learning.	3. The environment for learning is physically comfortable; offers an atmosphere of mutual helpfulness, trust, respect, and acceptance; and allows for free expression of ideas.
4. Involve clients throughout the learning process.	4. Clients actively participate. They assess needs, establish goals, and evaluate their learning progress.
5. Make subject matter relevant to clients' interest and use.	5. Clients feel motivated to interest and learn.
6. Ensure client satisfaction during the teaching–learning process.	6. Clients sense progress toward their goals.
7. Provide opportunities for clients to apply material taught.	7. Clients integrate the learning through application.

Adapted from Knowles, M. (1980). *The modern practice of adult education: Andragogy versus pedagogy* (2nd ed.). Chicago, IL: Follett; Knowles, M. S., Holton, E. F., & Swanson, R. A. (2015). *The adult learner: The definitive classic in adult education and human resource development* (8th ed.). New York, NY: Routledge.

For instance, one community health nurse found that a young primipara was not ready for prenatal teaching on fetal growth and development. She had strong fears that she would be unable to lose her baby weight and that this would make her sexually unattractive to her partner. Until these anxieties were addressed, the teaching would remain ineffective. Clients' needs, interests, motivation, stress, and concerns determine their readiness for learning.

Another factor that influences readiness is educational background. If a group of women who never completed grade school meet to learn how to care for a sick person in the home, material should be presented in a factual and easily accessible manner and in terms that they understand. To discuss complex concepts of health, illness, and scientific research would be above their level of readiness. However, you can begin to introduce more complex concepts as you work with the women and assess their readiness for additional knowledge.

Maturational level also affects readiness. An adolescent mother who is still working on the normal developmental tasks of her age group, such as seeking independence or selecting a career path, may not be ready to learn parenting skills. Readiness of the client determines the amount of material presented in each teaching session. The pace or speed with which information is presented must be manageable. A small amount of anxiety often increases client receptivity to learning; however, high levels of anxiety can have the opposite effect.

Client Perceptions

Clients' perceptions also affect their learning, serving as a screening device or filter through which all new information must pass. Individual perceptions help people interpret and attach meaning to things. A wide range of variables affects human perception. These variables include values, past experiences, culture, religion,

personality, developmental stage, educational and economic level, surrounding social forces, and the physical environment. One client may view the experience of parenting as a positive, growth-producing relationship; another may see it as a conflict-ridden, unhappy experience to avoid. Each kind of perception has a different consequence for teaching and learning (Wesely, 2012).

Frequently, clients use selective perception. They screen out some statements and pay attention to those that fit their values or personal desires. For example, a PHN is teaching a client about the various risk factors in coronary disease; the individual screens out the need to quit smoking and lose weight, paying attention only to factors that would not require a drastic change in lifestyle. Nurses must know their clients, understand their backgrounds and values, and learn about their perceptions before health teaching can influence their behavior (Kitchie, 2011).

Davies (2011, p. 22) describes motivational interviewing skills (e.g., empathy, overcoming resistance, promoting self-efficacy, active listening, empowerment) and effective strategies, such as:

- Communication (using open-ended questions; affirmations; reflective listening; summarizing to ensure understanding)
- Tools and strategies (setting the scene; agreeing on the agenda; exploring a client's typical day; assessing confidence level; exploring two possible futures; looking back and looking forward; exploring options; agreeing on goals; agreeing on a plan)

Educational Environment

The setting in which the educational experience takes place has a significant impact on learning (Kitchie, 2011). Students probably have had the experience of sitting in a cold room and trying to concentrate during a lecture or of being distracted by noise, heat, or uncomfortable seating. Physical conditions such as ventilation, lighting, room temperature, view of the speaker, and noise level should be controlled to provide an environment that is conducive to learning.

Equally important for learning is an atmosphere of mutual respect and trust. The nurse needs to convey this attitude both verbally and nonverbally. The way the PHN addresses clients, shows concern, and gives recognition makes a considerable difference in establishing clients' rapport and trust. Both nurse and clients need to be mutually helpful and considerate of one another's needs and interests. All participants in the educational experience should feel free to express ideas, should know that their views will be heard, and should feel accepted despite differences of opinion and perspective. According to the adult learning theorist Knowles, this requires that the nurse refrain from seeming judgmental or inducing competitiveness among learners. Knowles (1980, p. 58) adds that teachers should share their own feelings and knowledge "as a colearner in the spirit of inquiry."

Client Participation

The degree of participation in the educational process directly influences the amount of learning (Moffett, Berezowski, Spencer, & Lanning, 2014). One nurse discovered this principle while working with a group of clients who were nearing retirement. After talking to them about the changes they would face and receiving little response, the nurse shifted to a different method of teaching. Handouts on Social Security benefits were distributed, and everyone was asked to read them during the week and come the next week with questions generated by the pamphlets. The PHN began the next session with a story about an older couple unprepared for retirement and the problems that they incurred. He then asked the group to share questions and concerns they had about retirement. This strategy prompted the group to slowly begin to participate in their own learning.

When the nurse works with clients in a learning context, one of the first questions to discuss is: What does the client want to learn? PHNs should begin from the client's place of interest. Learning is facilitated when the student is engaged and fully participates in the learning process. When the client chooses own directions, helps to discover own learning resources, formulates own problems, decides own course of action, and lives with consequences of each of these choices, then the client has significantly maximized his or her learning.

The amount of learning is directly proportional to the learner's involvement. In another example, a group of senior citizens attended a class on nutrition and aging yet made few changes in eating patterns. It was not until the members became actively involved in the class, encouraged by the nurse to present problems and solutions for food purchasing, understanding how to read nutrition labels, and preparation of meals on limited budgets, that any significant behavioral changes occurred.

Contracting, in which the client participates in the process as a partner to determine goals, content, and time for learning, can contribute to client learning (see Chapter 10). Contracting in the context of teaching assists clients to develop a sense of accountability for their own learning (Richards & Digger, 2011) (Fig. 11–12).

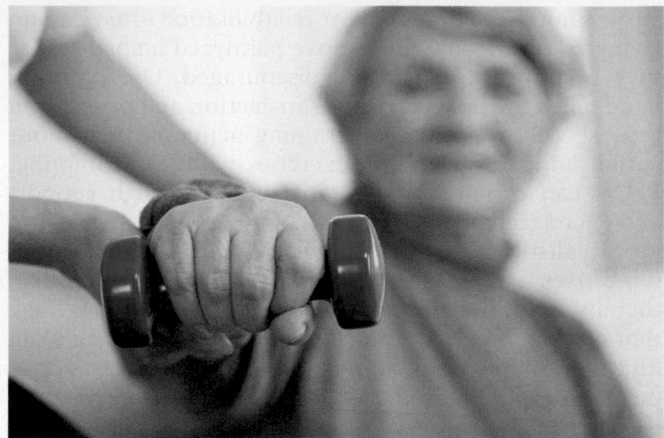

FIGURE 11–12 Client participation is a key to successful health promotion programs.

Subject Relevance

Subject matter that is relevant to the client is learned more readily and retained longer than information that is not meaningful. Our interest in a subject can predict our attention, processing speed, and retention of the material (Paul, 2013). Learners gain the most from subject matter that is immediately useful to their own purposes. This is particularly true for adult learners, who have more life experiences that can be related to learning and who tend to see the immediate relevance of the material taught (Bastable et al., 2011; Knowles, 1980).

Consider two middle-management men taking a physical fitness course offered by their employer. One, the father of a Boy Scout, has agreed to colead his son's troop on a 2-week backpacking trip in the mountains. He wants to get in shape. The second man is taking the course because it is a requirement of his company. Its only relevance to his own purposes is that it demonstrates his willingness to go along with company policies. There is little question about which man will learn and retain the most. The course has considerable relevance and meaning to the first man and little to the second.

Relevance also influences the speed of learning. Many adolescents complain that they will never use high school algebra; it holds no relevance for them. However, diabetic clients, who must give themselves daily injections of insulin in order to live, often learn that skill quickly. When clients see the relevance in learning, they accomplish it more promptly. When the subject matter is relevant to the learner, more knowledge is retained. On seeing the usefulness of the material, the learner develops a strong motivation to acquire and use it, and he is less likely to forget it (Bastable et al., 2011). Even in instances when a previously learned motor skill has not been used for years, it often is quickly recaptured when it is needed.

Client Satisfaction

To maintain motivation and increase self-direction, clients must derive satisfaction from learning. Learners need to feel a sense of steady progress in the learning process. Obstacles, frustrations, and failures along the way discourage and impede learning. Many clients who have had strokes and have potential for rehabilitation often give up trying to regain speech or move paralyzed limbs because they become frustrated and discouraged. On the other hand, clients who experience satisfaction and progress in their speech and muscle retraining maintain their motivation and may work on exercises without prompting. PHNs can promote client satisfaction through support and encouragement.

Realistic goals contribute to learner satisfaction. Objectives should be set within the learner's ability, thereby avoiding the frustration resulting from a task that is too difficult and the loss of interest resulting from one that is too easy. Setting objectives requires agreement on goals, periodic reviews, and revision of goals if they become too easy or too difficult (Bastable et al., 2011). PHNs further promote client's learning satisfaction by designing tasks with rewards. One school nurse led a class for obese adolescents, and together, they set the goal of a weekly 2-lb weight loss. The nurse helped the group design a plan that included counting calories, reducing fast food in their diets, increasing physical activity, and a buddy system to bring about behavior change. As members in the group achieved monthly goals, they were encouraged to reward themselves with a pair of earrings, new nail polish, time playing a favorite video game, or a special outing as a group. These students found this learning experience satisfying because goals were attainable, and their progress was rewarded. Instead of competing with one another, the group members set out to help each member achieve the goal. As a result, most kept the weight off after the class finished.

Client Application

Learning is reinforced through application (Bastable et al., 2011). Learners need as many opportunities as possible to apply the knowledge in daily life. If such opportunities arise during the teaching–learning process, clients can try out new knowledge and skills under supervision. Learners are given an opportunity to begin integrating the learning into their daily lives at a time when the teacher is there to help reinforce that pattern. Take a prenatal class as an example. The learning begins with explanations of proper nutrition and exercise during pregnancy, breathing techniques, hygiene, and avoidance of alcohol and tobacco. More learning occurs as the group members discuss these issues and apply them intellectually, exploring ways to practice them at home. Additional reinforcement comes by demonstrating how to do these activities. Sample diets, demonstrations of exercises, posters, pamphlets, or models may be used. The group can begin application in the classroom by making weekly diet plans, exercising, group role-play of parenting behavior, or engaging in problem-solving activities. The members then can be encouraged to apply these activities on a daily basis at home and to share their results with the group at future sessions.

Frequent use of newly acquired information fosters transfer of learning to other situations. The major goal of illness prevention and health promotion depends on such a transfer. For instance, mothers who learn and practice a well-balanced diet that is free of nonnutritious snacks can be encouraged to offer more nourishing foods to other family members. A family that practices good hand washing and sterile technique when caring for a family member's postsurgical wound can learn to transfer this same principle to prevention of infection in daily living.

Teaching Process

The process of teaching in community health nursing follows steps similar to those of the nursing process:

- *Interaction:* Establish basic communication patterns between clients and nurse.
- *Assessment and diagnosis:* Determine client's present status and identify client's need for teaching (keeping in mind that clients should determine their own needs).
- *Setting goals and objectives:* Analyze needed changes and prepare objectives that describe the desired learning outcomes.
- *Planning:* Design a plan for the learning experience that meets the mutually developed objectives; include content to be covered, sequence of topics, best conditions for learning (place, type of environment), methods, and materials (e.g., visual aids, exercises). A written plan is best; it may be part of the written nursing care plan.
- *Teaching:* Implement the learning experience by carrying out the planned activities.
- *Evaluation:* Determine whether learning objectives were met, and if not, why not. Evaluation measures progress toward goals, effectiveness of chosen teaching methods, or future learning needs.

Interaction

Reciprocal communication must occur between nurse and client. It is essential in the nurse–client relationship and requisite to effective use of the nursing process. Community health nurses need to develop good questioning techniques and listening skills to determine clients' learning needs and levels of readiness (Davies, 2011).

Assessment and Diagnosis

Identifying client's learning needs presents a challenge to the nurse. Too often, teaching occurs based on the nurse's assumption of what the learner needs to know. In client education, nurses have a responsibility to tailor their teaching to client's real and perceived needs. Knowles (1980, 1984, 1989) and Knowles et al. (2015) described educational needs as gaps between what people know and what they need to know in order to function effectively. He related that the potential learners, the sponsoring organization, and the community all help to determine the needs to be addressed in the teaching–learning situation.

Assessing educational needs may be accomplished in several ways. The nurse can use surveys, interviews, open forums, or task forces that include representative clients as members. The principle to remember is that clients should be involved in identifying what they want to learn. When a "need" to learn something, such as the importance of immunizing children, is identified by the nurse rather than by clients, the nurse may need to "sell" clients on the importance of the topic in order to gain interest. Nurses may need to use approaches that assist clients toward their own awareness needs; however, it is usually best to begin with the client's most pressing needs or interests.

Setting Goals and Objectives

Once a need has been clearly identified, the nurse and clients can establish mutually agreed-on goals and objectives. *Goals* are broad statements of intent, and *objectives* are more specific descriptions of intended outcome (Miller et al., 2012). Sometimes, in a teaching situation, an objective may be broken down into short- as well as long-term goals. For example, the nurse may have identified a group's desire to stop smoking. The need and teaching goals might be stated as follows:

> *Need:* A group of smokers wish to end their addiction to nicotine.
>
> *Short-term goal:* Within 1 month, all members of the group will reduce the number of cigarettes smoked.
>
> *Long-term goal:* Ninety percent of group members will remain tobacco-free for 6 months.

Objectives should be stated in measurable behavioral terms, using a grammatical structure that contains a subject, verb, condition/criterion, and time frame. That is, each objective should include a single idea that describes an outcome that can be measured within a certain time frame. To accomplish the short- and long-term goals of smoking cessation, educational objectives are developed from the levels of cognitive learning covered earlier in this chapter. Each behavioral objective is stated in measurable terms and includes a verb that describes with one of the six levels within the cognitive domain, discussed earlier (11.3). Objectives might appear in the following format.

At the end of the program, all clients should be able to do the following:

- *List* three reasons why smoking is unhealthy.
- *Identify* at least two factors that influence their smoking habit.
- *Apply* a series of action steps leading to smoking cessation within 1 month.
- *Examine* the steps as they work to live tobacco-free in the first 3 months.
- *Design* a way to live a fulfilled, tobacco-free life.
- *Evaluate* successful strategies to remain tobacco-free for 6 months.

Each of these objectives (a) refers to a subject; (b) can be readily measured, because each describes a specific outcome, condition, criterion, or expected behavior; (c) uses a verb for stating cognitive outcomes; and (d) includes a specific time frame (see Display 11–5). Well-written objectives meet these four criteria and enhance evaluation of the success of the educational effort.

Planning

Teaching preparation and planning for it are all-important to successful educational experiences (Bastable et al., 2011). Although nurses teach individuals and families informally, it is generally a good idea to have a written lesson plan. The formalization of creating a written plan provides a framework and permits organization of the topic in a well-thought-out manner that has been individualized for a specific client group. This plan should include the

---

DISPLAY 11–5 SAMPLE VERBS FOR STATING COGNITIVE OUTCOMES

Knowledge	Comprehension	Application	Analysis	Synthesis	Evaluation
Define	Translate	Interpret	Analyze	Compose	Judge
Repeat	Restate	Apply	Distinguish	Plan	Appraise
Record	Describe	Employ	Appraise	Propose	Evaluate
List	Discuss	Use	Calculate	Design	Rate
Recall	Recognize	Practice	Experiment	Formulate	Value
Name	Explain	Operate	Differentiate	Arrange	Revise
Relate	Express	Schedule	Test	Assemble	Score
Underline	Identify	Sketch	Compare	Collect	Select
	Locate	Shop	Contrast	Construct	Choose
	Report	Practice	Criticize	Create	Assess
	Review	Demonstrate	Diagram	Set up	Estimate
	Tell		Inspect	Organize	Measure
			Debate	Manage	
			Inventory	Prepare	
			Question		
			Relate		
			Categorize		
			Examine		

Adapted from Miller, D. M., Linn, R., & Gronlund, N. E. (2012). *Measurement and assessment in teaching* (11th ed.). Upper Saddle River, NJ: Pearson.

following eight items: (1) purpose, (2) statement of the overall goal, (3) list of objectives, (4) outline of the related content, (5) instructional methods, (6) time allotted for the teaching of each objective, (7) instructional resources, and (8) evaluation methods and criteria.

Teaching

The class, seminar, workshop, or small-group teaching should be conducted according to the plan described earlier. Even with one-on-one teaching, these eight steps should be planned in advance, because each client has a different cultural background, educational and intellectual level, as well as learning need. Use of a variety of teaching methods addresses the unique needs of learners and makes the teaching more engaging and interesting. Include and combine such methods as lectures, discussions, role-playing, demonstrations, and videos (see "Teaching Methods and Materials").

If necessary, assignments can be made, such as readings, watching suggested videos on the Web, presentations, or journaling, and practice experiences (or return demonstrations) can be used to reinforce and synthesize the learning. The teaching methods used and activities selected are important parts of the teaching plan. A well-designed plan enhances the flow of knowledge in the teaching situation. Poorly thought-out or unorganized plans may lead to inferior outcomes.

Evaluation

The final step of evaluation is critical in the teaching–learning process. Evaluation is the process for verifying the degree to which behavioral changes are actually occurring. At this point, the nurse determines whether the goals and objectives for the educational experience have been met and, if not, why they have not been met. Clear, measurable objectives facilitate evaluation.

If objectives have not been met or have been met only partially, the nurse should explore this outcome with clients to determine what factors hindered their success and what actions might be helpful. Client evaluation is very important to the PHN organizing the session. It is helpful to know that clients found it helpful and interesting and were engaged or not. Partially met objectives can be addressed at the start of the next meeting.

Teaching Methods and Materials

Teaching occurs on many levels and incorporates various types of activities. It can be formal or informal, planned or unplanned. Formal presentations, such as group lectures, usually are planned and fairly structured. Some teaching is less formal but still planned and relatively structured, as in group discussions in which questions stimulate the exploration of ideas and guide thinking. Informal levels of teaching, such as counseling or **anticipatory guidance** (in which the client is assisted in preparing for a future role or developmental stage), require the teacher to be prepared, but there is no defined presentation plan. The PHN may use a handout or agency protocol steps as a guide. PHNs use one or a combination of methods, along with a variety of materials, to facilitate the teaching–learning process. However, nurses need to expand their diversity of teaching techniques and avoid relying on only one or two

methods (Bastable et al., 2011). Generating variability of teaching methods stimulates creative thinking. Nurses use knowledge from physiology, pathology, sociology, and psychology in their practice, and, when teaching, nurses can benefit from using concepts, principles, and teaching methods derived from education, especially adult education. Four commonly used teaching methods (lecture, discussion, demonstration, and role-playing), along with teaching materials for enhanced learning, follow.

Lecture

The community health nurse sometimes presents information to a large group, such as a local parent–teacher association, a senior citizen's group, or a county board of commissioners. Under such circumstances, the lecture method, a formal kind of presentation, may be the most efficient way to communicate general health information. However, lecturers tend to create a passive learning environment for the audience unless strategies are devised to involve the learners. Many individuals are visual rather than auditory learners. To capture their attention, computer-generated slide programs or video presentations can supplement the lecture. Allowing time for questions and discussion after a lecture also actively involves learners. This method is best used with adults, but even they have a limited attention span, and breaks should be given every 30 to 60 minutes. Distributing printed material that highlights and summarizes, or supplements, the shared content also reinforces important points. Excellent suggestions for giving dynamic lectures and presentations may be found by searching the Web.

DISCUSSION

Two-way communication is an important feature of the learning process. Learners need an opportunity to raise questions, make comments, reason out loud, and receive feedback to develop deeper understanding. When discussion is used in conjunction with other teaching methods, such as demonstration, lecture, and role-playing, it improves their effectiveness. During group teaching sessions, discussion enables clients to learn from one another as well as from the nurse. The nurse must exercise leadership in controlling and guiding the discussion so that learning opportunities are maximized and objectives are met. Discussions that are organized around specific questions or topics are generally a good way to begin discussion.

Demonstration

The demonstration method often is used for teaching psychomotor skills and is best accompanied by explanation and discussion, with time set aside for return demonstration by the client or caregiver. It gives clients a clear sensory image of how to perform the skill. Because a demonstration should be within easy visual and auditory range of learners, it is best to demonstrate in front of small groups or a single client. Use the same kind of equipment that clients will use, show exactly how the skill should be performed, and provide learners with ample opportunities to practice until the skill is perfected.

This is an ideal method to use in a client's home, as well as in groups. The materials and supplies that the client will use when unaided by the PHN should be employed in the demonstration. But, you may need to use improvising skills. Helping families figure out ways to accomplish goals with materials found at home often becomes the hallmark of an experienced community health nurse. The new mother learns how to bathe her baby safely in the kitchen sink. The PHN assists several low-income parents in using household items to make inexpensive toys (e.g., mobiles from plastic coat hangers, string, and pictures from a magazine; bean bags using dry beans and scraps of fabric). The husband learns how to change dressings over the site of his wife's central venous line using sterile technique while conserving supplies purchased on their fixed income. Each activity takes a different type of psychomotor skill and ingenuity on the part of the PHN.

Role-Playing

At times, having clients assume and act out roles maximizes learning. A parenting group, for example, found it helpful to place themselves in the role of their children. In doing so, their feelings about various ways to respond became more apparent. Reversing roles can effectively teach conflicting spouses better ways to communicate. To prevent role-playing from becoming a game with little learning, it should be planned with clear objectives in mind. What behavioral outcomes should be achieved? Define the context (the "stage") clearly, so that everyone shares in the situation. Then define each role ahead of time, making sure that participants understand their performance roles. Emphasize that no wrong or right performance exists and that participants should behave the way people behave in everyday life. Avoid having people play themselves, because it can embarrass them and make it difficult for them to achieve objectivity. After the drama has concluded, begin discussion with carefully prepared questions. This technique can be used with staff, coworkers, young children, teenagers, and adults. However, it can be a risk-taking experience for some people, and they may be reluctant to participate. The nurse should use judgment, begin with volunteers, and avoid pushing this technique on unwilling or nonreceptive people. It is best to build up to full participation.

Teaching Materials

Many different kinds of teaching materials are available to the nurse. They often are employed in combination and are useful during the teaching process. Visual images—such as PowerPoint presentations (using graphics, photos), pictures, posters, chalkboards, flannel boards, DVDs, online videos, bulletin boards, flash cards, pamphlets, flyers, charts, and gestures—can enhance most learning. Americans readily learn from television and the Web, as there is visual and auditory appeal. Learning of both positive and negative health behaviors through television or the Web can be more effective and efficient than traditional teaching methods. Other tools, such as anatomic models and improvised or purchased equipment, provide clients with both visual and tactile learning experiences. Still others, such as interactive computer games or instruction, actively involve the learners (Fig. 11–13).

The choice of teaching materials varies with the client's interests and abilities and the resources available. Teaching often occurs in casual conversations, spontaneously in situations when clients raise unexpected questions, or when a

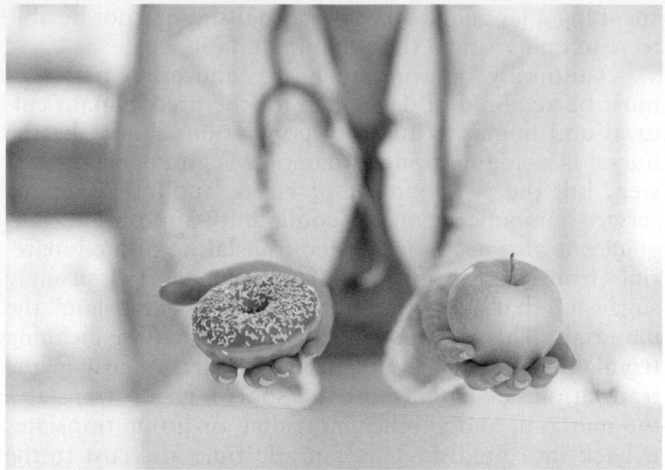

FIGURE 11–13 Teaching materials help to make your point.

crisis arises. In these instances, PHNs draw on their background of knowledge and exercise professional judgment in their selection of content, methods, and materials.

Printed educational support materials are available, such as pamphlets, brochures, booklets, flyers, and informational sheets. Each should be evaluated for appropriateness and effectiveness with particular individuals, families, or groups. Many come from state and local public health sources. Nurses can create their own handouts, customizing them to the needs of individual clients. The nurse can get educational information from state, federal, and international health agencies such as state health departments, the U.S. Food and Drug Administration (FDA), the Centers for Disease Control and Prevention (CDC), the National Institutes of Health (NIH), and the World Health Organization. Other materials come from nonprofit national agencies such as the American Diabetes Association (ADA), the March of Dimes, the American Association for Retired Persons (AARP), and the American Heart Association (AHA).

Factors to be considered with all educational literature include the material's content, complexity, and reading level. There are several ways to assess the readability of the printed word. One easy way is to use the Fry Readability Graph or the Gunning-Fog formula. These tools are rough way of determining the years of schooling needed to understand printed material. It works by analyzing words and sentence length; the higher the number, the more difficult the reading level. A Gunning-Fog Index of 6 is a sixth-grade reading level, and a score of 11 is at the junior year in high school. Fortunately, most word processing programs now include a feature to allow assessment of the reading level in text. Another very common tool is the Flesch Reading Ease program, available in Microsoft Word grammar checker, which evaluates reading material. Similar to the Fry Graph, the Flesch-Kincaid Grade Level readability score rates the material in terms of typical grade level; however, it may not be as accurate and you may need to adjust results downward (Medline Plus, 2015). The nurse should always consider the population when selecting a reading level, as many individuals cannot understand materials at even the 6th grade level. Also, clients, including those speaking a language other than English, may not be able to read and write in their dominant language.

Culturally appropriate health education materials must be acquired or developed for the predominant cultural and linguistic minority populations taught by the nurse. Developing printed materials is an important first step, but the development of video, audio, and public service announcements in community-appropriate languages is also necessary. When translating printed materials from English into another language, it is strongly suggested that a separate translator "back-translate" the materials. This added step helps assure that the meaning from the original has not been distorted or lost in the translation. Essentially one person or group translates the material, and another individual or group translates it back into English. This can add time and cost to the project, but it may prevent inaccuracies in the final material (Huff, Klein, & Peterson, 2015).

Finally, nurses teach by example. Actions speak louder than words. If a nurse teaches the importance of washing hands to reduce disease transmission and then begins a newborn assessment without hand washing, the message of observed actions carries more impact than the words. Nurses who exhibit healthy practices use themselves as teaching tools and serve as role models as well as health teachers.

Clients with Special Learning Needs

At times, the nurse experiences a challenging teaching situation with an individual, family, or group. These challenges may involve clients who have cultural or language differences, hearing impairments, developmental delays, memory losses, visual perception distortions, and problems with fine or gross motor skills, distracting personality characteristics, or demonstrations of stress or emotions. Regardless of the situation, the PHN will feel most comfortable and confident if he is prepared to deal with these situations before they are experienced.

Before beginning to teach a client, family, or aggregate, thorough preparation is important for successful learning to occur. This includes finding out whether it is possible to teach in English or whether other modifications are needed as the teaching plan is being developed. Community health nurses should never assume anything, including the primary language spoken by clients, their visual or hearing ability, or their capacity to understand. When teaching unfamiliar groups, the nurse can obtain information regarding the interests and abilities of the members from a center manager, caretaker, or program director. These human resources are invaluable in planning any teaching when English may be a second language or when other barriers exist that may impede success if they are not known by the nurse. Interpreters may be needed, and the PHN should work closely with the interpreter to assure that the intended message is sent and received by the clients (Huff et al., 2015). The phases of the nursing process continue to guide the nurse as a teacher.

Another difficulty that can arise is unexpected behavior from a client who disrupts the group process. The client may monopolize the discussion, answer questions asked of others, burst out with personal experiences that have no relevance to the topic, become irate at the comments of others, or sit silently and never speak. This can be unnerving to even the most experienced nurse. The PHN must tactfully diffuse any behavior that has the potential to distract the other learners. This is accomplished by considerately giving the recognition sought by the person while also setting limits.

SUMMARY

The purpose of health education is to effect change, which alters the equilibrium in a system. Change may occur gradually, with time for people involved to adjust, or it may occur in a drastic fashion, such as in a crisis or natural disaster. Change occurs in three stages: *unfreezing* when the system is ready for change, *changing* when the innovation is implemented, and *refreezing* when the change is stabilized.

Planned or managed change is a purposeful, designed effort to effect improvement in a system with the help of a change agent. It involves a process of eight steps, similar to the nursing process, which nurses can use to create change. These steps include assessing symptoms, diagnosing need, analyzing alternative solutions, selecting a change, planning the change, implementing the change, evaluating the change, and stabilizing the change. During planned change, the nurse can use one or a combination of several change strategies. However, the three major change strategies—a rational approach of providing information to influence people to change, an educative approach of combining new information with persuasion to effect change, and a coercive approach of enforcing compliance—are encompassing strategies. Several important principles serve as guidelines for community health nurses to effect change. They include involving all persons affected by the change, introducing change in a timely fashion, considering the impact of the change on other systems, being flexible, and understanding oneself and one's own qualities, which can be groomed to provide the most effective leadership.

Much of community health nursing practice involves teaching. More than simply giving health information to clients, the purpose of teaching is to change client behavior to healthier practices. If these practices are internalized and implemented regularly, years of morbidity and premature mortality can be avoided, thus contributing to the quality and length of the human lifespan.

Healthy People 2020 objectives foster recognition that social determinants of health must be factored into any educational or health promotion effort.

Understanding the nature of learning contributes to the effectiveness of teaching in community health. Learning occurs in three domains: cognitive, affective, and psychomotor. The cognitive domain refers to learning that takes place intellectually. It ranges in levels of learner functioning from simple recall to complex evaluation. As learners move up the scale of cognitive learning, they become more self-directed; the nurse then assumes a more facilitative role.

Affective learning involves the changing of attitudes and values. Learners may experience several levels of affective involvement, from simple listening to adopting the new value. Again, as the client increases involvement, the nurse uses a less directive approach.

Psychomotor learning involves the acquisition of motor skills. Clients who learn psychomotor skills must meet three conditions: they must be capable of the skill, they must develop a sensory image of the skill, and they must practice the skill.

Learning theories can be grouped into four broad categories: (1) behaviorist theories, which view learning as a behavioral change accomplished through stimulus–response or conditioning; (2) cognitive learning theories, which seek to influence learners' understanding of problems and situations through promoting their insights; (3) social learning theories, which explain dysfunctional behavior and facilitate learning; and (4) humanistic theories, which assume that people have a natural tendency to learn and that learning flourishes in an encouraging environment. Knowles' adult learning theory provides a framework for understanding adult characteristics and appropriate teaching interventions.

Health teaching models work together with the learning theories to give nurses a more accurate picture of the client and the client's learning needs. Four models were explored in this chapter. The HBM is useful in explaining the behaviors that are triggered by people with an interest in preventing diseases, and the revised HPM focuses on predicting behaviors that influence health promotion. The Health Promotion Model helps to predict behaviors that lead to health promotion and includes concepts about the interpersonal influence of others, such as health professionals, friends, and family. The Transtheoretical or Stages of Change Model is not a linear model, but recognizes that behavior change occurs more like a spiral, with plateaus, relapses, and false starts. Determining the current stage of the client (individual, group, or population) helps the PHN target education and health promotion efforts more accurately. The PRECEDE–PROCEED model is designed to guide health educational program development. The model has a strong focus on the perceived problems and priorities of a particular individual or group as they impact quality of life. Educational interventions are developed following a thorough assessment, which includes administrative and policy issues, and evaluation is conducted at three levels: process, impact, and outcome.

Teaching in community health nursing is the facilitation of learning that leads to behavioral change in the client. Ideally, this is done at the primary level of prevention. However, much of the nurse's work is done at the secondary and tertiary levels. The nurse uses several teaching–learning principles to facilitate the learning process, such as client's readiness for learning, client's perceptions, learner's physical and emotional comfort within an educational setting, degree of client participation, relevant subject matter, allowing clients to derive satisfaction from learning, and reinforcing learning through application. PHNs can incorporate behaviors associated with characteristics of effective instructors in an effort to better address learner needs.

The teaching process in community health nursing is similar to the nursing process, including steps of interaction, assessment and diagnosis, goal setting, planning, teaching, and evaluation. The teaching may be formal or informal, planned or unplanned, and methods may range from structured lecture presentations and discussions to demonstration and role-playing.

Selection of teaching materials depends on how well they suit learners and help to meet the desired objectives. Sources of teaching materials that are free or inexpensive can enhance the nurse's teaching efforts, but need to be evaluated for effectiveness and appropriateness. The nurse needs to know how to help learners with special needs, those with physical or mental disabilities, and those who are from a different culture or who speak a different language, as well as those who monopolize the discussion, become emotional, or are hostile. The nurse must be prepared for each situation to effectively teach the individual, family, or group.

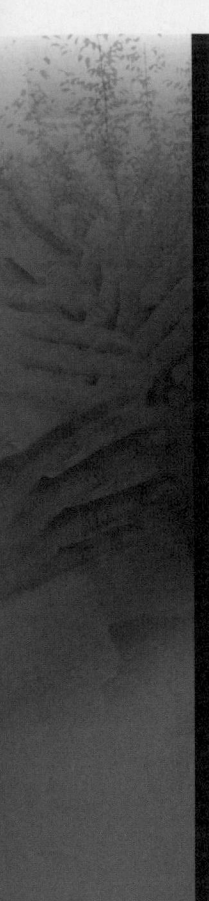

ACTIVITIES TO PROMOTE **CRITICAL THINKING**

1. As a staff public health nurse, you have been asked to chair an ad hoc committee in your health department made up of interdisciplinary colleagues and community members. The committee's task is to plan a health fair for the local community.
   a. Outline the specific planned-change steps that your committee needs to ensure a successful health fair with outcomes that promote improved levels of community health.
   b. Select one specific objective of your health fair (e.g., cholesterol screening of an at-risk aggregate with the goal of reduced cholesterol levels in a year). Does the proposed objective require an evolutionary or revolutionary change in citizen's health-related behaviors? Justify your choice of the type of change.
   c. Explain the strategies that you would use to effect the change.
   d. Six principles for effecting positive change are presented in this chapter. Briefly discuss how you would use each one as you and your committee develop the health fair.
2. What learning theories discussed in this chapter most closely resonates with you? How can they be applied in your practice?
3. Your city governmental officials often make decisions that appear to reflect a lack of knowledge regarding health and health care. How might you "educate" them using the concepts and principles described in this chapter?
4. Using behavioral objectives that match the learning level desired, develop a flyer or program for an educational presentation for clients.
5. Select one of the health teaching models. Use the model to plan an educational program for a group of teenagers. How did the use of the model enhance your teaching?
6. You are teaching an aggregate of middle-aged women about menopause. One woman monopolizes the class by telling stories and talking negatively about her husband. The other women are getting upset with her. How do you tactfully resolve the situation?
7. Interview an adolescent, a young adult, and a middle-aged as well as an older adult about their thoughts on health and what makes people healthy. What do they do to maintain their health? Do they have any dietary or other restrictions? What do they find the most difficult thing to do on a regular basis and why? Do you notice differences between the younger and older subjects? Is there a consistent theme among all of those that you interviewed? Compare your results with a peer's results.

REFERENCES

American Nurses Association (ANA). (2015). *Executive summary: American Nurses Association Health Risk Appraisal (HRA) preliminary findings October 2013-October 2014.* Retrieved from http://www.nursingworld.org/HRA-Executive-Summary

Asadzandi, M., Sekarifard, M., Ebadi, A., Morovvati Sharif Abad, M. A., & Salari, M. M. (2015). Effects of anger management training based on Health Promotion Model on soldiers engaged in risky behavior. *Iranian Journal of Psychiatric Nursing, 2*(4), 68–79.

Aspen Institute. (2012). *Health in all policies.* Retrieved from http://www.aspeninstitute.org/policy-work/health-biomedical-science-society/health-stewardship-project/principles/health-all-policies

Bandura, A. (1977). *Social learning theory.* Englewood Cliffs, NJ: Prentice-Hall.

Bandura, A. (1986). *Social foundations of thought and action: A social cognitive theory.* Englewood Cliffs, NJ: Prentice-Hall.

Bartholomew, L. K., Markham, C., Mullen, P., & Fernandez, M. E. (2015). Planning models for theory-based health promotion interventions. In K. Glanz, B. K. Rimer, & K. Viswanath (Eds.), *Health behavior: Theory, research, and practice* (5th ed., pp. 359–388). San Francisco, CA: Jossey-Bass.

Bastable, S. B., Gramet, P., Jacobs, K., & Sopczyk, D. L. (2011). *Health professional as educator: Principles of teaching and learning.* Sudbury, MA: Jones & Bartlett Learning.

Bates, B. (2016). *Learning theories simplified and how to apply them to teaching.* Thousand Oaks, CA: Sage.

Belguzar, K. (2015). The efficacy of an educational intervention on health behaviors in a sample of Turkish female nursing students: A longitudinal, quasi-experimental study. *Nurse Education Today, 35*(1), 146–151.

Bergold, J., & Thomas, S. (2012). Participatory research methods: A methodological approach in motion. *Forum: Qualitative Social Research, 13*(1), art. 30. Retrieved from http://www.qualitative-research.net/index.php/fqs/article/view/1801/3334

Bloom, B. (Ed.). (1956). *Taxonomy of educational objectives: The classification of educational goals. Handbook I: Cognitive domain.* New York, NY: Longman.

Borwick, J. (2013, June 5). *Revolutionary vs. evolutionary organizational change.* Retrieved from http://www.heitmanagement.com/blog/2013/06/revolutionary-vs-evolutionary-organizational-change/

Boston University School of Public Health. (2013). *Diffusion of innovation theory.* Retrieved from http://sphweb.bumc.bu.edu/otlt/MPH-Modules/SB/SB721-Models/SB721-Models4.html

Burke, W. W. (2013). *Organization change: Theory and practice* (3rd ed.). Thousand Oaks, CA: Sage Publications.

Centers for Disease Control and Prevention (CDC). (2014). *Gateway to health communication and social marketing practice.* Retrieved from http://www.cdc.gov/healthcommunication/campaigns/index.html

Centers for Disease Control and Prevention (CDC). (2015). *Characteristics of an effective health education curriculum.* Retrieved from http://www.cdc.gov/healthyschools/sher/characteristics/index.htm

Centers for Disease Control and Prevention (CDC). (n.d.). *CDCynergy Lite: Social marketing made simple. A guide for creating effective social marketing plans.* Retrieved from http://www.cdc.gov/health-communication/pdf/cdcynergylite.pdf

Davies, N. (2011). Healthier lifestyles: Behaviour changes. *Nursing Times, 107*(23), 20–23.

DiClemente, R. J., Salazar, L. F., & Crosby, R. A. (2013). *Health behavior theory for public health: Principles, foundations, and applications.* Burlington, MA: Jones & Bartlett Learning.

Genberg, B. Lee, Y., Rogers, W. H., Wiley, C., & Wilson, I. B. (2013). Stages of change for adherence to antiretroviral medications. *AIDS Patient Care and STDs, 27*(10), 567–572.

Gielen, A. C., & Green, L. W. (2015). The impact of policy, environmental, and educational interventions: A synthesis of the evidence from two public health success stories. *Health Education & Behavior, 42*(Suppl. 1), 20s–34s.

Gilbert, G. G., Sawyer, R. G., & McNeill, E. B. (2015). *Health education: Creating strategies for school and community health* (4th ed.). Burlington, MA: Jones & Bartlett.

Glanz, K., Rimer, B. K., & Viswanath, K. (Eds.). (2015). *Health behavior: Theory, research, and practice.* San Francisco, CA: Jossey-Bass.

Goodenough, K., Galway, G., Badenhorst, C., & Kelly, R. (Eds.). (2013). *Inspiration and innovation in teaching and teacher education.* Lanham, MD: Lexington Books.

Goulston, M. (2013). *Practical tips for overcoming resistance.* Retrieved from https://hbr.org/2013/07/practical-tips-for-overcoming-r/

Green, L. W., & Kreuter, M. W. (1991). *Health promotion planning: An educational and environmental approach* (2nd ed.). Mountain View, CA: Mayfield.

Green, L. W., & Kreuter, M. W. (2005). *Health program planning: An educational and ecological approach* (4th ed.). New York, NY: McGraw Hill.

Green, L.W., Ottoson, J. M., & Roditis, M. L. (2014). Public health education and health promotion. In L. Shi & J. A. Johnson (Eds.), *Novick & Morrow's public health administration: Principles for population-based management* (3rd ed., pp. 477–504). Burlington, MA: Jones & Bartlett Learning.

Hales, D. (2014). *An invitation to health: Build your future* (8th ed.). Belmont, CA: Wadsworth, Cengage Learning.

Healthy Sonoma. (2015). *School nutrition policy initiative.* Retrieved from http://www.healthysonoma.org/index.php?controller=index&module=PromisePractice&action=view&pid=3307

Hendrickson, K. E. (2015). *The encyclopedia of the industrial revolution* (Vol. 3). Lanham, MD: Roman & Littlefield.

Hersey, P., Blanchard, K., & Johnson, D. E. (2012). *Management of organizational behavior: Leading human resources* (10th ed.). Upper Saddle River, NJ: Prentice-Hall.

Huff, R. M., Kline, M. V., & Peterson, D. V. (Eds.). (2015). *Health promotion in multicultural populations: A handbook for practitioners and students.* Thousand Oaks, CA: Sage.

Jalilian, F., Motlagh, F. Z., Solhi, M., & Gharibnavaz, H. (2014). Effectiveness of self-management promotion educational program among diabetic patients based on health belief model. *Journal of Education and Health Promotion, 3,* 14. doi: 10.4103/2277-9531.127580.

Jepson, R. G., Harris, F. M., Platt, S., & Tannahill, C. (2010). The effectiveness of interventions to change six health behaviors: A review of reviews. *BMC Public Health, 10,* 538.

Jerome, B., & Powell, C. (2016). *The disposable visionary: A survival guide for change agents.* Santa Barbara, CA: ABC-CLIO, LLC.

Kaminski, J. (2011). Theory applied to informatics: Lewin's change theory. *Canadian Journal of Nursing Informatics, 6*(1). Retrieved from http://cjni.net/journal/?p=1210

Kitchie, S. (2011). Determinants of learning. In S. B. Bastable, P. Gramet, K. Jacobs, & D. L. Sopczyk (Eds.). *Health professional as educator: Principles of teaching and learning* (pp. 103–150). Sudbury, MA: Jones & Bartlett Learning.

Knowles, M. (1980). *The modern practice of adult education: Andragogy versus pedagogy* (2nd ed.). Chicago, IL: Follett.

Knowles, M. (1984). *The adult learner: A neglected species* (3rd ed.). Houston, TX: Gulf.

Knowles, M. (1989). *The making of an adult educator: An autobiographical journey.* San Francisco, CA: Jossey-Bass.

Knowles, M. (1990). *The adult learner: A neglected species* (4th ed.). Houston, TX: Gulf Publishing.

Knowles, M. S., Holton, E. F., & Swanson, R. A. (2015). *The adult learner: The definitive classic in adult education and human resource development* (8th ed.). New York, NY: Routledge.

Koeppl, P., & Robertson, E. C. (2015). *The healthy choice: How behavioral factors create influential health campaigns.* Retrieved from http://dupress.com/articles/behavior-change-communications-in-health-care/

Kominiarek, M. A. (2014). A survey of health behaviors in minority women in pregnancy: The influence of body mass index. *Women's Health Issues, 24*(3), e291–e295.

Lewin, K. (1947). Frontiers in group dynamics: Concept, method, and reality in social science; social equilibria and social change. *Human Relations, 1*(1), 5–41.

Lewin, K. (1951). *Field theory in social science: Selected theoretical papers.* New York, NY: Harper & Row.

Liebergall-Wischnitzer, M., Buyum, M., & Ganz, F. D. (2015). Health promoting lifestyle among Israeli adult survivors of childhood cancer. *Journal of Pediatric Oncology Nursing.* doi: 10.1177/1043454215600177.

Lippitt, G. L. (1973). *Visualizing change: Model building and the change process.* La Jolla, CA: University Associates.

Lippitt, R., Watson, J., & Westley, B. (1958). *The dynamics of planned change.* New York, NY: Harcourt.

Maslow, A. H. (1970). *Motivation and personality* (2nd ed.). New York, NY: Harper and Row.

Mastellos, N., Gunn, L. H., Felix, L. M., Car, J., & Majeed, A. (2014). Transtheoretical model stages of change for dietary and physical exercise modification in weight loss management for overweight and obese adults. *Cochrane Database Systematic Reviews, 2,* CD008066. doi: 10.1002/14651858.CD008066.pub3.

Medline Plus. (2015). *How to write easy-to-read health materials.* Retrieved from https://www.nlm.nih.gov/medlineplus/etr.html

Miller, D. M., Linn, R., & Gronlund, N. E. (2012). *Measurement and assessment in teaching* (11th ed.). Upper Saddle River, NJ: Pearson.

Minnesota Department of Health. (n.d). *QI toolbox: Force field analysis.* Retrieved from http://www.health.state.mn.us/divs/opi/qi/toolbox/forcefield.html

Mirghafourvand, M., Baheiraei, A., Nedjat, S., Mohammadi, E., Charandabi, S. M. A., & Majdzadeh, R. (2014). A population-based study of health-promoting behaviors and their predictors in Iranian women of reproductive age. *Health Promotion International, 30*(3), 586–594.

Moffett, J., Berezowski, J., Spencer, D., & Lanning, S. (2014). An investigation into the factors that encourage learner participation in a large group medical classroom. *Advances in Medical Education and Practice, 5,* 66–71.

Morris, S. (2014, September 30). Explore the life of a public health specialist. *U.S. News & World Report.* Retrieved from http://www.usnews.com/education/blogs/medical-school-admissions-doctor/2014/09/30/explore-the-life-of-a-public-health-specialist

Muma, R. D., & Lyons, B. A. (2012). *Patient education: A practical approach* (2nd ed.). Sudbury, MA: Jones & Bartlett Learning.

National Heart Lung and Blood Institute. (2012). *Guide to behavior change.* Retrieved from http://www.nhlbi.nih.gov/health/public/heart/obesity/lose_wt/behavior.htm

Nigg, C. R., Geller, K. S., Horwath, C. C., Wertin, K. K., & Dishman, R. K. (2011). A research agenda to examine the efficacy and relevance of the transtheoretical model for physical activity behavior. *Psychology of Sport and Exercise, 12*(1), 7–12.

Paul, A. M. (2013, November 4). *How the power of interest drives learning.* Retrieved from http://ww2.kqed.org/mindshift/2013/11/04/how-the-power-of-interest-drives-learning/

Pavlov, I. P. (1957). *Experimental psychology and other essays.* New York, NY: Philosophical Library.

Pender, N. J., Murdaugh, C. L., & Parsons, M. A. (2015). *Health promotion in nursing practice* (7th ed.). Upper Saddle River, NJ: Prentice Hall.

Pew Charitable Trusts. (2015). *Health impact project.* Retrieved from http://www.pewtrusts.org/en/projects/health-impact-project

Piaget, J. (1966). *The origin of intelligence in children.* New York, NY: Norton.

Piaget, J. (1970). *Child's conception of movement and speed.* Abingdon, UK: Routledge.

Prochaska, J. O., Norcross, J. C., & DiClemente, C. C. (2007). *Changing for good: A revolutionary six-stage program for overcoming bad habits and moving your life positively forward* (Reprint Ed.). New York, NY: William Morrow Paperbacks.

Rector, C., Gilchrist, K., Camarena, E., & Cauthen, S. (2014). *Comparison of health promoting behaviors among working acute care nurses and public health nurses.* Poster session presented at the American Public Health Association Annual Conference, New Orleans, LA .

Reutter, L., & Kushner, K. E. (2012). Health equity through action on the social determinants of health: Taking up the challenge in nursing. *Nursing Inquiry, 17*(3), 269–280.

Reyes, D. J., Bekemeier, B., & Issel, L. M. (2014). Challenges faced by public health nursing leaders in hyperturbulent times. *Public Health Nursing, 31*(4), 344–353.

Richards, E., & Digger, K. (2011). Compliance, motivation, and health behaviors of the learner. In S. B. Bastable, P. Gramet, K. Jacobs, & D. L. Sopczyk (Eds.), *Health professional as educator: Principles of teaching and learning* (pp. 199–226). Sudbury, MA: Jones & Bartlett Learning.

Robert Wood Johnson Foundation. (2015). *A new way to talk about social determinants of health.* Retrieved from http://www.rwjf.org/en/library/research/2010/01/a-new-way-to-talk-about-the-social-determinants-of-health.html

Rogers, C. (1969). *Freedom to learn.* Columbus, OH: Merrill.

Rogers, C. (1989). *Freedom to learn for the eighties.* Columbus, OH: Merrill.

Rosenstock, I. M. (1966). Why people use health services. *Milbank Memorial Fund Quarterly, 44,* 94–127.

Roussel, L. A., Harris, J. L., & Thomas, T. (2016). *Management and leadership for nurse administrators* (7th ed.). Sudbury, MA: Jones & Bartlett.

Science Daily. (2015, November 16). *Population health promotion: Stratified approach for cardiovascular health.* Retrieved from http://www.sciencedaily.com/releases/2015/11/151116120814.htm

Simonds, V. W., Wallerstein, N., Duran, B., & Villegas, M. (2013). Community-based participatory research: Its role in future cancer research and public health practice. *Preventing Chronic Disease, 10,* 120205.

Singh, S., Pai, D., Sinha, N., Kaur, A., Soe, H. H., & Barua, A. (2013). Qualities of an effective teacher: What do medical teachers think? *BMC Medical Education, 13,* 128.

Skinner, B. F. (1974). *About behaviorism.* New York, NY: Knopf.

Skinner, B. F. (1987). *Upon further reflection.* Englewood Cliffs, NJ: Prentice-Hall.

Skinner, C. S., Tiro, J., & Champion, V. L. (2015). The health belief model. In K. Glanz, B. K. Rimer, & K. Viswanath (Eds.), *Health behavior: Theory, research, and practice* (5th ed., pp. 75–94). San Francisco, CA: Jossey-Bass.

Spradley, B. W. (1980). Managing change creatively. *Journal of Nursing Administration, 10*(5), 32–37.

Spradley, J., & McCurdy, D. (1994). *Conformity and conflict: Readings in cultural anthropology* (8th ed.). New York, NY: HarperCollins.

Thorndike, E. L. (1932). *The fundamentals of learning.* New York, NY: Teachers College Press.

Thorndike, E. L. (1969). *Educational psychology.* New York, NY: Arno Press.

Trickett, E. J., Beehler, S., Deutsch, C., Green, L. W., Hawe, P., McLeroy, K., ... Trimble, J. E. (2011). Advancing the science of community-level interventions. *American Journal of Public Health, 101*(8), 1410–1419.

U.S. Department of Health and Human Services (USDHHS). (2016a). *Healthy People 2020: About Healthy People.* Retrieved from http://www.healthypeople.gov/2020/About-Healthy-People

U.S. Department of Health and Human Services (USDHHS). (2016b). *Healthy People 2020: Education and community based programs.* Retrieved from http://www.healthypeople.gov/2020/topics-objectives/topic/educational-and-community-based-programs

U.S. Department of Health and Human Services (USDHHS). (2016c). *Healthy People 2020: Social determinants of health.* Retrieved from http://www.healthypeople.gov/2020/topicsobjectives2020/overview.aspx?topicid=39

U.S. Department of Health and Human Services (USDHHS). (2016d). *Secretary's advisory committee on health promotion and disease prevention objectives for 2020.* Retrieved from

U.S. Department of Health and Human Services (USDHHS). (n.d.). *Healthy People 2020 Framework: The vision, mission, and goals of Healthy People 2020.* Retrieved from http://www.healthypeople.gov/sites/default/files/HP2020Framework.pdf

Wertheimer, M. (Ed.). (1959). *Productive thinking.* New York, NY: Harper & Row. (Original work published 1945.)

Wertheimer, M. (1980). *Gestalt theory of learning.* In G. M. Gazda & R. H. Corsini (Eds.), *Theories of learning: A comparative approach.* Itasca, IL: Peacock.

Wesely, P. M. (2012). Learner attitudes, perceptions, and beliefs in language learning. *Foreign Language Annals, 45,* s98–s117.

Wills, J. (Ed.). (2014). *Fundamentals of health promotion for nurses* (2nd ed.). West Sussex, UK: John Wiley & Sons.

World Health Organization, Government of South Australia. (2010). *Adelaide statement on health in all policies.* Retrieved from http://www.who.int/social_determinants/hiap_statement_who_sa_final.pdf

World Health Organization. (2014). *Targeting both children and parents for better hygiene in India: Sesame Workshop's Galli Galli Sim Sim.* Retrieved from http://apps.who.int/iris/handle/10665/184990

thePoint: Everything You Need to Make the Grade!

thePoint® Visit http://thePoint.lww.com/Rector9e for selected readings, study aids for all learning styles, and more!

Planning and Developing Community Programs and Services

"True genius resides in the capacity for evaluation of uncertain, hazardous, and conflicting information."

—*Winston Churchill* (1874–1965), **British Prime Minister (1940–1945; 1951–1955)**

KEY TERMS

Advisory group
Authoritative knowledge
Benchmarking
Enabling factors

Geographic information
  system (GIS)
Grant
Grant writing

Letter of inquiry
Logic models
Predisposing factors
Quality indicators

Reinforcing factors
Request for proposal (RFP)
Social marketing

LEARNING OBJECTIVES

Upon mastery of this chapter, you should be able to:

- List sources of information that can be used to identify group and community health problems.
- Identify change strategies that maximize cooperation of target populations.
- Identify methods to gain input from target populations to define the scope of a health problem.
- Identify and evaluate the effectiveness of intervention methods targeting health problems.
- Classify health problems based on their changeability.
- Identify barriers to solving health problems.
- Discuss the role of the nurse within quality measurement and improvement programs in community/public health nursing.
- Recognize the role of social marketing in health promotion programs.
- Locate appropriate grant funding sources for select health promotion programs.

A public health nurse collaborates with the county housing authority to implement a comprehensive fall prevention program for community-dwelling seniors; another nurse works into the night to complete a multimillion-dollar grant to fund comprehensive human immunodeficiency virus (HIV) educational programs in Kenya; community health nursing students volunteer to assist the local public health department with a social marketing campaign on health promotion. The efforts described may seem very different, but each represents a health promotion program targeting populations, not just individuals. A fall prevention program could potentially reduce the number of hospitalizations in the community resulting from serious falls, the HIV program may ultimately save tens of thousands from contracting this disease, and the social marketing campaign may reach thousands in the community, prompting them to think about their own health habits and engage in health-promoting behaviors. Each of these examples represents the emerging role of the public health nurse and argues for the acquisition of a new set of skills. The skills of grant writing, social marketing, and collaborating with county officials all require new abilities that may require additional training or working with a mentor. These roles may seem foreign to you now, as you begin your career, but they may be the very skills needed to help bring vital health promotion programs to fruition.

In many communities across the country, local health departments struggle to recruit nurses to provide much-needed services. With shrinking budgets, many communities are forced to change long-held views on the scope and nature of services provided by public health nurses. The home visiting model, once a mainstay of public health nursing, has been eliminated in many communities. Increasingly, public health nurses find themselves providing health promotion and educational programs to larger and larger audiences. To meet this need, public health nurses must become skilled at planning and implementing health promotion programs. As with any activity, the need for the program must be justified, and with limited resources, the benefit to the community must be demonstrated. Additionally, communities are rarely in a position to fund the entire realm of needed health programs and must turn to outside agencies for funding, through either grants or contracts. The public health nurse often assumes responsibility for locating, securing, and maintaining grant funding.

Whether or not program funding comes from the county or an outside agency, program results must be assessed. Evaluation of programs is vital for their continuation and is a requirement of most funders, whether public or private. A nurse who receives $500 to start an emergency preparedness program with low-income families may not be expected to provide the level of evaluation data that a million-dollar effort to address methamphetamine use in the community would likely require. However, some level of evidence that demonstrates the impact of the program will be needed. Even the populations served want to know whether the programs were successful and why. For instance, a mother agrees to have her daughter enrolled in an after-school program to increase self-esteem. At the end of the first 6-week session, the mother is asked to give permission for her daughter to attend the second session. Her daughter says she enjoys the sessions but would also like to go to a dance class that is held at the same time. With competing demands on the daughter's time, the mother may ask for details on what was accomplished in the first session

and what expectations the providers have for this second session. With this information, she can discuss various options with her daughter. The funders, consumers, and the nurse all need to be aware of the demonstrated outcomes of programs.

In Chapter 11, you were introduced to the concept of change—how it influences the adoption of health behaviors and what factors impede change in individuals. Educational methods are often used to influence change in behaviors and play a vital role in those efforts. In this chapter, we build on the concepts of change and appropriate educational techniques and apply them to larger groups and populations. The discussion of the PRECEDE–PROCEED model (Green & Kreuter, 1999, 2005; Green, Ottoson, & Roditis, 2014; Ottoson & Green, 2008) will be expanded upon as you are introduced to the basics of health program planning, intervention, and evaluation to maximize successful results. Meeting the Institute of Medicine's (IOM, 2003, 2011) call for enhanced quality and safety in nursing education and the impact this has on performance and outcome assessment of community health programs and services will be addressed, as well as the Quality and Safety Education for Nurses (QSEN, 2014) project that evolved from this call for action. Within this overall context, the subsequent IOM reports, the *Future of Nursing* (IOM, 2011) and *For the Public's Health* (IOM, 2012), will build on the challenges specific to public health and public health nursing. *Social marketing*, a tool for reaching large audiences with health information will be presented. Several well-known models familiar to nurses will be explored in terms of facilitating the evaluation of programs and services. Finally, as the need for grant funding becomes increasingly important, information on the various types of available funding will be provided.

PROGRAM PLANNING: THE BASICS

In the classic text by Ottoson and Green (2008, p. 590), public health education programs are defined as interventions "designed to inform, elicit, facilitate, and maintain positive health practices in large numbers of people." Even the American Nurses Association (ANA), *Public Health Nursing: Scope and Standards of Practice* (2013), is centered on the role of the nurse in planning, implementing, and evaluating population-focused health promotion/health education programs. Specifically, Standard 5B calls on the public health nurse to "employ multiple strategies to promote health, and a safe environment" (p. 37), through programs and services that include appropriate teaching–learning methods, that are culturally and age appropriate, and that also include an evaluation component. Advanced PHNs plan "evidence-based health promotion programs and services" and engage with consumers and advocacy groups in promoting health and modifying programs (p. 38).

With so much emphasis on planning and developing health education/health promotion programs, the process can seem overwhelming to the new public health nurse or even to the acute care nurse who may be involved in some aspect of health initiative development within an agency. The first part of this chapter is designed to take some of the mystery out of the process. You will be guided through the complex problem of obesity in school-aged children. This particular issue is of great importance to the health of our children, and the principles applicable to this example can be utilized in other situations and other programs, even those that are very broad in scope and involve many practice partners. In your nursing program, you may even have been tasked with developing a health program, working on an existing community program, or simulating the process in a written assignment. Whatever your experience level, the essential elements are the same. As you begin this next section, think about past experiences you have had, such as taking blood pressures at a local health fair or developing a pamphlet on the need for prostate screening for non–English-speaking residents. Did these actions have the impact you hoped for? Successful health promotion programs do not occur by accident; they take skill, time, patience, and most of all listening to and understanding the needs and opinions of the individuals who are the focus of your program (the target population) (Fig. 12–1).

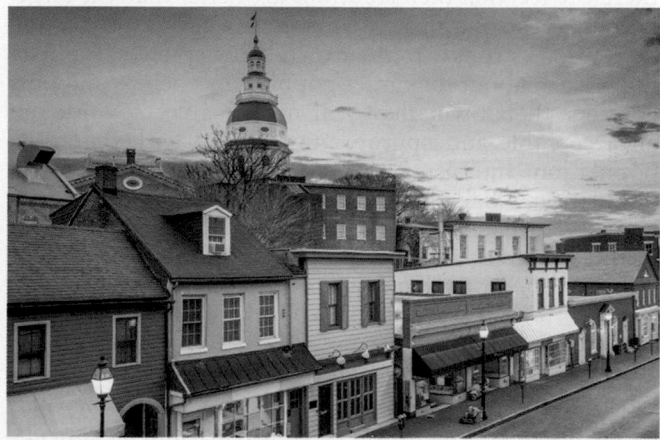

FIGURE 12–1 Every community has unique health problems that need to be identified.

IDENTIFYING GROUP OR COMMUNITY HEALTH PROBLEMS

Nursing education emphasizes practice with a focus on individuals, families, and communities, yet nurses often practice at the individual and family level. When is it appropriate for a nurse to expand his or her practice to the community level? Perhaps the most natural time is when a nurse identifies an ongoing issue that does not change with traditional interventions. Examples might include overuse of the emergency room for urgent care; recurrent hospitalization of the elderly from several nursing homes for dehydration, sepsis, and malnutrition; or hospitalization of 6- to 8-year-olds for injuries caused by insufficient car seat restraint. These types of recurrent problems might lead the nurse to investigate the feasibility of a community-based intervention.

Individually or in a group, identify a possible issue to explore—one that you believe is leading to poor health outcomes in your community. How do you know if this problem is widespread or if others also find it to be a problem? Several methods can be used to validate the importance of the issue. One method would be to consider *Healthy People 2020* objectives for the nation (U.S. Department of Health and Human Services [USDHHS], 2016). What are the major issues that are of concern to improving health outcomes for the United States? What are the priorities of the state in which you live? You might take some time to review Web sites for federal agencies to identify the programs they are promoting to meet the *Healthy People 2020* goals and objectives. Your state department of health may also have a Web site with information on achievement of *Healthy People 2020* objectives, including those objectives that remain challenging. Local communities also establish priorities that reflect the *Healthy People 2020* objectives for the nation. These overarching national goals are as follows:

- Attain high-quality, longer lives free of preventable disease, disability, injury, and premature death.
- Achieve health equity, eliminate disparities, and improve the health of all groups.
- Create social and physical environments that promote good health for all.
- Promote quality of life, healthy development, and healthy behaviors across all life stages (USDHHS, 2016, para. 5).

Community agencies and organizations frequently network to establish community-wide goals, and the local health department often spearheads this effort. It may also be organized by community-based health agencies and volunteer organizations. Improved outcomes for individuals who have diabetes or asthma are issues a local community might want to address. Another topic of concern is childhood obesity. Nurses can work collaboratively with these types of special interest groups to find solutions for individuals and families with identified problems.

As a specific problem is identified, it is crucial to analyze the extent to which individuals and families are affected by the problem. It is a poor use of resources to set up a program if there is a very small incidence of the condition or situation. For example, it would be a waste of resources to establish a program on diabetes and pregnancy for a local homeless shelter that only serves 35 women a year. Of those 35 women, none may be pregnant, and because 4.6% to 9.2% of the population of pregnant women develops gestational diabetes, it may be a number of years before an eligible client is found (DeSisto, Kim, & Sharma, 2014). A better use of resources would be to target a community with a higher proportion of individuals at risk for diabetes during pregnancy (Hedderson et al., 2012). An example might be a program targeting a community with a large population of young Asian/Pacific Islander or Hispanic mothers, as the incidence of gestational diabetes is higher in this population (16.3% and 12.1%, respectively) than for non-Hispanic Whites (6.8%). Yet another target group may be older women who are also at increased risk (DeSisto et al., 2014). There are many ways a nurse can decide if a problem has affected a sufficient percentage of the population to warrant intervention. The best way to start is by reviewing the local, state, and national data available through government repositories. This can be done by searching the Internet, by going to a university library for assistance, and by asking for sources of specific data from your local health and social service agencies, police and judicial departments, and local school districts. Hospital discharge data are also reported to state agencies, and this information is sometimes available at the local level.

As nurses and other community groups narrow their focus, they can often map data by zip codes and neighborhoods, which helps to identify the best places to target groups and communities. Currently, many organizations have this ability and are able to identify target groups by race, age, and family status. These types of data, known as **geographic information system (GIS)** information, are widely available. At the federal level, the National Center for Health Statistics (NCHS) Web site maintains GIS maps on the major causes of mortality in the country. Additional GIS data can be found through a variety of federal sources, including the CDC, the National Cancer Institute, the Center for Mental Health Services, the National Library of Medicine, and the Environmental Protection Agency (Public Health Partners, 2016) (see Chapter 10; Fig. 12–2).

Another effective approach is to talk to other nurses and other health care professionals within and outside of your organization. Get their ideas about the problem and ideas about what should be done to alleviate the problem. In addition, find out what has been tried in the past and get their input on why past interventions failed. One very helpful source of information is the *Guide to Community Preventive Services: What Works to Promote Health?* (Community Preventive Services Task Force, 2014), a federally sponsored initiative that provides recommendations regarding population-based interventions, including which are recommended, which need more evidence to determine effectiveness, and which are not recommended. The interventions with limited evidence may actually be very effective but need to be demonstrated by more studies; perhaps your idea is among those listed. Publication of program results not only is professionally gratifying but adds to the body of evidence on which health promotion programs can be evaluated. For example, in Chapter 6 of the guide, recommendations to increase community demand for vaccinations include client reminder and recall systems, yet there is not enough evidence to support client or family incentives, or the use of patient-held medical records (see pp. 223–224) (see Chapter 15).

The next step of intervention is the most important of all, as it will determine whether your interventions succeed or fail. A nurse may think, "I know what the problem is—now I will think up an intervention to alleviate it!" This approach may be well intentioned but will lead the nurse down the path of failure. At this point, only part of the assessment is completed; the most important part of the assessment is to find out the views of the target population about the identified problem. What do they think may be causes for this? What ideas do they have about solving it? Which approaches do they think will work, and which are doomed to failure? These are all important questions the nurse needs to ask. It is crucial that the views of the target population be heard and respected. Anthropologists talk about a concept called **authoritative knowledge**. This is based not on whose knowledge may be right but rather on what is "accepted as legitimate and accurate" because it may come from medical experts, for instance (McCoyd, 2010, p. 591). Nurses may think that they know more about a topic than their target population does (e.g., diabetes), and therefore feel that their solutions are better than the target population's solutions. Members of a target population hold just as strongly to their own belief systems. If nurses don't learn about the target population's beliefs and only consider their own, they will not be able to work out an acceptable and appropriate solution with the target population. Interventions that fail to engage the target population will likely be unsuccessful because of this. It is crucial that chosen interventions involve effective use of health resources and that positive working relationships be established with high-risk target communities.

Getting Started

When working with target groups, it's important to get as much information about the population as possible. Start by asking those you know, as colleagues and as patients/clients, about their local community. What do they see as issues regarding the problem about which you are

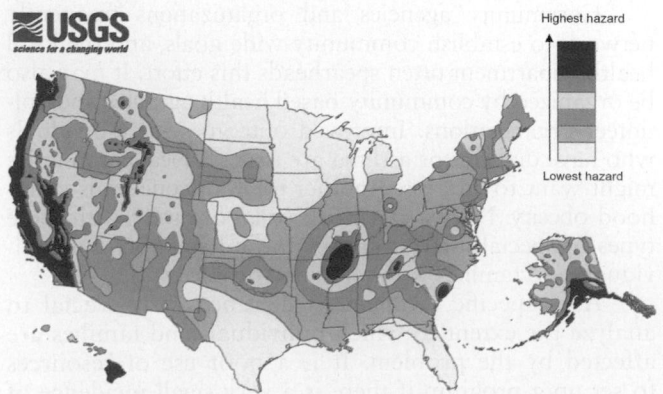

FIGURE 12-2   2014 USGS earthquake hazard map.

concerned? What do they think about the quality of services currently available? What do they see as barriers to services? What about barriers to adherence to treatment and other health care recommendations?

Additional issues to explore include the following: Who else do they think you should speak with to gain insight about the issues relevant to this problem? Who are key people with whom you should build relationships? What are their customs in regard to health care? Who are the leaders within a family? If you want to establish linkages with this population, what is the best method? Who are their *formal* and *informal leaders*? What types of events bring them together? What are the roles of family, church, and health care providers within their community? Should you go through church groups, school groups, or other organizations? What radio stations do they listen to, and what television stations are they most likely to watch? What are the most common Web sites used by this population when accessing health topics? This information will not only help you gain insight into factors influencing the health problem, it will also give you information about how most effectively to reach out to the target population. Concepts from community-based participatory research and health promotion are useful (Kulbok, Thatcher, Park, & Meszaros, 2012) (see Chapter 4).

As you start to gain insight into the environmental and social factors that influence the problems about which you are concerned, you are also building interest in the issue. As you participate in discussions with others, be open to their input. It may be that the ideas you start out with need to change in response to feedback from members of the target and service communities. For example, an experienced public health nurse was involved in a project developed to serve Hispanic women with gestational diabetes. When interviewed, the monolingual Spanish-speaking women expressed concern that they were told to go on a diabetic "diet" and were then chastised for not eating enough. To these women, going on a "diet" meant they should eat less. They were also told that if they followed the diabetic diet, they wouldn't have such "big babies." They thought a "big" baby was a healthy baby and couldn't understand why they were being told to avoid having a larger baby. These were simple issues to fix but required knowledge of how the "diabetic teaching plan" was interpreted by the target audience. Another key factor was that the clinic was a family event; thus, all of the children were brought along. The clinic staff had been consistently irritated by the presence of large groups of children but learned that they needed to alter the clinic setup and resources to accommodate the expectations of their clients. Modifications were made based on dialogue with members of the target population that positively influenced the eventual success of the clinic's program.

This example demonstrates how use of *local knowledge* can increase the effectiveness of a community-based intervention. The participation of members of the target population also builds greater community capacity for resolution of health problems within target communities. Working with community partners, including members of the target populations, is a technique that has been used in providing services within developing countries. This type of approach ensures community *buy-in* for an intervention. It also builds networks that can continue to increase the capacity of communities to resolve other health care issues, both current and emerging (Bolton, Moore, Ferreira, Day, & Bolton, 2016; Buta et al., 2011; Kulbok et al., 2012; Zlotnick, Wright, Sanchez, Kusnir, & Te'o-Bennett, 2010).

It is essential to review literature regarding health problems, factors influencing the outcomes of interventions, and the role of families and communities in adherence to interventions. The search for evidence-based practice is important to program success. The literature review can offer the opportunity to develop additional insights that may shape interviews with members of the target and service communities. How does this target group compare to other target groups? What else should be addressed that wasn't found in the literature? For instance, a public health nurse wanted to know why parents were using emergency rooms for after-hours urgent care. A literature review found studies focused heavily on the "misuse" of emergency rooms by parents to treat urgent ambulatory care health problems, such as otitis media. Based on input from an emergency room nurse, the PHN decided to go directly to the source and asked families what their doctors had told them to do if their child became ill at night. The families indicated that they were told to take their children to the emergency room! None of the literature addressed what the families had been told to do for after-hours care. This is an example of how being open to information from a variety of sources (in this case the emergency room nurse) enhanced the PHN's understanding of the problem beyond what could be learned by solely relying on the literature.

As nurses work with community members to identify factors contributing to a health problem, individuals will begin to stand out because of their knowledge, their network capabilities, and their interest in the subject. A key factor for ensuring the success of any intervention is to appoint an **advisory group** that includes representatives from the target and service communities. Findings from interviews, literature reviews, and data analyses need to be reviewed with this advisory group. To ensure success of the advisory group, all meetings should be carefully planned, so that they are well organized, punctual, and efficient. Strategies to encourage input from the advisory group should be employed; meetings should focus on getting the advisory group to interpret findings and community feedback and to develop possible solutions. Contributions from each member should be sought and valued equally. Depending on the size of the group, it may be most effective to have some breakout sessions as well as larger group sessions. Every member should do an evaluation at the conclusion of each meeting, so that any problems can be addressed before the next meeting. Maintaining a record of these meetings—in the form of either minutes or a brief written overview—is also very helpful. Be certain to also keep a record of attendees. Maintaining a *paper trail* is always important (Fig. 12–3).

Delineating the Problem to be Addressed

With the help of the advisory group, it's important to delineate the problem or problems to be addressed. The following is a case example. A group of nurses identified

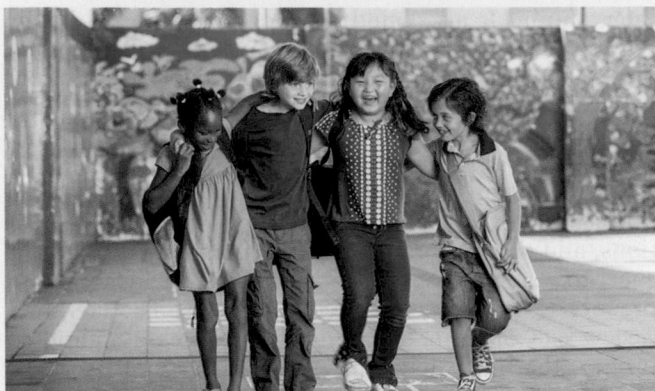

FIGURE 12-3 Educational programs for schoolchildren can address problems such as childhood obesity.

childhood obesity as a problem. Input from community members, as well as a review of data, demonstrated a greater rate of childhood obesity in a local elementary school where a high proportion of the children were African American. Although the original plan made by the nurses was to establish a special educational program for overweight children, ages 10 to 12, input from members of the service and target community indicated major problems with this approach:

1. It would be embarrassing for any child identified as needing the program.
2. Children this age usually don't pick the menu for their home or school.
3. Diet is culturally dependent, and the nurses knew very little about the dietary practices of African American families within the targeted community.

The use of an advisory group helped the nurses first identify what behavioral factors contributed to childhood obesity in the target population. These behavioral factors included the following:

- School breakfasts and lunches served were high in fat and salt, with limited fresh vegetable and fruit choices.
- Physical education classes were conducted for 45 minutes, once a week.
- No sports equipment was available for use during school recess and lunch periods.
- Participation in after-school sports cost $150 per student for uniforms and fees.
- The students aged 10 to 12 preferred to drink sodas and eat French fries for lunch.
- Most parents were working and often bought "fast food" for their children for dinner.
- Local parks were unsafe for children to play in, and there were no outdoor recreational activities that were free (at no cost).
- Children in the target group described feeling very stressed because of high homework demands and expectations to score well on national tests.
- Children in the target group indicated that they went home after school and watched TV or played video games because their parents wouldn't allow them to play outside while they were at work.

- When asked what they did when stressed, children in the target group indicated they watched TV, listened to music, played video games, and had snacks.
- The favorite after-school snacks eaten by children in the target group were macaroni and cheese from a box or packaged noodles—both of which are high in fat, carbohydrates, and salt.

Rating the Importance and Changeability of Identified Behavioral Factors

To achieve success, programs must narrow their focus to a limited number of health behaviors that can be addressed successfully within a specific time frame (Green & Kreuter, 2005; Green et al., 2014). To prioritize which behaviors to address, the authors suggest that they be rated in terms of importance and changeability. The final list should include problems that are both important and easy to change.

Importance is determined by rating how frequently the identified behavior occurs and how strongly it is linked to a health problem. The advisory group for childhood obesity ranked the importance of the identified behaviors; their ranking and rationale (basis) for the ranking can be seen in Table 12–1. For instance, the lack of available sports equipment was not rated very highly because the advisory group observed that children could be physically active without sports equipment. A highly rated item was the poor quality of the school-provided breakfasts and lunches; as a primary source of nutrition for many of the school's children, it could contribute to obesity in this population.

The advisory group was then asked to rate the changeability of the behaviors. In their classic book, Green and Kreuter (2005) indicate that those behaviors that are easiest to change:

- Are usually still developing
- Are more recently adopted
- Do not have deep roots in culture or lifestyle
- Have been attempted before with some success

The advisory group's changeability ratings for the behaviors can be seen in Table 12–2. In this round of assessments, the advisory group found that the lack of sports equipment, although not as important, could be potentially changed. This rating was based on the fact that the underfunding of the play equipment was a relatively new occurrence, and funding might be redirected if attention was brought to the problem. The poor nutritional quality of the breakfasts and lunches was seen as less changeable because of existing contracts with outside businesses to provide the meals.

After rating the identified problems based on changeability and importance, the nurses and advisory group sought to narrow their focus to specific goals. Ranking the behaviors in a simple table, as seen in Table 12–3, is suggested (Green & Kreuter, 2005; Green et al., 2014). This effort yielded a table with the problems categorized in four groups: more important/more changeable, less important/more changeable, more important/less changeable, and less important/less changeable. The issues seen as most important and changeable included fifth and sixth grade students choosing high-fat, high-sugar foods for lunch and breakfast; children feeling stressed by homework demands; and children engaging in sedentary activities.

Table 12-1 Importance of Behaviors Contributing to Childhood Obesity at Stevens Place Elementary School

Important	Basis for Rating
• School breakfasts and lunches were served that were high in fat and carbohydrate, with limited fresh vegetable and fruit choices.	A number of children ate their main meals at school, and studies have shown that high-fat, high-carbohydrate diets contribute to childhood obesity.
• Physical education classes were conducted for 45 min once a week.	Increasing exercise frequency will increase muscle mass as well as metabolic rates.
• The students aged 10–12 preferred to drink sodas and eat French fries for lunch.	Peer pressure can adversely influence food choices.
• Most parents were working and often bought "fast food" for their children for dinner.	Fast foods are high in carbohydrates and fat.
• Children in the target group described feeling very stressed because of high homework demands and expectations to score well on national tests.	High stress levels in adults contribute to obesity by increasing cortisol levels.
• Children in the target group indicated they went home after school and watched TV or played video games because their parents wouldn't allow them to play outside while they were at work.	Sedentary activities contribute to childhood obesity.
• When asked what they did when stressed, children in the target group indicated they watched TV, listened to music, played video games, and had snacks.	Sedentary activities contribute to childhood obesity.
• The favorite after-school snacks eaten by children in the target group were macaroni and cheese from a box or packaged noodles—both of which are high fat, high carbohydrate, and high salt.	These foods are high in fat and carbohydrates.
Less Important	
• There was no sports equipment available for use during school recess and lunch periods.	Children can be physically active without sports equipment.
• Participation in after-school sports cost $150 per student for uniforms and fees.	High costs for participation in sports are a deterrent for low-income children.
• Local parks were unsafe for children to play in, and there were no outdoor recreational activities that were free.	Although important, there isn't a direct linkage between the lack of safe parks and free recreation and childhood obesity.

The use of this grid enabled the advisory group to focus on more changeable and important issues. They wrote behavioral objectives for each identified factor they hoped to change. These objectives identified *who* was targeted, *what* they hoped would change or what action would be taken, *how* the change would be measured, and what the *time frame* was for achieving the expected outcome. The following are their behavioral objectives:

1. By the end of the fall semester, 75% of the fifth and sixth grade students will choose a breakfast and lunch diet that includes fruit, vegetables, protein, dairy, and starch (bread, potatoes) at each meal.
2. By the end of the school year, the teachers will schedule homework that can easily be done by a low-average student within a half hour.
3. By the end of the fall semester, all fifth and sixth grade students will be provided physically interactive games free of charge.

Factors That Influence Behavior Change: Predisposing, Reinforcing, and Enabling Factors

Three categories of factors affecting individual behavior can be addressed, as factors are delineated that contribute to successful behavioral change and create barriers to behavioral change (Green & Kreuter, 2005; Green et al., 2014). Per the PRECEDE–PROCEED model, these factors are as follows:

- **Predisposing factors** provide the rationale or *motivation* for subsequent behavior.
- **Reinforcing factors** provide a continued motivation to repeat or persist in the behavior.
- **Enabling factors** promote or facilitate the behavior based upon availability.

Predisposing factors include the knowledge, beliefs, values, attitudes, and confidence of the target population that influence their behavioral choices. Reinforcing

Table 12-2   Changeability Ratings of Behaviors Contributing to Childhood Obesity at Stevens Place Elementary School

More Changeable	Basis for Rating Behavior
There was no sports equipment available for use during school recess and lunch periods.	Trends in underfunding school play equipment are relatively recent.
The students aged 10–12 preferred to drink sodas and eat French fries for lunch.	Peer pressure often changed student behavior and could be used to encourage healthy choices.
Children in the target group described feeling very stressed because of high homework demands and expectations to score well on national tests.	Pressure for children to perform well on standardized tests is a recent phenomenon of questionable value.
When asked what they did when stressed, children in the target group indicated they watched TV, listened to music, played video games, and had snacks.	This was rated as easier to change because of the newer interactive video games that include movement.
Less Changeable	
Physical education (PE) classes were conducted for 45 min once a week.	Trends to decrease PE time per week are relatively recent—limited funding creates barriers to PE.
School breakfasts and lunches were served that were high in fat and salt, with limited fresh vegetable and fruit choices.	For a number of years, schools have contracted out for lunch services from businesses based on bids.
Participation in after-school sports cost $150 per student for uniforms and fees.	Sports have been privately funded for a number of years.
Most parents were working and often bought "fast food" for their children for dinner.	Most parents are working, and fast food restaurants have become part of the American culture.
Local parks were unsafe for children to play in, and there were no outdoor recreational activities that were free.	Funding for parks and recreation has steadily declined for a number of years.
Children in the target group indicated they went home after school and watched TV or played video games because their parents wouldn't allow them to play outside while they were at work.	This has become commonplace in the modern culture.
The favorite after-school snacks eaten by children in the target group were macaroni and cheese from a box or packaged noodles—both of which are high fat, high carbohydrate, and high salt.	These are cheap and easy foods to fix.

factors include the knowledge, values, beliefs, and attitudes of the family and friends of the target population. It also includes authority figures such as teachers or managers, as well as agency and community decision-makers, as these individuals also influence the target population. Finally, enabling factors include the availability of resources; the accessibility of resources, laws, and government support for the health behaviors or for the health program; as well as skills (Green & Kreuter, 2005; Green et al., 2014).

Table 12-3   Rankings of Behaviors Contributing to Childhood Obesity at Stevens Place Elementary School by Importance and Changeability

	More Important	Less Important
More Changeable	Fifth and sixth grade students chose high-fat, high-sugar foods for lunch and breakfast. Children stressed by homework demands Children engaged in sedentary activities (watch TV, play video games) after school.	Limited sports equipment
Less Changeable	High-fat and high-carbohydrate school food Limited physical education classes Favorite after-school snacks high fat, high carbohydrate, and high salt	Participation in after-school sports cost $150 per student. Parents often bought "fast food" for dinner. Local parks unsafe; lack of free recreational activities

The advisory group, following the PRECEDE–PROCEED model, identified the predisposing, enabling, and reinforcing factors that affected each behavioral objective. Table 12–4 shows the grid they developed for the first behavior objective—"By the end of the fall semester, 75% of the fifth and sixth grade students will choose a breakfast and lunch diet that includes fruit, vegetables, protein, dairy and starch (bread, potatoes) at each meal." For example, one enabling factor that supported the change was the identification of a community group that agreed to provide incentives to students making positive food choices. On the other hand, the lack of school funding for educational intervention programs for obese children was seen as inhibiting change.

The advisory group decided to establish a peer-mentoring program, in which student leaders would work with the advisory group and model food choices from all food groups. The advisory group had teachers nominate students for this intervention. The principal allowed the nominated students to attend special educational classes conducted by the nurses to increase their knowledge about the food groups. The nurses worked collaboratively with the students to ensure their teaching approaches were effective. Students suggested rewards that the students could work for that would encourage them to eat more balanced meals. One of the rewards that students felt should be offered is sports equipment for student use during recess and lunch periods. One local community-based organization offered to sponsor a fund-raising event that would allow them to purchase sports equipment for the school.

Grids similar to that shown in Table 12–4 were developed for the remaining two objectives. This process allowed the nurses and the advisory group to develop program intervention strategies that maximized their potential to achieve desired outcomes. Working with the advisory group, the nurses developed a program plan map outlining activities for each objective, as well as the individual responsible for the activity, the date by which the activities were to be accomplished, and how outcomes would be documented. Display 12–1 shows the program plan that was developed for the first objective. This type of mapping allows the group to stay focused, share responsibilities, and monitor outcomes. For instance, student leaders were tasked with modeling balanced food choices at breakfast and lunch and completing a checklist of their food choices each day. The nurses were tasked with meeting each week with the student leaders to provide peer-mentoring training sessions.

Working with the advisory group allowed the nurses to contextualize the problem about which they were concerned within the target community. The advisory group ensured that the nurses identified solutions that were culturally acceptable, appropriate, and ultimately effective. This process also helped them to develop outcome measures that were consistent with the concerns of the community. As data were gathered, findings could be interpreted with input from the advisory group. This approach grounded the findings and ensured that interpretations were culturally consistent with the target population. Evaluation was facilitated by clearly defined goals that could be measured against actual results.

Table 12–4   Predisposing, Enabling, and Reinforcing Factors That Influence Meal Choices of Fifth and Sixth Grade Students Attending Stevens Place Elementary School

Factors That Support the Change	Factors That Inhibit the Change
Predisposing	
Fifth and sixth grade students tend to believe what they are taught by teachers; thus educating them on food choices could positively affect their choices. Fifth and sixth grade students like to be similar to other children their age.	Fifth and sixth grade students are beginning to feel some independence from adults and may like to eat what they want vs. what adults tell them they should do. Students like the taste of sodas and French fries more than balanced food choices.
Reinforcing	
Students emulate behavior of popular students. Teachers and parents are concerned about poor food choices being made by fifth and sixth grade students. Local community leaders expressed outrage about the obesity rates of African American children at Stevens Place Elementary School.	Media shows teens eating French fries and drinking sodas.
Enabling	
A local community-based organization has offered to provide incentives to students who model positive food choices. The principal has offered to allow time for the nurses to work with an identified group of student leaders to educate them about modeling better food choices. The local Parent–Teacher Association has offered to help monitor student behavioral changes.	The school has no funding for educational intervention programs for obese children.

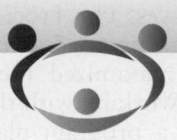

DISPLAY 12-1 SAMPLE PROJECT PLAN MAP

Goal: Fifth and sixth grade students attending Stevens Place Elementary School will engage in behaviors designed to decrease their obesity levels.

Objective	Activity	Who Is Responsible	Due Date	Evaluation
1. By the end of the fall semester, 75% of the fifth and sixth grade students will choose a breakfast and lunch diet that includes fruit, vegetables, protein, dairy, and starch (bread, potatoes) at each meal.	1a. Teachers will identify student leaders from the fifth and sixth grade classes who can participate in leadership training for peer mentoring.	1a. J. Jamison, school principal	September 20, 2012	1a. A list of student leaders will be available for review.
	1b. Students will be approached to participate in the program.	1b. J. Jamison, school principal	September 25, 2012	1b. Student response will be documented.
	1c. Permission slips for student leaders to participate will be sent home to parents.	1c. J. Jamison, school principal	September 27, 2012	1c. Copies of permission slips will be maintained by the principal.
	1d. Nurses will meet with the student leaders weekly during the designated time period to provide them training for their peer mentoring.	1d. Nurses	September 28–October 31, 2012	1d. Copies of the meeting notes and educational plans will be maintained by the nurses.
	1e. Student leaders will model balanced food choices during breakfast and lunch meals.	1e. Student leaders	November 1–December 22, 2012	1e. Student leaders will provide a checklist of their food choices to the principal at the end of each day.
	1f. A checklist of possible food choices for students' breakfast and lunch meals using the school menus will be developed.	1f. Nurses	December 1, 2012	
	1g. PTA volunteers will monitor student food choices during breakfast and lunch meals 1 day each week for 3 weeks.	1g. PTA volunteers	December 3, 12, and 17, 2012	1g. Results of checklists will be tabulated and available for review.

This particular case study is an example of the program development needed in schools to address obesity and overweight. The *Guide to Community Preventive Services* (Community Preventive Services Task Force, 2014) systematic review of published school-based programs indicated that more evidence was needed to determine the effectiveness of these types of programs. Although they noted some positive effects in the studies reviewed, the results were too varied to make any conclusions. Their review supports continued efforts to demonstrate program effectiveness in school-based programs. Clear and verifiable outcome measures are needed.

EVALUATION OF OUTCOMES

The IOM (2002) report, *The Future of the Public's Health in the 21st Century*, called for examining the benefits that accreditation of governmental public health departments might bring. Responding to this challenge, the Exploring Accreditation Steering Committee published *Final Recommendations for a Voluntary National Accreditation Program for State and Local Public Health Departments* in 2006, outlining this first-ever accreditation program for health departments (Benjamin, Fallon, Jarris, & Libbey, 2006). Later, participating health departments characterized the benefits of accreditation as:

- Helping them to identify their strengths
- Documenting their capacity for delivery of core public health functions and 10 Essential Public Health Services
- Promoting transparency in government and accountability to the community, policy-makers, and stakeholders, as well as communication with governing body
- Improving the processes of management and competitive abilities in opportunities for funding
- Stimulating quality improvement and organizational performance (Centers for Disease Control and Prevention [CDC], 2016b).

In 2008, 17 states were selected to lead a national initiative that would advance accreditation and quality improvement among public health departments (Robert Wood Johnson Foundation, 2014). Areas explored by these states in the initiative included culturally appropriate services, use of health data, and integration of customer service into health programs. The Public Health Accreditation Board is a nonprofit entity that is the independent accrediting body. With support from the Centers for Disease Control and Prevention, Office for State, Tribal, Local, and Territorial Support (2016); and the Robert Wood Johnson Foundation, the Public Health Accreditation Board was launched in 2011 and accredited the first cohort of health departments in 2013 utilizing Standards and Measures version 1.0. Version 1.5 of the Standards and Measures came into effect during July 2014, adding ethics, data management, communication science, workforce development, and equity as important new areas for evaluation. The National Association of County and City Health Officials (2016) offers resources that assist health departments to assess the feasibility of becoming accredited and tools to further support a successful accreditation process if departments choose to

seek accreditation. Of the 12 domains in Standards and Measures version 1.5 for accreditation, three are particularly applicable to program development and outcome measurement (Public Health Accreditation Board, 2014):

Domain 4: Engage with the community to identify and address health problems.

Domain 9: Evaluate and continually improve health department processes, programs, and interventions.

Domain 10: Contribute to and apply the evidence base of public health.

As more agencies seek accreditation, there will likely be increased pressure to achieve this status at all levels (local, county, or state) to demonstrate excellence. Public health nurses can work with state and local health departments to achieve accreditation. Accreditation not only serves to promote high-quality services to the public and demonstrate a commitment to meeting the specific needs in these communities but also supports the need for public health nursing services to meet those challenges.

The previous section of this chapter discussed the issues of program planning, implementation, and evaluation as they related to a small health program. This section focuses on the programs and services provided by agencies. Although the scope of the effort to address outcome evaluation is understandably broader, the concepts are essentially the same. The accreditation initiative has raised the issue of demonstrating in real and objective terms the outcomes resulting from health promotion programs provided through public health agencies. The principles discussed have relevance in many community settings and should be considered whenever health promotion programs and services are provided. Public health nurses at local, state, and global levels are instrumental to many of the health promotion programs and services offered through health departments; their expertise with and understanding of the communities served are invaluable to assuring ongoing quality assurance and outcome evaluation.

An important step in evaluating any program entails constructing a clear model of what the program is meant to achieve (Cornell University, 2016). **Logic models**, or pathway logic models, are often used to articulate the causal relationship between planned program activities and the expected outcome. Whereas community problems may be easy to recognize, it is harder to determine which strategies offer the highest likelihood for successful change and, more importantly, what evidence will indicate progress or success. In their seminal work for the Annie E. Casey Foundation, the Organizational Research Services (2004) report on community change theories and underscore that a helpful change theory can be used as a road map for planning and accomplishing individual and community change. Based on the change theory, logic models offer a clear picture of the desired impact, or outcome, the changes that need to be realized in order to achieve the outcome, the activities and resulting outputs that will affect the change, and the inputs necessary to carry out the planned activities. In other words, logic models provide a process for planning backward in order to implement forward (Allmark, Baxter, Goyder, Guillaume, & Crofton-Martin, 2013; Naimoli, Frymus, Wuliji, Franco, & Newsome, 2014).

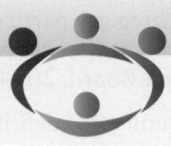

DISPLAY 12–2 CAUSAL PATHWAY FRAMEWORK

Plan backward; implement forward! Plan this way:

| Inputs | ← | Activities | ← | Outputs | ← | Outcome | ← | Impact |

Implement this way:

| Inputs | → | Activities | → | Outputs | → | Outcome | → | Impact |

Causal Pathway Framework hypothesizes that this set of inputs and activities will result in these products and services, which will facilitate these changes in the population, which will contribute to the desired impact (Kellogg Foundation, 2006). See Display 12–2 for a diagram of the causal pathway.

An example of the use of logic model for program planning, monitoring, and evaluation of a blood safety project in Kenya is shown in Display 12–3.

Use of these types of models can be very helpful in developing new programs and can help guide community health nurses who are not familiar with methods of

DISPLAY 12–3 CASE STUDY ON LOGIC MODELS FOR PROGRAM PLANNING, MONITORING AND EVALUATION

Overview
A logic model is a framework that graphically depicts causal relationships between elements of a program and is used for program planning, monitoring, and evaluation. When using a logic model for program planning, focus is placed on the ultimate outcomes or results, and planners work backward to determine the following key aspects:

Example of using a logic model to design, monitor, and evaluate a blood safety project in Kenya

Inputs	Activities	Outputs	Outcomes	Impact
• Human resource	• Blood donor mobilization, education, and recruitment	• Individuals reached with information on blood donation	• Improved equity and access to safe blood and blood products	• Reduced mortality related to blood and blood component issues
• ICT resources	• Blood collection	• Facilities for blood bank and transfusion	• 100% testing for TTIs	
• Financial support	• Blood testing and grouping	• Blood donors mobilized	• Increased proportion of repeat blood donors	• Reduced morbidity related to blood and blood product issues
• Test kits and consumables	• Preparation of blood components	• Blood units collection	• Increased knowledge on the importance of blood donation	
• Blood bags	• Training of staff	• Screening for transfusion transmissible infections (TTIs)	• Increased proportion of donors notified of their TTIs test results	• Reduced incidence and prevalence of TTIs
• Technical assistance	• Mentorship of staff	• Blood donor notification and referral		
	• On-site support of staff	• Blood components prepared, stored, and transported		
	• Blood donor notification	• Appropriate use of blood and blood components		
	• Stakeholder data review meetings	• Data review meetings held		
	• Surveillance	• Individuals trained in blood transfusion services		

(Contributing Authors: Missie Oindo, BA, MCHD and Serah Malaba-Kambale, Bsc, MPH, PRINCE2® Practitioner, both of Kenya)

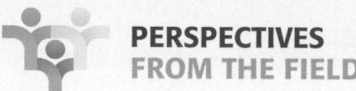

program planning, monitoring, and evaluation. See Perspectives: From the Field.

Setting Measurable Goals and Objectives

Using the logic model as a guide, planned programs should have specific goals to help identify who the program is supposed to serve, what services are provided, the length of time the services are to be provided, and the resources that are needed. Then, measurable objectives are developed that describe the expected outcomes. Use of selected verbs indicates the expected level of achievement, such as "clients will be able to demonstrate safe administration of insulin after three home visits" or "parents will have their infants' recommended immunizations

up to date by 24 months of age." Goal setting is imperative when developing an educational program for an entire health program or service (see Chapter 11). These statements of measurable goals are then examined during the program evaluation. Without such statements, accurate evaluations cannot be conducted.

One helpful acronym, SMART has been attributed to a number of authors since the 1960s including a 1981 publication by G.T. Doran (Morrison, 2010). Regardless of the original source, the acronym is frequently used in developing outcome measures. The general consensus is that SMART stands for *Specific, Measureable, Attainable, Relevant,* and *Timely,* and often, *Evaluate* and *Reevaluate* are added (SMARTER). Display 12–4 describes specific questions that must be asked and answered at each step of the SMART process.

In evaluating programs and care, outcomes must be measured against certain standards. *Standards* are generic guidelines of expected functioning. They can focus on the client, the caregiver, or the organization (finances). All care and services must also be measured against these guidelines. The core standards of care, practice, and finance must be integrated and compatible if they are to ensure quality care.

Evaluating Outcomes

The outcomes or results of care (having the right things happen) are the desired effect of the structure (having the right things) and the processes (doing the right things). The focus on client outcomes demands continued analysis of structure and process, because these two components produce the desirable or undesirable outcomes. With the focus on outcomes, there has been an impetus to include positive outcome terms such as improved health status, functional ability, perceived quality of life, and client satisfaction. Client satisfaction is measured by how closely a client's expectations of nursing care match the perception of the nursing care actually received (Gordon,

---

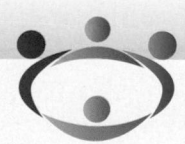

DISPLAY 12–4 DEVELOPING SMART OBJECTIVES

Specific
- What: What do we want to accomplish?
- Why: Specific reasons, purpose, or benefits of accomplishing the goal.
- Who: Who is involved?
- Where: Identify a location.
- Which: Identify requirements and constraints.

Measurable
- How much?
- How many?
- How will we know when it is accomplished?

Attainable
- How can the goal be accomplished?

Relevant
- Does this seem worthwhile?
- Is this the right time?
- Does this match our other efforts/needs?
- Are we the right group or agency?

Time-Bound or Timely
- When?
- What can we do 6 months from now?
- What can we do 6 weeks from now?
- What can we do today?

From Doran, G. T. (1981). There's a S.M.A.R.T. way to write management's goals and objectives. *Management Review (American Management Association Forum),* 70(11) 35–36; Meyer, P. J. (2003). *What would you do if you knew you couldn't fail? Creating S.M.A.R.T Goals. Attitude is everything: If you want to succeed above and beyond.* Waco, TX: Meyer Resource Group, Inc.; Wikipedia. (2016). *SMART criteria.* Retrieved from https://en.wikipedia.org/wiki/SMART_criteria

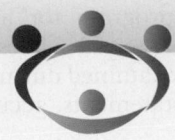

DISPLAY 12–5 CAUSAL PATHWAY FRAMEWORK EXAMPLE

Inputs	→	Where inputs available and utilized?
Activities	→	Were activities performed as planned?
Outputs	→	Were outputs produced?
Outcome	→	Were expected outcomes or effects observed?
Impact	→	Did the project achieve the desired long-term impact?

2016). Client satisfaction, as one outcome measurement, can be determined by a telephone survey or a mailed questionnaire as well as confidential online surveys.

Using the causal pathway logic model as a guide, it is easy to link between planned program implementation and evaluation of success at all levels. See Display 12–5 for an example using a causal pathway logic model.

If the responses indicate that a program is meeting its goals, maintaining set standards, and having positive client outcomes and satisfied clients, the program is providing quality care. However, the accuracy of using outcomes as a primary measure of quality care is limited, because some clients have unsatisfactory outcomes despite receiving good care. Factors other than specific health interventions influence outcomes. These factors include a client's adherence to medically prescribed treatments; the progress of chronic or terminal disease beyond the capabilities of medicine, nursing care, or client behaviors; and the client's ability to respond to care as a result of such situations as a compromised immune system. Public health nurses need to keep such factors in mind when evaluating care.

Quality indicators of client outcomes are the quantitative measures of a client's response to care (Gordon, 2016). Defining and quantifying client outcomes from these indicators are worthwhile processes that enable the nursing staff to evaluate the results of the care they provide. The goal of care in the community is successful client outcomes. By starting with measurable indicators, successful outcomes can be demonstrated in quantifiable terms. When client care meets the standards set, client satisfaction—another quality outcome indicator—is greater.

Quality indicators are part of the broader quality management program and are used to determine goal achievement. A chart audit is a useful method by which to measure the frequency of quality indicator occurrence. For example, an agency may have a quality indicator such as "all infants younger than 6 months of age are weighed on each home visit." Every fifth chart of infants visited in March, June, September, and December during a designated year is audited for documentation of the number of home visits and the number of infant weights recorded. A sampling of charts is sufficient to measure goal achievement and specific quality indicators. It is generally accepted that a sample of 20 randomly selected cases will provide useful information. If the population to be sampled numbers more than 200, some sources recommend that the sample include more than 20 cases.

Quantifying the indicators also can be accomplished through a rate or ratio of events for a defined population and time frame. Such indicators can be tailored to express almost any patient outcome. For example, in Display 12–6, the nursing staff sets a standard for the number of urinary tract infections (UTIs) the agency will tolerate in clients with indwelling urinary catheters (perhaps 5% to 7%, depending on client age,

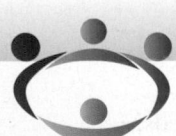

DISPLAY 12–6 QUANTIFYING OUTCOME INDICATORS

$$\text{Outcome indicators} = \frac{\text{Number of patient care events}}{\text{Total number of clients of total number of times at risk for event during a given period}}$$

Example:

$$\text{Occurrence of urinary tract infections in clients with indwelling urinary catheters} = \frac{\begin{array}{c}\text{Number of clients experiencing urinary tract infections related}\\\text{to long-term use of indwelling urinary catheters from}\\\text{January 1 to March 1, 2012}\end{array}}{\begin{array}{c}\text{Number of clients with long-term indwelling urinary catheters}\\\text{from January 1 to March 1, 2012}\end{array}}$$

diagnosis, family support, and home environment). In another situation, a community/public health nursing service has a standard to make home visits within 5 days of delivery to first-time mothers and babies born at one hospital 95% of the time. To evaluate this goal, the dates of initial home visits to first-time mothers and the birth dates of the infants are measured from a sample of client records during several measurement periods. These are both examples of assessing quality outcome indicators.

It is necessary to have indicators when setting standards in order to measure the success and quality of programs at home or in the community. The same types of indicators are used in acute care settings, with the focus appropriate to that population. If the standards are being met, but client outcomes are unacceptable, the process indicators are explored for possible areas of weakness. Such areas may need further study to identify the cause of the poor client outcomes. For example, a process indicator such as the catheter-care protocol used by an agency or the communication system between hospital and health department nurses may be examined to determine, respectively, the cause of infections or the reason why initial home visits are delayed. In addition, Medicaid and Medicare regulations in some states mandate that a percentage of records be audited each year.

While striving for excellence and best practices, agencies use the benchmarking process (Ettorchi-Tardy, Levif, & Michel, 2012). **Benchmarking** uses continuous, collaborative, and systematic processes for measuring and examining internal programs' strengths and weaknesses; benchmarking includes studying another's processes in order to improve one's own (Diffenderfer, Dunham-Taylor, & Malcolm, 2015). Internal benchmarking occurs within the organization, between departments or programs. External benchmarking occurs between similar agencies providing like services. For example, a home care agency may have developed a clinical pathway that has proved useful with clients with congestive heart failure; another agency could benefit by using the same clinical pathway. In another example, an agency may use clinical practice guidelines obtained from a specialty organization along with information from a national database; another agency could benefit from this knowledge. In this way, an agency identifies what is achievable while comparing and contrasting how others provide quality services. One example of benchmarking is a descriptive, comparative study of benchmark attainment by maternal and child health clients using the Omaha System (discussed later in this chapter and in Chapter 14). This study supported the use of benchmarking both to compare individual progress toward benchmark standards and to assess overall attainment of standards between programs offering similar services (Monsen et al., 2011a).

Role of the Nurse in Quality Measurement and Improvement

Although nurses who deliver care directly to clients are not managers, as such, improving quality is a "management" activity. This is not only true of administration personnel but of the practicing nurses, as members of the team (Fig. 12–4). Public health nurses may or may not be responsible for a staff or agency budget and functioning,

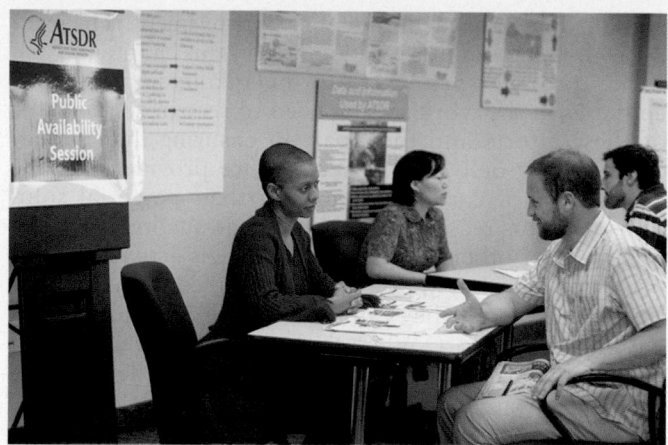

FIGURE 12–4 PHNs are team members in quality improvement.

but they may be responsible for managing a caseload of clients with needs of varying degrees of urgency. With judicious use of the resources available, they must provide priority services that promote the highest possible level of personal and group functioning and health. Any activities the public health nurse engages in to realize these goals contribute to the quality management program.

Some quality improvement activities for public health nurses include daily prioritizing of care needs for a caseload of clients, seeking supervision or skills development for a difficult case, systematizing charting so that needed documentation is efficiently completed (e.g., using flow sheets to chart maternal–child health visits), proposing better ways to organize care of chronically ill clients, and establishing new agency procedures. All of these actions demonstrate that nurses are evaluating their work and looking for ways to improve care. Staff meetings, peer review, and case conferences are common settings for nurses to bring the lessons of their practices to the larger group for examination and potential adoption.

It is the role of nursing administration to develop a formalized quality management program that includes a three-pronged focus, based on a classic approach to quality management: (1) review organizational structure, personnel, and environment; (2) focus on standards of nursing care and methods of delivering nursing care (process); and (3) focus on the outcomes of that care (Donabedian, 2003). These formal evaluations include peer review audits (documented care delivered by peers), client satisfaction assessments, review of agency policies and procedures, analysis of demographic information, and the like (American Nurses Association, 2013; Issel, 2014; Stubbs & Achat, 2011). The issue of quality and safety has more recently been addressed through the QSEN project (QSEN, 2014). Building on the IOM reports *To Err is Human: Building a Safer Health System* (1999), *Keeping Patients Safe: Transforming the Work Environment for Nurses* (2004), and *The Future of Nursing: Leading Change, Advancing Health* (2011), the QSEN project provides a framework for nursing education. It also forms a sound basis for community health program evaluation, especially as it relates to professional quality. The QSEN competencies are consistent with the

Donabedian approach to quality improvement. The project is discussed in more detail later in this chapter.

Nurses who are new to formal quality improvement activities in the work setting need to recognize the value of these efforts and their part in ensuring that quality care is being delivered. Direct service providers are the best judges of care problems and their potential solutions. For this reason, it is critical that quality assurance reviews and other quality improvement activities focus on issues relevant to staff and client concerns and be structured so that they can be accomplished quickly and with minimal effort. When these activities are clear, concise, and well integrated into daily routines, they become less time-consuming, and staff members can see the positive client outcomes as rewards for their contributions to the process. Moreover, when health care providers have the opportunity to systematically examine the care they provide, they can generate useful ideas for improving that care and can identify care issues sooner.

Whether small or large, health care agencies are complex organizations with interrelated components. The nursing staff has input into or some control over the quality of care delivered to clients who use the services of the agency. The following paragraphs review the nurse's role in each of the three areas of structure, process, and outcomes.

Structure

The organizational structure and financial stability of the agency should allow the mission statement or philosophy to be realized (Dunham-Taylor, 2015). The agency should be client focused, with sufficient resources to maintain present services and introduce additional services as needed. Public agencies need to operate within budget and also have a well-developed system of acquiring additional funding for new services through grants and contract expansion. Private agencies should operate efficiently enough to realize a profit that encourages the owners and boards of directors to continue to support the services. They should look for additional ways to solicit clients, in addition to employing highly motivated and qualified staff.

Process

The agency should maintain standards set by the professional staff that comply with or surpass those recommended by the relevant accrediting bodies (Sills, 2015). The staff is encouraged to contribute to the evaluation of the standards and to revise them as needed. Staff members need to keep themselves current by attending in-service training sessions and acquiring additional education appropriate to their job requirements. The staff members work collaboratively with others across disciplines to improve the quality of care given in the community by using a variety of participative management tools (e.g., audit instruments, peer review). The agency is supportive of its staff and the needs of individuals. Staff turnover is minimal because employee values are compatible with the goals of the agency. Administration and staff have a compatible working relationship. A system of quality review is in place, and each staff member contributes to this process as a member of a peer review committee or quality improvement or assurance committee. Staff members also listen to clients and provide an outlet to evaluate the care received (e.g., questionnaires, surveys, interviews), and the agency acts on client suggestions and comments.

Outcomes

All services an agency provides should be reviewed periodically to determine whether standards are meeting the present needs of their population and whether the nursing staff are implementing these standards (Dunham-Taylor, 2015). The nursing services used most frequently, such as well-child care, self-care education with chronically ill adults, and various screening programs, are excellent places to begin the review. Usually, these services involve the entire nursing staff and consume a significant amount of nursing care time.

The focus on commonly served high-risk groups presents an opportunity to optimize care delivery as well as to benefit high-risk clients. Children living in neighborhoods that are known to have high lead toxicity rates from leaded paint in older homes stand to benefit tremendously from a consistently implemented lead screening, treatment, and advocacy program. Without review, such a program may not achieve its goals of decreasing toxic levels of lead affecting the area's children.

Incidents of poor client outcomes are important areas for further study. Through clinic or home visit records, community nurses can routinely review documentation of deceased or hospitalized clients to assess whether any aspect of the clinic's care or home visit activities might have prevented these occurrences. For instance, the case of a child with repeated high serum lead levels that requires hospitalization for chelation might stimulate a clinic's examination of the adequacy of parent education regarding environmental sources of lead. The clinic could also explore the effectiveness of its advocacy with the area's lead-abatement staff to ensure needed repairs in leaded homes and the removal of families to safe housing while repairs are being made.

As another example, a review of the charts of hospitalized clients who take multiple medications can be conducted to ascertain whether teaching or compliance issues regarding medication contributed to each client's hospitalization. The results may prompt a change in home visit teaching techniques, an increase in the frequency of visits, or a change in vital sign parameters for notifying a physician. Persistence of problems and deficiencies could be a clue that the public health nurse needs additional education in this area or that the nurse's caseload is too heavy and therefore exceeds the ability of the nurse to provide minimally expected care. Once the cause is determined, implementation of appropriate changes can commence, after allowing adequate time for the staff to address critical issues. Should additional education be needed, it is the responsibility of the coordinating, in-service, or staff education nurse to provide or arrange for the needed education.

Given adequate resources, including sufficient time, information, and support, good care is the norm. Occasionally, quality-of-care problems result from an individual provider's performance. Recommendations are made for counseling or another type of intervention by that person's supervisor, and appropriate corrective action should be taken to resolve the problem and preserve the employee's potential contributions as a successful team member.

Identification of quality health care characteristics and "checkpoints" for quality helps the community/public health care practitioner recognize the quality indicators of best practice. These also give public health nurses direction for their role in quality measurement and improvement. This role is grounded in the structure, process, and outcomes of caregiving and services provided.

MODELS USEFUL IN PROGRAM EVALUATION

Models of client caregiving are based on structure, process, and outcome; ideally, they provide *structure* to guide nurses through the *nursing process* to reach desired *client outcomes*. Each of the following models has all three components; some work more effectively than others, depending on the agency and its philosophy.

Donabedian Model

Donabedian (1966, 1969, 1981, 1985, 2003), the country's premier researcher on health care quality, proposed a model for the structure, process, and outcome of quality that has been widely used as the framework for more elaborate models. The care environment structure—from philosophy to facility resources to personnel—is the first component. Next are the processes responsible for improving or stabilizing the client's health status, such as standards, attitudes, and effectiveness of tools used in caregiving (e.g., nursing care plans). Finally, the resultant outcomes are causally linked indicators of quality, such as client health care goals and effectiveness of service. The Donabedian model is recognized as a simplistic and basic method of measuring quality. Evaluation of this model found that the concepts were relevant to common domains of nursing and that it is helpful in program evaluation (Cohen & Shang, 2015). Structure, process, and outcome can be depicted in a box-shaped model (see Fig. 12–5).

Quality Health Outcomes Model

Mitchell, Ferketich, and Jennings (1998) took the time-tested Donabedian model a step further. The Quality Health Outcomes Model includes the client in the model and proposes a two-dimensional relationship among components. Interventions always act through the system and the client, creating a dynamic model. The uniqueness of this model is the postulate that there are dynamic reciprocal relationships, and it has been used in studies as varied as organizing variable choices in acute and community care research, large multistate studies examining nurse skill and staffing mix with adverse patient events, and nursing care/patient satisfaction in several report cards on acute care. Self-care studies in chronic disease management, health-related quality of life, and health promotion studies have also benefited from the use of this model (Mitchell & Lang, 2004). A major criticism of other models is that they do not lend themselves to the population focus of community/public health nursing. However, this model includes community as a client. Cohen and Shang (2015) found that assumptions of reciprocal relationships in the model, as well as its ability for multilevel analysis and culturally sensitive inputs, served to broaden its appeal and applicability in a variety of areas. Figure 12–6 depicts the Quality Health Outcomes Model.

Omaha System

Also discussed in Chapter 14, the Omaha System has measurement approaches that make it a useful model for determining the quality of nursing care provided to individuals, families, and communities. Evaluation focuses on process indicators, client outcome measures, and satisfaction with care (Martin, Leak, & Aden, 1997). With the use of this multifocal approach, measurement of nursing practice becomes comprehensive. Although originally designed to evaluate care to individuals and families, the model has been modified to include the community (Martin, 2005). This revision was prompted by the wider use of the model to document population-based and community-level interventions. Community is defined as "groups, schools, clinics, neighborhoods, or other larger geographic areas that share a common physical environment and ownership of a health-related problem" (Martin, 2005, p. 464). Examples of the application of this model to community settings include a study of

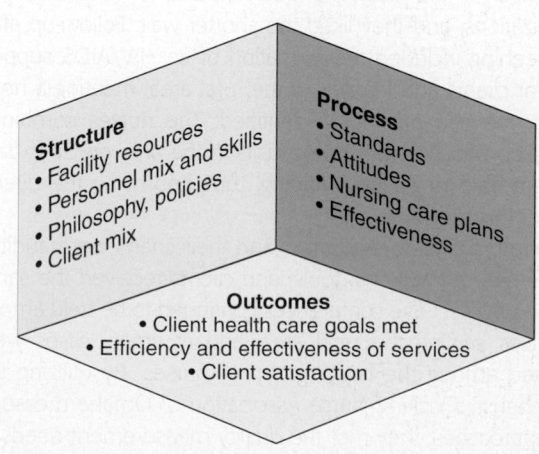

FIGURE 12–5 Structure, process, and outcome of quality model.

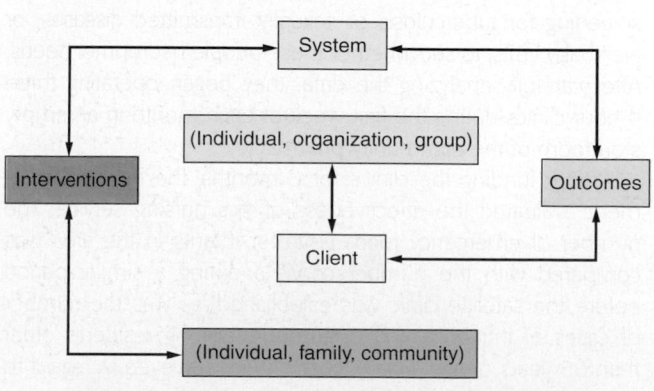

FIGURE 12–6 Quality Health Outcomes Model.

public health nursing interventions with at-risk families (Monsen, Radosevich, Kerr, & Fulkerson, 2011b), as well as nurse-managed wellness centers for vulnerable populations (Thompson, Monsen, Wanamaker, Augustyniak, & Thompson, 2012). In this model, outcomes are rated in terms of knowledge (what the client knows), behavior (what the client does), and status (how the client is). This approach allows for quantifying a range of severity, as well as progress either toward or away from optimal health. Ongoing monitoring of these aspects as they relate to individual, family, or community problems allows for evaluation of nursing interventions—a necessary component of both quality assurance and outcome assessment. For instance, individuals enrolled in a 6-week health promotion program on weight management can be assessed initially for their knowledge of healthy eating and exercise, their current behaviors relative to both, and their current health status (e.g., body mass index [BMI]). You can assess program outcomes by measuring those same indicators and then comparing the initially obtained individual and aggregated data with the data collected after the program is concluded. Whereas individual positive changes, such as decreased BMI, are a positive indicator, the impact on the entire group is of even more importance in terms of community-level health status. See From the Case Files I for an example using the Omaha System.

The Omaha System provides an organized method to assess individual-, family-, and community-level health. With ongoing research efforts, the utility of the model with respect to program evaluation will be enhanced. Program evaluation studies such as exploring the models utility in nondirect patient interventions by nurse managers (Monsen & Newsom, 2011); use of the system in acute care settings (Monsen, Schenk, Schyeler, & Schiavenato, 2015), as a method of quantifying care coordination (Popejoy et al., 2015); and the body of evidence created from this standardized data (Bowles, 2011) continue to support the broader use of the Omaha System to assess programmatic effectiveness in many settings, including community health.

The Quality Practice Setting Attributes Model

This model, developed by the College of Nurses of Ontario in Canada, provides the foundational framework for a unique quality improvement approach to creating quality practice environments. The College of Nurses of Ontario is the regulatory body for registered nurses and registered practical nurses in the Province of Ontario, Canada; it has functions similar to those of the Board of Registered Nursing in each state in the United States. The Quality Practice Setting Attributes Model is used as a tool to assist in ensuring the quality of nursing practice and the nursing profession by promoting continuing competence among nurses in Canada (MacKay & Risk, 2001). The model provided the framework of the Practice Setting Consultation Program (MacKay & Risk, 2001); later

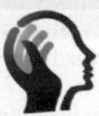

From the Case Files I

Using the Omaha System to Evaluate a Rural Satellite Clinic

A group of county health department public health nurses conducted an assessment of a community's need for a satellite health clinic in a rural part of the county. The nurses gathered data on population needs, age, health status, and accessibility to health care by surveying clients who lived in rural zip code areas and used the main health department. They also conducted a survey by mail of additional residents who were not presently using the health department clinic system for immunizations, screening for tuberculosis or sexually transmitted diseases, or well-baby visits, to see whether these people had unmet needs. After carefully analyzing the data, they began operating three 4-hour clinics during the first week of each month in an empty storeroom of the community pharmacy.

After funding the clinics for 6 months, the health department evaluated the effectiveness of this nursing service. The number of emergency room visits for infants in the area was compared with the number of visits during a similar period before the satellite clinic was established, as was the number of cases of influenza and pneumonia among residents older than 65 years of age. Finally, clients were surveyed in regard to

their satisfaction with nursing care and services and were asked if there were any additional services they needed. Survey outcomes were supportive of continuing the clinics and adding an additional well-baby clinic, a dental clinic, and a prenatal clinic. Clients liked the convenience—older residents did not have to drive the 35 miles to the main clinic, parents were able to keep more closely to the recommended schedule for their children's immunizations, and they liked the shorter wait. Follow-up after HIV screening included the formation of an HIV/AIDS support group for clients and families in the rural area, meeting a need that no one had previously identified. The nurses combined clinic responsibilities with home visits in the area on clinic days and were able to do case finding, thus improving the overall health of this rural area.

The nurses were evaluated, and their charts were audited with the use of traditional tools, and clients received the same periodic surveys. Case conferences continued to be held among the nurses serving the rural area, and at times, cases were presented among the larger group of nurses. By utilizing the comprehensive Visiting Nurse Association of Omaha measurement approaches, they met the quality measurement needs of a population.

known as the Quality Practice Environment Consultation Program (MacKay, 2007) of the College and Association of Registered Nurses of Alberta (CARNA), the program was developed to assist nurses and agencies in determining and advancing workplace characteristics that support the quality of professional nursing practice and certification (Brookes & Tansey, 2003; Patry, 2006; Saxe-Braithwaite, Carlton, & Bass, 2009).

This nurse-centered model of quality improvement is designed to contribute to the best possible health outcomes for the client, regardless of health care setting. The components of this quality assurance program include reflective nursing practice, practice review, and practice setting consultation. The first two components focus on nurses' individual responsibility for maintaining competence throughout their career; the practice setting consultation focuses on the practice environment in which nursing care is delivered. The governing body for nurses in Ontario, Canada, has relied on the Quality Practice Setting Attributes Model to improve nursing care quality in their province. As mentioned earlier, it also serves as a framework in Alberta (CARNA) in their nursing quality practice

program. The model identifies seven key systems attributes in the work environment that create a quality practice setting. Figure 12–7 portrays this model and its components.

Quality and Safety Education for Nurses

Both the Magnet Recognition Program and the Pathway to Excellence Program focus on quality outcomes (similar to nurse-centered quality improvement in the Quality Practice Setting Attributes Model just discussed). Magnet hospitals have been shown to provide better work environments for nurses and have better nurse staffing and satisfaction measurements as well as patient satisfaction and outcomes (Dunham-Taylor, 2015; Kutney-Lee et al., 2015). As was mentioned earlier, the issue of quality and safety in health care was brought to the public's attention with the groundbreaking IOM (1999) report on medical errors and the subsequent 2004 report that focused on nursing quality and safety. This recognition promoted the funding by the Robert Wood Johnson Foundation of what has become known as the QSEN project. The purpose of the project is "the challenge of preparing future nurses who will have the knowledge, skills and attitudes (KSAs) necessary to

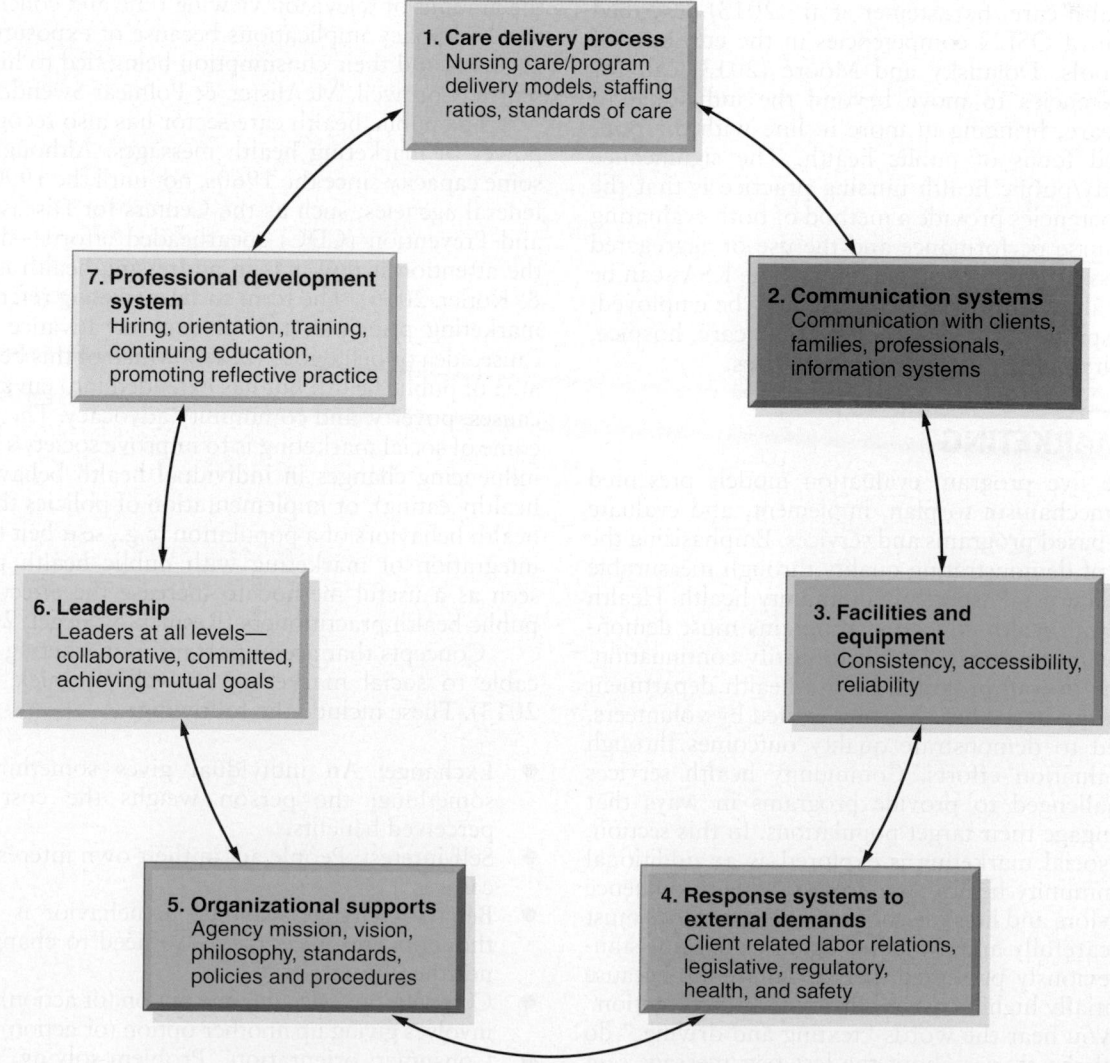

FIGURE 12–7 The Quality Practice Setting Attributes Model.

continuously improve the quality and safety of the health care systems within which they work" (QSEN, 2014, para. 1). Although QSEN is not presented in a diagrammatic form, it is nevertheless a model of quality improvement. Consistent with the taxonomy of educational objectives (Bloom, 1956; Miller, Linn & Gronlund, 2013) as discussed in Chapter 11, the foundational competencies delineated by KSAs can also be described as falling within the cognitive, psychomotor, and affective domains. The KSAs are also similar to the Omaha System outcome measures of knowledge (what the client knows), behavior (what the client does), and status (how the client is). Specific to QSEN (2014, para. 4), the prelicensure KSAs include:

- Patient-centered care
- Teamwork and collaboration
- Evidence-based practice
- Quality improvement
- Safety
- Informatics

Of most relevance to community/public health program assessment is quality improvement, which is defined as the use of data to monitor the outcomes of care and improving methods for changing quality and safety in health care. Barnsteiner et al. (2013) described the diffusion of QSEN competencies in the curricula of nursing schools. Dolansky and Moore (2013) call for these competencies to move beyond the individual to systems of care, bringing in more in line with the population-based focus of public health. The significance to community/public health nursing practice is that the QSEN competencies provide a method of both evaluating individual nurse performance and the use of aggregated data to assess programmatic outcomes. The KSAs can be used across all settings where a nurse may be employed, whether hospital, outpatient center, home care, hospice, or community/public health nursing services.

SOCIAL MARKETING

Each of the five program evaluation models presented provides a mechanism to plan, implement, and evaluate community-based programs and services. Emphasizing the importance of demonstrating quality through measurable outcomes is a crucial aspect of community health. Health promotion and health education programs must demonstrate achievement of stated goals to justify continuation. Likewise, the overall program, be it a health department or a community-based health center staffed by volunteers, is challenged to demonstrate quality outcomes through ongoing evaluation efforts. Community health services are also challenged to provide programs in ways that reach and engage their target populations. In this section, the role of social marketing is explored as an additional tool for community health care professionals to influence health behaviors and lifestyle choices. These methods must be selected carefully and evaluated against the same standards as previously presented, perhaps more so, because of the potentially higher costs of this type of intervention.

When you hear the words "texting and driving," do you think of the stories about the last text message sent by someone before a fatal crash? Or, have you watched the story of the woman showing her high school photo at age 16 when she started smoking and who now walks around her house dragging oxygen tubing because of her COPD? If you remember these, or ones like them, then social marketing has achieved its goal. Businesses have long recognized that providing "catchy" advertisements in a way that is memorable to the potential customer is vital to their success. Marketing can literally make or break their business. If the message is effective, they often have more business; if not, they may lose customers. The military has recognized the effectiveness of these advertising methods (e.g., military video games), using those same techniques in television and print advertising to increase recruitment. Children as young as 3 years have been found to be "branded" with current fast food items and beverages, meaning they recognize and prefer one particular brand or logo over another (Bryner, 2010; McAlister & Cornwell, 2010). The techniques used by some of these businesses and corporations have in many ways contributed to health issues we currently face as a nation (i.e., obesity in children, teenage smoking). A line of research examining knowledge of brands with products high in salt, fat, and sugar among 3- to 6-year-old children found that this brand knowledge was a significant predictor of the child's BMI. Researchers controlled for gender, age, and the amount of television viewing time and concluded that this had policy implications because of exposure to these products and their consumption being tied to higher BMI scores (Cornwell, McAlister, & Polmear-Swendris, 2014).

The public health care sector has also recognized the power of marketing health messages. Although used in some capacity since the 1960s, not until the 1990s—when federal agencies, such as the Centers for Disease Control and Prevention (CDC) spearheaded efforts—did it gain the attention it now has in addressing health issues (Lee & Kotler, 2016). The term **social marketing** refers to using marketing principles to influence or advance "a social cause, idea or behavior" (p. 14). Much of this began in the area of public health but has extended into environmental causes, poverty, and community advocacy. The main outcome of social marketing is to improve society's health, by influencing changes in individual health behaviors (e.g., healthy eating), or implementation of policies that impact health behaviors of a population (e.g., seat belt laws). The integration of marketing with public health practice is seen as a useful method to increase the effectiveness of public health practitioners (Resnick & Siegel, 2013).

Concepts that are important in marketing are applicable to social marketing as well (Resnick & Siegel, 2013). These include the following:

- Exchange: An individual gives something to get something; the person weighs the cost and the perceived benefits.
- Self-interest: People act in their own interests in most cases.
- Behavior change: Change in behavior is the focus; thoughts and ideas may also need to change but are not the ultimate goal.
- Competition: Selecting one option (or action) inherently involves giving up another option (or action).
- Consumer orientation: Problem-solving process is directed at the target—the consumer (could be an individual, group, or organization).

- Four P's (product, price, place, and promotion): Also called the marketing mix; each can be altered to increase market share.
- Partners and policy: Other organizations that share similar interests and could provide opportunities to work together; identification of policy changes necessary for behavioral change, those supportive of the change, and those that the organization could help influence.

These principles seem rather straightforward, yet public health practitioners are often at a disadvantage when attempting to implement social marketing campaigns (Resnick & Siegel, 2013). They often lack training in the necessary skills, may be outspent by the competition (e.g., the fast food industry), or have limited access for the distribution of their message (e.g., public service announcements). One example of a very successful social marketing campaign is the *Go Red for Women* initiative begun in 2004 by the American Heart Association (2016). Using a red dress as the symbol of the program, the initiative seeks to raise awareness of heart disease among women. These health issues are equally important, but one has a more broadly recognized campaign; the other was humorous but not necessarily well received. Ultimately, the issue is whether or not behaviors have been changed and health outcomes improved as a result of these social marketing campaigns. Time will be the judge of all these efforts (see Chapter 11; Fig. 12–8).

Cates, Ortiz, Shafer, Romocki, and Coyne-Beasley (2012) reported on a qualitative study to explore messaging that was most effective in promoting vaccination for human papillomavirus (HPV) of preteen age boys. Focus groups of parents were conducted and transcripts coded using a constant comparison method to interpret themes. Although the parents knew little about HPV and the vaccine, they supported vaccination of their children, yet did express concern about safety and cost. From a social marketing perspective, the messages that were most motivating focused on infection risk and those that included images of the parents with their sons, providing a visual and more personal link to the parental role (Cates et al., 2012). This study exemplifies the importance of framing health-related messages in a manner that is appealing, relevant to the situation, and acceptable to the audience.

How can social marketing principles be utilized when you have a limited budget, limited time, and limited creativity? See From the Case Files II.

When planning for and beginning development of a social marketing approach, there are many resources available to the public health nurse and other public health professionals. The Centers for Disease Control and Prevention offers an excellent Web site, *Gateway to Health Communications and Social Marketing* (CDC, 2016a) that includes links to a wide variety of resources. For instance, one of the social marketing resources, *Social Marketing for Nutrition and Physical Activity Web Course*, is available through the Division of Nutrition, Physical Activity, and Obesity (CDC, 2011). The European Centre for Disease Prevention and Control (2014) offers a comprehensive *Social Marketing Guide for Public Health Programme Managers and Practitioners*. Another very helpful publication is *Using Social Media Platforms to Amplify Public Health Messages* (Ogilvy Washington & the Center for Social Impact Communication at Georgetown

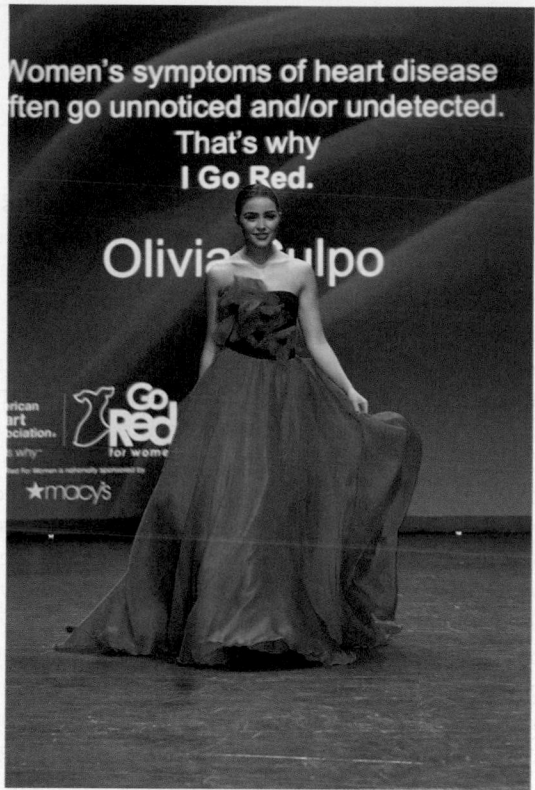

FIGURE 12–8 *Go Red for Women*, the American Heart Association's social marketing campaign about heart disease in women, has successfully raised awareness about heart disease among women.

University, 2010). Heldman, Schindelar, and Weaver (2013) provide information that goes beyond mass dissemination of public health information and shows the benefits of engaging your targeted audience in "true multiway conversations and interactions" as a means of providing more powerful social media impact (para. 1). There are also downsides to this approach.

The plethora of social marketing campaigns have raised a spotlight on ethical issues that need to be carefully considered when designing, implementing, and evaluating social marketing programs (Carter et al., 2011). The International Union for Health Promotion and Education (2016) is dedicated to seeing optimum health and well-being globally. Their values highlight the importance of ethics in this arena:

- Respect—for the innate dignity of all people; for cultural identity; for cultural diversity; and for natural resources and the environment
- Inclusion and involvement of people in making the decisions that shape their lives and impact upon their health and well-being
- Equity in health, social and economic outcomes for all people
- Accountability and transparency—within governments, organizations and communities
- Sustainability
- Social justice for all people
- Compassion and empowerment (International Union for Health Promotion and Education, 2016, para. 3)

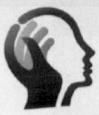

From the Case Files II

Nursing Students and a Social Marketing Campaign

University campuses hold a wealth of often-untapped expertise. For nursing students working on a health promotion program, the substance of the effort (the health issue) is often pretty straightforward, but the presentation is more challenging. Many schools of nursing are providing collaborative experiences for students, supporting partnering with nonnursing students and faculty in addressing health education needs. The following is one example of how collaboration can be effective: Two nursing students recognized that off-campus housing lacked sufficient smoke detectors because of a "loophole" in state and local building codes. This meant that students living in the most high-risk housing for fires (older buildings) might only have one smoke detector in the entire apartment; this was clearly inadequate. After discussing the issue with their faculty member, they sought input from several student organizations. From those discussions, they identified a low level of knowledge about the issue and modest concern by the students present. Recognizing that college students are not prone to worrying about how many smoke detectors they have, the nursing students sought help from the university housing department. The staff of housing agreed that this was an important issue, and they were willing to post information on the housing Web site regarding the need to install additional smoke detectors. The students didn't know how to develop online materials, but based on input from the student groups, they knew that it had to be eye-catching and

quickly present a message. In conjunction with their faculty advisor, they contacted the graphic arts department and found an instructor who was willing to include the development of an online smoke detector campaign as part of a class assignment. The nursing students provided the educational information that needed to be included, and the graphic arts students proceeded to develop a campaign within those parameters. In the end, several outstanding examples were submitted, and one was selected and posted on the housing Web site. The campaign was particularly effective with parents who saw the campaign on the Web site as they helped in apartment searches. Many messages were sent to the Web site by the parents regarding the campaign, and the responses were handled by the nursing students. The campaign was not expensive, and it identified the most skilled individuals for each task (health information, nursing students; Web-based campaign, graphic arts students). It also provided much-needed health and safety information to the university students and their parents. Even though they had targeted the college students, the nursing students found that the parents were much more interested in the campaign. The results of this initial effort provided vital information for future campaigns that might target parents, students, apartment management, and the local building code enforcement office.

Can you think of an issue on your university campus that could benefit from social marketing? Do you recognize any social marketing efforts sponsored by your university or your school of nursing?

As Carter et al. (2011) point out "the need to integrate evidence and ethics in health promotion becomes especially critical when large-scale intervention for a problem is urged, but guidance for action is limited" (para. 4).

Social marketing is not a panacea, but it does provide techniques that can support health education and health promotion programs. The method can be very expensive and very elaborate, or it can provide simple, straightforward messages. The point is that well-presented marketing can be the difference in whether behavior changes are made or not. Media messages are not a replacement for a sound health promotion program; they are just one tool that can be used for great impact.

GRANTS

Grants are a reality in public health efforts. They are not easy to locate, easy to secure, or easy to manage once you have one, but they are vital to providing a wide range of programs and services in the community. Many local and county health departments see them as an integral part of their service delivery, even hiring grant writers and grant managers in some cases. For most health departments, community agencies, and volunteer service providers, the task of locating grant funds, writing the grant application, and doing the work stipulated by the grant all falls

on the nurses and other professionals within those agencies. On the positive side, it provides an opportunity for community health nurses to explain to others what they can provide to the community in terms of services and programs targeting the community's health. Some basic knowledge about grants can demystify the topic.

Even if you aren't ever required to write a grant, you will likely be involved in some part of a programmatic grant at some point in your career, either in the delivery of services stipulated by the grant (product) or in evaluating the outcomes of the services provided (i.e., satisfaction surveys). You may even be asked to provide ideas for specific services to be included in the grant application; take advantage of these opportunities. The experience you gain will enhance your knowledge of the process and may prove instrumental in future efforts you may be involved with. The grant process, although arduous, provides the opportunity to focus clearly on what you intend to accomplish, why it is needed, and what part you will play in the successful outcome of the project. This is similar to a job interview, in which your prospective employer asks you *"Why should we hire you? What will you contribute to this organization?"* You have a limited amount of time to express your worth. You have to be very specific and concise about what you and your organization or group will be doing to address a specific need. You are making the case that providing you with support is the best choice.

What exactly is a grant? A **grant** is, very simply, one individual or group providing another individual or group with the support (i.e., money) for a specified purpose. In health promotion and education, it generally means funding for program development or project support. These types of grants fall into the following common categories: planning grants (i.e., initial project development), start-up grants (i.e., seed money), management or technical assistance grants (e.g., for fund raising or marketing), research grants, and facilities or equipment grants (National Institutes of Health, 2016). This money doesn't typically need to be paid back; however, it is a contractual agreement, and the terms and conditions are usually clearly delineated. Federal grants award government funds to implement projects that provide public service and stimulate the economy (Grants. gov, 2016). Federal grants are available from 26 grant-making agencies. The funding categories most applicable to community health include community development, disaster preparation and relief, food and nutrition, and health. Federal grants are available to a wide variety of groups, but typically, health-related grants are available to state or local governments, which include public health departments, public housing organizations, educational organizations, and nonprofit organizations (Grants.gov, 2016).

What is a *nonprofit organization*? Nonprofit means that the organization was not established to earn a profit. This does not mean that it doesn't generate income, only that there are restrictions on how those funds can be used. Of particular importance to the discussion of grants is the term *501c3*. This is a designation that refers to the Internal Revenue Service (IRS) tax-exempt status granted to certain nonprofit organizations. To be granted this designation, an organization must be organized and operated exclusively for specific purposes, which include charity, science, education, or the prevention of cruelty to children or animals (Internal Revenue Service, Department of the Treasury, 2016). Some grants are only available to 501c3 organizations, and the funders will request proof of this in the grant application. Only corporations, community chests, funds, or foundations can receive this designation; individuals or partnerships do not qualify (Internal Revenue Service, Department of the Treasury, 2016). Essentially, the 501c3 organization can be the provider of the grant funding or the organization seeking the funding.

Grants are available from government sources, private philanthropic sources, and corporations. Federal grants can be found on the Web site www.grants.gov or on individual federal agency Web sites. Private organizations often have sections on their Web sites with information on available grant funding. This is likewise the case with corporations. This broad search approach is not a terribly effective way to find grants; to improve search efficiency, a number of proprietary grant-locating programs are available. These programs are very expensive and, because of cost considerations, often are licensed only to large organizations, such as universities and medical centers. They allow the user the ability to limit the search (e.g., type of funder, health issue, age group,

program or research grant, funding limits, and time frame for submission). For the small nonprofit organization seeking funding, one effective approach is to partner with a local university, which allows for more access to grant-locating programs, as well as the expertise offered on the campuses (e.g., content area experts, experienced researchers, statisticians, business plan experts). These partnerships are becoming more attractive, as they meet the needs not only of the nonprofit agency but of the university's school of nursing. An integrative review of over 300 articles on academic-service partnerships found common themes (Beal, 2012). These included:

- Recognize the prerequisites for successful partnerships (e.g., acknowledge difficulty/time-intensiveness, assessment of both individual and mutual opportunities/strengths, base on shared trust/respect/commitment/goals/vision, commit to open/ongoing communication/problem-solving, develop structured leadership and accountability).
- Understand the benefits of partnerships (e.g., nursing esteem and visibility increased, resources maximized, opportunities for nursing student learning/faculty practice, benefits of greater retention/recruitment).

Many grants require proof of some type of interdisciplinary or community involvement. Some grant funders allow letters of inquiry to be submitted prior to an actual full grant application. The letter of inquiry may be by invitation-only or be part of the original advertisement of the grant funding. In any case, this letter is normally only two or three pages in length and includes a concise overview of the project. For example, Karsh and Fox (2014) note that a **letter of inquiry** would likely include an overview of your organization and its purpose, the reason for the funding request, clearly stated need or problem to be addressed, overview of the proposed project or program, and other funding sources for your project or program (prospective and committed). This letter is brief, yet clearly lays out your plan. Your goal is to be invited to submit a full proposal for consideration. If this approach is successful, you will be asked to complete the organization's application process (the proposal), which can vary in length and complexity depending on the organization.

Crucial to either the letter of inquiry or the full proposal is that you have selected a funder that is a good match for your organization and your program/project. For instance, applying to a faith-based organization that supports abstinence-only educational programs would not be a good fit for your program that seeks to provide contraceptive information in an after-school program for teens. Before you spend valuable time and energy writing a letter of inquiry or a grant application, be sure to do your homework. The Internet provides a quick method for reviewing potential funders, their vision, mission, and types of previous funding. You may even be able to find out the monetary range of grants funded by the organization. Perhaps you have a small grant request and find that the organization you are reviewing only funds large multimillion-dollar projects; it might be best to look for other options. The Web site will likely have contact information; making a phone call can assure you that this organization is a good match for your project and can give you an opportunity to start building a relationship with their staff.

Grants are most often competitive—which means you can expect to have competition from other deserving groups—so be prepared. A well-prepared grant—one that carefully follows the application guidelines specified in the request for proposals (RFPs) and very clearly describes the program you are seeking support for—is more likely to be funded. The **request for proposals (RFPs)** outlines the specific requirements of the application, the information to include and in what order, and what supplemental forms to include, if any. Submitting a grant after the deadline and not including all required items will mean that your grant application is not likely to be reviewed. If your grant is not selected, make certain to contact the funder to see if they will provide you with a review of your submission; this is common with government-sponsored grants. With knowledge of what hampered your selection, you will be in a much better position to resubmit to this funding source again or to be more prepared for other grant opportunities. Another suggestion for new grant writers is to seek the help of an experienced mentor—someone who has been successful in **grant writing**—as they can critique your proposal prior to submission and offer suggestions.

The following tips may be helpful as you begin the process of seeking grant funding (Federal Grants Wire, 2016):

- Gain a sound understanding of the grant and specific criteria required, ensuring that your interests and intensions are in line with the grantor agency.
- Seek input from the community that services are meant to benefit.
- Compile all required documents, such as articles of information, tax exemption certificated, etc.
- Organize the proposal to conform to the requirements of the call for applications. The order of contents may vary but in general include a proposal summary, problem statement, project goal and objectives, project methods or designing, project evaluation, and budget.

- Review, proofread, and ensure all requirements met prior to submitting your proposal.
- Ensure the proposal is submitted prior to the deadline.

One reality of grant funding is that experience counts. If you have a proven record in securing grants and completing the requirements specified in those grants, you or your organization will have an easier time securing additional funding. For the new grant seeker, this can be a bit discouraging. So, where to begin? Don't start with the most complicated grants available. Look for small local grants with a proven track record in grant management, and build your reputation. Work with partners. A school of nursing could partner with a home health agency to write a grant to provide worksite wellness programs for uninsured agricultural workers. Or several faith-community groups could partner in a grant application to provide free health screenings for uninsured adults in their area. Finally, be certain that the grant will allow you to meet the mission and goals of your program. The grant funder will also be looking to see if their support will enable you to provide a service that you have both the skill and expertise to accomplish. With limited funds available, funders are looking for proof of the sustainability of your program after their support ends. For instance, a breast-feeding support program sought funding in a high-risk area where there was a clear need. Although the need was demonstrated, the agency had no plan for continuing the program after the funding ended; they did not receive funding. Grant support is often seen as funding to get programs started—not to provide for long-term operations (Karsh & Fox, 2014).

Many courses are available to assist you in understanding how to locate grants, write them, and be successful in your attempts. Your local library is another source of information, and a wide variety of information is available on the Internet. Some examples of helpful Web sites are included in the Internet Resources found on *thePoint*.

SUMMARY

Successful community health programs require that the nurse listen to the target population and not determine the problem and solution without their assistance. Awareness of predisposing, reinforcing, and enabling factors facilitates the assessment of health-related behaviors. Importance and changeability are important considerations when determining priorities among competing behavioral targets. Community-based participatory research is an effective method to increase engagement. An advisory group, with representation from the target and service communities, is an effective tool in helping to identify the problem, select appropriate interventions to address the problem, and evaluate the outcomes of the interventions chosen. Outcome measures should be consistent with the concerns of the community. Evaluation can be facilitated by clearly defined goals that can be measured against actual results.

The multiple models or frameworks on which quality management systems are based include a classic way of looking at programs through organizational structure, process, and outcomes, along with the interrelatedness of each component. The six models presented in this chapter are structured in unique ways that enable them to meet the differing needs of community agencies. Whether quality measurement and improvement techniques are formally or informally practiced, whenever nurses monitor, assess, and judge the quality and appropriateness of care as measured against professional standards, the interests of clients are being served.

Social marketing is one tool that can enhance health promotion efforts in the community. Media messages are particularly helpful in reaching large audiences. The basis of social marketing is similar to product marketing to consumers. The goal of consumer marketing is not necessarily to change the way people think but the way they behave. Social marketing seeks to first change behavior and then to influence how people think about health, lifestyle, and the choices they make every day that influence their health. One example of social marketing is the American Heart Association *Go Red for Women* campaign, which seeks to bring attention to heart disease risk among women. Social marketing, like any consumer-focused marketing, must consider the target population in the design, implementation, and evaluation of the effort. Successful outcomes are imperative for continuation of this type of program, as with any other health promotion campaign.

Grants are increasingly vital to providing health promotion programs and services in the community. Community health nurses frequently are involved in some aspect of a grant program, whether in the writing, in implementation of the program or services stipulated in the grant, or in the evaluation of the outcomes for the grant. Grants are available from government sources, private philanthropic sources, and corporations. Successful grant proposals comply with the instructions provided in the RFPs. Community agencies and academic programs can collaborate in providing community services and evaluation research that seeks to improve the lives of the target population. Mastering the grant process, from formulating the goal to defining the evaluation methods, is a skill that can benefit all manner of health promotion programs, whether funded or not.

Community/public health nurses are in a key position to plan, implement, and evaluate all types of health promotion/health education programs. Knowledge of the target population and engaging the target population in determining the problem and solutions are vital to successful outcomes. Ongoing use of quality measurement techniques and application of recognized professional standards help assure effective and appropriate service delivery. Social marketing is a tool that can be effective in reaching large audiences with valuable health messages. Finally, the skills gained in working on any portion of a grant effort can be utilized in future programmatic efforts, whether supported through funding or not.

ACTIVITIES TO PROMOTE **CRITICAL THINKING**

1. Evaluate examples of community assessments and subsequent program planning and implementation based upon them (from local or state public health departments, community agencies, or the Web site: https://www.healthypeople.gov/2020/LHI/whosleading.aspx). Which *Healthy People 2020* topics and objectives, or leading health indicators, are represented in this assessment/program plan? How were the program objectives achieved? How effective was the program in meeting the assessed needs of the population?

2. A faculty member who teaches acute care nursing approaches a group of nursing students about a problem she has identified. She informs them that there is a high incidence of *Chlamydia* infection in a local community among Spanish-speaking people. The hospital where she and her students have clinical rotations wants to do something to reduce the incidence of *Chlamydia*. The faculty member has found a pamphlet online that describes *Chlamydia* infection, how it's diagnosed, and how it's treated. She thinks it would be a wonderful idea for the student PHNs to translate the pamphlet into Spanish.
   a. Do you feel that this is an appropriate intervention?
   b. What data should be gathered? What literature should be reviewed?
   c. What agencies, organizations, and groups should the students contact?
   d. Who is the target population?
   e. What outreach should be done with this population? What information should be gathered from the population prior to developing any educational materials?
   f. What steps should the students take to ensure that the target population finds the educational materials they develop to be appropriate, acceptable, and understandable?

3. A school nurse works in a rural agricultural community. The main crop is rice. Every year after harvesting the rice, the local farmers burn their rice fields. The school nurse notes a significant increase in absences during this period for respiratory problems, especially asthma. She notes that even the teachers have increasing respiratory

problems. She believes that the burning rice fields may aggravate the respiratory problems. She mentions her concerns about the relationship between the fields burning and increased respiratory-related illnesses to the school principal. He responds that while it may be true, the local farmers control the local community—without them, the community would collapse. He states that kids and adults will just have to adjust.

   a. What can the nurse do to determine if the burning rice fields are a threat to the health of children and adults in the local area? (What data should be gathered, what literature should be reviewed, to whom should she talk?) See Chapter 9.

   b. What steps should she take to increase interest in addressing this problem?

   c. What agencies, organizations, and groups should she contact? Who are the stakeholders?

4. Identify a health-related social marketing campaign that you viewed recently on television, social media sites, or in print. Who is the target audience? What is the main message it is sending? What is the target behavior or problem? Does it reach the target audience? How effective is it?

5. Organize a group of nursing students and meet with other students on campus about public health issues that affect them (e.g., housing, safety on campus, lack of healthy food choices, health issues). Brainstorm possible ways social marketing could be helpful in addressing this issue. Identify who you might work with to address this issue. What message do you want to send and what is the most cost-effective and practical way to do this?

6. Search for examples of social marketing campaigns (e.g., Red Dress campaign) and discuss them in your clinical group. What works? What doesn't seem to be effective? How could you improve on methods to reach the target audience?

7. Talk with PHNs at your local or state public health department. How many and what types of grants do they have? What programs do they fund exclusively from grant writing? How do they manage grant funding and data gathering to justify outcomes for grant funders?

REFERENCES

Allmark, P., Baxter, S., Goyder, E., Guillaume, L., & Crofton-Martin, G. (2013). Assessing the health benefits of advanced services: Using research evidence and logic model methods to explore complex pathways. *Health and Social Care in the Community, 21*(1), 59–68. doi: 10.1111/j.1365-2524.2012.01087.x.

American Heart Association. (2016). *Go red for women: About go red*. Retrieved from https://www.goredforwomen.org/home/about-go-red/

American Nurses Association. (2013). *Public health nursing: Scope and standards of practice* (2nd ed.). Silver Spring, MD: Nursesbooks.org.

Barnsteiner, J., Disch, J., Johnson, J., McGuinn, K., Chappell, K., & Swartwout, E. (2013). Diffusing QSEN competencies across schools of nursing: The AACN/RWJF Faculty Development Institutes. *Journal of Professional Nursing, 29*(2), 68–74.

Beal, J. A. (2012). Academic-service partnerships in nursing: An integrative review. *Nursing Research and Practice*, Article ID 501564. Retrieved from http://www.hindawi.com/journals/nrp/2012/501564/

Benjamin, G., Fallon, M., Jarris, P. E., & Libbey, P. M. (2006). *Final recommendations for a voluntary national accreditation program for state and local public health departments*. Retrieved from http://www.rwjf.org/pr/product.jsp?id=23495

Bloom, B. S. (1956). *Taxonomy of educational objectives: Handbook I. Cognitive domain*. New York, NY: D. McKay.

Bolton, M., Moore, I., Ferreira, A., Day, C., & Bolton, D. (2016). Community organizing and community health: Piloting an innovative approach to community engagement applied to an early intervention project in south London. *Journal of Public Health, 38*(1), 115–121. doi: 10.1093/pubmed/fdv017.

Bowles, K. H. (2011). Achieving meaningful use with standardized data. *Online Journal of Nursing Informatics, 15*(2). Retrieved from http://ojni.org/issues/?p=574

Brookes, N. L., & Tansey, M. R. (2003). Visionary leadership in psychiatric and mental health nursing. Paper presented at the 2003 Sigma Theta Tau International Biennial Convention, Toronto, Ontario.

Retrieved from http://www.nursinglibrary.org/vhl/handle/10755/148157?mode=full&submit_simple=Show+full+item+record

Bryner, J. (2010, March 9). *Even a 3-year old understands the power of advertising*. Retrieved from http://www.livescience.com/6181-3-year-understands-power-advertising.html

Buta, B., Brewer, L., Hamlin, D. L., Palmer, M. W., Bowie, J., & Gielen, A. (2011). An innovative faith-based healthy eating program: From class assignment to real-world application of PRECEDE/PROCEED. *Health Promotion Practice, 12*, 867–875. doi: 0.1177/1524839910370424.

Carter, S. M., Rychetnik, L., Lloyd, B., Kerridge, I. H., Baur, L., Bauman, A., ... Zask, A. (2011). Evidence, ethics, and values: A framework for health promotion. *American Journal of Public Health, 101*(3), 465–472. doi: 10.2105/AJPH.2010.195545.

Cates, J. R., Ortiz, R., Shafer, A., Romocki, L. S., & Coyne-Beasley, T. (2012). Designing messages to motivate parents to get their preteenage sons vaccinated against human papillomavirus. *Perspectives on Sexual and Reproductive Health, 44*(1), 39–47. doi: 10.1363/4403912.

Centers for Disease Control and Health Promotion (CDC). (2011). *Social marketing resources*. Retrieved from http://www.cdc.gov/nccdphp/DNPAO/socialmarketing/index.html

Centers for Disease Control and Prevention (CDC). (2016a). *Gateway to health communication & social marketing practice*. Retrieved from http://www.cdc.gov/healthcommunication/

Centers for Disease Control and Prevention (CDC). (2016b). *National voluntary accreditation for public health departments*. Retrieved from http://www.cdc.gov/stltpublichealth/hop/pdfs/nvaph_factsheet.pdf

Centers for Disease Control and Prevention, Office for State, Tribal, Local, and Territorial Support. (2016). *National voluntary accreditation for public health departments*. Retrieved from http://www.cdc.gov/stltpublichealth/hop/pdfs/nvaph_factsheet.pdf

Cohen, C. C., & Shang, J. (2015). Evaluation of conceptual frameworks applicable to the study of isolation precautions effectiveness. *Journal of Advanced Nursing, 71*(10), 2279–2292.

Community Preventive Services Task Force. (2014). *The community guide: What works to promote health*. Retrieved from http://www. thecommunityguide.org/library/book/index.html

Cornell University. (2016). *Modeling the program: Conceptualization, logic models, & pathway models*. Retrieved from https://core. human.cornell.edu/resources/modeling.cfm

Cornwell, T. B., McAlister, A. R., & Polmear-Swendris, N. (2014). Children's knowledge of packaged and fast food brands and their BMI. Why the relationship matters for policy makers. *Appetite, 81*(1), 277–283.

DeSisto, C. L., Kim, S. Y., & Sharma, A. J. (2014). Prevalence estimates of gestational diabetes mellitus in the United States, Pregnancy Risk Assessment Monitoring System (PRAMS), 2007-2010. *Preventing Chronic Disease, 11*, 130415. Retrieved from http://www.cdc.gov/ pcd/issues/2014/13_0415.htm

Diffenderfer, S. K., Dunham-Taylor, J., & Malcolm, D. (2015). Providing value-based service. In J. Dunham-Taylor and J. Z. Pinczuk (Eds.), *Financial management for nurse managers: Merging the heart with the dollar* (3rd ed.; pp. 167–222). Burlington, MA: Jones and Bartlett.

Dolansky, M. A., & Moore, S. M. (2013). Quality and Safety Education for Nurses (QSEN): The key is systems thinking. *Online Journal of Issues in Nursing, 18*(3), Manuscript 1.

Donabedian, A. (1966). Evaluating the quality of medical care. *Milbank Memorial Fund Quarterly, 44*, 166–206.

Donabedian, A. (1969). *Medical care appraisal: Quality and utilization. In guide to medical care administration*. New York, NY: American Public Health Association.

Donabedian, A. (1981). *The criteria and standards of quality*. Ann Arbor, MI: Health Administration Press.

Donabedian, A. (1985). *Explorations in quality assessment and monitoring* (Vol. 3). Ann Arbor, MI: Health Administration Press.

Donabedian, A. (2003). *An introduction to quality assurance in health care*. New York, NY: Oxford University Press.

Doran, G. T. (1981). There's a S.M.A.R.T. way to write management's goals and objectives. *Management Review (American Management Association Forum), 70*(11), 35–36.

Dunham-Taylor, J. (2015). Organizations: Surviving within a chaotic, complex, value-based environment. In J. Dunham-Taylor & J. Z. Pinczuk (Eds.), *Financial management for nurse managers: Merging the heart with the dollar* (3rd ed.; pp. 81–165). Burlington, MA: Jones and Bartlett.

Ettorchi-Tardy, A., Levif, M., & Michel, P. (2012). *Benchmarking: A method for continuous quality improvement in health*. Retrieved from http://www.ncbi.nlm.nih.gov/pmc/articles/PMC3359088/

European Centre for Disease Prevention and Control. (2014). *Social marking guide for public health programme managers and practitioners*. Retrieved from http://ecdc.europa.eu/en/publications/ Publications/social-marketing-guide-public-health.pdf

Federal Grants Wire. (2016). *How to write a federal grant proposal*. Retrieved from http://www.federalgrantswire.com/writing-a-federal-grant-proposal.html#.Vr2CePkrL3Q

Gordon, M. (2016). *Manual of nursing diagnosis* (13th ed.). Burlington, MA: Jones & Bartlett Learning.

Grants.gov. (2016). *Grants 101: A short summary of federal grants*. Retrieved from http://www.grants.gov/web/grants/learn-grants/ grants-101.html

Green, L. W., & Kreuter, M. W. (1999). *Health program planning: An educational and environmental approach* (3rd ed.). Mountain View, CA: Mayfield Publishing Company.

Green, L. W., & Kreuter, M. W. (2005). *Health program planning: An educational and ecological approach* (4th ed.). New York, NY: McGraw-Hill.

Green, L. W., Ottoson, J. M., & Roditis, M. L. (2014). Public health education and health promotion. In L. Shi & J. A. Johnson (Eds.), *Novick & Morrow's public health administration: Principles for population-based management* (3rd ed.; pp. 477–504). Burlington, MA: Jones & Bartlett Learning.

Hedderson, M. M., Ehrlich, S., Sridhar, S., Darbinian, J., Moore, S., & Ferrara, A. (2012). Racial/ethnic disparities in the prevalence of gestational diabetes mellitus by BMI. *Diabetes Care, 35*(7). doi: 10.2337/dc11-2267.

Heldman, A. B., Schindelar, J., & Weaver, J. B. (2013). Social media engagement and public health communication: Implications for

public health organizations being truly "social." *Public Health Reports, 35*(1), 1–18.

Institute of Medicine (IOM). (1999). *To err is human: Building a safer health system*. Washington, DC: National Academies Press.

Institute of Medicine (IOM). (2002). *The future of the public's health in the 21st century*. Washington, DC: National Academies Press.

Institute of Medicine (IOM). (2003). *Health professions education: A bridge to quality*. Washington, DC: National Academies Press.

Institute of Medicine (IOM). (2004). *Keep patients safe: Transforming the work environment of nurses*. Washington, DC: National Academies Press.

Institute of Medicine (IOM). (2011). *The future of nursing: Leading change, advancing health*. Washington, DC: National Academies Press.

Institute of Medicine (IOM). (2012). *For the public's health: Investing in a healthier future*. Washington, DC: National Academies Press.

Internal Revenue Service, Department of the Treasury. (2016). *Tax-exempt status for your organization*. Retrieved from http://www.irs. gov/publications/p557/index.html

International Union for Health Promotion and Education. (2016). *Mission and values*. Retrieved from http://www.iuhpe.org/index.php/en/

Issel, L. M. (2014). *Health program planning and evaluation: A practical, systematic approach for community health* (3rd ed.). Burlington, MA: Jones & Bartlett Learning.

Karsh, E., & Fox, A. S. (2014). *The only grant-writing book you will ever need* (4th ed.). New York, NY: Basic Books.

Kellogg Foundation. (2006). *W. K. Kellogg Foundation logic model development guide*. Retrieved from https://www. wkkf.org/resource-directory/resource/2006/02/wk-kellogg-foundation-logic-model-development-guide

Kulbok, P. A., Thatcher, E., Park, E., & Meszaros, P. S. (2012). Evolving public health nursing roles: Focus on community participatory health promotion and prevention. *Online Journal of Issues in Nursing, 17*(2), Manuscript 1.

Kutney-Lee, A., Stimpfel, A. W., Sloane, D. M., Cimiotti, J. P., Quinn, L. W., & Aiken, L. H. (2015). Changes in patient and nurse outcomes associated with Magnet hospital recognition. *Medical Care, 53*(6), 550-557.

Lee, N. R., & Kotler, P. (2016). *Social marketing: Changing behaviors for good* (5th ed.). Thousand Oaks, CA: Sage Publications, Inc.

MacKay, S. A. (2007). President's update. *Alberta RN, 63*(1). Retrieved from http://nurses.ab.ca/carna-admin/Uploads/AB_RN_jan_07_web.pdf

MacKay, G., & Risk, M. (2001). Building quality practice settings: An attributes model. *Canadian Journal of Nursing Leadership, 14*(3), 19–27.

Martin, K. S. (2005). *The Omaha System: A key to practice, documentation, and information management* (2nd ed.). Omaha, NE: Health Connections Press.

Martin, K., Leak, G., & Aden, C. (1997). The Omaha system: A research-based model for decision making. In B. W. Spradley & J. A. Allender (Eds.), *Readings in community health nursing* (5th ed.; pp. 316–324). Philadelphia, PA: Lippincott-Raven.

McAlister, A. R., & Cornwell, T. B. (2010). Children's brand symbolism understanding: Links to theory of mind and executive functioning. *Psychology & Marketing, 27*(3), 203–228.

McCoyd, J. L. M. (2010). Authoritative knowledge, the technological imperative and women's responses to prenatal diagnostic technologies. *Culture, Medicine, & Psychiatry, 34*, 590–614.

Miller, M., Linn, R. L., & Gronlund, N. E. (2013). *Measurement and assessment in teaching* (11th ed.). Upper Saddle River, NJ: Pearson.

Mitchell, P. H., Ferketich, S., & Jennings, B. M. (1998). Quality health care outcomes model. *Image: Journal of Nursing Scholarship, 30*, 43–46.

Mitchell, P. H., & Lang, N. M. (2004). Framing the problem of measuring and improving healthcare quality: Has the quality health outcomes model been useful? *Medical Care, 42*(2 Suppl), II4–II11.

Monsen, K. A., & Newsom, E. T. (2011). Feasibility of using the Omaha System to represent public health nurse manager interventions. *Public Health Nursing, 28*, 421–428. doi: 10.1111/j.1525-1446.2010.00926.x.

Monsen, K. A., Radosevich, D. M., Johnson, S. C., Farri, O., Kerr, M. J., & Geppert, J. S. (2011a). Benchmark attainment by maternal and child health clients across public health nursing agencies. *Public Health Nursing, 29*, 11–18. doi: 10.1111/j. 1525-1446.2011.00967.x.

Monsen, K. A., Radosevich, D. M., Kerr, M. J., & Fulkerson, J. A. (2011b). Public health nurses tailor interventions for families at risk. *Public Health Nursing, 28,* 119–128.

Monsen, K. A., Schenk, E., Schyeler, R., & Schiavenato, E. (2015). Applicability of the Omaha System in acute care nursing for information interoperability in the era of accountable care. *American Journal of Managed Care, 3*(3), 53–61.

Morrison, M. (2010). *History of SMART objectives. Introduction to SMART objectives and SMART goals.* Retrieved from http://rapidbi.com/history-of-smart-objectives/

Naimoli, J. F., Frymus, D. E., Wuliji, T., Franco, L. M., & Newsome, M. H. (2014). *A community health worker "logic model": Towards a theory of enhanced performance in low- and middle-income countries.* doi: 10.1186/1478-4491-12-56.

National Association of County & City Health Officials. (2016). *Accreditation preparation.* Retrieved from http://naccho.org/programs/public-health-infrastructure/accreditation-preparation

National Institutes of Health. (2016). *Grants & funding: Types of grant programs.* Retrieved from http://grants.nih.gov/grants/funding/funding_program.htm

Ogilvy Washington & the Center for Social Impact Communication at Georgetown University. (2010). *Using social media platforms to amplify public health messages: An examination of tenets and best practices for communicating with key audiences.* Retrieved from http://smexchange.ogilvypr.com/wp-content/uploads/2010/11/OW_SM_WhitePaper.pdf

Ottoson, J. M., & Green, L. W. (2008). Public health education and health promotion. In L. F. Novick, C. B. Morrow, & G. P. Mays (Eds.), *Public health administration: Principles for population-based management* (2nd ed., pp. 589–619). Sudbury, MA: Jones & Bartlett Publishers.

Organizational Research Services. (2004). *Theory of change: A practical tool for action, results and learning.* Retrieved from http://www.aecf.org/m/resourcedoc/aecf-theoryofchange-2004.pdf#page=3

Patry, L. A. (2006). Certification: Building on what you know. *Canadian Nurse, 102*(2), 17–21.

Popejoy, L. L., Khalilia, M. A., Popescu, M., Galambos, C., Lyons, V., Rantz, M., Hicks, L., & Stetzer, F. (2015). Quantifying care coordination using natural language processing and domain-specific ontology. *Journal of the American Medical Informatics Association, 22*(e1), e93–e103.

Public Health Accreditation Board. (2014). *Standards and measures: Summary of version 1.5 revisions and clarifications.* Retrieved from http://www.phaboard.org/wp-content/uploads/Version-1.5-changes-and-clarifications-FINAL1.pdf

Public Health Partners. (2016). *Statistical information by subject. Geographic Information Systems (GIS).* Retrieved from http://phpartners.org/tutorial/03-hs/3-sources/3.3.6.html

Quality and Safety Education for Nurses (QSEN). (2014). *Pre-licensure KSAs.* Retrieved from http://qsen.org/competencies/pre-licensure-ksas/

Resnick, E. A., & Siegel, M. (2013). *Marketing public health: Strategies to promote social change.* Burlington, MA: Jones & Bartlett Learning.

Robert Wood Johnson Foundation. (2014). *Lead states in public health quality improvement (originally called the Multistate Learning Collaborative).* Retrieved from http://www.rwjf.org/en/library/research/2010/07/multistate-learning-collaborative-.html

Saxe-Braithwaite, M., Carlton, S., & Bass, B. (2009). Aligning career development with organizational goals: Working towards the development of a strong and sustainable workforce. *Nursing Leadership, 22*(1), 56–69.

Sills, F. W. (2015). Contemporary legal issues for the nurse administrator. In J. Dunham-Taylor & J. Z. Pinczuk (Eds.), *Financial management for nurse managers: Merging the heart with the dollar* (3rd ed., pp. 347–378). Burlington, MA: Jones and Bartlett.

Stubbs, J. M., & Achat, H. M. (2011). Monitoring and evaluation of a large-scale community-based program: Recommendations for overcoming barriers to structured implementation. *Contemporary Nurse, 37*(2), 188–196.

Thompson, C. W., Monsen, K. A., Wanamaker, K., Augustyniak, K., & Thompson, S. L. (2012). Using the Omaha System as a framework to demonstrate the value of nurse managed wellness center services for vulnerable populations. *Journal of Community Health Nursing, 29,* 1–11.

U. S. Department of Health and Human Services. (2016). *Healthy People 2020: About Healthy People.* Retrieved from http://www.healthypeople.gov/2020/About-Healthy-People

Zlotnick, C., Wright, M., Sanchez, R. M., Kusnir, R. M., & Te'o-Bennett, I. (2010). Adaptation of a community-based participatory research model to gain community input on identifying indicators of successful parenting. *Child Welfare, 89*(4), 9–27.

thePoint: Everything You Need to Make the Grade!

thePoint® Visit http://thePoint.lww.com/Rector9e for selected readings, study aids for all learning styles, and more!

Policy Making and Community Health Advocacy

"Never doubt that a small group of thoughtful citizens can change the world. Indeed, it is the only thing that ever has."

—*Margaret Mead*

KEY TERMS

Advocacy
Community health advocacy
Distributive health policy
Empowerment
Grassroots

Health policy
Lobbying
Lobbyists
Polarization
Policy

Policy analysis
Political action
Political action committee (PAC)
Politics
Power

Public policy
Redistributive health policy
Regulatory health policies
Special interest groups

LEARNING OBJECTIVES

Upon mastery of this chapter, you should be able to:

- Identify three measures of population health relevant for national comparisons.
- Describe the relationship between social policy and health outcomes.
- Define health policy and explain how it is established.
- Provide one health-relevant example of each of the four types of policy.
- Discuss policy examples for legislation, regulation, and policy modification.
- Identify a health policy issue for each level of jurisdiction (local, state, national).
- Identify one current health policy issue of interest to public health nursing in terms of the policy problem, the solution, interested parties, and their relative power and influence.
- Describe the five components of the rational framework for policy analysis and identify when it would be most useful for PHNs.
- Define the three components of Kingdon's framework for policy analysis and identify when it would be most useful for PHNs.
- Identify three possible ways a PHN could engage in policy activism.
- Explain the role of special interest groups in health care legislation and policy making.
- Identify the difference between advocacy and lobbying, as well as the influence of both on policy.
- Discuss power and empowerment and the roles these concepts play in policy development.
- Describe three new Affordable Care Act (ACA) policies that impact the health of the public.
- For each ACA policy, identify one PHN policy-relevant activity that could improve the health of the public.
- Identify two methods of communicating with legislators on advocacy or policy issues.

Behind all legislation and health care regulation lie power struggles. Only the very naive think that others will be persuaded by facts alone. In all legislative activities and reforms, social and political factions are at work—special interest groups, business, and industry each bring their power into play. Because the outcomes of these struggles determine the availability and quality of all health and social services, nurses need to develop a working knowledge of the political process and health policy in order to protect the individuals, families, and communities they serve, as well as their own nursing practice. This chapter examines health policy, the political process involved in determining health policy, and the role of public health nursing in the process. Community health nurses should provide not only input to policy circles through advocacy but also leadership at decision-making tables. Nurses must understand and emphasize their powerful role in providing an essential influence and unique perspective in health care.

Health policy consists of the rules, regulations, legislation, and funding that we, as members of the public, choose to invest in providing, regulating, and researching health care for our fellow Americans. Although we may often be unaware of policy specifics, by virtue of our rights to vote, and the way our governmental system is designed, we are responsible for policy outcomes. For public health nurses, these outcomes affect us personally, but also impact the communities in which we practice—and the health of our neighbors. If we define public health nursing as being related to impacting the health of populations, then the public health nurse needs to understand how health policy impacts health outcomes. In this chapter, we will discuss the current state of the health of Americans, how policy impacts health, how policy is developed, and how PHNs can be involved in health policy formation. We will discuss specific examples of PHN policy involvement and potential action, given the current health care policy changes in the United States.

HEALTH IN THESE UNITED STATES: HOW HEALTHY ARE WE?

The United States is often touted as having the best health care system in the world. It is recognized worldwide for achievements in the medical and auxiliary sciences that have contributed to the mapping of the genome, advances in biomedical technologies, and increasing numbers of pharmaceuticals that hold promise for addressing the myriad chronic and acute illnesses that affect the world's populations. People often come from other countries to the United States to access our high-quality medical care.

It is well understood that the U.S. health care system is expensive. Current data indicate that the United States spends 17.5% of its gross domestic product (GDP) on health care costs; this is twice as much as the average health care expenditures from countries with similar levels of economic development (Center for Medicare and Medicaid Services [CMS], n.d.; Organization for Economic Cooperation & Development, 2015). High expenditures are not necessarily problematic. Two questions need to be asked: (1) Can the country afford this amount of expenditure for health care? That is, do these expenditures prevent the country from spending resources on other necessities or socially desirable goods? (2) Are the costs worth it? That is, are we getting what we want from these expenditures? The first question is a larger political question, as the nation grapples with where to spend its public funds, because any increase in one area necessarily causes a decrease in another, as resources are never without limits. The government is responsible for debating and deciding these trade-offs, and that debate is not going to be addressed here. However, the second question is relevant to discuss in this chapter. For

the amount the United States spends on health care, are we achieving the results we desire? In other words, how healthy is the public? See What Do You Think?

Chapter 6 presented outcomes for health in the United States and comparison countries. As stated earlier, the U.S. health outcomes are very mixed, especially given the cost of the overall health care system. The United States does not compare well to countries at similar levels of economic development in the areas of life expectancy, mortality rates for chronic illnesses, mortality rates for communicable disease, and infant mortality, among other health measures. The recent Institute of Medicine report, *Shorter Lives, Poorer Health* (IOM, 2013), presents additional analyses to explain these disparities in health outcomes. The IOM report corrects the international health outcome comparisons for racial/ethnic diversity, income, and educational levels, among other factors, and proceeds to present additional explanations of why these disparities exist, including environmental, social, and policy factors.

The IOM report also documents areas where the United States compares favorably to other Office of Economic Cooperation and Development countries. These areas include

- Cancer mortality
- Stroke mortality
- Control of blood pressure and cholesterol levels
- Suicide
- Elderly survival
- Self-rated health

Cancer and stroke mortality, and control of blood pressure and cholesterol, are areas of strength for the U.S.

What do *you* think?

Martin Luther King, Jr. Memorial. (Photo courtesy of NPS.org)

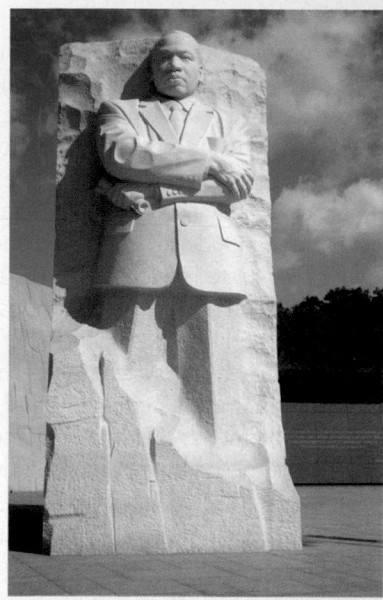

Of all the shocking and inhumane in society; the lack of access to health care is the most inhumane.

—Dr. Martin Luther King

In the decade or so leading up to President Clinton's attempt at health care reform, the debate about access to health care centered on whether health care was a *right* or a *privilege*. What do you think? Given that so many millions of Americans were without any access to insurance or health care before the Patient Protection and Affordable Care Act (ACA) was passed, should there be some basic rights regarding access to services as found in most other developed nations (e.g., a safety net)? Or is this a privilege that should be earned? What are your thoughts on President Obama's health care reform and how it is being implemented? Has it affected you or someone you know?

health care system, with advances in early diagnosis, and development of new and effective pharmaceutical treatments. In the area of suicide, although the United States does well overall, the one facet of suicide rates where the U.S. population does not compare favorably is suicide using a gun; our numbers far exceed those in our peer countries. Elderly survival is also potentially related to medication therapy and technological advances in old age, so that for those who live to age 75, their odds of living longer are greatly increased. Lastly, self-rated health is high in the United States, possibly because of our technological developments, which provide consumers with the perception of great medical advances from which

it is logical to conclude that one's health outcomes are positive.

By comparison, the IOM report cites areas where U.S. health outcomes do not compare favorably with peer countries, including

- Infant mortality and low birth weight
- Injuries and homicides
- Adolescent pregnancy and STIs
- HIV and AIDS
- Drug-related deaths
- Obesity and diabetes
- Cardiovascular disease
- Chronic lung disease
- Disability

These are all conditions that are chronic or have strong behavioral and social components, and where prevention and management of long-term conditions are equally as important as diagnosis and treatment in the improvement of overall health outcomes. The IOM presents a variety of explanations for these health inequities in the United States, including a lack of attention within the current health care system to the social determinants of health, or the challenges with access to health care and social policies that do not address the nonclinical causes of poor health.

From the Case Files I: Obesity in America is an exemplar of the way in which the U.S. health care system addresses the social and nonclinical determinants of health in the area of obesity.

This raises the question that is the focus of this chapter—what is health policy and how it is relevant to community health nursing practice? How are politics and health policy intertwined? If PHNs are to promote and protect the health of populations (APHA, PHN Section, 2013), they need to understand health policy as it relates to the health of the public. Policies affect our daily lives, regardless of whether they are health or work related. So, public health nurses must have an understanding of health policy to better understand the issues affecting the communities they serve. It must be recognized that nurses have differing opinions on health policy, even down to the basic premise of whether nurses should become involved in political issues and the political process. But, according to Plato, "One of the penalties for refusing to participate in politics is that you end up being governed by your inferiors." So it is helpful for nurses to have a better understanding of the political process and health policy. Some questions to ask include the following:

- What do we need to understand about health policy?
- How can it be critical to the overall health of our nation?
- How is policy important in addressing both issues of access to care and of creating and supporting the social conditions that support health?
- What is the relationship of politics and health policy?
- How can nurses become involved in the political process and in promoting meaningful health policies?

In the remainder of the chapter, we will discuss policy, how it is formed, the stages of the policy process, how public health nurses can learn to be policy competent and

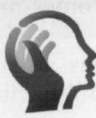

From the Case Files I

Obesity in America

Obesity and overweight are defined as weight higher "than what is considered as generally healthy for a given height," and body mass index (BMI) is a common screening tool to determine if someone is overweight or obese (CDC, 2016, para. 1). Factors related to obesity include "a combination of causes and contributing factors, including individual factors such as behavior and genetics" (CDC, 2016, para. 1). Behaviors can include one's patterns of eating, physical activity or inactivity, and the medications taken, as well as other exposures. In the larger community and society, there are also physical activity and food environments (e.g., access to fast food, safe walking environments), as well as education and how food is promoted and marketed. These latter factors are in large part, public policy issues, as defined earlier in the chapter.

John, a 6-year-old boy, is brought by his mother to see their primary care provider. The nurse practitioner (APRN) notes that John is overweight as defined by the CDC, and talks to his mother about the consequences of being overweight for lifelong health. His mother is interested in helping John achieve a healthy weight, and the APRN provides her with guidance to address John's weight; the mother is asked to return with her son in 6 weeks to see how John is progressing with the changes they discuss. The health care system, in this case, functioned well in that John had access to care, and the primary care provider recognized the potential weight problem early and spent time with John's mother to discuss ways to address helping John achieve a healthy weight. However, when John leaves the clinic, there are additional resources necessary to help his mother implement the plan she discussed with the provider. Does John's family have access to healthy, affordable foods? Such access could be related to where they live, their income level, cultural influences on food choices that also include marketing and advertising, as well as agricultural policy related to food subsidies and what is grown locally or imported and exported. Also, policies on regulating food safety, additives, and labeling, among other thing, have an effect. How does the health care system use its knowledge to influence such policies in ways that promote health?

The APRN also recommends that John increase his physical activity through active play and recreational activities. Does John's family have access to such opportunities? Is it safe to play in their community? Are there recreational opportunities available at school (do they even offer physical education classes)? Does John's family live in a manner where John has time to be outside and active? Are his parents available to supervise his play when necessary, depending on his age? Again, these factors relate to such policy concerns as tax funding for parks and schools, the income and job opportunities available to John's family, and street safety in their wider neighborhood, among other things. How can and should health professionals be involved in the development or implementation of policies to promote healthy physical activity?

---

impact policy in their practice, and the policy changes resulting from the ACA and how they impact public health nursing practice (U.S. Department of Health and Human Services [USDHHS], 2015).

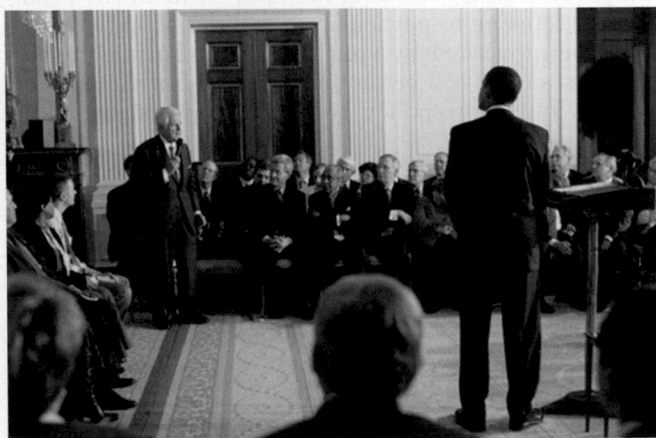

White House forum on health care reform. (Photo courtesy of USA.gov)

We will also discuss the relationship of politics and health policy. Your role as a public health nurse is to be responsive to the needs of the community you serve and its attendant politics. **Politics** is defined as the art or science of government, or governing of a political entity. It can be and is often defined as the art of using influence to bring about change. However, you may already be aware that politics can represent the machinations in which groups or individuals engage to influence, gain power, or get their way. Politics can also be labeled as the relationships between elected officials and their constituents; it can also be seen as the interplay between staff nurses and their head nurse or nursing supervisor. Politics can be described as the practice of public ethics. A clear example of this is the conflict between individual needs and the needs of a community—such as the debate around assisted suicide or the continuing debate regarding universal health care. Within communities, it may be the debate on whether to have and/or where to locate a family planning clinic or the most appropriate and effective methods to address teen pregnancy issues. As stated by the late Massachusetts Congressman and former Speaker of the House, Tip O'Neill, "*All politics is local.*"

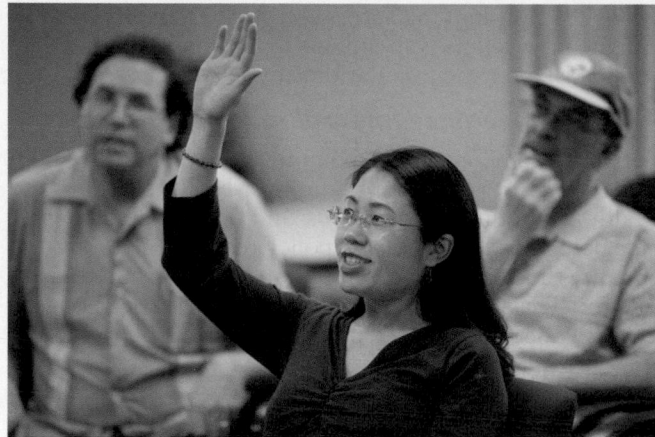

Town hall meetings promote community participation. (Photo courtesy of CDC Photo Image Library.)

HEALTH POLICY ANALYSIS

What Is Policy?

Nancy Milio, a well-known public health nurse, wrote extensively on policy and public health nursing practice, coining the term *healthy public policy*. Milio (1981) defined policy as option setting:

> To bring about the largest improvement in health requires the development of policies that will change the options that organizations and individuals face today. A health-making policy strategy would eliminate or increase the cost of those options that now result in health-damaging situations. It would provide new, easier opportunities, or reduce the cost of current options, in areas that now lack health-promoting resources. It would increase the cost of opportunities where health-promoting resources exist in deleterious excess (p. 76).

From Milio's perspective, **public policy** was a method for gaining consensus on which options a society would choose in order to meet social goals. Taking this approach, our health care system was guided for most of the 20th century on policy options including:

- Focus on medical treatment
- Fee-for-service financing
- Employment-based insurance
- Significant investment in medical technology and pharmaceuticals
- Limited financial support for prevention and public health

These options differ from what many peer countries select and, according to the Institute of Medicine report, might be a significant factor in U.S. health care disparities. Recent policy changes, primarily the ACA, are changing these options dramatically (USDHHS, 2015), as we shall discuss later in this chapter. Policy analysts define **policy** as (Anderson, 2015)

- A relatively stable, purposive course of action to deal with a problem or matter of concern
- A set of purposive actions taken over time

- Actions that emerge in response to needs or demands
- Actions that relate to government action, not stated intention
- Actions that can be negative or positive
- Actions that are based on law/regulation
- Actions that are authoritative

This definition focuses attention on purposive action based on law or regulations. We will talk later about how implementation and evaluation of these actions is also a critical component of the policy process. There are also different types of policies (Birkland, 2015). These include

- *Substantive policy*: This refers to policy that involves an action or activity, such as funding for a health program or health-related agency. One example would be federal funding for the Indian Health Service and its activities.
- *Procedural policies*: These involve how something is done, the procedure by which an outcome is sought. An example of this would be voting rights policies, which stipulate the process for voting eligibility.
- *Distributive policies*: Include those that allocate services or benefits to specific groups of people, for example, Medicare, which is also a substantive policy as it distributes resources to people who meet age and/or physical condition criteria.
- **Regulatory health policies**: These put limitations on the activities or behaviors of certain groups or individuals, such as age limits for purchase of alcohol or health professional licensing regulations.

These types can be defined in varying ways and the definitions are descriptive, but not necessarily mutually exclusive.

Policy and Public Health Nursing Practice

Now that we have some basic definitions of policy, we can consider how policy is relevant to public health nursing practice. The definition of PHN practice used in this text can be found in Chapter 1. This definition, developed and disseminated by the PHN Section of the American Public Health Association (APHA) in 1996 and reaffirmed in 2013 is as follows:

> Public health nursing is the practice of promoting and protecting the health of populations using knowledge from nursing, social, and public health sciences (APHA, PHN Section, 2013, para. 5).

The definition is further described as consisting of several key elements: (a) a focus on the health needs of an entire population; (b) assessment of population health using a comprehensive, systematic approach; (c) attention to multiple determinants of health; (d) an emphasis on primary prevention; and (e) application of interventions at all levels—individuals, families, communities, and the systems that impact their health. This definition is very consistent with the earlier discussion on health outcomes in the United States and the need for health care services. It also relates to health and social policies that create conditions in which people can be healthy by addressing the social factors determinants of health in addition to the physiological and behavioral determinants. Assessing

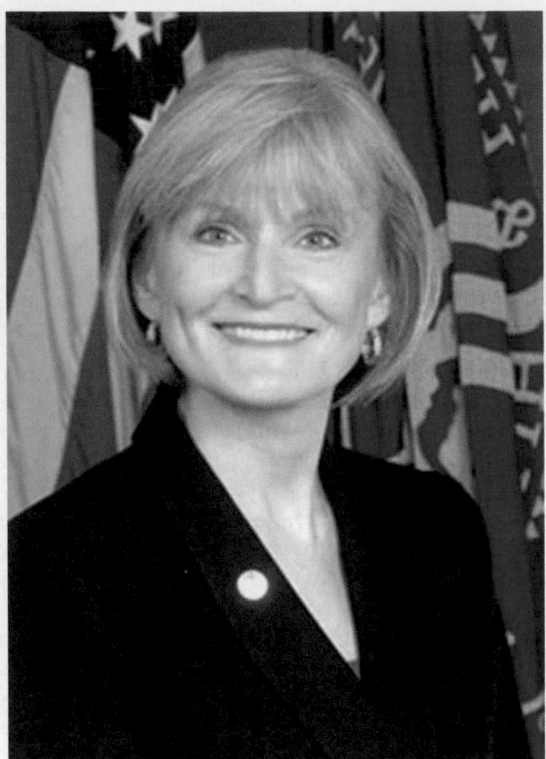

Mary Wakefield, PhD, RN, was appointed Administrator of the Health Resources and Services Administration (HRSA) by President Obama in 2009. (Photo courtesy USA.gov).

and treating the social determinants of health includes working with communities to develop policies that impact living conditions for families and communities. Thus, PHN practice must address policy implications of health needs and conversely look at creating policies to promote and maintain health for communities and populations. A recent movement in public health of interest to nurses is that of *Health in All Policies* (APHA, 2013). The APHA presents this as embedding health considerations into decision-making processes across all sectors.

An example of a *Health in All Policies* approach is a city planning policy for zoning and deciding on a site for a new retirement community for seniors. In the planning phase for the project, a health impact assessment would be done. A health impact assessment (HIA) is a "process that helps evaluate the potential health effects of a plan, project or policy before it is built or implemented. An HIA can provide recommendations to increase positive health outcomes and minimize adverse health outcomes. HIA brings potential public health impacts and considerations to the decision-making process for plans, projects, and policies that fall outside the traditional public health arenas, such as transportation and land use" (CDC, 2016, para. 2). In this case, the HIA would look at health implications of different site options. For example, what are the health implications for the residents if the facility is built just off a major highway? Is the population being served particularly vulnerable to noise or auto exhaust? What about building the facility on the outskirts of a town? Does this population have unique transportation needs? *Health in all Policies* as an approach helps

guide decision-making across sectors to maximize health-enhancing options and minimize options that increase health risks for the populations involved.

Policy Competence Integral to PHN Practice

For PHNs to practice to maximum effectiveness, they need to be aware of policy implications of health planning and health-promoting interventions and be prepared to provide data in order to support policy recommendations that enhance the health opportunities of a target group or community. This is called being *policy competent* (Longest, 2016). Policy competence means being able to

- Assess the impact of public policies on one's domain of interest/responsibility
- Understand policy and the policy process sufficiently to be able to exert influence on the process and impact policy
- Exert influence on the policy-making process

For public health nursing practice, this means that the PHN is able to assess which policies are relevant to his/her practice focus and understand the policy process sufficiently to be able to determine where the relevant policy is in the process. The PHN must also be able to determine where action is needed to influence the policy process and determine the role to take in lobbying for new legislation. Depending on the PHN practice role, the nurse (working for a government agency, for instance) may not be able to lobby for new legislation, but may choose to be policy active in private life. Deschaine and Schaffer, in a classic 2003 qualitative study of public health nurse leaders' role in policy development, used Longest's framework to describe political competence. The three areas included policy formulation (defining issues and setting policy agendas), policy implementation (development of potential solutions to identified problems), and policy implementation/modification (creating political circumstances that turn problem-solving into policy action). The study participants identified barriers to development of health policies as political and financial and could often be explained by the public's lack of knowledge about public health and its mission. Having only a few women in politics was also mentioned, along with the need for more in-depth training in policy development for PHN administrators and better access to research materials, trending data, and demographic information. A more recent study of African nurse leaders found that having knowledge of policy and practicing health policy development enhanced nursing's image, whereas a lack of policy involvement promoted a more negative nursing image and promoted processes and structures that excluded nurses (Shariff, 2014). As we shall see later in the chapter, there are many activities relevant to the policy process in addition to lobbying for legislation.

Local, State, and National Level Policy

Policies are laws, regulations, or administrative rulings; when issued by national, state, or local governments, they are called public policy. Health policy refers to specific policies involving health care. The legislative and regulatory process may start with lofty goals, but the final product is usually the result of compromise often encouraged by special interest groups, coalition groups, political realities, or the current economic environment. Although the study of politics has a long history, the systematic study of public policy, on the other hand, can be said to be a 20th-century creation. According to Daniel McCool, in his classic treatise on policy (1995), the study of public policy dates to 1922, when political scientist Charles Merriam sought to "connect the theory and practices of politics to understanding the actual activities of government, which is public policy" (p. 4).

Health policies can be distributive or redistributive. A **distributive health policy** promotes nongovernmental activities that are thought to be beneficial to society as a whole. An example of a distributive policy is the Nurse Training Act, Title VIII of the Public Health Service Act, which was established in 1965 and provided federal subsidies for nursing education in an effort to address the need for more nurses. A **redistributive health policy** changes the allocation of resources from one group to another, usually to a broader or different group. Medicare is an example of redistributive policy, in that provisions under Medicare were expanded to provide a broader range of benefits and coverage to needy groups—such as those older than age 65 and the permanently disabled of any age (Frederick, Saguy, & Gruys, in press).

One of the first policy questions to address is that of jurisdiction. Public policy impacts health and well-being at community, state, and national levels, so looking at policy jurisdiction is critical. The first step in understanding a policy issue is to know whether the key decision makers are local policy makers, state policy makers, or national policy makers.

Local Policy

Many policies that impact health care are developed and implemented at the local level, such as tobacco use in public places, availability of facilities for exercise and farmers markets, or access to locally funded health and social services. Although such policies may also be subject to guidelines from other jurisdictions (e.g., state, federal), a hallmark of the U.S. governmental system has been to have robust local policy authority (National League of Cities, 2013). Although the U.S. Constitution specifically talks about state authority, each state also gives powers to local governments, and so the policy-competent PHN needs to know what jurisdiction governs the issue of interest to the health of the community. Such public health–relevant policies as requirements for gun ownership or speed limits on public roads are often made by local level governing bodies. At the local level, these policies are very open to public involvement, because often the legislative and regulatory bodies are close by and composed of neighbors and community residents. The PHN is often able to collect or interpret data relevant to the health impact of local policies, and can talk directly to these people about local policy concerns.

State Policy

There is a limit to municipal powers and some policies are developed and regulated at the state level. Longest (2016) notes that the role of states in health policy includes being public health guardians (e.g., protect public health and welfare through laws and regulations), health care service purchasers (often in conjunction with the federal level; safety-net providers), and as providers of education and public health laboratory services. Health and related policies such as Medicaid eligibility and services, health professional license regulation and scope of practice, and public health codes including immunization regulations are some of the functions that fall within state powers. With the recent passage of the ACA, participation in the marketplace of insurance plans and expanded federal funding for Medicaid were decisions made by state legislatures and had significant impacts on access to care (Callow, 2015).

National Policy

Funding for the health insurance plan Medicare, the ACA, parts of Medicaid, and health research are all national level policies. This level of policy has the advantage of being broadly applicable across the country, with the potential for significant impact on population health. It is challenging, however, to work at this level because there are a large number of stakeholders and an enormous political and policy bureaucracy for creation of legislation, as well as for implementation and evaluation. However, federal funding and regulatory requirements impact the role and practice of public health nurses, and PHN practice includes being aware of, and in compliance with, federal policies. See Perspectives: Policy Impacts at Local, State, and National Levels.

PERSPECTIVES: POLICY IMPACTS AT LOCAL, STATE, AND NATIONAL LEVELS

Local policy—In January 2016, the mayor of the city of Chicago called for legislation to increase the minimum age for purchasing of tobacco from 18 to 21 years. Teenagers are the largest group of new smokers, and research suggests that increasing the legal age to purchase tobacco is part of an overall strategy to discourage teens from using tobacco products (Rhodes, 2016).

State policy—As of 2015, 22 states and the District of Columbia require that public schools teach sex education; and 20 districts mandate sex education and HIV education. Three states require parental consent before a child can receive instruction. A total of 35 states and the District of Columbia allow parents to opt out on behalf of their children (i.e., if parents sign the form stating that they don't want their child to participate, the school district will exclude them; but, if no form is returned, the child has tacit permission to attend). Clearly, the PHN working in school health needs to be aware of the state policies in this area before planning interventions with school age children on sex education, including HIV education (National Council of State Legislatures, 2015).

National policy—Data indicate that climate change can have detrimental health effects on populations including increased respiratory and cardiovascular disease, injuries and premature deaths related to extreme weather events, changes in the prevalence and geographical distribution of food- and water-borne illnesses and other infectious diseases, and threats to mental health (CDC, 2015a). National policy efforts, implemented by the Environmental Protection Agency (2016), include monitoring greenhouse gas emissions and developing regulatory policies, in conjunction with private sector corporations, to reduce such emission.

LEGISLATIVE PROCESS AT THE NATIONAL LEVEL

How does legislation get passed at the federal level? The federal model for how an idea becomes a bill and how a bill is passed into legislation is relevant across the country. States each have their own mechanism. The first step in becoming policy competent on any issue is to know under which jurisdiction the issue falls (local, state, or federal) and then know how policy is developed and regulated at that level. There are a wide variety of Web sites and descriptions of the legislative process, but the definitive version can be found on the house of representatives Web site: http://www.house.gov/content/learn/legislative_process/. It is estimated that only 5% or less of bills introduced into any session of Congress actually become laws (Braun, 2013). The two session of Congress between 2011 and 2015 only enacted 2% to 3% of bills into law (Civic Impulse, 2015).

How a Bill Becomes a Law

This section will review the process for how a bill becomes a law at the federal level, but the process is very similar at the state level. See Figures 13–1 and 13–2 for state and federal examples.

Ideas for legislation can originate anywhere and be introduced as legislation at the state and federal levels. For federal legislation, the bill is introduced in either the house of representatives or the senate. Individuals or groups may call their local congressman or senator and propose an idea, or lobbyists working for the APHA,

for instance, can ask for changes to existing laws that promote their members' interests. Only budget bills must originate in the house of representatives. This was done to keep the budget process closest to the "people's house," the body of the legislature where members represent relatively small numbers of constituents for 2-year terms and thus are thought to be more responsive to their constituents. This structure, built into the U.S. Constitution, was designed to avoid too much control of government by moneyed classes and to enhance representation of the majority (Jensen, 2011; Longest, 2016). When a bill is introduced to either house, it is assigned to a committee based upon the general area of focus (e.g., appropriations, agriculture). The committee structure is designed to allow members of each house to focus on a smaller number of issues in depth and then vote, as a whole, on issues that are deemed worthy of going before the whole legislature (i.e., going to the "floor") for a vote. Often, bills never leave the committee, stalling there because of lack of interest from the majority party, whose members chair committees and thus set the committee's agenda, in both houses. Some bills have hearings, where experts are brought in to testify to facets of the bill, and answer questions from the committee members. For bills where there is sufficient interest or political will, the bill will be discussed, amended as needed, and voted upon in the committee. If the bill passes in committee, it is sent to the full house for further discussion, possible amendments, and an ultimate vote (Longest, 2016).

If the bill passes the full house, it is sent to the other chamber, and the process begins again. Sometimes, bills are introduced simultaneously to both houses, which can speed the process, as each committee and house reviews and votes on the bill during the same time period. If the

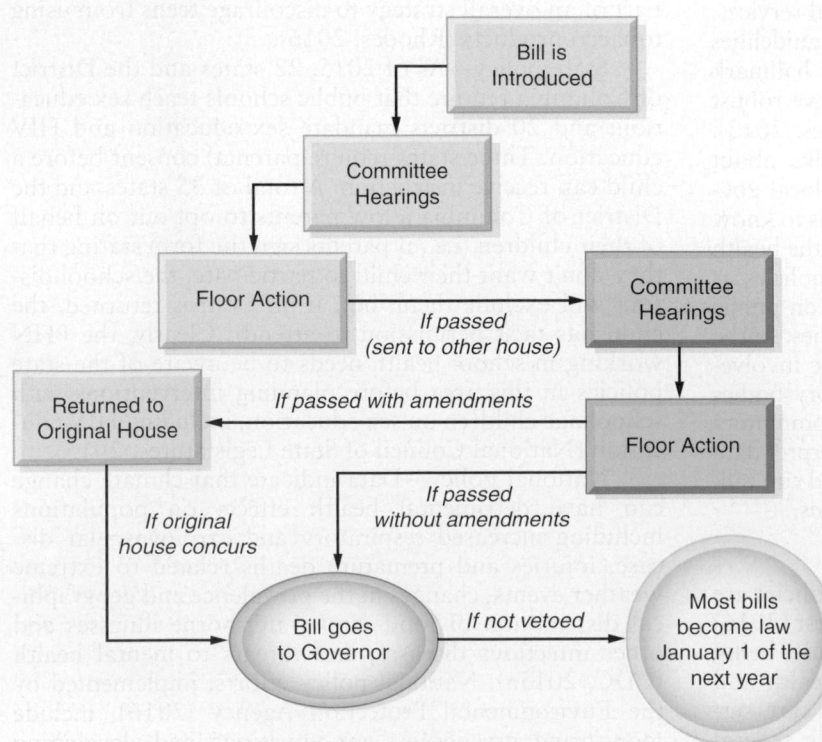

FIGURE 13–1 How a bill becomes a law—state process. The process may vary by state, but generally the schematic shows how the process unfolds. (Source: California Legislative Counsel.)

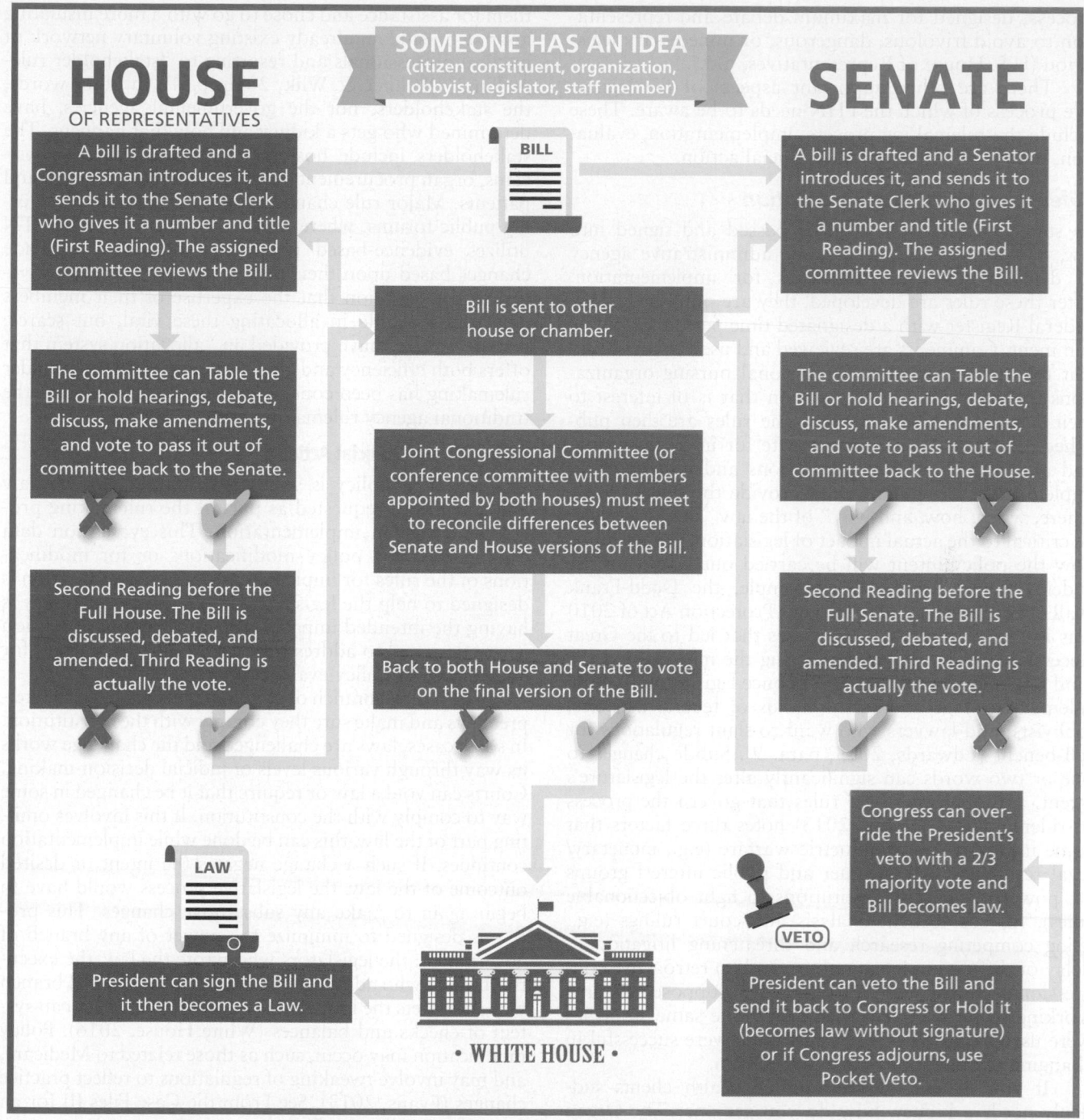

HOUSE
OF REPRESENTATIVES

SOMEONE HAS AN IDEA
(citizen constituent, organization,
lobbyist, legislator, staff member)

SENATE

BILL

A bill is drafted and a Congressman introduces it, and sends it to the Senate Clerk who gives it a number and title (First Reading). The assigned committee reviews the Bill.

A bill is drafted and a Senator introduces it, and sends it to the Senate Clerk who gives it a number and title (First Reading). The assigned committee reviews the Bill.

Bill is sent to other house or chamber.

The committee can Table the Bill or hold hearings, debate, discuss, make amendments, and vote to pass it out of committee back to the Senate.

Joint Congressional Committee (or conference committee with members appointed by both houses) must meet to reconcile differences between Senate and House versions of the Bill.

The committee can Table the Bill or hold hearings, debate, discuss, make amendments, and vote to pass it out of committee back to the House.

Second Reading before the Full House. The Bill is discussed, debated, and amended. Third Reading is actually the vote.

Back to both House and Senate to vote on the final version of the Bill.

Second Reading before the Full Senate. The Bill is discussed, debated, and amended. Third Reading is actually the vote.

Congress can override the President's veto with a 2/3 majority vote and Bill becomes law.

LAW

VETO

President can sign the Bill and it then becomes a Law.

· WHITE HOUSE ·

President can veto the Bill and send it back to Congress or Hold it (becomes law without signature) or if Congress adjourns, use Pocket Veto.

FIGURE 13–2   How a bill becomes a law—federal level. (Adapted from http://beyond5.org/wp-content/uploads/infographics/Bill_to_Law.jpg. Used with permission.)

bill is passed in each house, but in a slightly different version, a conference committee, composed of members of both houses, is convened to discuss, amend, and vote on the bill. The bill can stall in the conference committee until the session of Congress ends, and then it would need to be reintroduced in the next session, as bills do not carry over from one session to the next. Alternatively, the bill may be passed by the conference committee and then be returned to each chamber for a final vote. At this point, amendments would not be added or the bill would be stalled again and have to go back through

the process once again (Longest, 2016; U.S. House of Representatives, n.d.).

After both chambers of Congress pass the same version of a bill, it then goes to the president for signature. The president can sign the bill, in which case it becomes law and is sent to the appropriate administrative agency for rule making, or the president can actively or passively veto the legislation, in which case the bill needs to be sent back to each chamber for a 2/3 vote to override the president's veto, or the bill stalls again, and the process begins anew. In summary, passing legislation is a complex process, designed for maximum debate and representation to avoid frivolous, dangerous, or unnecessary legislation (U.S. House of Representatives, n.d.).

There are other important aspects of the legislative process of which the PHN needs to be aware. These include the rulemaking process, implementation, evaluation, policy modification, and judicial action.

Rulemaking and Implementation

As stated earlier, after a bill is passed and signed into law, it is sent to the appropriate administrative agency to develop rules and processes for implementation. After these rules are developed, they are published in the Federal Register with a designated time period for public comment. Comments are reviewed and used to revise and edit the rules as needed. Professional nursing organizations monitor rules and legislation that is of interest to their members (ANA, 2016a). The rules are then published, along with an effective date for implementation, and are used to guide organizations and individuals in implementing the policy; rules provide the "who, what, where, when, how, and why" of the law. These rules can be critical to the actual impact of legislation, as they guide how the policy intent will be carried out (Office of the Federal Register, n.d.). For example, the Dodd-Frank Wall Street Reform and Consumer Protection Act of 2010 was intended to reform the abuses that led to the Great Recession. However, "manipulating the minutiae" is the kind of game playing that occurs once legislation is at the rulemaking stage and in the hands of federal agencies, lobbyists, and lawyers who want to slant regulations for self-benefit (Edwards, 2013, para. 9). Subtle changes to one or two words can significantly alter the legislature's intent. Although there are rules that govern the process of rulemaking, Edwards (2013) notes three factors that come into play: (a) asymmetric warfare (e.g., monetary/legal resources for consumer and public interest groups vs. powerful financial institutions to fight objectionable rules), (b) cost–benefit analysis and court rulings (e.g., using competing research and threatening litigation to delay or diffuse implementation), and (c) retroactive congressional attacks (e.g., legislators who opposed the law working to retroactively weaken it). The same strategies were used against the ACA, and some were successful in changing the intent of health care reform.

If you or one of your public health clients suddenly needs a kidney, how do you get one? The Organ Procurement and Transplantation Network (OPTN) allocates kidneys and other organs. Donated-organ allocation provides an example of rulemaking that was not done through a government agency. When organ transplants became more feasible after immunosuppressive medications were developed in the 1980s, the National Organ Transplant Act (PL 98-507) created the OPTN and the Scientific Registry of Transplant Recipients (SRTR) to monitor and "predict the consequences of rule changes" and provide feedback from stakeholders on the consequences of any rule changes (Weimer & Wilk, 2016, p. 2). With such a sensitive issue as shortages or organs available for transplant and deciding who gets one first, legislators wanted to avoid the usual government agency rulemaking that could have their constituents continually badgering them for assistance and chose to go with a more insulating approach using an already existing voluntary network of medical professionals and resorting to "stakeholder rulemaking" (Weimer & Wilk, 2016, p. 4). In other words, the stakeholders, not the governmental agencies, have determined who gets a kidney and how that happens. The stakeholders include hospital transplant centers, physicians, organ procurement organizations, laboratories, and patients. Major rule change proposals are presented during public forums, where feedback is elicited. The OPTN utilizes evidence-based policy making and has made changes based upon their definition of medical effectiveness and the notion that the expertise of their members has been valuable in allocating these vital, but scarce, resources. They have provided an "allocation system that offers both efficiency and greater equity," and stakeholder rulemaking has been considered more successful than the traditional agency rulemaking in this example (p. 27).

Evaluation and Judicial Action

Evaluation of policy is sometimes written into the law and sometimes requested as part of the rulemaking process as a step in implementation. This evaluation data can be used for policy modifications or for modifications of the rules for implementation. Policy evaluation is designed to help the legislature know whether a policy is having the intended impact on the problem or condition it was designed to address. See From the Case Files II for an example of policy evaluation.

The judicial branch of government is designed to interpret laws and make sure they comply with the constitution. In some cases, laws are challenged and the challenge works its way through various levels of judicial decision-making. Courts can void a law or require that it be changed in some way to comply with the constitution. If this involves omitting part of the law, this can be done while implementation continues. If such a change negates the intent or desired outcome of the law, the legislative process would have to begin again to make any substantive changes. This process is designed to minimize the power of any branch of government: the legislators who wrote the law, the executive branch who administers the law, or the judicial branch who interprets the law. This is known as the American system of checks and balances (White House, 2016). Policy modification may occur, such as those related to Medicare, and may involve tweaking of regulations to reflect practice changes (Evans, 2013). See From the Case Files III for an example of policy modification.

POLICY ANALYSIS FOR THE PUBLIC HEALTH NURSE

Once the PHN understands how an idea becomes law, and how that law is implemented, she or he can begin to analyze the policy process to determine where they might become involved to create "healthy public policy" (Bowman et al., 2012, p. 2). **Policy analysis** is the technique of understanding a policy from a variety of perspectives. Such analysis can provide results for better understanding policy, finding ways to impact policy development, understanding the values behind policy, tracking the history of policy in specific areas, and other policy-relevant research and practice questions. Policy analysis can be

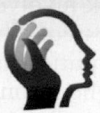

From the Case Files II

An Example of Evaluating Policy Changes: California's Safe Patient Handling Legislation

California's Hospital Patient and Health Care Worker Injury Protection Act (or Safe Patient Handling) went into effect in 2012 and directed acute care hospitals to implement policies and procedures for safe patient handling with the hope of reducing musculoskeletal injuries in nurses and other health care workers (State of California, 2012). Researchers completed an epidemiological assessment of 220 nurses with patient handling duties working in California hospitals and found, over a 1-year period, that 69% had musculoskeletal symptoms that were work related. Of those, 37% reported that their hospitals had lift teams, 61% had mechanical lift equipment available, and 22% noted that their hospitals had a "no-lift" policy (Lee, Lee, & Gershon, 2015). Nurses working in hospitals with lift teams had a significantly lower proportion of reported low back pain, and those with ceiling lifts had significantly lower reports of shoulder pain than those working in hospitals without lift teams and ceiling lifts. About 60% of nurses in the study had some

knowledge of the new law, and about one third said that their hospitals had made changes regarding patient handling policies and procedures. Lee et al. (2015) concluded that this evaluation of the impact of this legislation and policy change had both positive and "suboptimal" elements and that safe patient handling practices should continue to be monitored.

Do you think nurses are generally aware of legislation that affects their workplace, practice, and patient outcomes? Why? Why not?

How could nurses become involved in the implementation of new laws/regulations and policy evaluation?

Lee, S. J., Lee, J. H., & Gershon, R. R. (2015). Musculoskeletal symptoms in nurses in the early implementation phase of California's Safe Patient Handling legislation. Research in Nursing and Health, 38(3), 183–193

State of California, Department of Industrial Relations. (2012, January 25). Frequently asked questions: Cal/OSHA AB 1136 Safe Patient Handling. Retrieved from https://www.dir.ca.gov/dosh/ Safe%20Patient%20Handling%20FAQ.pdf

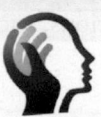

From the Case Files III

How to Solve a Problem: Pseudoephedrine Legislation and Methamphetamine

Because pseudoephedrine (PSE; a nasal decongestant often used for allergies, colds, and sinus congestion) is a main ingredient in the production of meth (methamphetamine), Congress passed the Combat Methamphetamine Epidemic Act of 2005 to help limit the sale of medications containing PSE. It is now sold only from behind the counter, and daily/monthly limits are mandated. Purchasers are required to show photo identification, and the seller must keep a logbook of customer identification and sales. However, PSE remains an over-the-counter drug, with no prescription necessary for its purchase. Because of the spread of methamphetamine throughout this country, into rural/suburban and urban areas, some states have gone further. Both Mississippi and Oregon have now passed laws requiring that a customer must have a physician's order for any medication containing PSE and have classified these medications as Schedule III. Many other states have introduced legislation requiring prescriptions for PSE-containing medications, some classifying PSE as a controlled substance.

Indiana proposed legislation that would have permitted local governments to tighten rules on PSE or allow counties or cities to require prescriptions for PSE or ephedrine products. Several cities in Missouri and Tennessee have passed laws making PSE medications available by prescription only.

This is an example of policy modification. A federal policy was modified by state and local governments, who chose to tighten regulations on PSE in order to try to control the supply of methamphetamine and better meet the needs of their citizens (Longest, 2016).

Can you think of an example of federal legislation that might be better implemented in your area through policy modification (e.g., environmental, occupational, health/safety)? Or state legislation that should be modified to better serve the needs of your county or city population?

Centers for Disease Control, Office for State, Tribal, Local and Territorial Support Centers for Disease Control and Prevention. (2013, August 17). Pseudoephedrine: Legal efforts to make it a prescription-only drug. Retrieved from http://www.cdc.gov/phlp/docs/ pseudo-brief112013.pdf.

done using a variety of approaches and methods. Here, we will present policy analysis for practicing PHNs to help them develop policy competence.

Policy competence, as discussed earlier, means understanding policy and the policy process sufficiently to be able to exert influence on the process and impact policy (Longest, 2016). In order to be policy competent, the PHN must be able to assess the impact of public policies on one's domain of interest/responsibility and exert influence on the policy-making process. This can be done at a variety of levels. Because policy sets the context for much of PHN practice, policy competence is particularly important for PHNs, but all nurses should have some concept of how policy affects nurses, patients, and communities. For example, changes in Medicaid funding, at either the national or state level, might directly impact which clients the PHN is allowed to include in certain health promotion/disease prevention programs. Therefore, the PHN should understand this impact, the reasons for the Medicaid changes, and where useful input might be provided. This might be as straightforward as explaining to agency administrators what the impact of these changes will be on individuals in the community, or it may be more complicated and involve policy evaluation mechanisms or development of alternative policy solutions to meet the health goals of the community.

For the purposes of policy competence in PHN practice, we will discuss two frameworks for policy analysis, the rational framework and John Kingdon's framework. These frameworks provide two interrelated mechanisms for looking at the policy process and are combined into a useful diagram by Longest (2016). See Figure 13–3.

The rational framework is commonly found in policy texts as a straightforward way to comprehend the intent and effect of a particular policy. The framework involves first, defining the policy problem to be addressed. The more clear and measurable this problem definition is, the more specific any policy response can be. The second step in this framework is to understand possible solutions to this policy problem and compare and contrast them to each other in order to determine which is optimal in terms of being politically feasible, easily implemented, and likely to result in the desired outcome. The third step, based on comparing and contrasting the possible policy alternatives, is to select an alternative, after which the alternative is implemented and evaluated for its effectiveness (Kingdon, 2011). This logical analytic framework is very similar to the nursing process, in its structure and components, and as such is easily understood by PHNs (ANA, 2016b). An example from Sri Lanka involves achieving a consensus on the public health problem of high rates of suicide (47 overall and 80 for males per 100,000—the highest in the world at that time). The initial policy change restricted toxic pesticide access and resulted in some reduction in mortality rates. Further reductions were sought, so a presidential committee of experts was convened to examine and make recommendations about the problem, using the rational framework approach. A large proportion of suicides were deemed self-poisoning, and suggestions ranged from reducing access to lethal pesticides, research to decrease the lethality level of pesticides, changing the culture to discourage suicides, repackaging pesticides into nonlethal doses, and increasing access to care to improve survival rates after suicidal poisoning. Once the data and the potential interventions were discussed, policy analysis was used to determine weaknesses, strengths, and costs of options. Interventions that required further political actions, such

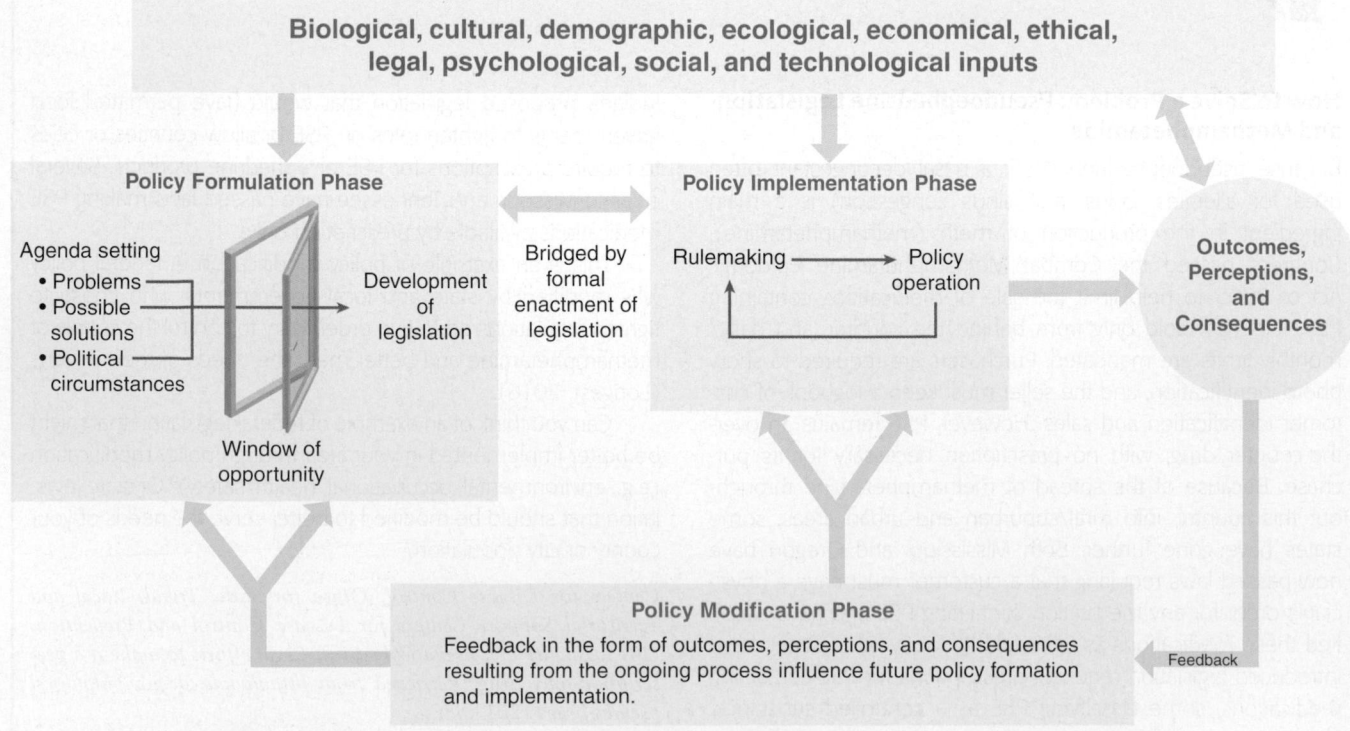

FIGURE 13–3 Longest's model. (Adapted from Longest, B. B. (2016). *Health policymaking in the United States* (5th ed.). Chicago, IL: Health Administration Press, p. 82, with permission.)

as taxation, new programs, or private sector self-interest, were weighed. The influence of expert evidence and data are not sufficient to change policies—**political action** is needed with an understanding of "context, networks, knowledge, implementation, and impact" (Pearson, Anthony, & Buckley, 2010, para. 37). Understanding of technical feasibility, budgets, marketability, and dominant cultural values are necessary to incorporate, along with evidence and data, in order to exert political influence and change cultural practices.

There are several challenges to using this framework. Again, much like the nursing process, it examines policy as a structured, linear process, and that is often not the case. Challenges in defining the problem or in comparing viable solutions might often influence policy to be formed with insufficient data or based on the power and influence of specific stakeholders, meaning that all elements may not be considered carefully and in the order presented in the framework (Kingdon, 2010, 2011). Additionally, this framework doesn't assist the PHN in addressing the politics involved or in determining why one issue might be addressed when another—equally important to the community—might languish with no policy activity taking place.

The second framework to be discussed here is that developed by John Kingdon (2010, 2011). Kingdon set out in his research to address the question of why some issues came to the forefront in policy development and others did not. Kingdon argued, based on his research results, that policy was enacted when a *window of opportunity* was opened. During the period of this open window, bills could be voted on and new legislation made. The window of opportunity opened when there was a confluence of a *policy problem*, a *viable solution* or solutions, and *political will* on this issue. This confluence opened a window of opportunity for the issue to be acted upon (however briefly). See Figure 13–4, Kingdon's Model of the Policy Process.

Kingdon presented each component of the framework specifically. The *problem*, he contended, should be defined using *indicators*, that is, data to document its existence. However, he also said problems could be defined by *focusing events*, or attention getting incidents, which highlighted a problem for a large portion of the population. An example of a focusing event would be the terrorist attacks on the World Trade Center and Pentagon in September 2001, which brought national and international attention to the problems of terrorism and airline safety. Kingdon also argued that it was important to

understand the problem from multiple perspectives; that is, how would others see the same problem and data? In this way, he contended that the analyst could understand multiple perspectives and how they might impact the solutions and politics (Kingdon, 2010, 2011).

Identifying a *policy solution* was the next component of the Kingdon framework. Kingdon stated that there are always policy solutions floating around in what he called the "policy primeval soup" (2010, para. 10). He provided some parameters for assessing solutions: Are they technically feasible (can they be implemented)? Are they acceptable in terms of public values? Are they within acceptable costs? Do they comply with the current size and role of government? Would they be considered fair and equitable? He used these questions to compare solutions for those most likely to align with problems and politics (Kingdon, 2011).

When analyzing the *politics* of an issue, Kingdon had several facets to consider. First, what is the political climate at the current time? For example, immediately after the 9/11 terrorist attacks, the U.S. political climate was focused almost entirely on safety and security, and very few other issues were being seriously addressed. Kingdon (2011) also advised looking at stakeholders on both sides of an issue and assessing relative power and influence. This can be done by looking at the numbers of people they represent, resources available for lobbying, and political reputation and past achievements.

When a *window of opportunity* does open, Kingdon (2011) cautioned that it does not remain open forever. Sometimes, other issues arise and take precedence. Sometimes, partial action is taken, and the public perceives the problem has been resolved, at least in the near term. And, other times, a window closes because the public loses interest in unresolved issues that have been around for a long time. In Kingdon's terms, policy activists should look for opportunities to open windows and, when windows are open, should act to capitalize on the opportunity. A global example involves tobacco control. As the United States utilized decades of research and began legislating no-smoking ordinances and tax increases on tobacco products and rates of tobacco-related morbidity and mortality dropped, a window of opportunity opened for countries around the world to enact tobacco control policies (Gneiting, 2016). Employing Kingdon's framework and an international treaty on tobacco control (Framework Convention on Tobacco Control) established by the World Health Organization, the Framework Convention Alliance (FCA) began working globally toward raising awareness of tobacco as a public health threat and utilizing new funding sources (e.g., Gates Foundation, Bloomberg Initiative) to shape national policy agendas. Smoke-free legislation gained the most "advocacy momentum and policy traction," with 120 member countries on board (Gneiting, 2016, p. i80). The tobacco industry has responded by marketing e-cigarettes, influencing trade and governmental partnership agreements, and aggressively lobbying against tobacco tax increases. Some of these measures are not part of the original treaty and now must be addressed. Measures to increase tobacco taxes have not been as successful as smoke-free initiatives. The relative political power of the tobacco industry has been difficult to overcome, but the alliance members continue their work.

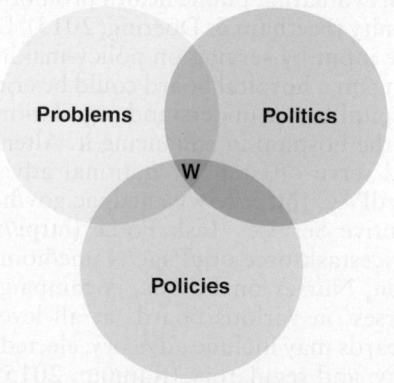

FIGURE 13–4 Kingdon's model of the policy process.

Drawbacks to Kingdon's framework include the fact that his framework analyzes policy to the point of passing a bill into law. His framework doesn't address the issue of implementation, evaluation, or policy modification. As mentioned earlier, Longest combined the rational framework and Kingdon's framework into a figure encompassing all facets of policy making.

For the policy analyst, both frameworks present important components of understanding an issue. The rational framework allows the analyst to look post hoc at an issue and learn from the process as it unfolded. For policy activists, or PHNs who want to use policy effectively in practice (policy competence), the Kingdon framework allows you to examine a current issue in real time and determine if a window of opportunity exists or if one could be created. This helps the PHN, or a public health organization, to prioritize its time and resources and focus policy efforts where they can be most effective.

Policy Analysis for Activism

Now, we will put this altogether—how can a PHN use this information to be policy active in practice? The first step is to select a policy issue to address. What health concern in your community or target population has policy implications or is being impacted by current health policy or the lack thereof? Perhaps there are water quality concerns in the community, or the most recent community assessment has identified an increase in sexually transmitted infections (STIs) among adolescents and young adults. Are these public policy issues? That is, does it involve public decisions about laws and regulations related to funding, services, or rights and behaviors?

The second step, once the PHN has determined that the issue is indeed one of public policy, is to conduct a brief policy analysis using Kingdon's framework initially: What is the *problem*? Are there *solutions*, and are they adequate and appropriate? What are the *politics*—or who are the stakeholders and what is their level of influence? This preliminary analysis will inform the PHN whether this is a new issue on the agenda or whether it is an issue of *implementation* or *evaluation* of existing legislation or regulations.

Given this, what does the PHN want in relation to this issue? And under what policy jurisdiction does the issue fall (local, state, federal)? Perhaps the key concern is the problem: Is it not well defined, or does the definition need to be expanded? Is the main goal to get the issue on the policy agenda via outreach to policy makers? Are better data needed to more clearly define the problem? Is there a viable solution available, or do solutions need to be tested and developed based on practice standards and population needs? Is this an issue of the way a regulation is being implemented, and thus, can change be made by working with legislators to identify the problem and develop implementation modifications? Is there a policy in place that lacks clarity about whether it is working, or if it needs expansion or contraction? Who would be the key stakeholders and target audience for any action?

Once the PHN has answered these questions, then the level of involvement necessary can be determined. And given constraints on time, lobbying, access to data, and the priority of the issue, the level of engagement can then be determined. A number of avenues for activism are available, based on the above criteria. Table 13–1 demonstrates how the analysis framework relates to concerns of the PHN and possible actions in response.

POLITICAL ACTION AND ADVOCACY FOR PHNS

The definition of PHN practice describes efforts to promote and protect the public's health. When looking at *Healthy Public Policy*, PHN efforts to do so can take many forms from active participation as an informed citizen to actions taken as part of PHN practice to promote *Healthy Public Policy* (Bowman et al., 2012; Gottlieb, Fielding, & Braveman, 2012; National Collaborating Centre for Healthy Public Policy, 2010).

The PHN as an informed citizen, who has valuable knowledge and experience in health and health promotion, can be involved at a basic level by being aware of health policy and using this awareness for informed voting in elections across levels of jurisdiction. Individual PHNs might choose to increase their involvement by serving in a campaign to support a legislator that espouses public policies promoting health and preventing disease. Additionally, the PHN might choose to share their expertise with others, as a means to inform their voting and citizen involvement. The PHN could also choose to be involved in professional organizations or citizen organizations to advocate for *Healthy Public Policies* and the legislators who promote them. PHN practice, looking broadly at health and the social determinants of health, can provide background that is valuable in any number of professional and civic organizations. For example, at the state level, the PHN can ensure that the state nursing organizations maintain a broad-based focus on the health of the public. And locally, PHNs can serve on health boards, but can also provide valuable input into health and education by serving on school boards or parent–teacher organizations. Working toward eliminating health inequities, healthier built environments, HIAs, and sharing knowledge are all worthwhile endeavors for nurses who want to affect population through health policy work (Kostas-Polston, Thanavaro, Arvidson, & Taub, 2015; National Collaborating Centre for Healthy Public Policy, 2010).

PHN researchers can provide policy-relevant input by focusing on research questions related to the social determinants of health or health in all policies and sharing results in a clear and persuasive manner with policy makers and legislators. PHN research might include assessing the impact of public policies on community health outcomes or on evaluating public health promotion efforts in the community (Feetham & Doering, 2015). Lastly, PHNs can provide input by serving on policy-making bodies. A PHN serving on a hospital board could be critical in helping the hospital better understand population health and the role of the hospital in enhancing it. Alternatively, the PHN could serve on state or national advisory groups such as MedPAC (http://www.medpac.gov/home) or the U.S. Preventive Services Task Force (http://www.uspreventiveservicestaskforce.org/Page/Name/home). The organization, Nurses on Boards, is campaigning to put 10,000 nurses on various boards at all levels by 2020. Types of boards may include advisory, elected, appointed, constituency, and regulatory (Rambur, 2015). The organization provides a wide variety of examples across each

Table 13–1 PHN Practice Mechanisms to Address Policy Issues

Component of Analysis Framework	Action Needed	Mechanisms of Action
Problem	Data to define	• Collect or analyze evaluation data; assessment data • Collaborate with researchers on problem definition
	Expand definition	• Collaborate with researchers on problem definition
Policies/solutions	Develop/pilot possible solutions	• Develop and implement model projects
	Change context to increase solution viability	• Evaluate/collect outcome data on projects to evaluate process of implementation
Politics	Educate public or other stakeholders	• Letters, phone call, e-mails, office visits to key stakeholders • Communicate via letters to the editor or social media • Present program results or assessment results in public forum • Disseminate reports on service outcomes or new conditions to key stakeholders
Implementation	Revise regulations to improve implementation	• Work with regulators to revise regulations and rules
	Expand implementation to others affected	• Work with legislators and/or regulators to expand eligible populations for interventions
Evaluation	Data needed to measure impact	• Evaluate services provided
	Disseminate evaluation results	• Present program results or assessment results in public forum • Disseminate reports on service outcomes or new conditions to key stakeholders
	Policy modification needed (see Problem)	• Collaborate to collect data for problem definition

state, along with guidance on how to prepare to serve on a board (http://nursesonboardscoalition.org/).

Public Health and Social Justice

The concept of social justice is seen as the very foundation of public health and public health nursing (deChesnay & Anderson, 2016; Donohoe, 2013). The American Association of Colleges of Nursing (n.d.) emphasizes that the guiding values of nursing include social justice at all levels of preparation, and the ANA *Code of Ethics with Interpretative Statements* (2015, preface) states that nurses should "act to change those aspects of society that detract from health and wellbeing." The ANA's *Public Health Nursing: Scope and Standards of Practice* document also highlights the basic value of social justice in community health nursing (2013). The many definitions of social justice depend on the discipline involved; for purposes of this chapter, social justice is a fair allocation of both the costs and rewards of being a member of a group focusing on the processes, perceptions, and roles (Barusch, 2012). This could also be characterized as balancing or equalizing societal costs and benefits. However, nurses are not always consistent in their abilities to fully comprehend or develop strategies to address injustice.

We often want things to be fair, but do not always clearly define what that means, or sufficiently promote specific actions needed to ensure it. We may feel frustrated about situations we see every day, but need to be better equipped to address them (Paquin, 2011). You may be caught in a "Catch-22" situation, working within a market-based system that is inherently unfair and often leads

to health and social disparities for ethnic and other disadvantaged groups while having pledged to alleviate suffering within the groups you serve (ANA, 2013, 2015).

As a public health nurse, you are expected to give voice to the disparities found in the communities you serve (e.g., substandard housing, high rates of unemployment, death, and disability)—disparities that often could be prevented or alleviated at early stages. Your efforts through nursing interventions can address not only health issues but also the educational, social, and economic issues that give rise to these disparities (deChesnay & Anderson, 2016; Donohoe, 2013). The Minnesota Department of Public Health Nursing Section has developed a public health interventions model that gives a broad overview of public health nursing. The model is based on the type of intervention and practice levels that allows a range of activities, such as advocacy, community organizing, coalition building, case management, and policy development, which you as a public health practitioner can activate (see Chapter 14). The nexus between social justice, advocacy, and policy is interrelated, complex, and one that will affect every aspect of your community health nursing career.

History of Public Health Nursing Advocacy

Nurses have a long history of action in social justice and **advocacy**, which can be defined as pleading the case of another or championing a cause (see Chapter 2). Developing policy solutions is a fundamental role for nurses—for the welfare of patients and communities, as well as the profession (Mason, Gardner, Outlaw,

& O'Grady, 2016). To advocate is to try to influence outcomes that affect people, communities, and systems. Additionally, advocacy is a process, not an outcome, one that includes identifying an issue, collecting information, identifying who can be influenced/who can make the decision sought, building support, and taking action. Advocacy can present itself in a variety of ways—self-advocacy, which is advocating for oneself; individual advocacy, which is pleading the case of others; and legislative advocacy, which is changing or modifying state or federal laws. Advocacy also includes litigation and public education campaigns. Finally, advocacy is also the process of empowering those less able to present their views or needs, with the goal of giving them a voice and/or achieving their objectives. Nurses have long been advocates for their patients, and advocacy can and does affect the larger systems of care (deChesnay & Anderson, 2016; Donohoe, 2013; Paquin, 2011). **Community health advocacy** refers to efforts aimed at creating awareness of and generating support for meeting the community's health needs. Both nurses and communities have a common goal—the best possible health services for all.

The term and concept of *public health nursing* was coined in 1893 by Lillian Wald, who described PHNs as nurses who worked outside the hospital "to provide decent health care" to those people living in poor communities and tenements (Jewish Women's Archive, 2016, para. 2). These nurses specialized in both preserving health and prevention measures as they responded to referrals from patients and physicians and they were only paid if the patient was able to afford payment. In 1893, Lillian Wald and Mary Brewster established the Visiting Nurses Service, and a year later, the famed Henry Street Settlement House was established. Wald's exposure to the plight of newly arrived immigrants to the Lower East Side and the appalling living conditions there spurred her to action. She was determined that these immigrants and other poor people, regardless of ethnicity or religious affiliation, would have access to health care and adequate housing. Wald went on to encourage the establishment of the Department of Nursing and Health at Columbia University's Teachers College through a series of lectures she presented starting in 1910. She also was instrumental in creating the U.S. Children's Bureau in 1912, an agency that oversaw fair child labor laws (see Chapter 2).

The importance of these nurses—Lillian Wald and her compatriots, Sojourner Truth, Margaret Sanger, Clara Barton, Mary Seacole, Susie King Taylor, Mary Mahoney, and others—is that they wielded influence at a time when women were not even allowed to vote. In fact, many women in the 1800s, regardless of socioeconomic status, did not attend school. African American women in the early 20th century were legally forbidden to learn to read and write (Foreman, 2009; Nickitas, Middaugh, & Aries, 2016). Historically, women—both Black and White—volunteered their services during crises although nursing, as a profession, didn't exist (Whitfield, 2015). For these women to be successful and influential during the 19th century is a tribute to their ability to take on the system in which they lived and to triumph over it. Women during these times rarely, if ever, voiced their opinions about issues affecting their lives, the lives of their children, their families, or their communities; it was neither expected nor accepted. These early pioneers also are seen as feminists, and the entrance of these women into the political arena opened the way for others, such as Nancy Pelosi, former (and first-ever) Speaker of the house of representatives, and the four women Supreme Court justices (including one retired). In 2016, there 20% of members of the senate were women, and close to that number served in the house. In state legislatures, those numbers were 22.6% and 24.6%, respectively (Rutgers Center for American Women and Politics, 2016).

Professional Advocacy

One of the chief ways in which nurses have been successful in advocating is through membership in their professional organizations. The late 19th century may be seen as the beginning of nurse activism. The Nurses Associated Alumnae of the United States and Canada and the American Society of Superintendents of Training Schools of the United States and Canada were formed in 1890s (ANA, n.d.; National League for Nursing, 2016). Out of these groups came the ANA and the National League for Nursing. However, in the 1980s, with the stratification of nursing into various specialties and organizations, representing an assortment of specialty groups, came the realization that the many nursing groups needed to coordinate efforts in order to be more successful (Cohen et al., 1996). Throughout the next few decades, the nursing organizations realized, regardless of internal differences and competition, that to be politically successful, they must join together to work toward their common political goals. The formation of the following coalitions occurred:

> *Tri-Council for Nursing*—comprising ANA, the American Association of Colleges of Nursing, National League for Nursing, and the American Organization of Nurse Executives
> *American College of Nurse Practitioners (NPs)*—state and national NP groups initially met for a national forum and eventually to influence health policy
> *Nursing Organizations Alliance (The Alliance)*—an alliance of National Federation of Specialty Nursing Organizations and Nursing Organizations Liaison Forum

These and other coalitions permitted the organizations to lobby for common nursing issues (e.g., maintenance of federal funding for nursing education and research) and ultimately the establishment of the National Institute of Nursing Research within the National Institutes of Health (Milstead, 2016). Many of the current state nurse practice acts and expanded responsibilities for NPs are the result of these new coalitions. But more significantly, nursing now has a better understanding that there is a difference between "self-interest" and "selfishness" (Matthews, 2012; Milstead, 2016). One of the most significant outcomes of this time was the development of *Nursing's Agenda for Health Care Reform* (ANA, 1994), this document exemplified the maturing of nursing as a special interest group, but more importantly demonstrated consensus building and collaboration among the more than 60 nursing and various health care provider organizations. Despite nursing's early history of political activism and the fact that nurses are the largest group of health care providers in the United States, widespread political involvement has yet to be fully realized (Nickitas et al., 2016). Nursing has the potential to be a major player in Washington when discussing health care policy. Currently, the call for political action and participation in health policy work among nurses encompasses the global view of "One World, One Health" (Premji & Hatfield, in press, para. 1). For a more recent example of successful professional advocacy, see From the Case Files IV: Nurse Practitioners.

Large professional organizations have the resources, relationships with policymakers, success at coalition building, and reputation for the ability to compromise needs to assure viable outcomes. Being a part of your

---

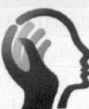 ## From the **Case Files** IV

Nurse Practitioners

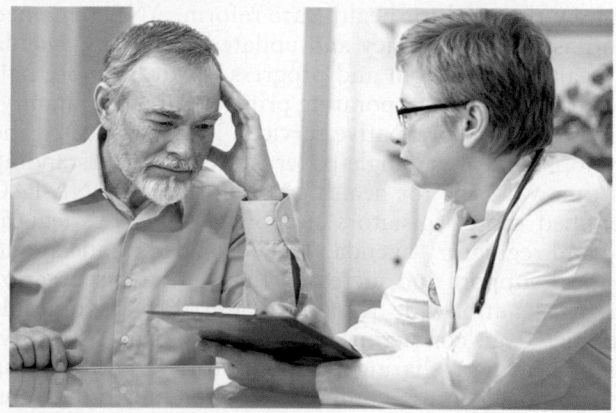

With full implementation of the Patient Protection and ACA, it is estimated that 32 million more Americans will have access to primary health care; by 2020, there is an expected shortage of 45,000 primary care physicians (Poghosyan, Lucero, Rauch, & Berkowitz, 2012). The demand for nurse practitioners (NPs) or advanced practice nurses (APNs) is increasing; nationally, it is expected to reach an increase of 30% between 2016 and 2020 (Xue & Intrator, 2016). NPs are often thought by patients to be better communicators and provide clearer education about self-management of chronic conditions (e.g., diabetes), but the terms "physician extender," "midlevel practitioner," and "non-physician provider" are thought to lead to misconceptions about the quality of their care (Poghosyan et al., 2012, p. 147). Many new policies and programs related to the ACA are beneficial to NPs, including

- Graduate Nurse Education funding for demonstration awards to expand NP education programs.
- Increased funds for hiring NPs into the National Health Service Corps; about 1,900 have been hired to practice in medically underserved areas with increasing levels of retention and extension of their contracts.
- Both Federally Qualified Health Centers (FQHC) and Nurse-Managed Health Clinics (NMHCs) have received increased support, as safety-net providers, to hire NPs to care for their often vulnerable, high-risk clients.
- Medicare beneficiaries with functional limitations and chronic illnesses are able to receive home-based primary care from

NPs through a 3-year project, Independence at Home Demonstration (Carthon, Barnes, & Sarik, 2015).

Although these gains have been the hard won result of consistent lobbying and advocacy efforts on the part of professional nursing organizations and individuals, the bright future on the horizon for NPs is at risk because of inconsistent scope of practice laws at the state level (Poghosyan, Boyd, & Clarke, 2016). In 2015, only 21 states and the District of Columbia had full autonomy rules for NPs (e.g., NPs could evaluate/treat patients, order/interpret diagnostic tests, prescribe medications). That leaves 29 states with laws for NPs that restrict or reduce their scope of practice; often, this involves requiring physician oversight or collaboration (Xue & Intrator, 2016). Some states prohibit NPs from certifying home health or long-term care, and limit their admitting privileges to hospitals. This practice leads to barriers to practice and uneven distribution of primary health care providers, with per capita rates for NPs ranging from 1.7 to 8 per 10,000 people in rural areas of the country. Most are working in large cities and urban areas (Xue & Intrator, 2016). Those states with fewer restrictions on NP practice have 30% higher enrollments in advanced practice nursing (APN) programs (Poghosyan et al., 2012).

Another important consideration is the fact that NPs often work with the most vulnerable populations in areas where other health care providers are scarce, and "their active participation in advocating for both health and social policies" for their clients is helpful in promoting health equity in access and quality (Xue & Intrator, 2016, p. 5). Although NPs are achieving success in the area of policy making and expanded practice opportunities, it is still vitally important for them to advocate and politically support health policies that benefit the clients they serve.

Carthon, J. M. B., Barnes, H., & Sarik, D. A. (2015). *Federal policies influence access to primary care and nurse practitioner workforce. Journal for Nurse Practitioners, 11(5),* 526–531.

Poghosyan, L., Boyd, D. R., & Clarke, S. P. (2016). *Optimizing full scope of practice for nurse practitioners in primary care: A proposed conceptual model. Nursing Outlook, 64(2),* 146–155.

Poghosyan, L., Lucero, R., Rauch, L., & Berkowitz, B. (2012). *Nurse practitioner workforce: A substantial supply of primary care providers. Nursing Economics, 30(5),* 268–274.

Xue, Y., & Intrator, O. (2016). *Cultivating the role of nurse practitioners in providing primary care to vulnerable populations in an era of health-care reform. Policy, Politics, & Nursing Practice, 17(1),* 24–31.

professional organization demonstrates your professionalism, promotes your organization's viability, and demonstrates your social responsibility to advocate for the needs of your patients. Nurses must take advantage of how the public views the profession. For more than a decade, nurses have ranked highest in a Gallup poll for honesty and ethical standards (Gallup, 2016). Clearly, there is favorable impression of nursing as a profession among the general public. Despite criticism about special interest and professional organizations "protecting their turf," professional nursing organizations demonstrate how a critical mass can be influential and successful in moving the discussion forward on health care and the public's perception of nursing. It is the professional nursing organizations that have elevated nursing professionalism, given voice to the inequities that affect our society, and developed the paradigms that influence and affect public health at the institutional, state, and national level in the 21st century. A united voice on public policy is more powerful than individual nurses pleading with their legislators (Duncan, Thorne, & Rodney, 2015; Taylor, 2016).

The pursuit of personal agendas over the common good results in a piecemeal approach to problems and promotes polarization. **Polarization** is the process by which a group is severely split into two or more factions over a political issue. Polarization can be so intense that people perceive one another as good or wicked, depending on their ideological opinions. One of the primary goals of a professional nursing association is to build a collective voice for nurses. A strong professional association limits polarization by developing the political skills of its members and ensures that its structure and processes equitably meet the needs of its constituencies. This is the essence of politics: people must listen to each other, learn from others' viewpoints, and compromise to ensure the most positive outcomes from their endeavors (Nickitas et al., 2016).

Nursing's Role in Health Care Reform

Since the 1950s, the ANA has advocated for reforms in health care that will benefit both nurses and their patients. Their involvement in federal health care reform began in the 1960s with the passage of Medicaid and Medicare. In the 1970s, ANA formed a **political action committee (PAC)**. PACs are organizations that raise money to contribute to political parties or candidates, with the understanding that those receiving financial and political support will be sympathetic toward issues of interest to members of the PAC.

In 1991, ANA released *Nursing's Agenda for Health Care Reform: A Call to Action*—a plan so ambitious and forward looking that Senator Kennedy referenced this document when introducing his legislation on health care reform. Even though this legislation failed to pass, ANA and other nursing organizations gained wide recognition for their policy acumen and leadership abilities. During the Clinton-era health care debate, ANA continued to play a key role in the policy and political discussions on health care reform. As research and experience continued to show the need for health care reform, ANA remained steadfast in its advocacy and updated the policy agenda on health care reform and progress toward a more balanced approach incorporating primary care, community-based care, and preventive services. ANA supported the development of a single-payer system. Understanding the time was ripe for health care reform, the ANA-PAC identified those legislators supportive of ANA's legislative and regulatory agenda. They provided financial and political support and increased their **grassroots** organizing. RNs nationwide responded and through multiple activities (e.g., contacting members of Congress, testifying at hearings, sharing personal stories, participating in high-profile press conferences, attending rallies and events) lobbied for action (see Display 13–1). The frontline nurses also joined ANA's health care reform team, and through these concentrated efforts and collaborations, health care reform became a reality in March 2010 (Lewenson, 2015).

Nurses are increasingly becoming shapers of policy on both the local and federal level; this is occurring because of our experience, perspective, and expertise in health care. The realization that improving conditions for nursing also improves conditions for the communities we serve and the larger society in which we live and work has enhanced our ability to organize. This increases our visibility, access

---

DISPLAY 13–1 AMERICAN NURSES ASSOCIATION (ANA) LOBBYING EFFORTS TOWARD HEALTH CARE REFORM

ANA and its members played a critical role in advocating for health reform. Below is a list of their activities, over a 15-month period:

- Participated in hundreds of media interviews
- Participated in dozens of local media events
- Testified before three Congressional Committees
- Met with White House and Congressional health care reform staff
- Participated in two presidential press conferences at the White House: ANA was one of only 150 representatives invited to participate in the White House Health Care Summit on March 5, 2009
- Participated in the June 25, 2009 rally—*Health Care for America Now*
- Gathered at the July 15, 2009, Rose Garden event where President Obama personally thanked ANA for its involvement in health care reform efforts
- Helped organize America's national-call-in day to Congress in October 2009 (ANA, 2011).

to policy makers, and, more importantly, our capacity to influence the political process (Kostas-Polston et al., 2015). See From the Case Files V: Nurses Lobby Congress.

Nurses represent the largest number of health care practitioners in America—more than 3 million—and are poised at the frontline in patient care to play a major role in implementing of health care reform. Being fully involved in the regulatory framework development (e.g., how the law will be implemented) will further demonstrate the advocacy of nurses as they work to improve the health care delivery system and remove barriers that prevent nurses from providing high-quality, competent, appropriate care. However, to change the existing system, the barriers to competent, quality care (e.g., nursing shortages, faculty shortages, a lack of proper education and training) that prevent nursing from taking its rightful place among the cadre of providers must be addressed. To that end, the Robert Wood Johnson

Foundation (2010) in collaboration with the IOM began the activities necessary to "assess and transform" nursing. The document resulting from this evaluation is *The Future of Nursing: Leading Change, Advancing Health* (IOM, 2011). To encourage and assure public participation, three forums were held around the country.

The Future of Nursing is a seminal document that addresses the need to reform the health care and public health system of the 21st century and outlines nursing's pivotal role in this. This is the first time *nurses* are seen as key to "meeting current and future health care needs" (Schultz, 2010, p. 345). In the development of this document, the process was open to all. This allowed nursing to address challenges to the profession while simultaneously putting forth solutions that result in a rationale and a comprehensive approach to the delivery of high-quality health care for all. It also encourages system responsiveness to the needs of those accessing care.

As expected, the nursing organizations were active in the process of developing this document and participated in the National Summit on Advancing Health through Nursing held in late 2010 to discuss the implications of the recommendations for the future of health care and the future role of nurses in America (Robert Wood Johnson Foundation, 2010). Four key messages from *The Future of Nursing: Leading Change, Advancing Health* (IOM, 2011, p. 4) include the following:

1. Nurses should practice to the full extent of their education and training.
2. Nurses should achieve higher levels of education and training through an improved education system that promotes seamless academic progression.
3. Nurses should be full partners, with physicians and other health professionals, in redesigning health care in the United States.
4. Effective workforce planning and policy making require better data collection and an improved information infrastructure.

The resulting eight recommendations are

Recommendation 1—*Remove scope of practice barriers.* Advanced practice RNs should be able to practice to the full extent of their education and training (p. 9). Lewenson (2015) notes the historical and current documents that call for nurses to practice to the full extent of their education and to remove barriers to practice.

Recommendation 2—*Expand opportunities for nurses to lead and diffuse collaborative improvement efforts.* Private and public funders, health care organizations, nursing education programs, and nursing associations should expand opportunities for nurses to lead and manage collaborative efforts with physicians and other members of the health care team to conduct research and to redesign and improve practice environments and health systems. These entities should also provide opportunities for nurses to diffuse successful practices (p. 11).

Recommendation 3—*Implement nurse residency programs.* State boards of nursing, accrediting

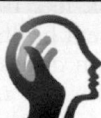

From the Case Files V

Nurses Lobby Congress

Over 260 nurses came to Washington, DC, in June 2015 to meet and talk with over 200 members of Congress. They learned that legislators want them to participate and share their professional perspective on issues related to health, and Rep. Michelle Lujan Grisham noted that nurses have been "the best champions for health care" and have tirelessly advocated for "long-term care, public health, and greater access to care" (ANA, 2016, para. 6). At the same time, over 1,500 nurses participated in virtual Lobby Day by tweeting, posting on Facebook, and sending e-mails to their members of Congress. Some also visited their local legislator's district offices. The nurses advocated for passing legislation—specifically the Registered Nurse Safe Staffing Act (H.R. 876/S.58), the Veterans Access to Care Act (H.R. 1247), and the Home Health Care Planning Improvement Act (H.R. 2267/S. 227), as well as asking for increased funding for Nursing Workforce Development. Through their earlier efforts, 100 new cosponsors for the nurse staffing and home health bills were found. This is an annual event sponsored by the American Nurses Association.

Do you know about Lobby Days at your local state capitol? Do nurses participate? Which nursing organizations or groups have lobbyists working with your state legislators?

Look up the three bills mentioned above (www.thomas. gov) and analyze how this legislation might improve nursing care and patient outcomes.

American Nurses Association (ANA). (2016). ANA Lobby Day: Let the advocacy begin. The American Nurse. Retrieved from http://www.theamericannurse.org/index.php/2015/08/31/ana-lobby-day-let-the-advocacy-begin-2/

bodies, the federal government, and health care organizations should take actions to support nurses' completion of a transition-to-practice program (nurse residency) after they have completed a prelicensure or advanced practice degree program or when they are transitioning into new clinical practice areas (p. 11).

Recommendation 4—*Increase the proportion of nurses with a baccalaureate degree to 80% by 2020.* Academic nurse leaders across all schools of nursing should work together to increase the proportion of nurses with a baccalaureate degree from 50% to 80% by 2020. These leaders should partner with education accrediting bodies, private and public funders, and employers to ensure funding, monitor progress, and increase the diversity of students to create a workforce prepared to meet the demands of diverse populations across the lifespan (p. 12).

Recommendation 5—*Double the number of nurses with a doctorate by 2020.* Schools of nursing, with support from private and public funders, academic administrators and university trustees, and accrediting bodies, should double the number of nurses with a doctorate by 2020 to add to the cadre of nurse faculty and researchers, with attention to increasing diversity (p. 13).

Recommendation 6—*Ensure that nurses engage in lifelong learning.* Accrediting bodies, schools of nursing, health care organizations, and continuing competency educators from multiple health professions should collaborate to ensure that nurses and nursing students and faculty continue their education and engage in lifelong learning to gain the competencies needed to provide care for diverse populations across the lifespan (p. 13).

Recommendation 7—*Prepare and enable nurses to lead change to advance health.* Nurses, nursing education programs, and nursing associations should prepare the nursing workforce to assume leadership positions across all levels, whereas public, private, and governmental health care decision-makers should ensure that leadership positions are available to and filled by nurses (p. 14).

Recommendation 8—*Build an infrastructure for the collection and analysis of interprofessional health care workforce data.* The National Health Care Workforce Commission, with oversight from the Government Accountability Office and the HRSA, should lead a collaborative effort to improve research and the collection and analysis of data on health care workforce requirements. The Workforce Commission and the HRSA should collaborate with state licensing boards, state nursing workforce centers, and the Department of Labor in this effort to ensure that the data are timely and publicly accessible (p. 14).

Nurses are realizing that they are an important force in health care and should be at the table with other stakeholders when important decisions are being made. The IOM report on nursing is a clear hallmark of our growth in the area of health policy and health reform. Health care reform legislation has the potential to transform the current system to be more responsive to the least among us, is more focused on primary care and prevention, and encourages wellness and disease prevention. The resulting system change will be based on research and data collection that fosters better patient outcomes and high-quality care, but more importantly, without the anticipated transformation of nursing, it cannot occur. "Nurses' regular, close proximity to patients and scientific understanding of care processes across the continuum of care give them a unique ability to act as partners with other health professionals and to lead in the improvement and redesign of the health care system and its many practice environments, including hospitals, schools, homes, retail health clinics, long-term care facilities, battlefields, and community and public health centers" (IOM, 2011, p. S-3). This is a mandate for community health nurses to be actively involved in advocacy and influencing the future development of our health care system.

CURRENT U.S. HEALTH POLICY OPTIONS

What does the current health care system look like for PHNs? Earlier in this chapter, we discussed current health outcomes and the need for an increased focus on disease prevention and addressing the social determinants of health. The ACA has changed the policy options for health care on a national level. The United States had a long history of private support for medical care dating back to the early 20th century. Initially, most care was provided in the home, and families paid for any outside services they required. With the development of the germ theory, and the professionalization of medicine and nursing, people began to call on outside professionals to provide health care, primarily financed by individuals and families. As care began to shift to hospitals, and expenses increased, organizations that provided group insurance to cover hospital expenses became more common (Rambur, 2015).

During the First World War, the government recognized that many men of draft-eligible age had health conditions that prevented them from serving in the military. This prompted the first proposal for some type of national health insurance or coverage for health services. This proposal was not successful, but the issue continued to be discussed among policy makers for the next 100 years, with laws passed and regulations developed addressing health insurance coverage and health care regulation along the way. During the New Deal efforts of the Roosevelt administration, national health insurance coverage was originally included, but later bargained away, as part of compromise to get the legislation passed. With the beginning of World War II, the issue was dropped in favor of legislation to keep the country united and prepared for wartime sacrifices. Also during this period, many wartime industries had difficulty finding an appropriate labor source, as so many men were being drafted into the armed services. National cost control measures prevented industries from raising salaries to compete for workers, so industries began to offer benefits to recruit a capable workforce. These benefits included health insurance coverage (Rambur, 2015).

When World War II ended, and servicemen returned to their jobs, they found wartime industries converting to peacetime purposes, but the benefits like health insurance coverage had become an established part of worker benefits. Again, these benefits served to help companies attract and retain the best workers and created an expectation of health care coverage for workers and their families. However, for those who couldn't find work or those who were old enough to retire, there was a question of how their health insurance coverage would be managed. This led to a national policy debate focused on health insurance coverage for the unemployed and poor and for the elderly. This debate culminated in the 1965 enactment of Medicare that provides health insurance coverage for the elderly and Medicaid that offers coverage for the poor and unemployed (CMS, 2015).

Medicare and Medicaid were huge changes in the way health care had been financed. The options for financing were seen as employer-provided insurance, Medicare or Medicaid, which ideally covered most of the population. And there was consensus on services to be covered. During the first half of the 20th century, medical technology and innovation proliferated—often because of advances in treatment developed during wartime in response to battle injuries and communicable illnesses. Simultaneously, economic prosperity led to improved living conditions and social policy changes, which had beneficial health effects for the population, including the development of vaccines, clean water and sewage treatment extended to most of the country, refrigeration and preservation of food, worker safety policies and the elimination of child labor, development and use of antibiotics, and improved nutrition. These medical and public health advances led to an increase in life expectancy of over 30 years between 1900 and 1965 when Medicare and Medicaid were enacted (CMS, 2015).

Thus, to use Milio's language, the health policy options of the late 1960s were focused on an assumption of continued access to safe water, good food, immunizations, antibiotics, and medical treatment. Medicare and Medicaid were designed to ensure that most American would have access to medical treatment. Once these were enacted, the policy challenges shifted to new and emerging treatments, and coverage under insurance, whether privately or governmentally supported. Physicians were the primary providers of medical treatments, and increasingly, such treatments were provided in hospitals. The policy challenge then came in the form of costs. With new medical technologies, pharmaceuticals, and innovations, along with new coverage for many people, medical costs began to rise. Ethical dilemmas arose, such as, should Medicare coverage be provided for the new procedure of renal dialysis? This issue became very controversial, as it was a policy debate addressing the intersection of costs and ethics. Who should be covered for this procedure? Those who had the greatest need (either medical or financial), or those with the most potential for productive life moving forward? In the end, the policy decision for that issue was that Medicare and Medicaid would cover renal dialysis costs for all eligible clients, which lead to a large number of people surviving end-stage kidney disease who previously would have died and a new and expensive innovation being used for a large number of people, thus increasing costs greatly (Swaminathan, Mor, Mehrotra, & Trivedi, 2012). This scenario arose for numerous new medical procedures and pharmaceuticals leading to a crisis in rising costs.

Other policy concerns addressed included funding for long-term care, for the increase in the population living longer, and debates on specific services to be covered by insurance. Medicare and Medicaid, as the largest insurers with one payer, became the standard setters for such decisions, and big private insurers followed their direction. Medical specialties proliferated to address new care needs brought about by technological advances, driving costs even higher. The policies leading to coverage for medical care spurred technological and pharmaceutical innovations, which had individual impacts on specific diseases, but led to ever-increasing costs. During this time, outcomes were examined for individuals, with dramatic successes of people with previously fatal illnesses, saving infants born earlier, and an increasing demand for high-end, technological services to extend life, despite the cost. Policy makers talked about providing all Americans with the same access to services that were affordable for the very wealthy, and research funds supported development of increasingly technological, specialized treatments. Additional concerns came about when people lost their jobs and thus lost insurance or had jobs that didn't provide insurance coverage. National health insurance continued to be discussed, but was opposed by a wide variety of groups including fiscal conservatives, those who wanted limited government, some physician provider groups, and insurance companies (Nickitas et al., 2016; Rambur, 2015).

This debate continued until the passage of the ACA, and since its enactment, concerns persist regarding whether this is the best solution to ensuring access and controlling costs of care. However, in the past decade, policy and public health researchers have begun to examine seriously the health outcomes that have derived from the U.S. health care system as configured, with access to care largely through employer-based insurance and a focus on medical treatment. Although the system has spawned innovations in pharmaceuticals and technological innovations, these services have often been effective for a small number of people, in acute need and at a large cost. Thus, the system has developed to be expensive and largely ineffective for the overall population and more widespread disease prevention and chronic disease management needs. As mentioned earlier, the U.S. health care system options included

- Fee-for-service care
- Choice among physician providers
- Employment-based insurance
- Development and use of innovative technological and pharmacological interventions
- Individual responsibility for health promotion
- Prevention not cost-effective for consumers
- Focus on medical treatment

These options have been very successful as measured in terms of education of medical specialists, pharmacological treatments for many illnesses, surgical innovations, and diagnostic technologies. As discussed earlier, however, these options have not led to overall positive health outcomes for the population as a whole. Recent passage of the ACA (Medicaid.gov, n.d.) has led to policy changes designed to address these concerns.

The Affordable Care Act (ACA) and PHN Practice

The Patient Protection and ACA provided a dramatic change in U.S. policy options. Recognizing that the U.S. health care system was not addressing all the factors necessary to improve the health of the public, and that it was costing U.S. taxpayers an ever-increasing and sustainable proportion of the national budget, the Obama administration moved to pass health care reform legislation in 2010. The focus of the ACA, in the minds of the public, was to mandate health insurance coverage for all U.S. citizens, via a required minimal health insurance package, a mandate on employer provision of health insurance or employer contribution to a marketplace of insurance options for individuals to access, and government provision of subsidies for long income people without employer insurance coverage. Indeed, data indicate that the ACA has been successful at insuring those previously uninsured, with a recent Rand Corporation study indicating that the number of newly insured has risen by 16.9 million people as of 2015 (Rand Corporation, 2015). Provisions in health care reform also limit insurance companies from excluding persons because of preexisting conditions and provide for a broader array of coverage for preventive services, such as wellness programs and making nutritional information a requirement for chain restaurants. However, lesser known, but equally critical, changes in options available to people included regulations to improve quality of care provided, cost control mechanisms including future plans for moving from paying for services provided to paying for health outcomes achieved, and beginning efforts to focus health care policy and services on prevention of disease and health promotion (Knickman & Kovner, 2015).

As part of the ACA efforts to move to a culture of disease prevention, the ACA mandated formation of a National Prevention Council, composed of cabinet officials representing the social determinants of health, chaired by the Surgeon General of the United States. The council is charged with development of a National Prevention Strategy (Surgeon General, n.d.a). This strategy was introduced in June 2011 and addressed core strategic directions and priorities for an increased focus on public health and well-being. See Figure 13–5 for the National Prevention Strategy model.

At the core of the strategy is the overall goal of "increasing the number of Americans who are healthy at every stage of life" (para. 5). To achieve this, the strategy outlines four strategic directions, which address health care, health equity, and the social determinants of health and include

- Healthy and safe community environments: This strategy encompasses access to care, community health and development, neighborhood safety, environmental health and all the various social conditions that impact health.
- Clinical and community preventive services: Included in this strategy are those clinical screening and prevention services that are evidence based, with the goal of making these services accessible and affordable for all Americans.
- Empowered people: This addresses the need for community involvement in health and health care,

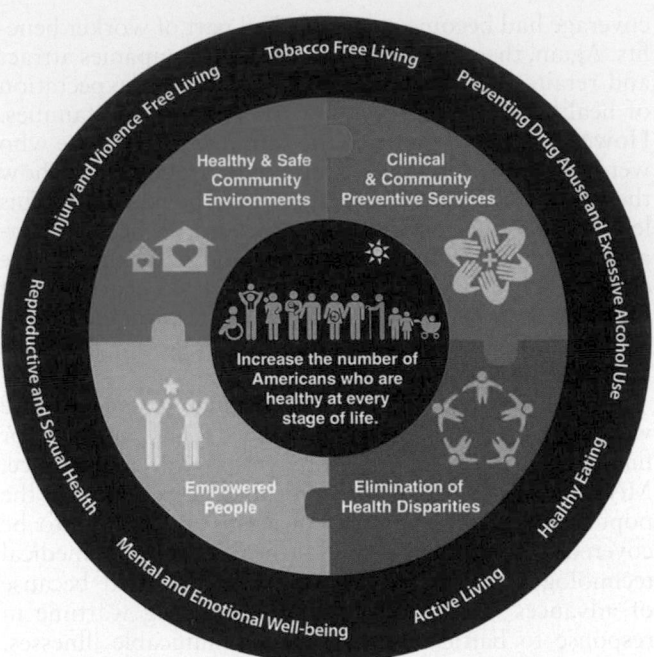

FIGURE 13–5 National Prevention Strategy model. (Adapted from Surgeon General. (n.d.). Retrieved from http://www. surgeongeneral.gov/priorities/prevention/strategy/)

from the level of schools and businesses being able to see the importance of health to their work to individuals and families being empowered to act to improve their health and well-being.

- Elimination of health disparities: This strategy examines health inequities and recommends beginning prevention efforts in communities where disparities are greatest (para. 7).

Each of these four strategic directions included seven strategic priorities, based on data indicating that two thirds of premature deaths are due to chronic illnesses that can be prevented or controlled with prevention measures. For each strategic direction and priority, evidence-based recommendations are provided for all partners/stakeholders to address, including clinicians, businesses, elected officials and local/state/national government, church leaders and community service providers, educators, and individuals and families, thus highlighting that health promotion and disease prevention are the business of all Americans in every walk of life. The seven strategic priorities include (para. 9)

- Tobacco-free living
- Preventing drug abuse and excessive alcohol use
- Healthy eating
- Active living
- Mental and emotional well-being
- Reproductive and sexual health
- Injury and violence-free living

Subsequent work by the National Prevention Council and the federal advisory group appointed to advise and guide these efforts has included work to disseminate the strategies, document successes and lessons learned, and assist in promotion of model and exemplary interventions and policies to promote health and prevent disease across all levels of government (Surgeon General, n.d.a). The federal advisory group, appointed by the president, includes two nurses, who have worked to disseminate the NPS to PHNs across the country so that it may be incorporated as part of their practice initiatives (Surgeon General, n.d.b).

Additional components of the ACA that have the potential for great changes in health and health policy at the community level include value-based purchasing and accountable care organizations (ACOs), along with the expanded Internal Revenue Service (IRS) requirement for nonprofit hospitals to conduct regular community health needs assessments and develop implementation plans based on this data for improving the health of their communities (Knickman & Kovner, 2015). Nonprofit hospitals have a long history of providing care in the United States as part of a community or charitable mission. Often run by religious organizations, these facilities served communities, often caring for patients with no reimbursement for services. To support and encourage such work, local municipalities provided tax exemptions for such organizations, because of their benefit to the community. The U.S. Government Accountability Office (GAO) has estimated that tax-exempt status saved hospitals $12.6 billion in federal, state, and local taxes in 2002 ($16.1 billion in 2012 dollars). With implementation of the ACA, medical insurance coverage has been achieved for an additional 16.9 million Americans who previously would have required charity care and now will have their care reimbursed (Rand Corporation, 2015). Hence, the ACA includes new IRS regulations to guide nonprofit hospitals in using their savings from the decrease in uninsured patients to conduct regular community assessments and develop a plan to work with others in their community to improve overall community health (Horwitz & Cutler, 2015). This process has great potential for PHN involvement, to assist local hospitals in conducting such assessments and being involved in planning for implementation of interventions to improve community health. Indeed, this is the cornerstone of public health practice, and PHNs can play key roles in this work.

Value-Based Purchasing and Accountable Care Organizations

The ACA began a movement away from the traditional fee-for-service care where health providers diagnose and treat individuals and are paid for each service provided (e.g., office visits, lab fees, prescriptions, follow-up visits) and that has thought to have led to increasing health care costs (James, 2012). This style of reimbursement for care has had the problem of indirectly encouraging additional care, as each service is reimbursed separately. National health policy has begun to reverse this by mandating no reimbursement for specific services required because of medical error. The ACA expands this with a move toward *value-based purchasing*, or reimbursing a specific amount based on achieving the likely outcome for clients within specific diagnostic categories. For example, instead of fees for office visits, lab fees, and prescriptions, the federal government is proposing

paying for achievable health outcomes in a bundled manner based on the client's demographics and diagnosis. A diabetic would not have each service reimbursed, but rather a lump sum reimbursement would be provided upon the client achieving a level of stability in the disease (e.g., lab values for hemoglobin A1c within normal limits). This reimbursement would cover whatever services were required to achieve this outcome, which might be lab tests and medications, but might also include PHN-provided chronic disease self-management training or clinical nutrition counseling. Such a change in reimbursement mechanisms would have a large impact on health care services, as clinical agencies would need to begin looking at what services and providers were most effective at achieving the desired outcomes. This would provide an opportunity for PHNs to demonstrate the effectiveness of their practice interventions in improving health outcomes for individuals and populations (California Directors of Public Health Nursing, 2015; Knickman & Kovner, 2015; Kulbok, 2013; Porter & Lee, 2013; Rambur, 2015; Washington State Nurses Association, 2011). When a national sample of public health nurses were asked about their involvement with components of the ACA, over 65% responded that they were actively involved with integration of public and primary health care, and nearly as many were working in clinical preventive services. Almost 60% noted activity with patient navigation, care coordination, and establishing public/private collaborations. Slightly fewer mentioned involvement with population health strategies and data, along with community health assessments (Edmonds, Campbell, & Gilder, 2015).

Accountable Care Organizations (ACOs) are another feature of health care reform that is intended to emphasize quality over quantity. Physicians and other health care providers are forming groups, sometimes in conjunction with hospitals, and will be paid based on patient's treatment outcomes (not the number of visits or tests). Thus, duplicative tests or procedures should be avoided, as a more coordinated form of treatment is available. One goal of ACA is to provide 30% of Medicare services to alternative payment models, such as ACOs, and away from fee-for-service models. In addition to cost savings, quality is also a focus. In 2014, Medicare ACOs demonstrated $411 million in cost savings, while 27 out of 33 quality measures were improved between 2013 and 2014 (USDHHS, 2016). Newer types of ACOs not only pay based on quality outcomes but also penalize for negative outcomes, shifting risk to providers and away from the government. The number of ACOs is growing, with 121 new participating groups in 49 states announced in 2016.

Policy Competence as an Integral Part of PHN Practice

The U.S. health care system is undergoing significant changes to improve the health of the public and contain costs. These changes are impacting health care across the system, but are particularly critical for those who work in communities with the increased emphasis on population health and disease prevention. The PHN can be an integral part of these efforts and help lead the way in addressing the social determinants of health and focusing efforts on prevention and long-term health promotion for families and communities. Along with other public health professionals, PHNs need to do this by understanding the policy process and then determining where their efforts would be most effective in improving overall population health (Haughton & Stang, 2012). This is a critical time for nursing in general, and PHN specifically, as the health care system focuses attention on what has always been at the core of PHN concern—health where people live, work, play, and pray.

POWER AND EMPOWERMENT

Eliciting services and programs for underserved populations is a never-ending issue. Citizen participation is never particularly easy in communities that are excluded from political or economic resources. Sherry Arnstein, in her classic 1969 treatise *A Ladder of Citizen Participation*, stated that "citizen participation is citizen power," and without access to information about how the system functions, these populations cannot obtain the resources they need to make their communities livable and nurturing (p. 217). Arnstein goes on to point out that those in power prevent those in need from accessing the process:

> The idea of citizen participation is a little like eating spinach: no one is against it in principle because it is good for you. Participation of the governed in their government is, in theory, the cornerstone of democracy—a revered idea that is vigorously applauded by virtually everyone. The applause is reduced to polite handclaps, however, when this principle is advocated by the have-not Blacks, Mexican Americans, Puerto Ricans, Indians, Eskimos, and Whites. When the have-nots define participation as redistribution of power, the American consensus on the fundamental principle explodes into many shades of outright racial, ethnic, ideological, and political opposition (p. 216).

Although Arnstein writes about the anger that disenfranchised populations feel, she does offer possible solutions that allow each party to "share power through partnership," as outlined by engaging in the process discussed in her treatise (p. 217). See more on this in Chapter 15. **Power** can be defined as the ability to act or produce an effect, possession of control, or authority or influence over others. As public health professionals, nurses have a commitment to social justice and working with disadvantaged communities. This means that nurses have a responsibility to ensure community participation in issues affecting them, and they must continually examine the relationship and position they hold within these communities. The term **empowerment** has been used to explain a process of assisting communities to come together to express their values and ideas to those outside the community (Cawley & McNamara, 2011). Generally, the issue of empowerment comes up when outside forces are behaving in a way that the community considers detrimental to its well-being. The various

definitions of empowerment and the expansion of the definition of health, which now includes the social, political, and economic determinants of health, have changed our thinking on how best to interact with the communities we serve. Theorists have suggested that if power is the ability to control, predict, and participate in one's environment, then empowerment is the process whereby individuals and communities take power and transform their lives (Baffour, 2012; Petit, 2012; Turner & Maschi, 2015). This also suggests a change in the relationship between professionals and communities—a change from the customary hierarchical patient–provider relationship to one of a partnership. How does the PHN make sure that preconceived ideas about certain communities are not forced on the community in order to meet the goals and objectives of the public health agency? In the past, community health promotion practice often only met the bottom rung of Arnstein's ladder by using the rhetoric of community participation while the professionals working with the community actually set the agenda. Health promotion may best be facilitated by the use of empowerment and assisting individuals and communities in articulating their problems and solutions. Discovering what is most important to the community and providing access to that information while supporting leadership from within the community and encouraging them to overcome bureaucratic hurdles to action are important parts of community empowerment. This helps to improve problem-solving skills and abilities (Kulbok, Thatcher, Park, & Meszaros, 2012; Piper, 2011; Wong, Zimmerman, & Parker, 2010). Maryland and Gonzalez (2012) note that sharing personal experiences and stories with legislators is one effective method of advocacy. Real stories about clients having problems gaining access to services or resources, not receiving adequate or timely treatment, or about the need for more school nurses who are currently spread so thin that they cannot adequately perform their assigned roles and functions. Firsthand knowledge of how our health care system works (or doesn't work) can be very persuasive when a nurse shares personal examples in a way that demonstrates a passion for clients and communities.

So, how can PHNs influence policies that affect the clients and communities they serve? And, how do we influence policymakers to hear our concerns and act on them? Seasoned advocates have developed skills in influencing policy decisions; ground rules also exist by which to play the game. Some call them the "ten commandments of lobbying." However these steps are described, advocates adhere to the basic ideas inherent in the following:

1. **Honesty is the best policy.** Being known as someone who has integrity is a lasting virtue. Never mislead a legislator or someone who is likely to support your interests, as it is difficult to regain credibility once you lose it. Speaking beyond your level of expertise gets advocates into trouble. If you don't know the answer, say so; but if you promise to get the answer, then do so. Do not promise what you can't deliver.
2. **Start early.** Planning always takes longer than you think it will. Your interests are not everyone's interests

and convincing others they should be involved always involves time. If you are planning policy change at the state or federal level, it is vital to know the legislative process and the critical time lines.

3. **Know what you want.** Be aware of all sides of the issue prior to approaching a policy maker, know the pros and cons, and be prepared to answer questions and provide data on both sides of the issue. Understand the role politics plays in getting what you want and how policy makers may respond to your issue. Targeting your story to the goals, emotions, and interests of the legislator is important and may result in a positive outcome. Be *clear* about what you are asking the legislator for—to carry legislation, or to vote no or yes on specific legislation. Asking your legislator to vote a certain way is perfectly legitimate, and if you don't ask, the opposition will.

4. **KISS** (Keep it simple, stupid). Be able to articulate your issues in a clear and concise manner. Do not confuse possible supporters with complicated arguments. Key issues should be concise and clear and on one page, no more than two. Leave behind an informational packet with pertinent information about the community and/or services and programs.

5. **No permanent enemies, no permanent friends.** Political affiliation doesn't always determine what interests a person has or whether they are likely to support your interests. It behooves you to speak with everyone on your issue; if nothing else, you may find out who they are and why they may oppose your concerns. Remember, in politics, there are only permanent interests.

6. **Know your opponents.** Visit with all possible supporters—just because someone opposed you in the past doesn't mean they won't support you on a current issue. Respectful disagreement keeps the door open for future agreement and compromise.

7. **Compromise.** Ask for much more than you think you can get. When negotiating, you can give up something without hurting your priorities or your bottom line. In politics, rarely does anyone get all they want, but priority setting is key: What do we expect to accomplish with this activity?

8. **There is strength in numbers.** The more groups involved, the more likely you are to be successful. Any opportunity for networking is an opportunity to enlarge your coalition. Including disparate groups means you may have accessed conflicting political persuasions. Additionally, it is useful to have groups who can speak with those who are not viewed as "friends." Cross-fertilization of groups is politically expedient, but understand that next time you or they may be in opposition.

9. **Work at the local level.** Legislators are interested in their constituents—these are the people who elected them to office and who will keep them in office. To be noticed by policy makers, sharing information with them about their constituents is the surest way to capture their attention. Information sharing should occur on issues both in the community where you live and in the one where you work.

10. **Thank you.** Everyone loves to be told, "Job well done." To maintain your coalitions, always recognize the work of others. Spreading the credit is like sowing seeds: the wider the spread, the more bountiful the crop.

Common methods of generating a conversation with legislators are by e-mail, over phone, or in person. Often, your first contact will be a staff member. It is important to organize your thoughts and carefully craft an "Ask" or what legislation you want the legislator to support that is also something of interest to them and their constituents (Kostas-Polston et al., 2015, p. 12). If possible, you can prepare a "one-pager," with your contact information and credentials listed, along with brief bulleted points on the subject of interest that includes current statistics and research (p. 13). If you meet with a legislator, it is important to remember that they are not allowed to discuss campaign contributions in their legislative offices. Finally, it is important for those new to advocacy to understand that the thing with the most critical influence on policy is *money*. Nurses, even with the passage of the recent health care reform legislation, must become even more actively involved in the process of influencing policy. How many nurses understand that the nurse practice acts, or portions thereof, under which they work are developed by legislators or special interest groups who don't have a background in health care? How many nurses know who their legislators are at either the state or federal level? How many nurses have written their legislators about pending health care legislation or legislation that affects nursing?

Political Action Committees

One reason why nurses are less politically active can be tied to a lack of money. Nurses don't earn as much money or appear not to have access to as much money as other health care interests (e.g., hospitals, physicians, insurance companies, and health care plans), and as such, there is much less money for nursing organizations to use for lobbyists or to assist chosen candidates. As mentioned earlier, the ANA has a PAC that supports federal candidates on a nonpartisan basis; candidates must demonstrate an interest in and willingness to vote for nursing issues or issues that nurses support. To participate in the PAC, you must be a member of ANA (this also allows your family to contribute to the PAC). By giving to the ANA-PAC, one maximizes their contribution by joining with other nurses—this power in numbers increases our influence with those candidates we choose to endorse. ANA-PAC has the "Race for the Million" campaign to raise money in support of candidates and legislators who back nurses' issues (Song, n.d.). However, giving to your personal legislator can keep you on their mailing list, and it may get you invited to local legislative activities. It also lets your legislator know you are interested in whether she remains in office. Being in regular contact with your legislators provides an avenue for introducing legislation that impacts nursing or other health-related issues, and when you call to ask for a vote "for" or "against" an issue, the legislator is more likely to entertain your request. Aren't you more likely to respond to someone you know, rather than someone who comes to you out of the blue to ask for a favor?

Lobbyists may work for PACs or independently represent various special interests or groups. **Lobbying** is the process of influencing legislators or other policy makers to make decisions on policy issues. Professional organizations or other **special interest groups** (individuals who share a common interest and work politically to make their goals a reality) may retain paid lobbyists. **Lobbyists** are professionals who know the rules governing the state or federal political process, have or develop relationships with policy makers, provide guidance for members of the organizations employing them on how to impact public policy decisions, and work behind the scenes to influence policy discussions and outcomes. States and the federal government have laws and regulations that determine the legal actions of lobbyists as well as the organizations that employ them (Mason et al., 2016; Milstead, 2016). However, some lobbyists are former legislators or staff members who "take lucrative jobs representing the very industries" they formerly regulated, and this "revolving door" lobbying is disconcerting to most citizens as they are often seen as selling their access to current key legislators (LaPira & Thomas, 2014, p. 4).

Volunteering

Money is *not* the only way to build a relationship with your legislator. Volunteering your time can be just as important (see *Perspectives—Voices from the Community*). Candidates for office need people to get things done (e.g., phone banking, stuffing mailers, answering phones, putting up flyers and campaign posters, walking door to door to spread the message, and assisting in the development of issue papers). Candidates develop issue papers to tell their constituents where they stand on key campaign concerns. Nurses have the expertise to assist legislators in developing an agenda on health care policy or at the least to review and comment on issue papers.

Relationships are critical in policy development and in affecting public policy. As demonstrated earlier, being a friend can reap huge benefits when health care policy is on the line. Being involved in local and state elections can take many forms. Voting, for instance, is vital—RNs represent a substantial block of potential voters (Nickitas et al., 2016). Joining your local and state professional organizations is vital to having the voice of nursing heard at all levels. You can become more actively involved by writing legislators about the health care issues that impact the communities, both where you live and work. It is also vital to understand the importance of critically timing those communications. Effective communications with legislators should be tied to times when the issues are being heard in policy committee—thus, you must know when your issue is scheduled to be discussed in

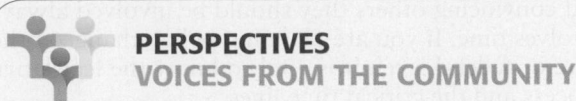

PERSPECTIVES
VOICES FROM THE COMMUNITY

Volunteer Service for the Long Term

A registered nurse (RN) who had been through what I called the women's legislative career ladder—School Board, City Council, and the County Board of Supervisors—was now posed to run for the state legislature. Because we had had numerous contacts and I believed she would make a good state legislator and a voice for nursing and health care, I volunteered to work in her campaign office. I primarily answered the phones on the evenings I worked, but I met the office staff—many of them were much younger than me. And, even once, she came in while I was there. I talked with the staff about some of my experiences as a lobbyist, and they shared their experiences; many of them were fresh out of college.

She was successful in her run for office, and whenever I needed to meet with her or her staff, I was shown right in. I was also asked my opinion about the hiring of certain staff. Her staff knew me by name—many of them did not work on her campaign, but they were told about me by those campaign staff who were still around. After 3 years in office, she was appointed chairperson of a key committee, and I maintained access to her committee consultants and to her when necessary. We were able to work together quite successfully, and although we didn't always agree on every policy issue, I think the weeks I put in volunteering 3 years earlier really paid off for the clients and the issues I was representing.

—L.B., Professional Lobbyist

committee. For example, it is prudent to send letters on your issue—via fax or regular mail—close to the time of the committee hearing. Holding a press conference or getting other media coverage when the bill is introduced, or on the day it will be heard in committee, is quite effective in drawing attention to your issue. Writing letters to the editor of your local newspaper on health issues and writing articles for various publications are also effective methods of persuading others to back your issue. Other methods for influencing health policy or nursing issues include applying for positions on boards and commissions; each local area has advisory committees for their locally elected officials at the city and county level. The state board of RNs needs nurses willing to sit on their board or to serve on various advisory committees and task forces. At your state capitols, there are usually vacancies on policy committees, or legislators may be looking for new staff—either personal or policy. And, who better to serve in this capacity than a nurse! Who else has more knowledge about health issues than nurses? When all else fails, *run for office.*

SUMMARY

This chapter has reviewed briefly the disparities in health outcomes and discusses the relationship between health policies and population health outcomes. Public health policy is explained, and types of policies (e.g., substantive, procedural, distributive, redistributive, regulatory) are described. Policy competence, or an understanding of policy formulation, implementation, and modification, is important for public health nurses because of the ability to influence both the policy process and the impact of policies on the clients. PHNs need to determine first the level at which policies are considered (e.g., local, state, national). The legislative process (i.e., how a bill becomes law, rulemaking, implementation, evaluation, judicial action) occurs in similar ways at the state and national levels. Policy analysis requires the ability to comprehend policy from various viewpoints, and the rational framework and Kingdon's framework, along with Longest's model, provide guidance in determining windows of opportunity upon which public health nurses may act to initiate policy changes.

The political process is inherent in the development of health policies, and the public health nurse has a role in policy and advocacy within those processes. Lillian Wald, and others like her, provided a rich history of political action and advocacy in public health nursing as they worked to provide a voice for vulnerable and disenfranchised populations. Social justice remains a pillar of our current practice.

Advocacy for our clients is always important, but professional advocacy through affiliation and activity in our professional nursing organizations is also vital so that we, as PHNs, may have a "collective voice." Politics may be uncomfortable and foreign to many of us, yet it provides the methods for needed change through lobbying or influencing legislators. Nurses and special interests groups can gain access to legislators individually or through the services of a professional lobbyist or PACs. Nurses can also serve on various advisory and community boards, and provide input on policy matters by sharing expertise, research/evidence, and personal experiences.

Policies are actions or agendas that can be used to implement important goals and objectives, such as the health objectives found in *Healthy People 2020*, and PHNs can use processes to impact policy formulation, adoption, implementation, and evaluation. Tips on how to influence policy makers were outlined, and nurses may consider volunteering time to a candidate of their choice as a means of gaining greater access to the political process. Nurses' role in health care reform was discussed, along with IOM's *The Future of Nursing* and examples of lobbying efforts. Current U.S. policies, including the ACA and the National Prevention Strategy, provide opportunities for PHNs to improve the health of populations and share with policy makers and legislators the importance of social determinants of health.

Community health nursing is by nature political because we deal with many issues that affect the health and well-being of the diverse populations we serve. Power and empowerment are important concepts to both public health nursing and politics; Arnstein's ladder provides guidance on citizen participation. Every community health nurse should hone political action and advocacy skills.

ACTIVITIES TO PROMOTE **CRITICAL THINKING**

1. Investigate a major health policy system in your community or state, discover how it works, and determine whether public health nurses are represented in this system. Areas to investigate include the boundaries of the system, the authority by which the system generates health policy, how the system receives input (formally and informally), resources the policy system uses and allocates to others, and the system's output over the past few years.

2. Describe a legislative bill related to health at either the state or federal level and the issues involved in it. Identify who is sponsoring the bill, who is opposing it, and why. Determine the population that will be affected by the bill if it passes and in what ways they will be affected. Discuss what you, as a community health nurse, could do to be involved in this bill and then develop a political action plan to support or oppose the bill. E-mail your legislator regarding your position.

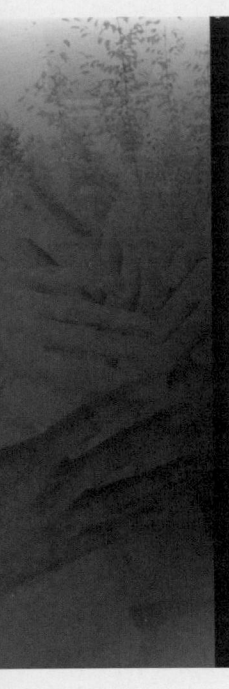

3. Attend a meeting of a professional organization, board of directors, government agency, or council when a health policy or health care issue is on the agenda. Analyze the positions of the major interest groups involved and describe to what extent economics comes into the discussion. Describe who controls the discussion and how this is done.

4. What issues or events occurred in the United States that reduced the willingness of nurses to speak out about health care issues? Examine the years starting with the 1930s. What events or issues changed, if any, to reinvigorate nurses serving as political activists?

5. Are nurses the most qualified group to articulate national health care issues? If so, why? If not, why not?

6. Who are your state legislators? What are the critical health issues in your state, and how have your legislators responded to the issues? If there has been health care–related legislation introduced:
   - What is the issue?
   - What political party introduced the bill?
   - At the current time, where is the bill in the legislative process?
   - What groups support or oppose the legislation?
   - What is the reasoning for the groups' support or opposition?

7. How active is your state professional nursing organization in policy issues? Are you a member of the organization? If not, why not? What are the public policy issues the organization is involved in? How successful have they been? Does the group have a paid lobbyist or does it rely on volunteer lobbyists?

REFERENCES

American Association of Colleges of Nursing. (n.d.). *Crosswalk of the Master's Essentials with the Baccalaureate and DNP Essentials.* Retrieved from http://www.aacn.nche.edu/faculty/faculty-tool-kits/masters-essentials/Crosswalk-of-Masters.pdf

American Nurses Association (ANA). (n.d.). *ANA historical review.* Retrieved from http://www.nursingworld.org/history

American Nurses Association (ANA). (1994). *Nursing's agenda for healthcare reform.* Washington, DC: American Nurses Association.

American Nurses Association (ANA). (2011). *At the health system reform table.* Retrieved from http://www.nursingworld.org/MainMenuCategories/HealthcareandPolicyIssues/HealthSystemReform/What-ANA-is-Doing/At-the-Table.aspx

American Nurses Association (ANA). (2013). *Public health nursing: Scope and standards of practice* (2nd ed.). Silver Spring, MD: Author.

American Nurses Association (ANA). (2015). *Code of ethics for nurses with interpretive statements (revised).* Silver Spring, MD: Author.

American Nurses Association (ANA). (2016a). *Agencies and regulations.* Retrieved from http://www.nursingworld.org/Agencies-RegulatoryAffairs

American Nurses Association (ANA). (2016b). *The nursing process.* Retrieved from http://www.nursingworld.org/EspeciallyforYou/StudentNurses/Thenursingprocess.aspx

American Public Health Association (APHA). (2013). *Health in all policies: A guide for state and local governments.* Retrieved from http://www.apha.org/~/media/files/pdf/factsheets/health_inall_policies_guide_169pages.ashx

American Public Health Association, PHN Section (2013). *Definition of public health nursing.* Retrieved from https://www.apha.org/~/media/files/pdf/membergroups/nursingdefinition.ashx

Anderson, J. E. (2015). *Public policymaking: An introduction* (8th ed.). Stamford, CT: Cengage Learning.

Arnstein, S. (1969). A ladder of citizen participation. *Journal of American Planning Association, 35*(4), 216–224.

Baffour, J. M. (2012). Do empowerment strategies facilitate knowledge and behavioral change? The impact of family health advocacy on health outcomes. *Social Work in Public Health, 27*(5), 507.

Barusch, A. S. (2012). *Foundations of social justice in human perspective* (4th ed.). Belmont, CA: Brooks/Cole, Cengage Learning.

Birkland, T. A. (2015). *An introduction to the policy process* (4th ed.). London, UK: Routledge.

Bowman, S., Unwin, N., Critchley, J., Capewell, S., Husseini, A., Maziak, W., ... Ahmad, B. (2012). Use of evidence to support healthy public policy: A policy effectiveness-feasibility loop. *Bulletin of the World Health Organization*, Article ID BLT.12.104968. Retrieved from http://www.who.int/bulletin/online_first/12-104968.pdf

Braun, A. (2013, August 10). *Out of 5,000 bills in every Congress, guess how many become law?* Retrieved from https://mic.com/articles/59033/out-of-5-000-bills-in-every-congress-guess-how-many-become-law#.i11yerh29

California Directors of Public Health Nursing. (2015, November). *Position paper on the role of public health nurses in healthcare reform.* Retrieved from http://phncalifornia.org/resources/Role%20of%20Public%20Health%20Nurses%20in%20Healthcare%20Reform.pdf

Callow, A. (2015). *Census report shows that states that expand Medicaid see lower uninsured rates.* Retrieved from http://familiesusa.org/blog/2015/09/census-report-shows-states-expand-medicaid-see-lower-uninsured-rates

Cawley, T., & McNamara, P. (2011). Public health nurse perceptions of empowerment and advocacy in child health surveillance in West Ireland. *Public Health Nursing, 28*(2), 150–158.

Centers for Disease Control and Prevention (CDC). (2015a). *Climate change and public health.* Retrieved from http://www.cdc.gov/climateandhealth/effects/

Centers for Disease Control and Prevention (CDC). (2015b). *Healthy Places: Health Impact Assessment.* Retrieved from http://www.cdc.gov/healthyplaces/hia.htm

Centers for Disease Control and Prevention (CDC). (2016). *Disability and obesity.* Retrieved from http://www.cdc.gov/ncbddd/disability-andhealth/obesity.html

Center for Medicare and Medicaid Services (CMS). (n.d.). *National health data: Historical.* Retrieved from https://www.cms.gov/research-statistics-data-and-systems/statistics-trends-and-reports/nationalhealthexpenddata/nationalhealthaccountshistorical.html

Center for Medicare and Medicaid Services (CMS). (2015, July). *Medicare and Medicaid milestones 1937-2015.* Retrieved from https://www.cms.gov/About-CMS/Agency-Information/History/Downloads/Medicare-and-Medicaid-Milestones-1937-2015.pdf

Civic Impulse. (2015). *Statistics and historical comparison: Bills by final status.* Retrieved from https://www.govtrack.us/congress/bills/statistics

Cohen, S. S., Mason, D. J., Kovner, C., Leavitt, J. K., Pulcine, J., & Sochalshi, J. (1996). Stages of nursing's political development: Where we've been and where we ought to go. *Nursing Outlook, 44*(6), 259–266.

deChesnay, M., & Anderson, B. A. (2016). *Caring for the vulnerable: Perspectives in nursing theory, practice, and research* (4th ed.). Burlington, MA: Jones & Bartlett Learning.

Deschaine, J. E., & Schaffer, M. A. (2003). Strengthening the role of public health nurse leaders in policy development. *Policy, Politics, & Nursing Practice, 4*(4), 266–274.

Donohoe, M. T. (Ed.). (2013). *Public health and social justice.* San Francisco, CA: Jossey-Bass/Wiley.

Duncan, S., Thorne, S., & Rodney, P. (2015). Evolving trends in nurse regulation: What are the policy impacts for nursing's social mandate? *Nursing Inquiry, 22*(1), 27–38.

Edmonds, J. K., Campbell, L. A., & Gilder, R. E. (2015). *Public health nursing and the Affordable Care Act: Survey results.* Presented at the 143rd meeting of the American Public Health Association, 3393.0, Health Systems and Practice Reform Round Table, Chicago, IL.

Edwards, H. S. (2013, March/April). He who makes the rules. *Washington Monthly: The Magazine.* Retrieved from http://www.washingtonmonthly.com/magazine/march_april_2013/features/he_who_makes_the_rules043315.php?page=all

Environmental Protection Agency. (2016). *What EPA is doing about climate change.* Retrieved from http://www3.epa.gov/climatechange/EPAactivities.html

Evans, K. A. (2013, June 9). *Health policy: What's your role?* Retrieved from http://nurse-practitioners-and-physician-assistants.advanceweb.com/Columns/Role-Growth/Health-Policy-Whats-Your-Role.aspx

Feetham, S., & Doering, J. J. (2015). Career cartography: A conceptualization of career development to advance health and policy. *Journal of Nursing Scholarship, 47*(1), 70–77.

Foreman, P. G. (2009). *Activist sentiments: Reading Black women in the 19th century.* Chicago, IL: University of Illinois Press.

Frederick, D. A., Saguy, A. C., & Gruys, K. (2016). Culture, health, and bigotry: How exposure to cultural accounts of fatness shape attitudes about health risk, health policies, and weight-based prejudice. *Social Science & Medicine, 165,* 271–279.

Gallup. (2016). *Honesty/ethics in professions.* Retrieved from http://www.gallup.com/poll/1654/honesty-ethics-professions.aspx

Gneiting, U. (2016). From global agenda-setting to domestic implementation: Successes and challenges of the global health network on tobacco control. *Health Policy & Planning, 31,* i74–i86.

Gottlieb, L. M., Fielding, J. E., & Braveman, P. A. (2012). Health impact assessment: Necessary but not sufficient for healthy public policy. *Public Health Report, 127,* 156–162.

Haughton, B., & Stang, J. (2012). Population risk factors and trends in health care and public policy. *Journal of the Academy of Nutrition & Dietetics, 112*(Suppl 3), s35–s46.

Horwitz, J., & Cutler, D. (2015). *The ACA's hospital tax-exemption rules and the practice of medicine.* Retrieved from http://healthaffairs.org/blog/2015/03/03/the-acas-hospital-tax-exemption-rules-and-the-practice-of-medicine/

Institute of Medicine (IOM). (2011). *The future of nursing: Leading change, advancing health.* Washington, DC: National Academies Press.

Institute of Medicine (IOM). (2013). *Shorter lives, poorer health: US health in international perspective.* Washington, DC: National Academies Press.

James, J. (2012). *Pay for performance: Health Affairs policy brief.* Retrieved from http://www.healthaffairs.org/healthpolicybriefs/brief.php?brief_id=78

Jensen, E. M. (2011, January 27). *Hands off my purse! Why money bills originate in the House.* Retrieved from http://www.heritage.org/research/reports/2011/01/hand-off-my-purse-why-money-bills-originate-in-the-house

Jewish Women's Archive. (2016). *Women of valor: Lillian Wald.* Retrieved from http://jwa.org/womenofvalor/wald

Kingdon, J. W. (2011). *Agendas, alternatives and public policies* (2nd ed.). Boston, MA: Pearson/Longman.

Kingdon, J. W. (2010). *Agendas, alternatives and public policies.* Retrieved from http://marieljohn.blogspot.com/2010/02/agendas-alternatives-and-public.html

Knickman, J. R., & Kovner, A. R. (Eds.). (2015). *Jonas & Kovner's health care delivery in the United States* (11th ed.). New York, NY: Springer Publishing Company.

Kostas-Polston, E. A., Thanavaro, J., Arvidson, C., & Taub, L. M. (2015). Advanced practice nursing: Shaping health through policy. *Journal of the American Association of Nurse Practitioners, 27,* 11–20.

Kulbok, P. (2013, September 29). Public health nurses must rise to growing care need. *The Daily Progress.* Retrieved from http://www.dailyprogress.com/opinion/guest_columnists/public-health-nurses-must-rise-to-growing-care-need/article_8285ddce-290b-11e3-8b65-0019bb30f31a.html

Kulbok, P. A., Thatcher, E., Park, E., & Meszaros, P. S. (2012). Evolving public health nursing roles: Focus on community participatory health promotion and prevention. *Online Journal of Issues in Nursing, 17*(2), Manuscript 1.

LaPira, T. M., & Thomas, H. F. (2014). Revolving door lobbyists and interest representation. *Interest Groups & Advocacy, 3*(1), 4–29.

Lewenson, S. B. (2015). Overview and summary: Cornerstone documents in healthcare: Our history, our future. *Online Journal of Issues in Nursing, 20*(2). Retrieved from http://www.nursingworld.org/MainMenuCategories/ANAMarketplace/ANAPeriodicals/OJIN/TableofContents/Vol-20-2015/No2-May-2015/OS-Cornerstone-Documents.html

Longest, B. B. (2016). *Health policymaking in the United States* (6th ed.). Chicago, IL: Health Administration Press.

Maryland, M. A., & Gonzalez, R. I. (2012). Patient advocacy in the community and legislative arena. *Online Journal of Issues in Nursing, 17*(1). Retrieved from http://www.nursingworld.org/MainMenuCategories/ANAMarketplace/ANAPeriodicals/OJIN/TableofContents/Vol-17-2012/No1-Jan-2012/Advocacy-in-Community-and-Legislative-Arena.html

Mason, D. J., Gardner, D. B., Outlaw, F. H., & O'Grady, E. T., (Eds.). (2016). *Policy and politics in nursing and health care* (7th ed.). St. Louis, MO: Elsevier.

Matthews, J. H. (2012). Role of professional organizations in advocating for the nursing profession. *Online Journal of Issues in Nursing, 17*(1). Retrieved from http://www.medscape.com/viewarticle/766817_4

McCool, D. (1995). *Public policy theories, models and concepts: An anthology.* Old Tappan, NJ: Prentice Hall.

Medicaid.gov. (n.d.). *Affordable Care Act.* Retrieved from https://www.medicaid.gov/affordablecareact/affordable-care-act.html

Milio, N. (1981). *Promoting health through public policy.* Philadelphia, PA: F. A. Davis.

Milstead, J. A. (Ed.). (2016). *Health policy and politics: A nurse's guide* (5th ed.). Burlington, MA: Jones & Bartlett Learning.

National Collaborating Centre for Healthy Public Policy. (2010). *How can we make healthy public policies?* Retrieved from http://www.ncchpp.ca/en/

National Council of State Legislatures. (2015). *State policies on sex education in schools.* Retrieved from http://www.ncsl.org/research/health/state-policies-on-sex-education-in-schools.aspx

National League of Cities. (2013). *Local government authority.* Retrieved from http://www.nlc.org/build-skills-and-networks/resources/cities-101/city-powers/local-government-authority

National League for Nursing. (2016). *Overview.* Retrieved from http://www.nln.org/about

Nickitas, D. M., Middaugh, D. J., & Aries, N. (2016). *Policy and politics for nurses and other health professionals* (2nd ed.). Burlington, MA: Jones & Bartlett Learning.

Office of the Federal Register. (n.d.). *A guide to the rulemaking process.* Retrieved from https://www.federalregister.gov/uploads/2011/01/the_rulemaking_process.pdf

Organization for Economic Cooperation & Development. (2015). *Focus on health spending: OECD statistics, 2015.* Retrieved from http://www.oecd.org/health/health-systems/Focus-Health-Spending-2015.pdf

Paquin, S. O. (2011). Social justice advocacy in nursing: What is it? How do we get it? *Creative Nursing, 17*(2), 63–67.

Pearson, M., Anthony, Z. B., & Buckley, N. A. (2010). Prospective policy analysis: How an epistemic community informed policymaking on intentional self poisoning in Sri Lanka. *Health Research Policy & Systems, 8,* 19. doi: 10.1186/1478-4505-8-19.

Petit, J. (2012). *Empowerment and participation: Bridging the gap between understanding and practice.* Retrieved from http://www.un.org/esa/socdev/egms/docs/2012/JethroPettit.pdf

Piper, S. M. (2011). Community empowerment for health visiting and other public health nursing. *Community Practitioner, 84*(8), 28–31.

Porter, M. E., & Lee, T. H. (2013). The strategy that will fix health care. *Harvard Business Review.* Retrieved from https://hbr.org/2013/10/the-strategy-that-will-fix-health-care

Premji, S. S., & Hatfield, J. (2016). Call to action for nurses/nursing. *BioMed Research International*. Article ID 3127543. http://dx.doi.org/10.1155/2016/3127543

Rambur, B. (2015). *Health care finance, economics, and policy for nurses: A foundational guide*. New York, NY: Springer Publishing Company.

Rand Corporation. (2015). *Health coverage grows under Affordable Care Act*. Retrieved from http://www.rand.org/news/press/2015/05/06.html

Rhodes, D. (2016, January 17). Raising cigarette-buying age to 21 a new strategy in fighting addiction. *Chicago Tribune*. Retrieved from http://www.chicagotribune.com/news/ct-minimum-tobacco-age-emanuel-met-20160117-story.html

Robert Wood Johnson Foundation. (2010, November 30). *Robert Wood Johnson Foundation launches national campaign to advance health through nursing*. Retrieved from http://www.rwjf.org/pr/product.jsp?id=71510

Rutgers Center for American Women and Politics. (2016). *Current numbers*. Retrieved from http://www.cawp.rutgers.edu/current-numbers

Schultz, C. (2010). Transformation: The Institute of Medicine report on the future of nursing. *Nursing Education Perspectives*, 31(6), 345.

Shariff, N. (2014). Factors that act as facilitators and barriers to nurse leaders' participation in health policy development. *BMC Nursing*, 13, 20.

Song, A. (n.d.). ANA-PAC wraps up first half of the "Race for the Million" campaign. ANA Capitol Update. Retrieved from http://www.rnaction.org/site/PageServer?pagename=CUP_Arch_022908_en1_racemillion&ct=1

Surgeon General. (n.d.a). *National Prevention Strategy*. Retrieved from http://www.surgeongeneral.gov/priorities/prevention/strategy/

Surgeon General. (n.d.b). *Prevention advisory group members*. Retrieved from http://www.surgeongeneral.gov/priorities/prevention/advisorygrp/advisory-group-members.html

Swaminathan, S., Mor, V., Mehrotra, R., & Trivedi, A. (2012). Medicare's payment strategy for end-stage renal disease now embraces bundled payment and pay-for-performance to cut costs. *Health Affairs*, 31(9), 2051–2058.

Taylor, M. R. (2016). Impact of advocacy initiatives on nurses' motivation to sustain momentum in public policy advocacy. *Journal of Professional Nursing*, 32(3), 235–245.

Turner, S. G., & Maschi, T. M. (2015). Feminist and empowerment theory and social work practice. *Journal of Social Work Practice: Psychotherapeutic Approaches in Health, Welfare and the Community*, 29(2), 151–162.

U.S. Department of Health and Human Services. (2015). *Read the law: The Affordable Care Act, section by section*. Retrieved from http://www.hhs.gov/healthcare/about-the-law/read-the-law/index.html

U.S. Department of Health and Human Services. (2016, January 11). *New hospitals and health care providers join successful, cost-cutting federal initiative that cuts costs and puts patients at the center of their care*. Retrieved from http://www.hhs.gov/about/news/2016/01/11/new-hospitals-and-health-care-providers-join-successful-cutting-edge-federal-initiative.html

U.S. House of Representatives. (n.d.). *The legislative process*. Retrieved from http://www.house.gov/content/learn/legislative_process/

Washington State Nurses Association. (2011, June 6). *Public health and public health nursing: Position paper*. Retrieved from http://www.wsna.org/assets/entry-assets/Nursing-Practice/Publications/Position-Paper-on-Public-Health-r2.pdf

Weimer, D. L., & Wilk, L. (2016). Allocation of indivisible life-saving goods with both intrinsic and relational quality: The new deceased-donor kidney allocation system. *Administration & Society*. doi: 10.1177/0095399716647156.

White House. (2016). *The judicial branch*. Retrieved from https://www.whitehouse.gov/1600/judicial-branch

Whitfield, S. (2015). *Black nurses in history: A bibliography and guide to web resources*. Retrieved from http://libguides.rowan.edu/blacknurses

Wong, N. T., Zimmerman, M. T., & Parker, E. A. (2010). A typology of youth participation and empowerment for child and adolescent health promotion. *American Journal of Community Psychology*, 46(1–2), 100–114.

thePoint: Everything You Need to Make the Grade!

thePoint® Visit http://thePoint.lww.com/Rector9e for selected readings, study aids for all learning styles, and more!

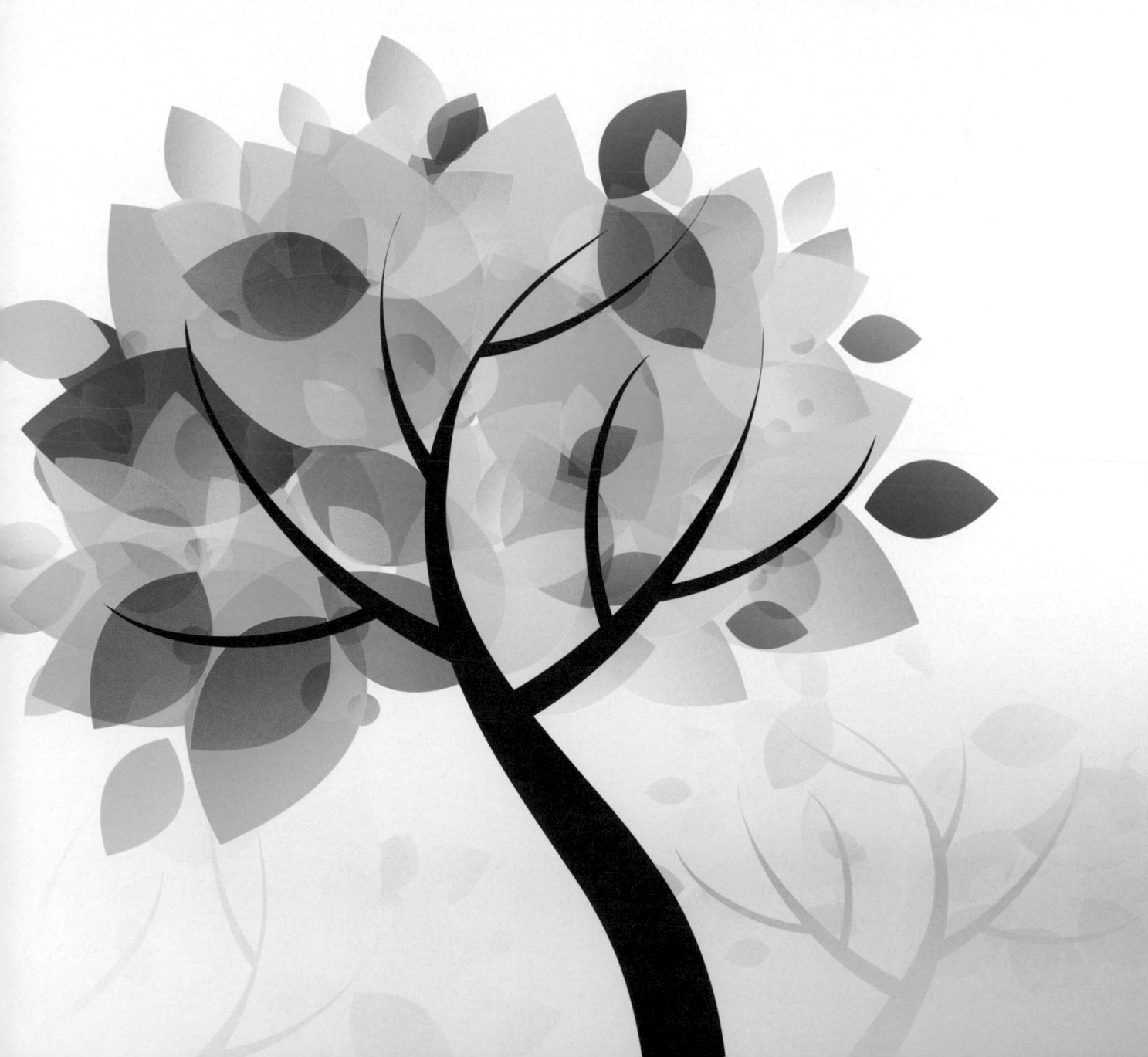
THE COMMUNITY AS CLIENT

Theoretical Basis of Community/Public Health Nursing

"We know a great deal more about the causes of physical disease than we do about the causes of physical health."

—**M. Scott Peck,** The Road Less Traveled

KEY TERMS

Bioterrorism
Community-oriented, population-focused care
Conceptual model

Genetics
Genomics
Genetic engineering
Global economy

Intersectionality
Migration
Model
Nursing theory

Principle
Technology
Theory

LEARNING OBJECTIVES

Upon mastery of this chapter, you should be able to:

- Discuss three essential characteristics of nursing service when a community is the client: community-oriented, population-focused care and relationship-based care.
- Describe the contributions of at least five models of nursing practice to community/public health nursing practice.
- Describe four programs or initiatives that demonstrate application of the eight principles of public health nursing to community/public health nursing.
- Identify at least five social issues that influence contemporary community/public health nursing care.

When you open the door of a senior center where you will be promoting cardiovascular fitness, advocating for exercise equipment, and suggesting changes in the on-site meal program, how might theories of public health nursing contribute to your success? When you approach your city council about the need to increase staffing for public health services, what models of public health nursing practice might support your argument? What are *theories, models,* and *principles,* and what is their relevance to day-to-day public health nursing practice? These are the key issues explored in this chapter. First, however, we revisit some of the fundamental characteristics of community/public health nursing that we began to explore in Unit 1.

WHEN THE CLIENT IS A COMMUNITY: CHARACTERISTICS OF COMMUNITY/PUBLIC HEALTH NURSING PRACTICE

Nursing exists to address people's health care needs, and nurses fulfill this purpose through their work in various specialty areas. Specialties are characterized by the unit of care for which the specialty is responsible and by the goal of the specialty. Each specialty requires a particular area of knowledge and a set of skills for excellence in practice.

Public health nursing is a specialty in which the unit of care is a specific community or aggregate, and the nurse has responsibility to promote group health. The goal of this specialty is health improvement of the community. Some of the skills required for excellence in public health nursing practice include epidemiology, research, teaching, community organizing, and interpersonal relational care.

In summary, community/public health nursing is characterized by community-oriented, population-focused care and is based on interpersonal relationships. In the following sections, each of these characteristics is examined in more depth.

Community-Oriented, Population-Focused Care

As was discussed in Chapter 1, a *community* is a group of people who have some characteristics in common, are bounded by time, interact with one another, and feel a connection to one another. For example, members of an Internet-based support group for people with colitis are a community. They share similar experiences and concerns, and they often influence one another's behavior. For instance, they may recommend food choices or complementary therapies to one another. Members of a class of community/public health nursing students are also a community. Because they begin and end their studies in a particular month and year, they are bonded by time, and they most likely share certain values and feel a sense of connection to one another.

Community orientation is a process that is actively shaped by the unique experiences, knowledge, concerns, values, beliefs, and culture of a given community. For example, when an outbreak of hepatitis occurs, the public health nurse does more than simply treat infection in individuals. The nurse also:

- Uses disease investigation skills to locate possible sources of infection
- Determines how the community's knowledge, values, beliefs, and prior experiences with infectious disease may influence its interpretation of the disease, response to the outbreak, and treatment preferences
- Uses knowledge and suggestions gathered from the community to develop, in collaboration with other health professionals, a community-specific program to prevent future outbreaks

A community-oriented nurse who provides education about sexually transmitted diseases to a group of students at a Catholic university includes consideration of community values regarding sexual behavior. Similarly, a community-oriented nurse who provides nutritional counseling to a community of Hispanic seniors considers the meaning of food in this culture, the types of food most commonly consumed, and the cooking methods most commonly used.

A *population* is any group of people who share at least one characteristic, such as age, gender, race, a particular risk factor, or disease. Smokers and breast cancer survivors are two populations. The concept of population may also include delineation by time (e.g., all infants born in the year 2017). The nurse's place of employment commonly limits the population that the nurse serves. For example, a nurse who works for a county health department is limited professionally to caring for the population residing in that county.

A *population focus* implies that a nurse uses population-based skills such as epidemiology, research in community assessment, and community organizing as the basis for interventions. For example, a population-focused nurse employed by an autoworkers' union may study all cases of repetitive-use injury occurring in the auto industry in the United States in the past 5 years, develop a program for reducing repetitive-use injury, and lobby industry executives for adoption of the program.

Community-oriented, population-focused care employs population-based skills and is shaped by the characteristics and needs of a given community. Public health nurses provide community-oriented, population-focused care when they count and interview homeless people sleeping in a park and, based on these data, help develop a program to provide food, clothing, shelter, health care, and job training for this population.

THEORIES AND MODELS FOR COMMUNITY/PUBLIC HEALTH NURSING PRACTICE

A **theory** is a set of systematically interrelated concepts or hypotheses that seek to explain or predict phenomena. For example, the "big bang theory" seeks to explain the series of events that occurred during the earliest moments in the history of our universe. A theory is based either explicitly or philosophically on a conceptual model (also referred to as a conceptual framework, a conceptual system, or a paradigm). A **conceptual model**, as defined by Bigby and Issel (2012, p. 371), is "an integrated set of concepts and relational statements that provide direction for clinical assessment, analysis, planning and evaluation." These concepts are presented in a framework format, used to explain the relationships between variables.

Nurses can enhance their practice in an ever-changing clinical environment by embracing nursing theories and incorporating them with empirical evidence from the research (McCrea, 2012). In response to a wide gap between what was known through research and what was implemented in practice, a movement had begun to implement evidence-based practice (EBP) into nursing care to improve patient outcomes. The Quality and Safety Education for Nurses (QSEN) project identified EBP as one of the six competencies recommended for safe, high-quality nursing care (Case Western Reserve University, 2014). Evidence-based nursing practice brings together empirical evidence obtained through research, nursing expertise, and patient values (Stevens, 2013). Theory plays a critical role in each of these three legs of the EBP triangle. Theoretical frameworks are used to guide the research process. In addition, theory can be used to understand patient values and behaviors, and theory can describe nursing practice.

Nursing theorists have sought to present nursing practice constructs in comprehensive and systematic ways. The evolution of conceptual model and theory development in nursing dominated the last half of the 20th century. The scholarly and creative efforts of those nurse leaders and researchers sought to explain what nursing is and how it influences individuals, families, or communities and provide a basis for building nursing knowledge. From those early efforts came more testable theories, many from those same nurse researchers; those theories are typically referred to as middle-range theories. Although less abstract than conceptual models, the need for an even more practical approach to theory use and testing led ultimately to practice-based theories (Alligood, 2014; McCrea, 2012).

To more fully understand the elements inherent in a **nursing theory** and the underlying conceptual model, a pictorial representation, or graphic model, is often used. These models provide a visual means to understand the relationships between, for instance, the nurse and the environment, the nurse and the client, or the client and stressors. However complex these models are, comprehension of the entire work can only be derived from reading the theorist's descriptions of the conceptual models, the theories, and the subsequent research testing those theories. Concepts, when fully defined, related/linked, and measured, describe the building blocks of the theory. Both theories and conceptual models have been developed to describe, clarify, and guide nursing practice (Alligood, 2014). Theories and conceptual models that have particular relevance to the practice of community/public health nursing are described here.

Nightingale's Theory of Environment

Florence Nightingale's environmental theory has great significance to nursing in general and to public health nursing specifically, because it focuses on preventive care for populations. While organizing and supervising a nursing service for soldiers in the Crimean War, Nightingale kept meticulous records. Her observations suggested that disease was more prevalent in poor environments and that health could be promoted by providing adequate ventilation, pure water, quiet, warmth, light, and cleanliness. In fact, 420 soldiers per 1,000 died within the first 2 months of Nightingale's arrival, and she was able to reduce that rate to 22 per 1,000 soldiers within 6 months time. The crux of her theory was that poor environmental conditions were bad for health and that good environmental conditions reduced disease (Johnson & Webber, 2015; Nightingale, 1859/1992).

As current-day public health practitioners look upstream to identify the root causes of poor health, physical, social, and economic factors have been identified as influencing health outcomes. Where people live, work, and play impacts their overall health (U.S. Department of Health and Human Services [USDHHS], 2016d). Examples of these determinants of health include segregation, the design of a home or a community, the availability of green spaces and light, access to healthy foods, and much more. These same observations were made generations ago by Florence Nightingale as she provided care to those living and dying in unhealthy environments.

A more expansive list of social and physical determinants of health can be seen in greater detail in Displays 14–1 and 14–2 (USDHHS, 2016d). As you

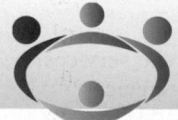

DISPLAY 14–1 EXAMPLES OF SOCIAL DETERMINANTS OF HEALTH

- Availability of resources to meet daily needs (e.g., safe housing and local food markets)
- Access to educational, economic, and job opportunities
- Access to health care services
- Quality of education and job training
- Availability of community-based resources in support of community living and opportunities for recreational and leisure-time activities
- Transportation options
- Public safety
- Social support
- Social norms and attitudes (e.g., discrimination, racism, and distrust of government)
- Exposure to crime, violence, and social disorder (e.g., presence of trash and lack of cooperation in a community)
- Socioeconomic conditions (e.g., concentrated poverty and the stressful conditions that accompany it)
- Residential segregation
- Language/literacy
- Access to mass media and emerging technologies (e.g., cell phones, the Internet, and social media)
- Culture

From U.S. Department of Health and Human Services. (2016). *Healthy People 2020: Social determinants of health*. Retrieved from http://www.healthypeople.gov/2020/topicsobjectives2020/overview.aspx?topicid=39

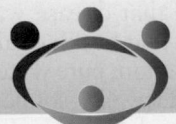

DISPLAY 14–2 EXAMPLES OF PHYSICAL DETERMINANTS OF HEALTH

● Natural environment, such as green space (e.g., trees and grass) or weather (e.g., climate change)
● Built environment, such as buildings, sidewalks, bike lanes, and roads
● Worksites, schools, and recreational settings
● Housing and community design
● Exposure to toxic substances and other physical hazards
● Physical barriers, especially for people with disabilities
● Aesthetic elements (e.g., good lighting, trees, and benches)

From U.S. Department of Health and Human Services. (2016). *Healthy People 2020: Social determinants of health*. Retrieved from http://www.healthypeople.gov/2020/topicsobjectives2020/overview.aspx?topicid=39

think about services included in Display 14–1, it is useful to consider:

● Why these services were created?
● Who benefits from the services?
● Who pays for the services?
● What is the cost to the people using the services?
● What is the public perception of the services?

For example, if ventilation in a city's homeless shelter is inadequate, the public health nurse who plans to advocate for capital improvements to the shelter needs to consider who pays for the shelter as well as the public's perception of the shelter.

One contemporary example of the utility of Nightingale's theory is the work done by public health nurses in Cook County, Illinois. These nurses used geographic information system (GIS) technology to create maps that indicated the level of walkability in low-income neighborhoods. Features that were identified included availability of sidewalks and accessibility to grocery stores and health services (DeGuzman & Kulbok, 2012). Using the evidence that demonstrates the link between environment and poor health, these nurses were able to advocate for changes to be built into those communities identified as having poor walkability. Nightingale's influence on the way nurses approach health issues that impact the communities of today remains a powerful force, as noted by Zborowsky (2014) in a study about the influence of Nightingale's theory on nursing research.

Orem's Self-Care Model

Dorothy Orem (1914–2007), a nurse administrator and educator, focused on the concept of *self-care*—learned, goal-oriented actions to preserve and promote life, health, and well-being. She described people who need nursing care as those who lack ability in self-care and discussed three systems of self-care: fully compensatory system

where the nurse needs to provide care as the patient is unable to do any self-care, partially compensatory system where both the patient and the nurse work together in care provision, and the supportive–educative system where the nurse reinforces the patient's self-care efforts (Johnson & Webber, 2015; Orem, 2001). If a demand for self-care exceeds the client's ability, the client experiences a self-care deficit, and nursing intervention becomes appropriate. The goal of nursing action is to help people recognize their self-care demands and limitations and increase their self-care ability. Nursing care also functions to meet clients' self-care needs until they are able to care for themselves. Orem further described three types of requirements that influence people's self-care abilities:

● Universal requirements are activities common to all human beings, which are essential to meet physiologic and psychosocial needs.
● Developmental requirements are activities necessary to help people progress developmentally.
● Health-deviation requirements are activities needed to help people deal with a diminished level of wellness.

Although Orem's model focused primarily on individuals, it can be applied to public health nursing practice. Populations and communities can be considered to have a collective set of self-care actions and requirements that affect the well-being of the total group. If an aggregate's demands for self-care exceed its ability, the aggregate experiences a self-care deficit, and public health nursing intervention is indicated. According to this interpretation, the goal of nursing is to promote a community's collective independence and self-care ability. Kagan expanded on Orem's interpretation of self to reflect a more unitary link between humans and their environment; considering human–environment as one entity. With this worldview, she emphasized that nurses "can learn new information, make ethical and political decisions, and act to take care of the environment including regulation of human interaction with, and impact on, the environment" (Kagan, 2011, p. 73).

Green (2013) described how Orem's Self-Care Deficit Theory can be applied at the population level by school nurses who develop care plans for children with disabilities to help them meet their self-care requisites. Orem's constructs of conditioning factors and universal self-care requisites correlate to the public health concepts of social determinants of health and the World Health Organization's (2016) definition of health, not as the absence of disease, but as physical, mental, and social well-being. Orem's basic conditioning factors can be related to the compounding effect that overlapping factors of inequality such as access issues, discrimination, and racism present. This is known as *intersectionality* (Green, 2013). Children with disabilities are an example of a vulnerable population because of accessibility challenges, discrimination, and their young age, which is further compounded by health risks related to their preexisting medical condition. Health outcomes are likely to differ between students even though they may have similar diagnoses. One child may be from a mainstream culture and have a stable, middle-income family, whereas another may be a minority, experiencing racism and living in poverty. To ensure optimal health for all, school nurses must be mindful that children may experience confounding factors beyond their physical disability that further threaten their self-care agency to ensure health (Green, 2013).

Neuman's Health Care Systems Model

Betty Neuman, a leader in mental health nursing and nursing education, proposed a systems model first used in a graduate community mental health clinical specialist program (Neuman, 1982; Neuman & Fawcett, 2011) and can be adapted to view clients as aggregates. In this model, people are seen as open systems that constantly and reciprocally interact with their environments. Each system is greater than the sum of its parts, and wellness exists when the parts of the system interact in harmony with each other and with the system's environment. Four sets of variables, or influences, make up each system's "whole." These are physiologic, psychological, sociocultural, and developmental variables. Given these variables, each system has a unique response to environmental stressors and to those tension-producing stimuli that may cause disequilibrium or illness (Alligood, 2014; Johnson & Webber, 2015).

A system's response to stressors may be envisioned as a series of concentric circles (Fig. 14–1). In the center is a core of basic survival abilities, such as a community's ability to make the best use of its natural resources. Surrounding this core are three boundaries. The innermost boundary is a flexible line of resistance that encompasses internal defenses, such as a community's collective sense of responsibility for raising healthy children. The second boundary is the system's normal line of defense, such as a community's police force or voluntary fire

brigade. The third boundary is a dynamic, flexible line of defense, a buffer that prevents stressors from invading the system's normal line of defense (Alligood, 2014; Johnson & Webber, 2015). An example is regular maintenance of a community's roads and bridges.

In Neuman's model, stressors can originate from the internal environment or the external environment. Examples of internal stressors include a high proportion of low-income residents or an inadequate system of water purification. External stressors might include natural disasters, war, or a downturn in the global economy. The role of public health nursing, then, is to assist communities in remaining stable within their environments.

Olowokere and Okanlawon (2015) used the concepts from Neuman's Healthcare Systems Model to guide population-level interventions for school children in Nigeria. Neuman's model is a good fit for population-level nursing interventions because it provides a systems perspective on the relationships between people, the environment, nursing care, and health. This intervention focused on addressing the psychosocial needs of children who had chronic illnesses such as HIV/AIDS, had one or both parents die, were victims of abuse or traumatized by conflict, or were in need of legal protection or alternative care. The nurses caring for the children had little time and no training to provide psychosocial support to these children. Neuman's model provided the framework for public health nurses to help the students develop a line of resistance to prevent stress (primary prevention) or to help them cope with the stressors they faced (secondary prevention) to protect their inner core. Examples of resistance resources included participation in support groups and resilience training (Olowokere & Okanlawon, 2015). Public health nurses also helped develop protective resources within the

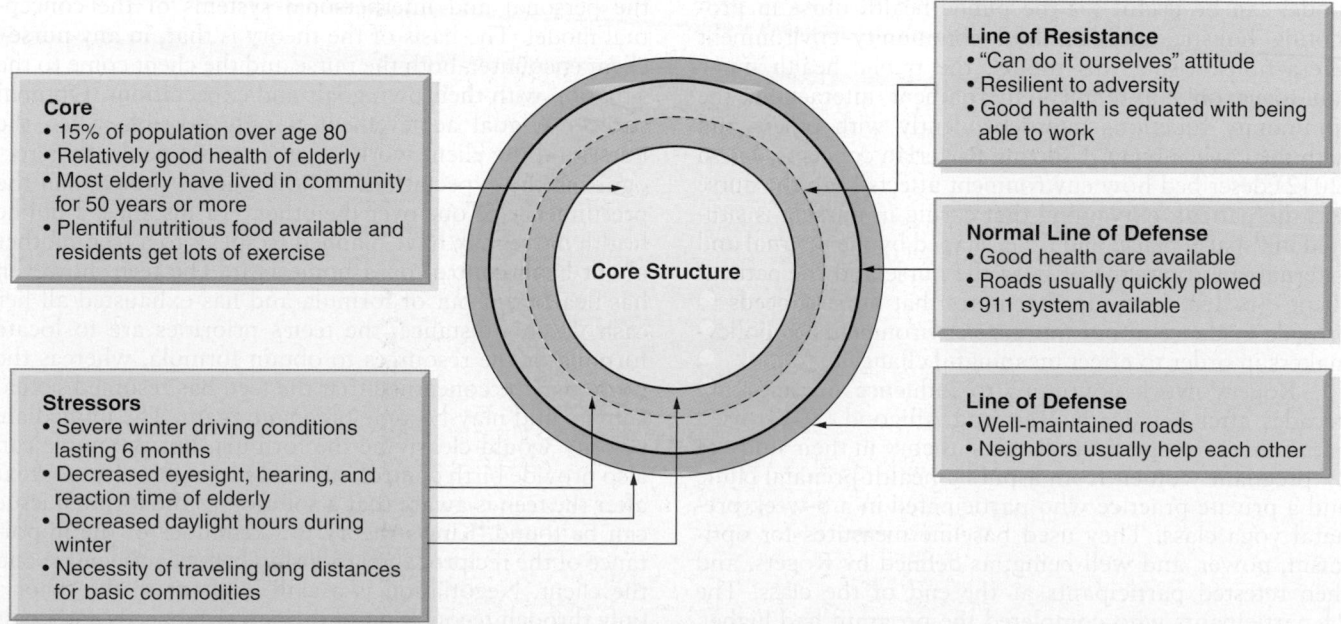

FIGURE 14–1 Neuman's Health Care Systems Model applied to a rural county regarding traffic safety issues concerning the elderly by D. Block. (From Allender, J., & Spradley, B. (2001). *Community health nursing: Concepts and practice* (5th ed.). Philadelphia, PA: Lippincott, with permission.)

family and the community by serving as case managers to help the children access needed resources. At the tertiary level, the nurse facilitated access to needed services such as counseling to prevent regression (Olowokere & Okanlawon, 2015).

Rogers' Model of the Science of Unitary Human Beings

Martha Rogers (1914–1994) created the Science of Unitary Human Beings Model. She had a strong public health nursing background. She worked as a public health nurse in 1937 to 1939 and was on staff as a home visiting nurse from 1940 to 1945 and established the first visiting nursing service in Arizona in the mid-1940 to 1951; it was one of the first in the nation (American Nurses Association [ANA], 2016; Tomasson, 1994). In 1954, she obtained a public health master's degree from Johns Hopkins University (ANA, 2016). A nursing administrator and long-time nurse educator, Rogers is responsible for modern nursing's emphasis on the whole person. In 1970, she developed a nursing conceptual model based on systems theory. Her model emphasized that the individual and environment should be viewed as one unit; that is, focusing on the individual without examining their environment, or examining parts of a community, such as its health care or housing, does not provide an adequate picture of its totality in relation to the person (Johnson & Webber, 2015).

Rogers also incorporated developmental theory into her model by describing the development of "unitary" persons or systems according to three principles: (1) life proceeds in one direction along a rhythmic spiral, (2) energy fields follow a certain wave pattern and organization, and (3) human and environmental energy fields interact simultaneously and mutually, leading to completeness and unity (Rogers, 1990). Not typically linked with community/public health nursing practice, this model can be useful for the public health nurse in promoting holistic and healthful community–environment interactions. Using this model, the public health nurse can focus on community–environment interaction; the community functions interdependently with others and with the environment. Utilizing Rogerian concepts, Jarrin (2012) described how environment affects both the nurse and the patient, explaining that caring in nursing is situated in "space, place, and time, shaped by the internal and external environments of both the nurse and the patient/client" (p. 15). Jarrin further notes that nursing needs to provide evidence about our care environments to policymakers in order to effect meaningful changes.

Rogers' work continues to influence nursing care decades after her death. Reis and Alligood (2014) used patterning concepts from Rogers' theory in their study of 27 pregnant women from a public health prenatal clinic and a private practice who participated in a 6-week prenatal yoga class. They used baseline measures for optimism, power, and well-being, as defined by Rogers, and then retested participants at the end of the class. The 21 participants who completed the program had higher, statistically significant scores on all three measures at the conclusion of the yoga classes that were viewed by the researchers as a "holistic practice" consistent with a "holistic Rogerian view" (p. 35).

Guided by Rogers' concepts of human–environment and the effect of environmental stressors on human–environment energy field, Greene and Greene (2012) provided Internet-based guided imagery to a convenience sample of adults. Guided imagery uses visual stimuli and a calming story or fantasy journey that encourages relaxation and may integrate "suggestion and affirmations" (p. 152). It has been found to be helpful with chemotherapy patients and those patients experiencing pain. This pilot study provided a 7-minute session that was available on demand to participants by accessing a specific Web site. No limits were set on the number of times a person could participate in the guided imagery session, and participants took a brief pretest as a baseline measure of stress and anxiety and then completed a posttest. Researchers found participants by sending email invitations to known subjects, who in turn forwarded the email invitations to others (e.g., a snowball sample). Results revealed a significant difference in pre- and posttest scores, indicating reduction in self-reported levels of stress. This research has implications for population health, especially for those living in remote areas.

King's Theory of Goal Attainment

Imogene King (1923–2007), nursing scholar and educator, was one of the early nurse theorists to provide a conceptual model of nursing (Messmer & Palmer, 2008). Her groundbreaking work *Toward a Theory for Nursing* (1970) and the subsequent *A Theory for Nursing: Systems, Concepts, Process* (1981) were both designed to "promote conceptual learning in undergraduate and graduate nursing programs" (1981, p. vii) and can be utilized by the public health nurse to define the nurse–client relationship. From the original general systems model that demonstrated the interrelationship between social, interpersonal, and personal systems (Killeen & King, 2007), King formulated the Theory of Goal Attainment. The theory focuses on the personal and interpersonal systems of the conceptual model. The basis of the theory is that, in any nurse–client encounter, both the nurse and the client come to the situation with their own goals and expectations. Optimal success at goal achievement is only possible when the nurse and the client work together to set goals, thus recognizing the expectations of both parties rather than the preeminence of one over the other. For instance, a public health nurse may have planned to speak to a teen mother about birth control on a home visit. The teen, however, has nearly run out of formula and has exhausted all her cash. In this instance, the teen's priorities are to locate formula or the resources to obtain formula, whereas the nurse may be concerned that the teen has resumed sexual activity and may become pregnant again. The immediate priority would clearly be the formula, but the nurse can also provide birth control information within that context after the teen is aware that a solution to the formula issue can be found. King's theory is a reminder of the importance of the reciprocal relationship between the nurse and the client. Negotiation is a skill inherent in the theory; only through recognition of the perceived needs and goals of the client can the public health nurse help maintain or improve the client's health and well-being.

Another example is seen with Housing First programs where the primary focus is on housing those who experience chronic homelessness, rather than on enforcement of strict abstinence rules among those who struggle with addition (Collins et al., 2012). The traditional abstinence-only programs were found to not be in alignment with the needs of this population. Collins et al. (2012) sought to understand the barriers to abstinence and identified that chronic alcohol use served to hold off withdrawal symptoms, was used as self-medication for psychiatric conditions, and also served as a social convener. Through the program, instead of only recognizing total abstinence, any positive change was rewarded. Ultimately, residents reported that having housing allowed them to have control over their own goals and most were able to reduce their substance use (Collins et al., 2012). The results of this program serve as a reminder of the importance of treating the client as an equal partner in their own goal setting.

Community engagement and empowerment are key concepts in international public health practices as well. An example of the importance of this approach can be seen during an Ebola outbreak where community participation can play a critical role in the control of this disease (Shrivastava, Shrivastava, & Ramasamy, 2015). Fear and lack of information contribute to the rapid spread of this deadly disease. Culturally sensitive approaches are needed to counter misunderstandings about the disease, ineffective treatments through traditional healers, and exposures to reservoir species (e.g., bats). Community-based approaches where public health nurses and community members are working toward common goals can result in collaboration in contact investigations, improved cooking methods, and even changes in funeral practices (Shrivastava et al., 2015). These and many other examples demonstrate the utility of King's work to current practice in public health.

Parse's Theory of Human Becoming

Rosemarie Rizzo Parse developed her theory, initially called the "man-living-health" theory, in 1981. In 1992, she changed the name to Human Becoming Theory to better reflect all people. The theory posits quality of life from each person's own perspective as the goal of nursing practice (Johnson & Webber, 2015). The theory is structured around three themes (Parse, 1981, 1998):

Meaning. People coparticipate in creating what is real for them through self-expression by living their values in their own chosen way.

Rhythmicity. The unity of life encompasses apparent opposites in rhythmic patterns of relating. While living moment to moment, one shows and does not show the self, creating both opportunities and limitations that emerge as moving with and moving apart from others.

Transcendence. Viewed as moving beyond the moment and forging a unique personal path for oneself in the midst of ambiguity and continuous change.

These three themes apply effectively to the community. The nurse must know what the community means to its inhabitants, identify and be aware of the rhythmicity of the people as attempts are made to create positive health changes in the community, and realize the transcendence that occurs when people work in the presence of ambiguity and continuous change, characteristics

inherent in a community. Use of this theory as a guide enhances the ability of community members to work together to accomplish identified goals. Examples of the use of the theory most applicable to public health nursing practice include nursing's engagement in health policy (Poirier, 2012), the act of being "present" in professional practice (Zyblock, 2010), and supporting caring–healing–sustainable nursing practices (Clark, 2012).

Building on her research, Parse has developed what she terms a Human Becoming Community Model (Parse, 2012). The model emphasizes the change concepts of moving–initiating, anchoring–shifting, and pondering–shaping. She clarifies the significance of community such that "when people come together as a group, the individual communities bring their histories to the emerging now, and this creates an entity of coevolving histories, which confirms individual as community and group as community" (pp. 44–45). The work of Parse and others brings a unique and holistic perspective to community/public health nursing practice.

This theory can serve as a guide for nurses advocating for health care policy change. Milton (2015) noted that the constructs of freedom and choice are often overridden when policies and protocols are implemented in health care settings. People often become labeled as noncompliant if they do not agree with set protocols. However, Parse's theory described freedom and choice as woven into the fabric of being human (Milton, 2015). Milton called for nurses to honor the importance of freedom and choice when creating and implementing policies rather than dehumanize the health care process.

Pender's Health Promotion Model

As we have noted throughout this text, health promotion is a priority in community/public health nursing practice. Pender defined health promotion as actions that are directed toward increasing the level of well-being and self-actualization in individuals or groups (Pender, Murdaugh, & Parsons, 2015). It is a proactive set of behaviors in which people act on their environment rather than react to stressors arising from the environment.

Pender's *Health Promotion Model* seeks to explain this proactive behavior. The model, based on social learning theory, stresses cognitive processes that help regulate behavior such as perceptions people have that directly influence their motivation to begin or continue health-promoting behaviors. These include, for example, perceptions of control of health, health status, benefits of health-promoting behaviors, and barriers to engaging in health-promoting behaviors (Pender et al., 2015; Sakraida, 2014).

Five types of modifying factors influence people's perceptions about pursuing health-promoting behaviors:

- Demographic factors, such as age and race
- Biologic characteristics, such as height and weight
- Interpersonal influences, such as the expectations of others
- Situational factors, such as availability of healthful foods
- Behavioral factors, such as stress-coping patterns

Using Pender's model, a public health nurse might interview the residents of a low-income housing project to determine their perceptions about improving health and safety. Research of demographic, situational, and other factors that might influence the residents' motivation and ability to change their circumstances could then be conducted.

Pender's model was validated as a motivational model during a program that incorporated exercise and physical activity for people with spinal cord injuries (Keegan, Chan, Ditchman, & Chiu, 2012). People who have sustained a spinal cord injury are at a greater risk of secondary health complications and chronic conditions related to inactivity. Nurses designed exercise and physical activity plans taking into consideration the four predictor variables described in Pender's model including individual factors, interrelational and situational factors, behavior-specific cognition, and commitment to the plan (Keegan et al., 2012). Self-efficacy and sense of control were found to be strong predictors of commitment resulting in engaging in health-promoting behavior. Beliefs about control and support and encouragement from family and friends were also linked to increased motivation. Perceived barriers had a low prediction correlation. To promote long-term health among people with spinal cord injuries, rehabilitation plans should include these factors to increase motivation (Keegan et al., 2012).

Although pertinent to public health nursing practice, the model is not strictly speaking of a conceptual model of nursing, as was discussed earlier in this chapter. The metaparadigm concepts of patient/client, health, and environment are present, but the model does not stipulate that the provider of health educational services be a nurse and can in fact be from other disciplines. Pender's model is further discussed in relation to client education in Chapter 11.

Roy's Adaptation Model

Sister Callista Roy's model describes people as open and adaptive systems that experience stimuli, develop coping mechanisms, and produce responses. These responses, which may be adaptive or maladaptive, provide feedback that influences the amount and type of stimuli that can be handled in the future. Nursing works, using four modes (i.e., basic physiologic needs, role mastery, self-concept, interdependence) to bring about environmental changes that permit the client to adapt (Andrews & Roy, 1991; Johnson & Webber, 2015; Roy, 2009; Roy & Andrews, 1999). This model helps the public health nurse understand how a community's ability to adapt to stressors will affect the health of the community (Fig. 14–2).

Roy describes two response processes. In the *regulator* or focal stimulus process, stimuli from the internal and external environments are received, and this combination of information is then processed to produce a response. In the *control* or contextual stimulus process, perceptions, learning, judgment, and emotion are considered in formulating a response to stimuli. An example of the regulator process might begin with a community's desire to keep adolescents from smoking (internal stimulus) and new state regulations prohibiting the sale of tobacco products to minors (external stimulus). These combined

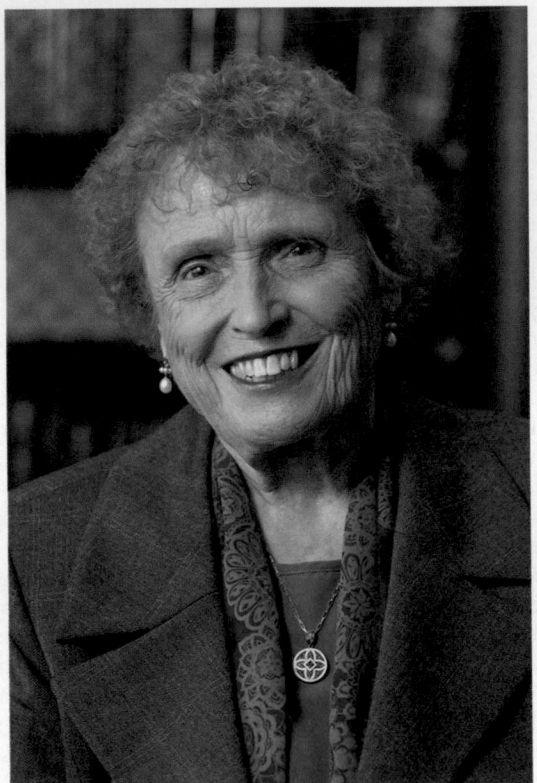

FIGURE 14–2 Sister Callista Roy. (Courtesy of Christopher Sold.)

stimuli lead to a city ordinance that prevents the sale of cigarettes to minors (coping mechanism), resulting in reduced levels of smoking (response) among this population. A regulator process might begin with the stimulus of heavy rainfall in a riverside community. Residents' perceptions of the amount of rainfall, memories of past floods, insights about preventing or managing floods, and the level of anxiety all contribute to their plans for evacuation, sandbagging, and soliciting county or state assistance (Phillips & Harris, 2014).

In applying Roy's conceptual model to public health nursing, it is important to remember that a community is made up of many parts and is influenced by many variables. The community's collective adaptation level is constantly changing. The public health nurse must assess a community's coping mechanisms and help its members use these collective abilities in adapting to challenges. For example, if a community is doing nothing to respond to the increased number of obese children, nursing actions can be designed to encourage more healthful coping patterns and adaptive responses.

Roy's Adaptation Model is well designed to help guide public health nursing practice as demonstrated with nurses working with newly diagnosed HIV/AIDS clients. Perrett and Biley (2013) found the model constructs of adaptation to be applicable. The diagnosis serves as the stimulus, triggering a level of uncertainty. Adaptation was not a passive event, rather it was noted to be a conscious effort. Factors such as the optimism gained from the availability of antiretroviral medications and new relationships triggered steps toward adaptation. Ineffective adaptation would present as anxiety, powerlessness, and loneliness (Perrett & Biley, 2013). Nurses need to assess the client's sense of self, including their perception of their health and their role within society. This can guide nursing interventions to support clients as they move toward effective adaptation (Perrett & Biley, 2013).

Salmon's Construct for Public Health Nursing

Marla Salmon, a leader in public health nursing administration, nursing education, and public health policy in the United States, has proposed a model to specifically guide community health nursing practice. In *Construct for Public Health Nursing*, Salmon (1982, 1993) described public health as an organized societal effort to protect, promote, and restore the health of people and public health nursing as focused on achieving and maintaining public health.

The model describes three practice priorities. These priorities are prevention of disease and poor health, protection against disease and external agents, and promotion of health. There are three general categories of nursing intervention:

- Education that is directed toward voluntary change in the attitudes and behavior of the subjects
- Engineering that is directed at managing risk-related variables
- Enforcement that is directed at mandatory regulation to achieve better health

The scope of practice spans individual, family, community, and global care. Interventions target determinants in four categories: human/biologic, environmental, medical/technologic/organizational, and social.

The Centers for Disease Control and Prevention included the three E's in the 2012 National Action Plan for Child Injury Prevention. In their work to prevent drowning among young children, public health nurses could engage in education outreach to families with small children about potential risks of drowning and safety measures they could implement. In addition, nurses could advocate for policies mandating fences around pools and natural bodies of water. Finally, nurses can help families find affordable fencing resources if they were struggling to pay for a fence installation (CDC, 2012). These examples of client advocacy on several levels are an important component of public health nursing and represent the types of activities common to early nurses who saw social problems resulting in poor health and worked on local and national levels to address them (see Chapter 13 for more on advocacy and policy making). Kelley, Connor, Kun, and Salmon (2008, p. 4) described social responsibility as a foundational professional duty that is "woven into the fabric of nursing's history."

Using Salmon's approach, a public health nurse attempting to reduce the transmission of tuberculosis would use education, engineering, and enforcement in working with the population of affected individuals and families. Strategies could include collaboration with the client community on a variety of interventions, from mandating isolation precautions to providing education about medications and connecting the client and their family to social support: all in an effort to prevent further disease in the community and to promote global health.

PUBLIC HEALTH PRACTICE MODELS

Minnesota Wheel—The Public Health Interventions Model

The Minnesota Department of Health, Division of Community Health Services, Public Health Nursing Section, devised a **model** that depicts public health interventions and applications for public health practice. In the form of a wheel, the model presents 17 different interventions within three levels of public health practice: population-based community-focused practice, systems-focused practice, and individual-focused practice. The "Minnesota Wheel" (Public Health Nursing Section, Minnesota Department of Health, 2001) is depicted in Figure 14–3.

The intervention wheel was first proposed in 1998 (Keller, Strohschein, Lia-Hoagberg, & Schaffer, 1998) as a practice model for population-based public health nursing. It presents public health nursing as a specialty practice within the field of nursing (Public Health Nursing Section, Minnesota Department of Health, 2001). It can be applied in a variety of venues including public health practice, nursing education, and management. Keller and colleagues emphasized that the "use of the Wheel has empowered nurses to explain in a better way how their practice contributes to the improvement of population health" (Keller, Strohschein, Lia-Hoagberg, & Schaffer, 2004, p. 454). The wheel is useful for public health nurses because it visually depicts the comprehensive list of interventions nurses must consider in the scope of practice. Schaffer, Anderson, and Rising (2015) described how school nurses using the interventions presented within the model in their day-to-day work. Including nurses who were not even aware of the model, school nurses identified screening, referrals, and case management as the interventions they most commonly implement (Schaffer et al., 2015). This example shows how well the model describes and guides community health nursing interventions.

Public Health Nursing Practice Model

The Los Angeles County Public Health Nursing Practice Model (LAC PHN Practice Model) was developed in response to an identified need for a model that could blend public health nursing practice and the principles of public health, which could be applicable to both the generalist nurse and nurses working in specific programs (Smith & Bazini-Barakat, 2003). Public health nurses at the Los Angeles County Department of Health Services (LAC-DHS) created the model, with input from the California Conference of Local Health Department Nursing Directors (CCLHNDN) Southern Region and other public health nurse leaders. The LAC PHN Practice Model (Public Health Nursing, Los Angeles County Department of Health Services [PHN, LAC-DHS], 2013) integrates foundational nursing and public health guiding documents including the Public Health Nursing Standards of Practice, the 10 Essential Public Health Services, the 12 Leading Health Indicators from *Healthy People 2020*, and the Minnesota Public Health Nursing Interventions Model. The LAC PHN Practice Model provides a "conceptual framework that assists in clarifying the role of the public health nurse and presents a guide

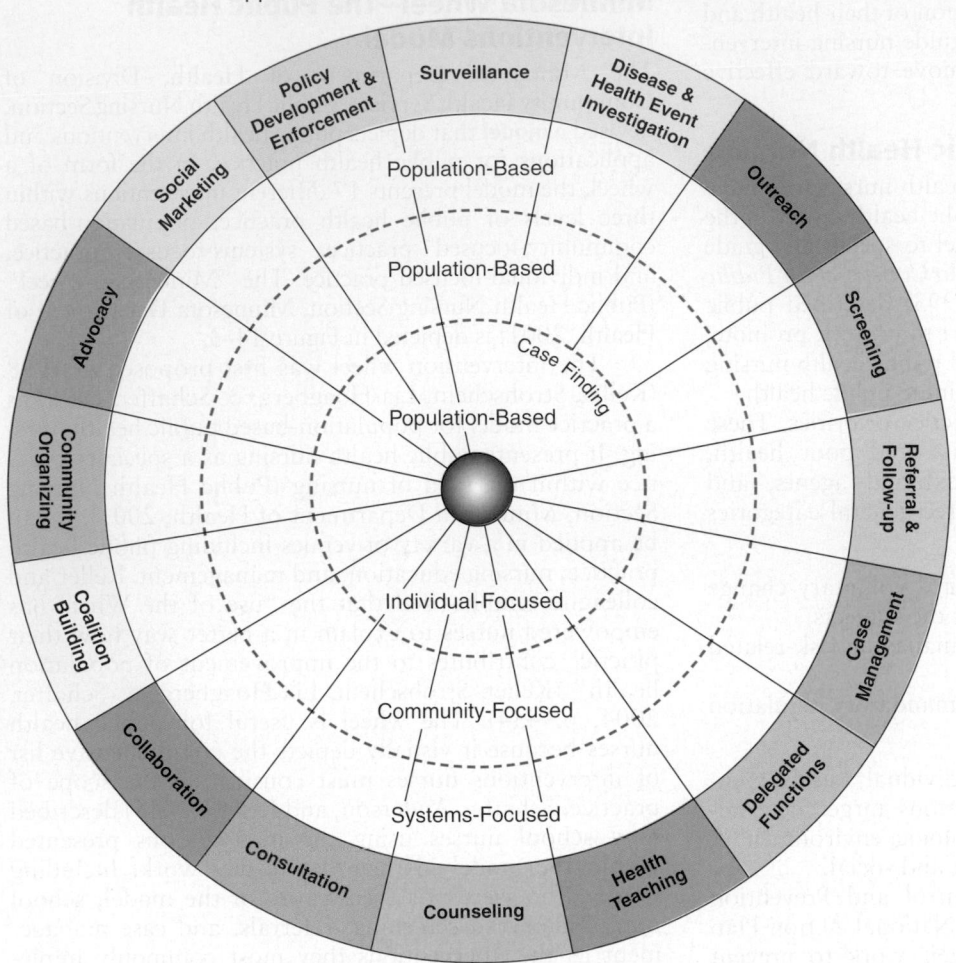

Public Health Interventions
Applications for Public Health Nursing Practice

FIGURE 14-3   The Minnesota Wheel. (Source: Minnesota Department of Health, Division of Community Health Services, Public Health Nursing Section.)

for public health practice applicable to all public health disciplines" (Smith & Bazini-Barakat, 2003, p. 42). It establishes that public health nursing is population based and was created to "describe the building blocks of PHN practice and to delineate their relationship to each other" (PHN, LAC-DHS, 2013, para. 1).

As described by Smith and Bazini-Barakat (2003) and Public Health Nursing (PHN, LAC-DHS, 2013), the principles of population-based practice are included in the LAC PHN Practice Model. Public health nurses integrate assessment, policy development, and assurance into their work. The three levels of population-based practice—individuals and families, community, and systems—are addressed, with the nursing process applied throughout the model. The 17 interventions, as first presented in the Minnesota Public Health Nursing Model described above, are also incorporated into the LAC PHN Practice Model. The LAC PHN Practice Model promotes the concepts of an interdisciplinary public health team working together, with an emphasis on primary prevention. It also recognizes the importance of active participation of the individual, family, and community (PHN, LAC-DHS, 2013; Smith & Bazini-Barakat, 2003). See Figure 14–4 for a depiction of the LAC PHN Model.

Omaha System

The Omaha System is a multidisciplinary standardized interface that incorporates documentation of nursing assessment and interventions (Thompson, Monsen, Wanamaker, Augustyniak, & Thompson, 2012). It was developed and refined during four research projects conducted between 1975 and 1992 with the Omaha Visiting Nursing Association. It was designed to increase the effectiveness and efficiency of nursing practice in the agency (Bowles & Naylor, 1996; Martin, Leak, & Aden, 1992). The system is now finding increasing utility in facilitating EBP, documentation, and information management, all of which are critical to contemporary public health care systems. It is a comprehensive system, including the following components (Martin, 2005):

- *Problem classification scheme* that offers nurses a holistic, comprehensive method for identifying clients' health-related concerns. It includes domains, problems, modifiers, and signs/symptoms. Problems can be identified at the individual, family, or community level.
- *Intervention scheme* that provides a framework for documenting plans and interventions in the client

Public Health Nursing Practice Model*

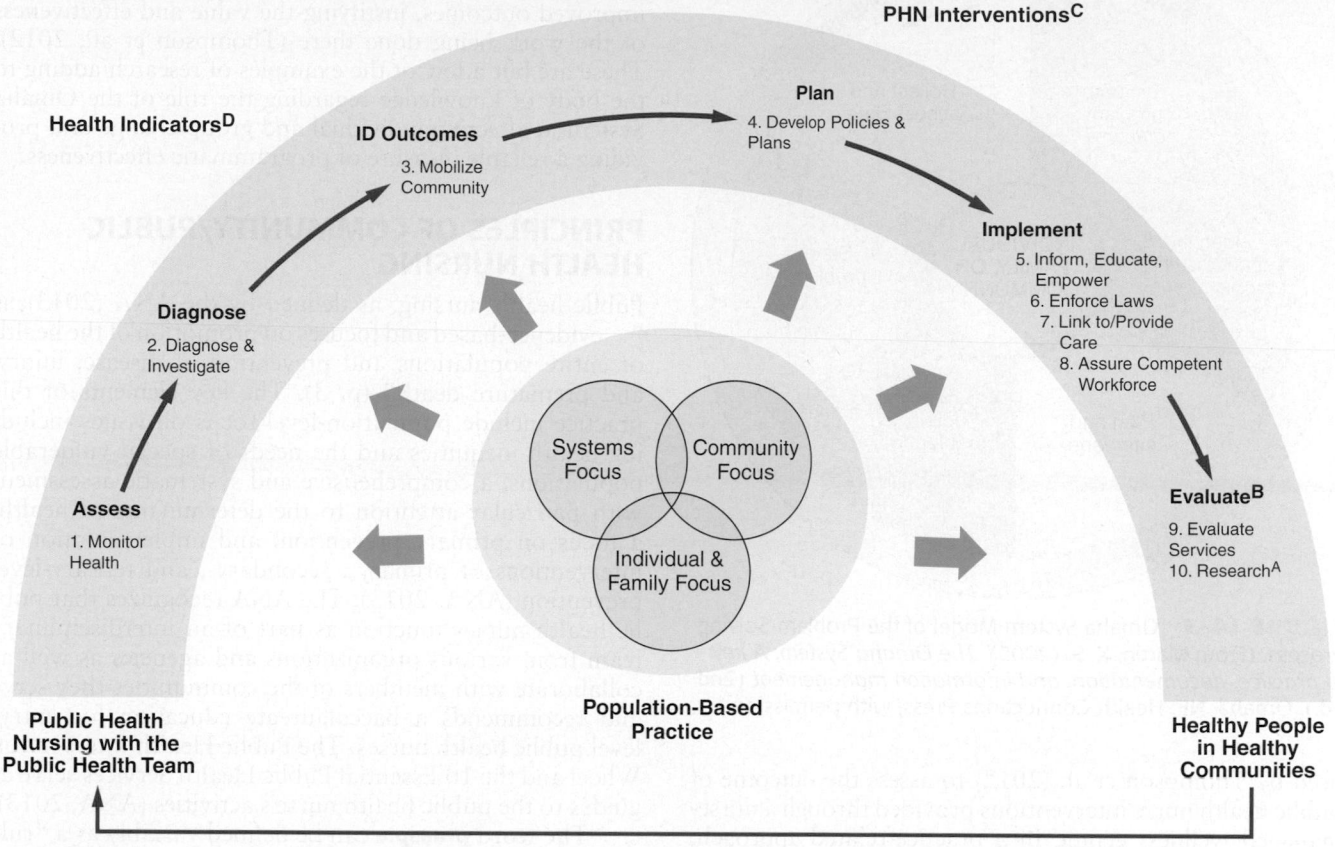

PHN Interventions[C]

Health Indicators[D]

Plan
4. Develop Policies & Plans

ID Outcomes
3. Mobilize Community

Implement
5. Inform, Educate, Empower
6. Enforce Laws
7. Link to/Provide Care
8. Assure Competent Workforce

Diagnose
2. Diagnose & Investigate

Systems Focus

Community Focus

Individual & Family Focus

Assess
1. Monitor Health

Evaluate[B]
9. Evaluate Services
10. Research[A]

Population-Based Practice

Public Health Nursing with the Public Health Team

Healthy People in Healthy Communities

References:
(A) Public Health Functions Steering Committee. (1994, Fall). *Public Health in America*. Retrieved May 7, 2001,from the World Wide Web: http://health.gov/phfunctions/public.htm
(B) Quad Council of Public Health Nursing Organizations. (2007). *Public Health Nursing: Scope & Standards of Practice*. Washington D.C.: American Nurses Association.
(C) Minnesota Department of Health, Public Health Nursing Section. (2000). *Public Health Nursing Practice for the 21st Century: National Satellite Learning Conference; Competency Development in Population-based Practice October 5, November 2, December 7, 2000*. St. Paul, MN: Minnesota Department of Health Nursing Section. Retrieved May 7, 2001, from the World Wide Web: http://www.health.state.mn.us/divs/chs/phr/material.htm.
(D) U.S. Department of Health and Human Services. (2000). Healthy People 2010. (Vol. 1). McLean, VA: International Medical Publishing, Inc.

*Created by Los Angeles County DPH, Public Health Nursing with input from CCLHDND-Southern Region. This model serves as the basis for the CCLHDND California PHN Practice Model (05-2002).

FIGURE 14–4 Public Health Nursing Practice Model. (Used with permission from the Los Angeles County Department of Public Health, Public Health Nursing. Retrieved from http://publichealth.lacounty.gov/phn/docs/PracticeModelfinal2.pdf)

record in the areas of health teaching, guidance, and counseling; treatments and procedures; case management; and surveillance.

- *Problem rating scale* for outcomes that consists of a Likert-type scale that is a systematic and recurring method used to document the progress of clients in the record and in case conferences during their time of service in the agency. It is used in conjunction with any problem in the Problem Classification Scheme. Central to problem rating is quantifying outcomes in three dimensions: knowledge (what the client knows), behavior (what the client does), and status (how the client is).

The Omaha System is based on universal principles of nursing practice. The model was judged to be consistent with the Nightingale model of environmental health (Zurakowski, 2005). Citing some variations in language use, Griffin and Landers (2014) found that Orem's model

of self-care was also consistent with the premises of the Omaha System. The *Omaha System Model of the Problem-Solving Process* (Fig. 14–5) shows the interrelationship between the practitioner and the client in addressing health problems. The model guides the nurse through the six steps in the process: (1) collecting and assessing data, (2) stating the problem, (3) identifying the problem rating on admission, (4) planning and actual interventions, (5) identification of interim or dismissal problem rating, and, finally, (6) evaluating the problem outcome. The model is applicable to individuals, families, and communities and provides a mechanism to evaluate both individual and group change over time. With ongoing pressure for public health program funding, outcome data is vital and can be achieved through the application of the Omaha System.

Research regarding the contribution of the Omaha System to program evaluation has included. This model was

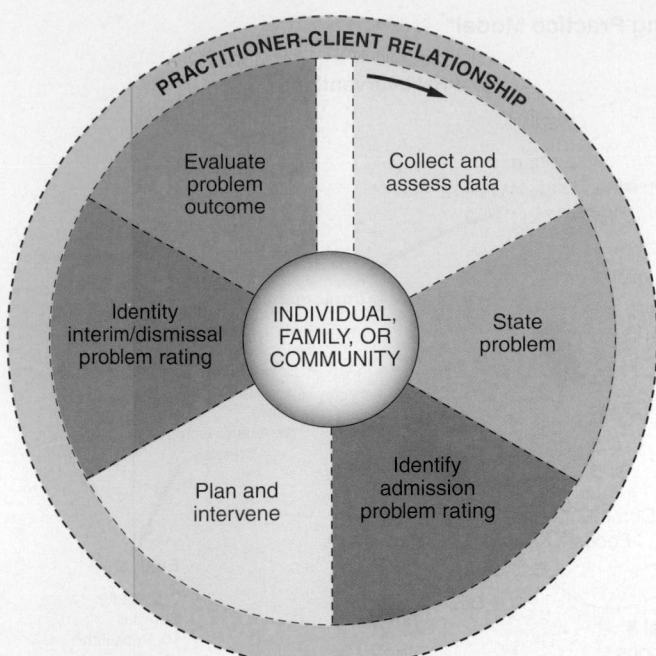

FIGURE 14–5 Omaha System Model of the Problem-Solving Process. (From Martin, K. S. (2005). *The Omaha System: A key to practice, documentation, and information management* (2nd ed.). Omaha, NE: Health Connections Press, with permission.)

used by Thompson et al. (2012) to assess the outcome of public health nurse interventions provided through a nurse-managed wellness center. In a practice-related approach, health promotion lifestyle profiles and quality of life in Turkish women were explored using the Omaha System (Erci, 2012). The findings of this study demonstrated that application of system interventions improved measurements of self-actualization, health responsibility, interpersonal support, and stress management. Thompson et al. (2012) utilized the Omaha System to gather data regarding the effectiveness of a nurse-managed wellness center. Students documented their interventions in the system that

allowed the researchers to access and analyze the data. The results indicated that the nurse-managed center saw improved outcomes, justifying the value and effectiveness of the work being done there (Thompson et al., 2012). These are but a few of the examples of research adding to the body of knowledge regarding the role of the Omaha System in affecting individual and group change and providing a reliable measure of programmatic effectiveness.

PRINCIPLES OF COMMUNITY/PUBLIC HEALTH NURSING

Public health nursing, as defined by the ANA (2013), is "...evidence-based and focuses on promotion of the health of entire populations and prevention of disease, injury, and premature death" (p. 3). The key elements of this practice include population-level focus on issues including health inequities and the needs of special vulnerable populations, a comprehensive and systematic assessment with particular attention to the determinants of health, a focus on primary prevention, and implementation of interventions of primary-, secondary-, and tertiary-level prevention (ANA, 2013). The ANA recognizes that public health nurses function as part of an interdisciplinary team from various organizations and agencies as well as collaborate with members of the communities they serve and recommends a baccalaureate education for entry-level public health nurses. The Public Health Intervention Wheel and the 10 Essential Public Health Services serve as guides to the public health nurse's activities (ANA, 2013).

The word **principle** can be defined variably as a "rule or code of conduct" or an underlying aptitude or ability (Merriam-Webster, n.d., para. 2). Whatever the definition, there are universals in practice that can guide public health nursing practice in a way that can help achieve the most beneficial outcomes. The goals of public health nursing, to promote and protect the health of communities, are facilitated by adhering to eight principles identified by the ANA (2013) for public health nursing practice. These principles are summarized in Display 14–3 (ANA, 2013).

DISPLAY 14–3 PRINCIPLES OF PUBLIC HEALTH NURSING

1. **Focus on the Community.** The client or unit of care is the population.
2. **Give Priority to Community Needs.** The primary obligation is to achieve the greatest good for the greatest number of people or the population as a whole.
3. **Work in Partnership with the People.** The processes used by public health nurses include working with the client as an equal partner.
4. **Focus on Primary Prevention.** Primary prevention is the priority in selecting appropriate activities.
5. **Promote a Healthful Environment.** Public health nursing focuses on strategies that create healthy environmental, social, and economic conditions in which populations may thrive.

6. **Target All Who Might Benefit.** A public health nurse is obligated to actively identify and reach out to all who might benefit from a specific activity or service.
7. **Promote Optimum Allocation of Resources.** Optimal use of available resources to ensure the best overall improvement in the health of the population is a key element of the practice.
8. **Collaborate with Others in the Community.** Collaboration with a variety of other professions, populations, organizations, and other stakeholder groups is the most effective way to promote and protect the health of the people.

Adapted from American Nurses Association. (2013). *Public health nursing: Scope and standards of practice* (2nd ed., pp. 8–9). Silver Spring, MD: Nursesbooks.org.

Principle 1: Focus on the Community

The first principle reminds us that the ultimate responsibility of public health nursing is to direct services to the population as a whole. Even though public health nurses may intervene to address individual, family, or group needs, the entire community is the client (Kulbok, Thatcher, Park, & Meszaros, 2012).

Principle 2: Give Priority to Community Needs

The second principle deals with the ethical obligation of the public health nurse to give priority to the needs and preferences of the whole community over those of one individual. This means that the nurse must consider interventions that will lead to the greatest good for the most people (Rushton & Broome, 2015). For example, programs that make mammograms for early detection of breast cancer available to all women regardless of income level are given priority over those that provide bone marrow transplantation for women with advanced metastatic breast cancer.

Principle 3: Work in Partnership with the People

The third principle requires the public health nurse to work in partnership with the community. The nurse and the community members (or groups) each bring their own values, beliefs, and expertise to the partnership (Kulbok et al., 2012). Policy development and assurance are more likely to be accepted and applied if there is mutual consideration of and respect for these elements. Developed policies need to be communicated in language that reflects an understanding of the community. For these reasons, an essential part of establishing a partnership with a community is getting to know the members and groups within that community.

Principle 4: Focus on Primary Prevention

The fourth principle of public health nursing underscores the importance of primary prevention in promoting the health of people. Most fields of medicine, including acute care nursing, are primarily concerned with illness and with efforts to prevent complications from and reoccurrence of the illness. In contrast, public health nursing has an obligation to prevent health problems and to promote a higher level of wellness. Public health nurses take the initiative to seek out high-risk groups, potential health problems, and situations that contribute to health problems. They then institute preventive programs (Kulbok et al., 2012). For example, if community assessment revealed a large number of new mothers with postpartum depression, public health nurses would address secondary prevention by establishing mental health programs. Equally as important, they would attend to primary prevention by working to change the conditions in the community that increase the risk for postpartum depression.

Principle 5: Promote a Healthful Environment

The fifth principle recognizes the importance of ensuring that people live in conditions conducive to health. Therefore, it is aligned with Nightingale's Environmental Theory of Health. People are less likely to be healthy if they live in a community with high unemployment, crowded housing, and dirty air or where it is difficult to obtain inexpensive, healthful food. They are also less likely to be healthy if the community's norms include acceptance or even encouragement of activities such as smoking, binge drinking, drug use, or unsafe sex. To change these conditions requires commitment, perseverance, patience, resourcefulness, and a long-range view. Public health nurses, along with other public health professionals, understand the effects of social determinants of health and work to improve them (Braveman & Gottlieb, 2014).

Principle 6: Target All Who Might Benefit

The sixth principle involves outreach strategies to meet the obligation to serve all people who might benefit from an intervention. This tenet requires that the nurse examine policies or programs to determine whether they are accessible and acceptable to the entire population in need and advocate for change if necessary (Maryland & Gonzalez, 2012).

Public health nurses can advocate for clients on many levels. For instance, for those clients who have limited economic resources and need regular medications to maintain normal blood pressure and other common health problems, PHNs can recommend a program available through Walmart stores that offers 30-day supplies of medications for as low as $4.00 (Maryland & Gonzalez, 2012). They can also work with local, state, and national legislators to promote health and necessary services for vulnerable populations.

The questions in Display 14–4 can help the nurse evaluate a planned program's success in reaching people who might benefit. These questions should guide the design, implementation, and evaluation of outreach strategies.

Principle 7: Promote Optimum Allocation of Resources

The seventh principle addresses resource allocation decisions. In most communities, the available resources are not sufficient to meet all the needs of all the people.

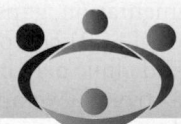

DISPLAY 14–4 DETERMINING WHETHER PROGRAMS SERVE INTENDED POPULATIONS

- Is the service offered in a manner that encourages utilization?
    Are the services located conveniently?
    Do the hours of the service fit with the work or school life of the people?
    Are the services offered in a manner that is respectful of the values, beliefs, mores, and traditions of the people?
    What kind of marketing strategies has been used to inform the people of the service?
- What is the satisfaction level of users of the service?
- Why are some people not using the services?

The nurse must ensure that the community is using limited resources in ways that lead to the greatest improvement in health (Bekemeier, Chen, Kawakyu, & Yang, 2013). To promote optimum allocation of resources, the nurse must:

- Know the latest research on the effectiveness of various programs in addressing needs
- Collect information about the short- and long-term costs of programs
- Evaluate existing programs and policies for ways to improve or discontinue them
- Communicate this information to community decision makers, so that they can make resource allocation decisions that are most likely to improve the community's health.

In current research on resource allocation in public health agencies, the majority of agencies in one study reported little impact resulting from public input, but more influence from boards of health. Most agencies did not conduct needs assessments or use economic analyses in their decision making about how to allocate resources (Baum, DesRoches, Campbell, & Goold, 2011). The realities of constrained budgets and mandated and categorically determined services, along with workforce capacity and local stakeholder input, had greater influence than EBP research and recognized community needs. What "should" happen and what "does" happen are often at odds, as noted in one Washington state study of quantitative data and interviews with public health leaders (Bekemeier et al., 2013). Public health nurses should continue to work on all levels to promote greater funding for public health programs and more effective allocation of resources.

Principle 8: Collaborate with Others in the Community

The eighth principle underscores the importance of collaboration with other nurses, health care providers, social workers, educators, spiritual leaders, business leaders, and government officials within the community. This interdisciplinary collaboration is essential to establish and maintain effective programs. Programs that are planned and implemented in isolation can lead to fragmentation, gaps, and overlaps in health services (Kulbok et al., 2012). For instance, without collaboration, a well-child clinic may be started in a community that already has a strong developmental screening program but does not have community prenatal services. Without collaboration, programs may also fail to be effective. Another example, a Saturday-morning cardiovascular fitness program designed without consultation with spiritual leaders may be totally ineffective in a devout Jewish community, where members devote Saturdays to religious observances.

SOCIETAL INFLUENCES ON COMMUNITY-ORIENTED, POPULATION-FOCUSED NURSING

Society is constantly changing, and these changes influence a community's health, either positively or negatively. For this reason, public health nurses need to continually alter their strategies to respond to these changing conditions.

An example is international air travel combined with reduced levels of immunizations among school-age children, which increases risk for transmission of measles at a world-renowned amusement park (Halsey & Salmon, 2015). Public health nurses must be proactive in developing strategies to control the spread of communicable disease through primary prevention interventions such as launching an immunization campaign. Social changes may also affect the availability of resources necessary to ensure that effective intervention strategies are available, for example, mistrust of vaccines and communities of under- or unvaccinated children.

Contemporary public health nurses must be especially aware of the mutual interaction between nursing and technology. The term **technology** refers to the application of science to change processes of production or industry or simply the practical application of knowledge (Merriam-Webster, n.d.). Ideally, technologic innovations lead to improvements in processes for creating products or services. The 20th century was filled with technologic innovations that simultaneously disrupted old patterns of production and created new opportunities to increase production, but new technology also presents new challenges. Two technologic changes that are highly relevant to contemporary public health nursing are communication technology and genetic engineering (Fig. 14–6).

Communication Technology

The rapid changes in communication technology present new opportunities and challenges for community-oriented, population-focused care. Because of advances in satellite and telecommunications technology, communication is possible anywhere in the world where resources are available to purchase equipment and services. This means that a public health nurse, whether working in the Australian outback or at a public health clinic in Anchorage, Alaska, can contact clients, consultants, and agencies worldwide, if resources are available to take advantage of the technologies. Community members can become more involved in the decision-making process on issues that impact them or their communities, self-management tools can be personalized, clients can access online support networks and resources, health

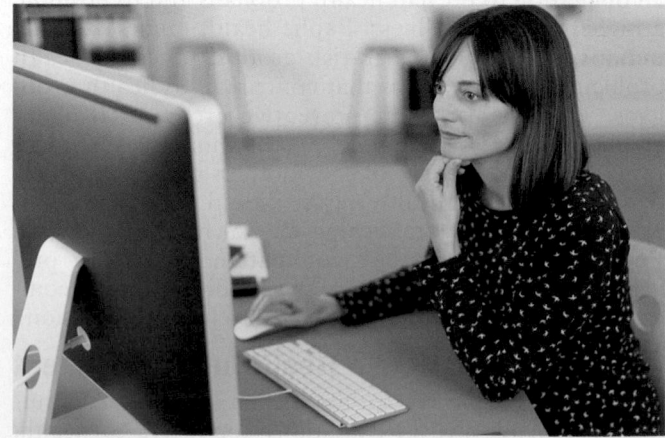

FIGURE 14–6 Communication technology offers many benefits for population health.

literacy can increase, and culturally isolated populations may be more readily accessed (USDHHS, 2016a).

In addition, Internet technology has made it possible to access local, state, national, and international data for community assessment, planning, and evaluation. Nurses who require data for a new intervention strategy, for example, can search the Internet for information from consumer groups, researchers, and other experts worldwide. To keep apprised of emerging issues and trends in public health, the nurse can join numerous Internet-based electronic discussion groups or LISTSERV (electronic discussions distributed by way of email). The challenge to the nurse is to manage the volume of information and to critically evaluate the validity and credibility of this information.

Health care consumers face similar opportunities and challenges. Most diseases and disabilities can be researched online; information is available on the Internet, and consumers are increasingly searching the Net for health-related data. Certainly, the validity and reliability of information on the Internet can vary widely. Research is needed to understand how people decide what information to use from the Internet, how they use it, and how its use affects their health. As health educators, public health nurses can provide guidelines to help people decide how to use health information found on the Internet (Display 14–5). At the same time, public health nurses need to be actively involved in creating technology resources, such as Internet sites, to provide health information specific to their targeted communities. Public health nurses must bear in mind that disparities exist among those who have access to new technology and those who do not. This could present a barrier to accessing critical information to protect and promote health (USDHHS, 2016a). Alternate modes of information sharing need to be in place. See Chapter 10 for more on technology.

The Internet is a superb vehicle for rapidly tracing the international spread of infectious diseases. For example, the World Health Organization has an Internet site for countries to report epidemiologic and laboratory data on influenza. The Centers for Disease Control and Prevention (CDC) offers current data on communicable diseases through the online publication *Morbidity and Mortality Weekly Report*. In addition, many local health departments and health agencies have their own Web sites that can provide information and resources specific to the needs of the local communities. In addition, health care providers are integrating electronic medical records into their practices. Between 2007 and 2013, the number of medical practices that implemented electronic health records increased by 175.6% (USDHHS, 2016c). This can improve health care efficiency and care delivery, increase health care quality and safety and support clinical and consumer decision making (USDHHS, 2016b). See Chapter 8 for more on communicable diseases.

New forms of technology continue to be introduced. Today, forms of communication can range from cell phones and text messages to instant messaging and social networking. This new technology provides innovative ways to enhance health communication and social marketing. Nurses can utilize social media such as Web blogs, Facebook, and Twitter to disseminate health messages to specific target populations (CDC, 2015). Health messages distributed through a variety of modalities including mass media such as television and radio, small media such as brochures, social media such as computer networking, and interpersonal communication such as face-to-face interactions increase the exposure of the message to a wider swath of the population (CDC, 2015).

As technology advances, nurses must keep up to date on new ways information can be shared. In addition, the lines between professional recommendations and peer advice can become blurred, leading to the risk of decisions being made on information that is not based on empirical evidence (USDHHS, 2016b).

Genetics, Genomics, and Genetic Engineering

Genetics, the science of heredity and **genomics**, the study of the entire genome, are terms that have gained increased attention from nurses over the past decade. An outgrowth of this knowledge is **genetic engineering**, which can be defined as "the group of applied techniques of genetics and biotechnology used to cut up and join together genetic material and especially DNA from one or more species of organism and to introduce the result into an organism in order to change one or more of its characteristics" (Merriam-Webster, n.d., para. 2). The development of the field was made possible by the discovery of certain enzymes that can "cut" DNA from two or more different sources into pieces that can be recombined in a test tube. Gene manipulation also required the development of methods for inserting these recombinant DNA molecules into cells by the use of so-called *vectors* such as viruses (Fig. 14–7).

The topic of genomics is a new area that included *Healthy People 2020*. This topic was added because genomics is associated with nine of the 10 leading causes of death. Genetic testing might help to reduce the risk for certain types of cancer (USDHHS, 2016a). *Healthy People 2020* objectives currently include two

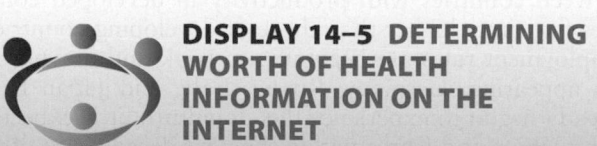

DISPLAY 14–5 DETERMINING WORTH OF HEALTH INFORMATION ON THE INTERNET

- What are the credentials and affiliation of the author?
- Is it easy to determine who is the publisher or sponsor of the Web site? Evaluate how the publisher or sponsor might gain economically through your use of the information.
- Is the date of publication of the Web site included? Is the information current?
- Are both sides of an issue described? Does the author discuss pros and cons of information presented?
- What references are included to substantiate the information in the article?

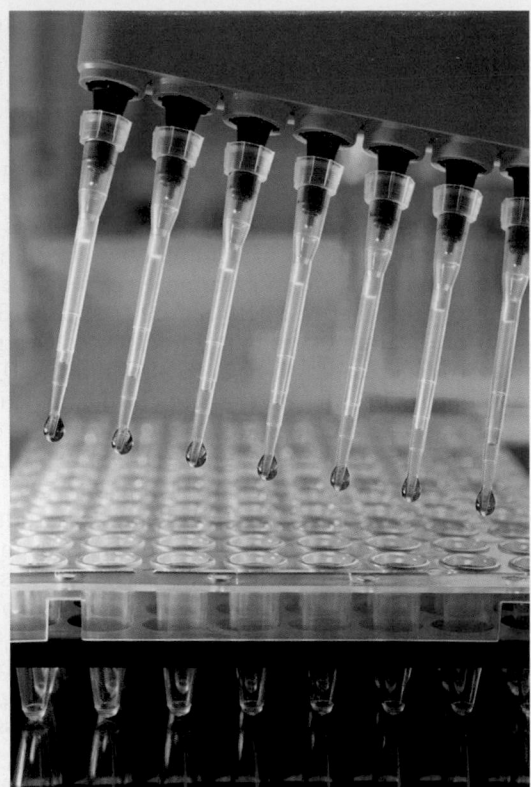

FIGURE 14–7 DNA discoveries have changed health care.

recommendations related to genomics. The first genomics recommendations are for women at increased risk for breast, ovarian, tubal, or peritoneal cancer to receive genetic counseling and obtain information about BRCA-12 testing options. The second recommendation is for people who are newly diagnosed with colorectal cancer to receive counseling and information about genetic testing (USDHHS, 2016a).

Genomics is another rapidly changing field. There is a lull of research regarding genetic tests and family health history tools and the risk versus benefits of using genomics in health care decision making. This is an area that needs further exploration. Issues of future exploration include assuring privacy and confidentiality of information acquired through genomics, including this information in electronic health records, implementation of testing, and exploration of how practitioners can use this information for patient education and recommendations (USDHHS, 2016a).

The Human Genome Project has opened dramatic possibilities for health and well-being, as well as created ethical challenges in the near future. The potential scientific capacity to alter methods of human reproduction raises concerns about creating unintended consequences for the human race. Another source of concern is that science is "playing God." For some people, the possibility of being able to select the gender, intelligence, or eye color of a child raises concerns about interfering with nature and creates conflict with religious or ethical views. In addition, genetic screening could be used to deny rights and opportunities to people. For example, someone who is found to carry a gene that increases the risk for heart disease might be denied health insurance coverage. Another source of concern has been the distrust many people have of government, large commercial enterprises, and the scientific community. Some people believe that they are not being told the truth about scientific or other issues.

In dealing with these concerns, it is the public health nurse's responsibility to be aware of the latest scientific information when educating communities, so that the decisions made best fit the community's value system. Advocating for the highest scientific rigor in genetic engineering research is another important role of public health nurses. Public health nurses need to advocate for research that not only maps DNA but also identifies interventions that can change the outcome for people at risk for genetic disorders. Nurses need to balance what is good for the community as a whole against potential costs to people at risk, advocating for policies and regulations that ensure such a balance. The *Essentials of Baccalaureate Education for Professional Nursing Practice* (American Association of Colleges of Nursing, 2008) emphasized the impact of advances in genetics and genomics. Specifically, Essential VII: Clinical Prevention and Population Health stresses that the graduate be prepared to (1) "Assess protective and predictive factors, including genetics, which influence the health of individuals, families, groups, communities, and populations" and (2) "Conduct a health history, including environmental exposure and a family history that recognizes genetic risks, to identify current and future health problems" (p. 24).

Global Economy

The **global economy** has grown exponentially over the past half century. It expanded six times more than the world's population. Per capita income tripled while the population doubled in size (Executive Summary, 2015). The rapid rate of growth is attributed to two factors, a growing labor force and increased productivity. The labor force grew due to reductions in high fertility rates, infant mortality rates, and expanded life expectancy. This resulted in a bulge of people of working age from 58% in 1964 to 68% in 2014 (Executive Summary, 2015). Productivity varied between countries with productivity in developed countries five times higher than those of developing countries. Employment rates are beginning to peak and downturns are appearing. Germany, Russia, Italy, and Japan have already begun to experience this downturn, it is expected to hit China and Korea within the next decade, and other countries will follow over the next half century (Executive Summary, 2015). Steps have been identified by economists to boost the world's economy, they include enabling catch-up through transparency and competition, especially in emerging markets; using incentivizing innovation to push the frontier; mobilizing labor, particularly among women and young people; and allowing cross-border economic flow for goods and trade services (Executive Summary, 2015). Figure 14–8 depicts a European Central Bank.

The United Nations adopted the Millennium Development Goals (MDGs) in an effort to counter the impact of global poverty and hunger. Interventions would focus on universal primary education, improved maternal and child health, address gender inequalities, promote environmental stability, and reduced rates of

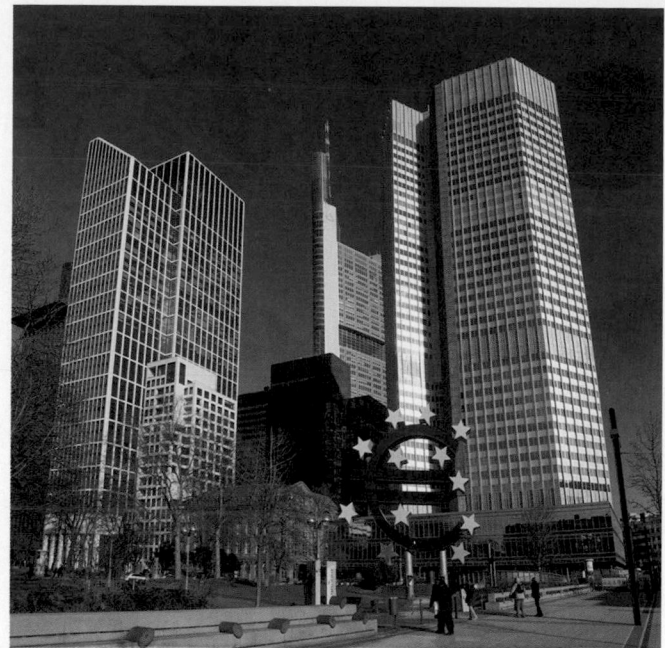

FIGURE 14-8 European Central Bank in Frankfurt, Germany.

HIV/AIDS and other communicable diseases. Progress on these goals varied, and areas such as the sub-Saharan African and South Asian regions did not experience much progress at all (Sridhar et al., 2013). In 2015, the 2030 Agenda for Sustainable Development was developed as an extension of the MDGs (WHO, 2015). This initiative focuses on economic, social, and environmental issues with 17 Sustainable Development Goals (SDGs). Financing for global health and shifts in governance have potential to impact these goals. Rising economies are developing in Brazil, China, and India. These countries have the potential to assume more influence in global governance. Countries that have traditionally held dominance, such as the United States and European countries, may not hold the same influence. These shifts in influence can impact global health decisions. Health issues have dropped off the agenda of international meetings such as G8 and G20. Historically, the G8 meetings resulted in global strategies on tuberculosis and HIV/AIDS. These topics are no longer part of the conversations. Universal goals may be needed to address the interests of emerging economies (Sridhar et al., 2013). Shifts have occurred in funding at the World Health Organization and World Bank. Funding through these organizations has flattened and is earmarked for special project. New funding organizations have emerged, such as the Global Fund and the GAVI Alliance. The Global Fund is becoming the largest donors at $3.2 billion in 2010. The Bill and Melinda Gates Foundation and other private sector and nongovernmental organizations have voting rights on this board. They narrow down on a few health topics such as immunizations, bed netting, or access to antiretroviral medication. They also measure their success based on outcomes on specific topics rather than a wide range of countries around the globe. Their funding is more discretionary and based on donations rather than through government funds. Unfortunately, donations have been

dropping (Sridhar et al., 2013). Philanthropic organizations are becoming more of a force in global health issues. It is important that these various organizations align goals and work together rather than having competing projects (Sridhar et al., 2013). For more on global health, see Chapter 16.

The increase in noncommunicable diseases impacts social and economic opportunity and result in greater inequality (Sridhar et al., 2013). More than 80% of noncommunicable diseases are occurring in middle- to low-income countries. For example, the increased consumption of high-sugar beverages in low-income nations results in increased chronic illnesses and more years lost to disability while rates of heart disease is dropping in the United States. Other factors impacting chronic illness are climate change and increased numbers of people living in urban settings (Sridhar et al., 2013).

Universal health coverage (UHC) is another economic issue that impacts the global economy. In 2012, the United Nation General Assembly voted to adopt a resolution on UHC that would encourage governments to move forward with promoting this initiative for affordable access to quality health care. The risk is that various countries may interpret differing meanings to the term UHC (Sridhar et al., 2013). The World Health Organization is moving toward promoting UHC globally rather than a state level; however, this is very difficult to achieve as every situation is different, requiring individual solutions (Sridhar et al., 2013). See Chapter 16 for more on global health issues.

Migration

Migration is the act of moving from one region or country to another, temporarily, seasonally, or permanently. Throughout history, people have migrated from place to place to seek improved opportunities or to escape intolerable conditions in their home countries. In the late 20th century and the early years of the 21st century, a dramatic increase occurred in the number of *refugees* who migrated from their homes to escape invasion, oppression, or persecution (WHO, 2012). For example, recent displacement of Syrian refugees who are escaping civil unrest and violence has impacted neighboring countries. The crisis in Syria began in 2011, and as of October of 2014, more than 3.2 million refugees had entered Lebanon, Turkey, and Jordan (Doocy, Lyles, Delbiso, & Robinson, 2015). These refugees are poor and vulnerable. The receiving countries have limited resources to assist them. As new refugees enter, their needs differ from those who have been already in the country for 1 to 4 years. The type of violence that they escaped can also impact their specific needs (Doocy et al., 2015). This type of ongoing mass exodus puts extraordinary strain on resources and requires ongoing assessment of needs (Doocy et al., 2015). See Chapter 16.

We also saw an increased reliance on migrant farmworkers, people who move from one region to another seasonally, following the crops. The health care needs of migrants and migrant refugees are enormous. Environmental factors are a primary reason for compromised health and include inadequate waste disposal, crowded and unsanitary living conditions, lack of access to healthful foods, and air pollution from an increased concentration of vehicles used for moving refugees. Compounding these problems are language and cultural barriers, as well as distrust and fear that may interfere with meeting the needs of these vulnerable populations. The potential detriments to health associated with migration require that public health nurses ensure that surveillance systems able to detect emerging health problems are in place; programs to prevent health problems and treat existing conditions also need to be developed (Ruiz-Casares et al., 2013). See Chapter 29 for more on migrant health issues.

Terrorism and Bioterrorism

Terrorism is one way in which a small number of people who perceive that they have been unfairly treated can exert influence on a larger group or nation. Groups wishing to harm other countries need sophisticated skills and coordination for most conventional weapons. Terrorists may also use unconventional weapons when highly motivated, such as flying planes into buildings, strapping bombs to their bodies, or even allowing bombs to be implanted in their bodies.

Some methods of bioterrorism may be even cheaper and easier to use. **Bioterrorism** is the use of living organisms, such as bacteria, viruses, or other organic materials, to harm or intimidate others, in order to achieve political ends. Some of the possible biologic agents used include *Bacillus anthracis*, smallpox virus, *Brucella*, and botulinum toxin (see Chapters 8 and 17). The federal government has adopted an increasingly proactive approach to reduce the risk of both natural-occurring and deliberate outbreaks of disease. This approach requires a melding of biodefense needs with an increased emphasis on biosecurity, balancing both public health and national security interests (Koblentz, 2012).

Because of escalating concerns about bioterrorism, public health workers increasingly recognize the need for skills in dealing with a bioterrorist attack. They need to engage in emergency preparedness activities and be prepared to initiate response activities in the event of an actual bioterrorism attack (CDC, 2011). Preparedness includes the following:

- Establish relationships with mutual aid partners.
- Conduct hazard vulnerability and risk assessment.
- Identify resources.
- Acquire resources.
- Develop objectives and a plan.
- Put plans into place to mass casualties.
- Develop plan for communicating with members of the community.
- Train personnel.
- Conduct training exercises and engage in after-action reviews.

Response includes the following:

- Assess the situation.
- Activate key personnel.
- Develop objectives and action plan.
- Participate in the Emergency Operations Center (EOC).
- Coordinate with the safety officer to identify hazards.
- Communicate with key partners.
- Deploy resources.
- Respond to health-related requests.
- Communicate with the public.
- Involve legal counsel.
- Document all activities.

Engagement in ongoing public health response duties incorporates:

- Surveillance
- Meeting the needs of the community
- Addressing needs of special populations
- Engaging in the recovery phase

Perhaps more importantly, public health nurses need to be involved in primary prevention of bioterrorism through advocating for the elimination of biologic weapons and addressing the root causes of terrorism, such as poverty, hunger, poor housing, limited educational opportunities, lack of clean water, and inadequate or no health care. See Chapter 17.

Climate Change

Climate change can be considered societal changes because they may be influenced by economics. Since the Industrial Revolution, increased amounts of carbon dioxide, methane, and nitrous oxide created by manufacturing industries, automobile emissions, and consumer products have been introduced into the earth's atmosphere. These increases have contributed to climate changes that are expected to affect sea level; the production of food, fiber, and medicines; and the spread of infectious diseases. Conversely, significant increases in fuel efficiency and efforts to reduce pollution could avoid millions of deaths around the world. Population-focused nurses need to educate the public about the potential dangers of continuing to contaminate the environment and to advocate for changes in public policy that reduce air and water contaminants. In 2008, the American Nurses Association's House of Delegates passed a Global Climate Change initiative that encourages nurses to "advocate for change on both individual and policy levels; to support local public policies that endorse sustainable energy sources and reduce greenhouse gas emissions; and ... to support initiatives to decrease the contribution to global warming by the healthcare industry" (ANA, 2012). This built on elements of the 2007 Public Health Nursing: Scope and Standards of Practice most notably in terms of ethics in practice, challenging nurses to contribute to "resolving social and environmental issues and barriers to healthy living conditions" (p. 34). Chapter 9 explores health-related environmental issues in more detail.

SUMMARY

Public health nursing is a community-oriented, population-focused nursing specialty that is based on interpersonal relationships. The unit of care is the community or population rather than the individual, and the goal is to promote healthy communities.

Theories and models of community/public health nursing practice aid the nurse in understanding the rationale behind community-oriented care. Florence Nightingale's environmental theory emphasizes the importance of improving environmental conditions to promote health. Orem's self-care model provides a framework, within which the public health nurse can promote a community's collective independence and self-care ability. Neuman's Health Care Systems Model describes the nurse's role as one of assisting clients to remain stable within their environment, whereas Rogers' model of the science of unitary man focuses on client–environment interaction and holistic health. King's Theory of Goal Attainment reminds nurses to work in partnership with clients to achieve the best health outcomes. Parse's Human Becoming Theory posits quality of life from each person's own perspective as the goal of nursing practice. Pender's model focuses on the promotion of health behaviors in people; the goal of nursing is to enhance the likelihood that people will engage in health-promoting behaviors by assessing and influencing perceptual and modifying factors. Roy's adaptation model describes the nurse's goal as one that promotes healthful coping mechanisms and adaptive responses to stressors. Salmon's construct for public health nursing prescribes education, engineering, and enforcement with individuals, families, communities, and nations. Finally, the models used in public health nursing practice, the Minnesota Intervention "Wheel," the Los Angeles County–Public Health Nursing Practice Model, and the Omaha System Model of the Problem-Solving Process provide a mechanism for public health nurses to assess, plan, intervene, and evaluate the care they provide in their communities.

The eight principles of public health nursing applied to community/public health nursing practice provide a framework within which the nurse works to promote and protect the health of populations. They emphasize the primacy of prevention, the need for outreach, and the importance of working in collaboration for the greatest good of the greatest number of people.

Nurses must anticipate and adapt to societal changes in order to fulfill their mission of promoting the health of all people. Contemporary societal influences on public health nursing include communication technology, genetic engineering, the global economy, migration, terrorism, and climate changes.

ACTIVITIES TO PROMOTE **CRITICAL THINKING**

1. Search your local public health agency's Web site to determine what population-focused programs are offered in your locality. Talk with the public health nursing director or a program manager to explore nursing's role in the assessment, development, implementation, and evaluation of these programs. Discuss how public health nurses might expand their population-focused interventions.
2. Describe a situation in community/public health nursing practice in which the use of an educational intervention would be most appropriate. Do the same with engineering (Salmon) and enforcement interventions. Discuss your rationale for matching each situation with that intervention.
3. Assume you have been asked to make a home visit to a 75-year-old man, living alone, whose wife recently died. In addition to assessing his individual needs, what factors should you consider for assessment and intervention that would indicate an aggregate- or community-focused approach?
4. Select one of the societal influences on a community or population. How would the theories or models for community/public health nursing practice that were discussed in this chapter guide your practice concerning that societal issue? Choose three models or theories to apply and examine main concepts in relation to your chosen issue. Search for current research studies that utilize this model or theory and critique its applicability.
5. Search online to explore one of the societal influences on community or population. Using the information in Display 14–5, try to determine the worth of the information available on several Internet sites.
6. Select five or six conceptual models used in nursing research with a community/public health focus. Develop a chart showing how each model defines the nursing metaparadigm concepts: nurse, client/patient, health, and environment. Which of these conceptual models include all of these concepts? In instances where the provider of services is defined, can public health nurse be substituted for another provider of services?

REFERENCES

Alligood, M. R. (Ed.). (2014). *Nursing theorists and their work* (8th ed.). St. Louis, MO: Mosby/Elsevier.

American Association of Colleges of Nursing. (2008). *The essentials of baccalaureate education for professional nursing practice.* Washington, DC: Author.

American Nurses Association (ANA). (2012). *Climate change.* Retrieved from http://nursingworld.org/MainMenuCategories/WorkplaceSafety/Environmental-Health/Issues/Climate

American Nurses Association (ANA). (2013). *Public health nursing: Scope and standards of practice* (2nd ed.). Silver Spring, MD: Nursesbooks.org.

American Nurses Association (ANA). (2016). *ANA hall of fame inductee: Martha Elizabeth Rogers (1914–1994) 1996 inductee.* Retrieved from http://www.nursingworld.org/MarthaElizabethRogers

Andrews, H. A., & Roy, C. (1991). *The Roy adaptation model: The definitive statement.* Norwalk, CT: Appleton-Lange.

Baum, N. M., DesRoches, C., Campbell, E. G., & Goold, S. D. (2011). Resource allocation in public health practice: A national survey of local public health officials. *Journal of Public Health Management & Practice, 17*(3), 265–274.

Bekemeier, B., Chen, A. L., Kawakyu, N., & Yang, Y. (2013). Local public health resource allocation: Limited choices and strategic decisions. *American Journal of Preventive Medicine, 45*(6), 769–775.

Bigby, J. L., & Issel, L. M. (2012). Conceptual models for population-focused public health nursing interventions and outcomes: The state of the art. *Public Health Nursing, 29*(4), 370–379. doi: 10.1111/j.1525-1446.2011.01006.x.

Bowles, K. H., & Naylor, M. D. (1996). Nursing intervention classification systems. *Journal of Nursing Scholarship, 28*(4), 303–308.

Braveman, P., & Gottlieb, L. (2014). The social determinants of health: It's time to consider the causes of the causes. *Public Health Reports, 129*(Suppl. 2), 19–31.

Case Western Reserve University. (2014). *Competencies: Pre-licensure KSAs.* Retrieved from http://qsen.org/competencies/pre-licensure-ksas/

Centers for Disease Control and Prevention (CDC). (2011). *Public health emergency response guide for state, local, and tribal public health directors: Version 2.0.* Retrieved from http://emergency.cdc.gov/planning/pdf/cdcresponseguide.pdf

Centers for Disease Control and Prevention (CDC). (2012). *National action plan for child injury prevention: An agenda to prevent injuries and promote the safety of children and adolescents in the United States.* Retrieved from http://www.cdc.gov/safechild/pdf/National_Action_Plan_for_Child_Injury_Prevention.pdf

Centers for Disease Control and Prevention (CDC). (2015). *Social media at CDC.* Retrieved from http://www.cdc.gov/socialmedia/

Clark, C. S. (2012). Beyond holism: Incorporating an integral approach to support caring-healing-sustainable nursing practices. *Holistic Nursing Practice, 26*(2), 92–102, doi: 10.1097/HNP.0b013e3182462197.

Collins, S. E., Clifasefi, S. E., Dana, E. A., Andrasik, M. P., Stahl, N., Kirouac, M., Malone, D. K. (2012). Where harm reduction meets housing first: Exploring alcohol's role in a project-based housing first setting. *International Journal of Drug Policy, 23*(2), 111–119. doi: 10.1016/j.drugpo.2011.07.010.

DeGuzman, P. B., & Kulbok, P. A. (2012). Changing health outcomes of vulnerable populations through nursing's influence on neighborhood built environment: A framework for nursing research. *Journal of Nursing Scholarship, 44*(4), 341–348. doi: 10.1111/j.1547.5069.2012.01470.x.

Doocy, S., Lyles, E., Delbiso, T. D., & Robinson, C. W. (2015). Internal displacement and the Syrian crisis: An analysis of trends from 2011–2014. *Conflict and Health, 9*(33). doi: 10.1186/s13031-015-0060-7.

Erci, B. (2012). The effectiveness of the Omaha System intervention on the women's health promotion lifestyle profile and quality of life. *Journal of Advanced Nursing, 68,* 898–907.

Executive Summary. (2015). *McKinsey Quarterly,* (1), 1–12.

Green, R. (2013). Application of the self-care deficit nursing theory: The community context. *Self-Care & Dependent-Care Nursing, 20*(1), 5–15.

Greene, C., & Greene, B. A. (2012). Efficacy of guided imagery to reduce stress via the Internet: A pilot study. *Holistic Nursing Practice, 26*(3), 150–163.

Griffin, M.T. Q. & Landers, M. G. (2014). Extant nursing models and theories: Grand and middle range theories in nursing. In J. J. Fitzpatrick & G. McCarthy (Eds.), *Theories guiding research and practice: Making nursing knowledge development explicit* (pp. 15–34). New York, NY: Springer Publishing Company.

Halsey, N. A., & Salmon, D. A. (2015). Measles at Disneyland, a problem for all ages. *Annals of Internal Medicine, 162*(9), 655–656.

Phillips, K. D., & Harris, R. (2014). Sister Callista Roy: Adaptation model. In M. R. Alligood (Ed.), *Nursing theorists and their work* (8th ed., pp. 303–331). St. Louis, MO: Elsevier.

Jarrin, O. F. (2012). The integrality of situated caring in nursing and the environment. *Advances in Nursing Science, 35*(1), 14–24.

Johnson, B. M., & Webber, P. B. (Eds.). (2015). *An introduction to theory and reasoning in nursing* (4th ed.). Philadelphia, PA: Wolters Kluwer.

Kagan, P. N. (2011). Catastrophe and response: Expanding the notion of 'self' to mobilize nurses' attention to policy and activism. *Nursing Science Quarterly, 24*(1), 71–78. doi: 10.1177/0894318410389076.

Keegan, J. P., Chan, F., Ditchman, N., & Chiu, C. (2012). Predictive ability of Pender's Health Promotion Model for physical activity and exercise in people with spinal cord injuries: A hierarchical regression analysis. *Rehabilitation Counseling Bulletin, 56*(1), 34–47. doi: 10.1177/0034355212440732.

Keller, L. O., Strohschein, S., Lia-Hoagberg, B., & Schaffer, M. A. (1998). Population-based public health interventions: A model from practice. *Public Health Nursing, 15,* 207–215.

Keller, L. O., Strohschein, S., Lia-Hoagberg, B., & Schaffer, M. A. (2004). Population-based public health interventions: Practice-based and evidenced-supported. Part I. *Public Health Nursing, 21,* 453–468.

Kelley, M. A., Connor, A., Kun, K. E., & Salmon, M. E. (2008). Social responsibility: Conceptualization and embodiment in a school of nursing. *International Journal of Nursing Education Scholarship, 55*(1), 1–16.

Killeen, M. B., & King, I. M. (2007). Viewpoint: Use of King's conceptual system, nursing informatics, and nursing classification systems for global communication. *International Journal of Nursing Terminologies and Classifications, 18*(2), 51–57.

King, I. M. (1970). *Toward a theory for nursing.* New York, NY: John Wiley & Sons.

King, I. M. (1981). *A theory for nursing: Systems, concepts, process.* Albany, NY: Delmar Publishers, Inc.

Koblentz, G. D. (2012). From biodefense to biosecurity: The Obama administration's strategy for countering biological threats. *International Affairs, 88*(1), 131–148.

Kulbok, P. A., Thatcher, E., Park, E., & Meszaros, P. S. (2012). Evolving public health nursing roles: Focus on community participatory health promotion and prevention. *Online Journal of Issues in Nursing, 17*(2), 1. Retrieved from http://nursingworld.org/MainMenuCategories/ANAMarketplace/ANAPeriodicals/OJIN/TableofContents/Vol-17-2012/No2-May-2012/Evolving-Public-Health-Nursing-Roles.html

Martin, K. S. (2005). *The Omaha system: A key to practice, documentation, and information management* (2nd ed.). Omaha, NE: Health Connections Press.

Martin, K., Leak, G., & Aden, C. (1992). The Omaha System: A research-based model for decision making. *Journal of Nursing Administration, 22*(11), 47–52.

Maryland, M. A., & Gonzalez, R. I. (2012). Patient advocacy in the community and legislative arena. *Online Journal of Issues in Nursing, 17*(1), 2. Retrieved from http://www.nursingworld.org/MainMenuCategories/ANAMarketplace/ANAPeriodicals/OJIN/TableofContents/Vol-17-2012/No1-Jan-2012/Advocacy-in-Community-and-Legislative-Arena.html

McCrea, N. (2012). Whither nursing models? The value of nursing theory in the context of evidence-based practice and multidisciplinary health care. *Journal of Advanced Nursing, 68*(1), 222–229. doi: 10.1111/j.1365-2648.2911.05821.x.

Merriam-Webster. (n.d.). *Merriam-Webster online dictionary.* Retrieved from http://www.merriam-webster.com

Messmer, P., & Palmer, J. (2008, First Quarter). In honor of Imogene M. King. *Reflections on Nursing Leadership.* Retrieved from http://nursingsociety.org/RNL/Current/in_touch/tribute_king.html

Milton, C. L. (2015). The ethics of human freedom and healthcare policy: A nursing theoretical perspective. *Nursing Science Quarterly, 28*(1), 192–194. doi: 19.1177/0894315585630.

Neuman, B. (1982). *The Neuman systems model: Application to nursing education and practice*. Norwalk, CT: Appleton-Lange.

Neuman, B., & Fawcett, J. (2011). *The Neuman systems model* (5th ed.). Upper Saddle River, NJ: Pearson.

Nightingale, F. (1992). *Florence Nightingale's notes on nursing*. In: V. Skretkowicz (Ed.). London, UK: Scutari Press. (Original work published 1859.)

Olowokere, A. E., & Okanlawon, F. A. (2015). Application of Neuman System Model to psychosocial support of vulnerable school children. *West African Journal of Nursing, 26*(1), 14–25.

Orem, D. E. (2001). *Nursing: Concepts of practice* (6th ed.). St. Louis, MO: Mosby.

Parse, R. R. (1981). *Man-living-health: A theory of nursing*. New York, NY: Wiley & Sons.

Parse, R. R. (1998). *The human becoming school of thought: A perspective for nurses and other health professionals*. Thousand Oaks, CA: Sage.

Parse, R. R. (2012). New human becoming conceptualizations and the human becoming community model: Expansions with sciencing and living the art. *Nursing Science Quarterly, 25*(1), 44–52. doi: 10.1177/0894318411429068.

Pender, N. J., Murdaugh, C. L., & Parsons, M. A. (2015). *Health promotion in nursing practice* (7th ed.). Upper Saddle River, NJ: Pearson Education, Inc.

Perrett, S. E., & Biley, R. C. (2013). A Roy Model study of adapting to being HIV positive. *Nursing Science Quarterly, 26*(4), 337–343. doi: 10.1177/0894318413500310.

Poirier, P. A. (2012). Human becoming: Transcending the now to explore the possibilities in health policy. *Nursing Science Quarterly, 25*(1), 104–110. doi: 10.1177/0894318411429036.

Public Health Nursing, Los Angeles County Department of Health Services (PHN, LAC-DHS). (2013). *Public health nursing practice model*. Retrieved from http://publichealth.lacounty.gov/phn/docs/Narrative%20of%20Revised%20PHN%20Practice%20Model%202013.pdf

Public Health Nursing Section, Minnesota Department of Health. (2001). *Public health interventions—applications for public health nursing practice (Minnesota Wheel)*. Retrieved from http://www.health.state.mn.us/divs/opi/cd/phn/wheel.html

Reis, P. J., & Alligood, M. R. (2014). Prenatal yoga in late pregnancy and optimism, power, and well-being. *Nursing Science Quarterly, 27*(1), 30–36.

Rogers, M. (1990). Nursing: Science of unitary, irreducible human beings: Update 1990. In E. A. M. Barrett (Ed.), *Visions of Rogers' science-based nursing* (pp. 5–11). New York, NY: National League for Nursing.

Roy, C. (2009). *The Roy adaptation model* (3rd ed.). Upper Saddle River, NJ: Pearson.

Roy, C., & Andrews, H. A. (1999). *The Roy adaptation model*. Stamford, CT: Appleton-Lange.

Ruiz-Casares, M., Rousseau, C., Laurin-Lamothe, A., Rummens, J. A., Zelkowitz, P., Crépeau, F., & Steinmetz, N. (2013). Access to health care for undocumented migrant children and pregnant women: The paradox between values and attitudes of health care professionals. *Maternal Child Health Journal, 17*, 292–298.

Rushton, C. H., & Broome, M. E. (2015). Safeguarding the public's health: Ethical nursing. *Hastings Center Report, 45*(1). doi: 10.1002/hast.410.

Salmon, M. E. (1982). Construct for public health: Where is it practiced, in whose behalf, and with what desired outcome. *Nursing Outlook, 30*(9), 527–530. (Originally published under the author name Marla Salmon White.)

Salmon, M. E. (1993). Public health nursing: The opportunity of a century. *American Journal of Public Health, 83*(12), 1674–1675.

Sakraida, T. J. (2014). Health promotion model. In M. R. Alligood (Ed.), *Nursing theorists and their work* (8th ed., pp. 396–416). St. Louis, MO: Elsevier.

Schaffer, M. A., Anderson, L. J., & Rising, S. (2015). Public health interventions for school nursing practice. *The Journal of School Nursing*. Retrieved from http://eds.b.ebscohost.com.mantis.csuchico.edu/eds/detail/detail?vid=1&sid=da79ded8-f8a6-4798-a25c-bda97588d642%40sessionmgr198&hid=108&bdata=JnNpdGU9ZWRzLWxpdmU%3d#AN=26404552&db=cmedm

Sridhar, D., Brolan, C. E., Durrani, S., Edge, J., Gostin, L., Hill, P. E., McKee, M. (2013). Governance and financing of global public health: The post-2015 agenda. *Brown Journal of World Affairs, 20*(1), 69–86.

Shrivastava, S. R., Shrivastava, P. S., & Ramasamy, J. (2015). Public health strategies to ensure optimal community participation in the Ebola outbreak in West-Africa. *Journal of Research in Medical Sciences, 20*(3), 318–319.

Smith, K., & Bazini-Barakat, N. (2003). A public health nursing practice model: Melding public health principles with the nursing process. *Public Health Nursing, 20*, 42–48.

Stevens, K. R. (2013). The impact of evidence-based practice in nursing and the next big ideas. *Online Journal of Issues in Nursing, 18*(2), 4. Retrieved from http://nursingworld.org/MainMenuCategories/ANAMarketplace/ANAPeriodicals/OJIN/TableofContents/Vol-18-2013/No2-May-2013/Impact-of-Evidence-Based-Practice.html

Thompson, C. W., Monsen, K. A., Wanamaker, K., Augustyniak, K., & Thompson, S. L. (2012). Using the Omaha system as a framework to demonstrate the value of nurse managed wellness center services for vulnerable populations. *Journal of Community Health Nursing, 29*(1), 1–11.

Tomasson, R. E. (1994, May 24). Martha Rogers, 79, an author of books on nursing theory. *New York Times*. Retrieved from http://www.nytimes.com/

U.S. Department of Health and Human Services (USDHHS). (2016a). *Healthy People 2020: Genomics*. Retrieved from http://www.healthypeople.gov/2020/topics-objectives/topic/genomics

U.S. Department of Health and Human Services (USDHHS). (2016b). *Healthy People 2020: Health communication and health information technology*. Retrieved from http://www.healthypeople.gov/2020/topics-objectives/topic/health-communication-and-health-information-technology

U.S. Department of Health and Human Services (USDHHS). (2016c). *Healthy People 2020: Health communication and health information technology, national snapshot*. Retrieved from http://www.healthypeople.gov/2020/topics-objectives/topic/health-communication-and-health-information-technology/national-snapshot

U.S. Department of Health and Human Services (USDHHS). (2016d). *Healthy People 2020: Social determinants of health*. Retrieved from http://www.healthypeople.gov/2020/topics-objectives/topic/social-determinants-of-health

World Health Organization (WHO). (2012). *Humanitarian health action*. Retrieved from http://www.who.int/hac/en/

World Health Organization (WHO). (2015, September 25). *New agenda for sustainable development: Towards a healthier, equitable, and peaceful future for all*. Retrieved from http://www.euro.who.int/en/health-topics/health-determinants/millenium-development-goals/news/news/2015/09/new-agenda-for-sustainable-development-towards-a-healthier,-equitable-and-peaceful-future-for-all

World Health Organization (WHO). (2016). *Health*. Retrieved from http://www.who.int/trade/glossary/story046/en/

Zurakowski, T. L. (2005). In J. J. Fitzpatrick, & A. L. Whall (Eds.), *Conceptual models of nursing: Analysis and application* (4th ed., pp. 21–45). Upper Saddle River, NJ: Pearson Education, Inc.

Zyblock, D. M. (2010). Nursing presence in contemporary nursing practice. *Nursing Forum, 45*(2), 120–124.

Zborowsky, T. (2014). The legacy of Florence Nightingale's environmental theory: Nursing research focusing on the impact of health care environments. *Health Environments Research & Design Journal, 7*(4), 19–34.

thePoint: Everything You Need to Make the Grade!

Community as Client: Applying the Nursing Process

"A community needs a soul if it is to become a true home for human beings. You, the people, must get it this soul."

—*Pope John Paul II* (1920–2005)

KEY TERMS

Assets assessment
Coalition
Community as client
Community development
Community diagnoses
Community assessment
Community subsystem
   assessment

Comprehensive assessment
Descriptive epidemiologic
   study
Evaluation
Familiarization assessment
Goals
Implementation
Interaction

Key informants
Location variables
Objectives
Outcome criteria
Partnerships
Planning
Population variables
Priority setting

Problem-oriented
   assessment
Social class
Social determinants of
   health
Social system variables
Survey
Windshield survey

LEARNING OBJECTIVES

Upon mastery of this chapter, you should be able to:

- Describe the characteristics of a healthy community.
- Describe the meaning of community as client.
- Articulate three specific considerations of each of the three dimensions of the community as client.
- Explain methods the community health nurse might use to interact with the community.
- Discuss methods of community health assessment.
- Compare and contrast five types of community assessment.
- Delineate five sources of community data.
- Describe the role of the community health nurse as a catalyst for community development.

By this point in your nursing education, you are familiar with the use of the nursing process in caring for individuals in the acute care setting. It is a new experience to think of an entire community as your focus of care, but similar principles apply. Although community health nursing practice involves the care of individuals, families, and populations, the care of communities is vital to promoting health and preventing disease. The term community has been well defined in the nursing literature. A community is a collection of people interacting with one another because of geography, common interests, characteristics, or goals. These interactions include social institutions, such as schools, government agencies, and social services. The concept of **community as client** refers to a group or population of people as the focus of nursing service (Anderson & McFarlane, 2015). As described in Chapter 1, understanding the concept of the community as client is a prerequisite for effective service at every level of community nursing practice. In this era of increased emphasis on population health and public health improvement, the demand for related skills is increasing (Michener, Koo, Castrucci, & Sprague, 2015). It is this population-focused practice that distinguishes community health nursing from other nursing specialties (American Nurses Association [ANA], 2013; American Public Health Association, Public Health Nursing Section, 2013).

WHAT IS A HEALTHY COMMUNITY?

What is a healthy community? Just as health for an individual is relative and will change, all communities exist in a relative state of health. A community's health can be viewed within the context of health being more than just the absence of disease and including things that promote the maintenance of a high quality of life and productivity. A key vision for healthy communities is presented in *Healthy People 2020*, the national health promotion and disease prevention agenda published by the U.S. Department of Health and Human Services (USDHHS). Its four overarching goals for the health of the nation are

- To attain high-quality, longer lives free of preventable disease, disability, injury, and premature death
- To achieve health equity, eliminate disparities, and improve the health of all groups
- To create social and physical environments that promote good health for all
- To promote quality of life, healthy development, and healthy behaviors across all life stages (USDHHS, 2016, para. 5)

The 42 topic areas and 1,200 objectives are discussed in more detail elsewhere (see Chapter 1 describing *Healthy People 2020*). These objectives and targets provide guidelines for communities to follow in order to promote the health of their members. By encouraging collaboration across communities, empowering individuals to make better choices, and measuring progress toward set benchmarks, *Healthy People 2020* can be used as a road map for achieving longer and healthier lives for all Americans.

The National Prevention Strategy (NPS), largely based on *Healthy People 2020* priorities, was developed in 2011 to further national health improvement efforts. The NPS aims to guide national efforts in the most effective and achievable means for improving health and well-being. The strategy prioritizes prevention by integrating recommendations and actions across multiple settings in order to improve health and save lives. To realize this vision and achieve this goal, the strategy identifies four strategic directions and seven targeted priorities (National Prevention Council, 2011).

The *strategic directions* provide a strong foundation for all of our nation's prevention efforts and include core recommendations necessary to build a prevention-oriented society. They include

- Healthy and safe community environments: Create, sustain, and recognize communities that promote health and wellness through prevention.
- Clinical and community preventive services: Ensure that prevention-focused health care and community prevention efforts are available, integrated, and mutually reinforcing.
- Empowered people: Support people in making healthy choices.
- Elimination of health disparities: Eliminate disparities, improving the quality of life for all Americans.

Within this framework, the *priorities* provide evidence-based recommendations that are most likely to reduce the burden of the leading causes of preventable death and major illness, and include

- Tobacco-free living
- Preventing drug abuse and excessive alcohol use
- Healthy eating
- Active living
- Injury- and violence-free living
- Reproductive and sexual health
- Mental and emotional well-being

The NPS serves as a road map for community health nurses collaborating with stakeholders and community partners, to address priority areas such as healthy eating, active living, and tobacco control through the prioritization of prevention and integration of recommendations and actions across multiple settings. By working on shared priorities, community health nurses can serve as a valuable partner in identifying community health needs and connecting communities with available resources (Jarris & Schneider, 2013). Nurses can also serve as community educators, empowering people with information to make healthy choices while working to create environments where healthy choices are more accessible and affordable, which is the ultimate intent of the strategy (Lushniak, Alley, Ulin, & Graffunder, 2015).

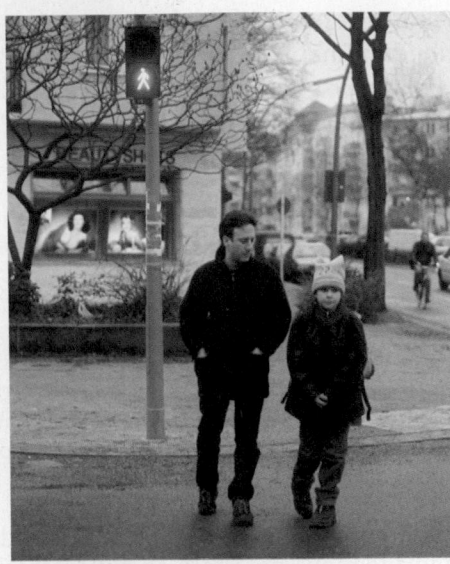

Healthy communities promote productivity and a good quality of life for their residents.

DIMENSIONS OF THE COMMUNITY AS CLIENT

The health of a community can be characterized through a number of perspectives. Donabedian's classic theory of structure, process, and outcomes provides unique insight into the health status of the community (Donabedian, 2005).

Status/people is the most common measure of the health of a community. It typically comprises morbidity and mortality data identifying the physical, emotional, and social determinants of health (SDH). Physical and social indices include vital statistics, leading causes of death and illness, suicide rates, and rates of drug and alcohol addiction. Social determinants can be identified by crime rates and functional ability level or by high school dropout rates or average income levels. Other demographic characteristics, such as single, female-headed households, are also helpful status measures. Informal leaders and resource persons can impact the health of communities outside the formal health care system.

Structure of a community refers to its services and resources. Community associations, groups, and organizations provide a means for accessing needed services. Adequacy and appropriateness of health services can be determined by examining patterns of use, number and types of health and social services, and quality measures. Classification as a medically underserved area is indicative of a lack of sufficient health care providers (e.g., nurses, physicians, dentists) and is determined by the federal government (Health Resources & Services

Administration [HRSA], 2014). Demographic data, such as socioeconomic and racial distribution, age, gender, and educational level, are also important indicators of community structure. These measures provide key information and correlate to health status.

Process reflects the community's ability to function effectively. It includes processes within the community (collaboration between subsystems of education and health, for instance) and between the community and the state or national levels. Social capital (i.e., the networks of relationships among people who live and work in a particular society, enabling that society to function effectively) is a key component to the process dimension (Murayama, Fujiwara, & Kawachi, 2012). Just as nurses assess the strengths and limitations of clients when working with individuals, the community health nurse must assess the strengths and limitations of the community when working with the community as client. Strengths must be enhanced and limitations addressed to achieve agreed-upon goals. Communities with social capital are able to:

● Collaborate effectively in identifying community needs and problems
● Achieve a working consensus on goals and priorities
● Induce collective action to implement agreed-upon goals
● Collaborate effectively to take the required actions

These characteristics are discussed in more detail later in this chapter under the discussion on "Planning to Meet the Health Needs of the Community." See Chapter 1 for more information on healthy communities.

Addressing community health by examining the process, in addition to the structure and status dimensions, provides a broader view into the complexities of community health and community actions for change. It is key not only to examine health outcomes but also to consider how the interactions between processes and structure impact health outcomes (Public Health Accreditation Board, 2013).

Another perspective identifies the community as having three features: a location, a population, and a social system. Figure 15–1 presents a visual interpretation of this perspective. Each of these features has several components that need to be addressed and represents further information that must be collected and analyzed when assessing the health of a community. These are detailed in Tables 15–1 to 15–3.

Location

Every physical community carries out its daily existence in a specific geographic location. The health of a community is affected by location, because placement of health services, geographic features, climate, plants, animals, and the human-made environment are intrinsic to geographic location. The location of a community places it in an environment that offers resources and also poses threats (Nykiforuk et al., 2012; Thomas, DiClemente, & Snell, 2013). The healthy community is one that makes wise use of its resources and is prepared to meet threats and dangers. In assessing the health of any community, it is necessary to collect information not only about variables specific to location but also about relationships

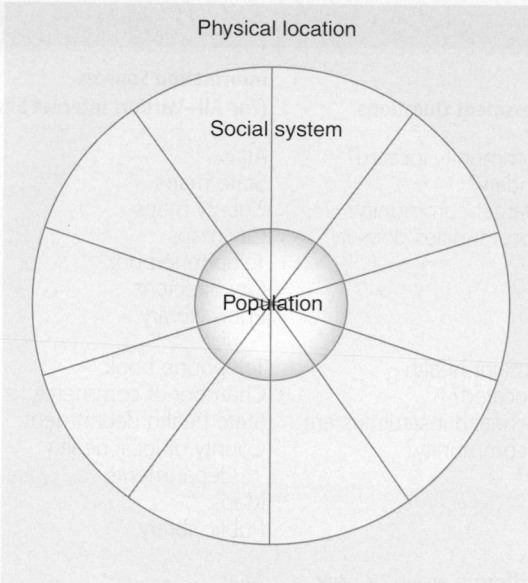

FIGURE 15–1 Three features of a community. The community has (1) a physical location, represented here by the square boundary; (2) a population, shown here by the central circle; and (3) a social system, divided here into subsystems.

between the community and its location. Do groups cooperate to identify threats? Do health agencies cooperate to prepare for an emergency such as a flood, tornado, or earthquake? Does the community make certain that its members are given available information about resources and dangers? Table 15–1 describes the location perspective of the Community Profile Inventory, including the six **location variables:** community boundaries, location of health services, geographic features, climate, flora and fauna, and the human-made environment.

Community Boundaries

To talk about the community in any sense, one must first describe its boundaries (Schildkraut, 2014). Measurements of wellness and illness within a community depend on defining the outer geographic limits of the unit under consideration and also the more informal boundaries that are present (Swarts, 2011). Nurses need to be clear, for example, that a target community of the elderly includes a description of age and location (e.g., all persons age 65 and older in a given city or county). Some communities are distinctly separate, such as an isolated rural town, whereas others are closely situated to one another, such as the suburbs of a large metropolis. Therefore, it is important for the nurse to know the nature of each location and clearly define its boundaries.

Location of Health Services

If the members of a town must travel 200 miles to the nearest clinic or dental office, the health of the community will be affected. When assessing a community, the community health nurse needs to identify the major health centers and know where they are located (Barnett, 2012). For example, an alcoholism treatment center for indigent alcoholics was located 30 miles outside one city. This location presented transportation problems and profoundly affected the

length of time they remained at the center and the willingness of clients to voluntarily seek treatment there. If a well-baby clinic is located on the edge of a high-crime district, parents may be deterred from using it. It is often helpful to plot the major health institutions, both inside and outside the community, on a map that shows their proximity and relationship to the community as a whole.

Geographic Features

Communities have been constructed in every conceivable physical environment, and environment certainly can affect the health of a community (see Chapter 9). A healthy community is one that takes into consideration the geography of its location, identifies possible problems and likely resources, and responds in an adaptive fashion (Kindig & Isham, 2014). For example, Anchorage, Alaska, and San Francisco, California, are both located on a geologic fault line and are subject to major earthquakes. In such places, the health of the community is determined, in part, by its preparedness for an earthquake and its ability to cope and respond quickly when such a crisis occurs.

Soil and water pollution pose a serious threat to food safety, and both represent an important threat to human health. Concerns of this kind have become increasingly problematic in China, where a combination of pollution and an increasing food safety risk has affected a large part of the population. Clean water shortages in the country have forced residents to use wastewater irrigation to fulfill the water requirements for agricultural production. Water shortages, coupled with the overapplication of pesticides and chemical pollutants, have caused serious agricultural land and food pollution leading to increased health risks for those living in affected areas (Lu et al., 2015; Starks et al., 2011).

Climate

Winter weather patterns are expected to become more variable as average global temperatures continually increase. Research findings indicate that there is a relationship between temperature variability and health outcomes, including cardiovascular, respiratory, cerebrovascular events, and all-cause morbidity and mortality. Epidemiologic studies indicate that the populations most vulnerable to variations in cold winter weather are the elderly, rural, and, generally, populations living in moderate winter climates (Conlon, Rajkovich, White-Newsome, Larsen, & O'Neill, 2011).

The intense summer heat of a location such as Phoenix, Arizona, can create many health problems (e.g., heatstroke, heat exhaustion). Skin cancer incidence is associated with unprotected sun exposure, which increases the risk for people who live in warm, sunny regions (Townsend et al., 2011). Asthma and other lung diseases are exacerbated in the Central San Joaquin Valley of California because mountains surround this area and create an air inversion, trapping vehicle and agricultural by-products in what can be described as a "large bowl," causing smog during many months of the year. Asthmatic children in densely populated areas of Baltimore, Maryland, have been found to experience exacerbations of asthma symptoms in both the summer and winter months (Teach et al., 2015). Climate can

Table 15–1 Community Profile Inventory: Location Perspective

Location Variables	Community Health Implications	Community Assessment Questions	Information Sources (For All—Various Internet Sites)
Boundary of community	Community boundaries serve as basis for measuring incidence of wellness and illness and for determining spread of disease.	Where is the community located? What is its boundary? Is it a part of a larger community? What smaller communities does it include?	Atlas State maps County maps City maps Telephone book City directory Public library
Location of health services	Use of health services depends on availability and accessibility.	Where are the major health institutions located? What necessary health institutions are outside the community? Where are they?	Telephone book Chamber of commerce State health department County or local health departments Maps Public library
Geographic features	Injury, death, and destruction may be caused by floods, earthquakes, volcanoes, tornadoes, or hurricanes. Recreational opportunities at lakes, seashore, and mountains promote health and fitness.	What major landforms are in or near the community? What geographic features pose possible threats? What geographic features offer opportunities for healthful activities?	Atlas Chamber of commerce Maps State health department Public library
Climate	Extremes of heat and cold affect health and illness. Extremes of temperature and precipitation may tax community's coping ability.	What are the average temperature and precipitation? What are the extremes? What climatic features affect health and fitness? Is the community prepared to cope with emergencies?	Weather atlas Chamber of commerce State health department Maps Local government Weather bureau Public library
Flora and fauna	Poisonous plants and disease-carrying animals can affect community health. Plants and animals offer resources as well as dangers.	What plants and animals pose possible threats to health?	State health department Poison control center Police department Emergency rooms Encyclopedia Public library
Human-made environment	All human influences on environment (housing, dams, farming, type of industry, chemical waste, air pollution, and so forth) can influence levels of community wellness.	What are the major industries? How have air, land, and water been affected by humans? What is the quality of housing? Do highways allow access to health institutions?	Chamber of commerce Local government City directory State health department University research reports Public library

also affect infectious disease rates (McMichael, 2015). A healthy community encourages physical activity among its members, but the climate affects this activity. Although long, cold winters can restrict activity, one community, St. Paul, Minnesota, holds an annual Winter Carnival. Sporting events, parades, ice sailing, dog sledding, a treasure hunt, and hot air balloon races bring thousands of Minnesotans outdoors at a time when they might otherwise be confined by the weather.

Flora and Fauna

Plant and animal populations in a community are often determined by location. The way a community responds to these populations, whether wild or domesticated, can affect the health of the community. More than 26 million American children and adults live with asthma. Evidence of a connection between asthma attacks and community environments has been demonstrated both in the United States and abroad (Iqbal, Oraka, Chew, & Flanders, 2014). Inner-city children have been shown to demonstrate higher rates of asthma, and research has shown strong allergic reactions, especially to rat and cat allergens (Rao et al., 2015).

Public health officials note chronic environmental factors as a possible cause for increased asthma cases: pollution from high-traffic areas, secondhand smoke in homes, and poor living conditions characterized by dust mites, mold, industrial air pollution, mouse and cockroach droppings, and animal dander. However, research completed at Johns Hopkins University in 2015 counters that claim. Researchers examined records for 23,065 children living in 5,853 census tracts and found asthma prevalence of 12.9% for inner-city children and 10.6% for those living outside of inner cities. When they statistically adjusted for age, gender, region, and race/ethnicity, no statistical difference was found. They noted that poverty increased the risk of asthma for children (Keet et al., 2015).

For 2015, the city named "asthma capital" of the United States was Memphis, Tennessee (Asthma and Allergy Foundation of America, 2015). Many of the asthma capitals that year were in the South, largely because of the lack of smoke-free legislation in many tobacco-producing states, along with poor air quality and high pollen counts. To further make the case for a connection between environment and asthma, in Atlanta, the 1996 Olympics brought an unexpected benefit: a 42% reduction in asthma-related emergency room visits. With the Olympic congestion downtown, Atlanta restricted traffic and thus improved air quality. The same outcomes were experienced with the Beijing Olympics. Internationally, Singapore also noticed a reduction in emergency room visits for asthma after it restricted automobile traffic in its central business district (Li et al., 2011).

Poison oak, ivy, and sumac can be found across the United States, and these plants produce an allergic contact dermatitis in many people who come in contact with it (Petersen, 2011). In the Sierra foothill communities of central California, black widow and tarantula spiders, scorpions, and rattlesnakes are resident populations that pose potential health threats. The poison from a single snakebite may cause serious injury or death (Gras, Plantefève, Baud, & Chippaux, 2012). In the south–central Midwest, the bite of the brown recluse spider injects a toxin that can lead to necrotic skin ulcers as well as systemic symptoms (Quan, 2012). In the Northeast and Mid-Atlantic states, increased deer populations—and consequently deer ticks—bring with them an increased incidence of Lyme disease (Tran & Waller, 2013).

Public health nurses need to know about the major sources of danger from plants and animals affecting the community under study. Are there community agencies that provide educational information about these dangers? Does the populace understand their significance? Are emergency services, such as a poison control center, available to community members?

The Built Environment

Every community is located in the midst of an environment created and transformed by human ingenuity. People build houses and factories, dump wastes into streams or vacant lots, fill the air with gases, and build dams to control streams. All of these human alterations of the environment have important implications for community health (Trowbridge & Schmid, 2013). A Public Health Nursing (PHN) might improve the health of a community by working with community members, legislators, and stakeholders to improve the design of the built environment to promote health and well-being. Such initiatives have become an emerging priority within public health, particularly as the ongoing epidemics of childhood and adult obesity persist (Trowbridge et al., 2013). Evidence-based environmental design guidelines and evaluation tools are available to promote physical activity and healthy eating.

The promotion of walking has become a common and effective intervention for increasing physical activity, both as recreational exercise and as a daily activity to prevent and control obesity (Trowbridge & Schmid, 2013). Other modifications of the built environment that have been found effective in promoting healthy behaviors include the designation of exercise areas and building safe walking and biking paths (Simiyu, Njororai, & Jivetti, 2015).

Population Characteristics

When one considers the community as the client, examining the health status of the total population in a given community is a critical component. The population consists not of a specialized aggregate but of all the diverse people who live within the boundaries of the community. The health of any community is greatly influenced by the attributes of its population. Various features of the population suggest health needs and provide a basis for health **planning** (Nguyen, Knight, Roughead, Brooks, & Mant, 2015; Schoenbaum, Schoen, Nicholson, & Cantor, 2011). A healthy community has leaders who are aware of the population's characteristics, know its various needs, and respond to those needs. Community health nurses can better understand any community by knowing about its **population variables**: size, density, composition or demography, rate of growth or decline, cultural characteristics, social class structure, and mobility. Table 15–2 presents the population perspective section of the Community Profile Inventory.

Size

Dover, Delaware (with about 35,000 people), and the city of Los Angeles, California (with around 4 million people), have radically different health problems. If a single case of *Salmonella* poisoning occurred in Dover, health officials would probably quickly learn of it. It would be relatively easy to trace the course, check the few restaurants in town, and interview people about sanitation practices. However, many cases might occur in Los Angeles without the health department's knowledge. Moreover, once the cases were discovered, tracing the source of contamination might involve a long and complicated search. This is only one small way in which population size can affect the health of a community. The size of a community also influences the presence of inadequate housing, the heterogeneity of the population, and almost every conceivable aspect of health needs and services (Nauenberg, Laporte, & Shen, 2011). Knowing a community's size provides community health nurses with important information for planning. See Chapter 29 for issues related to rural and urban population health.

Density

In some communities, thousands of people are crowded into high-rise apartment buildings. In others, such as farm communities, people live great distances from one another. Population density, or the number of people residing within a square mile area, is used to describe

Table 15–2   Community Profile Inventory: Population Perspective

Population Variables	Community Health Implications	Community Assessment Questions	Information Sources (For All–Various Internet Sites)
Size	The number of people influences number and size of health care institutions. Size affects homogeneity of the population and its needs.	What is the population of the community? Is it an urban, suburban, or rural community?	State health department Census data Maps City or town officials Chamber of commerce
Density	Increased density may increase stress. High and low density often affects the availability of health services.	What is the density of the population per square mile?	Census data State health department
Composition	Composition of the population often determines types of health needs.	What is the age composition of the community? What is the sex composition of the community? What is the marital status of community members? What occupations are represented and in what percentages?	Census data State health department Chamber of Commerce U.S. Department of Labor Statistics
Rate of growth or decline	Rapidly growing communities may place excessive demands on health services. Marked decline in population may signal a poorly functioning community.	How has population size changed over the past two decades? What are the health implications of this change?	Census data State health department
Cultural differences	Health needs vary among subcultural and ethnic populations. Utilization of health services varies with culture. Health practices and extent of knowledge are affected by culture.	What is the ethnic breakdown of population? What racial groups are represented? What subcultural populations exist in the community? Do any of the subcultural groups have unique health needs and practices? Are different ethnic and cultural groups included in health planning?	Census data State health department Social and cultural research reports Human rights commission City government Health planning boards
Social class	Class differences influence the utilization of health services. Class composition influences cost of public health services.	What percentage of the population falls into each social class? What do class differences suggest for health needs and services?	State health department Census data Sociological reports
Mobility	Mobility of the population affects continuity of care. Mobility affects availability of service to highly mobile populations.	How frequently do members move into and out of the community? How frequently do members move within the community? Are there any specific populations, such as migrant workers, that are highly mobile? How does the pattern of mobility affect the health of the community? Is the community organized to meet the health needs of mobile groups?	State health department Census data Health agencies serving migrant workers Farm labor offices Program serving transients and the homeless
Poverty level	Economic disparities may lead to health disparities.	What percentage of the population is below federal poverty levels? How many children qualify for free or reduced cost school lunch?	Census data State data Local data (schools)

Table 15–2   Community Profile Inventory: Population Perspective (*Continued*)

Population Variables	Community Health Implications	Community Assessment Questions	Information Sources (For All–Various Internet Sites)
Education level	Education disparities may lead to health disparities.	What percentage of the population has less than high school education? What is the literacy rate?	State data Local data (schools)
Unemployment rate	Health insurance is often tied to employment. Lack of regular income can be a family stressor. Both can lead to health disparities.	What is the rate of unemployment? How variable is this rate?	U.S. Department of Labor State data Local data
Population by age	A high proportion of children and elderly can overburden health care and social systems.	What is the dependency ratio? Has this rate changed dramatically? What is the trend?	Census data State data Local data
Health status	Community members' status relative to the 10 Leading Health Indicators can impact overall community health.	What is the rate of obesity/overweight? What are the rates of tobacco use and substance abuse? What is the immunization rate? What are rates of injury and violence? What are the STD and HIV/AIDS rates?	State data Local data Centers for Disease Control and Prevention (CDC) data Vital statistics—numbers of births, deaths, marriages, and infant mortality rate. (Compare local to state data; state to national data.)
Environmental health status	Poor environmental health (e.g., presence of coliform bacteria in well water, toxic chemicals, or poor air quality) can lead to increased incidence of communicable or chronic diseases.	What are rates of communicable or chronic diseases (e.g., *E. coli* infections, asthma)? What is the Toxic Release Inventory?	CDC data State data Local data

how many people live within a community. Using our example of Dover, Delaware, at 1,566 people per square mile, and the greater Los Angeles area with 23,557 people per square mile, it is readily apparent which one is more densely populated. The full impact of living in high-density communities is being researched, and some research has already shown that crowding affects individual and community health. Motor vehicle exhaust from highways has been shown to be associated with higher risk of asthma and reduced lung function in children, as well as higher pulmonary and cardiac mortality in adults (Cesaroni et al., 2013). When compared with rural populations, urban populations in some countries have a higher incidence of allergic diseases and respiratory symptoms, thought to be associated with higher air pollution levels (Shpakou, Brożek, Stryzhak, Neviartovich, & Zejda, 2012).

A low-density community, however, may have problems. When people are spread out, provision of health care services can become difficult. There may not be enough resources in the form of taxes to support public health services. Rural communities often suffer from inadequate distribution of health care personnel, including private physicians and community health nurses. A national study of rural–urban health disparities found a higher prevalence of poverty, premature death, and all-cause

mortality in rural areas than in more densely populated metropolitan areas (Singh & Siahpush, 2014). Artnak, McGraw, and Stanley (2011) noted "quality health care services in rural communities for the chronically ill and dying remain problematic" (p. 140). One large study found that populations using critical access rural hospitals had higher mortality rates for acute myocardial infarction (MI), congestive heart failure, and pneumonia when compared with patients at nonrural hospitals (Joynt, Harris, Orav, & Jha, 2011). Other rural health risks include greater rates of injuries from traffic accidents (Burrows, Auger, Gamache, & Hamel, 2013) and illnesses related to agricultural pesticide exposure. Recent studies have also found an association between increasing pesticide exposure and attention-deficit hyperactivity disorder (ADHD) that may be stronger for hyperactive–impulsive symptoms compared to inattention and in boys compared to girls. Given the growing use of pesticides, these results may be of considerable public health importance (Wagner-Schuman et al., 2015).

A healthy community takes into consideration the density of its population. It organizes to meet the differing needs created by its density levels (e.g., it recognizes differences in density between the inner city and the suburbs and allocates services accordingly). See Chapter 29 for more on health risks specific to rural and urban areas.

Composition/Demographics

Communities differ in the types of people who live within their boundaries. A retirement community in Florida whose members are mostly older than age 65 has one set of interests and concerns, whereas a city with a large number of women in their childbearing years will have another set of concerns. A healthy community is one that takes full account of the needs of its constituents and provides for their differences. Age, sex, educational level, occupation, and many other demographic variables affect health concerns (Zheng, Tumin, & Qian, 2013). In communities with a high proportion of low-income families, considerations must be made to accommodate the needs of the poor (Lee et al., 2011). Occupation can also affect health. For example, in a town where 75% of the workers are employed in a textile mill, the community lives with the threat of brown lung disease, which is caused by cotton dust. In areas where tobacco is the main source of income and a large proportion of the population is engaged in its production, green tobacco sickness—or acute nicotine poisoning—is a concern because workers can absorb nicotine through the skin, and precautions must be taken to prevent this from happening (Fassa et al., 2014). Understanding a community's composition is an important early step in determining its level of health.

Rate of Growth or Decline

Community populations change over time. Some grow rapidly. The growth of Las Vegas, Nevada, as a popular place to live has placed extreme demands on the environment, along with the provision of health care and other services. Other populations may experience a decline because of economic change, for example, those areas of the United States where steel and auto manufacturing have declined. Any significant fluctuation in population size can affect the health of the community, much like the size of a hospital is often correlated with rates of drug-resistant infections (Kouyos, Wiesch, & Bonhoeffer, 2011). As people leave to find new employment or better living conditions, consumption of goods and services drops. Community morale may suffer, and community leadership may decline. Even a stable community can have problems (e.g., members may resist needed change because they notice little fluctuation in their population; commercial and residential properties may be abandoned or left vacant).

Cultural Characteristics

A community may be composed of a single cultural group, such as Ojibway Indians on their reservation in Wisconsin, or it may be made up of many cultures or subcultures. For instance, if a city has a large Hispanic population, along with a group of Native Americans living in the inner city and a cluster of Vietnamese refugees, the cultural differences among these members will influence the health of the community. These differences can create conflicting or competing demands for resources and services or create intergroup hostility. A healthy community is aware of such cultural differences and acts to promote understanding among cultural subgroups (Spector, 2013). See Chapter 5 for more about transcultural nursing in the community.

Social Class and Educational Level

Social class refers to the ranking of groups within society by income, education, occupation, social class, or a combination of these factors. There is no absolute agreement on income levels or other criteria to designate social class categories (upper, middle, lower), other than the government formula used to compute poverty level (USDHHS, 2015). Although class distinctions are not clearly defined, class rankings based on occupation, education, and wealth (income plus assets) seem to correlate with many different health outcomes and are used frequently in research (Mondal & Shitan, 2014). Occupational level, in particular, has historically and consistently proven to be a reliable measure, with surprisingly similar rankings among all societies for which data exist (Adcock & Brown, 1957). This classic research has shown that people with higher occupational levels generally have higher incomes and education, exert greater political influence, and are more highly esteemed by others. More recent research, linking educational attainment with mortality, indicates that income (linked to education and occupation) is often the best predictor for mortality (Hummer & Hernandez, 2013; Lantz, Golberstein, House, & Morenoff, 2010). *Healthy People 2020* identified the relationship between these factors and others by defining **social determinants of health**:

> Social determinants of health reflect social factors and the physical conditions in the environment in which people are born, live, learn, play, work, and age. Social and physical determinants of health impact a wide range of health, functioning, and quality of life outcomes. (USDHHS, 2016, para. 10)

For example, socioeconomic conditions (e.g., poverty), resources to meet daily needs (e.g., opportunities for quality education and employment; access to healthy food), social norms and attitudes (e.g., segregation, discrimination), public safety and transportation (e.g., crime, violence, sanitation, mass transit), and social support/interactions (e.g., cell phones, mass media, families/friends) are part of the larger construct of SDH. Physical determinants of health include things like the natural environment (e.g., climate, plants), the built environment (e.g., transportation, buildings), housing and neighborhoods (e.g., density, condition), exposure to hazards (e.g., physical, toxic), barriers (e.g., being disabled), and aesthetic elements (e.g., green belts, lighting). While health promotion and preventive health services can be beneficial to all social and economic groups, low-income groups and people with fewer years of education who are most likely to be affected by health disparities can gain particular benefit from targeted community health improvement efforts. Frieden's (2010) influential Health Impact Pyramid has as its base socioeconomic factors (or SDH), as these can have the greatest impact on populations, followed by changing context to make default decisions more healthy (e.g., when most people don't smoke, it is easier to be a nonsmoker), then protective interventions that are long lasting (e.g., immunizations, colonoscopies), and finally clinical interventions (e.g., ongoing monitoring for chronic conditions like heart disease) and counseling/education (e.g., health education to improve diet/exercise) (see Fig. 15–2).

Increasing
Population
Impact

Increasing
Individual
Effort Needed

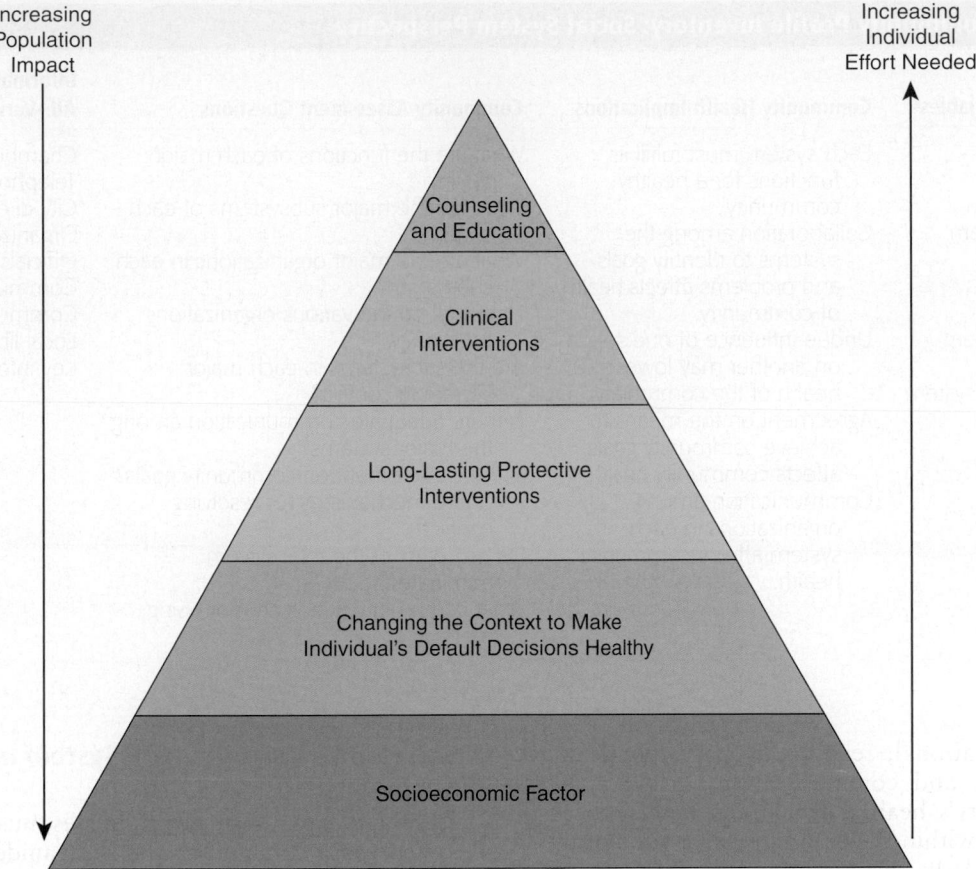

Counseling
and Education

Clinical
Interventions

Long-Lasting Protective
Interventions

Changing the Context to Make
Individual's Default Decisions Healthy

Socioeconomic Factor

FIGURE 15–2   Health Impact Pyramid. (Source: http://www.ncbi.nlm.nih.gov/pmc/articles/
PMC2836340/figure/fig1/)

It is generally known that different social classes have different health problems, as well as a variety of resources for coping with illness and diverse ways of using health services. A healthy community recognizes these differences and creates health care services to meet these varied needs.

Mobility

Americans are a mobile population. Between the 2007 to 2009 period of recession and the 2010 to 2012 post-recession period, 15.7% of Americans moved. However, that is a record low compared to 20.2% in 1985, and these fluctuations have been linked to social and economic factors (U.S. Census Bureau, n.d.). People move to go to college, take a new job, join other family members or friends, or seek a new climate after retirement. This mobility has a direct effect on the health of communities (Gushulak & MacPherson, 2011). If the population turnover is extensive, continuity of services may suffer. Leadership for improving the health of the community may change so frequently that concerted action becomes difficult. High turnover may necessitate special attention to health education about local conditions.

Population groups may arrive and depart in seasonal swings; fluctuations in the number of migrant farm workers, tourists, or college students can affect a community. Border health issues are of special concern, as people continually move across borders, bringing with

them health issues such as vaccine-preventable diseases and chronic illnesses (Matthews et al., 2015). Immigrants and refugees may represent a significant population subgroup in many areas of a country, and public health officials must meet their unique needs. The community health nurse also needs to identify those populations that are seasonally mobile. These subgroups present special health needs and place an added burden on a community (e.g., migrant workers). If a town of 3,000 people has an annual influx of 10,000 students who disappear in the summer, residents must prepare to meet this population instability. The small towns of the San Juan Islands in Puget Sound, Washington, can command such high prices for accommodations in the summer that some low-income, year-round residents camp in tents during those months because they are unable to pay the high rents. Thus, the lives of many families are disrupted each year. A healthy community neither ignores nor overreacts to this kind of mobility. Rather, it identifies the nature of the population change, determines the needs created by such change, and organizes to meet those needs.

Social System

In addition to location and population, every community has a third feature—a social system. The various parts of a community's social system that interact and influence the health of a community are called **social system variables**. These variables include health, family,

Table 15-3   Community Profile Inventory: Social System Perspective

Social System Variables	Community Health Implications	Community Assessment Questions	Information Sources (For All–Various Internet Sites)
Health system Family system Economic system Educational system Religious system Welfare system Political system Recreational system Legal system Communication system	Each system must fulfill its functions for a healthy community. Collaboration among the systems to identify goals and problems affects health of community. Undue influence of one system on another may lower the health of the community. Agreement on the means to achieve community goals affects community health. Communication among organizations in each system affects community health.	What are the functions of each major system? What are the major subsystems of each system? What are the major organizations in each subsystem? How well do the various organizations function? Are the subsystems in each major system in conflict? Is there adequate communication among the major systems? Is there agreement on community goals? Are there mechanisms for resolving conflict? Do any parts of the total system dominate the others? What community needs are not being met?	Chamber of Commerce Telephone book City directory Organizational literature Officials in organizations Community self-study Community survey Local library Key informants

economic, educational, religion, welfare, political, recreational, legal, and communication. Whether assessing a community's health, developing new services for the mentally ill within the community, or promoting the health of the elderly, the community health nurse needs to understand the community as a social system. A community health nurse working in a tiny village in Alaska needs to understand and work with the social system of that village no less than a nurse practicing in New York City. Table 15–3 guides the nurse in assessing a community's social system variables.

The Concept of a Social System

A social system is an abstract concept and can be more readily understood by first considering the people who make up the community's population. Each person enacts multiple roles, such as parent, spouse, employee, citizen, church member, and/or political volunteer. People in certain roles tend to interact more closely with others in related roles, such as a nursing supervisor with a staff nurse or a customer with a sales clerk. The patterns and communication that emerge from these interactions form the basis of organizations. Some organizations are informal (e.g., an extended family group). Other organizations, such as a city police department or a software business, are more formal. However, all organizations are constructed from roles that are enacted by individual citizens. Organizations, in turn, interact with one another, forming linkages. For example, a medical equipment company and a laboratory establish contracts (linkages) with a home care agency. When a group of organizations are linked and have similar functions, such as all those providing social services, they form a community system or subsystem (Fig. 15–3). The various community systems have a profound influence on one another. Because this interaction among parts determines the health of the whole, it is the total social system that concerns community health nurses.

The Health Care Delivery System as Part of the Social System

Although community health nurses must examine all the systems in a community and must understand how they interact, the health system is of particular importance. The major function of the health system is to promote the health of the community. **Community assessment** asks not only whether but also how well the system is functioning. What is the level of health promotion carried out by the

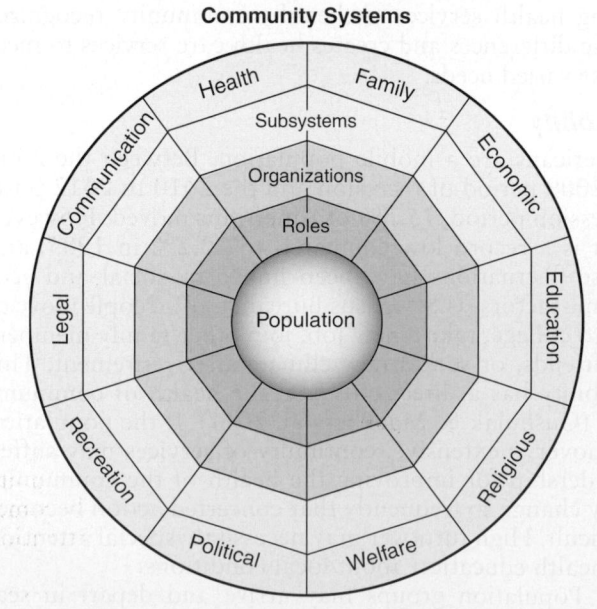

FIGURE 15-3   The community as a social system. Each of the 10 major systems of a community includes a number of subsystems that are made up of organizations. Members of the community occupy roles in these organizations.

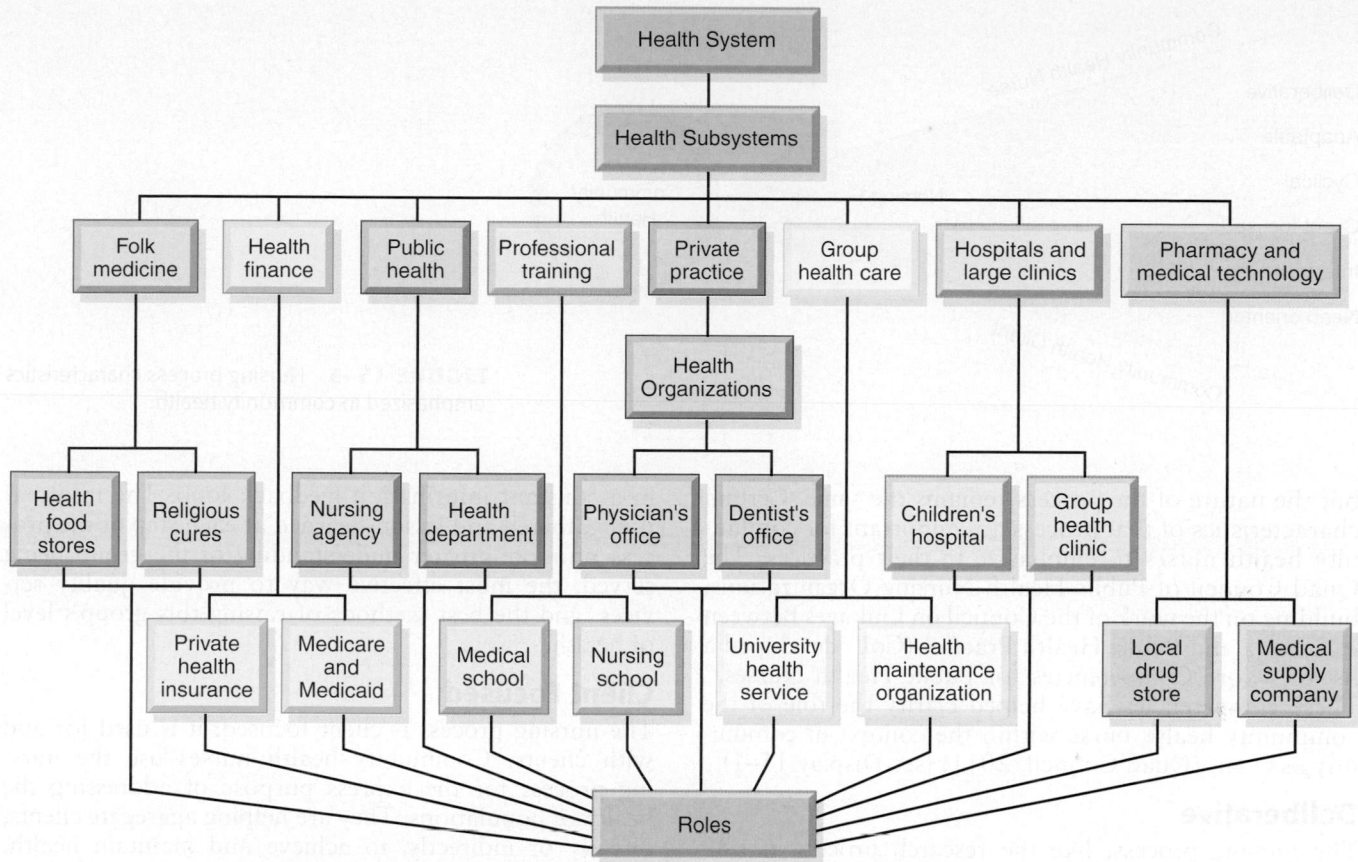

FIGURE 15–4 Components of the health system. This figure shows some representative types of organizations for each of the major subsystems. In turn, each of these organizations also has members with many different roles, and the health of the entire system depends, in part, on how well these roles are carried out.

health system of a community? To answer this question—one that can be applied to any system—the PHN needs a clear notion about the subsystems, organizations, and roles that make up the system. Any evidence of inadequate functioning becomes a warning signal for more careful assessment. For example, a high rate of teenage pregnancies in a city may signal inadequate functioning of several systems (e.g., family, educational, religious, health), so a closer look is in order. What community values influence sexual behavior among adolescents? What sex education programs are available to this population? Does the health system provide information and counseling?

The components of the health system, described in Figure 15–4, include eight major subsystems—each with one or more organizations. Although the community health nurse must be aware of all the systems in a community, the health system is of central importance. Figure 15–4 represents an organizational view of health system components.

THE NURSING PROCESS APPLIED TO THE COMMUNITY AS CLIENT

Consisting of a systematic, purposeful set of interpersonal actions, the nursing process provides a structure for change that remains a viable tool employed by the

community health nurse. This chapter examines the use of the nursing process as applied at the aggregate or community level. Five components—assessment, diagnosis, planning, implementation, and evaluation—give direction to the dynamics for solving problems, managing nursing actions, and improving the health of communities and community health nursing practice.

Three characteristics support the use of the nursing process in community health nursing. First, the nursing process is a problem-solving process that addresses community health problems at every aggregate level with the goals of preventing illness and promoting public health. Second, it is a management process that requires situational analysis, decision-making, planning, organization, direction, and control of services, as well as outcome evaluation. As a management tool, the nursing process addresses all aggregate levels. Third, it is a process for implementing changes that improve the function of various health-related systems and the ways that people behave within those systems. A representation of nursing process characteristics used in community health nursing is seen in Figure 15–5.

The nursing process provides a framework or structure on which PHN actions are based (ANA, 2013). Application of the process varies with each situation,

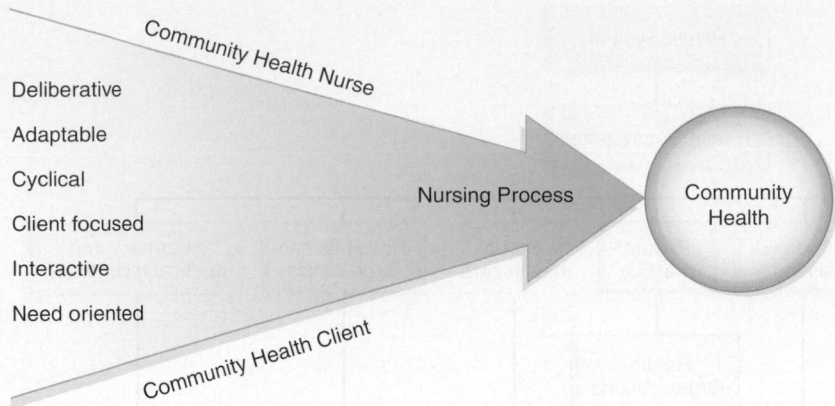

Deliberative

Adaptable

Cyclical

Client focused

Interactive

Need oriented

Community Health Nurse

Nursing Process

Community Health

Community Health Client

FIGURE 15–5 Nursing process characteristics emphasized in community health.

but the nature of the process remains the same. Certain characteristics of that process are important for community health nurses to emphasize in their practices. The Quad Council of Public Health Nursing Organizations, building on the work of the Council on Linkages Between Academia and Public Health Practice (CoL) developed a list of "Core Competencies for Public Health Nurses." These competencies have helped clarify the role of the community health nurse within the context of community as client (Quad Council, 2011) (see Display 15–1).

Deliberative

The nursing process, like the research process in EBP (evidence-based practice), is deliberative—purposefully, rationally, and carefully thought out. It requires the use of sound judgment that is based on adequate information. Community health nurses often practice in situations that demand the ability to think independently and make difficult decisions. Furthermore, thoughtful, deliberative problem solving is a necessary skill for working with the community health team to address the needs and problems of aggregates in the community. The nursing process is a decision-making tool to facilitate these determinations.

Adaptable

The nursing process is adaptable. Its dynamic nature enables the community health nurse to adjust appropriately to each situation and to be flexible in applying the process to aggregate health needs. Furthermore, its flexibility is a reminder to the nurse that each client group and each community situation is unique. The nursing process must be applied specifically to the individual situation and group of people. Based on assessment and sound planning, the nurse adapts and tailors services to meet the identified needs of each community client group.

Cyclical

The nursing process is cyclical and in constant progression. Steps are repeated over and over in the nurse–aggregate client relationship. The nurse engages in continual interaction, data collection, analysis, intervention, and evaluation. As interactions between nurse and client group continue, various steps in the process overlap with one another and are used simultaneously. The cyclic nature of the nursing process enables the nurse to engage

in a constant information feedback loop: The information gathered and lessons learned at each step of the process promote greater understanding of the group being served, the most effective way to provide quality services, and the best methods of raising this group's level of health.

Client Focused

The nursing process is client focused; it is used for and with clients. Community health nurses use the nursing process for the express purpose of addressing the health of populations. They are helping aggregate clients, directly or indirectly, to achieve and maintain health. Clients as total systems—whether groups, populations, or communities—are the targets of the PHN's nursing process (ANA, 2013).

Interactive

The nursing process is interactive, in that nurse and clients are engaged in a process of ongoing interpersonal communication. Giving and receiving accurate information is necessary to promote understanding between nurse and clients and to foster effective use of the nursing process. Furthermore, because of the movement toward informed use of health care, demands for clients' rights and the concept of self-care have gained emphasis. Client groups and community health nurses have increasingly joined forces to assume responsibility for promoting community health. The nurse–aggregate client relationship can and should be a partnership, a shared experience by professionals (nurses and others) and client groups (Tucker, Arthur, Roncoroni, Wall, & Sanchez, 2015).

Need Oriented

The nursing process is need oriented. A long association with problem solving has tended to limit the focus of the nursing process to the correction of existing problems. Although problem solving is certainly an appropriate use of the nursing process, the community health nurse can also use the nursing process to anticipate client needs and prevent problems. The nurse should think of nursing diagnoses as ranging from health problem identification to primary prevention and health promotion opportunities. This focus is needed if the goals of community health—to protect, promote, and restore the people's health—are to be realized.

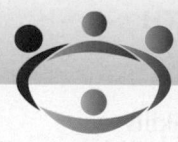

DISPLAY 15–1 QUAD COUNCIL CORE COMPETENCIES OF PUBLIC HEALTH NURSING (2011)

Tier 2 Community Based, Population Focused

1. **Analytic and Assessment Skills**
   - Assesses health status of populations and related determinants of health and illness. Partners with populations, health professionals, and other stakeholders to attach meaning to collected data.
   - Develops PHN diagnoses for individuals, families, communities, and populations. Uses a synthesis of nursing, public health, and system science/theory when characterizing population-level health risks. Assures that assessments identify population assets and needs, values and beliefs, resources, and relevant environmental factors. Derives population diagnoses and priorities based on assessment data, including input from populations.
   - Utilizes a wide variety of relevant variables to measure health conditions for a community or population.
   - Develops a data collection plan using models and principles of epidemiology, demography, and biostatistics, as well as social, behavioral, and natural sciences to collect quantitative and qualitative data on a community or population. Uses methods and instruments for collecting valid and reliable quantitative and qualitative data.
   - Uses multiple methods and sources when collecting and analyzing data for a comprehensive community/population assessment. Assures that assessments are documented and interpreted in terms that are understandable to all who were involved in the process, including communities.
   - Critiques validity, reliability, and comparability of data collected for communities/populations.
   - Identifies gaps and redundancies in data sources used in a comprehensive community/population assessment. Examines the effect of gaps in data on PH practice/program planning.
   - Assures the application of ethical, legal, and policy principles in the collection, maintenance, use, and dissemination of data and information.
   - Synthesizes qualitative and quantitative data during analysis for a comprehensive community/population assessment. Uses various data collection methods and qualitative and quantitative data sources to conduct a comprehensive, community/population assessment.
   - Incorporates an ecological perspective when analyzing data from a comprehensive community/population assessment. Partners with groups, communities, populations, health professionals, and stakeholders to review and evaluate data collected.
   - Utilizes information technology effectively to collect, analyze, store, and retrieve data related to care of communities and populations.

   - Practices evidence-based PHN to promote health of communities and populations.
   - Collects data related to SDH and community resources to plan for community-oriented and population-level programs. Analyzes those data. Incorporates the results of those analyses into program planning.

2. **Policy Development/Program Planning Skills**
   - Identifies valid and reliable data relevant to health policies targeted to communities and populations. Conducts and uses policy analysis to address specific public health issues.
   - Plans population-level interventions guided by relevant models and research findings.
   - Conducts and uses policy analysis to address public health issues. Incorporates a wide range of policy options into the planning and delivery of health services and interventions to groups, communities, and populations.
   - Plans population-level interventions guided by relevant theories, concepts, models, policies, and evidence. Uses planning models, epidemiology, and other analytical methods in evaluating population-level interventions. Critiques the evidence for population-level interventions. Conducts and uses policy analysis to address specific public health issues.
   - Selects an appropriate method of decision analysis for an issue relevant to an identified group, community, or population. Uses planning models, epidemiology, and other analytical methods in the development and implementation of population-level interventions.
   - Manages the delivery of community/population-based health services. Evaluates and ensures compliance with public health laws and regulations.
   - Develops plans to implement programs and organizational policies. Works as part of an interdisciplinary team to implement relevant policies into community/population-level interventions.
   - Manages the implementation of organizational policies and programs for areas of responsibility.
   - Designs an evaluation plan that addresses multiple variables, includes both process and outcome measures, and uses multiple data collection methods. Conducts evaluation of care delivery to communities and populations served by the organization. Provides feedback on the organization's quality improvement program. Establishes methods to utilize technology to collect data to monitor and evaluate the quality and effectiveness of programs for communities and populations.
   - Identifies a variety of sources and methods to access public health information for a community/population. Utilizes technology to collect

(continued)

DISPLAY 15–1 QUAD COUNCIL CORE COMPETENCIES OF PUBLIC HEALTH NURSING (2011) *(Continued)*

data to monitor and evaluate the quality and effectiveness of programs for populations.

- Develops quality improvement indicators and core measures as part of the process to improve public health programs and services. Utilizes quality improvement indicators and core measures as part of the process to improve public health programs and services.

3. Communication Skills

- Assesses the health literacy of communities/populations served.
- Communicates effectively in writing, orally, and electronically. Communications are characterized by critical thinking and complex decision-making.
- Solicits input from community/population members and stakeholders when planning health care programs.
- Utilizes a variety of methods to disseminate public health information tailored to communities/populations.
- Demonstrates presentation of targeted health information and outcomes of evidence-based practice (EBP) to multiple audiences, including community and professional groups.
- Communicates effectively with community groups, partners, and interprofessional teams.
- Articulates role of public health within the overall health system to internal and external audiences.

4. Cultural Competency Skills

- Utilizes social and ecological determinants of health to develop culturally responsive interventions with communities and populations.
- Uses epidemiological data, concepts, and other evidence to analyze the SDH when developing and tailoring population-level health services. Applies multiple methods and sources of information technology to better understand the impact of SDH on communities and populations.
- Plans health services to meet the cultural needs of diverse communities and populations.
- Explains the interplay of multiple forces contributing to cultural diversity.
- Serves as an advocate to build a diverse public health workforce.
- Uses evidence and awareness of cultural models to tailor interventions to diverse populations. Evaluates current population health programs for evidence of cultural tailoring. Evaluates staff development needs related to cultural competency.
- Uses evidence and cultural models to tailor program level interventions.

5. Community Dimensions of Practice Skills

- Utilizes an ecological perspective in health assessment, planning, and interventions with communities and populations.
- Provides population health expertise for community-based participatory research (CBPR) teams.
- Identifies need for community involvement and partners to create community groups/coalitions.
- Identifies mechanisms for enhancing collaboration among stakeholders in population-focused health interventions. Develops partnerships with key stakeholders and groups.
- Partners effectively with key stakeholders and groups in care delivery to communities/populations.
- Identifies areas for community involvement in agency programs and initiatives. Critiques the evidence on approaches to fostering community partnerships and involvement. Uses evidence-based guidelines and effective group processes to partner with community members and groups.
- Explains to community groups and partners the role of government and the private and non-profit sectors in the delivery of community health services.
- Utilizes community assets and resources to promote and deliver care to communities/populations.
- Uses input from a variety of community/aggregate stakeholders in development of public health programs and services.
- Advocates for public health policies, programs, and resources that better serve populations.

6. Basic Public Health Sciences Skills

- Utilizes public health and nursing science to practice at population and community level.
- Describes the influence of sentinel events on current PHN practice.
- Uses EBP to assure population-level programs contribute to meeting core public health functions and the 10 essential services.
- Uses descriptive and analytical methods and public health sciences to design, implement, and evaluate interventions at community and population level.
- Synthesizes research across disciplines related to public health concerns and population-level interventions.
- Identifies gaps in the scientific evidence related to public health issues, concerns, and population-level interventions.
- Identifies a wide variety of sources and methods to access public health information, for example, geographic information system (GIS) mapping. Identifies gaps and inconsistencies in research evidence for practice.

DISPLAY 15–1 QUAD COUNCIL CORE COMPETENCIES OF PUBLIC HEALTH NURSING (2011) *(Continued)*

- Incorporates the requirements of patient confidentiality, human subject protection, and research ethics into data collection and processing.
- Disseminates theory-guided and/or EBP outcomes in peer-reviewed journals and national level meetings. Facilitates research projects with organizations.

7. **Financial Management and Planning Skills**
   - Collaborates with relevant public and/or private systems for managing programs in public health.
   - Supervises the operations of health programs within federal, state, tribal, and local public health agencies.
   - Develops partnerships with communities and agencies within federal, state, tribal, and local levels of government that have authority over public health situations, such as emergency preparedness.
   - Implements the judicial and operational procedures of the governing body and/or administrative unit designated with oversight of public health organizational operations.
   - Develops a programmatic budget.
   - Manages care delivery to communities/populations within current and forecasted budget constraints.
   - Develops strategies for determining budget priorities based on financial input from federal, state, tribal, and local sources.
   - Assesses impact of organizational budget priorities on PHN programs and practice. Establishes organization PHN resource priorities that assure effective PHN practice.
   - Designs evaluation plans for population-focused programs. Implements evaluation plans for population-focused programs.
   - Leads revisions to population-focused programs based on formative and summative evaluation results.
   - Develops proposals for funding from external sources.
   - Applies basic human relations and conflict management skills in interactions with direct reports, other professionals, and health care team members.
   - Identifies opportunities to use health care technologies and informatics to improve public health program and business operations. Incorporates health care technology and informatics to improve public health program and business operations.
   - Assists in the development of contracts and other agreements for the provision of services.
   - Describes how cost-effectiveness, cost–benefit, and cost–utility analyses affect programmatic prioritization and decision-making. Employs cost-effectiveness, cost–benefit, and cost–utility analyses for programmatic prioritization and decision-making.
   - Participates in implementation and evaluation of performance management systems.

8. **Leadership and Systems Thinking Skills**
   - Addresses ethical issues related to the PHN care of communities/populations.
   - Applies system theory to PHN practice with communities and populations.
   - Leads team and community partners in identifying vision, values, and principles for community action.
   - Analyzes internal and external factors that may impact the delivery of essential public health services. Implements strategies to assure quality, collaboration, and coordination in delivery of PHN services.
   - Leads interprofessional team and organizational learning opportunities. Provides leadership in staff development.
   - Implements opportunities to mentor, advise, coach, and develop peers, direct reports, and other members of the public health workforce.
   - Uses evidence-based models to design and implement quality initiatives. Establishes indicators to monitor organizational performance.
   - Adapts program delivery to communities/populations in consideration of changes in the public health system and larger social, political, and economic environment. Assesses outcomes of current health policy relevant to public health/PHN practice.

Note: Tier 1 competencies cover generalist PHNs, and tier 2 competencies cover PHNs with program implementation and supervisory/management duties that may include clinical services, home visiting, and community-based and population-focused programs. Tier 3 competencies refer to senior management or executive level PHNs in administrative/leadership roles at public health agencies or organizations. Refer to the complete document for a total list of competencies at all three levels.

From Swider, S., Krothe, J., Reyes, D., & Cravetz, M. (2013). The Quad Council practice competencies for public health nursing (pp. 525–536). *Public Health Nursing, 30*(6), 519–536. Used with permission.

Interacting with the Community

All steps of the nursing process depend on **interaction**, reciprocal exchange, and influence among people. Although nurse–client interaction is often an implied or assumed element in the process, it is an essential first consideration for community health nursing (see Chapter 10 for more details). Listening to a group of elderly people, teaching a class of expectant mothers, lobbying in the legislature for the poor, working with parents to set up a dental screening program for children—all these involve

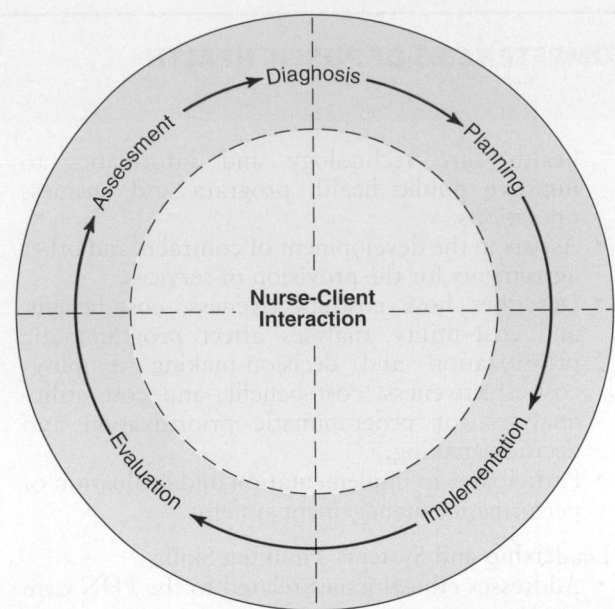

FIGURE 15–6 NURSING process components. Nurse–client interaction, a preamble structure, forms the core of the process. As a nurse and client maintain a reciprocal exchange of information and trust through interaction, they can effectively assess client needs, diagnose needs, and plan, implement, and evaluate care.

relationships, and relationships require interaction. Mutual give and take between nurse, clients, and community stakeholders—whether a family, a group of mothers on a Native American reservation, or representatives from resource agencies within the community—is an expected and much needed skill that should be integrated throughout the nursing process (see Fig. 15–6).

Need for Communication

When a community health nurse initially contacts a group of community leaders, for example, any information the nurse may have in advance can give only partial clues to that group's needs and wants. Unless everyone involved talks and listens, the steps of the nursing process will go awry (LeBan, 2011). PHNs can serve as effective liaisons—facilitating communication between stakeholders and clients to ensure that health needs both identified and adequately addressed (University of Michigan Center of Excellence in Public Health Workforce Studies, 2013).

Interaction and Effective Communication

Through open and honest sharing, the nurse (and others on the health team) will begin to develop trust and establish lines of effective communication. For instance, the nurse explains who he is and why he is there. The nurse encourages the group members to talk about themselves. Nurse and group members together discuss their relationship and clarify the desired nature of that alliance (Pavlish & Pharris, 2012). Does the group want help to identify and work on its health needs? Would its members like this nurse to continue regular contacts? What will their respective roles be? Effective communication, as a part of interaction, is essential to develop understanding and facilitate a free exchange of information between nurse and client.

Interaction is Reciprocal

Sharing of information, ideas, feelings, concerns, and self goes both ways. Nurses must avoid the temptation either to do all the talking or merely to listen while a few group members monopolize the conversation (Rost & Wilson, 2013). A dynamic exchange must exist between two systems. The community health nurse (and other collaborating health professionals) represents one system and the client group represents the other. Health care professionals tend to prioritize based on their own perspective and many times neglect to take the clients' wishes into account. Whether the client is a parent group, a homeless population, or an entire community, this exchange involves a two-way sharing between the nurse and client group. The key elements of interaction are mutuality and cooperation.

Consider the following example: Members of a disadvantaged community met for several weeks at a community center to discuss disease management, physical activity, and healthy diets. After their agreed-upon goals had been accomplished, the nurse wondered whether further meetings were needed. After several discussions, the residents verbalized concern about unsafe conditions within the neighborhood that limited physical activity of the residents and the lack of fresh food availability within the community. These external conditions would limit the residents' ability to adopt the healthy behaviors they had learned in the group. The nurse initially felt unprepared to address these issues, but after consulting with other support agencies within the community, she realized that resources were available and was able to work with community members and local agencies to develop a feasible physical activity plan for residents. Engagement with community members and communication were the first step in reapplying the nursing process and allowed goals for the group to be accomplished.

Interaction Paves the Way for a Helping Relationship

As nurse and client interact, each learns about the other. A test period occurs before trust can be fully established (Summach, 2011). For the female school nurse working with middle school students about health education and human sexuality, establishing interaction was more difficult at the time of the initial contact with the boys than with the girls. They had been reluctant to talk and felt embarrassed to discuss personal subjects with an adult they did not know. Nonetheless, their interests in body-building and personal appearance were strong enough to them to these optional sessions. Interaction began with a friendly exchange on nonthreatening topics and gradually deepened, as the boys seemed ready to discuss personal subjects. Eventually, it was relatively simple to talk about a new "problem" (and start the nursing process over again), because a helping relationship had already been developed. The nurse had a track record. The boys trusted, respected, and liked the nurse, so they were happy to interact around a newly stated need.

Aggregate Application

As noted in earlier chapters, community health practice focuses largely on the health of population groups; therefore, interaction goes beyond the one-on-one with individual patients. The challenge that the community health nurse faces is a one-to-aggregate approach. A group of parents concerned about teenage alcohol abuse, physically disabled people needing access ramps, and a neighborhood's older adult population frightened by muggings and thefts are all aggregates or clients with different concerns and opinions. As defined in Chapter 1, an aggregate refers to a mass or grouping of distinct individuals who are considered as a whole and who are loosely associated with one another. Each person in an aggregate is influenced by the thoughts and behavior of other group members. Nursing interaction with an aggregate client demands an understanding of group behavior, group dynamics, and group-level decision-making. It requires interpersonal communication skills applied at the group level. Interaction is more complex with an aggregate than with an individual, but it also can be challenging and rewarding. Once community health nurses acquire an understanding of aggregate behavior, they can capitalize on the potential of group influence to make a far-reaching impact on the health of the total community (see Perspectives for an example of a public health nurse partnering with law enforcement to provide preventive health care to gang youth). Chapter 10 more closely examines communication and interaction with groups.

Forming Partnerships and Building Coalitions

Another important consideration in community-level nursing practice requires teamwork. The job of planning for the health of an entire community or a community subsystem requires that the nurse collaborate with other professionals. Usually, the nurse is part of an organized team, separate from the agency that employs the nurse. The team is brought together with the goal of improving the health of the community. Each group member brings expertise and a particular view of the problem. These interprofessional work groups are often formed as either partnerships or coalitions (Wyer, Umscheid, Wright, Silva, & Lang, 2015).

Partnerships are agreements between people (and agencies) that support a joint purpose (Beal, 2012). A partnership can be large (e.g., a multinational corporation and several high schools; a city government and the county jail system), or it can be a more modest endeavor (e.g., a group of senior citizens and a preschool program; a Girl Scout troop and a community recycling program). Community-wide partnerships require more planning and coordination than do small partnerships. For example, because of increased student enrollment, a college may need two additional temporary and part-time faculty members who can teach the PHN course. The county public health department is interested in more new graduate nurses coming to work in the agency. The nursing program and the health department form a partnership and design a plan to solve both problems. The health department selects two staff nurses who have master's degrees and are qualified to teach undergraduate clinical courses in PHN one day a week for two semesters. The benefits for everyone are numerous. The nursing program solves a temporary staffing problem; the nurses from the health department share their expertise with students, enhancing their practice and the students'

learning experience; and the health department successfully introduces a pool of students, who may be potential staff members, to the agency and the services that it provides for the community.

A **coalition** is an alliance of individuals or groups that work together to influence the outcomes of a specific problem (Clark et al., 2011; Trinh-Shevrin et al., 2011). Coalitions are an effective means to achieve a collaborative and coordinated approach to solving community problems (Anderson, Adeney, Shinn, Krause, & Safranek, 2012). Steps to coalition building include defining goals and objectives, conducting a community assessment, identifying key players or leaders, and identifying potential coalition members (CDC, 2015c). Once these steps have been accomplished, the leader needs to keep the coalition active. This is best done by knowing and staying in touch with the coalition members, running effective meetings, and keeping every participant involved. An example of a successful coalition is an Asian American hepatitis B program using CBPR as a means of community assessment and providing pooled resources for this community in New York City (Trinh-Shevrin et al., 2011).

Sound public health practice depends on pooling resources—including people—in ways that will best serve the public. Whether health service is aimed at families, groups, subpopulations, populations, or communities, the consumers of that service are equally important members of the team. In planning for a community's health, the community (represented by appropriate individuals and agencies) must be involved. Community health nurses cannot lose sight of the need for client involvement at all levels and in all stages of community health practice (see Perspectives: Voices From the Community).

Types of Community Needs Assessment

After considering the importance of community partnerships and coalitions, the community health nurse is ready to determine the community's health status, resources, and needs. Assessment is the key initial step of the nursing process. Assessment for nurses means collecting and evaluating information about a community's health status to discover existing or potential needs and assets as a basis for planning future action (Anderson & McFarlane, 2015). Assessments are also a critical requirement for public health department accreditation (Public Health Accreditation Board, 2013) and are now a requirement for nonprofit hospitals under the Affordable Care Act, or health care reform, a program supported by nurses (Rice et al., 2014; ANA, 2014).

Several models or frameworks can be used for assessment. Three such models are Mobilizing for Action through Planning and Partnerships (MAPP) and Protocol for Assessing Community Excellence in Environmental Health (PACE EH). These models have been developed through partnership with the Centers for Disease Control and Prevention (CDC) to improve community assessment in relation to Healthy People goals (CDC, 2015a). An earlier tool, the Planned Approach to Community Health (PATCH), was developed to assist communities in assessing health promotion and chronic disease prevention programs (NACCHO, 2012). The *Healthy People 2020* website also provides planning tools and toolkits to assist local communities (see Internet

PERSPECTIVES
VOICES FROM THE COMMUNITY

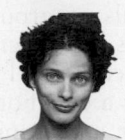

Public Health Nurse

I am a public health nurse, married to a Los Angeles–area police officer. His job with a juvenile diversion program for 13- to 18-year-old offenders (gang youth or those at risk of gang involvement) includes organizing a semester-long course to build confidence and self-esteem, as well as physical training and education in a classroom setting. Various officers teach the course, and they invite guest speakers. I ended up being a guest speaker for three 3-hour sessions and loved it! In order to prepare, I examined statistics and other assessment information about gangs as an aggregate. I noted that they have been found to have higher drug and alcohol use, earlier sexual initiation, and unsafe sexual practices with attendant higher rates of STIs (sexually transmitted infections). Higher rates of mental disorders, drug-related crime, and violent victimization are also hallmarks of gang membership. Basically, they are more likely to engage in high-risk behaviors, and I wanted to try to reach this aggregate that often has little access to health care. I thought this was a great opportunity to reach a vulnerable population and generate a discussion with them on health-related issues. I wanted it to be interactive and used examples they could identify with; I also spoke with some of their slang terms. The first session addressed major causes of morbidity and mortality among their age group. I showed them a photograph of a car involved in a crash due to driver texting and discussed the dangers of racing cars, driving drunk, and driving while distracted (as this driver had done). I started a discussion with them about homicide statistics and asked how this has personally affected them. I also gave them information about suicide and hotline numbers. At the second session, I wanted to focus on major health issues (e.g., obesity, drug use, mental and sexual health) and addressed each by highlighting the health consequences, behaviors that needed to change, and how they could prevent problems and access care when needed. We discussed obesity, and I brought examples of food nutrition labels, especially from fast food restaurants they frequented. They were amazed at the calories and fat levels, so we discussed healthier alternatives. At the last session, I focused on health promotion and risk prevention. I emphasized testicular and breast self-exams (yes, there were girls) and encouraged medical screening for STIs, with information on free clinics in their areas.

Although no formal evaluation of the program was done, I got great feedback from parents of the youth involved, who reported that their child's attitudes improved. Also, a good number of graduates of the program came back to work as student volunteers with subsequent cohorts. I felt a sense of accomplishment, having reached this difficult yet vulnerable population. I think that my openness and frankness in answering their questions and comfortable use of their slang terms developed rapport with them and permitted me to reach them with health information that they really needed to hear. I would encourage you to look for opportunities to do the same!

Alisha, BSN

Adapted from Sanders, B., Schneiderman, J., Loken, A., Lankenau, S., & Bloom, J. (2009). Gang youth as a vulnerable population for nursing intervention. Public Health Nursing, 26(4), 346–352.

Resources on *thePoint*). These are all valuable resources that provide specific guidelines focusing on local-level strategies to improve the health of communities.

Assessment involves two major activities. The first is collection of pertinent data, and the second is analysis and interpretation of data. These actions overlap and are repeated constantly throughout the assessment phase of the nursing process. While assessing a community's ability to enhance its health, the nurse may simultaneously collect data on community lifestyle behaviors and interpret previously collected data on morbidity and mortality.

Community health assessment is the process of determining the real or perceived needs of a defined community. In some situations, an extensive community study may be the first priority; in others, all that is needed is a study of one system or even one organization. At other times, community health nurses may need to perform a cursory examination or windshield survey to familiarize themselves with an entire community without going into any depth (Anderson & McFarlane, 2015).

Familiarization or Windshield Survey

A familiarization assessment is a common starting place in evaluation of a community. **Familiarization assessment** involves studying data already available on a community and then gathering a certain amount of firsthand data in order to gain a working knowledge of the community. Such an approach may utilize a **windshield survey**—an activity often used by nursing students in public health courses and by new staff members in community health

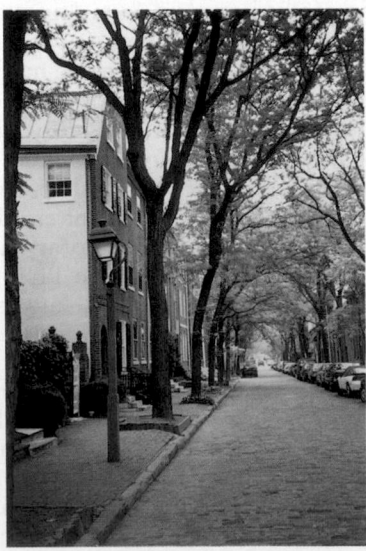

Windshield surveys are a quick way to become familiar with a new community and its residents.

agencies. Nurses drive (or walk) around the community of interest; find health, social, and governmental services; obtain literature; introduce themselves and explain that they are working in the area; and generally become familiar with the community and its residents. This type of assessment is needed whenever the community health nurse works with families, groups, organizations, or populations. The windshield survey provides knowledge of the context in which these aggregates live and may enable the nurse to better connect clients with community resources (Table 15–4). See an example in From the Case Files I.

Problem-Oriented Assessment

A second type of community assessment, **problem-oriented assessment**, begins with a single problem and assesses the community in terms of that problem. Suppose that Jean, the nurse who explored services available for the Angelo family's deaf child in From the Case Files I, had discovered that there were none. Confronted with this problem—one family with one deaf child—she could make a problem-oriented community assessment. Her first step would be to discover the incidence of childhood deafness, both in the community and in the state. Second, she might begin interviewing officials in the schools and

Table 15–4   Community Familiarization (Windshield) Survey

This is often done to help you become familiar with a new community or public health service area. Walking/driving around neighborhoods and interacting with community members can provide a context for further community assessment. You might begin at the local Chamber of Commerce or government building to determine history, current statistics, and demographics and to access maps and further resources for data you might use for a more formal community health assessment.

Physical
- Look at the age and conditions of the buildings, the density (apartments, houses on large lots) and materials used (bricks, plywood), and the zoning and maintenance of yards/empty lots. What clues does that give you about the community as a whole?
- How similar are the houses (are some neighborhoods very rich, others very poor)? Are there abandoned vehicles, piles of excess trash, large numbers of stray animals/for sale signs, or vacant houses?
- Are there open spaces (parks, agricultural areas, public/private areas like golf courses) and are they being used; by whom?
- Are there boundaries separating the community (e.g., natural boundaries like rivers, economic boundaries, commercial/residential boundaries)?
- What about air/water quality, signs of pollution?

Economic
- Does the area look like it is a thriving community?
- Are there areas where homeless gather? Soup kitchens?
- Is there adequate shopping (e.g., grocery stores, shopping centers)?
- Does it appear that food stamps are accepted/welcomed?
- Are there businesses, industries, manufacturing, and adequate places for employment? What is the unemployment rate?

Services
- Are there schools (how many, in what condition)? School nurses? What are the main concerns or problems with the educational system here (e.g., dropout rates)?
- Are there libraries? Do they provide additional services (e.g., Internet)? Are they well used?
- Are there recreational facilities (e.g., gyms, playgrounds, soccer fields, baseball diamonds)? Are these being used and by whom?
- How many churches do you see? What denominations?
- Is there adequate health care? Does the community have a hospital? Are there adequate health care services (e.g., physicians, clinics, nurses, mental health/substance abuse facilities, PH department services, nursing homes, traditional health care providers)? Is it a medically underserved area or a health professions shortage area?
- What types of social services are available (e.g., welfare/social workers, shelters, mental health counseling)? Do you see one main location for social services (e.g., government center) or are they dispersed around the community?
- What types of public/private transportation are available? Are highways and roads crowded with traffic? Accident rate? Are there bike paths/trails and adequate sidewalks? How is transportation access for the disabled?
- Does the community "feel" safe to you? Is there adequate fire and police protection? What is the crime rate? What are the most common types of crimes?
- Are there signs of political activity (e.g., posters, notices of meetings, predominant party affiliations)? Do people feel that they can be involved in decisions made by their local government?

Social
- Are there common "hangouts" (e.g., teen gathering spots, chess playing for older adults)? What about local newspapers, radio, and TV (e.g., satellite dishes)?
- Who do you see on the streets? Are there indications of homogeneity or diversity of ethnicities, languages spoken, SES (socioeconomic status), and occupations? How are people dressed?
- How do people feel about living in this community? What problems or concerns do they express? What strengths do they note? How "healthy" is their community?
- What are your impressions of this community?

Adapted from Anderson, E. T., & McFarlane, J. (2015). *Community as partner: Theory and practice in nursing* (7th ed.). Philadelphia, PA: Lippincott Williams & Wilkins.

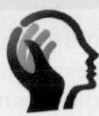

From the Case Files I

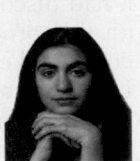

The Angelo Family and a Familiarization Assessment

A community health nurse named Jean visited the Angelo family on the outskirts of Philadelphia. During the initial visit, she gathered information, learning that the family was Italian American and that there were four children, ranging in age from 15 to 3. The father had been out of work for 6 months; the mother worked on weekends as a maid in a motel; the oldest boy had been in trouble with the juvenile authorities; the 13-year-old girl was deaf; and their house appeared rundown. Jean assessed this family, trying to determine its coping ability and its level of health. Furthermore, because community health nursing is population focused, her concern was not only for the Angelo family but also for the population of families with similar problems that this family represented.

However, the nurse's assessment was almost impossible without further knowledge of the community. Was theirs an Italian American neighborhood with specific cultural influences? What was the extent of unemployment in this city? What were the services for the deaf? Were all the houses in this part of town old and in need of repair? Once the nurse began working with the family, familiarity with the community became even more imperative. She discovered that, as a result of the Angelos'

low income, family conflicts were intense. The family members seldom got out; they made almost no use of the community's recreational system. Before she could help them make use of it, however, the nurse had to find out what resources were available. As she familiarized herself with the community, she discovered Friends of the Deaf, which sponsored a group for parents of deaf children. The nurse could now help Mr. and Mrs. Angelo become part of that group. A quick survey of the religious system in the community revealed two job-transition support groups, one of which would welcome Mr. Angelo. In the meantime, the nurse chose to find out about the public assistance or welfare system and how this family and other similar families could benefit from its services. Even her own attitude changed as she studied the community. For instance, she discovered that a strike had closed down the plant where Mr. Angelo worked for 20 years and could view his and others' unemployment from a broader perspective. Using a familiarization assessment helped this nurse to enhance her practice.

Whatever role nurses play in community health promotion, they will want to be making a continuous study, an ongoing assessment. Whether nurses become client advocates, work with the local government, or operate from a nursing agency serving the elderly, a familiarization assessment is prerequisite for their work.

---

health institutions to find out what had been done in the past to assist deaf children. She could do an Internet search to locate available resources on the subject of deafness. Are there interpreters available for people who use sign language? How do hospitals and courts approach deafness? Are there any clubs or other organizations for deaf people? Are there school programs for the deaf, and if so, where are they located?

The problem-oriented assessment can be used when familiarization is not sufficient and a comprehensive assessment is not feasible. This type of assessment is responsive to a particular need and should also seek to describe contextual issues associated with the need. The data collected can support community efforts to address specific problems. Data should address the magnitude of the problem to be studied (e.g., prevalence, incidence), the precursors of the problem, and information about population characteristics (e.g., community resources, strengths, and weaknesses), along with the attitudes and behaviors of the population being studied (Kirst-Ashman, 2014).

Community Subsystem Assessment

In **community subsystem assessment**, the community health nurse focuses on a single dimension of community life. For example, the nurse might decide to survey churches and religious organizations to discover their roles in the community. What kinds of needs do the leaders in these organizations

believe exist? What services do these organizations offer? To what extent are services coordinated within the religious system and between it and other systems in the community? For example, churches and other cultural leaders were instrumental in providing information to address a public health department's concerns. A small county health department worked with the nearby university PHN clinical instructor and her students to determine why two specific racial/ethnic groups were not using the health department's free women's health clinics. One group of students led by a Black student met with local pastors from several Black churches, and the other group, who was led by a Hmong student, met with Hmong leaders. Students attended the local Black churches on a particular Sunday and met with the congregation after the services to ask them about their knowledge and use of the health department's clinics. The students let them know about the available health services and answered questions. The health department followed up with the pastors, and it was determined that most of the members of the congregations were unaware of the services provided through the county health department. PHNs and other staff made efforts to regularly meet with members of the congregations to encourage their attendance at various clinics. For the Hmong population, students met with a local clan leader and several members of the community to inquire about the lack of attendance at the women's clinic. They were told that, with the Hmong culture, husbands generally accompanied their wives when getting prenatal care or family planning services. Also, they felt more comfortable with Hmong health care personnel than those from outside their group, and there happened to be a Hmong physician available to them in a larger neighboring county. The health department staff later met with members of the Hmong community to discuss their concerns, and it was determined that this population felt more comfortable not using health department services for women's health but would participate in well-child and immunization clinics. Working with and through these subsystems facilitated this process.

Community subsystem assessment can be a useful way for a team to conduct a more thorough community assessment. If five members of a nursing agency divide up the ten systems in the community and each person does an assessment of two systems, they could then share their findings to create a more comprehensive picture of the community and its needs.

Comprehensive Assessment

Comprehensive assessment seeks to discover all relevant community health information. It begins with a review of existing studies and all the data presently available on the community. A survey compiles all the demographic information on the population, such as its size, density, and composition. **Key informants** are interviewed in every major system—education, health, religious, economic, and others. Key informants are experts in one particular area of the community or they may know the community as a whole. Examples of key informants would be a school nurse, a religious leader, key cultural leaders, the local police chief or fire captain, a mail carrier, or a local city council person. Then, more detailed surveys and intensive interviews are performed to yield information on organizations and the various roles in each organization. A comprehensive assessment describes the systems of a community and also how power is distributed throughout the system, how decisions are made, and how change occurs (Anderson & McFarlane, 2015; LeBan, 2011).

Because comprehensive assessment is an expensive, time-consuming process, it is not often undertaken. Performing a more focused study, based on prior knowledge of needs, is often a better and less costly strategy. Nevertheless, knowing how to conduct a comprehensive assessment is an important skill when designing smaller, more focused assessments (see Perspectives: Public Health Nursing Instructor).

PERSPECTIVES
PUBLIC HEALTH NURSING INSTRUCTOR

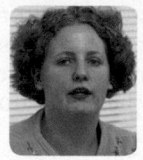

I have worked for many years in community and public health settings. I had been teaching community health nursing at a state university for 5 or 6 years when I decided to break from the "usual procedure" of having students do a comprehensive type of community assessment (all subsystems, vital statistics, etc.). This information did not change dramatically from the previous semester or the prior 2 to 3 years for that matter. Students hate busy work and I do, too! They had complained to instructors about this repetitive assignment (a classic learning activity in PHN coursework) for many years, and some were tempted to just repackage previous groups' assessments. I felt it would be more meaningful, but still have a population focus, if we could actually gather data and information for the small country health department where we were assigned. I asked several department heads to come up with ideas of aggregate or population assessment data that they needed (often related to grants they were writing or state-directed program evaluations). Several of them "pitched" these ideas and projects to our student group. The students then voted on the one they found most interesting or viable, and we set about creating our own community assessment template, usually drawing from standardized assessment tools. Each semester was different, depending upon the need. They would gather data, analyze it, and present it to the department head. From that assessment, they would create a project (often an educational intervention) that could be completed and evaluated within their time frame. They were excited to gather this information; it was like a bunch of detectives chasing down leads! They problem-solved

and worked together to achieve their goals. They worked with other agencies and NGOs; they spoke with local health care providers and members of the community. Once, the program director for a teen pregnancy program asked them to help with getting questionnaires distributed to local teens to gather information on sexual activity and attitudes. At that time, the county had the highest rate of teen pregnancies in the state, and one of the large universities in a metropolitan area was developing a survey to gather data on teen pregnancy and sexual activity in the state. This was a conservative county, and many parents opposed *Sex Ed*. However, students were able to gather information and statistics on teen pregnancies in this county and compared it with state and national data. They investigated best practices for teen pregnancy prevention programs. Forming into smaller work groups, some met with school officials, high school students, teachers, and parents in order to educate them about this project. Others worked with the program director and local school nurses and counselors. They were able to convince one school superintendent to distribute this survey to high school students in his district. The nursing students strategized about the best methods for distributing and collecting the surveys. The day came for the survey, and it was a rousing success, with no major roadblocks. They felt that their community assessment and project were worthwhile and very meaningful to this community. The health department and the university heartily agreed! I never went back to the "usual procedure," and I always encourage other instructors to try this approach.

Debbie, PHN Instructor

Community Assets Assessment

The final form of assessment presented here is **assets assessment**, also known as asset mapping. This method of assessment focuses on the strengths and capacities of a community rather than its problems (Jakes, Hardison-Moody, Bowen, & Blevins, 2015) and evaluates variables such as the needs that exist, the goals to be achieved, and the resources available for carrying out the study. Although it is difficult to determine the type of assessment needed in advance, understanding the various types of community assessment in advance helps to facilitate your decision. Based on a classic model developed by McKnight and Kretzmann in the 1980s (Kretzman & McKnight, 1993), the assets assessment provides a framework for conducting a complete functional community assessment and serves as a guide to the community for the nurse, as well as the foundation for community development. The previously mentioned methods are needs oriented and deficit based—in other words, they are *pathology* models, in which the assessment is performed in response to needs, barriers, weaknesses, problems, or perceived scarcity in the community. This may result in a fragmented approach to solutions for the community's problems rather than an approach focused on the community's possibilities, strengths, and assets. The assets assessment also provides the community the ability to "identify a variety and richness of skills, talents, knowledge, and experience of people" and "provides a base upon which to build new approaches and enterprises" (p. 4).

Assets assessment begins with what is present in the community (Jakes et al., 2015). The capacities and skills of community members are identified, with a focus on creating or rebuilding relationships among local residents, associations, and institutions to multiply power and effectiveness. This approach requires that the assessor look for the positive or see the glass as half full. The nurse can then become a partner in community intervention efforts, rather than merely a provider of services. Assets assessment includes three levels (Kramer, Seedat, Lazarus, & Suffla, 2011):

1. Specific skills, talents, interests, and experiences of individual community members such as individual businesses, cultural groups, and professionals living in the community.
2. Local citizen associations, organizations, and institutions controlled largely by the community such as libraries, social service agencies, voluntary agencies, schools, and police.
3. Local institutions originating outside the community controlled largely outside the community such as welfare and public capital expenditures (p. 14).

The key, however, is linking these assets together to enhance the community from within. The community health nurse's role is to assist with those linkages.

COMMUNITY ASSESSMENT METHODS

The health status of the community may be assessed using a variety of methods. Regardless of the assessment method used, data must be collected. Data collection in community health requires the exercise of sound professional judgment, effective communication techniques, and special investigative skills. Four important methods are discussed here: surveys, descriptive epidemiologic studies, community forums or town meetings, and focus groups.

Surveys

A **survey** is an assessment method in which a series of questions is used to collect data for analysis of a specific group or area. Surveys are commonly used to provide a broad range of data that will be helpful when used with other sources or if other sources are not available. To plan and conduct community health surveys, the goal should be to determine the variables (selected environmental, socioeconomic, and behavioral conditions or needs) that affect a community's ability to control disease and promote wellness. The nurse may choose to conduct a survey to determine such things as health care use patterns and needs, immunization levels, demographic characteristics, or health beliefs and practices. The survey method involves self-report, or response to predetermined questions, and can include questionnaires, telephone, or in person interviews (Polit & Beck, 2014). Survey findings can be combined with other health data in order to better understand the health status of the community and the determinants of health. These data include reports of health risks and outcomes by zip code (Agarwal, Menon, & Jaber, 2015; Wang, Ponce, Wang, Opsomer, & Yu, 2015) and CDC Environmental Health Tracking Network reports of local environmental health exposures (Charleston, Wilson, Edwards, David, & Dewitt, 2015). Consideration of these data along with survey results allows for a more comprehensive understanding of the communities health status and the conditions impacting health.

Descriptive Epidemiologic Studies

A second assessment method is a **descriptive epidemiologic study**, which examines the amount and distribution of a disease or health condition in a population by person (Who is affected?), by place (Where does the condition occur?), and by time (When do the cases occur?). In addition to their value in assessing the health status of a population, descriptive epidemiologic studies are useful for suggesting which individuals are at greatest risk and where and when the condition might occur. They have also long been known to be useful for health planning purposes and for suggesting hypotheses concerning disease etiology (Merrill, 2013). Their design and use are detailed in Chapter 7.

Geographic Information System Analysis

In Chapter 10, the concept of GIS was introduced as a health information technology. GIS technology is an integration of research methods and analytic techniques from both medical geography and spatial epidemiology. It has been well documented as a tool that can collect, organize, and display public health data (Graham, Carlton, Gaede, & Jamison, 2011), and it is widely used in assessment and research of health disparities, resources availability, and health-related behaviors (Auchincloss, Gebreab, Mair, & Roux, 2012).

Harvard's T.H. Chan School of Public Health offers a Web site designated to the use of GIS in public health, including particular research studies. For instance, one line of research examines effects of air pollution on MI rates within the community of Worcester and spatial mapping of incidence and levels of pollution. Researchers are also working on developing a predictive model for pollution's effect on death rates in Eastern Massachusetts. A prospective study of normative aging began with data collected from healthy cohort of 2,500 individuals in the 1970s; and GIS data on exposure is used to estimate cumulative exposure to pollution and its association with COPD, MI, and death (Harvard University, 2013). Earlier research has been useful in identifying air pollutant risk exposure (Hammond et al., 2011), and another common use of GIS is in planning for disaster response and support (Kawasaki, Berman & Guan, 2013; Wheeler & Basch, 2014).

Community Forums and Social Media

The community forum or town hall meeting is a qualitative assessment method designed to obtain community opinions (Fig. 15–7). It takes place in the neighborhood of the people involved, perhaps in a school gymnasium or an auditorium. The participants are selected to participate by invitation from the group organizing the forum. Members come from within the community and represent all segments of the community that are involved with the issue. For instance, if a community is contemplating building a swimming pool, the people invited to the community forum might include potential users of the pool (residents of the community who do not have pools and special groups such as the Girl Scouts, elders, and disabled citizens), community planners, health and safety personnel, and other key people with vested interests. They are asked to give their views on the pool: Where should it be located? Who will use it? How will the cost of building and maintaining it be assumed? What are the drawbacks to having the pool? Any other pertinent issues the participants may raise are included. This method is relatively inexpensive, and results are quickly obtained. A drawback of this method is that only the most vocal community members, or those with the greatest vested interests in the issue, may be heard. This format does not provide a representative voice to others in the community who also may be affected by the proposed decision.

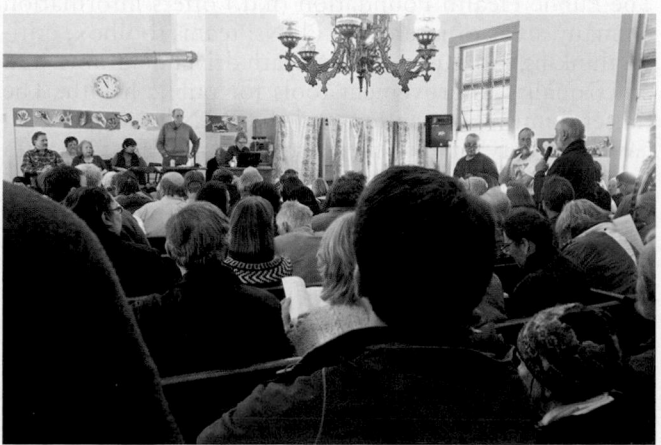

FIGURE 15–7   A town hall meeting in Vermont.

This method is used to elicit public opinion on a variety of issues, including health care concerns, political views, and feelings about issues in the public eye, such as school safety. Frequently, local cable television channels air important city government or school board meetings. Local news programs may hold town meetings, soliciting public opinion on regional issues. Other methods of opinion gathering include e-mailing (e.g., to a television news program) to support a particular view, Web-based survey sites (e.g., Survey Monkey), and using a toll-free phone number set up especially for text messaging a Yes or No vote on an issue.

Social media sites, like Facebook and Twitter, are also popular forums for opinion sharing. Digital media is often used to elicit grassroots opinions from local community members and has been utilized by many entities to enable political organization, including those in favor of health care reform and other social and political agendas (Howard & Parks, 2012; Gil de Zúñiga, Jung, & Valenzuela, 2012). See more ideas on the use of social media in Chapter 10.

Focus Groups

This fourth assessment method, focus groups, is similar to the community forum or town hall meeting in that it is designed to obtain grassroots opinion. However, it has some differences. First, only a small group of participants, usually 5 to 15 people, is present (Polit & Beck, 2014). The members chosen for the group are homogeneous with respect to specific demographic variables. For example, a focus group may consist of female community health nurses, young women in their first pregnancy, or retired businessmen. Leadership and facilitation skills are used in conjunction with the small group process to promote a supportive atmosphere and to accomplish set goals. The interviewer guides the discussion according to a predetermined set of questions or topics. The best use of focus group data includes not only an analysis of verbal messages but also behavioral data such as facial expressions (Stewart & Shamdasani, 2014). Major advantages of focus groups are their efficiency and low cost, similar to the community forum or town hall meeting format. A focus group can be organized to be representative of an aggregate, to capture community interest groups, or to sample for diversity among different population groups. One example is a research study involving adult e-cigarette users. Eleven focus groups were held to determine perceptions of e-cigarette efficacy in smoking cessation (Barbeau, Burda, & Siegel, 2013). Whatever the purpose, however, some people may be uncomfortable expressing their views in a group situation (Polit & Beck, 2014).

The choice of assessment method varies depending on the reasons for data collection, the goals and objectives of the study, and the available resources. It also varies according to the theoretical framework or philosophical approach through which the nurse views the community. In other words, the community health nurse's theoretical basis for approaching community assessment influences the purposes for conducting the assessment and the selection of methodology. For example, Neuman's health care systems model forms the basis for the "community-as-partner" assessment model developed by Anderson and

McFarlane (2015). Additional resources on methodologies for assessing community health (e.g., list of Internet resources, selected readings) are available on *thePoint*.

SOURCES OF COMMUNITY DATA

The community health nurse can look in many places for data to enhance and complete a community assessment. Data sources can be primary or secondary, and they can be from international, national, state, or local sources. Websites for many primary and secondary data sources are included in Internet resources on *thePoint*.

Primary and Secondary Sources

Community health nurses make use of many sources in data collection. Community members, including formal leaders, informal leaders, and community members, can frequently offer the most accurate insights and comprehensive information. Information gathered by talking to people provides primary data, because the data are obtained directly from the community. Secondary sources of data include people who know the community well and the records such people create in the performance of their jobs. Specific examples are health team members, client records, community health (vital) statistics, census bureau data, reference books, research reports, HEDIS measures, and community health nurses. Because secondary data may not totally describe the community and do not necessarily reflect community self-perceptions, they may need augmentation or further validation through focus groups, surveys, and other primary data collection methods.

International Sources

International data are collected by several agencies, including the World Health Organization (WHO) and its six regional offices and health organizations, such as the Pan-American Health Organization. The WHO publishes an annual report of their activity, and international statistics for diseases and illness trends can be found on the Internet (WHO, 2015). The WHO also publishes health statistics by country and information about specific diseases and health measures in their annual Global Health Observatory. This report tracks progress toward Millennium Health Goals that include poverty reduction, education improvements, and increased access to safe drinking water (WHO, 2014). Information from these official sources can give the nurse in the local community information about immigrant and refugee populations he serves. More information on international health agencies can be found in Chapter 16.

National Sources

Community health nurses can access a wealth of official and nonofficial sources of national data (see Chapter 6 for more information). Official sources develop documents based on data compiled by the government. The following are the major official agencies:

- **USDHHS.** This is the main agency from which data can be retrieved, and the National Center for Health Statistics (NCHS) at the **Centers for Disease Control and Prevention (CDC)** was specifically established under its auspices for the collection and dissemination of health-related data. This agency is the nation's principal health statistics agency, compiling data from many sources. These data provide information for many functions, including health status for various populations and subgroups, identification of disparities, monitoring trends, identifying health problems, and supporting research.
  - USDHHS also developed *Healthy People 2020* (USDHHS, 2016), designed to focus America's attention on the major national health problems, including realistic goals for national, state, and local agencies to work toward over one decade. Data from *Healthy People 2010* is available for analysis. Other data sources available through the CDC include Health Indicators Warehouse, Health Data Interactive, Surveillance Resource Center, Community Health Status Indicators, and VitalStats (CDC, 2015b).
- **U.S. Census Bureau.** This agency undertakes a major survey of American families every 10 years, gathering data on health, socioeconomic, and environmental conditions. This information is available on the Web or on a CD-ROM, allowing numerous variables to be viewed in combination, for easier development of a community profile (U.S. Census Bureau, n.d.).
- **National Institutes of Health (NIH).** This system of 27 institutes and centers, a part of the USDHHS, focuses on improving the health of the nation. An emphasis is placed on discovery of new cures or treatments and preventing disease. Employees of these agencies prevent, diagnose, and treat diseases and conduct research and disseminate research findings (NIH, 2015).

Nonofficial agencies have data sources generated from research they conduct that focuses on the population, disease, or condition they were developed to serve. Each agency collects data at the national level; however, the more accessible arm for services functions at state, county, and local levels. Examples of these agencies are the American Cancer Society (ACS), American Heart Association (AHA), the American Association of Retired Persons (AARP), Mothers Against Drunk Drivers (MADD), and Students Against Drunk Drivers (SADD). The Public Health Foundation (n.d.) offers information on many areas of interest to PHNs: teams toolbox, critical thinking tools, population heath driver diagrams, and other quality improvement tools for public health. The Kaiser Family Foundation and the RAND Corporation have a variety of fact sheets and compilations of data from various sources. The Gallup Poll provides national survey information on various topics, including health. Information from such national sources allows community health assessment teams to compare local data with national and state statistics and trends—a very valuable function. The Robert Wood Johnson Foundation's (2015) County Health Rankings and Roadmaps is based on a model of population health that emphasizes the many factors that, if improved, can help make communities healthier places to live, learn, work, and play. Proprietary data sources include the American Hospital

Association, the American Medical Association, or various health insurance companies. See Chapter 6 for a list of data collection systems.

State and Local Sources

For nurses, the most significant state source of assessment data comes from the state health department. This official agency is responsible for collecting state vital statistics and morbidity data. The Behavioral Health Surveillance System (BRFSS) is the world's largest telephone health survey that monitors health risk at the state level (CDC, 2012). Supported by the CDC, the information is used at various levels to identify risk and prevent disease. As a resource to local health departments, the state health department provides invaluable support services, and it is the main source of health-related data on the state level. Nonofficial agencies have state chapters or headquarters and compile their information at the state level. Local nonofficial agency chapters have documents of compiled state and national data on the population, disease, or condition they address.

State and county budgets or public health agency Web sites may also provide helpful information. All states collect vital statistics (e.g., births, deaths), and many collect information on hospitalization and morbidities related to infectious diseases, cancer, or cardiovascular disease. State departments of education may have school-based data on immunizations and overall school health. Information on traffic accidents, mental health, and environmental hazards are often available at the state level. States may also organize their statistics by county level, making it easier to compare your county's data with others.

Many sources of information may be obtained at the local level. Some key sources are the local visitor's bureau, city chamber of commerce, city planner's office, health department, hospitals, social service agencies, county extension office, school districts, universities or colleges, libraries, clergy, business and service organizations, and community leaders and key informants. Some of these sources compile their own statistics, but all have views of the community particular to their discipline, interest, or knowledge base. Some agencies at the local level develop city or county directories. These are updated periodically and are valuable resources for community health assessment teams and community health nurses. More detailed information on national, state, and local health agencies, and information available from them, can be found in Chapter 6.

Data Analysis and Diagnosis

This stage of assessment requires analysis of the information gathered, so that inferences or conclusions may be made about its meaning. Such inferences must be validated to determine their accuracy, after which a nursing diagnosis can be formed.

The Analysis Process

First, the data must be validated: Are they accurate, complete, representative of the population, and current? Several validation procedures may be used (Northwest Center for Public Health Practice, n.d.):

- Data can be rechecked by the community assessment team.

- Data can be rechecked by others.
- Subjective and objective data can be compared.
- Community members can consider the findings and verify them.

Validated data are then separated into categories such as physical, social, and environmental data. In many instances, data spreadsheets are used to provide a structure for data organization. Next, each category is examined to determine its significance. At this point, there may be a need to search for additional information to clarify the meaning of the data. Only then can inferences be made and a tentative conclusion about the meaning of the data be reached (Anderson & McFarlane, 2015).

Some computer programs are designed to analyze community assessment data. For large, complex, or ongoing community assessment plans, this may be the best method. For smaller, one-time assessments, the paper-and-pencil method may be sufficient and less unwieldy. Some communities may hire an outside professional assessment service. These teams often use the latest technology when analyzing data. Not all communities can afford such a service, and if key leaders become familiar with assessment, analysis, and diagnostic processes, an investment in a computer program may be worthwhile. GIS technology, as noted earlier, is proving very useful in community assessment. These tools are becoming more user friendly and cost-effective and have been used to pinpoint incidences of various diseases, display environmental risks, note the location of health care facilities, and determine accurate community boundaries (Auchincloss et al., 2012; McEntee & Agyeman, 2010). Regardless of the analysis method used, data interpretation remains a critical phase of the process.

In data interpretation, the ever-present danger exists of making inaccurate assumptions and diagnoses. The importance of validation cannot be overemphasized. Before making a diagnosis, all assumptions must be validated: Are they sound? Community members should participate actively in validation efforts by clarifying perceptions, explaining the circumstances surrounding the situation, and acting as sounding boards for testing assumptions. Other resources, such as the health team members and community leaders, are used to explore and confirm inferences. Data collection, data interpretation, and nursing diagnosis are sequential activities, with validation serving as the bridges between them (Fig. 15–8). When performed thoroughly, these steps lead to accurate diagnoses.

Community Diagnosis Formation

The next step of the nursing process, after analysis, is the development of the community diagnosis. Community diagnoses stems from analysis of assessment data. The diagnosis "describes a situation" and "implies a reason" or etiology focusing on a specific community (Anderson & McFarlane, 2015). Various taxonomies and classification systems are used in nursing to describe specific nursing problems, and each one has its limitations when dealing with community-level diagnoses. The North American Nursing Diagnosis Association (NANDA) is much more oriented to nursing diagnoses of individuals

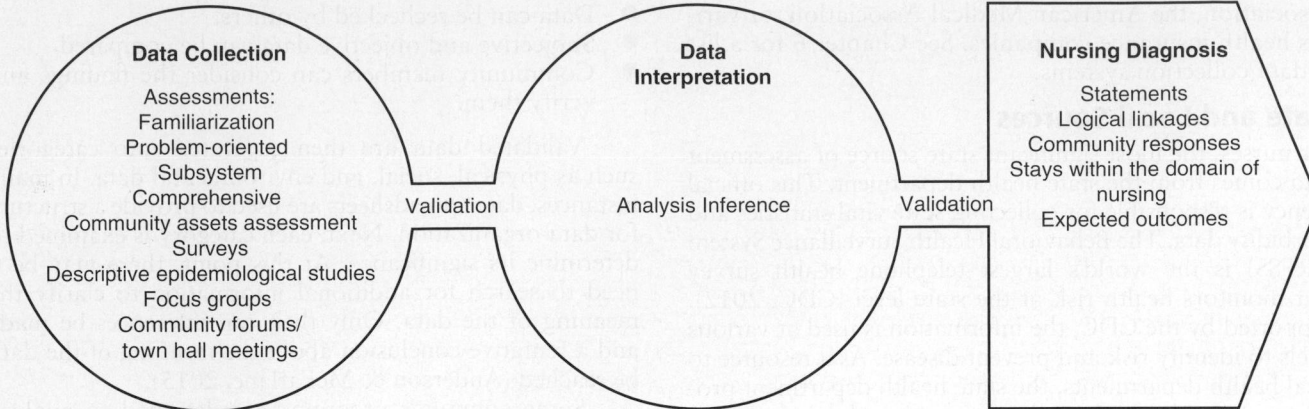

FIGURE 15-8   Assessment and Diagnosis Phases of the Nursing Process. Interpretation of data leads to diagnosis of a community's needs, the community responses, and expected outcomes.

and families than to community-level problems. Nursing Outcomes Classification (NOC) is also generally individual oriented. The Omaha System, originally designed by the Omaha Visiting Nurse Association, is again primarily used in nursing diagnoses of individuals, families, and small groups, and some community health applications have been developed (Omaha System, 2015).

This chapter discusses nursing diagnosis as characterized by Neufeld and Harrison (1996), based on the classic work of Mundinger and Jauron (1975). These authors proposed the use of nursing diagnoses in the community by substituting the term *client, family, group,* or *aggregate* for the word *patient.* Their definition of a nursing diagnosis is (Neufeld & Harrison, 1996, p. 221)

> The statement of a [client's] response which is actually or potentially unhealthful and which nursing intervention can help to change in the direction of health. It should also identify essential factors related to the unhealthful response.

Neufeld and Harrison (1996, p. 221) built on this work to form a wellness diagnosis by using the phrase *healthful response* instead of *unhealthful response.* Their definition of a wellness diagnosis is

> ...the statement of a client's [or community's] healthful response which nursing intervention can support or strengthen. It should also identify the essential factors related to the healthful response.

In 1996, Stolte developed a manual dedicated solely to nursing wellness diagnosis. Carpenito (2012) incorporated both community diagnosis and wellness diagnosis into her well-known handbook on applying nursing diagnosis to clinical practice. By substituting the term *community* for client, family, group, or aggregate, the nursing or wellness diagnosis can be applied to the community as a whole. These diagnoses identify the conclusion the nurse draws from interpretation of collected data and describe a community's healthy or unhealthy responses that can be influenced or changed by nursing interventions. Change comes about through collaboration with other community and health team members.

In community health, nurses do not limit their focus to problems; they consider the community as a total system and look for evidence of all kinds of responses that may influence the community's level of wellness (as shown in Fig. 15-6). Responses encompass the whole health–illness continuum, from specific deficits, such as a lack of senior centers or day care programs, to opportunities for maximizing a community's health, such as promoting farmer's markets for better access to fresh fruits and vegetables or improving the safety of the roadways. The statement of community response—the diagnosis—can focus on a wide range of topics.

Community Diagnoses

Data have been gathered from a variety of sources and have been validated by several means. The data have been recorded, tabulated, analyzed, and synthesized, so that patterns and trends can be seen. The use of charts, graphs, and tables assists in visualizing the synthesized data. The community assessment team should present their findings to peers and colleagues and use their expertise to assist in the formulation of the community diagnoses. Inferences are drawn from the data, and these statements refer to *actual* or *potential* problems. Additional statements involve *etiology,* by stating that this condition is *related to* certain conditions or problems. There may be a number of these statements, involving several subsystems, for every one diagnosis. Signs and symptoms of the diagnosis relate to the *magnitude* or *duration* of the problem, usually documented "as manifested by" (Anderson & McFarlane, 2015).

Continuing with the nursing process format, nursing diagnoses for the community are developed. **Community diagnoses** refer to nursing diagnoses about a community's ineffective coping ability and potential for enhanced coping. The statements about the community should include the strengths of the community and possible sources for community solutions, as well as the community's weaknesses or problem areas. Using the standard nursing diagnosis format, community-level diagnoses can be developed (Carpenito, 2012). These diagnoses are used as tools as the community begins to plan, intervene, and evaluate outcomes. Diagnostic categories for individuals (e.g., knowledge deficit of senior services, high risk for injury or falls) can often be applied at the community level. Community-level nursing diagnoses should portray a community focus, include the community response, and identify any related factors that have potential for change through community health nursing. These may also include wellness diagnoses, which indicate maintenance or potential change responses (due to growth and development), when no deficit is present. Community nursing diagnoses must also include statements that are narrow enough to guide interventions, have logical linkages between community responses and related factors, and include factors within the domain of community health nursing intervention.

Examples of wellness and deficit community nursing diagnoses and several diagnoses for a specific community follow:

1. *Wellness nursing diagnosis for an assisted living community of elders.* The senior residents of an assisted living center (*community focus*) have the potential for achieving optimal functioning related to (*host factors*) their expressed interest in exercise, diet, and meaningful activities and to (*environmental factors*) their access to exercise opportunities, nutritional information, and social outlets.

2. *Deficit community nursing diagnosis for a rural farmworker community.* The inhabitants of (*name of the town*) in (*name of the state*) are at risk for illness and injury related to (*host factors*) exposure to pesticides, lack of motivation to add or use safety devices on farm machinery, lack of safety knowledge, choice to take unnecessary risks (*environmental factors*), lack of family income to purchase newer equipment, and long hours of work that lead to stress and exhaustion.

3. *Community diagnoses for Anytown, Kansas.* Anytown, Kansas, is experiencing an increase in crime, a problem compounded by the small size of the police force and an influx of many new community members. The community has worked together constructively in the past, communicates well, and has strong recreational outlets for community members. The community:

   • Has expressed vulnerability and feels overwhelmed related to threats to community safety
   • Has failed to meet its own expectations related to inadequate law enforcement services
   • Has expressed difficulty in meeting the demands of change related to an influx of new community members
   • Has a successful history of coping with a previous crisis of teenage pregnancy
   • Has positive communication among community members
   • Has a well-developed program for recreation and relaxation

Such diagnoses can guide communities toward maximizing or improving their health as they plan, implement, and evaluate changes to be measured by established outcome criteria. Broad goals can form the basis for planning

interventions. From these goals, more specific activities, interventions, and targeted programs can be designed. Measurable objectives can be written and evaluated (Anderson & McFarlane, 2015; Issel, 2014). **Outcome criteria** are measurable standards that community members use to measure success as they work toward improving the health of their community. Outcome-based or evidence-based nursing practice applies to aggregates in the community as well as to patients in acute care settings.

Nursing diagnoses change over time because they reflect changes in the health status of the community; therefore, diagnoses need to be periodically reevaluated and redefined. The changing diagnosis can be a useful means of moving a community toward improved health because it gives community members a clear standard against which to measure progress.

PLANNING TO MEET THE HEALTH NEEDS OF THE COMMUNITY

Planning is the logical decision-making process used to design an orderly, detailed series of actions for accomplishing specific goals and objectives. Planning for community health is based on assessment of the community and the nursing diagnoses formulated, but assessment and diagnosis alone do not prescribe the specific actions necessary to meet clients' needs (Anderson & McFarlane, 2015; Minnesota Department of Health, n.d.a). Knowing that a group of mothers at the well-child clinic need emotional support does not tell the nurse what further action is indicated. A diagnosis of culture shock (adjustment deficit to a contrasting culture) for a family newly arrived from Cuba does not reveal what action to take. The nurse must systematically develop an appropriate plan (see Levels of Prevention Pyramid).

Tools to Assist with Planning

A wide variety of tools are available to enhance community health improvement planning; these include activity descriptions, templates, and models (Minnesota Department of Health, n.d.a; NACCHO, 2015). Such tools help prioritize health issues, develop goals and objectives, specify interventions, and anticipate client outcomes. Tools that assist with planning also enable the nurse to test ideas and adjust solutions before actual implementation. Finally, the use of standardized tools enhances the planning process and promotes effectiveness of services, as well as professional standards of practice.

In addition to using tools, a systematic approach guides the community health nurse in the development of a feasible plan that adequately and appropriately addresses the needs of the community (Anderson & McFarlane, 2015). As they do in the rest of the nursing process, community health nurses collaborate with clients and other appropriate professionals throughout each of these planning activities.

The Health Planning Process

The health planning process is a four-stage system used to design new health-related programs or services in the community. The process is often used by health educators when designing educational programs or by

LEVELS OF PREVENTION PYRAMID

THE PROBLEM OF CHILD ABUSE

SITUATION: Desire to reduce the incidence of child abuse in a given community by 50% within 2 years.
GOAL: Using the three levels of prevention, negative health conditions are avoided, or promptly diagnosed and treated, and the fullest possible potential is restored.

TERTIARY PREVENTION

Rehabilitation	Primary Prevention	
	Health Promotion and Education	*Health Protection*
• Establish rehabilitation programs for abused children, including safe home placement, physical and emotional treatment, and self-esteem building • Rebuild the family unit if appropriate or possible	• Provide family life education programs for families • Develop resources to support health promotion programs	• If unable or inappropriate to rehabilitate the abuser or family, keep abuser away from victim through incarceration or court order

SECONDARY PREVENTION

Early Diagnosis	Prompt Treatment
• Develop early detection programs through schools, clinics, and physicians' offices • Promote enforcement of child protection laws	• Establish programs to provide prompt treatment for abused children and abusing parents

PRIMARY PREVENTION

Health Promotion and Education	Health Protection
• Assess factors contributing to child abuse • Institute family life education programs through schools and community groups • Develop community resources to support health protection programs	• Identify families in the community who are at greatest risk (e.g., parents with history of child abuse, families under great stress) • Develop community resources to support health promotion programs

administrators in community health agencies when initiating new services. The nursing process is similar to the health planning process (Table 15–5). Each model helps to promote service effectiveness in addition to maintaining standards of practice. Community health nurses familiar with both the health planning process and the nursing process should be able to work collaboratively with community health professionals using either model.

Setting Priorities

Priority setting involves assigning rank or importance to the identified needs to determine the order in which goals should be addressed. There are numerous ways to set priorities in the planning process. Many have identified useful criteria that can guide ranking problems for order of action (CDC, n.d.; Issel, 2014; McGregor, Henderson, & Kaldor, 2014; National Association of County & City Health Officials, n.d.; Office of the Assistant Secretary for Planning and Evaluation, n.d.; Public Health Institute, 2012). They are presented here as a combination of criteria:

1. Significance of the problem or the number of people affected in the community

2. Level of community awareness of the problem
3. Community motivation to act on the problem (or, Is this important to the community?)
4. Nurse and partnership's ability to reduce risk and/or influence the solution
5. Cost of risk reduction in terms of financial, social, and ethical capital
6. Ability to identify a specific target population for an intervention
7. Availability of expertise to solve the problem within the partnership, coalition, or community
8. Severity of the outcome if left unresolved or the consequences of inaction
9. Speed with which the problem can be resolved

A common test for priority setting is called PEARL, an acronym for "propriety, economics, acceptability, resources, and legality" (Public Health Institute, 2012, p. 50). A priority matrix may also be developed, but decisions must not be unilateral and should include input from all stakeholders, including community members. For example, a community assessment revealed that a group of elderly residents living within a specific zip

Table 15–5 **Comparison Between the Health Planning Process and the Nursing Process**

Health Planning Process	Nursing Process
1. ASSESSMENT STAGE Determine data needed and collect data. Interpret data and identity needs. Set goals based on needs.	**1. ASSESSMENT** Determine data needed and collect data. Interpret data and identity needs. Set goals based on needs.
2. ANALYSIS AND DESIGN Analyze findings and set specific objectives. Design alternative interventions. Analyze and compare pros and cons of various solutions.	**2. DIAGNOSIS** Analyze findings and set specific objectives. Design alternative interventions. Analyze and compare pros and cons of various solutions. Formulate nursing diagnoses.
Create a plan.	**3. PLANNING** List needs in order of priority. Establish goals and objectives. Write an action plan.
3. IMPLEMENTATION STAGE Describe how to operationalize the plan. Design a method for monitoring progress.	**4. IMPLEMENTATION** Describe how to operationalize the plan. Design a method for monitoring progress.
4. EVALUATION STAGE Examine costs and benefits of proposed solution. Judge the potential outputs, outcomes, and impact of plan. Modify to achieve the best plan. Present plan to sponsoring group or agency. Obtain acceptance (and funding).	**5. EVALUATION** Examine costs and benefits of proposed solution. Judge the potential outputs, outcomes, and impact of plan. Modify to achieve the best plan. Present plan to sponsoring group or agency. Obtain acceptance (and funding).

code were fearful of crime, but also identified the lack of public transportation as issues to be addressed. Using the above criteria, the community health nurse working in this community identified that 85% of residents of the community had fears about crime but did not see transportation as an issue. The residents saw crime as an important concern and were also motivated to act on the crime issue, but were not willing to explore the transportation issue at the current time. The nurse, along with the community coalition partners, would be better able to influence the crime problem by helping to form town watch groups and getting the local police district to provide increased patrols during evening hours when robberies were more likely to occur. However, the partners had little influence to extend the hours of operation on buses or influence the creation of new bus routes. Members of the coalition included the local police chief and chamber of commerce director. If the crime problem was left unchecked, more people could be adversely affected, including businesses, because people would not be willing to leave their homes to shop or might even be forced to move away. Finally, these initiatives could be put in place rather quickly and inexpensively after the formation and training of volunteer town watch groups. There certainly are no adverse social, economic, or ethical consequences attached to addressing this problem. Therefore, it would seem that the crime issue would take priority over the transportation issue. It is important to remember that each community diagnosis is examined separately and then compared. Priorities for action are discussed, ranked, and then prioritized for action (Hauck & Smith, 2015) (Fig. 15–9).

Establishing Goals and Objectives

Goals and objectives are crucial to planning and should be feasible, specific, and measurable (Anderson & McFarlane, 2015; CDC, n.d.). The diagnosis that identifies needs must be translated into goals to give focus and meaning to the nursing plan. **Goals** are broad statements

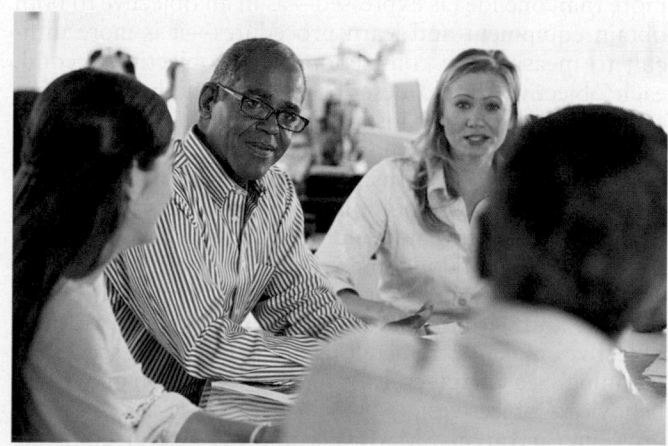

FIGURE 15–9 A team meeting held to develop goals and objectives.

of desired outcomes. **Objectives** are specific statements of desired outcomes, phrased in behavioral terms that can be measured. Target dates for expected completion of each objective are also stated. Objectives are the stepping-stones to help one reach the end results of the larger goal. For the elderly group concerned about crime in the neighborhood, the need, the goal, and the objectives were defined as follows:

- *Need*: The group of elderly people has altered coping ability related to their fear of crime.
- *Goal*: Within 6 months, this group of elderly people will feel comfortable to walk the streets of their neighborhood without experiencing any incidents of criminal assault.
- *Objectives*:
  1. By the end of the first month, a safety committee (composed of senior citizens, nurses, police, and other appropriate community members) will be established to study the crime patterns in the neighborhood.
  2. The safety committee will develop strategies for crime reduction and elder protection, which will be presented to the city council for approval by the end of the third month.
  3. Safety strategies, such as increased police surveillance, town watch patrols, and escort services, will be implemented by the end of the fifth month.
  4. By the end of the sixth month, nursing assessment will determine that senior citizens feel free to walk about the neighborhood.
  5. By the sixth month, there will be fewer reported incidents of criminal assault.

Development of objectives depends on a careful analysis of all the ways in which one could accomplish the larger goal. PHNs should first select the course of action that is best suited to meet the goal and then build objectives. For the group of elderly people, other alternatives, such as staying indoors or always walking in pairs, were considered and rejected. The ultimate choice was to find a way to make their environment safe and enjoyable.

Some rules of thumb are helpful when writing objectives. First, each objective should state a single idea. When more than one idea is expressed—as in an objective to both obtain equipment and learn procedures—it is more difficult to measure the completion of the objective. Second, each objective should describe one specific behavior that can be measured. For instance, the fourth objective from the list states that the seniors will report feeling free to walk outdoors within 6 months. It describes a behavior that can be measured at some point in time. One can more readily evaluate objectives that include specifics—such as what will be done, who will do it, and when it will be accomplished. Then it is clear to everyone involved exactly what has to be done and within what time frame. Writing measurable objectives makes a tremendous difference in the success of planning. See Chapter 11 for more information on writing behavioral objectives.

The acronym SMART is another useful guideline when writing objectives (Minnesota Department of Health, n.d.b). SMART objectives are

- **Specific:** Concrete, detailed, and well defined so that you know where you are going and what to expect when you arrive.
- **Measurable:** Numbers and quantities provide means of measurement and comparison.
- **Achievable:** Feasible and easy to put into action.
- **Realistic:** Considers constraints such as resources, personnel, cost, and time frame.
- **Time bound:** A time frame helps to set boundaries around the objective.

Planning means thinking ahead. The nurse looks ahead toward the desired end and then decides what intermediate actions are necessary to meet that goal. Sometimes, an objective itself describes the intermediate actions. At other times, an objective may be further broken down into several activities. For example, the second objective states that the safety committee will be charged with developing strategies, presenting them to the city council, and gaining their approval. Good planning requires this kind of detail.

Making decisions is an important part of planning. Decisions must be made during the process of establishing priorities. Decisions are necessary for selecting goals and for choosing the best course of action from many possible courses. Further decision-making is involved in selecting objectives and taking action to accomplish the objectives.

To facilitate planning and decision-making, the community health nurse involves other people. Clients must be included at every step because they are the ones for whom the planning is being done. Without their insight and cooperation, the plan may not succeed. Additionally, the involvement of other nurses may be important. Team meetings, nurse–supervisor conferences, and nurse–expert consultant sessions are all useful resources for planning. In addition, it is essential that you confer with members of other health and professional disciplines (e.g., teachers, social workers, mental health professionals, hospital representatives, city planners). Interdisciplinary team conferences are valuable for gaining a broader perspective and enlisting wider support for the evolving plan.

IMPLEMENTING HEALTH PROMOTION PLANS FOR THE COMMUNITY

Implementation is putting the plan into action. The nurse, other professionals, or clients carry out the activities of the plan. Implementation is often referred to as the action phase of the nursing process. In community health nursing, implementation includes not just nursing action or nursing intervention, but collaboration with clients, stakeholders, and other professionals. When bringing about change in a community organization, implementation involves the greatest commitment of time and planning. This often includes an implementation timetable, as well as funding or organizing physical/informational/staff/management resources, collaboration with outside agencies, training staff and working with community volunteers as needed for program implementation, and actually putting into action those interventions created during the planning phase (Anderson & McFarlane, 2015; Issel, 2014; Public Health Institute, 2012). Certainly, the nurse's professional expertise and judgment provide a necessary resource to the client group. The nurse is also a catalyst and facilitator in planning and activating the action plan. However, a primary goal in community health is to help people learn to help themselves in achieving their optimal level of health. To realize this goal, the nurse must constantly involve clients in the deliberative process and encourage their sense of responsibility and autonomy. Other health team members may also participate in carrying out the plan. All are partners in implementation.

Preparation

The actual course of implementation, outlined in the plan, should be fairly easy to follow if goals, expected outcomes, and planned actions have been designed carefully. Professionals and clients should have a clear idea of *who, what, why, when, where,* and *how.* Who will be involved in carrying out the plan? What are each person's responsibilities? Do all understand why and how to do their parts? Do they know when and where activities will occur? As implementation begins, nurses should review these questions for themselves, as well as for clients. This is the time to clarify any doubtful areas, thereby facilitating a smooth implementation phase. An operations manual may be needed, as well as organizational charts, clear budgets, and social marketing plans (Anderson & McFarlane, 2015; Issel, 2014).

Even the best planning may require adjustments. For example, some nurses who planned a health fair for seniors discovered that the target group would not have transportation to the site because the volunteering bus company had withdrawn its offer. To smoothly implement the plan, the nurses arranged for volunteers from local churches to pick up the seniors, bring them to the health fair, and deliver them afterward to their homes. Implementation requires flexibility and adaptation to unanticipated events.

Activities or Actions

The process of implementation requires a series of nursing actions or activities:

- The nurse applies appropriate theories, such as systems theory or change theory, to the actions being performed.
- The nurse helps to facilitate an environment that is conducive to carrying out the plan (e.g., a quiet room in which to hold a group teaching session or solicitation of support from local officials for an environmental cleanup project).
- The nurse and other health team members prepare clients to receive services by assessing their knowledge, understanding, and attitudes and by carefully interpreting the plan to clients. This interaction nurtures open communication and trust between nurse and clients. Professionals and clients (or representatives if the aggregate is large) form a contractual agreement about the content of the plan and how it is to be carried out.
- The plan is carried out, or modified and then carried out, by professionals and clients. Modification requires constant observation and interchange during implementation, because these actions determine the success of the plan and the nature of needed changes.

- The nurse and the team monitor and document the progress of the implementation phase by process evaluation, which measures the ongoing achievement of planned actions (Anderson & McFarlane, 2015; Issel, 2014).

EVALUATING IMPLEMENTED COMMUNITY HEALTH IMPROVEMENT PLAN

Evaluation is usually seen as the final step, but because the nursing process is cyclic in nature, the nurse is constantly evaluating throughout the entire process. For instance, in the assessment phase, the nurse must evaluate whether the collected data are sufficient and appropriate to beginning planning. Evaluation methods must be addressed during the planning phase as goals and objectives as well as interventions are identified (Anderson & McFarlane, 2015; Issel, 2014). **Evaluation** refers to measuring and judging the effectiveness of goal or outcome attainment. Too often, emphasis is placed primarily on assessing client needs and on planning and implementing service. The nursing process is not complete until evaluation takes place. Ideally, the nursing process should be observed as cyclical instead of linear, and when this occurs, it is obvious that evaluation guides the next assessment (Issel, 2014). The Community Toolbox (2015) provides suggestions for participatory evaluation that includes examination of the process (e.g., how the assessment was conducted), implementation (e.g., how the program was designed and executed), and outcomes (e.g., if desired results were accomplished). Appropriate questions include the following: Was all potential information assessed? How effective was the service provided? Were client needs truly met? How has health status changed? Professional practitioners owe it to their clients, themselves, and other health service providers to fully and effectively evaluate a program (see From the Case Files II).

As stated earlier, evaluation is an act of appraisal in which one judges value in relation to a standard and a set of criteria. Evaluation requires a stated purpose, specific standards, and criteria by which to judge and judgment skills.

Types of Evaluations

To determine the success of their planning and intervention, community health nurses use two main types of evaluation: formative and summative evaluation. The focus of *formative* evaluation is on process during the actual interventions. *Summative* evaluation focuses on the outcome of the interventions: Did you meet your goals? In formative evaluation, performance standards are developed and used to determine what is and is not working throughout the process. These could include the physical and organizational structure of the agency, as well as resources that provide a foundation for any interventions. Formative evaluation essentially looks at the step-by-step process of program implementation (Green, Sim, & Breiner, 2013). Could I do anything better or differently to increase my desired outcome? An example would occur when looking at the poor attendance at two sessions of an evening health promotion class for senior citizens. The nurse identifies the reason for poor attendance as being seniors' reluctance to attend an evening

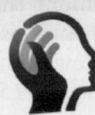

From the **Case Files II**

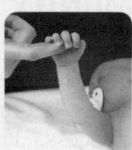

Evaluating Outcomes of a Home Care Postpartum Program

As a nurse working as the liaison between Capitol City Hospital and its home health agency, you are given the job of reviewing your early postpartum discharge program. Your program has been in effect for 18 months. Client satisfaction is high. The program has increased revenue for the hospital as many clients choose to deliver at Capitol City Hospital because of the early discharge program.

The protocol for your early discharge program includes a postpartum home visit by an RN from the home health agency. These visits are provided as a service to the client. In some cases, visits are billable to insurance companies. Medicaid authorizes payment for one postpartum visit.

You have gathered the following information about the early discharge program:

I. Protocol: Standard is one visit within 48 hours after discharge, which includes
   A. Education:
      1. Newborn care
      2. Breast-feeding
      3. Warning signs warranting follow-up (mother and baby)
         – Infection
         – Hemorrhage
      4. Comfort
      5. Parenting
      6. Sexuality
         – Resumption of sexual activity
         – Contraception
      7. Community resources
      8. Nutrition
      9. Well and sick baby care
   B. Assessment:
      1. Infant: Jaundice (heel stick performed if necessary) Mother: Hemorrhage, perineal lacerations, hematomas
         Both: Nutrition
         – Weight
         – Hydration
         – Breast-feeding
      2. Elimination

II. Cost:
   A. Fully reimbursed by some insurance companies.
   B. All mother/baby dyads receive postpartum visits, regardless of insurance coverage.
   C. Optional or additional methods of reimbursement have not been explored by the agency.
   D. Agency makes money on reimbursed visits, loses money on non-reimbursed, but additional revenue generated by clients choosing the hospital because of the positive public perception. The program is thought to balance out cost of nonreimbursed visits.

Outcomes of postpartum early discharge with accompanying home visit (as compared to traditional length of postpartum stay):

I. Positive:
   A. Higher percentage of successful (at least 2 months) breast-feeding
   B. Higher rate of immunization compliance
   C. Fewer inappropriate emergency room visits
   D. High client satisfaction
   E. Lower levels of maternal stress reported to pediatricians
II. Negative:
   A. Higher incidence in jaundice in babies whose mothers participated in the early discharge program

   1. What, if any, additional information do you need to make a recommendation regarding the program?
      • How will you obtain this information?
   2. As the nurse making a recommendation for the continuation or termination of the postpartum early discharge program, what are your recommendations?
      • Should the program be abandoned?
      • Should the program be maintained?
   3. What, if any, alterations would you make in the following areas:
      • Funding
      • Protocol
      – Client education
      – Assessment
      – Timing of visit
   4. Outcome measurements are critical to demonstrate the efficacy of this program.
      • What will you evaluate?
      • How often?
      • Why?

class because they either don't drive at night, have low vision at night, or fear coming out in the dark. The class is rescheduled for midmorning, and the attendance dramatically increases.

Summative evaluation examines outcomes of the interventions. The *effect*, or degree to which an outcome objective has been met, informs the agency or program leader of the program's impact on clients' health. As an example, one manufacturing company had an 80% adherence rate for employees who were supposed to wear proper protective devices (goggles, safety shoes, and hard hats) in the plant. Noncompliance on the part of some workers was a concern to union representatives, the health and safety team, and the company management. They were concerned that 20% of their employees were at risk for injury that would cause pain, suffering, loss of work time, disruption to the manufacturing process, and reduced profitability. The occupational health nurse along with the safety officer began a month-long safety campaign that included safety miniclasses, posters, and incentives for departments with 100% safety equipment adherence. Three months after the program, 95% of the employees were adhering to the safety regulations. This 15% increase was attributed to the effect of the safety program.

The *impact* of a program determines how close it comes to attaining its goals. In the earlier example, the objective of the safety campaign was to increase safety equipment use, and use was significantly increased as a result of the program. However, if the goal of the program had been to decrease accidents and save the company money, the result could be determined only with additional information. Were there fewer injuries caused by accidents? Were there fewer days lost to injuries? Did the company save money as the direct result of employee safety adherence? What was the cost–benefit ratio? Depending on the answers to these questions, the overall goal of the program may or may not have been met, even though the objective of the program was met. The full impact of the program cannot be determined without additional data. See Chapter 12 for more on program evaluation.

Community Development Theory

An outcome of effective community-level nursing practice is **community development**. Community development is the process of collaborating with community members to assess their collective needs and desires for positive change and to address these needs through problem solving, collaboration with community stakeholders, and resource development (Leigh & Blakely, 2013). A community development perspective assumes that community members participate in all aspects of change—assessment, planning, development, delivery of services, and evaluation. With this approach, the focus is on healthful community changes generated from within the community, as a partnership between health care providers and inhabitants, rather than a commodity dispensed by health care providers. The community as partner model exemplifies this approach (Anderson & McFarlane, 2015). Chapter 11 details community change theory.

The outcomes are more positive when community members have a sense of ownership in the health programs and services that address their needs. This enhances empowerment among members of the community and enables them to more effectively control and participate in transforming their environment and their personal circumstances. This implies that health care agency infrastructures are appropriate additions to services that are planned and delivered in an acceptable manner to the community (see Fig. 15–10, Arnstein's Ladder). This empowerment leads to greater resilience and ultimately, wellness (RAND Corporation, 2015) (see Chapter 13).

When applying community development theory, the agent of change (often the public health nurse) is considered a partner rather than an authority figure responsible for the community's health. To achieve acceptance as a partner, the nurse must listen and learn from the community members, because they are the experts with respect to their health care needs, culture, and values (Michener et al., 2012). They have mastered adaptation to the community, and they have firsthand knowledge of prevention methods and interventions that are appropriate to their lifestyles. For example, a randomized controlled trial with 285 women having chronic health conditions and receiving Temporary Aid for Needy Families (TANF), and utilizing a CBPR approach, found that 9 months of PHN case management improved health outcomes for those in the intervention group (Kneipp et al., 2011). Medicaid knowledge and skills improved for both the intervention and control groups, but those in the intervention group had improved depression and functional status; they were also more likely to have a new mental health visit (Kneipp et al., 2011). The PHNs developed rapport with their clients and formed a partnership with them. The principles of CBPR involve this type of partnership

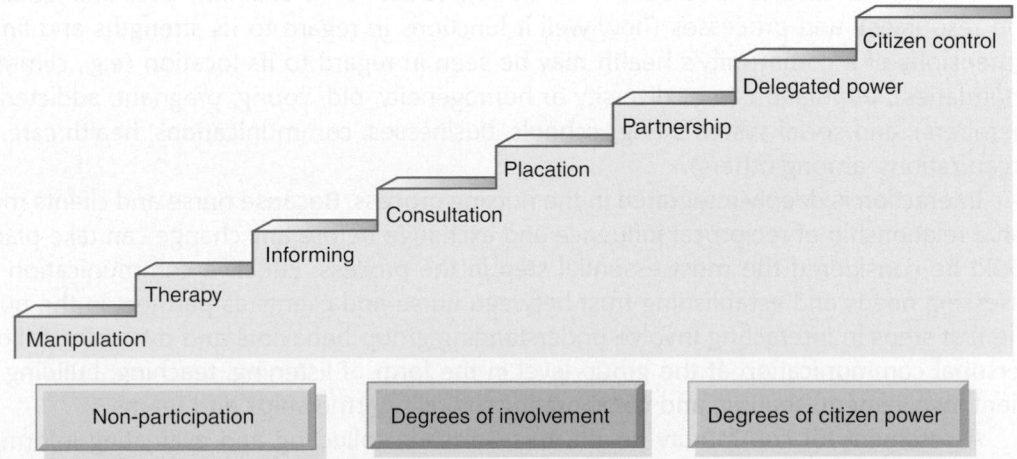

FIGURE 15-10 Arnstein's Ladder—Eight steps of citizen participation. (Adapted from Arnstein, S. R. (1969, July). A ladder of citizen participation. *Journal of the American Institute of Planners, 35*(4), 217–224.)

(see Chapters 4, 13, and 25 for more information on CBPR). Members of the community are engaged as coresearchers, and time is spent building trust and developing collaborative relationships with community members, stakeholders, and neighborhood health care providers. The expertise of community members is valued and can be useful in designing recruitment strategies, as well as in data analysis (Perry & Hoffman, 2010). This experience can enrich the community as a whole, as well as the actual participants.

The outcomes of the services provided by any organization can be benchmarked against those of other groups. *Benchmarking* involves comparing an organization's outcomes against those of a similar organization or an organization that is known for its excellence in a particular area of client care (Haustein et al., 2011). Information from this comparison can be used to identify an organization's areas of weakness and to focus attention on specific outcomes. The establishment of *best practice* activities entails constant comparisons between high- and low-performance programs and interventions (Ettorchi-Tardy, Levif, & Michel, 2012).

From a global perspective, the Conference on Primary Health Care held at Alma-Ata in 1978 concluded that people have little control over their own health care services and that the emphasis should be on health problems identified by the members of the community in their attempts to attain a state of wellness (WHO, 1998). Since that time, the WHO, along with other agencies and groups, has been providing leadership in the use of community development methods to improve global health, based on the following concepts (Brennan, Birdger, & Alter, 2013):

- Promote active, representative participation to influence decisions affecting community members' daily lives
- Engage community members in economic, social, political, environmental, psychological, and other issues that impact them
- Interest them in learning more about alternative courses of action
- Incorporate diverse cultures, ethnic and racial groups, and varied interests in the process of community development
- Refrain from supporting efforts that are likely to adversely affect disadvantaged members of the community
- Actively work to build leadership capacity of community leaders and groups, and individuals
- Work toward long-term sustainability and community well-being

SUMMARY

Characteristics of healthy communities include those elements that enable people to maintain a high quality of life and productivity by increasing health and decreasing disease and disparities in health and health care delivery. The effectiveness of community health nursing practice depends on how well the nursing process is used as a tool to enhance aggregate or population health. The nursing process involves appropriate application of a systematic series of actions with the goal of helping clients achieve their optimal level of health. The components of this process are assessment, diagnosis, planning, implementation, and evaluation.

The concept of community as client refers to a group or population of people as the focus of nursing service. The community's health is reflected in its status (e.g., morbidity and mortality rates, crime rates, educational and economic levels), structure (availability, use, and quality of services and resources), and processes (how well it functions in regard to its strengths and limitations). The dimensions of a community's health may be seen in regard to its location (e.g., climate, vegetation, boundaries), population (e.g., diversity or homogeneity, old, young, pregnant, addicted, or academic members), and social systems (e.g., schools, businesses, communications, health care, and religious organizations, among others).

Interaction is deeply integrated in the nursing process. Because nurse and clients must first establish a relationship of reciprocal influence and exchange before any change can take place, interaction could be considered the most essential step in the process. Effective communication is inherent in assessing needs and establishing trust between nurse and clients as partners in the nursing process. The first steps in interacting involve understanding group behaviors and dynamics, followed by interpersonal communication at the group level in the form of listening, teaching, building trust, seeking client involvement, sharing, and collaborating to build partnerships and teams.

Assessment for community health nurses means collecting and evaluating information about a community's health status to discover existing or potential needs and assets as a basis for planning future action. Assessment involves two major activities. The first is collection of pertinent data, and the second is analysis and interpretation of that data.

Community health nurses may use various assessment methods to determine a community's needs. They include *familiarization assessments*, such as windshield surveys, which involves studying data already available on a community; *problem-oriented assessment*, which focuses on a single problem and looks at the community in terms of that problem; *community subsystem assessment*, by which the community health nurse focuses on a single dimension of community life; a complicated and often time-consuming *comprehensive assessment*, to discover *all* relevant community health information; or an *assets assessment* that focuses on the strengths of a community as opposed to its deficits. Combinations may also prove useful (e.g., problem oriented and assets assessments).

Community data may be provided by many means—surveys, descriptive epidemiologic studies, community forums, and town meetings. Focus groups as well as primary and secondary sources (e.g., people who are familiar with the community and its character and history) are also common sources of data, along with Web sites, and government departments and agencies that compile statistics (e.g., U.S. Census Bureau, state or county health departments). Sources can include national, international, state, county, and local agencies, as well as business and social organizations.

Using the nursing process in the community would not be complete without looking at the role of the public health nurse as a catalyst for community health improvement. Community development theory is the foundation that supports citizen empowerment and use of key players in the community to plan for the health and safety of that community.

ACTIVITIES TO PROMOTE **CRITICAL THINKING**

1. Explain to a nonnursing friend why it is important to understand and work with the community as a total entity, in addition to individuals and families.
2. How does defining the community as the client change the community health nurse's practice? List some specific examples of how this concept can be applied.
3. If you were part of a health planning team concerned about the health needs of senior citizens in your community, what are some location, population, and social system variables you would want to assess? Name some of the sources from which you might collect the data.
4. Discuss under what circumstances you might choose to conduct a problem-oriented community health assessment. What method would you consider using to conduct this assessment, and how would you carry it out?
5. If possible, interview someone from your state or local health department or from a nonprofit hospital who has recently conducted a community health assessment survey. Or, access one on a state or hospital Web site. Analyze the process used, and compare it with the steps for conducting a survey described in this chapter. How are they similar? Different?
6. Critically reflect on the community in which you were raised. Who were the "haves" and "have-nots" in your community? What characterized them as that (e.g., money, education/position, race/ethnicity)? Verify this by examining current vital statistics by income, education, and ethnicity. How has your community changed since you were in grade school? Speak with a few people from older generations about their views on the community (e.g., causes of morbidity/mortality, general population health). How do their views differ from your? How are they similar? Compare current vital statistics with those of your birth year. Do the results follow the expected patterns based upon your interviews? Compare your community to a peer's community. Which one might be seen as healthier? Why?

REFERENCES

Adcock, C., & Brown, L. (1957). Social class and the ranking of occupations. *British Journal of Sociology, 8*(1), 26–32.

Agarwal, S., Menon, V., & Jaber, W. (2015). Outcomes following acute ischemic stroke in the United States: Does residential zip code matter? *Journal of the American College of Cardiology, 65*(10S).

American Nurses Association. (2013). *Public health nursing: Scope and standards of practice* (2nd ed.). Washington, DC: American Nurses Publishing.

American Nurses Association (ANA). (2014). *Health care reform. Health care transformation: The Affordable Care Act and more.* Retrieved from http://www.nursingworld.org/MainMenuCategories/Policy-Advocacy/HealthSystemReform/AffordableCareAct.pdf

American Public Health Association, Public Health Nursing Section. (2013). *The definition and practice of public health nursing: A statement of the public health nursing section.* Washington, DC: American Public Health Association.

Anderson, L. M., Adeney, K. L., Shinn, C., Krause, L. K., & Safranek, S. (2012). Community coalition-driven interventions to reduce health disparities among racial and ethnic minority populations. *The Cochrane Library.* Retrieved from http://www.cochrane.org/CD009905/PUBHLTH_community-coalition-driven-interventions-to-improve-health-status-and-reduce-disparities-in-racial-and-ethnic-minority-populations

Anderson, E. T., & McFarlane, J. (2015). *Community as partner: Theory and practice* (7th ed.). Philadelphia, PA: Lippincott Williams & Wilkins.

Artnak, K. E., McGraw, R. M., & Stanley, V. (2011). Health care accessibility for chronic illness management and end-of-life care: A view from rural America. *The Journal of Law, Medicine, and Ethics, 39*(2), 140–155.

Asthma and Allergy Foundation of America. (2015). *Fall allergy capitals.* Retrieved from http://www.aafa.org/media/Fall-Allergy-Capitals-List-2015.pdf

Auchincloss, A. H., Gebreab, S. Y., Mair, C., & Roux, A. V. D. (2012). A review of spatial methods in epidemiology, 2000–2010. *Annual Review of Public Health, 33,* 107.

Barbeau, A. M., Burda, J., & Siegel, M. (2013). Perceived efficacy of e-cigarettes versus nicotine replacement therapy among successful e-cigarette users: A qualitative approach. *Addiction Science & Clinical Practice, 8*(1), 5.

Barnett, K. (2012). *Best practices for community health needs assessment and implementation strategy development: A review of scientific methods, current practices, and future potential public forum.* Retrieved from http://www.cdc.gov/policy/ohsc/chna/

Beal, J. A. (2012). Academic-service partnerships in nursing: An integrative review. *Nursing Research and Practice, 2012.* doi: 10.1155/2012/501564.

Brennan, M., Birdger, J., & Alter, T. R. (2013). *Theory, practice, and community development.* New York, NY: Routledge.

Burrows, S., Auger, N., Gamache, P., & Hamel, D. (2013). Leading causes of unintentional injury and suicide mortality in Canadian adults across the urban-rural continuum. *Public Health Reports, 128*(6), 443.

Carpenito, L. J. (2012). *Nursing diagnosis: Application to clinical practice* (14th ed.). Philadelphia, PA: Lippincott Williams & Wilkins.

Centers for Disease Control and Prevention (CDC). (2012). *Behavioral risk factor surveillance system.* Retrieved from http://www.cdc.gov/brfss/

Centers for Disease Control and Prevention (CDC). (2015a). *Assessment & planning models, frameworks & tools.* Retrieved from http://www.cdc.gov/stltpublichealth/cha/assessment.html

Centers for Disease Control and Prevention (CDC). (2015b). *Data & statistics.* Retrieved from http://www.cdc.gov/datastatistics/

Centers for Disease Control and Prevention (CDC). (2015c). *Developing program goals and measurable objectives.* Retrieved from http://www.cdc.gov/std/Program/pupestd/Developing%20Program%20Goals%20and%20Objectives.pdf

Centers for Disease Control and Prevention (CDC). (n.d.). *Prioritization.* Retrieved from http://www.cdc.gov/od/ocphp/nphpsp/documents/Prioritization.pdf

Cesaroni, G., Badaloni, C., Gariazzo, C., Stafoggia, M., Sozzi, R., Davoli, M., & Forastiere, F. (2013). Long-term exposure to urban air pollution and mortality in a cohort of more than a million adults in Rome. *Environmental Health Perspectives, 121*(3), 324–331.

Charleston, A. E., Wilson, H. R., Edwards, P. O., David, F., & Dewitt, S. (2015). Environmental public health tracking: Driving environmental health information. *Journal of Public Health Management & Practice, 21,* S4–S11.

Clark, C. R., Baril, N., Hall, A., Kunicki, M., Johnson, N., Soukup, J., ... Bigby, J. (2011). Case management intervention in cervical cancer prevention: The Boston REACH coalition women's health demonstration project. *Progress in Community Health Partnerships, 5*(3), 235–247.

Community Toolbox. (2015). *Section 6: Participatory evaluation.* Retrieved from http://ctb.ku.edu/en/table-of-contents/evaluate/evaluation/participatory-evaluation/main

Conlon, K. C., Rajkovich, N. B., White-Newsome, J. L., Larsen, L., & O'Neill, M. S. (2011). Preventing cold-related morbidity and mortality in a changing climate. *Maturitas, 69*(3), 197–202.

Donabedian, A. (2005). Evaluating the quality of medical care. *Milbank Quarterly, 83*(4), 691–729.

Ettorchi-Tardy, A., Levif, M., & Michel, P. (2012). Benchmarking: A method for continuous quality improvement in health. *Healthcare Policy, 7*(4), e101.

Fassa, A. G., Faria, N. M., Meucci, R. D., Fiori, N. S., Miranda, V. I., & Facchini, L. A. (2014). Green tobacco sickness among tobacco farmers in southern Brazil. *American Journal of Industrial Medicine, 57*(6), 726–735.

Frieden, T. R. (2010). A framework for public health action: The health impact pyramid. *American Journal of Public Health, 100*(4), 590–595.

Gil de Zúñiga, H., Jung, N., & Valenzuela, S. (2012). Social media use for news and individuals' social capital, civic engagement and political participation. *Journal of Computer-Mediated Communication, 17*(3), 319–336.

Gras, S., Plantefève, G., Baud, F., & Chippaux, J. P. (2012). Snakebite on the hand: Lessons from two clinical cases illustrating difficulties of surgical indication. *Journal of Venomous Animals and Toxins including Tropical Diseases, 18*(4), 467–477.

Graham, S. R., Carlton, C., Gaede, D., & Jamison, B. (2011). The benefits of using geographic information systems as a community assessment tool. *Public Health Reports, 126*(2), 298–303.

Green, L. W., Sim, L, & Breiner, H. (Eds.). (2013). *Evaluating obesity prevention efforts: A plan for measuring progress.* Washington, DC: National Academies Press.

Gushulak, B. D., & MacPherson, D. W. (2011). Health aspects of the pre-departure phase of migration. *PLoS Medicine, 8*(5), e1001035. doi: 10.1371/journal.pmed.1001035.

Hammond, D., Conlon, K., Barzyk, T., Chahine, T., Zartarian, V., & Schultz, B. (2011). Assessment and application of national environmental databases and mapping tools at the local level to two community case studies. *Risk Analysis, 21*(3), 475–487.

Harvard University. (2013). *Geographic information systems (GIS) in public health research.* Retrieved from http://www.hsph.harvard.edu/gis/gis-research/eer-program/

Hauck, K., & Smith, P. C. (2015). *The politics of priority setting in health: A political economy perspective—working paper 414.* Retrieved from http://www.cgdev.org/publication/politics-priority-setting-health-political-economy-perspective-working-paper-414

Haustein, T., Gastmeier, P., Holmes, A., Lucet, J., Shannon, R. P., Pittet, D., & Harbarth, S. (2011). Use of benchmarking and public reporting for infection control in four high-income countries. *The Lancet Infectious Diseases, 11*(6), 471–481.

Health Resources & Services Administration (HRSA). (2014). *Shortage designation: Health professional shortage areas and medically underserved areas/populations.* Retrieved from http://www.hrsa.gov/shortage/

Howard, P. N., & Parks, M. R. (2012). Social media and political change: Capacity, constraint, and consequence. *Journal of Communication, 62*(2), 359–362.

Hummer, R. A., & Hernandez, E. M. (2013). *The effect of educational attainment on adult mortality in the US.* Retrieved from http://www.prb.org/Publications/Reports/2013/us-educational-attainment-mortality.aspx

Issel, L. M. (2014). *Health program planning and evaluation: A practical, systematic approach for community health* (3rd ed.). Sudbury, MA: Jones & Bartlett Publishers.

Iqbal, S., Oraka, E., Chew, G. L., & Flanders, W. D. (2014). Association between birthplace and current asthma: The role of environment and acculturation. *American Journal of Public Health, 104*(S1), S175–S182.

Jakes, S., Hardison-Moody, A., Bowen, S., & Blevins, J. (2015). Engaging community change: The critical role of values in asset mapping. *Community Development, 46*(4), 392–406.

Jarris, P. E., & Schneider, J. P. (2013). Engaging partners to support the national prevention strategy. *Journal of Public Health Management & Practice, 19*(4), 386–387.

Joynt, K. E., Harris, Y., Orav, J., & Jha, A. (2011). Quality of care and patient outcomes in critical access rural hospitals. *The Journal of the American Medical Association, 306*(1), 45–52.

Kawasaki, A., Berman, M. L., & Guan, W. (2013). The growing role of web-based geospatial technology in disaster response and support and describing the prevalence of cancer disparities. *Disasters, 37*(2), 201–221.

Keet, C. A., McCormack, M. C., Pollack, C. E., Peng, R. D., McGowan, E., & Matsui, E. C. (2015). Neighborhood poverty, urban residence, race/ethnicity, and asthma: Rethinking the inner-city asthma epidemic. *Journal of Allergy and Clinical Immunology, 135*(3), 655–662.

Kindig, D. A., & Isham, G. (2014). Population health improvement: A community health business model that engages partners in all sectors/response from feature authors. *Frontiers of Health Services Management, 30*(4), 3.

Kirst-Ashman, K. (2014). *Human behavior in the macro social environment.* (4th ed.). Belmont, CA: Brooks/Cole–Cengage Learning.

Kneipp, S. M., Kairalia, J., Lutz, B., Pereira, D., Hall, A. G., Flocks, J., ... Schwartz, T. (2011). Public health nursing case management for women receiving temporary assistance for needy families: A randomized controlled trial using community-based participatory research. *American Journal of Public Health, 101*(9), 1759–1768.

Kouyos, R. D., Wiesch, P. A., & Bonhoeffer, S. (2011). On being the right size: The impact of population size and stochastic effects on the evolution of drug resistance in hospitals and the community. *PLOS Pathogens, 7*(4):e1001334.

Kramer, S., Seedat, M., Lazarus, S., & Suffla, S. (2011). A critical review of instruments assessing characteristics of community. *South African Journal of Psychology, 41*(4), 503–516.

Kretzman, J., & McKnight, J. (1993). *Building communities from the inside out: A path toward finding and mobilizing a community's assets.* Chicago, IL: ACTA Publications.

Lantz, P. M., Golberstein, E., House, J., & Morenoff, J. (2010). Socioeconomic and behavioral risk factors for mortality in a national 19-year prospective study of U.S. adults. *Social Sciences and Medicine, 70*(10), 1558–1566.

LeBan, K. (2011). *How social capital in community systems strengthens health systems: People, structure, processes.* Retrieved from http://core-group.org/storage/Program_Learning/Community_Health_Workers/Components_of_a_Community_Health_System_final10-12-2011.pdf

Lee, B. Y., Brown, S. T., Bailey, R. R., Zimmerman, R. K., Potter, M. A., & McGlone, S. M. (2011). The benefits to all of ensuring equal and timely access to influenza vaccines in poor communities. *Health Affairs, 30*(6), 1141–1150.

Leigh, N. G., & Blakely, E. J. (2013). *Planning local economic development: Theory and practice* (5th ed.). Thousand Oaks, CA: Sage Publications, Inc.

Li, Y., Wang, W., Wang, J., Zhang, X., Lin, W., & Yang, Y. (2011). Impact of air pollution control measures and weather conditions on asthma during the 2008 Summer Olympic Games in Beijing. *International Journal of Biometeorology, 55*(4), 547–554.

Lu, Y., Song, S., Wang, R., Liu, Z., Meng, J., Sweetman, A. J., ... Wang, T. (2015). Impacts of soil and water pollution on food safety and health risks in China. *Environment International, 77*, 5–15.

Lushniak, B. D., Alley, D. E., Ulin, B., & Graffunder, C. (2015). The National Prevention Strategy: Leveraging multiple sectors to improve population health. *American Journal of Public Health, 105*(2), 229–231.

Matthews, C. E., Wooten, W., Gomez, M. G. R., Kozo, J., Fernandez, A., & Ojeda, V. D. (2015). The California border health collaborative: A strategy for leading the border to better health. *Frontiers in Public Health, 3*, 141.

McEntee, J., & Agyeman, J. (2010). Towards the development of a GIS method for identifying rural food deserts: Geographic access in Vermont, USA. *Applied Geography, 30*(1), 165–176.

McGregor, S., Henderson, K. J., & Kaldor, J. M. (2014). How are health research priorities set in low and middle income countries? A systematic review of published reports. *PLoS One, 9*(10), E108787.

McMichael, A. J. (2015). Extreme weather events and infectious disease outbreaks. *Virulence, 6*(6), 543–547.

Merrill, R. M. (2013). *Introduction to epidemiology* (6th ed.). Sudbury, MA: Jones & Bartlett Learning.

Michener, L., Cook, J., Ahmed, S. M., Yonas, M. A., Coyne-Beasley, T., & Aguilar-Gaxiola, S. (2012). Aligning the goals of community-engaged research: Why and how academic health centers can successfully engage with communities to improve health. *Academic Medicine, 87*(3), 285–291. http://doi.org/10.1097/ACM.0b013e3182441680

Michener, J. L., Koo, D., Castrucci, B. C., & Sprague, J. B. (Eds.). (2015). *The practical playbook: Public health and primary care together.* New York, NY: Oxford University Press.

Minnesota Department of Health. (n.d.a). *Local public health assessment and planning.* Retrieved from http://www.health.state.mn.us/lphap/

Minnesota Department of Health. (n.d.b). *SMART and meaningful objectives.* Retrieved from http://www.health.state.mn.us/divs/opi/qi/toolbox/objectives.html

Mondal, M. N. I., & Shitan, M. (2014). Relative importance of demographic, socioeconomic and health factors on life expectancy in low-and lower-middle-income countries. *Journal of Epidemiology, 24*(2), 117.

Mundinger, M. O., & Jauron, G. D. (1975). Developing a nursing diagnosis. *Nursing Outlook, 23*(2), 94–98.

Murayama, H., Fujiwara, Y., & Kawachi, I. (2012). Social capital and health: A review of prospective multilevel studies. *Journal of Epidemiology, 22*(3), 179–187.

National Association of County & City Health Officials (NACCHO). (2012). *Integrating MAPP with other national initiatives: Questions and answers.* Retrieved from http://www.naccho.org/topics/infrastructure/mapp/QAnationalinitiatives.cfm

National Association of County & City Health Officials (NACCHO). (2015). *Developing a community health improvement plan.* Retrieved from http://www.naccho.org/topics/infrastructure/CHAIP/chip.cfm

National Association of County & City Health Officials (NACCHO). (n.d.). *First things first: Prioritizing health problems.* Retrieved from http://chfs.ky.gov/NR/rdonlyres/B070C722-31C1-4225-95D527622C16CBEE/0/PrioritizationSummariesandExamples.pdf

National Institutes of Health (NIH). (2015). *About NIH.* Retrieved from https://www.nih.gov/about-nih

National Prevention Council. (2011). *National prevention strategy.* Washington, DC: U.S. Department of Health and Human Services, Office of the Surgeon General.

Nauenberg, E., Laporte, A., & Shen, L. (2011). Social capital, community size, and utilization of health services: A lagged analysis. *Health Policy, 103*(1), 38–46.

Neufeld, A., & Harrison, M. J. (1996). Educational issues in preparing community health nurses to use nursing diagnosis with population groups. *Nurse Education Today, 16*, 221–226.

Nguyen, T. A., Knight, R., Roughead, E. E., Brooks, G., & Mant, A. (2015). Policy options for pharmaceutical pricing and purchasing: Issues for low- and middle-income countries. *Health Policy & Planning, 30*(2), 267–280.

Northwest Center for Public Health Practice. (n.d.). *Module one: An overview of public health data.* Retrieved from http://www.nwcphp.org/docs/bcda_series/data_analysis_mod1_transcript.pdf

Nykiforuk, C., Schopflocher, D., Vallianatos, H., Spence, J. C., Raine, K. D., Plotnikoff, R. C., ... Nieuwendyk, L. (2012). Community health and the built environment: Examining place in a Canadian chronic disease prevention project. *Health Promotion International, 28*(2), 257–268. doi: 10.1093/heapro/dar093

Office of the Assistant Secretary for Planning and Evaluation. (n.d.). *Setting priorities and objectives.* Retrieved from http://aspe.hhs.gov/ezec/planning/setting.htm

Omaha System. (2015). *The Omaha System: Solving the clinical data-information puzzle.* Retrieved from http://www.omahasystem.org/overview.html

Pavlish, C. P., & Pharris, M. D. (2012). *Community-based collaborative action research: A nursing approach.* Sudbury, MA: Jones & Bartlett Learning.

Perry, C., & Hoffman, B. (2010). Assessing tribal youth physical activity and programming using a community-based participatory research approach. *Public Health Nursing, 27*(2), 104–114.

Petersen, D. D. (2011). Common plant toxicology: A comparison of national and southwest Ohio data trends on plant poisoning in the 21st century. *Toxicology and Applied Pharmacology, 254*(2), 148–153.

Polit, D. F., & Beck, C. T. (2014). *Essentials of nursing research: Appraising evidence for nursing practice* (8th ed.). Philadelphia, PA: Lippincott Williams & Wilkins.

Public Health Accreditation Board. (2013). *Standards & measures, version 1.5. 2013.* Retrieved from http://www.phaboard.org/wp-content/uploads/SM-Version-1.5-Board-adopted-FINAL-01-24-2014.docx.pdf

Public Health Foundation. (n.d.). *Resources and tools.* Retrieved from http://www.phf.org/resourcestools/Pages/default.aspx

Public Health Institute. (2012). *Best practices for community health needs assessment and implementation strategy development: A review of scientific methods, current practices, and future potential.* Retrieved from http://www.phi.org/uploads/application/files/dz9vh55o3bb2x56lcrzyel83fwfu3mvu24oqqvn5z6qaeiw2u4.pdf

Quad Council. (2011, Summer). *Quad Council PHN competencies for public health nurses.* Retrieved from http://www.resourcenter.net/images/ACHNE/Files/QuadCouncilCompetenciesForPublicHealthNurses_Summer2011.pdf

Quan, D. (2012). North American poisonous bites and stings. *Critical Care Clinics, 28*(4), 633–659.

RAND Corporation. (2015). *Healthy populations and communities: In depth.* Retrieved from http://www.rand.org/health/key-topics/populations-communities/in-depth.html

Rao, D. R., Sordillo, J. E., Kopel, L. S., Gaffin, J. M., Sheehan, W. J., Hoffman, E., ... Phipatanakul, W. (2015). Association between allergic sensitization and exhaled nitric oxide in children in the School Inner-City Asthma Study. *Annals of Allergy, Asthma & Immunology, 114*(3), 256.

Rice, T., Unruh, L. Y., Rosenau, P., Barnes, A. J., Saltman, R. B., & van Ginneken, E. (2014). Challenges facing the United States of America in implementing universal coverage. *Bulletin of the World Health Organization, 92,* 894–902.

Robert Wood Johnson Foundation. (2015). *County health rankings & roadmaps.* Retrieved from http://www.countyhealthrankings.org/

Rost, M., & Wilson, J. J. (2013). *Active listening.* New York, NY: Routledge.

Schildkraut, D. J. (2014). Boundaries of American identity: Evolving understandings of "us." *Annual Review of Political Science, 17,* 441–460.

Schoenbaum, S., Schoen, C., Nicholson, J., & Cantor, J. (2011). Mortality amenable to health care in the United States: The roles of demographics and health systems performance. *Journal of Public Health Policy, 32,* 407–429.

Shpakou, A., Brożek, G., Stryzhak, A., Neviartovich, T., & Zejda, J. (2012). Allergic diseases and respiratory symptoms in urban and rural children in Grodno Region (Belarus). *Pediatric Allergy and Immunology, 23*(4), 339–346.

Simiyu, W. W. N., Njororai, F., & Jivetti, B. A. (2015). Walkable scores for selected three east Texas counties: Physical activity and policy implications. *International Journal of Human Sciences, 12*(2), 674–687.

Singh, G. K., & Siahpush, M. (2014). Widening rural–urban disparities in all-cause morbidity and mortality from major causes of death in the USA, 1969–2009. *Journal of Urban Health, 91*(2), 272–292.

Spector, R. E. (2013). *Cultural diversity in health and illness* (8th ed.). Upper Saddle River, NJ: Prentice-Hall Allied Health.

Starks, S. E., Gerr, F., Kamel, F., Lynch, C. F., Alavanja, M. C., Sandler, D. P., & Hoppin, J. A. (2011). High pesticide exposure events and central nervous system function among pesticide applicators in the Agricultural Health Study. *International Archives of Occupational and Environmental Health, 85*(5), 505–515. doi: 10.1007/s00420-011-0694-8.

Stewart, D. W., & Shamdasani, P. N. (2014). *Focus groups: Theory and practice* (Vol. 20). Thousand Oaks, CA: Sage Publications.

Summach, A. H. (2011). Facilitating trust engenderment in secondary school nurse interactions with students. *The Journal of School Nursing, 27*(2), 129–138.

Swarts, H. (2011). Drawing new symbolic boundaries over old social boundaries: Forging social movement unity in congregation-based community organizing. *Sociological Perspectives, 54*(3), 453–477.

Teach, S. J., Gergen, P. J., Szefler, S. J., Mitchell, H. E., Calatroni, A., Wildfire, J., ... Busse, W. W. (2015). Seasonal risk factors for asthma exacerbations among inner-city children. *Journal of Allergy and Clinical Immunology, 135*(6), 1465–1473.

Thomas, T. L., DiClemente, R., & Snell, S. (2013). Overcoming the triad of rural health disparities: How local culture, lack of economic opportunity, and geographic location instigate health disparities. *Health Education Journal.* doi: 0017896912471049.

Townsend, J. S., Pinkerton, B., McKenna, S., Higgins, S., Tai, E., Steele, C. B., ... Brown, C. (2011). Targeting children through school-based education and policy strategies: Comprehensive cancer control activities in melanoma prevention. *Journal of the American Academy of Dermatology, 65*(5, Suppl. 1), s104–s113.

Tran, P. M., & Waller, L. (2013). Effects of landscape fragmentation and climate on Lyme disease incidence in the northeastern United States. *Ecohealth, 10*(4), 394–404.

Trinh-Shevrin, C., Pollack, H., Tsang, T., Park, J., Ramos, M. R., Islam, N., ... Kwon, S. C. (2011). The Asian American hepatitis B program: Building a coalition to address hepatitis B health disparities. *Progress in Community Health Partnerships, 5*(3), 261–271.

Trowbridge, M. J., Huang, T. T. K., Botchwey, N. D., Fisher, T. R., Pyke, C., Rodgers, A. B., & Ballard-Barbash, R. (2013). Public health and the green building industry: Partnership opportunities for childhood obesity prevention. *American Journal of Preventive Medicine, 44*(5), 489–495.

Trowbridge, M. J., & Schmid, T. L. (2013). Built environment and physical activity promotion: Place-based obesity prevention strategies. *The Journal of Law, Medicine & Ethics, 41*(s2), 46–51.

Tucker, C. M., Arthur, T. M., Roncoroni, J., Wall, W., & Sanchez, J. (2015). Patient-centered, culturally sensitive health care. *American Journal of Lifestyle Medicine, 9*(1), 63–77.

University of Michigan Center of Excellence in Public Health Workforce Studies. (2013). *Enumeration and characterization of the public health nurse workforce: Findings of the 2012 Public Health Nurse Workforce Surveys.* Ann Arbor, MI: University of Michigan.

U.S. Census Bureau. (n.d.). *Data.* Retrieved from http://www.census.gov/data.html

U.S. Department of Health and Human Services (USDHHS). (2015). *The 2015 HHS poverty guidelines.* Retrieved from http://aspe.hhs.gov/poverty/05poverty.shtml CHANGE

U.S. Department of Health and Human Services (USDHHS). (2016). *Healthy People 2020.* Retrieved from http://www.cdc.gov/nchs/healthy_people/hp2020.htm

Wagner-Schuman, M., Richardson, J. R., Auinger, P., Braun, J. M., Lanphear, B. P., Epstein, J. N., ... Froehlich, T. E. (2015). Association of pyrethroid pesticide exposure with attention-deficit/hyperactivity disorder in a nationally representative sample of US children. *Environmental Health, 14*(1), 44.

Wang, Y., Ponce, N. A., Wang, P., Opsomer, J. D., & Yu, H. (2015). Generating health estimates by zip code: A semiparametric small area estimation approach using the California health interview survey. *American Journal of Public Health, 105*(12), 2534–2540.

Wheeler, S. B., & Basch, E. (2014). Cancer care research in North Carolina: The state of the state. *North Carolina Medical Journal, 75*(4), 248–252.

World Health Organization (WHO). (1998). *Primary health care in the 21st century is everybody's business.* Geneva, Switzerland: Author.

World Health Organization (WHO). (2014). *Global Health Observatory (GHO).* Retrieved http://www.who.int/gho/en/

World Health Organization (WHO). (2015). *The world health report.* Retrieved from http://www.who.int/gho/publications/world_health_statistics/2015/en/

Wyer, P. C., Umscheid, C. A., Wright, S., Silva, S. A., & Lang, E. (2015). Teaching evidence assimilation for collaborative health care (TEACH) 2009–2014: Building evidence-based capacity within health care provider organizations. *eGEMs, 3*(2).

Zheng, H., Tumin, D., & Qian, Z. (2013). Obesity and mortality risk: New findings from body mass index trajectories. *American Journal of Epidemiology, 178*(11), 1591–1599.

thePoint: Everything You Need to Make the Grade!

Global Public Health Nursing: Population Health Around the Globe

"When it comes to global health, there is no 'them'... only 'us.'"

—**Global Health Council** (2010)

KEY TERMS

Community health worker (CHW)
Control
Disability-adjusted life year (DALY)
Elimination
Era of Chronic, Long-Term Health Conditions
Era of Infectious Diseases

Era of Social Health Conditions
Eradication
Global burden of disease (GBD)
Global nursing
Health for All
Integrated management of childhood illness (IMCI)

Jakarta Declaration
Multilateral agencies
Oral rehydration therapy (ORT)
Ottawa Charter for Health Promotion
Pluralistic health care systems
Primary health care (PHC)

Universal imperatives of care
World Bank (WB)
World Health Assembly (WHA)
World Health Organization (WHO)
World Health Organization Collaborating Centers

LEARNING OBJECTIVES

Upon mastery of this chapter, you should be able to:

● Describe a context and framework for delivering community-based nursing within the context of international community health nursing.

● Describe the major health care conditions currently affecting the world's populations and the types and preparation of health care workers addressing them.

● Describe the community health nursing interventions and strategies commonly used within an international context.

● Recognize the factors that influence populations' perceptions of health and health status and their receptivity to community health nursing programs.

● Describe the personal and professional perceptions and biases you bring to providing community health nursing interventions within an international context.

● Identify the major international, national, regional, and local organizational structures and organizations that affect the ways in which community health nursing is practiced.

● Locate relevant resources as a basis for planning the assessment, implementation, and evaluation of community health nursing within an international context.

Let us suppose that you have completed your schooling and are ready to embark on a career in global community health nursing. **Global nursing** can range from providing clinical services to policymaking at an international level. Perhaps you engaged in several years of successful clinical practice and are interested in pursuing an international opportunity to practice nursing in another country. You undertake a search of the Internet, you talk to professional colleagues, and you read articles in nursing and other professional and popular journals.

You quickly realize that researching health care is a rather awesome undertaking, and the search for health care opportunities within a global context yields a plethora of Web sites, universities, and organizations going global. We can connect to almost anyone, anywhere, by computer or cell phone. We can access ancestral records that are centuries old, talk to colleagues in the far reaches of Africa or Asia, and instantly learn about global health issues occurring on the opposite side of the globe.

You also learn that community health care is complex and that it affects and is affected by multiple factors that have to do with geography, history, politics, culture, religion, and a nation's wealth. Your searches will be informative. You will notice that some countries' data are difficult to access, and you realize that this may be because a country has been involved in a long, protracted civil war or has experienced continuous cycles of disasters or financial collapse.

In your search, you also find that people's conception of health, wellness, and illness varies from culture to culture and that the ways in which they view nurses and other health care providers is affected by their attitudes toward women, their culture, and belief systems. You will also notice patterns of privilege across countries and regions regarding who lives, who dies, the way people function on a day-to-day basis, the health care decisions they make, and the cost of the care they receive.

In your search, you also will learn a great deal about the health care providers that countries look to for nursing care and medical treatment. You will notice a disparity between the health status and health conditions of people in a country, as well as the kind of health care providers who are educated practicing in that country. For example, if you were to travel to mountainous areas, such as Nepal, you would see medications and treatments being administered without questions asked about the provider's credentials. The closest **primary health care (PHC)** station might be 20 miles away, and any relief from pain is welcome.

You may become sensitized to the difference between your kind of nursing education and that of the nurses in countries different from your own. The ways in which one is recruited and educated varies from country to country, as does legislation regarding licensure and entry to practice. For example, midwifery in the United States is based on a baccalaureate degree in nursing, whereas in Denmark, students have been admitted directly into a midwifery program without a nursing background and foundation. In France, midwives are aligned with the field of medicine and see their practice from that standpoint rather than from a nursing perspective.

You will come across hundreds of references to international, national, and regional agencies that work in health care internationally. These references will be organized according to international agencies, national governments, universities, churches, and nongovernmental organizations (NGOs), including those with religious affiliations and those that are nondenominational.

Most importantly, you will become aware of your own approach to community health nursing. The ways in which practice takes place in an international context are influenced by all these factors and by your own personal background, your religious beliefs and attitudes, your orientation toward the theory of community health nursing practice, as well as your values and cultural beliefs. These factors and issues constitute a global framework for community health nursing, and they are the foci of this chapter. The question arises: How to put all of this in perspective, to apply a way of thinking to assist you in achieving your goal of an international nursing experience?

This chapter begins with a framework you can use to organize your thinking and around which you can structure your search as you expand your repertoire of knowledge and understanding. Those of us who work abroad need a framework in which to place our searches, professional dialogues, and readings. We need a compass to guide us as we conduct these searches to help match us with the people we hope to serve. We also need a way of thinking about the communities, regions, or countries of the world and about the kinds of community health nursing interventions a country may need, given the elements described here.

A FRAMEWORK FOR GLOBAL PUBLIC HEALTH NURSING

The Three P's

To guide your thinking, consider a global framework that includes three parts, the three "P's": the population, the provider, and the procedure. In community health nursing, our focus is on populations rather than individual patients. The provider refers to the health care team, which may include a community health nurse, a physician, a midwife, an "injector" (someone who is trained to only give injections), or a **community health worker (CHW)**. The procedure refers to the interventions health care providers implement for or with populations.

In this global framework, alongside the three P's, think about three *eras* of health and health conditions, as described in a classic article by Breslow (2006). During our ancestors' time, populations of people died from the plague, tuberculosis (TB), puerperal fever, and other infectious diseases. Entire populations were sometimes eliminated through these infections. During this first era, families had many children, as they knew that most children would die before adulthood, and without any form of social security, children were their parents' only source of livelihood. Sons were preferred over daughters as sons ensured the family's livelihood and were capable of defending the community from enemies. This is referred to as the **Era of Infectious Diseases**. With the advent of antibiotics, people survived common infections. The lifespan of children was longer than that of their parents, but often, they suffered from chronic, long-term illnesses such as heart disease, cancer, and debilitating arthritis (Remington & Brownson, 2011). This is referred to as the **Era of Chronic, Long-Term Health Conditions**. Despite changes and advances in health care, people continued to produce large families because of the cost or absence of birth control measures, persistent religious beliefs that influenced families regarding birth, and the intent of countries—such as Romania (before 1989)—to increase their populations for financial reasons. More recently, a new array of health conditions is affecting world populations, including addictions and obesity, and social conditions such as prostitution, sexual abuse, and deviant behavior. These are examples from the **Era of Social Health Conditions**. The popular press has exposed many of these conditions through documentaries on the effects of methamphetamine on entire communities, the abuse of prescription painkillers, the obesity epidemic sweeping countries throughout the world, and the exploitation of children.

Continuing Emerging Health Conditions

Today, the communities of the world are experiencing all three eras of health conditions simultaneously. In one community, a population may be dealing with the Ebola virus, heart disease, cancer, adolescent prostitution, and mental illness. Some of these health conditions have been present for many years, some for thousands of years, and some are relatively new. Although significant progress has been made in controlling infectious diseases, the recent globalization of our world has increased opportunities for the spread of known and emerging infectious diseases (Centers for Disease Control and Prevention, [CDC], 2015c). This trend is attributed, in part, to the increase in travel, the massive migration of populations occurring because of wars and civil uprising, and the economic situation forcing people to leave their home countries for employment. This chapter examines the context where these conditions occur, the health care providers who work with them, and the ways in which interventions are applied through the work of many sponsoring global health organizations.

Universal Imperatives of Care

In addition to the three P's and the three eras of health conditions, community health nurses need to consider the current status of health in the community of interest. One useful paradigm is the **universal imperatives of care**. When we ask the question, how many nurses does a community need, part of answer has to do with these imperatives. These imperatives include mortality, morbidity, daily functioning, decision-making, and cost of and access to health care. This paradigm underscores the notion of *first things first*. That is, one must be alive and well before interventions can focus on functioning or decision-making (Fig. 16–1).

Mortality

A government's first priority is to keep its population alive and free from illness. This is critical if a country is to survive, protect itself, and feed its population. In this regard, community health nurses may be frustrated that the disabled are going without community resources, programs are not created to help couples make informed decisions about abortion and birth control, or the mentally ill have no possibilities for therapy. However, when countries are poor, they will focus on preventing mortality and the evidence-based interventions that will ensure the survival of

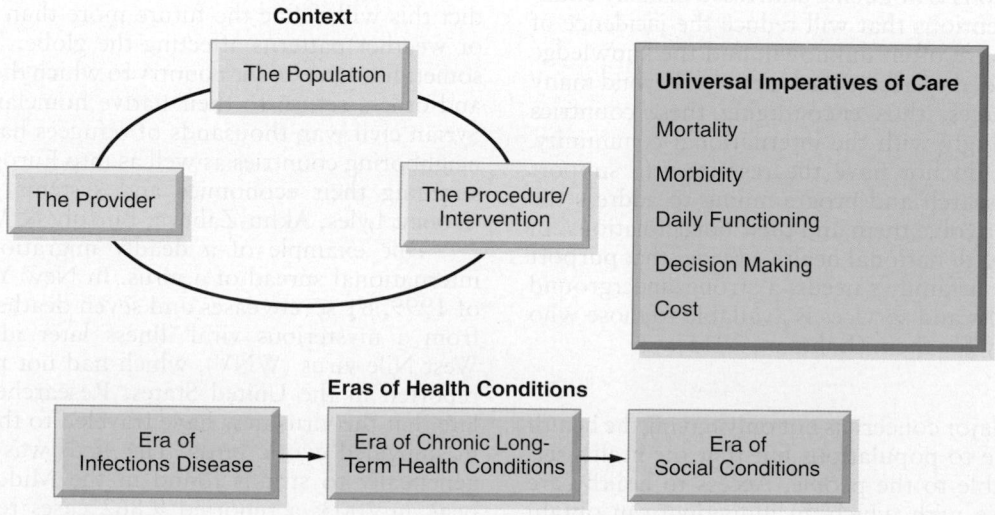

FIGURE 16–1 Framework for global community health nursing. (M. Farrell, 2012.)

the people (World Bank, 2014). The health care team member required when mortality is a priority is the physician.

Morbidity

When people are not dying, a country can focus on its population's morbidity—the conditions that make people sick—and will look to physicians and nurses for assistance. Sickness derives from infectious diseases, long-term chronic health conditions, and the social conditions introduced above and will be discussed in more detail in upcoming sections.

Daily Functioning

In many countries, the ability to care for oneself—to bathe, secure food, and carry out other activities of daily living for fragile elderly or the disabled—is the purview of nurses, physical therapists, social services, and social workers. However, in some countries, certain health care team members that nurses in the United States take for granted do not exist. Caring for an autistic child or a severely disabled parent is left entirely to the family. This is not because the government is negligent. It is because the universal imperatives in a country with constrained resources must focus on the necessities first.

Decision-Making

In order to choose, one needs options. In countries with only one health care delivery system, there are no other options. As countries have expanded to include privatization, and as people increasingly have access to the Internet, they have generally evolved in their decision-making processes about the providers they will use and the sources of their health information.

Cost

In many countries in the past, the state provided all health care, and all costs were the burden of the community. Increasingly, these health services are being rationed, restricted, or placed under insurance schemes. Nations are forced to weigh the cost of managing some health conditions over others. Most of the time, they opt for those that can be addressed with the least input and the maximum benefit. This is, in part, the reason that the Era of Social Conditions is not being addressed in many countries. The interventions that will reduce the incidence of these conditions are often unknown, and the knowledge and research needed to access them are well beyond many countries' resources, thus encouraging these countries to work increasingly with the international community. Many countries do not have the resources to support the necessary research and programming to address the issues that may involve them and their border nations. In some countries with national health services that purport to provide all of a family's needs, a strong underground of health products and services is available to those who can afford to pay for them (Lohman, 2015).

Access

Increasingly, a major concern is not only having the health services available to populations but that the health services are accessible to the people. Access to health care refers to the ease with which an individual can obtain needed (health care) services. Several factors influence access worldwide. For example, people who speak the language, people who have insurance, and those who are part of the military establishment may have priority in some countries. Most often, the particular groups who go wanting include the poor, the illiterate, those living in rural or remote areas, and, in some places, women (because of religious taboos).

THE CONTEXT

A Context of Interdependency

The context of community health nursing suggests considering one planet of interdependent nations. This interdependence relates to virtually all areas of life, including health. As of July 2015, the world's population reached 7.325 billion, with an estimated 8.501 billion by 2030 and 9.925 billion by 2050 (United Nations, Department of Economic and Social Affairs, Population Division, 2015). As systems theory suggests and Friedman (2005) reiterates in his definitive book, "The World Is Flat," what happens in one country affects many others in important ways. For example, air travel can transport health problems from a country halfway around the world to new communities in less than a day.

> On our one Earth, "water tables are falling, soil is eroding, glaciers are melting, and fish stocks are vanishing. Close to a billion people go hungry each day. Decades from now, there will be most likely two billion more mouths to feed, mostly in poor countries. There will be billions more people wanting and deserving to boost themselves out of poverty. If they follow the path blazed by wealthy countries—clearing forests, burning coal and oil, freely scattering fertilizers and pesticides—they too will be stepping hard on the planet's natural resources" (p. 43).

In addition to the number of people, the location and movement of populations is a major consideration. The number of migrants internationally has doubled over the past 25 years to 231 million people (United Nations Department of Economic Affairs, Population Division, 2013), and Goldin, Cameron, and Balarajan (2011) predict this will define the future more than environmental or weather patterns affecting the globe. These migrants sometimes settle in the country to which they have moved, and others return to their native homeland. During the Syrian civil war, thousands of refugees have poured into neighboring countries as well as into European countries, straining their economies and systems of health care (Doocy, Lyles, Akhu-Zaheya, Burtob, & Weiss, 2016).

One example of a deadly migration involves the international spread of a virus. In New York, in the fall of 1999, 61 severe cases and seven deaths were reported from a mysterious viral illness later identified as the West Nile virus (WNV), which had not previously been reported in the United States. Researchers now speculate that the virus may have traveled to the United States in smuggled exotic birds. The virus was closely related genetically to strains found in the Middle East. At its peak in 2003, a reported 9,862 cases related to WNV and 264 deaths had occurred in 46 states (CDC, 2015e,

2015f). By 2014, over 2,200 total cases were reported (CDC, 2015f). A new threat emerged in 2015; the Zika virus was found in Brazil and travelers returning to the United States were reported to have cases of the virus, known to be a danger for pregnant women because of its link with birth defects (CDC, 2016).

The globalization of food commodities and food safety also affects health. For example, researchers suggest that a causal relationship exists between ongoing outbreaks in Europe of bovine spongiform encephalopathy, or *mad cow disease*, and the human disease called new variant Creutzfeldt-Jakob disease (vCJD). Of the worldwide total of 153 vCJD cases, 143 have occurred in the United Kingdom. Cattle are considered the only source of the disease (CDC, 2011).

The 2014 Ebola outbreak in West Africa was bigger and more extensive than any prior Ebola epidemic. Numerous responders from a variety of disciplines, including nursing, rushed to help as teams tried to contain the spread of the deadly virus. Responders later reported tales of challenges and ingenuity as they struggled to overcome hardships and obstacles. Visit the following Web site for further stories of what it is really like to work under harsh conditions in the face of deadly epidemics (http://www.cdc.gov/about/ebola/overcoming-challenges.html).

It wasn't long before the virus reached U.S. soil, including two imported cases and two locally acquired cases among health care workers (CDC, 2015b). Standard screening protocols are now in place in the United States to guide screening and management of travelers from West Africa with suspected symptoms (see Fig. 16–2).

> *"…Creativity is possibly just as valuable as all the hard facts and materials. When there is no money, people are working beyond exhaustion and options are limited, thinking creatively can be the thing to pull you through."*
>
> —Leisha Nolen, Ebola responder, Sierra Leone

Global health issues become everyone's concerns when they spread within or beyond one's borders, when we commit resources to a country in need, when we make a personal commitment to improve the health of a population beyond our shores, and when we import or export food.

These trends and examples underscore both the ways in which people are being exposed to the health conditions, food, and environmental effects that may originate in one part of the world and to the uniqueness of local communities with their own geography and environment, history, cultural traditions, religion, and ideas about health, wellness, disease, and death. The notion to *think globally and act locally* captures the essence of this seeming dichotomy. Each of these elements constitutes entire disciplines of study and requires years of interacting with people to understand the ways in which they affect health care in a particular country.

Geography and Environment

The environment in which people live includes air, climate, soil, and water, and each of these may undergo changes that turn natural elements into hazardous ones. Humans are exposed to pollutants in two basic ways: by exposure to the source or by release of the pollutant into air or water. See Chapter 9 for more on environmental health issues.

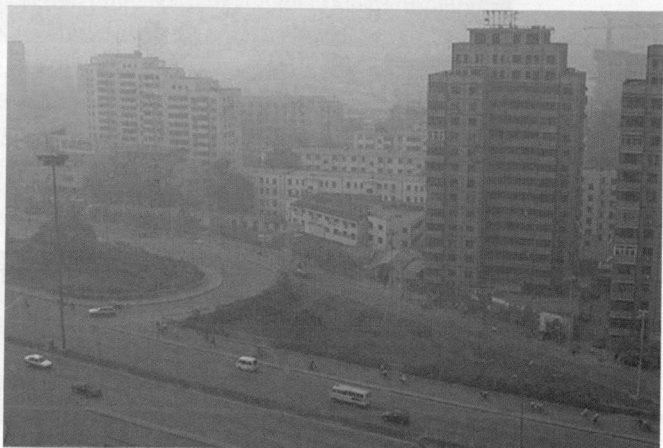

Air pollution in China. (Photo courtesy of CDC Photo Image Library.)

When people use streams and rivers to dispose of body wastes and then use the same body of water for cleaning and washing their clothes, they expose themselves to infections from those waters. For example, countries such as India, Indonesia, and Bangladesh—countries with large populations—have no choice as sewerage and clean water sources are not available in some parts of these countries. When people in villages build their homes around sources of water, they also invite mosquitoes that carry malaria, for instance. In this environment, community health nurses' interventions might include teaching people the steps to preventing malaria, such as placing netting around a bed during the night, cleaning pools of stagnant water around the home, and covering the body with light cotton clothes (Amoran, 2013), and advising on the placement and maintenance of latrines. See From the Case Files: Addressing Malaria in the Community.

People throughout the world are affected by the impact of major developments that may occur in their communities over which they have no control. For example, populations in Ethiopia were moved from one part of the country to another as colonial rulers developed crops for their own use. In the process, they displaced farmers to other areas to grow crops about which they knew little and which were not appropriate for the soil and weather conditions. In the aftermath of a 6.9 magnitude earthquake in Armenian Soviet Socialist Republic (SSR), Union of Soviet Socialist Republics (USSR), an Italian corporation built temporary housing in the available surrounding areas. The government provided basic metal enclosures for housing that later were destroyed to provide long-term structures and roads, along with many other donations of goods and services from countries around the world (ReliefWeb, 2011).

Environmental experts have focused on these and other issues, such as the effects on communities when climate changes occur or when weather conditions affect entire regions. The volcano eruption in Iceland, the tsunami and subsequent damage to the nuclear reactors in

Ebola Virus Disease (Ebola)
Algorithm for Evaluation of the Returned Traveler

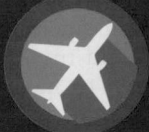

FEVER (subjective or ≥100.4°F or 38.0°C) or compatible Ebola symptoms* in a patient who has resided in or traveled to a country with wide-spread Ebola transmission** in the 21 days before illness onset
* headache, weakness, muscle pain, vomiting, diarrhea, abdominal pain, or hemorrhage

NO → **Report** asymptomatic patients with high- or low-risk exposures (see below) in the past 21 days to the health department

YES
1. Isolate patient in single room with a private bathroom and with the door to hallway closed
2. Implement standard, contact, and droplet precautions
3. Notify the hospital Infection Control Program and other appropriate staff
4. Evaluate for any risk exposures for Ebola
5. IMMEDIATELY report to the health department

HIGH-RISK EXPOSURE

Percutaneous (e.g., needle stick) or mucous membrane contact with blood or body fluids from an Ebola patient

OR

Direct skin contact with, or exposure to blood or body fluids of, an Ebola patient

OR

Processing blood or body fluids from an Ebola patient without appropriate personal protective equipment (PPE) or biosafety precautions

OR

Direct contact with a dead body (including during funeral rites) in a country with wide-spread Ebola transmission** without appropriate PPE

LOW-RISK EXPOSURE

Household members of an Ebola patient and others who had brief direct contact (e.g., shaking hands) with an Ebola patient without appropriate PPE

OR

Healthcare personnel in facilities with confirmed or probable Ebola patients who have been in the care area for a prolonged period of time while not wearing recommended PPE

NO KNOWN EXPOSURE

Residence in or travel to a country with wide-spread Ebola transmission** without HIGH- or LOW-risk exposure

Review Case with Health Department Including:
- Severity of illness
- Laboratory findings (e.g., platelet counts)
- Alternative diagnoses

Ebola suspected ⟷ **Ebola not suspected**

TESTING IS INDICATED

The health department will arrange specimen transport and testing at a Public Health Laboratory and CDC

The health department, in consultation with CDC, will provide guidance to the hospital on all aspects of patient care and management

TESTING IS NOT INDICATED

If patient requires in-hospital management:

- Decisions regarding infection control precautions should be based on the patient's clinical situation and in consultation with hospital infection control and the health department

- If patient's symptoms progress or change, re-assess need for testing with the health department

If patient does not require in-hospital management:

- Alert the health department before discharge to arrange appropriate discharge instructions and to determine if the patient should self-monitor for illness

- Self-monitoring includes taking their temperature twice a day for 21 days after their last exposure to an Ebola patient

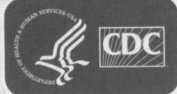

U.S. Department of Health and Human Services
Centers for Disease Control and Prevention

** CDC Website to check current countries with wide-spread transmission:
http://www.cdc.gov/vhf/ebola/outbreaks/2014-west-africa/case-counts.html

This algorithm is a tool to assist healthcare providers identify and triage patients who may have Ebola. The clinical criteria used in this algorithm (a single symptom consistent with Ebola) differ from the CDC case definition of a Person Under Investigation (PUI) for Ebola, which is more specific. Public health consultation alone does not imply that Ebola testing is necessary. More information on the PUI case definition: **http://www.cdc.gov/vhf/ebola/hcp/case-definition.html**

CS251958-A

FIGURE 16–2 Ebola virus disease algorithm for evaluation of returning travelers. (From Centers for Disease Control and Prevention (CDC). (2016). *Ebola (Ebola virus disease)*. Retrieved from http://www.cdc.gov/vhf/ebola/pdf/ebola-algorithm.pdf)

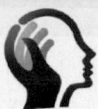

From the Case Files I

Addressing Malaria in the Community

Background: The Kenya Strategy for Community Health 2014 to 2019 includes an objective to "enhance community access to health care in order to improve productivity and thus reduce poverty, hunger, and child and maternal deaths, as well as improve education performance across all stages of life" (Kenya Ministry of Health, 2014, para. 1). In other words, it aims to empower Kenyan communities to take charge of improving their own health. One of the ways the community strategy intends to improve the health status of communities is by building the capacity of the community health extension workers (CHEWs) and community-owned resource persons (CORPs) to recognize and respond to emerging trends in the community.

Case: Atieno is a community nurse engaged as a CHEW in Siaya County. Over the past 3 months, she has observed a rise in the number of malaria cases involving children. In some cases, she herself made referrals during home visits in response to fever-related complaints. Though the county is a malaria endemic area, Atieno is concerned about the trend and begins to have conversations with the mothers/guardians. She soon learns that most of the patients are from a particular location in the community.

During one of the facility staff meetings, she raises the issue and proposes an explorative visit to the location by the extension team. During the visit, the team observes that almost every home compound has freshly dug pits that subsequently formed small, stagnant ponds. Some of the homes also have furnace-like structures. They learn that the local administration had recently hosted an organization promoting brick making as an income-generating venture. The venture had modest returns and was gaining popularity.

The team also noted that the start of the long rainy season had recently begun, which was accompanied by a steady rise in the number of children 0 to 5 years of age with fever-related symptoms. Some of the locals attribute the fever cases to the children playing in the stagnant ponds and catching cold. The team sought permission to check sleeping areas and realized that most do not have bed nets, and even for those who do, parents don't ensure that their children sleep under the net. The extension team heads back to their station to review their findings and discuss the next course of action.

In liaison with the local administration and the CHWs, the team participates in a community "baraza" (public meeting) to highlight the worrying trend in malaria morbidity and the findings of the explorative visit.

Together, the team and the community discuss the link between the findings and malaria morbidity. The community acknowledges that the brick-making venture has contributed to increase in stagnant water pools that have turned into breeding grounds for malaria-transmitting mosquitoes and that households have not adhered to protection measures to control malaria transmission. A number of immediate actions to address the problem without compromising their newfound source of income were identified:

- Draining stagnant water around the homesteads
- Monitoring fever, particularly in the children
- Seeking immediate medical attention at the local dispensary

Through collaboration, the community identifies and agrees on further steps to stem the problem:

- A community leader agrees to advocate for the distribution of free insecticide-treated bed nets, especially to households with pregnant women and children <5 years of age, because these are the most vulnerable.
- In the meantime, households were advised to buy locally available bed nets and treat them with approved insecticides.
- The household heads commit to identifying other areas for harvesting soil for brick making that would be away from the immediate home compounds.
- The local administration leader promises to work with the dispensary officials to access approved insecticides to fumigate the existing breeding grounds.
- The CHEW commits to providing ongoing community-based health services including health education, outreach services, and effective community–facility referrals
- One of the community nurses provides information on the causes, symptoms, and the importance of early treatment of malaria and demonstrated how to properly treat and use bed nets.

This case demonstrates highly effective, community-owned action, all spurred by one community nurse's observations and follow-up actions.

Contributing Authors: Missie Oindo, BA, MCHD and Serah Malaba-Kambale, BSc, MPH, PRINCE2® Practitioner, Kenya.
Kenya Ministry of Health. (2014, January 1). Strategy for community health 2014–2019. Retrieved from http://guidelines.health.go.ke/#/category/12/90/meta

Japan, the tsunami in Asia, and Hurricane Katrina in the United States are examples where entire communities were swept away (National Geographic Daily News, 2011). Over the past 5 years, the international meeting on the environment held in Copenhagen, Denmark, brought these issues to the forefront as did former United States Vice President and Nobel Prize winner, Al Gore, in his focus on global warming through his provocative and moving film, *An Inconvenient Truth*. In that film, Gore examined the ways in which our current habits and beliefs are affecting the world's temperature and environmental conditions (Parker, 2014; Takepart, n.d.).

Sometimes, change is intentional and is made in the interests of survival and daily functioning. For example, when governments address energy concerns for transportation and industry, they may move to nuclear sources of that energy—clearly as an effort to secure a local resource but also with some risk. The people in New Orleans experienced the aftermath of an oil rig disaster in the Gulf of Mexico as did the people of Chernobyl who found their homes a wasteland when the nuclear plant disaster polluted the region with cesium and iodine (Boston Globe, 2011). In a follow-up meeting to the Chernobyl accident, held a few years later in the Netherlands, representatives spoke of the population's fears and actions, including possessing machines that would measure the radioactivity near their homes. This accident prompted the discussion of disaster-preparedness strategies to evacuate entire cities of people after a nuclear environmental accident.

Environmental Hazards

Environmental health is about human health as determined by physical, chemical, biological, social, and psychosocial factors in the environment. Environmental risk factors are of increasing importance and have been influences by increased urbanization, a rise of employment in informal sectors, growth of the chemical industry, increased oil consumption, and climate change (WHO, 2011). Broad categories of environmental hazards include water, sanitation, and hygiene, chemical exposure, occupational health hazards, radiation exposure, air pollution, and climate change (Maxwell, 2014). Our job, as public health nurses, is to assess, correct, **control**, and prevent factors in the environment that have potential adverse effects.

Water and Sanitation

Worldwide, 780 million people lack access to safe water and 2.5 billion do not have improved sanitation; the implications for health are considerable (CDC, 2015f). Up to 90% of wastewater in developing countries is discharged untreated, polluting rivers, lakes, and coastal areas (Fuhrmeister, Schwab, & Julian, 2015). In places such as Peru, Egypt, Bangladesh, India, Indonesia, and Thailand, raw sewage is released into rivers that are used for drinking and bathing. In Western Africa, parts of the ocean are contaminated with raw sewage. Such practices often result in diarrheal diseases, including cholera. The International Centre for Diarrhoeal Diseases Control Research (ICDDR) in Bangladesh specializes in those illnesses, including cholera that results from these practices, for which residents know of no alternative.

Six to eight million people die annually from illnesses linked to unsafe drinking water, poor household hygiene, and improper human and animal waste disposal. Diarrheal diseases are the second leading cause of death in children >5 years of age, predominantly in developing countries (World Health Organization [WHO] Media Centre, 2013) (see Display 16–1, Environmental-Related Killers in Children Under Age 5). Half of the population in the poor countries of the world suffers from one or more of the five main diseases associated with water and sanitation—diarrhea, ascariasis, hookworm, schistosomiasis, and trachoma—and 35% of the world's population is without access to improved sanitation (CDC, 2015b).

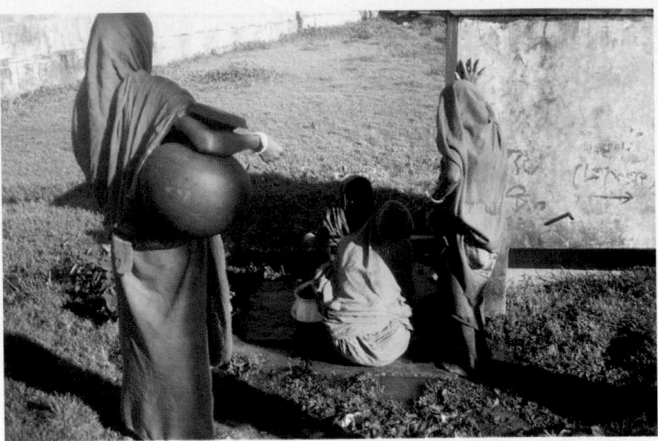
Women in a Bangladeshi village getting water from a communal well. (Photo courtesy of CDC Photo Image Library.)

Millions of people worldwide are infected with neglected tropical diseases, many of which are water and/or hygiene related. Diseases such as Guinea worm disease, Buruli ulcer, trachoma, and schistosomiasis thrive where there is unsafe drinking water, poor sanitation, and insufficient hygiene practices. Improving water, sanitation, and hygiene has the potential to prevent 9.1% of the disease burden globally. Improved water sources alone can reduce diarrheal morbidity by 21%. Improving sanitation reduces diarrheal morbidity by 37.5% (CDC, 2015e). In short, prevention is a key intervention for the public health nurse. See Display 16–1 about environmental-related child deaths.

Climate Change

There is a growing body of evidence supporting global warming. Data indicate that the global average combined land and ocean surface temperature has warmed by 0.85°C

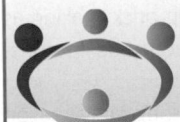

DISPLAY 16–1 ENVIRONMENTAL-RELATED KILLERS IN CHILDREN UNDER AGE 5

- Diarrhea kills 1.6 million children each year (mainly because of unsafe water and poor sanitation).
- Indoor air pollution kills 1 million children each year as a result of acute respiratory infections (because of use of biomass fuels for indoor cooking and heating).
- Malaria kills around 1 million children, mostly in Africa (exacerbated by poor management and storage of water, deforestation, and inadequate housing).
- Unintentional physical injuries account for 300,000 annual deaths due to drowning, fires, falls, poisoning, traffic accidents, and other causes (often related to community or household hazards).

From World Health Organization (WHO). (2016). *The environment and health for children and their mothers.* Retrieved from http://www.who.int/ceh/publications/factsheets/fs284/en/

between 1880 and 2012. Climate change, and the resulting variations in weather patterns, has the potential to impact our health. Predicted extreme weather events and longer-term impacts of drought are likely to lead to malnutrition and an increase in the spread of some infectious diseases such as malaria and dengue fever. Not surprisingly, the poorest and most vulnerable population are likely to experience the most dramatic impacts, often worsened by forced migration, unplanned urbanization, and contamination of air and water. Those of us in the health sector need to ensure that health facilities have access to clean energy and play our part in lowering the climate footprint of the health sector in developed countries (WHO, 2015a).

The Ozone Layer

As the challenge of a depleted ozone layer is addressed, the incidence of cataracts and cancer (especially melanoma and basal cell carcinoma) is reduced. It is believed that human activities are contributing to the depletion of the ozone layer; these activities include the use of chlorofluorocarbons (CFCs) (used in the manufacture of air conditioners, refrigerators, aerosol propellants, and other products) and methyl bromides (found in pesticides and herbicides). Efforts are under way to phase out CFCs in 13 countries, including the United States (Ozone Hole, n.d.). While the hole is still present, new ways of measuring ozone in the atmosphere and some weather changes have caused it to shrink slightly over Antarctica, thought to be a normal phenomenon of waxing and waning. But scientists are now hopeful that it may close entirely by 2070 (Heffernan, 2013).

History

If you have tea with a group of health care providers in Moscow, the conversation inevitably turns to the devastating effects of the major historical event that faced that country—World War II, or the Great Patriotic War. Despite the fact that this war occurred over 60 years ago, it remains in the collective memory of the Russian people, their leaders, and many others in Eastern Europe, as 20 million Russians died along with thousands of people in other countries. That war, and the war that involved Bosnia–Herzegovina and Serbia, will affect the health of people for decades to come and will influence the ways in which the health care systems of these countries will partner and collaborate with each other in the future (Ringdal & Ringdal, 2016).

The ways in which mental health was viewed historically was strongly influenced in England by leprosy as a reminder of death and the need to rid the community of those infected with this disease. Like lepers, the mentally ill were cast out of society. The response was to rid the community by first sending the insane outside the gates of the cities, then on ships out to sea (Ships of Fools), only later to be turned over to doctors and housed in buildings referred to as "madhouses," through a process of incarceration enforced by the law. In this way, the mentally ill became inextricably linked to law enforcement (as described in the classic book by Foucault, 1965), and this link persists today (Shimmon, 2011). This form of power was expressed through laws that controlled not only the mentally ill but the poor and the unemployed.

Throughout the past century, other forms of power and control occurred throughout the world as countries were colonized and sometimes purged of their wealth. The relationship between those colonized and their colonizers persists today. These political relationships also affect the ways in which community health nurses might be recruited and practice. For example, given a country's history, health care providers with particular nationalities or religious backgrounds might not be acceptable to a country. Whereas people in one country might consider these biases unacceptable, they remain as policy in other places, determining whether or not care providers of a particular nationality are allowed to enter and work in a country. These biases are often unexpected and may be puzzling. At first glance, one may wonder why Italy might want to support a disaster-preparedness program in Ethiopia. But a review of the historical relationship between Italy and Ethiopia reveals a relationship that preceded the program initiative. In a similar way, for example, Chad has a past relationship with France, Mozambique with Portugal, the Congo with Belgium, Albania with Italy, and Indonesia with the Netherlands, to name just a few (MacQueen, 2014). In addition to past relationships with other countries, communities also develop within the context of other relationships as well.

Public health nurses are involved in designing and implementing projects in collaboration with international governmental organizations and NGOs. In summary, the historical context of a country is paramount as people are selected for international positions and projects, for interventions that a community is willing to adopt, and organizations are chosen to intervene in a region.

Language

Often, a language connection exists between countries, and this linkage prompts health officials to seek nurses who speak the same language. For example, common history and language often connect Mozambique, Portugal, and Brazil, which are all Portuguese-speaking countries. Many people from Mozambique immigrated to Portugal during the 1970s, and the shared historical past affects current perceptions about the two countries' relationship with each other (MacQueen, 2014). Knowing that a shared language exists among countries may suggest ways of learning about cultural practices and about gathering existing health-related teaching and learning materials and can reduce the costs of production and language validation.

Political, Cultural, Religious Practices, and Context

A country's political orientation and practices affect the ways in which community health nurses are educated and function daily. For example, in some countries, nurses and midwives were not exposed to the emerging knowledge and practices concerning the HIV/acquired immunodeficiency syndrome (AIDS) epidemic. This happened, in part, because countries whose economies depended on tourism were fearful that public knowledge of high numbers of HIV-infected people would frighten away tourists. In other countries with closed borders and totalitarian regimes, health authorities were left out of the latest information on the epidemiology of diseases.

In some countries, tribal practices took precedence over protection from the virus, and in other countries, the custom of visiting brothels resulted in epidemic rates of the virus. Consequently, national health policies and announcements denied the presence of the virus, people by the hundreds were infected, and nurses and midwives were not protected as they collected blood samples, administered injections, and delivered babies. One large international study examined the differences in national response to HIV/AIDS and also noncommunicable diseases among four countries (Haregu, Setswe, Elliott, & Oldenburg, 2014). Two countries considered as upper middle-income (South Africa, Malaysia) and two lower-income countries (Sri Lanka, Ethiopia) were evaluated for prevalence of HIV (17.3% South Africa, 0.4% Malaysia, 0.1% Sri Lanka, 1.4%, Ethiopia) and diabetes (6.5% South Africa, 11.7% Malaysia, 7.8% Sri Lanka, 3.4% Ethiopia). Researchers noted differences in process and internal constituents.

The culture and religion of a community represent the frame within which people understand who they are, why they are on the earth, and what their purposes are in life (Spector, 2013). Culture and religion influence the knowledge, attitudes, and practices of people about what they think will kill them or make them sick, will help them function or make decisions, or will affect their financial status. People in different cultures manage these in ways that may seem peculiar, ill advised, immoral, or even criminal to someone outside the society. For example, Illyes (1979), in the classic book *People of the Puszta*, discussed the cultural practice of suicide in a part of Hungary, the Puszta, where people are characterized as "dirt poor." Yet, suicide is not a socially accepted option for people in other cultures. In the Philippines, some prostitutes see their activities as simply their "daily work," not as a moral act. Efforts to dismantle the country's prostitution business have met with negative reactions from the prostitutes themselves, as this is their way of feeding their children and caring for their families. However, as younger females are becoming more involved, often as unwilling victims, there is more momentum to address this problem (Tupas, 2015).

Community health nurses will face their own beliefs when confronting female circumcision, the use of non-licensed personnel to carry out medical treatments, and the use of Western interventions used simultaneously with local treatments. For example, in Chad, clients in a Chadian hospital received Western-style medical treatment and nursing care through the interventions of French physicians and nurses whereas lines wound around the grounds of the hospital to the offices of the two Chinese acupuncturists. In rural villages in India, untrained midwives, or *dais*, may fail to treat a fever in women during the postpartum period regardless of its etiology. Some of these alternatives are deemed helpful, whereas others have garnered mixed reviews in research studies (Das et al., 2012).

Cultural issues are of concern when individuals and groups of a particular background from one country are often fiercely committed to "helping" their homeland. Here, both donors and recipients need to understand each other and their reasons for entering collaborative relationships. When this is thought through, the results can be most positive. In this regard, Armenian communities benefited enormously from the fund-raising efforts of U.S. community health nurses and physicians who knew well the Armenian communities in Boston, parts of Canada, and Los Angeles. Similarly, the American Albanian community was mobilized after the economic collapse of Albania in 1991. The same thing occurred after the "Arab Spring" uprisings in Egypt, with calls for wealthy Egyptian Americans to help support postrevolution Egypt (Eishinnawi, 2011).

Women and Culture

Women in most societies are viewed in ways that require close scrutiny. Historically, women in Western society during the Middle Ages and the Renaissance had an incentive to marry early as they had no legal status before the courts and had to generally be represented by a male proctor (Blanton, 2014). These practices persist today in some European countries and in other parts of the world. For example, in Saudi Arabia, a male family member must accompany a female going to receive health care. Historically and today, poor women were and are particularly marginalized because of few opportunities for work. They were raised to produce children and were kept relatively secluded until marriage. If their spouses died, they had few options; typically, they entered a nunnery or prostituted themselves.

Women are seen as Madonnas, superheroes, warriors, nurturers, slaves, income producers, objects of sexual desire, concubines, negotiators, angels of mercy, and assistants. Although these characterizations may be repulsive to some, to others, women in their communities have played these roles for so long that they are considered immutable and acceptable. In many countries, nurses are exclusively women and experience these projections as they carry out their daily work. In some places, women have no or little voice and are viewed as weak or ineffectual, despite their physiological hardiness and ability to survive above their male counterparts. Kirk and Okazawa-Rey (2013) have documented the harmful economic, social, and military policies that they suggest have been imposed on the South and have wreaked havoc on U.S. working class and poor people of color as well as immigrant communities.

Community health nurses may perceive themselves as excellent practitioners with excellent theoretical and clinical backgrounds and expect to be respected for these qualities. Yet, in another country, their nursing notes may be torn up (who will read them?), their projects taken over by others (a nurse can't possibly lead a project), and their research may be published under someone else's name (anyone can write hypotheses, so what makes these so special?). In some countries, women (and nurses) are not expected to argue with authority, assume a team leadership role, or attend important meetings at high levels. In some circumstances, women have learned to succeed by the use of "feminine charm" in the workplace or to combine friendly approaches and a degree of flirtation (Kray, Locke, & Van Zant, 2012).

Globally, nurses strive for autonomy, and this is especially true when working in resource-limited settings.

Research has shown the profession of nursing is viewed differently in different cultural settings. Some nurses perceive a wide hierarchical distance from physicians that promotes subservience on the part of the nurse. Other factors that have been reported as having a negative impact on professional relationships are generational differences and gender biases (Ng'ang'a & Byrne, 2015).

These are challenging situations, some of which become teachable moments. Some may be events that alter the duration of one's assignment or provide an opportunity to reframe interactions with others of differing persuasions, beliefs, and practices. Community health nurses need to determine their own position on these issues and come to terms with being placed in subservient positions or in roles that detract from their level of academic preparation, expectations for learning and developing, and, ultimately, their sense of self. Yet, as noted below, women have played critical activist roles in the situations of crisis, conflict, and genocide.

Women carry the culture of a society, and they are inextricably linked with a country's history, conflicts, and their solutions. Here, women's issues intersect with issues of armed conflict, militarism, and their activism. In this section of this chapter, as in their lives, women provide a link between a society's culture and the wars in which the society engages. For example, Gallimore (2008) notes "women all over the African region have not only participated in, survived and resisted violent conflict, but played key roles in facilitating negotiations and peace-brokering efforts" (p. 6). Women have also joined together to campaign for an end to all violence against women and girls (Raab & Rocha, 2011).

Armed Conflict, Uprisings, Wars, and Humanitarian Emergencies

An armed conflict is defined as major if the number of deaths has reached 1,000. Increasingly, conflicts are internal rather than between states. In their quest for economic and political power, the combatants target the lives and livelihoods of civilians associated with opposing factions (Themnér & Wallensteen, 2013). Typically, armed conflicts and uprisings initially cause governments and agencies to place a high priority on health care, but their ability to sustain health care is reduced as time goes on. Countries engaged in armed conflict form internal factions, including those supporting the government and those in conflict against them. Most conflicts occur between states for economic and political power. Currently, the world is experiencing another sea change as rebel forces in Egypt, Libya, Yemen, Syria, and other countries reject the existing regimes in power. Sometimes, outside nations support a country's factions, and fighting escalates and continues until the supporting powers win, lose interest, change their political orientation, or exhaust their financial sources (Critchlow, 2015). In this regard, community health nurses need to be aware of those involved in the immediate situation and of those who are influencing the situation from abroad. In turn, funding and sustaining nursing projects may depend ultimately on a variety of factors, not the least of which is being able to participate in situations that may be a threat to the nurse's safety and survival.

Countries that have long-standing conflicts suffer as current health care needs are unaddressed, and the long-term health status of an entire country may be affected—sometimes for decades. For example, Mozambique had endured a national conflict for over two decades. Two generations of young people had no formal education and were prepared only to fight. Children were forced to be soldiers and prompted to commit horrible atrocities within their communities and often within their own families. Countries in conflict deflect resources to the battlefield, and those fighting, identified as the males in the society, receive whatever resources are available despite the fact that women and children experience extreme devastation during these times. These conflicts are extremely complex social phenomena, for which the most rooted causes are inequity, cultural and religious intolerance, and ethnic discrimination (Ringdal & Ringdal, 2016).

The health infrastructure during conflicts and uprisings becomes vulnerable because of the instability. Often, opposing factions raid hospitals and clinics. For example, during the 1989 Romanian uprising, health providers told of instances in which the underground secret police feigned injury, transported themselves in rigged ambulances, and entered the emergency room areas of the capitol's major hospitals, all in an effort to kill or wound the hospitals' health care providers. Also, refugees fleeing war-torn areas are often unable to receive adequate health care, shelter, and other necessities of life (Doocy et al., 2016).

The community interventions that nurses develop are informed by the situation and the layers of conflict that have occurred in the past and those that may be continuing (see From the Case Files I). During national conflicts, health services become disorganized and experience decreased resources. Outside help is needed in these instances, and international help is often available. For example, during the Romanian uprising, members of WHO/EURO international disaster-preparedness team, along with the country's health officials, established an Interim Ministry of Health and identified key areas that required attention. Members of the team, including the Regional Nursing Advisor, met with NATO and COMECON ambassadors in the capitol and communicated the health needs of the population. They remained in Romania and established a WHO office, participating with groups, universities, and organizations to assist the country during this difficult period. These actions have been repeated in numerous other areas over the years as conflicts have emerged. See Perspectives: WHO Regional Advisor.

During wars and other man-made disasters, epidemics are almost inevitable. As conflict goes on, the health care needs of the combatants often take priority over those of civilians; consequently, thousands of children may be injured, orphaned, and at risk for disease. Additionally, conflict disrupts food cultivation, harvest, and distribution, leaving populations at risk for malnutrition and setting the stage for disease. In the Syrian conflict, 6.5 million have been displaced, and infection outbreaks have increased in Syria and its neighbor countries (Sharara & Kanj, 2014). Refugees from such events have special health and social needs. Often, refugee camps are developed by international organizations on the fringe of such conflicts to temporarily assist refugees with shelter, food, and the rudiments of health care. Such camps place a strain on the resources of neighboring countries, as illustrated during the recent conflicts in the Middle East and the civil war in Syria (Doocy et al., 2016). It is estimated that by the start of 2015, over 3.7 million Syrians had fled and another 11.6 million were considered displaced (Ostrand, 2015). Sweden and Germany had accepted the largest proportion of refugees, and many other countries also opened their borders to them.

All of these factors can lead to complex humanitarian emergencies. The CDC describes complex humanitarian emergencies as situations that involve large civilian populations and factors related to war or civil strife, shortage of necessities such as food, and the dislocation of local populations. These situations and these factors result in mortality beyond that expected under normal circumstances (United Nations High Commissioner for Refugees, 2010).

Recovery after war is a long-term project. Any postwar recovery effort must deal with the disabled, the mentally ill, prisoners, widows, orphans, abandoned children, homeless and displaced persons, refugees, and the unemployed (Levy & Sidel, 2015). In addition, livestock and domestic animals must be cared for or their carcasses buried or incinerated. These issues are complex; for example, in some African countries, if a family loses its land and its members cannot plant and harvest crops, the family has no source of food and may become malnourished—leading to death. During the long conflict in that region, many women lost their husbands and their land. They required care from others who had very little to offer them. At times, the rebel forces in conflict countries are poorly equipped and have experienced severe injuries, and they require interventions from a population also under siege.

Health Promotion

It is not enough to strive to protect individuals from disease or adverse events, but health promotion is also vital. This paradigm shift was exemplified in the **Ottawa Charter**

for Health Promotion. The first international conference on health promotion took place there in 1986, and prerequisites were outlined: peace, shelter, food, income, education, a stable ecosystem, sustainable resources, and social justice/equity (WHO, 2016o). The participants acknowledged that individuals create their health each day as they care for themselves and others. The conference ended with this pledge to:

- Move into the arena of healthy public policy and to advocate a clear political commitment to health and equity in all sectors
- Counteract the pressures toward harmful products, resource depletion, unhealthy living conditions and environments, and bad nutrition and to focus attention on public health issues such as pollution, occupational hazards, housing, and settlements
- Respond to the health gap within and between societies; to tackle the inequities in health produced by the rules and practices of these societies; to acknowledge people as the main health resource; to support and enable them to keep themselves, their families, and friends healthy through financial and other means; and to accept the community as the essential voice in matters of its health, living conditions, and well-being
- Reorient health services and their resources toward the promotion of health and to share power with other sectors, other disciplines, and, most importantly, people themselves
- Recognize health and its maintenance as a major social investment and challenge and to address the overall ecological issue of our ways of living (WHO, 2016o, p. 3)

At the fourth international conference on health promotion in 1997, the **Jakarta Declaration** on Leading Health Promotion Into the 21st Century was developed (WHO, 2016i). This was the first health promotion conference held in a developing country (Jakarta, Indonesia). Participants acknowledged "health is a basic right and is essential for social and economic development" (p. 1). They noted that comprehensive approaches are most effective, that specific settings (e.g., workplaces, schools, cities, health care facilities) are best for implementation of these strategies, and that individual participation is critical and can be facilitated by proper information and education. Priorities for 21st century health promotion include the following:

- Promote social responsibility for health.
- Increase investments for health development.
- Consolidate and expand partnerships for health.
- Increase community and empower the individual.
- Secure an infrastructure for health promotion (p. 3).

Governments were called on to promote health within their own countries and work together to create alliances, and this was again emphasized at the Global Conference on Health Promotion (8GCHP) held in Helsinki, Finland, in 2013. This conference promoted the concept to *health in all policies*: a drive to inspire countries to think about health as they refine policies within all sectors.

Many countries have agencies that promote health within their boundaries and assist in health and development in other countries (e.g., Canadian International Development Agency [CIDA], National Primary Healthcare Development Agency [NPHCDA] in Nigeria, U.S. Centers for Disease Control and Prevention [CDC]). NGOs from many countries also work together to promote health and assist in community development (e.g., Aga Khan Development Network, Oxfam, Project HOPE).

Health Care Systems

Countries throughout the world have developed health care systems that they organize and structure in particular ways. When community health nurses find themselves in locations different from their own, they notice differences immediately, and their ability to practice within the context of these different ways of delivering health care services is critical to their success. The capacity to reflect on one's consciousness is an essential skill as one considers the ways in which people expect to govern others, provide people with what they need, determine who gets served and who does not, establish lines of authority and communication, and establish payment systems for health care services.

Important questions arise as one delivers community health nursing services within a country's health care system. For example, if a client has to wait 6 months for elective surgery, what does he or she do in the meantime? If a government provides all prenatal and obstetrical services but will not instruct couples on birth control, how do couples manage, and how do health authorities deal with prevalent practices that result in an abortion rate that is three times the birth rate (as documented in a classic article by Farrell et al., 1994) or that allow *under the table* reimbursement for these services? If a ministry of health is administered through a centrally governed model of decision-making, how do decisions get made that require local rather than district or national answers? If a local nursing group is interested in developing community health nursing standards of practice, and yet all nursing actions are reviewed by only a medical board of physicians, on what are the nursing standards based?

Pluralistic health care systems are found in many countries (see Chapter 6). They often consist of traditional healing systems, lay practices, household remedies, transitional health workers, and practitioners of Western medicine (Davis, Stremikis, Squires, & Schoen, 2014). Traditional healing may be all that is available to populations in some rural areas and in some cities.

Western medicine was introduced to some countries during colonial times, and systems were operated either by colonial administrations or by missions. After independence, health systems tended to vary in their development. Some continue their colonial practices; others followed tax-financed government insurance or socialist health care systems (Davis et al., 2014).

During the second half of the 20th century, curative health care expanded rapidly in urban areas, and the level of health care was raised in those areas. In the late 1970s, many countries adopted the PHC approach and the WHO regions of the world developed their own set of targets, for example, in the United States, *Healthy People 2000*, followed by *Healthy People 2010*, and now *Healthy People 2020* (USDHHS, 2016); through regional consultation, WHO (2016m) member states

developed objectives and targets for its *Health 2020*. Throughout the world, countries used this approach to serve their urban and rural populations. Four major types of health care systems are currently operational throughout the world. These systems are entrepreneurial, welfare-oriented, comprehensive, and socialist systems.

- *Entrepreneurial health care systems.* A country's health care system is based, in part, on its political economy. An entrepreneurial health system is typically found in industrialized countries with free-market economies, abundant resources, large amounts of money allocated to health care, and decentralized governments. These countries operate from a highly individualistic perspective. For example, the health care system in the United States is typical of the entrepreneurial system (Shi & Singh, 2016).
- *Welfare-oriented health care systems.* Statutory programs drive these systems that support the cost of health care for all, or almost all, of the population through their "national health insurance." In these, half of the health-related expenditures are covered by government sources, but most physicians and dentists remain in private practice. Western Europe, Japan, and Australia subscribe to welfare-oriented health care systems (Davis et al., 2014).
- *Comprehensive health care systems.* These systems are a step away from the welfare-oriented types in that substantial modifications exist in delivery and financing that result in universal entitlements. These systems abandon the separate and complex sources of financing found in the previous two systems. The Scandinavian countries, Great Britain, and New Zealand use a comprehensive health care delivery system (Davis et al., 2014).
- *Socialist health care systems.* These systems came about through social revolutions that abolished free-market economies and replaced them with socialism, in which the health care system is also socialized. The first overthrow of capitalism was in Russia in 1917, followed by Eastern Europe, Albania, Bulgaria, Czechoslovakia, Hungary, Poland, Romania, and later China, Cuba, and Korea. In these systems, health services were viewed as a social entitlement and a government responsibility. They emphasized prevention and engaged in central planning for health resources and services with one central health authority. They also prioritized special groups, such as industrial workers and children, and based health care work on scientific principles. Nonscientific and cultist practices were not permitted. Many of these countries have begun the process of democratization and redesign of their administrative and health care systems (Liebert, Condrey, & Goncharov, 2013).

The four health systems described above apply to industrialized countries. The renowned health system researcher Roemer (1993) used the same typology for transitional and very poor countries. Countries that are in the process of development are referred to as "transitional." Such countries and their health care systems are moving effectively toward economic and social development. The global median gross domestic product

(GDP) of these countries was $1,500 per capita. It should be noted that some might object to this classification system that considers being financially poor synonymous with being socially underdeveloped. This suggests a bias in thinking and a Western perspective that determines what is "developed" and what "needs developing."

Very poor countries are even less economically developed and have lower per capita GDPs than do the industrialized or transitional countries. Areas classified by the World Bank Group (2016) as poor have a large proportion of their population living on $1.90 or less per day. Some countries in sub-Saharan Africa have almost 43% of their population that meets this standard, as do almost 40% of people living in areas of conflict. South Asian regions have almost 19% of the population falling into this category.

Trends Affecting Health Care Systems

Health care systems are affected by major social factors such as urbanization, industrialization, education, government structure, international trade, and demographic changes. Many national health systems have undergone major changes during the last few decades of the 20th and into the 21st century. Specifically, these health care systems have changed the way they organize and are managed. For example, in England, health care has traditionally been provided through the National Health Service. People who can afford to pay for services outside the system are becoming more prevalent. Some health care systems that were totally funded by national health services are moving toward privatization of their services, whereas the United States has moved toward health care reform. See Chapter 6 for more on health care systems.

Health care systems also expanded their resources and added personnel, facilities, and equipment. Meanwhile, populations grew, migrated, and became more educated. They demanded more and better health care services. Over the past decade, hospitals worldwide have shifted to outpatient services and home care, expanding the roles and positions of community health nurses. Currently, in the United States, this trend has resulted in the closing of small community hospitals, to the consternation of many residents of smaller towns and rural areas (Tribble, 2011).

Hospitals in Denmark benefited from a surgical procedure for hip replacement that would allow a patient to be discharged from hospital to home in a much shorter time period than previously experienced. This meant that home care had to be ready to accept the patient within an abbreviated time frame, thus requiring innovations in discharge planning and teaching protocols. In addition to these advances, the PHC movement supported efforts to reduce the number of hospital buildings and to increase community-based nursing services (Husted et al., 2011).

Technological advances occurred to support this move, and ways of thinking about health promotion emerged with a variety of quality measures and, more recently, evidence-based practices that support nursing interventions on an outpatient basis and at lowered costs. The depopulation of some communities and the increasing number of empty beds has also been related to these closings.

Most importantly, people have begun to educate themselves through the use of the Internet. Ministries of health are training community care workers in communication, observation, and technical skills for telehealth systems that link remote areas to academic health centers. For example, a health center in Almaty, Kazakhstan, is now connected through the Internet, even though it began as a relatively isolated center in what was referred to as Alma-Ata. Now, groups with relatively rare health care conditions can receive support and information from others in parts of the world formerly unknown to them. See Chapter 10 for more on technology and telehealth.

THE POPULATION

The populations that community health nurses serve are complex and include clients' concerns, values, beliefs, physical symptoms, and health history. As described earlier, the framework that provides some boundaries for considering these issues focuses on context, the three eras of health conditions, and the universal imperatives of care.

Era of Infectious Diseases

Infectious diseases and conditions have killed people, made them sick, altered their daily functioning, influenced their decision-making, and affected the costs of care. Thus, these infections and infectious processes involve all the universal imperatives of care but do so differently, depending on a variety of factors (Davies, 2012). These factors include the climate, geography, and other conditions infectious organisms need to survive and thrive and the populations the infectious agents invade–often infants and children. Surveillance and response networks are key to containing infectious diseases, and this can be difficult for countries with underfunded health systems to accomplish. Thus, it is not surprising that 83% of all worldwide deaths in children younger than 5 years are due to infectious diseases, nutrition, or neonatal conditions. A good percentage of the almost 6 million deaths in children below the age of 5 in 2015 were due to infectious diseases (WHO, 2014b, 2016e). Three of the ten leading causes of death are communicable diseases that largely affect children. Most of these are preventable.

Almost 200 nations, and all member states of the World Health Organization (2016n), agreed to International Health Regulations (IHRs) regarding surveillance and notification about infectious diseases that may spread globally. Public Health Emergencies of International Concern (PHEIC) procedures clarify steps countries need to take in order to comply with the IHRs. Some of these include not only controlling borders but containing the source of infectious diseases and all public health threats, as well as allowing for adaptive responses (Davies, 2012). Three categories of concerns include:

1. Cholera, pneumonic plague, yellow fever, viral hemorrhagic fevers (Ebola, Lassa, Marburg), West Nile fever, and others of specific regional concern (e.g., dengue fever, Rift Valley fever, meningococcal disease)
2. Unusual or unexpected outbreaks and especially the following diseases: poliomyelitis, SARS, new human influenza subtype, and smallpox (all require immediate notification)
3. Novel outbreaks of diseases not noted above (Davies, 2012, p. 698)

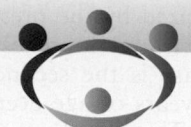

DISPLAY 16–2 GLOBAL DEATH RATE PER 100,000: SELECTED CAUSES, 2013

Causes	2013 Death Rate	Median % Change From 1990
All Causes	879.7	−24.2
Communicable, maternal, neonatal, and nutritional diseases	172.2	−40.5
Diarrhea, lower respiratory infections, and other common infectious diseases	72.4	−49.4
Malaria and neglected tropical diseases	13.9	−24.9
Noncommunicable diseases	637.5	−18.6
Neoplasms	133.8	−14.7
Cardiovascular disease	293.2	−22.0
Chronic respiratory diseases	73.0	−30.4
Neurological disorders	35.0	2.3
Behavioral health disorders	4.0	−5.7
Diabetes, urogenital, blood, and endocrine diseases	48.3	14.4
Injuries	70.0	−21.0

Adapted from Global Burden of Disease Mortality and Causes of Death Collaborators. (2015). Global, regional, and national age-sex specific all-cause and cause-specific mortality for 240 causes of death, 1990–2013: A systematic analysis for the Global Burden of Disease Study, 12013. *Lancet, 385*, 117–171.

The major preventive measure, immunization, is described here, followed by brief descriptions of some of the major infectious diseases. (See Display 16–2 for global death rates by selected causes worldwide.)

Immunization

The CDC estimates that vaccines prevent 2.5 million deaths among children younger than 5 years of age every year. Regardless, one child dies every 20 seconds from a disease that could have been prevented by a vaccine (CDC, 2015d). Vaccines are one of the most cost-effective interventions found in public health. Today, almost 75% of the world's children are being reached with essential vaccines, but many barriers make it difficult to maintain high levels of immunization in low- and middle-income countries. Scaling up vaccines in 73 of the poorest countries by 2020 could have 6.4 million lives and $6.2 billion in treatment costs and $145 billion in productivity losses (UNICEF, 2014).

Historically, a lot has been accomplished: smallpox has been eradicated; polio is close to being eradicated; measles deaths have declined by 75% since 2000; and deaths from maternal/neonatal tetanus dropped by 90% over the past 20 years.

Barriers persist and include limited finances, lack of trained health care workers, physical obstacles to reaching remote areas, and civil wars; these factors have prompted the development of an interagency vaccine initiative, which is now called GAVI—The Global Alliance (formerly the Global Alliance for Vaccine and Immunization). This initiative seeks to protect every child against vaccine-preventable diseases (WHO, 2016d). Strategies include funding, research, development, distribution of vaccines, and program sustainability. These approaches are expected to result in more immunized children and to move newer vaccines into developing

countries more quickly. See Chapter 8 for more on vaccine-preventable diseases.

Measles

Measles is a vaccine-preventable communicable disease. In 2014, the number of measles deaths was 114,900. The largest number of deaths—95%—occurred in low-income countries with inadequate health infrastructures (WHO Media Centre, 2015e). The intervention considered to have the greatest impact in reducing measles is the **integrated management of childhood illness (IMCI)**. This intervention promotes wide immunization coverage, rapid referral of serious cases, prompt recognition of secondary conditions, improved nutrition including breast-feeding, and vitamin A supplementation. Three main foci include improving health systems and case management skills, along with community and family health practice improvement. A WHO/UNICEF Measles Mortality Reduction and Regional Elimination Strategic Plan sought a 50% reduction in measles mortality worldwide by 2005—hoping eventually to eradicate the disease. Measles deaths actually fell worldwide by 79% between 2000 and 2014 worldwide (WHO Media Centre, 2015e).

Poliomyelitis

In 1988, there were 350,000 cases of poliomyelitis (polio) in the world. By 2013, there were only a total of 407 cases worldwide (CDC, 2014). Polio is now almost eliminated worldwide, even in densely populated and war-torn countries. Since the inception of the Global Polio Eradication Initiative, cases have fallen dramatically and there are now only three polio-infected countries remaining: Afghanistan and Pakistan (Global Polio Eradication Initiative, 2016). Still, as long as a single child remains infected with polio, children worldwide are at risk.

The CDC, WHO, UNICEF, and many national governments support the Global Polio Eradication Initiative.

Pandemic Influenza

The World Health Organization, in cooperation with many other agencies, prepared for the 2009 to 2020 H1N1 influenza pandemic. The United States has a pandemic influenza plan (see http://www.hhs.gov/pandemicflu/plan/) that outlines public health and medical support, guidance for state and local health departments, and an operational plan for the U.S. Department of Health and Human Services. The response to this novel virus may have seemed too many to be an overreaction—this was simply "the flu." But an H1N1 virus was responsible for the 1918 influenza pandemic that killed over 50 million people worldwide (much more than the 16 million lost in World War I), and it appeared without warning in late spring. It surfaced again in fall and was much more virulent, with some victims dying "within hours of their first symptoms" (National Archives and Records Administration, n.d., para 3). Young adults, along with children and the elderly, were most susceptible to complications and U.S. life expectancy "dropped by 12 years" during 1918 (para 4).

Because of this earlier pandemic experience with H1N1, WHO issued worldwide cautions and preparations, and scientists raced to produce enough specific vaccine to meet global demand. Researchers ran statistical models to predict transmissibility and control measures. Even though more recent reexaminations of preserved lung tissue samples from soldiers who died of influenza in 1918 found a majority of deaths due to bacterial pneumonia secondary to the flu, it was deemed important to take precautionary measures. This bacterial agent is commonly found in the nose and throat, but as H1N1 obliterated cells lining the bronchial tubes and lungs, it invaded the lungs causing pneumonia (Kash et al., 2011). Although we now have antibiotics to combat influenza complications, a pandemic of influenza can still wreak havoc on economies and societies. While WHO noted almost 18,500 laboratory-confirmed deaths from the 2009 to 2010 H1N1 flu epidemic, many believe that the actual number of deaths was closer to over 200,000 or more (Knox, 2013). The numbers are confusing, and this pandemic behaved very differently from most others; it had very varied responses in countries around the world. Whereas high numbers of deaths were not reported in Europe, Australia, and New Zealand, countries in the Americas were hit fairly hard. Even neighboring countries, like Chile and Argentina, had very different levels of severity and researchers have a difficult time explaining these regional variations. What was apparent, however, were the unusually high number of deaths among pregnant women and otherwise healthy children, teens, and young adults (Knox, 2013).

Diarrheal Diseases

Diarrhea is defined as the passage of more than three loose or liquid stools during a 24-hour period for individuals older than 3 months of age. The incidence of diarrheal diseases is somewhat elusive because it depends on the definition of diarrhea used, the frequency of surveillance, and the population. Sometimes, public health professionals use the term *diarrhea* to mean dysentery, although the latter is usually characterized by the presence of blood in the stool, with or without looseness or specified frequency. Diarrheal disease is the second leading cause of death in children <5 years of age even though it is preventable and treatable. The actual cause of death is generally severe dehydration and fluid loss. Children who are malnourished or immunocompromised are most at risk. The risk is highest among infants who are not breast-fed, and 88% of deaths associated with diarrhea poor sanitation, unsafe water supplies, or inadequate sanitation. Acute diarrhea due to rotavirus is responsible for 40% of hospitalizations for diarrhea in children under age 5 (CDC, 2015f). Each year, an estimated 1.2 million children die from diarrhea and related illnesses (Rehydration Project, 2016).

Reductions in mortality rates have occurred, and many international agencies and groups are working to make water safer to drink and to provide rotavirus vaccines for at-risk populations. One international nonprofit agency, PATH, has worked collaboratively with communities to provide low-cost rotavirus and pneumococcal vaccines and low-cost water treatment and storage products to low-income populations in India and Africa (and other countries) who have a higher burden of diarrheal diseases, pneumonia, and malnutrition (PATH, 2015). Actions need to prevent diarrheal disease include community programs that promote personal and domestic hygiene (especially hand washing), water supply and sanitation facility improvements, promotion of breast-feeding and improved weaning practices, zinc treatment, and immunizations for cholera, measles, and rotavirus (PATH, 2015). **Oral rehydration therapy (ORT)**, or the use of oral rehydration salts (ORS) are used to prevent or correct dehydration (not to treat the source of the diarrheal illness). A program to provide services of CHWs in three Indian states resulted in over 3 million children between 2 and 59 months reported and 84% were treated with both ORS and zinc. Researchers felt that CHWs could deliver timely care and appropriate supplies to deal with diarrheal illness (Kumar, Roy, & Dutta, 2015). ORS packets are available, but you can also make it yourself. See Display 16–3 for more information on this.

Wide implementation of seven preventive interventions: improved water sources; improved sanitation and household water treatments; exclusive breast-feeding for the first 6 months; hand washing with soap; good personal and food hygiene; health education; and rotavirus vaccination. Treatment interventions include oral rehydration salts, zinc supplements, rehydration with intravenous fluids in cases of severe dehydration, nutrient-rich foods, and seeking early treatment from a health professional (WHO Media Centre, 2015d).

Acute Respiratory Tract Infections

The most common illness in the world and a leading cause of mortality is acute respiratory tract infection (ARI). Pneumonia is the leading cause of death in children under 5 years of age, claiming nearly 1 million children annually. It is treatable, especially when caught early, and simple interventions such as vaccines, good nutrition, safe hygiene practices, and improved indoor

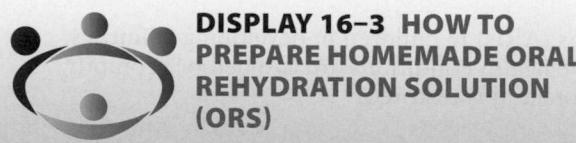

DISPLAY 16–3 HOW TO PREPARE HOMEMADE ORAL REHYDRATION SOLUTION (ORS)

- If ORS sachets are available: dilute one ORS sachet in 1 L of safe water.
- Otherwise, make your own:

  Use 1 L of safe water (clean or boiled and then cooled)—about 5 cups—and add:

  Salt—2.6 g (1/2 level teaspoon)

  Sugar (anhydrous glucose)—13.5 g (2 3/4 teaspoons)

  Potassium chloride—1.5 g (1/3 teaspoon)

  Trisodium citrate, dehydrate—2.9 g (1/2 teaspoon)
- Home remedy for watery diarrhea:

  ½ to 1 cup precooked rice baby cereal (or 1½ tablespoon granulated sugar)

  2 cups water

  ½ teaspoon salt

Note: Solutions should not taste saltier than human tears. Extra liquids are needed until diarrhea ceases.
From Rehydration Project. (2016). *Oral rehydration therapy*. Retrieved from http://rehydrate.org/ors/ort.htm

---

air quality can help reduce the impact (Nair et al., 2013). Risk factors include low birth weight, poverty, crowding, lower educational levels, poor nutrition, inadequate childcare practices, a lack of health education about ARI, and delays in seeking treatment. Additional risk factors include smoking and indoor and outdoor air pollution. Indoor air pollution is much higher among villages in poor areas than in homes in those countries of the world where people smoke. The source of pollution is largely indoor cook stoves that use organic fuel. Indoor cooking stoves kill 2 million people annually more than malaria (Sheridan, 2011). The risk of pneumonia is doubled with exposure to indoor air pollution (Burki, 2011). A threat to the reduction of pneumonia, however, is the increase in drug-resistant organisms. Measures to better control ARI include immunizations, birth spacing, and improvement in nutrition and living conditions (including use of smokeless cooking stoves). A global commitment to reduce ARI was realized by a resolution at the World Summit for Children in 1990 that called for a one-third reduction in deaths from the condition. The current trend is addressing community education to encourage mothers to seek care and treatment early and to empower CHWs to diagnose and treat signs of pneumonia early.

Human Immunodeficiency Virus Infection and Acquired Immunodeficiency Syndrome

HIV has claimed the lives of more than 34 million people so far. An estimated 36.9 million people worldwide are living with HIV by the end of 2014, with 1.2 million people dying from HIV-related causes globally. Sub-Saharan Africa accounts for nearly 70% of global new infections, with 25.8 million people living with HIV in 2014 (WHO Media Centre, 2015a).

Although there remains no cure for HIV infection, effective treatment can control the virus so people can live productive lives. Treatment also helps prevent transmission. Current trends in HIV prevention, treatment, and care focus on early testing, so people know their status and can take measure to either remain HIV negative or take measure to prevent transmission. HIV is diagnosed through rapid diagnostic tests that provide results the same day. Once HIV-positive status is known, treatment with antiretroviral therapy (ART) is initiated. Nearly 16 million people living with HIV were receiving ART globally as of mid-2015. Concurrent assessment and treatment for possible TB infections and prevention of mother-to-child transmission are also important interventions that have proved successful in improving health outcomes and reducing transmission to newborns. New HIV infections fell by 35% between 2000 and 2015, with 7.8 million lives saved as a result of global initiatives implementing evidenced-based practices (WHO Media Centre, 2015a).

The virus attacks young adults in productive age groups, requiring older people to care for and support their terminally ill adult children and, later, their orphaned grandchildren. Often, these elders are themselves impoverished and in poor health and are left without caregivers when they require assistance in their later years. For a time, the HIV/AIDS epidemic upset and destabilized entire societies in Africa, until medications were made available to make this more of a chronic illness than a death sentence (Kincaid, 2012; Smith, 2012). Reduced productivity of adult workers and early death are counterproductive to economic and social development.

Tuberculosis

TB is an infectious disease caused by the tubercle bacillus. The disease has been known for hundreds of years and was commonly referred to as *consumption*. The causative organism has become resistant to the medications used to treat it, and currently, a worldwide TB epidemic is under way. One third of the world's population is thought to be currently infected, but only 5% to 10% of those become ill or can spread this to others within their lifetime. In 2014, 9.6 million people fell ill with TB and it is estimated that 1.5 million people died from TB, with the highest number of deaths in Africa (50 per 100,000). TB is one of the illnesses that disproportionately affects poor people around the world, and it is estimated that the largest number of new cases of TB in 2008 were in Southeast Asia (WHO Media Centre, 2015h). Drug-resistant TB is a problem around the world. Globally, 480,000 people developed multidrug-resistant TB and the CDC estimates that there are a half a million new cases each year. In December 2015, President Obama announced the National Action Plan for Combating Multidrug-Resistant Tuberculosis, which provides urgent guidance for rapid, focused action. Although great progress has been made in tackling TB, MDR-TP threatens to reverse this progress and is a growing global health concern (CDC, 2016). WHO began the Stop TB Strategy in 2006, and 41 million people have

LEVELS OF PREVENTION PYRAMID

SITUATION: Prevent acute respiratory tract infections (ARIs) in children in developing countries.
GOAL: Using the three levels of prevention, negative health conditions are avoided or promptly diagnosed and treated, and the fullest possible potential is restored.

TERTIARY PREVENTION

Rehabilitation	Primary Prevention	
	Health Promotion and Education	*Health Protection*
• Restore child to optimal level of functioning through the recovery period.	• Continue to promote educational programs and individual teaching regarding practices that promote health and prevent diseases among family members.	• Educate on the prevention of recurrence and spread of disease.

SECONDARY PREVENTION

Early Diagnosis	Prompt Treatment
• Get a prompt diagnosis of an acute ARI.	• Collaborate with families to combine the best of folk and home remedies with established Western medical practices. • Diagnose and treat early • Provide culturally appropriate symptomatic care. • Teach caregiver signs and symptoms of complications.

PRIMARY PREVENTION

Health Promotion and Education	Health Protection
• Promote general health education among community members. • Good prenatal care • Advocate breast-feeding, child spacing, and adequate nutrition. • Teach good hygiene and childcare practices. • Teach when to seek medical attention. • Eliminate poverty and household crowding.	• Administer appropriate immunizations. • Eliminate indoor contaminants such as smoke from cook stoves without chimneys and cigarette, cigar, or pipe smoking. • Ventilate rooms to eliminate indoor smoke and allow fresh air in.

been treated using drug-observed therapy (DOTS). The newly adopted Sustainable Development Goals seek to end the TB epidemic by 2030 (WHO, 2013c).

Tuberculosis and Human Immunodeficiency Virus

TB alone is a pernicious illness. When TB and HIV occur in one individual, the combination is lethal, with each speeding the other's progress. TB is the leading cause of death among people who are HIV positive (WHO Media Centre, 2015h). In 2015, TB was the cause of one in three deaths among HIV-positive populations.

Malaria

Malaria is a disease caused by the presence of the protozoan parasite *Plasmodium* in human red blood cells; the parasite is usually transmitted to humans by the bite of an infected female *Anopheles* mosquito. Fifty percent of the world population lives in malaria endemic areas.

About 214 million new cases and 438,000 deaths occur per year because of malaria, most are among African children; however, mortality rates dropped by 66% over the last 15 years in all age groups from this region (WHO Media Centre, 2015i). As we have seen with other diseases, sub-Saharan Africa carries a disproportionately high share of the global burden, with 89% of malaria cases and 91% of malaria deaths in 2015 (WHO, 2015b). Those most at risk are young children, pregnant women, and people living with HIV. Malaria is resistant to multidrug therapy (MDT), and the mosquito, its tenacious vector, persists. Malaria is highly endemic in some areas, and its eradication depends on pesticides such as DDT. In addition, human and economic resources are not available to fully implement a malaria program. Perhaps, the major contributors to lack of success have been failure to integrate the malaria eradication effort into basic health services, inadequate efforts to exploit the effective involvement of communities, and the absence of political will. Also, climate has been shown to exacerbate malaria prevalence in one area of East Africa. Using predictive models, researchers found larger observed changes in malaria cases beyond the number expected by their predictive model and noted that climate change had an impact (Alonso, Bouma, & Pascual, 2011).

Current strategies to control malaria include community education programs, vector control (indoor and outdoor spraying to destroy mosquitoes and larvae), source detection through surveillance, early treatment-seeking behaviors, and reducing contact with mosquitoes through protective clothing and sleeping under insecticide-treated mosquito nets. In 2015, it was estimated that 55% of the population in sub-Saharan Africa were sleeping under the protection of these nets, up from 2% in the year 2000. Also, better and quicker diagnostic testing helps to discern malarial versus other nonmalarial fevers so that treatment can begin quickly; Artemisinin-based combination therapies (ACTs) have been used for the past decade and been found to be highly effective against the most common form of malaria. ACT, along with residual spraying inside homes and insecticide-treated mosquito net, have been the most impactful in preventing new cases—estimated at about 68% (WHO Media Centre, 2015i).

Over 500 partners, along with WHO, launched an initiative entitled the Roll Back Malaria (RBM) Program, which coordinates a worldwide action plan against malaria, and in 2015, a new 15-year plan for control of malaria in endemic regions was launched. Fifteen countries, largely in Africa, have the highest rates of malaria deaths (78%), and malaria cases and deaths have been slower to drop in these countries often due to health systems that are less than highly effective (WHO Media Centre, 2015f). There is currently no licensed malaria vaccine, but one research vaccine is being evaluated in seven African countries (WHO, 2015b). As with TB, malaria disproportionately affects the poor, and it has damaging effects on the economies of many poor countries.

West Nile Virus

WNV (*flavivirus: Flaviviridae*) is considered the most widespread *arbovirus* worldwide and is most often transmitted to humans through the bite of an infected mosquito (Moser, Lim, Styer, Kramer, & Bernard, 2015). This virus may cause a fatal neurological disease, but most of those individuals infected do not demonstrate any symptoms. In those that develop West Nile fever, symptoms often are comprised of fever, body aches, nausea and vomiting, headache, fatigue, and sometimes skin rash and enlarged lymph nodes. The severe disease, often termed West Nile encephalitis, is characterized by symptoms of headache, stiff neck, stupor, high fever, disorientation, coma, tremors, paralysis, and seizures. WNV can cause severe illness and death in horses, and contact with infected animals, their tissue or blood, can also be a source of transmission. It was first identified in the West Nile area of Uganda in 1937 and is commonly found in Africa, the Middle East, Europe, West Asia, and now North America. Birds are natural hosts (crows and jays may become ill and die), and mosquitoes most often transmit the infection from birds to humans. Sites for outbreaks are often on major migratory routes for birds (CDC, 2015e, 2015f, 2015g).

No vaccine is available for humans, but there is one for horses. Treatment is most often supportive in nature (e.g., IV fluids, hospitalization). Active animal surveillance and early warning from veterinarians and public health officials are being used to prevent transmission. Education and reducing mosquito transmission (e.g., use of nets, spraying, eliminating mosquito breeding sources) are also being used (WHO Media Centre, 2011). Research continues to find treatment for this illness and other mosquito-borne viruses such as yellow fever and dengue fever (Brecher et al., 2015).

Leprosy

Leprosy is a chronic granulomatous infection caused by *Mycobacterium leprae* (Hansen's bacillus). It affects various parts of the body including the skin of the face and the eyes and causes progressive and permanent damage even though it is not easily transmitted (WHO Media Centre, 2015b). In 2013, the prevalence was 180,618 cases for all types of leprosy. The World Health Organization (WHO Media Centre, 2015b) provides multidrug therapy (MDT) for this condition free of charge to all those infected. People with leprosy have had access to this free effective drug treatment since 1995. Communities can help eradicate this disease through proper diagnosis and treatment and provision of care without stigma or isolation. A change in the image of leprosy, so that people with the condition will more readily present themselves for treatment, is essential. Leprosy was considered eliminated around the world in 2000, because the prevalence rate of leprosy was <1 case per 10,000 persons globally. Over the past 20 years, nearly 16 million cases have been cured with MDT (WHO Media Centre, 2015b).

Guinea Worm Disease (Dracunculiasis)

Dracunculiasis, or guinea worm disease, is a parasitic disease that is transmitted to humans when a person drinks water containing a worm's intermediate host, a water flea that can ingest and harbor guinea worm larvae. Once in a human body, the larvae migrate through the tissue and the mature adult worm attempts to emerge, usually from the lower leg. Farmers are the most commonly affected. Although there is no cure, once the larvae are ingested, the eradication strategy includes interruption of transmission, surveillance, health education, and certification (Carter Center, 2016).

Guinea worm disease is nearly eradicated with incidents of Guinea worm reduced by more than 99.99% with only 22 cases in 2015. The Carter Center is an organization dedicated to the complete eradication of guinea worm and continues to work in the four remaining endemic countries of Chad, Ethiopia, Mali, and South Sudan (Carter Center, 2016).

Era of Infectious Disease and the Universal Imperatives of Care

The infectious diseases and processes carry the potential for death, illness, and compromised functioning but when addressed promptly can be prevented. When left unmanaged, they can result in sickness and lifelong consequences to daily functioning. Some of these conditions involve decision-making. For example, when national governments do not provide clear national policies or funding for immunization programs, entire populations are at risk for the consequences of diphtheria, pertussis, typhoid, measles, and polio. When families and communities are living in areas with infectious agents, or do not clear their land as needed, their members are exposed to malaria (Kremer, Leino, Miguel, & Zwane, 2011). When community health programs do not include sanitation and the building of latrines, the result is diarrheal diseases that affect an entire community (Turley, Saith, Bhan, Rehfuess, & Carter, 2013).

Eradication, Elimination, and Control of Communicable Diseases

The primary global health goals related to communicable disease are eradication, elimination, and worldwide control. **Eradication** means interruption of person-to-person transmission and limitation of the reservoir of infection so that no further preventive efforts are required; it indicates a status whereby no further cases of a disease occur anywhere. At times, the term **elimination** is used when a disease has been interrupted in a defined geographic area. In 1998, disease elimination was first defined as a reduction of prevalence in a certain area to zero, and disease eradication as a permanent worldwide incidence of zero (WHO, 2016b). In contrast, the term control indicates that a specific disease has ceased to be a public health threat. Control programs are aimed at reducing the incidence and prevalence of communicable and some noncommunicable conditions.

Although eradication is always the desired effect, extensive funding and much international cooperation are usually required to achieve such a goal (see What Do You Think?). The successful eradication of smallpox from the world came about because of the leadership of the WHO, and it was a tremendous accomplishment in public health. In 1959, several countries proposed the global eradication of smallpox, but progress was slow. The Intensified Smallpox Eradication Programme began in 1967, when smallpox was endemic in 31 countries, with 10 to 15 million individuals infected. Through enhanced surveillance and *ring vaccination* to prevent transmission between humans and control epidemics, progress improved. New cases were quickly identified and quarantined, and their close contacts were vaccinated and quarantined. Remarkably, by 1980, there were no cases in the world (Global Alert and Response, 2010). Clearly, if global eradication programs are to be successful, collaboration and partnerships are essential. The Global Outbreak Alert and Response Network helps to coordinate responses and deal with outbreaks (Mackenzie et al., 2014). Control of river blindness (onchocerciasis—the chief cause of blindness in many African countries) joined the growing list of global public health accomplishments (WHO, 2016k). These programs

are dependent on commitment from involved governments, international bodies, NGOs, and the affected communities themselves. Global eradication and elimination programs that are close to meeting the goal include poliomyelitis and guinea worm disease. Eradication programs for measles are continuing. Additional major efforts have increased to reduce, control, and prevent malaria, TB, HIV/AIDS, diarrheal diseases, and respiratory infections. Unfortunately, international terrorism threatens to reintroduce smallpox through acts of bioterrorism; in some instances, smallpox vaccination programs will need to be reestablished in order to protect health workers and the populations at risk (Adalja, Toner, & Inglesby, 2015).

New and Emerging Infectious Diseases and Conditions

Despite the advances made, new and emerging diseases, conditions, and syndromes have appeared in parts of the world. Health authorities thought that some of these were under control. Over the past 20 years, a number of previously unknown diseases have emerged, resulting in pandemics, economic losses, and travel restrictions. Among these emerging infectious diseases are severe acute respiratory syndrome (SARS), HIV/AIDS, H5N1 and H7N9 (bird flus) and H1N1 (swine flu) influenzas, Middle Eastern respiratory syndrome (MERS), and variant Creutzfeldt-Jakob disease, commonly known as mad cow disease (Kaiser Family Foundation, 2014; WHO, 2016p). See Table 16–1.

The development of antimicrobial-resistant organisms, mainly as a result of the overuse and misuse of antibiotics, has fueled a resurgence of some diseases that were under control, such as TB. Medication-resistant TB (MDR-TB) is now estimated to comprise almost 4% of new TB cases worldwide, and in previously treated patients, that proportion increases to 20% of cases (WHO, 2013c). Antimalarial medicines have become ineffective in some countries, and WHO (2013) estimates that 60% of the half million new cases of MDR-TB are in Russia, South Africa, Brazil, India, and China. About 9% of cases are classified as extensively drug-resistant TB (XDR-TB) and do not respond to two other classes of medication. A case–control study in Addis Ababa noted that first-line drug side effects, not using DOTS, and missing a daily dose of medication or a treatment lasting 2 to 7 months were all factors that were associated with MDR-TB (Hirpa et al., 2013). The easy availability of global air travel and subsequent rapid transmission of microbes pose real health threats. Despite the problems with MDR-TB, almost half of patients treated in 2009 were successful in their treatments (WHO, 2013c).

Another factor related to emergence of new and recycling conditions is migration (as discussed earlier in this chapter) and urbanization, which serves to concentrate large numbers of people in small geographic areas. With urbanization, deforestation continues, and the two phenomena may permit the infestation of microbes into human populations, as humans who move into the cleared forests may encounter previously unknown pathogens. Changes in agricultural practices, such as new dams and irrigation schemes, also present potential factors in transmission. The ability of microbes to change and adapt rapidly is a persistent threat as well.

What do *you* think?

Imagine today's world without any international cooperation related to communicable disease knowledge or control. What would be some of the health, social, political, and economic consequences of such inaction?

Table 16–1	**Examples of Emerging Pathogens Identified Since 1973**	
Agent	**Microbe**	**Disease**
V	Rotavirus	Major cause of infantile diarrhea globally
V	*Cryptosporidium parvum*	Acute and chronic diarrhea
V	Ebola virus	Ebola hemorrhagic fever (Africa)
B	*Legionella pneumophila*	Legionnaires' disease/pneumonia
V	Hantaan virus (Sin Nombre virus)	Hemorrhagic fever with renal syndrome
B	*Campylobacter jejuni*	GI infections (infants/children) globally
V	Human T-lymphotropic virus 1 (HTLV-1)	T-cell lymphoma and leukemia globally
B	Toxin producing strains of *Staphylococcus aureus*	Toxic shock syndrome
B	*Escherichia coli 0157:H7*	Mild to severe diarrhea, hemorrhagic colitis, hemolytic uremic syndrome (beef)
V	HTLV-II	Hairy cell leukemia and paraparesis globally
S	*Borrelia burgdorferi*	Lyme disease
V	Human immunodeficiency virus (I and II)	Acquired immunodeficiency syndrome (AIDS) worldwide
B	*Helicobacter pylori*	Peptic ulcer disease
V	Hepatitis C	Hepatitis, cirrhosis, carcinoma globally
V	Guanarito virus	Venezuelan hemorrhagic fever
V	Junin virus	Argentine hemorrhagic fever
B	*Vibrio cholerae 0139*	New strain associated with epidemic cholera
B	*Bartonella henselae*	Catscratch disease, bacillary angiomatosis
V	Sabia virus	Brazilian hemorrhagic fever
V	Machupo virus	Bolivian hemorrhagic fever
V	Human herpesvirus 6, 7, 8	Roseola infantum/mononucleosis in adults, febrile childhood illness, Kaposi's sarcoma in AIDS patients
V	Norovirus	Acute vomiting, cramps, diarrhea
V	Parvovirus B19	Fifth disease, arthropathy, anemia worldwide
V	Nipah virus	Encephalitis, coma, seizures
V	Hendra virus	Severe pneumonitis/meningitis
V	Marburg virus	Microvascular leakage/hemorrhages (Africa)
B	*Clostridium difficile*	Severe infections—toxic megacolon, sepsis, death (asymptomatic in healthy neonates, nosocomial adults)
V	Coronaviruses	Severe acute respiratory syndrome (SARS) and Middle Eastern respiratory syndrome (MERS)
V	Nairovirus *Bunyaviridae*	Crimean Congo hemorrhagic fever (India) and Rift Valley fever (Africa)

(continued)

Table 16-1	Examples of Emerging Pathogens Identified Since 1973 (*Continued*)

Agent	Microbe	Disease
V	Lassa virus *Arenaviridae*	Fever, mild to severe (Africa)
V	Dengue virus	Fever, headache, rash, bleeding, low white cell count (tropics/ subtropics, Texas outbreak)
V	West Nile virus	Fever, headache, myalgia, rash (United States 48 states)

From Blakemore, E. (2015, December 15). *These are the world's most dangerous emerging pathogens, according to WHO*. Retrieved from http://www.smithsonianmag.com/smart-news/these-are-worlds-most-dangerous-new-pathogens-according-who-180957541/?no-ist; Dong, J., Olano, J., McBride, J., & Walker, D. (2008). Emerging pathogens: Challenges and successes of molecular diagnostics. *Journal of Molecular Diagnostics*, 10(3), 185–197; Morens, D. M., & Fauci, A. S. (2013). Emerging infectious diseases: Threats to human health and global stability. *PLoS Pathogens*, 9(7), e1003467.
For information on emerging foodborne pathogens refer to Behravesh, C. B., Williams, I. T., & Tauxe, R. V. (2012). Emerging foodborne pathogens and problems: Expanding prevention efforts before slaughter or harvest. In Institute of Medicine (Ed.), *Improving food safety through a One Health approach: Workshop summary (Appendix 14)*. Washington, DC: National Academies Press. Retrieved from http://www.ncbi.nlm.nih.gov/books/NBK100665/

Era of Chronic Long-Term Health Conditions

Despite the programs of control, many infectious diseases persist, but people survive and live on to experience chronic, long-term conditions. These conditions, while averting mortality, persist through their ongoing etiology and affect people's daily functioning, decision-making, and cost. Adding to the burden is the escalating sale of tobacco and the use of cigarettes by young populations in developing countries. The long-term effects of these practices for people in these countries will undoubtedly follow a similar trajectory as has occurred in developed countries with increases in lung cancer, heart disease, and other illnesses related to tobacco use (WHO Media Centre, 2015g). Thus, the longevity that has resulted from meeting the challenges of the Era of Infectious Diseases compounds the more recent emergence of chronic diseases in the many countries. Here, a transition occurs. As infectious diseases decrease, life expectancy lengthens and the population experiences the degenerative diseases seen in developed countries.

The concept of epidemiologic transition explains the replacement of infectious disease morbidity and mortality with that of chronic disease. The ways in which people in remote areas will manage their heart disease or cope with the long-term effects of diabetes and cancer are yet to be understood. Formerly, those with mental illness, inborn genetic disorders, disabilities, or compromised activities of daily living were cared for by the family and were often hidden from the community. This was often because of religious and cultural beliefs, lack of knowledge, the availability of health providers with specialized expertise, and dedicated health care facilities or services for those chronic illnesses. However, it is difficult to gather precise statistics in many areas of the world. For instance, research on the global prevalence of mental illness is difficult, as many poorer nations do not conduct research in this area and definitions of various mental health conditions vary across regions (Baxter, Patton, Scott, Degenhardt, & Whiteford, 2013). The impact of mental illness on families and caregivers is also very difficult to ascertain.

As families change their composition, members of families migrate to seek employment; the care of those who require daily assistance will also have to change. It will require a change in the response of the health care system in terms of provision of care, planning, and allocation of resources. Addressing these concerns is considered a cost-effective investment in a nation's human capital (Yach, Mensah, Hawkes, Epping-Jordan, & Steyn, 2012).

Era of Social Health Conditions

The WHO researchers suggest that overall, dramatic changes in health-related needs will occur within the next 20 years. There is evidence that noncommunicable diseases are rapidly replacing infectious diseases as the major causes of disability and premature death. Noncommunicable diseases account for 8 of every 10 deaths in higher-income countries, compared with 6 of every 10 deaths worldwide (WHO Media Centre, 2016a; Yach et al., 2012). See Display 16–4 for differences in ranked causes of death between developed and developing countries.

Maternal and Perinatal Morbidity and Mortality

The WHO estimates that almost 303,000 women died in 2015 from complications of pregnancy and childbirth. Ninety-nine percent of these deaths are in economically poor countries. Pregnant women living in rural areas and adolescent mothers face higher mortality rates. The death of a mother profoundly affects the well-being of the entire family. Between 1990 and 2015, global rates of maternal mortality dropped by 44% (WHO Media Centre, 2015c).

Early pregnancy, high fertility, and close child spacing are common in developing countries and are known to be major determinants of poor health for mothers and children. Poverty, illiteracy, poor nutrition, and low weight gain in pregnancy are also risk factors. The leading causes of maternal death include severe bleeding and infections after childbirth, complications from delivery, high blood pressure during pregnancy, and unsafe abortions (WHO Media Centre, 2015c). As noted above, the added burden of long protracted civil wars has exacerbated these conditions, as have the factors associated with migration. As men leave home to seek employment abroad, women remain behind to care for children, often managing heavy workloads along with their pregnancies.

Prevention strategies include better general health for women through poverty alleviation, education, family planning guidance, prenatal care including food supplementation, immunization, local and regional care with referrals for complications, training of traditional birth attendants

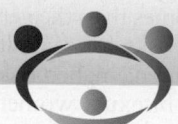

DISPLAY 16–4 RANKING OF 10 LEADING CAUSES OF DEATH WORLDWIDE: DEVELOPED AND DEVELOPING COUNTRIES, 2013

Developed Countries
1. Ischemic heart disease
2. Stroke
3. Lung cancer
4. Self-harm
5. Alzheimer's disease
6. Cirrhosis
7. COPD
8. Colorectal cancer
9. Lower respiratory infections
10. Road injuries

Developing Countries
1. Lower respiratory infections
2. Ischemic heart disease
3. Stroke
4. Diarrhea
5. HIV/AIDS
6. Preterm birth
7. Malaria
8. Road injuries
9. Neonatal encephalitis
10. Congenital

Adapted from Global Burden of Disease Mortality and Causes of Death Collaborators. (2015). Global, regional, and national age-sex specific all-cause and cause-specific mortality for 240 causes of death, 1990–2013: A systematic analysis for the Global Burden of Disease Study, 12013. *Lancet, 385*, 117–171.

(TBAs), and effective postpartum care. One pilot program in Malawi instituted community-linked maternal death reviews as a way to better understand causes of maternal death and implement community-planned actions to prevent them (Bayley et al., 2015). Researchers noted that 67% of district hospital and 65% of health centers completed actions to improve maternal care and reduce mortality rates. Another study examined strategies that had been developed and implemented by women's groups in an effort to improve maternal–child health and decrease mortality rates in Malawi (Rosato et al., 2012). Common strategies included birth attendant training, health education classes, cultivation of vegetable gardens, using bicycle ambulances, and distributing insecticide-treated bed nets.

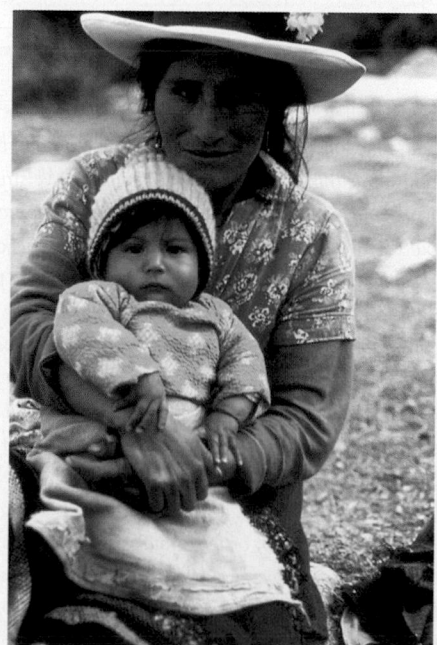

Maternal and perinatal morbidity and mortality are important global issues addressed by the World Health Organization. (Photo courtesy of CDC Photo Image Library.)

Mental Health Conditions

Mental illness has been thought of in a variety of ways over the centuries through drastic measures including exclusion from society, ridicule, and incarceration, as outlined in the classic book by Foucault (1965) and the writings of Shimmon (2011). In one review of 174 studies conducted in 63 countries, researchers found almost 18% of survey respondents met criteria for some type of common mental disorder within last year, and almost 30% had one at some point in their life (Steel et al., 2014). The recent civil wars and popular uprisings and the major wars in Iraq and Afghanistan have taken their toll on members of the armed forces resulting in posttraumatic stress among soldiers as well as the inhabitants who have experienced war (Levy & Sidel, 2013; Litz & Orsillo, 2015). These events and the recent financial downturn in the economies of the world have affected the mental health of people as they struggle to manage the multiple social, financial, and cultural issues facing them, not the least of which are the effects of unemployment and financial ruin for families throughout many parts of the world.

Tobacco

Over 100 million deaths were attributed to tobacco in the 20th century. Tobacco accounts for one death every 6 seconds in the world or about 6 million people annually. Without some form of intervention, this trend will continue ultimately resulting in over 8 million annual deaths by 2030 and over 1 billion deaths within the 21st century. Most of the world's 1 billion smokers live in low-income or mid-income countries where premature death and the burden of disease prevent economic growth (WHO Media Centre, 2015g). The statistics are startling when one considers the lifelong smoker who is as likely to die from tobacco as he/she is from all other causes of death combined (Schaffer Library of Drug Policy, 2011). Yet, it is difficult for smokers to stop smoking. With medication and counseling, however, the chances of success in quitting smoking are doubled (WHO Media Centre, 2015g).

The WHO Framework Convention on Tobacco Control took effect in 2005. The treaty's signatory parties (over 170 representing 87% of the world population) agreed to implement comprehensive tobacco control programs and strategies. WHO introduced a tobacco control package, MPOWER, to help implement the provisions of the treaty. The six components are as follows:

- Monitor tobacco use and prevention policies.
- Protect people from tobacco use.
- Offer help to quit tobacco use.
- Warn about the dangers of tobacco.
- Enforce bans on tobacco advertising, promotion, and sponsorship.
- Raise taxes on tobacco (WHO Media Centre, 2015g, para. 33).

This legally binding treaty and international effort represents an important step in global public health and is expected to reduce the impact of tobacco use in the decades to come.

Given that tobacco eventually kills about half of its users, this important global public health initiative should help save lives, improve standards of living and world economies, as well as improve global health.

Population Health of LGBT Globally

Amnesty International highlights the growing problems associated with the criminalization of homosexuality around the globe and the resulting systematic discrimination that compounds the risks and disadvantages already faced by lesbian, gay, bisexual, and transgender (LGBT) people (Amnesty International, 2015). In Uganda, for example, recently enacted, highly controversial, legislative bills have resulted in heightened repression and discrimination based on sexual orientation. According to a recent report, women believed to belong to the LGBT community based on their dress alone were attacked, stripped, and beaten, whereas other members of the community were "evicted from their homes, lost their jobs, and faced challenges accessing healthcare" (Amnesty International, 2014, para 5). As it is, LGBT individuals face poorer health outcomes than the general population globally, including higher risks for sexually transmitted infections and HIV for gay men; higher risks of obesity and breast cancer for lesbian, bisexual women; institutionalized prejudice, antihomosexual hatred, and violence; social exclusion and widespread stigmatization within health systems; and increased isolation for the aging LGBT population (U.S. Department of Health and Human Services [USDHHS], 2015; WHO, 2013a). The true extent of the problem is hard to measure, because there is limited health research on this population; but we do know that the LGBT community faces numerous barriers in accessing health care. These barriers include outright denial of care, substandard care, and fear of discrimination or criminal penalties. Moving forward, we, as nurses, need to engage in more rigorous research on the realities of discrimination toward the LGBT community globally and how this impacts their ability to achieve and maintain their full health potential. In addition, we need to contribute to the development of health standards and curricula that is designed to provide adequate training of health care professionals in the care of LGBT people (WHO, 2013a). Both populations we serve and health care professionals deserve respect in their choices. See Perspectives: One Nurse's Experiences Overseas.

Global Burden of Disease

If a member of your family dies, what does it cost? What does it cost if you miss a month of work or school because of an illness? What does it cost a country when the majority of adults smoke a package of cigarettes a day or when adults eat betel nut several times a day? These questions are often irritating and are sometimes considered in poor taste. Yet, insurance companies, governments, and community members do ask these questions—as they must carry the financial burden for them. But how does one go

PERSPECTIVES
ONE NURSE'S EXPERIENCES OVERSEAS

From an early age, I was exposed to nursing. My mother was a nurse, and I saw firsthand how she cared for us as a family and how she cared for her friends when they were in need. I also listened intently when she talked about the patients she helped over the years. Furthermore, I witnessed how she integrated her own faith with her nursing practice in the simplest of forms: genuine service to others. After I became a nurse, I also felt a deep calling to use my nursing skills in volunteer ways to serve others.

My first volunteer experience was in the rural mountains of Guatemala where I worked with indigenous women to improve birth practices. I thought I was going there to teach them how to safely deliver babies. But after spending 2 months caring for women during pregnancy and childbirth, they actually taught me more about the miracle of birth than I ever learned in my hospital-based experiences. We shared our knowledge with each other and both came away from the experience with a deeper understanding of what it means to become a mother.

Later in life, I met a nurse with the same deep passion for service to others. She was preparing to move to West Africa to serve women with childbirth injuries. She and I had both been raised within the same Christian faith and we both felt our nursing practice was very integrated into our values and beliefs. Then, we fell in love with each other. This was a challenging time for us, as we navigated the minority of being in a same-sex relationship within the Christian community. We struggled as some of our friends and family made it clear they did not approve of our relationship. But we also found new friends and family in the journey as well who were willing to see the greater value of who we were together.

In addition to navigating our home-front challenges, we also had to negotiate our relationship abroad. My wife was working for a faith-based organization in a predominately Muslim country, both of which do not condone same-sex relationships. In order for me to visit with her, to spend time together, and to also offer myself for service when I was there, we had to be silent about the depth of our relationship. We acted only as friends, with no public displays of affection. This was a compromise we both felt committed to in order to make a difference in the lives of the nurses and the women we cared for. Although some might find this compromise too costly, we continue to be grateful for the opportunities we had to serve and would do it again in a heartbeat.

Posted anonymously in order to protect future service opportunities.

about putting a value on a life? Or how can value be placed on the cost of a disability? To capture these concerns, the WHO coined the term the **global burden of disease (GBD)**.

The World Health Organization's GBD studies numerically verified numerous long-held assumptions about disparities in the burden of disease worldwide, especially in regard to children, through landmark studies that revealed startling statistics:

- 33% of worldwide deaths from neonatal encephalopathy occur in one country—India.
- 50% of diarrheal deaths in children/adolescents are in five countries—Ethiopia, Democratic Republic of Congo, India, Nigeria, and Pakistan (Global Burden of Disease Pediatrics Collaboration, 2016).

As more people around the world are living longer, the number of years lived with disability (YLD) increases.

Low back pain and depression are the most commonly cited causes of disability in countries worldwide, and most of increases in YLD are due to "musculoskeletal, mental, and substance use disorders, neurological disorders, and chronic respiratory distress" (Global Burden of Disease Study 2013 Collaborators, 2015, p. 743). In sub-Saharan Africa, the leading driver is HIV/AIDS. In addition to causes of mortality, the GBD study quantified the burden of disease with a measure that is used for cost-effectiveness analysis. To compare across conditions and risk factors, researchers developed a measure called the **disability-adjusted life year (DALY)**, which is the combination of years of life lost because of premature mortality and years of life lived with disability adjusted for the severity of disability (WHO, 2016j). The 2012 GBD study ranked the leading risk factor causes of DALYs overall (see Table 16–2). Another measure, years of life

Table 16–2 Worldwide Ranking of 20 Leading Risk Factor Causes of Disability-Adjusted Life Years (DALYs), 2012

Rank	Cause	DALYs (000s)	% DALYs	DALYs per 100,000 Population
	All causes	2,743,857	100.0	38,780
1	Ischemic heart disease	165,717	6.0	2,342
2	Lower respiratory infections	146,864	5.4	2,076
3	Stroke	141,348	5.2	1,998
4	Preterm birth complications	107,210	3.9	1,515
5	Diarrheal diseases	99,728	3.6	1,409
6	COPD	92,377	3.4	1,306
7	HIV/AIDS	91,907	3.4	1,299
8	Road injury	78,724	2.9	1,113
9	Unipolar depressive disorders	76,500	2.8	1,081
10	Birth asphyxia and trauma	74,600	2.7	1,054
11	Diabetes mellitus	59,258	2.2	838
12	Malaria	55,111	2.0	779
13	Back and neck pain	53,920	2.0	762
14	Congenital anomalies	52,532	1.9	742
15	Iron deficiency anemia	47,627	1.7	673
16	Tuberculosis	43,650	1.6	617
17	Falls	42,466	1.6	600
18	Neonatal sepsis and infections	39,646	1.4	560
19	Self-harm	39,358	1.4	556
20	Trachea, bronchus, and lung cancers	38,535	1.4	545

From World Health Organization. (2016). *DALY estimates, 200-2012: Global summary estimates.* Retrieved from http://www.who.int/healthinfo/global_burden_disease/estimates/en/index2.html

lost (YLL), is ranked by category of disease or condition (WHO, 2016g). Almost 40% are due to communicable diseases (e.g., TB, HIV/AIDS, diarrheal diseases) along with nutritional, maternal, and perinatal causes. Noncommunicable diseases are responsible for 47% (e.g., cardiovascular disease, diabetes, neoplasms).

The leading causes of death worldwide can be broken down by income level. For instance, the five most common cause of death among low-income countries are:

● Lower respiratory tract infections, HIV/AIDS, diarrheal diseases, stroke, and ischemic heart disease

Among lower middle-income countries, the top five are:

● Ischemic heart disease, stroke, lower respiratory tract infections, COPD, and diarrheal diseases

For upper middle-income countries, stroke, ischemic heart disease, and COPD remain, but lung cancer and diabetes are now in top five.

For high-income countries, the top five causes of death include:

● Ischemic heart disease, stroke, lung cancer, Alzheimer's/ other dementias, and COPD (WHO, 2016f).

About 44% of deaths in children occur during the neonatal period, and about 6.6 million children died in 2012. The major causes of death for those under age 5 were prematurity, birth trauma/asphyxia, pneumonia, and diarrheal diseases. Malaria is responsible for 15% of child deaths in sub-Saharan Africa (WHO, 2016e). See Table 16–3 for more on global monitoring of risk factors.

Table 16–3 Comprehensive Noncommunicable Disease Global Monitoring Framework, Risk Factors, Targets, and Indicators

Framework Element	Target	Indicator
Premature Mortality From Noncommunicable Disease	25% reduction in mortality from cancer, cardiovascular diseases, diabetes, chronic respiratory diseases	Unconditional probability of dying between ages 30 and 70 from these causes Cancer incidence per 100,000
Behavioral Risk Factors		
Harmful Use of Alcohol	10% reduction in harmful use of alcohol within national standards	Total alcohol consumption per capita; prevalence of heavy episodic drinking; alcohol-related morbidity/mortality
Physical Inactivity	10% reduction in physical inactivity prevalence	Prevalence defined as <60 min moderate to vigorous activity/day for adolescents; <150 min/wk for over 18 years
Sodium Intake	30% reduction in mean population intake of sodium	Mean population intake of sodium chloride in g/d for >18 (age standardized)
Use of Tobacco	30% reduction in current tobacco use prevalence in people over age 15	Prevalence of adolescent tobacco uses; prevalence of age-standardized tobacco use over age 18
Biological Risk Factors		
Hypertension	25% reduction in prevalence of hypertension, depending on national conditions	Prevalence of systolic blood pressure of ≥ 140 mm Hg systolic and/or ≥ 90 mm Hg diastolic blood pressure means
Obesity and Diabetes	Halt the rise in obesity and diabetes	Prevalence of fasting plasma glucose 126 mg/dL or on blood glucose medication (over age 18); prevalence of school-age and adolescent overweight and obesity per WHO growth reference; for adults ≥25 kg/m² for overweight and ≥30 kg/m² for obese
National Health Systems		
Availability of medications and treatments for risk factors	50%–80% availability	Proportion of those over age 40 with 10-year CVD risk ≥30% with access to medication and counseling; access to affordable medications and technologies for noncommunicable diseases

Adapted from World Health Organization (WHO). (2014). *Global status report on noncommunicable diseases, 2014.* Retrieved from http://apps.who.int/iris/bitstream/10665/148114/1/9789241564854_eng.pdf

The information obtained from the GBD and its analysis guides current decisions related to investments in health, research, human resource development, and physical infrastructure. Reassessment of global and regional information on diseases and injuries is expected to occur periodically.

PROVIDERS OF HEALTH CARE

The implications for community health nursing concerning the three eras of health conditions are many. The health provider most appropriate when death is a common occurrence, as it was during the Era of Infectious Diseases, is a physician. This category of health worker is best suited for saving lives and for delivering the medical interventions that keep people alive. Nursing and nursing personnel are health care providers who have traditionally served populations that experience long-term chronic illnesses. Nursing personnel worldwide serve populations in nursing homes, long-term care facilities, and community-based programs for the elderly and disabled. The nursing services in Slovenia and Germany are excellent examples of the latter practice in Europe.

The caregiver needed for the Era of Social Conditions is evolving. For example, community health nurses and primary care physicians are developing new competencies for HIV/AIDS prevention among adolescent prostitutes, but also needed is a host of other interventions that require collaboration with other social service. In addition, some communities, because of their former political persuasion and cultural beliefs, have viewed the state as the provider of all health care services. For example, during the earthquake in Armenia, international workers recognized the need for social supports for those whose homes and community had been destroyed. At that time, these social structures, as they existed in North America, were not available to that population. Although alcoholism has been rampant in parts of Eastern Europe, organizations such as Alcoholic Anonymous were not available. In other areas, such as South America, close-knit family structures are vital. Yet, few if any services are available to families living between the era of the close-knit family structure and one that requires outside help for emerging third era conditions.

In the future, community health care will be increasingly collaborative and experienced as participatory partnerships with clear shifts in ownership and leadership. Formerly, international workers and consultants went to a country as outsiders and delivered their ideas, programs, and projects. The philosophy, beliefs, practices, and values of this dominant group of outsiders prevailed, and the recipient groups were considered a success to the extent that they adopted the dominant group's ways of being, living, and caring for their health.

In the future, partnerships that are sensitive to the dynamics of power and oppression, and which honor the need for local groups to be in control of their own projects and the resources that are used to implement them, will prevail. Pablo Freire's (1970) well-known advocacy for using *generative themes* that support education and critical consciousness has been adopted as collaborative projects demonstrate innovative ways of learning and conducting research. For example, in many countries, local experts and community members are forming partnerships with outside consultants and are insisting on striking changes in responsibility, authority, and ownership of data and innovations. In these emerging models, action research projects are being adopted over positivist, empirical studies, where the community becomes the initiator of action. See more on community-based participatory research in Chapter 4.

Health Providers at District Levels

In earlier forms of PHC, the locus of decision-making was at the village level. However, after many years of effort, the WHO and other organizations realized that the power to sustain change required more than village-level involvement. Thus, the move to the district level of implementation is currently being practiced in many places.

Regardless of level, however, the essential point is the adage: Think globally, act locally. Specifically, this means that expertise is needed from those at international, national, regional, and district levels, but the ways in which communities interpret the issues and actually decides to use the solutions belong to them. In local areas, communities adopt the health centers or organizations created to address community concerns. For example, in one Greek community, a local mayor sat through a week of deliberations on ways to bring PHC to his island. He heard the comments of members of the local community, its health workers, and an international WHO PHC team. Ultimately, the mayor realized that rooms for health providers would be needed, and he declared the community's full support to provide these rooms to further the work of the health center. In this way, his community was fully active and responsible for its own health status.

Community Health Workers

In some countries, particularly those in which professional health providers are scarce, the community identifies a local, respected, responsible person most often called the CHW. This person is selected from the village and is approved by the committee to serve the village people in health matters. CHWs usually provide 1 to 2 hours of health service per day, for which they may or may not be compensated by the community. In Ethiopia, refugees in camps erected after disasters identify responsible adults to serve as their kind of CHWs; these adults are known to and are trusted by newly established communities.

The CHW is trained in the fundamentals of promoting health and preventing and treating the most common health care conditions. This includes basic first aid, advice and assistance on simple treatments, and health teaching on personal hygiene, safe water supplies, safe disposal of human waste and refuse, and nutrition. Community health nurses often serve as consultants to the CHW and, in some places, are expected to supervise their work and provide ongoing education. These CHWs, as noted above, have demonstrated their effectiveness in controlling communicable diseases (e.g., malaria treatment) and promoting health (e.g., cervical cancer/mammography screenings) in this country and around the world (Perry & Zulliger, 2012).

Village Midwife

The village midwife provides basic antenatal, intrapartum, and postnatal care and makes referrals as required. In India, the village midwife is referred to as a trained *dai*. These are most often older women who may have had training from professional nurses and who are expected to call on professionals when needed. However, they often make their own decisions even though they have a referral source to professionals. Many times, adverse effects occur because cultural practices take precedence over knowledge-based practices that require collaborative decision-making. In Africa and Sudan, village midwives deliver a good percentage of babies, often in isolated villages. In Indonesia, village midwives expanded these services to also provide family planning services and contraceptives (Weaver et al., 2013). In Sudan and other areas, training is provided and encouraged in order for midwives to perform infant resuscitation and other skills more effectively (Me Arabi et al., 2016).

In some countries, traditional health practitioners receive formal training and return to their villages to continue their services with new knowledge and skills to enhance their effectiveness. Countries such as Bangladesh implemented programs to train workers who would practice in ways similar to the "barefoot doctors" of China (Shah et al., 2014; Xu et al., 2014). WHO advisors examined the work of these barefoot doctors as the Ministry of Health in Bangladesh was challenged in its efforts during the 1980s to provide health care to rural population.

Because of cultural taboos, women were not allowed to leave their homes for training and, if they did, would rarely want to be posted in a village other than their own. This was because women were viewed as wayward if they were not with their families in their home environments. This issue also occurred in Indonesia, when community health nurses were placed in villages away from home. They did not have the respect of the local community, were not seen as experts, and were considered to be of dubious moral standing. This cultural barrier presents challenges to nursing education programs that focus on community rather than hospital-based experiences.

Midwives are considered an important resource in the effort to end preventable maternal deaths (Bergevin, Fauveau, & McKinnon, 2015). A recent systematic review found that women who used the services of midwives who provided "continuity models of care" were more satisfied and have fewer interventions than women who received "other models of care" (Sandall, Soltani, Gates, Shennan, & Devane, 2015, para. 10). The researchers also noted that care provided by midwives was often the only available maternal care in many areas of the world.

Community Health Nurses

Background and Age at Entry to Nursing Education

When community health nurses join their colleagues in a country other than their own, they often assume that "a nurse is a nurse, is a nurse." Nothing could be further

---

PERSPECTIVES
A NURSE–MIDWIFE IN SUDAN

I am a nurse–midwife in South Sudan. My husband, who works with local pastors, and I are Seventh-Day Adventist missionaries based out of Uganda. One evening, I got a call about a lady in labor. I had not seen her for prenatal care, and there was a terrible rainstorm that night. I was told this was a first baby for the young woman, and she had been in labor for more than 24 hours. They wanted to take her to a hospital but could not get a vehicle to transport her there. The dirt roads are slippery and awful in this area, and the girl was 11 miles away from me (5 miles were dirt roads). I rode my bike in the rain, watching children on the sides of the road trying to capture ants to eat. They were beating on tin cans to lure them out of the ant holes, in order to gather the fat, winged ants that are considered tasty treats. As my assistant and I got close to the girl's thatched hut, we noticed groups of people gathered nearby. Villagers were often concerned about mothers and babies, but we were quickly told that the baby had just been born and was dead. I went into the hut and noticed a limp baby girl. I began to examine the baby and felt a faint heartbeat on the umbilical cord (still connected to the mother). I grabbed my bag and mask and began resuscitating the baby. The baby was on the mat covering the dirt floor, and I finally found an oral airway to keep the baby's mouth open, as the air did not seem to be getting through. Air finally began going into the lungs, and I checked the heartbeat (normal). I kept

bagging the baby and watched the tiny chest rise and fall. The tiny hut was filled with concerned neighborhood women who had been wailing because they thought the baby had died. Now, they sat quietly, speaking softly to one another as they watched me intently. Other women were crowded around the doorway to the hut and still more sat outside. I looked over at the mother, who seemed to be alright, not bleeding too much. I asked the women for hot water so I could keep the baby warm, and I kept bagging the baby. Then, I tried shocking the baby with colder water, so that she would begin to breathe on her own. We went back and forth like this a few times, and the baby would take an occasional breath. I inserted a nasogastric tube to remove any excess air that may have accumulated, and her color improved and muscle tone increased. After awhile, the baby began to breathe on her own. I checked the mother for any tearing (none apparent) and stayed with them for several hours to make sure there were no further signs of respiratory distress or other problems. Because the next day was market day, the word about the baby's condition spread very fast. I don't know what will happen tomorrow, but I am grateful for the blessings of today!

Kristina, Nurse–Midwife

Adapted from Adventist Mission. (2012, February 1). *Reaching out to South Sudan: Meet the Muehlhausers.* Retrieved from https://itunes.apple.com/us/podcast/adventist-mission-podcast/id193856093?mt=2

from the truth. The ways in which women and men are socialized, recruited into, advanced through, and graduated from nursing programs vary considerably from country to country. So does the age at entry, the exposure that nursing students have to the social and behavioral sciences, the theoretical and clinical applications studied, and the kind and extent of supervision they receive. For example, in some countries, young people begin their study of nursing at age 15, studying nursing in programs designed, sequenced, and financed by the government. These graduates are expected to practice as fully experienced community health nurses by age 18. In some countries, the extent of responsibilities placed on these relatively young practitioners is beyond their ability or maturity levels; however, the expectations persist because the number of prepared health care personnel is often at a premium. Some American universities have relationships with students and health care professionals from other countries and work with them to provide additional skills and education (Anft, 2013).

Curricula of Nursing Programs

In the United States, curricula in nursing are designed to serve the community in which the nursing program is based. Thus, a community prone to hurricanes, for example, would provide enhanced curricula for delivering nursing care in this kind of natural disaster. However, in some countries, nursing education curricula are conceived and designed at national levels and, in this way, are not responsive to local situations. The opportunity this model provides is consistency of teaching and learning and the possibility to produce teaching–learning materials in a uniform way and in the language of the country. The risks are that local conditions are not included, and care practices essential for a region of a country may not be addressed. For example, during an earthquake in Armenia, a WHO European Regional Advisor requested that content related to earthquakes and disaster preparedness be added to the curriculum. Authorities declined, showing the consulting team and local nurse leaders the detailed content and hours developed for the curriculum designed in Moscow. No opportunities, at that time, were possible for this content to be added, despite the fact that 25,000 people had lost their lives in this natural disaster.

Around the world, nursing educational programs may still be based in hospitals or technical schools or offered in universities. Specialty areas may be introduced as part of the basic curriculum, as is the practice in Denmark where midwifery is a basic program offered and is seen as a discipline different from nursing. In France, midwifery is aligned with medicine. This design differs from other countries in which nursing is the basic preparation upon which mental health, midwifery, and other areas are built and considered as advanced practice. In some countries, mental health is not included as part of the basic curriculum. For the graduates of these programs, moving to and working in countries that require mental health theory and practice requires additional schooling before the candidate is allowed to sit for the licensing examination.

The World Health Organization (2013d) has developed guidelines to improve for health professions education and training that address the requirements for faculty and students, as well as the need for better educational pathways, accreditation, and interprofessional education. Also, there has recently been a focus on including curriculum that provides meaningful opportunities for students to learn about global health and cultural competency through study abroad courses. Often, these courses involve an emersion experience, whereby students learn the realities of health care challenges and about delivering culturally appropriate care in diverse settings. See Perspectives: From Faculty and Students.

International Migration of Nurses

Although this chapter often focuses on U.S. nurses working in other countries, another, sometimes ominous component of global nursing is the migration of nurses from less-developed nations to more industrialized countries offering higher wages. Conditions in sub-Saharan Africa are very problematic. Having an already weak and poorly developed health system, countries in this region are now facing a serious crisis due to nursing shortages and migration of nurses to South Africa or other countries within the region where a better standard of living exists. Although sub-Saharan Africa represents 25% of the global disease burden, it receives about 1% of the global financial resources and only 1.3% of the world's trained health care workers live in that area (Li, Nie, & Li, 2014). Filipino nurses are the largest group migrating to the United States, with nurses from the Caribbean, India, Korea, and other countries following. In fact, about 70% of nurses graduating from programs in the Philippines go abroad for higher-paying work (Li et al., 2014). Canada and the United Kingdom often recruit nurses from outside their countries, while at the same time losing Canadian nurses to the United States. The United States, with its history of nursing shortages and a large health care system, has often relied on foreign graduates of nursing schools to meet its demands. This has caused concern among other nations and exemplifies the uneven balance in economic and political might, along with questions of ethics.

Forces That Support Nursing Development

In many places, nursing has yet to distinguish itself with its own body of research, knowledge, managerial practices, standards of practice, and ethical tenets. In Saudi Arabia, only about 29% of the nursing workforce are citizens, and even though nursing education has existed for over 40 years there, no postgraduate advanced practice programs are offered there and very few advanced practice nurses work there. In Israel, limited programs and regulations have been developed for specific nurse specialists (e.g., palliative care, geriatrics, wound care), bur nurses practicing in a rural area kibbutz may function as a nurse practitioner when no physician is available (Kleinpell et al., 2014). However, it appears that nursing has thrived as a respected discipline in countries where, overall, women are respected and where those in leadership positions understand the value of the caring process and are willing to champion nursing at all levels, including at the national level. For example, Turkey stands out as a country with physicians that sponsored nurses so that they were able to pursue higher education through the doctoral level of preparation. Nursing has developed

PERSPECTIVES
FROM A NURSING PROFESSOR ON LEARNING ABROAD

As a public health nurse for many years and then as a Professor of Nursing in community health nursing, I have become aware of the need for a culturally competent nursing workforce. For the last 10 years, I have had the privilege of teaching nursing students in a 3-week cultural immersion course in Mexico and then in Ecuador. It is my belief based on the Essentials of Baccalaureate Education for Professional Nursing Practice (American Association of Colleges of Nursing, 2008) that learning abroad allows health care members to immerse themselves in cultures different from their own as a means to challenge beliefs and attitudes about cultures and better understands cultural differences. The aim of this class is to assist students in developing an awareness, understanding, and appreciation of the cultural factors and views that underlie a person's health and way of living. The course's goal is to assist and help increase the nurse's ability to make in-depth assessments of the cultural influences on individuals' health care and develop the ability to deliver culturally sensitive, safe, and effective care. Through study abroad, students gain knowledge, skills, and principles that will enable them to generalize to other cultural groups.

A cultural immersion experience for students adds to the effectiveness of the transfer of knowledge in cultural competent health care delivery. I believe that this teaching strategy assists students of all learning styles to gain knowledge in culturally appropriate care and is needed in light of the increasing population of Hispanics and in California and the United States in general. Students have come back from these experiences with renewed cultural understanding. Here is a sample of student comments after the immersion experience:

- *"Currently I work in a hospital setting, but I anticipate working in the community setting in the future. I hope that I will have more awareness of the Mexican culture with Spanish-speaking patients, and I will definitively have more empathy with potential language barriers and use a translator more readily."*
- *"I will most definitely appreciate the circumstances of health care in America and most definitely better understand the rationale of my Mexican patients."*
- *"A broader understanding of where they are coming from and what they deal with before we see them in the health care setting."*
- *"In many ways! I have a better understanding of habits and practices."*
- *"Oh—I'll always think twice when caring for all of my patients and consider culture in their care."*

As health professionals, we are always on the learning curve of cultural competency. The immersion experience is one very effective tool in teaching and assisting nursing students toward the goal of a more culturally competent workforce.

Judith Keswick, RN, PHN, MSN,
Associate Professor of Nursing

From American Association of Colleges of Nursing. (2008). *Essentials of baccalaureate education for professional nursing practice.* Washington, DC: Author.

in unusual ways in other countries as well. In the United Kingdom, home of Florence Nightingale, no national certification or regulations for advanced practice nursing exists, although many nurses and midwives practice in this capacity because of the "permissive approach to the scope of practice" there (Kleinpell et al., 2014, para. 16). In Australia, nurse practitioner practice is, at the present time, much less organized, despite a national board and standards, than what we have in the United States.

A major challenge to community health nurses who have undergone theory and clinical experiences as learners is working with nurses who have not had community health experience. As is well understood, functioning well in a fully equipped hospital is different from working in a community or village where resources are not easily available. Exploring these differences is an essential part of one's own needs assessment as one embarks on an experience with a team from locations other than one's own.

THE PROCEDURES/INTERVENTIONS

Community health nurses consider the population as their patient or client. A population might refer to all those living in a catchment area, in a neighborhood, village, a district, or city. Countries might refer to their populations at national, regional, or international levels. Regardless of location or level, community health nurses practice within the context of some kind of health care system or organization.

PERSPECTIVES
STUDENT NURSE IN ECUADOR

I never thought I would study abroad, but when the opportunity to take one of my nursing classes in Cuenca, Ecuador, arose, I decided to embrace it, expecting a great learning experience. Little did I imagine that it was going to be anything short of life changing. Simply stated, it was humbling to be a guest in a host family's home, accepted like family, and it was awesome to become immersed in a culture so different from our own. During our 1-month stay, our itinerary was packed with school as well as experiences in hospitals, clinics, school, and even an orphanage.

I recall a particular hospital where I assisted a compassionate nurse in giving bed baths with limited resources. I ripped three pairs of small-sized latex gloves before managing to keep a pair on my large hands. I learned that being a good nurse was not dependent on the availability of supplies but rather in maximizing the potential to deliver compassionate care in any circumstance.

I am happy I made the decision to study abroad. In addition to the learning experience, I gained insight, respect, humility, and gratitude for life and for others. It is as if I have become aware of what living fully is, something unattainable without the smells, sights, sounds, and interactions I encountered abroad.

Jaime Morga, SN

Nurses and midwives constitute a majority of the qualified workforce in many national health care systems, and they represent a powerful force for bringing health care to all populations. Nurses provide the spectrum of PHC services and conduct health research, and as the global population ages, average age of nurses is increasing; this further intensifies nursing shortages according to the most recent data from the International Centre for Human Resources in Nursing (ICHRN, 2008).

The interventions that community health nurses provide depend on the context in which they are working and on the population, its health status, and the health conditions it presents. These interventions also depend on the ways in which nursing is practiced in a country and on the organizations in which community health nurses are employed or with which they are collaborating. A key issue here is that community health nurses need to know the mission of the agencies with which they are working and the kinds of services and resources their employing organizations provide. This section describes selected organizations that provide interventions to address community health care issues and the ways in which community health nurses work within them.

Providing an intervention that "works" constitutes an achievement. Providing an intervention in community health constitutes a remarkable achievement. This is because interventions are complex and often costly and involve considerable knowledge, planning, and expert execution and evaluation skills. This section also focuses on the interventions community health nurses provide in a context different from their own within the context of a sponsoring organization.

As noted, the first step is to understand what the community's health needs are, who is involved in addressing them, the roles they play, and the contributions they are able to bring to the issue. Again, knowing the context in which one is working and understanding the population and their health status and health conditions are also critical elements (and have been addressed earlier). A second but often overlooked step is to understand the reasons the interventions are being delivered and one's reasons for being involved. Specifically, what does the sponsoring agency believe is its mission and why now, why here? What does the community have to say? Does the community see itself as a recipient of donations or as partners and collaborators? How do they see the intervention? Did they identify the need and ask for assistance? Have the recipients been involved in identifying the issue, in planning strategies for the intervention? Are they committed to the issue and to the outcome? What is their level of involvement in the issue?

These are complex questions. In some countries, the number and seriousness of challenges may be overwhelming, and despite outsiders' authoritative view of what should be tackled first, the community's perspective will often determine the intervention's effectiveness. For example, in Chad, of all the health information that the country could collect, Harvard University international consultants worked with the Ministry of Health and established an essential list that its people would find the most useful. At times, one's own interests may not be the ones the community needs to tackle.

Questions you need to ask yourself are the following: Why are you there? What motivates you and what is your commitment? How does this fit with the scope of the work you will be undertaking, and will your time commitment see the project through, and if not, what effect will your leaving have on its success? In some places, a custom has been established of exchanges where the international project staff is accommodated and where the local staff expects the same when they join the international staff in their home country. This commitment may represent a time and financial commitment you are not prepared to make. You will want to examine this issue before you commit to a project and its occasionally unwritten expectations.

Criteria for Support of Interventions

Sustainability. One of the most important criterions for donor support is sustainability: Can the recipient unit, a village health center, a regional health office, and a district hospital administer the projects after external funds are no longer available? For example, in one project slated for an African country, one consultant was instructed to avoid any project under $5 million, as the donor agency did not want to manage what they considered "small projects."

Absorptive capacity. Although many communities need support for their interventions, they often lack the personnel, structures, or processes to actually use the support. For example, in the project described above, the country's department requesting funding, although in dire need of help, was staffed at the national level with one full-time and one half-time person, with virtually no computer capability and no delivery system. In many countries, particularly after national disasters, well-intentioned donors flood a country with clothing, supplies, and equipment that go into warehouses as the infrastructure to receive, sort, transport, and deliver the goods are simply not functional.

Transferability. Many donor organizations and countries support pilot projects to assess their use in other places in the region, country, or throughout the world. For example, one country committed to its history of medicine requested funds from an international donor agency. The request was denied as this agency saw itself as promoting creative ideas and projects that might be applied to other places in the world.

When considering a project's funding, these questions need to be asked. Other questions need to be asked as well—about gender, political, and cultural issues. For example, if an organization plans to support the elimination of the practice of female circumcision, how will that be seen by the population? If a donor agency insists on a democratic process of decision-making, how do leaders implement this process when they have no background or skills in the democratic process and their positions are tied to their ability to make decisions without team input? How do CHWs implement sanitation programs that place farm animals in places segregated from humans when villagers see their cows as sacred and want to have them in the family compound? How does the community health nurse reduce the malaria fever of a newly delivered woman when the village midwife, the untrained *dais*, insists "you sponge her only on day three"? How do you provide international education for a country's highly intelligent practicing nurses when local physicians view the nurses as their assistants?

These and many other questions challenge the underlying assumptions about the process of change and the unplanned effects a well-intentioned intervention is designed to deliver. Yet another question relates to the way community health services are organized.

The most commonly involved organizations that provide health-related interventions and support are described here. An overall umbrella agency is the United Nations (UN). Most people know of the UN's work in peacekeeping. This body also focuses on working conditions through the International Labor Organization (ILO), educational issues through the United Nations Educational Scientific and Cultural Organization (UNESCO), and health issues, specifically, through WHO and UNICEF.

The World Health Organization

The leading global agency that focuses specifically on health is the **World Health Organization** (WHO, 2016q). The organization has regional offices in six parts of the world with its headquarters in Geneva, Switzerland (WHO, 2016s). The six regional offices include WHO Regional Office for Americas (PAHO), WHO Regional Office for the Eastern Mediterranean (EMRO), WHO Regional Office for Europe (EURO), WHO Regional Office for Southeast Asia (SEARO), WHO Regional Office for Africa (AFRO), and WHO Regional Office for the Western Pacific (WPRO).

The WHO, Its History, and Its Work

The UN began in 1945, and discussions about the need for a global health organization began. The WHO developed its own constitution that went into effect on April 7, 1948, although it has been closely associated with the UN since its inception. It is responsible for its own programs, funded by regular and extra budgetary funds, and also for health-related initiatives sponsored and funded by UN agencies and other international bodies. The WHO carries out its work through the policies it creates with its member states throughout the world. It provides leadership and technical support, monitors health trends, sets norms and standards, and helps to spur research worldwide (WHO, 2016h). It does this initially at its annual May meeting, the **World Health Assembly (WHA)**. World Health Day is celebrated annually on the anniversary of the WHO's inception (April 7th).

The World Health Assembly

The WHA is the highest governing body within the WHO and includes 193 member countries. Representatives from each of the world's regions attend this assembly and bring the policies and recommendations to their respective regional offices for implementation and expression at regional and local levels. Staff members at the regional offices then work with their member countries through their annual September Regional Committee Meeting held each year after the WHA (WHO, 2016s; WHO Media Centre, 2016b).

The WHO provides technical support and advises member states on strategies to meet their health care needs. The WHO serves as a catalyst to mobilize the resources of national governments, financial institutions and endowments, and bilateral partners for health development. Its six-point agenda includes promoting development, fostering health security, strengthening health systems, harnessing information/evidence/research, enhancing partnerships, and improving performance through its ongoing reforms (WHO, 2016a). The WHO is not the organization of choice when vehicles, equipment, and medicines are required; the WHO can help a member state determine the drugs that are essential and will assist in developing health policy, project plans, and programs.

The WHO employs many types of professionals, including nurses. However, the organization does not focus on professional issues to support the development of particular health-related practitioners, such as nurses, midwives, social workers, or physicians. Nurses interested in these types of issues should explore opportunities with the International Council of Nurses (ICN) or nursing organizations at national or state levels. In the United States, these would include the American Association of Colleges of Nursing, the American Nurses Association, or National Council of State Boards of Nursing.

The WHO does focus on providing technical support related to the interventions these health professionals deliver, and for these, considerable effort is expended on developing nursing, midwifery, social work, and physician-related knowledge and skills that are basic to these interventions. However, the WHO works closely with the ICN and with national nursing organizations on policies and programming issues.

WHO Collaborating Centers

The WHO generally uses a 5-year planning cycle that is divided into 2-year cycles of projects, documentation, publications, and the development of information systems. Community health nurses are employed at the international level in Geneva, and they hold regional level positions as Regional Nursing Advisors. However, one or two Regional Nursing Advisors cannot possibly carry out the work of a region that might be the home to thousands of nursing personnel. To address this issue, WHO developed a network of **World Health Organization Collaborating Centers**; these centers focus on specific areas of expertise and carry out the work of the member countries in these areas. For example, the collaborating center network in nursing of the European Region has focused on PHC and information systems. The European Regional also developed a collaborating center network on disaster preparedness that included a 30-member international team of experts, including the Regional Advisor for Nursing, Midwifery, and Social Work. The network in the United States has worked through universities in their respective areas of excellence. In the United States, early pioneer universities included the University of Illinois, the University of Pennsylvania, the University of Texas, the University of Alabama, and the University of California. Student nurses in these universities have the opportunity to participate in the research, nursing projects, and other international activities their universities sponsor, both in the United States and in their partnering countries. About 11% of WHO collaborating centers are in the United States. Sometimes, these collaborating centers represent the WHO and their countries at national and international meetings. They provide critical services that are recognized by but cannot be funded or staffed by the WHO. They also bring credibility to projects, as they come from the communities they represent, and they know the issues and interventions that have the greatest chances of succeeding (WHO, 2014a).

WHO and Its Collaborators

The WHO works closely with national governments, its collaborating center network, its universities, research centers, and NGOs. Experts from member countries are recruited throughout the year to deliberate on global health and health-related issues. For example, during the Chernobyl disaster, WHO/EURO called five internationally recognized nuclear experts to an emergency meeting to examine the issues and assist the member countries with next-step actions to protect their populations, livestock, and agricultural industries. Historically, the WHO has collaborated with centers of excellence throughout the world, including the CDC in the United States.

WHO as a Multilateral Agency

The WHO and other UN agencies are sometimes referred to as *multinational* or **multilateral agencies**. They support development efforts of governments, organizations, and universities in countries throughout the world. The WHO regional offices also collaborate with each other to address issues on which they can partner and provide resources. For example, during the civil wars in Africa, Chad, Angola, and Mozambique, WHO/AFRO and WHO/EURO collaborated to develop projects on rehabilitation for the countries with few nursing programs, no medical schools, and no comprehensive programs for the disabled. The WHO intervenes through its own staff's efforts and through those of its partnerships. In another example, the WHO's health-promoting schools is a collaborative effort with UNESCO and UNICEF. Still, another example is the Human Reproduction Program, a global research program on reproductive health. It collaborates with two programs of the UN as well as the World Bank (WB). Similarly, the WHO has joined with several other organizations to fight hunger and improve food standards and has collaborated with UNICEF, the WB, and other agencies on *Deliver Now for Women + Children*, a program launched in 2007 to promote advocacy for women and children in South America, Tanzania, India, and other areas of the world (WHO, 2016c).

Health for All: A Primary Health Care Initiative

In its earlier years, the WHO personnel watched as hospitals and costly health establishments were built throughout the world. One of the world's leading economists, Dr. Brian Abel Smith, noted that countries could not afford to erect costly buildings, nor could they add large numbers of health professional to their cadres of personnel. Rather, he suggested that the health personnel available work with the population to manage their health care needs. His major assertion is that health care needs and wants may expand infinitely, but resources do not, and all must manage with the resources currently available. Many health leaders throughout the world recognized the trends emerging and believed that a major change in thinking

and practice was needed. They met together in Alma-Ata, Kazakhstan, in the former Soviet Union and created a sweeping set of declarations that became the *Declaration of Alma-Ata* (see Chapter 1) or **Health for All**. The world body of 134 countries called on all members to reframe their expectations and implement PHC. In Europe, the 32-member countries developed its 38 regional targets for health. In the United States, health care professionals launched *Healthy People 2000*. After the year 2000, *Healthy People 2010* became the blueprint, and now, the *Healthy People 2020* document outlines our goals and objectives for the future (USDHHS, 2016).

PHC is sometimes called a philosophy, a movement, a way of thinking, a way of working, a setting for health services, or a set of principles. Making it operational at the national level, however, meant that communities would focus on health care services at the local level rather than building large, tertiary hospitals that cater exclusively to urban, financially secure populations. This also meant that the education of health care providers would be located at this level with a de-emphasis on high-cost medical interventions and technology available only to relatively few in the population.

Health for All emphasizes PHC that is affordable, culturally acceptable, appropriate, accessible, and delivered through partnerships between national health services system and local communities. The communities take the leading responsibility for identifying their own priority health concerns and planning and implementing their own PHC service. These PHC services include prevention, health promotion, and curative and rehabilitative care provided by the people themselves (WHO, 2012). See Figure 16–3 for an illustration of the organizational pattern of community-based PHC.

Functions of Primary Health Care

In 1978, Article VII of the *Declaration of Alma-Ata* (now Almaty) lists the eight basic elements of PHC (WHO, 2016r):

1. Education concerning prevailing health problems and the methods of preventing and controlling them
2. Promotion of food supply and proper nutrition
3. An adequate supply of safe water and basic sanitation
4. Maternal and child health, including family planning
5. Immunization against major infectious diseases
6. Prevention and control of locally endemic diseases
7. Appropriate treatment of common diseases and injuries
8. Provision of essential drugs

Public health care also involves related sectors concerned with national and community development, including agriculture, animal husbandry, food, industry, education, housing, public works, and communication (Article VI, Section 4). Health for All by the year 2000 was the goal, but the majority of global deaths occur in developing countries. Much assistance is needed there. Some have called for wealthy countries to devote a small percentage of their GDP to assist poor countries with their health issues. Also, low-income countries have been encouraged to devote a reasonable percentage of their own budgets to health. Access to PHN is also vital. Working

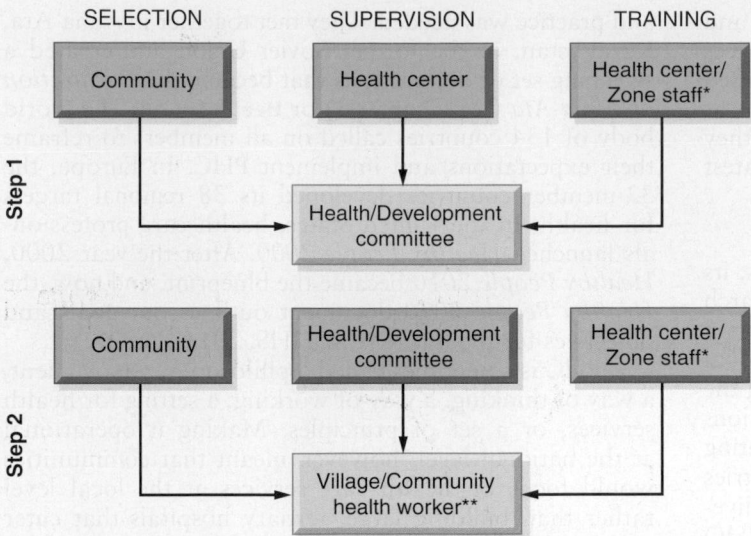

SELECTION SUPERVISION TRAINING

*Nurse, sanitarian, midwife, health education assistant
**Assistant midwife, traditional birth attendant, traditional practitioner

FIGURE 16–3 Community-based primary care.

with countries in various regions to address the social determinants of health through collaborative development of policies and priorities has shown some promise. This type of "intersectoral" approach to health problems has gained international support (WHO, 2013b, p. 3).

Deterrents to Primary Health Care

Fostering a PHC approach is one thing, implementing it is another. Initially, political reactions from professional groups, who felt threatened by a potential loss of income due to the shift away from specialists and tertiary hospitals in favor of primary care providers, were not supportive. Universities and teaching institutions lacked the experience of working in communities and did not know how to educate professionals for PHC. Textbooks were based on education for treating diseases and assumed the backup of well-equipped and, in some places, technically advanced hospital environments. Nursing faculty in developing countries adopted community health nursing textbooks from North America but did not understand the problems of placing student nurses in remote clinical areas with no faculty. Faculty was virtually nonexistent in rural areas and, if they were available, clients were not. Stationing young women in villages without supervision was seen in some countries as ill advised, and clients refused to appear at these health centers. In addition, populations in some rural areas were used to traditional methods and indigenous practitioners, and even when available, professional nurses or midwives were not consulted. Inadequate supervision and follow-up led to misapplication of theory learned, and those in rural areas were not prepared for the situations they faced daily. Health care workers did not understand their responsibilities for maintaining, restocking, and securing medical supplies on a regular basis, and many had no knowledge of community-based principles of case finding, record keeping, community monitoring of immunizations, prenatal care, disease prevention,

health promotion, and basic measures to ensure community sanitation. For example, in one rural health center in Southeast Asia, this author observed barrels of antibiotics, medicated creams, lotions, and other medications spoiled from running solutions that had not been sorted, shelved, or refrigerated.

In many places, referral systems to nearby hospitals were not effective, and health care workers were reluctant to place themselves in responsible positions without backup and accessible secondary and tertiary facilities. In one rural community in Spain, a nurse–physician pair who worked closely together confided that they worried that the distance between them and the nearest tertiary facility would threaten their success in securing help for those during periods of emergencies.

Natural environmental phenomena such as rain, floods, and poor or absent communication facilities periodically isolated areas and prevented transport of patients to nearby facilities. Other problems arose when expensive drugs were dispensed in place of less-expensive generic brands (or in some cases were given first to the family and friends of the health care workers) and when health centers failed to refer patients back to the referring CHW. See Evidence-Based Practice for comparison of physician-led and nurse-led patient care.

Achievements of Primary Health Care

In the almost 40 years since the 1978 proclamation of *Health for All* by WHO, there have been acknowledged significant global accomplishments. Childhood immunization rates have improved, as has the provision of safe water and sanitation. But the access to essential health care is still not available worldwide. Economic barriers, the shortage of health care personnel, and the worldwide HIV/AIDS epidemic have made it more difficult to achieve this worthwhile goal. One example of expansion of comprehensive services to their full population is Portugal

EVIDENCE-BASED PRACTICE
Substituting Physicians With Nurses

Researchers conducted a systematic review and meta-analysis of published randomized controlled trials (RCTs) that assessed nurse-led care with care by primary care physicians, on hospital admissions, costs of health care, mortality, quality of life, and patient satisfaction. Results from 28,974 participants across the 24 RCTs that met criteria for inclusion in the meta-analysis showed that "nurse-led care seems to have a positive effect on patient satisfaction, hospital admission, and mortality" (Martínez-González et al., 2014, para 4). Nurses in these studies worked in a variety of settings including general practice, health

care agencies, nurse clinics, community clinics, and nurse clinics.

This evidence is significant because of the growing concern about the global shortage of heath care providers, especially physicians. Many lower-income countries rely on nurses to provide some or most primary care to meet the growing demands of the aging population in health care environment where physicians are scarce.

From Martínez-González, N. A., Djalali, S., Tandjung, R., Huber-Geismann, F., Markun, S., Wensing, M., & Rosemann, T. (2014). *Substitution of physicians by nurses in primary care: A systematic review and meta-analysis.* Retrieved from http://www.biomedcentral.com/1472-6963/14/214

(Waddington, 2008). Portugal organized Family Health Units (FHU), where groups of physicians, nurses, and staff work to provide care to patients and families and make decisions together with them about health needs. Since the 1970s, Portugal's infant mortality rate has dropped by 50% every 8 years; the 2006 rate was 3 per 1,000. Life expectancy jumped 9.2 years in one generation. Patients register for government-sponsored health services through a family physician, and MD/RN salaries are based on productivity and performance (Waddington, 2008). Although Portugal has achieved provision of health care to most of its population and improved vital statistics, it still has a high out-of-pocket expenditure (about 22%). High-risk groups (e.g., pregnant women, children, people with diabetes) are exempt from these co-payments.

Many other nations need to achieve *Health for All* by making health care a right for all citizens and expanding services to meet the needs of rural populations and high-risk groups. Future action regarding PHC calls for strengthened collaboration among governmental agencies and NGOs in both the public and private sectors. Only then will the world have a realistic chance of achieving all the goals set out in the *Declaration of Alma-Ata* (WHO, 2016r).

The Way Forward

One of the greatest achievements of the WHO has been the eradication of smallpox. In 1967, this disease threatened 60% of the world's population. It is projected that 20 million people would have died in the next two decades if smallpox had not been eradicated. In 2010, a statue was erected to commemorate the 30th anniversary of smallpox eradication (WHO Media Centre, 2010). The WHO's other accomplishments include reduction of malaria, standardization of data collection systems, adoption of international standards for the control and reporting of morbidity and mortality, and publication of classic works for the prevention and management of disease. They have also partnered with Rotary International and UNICEF to provide measles, polio, and DPT immunizations to the world's children. In 1990, they reached the 80% mark. In addition, the WHO has been credited with preventing hundreds of millions of cases of tropical

diseases. As the 21st century begins, new eradication/elimination programs are under way for polio, guinea worm disease, and measles. Other initiatives include:

1. Reducing transmission and incidence of HIV/AIDS
2. Launching the *RBM* program
3. Stopping the transmission of TB
4. Increasing access to essential pharmaceuticals
5. Improving the poor quality of some pharmaceuticals
6. Preventing and treating iron deficiency
7. Reducing maternal morbidity and mortality
8. Promoting healthful lifestyles for all age groups, including elders (WHO, 2016l)

Dr. Gro Harlem Brundtland, former Director General of WHO, characterized the 20th century as one encompassing the biggest social transformations of history. Living conditions, she noted, have dramatically improved for the large majority of human beings, and she identified health as the key to improving the productivity of people and nations. She noted the persistence of excess mortality and morbidity that disproportionately affect poor people and underscored the need to focus on those interventions that can achieve the greatest health gains possible using available resources.

International Governmental Organizations With National Governments

Sometimes, the WHO is the first to describe a health-related situation requiring international support. It then contacts other groups or organizations with the requisite expertise, assembling members of its international disaster-preparedness teams from governmental organizations that represent various nations. Organizations such as church-related groups, universities, researchers, and governments provide international assistance.

Countries throughout the world are structured to fund within-country health issues and to contribute to the international agenda. The United States contributes internationally through its United States Agency for International Development (USAID). Some other countries' international arms include Denmark's DANIDA and Italy's Italian Cooperation. The European

Union (EU) is an organization that provides funding for many health-related projects.

United States Agency for International Development

The USAID is an independent, bilateral agency of the executive branch that is under the guidance of the Secretary of State. It works to enhance long-term and equitable economic growth and to advance U.S. foreign policy by supporting countries in their efforts to recover from disaster, escape poverty, and engage in democratic reforms. The agency provides support to developing countries for economic development, agriculture and trade, global health, democracy, conflict prevention, and humanitarian assistance and does this through its collaboration with many governmental and private agencies to implement its programs (Nichols, 2011). This agency also hires nurses and other health care providers and often provides workshops to brief grant writers on the interventions currently under exploration.

The Centers for Disease Control and Prevention

The CDC's Center for Global Health is a leading player in addressing global challenges such as HIV/AIDS, malaria, emergency and refugee health, noncommunicable diseases, injuries, and more. The center strives to protect and improve health globally through science, policy, partnership, and evidence-based public health action and has four broad goals:

Goal 1: Health Impact: Improve the health and well-being of people around the world

Goal 2: Health Security: Improve capabilities to prepare and respond to infectious disease or emerging health threats and public health emergencies

Goal 3: Health Capacity: Build country public health capacity

Goal 4: Organizational Capacity: Maximize potential of CDC's global program to achieve impact

The core of CDC's strength lies in its technical expertise and scientific rigor while working with partners around the globe to address pressing and emerging public health challenges (CDC, 2015a).

American International Health Alliance

The USAID often collaborates with other organizations to implement its programs. The American International Health Alliance (AIHA) is one of these and operates under a cooperative agreement with USAID. It establishes and manages hospital partnerships between health care institutions in the United States and their counterparts in Central and Eastern Europe and in the newly independent states of Central Asia. The AIHA is reportedly the U.S. hospital sector's most coordinated response to health care issues in those areas. AIHA manages programs and research in partnerships with countries in Eurasia (Central and Eastern Europe, Central Asia), Africa, Asia, and the Caribbean (AIHA, 2012).

World Bank

The **World Bank (WB)** is an agency that focuses on economic development, and it includes a health component (e.g., projects related to child health and health system performance). It partners with countries, the WHO, and

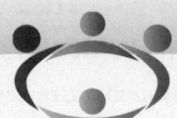

DISPLAY 16–5 WORLD BANK

The fight against poverty is not a fight for glory. It is about equity and social justice, about the environment and resources we all share, and about peace and security. It is a fight for a better life for all of us and for our children who will live in this very interconnected world.

From Wolfensohn, J. D., & Kircher, A. (2005). *Voice for the world's poor: Selected speeches and writings of World Bank President James D. Wolfensohn, 1995–2005.* Washington, DC: The World Bank. Quote excerpted from p. 167.

other organizations to address poverty, build capacity, transfer knowledge, provide resources, and forge partnerships in the public and private sectors (World Bank Group, 2016). See Display 16–5.

Nongovernmental Organizations

Countries throughout the world provide interventions through formal governmental organizations and through NGOs. These organizations are not under government sponsorship or control. In the United States, they are designated as private voluntary organizations (PVOs) that focus on humanitarian and professional issues related to global health. Examples of PVOs are the Global Health Council (GHC), the Center for International Health and Cooperation, Cooperative for American Remittances to Europe (CARE), the Carter Center, and the ICN.

These organizations contribute in their particular areas of expertise and work with other international organizations, research centers, and universities. Some focus on children, such as Save the Children and the International Society of Prevention of Child Abuse and Neglect (SPCAN); some on medically focused interventions, such as Doctors Without Borders; and some on logistics and supplies, such as Direct Relief International (DRI).

Global Health Council

The GHC (formerly known as the National Council for International Health) is the world's largest membership alliance dedicated to saving lives by improving health throughout the world. The GHC advocates for needed policies and resources, builds networks and alliances among those working to improve health, and shares innovative ideas, knowledge, and best practices in health (GHC, 2015a).

The GHC's membership includes hundreds of private and public organizations around the world, as well as several thousand professionals involved in global health. A multidisciplinary, cross-cultural board of directors, health professionals, student interns, volunteers, and members comprise its staff. Its mission is to "improve health globally through increased investment, robust policies and the power of the collective voice" (GHC, 2015a, para. 2).

Center for International Humanitarian Cooperation

The Center for International Humanitarian Cooperation (CIHC), founded in 1992, promotes peace and healing in countries shattered by war, regional conflicts, and ethnic violence, as well as natural disasters. Its belief is that health and other basic humanitarian actions often provide the only common ground for initiating dialogue and cooperation among warring parties. The center provides training in mental health issues, disaster management, and negotiation, as well as books on topics ranging from civil strife to epidemics (CIHC, n.d.).

CARE

The CARE was founded in 1945, when 22 American organizations joined together to rush lifesaving *care packages* from individual American citizens, churches, clubs, and businesses to survivors of World War II. Millions of CARE packages followed in the next two decades. In the 1950s, CARE expanded its program to developing nations, using surplus American food to feed the hungry. In the 1960s, it pioneered PHC. Now renamed the Cooperative for Assistance and Relief Everywhere, CARE is affiliated with foundations and other organizations, as well as the UN and the European Union (EU). CARE intervenes by responding to famines and disasters worldwide with emergency food, supplies, and rehabilitative efforts. It delivers programs in education, health, population, water and sanitation, agriculture, environmental preservation, economic development, and community building in over 90 countries (CARE, 2016).

The Carter Center

Former United States President, Jimmy Carter, and his wife, Roselyn, founded the Carter Center in 1986. The Carter Center intervenes in disease prevention and agriculture throughout the world and cites its fundamental mission as "human rights and alleviation of human suffering" (Carter Center, 2016, para 1). It is aligned with Emory University, and the particularly successful interventions include the guinea worm disease eradication program and the program to eradicate river blindness, as well as trachoma and schistosomiasis control. Lymphatic filariasis elimination, malaria control, and mental health issues, along with an international task force on disease eradication, are also components of its health program.

Bill & Melinda Gates Foundation

Bill Gates, the force behind popular computer software giant, Microsoft, and his wife Melinda operate a global foundation that provides assistance for those living in hunger and poverty. The foundation provides vaccines to prevent the spread of infectious diseases like malaria, polio, and HIV. They also work to improve maternal–child health and nutrition (Bill & Melinda Gates Foundation, 2015).

International Council of Nurses

As noted earlier, the ICN represents the global interests and concerns of the nursing profession. ICN's mission is to maintain the role of nursing in health care through its global voice. Its current membership includes nursing organizations from 130 countries representing 13 million nurses (ICN, 2014).

National Governments Working Alone

Individual nations have considerable experience working across agencies and organizations, and they have traditions that they honor as they intervene. For example, the Federal Republic of Germany has one of the largest voluntary sectors in the world and is known for its work with the International Red Cross. The Finnish Nursing Organization has an outstanding international reputation for its work during the Armenian earthquake and in other international efforts throughout Europe. The Danish Nurses Organization has provided funds, leadership, and expertise to numerous projects in collaboration with the WHO and with the ICN.

At times, however, governments facing a crisis or disaster prefer to operate alone, without international assistance. This position must be respected, and because of this expectation, international organizations will not appear in a country until a formal request is received from representatives of the country in crisis. Furthermore, some countries are more receptive to certain kinds of assistance than others. Some countries do not welcome foreign professionals, as they believe they have enough of their own. They may prefer help in the form of equipment, transport, medications, or vital supplies, such as water and food. Those in disaster preparedness are well aware of what some refer to as the "second disaster," when well-intentioned groups send in truckloads of used clothing and articles that are useless in some environments. The recent disasters in Haiti lead to an outbreak of cholera that was brought into the country by international workers. This experience has added another layer of concern for those involved in relief work. Further, these disasters have also spurred the removal of children from affected countries; some of these are characterized as rescue missions, some are reported to arise out of groups dedicated to religious objectives, and some have been shown to occur out of financial interests (receiving payment for couples wishing to adopt children). At times, governments would prefer to work alone but do not have the resources to do so, nor can their authorities provide the personnel to sort the kinds of contributions donors provide during emergencies.

Organizations With Religious Affiliations

Many religious groups sponsor organizations, and some of them include a religiously oriented agenda along with their interventions. Others, however, do not. Often, the work of these groups is similar to those with a nonreligious focus, and the source of funding for a particular project may be the only overt connection to any religious group. Catholic Charities and other Christian organizations provide critical interventions, as do Muslim, Jewish, and other religiously oriented organizations. These organizations often recruit community health nurses and other health care providers for short- and long-term assignments. See Perspectives: One Nurse's Experience Overseas.

COMMUNITY HEALTH NURSING OPPORTUNITIES

Let us suppose that, after reading this chapter and some of its references, you have decided to work in a location other than your own. You are not alone.

Global health programs are becoming increasingly prevalent at academic health centers. These programs range in scope from comprehensive, multidisciplinary, multiprofessional initiatives—with patient care, research, and

PERSPECTIVES
ONE NURSE'S EXPERIENCE OVERSEAS

I had always wanted to be a nurse and work in a foreign country, so when I heard of an organization that sent health workers overseas, I got involved while I was in college. The experiential cross-cultural training that my husband and I received before we left made all the difference in preparing us to have a positive transition. We learned that our goal would be to become "servant learners," serving the local population and learning from them rather than coming in to solve their problems with our superior ways of doing things. This was a hard lesson to learn, and we kept coming back to it in our 18 years abroad as we searched for the rationales behind customs that puzzled us. I also had to find a balance between "going native" in each new culture and keeping the parts of my own identity that were valuable.

When we first arrived, it was like nothing I expected. No one met us at the airport as planned, we did not speak the language, a luggage cart hit me from behind and cut my leg, and it was hot, crowded, and dirty. This was not a complete surprise as I had been prepared for the actual experience to differ from my expectations, but adjusting took conscious effort. I expected to go to a delta town and work in an established hospital. We were asked to go to a major seaport city and teach English! We did find an opportunity to work in community health with

the goal of "working ourselves out of a job" by training national workers who would be far more effective in their country than we could ever be.

Flexibility, comfort with ambiguity, being able to laugh at ourselves, and patience when results seemed few and far between were essential skills. I learned much about myself and grew in my ability to cross cultures. I learned to actually prefer other ways of doing and being. My faith deepened, and I learned to depend upon it like I never had before. We were accepted by people, who brought us into their culture, and treated us like family members. I consider that the most valuable part of the whole experience as I look back upon our time there. Our children were born overseas and grew up feeling at ease in many settings and with a particular sensitivity to differing perspectives. I know what it is to live with war, to celebrate life in impossibly difficult circumstances, and to stand truly in another's shoes—experiences I would never have had at home but which expanded my life. Although I had no idea when I first got off that airplane that I would spend most of my adult life in foreign countries, I am so grateful for the opportunity I have had to live my dreams.

Karin Urso, RN, PHN,
Missionary Nurse

---

education components—to individual courses. The larger initiatives may involve collaborative efforts among schools of medicine, public health, nursing, and dentistry and may have alliances with schools outside the health professions. This growth in the number of programs is accompanied by a surge of interest in every facet of global health among health science students and trainees (Pinto et al., 2014).

If you decide to pursue work abroad, you might begin your work at a local level, at a local health center in a village. You would be aware of your own issues and reasons for wanting this experience, and you would have selected the location because of some factors that draw you to it. How then might you go about preparing for the experience? In what kind of activities might you be involved? What might be the expectations and commitments you would make regarding the assignment?

Community health nurses, as shown in this chapter, carry major responsibility for managing health services in health centers, clinics, schools, workplaces, and community settings that range in population density and complexity from remote areas to major centers in large metropolitan areas. This work includes providing education, guidance, and professional supervision to other cadres of health care providers.

Before you travel, conduct your own preliminary needs assessment. You can use the logic of the thinking process developed in this chapter and move through the framework as a guide. Begin, as this chapter suggests, with a review of the context. Here, you would examine the location, climate, temperatures, weather conditions, travel routes, living arrangements, languages spoken, cultural patterns, religious beliefs, and religious holidays. Locate novels and literature from the country, as this source of data is often more revealing than many of the statistical charts

and information available from official sources. Interacting with people from the country often provides valuable insights not available from reading materials. In all probability, you will find enclaves of people living in the United States from the country in which you plan to work. For example, Armenian communities are located in Watertown, Massachusetts, and Los Angeles, California. There are many Ethiopian communities in Atlanta, Georgia; New York City, New York; and Los Angeles, California. There are groups and organizations of Albanian Americans, Polish Americans, Hungarian Americans, Romanian Americans, Indian Americans, Ethiopian Americans, and Mexican Americans. These groups maintain close contact with their mother country and receive and give support to their family members and organizations in those countries.

Next, examine the population's health status, at the regional levels (e.g., Europe, Asia, Africa), the country level (e.g., Chad, Nepal, India), and at the local level (e.g., Tete Provinces and villages in Tete Provinces, Mozambique). Here, you would review the data to identify the universals of care, that is, the causes of mortality and morbidity, the level of functioning in the community, decision-making (if available), and cost of health care.

Then, move on to review evidence of the three eras of health conditions in the country and determine the age of the population and the health conditions they experience, given their history, location, and experiences with natural or man-made disasters. Look at birth rates, death rates, infant mortality rates, and maternal mortality rates, asking the following: How many infants are born? How many of these die at birth, during the first month of life, during the first year of life? How long do people live? What kills them? What makes them sick? How do people function everyday? What kinds of decisions do they have to make and how do they make them? What community supports exist to help people with these processes? What is the average income per capita? What do people buy with their money?

Review the conditions and diseases that account for the three eras of health conditions as described in this chapter and determine the prevailing health conditions that you will encounter. Review the kinds of health conditions that are reported both in the professional literature and in the popular literature and media.

Next, it's helpful to review the organization with which you will be associated. Examine its philosophy, its mission, its ways of working, its relationship to the community of interest, and the ways in which community health nurses are considered, placed, and function. Query the nature of the health care team of which you would become a member, those to whom you report, and those who would report to you. Review their scope of practice, the interventions they provide, and their ways of delivering health services.

It is helpful to identify the international governmental and NGOs working in the area and obtain their publications for review and their addresses and contact numbers (when you arrive in the area, visit these organizations and request a briefing). Review the projects currently under way, and examine their track record for the factors that suggest ill-conceived outcomes and evidence of those that produced successful outcomes.

If you are considering further education, you will find many opportunities available to you. Universities throughout North America have developed partnerships with universities, governments, and agencies in other countries. The major universities and colleges that specialize in community health most often include schools of public health and graduate programs in nursing. Harvard's School of Public Health, Johns Hopkins University, Wayne State University, Duke University, the University of Illinois, the University of Pennsylvania, to name just a few, provide scholar practitioner education to those wishing to work toward providing access to health care, develop community partnerships to ensure health care for the uninsured, and serve as researchers, teachers, practitioners, community health administrators, or health information specialists. A world of challenges and a world of opportunity and self-learning are waiting—when you are ready.

Following this review, identify and remediate gaps in your knowledge of theory and practice. Most importantly, take the time to plan and to take care of yourself and your health, as your own health status is critical to your functioning in what may be a very different context from your own.

To explore specific opportunities, contact the organization of interest (see the listing of selected organizations at the end of the chapter). Some of the larger organizations, such as the WHO, require graduate education and at least 5 years of experience, but many organizations do not. Nurses can participate in numerous smaller organizations that are involved in health programs. Among such groups seeking nurses are the U.S. Peace Corps, religious and lay organizations, and private and governmental agencies, societies, and foundations. Health Volunteers Overseas (HVO) is an example of a private, nonprofit organization that seeks to improve health care quality and access in developing countries through education. Twelve professional organizations sponsor HVO, including the American Association of Colleges of Nursing (HVO, 2011). The GHC provides information on career opportunities in global health for community health nurses and others. It also offers career seminars and provides suggestions from global health experts for nurses interested in entering the field, as well as a newsletter (GHC, 2015b). University student nurses can also contact their campus office of global affairs for opportunities available overseas (see Perspectives: Voices From the Community).

PERSPECTIVES
VOICES FROM THE COMMUNITY

You cannot build a strong country on the backs of sick people.
> —Dr. Mohammad Akhter, Executive Director,
> American Public Health Association

Nurses and midwives play a crucial and cost-effective role in reducing excess mortality, morbidity, and disability and in promotion of healthy lifestyles.
> —Dr. Gro Harlem Brundtland, former Director
> General, World Health Organization

Global health nurses always receive far more than they give.
> —Cydne, former Peace Corps nurse

The developing world may be poor materially, but it is rich in hope and spirit.
> —Edith, missionary nurse

Nurses working in foreign lands make a big difference through their training and support of local nurses and others. Their professional dedication to quality health care and promotion of healthful living among their patients, families, and communities serves as an effective role model and has a profound impact on the well-being of the people they work with.
> —Tom, physician

Living overseas for many years was a challenging and rewarding experience. Raising a family was not always easy, but our six children, now adults, value the exposure they had to other cultures and the many interesting friendships they made.
> —Inez, spouse of a global health administrator

Nurses play an important role ministering to the health care needs of not only the indigenous population but also the sometimes-sizable population of expatriates and their families.
> —Jennifer, teacher

There is nothing so powerful as seeing a community that has changed through individuals taking responsibility for themselves and their own community.
> —Lydia, volunteer PHN with Medical Ambassadors

S U M M A R Y

Community health nursing is practiced throughout the world and can be considered within a useful, worldwide framework. This framework considers first the context within which the population, the provider, and the procedures interact.

The context reflects a location's geography, history, weather, culture, religious patterns, and belief systems. This context is a critical element that community health nurses appreciate for its influences on the populations, the providers, and the interventions they are able to deliver.

Community health nurses work with populations that vary from country to country, and to serve them appropriately requires an understanding of the ways in which the context in which they are located interacts with their health status and health histories. In this regard, an examination is required to assess the universal imperatives of care, to identify the population's current health status, and to determine the focus of nursing interventions. That is, when a population is experiencing high mortality, the interventions must be targeted to that level and not, say, at the level of functioning.

Community health nurses also examine the population to assess the kinds of health conditions they experience, and the three eras are helpful guides in this assessment. These are the Era of Infectious Diseases, the Era of Chronic Long-Term Health Conditions, and the Era of Social Conditions. The three P's (population, providers, and procedures) relate to the interventions community health nurses deliver as they serve populations and are informed by the organization with which the community health nurse works. A number of international, national, and local organizations intervene in communities. Some of these agencies are intergovernmental and multilateral, such as the UN and WHO; others are bilateral, such as the USAID and the Peace Corps. Many NGOs (or PVOs) also assist with global health.

The focus remains on delivering PHC to populations throughout the world. The world's communities deliver health care in different ways, depending on their political economies. The entrepreneurial, welfare-oriented, comprehensive, and socialist systems provide for the health of their citizens in unique ways.

Variations of these systems exist, depending on whether the country is considered industrialized, transitional, or very poor. The GBD study has provided important quantifiable information about morbidity and mortality in the world, as well as disability measurements. Primary global health concerns include the eradication, elimination, or control of communicable disease, as well as immunization, maternal and perinatal morbidity and mortality, tobacco-related diseases, chronic disease, environmental illness, and malnutrition. In addition to these age-old health problems, there are new, emerging, and reemerging diseases. Armed conflicts and political upheavals also adversely affect health; this is an important consideration because of the number of major armed conflicts occurring at any given time.

Community health nursing services are critical to the ultimate health of a community. They provide important primary, secondary, and tertiary levels of care and prevention throughout the world. In the future, community health nurses will continue as major contributors to global health.

ACTIVITIES TO PROMOTE **CRITICAL THINKING**

1. What infectious diseases are most commonplace around the world? What is being done to combat them?
2. Which of the worldwide leading risk factors also impact the United States? Why? What can you, as a public health nurse, do to address these risk factors?
3. Identify a country or community in which you would like to practice community health nursing. Before you begin a review of this country or community, write down your own knowledge, attitudes, and beliefs about the country or community, the people, and the culture. Examine your own reasons for wanting this experience. Identify the way you might feel if you were the recipient rather than the donor of the services you plan to provide.
4. Conduct your own needs assessment using the framework provided in this chapter. Given what you have found, what would you prioritize as the major focus of a community nursing intervention for that community? Provide your rationale for your choices.

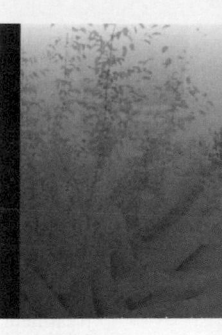

5. Given what you have found, what organizations, groups, or references would you access before you left on your assignment?

6. Based on your examination, what questions would you want to ask of the employing agency before you left on your assignment? What additional actions would you take to protect yourself and your health, given the review you conducted?

7. What sources of information appear to be most informative? What data are you seeking that are not reported? Why do you think this is the case?

REFERENCES

Adalja, A. A., Toner, E., & Inglesby, T. V. (2015). Clinical management of potential bioterrorism-related conditions. *New England Journal of Medicine, 372*(10), 954–962.

Alonso, D., Bouma, M. J., & Pascual, M. (2011). Epidemic malaria and warmer temperatures in recent decades in an East African highland. *Proceedings of the Royal Society B: Biological Sciences, 278*(1712), 1661–1669.

American Association of Colleges of Nursing. (2008). *Essentials of baccalaureate education for professional nursing practice.* Washington, DC: Author

American International Health Alliance (AIHA). (2012). *What we do.* Retrieved from http://www.aiha.com/en/WhatWeDo/

Amnesty International. (2014, October 16). *Rule by law: Discriminatory legislation and legitimized abuses in Uganda.* Retrieved from http://www.amnestyusa.org/sites/default/files/afr59062014en.pdf

Amnesty International. (2015). *Sexuality is not a crime.* Retrieved from http://www.amnestyusa.org/our-work/issues/lgbt-rights/decriminalizing-homosexuality

Amoran, O. (2013, March–April). *Impact of health education intervention on malaria prevention among nursing mothers in rural communities in Nigeria.* Retrieved from http://www.ncbi.nlm.nih.gov/pmc/articles/PMC3687863/

Anft, M. (2013, April 9). *In the wide world of global nursing, Johns Hopkins leads the conversation.* Retrieved from http://magazine.nursing.jhu.edu/2013/04/spring2013a-world-of-difference/

Baxter, A. J., Patton, G., Scott, K. M., Degenhardt, L., & Whiteford, H. A. (2013). Global epidemiology of mental disorders: What are we missing? *PLoS One, 8*(6), e65514.

Bayley, O., Chapota, H., Kainja, E., Phiri, T., Gondwe, C., King, C., … Colbourn, T. (2015). Community-linked maternal death review (CLMDR) to measure and prevent maternal mortality: A pilot study in rural Malawi. *BMJ Open, 5*(4), e007753.

Bergevin, Y., Fauveau, V., & McKinnon, B. (2015). Toward ending preventable maternal deaths by 2035. *Seminars in Reproductive Medicine, 33*(1), 23–29.

Bill & Melinda Gates Foundation. (2015). *What we do.* Retrieved from http://www.gatesfoundation.org/What-We-Do

Blanton, R. E. (2014). The changing role of medieval women. *Science, 343*(6170), 485–486.

Boston Globe. (2011, April 25). *Chernobyl disaster 25th anniversary.* Retrieved from http://www.boston.com/bigpicture/2011/04/chernobyl_disaster_25th_annive.html

Brecher, M., Chen, H., Li, Z., Banavali, N. K., Jones, S. A., Zhang, J., … Li, H. (2015). Identification and characterization of novel broad-spectrum inhibitors of the flavivirus methyltransferase. *ACS Infectious Diseases, 1*(8), 340–349.

Breslow, L. (2006). Health measurement in the third era of health. *American Journal of Public Health, 96*(1), 17–19.

Burki, T. K. (2011). Burning issues: Tackling indoor air pollution. *Lancet, 377*(9777), 1559–1560.

Carter Center. (2016). *Our mission: wage peace, fight disease, build hope. Overview.* Retrieved from http://www.cartercenter.org/about/index.html

Center for International Humanitarian Cooperation (CIHC). (n.d.). *About what we do.* Retrieved from http://www.cihc.org/whatwedo

Centers for Disease Control and Prevention (CDC). (2011). *Preliminary investigation suggests BSE-infected cow in Washington State was likely imported from Canada.* Retrieved from http://www.cdc.gov/ncidod/dvrd/bse/bse_washington_2003.htm

Centers for Disease Control and Prevention (CDC). (2014). *Our progress against polio.* Retrieved from http://www.cdc.gov/polio/progress/

Centers for Disease Control and Protection. (2015). *2014 Ebola outbreak.* Retrieved from http://www.cdc.gov/vhf/ebola/outbreaks/2014-west-africa/index.html

Centers for Disease Control and Prevention (CDC). (2015a). *Emerging infections program.* Retrieved from http://www.cdc.gov/ncezid/dpei/eip/

Centers for Disease Control and Prevention (CDC). (2015b). *Global health—Global immunization.* Retrieved from http://www.cdc.gov/globalhealth/immunization/

Centers for Disease Control and Prevention (CDC). (2015c). *Global water, sanitation, & hygiene (WASH): Global diarrhea burden.* Retrieved from http://www.cdc.gov/healthywater/global/diarrhea-burden.html

Centers for Disease Control and Prevention (CDC). (2015d). *West Nile virus activity in the United States, 2003.* Retrieved from http://www.cdc.gov/ncidod/dvbid/westnile/surv&controlCaseCount03_detailed.htm

Centers for Disease Control and Prevention (CDC). (2015e). *West Nile virus: Final cumulative maps and data for 1999-2014.* Retrieved from http://www.cdc.gov/westnile/statsmaps/cummapsdata.html

Centers for Disease Control and Prevention (CDC). (2015f). *West Nile virus: Virus history and distribution.* Retrieved from http://www.cdc.gov/ncidod/dvbid/westnile/background.htm

Centers for Disease Control and Prevention (CDC). (2016). *Zika-affected areas.* Retrieved from http://www.cdc.gov/zika/geo/index.html

Cooperative for American Remittances to Europe (CARE). (2016). *Our work: Where we work.* Retrieved from http://www.care.org/work

Critchlow, A. (2015, April 24). *Middle East civil war is now the biggest threat to the economy.* Retrieved from http://www.telegraph.co.uk/finance/newsbysector/energy/oilandgas/11561344/Instability-in-the-Middle-East-is-now-the-biggest-threat-to-the-economy.html

Das, J., Holla, A., Das, V., Mohanban, M., Tabak, D., & Chan, B. (2012). In urban and rural India, a standardized patient study showed low levels of provider training and huge quality gaps. *Health Affairs, 31*(12), 2774–2784.

Davies, S. E. (2012). The challenge to know and control: Disease outbreaks surveillance and alerts in China and India. *Global Public Health, 7*(7), 695–716.

Davis, K., Stremikis, K., Squires, D., & Schoen, C. (2014). *Mirror, mirror on the wall, 2014 update: How the U.S. health care system compares internationally.* Retrieved from http://www.commonwealthfund.org/~/media/files/publications/fund-report/2014/jun/1755_davis_mirror_mirror_2014.pdf

Doocy, S., Lyles, E., Akhu-Zaheya, L., Burton, A., & Weiss, W. (2016). Health service utilization and access to medicines among Syrian refugee children in Jordan. *International Journal of Health Planning and Management, 31*(1), 97–112. doi: 10.1002/hpm.2336.

Eishinnawi, M. (2011, June 7). *Egyptian Americans help post-revolution Egypt. Voice of America: North Africa.* Retrieved from http://www.voanews.com/english/news/africa/north/How-do-Egyptian-Americans-help-post-revolution-Egypt-123369318.html

Farrell, M., Harkless, G., Orzack, L. H., Houd, S., Oakley, A., & Socenyi, C. (1994). Hungarian midwives and their practice: A national survey. *Midwifery, 10*, 67–72.

Foucault, M. (1965). *Madness and civilization: A history of insanity in the age of reason.* New York, NY: Vintage.

Freire, P. (1970). *Pedagogy of the oppressed.* New York, NY: Continuum Publishing Company.

Friedman, T. L. (2005). *The world is flat: A brief history of the 21st century.* New York, NY: Farrar, Straus & Giroux.

Fuhrmeister, E. R., Schwab, K. J., & Julian, T. R. (2015). Estimates of nitrogen, phosphorus, biochemical oxygen demand, and fecal coliforms entering the environment due to inadequate sanitation treatment technologies in 108 low and middle income countries. *Environmental Science and Technology, 49*(19), 11604–11611.

Gallimore, R. B. (2008). Militarism, ethnicity, and sexual violence in the Rwandan genocide. *Feminist Africa, 10*, 9–25.

Global Alert and Response. (2010). *Scientific review of variola virus research, 1999–2010.* Retrieved from http://whqlibdoc.who.int/hq/2010/WHO_HSE_GAR_BDP_2010.3_eng.pdf

Global Burden of Disease Pediatrics Collaboration. (2016). Global and national burden of diseases and injuries among children and adolescents between 1990 and 2013: Findings from the Global Burden of Disease 2013 study. *JAMA Pediatrics, 170*(3), 267–287.

Global Burden of Disease Study 2013 Collaborators. (2015). Global, regional, and national incidence, prevalence, and years lived with disability for 301 acute and chronic disease and injuries in 188 countries, 1990–2013: A systematic analysis for the Global Burden of Disease Study 2013. *Lancet, 386*(9995), 743–800.

Global Health Council (GHC). (2015a). *About us.* Retrieved from http://globalhealth.org/about-us/mission-and-vision/

Global Health Council (GHC). (2015b). *Connections & coordination.* Retrieved from http://globalhealth.org/what-we-do/connections-coordination/

Global Polio Eradication Initiative. (2016). *Wild poliovirus cases, previous 6 months.* Retrieved from http://www.polioeradication.org/Dataandmonitoring/Poliothisweek/Poliocasesworldwide.aspx

Goldin, I., Cameron, G., & Balarajan, M. (2011). *Exceptional people: How migration shaped our world and will define our future.* Princeton, NJ: Princeton University Press.

Haregu, T. N., Steswe, G., Elliott, J., & Oldenburg, B. (2014). National responses to HIV/AIDS and non-communicable disease in developing countries: Analysis of strategic parallels and differences. *Journal of Public Health Research, 3*(1), 99.

Health Volunteers Overseas (HVO). (2011). *Improving global health through education.* Retrieved from http://www.hvousa.org/

Heffernan, O. (2013, December 13). Earth's ozone on bumpy road to recovery. *National Geographic.* Retrieved from http://news.nationalgeographic.com/news/2013/12/131212-ozone-hole-antarctica-recovery-2070/

Hirpa, S., Medhin, G., Girma, B., Melese, M., Mekonen, A., Suarez, P., & Ameni, G. (2013). Determinants of multidrug-resistant tuberculosis in patients who underwent first-line treatment in Addis Ababa: A case control study. *BMC Public Health, 28*(13), 782.

Husted, H., Lunn, T., Troelsen, A., Gaarn-Larsen, L., Kristensen, B., & Kehlet, H. (2011). Why still in hospital after fast-track hip and knee arthroplasty? *Acta Orthopaedica, 82*(6), 679–684.

Illyes, G. (1979). *People of the Puszta.* Budapest, Hungary: Franklin Printing House.

International Centre for Human Resources in Nursing (ICHRN). (2008). *An ageing nursing workforce.* Retrieved from http://www.icn.ch/images/stories/documents/publications/fact_sheets/2a_FS-Ageing_Workforce.pdf

International Council of Nurses (ICN). (2014). *Members.* Retrieved from http://www.icn.ch/members/members/

Kaiser Family Foundation. (2014, December 8). *The U.S. government and global emerging infectious disease preparedness and response.* Retrieved from http://kff.org/global-health-policy/fact-sheet/the-u-s-government-global-emerging-infectious-disease-preparedness-and-response/

Kash, J. C., Walters, K. A., Davis, A. S., Sandouk, A., Schwartzman, L. M., Jagger, B. W., … Taubenberger, J. K. (2011). Lethal synergism of 2009 pandemic H1N1 influenza virus and Streptococcus pneumonia coinfection is associated with loss of murine lung repair responses. *mBio, 2*(5), e00172-11.

Kincaid, M. M. (2012, July 13). *Health policy brief: Assistance for global HIV/AIDS.* Retrieved from http://healthaffairs.org/healthpolicybriefs/brief_pdfs/healthpolicybrief_71.pdf

Kirk, G., & Okazawa-Rey, M. (2013). *Women's lives: Multicultural perspectives* (6th ed.). New York, NY: McGraw-Hill.

Kleinpell, R., Sanlon, A., Hibbert, D., Ganz, F. D., East, L., Fraser, D., … Beauchesne, M. (2014). Addressing issues impacting advanced nursing practice worldwide. *Online Journal of Issues in Nursing, 19*(2), Manuscript 5.

Knox, R. (2013, November 26). *2009 flu pandemic was 10 times more deadly than previously thought.* Retrieved from http://www.npr.org/sections/health-shots/2013/11/26/247379604/2009-flu-pandemic-was-10-times-more-deadly-than-previously-thought

Kray, L. J., Locke, C. C., & Van Zant, A. B. (2012). Feminine charm: An experimental analysis of its costs and benefits in negotiations. *Personal and Social Psychology Bulletin, 38*(10), 1343–1357.

Kremer, M., Leino, J., Miguel, E., & Zwane, A. P. (2011). Spring cleaning: Rural water impacts, valuation, and property rights institutions. *Quarterly Journal of Economics, 126*(1), 145–205.

Kumar, S., Roy, R., & Dutta, S. (2015). Scaling-up public sector childhood diarrhea management programs: Lessons from Indian states of Gujarat, Uttar Pradesh and Bihar. *Journal of Global Health, 5*(2). doi: 10.7189/jogh.05.020414.

Levy, B. S., & Sidel, V. W. (2013). Adverse health consequences of the Iraq War. *Lancet, 381*(9870), 949–958.

Levy, B. S., & Sidel, V. W. (2015). Adverse health consequences of the Vietnam War. *Medicine, Conflict, and Survival, 31*(3–4), 162–170.

Li, H., Nie, W., & Li, J. (2014). The benefits and caveats of international nurse migration. *International Journal of Nursing Sciences, 1*(3), 314–317.

Liebert, S., Condrey, S. E., & Goncharov, D. (Eds.). (2013). *Public administration in post-communist countries: Former Soviet Union, Central and Eastern Europe, and Mongolia.* Boca Raton, FL: CRC Press.

Litz, B., & Orsillo, S. M. (2015). The returning veteran of the Iraq war: Background issues and assessment guidelines. In National Center for Post-Traumatic Stress Disorder (Ed.), *Iraq War clinician's guide* (2nd ed., pp. 21–32). Washington, DC: Department of Veteran's Affairs.

Lohman, D. (2015, April 29). *Venezuela's health care crisis.* Retrieved from https://www.hrw.org/news/2015/04/29/venezuelas-health-care-crisis

Maxwell, N. I. (2014). *Understanding environmental health: How we live in the world* (2nd ed.). Sudbury, MA: Jones & Bartlett.

Mackenzie, J. S., Drury, P., Arthur, R. R., Ryan, M. J., Grein, T., Slattery, R., … Bejtullahu, A. (2014). The global outbreak alert and response network. *Global Public Health, 9*(9), 1023–1039.

MacQueen, N. (2014). *Colonialism: A short history of a big idea.* New York, NY: Routledge.

Martínez-González, N. A., Djalali, S., Tandjung, R., Huber-Geismann, F., Markun, S., Wensing, M., & Rosemann, T. (2014). *Substitution of physicians by nurses in primary care: A systematic review and meta-analysis.* Retrieved from http://www.biomedcentral.com/1472-6963/14/214

Me Arabi, A., Ibrahim, S. A., Ahmed, S. E., MacGinnea, F., Hawkes, G., Dempsey, E., & Anthony Ryan, C. (2016). Skills retention in Sudanese village midwives 1 year following Helping Babies Breathe training. *Archives of Disease in Childhood, 101*(5), 439–442. doi: 10.1136/archdischild-2015-309190.

Moser, L. A., Lim, P. Y., Styer, L. M., Kramer, L. D., & Bernard, K. A. (2015). Parameters of mosquito-enhanced West Nile virus infection. *Journal of Virology, 90*(1), 292–299.

Nair, H., Simoes, E., Rudan, I., Gessner, B. D., Azziz-Baumgartner, E., Zhang, J., … Campbell, H. (2013). Global and regional burden of hospital admissions for severe acute lower respiratory infections in young children in 2010: A systematic analysis. *Lancet, 381*(9875), 1380–1390.

National Archives and Records Administration. (n.d.). *The deadly virus: The influenza epidemic of 1918.* Retrieved from http://www.archives.gov/exhibits/influenza-epidemic/

National Geographic Daily News. (2011, March 15). *Japan tsunami: 20 unforgettable pictures.* Retrieved from http://news.nationalgeographic.com/news/2011/03/pictures/110315-nuclear-reactor-japan-tsunami-earthquake-world-photos-meltdown/

Nichols, R. W. (2011). Moving USAID forward. *Science, 9*, 1381. doi: 10.1126/science.333.6048.1381-a.

Ng'ang'a, N., & Byrne, M. V. V. (2015). Professional practice models for nurses in low-income countries: An integrative review. *BCM Nursing, 14*, 44. doi: 10.1186/s12912-015-0095-5.

Ostrand, N. (2015). The Syrian refugee crisis: A comparison of responses by Germany, Sweden, the United Kingdom, and the United States. *Journal of Migration and Human Security, 3,* 255–279.

Ozone Hole. (n.d.). *Montreal Protocol on ozone-depleting substances effective, but work still unfinished says secretary general in message for International Day.* Retrieved from http://www.theozonehole.com/ozoneday2006.htm

Parker, C. (2014, June 23). *Changing world temperatures influence views on global warming Stanford scholar says.* Retrieved from http://news.stanford.edu/news/2014/june/climate-change-opinions-061914.html

PATH. (2015, June). *Protecting children from diarrheal diseases.* Retrieved from http://www.path.org/publications/files/GE_dd_fs_2015.pdf

Perry, H., & Zulliger, R. (2012). *How effective are community health workers? An overview of current evidence with recommendations for strengthening community health worker programs to accelerate progress in achieving the health-related Millennium Development Goals.* Retrieved from http://www.coregroup.org/storage/Program_Learning/Community_Health_Workers/review%20of%20chw%20effectiveness%20for%20mdgs-sept2012.pdf

Pinto, A. D., Cole, D. C., ter Kuile, A., Forman, L., Rouleau, K., Philpott, J., …, Muntaner, C. (2014). A case study of global health at the university: Implications for research and action. *Global Health Action, 7,* 24526.

Raab, M., & Rocha, J. (2011). *Campaigns to end violence against women and girls.* Retrieved from http://www.endvawnow.org/uploads/modules/pdf/1342724232.pdf

Rehydration Project. (2016). *What is diarrhea and how to prevent it.* Retrieved from http://rehydrate.org/diarrhoea/#65

ReliefWeb. (2011). *Armenia, USSR earthquake. 1988 UNDRO situation reports 1-14.* Retrieved from http://reliefweb.int/node/34437

Remington, P. L., & Brownson, R. C. (2011, October 7). Fifty years of progress in chronic disease epidemiology and control. *Morbidity and Mortality Weekly Report, 60*(4), 70–77.

Ringdal, G. I., & Ringdal, K. (2016). War experiences and general health among people in Bosnia-Herzegovina and Kosovo. *Journal of Traumatic Stress, 29*(1), 49–55.

Roemer, M. I. (1993). *National health systems of the world (Vols. I & II).* New York, NY: Oxford University Press.

Rosato, M., Malamba, F., Kuinyenge, B., Phiri, T., Mwansambo, C., Kazembe, P., Costello, A., & Lewycka, S. (2012). Strategies developed and implemented by women's groups to improve mother and infant health and reduce mortality in rural Malawi. *International Health, 4*(3), 176–184.

Sandall, J., Soltani, H., Gates, S., Shennan, A., & Devane, D. (2015, September 15). *Midwife-led continuity models versus other models of care for childbearing women.* Retrieved from http://onlinelibrary.wiley.com/doi/10.1002/14651858.CD004667.pub4/abstract

Schaffer Library of Drug Policy. (2011). *Worldwide trends in tobacco consumption and mortality.* Retrieved from http://druglibrary.net/schaffer/tobacco/who-tobacco.htm

Shah, R., Mullany, L. C., Darmstadt, G. L., Talukder, R. R., Rahman, S. M., Mannan, I., … ProjAHNMo Study Group in Bangladesh. (2014). Determinants and pattern of care seeking for preterm newborns in a rural Bangladeshi cohort. *BMC Health Services Research, 14,* 417.

Sharara, W. L., & Kanj, S. S. (2014). War and infectious diseases: Challenges of the Syrian civil war. *PLoS Pathogens, 10*(11), e1004438.

Sheridan, K. (2011, October 13). *Indoor cooking stoves kill 2 million yearly: Study.* Retrieved from http://www.google.com/hostednews/afp/article/ALeqM5ie2kolKAgQ65-FeWVnnWa9xNsr6A?docId=CNG.a3ab38cb5db8b5323b644de0172e361a.2b1

Shi, L., & Singh, D. A. (2016). *Essentials of the U.S. health care system* (4th ed.). Burlington, MA: Jones & Bartlett Learning.

Shimmon, S. A. (2011). *Treatment of the insane in modern Great Britain: A ship of fools.* Retrieved from http://www1.umassd.edu/euro/2011papers/shimmon.pdf

Smith, D. (2012, December 3). *AIDS drugs increase South African life expectancy by five years.* Retrieved from http://www.theguardian.com/world/2012/dec/03/aids-drugs-south-african-life

Spector, R. E. (2013). *Cultural diversity in health and illness* (8th ed.). Upper Saddle River, NJ: Pearson.

Steel, Z., Marnane, C., Iranpour, C., Chey, T., Jackson, J. W., Patel, V., & Silove, D. (2014). The global prevalence of common mental disorders: A systematic review and meta-analysis 1980–2013. *International Journal of Epidemiology, 43*(2), 476–493.

Takepart. (n.d.). *An inconvenient truth: About the film.* Retrieved from http://www.takepart.com/an-inconvenient-truth/film

Themnér, L., & Wallensteen, P. (2013). Armed conflict, 1946–2012. *Journal of Peace Research, 50*(4), 509–521.

Tribble, S. J. (2011, June 13). *East Cleveland's Huron Hospital closing despite best efforts of its longtime advocate.* Retrieved from http://www.cleveland.com/medical/index.ssf/2011/06/huron_hospital_closing_despite.html

Tupas, J. (2015, October 12). *In southern Philippines, victims are getting younger.* Retrieved from http://www.ucanews.com/news/in-southern-philippines-victims-of-prostitution-are-getting-younger/74404

Turley, R., Saith, R., Bhan, N., Rehfuess, E., & Carter, B. (2013). Slum upgrading strategies involving physical environment and infrastructure interventions and their effects on health and socio-economic outcomes. *Cochrane Database of Systematic Reviews, 2013*(1). doi: 10.1002/14651858.CD010067.pub2.

UNICEF. (2014, December). *Immunization: Keeping children alive and healthy.* Retrieved from http://www.unicef.org/immunization/files/Immunization_brochure.pdf

United Nations Department of Economic Affairs, Population Division. (2013). *International migration 2013.* Retrieved from http://www.un.org/en/development/desa/population/migration/publications/wallchart/docs/wallchart2013.pdf

United Nations, Department of Economic and Social Affairs, Population Division. (2015, July 29). *World population prospects: The 2015 revision.* Retrieved from http://esa.un.org/unpd/wpp/

United Nations High Commissioner for Refugees. (2010). *Public health equity in refugee and other displaced persons settings.* Retrieved from http://www.unhcr.org/cgi-bin/texis/vtx/home/opendocPDFViewer.html?docid=4bdfe1699&query=refugee%20health

U.S. Department of Health and Human Services (USDHHS). (2015). *Lesbian, gay, bisexual, and transgender health.* Retrieved from http://www.globalhealth.gov/global-health-topics/lgbt/index.html

U.S. Department of Health and Human Services (USDHHS). (2016). *About healthy people 2020.* http://www.healthypeople.gov/2020/About-Healthy-People

Waddington, R. (2008). Portugal's rapid progress through primary health care. *Bulletin of the World Health Organization, 86*(11), 817–908.

Weaver, E. H., Frankenberg, E., Fried, B. J., Thomas, D., Wheeler, S. B., & Paul, J. E. (2013). Effect of village midwife program on contraceptive prevalence and method choice in Indonesia. *Studies in Family Planning, 44*(4), 389–409.

World Bank (WB). (2014, September 16). *Newer data show mortality rates falling faster than ever.* Retrieved from http://www.worldbank.org/en/news/press-release/2014/09/16/new-data-child-mortality-rates-falling-faster

World Bank Group. (2016). *What we do.* Retrieved from http://www.worldbank.org/en/about/what-we-do

World Health Organization (WHO). (2011). *WHO public health & environmental global strategy.* Retrieved from http://www.who.int/phe/publications/PHE_2011_global_strategy_overview_2011.pdf?ua=1

World Health Organization (WHO). (2012). *Health for all: Focus on need for equity in reaching RMNCH goals.* Retrieved from http://www.who.int/pmnch/media/news/2012/201201_innocenti_centre/en/

World Health Organization (WHO). (2013a, May 14). *Improving the health and well-being of lesbian, gay, bisexual, and transgender persons.* Retrieved from http://www.ghwatch.org/sites/www.ghwatch.org/files/B133-6_LGBT.pdf

World Health Organization (WHO). (2013b). *Moving toward health in all policies: A compilation of experience from Africa, Southeast Asia, and the Western Pacific.* Retrieved from http://apps.who.int/iris/bitstream/10665/105528/1/9789241506595_eng.pdf?ua=1&ua=1

World Health Organization (WHO). (2013c). *Multidrug-resistant tuberculosis (MDR-TB): 2013 update.* Retrieved from http://www.who.int/tb/challenges/mdr/MDR_TB_FactSheet.pdf

World Health Organization (WHO). (2013d). *Transforming and scaling up health professionals' education and training: WHO guidelines 2013.* Retrieved from http://whoeducationguidelines.org./sites/default/files/uploads/WHO_EduGuidelines_20131202_web.pdf

World Health Organization (WHO). (2014a). *Collaborating centres: Fact sheet.* Retrieved from http://www.who.int/collaboratingcentres/Factsheet_WHO_CC_2014_English1.pdf?ua=1&ua=1

World Health Organization (WHO). (2014b). *ICMI chartbook.* Retrieved from http://www.who.int/maternal_child_adolescent/documents/IMCI_chartbooklet/en/

World Health Organization (WHO). (2015a). *Environmental context and health implications*. Retrieved from http://www.who.int/gho/publications/mdgs-sdgs/MDGs-SDGs2015_chapter2.pdf?ua=1

World Health Organization (WHO). (2015b). *Malaria vaccine development*. Retrieved from http://www.who.int/malaria/areas/vaccine/en/

World Health Organization (WHO). (2016a). *About WHO: Leadership priorities*. Retrieved from http://www.who.int/about/agenda/en/index.html

World Health Organization (WHO). (2016b). *Control, elimination, eradication, and re-emergence of infectious diseases: Getting the message right*. Retrieved from http://www.who.int/bulletin/volumes/84/2/editorial10206html/en/

World Health Organization (WHO). (2016c). *Deliver now for women + children*. Retrieved from http://www.who.int/pmnch/activities/delivernow/en/

World Health Organization (WHO). (2016d). *GAVI—The Global Alliance for Vaccines and Immunizations*. Retrieved from http://www.who.int/workforcealliance/members_partners/member_list/gavi/en/

World Health Organization (WHO). (2016e). *Global health observatory data: Child health*. Retrieved from http://www.who.int/gho/child_health/en/

World Health Organization (WHO). (2016f). *Health statistics and information systems: Estimates for 2000–2012*. Retrieved from http://www.who.int/healthinfo/global_burden_disease/estimates/en/index2.html

World Health Organization (WHO). (2016g). *Health topics: Global burden of disease*. Retrieved from http://www.who.int/topics/global_burden_of_disease/en/

World Health Organization (WHO). (2016h). *History of WHO*. Retrieved from http://www.who.int/about/history/en/index.html

World Health Organization (WHO). (2016i). *Jakarta Declaration on leading health promotion into the 21st century*. Retrieved from http://www.who.int/healthpromotion/conferences/previous/jakarta/declaration/en/

World Health Organization (WHO). (2016j). *Metrics: Disability-adjusted life year (DALY)*. Retrieved from http://www.who.int/healthinfo/global_burden_disease/metrics_daly/en/

World Health Organization (WHO). (2016k). *Priority eye diseases: Onchocerciasis (river blindness)*. Retrieved from http://www.who.int/blindness/causes/priority/en/index3.html

World Health Organization (WHO). (2016l). *Programmes and projects*. Retrieved from http://www.who.int/entity/en/

World Health Organization (WHO). (2016m). *Regional consultation on targets and indicators for Health 2020 monitoring: Report of results*. Retrieved from http://www.euro.who.int/en/data-and-evidence/equity-in-health-project/inequalities-in-health-system-performance-and-their-social-determinants-in-europe/regional-consultation-on-targets-and-indicators-for-health-2020-monitoring-report-of-results

World Health Organization (WHO). (2016n). *Strengthening health security by implementing the International Health Regulations (2005)*. Retrieved from http://www.who.int/ihr/about/en/

World Health Organization (WHO). (2016o). *The Ottawa Charter for Health Promotion*. Retrieved from http://www.who.int/healthpromotion/conferences/previous/ottawa/en/index.html

World Health Organization (WHO). (2016p). *Trade, foreign policy, diplomacy and health: Emerging diseases*. Retrieved from http://www.who.int/trade/glossary/story022/en/index.html

World Health Organization (WHO). (2016q). *What we do*. Retrieved from http://www.who.int/about/what-we-do/en/

World Health Organization (WHO). (2016r). *WHO called to return to the Declaration of Alma-Ata*. Retrieved from http://www.who.int/social_determinants/tools/multimedia/alma_ata/en/

World Health Organization (WHO). (2016s). *WHO regional offices*. Retrieved from http://www.who.int/about/regions/en/

World Health Organization (WHO) Media Centre. (2010). *Anniversary of smallpox eradication*. Retrieved from http://www.who.int/mediacentre/multimedia/podcasts/2010/smallpox_20100618/en/

World Health Organization (WHO) Media Centre. (2011). *West Nile virus: Fact sheet No. 354*. Retrieved from http://www.who.int/mediacentre/factsheets/fs354/en/

World Health Organization (WHO) Media Centre. (2013, April). *Diarrhoeal disease*. Retrieved from Media Center: http://www.who.int/mediacentre/factsheets/fs330/en/

World Health Organization (WHO) Media Centre. (2015a, November). *HIV/AIDS: Fact sheet No. 360*. Retrieved from http://www.who.int/mediacentre/factsheets/fs360/en/

World Health Organization (WHO) Media Centre. (2015b, May). *Leprosy: Fact sheet No. 101*. Retrieved from http://www.who.int/mediacentre/factsheets/fs101/en/

World Health Organization (WHO) Media Centre. (2015c, November 12). *Maternal deaths fell 44% since 1990*. Retrieved from http://www.who.int/mediacentre/news/releases/2015/maternal-mortality/en/

World Health Organization (WHO) Media Centre. (2015d, November). *Measles: Fact sheet No. 286*. Retrieved from http://www.who.int/mediacentre/factsheets/fs286/en/

World Health Organization (WHO) Media Centre. (2015e, November). *Maternal mortality. Fact sheet No. 348*. Retrieved from http://www.who.int/mediacentre/factsheets/fs348/en/

World Health Organization (WHO) Media Centre. (2015f, December 9). *New report signals country progress in the path to malarias elimination*. Retrieved from http://www.who.int/mediacentre/news/releases/2015/report-malaria-elimination/en/

World Health Organization (WHO) Media Centre. (2015g, July). *Tobacco: Fact sheet No. 339*. Retrieved from http://www.who.int/mediacentre/factsheets/fs339/en/index.html

World Health Organization (WHO) Media Centre. (2015h, October). *Tuberculosis: Fact sheet No. 104*. Retrieved from http://www.who.int/mediacentre/factsheets/fs104/en/

World Health Organization (WHO) Media Centre. (2015i). *Malaria: Fact sheet*. Retrieved from http://www.who.int/mediacentre/factsheets/fs094/en/

World Health Organization (WHO) Media Centre. (2016a). *The top 10 causes of death*. Retrieved from http://www.who.int/mediacentre/factsheets/fs310/en/index1.html

World Health Organization (WHO) Media Centre. (2016b). *World Health Assembly*. Retrieved from http://www.who.int/mediacentre/events/governance/wha/en/

Xu, H., Zhang, W., Gu, L., Qu, Z., Sa, Z., Zhang, X., & Tian, D. (2014). Aging village doctors in five countries in rural China: Situation and implications. *Human Resources for Health, 12*(36). doi: 10.1186/1478-4491-12-36.

Yach, D., Mensah, G., Hawkes, C., Epping-Jordan, J., & Steyn, K. (2012). Chronic diseases and risks. In M. H. Merson, R. E. Black, & A. J. Mills (Eds.), *Global health: Diseases, programs, systems, and policies* (3rd ed.). Sudbury, MA: Jones & Bartlett Learning.

thePoint: Everything You Need to Make the Grade!

thePoint® Visit http://thePoint.lww.com/Rector9e
for selected readings, study aids for all learning styles, and more!

Being Prepared: Impact of Disaster, Terrorism, and War

"In this dangerous world that we live in, where hatred and violence and natural disasters sometimes collide to almost overwhelm us, we each can help in some way."

—**Marsha Blackburn** (1952), American Politician

"I have an almost complete disregard of precedent, and a faith in the possibility of something better. It irritates me to be told how things have always been done. I defy the tyranny of precedent. I go for anything new that might improve the past."

—**Clara Barton,** Nurse Founder of the American Red Cross

KEY TERMS

Biologic warfare
Casualty
Chemical warfare
Complex emergency
Crisis intervention
Critical incident stress
  debriefing (CISD)
Directly impacted by disaster

Disaster
Disaster planning
Displaced persons
Incident command system
Indirectly impacted by
  disaster
Intensity
Man-made disaster

Mass-casualty incident
Moulage
Natural disaster
Nuclear warfare
Posttraumatic stress disorder
  (PTSD)
Refugee
Resilience

Scope
Shelter in place
Terrorism
Triage

LEARNING OBJECTIVES

Upon mastery of this chapter, you should be able to:

- Describe a variety of characteristics of disasters, including causation, number of casualties, scope, and intensity.
- Discuss a variety of factors contributing to a community's potential for experiencing a disaster.
- Identify the four phases of disaster management.
- Describe factors involved in disaster planning.
- Describe the role of the community health nurse in preventing, preparing for, responding to, and supporting recovery from disasters.
- Use the levels of prevention to describe the role of the community health nurse in relation to acts of chemical, biologic, or nuclear terrorism.

What would you do if your local news station broadcasts an announcement that your community was directly in the path of a hurricane that earlier in the day had caused extensive damage and loss of life in a neighboring state? What would you do if you were shopping at a local mall, suddenly heard an explosive noise followed by shouts and cries for help, and then noticed that a pungent odor was filling the air? In March of 2011, were you glued to your television watching live coverage of the earthquake and tsunami in Japan? When you hear news of riots and the civil war in Syria or other violence in the Middle East and bombings in Belgium or terrorist attacks in Paris or San Bernardino, do you think of it as a disaster? Even today, the impact of the 2005 hurricanes Katrina and Rita on the Gulf Coast continues to affect the lives of the residents of those communities devastated by the storms. This is also true for residents of New Jersey after Hurricane/Superstorm Sandy in 2012. As distant as some of these scenarios might seem from your own life, natural disasters and terrorism are ever-present possibilities, and nurses and other health care professionals have an obligation to respond appropriately. This chapter increases your understanding of the community health nurse's role in preparing for, responding to, and recovering from natural disasters and terrorism.

DISASTERS

A **disaster** is any natural or man-made event that causes a level of destruction or emotional trauma exceeding the abilities of those affected to respond without community assistance. The crash of a private plane over the Pacific Ocean in which no bodies are recovered and no environmental impact is felt is not a disaster by this definition, because no specific community-based response is required or even possible. Such a tragedy may, however, be felt for a lifetime by family members and friends who need emotional support and possibly long-term financial assistance. If a plane with 150 passengers crashes over land, destroying several homes in its path, the community affected is unable to cope with the resulting injuries, deaths, and property destruction without assistance; by the definition used here, this constitutes a disaster.

The geographic distribution of disasters varies because certain types of disasters are more common in some parts of the world. For example, California, Alaska, and Tennessee are associated with earthquakes and the Gulf Coast with hurricanes and oil spills. Similarly, it is not surprising to hear of drought in Ethiopia, floods in India during the monsoon season, or bombings in Afghanistan. When certain types of disasters are anticipated, communities are usually more prepared for them. For instance, California has strict building codes to prevent destruction of structures in the event of earthquakes, but most California homes lack the basements and insulation that characterize homes in Iowa and Oklahoma that are often visited by tornados or severe winter storms. Similarly, residents of Germany, Austria, and Russia are better prepared for blizzards than for heavy rain, which explains in part the devastation caused in some communities by floods there in 2002.

Because the local media in the United States do not typically report on disasters unless there are mass casualties, one may be unaware of the frequency and variety of both natural and technologic disasters worldwide. Here is a brief sampling of major disasters that occurred from 2007 to 2016 (Chuck & Kwong, 2015; Infoplease, 2008, 2009, 2012; International Charter, 2008; Littleton, Axsom, & Grills-Taquechel, 2009; Press Information Bureau, Government of India, 2008):

April 2007
- *Virginia*: Worst mass shooting in U.S. history at Virginia Tech University ended with 33 dead and 17 seriously wounded.

August 2007
- *Minnesota*. An eight-lane interstate bridge packed with cars broke into sections and collapsed into the Mississippi River, killing at least nine and injuring at least 60.

October 2007
- *California*: Wildfires burned more than 516,000 acres in Southern California. Seven died, and nearly ninety people were injured. Over 500,000 people were forced to evacuate their homes; 2,000 homes were destroyed.

November 2007
- *Bangladesh*: Cyclone killed nearly 3,500 people in southern Bangladesh; millions of people were left homeless.

January 2008
- *Kenya*: After an election, violent riots between tribes killed 300 people, and thousands of houses, farms, and businesses were burned.

February 2008
- *U.S. South*: Violent tornados struck Kentucky, Tennessee, Alabama, Mississippi, and Arkansas with little warning, resulting in 54 deaths and hundreds of injured, with widespread damage reported.

May 2008
- *China*: Earthquake struck eastern Sichuan, northwest of Chengdu. The tremor was felt throughout the region, with the death toll exceeding 65,000.

November 2008
- *India*: Terrorists attacked Mumbai with 10 coordinated bombings and attacks across the city. Terrorists killed 164 people and wounded over 300.

April 2009

- *International:* H1N1, also known as Swine Flu, outbreaks in more than 70 countries. CDC (2009) reported between April and October that 22 million Americans had contracted the virus, 98,000 required hospitalization, and about 3,900 people died from H1N1-related causes.

January 2010

- *Haiti:* Earthquake struck Port-au-Prince, Haiti. The tremor was felt throughout the region, with the death toll exceeding 222,570.

March 2011

- *Japan:* Earthquake and tsunami struck Pacific coastal areas of northeastern Japan. Estimates of over 9,000 dead and 18,000 missing.

October 2012

- *Hurricane Sandy:* Struck the east coast, killing 132 people and causing an estimated $82 billion dollars in damages to New York, New Jersey, and Connecticut.

December 2012

- *Newtown, Connecticut:* Sandy Hook Elementary School shooting, 26 people killed, including 20 children between the ages of six and seven. The lone gunman shot his mother prior to the school shooting.
- *U.S. Nationwide:* Meningitis outbreak traced back to contaminated steroid medication shipped to 23 states killed 36; 500 cases reported.

July 2012

- *Aurora, Colorado:* Mass shooting at a movie theater, 12 killed, 58 wounded. Lone gunman sentenced to life in prison after unsuccessful insanity defense.

March 2014

- *West Africa:* The largest outbreak of Ebola in history, with multiple countries affected (Liberia, Sierra Leone, and Guinea).

August to October 2015

- *Washington:* Wildfires and mudslides in the state of Washington killed three firefighters and damaged or destroyed hundreds of homes.

October 2015

- *United States:* Severe storms cause serious flooding in North and South Carolina, leading to 25 deaths and billions of dollars in property damage. Just prior to this, severe flooding in Kansas, Oklahoma, and Texas was responsible for 43 deaths and much destruction.

November 2015

- *Paris, France:* A coordinated, multisite terrorist attack kills 130 people and injures over 350 people. Earlier, in January, terrorists attacked offices of a magazine and a Jewish market, killing 17.

January 2016

- *United States:* Blizzard affected the northeast, mid-Atlantic, and southeast sections of the United States, killing 38 people.

March 2016

- *Belgium:* Coordinated terrorist attacks at the airport and metro system killed 35 and injured over 250 people.

Characteristics of Disasters

Disasters are often characterized by their cause. A **natural disaster** is caused by natural events, such as the earthquake and tsunami in Japan in 2011. A **man-made disaster** is caused by human activity, such as the 2008 shootings at Virginia Tech, the bombing of the World Trade Center in New York City in 2001, the displacement of thousands of Kosovars during their war with Serbia in 1999, or the riots in Kenya in 2008. Other man-made disasters include nuclear reactor meltdowns, industrial accidents, oil spills, construction accidents, and air, train, bus, and subway crashes. In fact, man-made disasters can and frequently do follow natural disasters, as occurred with the nuclear reactors in Japan following the earthquake and tsunami in 2011. A **complex emergency** is a multifaceted "humanitarian crisis in a country, region or society where there is a total or considerable breakdown of authority resulting from internal or external conflict and which requires a multi-sectorial, international response" (United Nations Inter-Agency Standing Committee, 2008, p. 9). Complex humanitarian emergencies disproportionately impact women and children.

A **casualty** is a human being who is injured or killed by, or as a direct result of, an accident or natural disaster. Although major disasters sometimes occur without any injury or loss of life, the number of casualties involved increases the likelihood of wider news coverage. If casualties number more than two people but fewer than 100, the disaster is characterized as a *multiple-casualty incident*. Although multiple-casualty incidents may strain the health care systems of small or midsized communities, a **mass-casualty incident**—often involving many casualties—can completely overwhelm the resources of even large cities. Preparedness for mass-casualty incidents is essential for all communities.

The possibility of being prepared is another characteristic that varies with different types of disasters. For instance, the path and time of landfall of a hurricane can be tracked, so that residents in the storm's path can be evacuated and families and businesses can be protected. Communities can also minimize devastation from flooding by building reservoirs or refusing to grant building permits in flood-prone areas and by reinforcing areas around waterways with sandbags during rainy weather. In fire-prone areas, communities can post notices to heighten awareness of fire danger and enforce regulations to cut back vegetation near structures in forested areas.

On the other hand, some disasters strike without warning. For example, the terrorist attacks in New York City caught thousands of civilians by surprise. They were trapped in buildings with limited escape routes and very little time to retreat to safety. For survivors of the 2015 Paris terrorist attacks, survival depended on being in the right place at the right time. Coworkers were trapped in a building during the 2015 San Bernardino terrorist attack. A total of 14 were killed and 27 were injured as a married couple sprayed them with automatic weapons fire. The number of wildfires across California in 2015 was not completely unanticipated, but was uncharacteristically large, and control was hindered by drought conditions, along with heat and high winds. Some residents were barred from reentering their communities for weeks, without any knowledge of whether they would have homes when they were allowed to return. The shootings at Virginia Tech in

2007 and in Tucson in 2011, which resulted in six deaths and seriously wounded Rep. Gabrielle Giffords, occurred without warning and were both the result of a mentally unstable individual acting alone. Some disasters, like the natural gas leak in a southern California community during 2015 to 2016, are at first unknown to the public. After residents began noticing headaches, nosebleeds, respiratory problems, and other symptoms, the Southern California Gas Company acknowledged that a deep well gas leak had occurred in a difficult-to-reach canyon miles away. The company assured the public that the leak did not pose an imminent health risk, although it had been occurring for months and would take several more months to stop. Many residents voluntarily moved their families to other areas because of the effects of the gas fumes. It was estimated that over 30,000 kg/hour of methane was released into the atmosphere, and the area became a no-fly zone per the Federal Aviation Administration (Reilly, 2016). It was finally stopped and "permanently sealed" in late February 2016 (Pamer, Wynter, & McDade, 2016, p. 4).

The **scope** of a disaster is the range of its effect, either geographically or in terms of the number of people impacted. The collapse of a 500-unit high-rise apartment building has a greater scope than the collapse of a bridge that occurs while only two cars are crossing.

The **intensity** of a disaster is the level of destruction and devastation it causes. For instance, an earthquake centered in a large metropolitan area and one centered in a desert may have the same numeric rating on the Richter scale yet have very different intensities in terms of the destruction they cause.

Persons Impacted by Disasters

Because disasters are so variable, there is no typical person impacted in a disaster. Nor can anyone predict whether he or she will ever become impacted by a disaster. **Directly impacted by disaster** are the people who experience the event, whether fire, volcanic eruption, war, or bomb. They are the dead and the survivors, and even if they are without physical injuries, they are likely to have health effects from their experience. Some may be without shelter or food, and many experience serious psychological stress long after the event is over (Display 17–1).

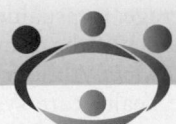

DISPLAY 17–1 DIRECTLY AND INDIRECTLY IMPACTED PEOPLE—HOW A DISASTER'S INFLUENCE LIVES ON

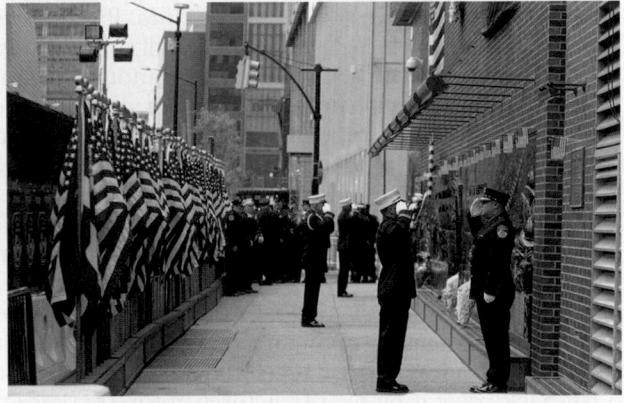

Anniversary observance of World Trade Center terrorist attack.

On September 11, 2001, almost 3,000 people died in the terrorist attacks on the World Trade Center in New York City. Although all of the employees and visitors in the two buildings were directly impacted by this disaster, the entire population of Manhattan can be considered indirectly impacted. Hotels, businesses, and apartments for blocks surrounding the Twin Towers suffered structural damage, blown-out windows, and interiors covered with inches of powdered cement and other debris. A year after this disaster, many residents in the surrounding areas still were unable to return home.

Many rescue workers who were survivors have lasting psychological effects from their own survival experiences and from losing close friends and colleagues. In addition, many rescuers inhaled the dust in the air for days and now are suffering from respiratory damage, which changes their status from indirectly impacted to directly impacted by the disaster.

All people working in or visiting Manhattan that day were affected by the closing of the bridges and tunnels and were stranded in New York City until transportation routes opened again, thus becoming indirectly impacted. Other indirectly impacted persons included were children attending school and living within sight of the Twin Towers. They received counseling in school for months, and in some cases years, after the disaster.

For 1 year after the attack, volunteer construction workers and rescue workers who lost fellow police officers, paramedics, or firefighters worked 24 hours a day. First, the efforts were geared to find survivors. Shortly after, workers knew that they were looking for the bodies or body parts of victims while removing thousands of tons of building pieces. Thousands of people involved in the recovery efforts can still be considered indirectly impacted.

Family members of the 2,980 deceased victims, who have been affected for a lifetime, also are indirectly impacted. Thousands of children lost a parent, some parents lost multiple children, and, in some cases, both spouses were lost because both the husband and wife were working in the World Trade Center. The ripples of tragedy extended beyond the borders of the United States, because hundreds of people from different countries were working in the Twin Towers whose family members remain indirectly impacted.

Depending on the cause and characteristics of the disaster, some direct survivors may become displaced persons or refugees. **Displaced persons** are forced to leave their homes to escape the effects of a disaster. Usually, displacement is a temporary condition and involves movement within the person's own country. A common example is relocation of residents of flooded areas to schools, churches, and other shelters on higher ground. Typically, the term **refugee** is reserved for people who are forced to leave their homeland because of war or persecution. For example, the catastrophic earthquake in Haiti in 2010 killed an estimated 316,000 people, and more than a million people were left homeless. Over 60,000 Haitian refugees reside in the United States today (Comas, 2013) escaping poverty and devastation. Returning refugees can place economic and social strains on the county of origin. Along with needs for employment and shelter, these influx situations raise concerns, especially regarding early or forced marriages, child labor, and human trafficking (United Nations Refugee Agency, n.d.). Whether the displacement of refugees is permanent or not, the lasting impact to both the country of origin and the host country is significant.

Indirectly impacted by disaster are the relatives and friends of persons directly impacted by disasters. Although these people do not experience the stress of the event itself, they often undergo extreme anguish from trying to locate loved ones or accommodate their emergency needs. If bodies cannot be found or are unidentifiable, indirectly impacted persons experience even greater anguish and may not be able to accept that a loved one has died. Family members of those killed on 9/11 in New York City worked with architects to develop a complex of buildings and a memorial that meets the expectations of most of those indirectly impacted by the attack and honors their loved ones. This effort, along with the Flight 93 National Memorial in Shanksville, PA, and the Pentagon Memorial, helps with the long healing process. They also serve as a reminder of the impact that day had on each of our lives.

Factors Contributing to Disasters

It is useful to apply the host, agent, and environment model (epidemiological triad) to understand the factors contributing to disasters, because manipulation of these factors can be instrumental in planning strategies to prevent or prepare for disasters.

Host Factors

The *host* is the human being who experiences the disaster. Host factors that contribute to the likelihood of experiencing a disaster include age, general health, mobility, psychological factors, and even socioeconomic factors. For instance, elderly residents of a mobile home community may be unable to evacuate independently in response to a tornado warning if they can no longer drive. Impoverished residents of a low-income apartment complex in a large city may notice that their building is not compliant with city fire codes, but may avoid alerting authorities for fear of being forced to move to more expensive housing.

Agent Factors

The *agent* is the natural or technologic element that causes the disaster. For example, the high winds of a hurricane and the lava of an erupting volcano are agents, as are radiation, industrial chemicals, biologic agents, and bombs. The Station nightclub fire and the apartment deck collapse in Chicago (both in 2003) demonstrated that the irresponsibility of contractors and inspectors and failure to adhere to safety policies can act as agents of disaster, resulting in death and destruction (Pemberton, 2013).

Environmental Factors

Environmental factors are those that could potentially contribute to or mitigate a disaster. Some of the most common environmental factors are a community's level of preparedness; the presence of industries that produce harmful chemicals or radiation; the presence of flood-prone rivers, lakes, or streams; average amount of rainfall or snowfall; average high and low temperatures; proximity to fault lines, coastal waters, or volcanoes; level of compliance with local building codes; and presence or absence of political unrest.

Agencies and Organizations for Disaster Management

In 1803, just 10 years after the Treaty of Paris, the United States first recognized the need to prepare for emergencies through law and dedicated organizations. The first law was written as a direct response to a major disaster, the Portsmouth, New Hampshire, fire of 1803. The majority of subsequent legislation was also in response to specific crises and created many different agencies to respond to those disasters. From 1803 until the passage of the Disaster Relief Act of 1950, there were 125 pieces of legislation related to disaster assistance and many of these pieces of legislation changed the roles and responsibilities of government agencies. The one constant was that the response of the federal government to disasters remained more reactive than proactive and was ad hoc in nature, only becoming coordinated with the establishment of the Federal Emergency Management Agency (FEMA) in 1979 and the passage of the Robert T. Stafford Disaster Relief and Emergency Assistance Act of 1988 (Haddow, Bullock, & Coppola, 2014). George Washington University has an Institute for Crisis, Disaster and Risk Management (n.d.) and offers resources and publications on this topic, as well as degrees in this area.

In response to World War II and the specter of all-out nuclear war with the Soviet Union, the United States created Civil Defense, a series of programs and agencies designed to protect the population from "counter-value" nuclear strikes and increase the survivability of a nuclear war. The Department of Health, Education, and Welfare (USDHEW) created the *Handbook for Civil Defense Emergency Planning in Welfare Institutions*, which was a guide to protect individuals and help staff prepare for fallout from a nuclear event (USDHEW, 1961). Significant in this handbook was the attention given to family responsibilities and the likelihood that staff, including nurses, would choose family responsibilities over professional responsibilities. To help alleviate the problems associated with absenteeism as a result of the nurses' conflicting responsibilities, the handbook recommended (1) reminding staff of their responsibility as public servants, (2) providing shelter for families within the institution, (3) planning for getting families to the shelter, and (4) planning for families to assist the staff during a crisis (USDHEW, 1961).

Under the 1950 version for the United States Civil Defense Plan, health services were to remain under the control of existing health agencies to avoid unnecessary duplication of services, but would now also be subject to the rules and regulations of civil defense. The U.S. Public Health Service was responsible for providing staffing for civil defense offices and would work for the state health officer who would have the lead. The roles have been in continual transition since that time, but the basic principles remain the same.

Public health has become recognized as a critical component of emergency planning, preparedness, and response. National public health response requires coordination with state and local authorities, to include nongovernmental agencies (CDC, 2011).

Among disaster-relief organizations, perhaps none is as famous as the Red Cross, which is referred to as the American Red Cross in the United States and the Red Crescent Societies in Islamic countries. The American Red Cross was founded in 1881 by Clara Barton and was chartered by the U.S. Congress in 1905. It is authorized to provide disaster assistance free of charge across the country through its more than half a million volunteers and staff. The duties assumed by the Red Cross in the event of a disaster are to provide shelter, food, basic health and mental health services, and distribution of emergency supplies (American Red Cross, n.d.). Even the role of this historic disaster response organization changed after September 11, 2001.

President George W. Bush sought to consolidate the roles and responsibilities of agencies and organizations involved in disaster response and to align them with the Emergency Support Functions (ESFs) (see Table 17–1). The Department of Homeland Security (DHS) was organized in 2002 and incorporates many of the nation's security, protection, and emergency response activities into a single federal department. In 2003, the Federal Emergency Management Agency (FEMA), along with parts of 23 agencies, became part of the DHS. The FEMA, established in 1979, is the federal agency responsible for assessing and responding to disaster events in the United States. It also provides training and guidance in all phases of disaster management. The DHS includes other widely known agencies including the Transportation Security Administration (TSA), U.S. Customs and Border Protection, U.S. Immigration and Customs Enforcement (ICE), U.S. Citizenship and Immigration Services (USCIS), U.S. Coast Guard, and U.S. Secret Service (DHS, 2006, 2011, 2015).

FEMA provides oversight of the National Incident Management System (NIMS), developed to allow responders from different jurisdictions and disciplines to work more cohesively in response to natural disasters, emergencies, and terrorist acts. The benefits of NIMS lie in its unified approach to incident management, standard command and management structures, and emphasis on preparedness, mutual aid, and resource management (FEMA, 2015). NIMS approach provides a proactive response system to terrorist attacks, natural disasters, and other emergencies (CDC, 2011). Among the elements of disaster preparedness that nurses must understand is the **incident command system** (ICS) that was created in the 1970s after catastrophic wildfires in California resulted in many deaths (see Fig. 17–1). Nurses and other health care professionals must understand this system and are encouraged to take courses dealing with the ICS; these courses are available free online from FEMA Emergency Management Institute at http://www.training.fema.

Table 17–1	**Emergency Support Functions (ESF) Responsibilities**	
ESF	**Scope**	**Coordinating Agency**
1. Transportation	Transportation modes management and control Transportation safety Stabilization/reestablishment of transportation infrastructure Movement restrictions Damage and impact assessment	Department of Transportation
2. Communications	Coordination with telecommunications and information technology industries Reestablishment/repair of telecommunications infrastructure Protection, reestablishment, and sustainment of national cyber and information technology resources Oversight of communications within the federal response structures	Department of Homeland Security (DHS)—National Communications System
3. Public works and engineering	Infrastructure protection and emergency repair Infrastructure reestablishment Engineering services and construction management Emergency contracting support for lifesaving and life-sustaining services	Department of Defense—U.S. Army Corps of Engineers

Table 17–1 Emergency Support Functions (ESF) Responsibilities (*Continued*)

ESF	Scope	Coordinating Agency
4. Firefighting	Support to wildland, rural, and urban firefighting operations	U.S. Department of Agriculture—U.S. Forest Service and DHS, FEMA, U.S. Fire Administration
5. Information and planning	Incident action planning Information collection, analysis, and dissemination	Department of Homeland Security—Federal Emergency Management Agency
6. Mass care, emergency assistance, temporary housing, and human services	Mass care Emergency assistance Disaster housing Human services	Department of Homeland Security—Federal Emergency Management Agency
7. Logistics	Comprehensive, national incident logistics planning, management, and sustainment capability Resource support (e.g., facility space, office equipment and supplies, contracting services)	General Services Administration and Department of Homeland Security, Federal Emergency Management Agency
8. Public health and medical services	Public health Medical surge support including patient movement Behavioral health services Mass fatality management	Department of Health and Human Services
9. Search and rescue	Structural collapse (urban) search and rescue Maritime/coastal/waterborne search and rescue Land search and rescue	Department of Homeland Security—Federal Emergency Management Agency
10. Oil and hazardous materials response	Environmental assessment of the nature and extent of oil and hazardous materials contamination Environmental decontamination and cleanup	Environmental Protection Agency
11. Agriculture and natural services	Nutrition assistance Animal and agricultural health issue response Technical expertise, coordination, and support of animal and agriculture emergency management Meat, poultry, and processed egg products safety and defense Natural and cultural resources and historic properties protection	Department of Agriculture
12. Energy	Energy infrastructure assessment, repair, and reestablishment Energy industry utilities coordination Energy forecast	Department of Energy
13. Public safety and security	Facility and resource security Security planning and technical resource assistance Public safety and security support Support to access, traffic, and crowd control	Department of Justice—Bureau of Alcohol, Tobacco, Firearms, and Explosives
14. Long-term community recovery	National Response Framework superseded by *National Disaster Recovery Framework*	Department of Homeland Security (FEMA)
15. External affairs	Public affairs and Joint Information Center Intergovernmental (local, state, tribal, and territorial) affairs Congressional affairs Private sector outreach Community relations	Department of Homeland Security

From The Department of Homeland Security. (2013). *National response framework*, pp. 32–35. Retrieved from http://www.fema.gov/media-library-data/20130726-1914-25045-1246/final_national_response_framework_20130501.pdf

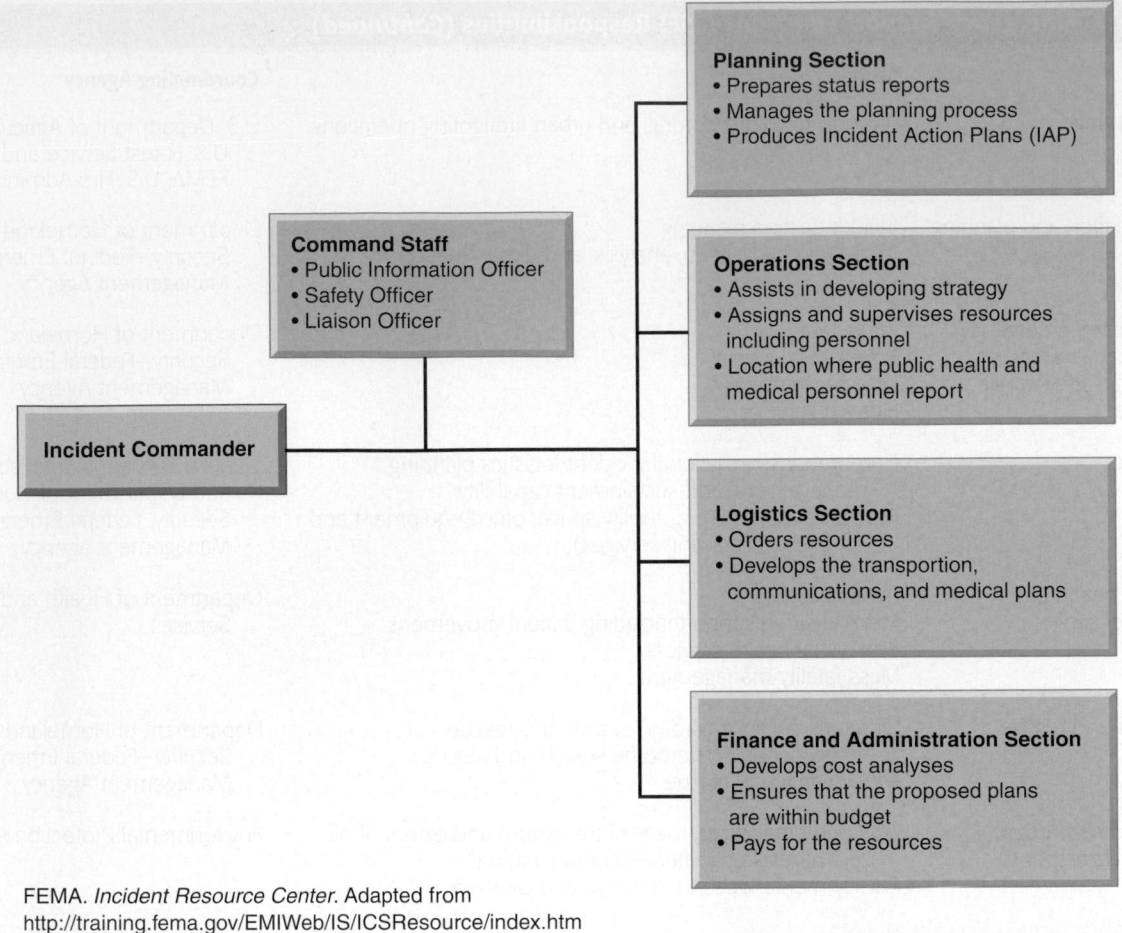

FEMA. *Incident Resource Center*. Adapted from
http://training.fema.gov/EMIWeb/IS/ICSResource/index.htm

FIGURE 17–1 Incident command system.

gov/EMI/. The most important courses for a nurse are (1) IS-100.HCb introduction to the ICS for health care/hospitals, (2) IS-700.a introduction to the NIMS, and (3) IS-800.b introduction to the nation response framework.

The USDHHS is the lead federal agency for public health and medical services during a public health or medical disaster. Supplemental services are provided to state, local, and territorial governments (USDHHS, 2014). The services may include Disaster Medical Assistance Teams (DMAT), U.S. Public Health Service officers, epidemiological personnel from the CDC, and veterinary support to name a few. The Assistant Secretary for Preparedness and Response leads the USDHHS preparedness and response efforts for public health and medical emergencies, and the Office of the Assistant Secretary for Public Health and Science leads recovery efforts. The USDHHS efforts to support human services needs, including disaster case management, are led by the Administration for Children and Families (n.d.). The surge of unaccompanied children (over 50,000) apprehended by DHS immigration officials in the summer of 2014 was an extraordinary challenge for law enforcement and health care providers. The children's safety and well-being was assured while their nutritional and basic human needs were immediately addressed upon apprehension by the Administration for Children and Families (Park, 2014).

When natural or man-made disasters are accompanied by civil disturbance, looting, or violent crime, the resources of local police departments in this country may be overwhelmed. In such cases, the National Guard is often called in to restore order. This action is typically accomplished within each individual state, under the jurisdiction of the governor.

The World Health Organization's (WHO) Emergency Relief Operations provide disaster assistance internationally, the Pan American Health Organization works to coordinate relief efforts in Latin America and the Caribbean, and the U.S. Agency for International Development (USAID) serves as the U.S. government agency responsible for directing contributions to nonprofit partners and international organizations that respond to disasters around the world. In addition, various international nongovernmental organizations (such as Doctors Without Borders, the International Medical Corps, and Operation Blessing), religious groups, and other volunteer agencies provide needed emergency care (see Chapter 16) (Fig. 17–2).

Governments often send their military personnel and equipment in response to international disasters.

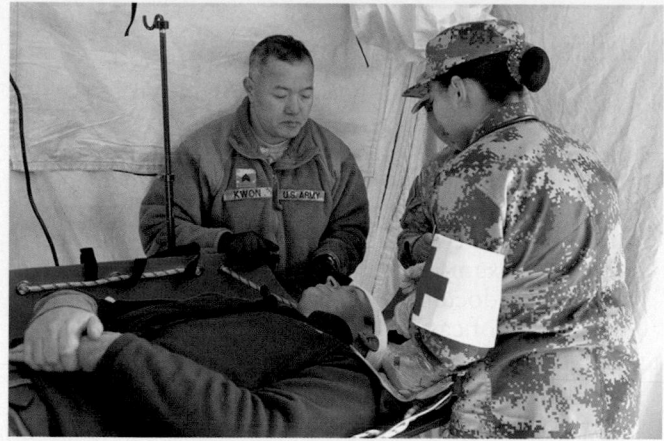

FIGURE 17–2 Mobile hospitals are often deployed during disasters.

For example, in May 2008, the U.S. Navy attempted for 3 weeks to provide much-needed supplies to the cyclone survivors in Myanmar (Burma). With limited options, the Navy had helicopters and landing craft on standby to deliver food, water, and medical supplies to the most remote areas of the country. The military junta in Myanmar refused to allow the shipments, further risking the lives of the millions of survivors. U.S. military planes were eventually allowed to land with supplies in the country's largest city, Rangoon (Kazmin, 2008). The government conducted the transport of vital supplies to the rural areas, and results were questionable.

In this situation, political agendas prevented the aid typically accepted by countries experiencing catastrophe. Fortunately, the Commissioned Corps of the U.S. Public Health Service (USPHS) was allowed to provide aid for the tsunami and earthquake survivors in Indonesia and Haiti. The USPHS has also worked collaboratively with the U.S. Navy to provide nursing and other medical care on combined humanitarian missions to South America and the South Pacific and was sent to Africa to assist with the Ebola crisis (USPHS, 2014). Chapter 30 contains additional information about the role of the USPHS Commissioned Corps Nurses and their role in emergency preparedness.

Phases of Disaster Management

In developing strategies to address the problem of disasters, it is helpful for the community health nurse to consider each of the four phases of disaster management: prevention, preparedness, response, and recovery. Additionally, some knowledge of the language typically used in disaster preparedness may be helpful and is included in Display 17–2.

Prevention Phase

During the *prevention phase*, no disaster is expected or anticipated. The tasks during this phase are to identify community risk factors, to develop and implement programs to prevent disasters from occurring or mitigate their impact, and to train personnel and educate citizens. Task forces typically include representatives from the community's local government, health care providers,

social services providers, police and fire departments, major industries, local media, schools, and citizens' groups. Programs developed during the prevention phase may also focus on strategies to mitigate the effects of disasters that cannot be prevented, such as earthquakes, hurricanes, and tornadoes (CDC, 2015).

The United States has strengthened the preparedness phase of disaster management since September 2001. This is most visible to the average citizen at airports, where airline passengers must now go through a more rigorous security screening before boarding the plane. Nonpassengers cannot go beyond the security area. Photographic identification is required at two or more points before boarding. Strict limits have been placed on liquids that can be in carry-on baggage. Random searches of hand-carried luggage occur, and passengers may be screened with advanced imaging technology. At more than 450 airports, over 1.8 million passengers are screened daily (TSA, 2012). In some airports, luggage is tested for radioactive material, police officials with trained dogs patrol the airport, or some people have credentials prescreened and are permitted to wear shoes and light jackets as part of the screening process. All of these measures have been initiated to prevent a terrorist attack.

Preparedness Phase

Disaster *preparedness* involves improving community and individual reaction and responses, so that the effects of a disaster are minimized. Disaster preparedness saves lives and minimizes injury and property damage. It includes plans for communication, evacuation, rescue, victim care, and recovery. Any plan must also address acquisition of equipment, personnel, supplies, medicine, and even food, clean water, blankets, and shelter. Semiannual disaster drills and tests of the Emergency Broadcast System are examples of appropriate activities during the preparedness phase (CDC, 2015).

Disaster preparedness activities occur locally, regionally, and nationally. A town keeps its warning system working and tests it each month. Sections of the country coordinate larger warning systems to notify communities in the path of a tornado or hurricane, and the country has a plan to stockpile vital pharmaceuticals such as smallpox vaccine for mass immunization. The Centers for Disease Control and Prevention (CDC, 2015) reports that the Strategic National Stockpile (SNS) contains doses of vaccines, medical countermeasures, and needed medical supplies stored around the country in various strategic locations. The CDC reports the SNS contains enough medications and medical supplies to manage a large public health emergency and protect the American public (CDC, 2016).

Response Phase

The *response phase* begins immediately after the onset of the disastrous event. Preparedness plans take effect immediately, with the goals of saving lives and preventing further injury or damage to property. Periodic notification drills are held, and 45-minute response time targets were recently met by 83% in the first drill, and 94% in the second drill of 2013 (CDC, 2015). Focused response teams (e.g., behavioral health, mortuary, social work)

DISPLAY 17–2 COMMON TERMS USED IN EMERGENCY PREPAREDNESS AND RESPONSE

All-hazards preparation: Preparedness for domestic terrorist attacks, major disasters, and other emergencies

Chain of command: A series of command, control, executive, or management positions in hierarchical order of authority

Credential: A health volunteer's qualifications. Credentials are used to determine a health volunteer's emergency credentialing level (i.e., nursing license).

Designated equivalent source: Selected agencies that have been determined to maintain a specific item or items of credential information that is identical to the information at the primary source

Disaster, major (federal): Any natural catastrophe, or, regardless of cause, any fire, flood, or explosion, in any part of the United States, which in the determination of the president causes damage of sufficient severity and magnitude to warrant major disaster assistance to supplement the efforts and available resources of states, local governments, and disaster relief organizations

Emergency declaration: Refers to the state (or local) government's capacity to declare a general emergency or public health emergency, or state of disaster

Emergency Management Assistance Compact (EMAC): An interstate mutual aid agreement that allows states to assist one another in responding to all types of natural and man-made disasters

Hospital emergency incident command system (HEICS): An emergency management system that employs a logical management structure, defined responsibilities, clear reporting channels, and a common nomenclature to help unify hospitals with other emergency responders

Incident command system (ICS): The combination of equipment, facilities, communication, personnel, and procedures that operates within a common organizational structure, designed to aid in the management of resources during incidents

***Just-in-time* training:** Concise, targeted training, normally provided on-site after a disaster or emergency has occurred. It provides a minimum level of exposure for volunteers regarding select issues in disaster response. Examples could be use of self-protection equipment, documentation, mental health triage, or registration of casualties.

National Electronic Disease Surveillance System (NEDSS): A CDC initiative promoting the use of data and information systems standards to improve disease surveillance systems at federal, state, and local levels

National Incident Management System (NIMS): The single all-hazards incident management system required by Homeland Security that governs the management of the National Response Plan

Public Health Information Network (PHIN): A framework providing the basis for information technology projects for CDC-funded programs including NEDSS, Health Alert Network (HAN), and others that improve public health

Shelter-In-Place: Used as alternative to evacuation; people may be asked to remain indoors in homes, businesses, schools, or public buildings (especially if there is limited time to react to a threat). People should plan on having 72 hours' worth of food, water, and medical supplies in order to remain indoors.

Strategic National Stockpile: A national cache of drugs, vaccines, and medical supplies that can be deployed to areas struck by disasters, including bioterrorism, in a matter of 12 to 36 hours

Surge capacity: The accommodation by the health system to a transient sudden rise in demand for health care following an incident with real or perceived adverse health effects or in some cases a more prolonged demand

Adapted from Blanchard, B. W. (2008). *Guide to emergency management and related terms, definitions, concepts, acronyms, organizations, programs, guidance, executive orders, & legislation: A tutorial on emergency management, broadly defined, past and present.* Retrieved from https://www.training.fema.gov/hiedu/docs/terms%20and%20definitions/terms%20and%20definitions.pdf

---

facilitate an effective, comprehensive response effort. Activities during the response phase include rescue, triage, on-site stabilization, transportation of injured, and treatment at local hospitals and clinics. Response also requires recovery, identification, and refrigeration of bodies, so that notification of family members is possible and correct, even weeks after a disaster. This care of the dead is demanding and time-consuming work that is often overlooked by people unfamiliar with disaster response. Persons trained in mortuary services are an essential part of any emergency planning efforts. The mortuary teams always have pastoral personnel with them to ensure that remains are always treated with respect and in accordance with religious traditions. Supportive care, including food,

water, and shelter for survivors and relief workers, is also an essential element of the total disaster response. The extent of care provided for animals is an additional area of concern that should be addressed in the overall plan. Veterinarian response teams are able to address the acute and long-term needs of the animals impacted by the disaster. Many shelters will not accept pets; those that do need to be identified as soon as possible to avoid unnecessary confusion and delays in sheltering (Fig. 17–3).

Recovery Phase

During the *recovery phase*, the community takes actions to repair, rebuild, or relocate damaged homes and businesses and restore health, social, and economic vitality

PERSPECTIVES
VOICES FROM THE COMMUNITY

It was 5:00 PM on October 17, 1989, in Santa Cruz, CA—a day that would change my view of life forever. I had just fed my newborn son and was rocking him in a soft, comfortable chair when the house began to shake. Without even thinking or being aware of what I was doing, I jumped up with my baby in my arms and headed for the nearest doorway, as I had done so many times before in an earthquake. I stood there holding my son in one arm and braced myself against the doorjamb with the other one as the house continued to shake all around us. It was not until the shaking stopped that I began to feel fear and worry as I surveyed the damage to my house.

In my kitchen, all of the cupboard doors were flung open and their contents spilled onto the floor, which was now a mess of spilled food, sticky sauces, dented tin cans, and broken glass. Tears came to my eyes as I saw my son's infant seat, where he had been seated only moments before the quake, covered with glass shards and fallen tin cans. I realized he could have been killed, and I had no control over it. I became afraid for the safety of my 10-year-old daughter, who was at dancing lessons across town. Fortunately, when I got to her, she was safe.

The next few days continued to be very stressful. We had no gas or electricity and no running water that was safe to drink. I went to the drug store in a panic to buy premixed formula to feed my son, since I could not boil the water to mix with the powdered formula. Both the drug store and the grocery store were "trashed," all of the items were thrown off of the shelves and laying on the debris-strewn floors. The grocery store was giving away the ice

cream because they had no power to keep it frozen. But who could eat ice cream?

There was something about seeing my favorite grocery store in such a disastrous condition that made me realize how little control I had over the consequences of what insurance companies call "acts of God." I couldn't just run to the grocery store for what I needed; it wouldn't be there for me. My family and I felt very unsafe as we all huddled together in the master bedroom at night. My son was in his bassinet at the foot of the bed and my daughter slept with me until she felt safe enough to return to her own room. I was attempting to regain control of my life as I cleaned up my house and waited for the water and electricity to be restored. Of all the losses, the greatest loss was the illusion of safety and the illusion that I had control over my life.

Over the next week, I experienced the loss of many services and products that made up my comfortable and safe lifestyle: homes were damaged, with their chimneys strewn across front lawns, there was no phone service for days, and a normal 10-minute drive took an hour and a half on clogged highways provided as an alternative route to highways and bridges damaged by the quake. As a community mental health nurse, I wanted to volunteer to help others who were experiencing the same feelings as I was, but I was told that they were not taking mental health volunteers from the immediate area because we, too, were victims of the disaster and needed to care for ourselves first. I think they were right, since I had many feelings that took a long while to heal and I have lost the illusion of control forever.

Nancy, age 32

---

to the community. Psychological recovery must also be addressed. The emotional scars from witnessing a traumatic event may last a lifetime. Both survivors and relief workers should be offered mental health services to support their recovery (see Perspectives: Voices From the Community). The Substance Abuse Mental Health Services Administration (SAMHSA) offers guides and a

disaster kit for managing stress in crisis for both professionals and victims (SAMHSA, 2015).

During the recovery phase, special attention should be given to the needs of children who are approximately 25% of the population in the United States and even higher in many countries. The Substance Abuse and Mental Health Services Administration has resources available for specific populations to assist with managing disasters (SAMHSA, 2015). One example is *Tips for Talking With and Helping Children and Youth Cope After a Disaster or Traumatic Event: A Guide for Parents, Caregivers, and Teachers.*

Role of the Community/Public Health Nurse

The public health nurse has a pivotal role in preventing, preparing for, responding to, and supporting recovery from a disaster (Association of Public Health Nurses [APHN] Public Health Preparedness Committee, 2013). After a thorough community assessment for risk factors, the community health nurse may initiate the formation of a multidisciplinary task force to address disaster prevention and preparedness in the community.

Preventing Disasters

Disaster prevention may be considered on three levels: primary, secondary, and tertiary. These are applied to a natural disaster in the Levels of Prevention Pyramid.

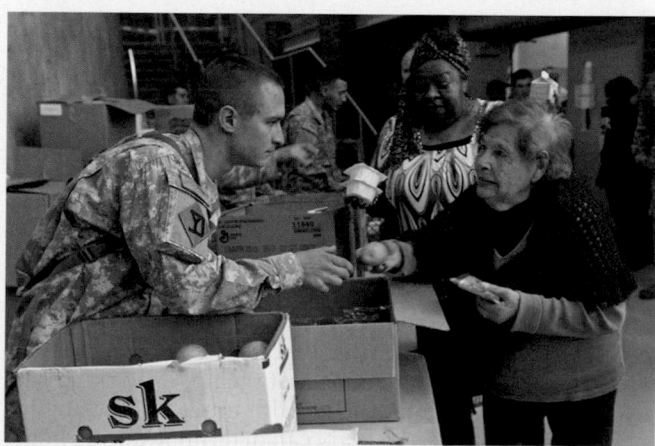

FIGURE 17–3 Victims of Superstorm Sandy receiving assistance at a temporary shelter.

LEVELS OF PREVENTION PYRAMID

SITUATION: A natural disaster—tornado
GOAL: By using the three levels of prevention, negative health conditions are avoided, promptly diagnosed, and treated, and/or the fullest possible potential is restored.

TERTIARY PREVENTION

Rehabilitation	Primary Prevention	
	Health Promotion and Education	*Health Protection*
• Remain safe during the immediate recovery period • Accept help from others—friends, family, and community services • Rebuild family lives through counseling and other services to reestablish stable life physically, emotionally, spiritually, and financially	• Educate community members about the need to enhance planning against damage from future natural disasters, based on experiences with the current disaster	• Keep recommended immunizations current • Community physical structures need rebuilding, with infrastructure planning and supports that improve ability to withstand natural disasters

SECONDARY PREVENTION

Early Diagnosis	Prompt Treatment
• Remain in your position of safety until a community all-clear warning signal is sounded or until rescued • Leave a damaged building cautiously, if able and not seriously injured, and do not return until it is declared safe	• Rescue individuals promptly and get appropriate care for those injured as soon as possible • The infrastructure of the community becomes/remains intact, keeping community members safe from hazards such as live wires, broken gas lines, and fallen debris

PRIMARY PREVENTION

Health Promotion and Education	Health Protection
• Increase community awareness • Increase community preparation through education • Each person is as prepared as possible both physically and emotionally	• Community members know what to do and where to go, whether at home, work, school, or elsewhere in the community • Get to safety before the impact—southwest corner of a home's basement or an interior room away from windows and under heavy furniture

Primary Prevention

Primary prevention of a disaster means keeping the disaster from ever happening by taking actions that completely eliminate its occurrence. This is the first aspect of primary disaster prevention. Although it is obviously the most effective level of intervention, both in terms of promoting clients' health and containing costs, it is not always possible. Tornadoes, earthquakes, terrorist attacks, and other disasters often strike without warning, despite the use of every available technologic device for prediction and tracking.

If possible, primary prevention of disasters can be practiced in all settings: in the workplace and home with programs to reduce safety hazards and in the community with programs to monitor risk factors, reduce pollution, and encourage nonviolent conflict resolution (CDC, 2015). Primary disaster prevention efforts should take into account a community's physical, psychosocial, cultural, economic, and spiritual needs. The community health nurse has a role in each of these areas. As a teacher, the community health nurse educates people at home, at work, at school, or in a faith community about safety and security focused on preventing a disaster. The community health nurse can teach community members how to protect themselves from the effects of a natural disaster. The nurse can be a part of a safety team, if working as a school nurse or occupational health nurse. If working for a health department, the PHN can determine during home visits whether a family has a personal disaster plan and help them develop one if none exists. Nursing students can work with low-income community–dwelling elders to ensure that they have enough food, water, and medical supplies to **shelter in place** for at least 72 hours. There are many actions the nurse can initiate (APHN Public Health Preparedness Committee, 2013).

The second aspect of primary disaster prevention is anticipatory guidance. Disaster drills and other anticipatory exercises help relief workers experience some of the feelings of chaos and stress associated with a disaster before one occurs (CDC, 2015). It is much easier to do this when energy and intellectual processes are at a high level of functioning. Anticipatory work can dissipate the impact of a disastrous event. The community health nurse has a role in these disaster drills through committee membership, organization of drills at the place of employment, or activism at the grassroots level to assist in holding community-wide disaster drills on a regular basis (see Quality and Safety Education for Nurses [QSEN] feature). In addition, the community health nurse could lead or participate with community health assessment programs seeking an understanding of the community needs predisaster and provide preventive education and preparation guidance.

Secondary Prevention

Secondary disaster prevention focuses on the earliest possible detection and treatment. For example, a mobile home community is devastated by a tornado. After the disaster, the local health department's community health nurses work with the American Red Cross to provide emergency assistance. Secondary prevention corresponds to immediate and effective response. For example, in a post-Katrina study of the emergency planning and response by home health providers serving the poor in New Orleans during the emergency, the successes and challenges of these providers were identified (Kirkpatrick & Bryan, 2007). Agencies that provided early evacuation, identified shelters for special-needs patients outside the high-risk area, implemented volunteer cascading communication systems, and conducted pre-event mock evacuation plans and those that included volunteers in their disaster plan were most successful. Recommendations to improve response include identification of patients who may be reluctant to evacuate, the provision of adequate security at special-needs shelters, and, most importantly, practice drills (DHS, n.d.). With appropriate planning, sound and easily understood emergency response can provide optimal care and services to those impacted by the disaster. New Orleans has developed a citywide preparedness program entitled *Are you Ready?*; this aims to inform, prepare, and ensure residents are ready for any type of man-made or natural disaster (City of New Orleans, 2016). Similar examinations are conducted after other disasters, for instance, after Hurricane/Superstorm Sandy (Ladislaw, Kostro, & Walton, 2013) and the Nepal earthquakes (Government of Nepal, National Planning Commission, 2015).

Tertiary Prevention

Tertiary disaster prevention involves reducing the amount and degree of disability or damage resulting from the disaster. Although it involves rehabilitative work, it can help a community recover and reduce the risk of further disasters. In this sense, it becomes a preventive measure.

An example from September 11, 2001, comes from a nurse living in the Boston area who, after that date, began to lose a sense of hope for her future. She often found it difficult to assist her patients with their needs because of her own insecurities and fears. She and a peer responded to a request from the Logan Airport Employee Assistance Program (EAP) asking for help with crisis counseling for United Airlines survivors of 9/11. The planes used in the attacks were from American and United Airlines, and the community of employees felt like survivors because they lived while fellow employees were lost in the disaster. Employees were in turmoil and their ability to function was affected. The most important intervention the nurses could provide was a listening ear and validation that what the employees were feeling and experiencing was normal, and often essential, for healthy grieving. Some employees needed to talk about good times, others were quiet and sad, and others expressed a fear of flying again but did so with the support of family and friends. All demonstrated courage and an ability to continue their lives with a sense of strength and hope. Since 9/11, the American Psychiatric Nurses Association has developed a profile that assists psychiatric nurses by providing clearer information for targeted assessments of those with significant emotional trauma (White, 2002) and provides access to many resources for nurses dealing with traumatic events (American Psychiatric Nurses Association, 2016).

Preparing for Disasters

Disaster planning is essential for a community, business, or hospital. It involves thinking about details of preparation and management by all involved, including community leaders, health and safety professionals, and lay people. A disaster plan need not be lengthy. Two weeks after the April 1995 Oklahoma City bombing of the Murrah Federal Building by two American citizens, one hospital distilled its 44-page manual into a 5-page disaster response guide. Despite many disaster drills and numerous iterations of disaster plans before Hurricane Katrina, some hospitals in New Orleans were better prepared for terrorism events than for the hurricanes and flooding that are not uncommon to this area. Memorial Medical Center was hit with massive flooding and electrical outages after Katrina, and their backup generators were in the basement and soon underwater (Fink, 2013). Unlike the Memorial disaster plan, the Oklahoma hospital plan was concise. Such a concise plan should still contain information on the elements discussed in this and the following section. Public health nurses can be very instrumental in disaster preparedness (APHN Public Health Preparedness Committee, 2013) (see Display 17–3 for a summary of these elements).

Personal Preparation

The preparation of a disaster plan for a community should be preceded by the need for all nurses to address their own personal preparedness to respond in a disaster. From the Case Files describes the tragic outcome of one nurse's lack of preparation when she attempted to

QSEN—How Can We Implement Quality Care During Mass-Casualty Incidents and Disasters?

Trauma centers in this country provide care to over 30 million people each year. In an effort to improve processes at their Level I trauma center, Jelinek, Fahje, Immermann, and Elsbernd (2014) report on strategies aimed at reducing the rate of undertriage reporting and providing more effective, safer, and quality care to their trauma patients. They piloted a program that implemented a new position, trauma report nurse (TRN), with the responsibility to assign trauma triage level for all injured patients and who could activate necessary trauma teams. Prehospital teams communicated by radio with the TRN, who in turn gave report to trauma team members about incoming trauma patients. New tools and flow sheets were implemented, and monthly case studies were used to provide ongoing education and feedback about the new system. Although some glitches were noted during the pilot, in the end, the TRN became a permanent position, and earlier trauma team notification provided quicker responses. The rate of undertriage dropped to 4.8% from the initial 14%, and a direct phone line to the trauma surgeon provided for improved prioritization and planning for care, especially with ICU and the operating room staff.

This is an example of quality improvement in a regularly functioning emergency department. But, what happens when hospitals become overwhelmed with patients?

Nurses from the emergency department at the University of Colorado Hospital describe what happened on the night of the Aurora, Colorado, movie theater shootings in July 2012 (Koehler, Scott, & Davis, 2014). It was a "typical summer night" with the hospital at capacity, a full emergency room (49 patients), and two people out sick; the staff had been diverting ambulances for the past 5 hours when "radio chatter" alerted the charge nurse to a shooting (p. 440). A few minutes later, police notified the hospital that they would receive between three and five gunshot wound patients, and four police cars arrived at the ambulance entrance carrying several patients—all bleeding and some unconscious. Two more groups of police cars arrived with patients over the next 15 minutes. There were 10 patients in less than 10 minutes, with some coming in private cars or walking in. One of these patients was dead on arrival, and there were four in critical condition. We then implemented disaster protocols (disaster triage, registration), as we were becoming overwhelmed with patients. During the next 11 minutes, we had eight additional patients. Patients filled our trauma area, the hallways, and some were placed in front of nurses' stations. In total, we received 23 of the 58 total victims. In less than 30 minutes from the first patient's arrival, the hospital implemented our full disaster plan. Staff from pharmacy, OR, radiology, and central supply, along with inpatient physicians, nurses, social workers, chaplains, and hospital directors and managers all pitched in to provide care for the injured and their families. The OR prepared nine rooms in under 2 hours, and radiology did 150 x-rays and 12 CTs in just the first hour. Our hospital command center responded to 1,500 calls during that night. We were probably the exception for most hospitals; in addition to the yearly hospital-wide disaster drill, the emergency staff engaged in two to three additional drills, we have a disaster committee that meets every month. Our hospital had "completed 45 emergency preparedness activities" just during 2012 (p. 443). Nonetheless, we found that our electronic medical record (EMR) system did not provide capacities to adequately track patients, so we resorted to taping patient stickers onto IV poles and documenting their conditions, pending tests, and potential dispositions. Electronic order entry was "nonfunctional during the surge event" (p. 444). We also found that we had problems with documentation, as there were not enough easily accessible computers for staff. We also had problems with external communications and were unaware that the other hospital on our campus, Children's Hospital of Colorado, had six adult patients. We also learned that trauma affects not only patients but also staff. Some members of our staff were diagnosed with PTSD, but we have become even closer because of this incident.

While this experience in Colorado demonstrates how quickly mass-shooting incidents can overwhelm a well-prepared hospital, how are quality and safety affected under dire conditions? What happens when a devastating natural disaster occurs?

Researchers in China conducted a qualitative study involving 12 hospital registered nurses who assisted with disaster relief after two major earthquakes, one with an 8.0 magnitude causing 87,456 deaths and over $85 billion in damages and the other having a magnitude of 7.1 causing 2,698 deaths and over 100,000 injuries (Wenji, Turale, Stone, & Petrini, 2014). The second one occurred in a mountainous Tibetan-inhabited area, about 2.5 miles above sea level. The nurses (11 female, 1 male) experienced numerous aftershocks, heavy rain, land/mudslides, and little sleep. Some nurses suffered from altitude sickness due to the high elevation. They also noted difficulties getting medical supplies, food, and water, and they experienced ethical challenges when some of the injured elderly refused to leave destroyed homes. There were cultural and language barriers, and they had no previous disaster nursing experience. Some of the competencies that participants felt were needed by disaster nurses included flexibility/adaptability, good clinical skills, ability to collaborate with diverse team members, good organizational/management skills, good ability to problem solve/think critically, and comprehensive education on disaster management. Their concerns included poor disaster planning/coordination and guidance, the levels of bureaucracy that impeded their work, as well as lack of emotional preparation and their daily needs being met (food, water, shelter, sleep). Some nurses had significant emotional health problems both during and following their disaster work, and one nurse, stating that she was "very fragile" even 4 years later, recognized she may have undiagnosed PTSD.

Given the desperate circumstances and lack of preparation that these nurses experienced, could they truly ensure safe nursing care and quality nursing practices?

Review the QSEN Web site (http://qsen.org/competencies/) and discuss the competencies needed in each of these three examples. How can you best ensure that you meet these competencies?

Jelinek, L., Fahje, C., Immermann, C., & Elsbernd, T. (2014). The trauma report nurse: A trauma triage process improvement project. *Journal of Emergency Nursing, 40*(5), e111–e117.

Koehler, A., Scott, R. A., & Davis, R. (2014). Surviving the dark night: The Aurora, Colorado mass shootings. *Journal of Emergency Nursing, 40*(5), 440–445.

Wenji, Z., Turale, S., Stone, T. E., & Petrini, M. A. (2014). Chinese nurses' relief experiences following two earthquakes: Implications for disaster education and policy development. *Nurse Education in Practice, 15*, 75–81.

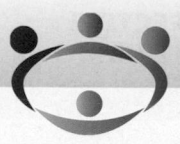

DISPLAY 17–3 ELEMENTS OF A DISASTER PLAN

A disaster plan should address all of the following:

Chain of authority
Lines of communication
Routes and modes of transport
Mobilization
Warning
Evacuation
Rescue and recovery
Triage
Treatment
Support of survivors and families
Care of dead bodies
Disaster worker rehabilitation

provide nursing care at the scene of the Oklahoma City bombing (see From the Case Files I).

Personal preparedness means that the nurse has read and understood workplace and community disaster plans and has developed a disaster plan for his or her own

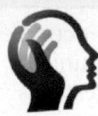

From the Case Files I

Nurses at Disaster Sites—Help or Hindrance?

On April 19, 1995, 37-year-old Rebecca Anderson, a registered nurse working in Oklahoma City, after hearing a televised report of the bombing of the Federal Building, went to the site wearing jeans and a sweatshirt. Along with firefighters and other rescue workers in hard hats and other protective gear, she was allowed to enter the scene. Within a short time, Rebecca was struck on the back of the head by a concrete slab that fell from the building's wreckage. She died 5 days later of massive cerebral edema. Nurses can learn the following lessons from this tragedy:

- Never enter a disaster scene unless you are directed to do so by an emergency medical technician, firefighter, or law enforcement official.
- Contact local hospitals and clinics to offer your help; your medical expertise is more useful in the clinical environment.
- Take courses in first aid and emergency care. Contact your local Red Cross for a list of courses.
- Contact your local health department to learn more about your community's disaster plan and how you can contribute in the event of a disaster in your area.

From McGuigan, P. B. (2010). Resolution honors nurse rescuer killed in the bombing's aftermath. Retrieved from http://www.capitolbeatok.com/reports/resolution-honors-nurse-rescuer-killed-in-the-bombing-s-aftermath

family (San Diego County Office of Emergency Services, n.d.). The prepared nurse also has participated in disaster drills and knows cardiopulmonary resuscitation and first aid. Finally, nurses preparing to work in disaster areas should bring copies of their nursing license and driver's license, durable clothing, and basic equipment, such as stethoscopes, flashlights, and cellular phones. In the event of an emergency, many who are unprepared or untrained often present at the site of a disaster or at local hospitals to volunteer. These "spontaneous volunteers" can be an additional burden to those in charge.

To increase understanding of and the ability to work within an emergency situation, every nurse should become familiar with the NIMS. The NIMS "is a systematic, proactive approach to guide departments and agencies at all levels of government, nongovernmental organizations, and the private sector to work together seamlessly and manage incidents involving all threats and hazards—regardless of cause, size, location, or complexity—in order to reduce loss of life, property and harm to the environment" (FEMA, 2015, p. 3). In essence, it provides a framework for management of incidents in support of the national preparedness system, using common language for disaster response, to reduce confusion as much as possible. Free online courses are offered through FEMA (see Display 17–4). Additionally, every nurse should have up-to-date vaccinations; many biologic threats have the same initial presentations, and reducing susceptibility to common illnesses such as influenza can help with initial identification.

Assessment for Risk Factors and Disaster History

As noted earlier in the chapter, the public health nurse is uniquely qualified to perform a community assessment for risk factors that may contribute to disasters (APHN Public Health Preparedness Committee, 2013).

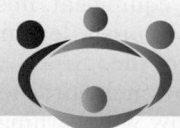

DISPLAY 17–4 FREE ONLINE EMERGENCY PREPAREDNESS TRAINING

CDC Emergency Preparedness and Response Training and Education: http://www.bt.cdc.gov/training/
Federal Emergency Management Agency (FEMA): http://training.fema.gov/emi.aspx
Public Health Foundation—Train.org: https://www.train.org
National Nurse Emergency Preparedness Initiative (NNEPI): http://www.nnepi.org/
National Institutes of Health—Radiation Emergency Medical Management: http://www.remm.nlm.gov/training.htm
University of Minnesota, School of Public Health: http://www.sph.umn.edu/academics/ce/tools/
Uniformed Services University of the Health Sciences Online Preparedness Education Program: http://opep.usuhs.edu/

In addition, the nurse should review the *disaster history* and preparedness plans of the community. Have earthquakes, tornadoes, hurricanes, floods, blizzards, riots, or other disasters occurred in the past? If so, what (if any) were the warning signs? Were they heeded? Were people warned in time? Did evacuation efforts remove all people in danger? What were the community's on-site responses, and how effective were they? What programs were put in place to rehabilitate the community?

Establishing Authority, Communication, and Transportation

In addition to assessing for preparedness, the effective disaster plan follows the NIMS model and establishes a clear chain of authority, develops lines of communication, and delineates routes of transport. Establishing a clear and flexible chain of authority is critical for successful implementation of a disaster plan (CDC, 2015). Usually, the chain is hierarchical, with, for example, the community's governmental head (e.g., mayor) initiating the plan, alerting the media to broadcast warnings, authorizing the police to begin evacuations, and so on. Within each level of the organization, the hierarchy continues. For example, at the local hospital, the hospital administrator may be responsible for alerting nurse managers to call in additional personnel. Flexibility is essential, because key authority figures may themselves be survivors of the disaster. If the home of the chief of police is destroyed in an earthquake, his or her second-in-command must have equal knowledge of the community's disaster plan and be able to step in without delay.

Effective communication is often a point of breakdown for communities attempting to cope with major disasters. After the terrorist attacks in Oklahoma City and New York City, phone lines were damaged and cellular sites were overwhelmed, making communication difficult. Communication was possible only through handheld radios or by way of couriers on foot. At times of heightened chaos and stress, as well as after physical damage to communication facilities and equipment, misinformation and misinterpretation can flourish, leading to delayed treatment and increased loss of life.

Again, clarity and flexibility are the watchwords for establishing lines of communication. How will warnings be communicated? What backups are available if the normal communication systems are destroyed in the disaster? How will communication between relief workers at the disaster site, hospital personnel, police, and governmental authorities be maintained? What role will local media play, both in keeping information flowing to the outside world and in broadcasting needs for assistance and supplies? Significant forms of communication have developed since the 9/11 terrorist attacks. Social media has become a critical method of communicating important health and safety information to the public since the 2001 terrorist attacks. Social media and disaster communication leaderships have collaborated and formed a partnership under the guidance of the FEMA Regional Interagency Steering Committee (2011). Finally, how will friends and family members be informed of the whereabouts or health status of loved ones? The characteristics of effective communication during disasters are summarized in Display 17–5.

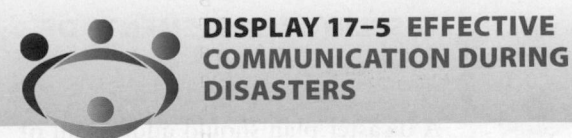

DISPLAY 17–5 EFFECTIVE COMMUNICATION DURING DISASTERS

To be effective, communication during disasters must elicit action. Communication that elicits action provides information that is

- Believable
- Current
- Unambiguous
- Authoritative
- Predictive of the probability of future events (what is going to happen next?)

Effective communication is

- Interactive—it allows for and addresses questions
- Conclusive—it eliminates room for speculation and *catastrophizing*
- Urgent—conveys seriousness without resorting to fear tactics
- Clear, simple, and repetitive
- Characterized by solutions and suggestions for success
- Personal—it uses people's names if possible and addresses their real and perceived needs

Finally, because rumors can hinder effective action or provoke premature action, effective communication includes rumor control. It provides suggestions for constructive activity, reducing time and energy spent on rumor generation and perpetuation.

Closed or inefficient routes of transportation can also increase injury and loss of life. For example, if a single, narrow mountainous road is the only means of transporting firefighters to or evacuating residents from the scene of a forest fire, then disaster planners should propose widening the road or clearing a second road. Disaster planners must also consider what routes emergency vehicles will take when transporting disaster survivors to local and outlying hospitals or health care workers to the disaster site. What if the chosen routes are inaccessible because of floodwaters, advancing fires, mountain slides, avalanches, or building rubble? Are alternative routes designated? Also, how will people move about after the disaster? After the Japanese earthquake and tsunami in 2011, Nakanishi, Matsuo, and Black (2013) examined planning methodologies and future hypothetical disaster scenarios to help answer these types of questions.

Mobilizing, Warning, and Evacuating

In many natural disasters, local weather service personnel, public works officials, police officers, or firefighters have the earliest information indicating an increasing potential for a disaster. These officials typically have a plan in place for providing community authorities with specific data indicating increased risk (CDC, 2015). They may also advise the mayor's office or other community leaders of their recommendations for warning or evacuating the public. Additionally, they may recommend actions the community can take to mitigate damage, such as spraying rooftops in the path of fires, sandbagging the banks of rising rivers, or imposing a curfew in times of civil unrest.

Disaster plans must specify the means of communicating warnings to the public, as well as the precise information that should be included in warnings (CDC, 2015). Planners should never assume that all citizens can be reached by radio or television or that broadcast systems will be unaffected by the disaster. Broadcast media may indeed be a primary means of communicating warnings, but alternative strategies, such as social media or police and volunteers canvassing neighborhoods, should be considered. Social media options such as Facebook, Twitter, and blogs are reliable methods used by news stations and public health agencies that must not be ignored. Over 20 million tweets were sent by utilities after Hurricane Sandy, and Google's Web application, *Person Finder*, was especially helpful during the Boston Marathon bombings (Maron, 2013). In multilingual communities, messages should be broadcast in multiple languages. Not only homes but also businesses must be informed. Information that should be communicated includes the nature of the disaster; the exact geographic region affected, including street names if appropriate; and the actions citizens should take to protect themselves and their property.

An evacuation plan is an essential component of the total disaster plan (CDC, 2015). The plan should include notification of the police, local military personnel, or voluntary citizens' groups of the need to evacuate people, as well as methods of notifying and transporting the evacuees. A plan should also be made for responding to citizens who refuse to evacuate. For example, will police authorities forcibly remove an elderly citizen from his home to a shelter? Will evacuation plans include household pets? If farms or ranches are in the path of fires or floods, will animals be evacuated? How? Who will do this and where will they be taken/sheltered?

Responding to Disasters

At the disaster site, police, firefighters, nurses, and other relief workers develop a coordinated response to rescue, triage, and treat disaster survivors. One of the first obligations of relief workers is to remove survivors from danger (Fig. 17–4).

Rescue

The job of rescue typically belongs to firefighters and urban search and rescue teams that have personnel with special training in search and rescue. Depending on the disaster agent, protective gear, heavy equipment, and special vehicles may be needed, and dogs trained to locate dead bodies may be brought in (Fig. 17–5). Sometimes, the immediate disaster site is not the best place for the disaster nurse, who can be far more effective in triage and treatment of survivors. The PHN's population-based approaches are needed, as well as knowledge of community resources and particularly vulnerable aggregates (APHN Public Health Preparedness Committee, 2013).

Rescue workers face the logistically and psychologically difficult task of determining when to cease rescue

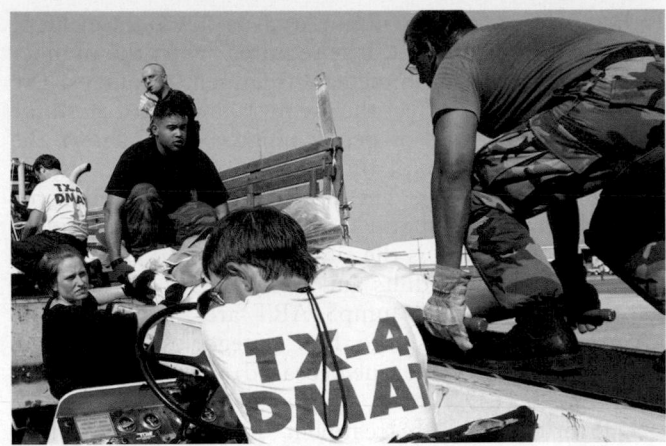

FIGURE 17–4 Rescue of Hurricane Katrina victim.

efforts. Some factors to consider include increasing danger to rescue workers, diminishing numbers of survivors, and diminishing possibilities for survival. For example, after a plane crash on a snowy mountain, rescue efforts may cease if it is deemed that anyone who might have survived the crash would subsequently have died of exposure.

Triage

Whereas emergency nurses daily determine which clients require priority care, the community health nurse may be at a loss as to where to start when faced with multiple persons impacted by a disaster. Knowing the principles and practice of triage allows the nurse to offer nursing skills most effectively (Wagner & Dahnke, 2015). **Triage**

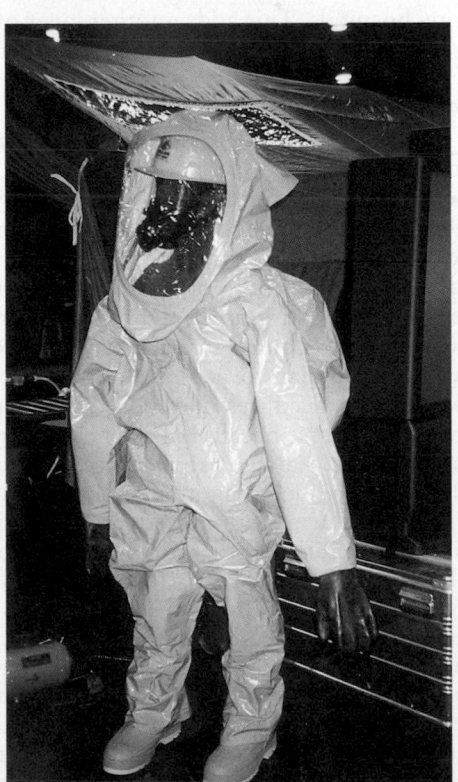

FIGURE 17–5 Hazardous materials suit used by the military and most fire departments. (Photo by Cynthia Tait.)

is the process of sorting multiple casualties in the event of a war or major disaster. It is required when the number of casualties exceeds immediate treatment resources. The goal of triage is to affect the greatest amount of good for the greatest number of people. Figure 17–6 shows the four basic categories of the international triage system, as well as a triage tag. The most common method of triage used by first responders at a mass-casualty incident in the United States is the simple triage and rapid treatment (START) for adults and JumpSTART for pediatric patients. START and JumpSTART are forms of triage used to sort victims into four categories (immediate, delayed, minor, or morgue/deceased) and are consistent with (Fig. 17–6).

Prioritization of treatment may be very different in a mass-casualty event as opposed to an average day in a hospital emergency department. Under normal circumstances, a person presenting to a hospital emergency department with a myocardial infarction and showing no pulse or respirations would receive immediate treatment and have a chance of recovery. At a disaster site, a person without a pulse or respirations would most likely be placed in the nonsalvageable category.

The term *mass casualty* refers to a number of persons impacted that is greater than that which can be managed safely with the resources the community has to offer, such as rescue vehicles and emergency facilities available to serve disaster survivors while also meeting the needs of the rest of the community (Culley & Svendsen, 2014; Lee, 2010). Frequently, in mass-casualty occurrences, the broader community needs to become involved, which necessitates calling in rescue vehicles, firefighters, and police officers from neighboring towns or the use of neighboring hospitals. This adds another layer of disaster management coordination that must be considered.

Immediate Treatment and Support

Disaster nurses provide treatment on-site at emergency treatment stations, at mobile field hospitals, in shelters, and at local hospitals and clinics (see Display 17–6). In addition to direct nursing care, on-site interventions might include arranging for transport once survivors are stabilized and managing the procurement, distribution, and replenishment of all supplies. Disposable items might be in short supply, requiring resterilization procedures that may be unfamiliar to a nurse not accustomed to fieldwork. These procedures may pose a challenge even to an experienced nurse because of the field environment. The nurse may also manage provision or distribution of food and beverages, including infant formulas and rehydration fluids, and arrange for adequate, accessible, and safe sanitation facilities, either on-site or in a shelter. Finally, the nurse often must also arrange for psychological and spiritual care of survivors of disasters (APHN Public Health Preparedness Committee, 2013).

Some survivors who seem physically uninjured may, in fact, be suffering from major injuries but be unable to relate their symptoms to a relief worker because of shock or anxiety. For instance, a father pulling debris away from his collapsed house after a tornado may be so worried about a missing child that he does not realize that he has a broken arm.

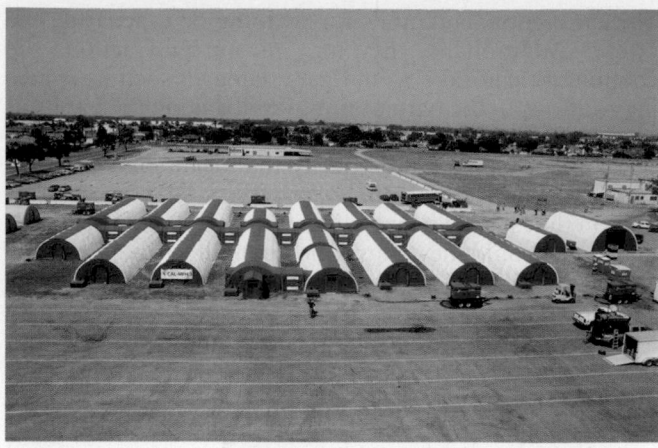

A

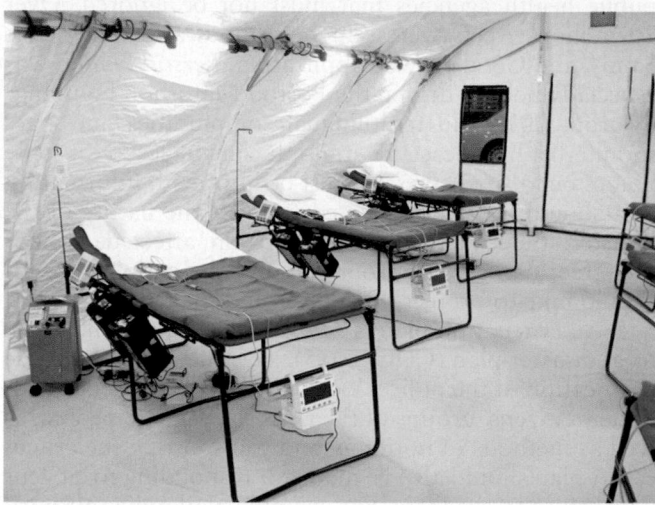

B

(A) Mobile field hospital, interior and exterior: CA Emergency Medical Services Authority 200-bed field hospital. **(B)** ICU with equipment. (With permission from BLU-MED Response Systems, Kirkland, WA.)

Other survivors may be so emotionally traumatized by a disaster that they act out, disrupting efforts to assist them and other survivors and even engaging in dangerous activities. This may cause relief workers to focus on emotional care; however, such survivors must be assessed for head trauma and internal injuries, because their behavior may have a physical cause. If they are physically able, such survivors may be given a simple, repetitive task to perform, which serves as both a distraction and a means to restore, to a small extent, their sense of control over their environment.

Care of Bodies and Notification of Families

Identification and transport of the dead to a morgue or holding facility are crucial, especially if contagion is feared though this is rare in mass-casualty situations. Toe tags make documentation visible and accessible. Records of deaths must be made and maintained, and family members should be notified of their loved ones' deaths as quickly and compassionately as possible. If feasible, a representative from each of the area's faith communities should be available to assist families awaiting news of

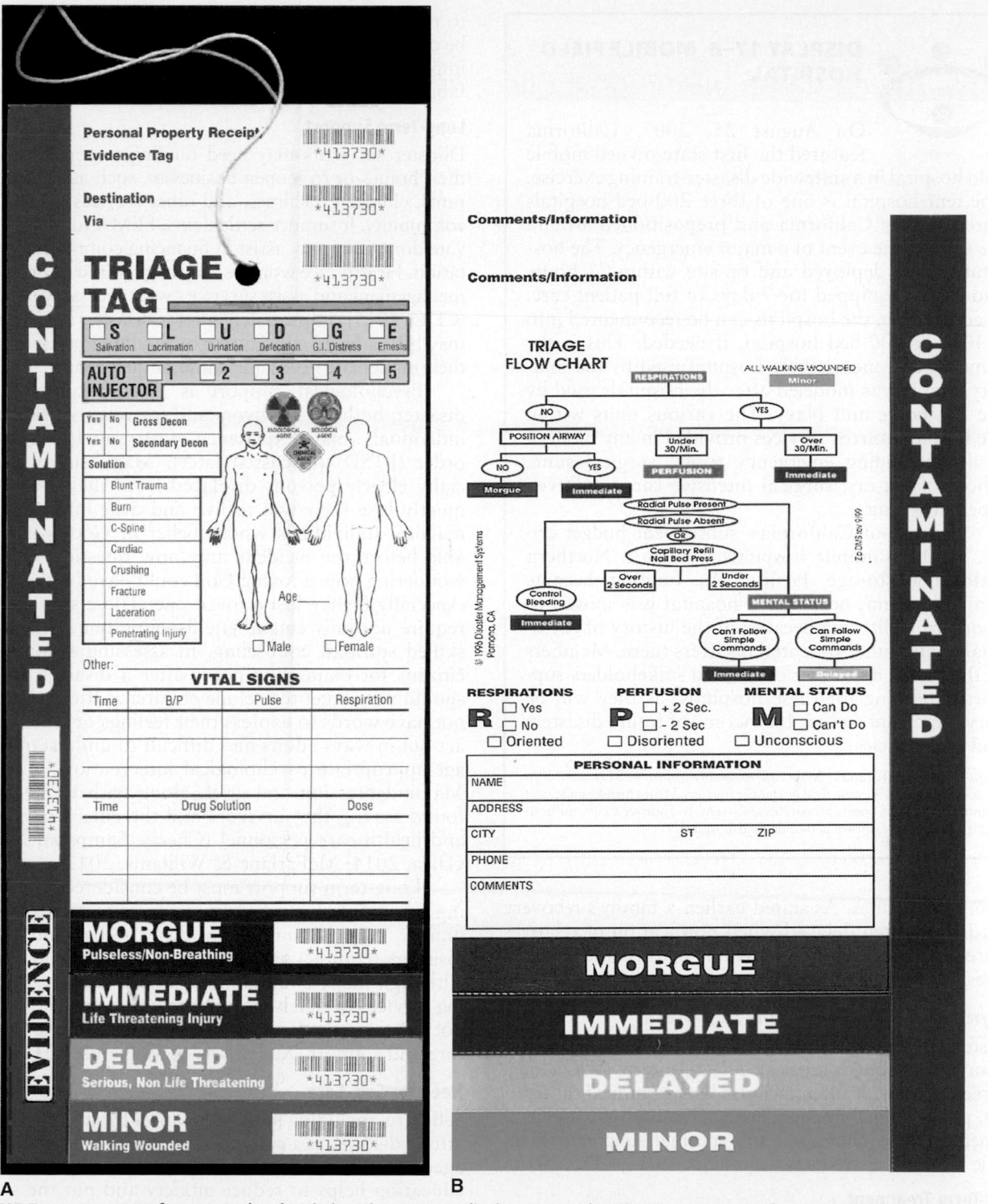

A   **B**

FIGURE 17–6   A and B. Example of a victim triage tag. Radio frequency identification (RFID) technology may be used, so that victim tags (barcodes) may be scanned with RFID readers in order to reduce triage time and provide better tracking of incident casualties. Four basic categories are applied when a medical system is overwhelmed with persons impacted by the incident: (1) *Red*: Urgent/Critical. Victims in this category have injuries or medical problems that will likely lead to death if not treated immediately (e.g., an unconscious victim with signs of internal bleeding). (2) *Yellow*: Delayed. Victims in this category have injuries that will require medical attention; however, time to medical treatment is not yet critical (e.g., a conscious victim with a fractured femur). (3) *Green*: Minor/Walking Wounded. Victims in this category have sustained minor injury or are presenting with minimal signs of illness. Prolonged delay in care most likely will not adversely affect their long-term outcome (e.g., a conscious victim with superficial cuts, scrapes, and bruises). (4) *Black*: Dead/Nonsalvageable. Victims in this category are obviously dead or have suffered mortal wounds because of which death is imminent (e.g., an unconscious victim with an open skull fracture with brain matter showing). Lifesaving heroics on this group of victims will only delay medical care on more viable victims. (From the U.S. Department of Homeland Security. (2013). *System assessment and validation for emergency responders (SAVER)*. Retrieved from https://upload.wikimedia.org/wikipedia/commons/9/97/Deconference-2002-triage-tag.jpg)

DISPLAY 17–6 MOBILE FIELD HOSPITAL

On August 25, 2007, California featured the first state-owned mobile field hospital in a statewide disaster-training exercise. The tent hospital is one of three 200-bed hospitals purchased by California and prepositioned around the state in the event of a major emergency. The hospital can be deployed and on-site within 72 hours and comes equipped for 7 days of full patient care. Used together, the hospitals can be reconfigured into a 400- or 600-bed hospital, if needed. This is the same type of mobile field hospital used by the military, and it was modeled after the hospitals used by the Air Force and Navy. The various units within the hospital mirror services provided in any modern facility including emergency room, surgical suite, laboratory, x-ray, surgical intensive care, and even a pediatric unit.

Because of California's subsequent budget crisis, all three mobile hospitals were in a Northern California storage facility. As funding became available again, one mobile hospital was moved to Southern California because of the history of earthquakes and other potential disasters there. Members of the public and other concerned stakeholders supported funding for these hospitals, as they will be very important to care for victims of future disasters and emergencies.

From Rodriguez, F. (2014, May 28). *Assembly approves $1.9 million to restore California's mobile field hospitals*. Retrieved from http://asmdc.org/members/a52/news-room/press-releases/assembly-approves-1-96-million-dollars-to-restore-californias-mobile-field-hospitals

---

missing loved ones. As stated earlier, a family's recovery from loss is often delayed when notification of relatives (indirectly impacted) is not possible because the persons' bodies are badly damaged or not found.

Supporting Recovery from Disasters

Disasters do not suddenly end when the rubble is cleared and the survivors' wounds are healed. Rather, recovery is a long, complex process. It often includes long-term medical treatment, physical rehabilitation, financial restitution, case management, and psychological and spiritual support (APHN Public Health Preparedness Committee, 2013; CDC, 2015).

Long-Term Treatment

Long-term treatment may be required for many survivors of disasters, straining the local rehabilitative care facilities and resources. Children who are survivors may have to deal with lifelong disabilities or scars from their ordeal, and families may be without adequate financial support for their child's medical care. Elderly citizens who had been in excellent health but who sustained serious injuries in the disaster might suddenly find that they can no longer live independently and must move to a long-term care facility. After floods, landslides, fires, or earthquakes, extensive property damage may cause some residents or businesses

to relocate rather than rebuild on land they now deem to be disaster prone. A disaster that creates numerous persons impacted in a small community may alter the entire social fabric of that community permanently.

Long-Term Support

Disaster survivors may need funding to repair or rebuild their homes or to reopen businesses, such as stores, restaurants, childcare facilities, and other services needed by the community. Insurance settlements, FEMA funding, and private donations may assist in financing community rehabilitation. Health care workers may be required to provide case management and assist survivors with necessary paperwork (CDC, 2015). Immediately after a disaster, some survivors may be unable to concentrate on anything beyond fulfilling their immediate needs and those of their family.

Psychological support is often required after a disaster, both for survivors and for relief workers. Some individuals may experience posttraumatic stress disorder (PTSD) (discussed later). Many survivors, especially elderly persons displaced from their homes, may quietly lose their will to live and drift into apathy and malaise. Individuals whose belief in God was unshakable before the incident may now question their faith, wondering how a loving God could have let this happen, especially if they lost a loved one. These survivors often require not only empathetic listening but also long-term skilled spiritual counseling. In assessing a community's citizens for counseling needs after a disaster, the nurse should not forget to include children. Often, children do not have words to express their feelings or fears and may act out in ways adults find difficult to understand, unless age-appropriate psychological intervention is provided. Major depression and grief, along with PTSD, may be found among the survivors and the emergency workers and health care personnel (Cherry, Sampson, Nezat, & Galea, 2014; McFarlane & Williams, 2012).

Long-term support must be considered when assessing a community and planning for disasters. Each community may be unique in their needs, and different disasters require a unique array of services and planning. Although many communities may be efficient in providing services in quick response to a disaster, they often do not factor in the long-term needs and provide the structure and support (McFarlane & Williams, 2012).

Need for Self-Care

Self-care, including stress education for all relief workers after a disaster, is a common practice and actively encouraged in many communities. Proponents report that stress education helps to reduce anxiety and put the situation into proper perspective. **Critical incident stress debriefing (CISD)** provides relief workers with professional debriefing in small groups or individually and becomes a mechanism for emotional reconciliation (Davis, 2013). CISD is generally provided between 24 and 72 hours after the disaster event. Proponents of CISD claim that it typically produces positive effects by:

- Accelerating the healing process
- Equipping participants with positive coping mechanisms
- Clearing up misconceptions and misunderstandings

- Restoring or reinforcing group cohesiveness
- Promoting a healthy, supportive work atmosphere
- Identifying individuals who require more extensive psychological assistance

A CISD addresses all components of the human response to trauma, including physiologic effects, emotions, and cognition (Pack, 2012). The research on CISD has been mixed, but Mitchell (n.d.) reports that if the personnel providing the intervention are well trained and follow acceptable CISD practice standards, the outcomes are more positive. Based on the conflicting research studies, nurses should be cautious about CISD, but should also be knowledgeable about it because it is so prevalent following a disaster. It can take years to end a popular practice even when it has been shown to be ineffective.

Self-care comes in many forms and is part of a prescription for emotional healing after a traumatic event. Self-care is not just for rescue workers; it is for everyone touched by trauma (Wall, 2012).

Psychological Consequences of Disasters

In addition to physical injury, potential loss of life, and destruction of property that can occur from a disaster, people affected by the disaster can also suffer from psychological consequences, such as acute stress disorder, depression, and PTSD (Cherry et al., 2014). The community health and community mental health nurses, through education, screening, assessment, and referral, have an important role in the primary, secondary, and tertiary prevention of psychological disturbances due to a disaster.

Primary Prevention

Although a disaster, by its very nature, is often unforeseen, people's ability to cope with the disaster can be determined in part by their previous level of coping and the resources available to help them. Stuart (2012) explains that primary prevention in behavioral health care has two basic objectives:

- To help people avoid stressors or cope with them more adaptively
- To change the resources, policies, or agents of the environment so that they no longer cause stress but rather enhance people's functioning

A community health nurse can engage in many activities to promote mental health and strengthen adaptive coping skills in individuals and the community. She or he can teach health education classes in positive stress adaptation, positive ways of coping, self-efficacy, and **resilience**, an important quality that enables people to cope with disaster. The American Psychological Association (2016) describes resilience as a process of behaviors, thoughts, and actions. The term resilience describes the personal and community qualities that enable us to rebound from adversity, trauma, tragedy, threats, or other stresses—and to go on with life with a sense of mastery, competence, and hope. We now understand from research that resilience can be a protective asset that may reduce the risk of mental health conditions (Mayo Clinic, n.d.). The building of competency or resilience is an important primary prevention strategy, since a competent person or

community can make informed decisions based on availability of resources and problem-solving skills. Boscarino, Hoffman, Pitcavage, and Urosevich (2015) noted the importance of the mental health team's alertness for psychological trauma behaviors after any type of disaster.

Community health nurses can contribute to primary prevention in the face of disaster by being active advocates for improving the social structure of the community, including housing, work, schools, child care, and economic conditions for community members. At a time when governments are reducing spending and services, it is important for the community health nurse to advocate for the resources necessary for the community to meet both the physical and psychological challenges of a disaster. Community disaster training must include information on resiliency and resources to support individual and community resilience (APHN Public Health Preparedness Committee, 2013).

Secondary Prevention

Despite community education and intervention, people involved in a disaster often feel anxious and overwhelmed. They are in a *mental health crisis*, defined as a state when people's usual coping mechanisms no longer are effective in the face of the overwhelming disaster (Stuart, 2012). A crisis or disaster, an event that is out of the ordinary in magnitude and personal experience, is called an *adventitious crisis*. Examples of adventitious crises are natural disasters, such as floods, earthquakes, and fires, and national disasters such as terrorist attacks, war, riots, mass shootings, and airplane crashes (Varcarolis & Halter, 2014). When the stress of these disasters causes overwhelming anxiety, *crisis intervention* is a secondary prevention intervention that the trained community health or community mental health nurse can employ to minimize the psychological consequences of the disaster (American Psychiatric Association, 2016).

Crisis intervention is a short-term intervention, no longer than 6 weeks, designed to return an individual or community to its predisaster level of functioning and solve immediate psychological problems. Interventions are provided on several levels: environmental manipulation, general support, generic approach, and the individual approach (Stuart, 2012). *Environmental manipulation* results in the change of a person's physical or interpersonal situation, providing situational support to relieve stress. An example of environmental manipulation is when a community health nurse coordinates the reunification of family members separated by the disaster. *General support* is defined as the caring, warmth, and concern the community health nurse conveys to the client as he or she delivers services (Stuart, 2012).

The *generic approach* is an aspect of crisis intervention that is particularly well suited to the community health nurse. This approach is designed to reach high-risk individuals and large groups who have experienced the same disaster, teaching them about the expected emotional reactions to the type of disaster they have experienced and promoting adaptive responses. Grief reactions follow a known pattern, and large groups can be taught what to expect in the face of severe loss while giving individual members of the group an opportunity to express their feelings of loss. This generic approach is sometimes called *debriefing*. Individual crisis intervention is reserved for high-risk individuals who need special treatment because of the severity of their symptoms and is best provided by nurses trained in mental health treatment and crisis intervention (Stuart, 2012).

Tertiary Prevention

People who have experienced or witnessed a disaster and have been unable to adequately cope with its consequences can develop long-term effects, such as *acute stress disorder* or **posttraumatic stress disorder (PTSD)**. According to the fifth edition of *Diagnostic and Statistical Manual of Mental Disorders* (DSM-5), text revision (American Psychiatric Association, 2013), both acute stress disorder and PTSD can occur after any traumatic event to which a person responds with intense fear, helplessness, or horror; this may be an actual or threatened death or serious injury to oneself or others. Both natural and man-made disasters fit into this definition.

The DSM-5 (American Psychiatric Association, 2013) defines PTSD more clearly as a traumatic or stress-related disorder activated by exposure to actual or threatened death or serious injury or social violation. The new diagnostic criteria includes "history of exposure to a traumatic event that meets specific stipulations and symptoms from each of four symptom clusters: intrusion, avoidance, negative alterations in cognitions and mood, and alterations in arousal and reactivity. The sixth criterion concerns duration of symptoms; the seventh assesses functioning; and, the eighth criterion clarifies symptoms as not attributable to a substance or co-occurring medical condition" (U.S. Department of Veterans Affairs, 2015, p. 3). It is important for the community health nurse to be aware of the symptoms of these disorders so that she or he can refer the client for treatment to the advanced practice mental health nurse and other mental health professionals.

TERRORISM AND WARS

At the start of the 21st century, the world is a global community. This is particularly evident with the increased incidence and sophistication of terrorist threats and acts around the world. Incidents occurring on U.S. soil, such as the initial bombing of the World Trade Center in 1993 and its destruction on September 11, 2001, alerted us to our vulnerability and dramatically emphasized the need for increased preparedness within our communities.

The July 2005 bombings in London that struck multiple transportation system sites and killed 56 while injuring over 700; the February 2008 bombings in Baghdad, by remotely controlled bombs carried by two mentally disabled women, that killed 98 and wounded 200; and the 2007 bombings in Karachi, Pakistan, that killed 136 and injured 387 all confirm that our vulnerability exists in many areas of the world. The Paris, France, and San Bernardino, California, terrorist attacks, mentioned earlier, also remind us of the global scope of this problem. Biologic, chemical, and nuclear terror attacks are tragically possible.

History of Terrorism

The U.S. Federal Bureau of Investigation (FBI, n.d.) has defined **terrorism** in three ways—international terrorism, domestic terrorism, and the federal crime of terrorism.

Generally, these involve dangerous acts, violating laws, and are injurious to human life. They also involve a type of coercion or intimidation that affects government (U.S. Department of Justice, 2011). A terrorist is overzealous and obsessed with an idea. Terrorism and terrorist acts are not new. The term *terrorism* can be traced to 1798, and the use of terrorist tactics precedes this date. A highly organized religious sect called the *Sicarii* attacked crowds of people with knives during holiday celebrations in Palestine at about the time of Christ. During the French and Indian War of 1763, British forces gave smallpox-contaminated blankets to Native Americans. During World War I, the German bioweapons program developed anthrax, glanders, cholera, and wheat fungus as weapons targeting cavalry animals. In World War II, the Japanese tested biologic weapons on Chinese prisoners, and the Nazi's conducted medical experiments with Jews forced into concentration camps (Spendlove & Simonsen, 2013).

Bioterrorism, Nuclear, and Chemical Warfare

Three major countries operated offensive bioweapons programs in recent years: the United Kingdom until 1957, the United States until 1969, and the former Soviet Union until 1990. Iraq started its bioweapons program in 1985 and continued to develop weapons until 2003. Bioweapons include mustard gas, sarin, and VX gas, as well as anthrax (Spendlove & Simonsen, 2013). Terrorists typically use biologic or chemical agents, explosives, or incendiary devices to deliver the agents to their targets.

Nuclear warfare involves the use of nuclear devices as weapons and can take several forms. Terrorists who gain access to nuclear power plants could cause a chain of events that lead to a meltdown of the nuclear core, thereby releasing radioactive particles for hundreds of miles around the site. Nuclear accidents have occurred, but no known terrorist attacks have yet involved the use of nuclear power plants as weapons (Spendlove & Simonsen, 2013). A terrorist attack using nuclear weapons or destruction of a nuclear plant would cause multiple and prolonged deaths with extensive damage and negative effects for decades.

Chemical warfare involves the use of chemicals such as explosives, nerve agents, blister agents, choking agents, and incapacitating or riot-control agents to cause confusion, debilitation, death, and destruction. Sarin and chlorine have been used most recently in Syria. They may be known as the "poor man's bomb" because of them being relatively inexpensive to create (Esfandiary, 2014, p. 1). Terrorists in the Middle East, willing to murder others and knowing they will be committing suicide, strap bombs to their bodies and detonate the explosives in or near targets. Others plant explosives at large outdoor events like the 2013 Boston Marathon (CNN Library, 2015) or crash vehicles loaded with explosives into crowds of people or into a building.

The aircraft used on September 11, 2001, were incendiary devices because they were carrying thousands of tons of jet fuel. The success of the mission depended on the surprise of the attack, severe damage to recognizable buildings, and the deaths of many people. Disaster responders and government officials did not expect the collapse of the buildings. If the planes had been low on fuel, the damage would have been less severe. The liquid fuel burned at such a high temperature that the internal structures of the buildings were weakened (National Institute of Standards and Technology, 2008).

Biologic warfare involves using biologic agents to cause multiple illnesses and deaths. Biological agents are graded as category A, B, or C by the CDC (see Table 17–2). Typical biologic agents are anthrax, botulinum, bubonic plague, Ebola, and smallpox. These agents could be used to contaminate food, water, or air. Deliberate food and water contamination remains the easiest way to distribute biologic agents for the purpose of terrorism (American Academy of Pediatrics, 2015; CDC, 2011).

The United States is very concerned about the possibility of biologic warfare or bioterrorism, as nations should be. The anthrax infections and deaths that occurred after September 11, 2001, added to these concerns. It was years before the government investigation led to a scientist at Fort Detrick as the cause of this terroristic act. Although charges were never filed because of the individual's suicide, the FBI

Table 17–2 Categories of Biologic Agents

Category	Definition	Agents/Diseases
Category A	• Pose highest risk to national security/public health: • Can be easily disseminated or transmitted from person to person • Result in high mortality rates and have the potential for major public health impact • Might cause public panic and social disruption • Require special action for public health preparedness	• Anthrax (*Bacillus anthracis*) • Botulism (*Clostridium botulinum* toxin) • Plague (*Yersinia pestis*) • Smallpox (variola major) and other pox viruses • Tularemia (*Francisella tularensis*) • Viral hemorrhagic fevers Arenaviruses (e.g., Lassas, Junin) Bunyaviruses (e.g., Hantaviruses) Flaviviruses (Dengue) Filoviruses (e.g., Ebola, Marburg)
Category B	• Second highest risk to national security: • Are moderately easy to disseminate • Result in moderate morbidity rates and low mortality rates • Require specific enhancements of CDC's diagnostic capacity and enhanced disease surveillance	• Q fever (*Coxiella burnetii*) • Brucellosis (*Brucella* species) • Melioidosis (*Burkholderia pseudomallei*) • Psittacosis (*Chlamydia psittaci*) • Ricin toxin (*Ricinus communis*) • Epsilon toxin of *Clostridium perfringens* • *Staphylococcus* enterotoxin B (SEB) • Typhus fever (*Rickettsia prowazekii*) • *Food and waterborne pathogens:* *Bacteria* (e.g., Diarrheagenic *E. coli*, Pathogenic Vibrios, Shigella species, salmonella, *Listeria monocytogenes*, *Campylobacter jejuni*, *Yersinia enterocolitica*) *Viruses*: (e.g., Calicviruses, Hepatitis A) *Protozoa*: (e.g., *Cryptosporidium parvum*, *Cyclospora cayetanensis*, *Giardia lamblia*, *Entamoeba histolytica*, *Toxoplasma gondii*, *Naegleria fowleri*, *Balamuthia mandrillaris*) *Fungi*: (Microsporidia) *Mosquito-borne encephalitis viruses*: (e.g., West Nile virus, LaCrosse/California encephalitis, Venezuelan/Eastern/Western equine encephalitis, Japanese/St. Louis encephalitis virus)
Category C	• Third highest priority agents include emerging pathogens that could be engineered for mass dissemination in the future because of: • Availability • Ease of production and dissemination • Potential for high morbidity and mortality rates and major health impact	• Nipah and Hendra viruses • Additional hantaviruses • Tick-borne hemorrhagic fever viruses • Tick-borne encephalitis complex flaviviruses • Yellow fever virus • Tuberculosis, including drug-resistant TB • Influenza virus • Other Rickettsias • Rabies virus • Prions • Chikungunya virus • Coccidioides spp. • SARS or MERS corona viruses • Antimicrobial resistance

From The U.S. Department of Health and Human Services, National Institute of Allergy and Infectious Disease. (2016). *NAIAD emerging infectious disease/pathogens: Category A, B, and C priority pathogens.* Retrieved from https://www.niaid.nih.gov/topics/biodefenserelated/biodefense/pages/cata.aspx.

believes that he was solely responsible for this act of domestic terrorism (FBI, 2008). Regardless of the source of terrorism, the outcomes are the same: fear, death, and destruction.

The Trauma of Warfare

Nurses, or men and women acting in that capacity, have provided comfort and care to soldiers long before Florence Nightingale arrived in the Crimea during the mid-19th century (see Chapter 2). Nurses helped during the Civil War and were part of the armed services during both World Wars; their influence has expanded with other conflicts and continues today (Brooks & Hallett, 2015; Judd & Sitzman, 2014). Military nurses often saw and experienced many sad and traumatic events. Nurses who have served in the military are themselves veterans and may experience some of the effects of this trauma long after their service (Aloi, 2011). Amputations, head injuries, and other physical problems are common in war. For Iraq and Afghanistan veterans, those who had early amputations had better psychological and physical outcomes than those who waited and had later amputations (Melcer, Sechriest, Walker, & Galarneau, 2013). For all combat veterans, the trauma of warfare can be devastating and may continue to affect them for many years after their active service (Magruder et al., 2016). Exposure to new traumatic events can cause additional problems for them (Hamblen & Sione, 2015). Studies have shown that many years after the close of the Vietnam conflict, PTSD prevalence for those over age 60 was close to 17% (Goldberg et al., 2016). It is estimated that about 271,000 Vietnam veterans (both men and women) currently suffer from PTSD, and about 33% have major depressive symptoms (Marmar et al., 2015). Others have noted that PTSD among this population of veterans is a risk factor for coronary heart disease (Vaccarino et al., 2013). Community health nurses should be aware of the needs of veterans, especially during disasters, terrorist attacks, and other traumatic events that may bring these past experiences to the forefront again. It is also important to know about services available to veterans and treatments that are effective (Jain et al., 2016). See From the Case Files II.

Factors Contributing to Terrorism

Political factors are the most common contributors to terrorism. Anti-American sentiment runs high in many foreign countries, especially those that perceive the United States as a threat to their military, economic, social, or religious self-determination. Terrorist acts against American military installations abroad, in airports, in airplanes, at American embassies, and even on American soil targeting civilian populations have occurred frequently in the last decade as an expression of political unrest. The war in Iraq in 2003 was based on information about suspected bioterrorism weapons and reports that Iraq was harboring anti-Western terrorists; these two pieces of information resulted in the toppling of the Saddam Hussein political regime. However, hundreds of military lives were lost and many thousands of civilians were killed, and no weapons of mass destruction were found. As of February 2016, more than 6,881 U.S. military and civilian personnel have lost their lives during conflicts in the Middle East. There have been 2,215 killed

---

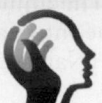

From the **Case Files** II

Missed Opportunities for an Older Veteran

Tom Walton is a 70-year-old retired salesperson from an equipment manufacturer and a Vietnam veteran who served in the U.S. Navy. He has been a widower for the past year, and his adult children live out-of-state. Tom's health has declined dramatically since his wife's death, and he is struggling to control his hypertension and diabetes. Tom is noncompliant with medications and diet restrictions, and he seems to have more frequent outbursts of anger than usual.

Sadly, Tom's case is not one that is rare or unusual. I work at a Veterans Administration (VA) clinic, and I often see cases like Tom's in our clinic. Many veterans do not deal with the traumas they experienced during warfare, and when support systems are weakened or they are no longer busy with work and family, these long-repressed feelings begin to reemerge. For Tom, his case could easily result in a deteriorating health care spiral that will ultimately lead to multiple hospitalizations or his demise. But, as a veteran, Tom may be a candidate for posttraumatic stress disorder (PTSD) treatment, mental health care treatment programs, or other proven treatment modalities offered by the VA. Unfortunately, many of our nation's veterans fail to take advantage of this resource or even acknowledge that they may have this type of problem. In this case, having a working knowledge of the resources available to veterans in your community provides an opportunity for you, as a public health nurse, to assist Tom in accessing services that meet his health care needs and may prolong his life.

—Bryan, VA Clinic Manager

---

in Afghanistan and 4,411 killed in Iraq (U.S. Department of Defense, 2016a). Many more have been wounded—to date, over 22,229 in Iraq (U.S. Department of Defense, 2016b). Additionally, there have been approximately 165,000 Iraqi civilian deaths due to "direct war-related violence" since the beginning of Operation Iraqi Freedom through 2015 (Watson Institute for International & Public Affairs, 2015, p. 1).

Within the United States, violence-prone members of militia movements, violent antiabortion activists, racial desegregation advocates, and other radical groups have committed terrorist acts, such as the bombing of health clinics offering abortions and bombings and shootings at Black churches. The variety of methods used is raising the level of fear in everyday lives of the average American citizen (Galhotra, 2012).

Role of the Community Health Nurse

Community health nurses need to be prepared for the possibility of terrorist activity. They have a role in primary, secondary, and tertiary prevention.

Primary Prevention

Community health nurses are in ideal situations within communities to participate in surveillance. They must look and listen within their communities for antigroup sentiments, for example, antireligion, antigay, or anti-ethnic feelings. The nurse should report any untoward activities accordingly.

Nurses should be alert to signs of possible terrorist activity. Specific indicators of possible chemical or biologic terrorism include unusual numbers of dead or dying animals; unexplained serious illnesses or deaths; an unusual liquid, spray, vapor, or odor; and low-lying clouds or fog unrelated to weather. Unusual swarms of insects might also indicate the use of biologic agents for terrorism. "It is imperative that each nurse acquire a knowledge base and minimum set of skills to enable them to plan for and respond to a disaster in a timely and appropriate manner" (Veenema, 2013, p. 17). Cox (2008), in a seminal article, presents a historical overview of terrorism and relating these to the current state of affairs that have become increasingly concerning for our government agencies as well as citizens. In addition, recommendations for pre- and postdisaster planning to include critical, specific nursing competencies and evidence-based practices are provided. The American Nurses Association (2016) has developed policies, resources, and educational opportunities for nurses on disaster preparedness acknowledging the importance of nurse preparation before a critical event (Fig. 17–7).

Secondary and Tertiary Prevention

Although prevention of terrorist incidents is primarily the responsibility of the Department of Defense, the DHS, and public health and law enforcement agencies, community health nurses must be ready to handle the secondary and tertiary effects of such attacks. Knowing the lethal and incapacitating chemical, biological, and radiological weapons that may be used by terrorists is important. Many of the communicable disease organisms that could be used by terrorists were discussed in Chapter 8.

Realizing that terrorist attacks may result in large numbers of casualties, the public health nurse must be prepared to act safely, access information rapidly, and use resources effectively. Specifically, the community health nurse may be called on to provide direct care to survivors, to volunteer as a hospital–community liaison, to set up and administer mass immunizations, to support shelters, to make home visits to affected families, to establish a case management system for survivors, or to serve on committees responding to terrorist acts. Formulating, updating, and following a disaster plan is one of the most effective community-based strategies to minimize injury and mortality from terrorism. However, recent survey research among working nurses and nursing students found that most participants were not very confident in their abilities related to disasters or managing violent or serious events. Prior experience with disasters and those who worked in emergency departments, especially during night shifts, resulted in higher scores on measures of disaster nursing competence (Baack & Alfred, 2013; Nilsson et al., 2015).

Most community health nurses will not be on the front line of uncovering or immediately responding to terrorist activities, but their skills will be needed with groups, families, or individuals who experience a terrorist-related event. Some of the activities listed earlier in this chapter to help people deal with the aftermath of a disaster would also be appropriate if terrorism is the cause of the disaster. In addition, community health nurses may work with people who need help coping or who want to do something to help. After experiencing a traumatic event such as a terrorist attack, people do not know how to cope. We are warned to expect more attacks. We are told to be vigilant. The terror we are fighting is often our own. This is a new experience for most people, and assistance from the community health nurse can help them cope effectively. Smith and Segal (2016) offer advice for those affected by traumatic events, such as disasters:

- Feeling scared, anxious, and worried about the future are common reactions to this type of stress.
- Deal with these feelings by taking care of yourself (acknowledge them, be patient with yourself, feel them without guilt or shame, try to reduce stress/promote relaxation and sleep, seek help).
- Recognize that people react to disasters and traumas in very different ways.
- Be aware of repetitive, obsessive thoughts about the incident and try to deflect them or find something to do that engages your mind in other ways (e.g., reading, watching a movie, visiting with family/friends).
- Understand that you will need to deal with your feelings and emotions regarding the event and that permitting yourself to feel these emotions will help you in the healing process.
- Talking about the experience, like dealing with your emotions, is also healing, as is expressing them through art or writing a journal.
- Seek comfort and support by establishing a routine, connecting with others, and challenging your sense of helplessness (e.g., comforting others, donating blood).
- Try to minimize your family's extended exposure to media coverage of the event (this is especially true for children).
- Provide support for children and opportunities for them to talk about the incident and their feelings and concerns.

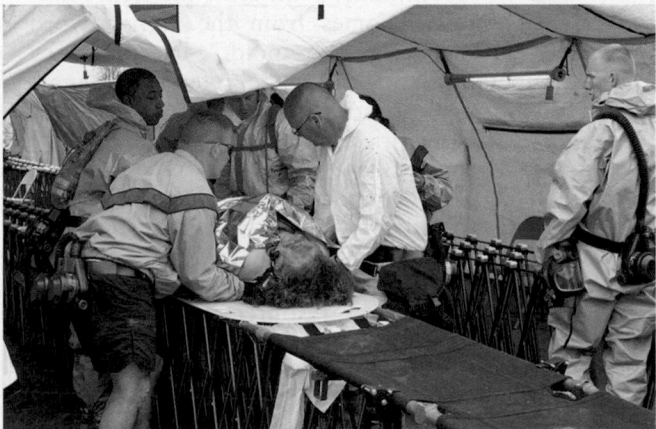

FIGURE 17–7   Disaster drills help prepare communities and health care workers.

DISPLAY 17–7 POPULATION FOCUS ON DISASTERS: USING A TABLETOP EXERCISE TO PLAN FOR POPULATION CARE

A tabletop exercise is an interactive drill typically used by emergency planners and responders. It is designed to allow personnel to gather in a semiformal setting, so that they can participate in open discussions regarding their role in the event of an emergency situation in their community. Participants typically assume their own role, but may be required to assume other key positions. A simulated disaster/emergency event that affects their population is used, called the *scenario*. A facilitator keeps participants on track with their scripts and any accompanying videos or other media. This type of activity:

- Does not require complete plans and procedures
- Allows for practice in coordinated emergency problem-solving
- Permits brainstorming gaps and discussion of response capabilities and plans
- Prepares personnel for larger, more costly exercises (i.e., mass-casualty exercises)
- Helps multidisciplinary teams to plan for services affecting their entire community, with attention given to specific vulnerable populations who are at risk

From the Federal Emergency Management Agency (FEMA). (2015). *Emergency planning exercises.* Retrieved from https://www.fema.gov/emergency-planning-exercises

---

Community health nurses can make major differences in grassroots efforts to bring about change, but on a day-to-day basis, the little things they say and do with peers and clients can make just as big a difference. For example, providing information on foods to avoid and nonmedical treatment options such as support groups, hypnosis, and biofeedback are a few examples of how nurses can assist with coping mechanisms.

Current and Future Opportunities

There are many ways in which nurses, especially nursing students, can prepare themselves both personally and professionally for emergency events in their own communities. Various governmental and educational programs have been developed to provide free online training covering a broad range of topics. A summary of some of those training opportunities is provided in Display 17–4. For the novice nurse, or nursing student, an important issue is your role, if any, in your local response plan. Many schools of nursing have now begun to formalize their emergency preparedness plans in coordination with local hospitals, public health departments, or faith institutions. Take some time to discuss with your faculty what role you have in the event of a local emergency. If no organized plan exists, then perhaps you can work with the nursing faculty or your local student nurses association to prepare one (Halstead, 2013).

Knowing your role in an emergency will give you the peace of mind of knowing where you should go and what you are expected to do. Doing a little extra work by completing some of the online courses listed will help you to feel more involved and less fearful if the unimaginable were to happen. FEMA offers four particular courses within the incident command system (ICS 100, ICS 200, IS 700, & IS 800B); these are recommended for all health care personnel. Students who are also employed at local hospitals as interns or salaried employees should find out what role they have in the hospital's emergency plan. Finally, make sure you have a family plan to reconnect with and care for children, spouses, and parents.

Increasingly, communities are conducting emergency preparedness exercises (e.g., mass-casualty exercises and tabletop exercises; see Display 17–7) in response to the need to prepare local resources to coordinate emergency response efforts for maximum effectiveness (CDC, 2016). As a student, you may be asked to participate in one of these exercises as a "victim." Take the opportunity; the knowledge you gain from this experience will enhance your understanding of the process, and you may be able to help identify gaps in services or areas in need of improvement. With your expertise in nursing, you are a much greater asset to the exercise than untrained individuals. You may be asked to have **moulage** applied to simulate injuries, and you will likely be given a brief description of your trauma (see Display 17–8 and Fig. 17–8). Your assigned health problem may be emotional and

DISPLAY 17–8 WHAT IS MOULAGE?

Pronounced *mü-läzh*, the term *moulage* comes from the French word *mouler*, which means "to mold." In emergency preparedness training, moulage refers to the art of applying mock injuries for use in mass-casualty exercises. These injuries can be very simple or more complex, depending on available resources and the skills of the person applying the moulage. The use of moulage typically provides a more realistic experience for personnel participating in mass-casualty exercises.

Of the many online resources for information regarding equipment needed and how-to advice, one such Web site is Community Emergency Response Team (CERT) Los Angeles: *Step-by-Step Moulage Instructions* at http://www.cert-la.com/education/moulage.htm

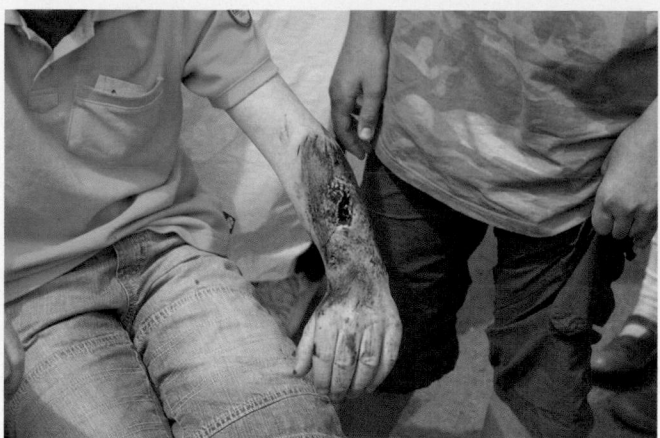

FIGURE 17–8 Moulage is often used to provide a more realistic experience for health care workers and "victims."

not physical, allowing you utilize your understanding of behavioral health issues and crisis intervention. Whatever your capacity, the experience will provide as close to a realistic event as possible. Just as immunizations help fight against infections, participating in an emergency preparedness drill can build your tolerance for responding appropriately in a real event.

Many organizations, both private and governmental, are seeking volunteers. As a student, you have more limited options; however, two major opportunities are available to you. Both require initial and ongoing training, but if you wish to become more active in emergency preparedness volunteer efforts, the American Red Cross and your local Medical Reserve Corps are two options. You can continue your relationship with these organizations after you receive your nursing license, and your role with them will likely evolve.

With your registered nurse license in hand, many more options are open to you. Each state is developing plans for a database of licensed health care providers who may be willing to volunteer in the event of local, state, or national emergencies. The exact criteria being developed for registration by each state may vary slightly, but as a licensed health care professional you may add your name to the registry along with your specialty training and contact information. Registration does not obligate you to any service; you agree only to be contacted if the need arises. The guidelines for these state-run databases were generated by the U.S. Department of Health and Human Services and can be reviewed in the document *Emergency Systems for Advance Registration of Volunteer Health Professionals* (ESAR-VHP; USDHHS, 2011). The professional volunteer registry in Wisconsin is named WEAVR (*Wisconsin Emergency Assistance Volunteer Registry*). Using similar guidelines, California launched its version of the registry (*Disaster Healthcare Volunteers*). Mississippi has the *Volunteers in Preparedness Registry* (VIPR), and Arkansas nurses can register with the *Arkansas Volunteer Registry*. Check with your state's office of emergency preparedness and response for the link to your particular registry or information on availability.

As you progress in your career, many other high-intensity efforts are available for your involvement. At both the national and state level are DMAT, groups of highly trained health professionals who can rapidly respond to emergencies within a state or nationally. The DMATs operate as part of the National Disaster Medical System (NDMS). Each DMAT has a sponsoring organization (i.e., major medical center, public health agency, nonprofit organization). Check to see if your organization has sponsored a DMAT; if so, you might want to interview one of the members to learn more about his training and experiences (Murray, 2012).

The APHN Public Health Preparedness Committee (2013) position paper, *The Role of the Public Health Nurse in Disaster, Preparedness, Response, and Recovery*, is based on the earlier work of Jakeway, LaRosa, Cary, Schoenfisch, and Association of State and Territorial Directors of Nursing (2008). They developed specific core competencies for public health nurses related to emergency preparedness, and these can serve as a guide for students and practicing public health nurses. These include the following:

1. Describe the public health role in responding to a range of likely emergencies.
2. Describe the agency's chain of command in emergency response.
3. Identify and locate the agency's emergency response plan.
4. Describe one's functional roles and responsibilities in emergency response and demonstrate those roles in regular drills.
5. Demonstrate the correct use of equipment (including personal protective equipment) and the skills required in emergency response during regular drills.
6. Demonstrate the correct use of all equipment used for emergency communication.
7. Describe communication role(s) in emergency response.
8. Identify the limits of one's own knowledge, skills, and authority, and identify key system resources for matters that exceed these limits.
9. Apply creative problem-solving skills and flexible thinking to unusual challenges within one's functional responsibilities, and evaluate the effectiveness of all actions taken.
10. Recognize deviations from the norm that might indicate an emergency and describe appropriate action.
11. Participate in continuing education to maintain up-to-date knowledge in areas relevant to emergency response.
12. Participate in planning, exercising, and evaluating drills.

An adapted version of the 2013 position paper's table of disaster phases and corresponding nursing process actions is found in Display 17–9. Many options are available to you as both a student and a practicing nurse. What is important is that you are prepared. Assuring that you understand the role you may assume in the event of a local disaster or emergency situation is critical to your own welfare as well as to your community. You decide your level of participation, but resources are available for you to become as prepared as possible.

DISPLAY 17-9 PHN USE OF THE NURSING PROCESS DURING DISASTERS

Disaster Cycle	Definition	Assessment	Planning	Implementation	Evaluation
PREPAREDNESS	Includes: Prevention, protection, mitigation. What is needed to prevent a disaster or reduce the impact of one (lives lost, property damage)?	Do you have specific populations in your service area that are vulnerable and at risk because of problems with access and functional needs during disaster (e.g., physically/mentally disabled, those with Alzheimer's, frail elderly)? Determine any hazards or threats that pose risks.	Plan for additional assistance and accommodations for those at-risk and vulnerable populations during disasters or other emergencies. Work with other stakeholders to meet their needs and the needs of your service area population (e.g., sheltering in place, evacuation, mass-casualty surge capabilities)	Conduct drills, trainings, and exercises regarding care of individuals, families, and communities during disasters. Focus on at-risk and vulnerable populations you have identified previously (e.g., physically/mentally disabled, those with Alzheimer's, frail elderly).	Evaluate the drills, trainings, and exercises in regards to care of at-risk and vulnerable populations. Identify gaps and any residual needs. Conduct evaluation of operational plans (e.g., preparedness, response, recovery for at-risk and vulnerable populations).
RESPONSE	Includes: Lifesaving. Protection of property. Meeting basic human needs post disaster. What services and personnel are needed to save lives and protect property in a disaster? What services and personnel are needed immediately after the disaster to meet basic needs?	Using population-based triage, assess the impact of any communicable disease outbreak. Who is susceptible? Who has been exposed? Who is infected?	Work with stakeholders to develop or choose triage plans and methods of patient flow based on present symptoms and known history (e.g., COPD).	Work to organize PHNs and other trained personnel to provide care per triage plans. Perform ongoing rapid needs assessments during this phase, and ensure planning for community care support.	During the disaster, take part in continuing response planning and service planning. Ensure that necessary PHN care is provided.
RECOVERY	Includes assistance in recovery after a disaster. What core skills and capacities are needed to ensure effective recovery?	Continue intermittent rapid needs assessment to ascertain health status and capacity for critical resources after the disaster (e.g., floods).	Together with stakeholders, make plans for any identified long-term health concerns, and pinpoint key resources needed for recovery.	Contribute to restoration of critical community services and sustaining the social and health infrastructures. Work to help the community achieve stabilization after the disaster.	Help with evaluation of disaster's long-term impact on the community. Through the work of PHNs, promote essential public health services.

Adapted from the Association of Public Health Nurses, Public Health Preparedness Committee. (2013). *The role of the public health nurse in disaster, preparedness, response, and recovery: A position paper* (2nd ed.). Retrieved from http://www.achne.org/files/public/APHN_RoleOfPHNinDisasterPRR_FINALJan14.pdf.

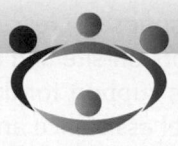

DISPLAY 17–10 *HEALTHY PEOPLE 2020*

PREP-1 (Developmental): Reduce the time necessary to issue official information to the public about a public health emergency.

PREP-2: Reduce the time necessary to activate designated personnel in response to a public health emergency. Baseline indicates that 66 minutes were needed for personnel to report to duty in 2009.

PREP-3: Increase the proportion of Laboratory Response Network (LRN) laboratories that meet proficiency standards.

　PREP 3.1 (Developmental) Proportion of LRN biological laboratories that meet proficiency standards for category A and B threat agents

PREP 3.2 Proportion of LRN chemical laboratories that meet proficiency standards for chemical threat agents

PREP-4: Reduce the time for state public health agencies to establish after action reports and improvement plans following responses to public health emergencies and exercises. Baseline indicates that it took state public health agencies 46 days to establish after action improvement plans in response to a public health emergency in 2009.

From the U.S. Department of Health and Human Services (USDHHS). (2016). *Healthy People 2020 topics & objectives: Preparedness.* Retrieved from https://www.healthypeople.gov/2020/topics-objectives/topic/preparedness/objectives

Healthy People 2020

Healthy People 2010 focused upon increasing quality and years of healthy life and to eliminating health disparities. Formulated in the years before January 2000, many disasters, both natural and man made, had yet to occur. The United States had not yet faced the national failures in the response to the hurricanes Katrina and Rita. We would also learn 18 months after the publication of *Healthy People 2010* that our nation was not immune from acts of terrorism. The objectives of *Healthy People 2020* directly address issues of emergency preparedness and response under the new topic of *Preparedness*.

Additional topics also include preparedness activities, such as the objectives for public health infrastructure. In the ensuing years, many of these objectives will help focus public's attention on health care during a disaster. The goal of the new topics and objectives are to improve our "ability to prevent, prepare for, respond to, and recover from a major health incident" (USDHHS, 2016, p. 1; see Display 17–10). Those specific objectives provide the support needed to enhance public health surveillance activities, laboratories, training, development of professional competencies, and performance standards for public health organizations.

S U M M A R Y

A disaster is any event that causes a level of destruction that exceeds the abilities of the affected community to respond without assistance. Disasters may be caused by natural or man-made/technologic events and may be classified as multiple-casualty incidents or mass-casualty incidents.

The scope of a disaster is its range of effect, and its intensity is the level of destruction it causes. Persons impacted by disasters include those directly impacted (those injured or killed) and indirectly impacted (the loved ones of directly impacted). Displaced persons are those who are forced to flee their homes because of the disaster, and refugees are those who are forced to leave their homelands, usually in response to war or political persecution.

Host factors that contribute to the likelihood of experiencing a disaster include age, general health, mobility, psychological factors, and socioeconomic factors. The disaster agent is the fire, flood, bomb, or other cause. Environmental factors are those that could potentially contribute to or mitigate a disaster.

In developing strategies to address the problem of disasters, it is helpful for the community health nurse to consider each of the four phases of disaster management: prevention, preparedness, response, and recovery.

Primary prevention of disasters means keeping the disaster from ever happening by taking actions to eliminate the possibility of its occurrence. Secondary prevention focuses on earliest possible detection and treatment. Tertiary prevention involves reducing the amount and degree of disability or damage resulting from the disaster.

In addition to assessing for preparedness, an effective disaster plan establishes a clear chain of authority, develops lines of communication, and delineates routes and modes of transport. Plans for mobilizing, warning, and evacuating people are also critical elements of the disaster plan. At the disaster site, police, firefighters, nurses, and other relief workers develop a coordinated response to rescue survivors from further injury, triage survivors by seriousness of injury, and treat survivors on-site and in local hospitals. Care and transport of dead bodies must also be managed, as well as support for the loved ones of the injured, dead, or missing. Long-term support includes both financial assistance and physical and emotional rehabilitation.

Physical injuries resulting from disasters are not the sole consequence; people also suffer psychological trauma that can affect them for life. The importance of prevention, early crisis intervention, and ongoing treatment for those in need is evident. The community health nurse plays a key role in assessing individuals for symptoms of psychological trauma and intervening to prevent long-term consequences. Self-care, including stress education for all relief workers after a disaster, helps to lower anxiety and put the situation into perspective. CISD provides relief workers with a mechanism for emotional reconciliation and healing.

Terrorism is the unlawful use of force or violence against persons or property to intimidate or coerce a government or civilian population in the furtherance of political or social objectives. Terrorism may be nuclear, biologic, or chemical and may involve the use of nerve agents and explosive devices. The community health nurse should be alert to signs of possible terrorist activity and prepared to address the secondary or tertiary effects of such attacks. Preparation includes knowledge of the effects of specific biologic or chemical agents and how to help people cope with the terror they personally feel. Around the world, wars and conflicts are a daily occurrence. Nurses have provided care and comfort in many conflicts. It is important for PHNs to understand both the physical and mental consequences of combat and the other traumatic events associated with conflicts. Many veterans continue to suffer from PTSD and other physical and mental conditions, even years after their participation in combat may have ended.

Many opportunities are available for both student nurses and experienced community health nurses to become involved in emergency preparedness and response efforts. Agencies such as the American Red Cross and the Medical Reserve Corps are options available to students and at a higher level of involvement, once licensed. Natural and man-made disasters are a too frequent occurrence. It is the obligation of all nurses to be involved in emergency preparedness and to seek training that will enable them to provide the best possible service if the unthinkable happens. With the development of *Healthy People 2020*, ongoing efforts to help communities prepare for disasters and emergencies will require more nurses willing and able to respond to a call for action.

ACTIVITIES TO PROMOTE CRITICAL THINKING

1. Think about your own community and its residents. What are some host factors that might increase its risk of experiencing a disaster? What environmental factors might be significant? In each case, identify the likely agent. What interventions could be included in a disaster plan to reduce these risk factors?
2. Current news sources show that at least 200 people have been injured in an explosion in a neighboring community. At the disaster site, survivors are still being recovered from the wreckage, and local hospitals are overwhelmed with patients who have fractures, lacerations, and burns. You want to offer your assistance as a registered nurse. How should you go about volunteering your services?
3. Think about your state and any sites that might be a target of terrorism. What is your state doing to address these issues? Examine Web sites (e.g., U.S. Homeland Security, Centers for Disease Control and Prevention, World Health Organization) for strategic planning or documents that could be helpful in assessing terror threats and preventing attacks. If an attack does occur, what should health professionals do to be most effective?
4. Check with your local and state health department. Are there plans in place for large-scale disasters or terrorist attacks? How often are they updated? Who is involved in the planning?
5. Check with your local hospital about their disaster plan. Do they collaborate with your local health department and other agencies in designing and executing this plan? How often do they hold "disaster drills"? Who is involved in these? How many types of emergency situations do they cover?
6. As a community health nurse practicing in an area with a high concentration of veterans, what knowledge and skills do you think are necessary to provide culturally competent, evidence-based care to this segment of the population? To become more familiar with this population, do the following activities:

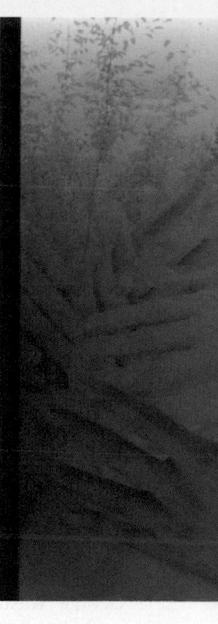

- *Talk to veterans* to find out what is meant by military culture or veteran culture. How does this relate to other aspects of culture for the individual, family, or population group?
- *Contact your state or county Veterans Commission* to find out about the veteran population in your community. In what ways are the members of this population similar, and how might they be different? Consider age, gender, exposure to combat, type of service (regular active duty, guard/reserve duty), physical or mental injury, trauma, sexual orientation, lifestyle, and other factors. Think about how gender plays a role in other areas of diversity for this population. What are some common assumptions about veterans or stereotypes that might impact the way veterans are viewed in the community?
- Access the U.S. Department of Veterans Affairs Public Health Web site to learn more about public health issues for the veteran population (http://www.publichealth.va.gov/PUBLICHEALTH/about/index.asp).

What health risk factors are common among this population? What are the health conditions and the accompanying risk factors and how does the local community address these needs? What facilitating actions or barriers do you see? How do health issues in the veteran population impact the community as a whole, or other individuals within the community? Based on the risks identified for this population, what would you anticipate to be important primary prevention strategies for a community with a large veteran population? What might be the most important health promotion and population health strategies for this community?

REFERENCES

Administration for Children and Families. (n.d.). *Unaccompanied children's services*. Retrieved from http://www.acf.hhs.gov/programs/orr/programs/ucs

Aloi, J. A. (2011). A theoretical study of the hidden wounds of war: Disenfranchised grief and the impact on nursing practice. *International Scholarly Research Notices*, Article ID 954081. Retrieved from http://www.hindawi.com/journals/isrn/2011/954081/

American Academy of Pediatrics. (2015). *Biological terrorism and agents*. Retrieved from https://www.aap.org/en-us/advocacy-and-policy/aap-health-initiatives/Children-and-Disasters/Pages/Biological-Terrorism-and-Agents.aspx

American Nurses Association. (2016). *Disaster preparedness & response*. Retrieved from http://www.nursingworld.org/disasterpreparedness

American Psychiatric Association. (2013). *Posttraumatic stress disorder*. Retrieved from http://www.dsm5.org/Documents/PTSD%20Fact%20Sheet.pdf

American Psychiatric Association. (2016). *What are anxiety disorders?* Retrieved from http://www.psychiatry.org/patients-families/anxiety-disorders/what-are-anxiety-disorders

American Psychiatric Nurses Association. (2016). *Resources for dealing with traumatic events*. Retrieved from http://www.apna.org/i4a/pages/index.cfm?pageid=5196

American Psychological Association. (2016). *The road to resilience*. Retrieved from http://www.apa.org/helpcenter/road-resilience.aspx

American Red Cross. (n.d.). *American Red Cross guide to services*. Retrieved from http://www.redcross.org/images/MEDIA_CustomProductCatalog/m3140117_GuideToServices.pdf

Association of Public Health Nurses (APHN) Public Health Preparedness Committee. (2013). *The role of the public health nurse in disaster preparedness, response, and recovery* (2nd ed.). Retrieved from http://www.achne.org/files/public/APHN_RoleOf PHNinDisasterPRR_FINALJan14.pdf

Baack, S., & Alfred, D. (2013). Nurses' preparedness and perceived competence in managing disasters. *Journal of Nursing Scholarship*, *45*(3), 281–287.

Boscarino, J. A., Hoffman, S. N., Pitcavage, J. M., Urosevich, T. G. (2015). Mental health disorders and treatment seeking among veterans in non-VA facilities: Results and implications from the veterans' health study. *Military Behavioral Health*, *3*(4), 244–254. Retrieved from http://www.ncbi.nlm.nih.gov/pubmed/26640743

Brooks, J., & Hallett, C. E. (Eds.). (2015). *One hundred years of wartime nursing practices, 1854–1953*. Manchester, UK: Manchester University Press.

Centers for Disease Control and Prevention (CDC). (2009). *What you should know about a smallpox outbreak*. Retrieved from http://www.bt.cdc.gov/agent/smallpox/basics/outbreak.asp

Centers for Disease Control and Prevention (CDC). (2011). *A national strategic plan for public health preparedness and response*. Retrieved from http://www.cdc.gov/phpr/publications/2011/a_natl_strategic_plan_for_preparedness_20110901a.pdf

Centers for Disease Control and Prevention (CDC). (2015). *A national snapshot of public health preparedness*. Retrieved from http://www.hhs.gov/about/news/2014/09/16/us-public-health-service-commissioned-corps-help-treat-ebola-patients-in-liberia.html

Centers for Disease Control and Prevention (CDC). (2016). *Office of Public Health Preparedness and Response*. Retrieved from http://www.cdc.gov/phpr/

Cherry, K. E., Sampson, L., Nezat, P. F., & Galea, S. (2014). Long-term psychological outcomes in older adults after disaster: Relationships to religiosity and social support. *Aging and Mental Health*, *19*(5), 1–14.

Chuck, E., & Kwong, H. (2015). *Tragic list: The deadliest mass shootings in U.S. history*. Retrieved from http://www.nbcnews.com/storyline/oregon-college-shooting/deadliest-mass-shootings-u-s-history-n437086

City of New Orleans. (2016). *Emergency preparedness*. Retrieved from www.nola.gov/health/emergency-preparedness

CNN Library. (2015). *Boston marathon terror attack fast facts*. Retrieved from http://www.cnn.com/2013/06/03/us/boston-marathon-terror-attack-fast-facts/

Comas, M. (2013). *Haitian refugees rebuild lives in U.S. after earthquake*. Retrieved from http://articles.orlandosentinel.com/2013-01-11/business/os-haiti-earthquake-central-florida-20130111_1_haitian-refugees-haitian-nationals-immigration-officials

Cox, C. W. (2008). Manmade disasters: A historical review of terrorism and implications for the future. *Journal of Online Issues in Nursing*, *13*(1). doi: 10.3912/OJIN.Vol13No01PPT04.

Culley, J. M., & Svendsen, E. (2014). A review of the literature on the validity of mass casualty triage systems with a focus on chemical exposures. *American Journal of Disaster Medicine*, *9*(2), 137–150.

Davis, J. A. (2013). *Critical incident stress debriefing from a traumatic event: Posttraumatic stress following a critical incident*. Retrieved from https://www.psychologytoday.com/blog/crimes-and-misdemeanors/201302/critical-incident-stress-debriefing-traumatic-event

Department of Homeland Security. (n.d.) *Hurricanes*. Retrieved from http://www.ready.gov/hurricanes

Department of Homeland Security (DHS). (2006). *Department of Homeland Security. Freedom of Information Act. Operational review and improvement plan*. Retrieved from http://www.dhs.gov/xlibrary/assets/foia/privacy_foia_improvement-plan_r.pdf

Department of Homeland Security (DHS). (2011). *Creation of the Department of Homeland Security*. Retrieved from http://www.dhs.gov/xabout/history/gc_1297963906741.shtm

Department of Homeland Security (DHS). (2015). *Operational and support components*. Retrieved from http://www.dhs.gov/components-directorates-and-offices

Esfandiary, D. (2014). *The five most deadly chemical weapons of war*. Retrieved from http://nationalinterest.org/feature/the-five-most-deadly-chemical-weapons-war-10897

Federal Bureau of Investigation (FBI). (n.d.). *Definitions of terrorism in the U.S. code*. Retrieved from https://www.fbi.gov/about-us/investigate/terrorism/terrorism-definition

Federal Bureau of Investigation (FBI). (2008). *Anthrax investigation: Closing a chapter*. Retrieved from http://www.fbi.gov/page2/august08/amerithrax080608a.html

Federal Emergency Management Agency (FEMA). (2015). *National Incident Management System (NIMS)*. Retrieved from https://www.fema.gov/national-incident-management-system

Federal Emergency Management Agency (FEMA) Regional Interagency Steering Committee. (2011). *Partners in preparedness*. Retrieved from https://www.fema.gov/pdf/about/regions/regionviii/risc_0311.pdf

Fink, S. (2013). *Five days at Memorial: Life and death in a storm-ravaged hospital*. New York, NY: Crown Publishers.

Galhotra, S. (2012). *Domestic terror: Are we doing enough to combat the threat from within?* Retrieved from http://www.cnn.com/2012/09/16/us/domestic-terrorism/

George Washington University Institute for Crisis, Disaster, and Risk Management. (n.d.). *Background*. Retrieved from http://www.gwu.edu/~icdrm/about/index.html

Goldberg, J., Magruder, K. M., Forsberg, C. W., Friedman, M. J., Litz, B. T., Vaccarino, V., ... Smith, N. L. (2016). Prevalence of posttraumatic stress disorder in aging Vietnam-era veterans. *American Journal of Geriatric Psychiatry*, 24(3), 181–190. doi: 10.1016/j.jagp.2015.05.004.

Government of Nepal, National Planning Commission. (2015). *Nepal earthquake 2014: Post-disaster needs assessment*. Retrieved from http://icnr2015.mof.gov.np/uploaded//PDNA_Executive_Summary_new.pdf

Haddow, G. D., Bullock, J. A., & Coppola, D. P. (2014). *Introduction to emergency management* (5th ed.). New York, NY: Elsevier.

Halstead, J. A. (2013). When disaster strikes: Are you and your nursing students prepared? *Nursing Education Perspectives*, 34(3), 213.

Hamblen, J., & Sione, L. B. (2015). *Research findings on the traumatic stress effects of terrorism*. Retrieved from http://www.ptsd.va.gov/professional/trauma/disaster-terrorism/research-findings-traumatic-stress-terrorism.asp

Infoplease. (2008). *2007 disasters*. Retrieved from http://www.infoplease.com/ipa/A0934966.html

Infoplease. (2009). *2008 disasters*. Retrieved from http://www.infoplease.com/ipa/A0001437.html

Infoplease. (2012). *News and events of 2012*. Retrieved from http://www.infoplease.com/year/2012.html

International Charter. (2008). *Charter activations*. Retrieved from http://www.disasterscharter.org/

Jain, S., McLean, C., Adler, E. P., & Rosen, C. S. (2016). Peer support and outcome for veterans with posttraumatic stress disorder (PTSD) in a residential rehabilitation program. *Community Mental Health Journal*. doi: 10.1007/s10597-015-9982-1.

Jakeway, C. C., LaRosa, G., Cary, A., Schoenfisch, S., & Association of State and Territorial Directors of Nursing. (2008). The role of public health nurses in emergency preparedness and response: A position paper of the Association of State and Territorial Directors of Nursing. *Public Health Nursing*, 25, 353–361. doi: 10.1111/j.1525–1446.2008.00716.x.

Judd, D., & Sitzman, K. (2014). *A history of American nursing* (2nd ed.). Burlington, MA: Jones & Bartlett Learning.

Kazmin, A. (2008). U.S. Navy ends bid to ferry storm relief into Burma. *The Washington Post*. Retrieved from http://www.washingtonpost.com/wp-dyn/content/article/2008/06/04/AR2008060400978.html

Kirkpatrick, D. V., & Bryan, M. (2007). Hurricane emergency planning by home health providers serving the poor. *Journal of Health Care for the Poor and Underserved*, 18, 299–314.

Ladislaw, S., Kostro, S. S., & Walton, M. A. (2013). *Hurricane Sandy: Evaluating the response one year later*. Retrieved from http://csis.org/publication/hurricane-sandy-evaluating-response-one-year-later

Lee, C. H. (2010). Disaster and mass casualty triage. *Virtual Mentor*, 12(6), 466–470.

Littleton, H., Axsom, D., & Grills-Taquechel, A. E. (2009). Adjustment following the mass shooting at Virginia Tech: The roles of resource loss and gain. *Psychological Trauma: Theory, Research, Practice, and Policy*, 1, 206–219.

Magruder, K. M., Goldberg, J., Forsberg, C. W., Friedman, M. J., Litz, B. T., Vaccarino, V., ... Smith, N. L. (2016). Long-term trajectories of PTSD in Vietnam-era veterans: The course and consequences of PTSD in twins. *Journal of Traumatic Stress*, 29(1), 5–16.

Marmar, C. R., Schlenger, W., Henn-Haase, C., Quian, M., Purchia, E., Li, M., ... Kulka, R. A. (2015). Course of posttraumatic stress disorder 40 years after the Vietnam War: Findings from the National Vietnam Veterans Longitudinal study. *JAMA Psychiatry*, 72(9), 875–881.

Maron, D. F. (2013). *How social media is changing disaster response*. Retrieved from http://www.scientificamerican.com/article/how-social-media-is-changing-disaster-response/

Mayo Clinic. (n.d.). *Resilience: Build skills to endure hardship*. Retrieved from http://www.mayoclinic.org/tests-procedures/resilience-training/in-depth/resilience/art-20046311

McFarlane, A. C., & Williams, R. (2012). Mental health services required after disasters: Learning from the lasting effects of disasters. *Depression Research and Treatment*, 2012(1), 1–14.

Melcer, T., Sechriest, V. F., Walker, J., & Galarneau, M. (2013). A comparison of health outcomes for combat amputee and limb salvage patients injured in Iraq and Afghanistan wars. *Journal of Trauma and Acute Care Surgery*, 75(Suppl. 2), s247–s254.

Mitchell, J. T. (n.d.) *Critical incident stress debriefing*. Retrieved from http://www.info-trauma.org/flash/media-e/mitchellCriticalIncidentStressDebriefing.pdf

Murray, J. S. (2012). Disaster care: National Disaster Medical System. *American Journal of Nursing*, 112(2), 58–63.

Nakanishi, H., Matsuo, K., & Black, J. (2013). Transportation planning methodologies for post-disaster recovery in regional communities: The East Japan earthquake and tsunami 2011. *Journal of Transport Geography*, 31, 181–191.

National Institute of Standards and Technology. (2008). *Federal building and fire safety investigation of the World Trade Center disaster: Answers to frequently asked questions*. Retrieved from http://wtc.nist.gov/pubs/factsheets/faqs_8_2006.htm

Nilsson, J., Johansson, E., Carlsson, M., Florin, J., Leksell, J., Lepp, M., ... Gardulf, A. (2015). Disaster nursing: Self-reported competence of nursing students and registered nurses, with focus on their readiness to manage violence, serious events, and disasters. *Nurse Education in Practice*, 17, 102–108.

Pack, M. J. (2012). Critical incident stress debriefing: An exploratory study of social workers' preferred models of CISM and experiences of CISD in New Zealand. *Social Work in Mental Health*, 10(4), 273–293.

Pamer, M., Wynter, K., & McDade, M. B. (2016). *SoCal Gas has permanently stopped leak in gas above Porter Ranch, state confirms*. Retrieved from http://ktla.com/2016/02/18/socal-gas-porter-ranch-leaking-well-announcement/

Park, H. (2014). Q & A: Children at the border. *The New York Times*. Retrieved from http://www.nytimes.com/interactive/2014/07/15/us/questions-about-the-border-kids.html?_r=0

Pemberton, P. (2013). *The Great White nightclub fire: Ten years later*. Retrieved from http://www.rollingstone.com/music/news/the-great-white-nightclub-fire-ten-years-later-20130715

Press Information Bureau, Government of India. (2008). *HM announces measures to enhance security*. Retrieved from http://pib.nic.in/release/release.asp?relid=45446

Reilly, K. (2016). *California residents fear long-term impact of gas leak*. Retrieved from http://time.com/4173516/california-gas-leak-resident-reaction/

San Diego County Office of Emergency Services. (n.d.). *Family disaster plan and personal survival guide*. Retrieved from http://www.sandiegocounty.gov/oes/docs/FamilyDisasterPlan.pdf

Smith, M., & Segal, J. (2016). *Traumatic stress: How to recover from disasters and other traumatic events*. Retrieved from http://www.helpguide.org/articles/ptsd-trauma/traumatic-stress.htm

Spendlove, J. R., & Simonsen, C. E. (2013). *Terrorism today: The past, the present, the future* (5th ed.). Boston, MA: Pearson Education, Inc.

Stuart, G. (2012). *Principles and practice of psychiatric nursing* (10th ed.). St. Louis, MO: Elsevier-Mosby.

Substance Abuse and Mental Health Services Administration (SAMHSA). (2015). *SAMHSA's efforts for disaster preparedness, response, and recovery.* Retrieved from http://www.samhsa.gov/disaster-preparedness/samhsas-efforts

Transportation Security Administration (TSA). (2012). *Testimony on TSA's use of technology to support a layered approach to security.* Retrieved from https://www.tsa.gov/news/testimony/2012/06/19/testimony-tsas-use-technology-support-layered-approach-security

United Nations Inter-Agency Standing Committee. (2008). *Civil-military guidelines and references for complex emergencies.* Retrieved from http://ochaonline.un.org/cmcs/guidelines

United Nations Refugee Agency. (n.d.). *Refugees: Overview of forced displacement.* Retrieved from http://www.un.org/en/globalissues/briefingpapers/refugees/overviewofforceddisplacement.html

U.S. Department of Defense. (2016a). *Operation Iraqi Freedom: Wounded in action, all.* Retrieved from https://www.dmdc.osd.mil/dcas/pages/report_oif_woundall.xhtml

U. S. Department of Defense. (2016b). *Total deaths.* Retrieved from http://watson.brown.edu/costsofwar/costs/human/civilians/iraqi

U.S. Department of Health and Human Services (USDHHS). (2011). *Emergency systems for advance registration of volunteer health professionals (ESAR-VHP).* Retrieved from http://www.phe.gov/esarvhp/pages/default.aspx

U.S. Department of Health and Human Services (USDHHS). (2014). *Disaster information management research center.* Retrieved from https://sis.nlm.nih.gov/enviro/chemicalwarfare.html

U.S. Department of Health and Human Services (USDHHS). (2016). *Healthy People 2020 topics & objectives: Preparedness.* Retrieved from https://www.healthypeople.gov/2020/topics-objectives/topic/preparedness/objectives

U.S. Department of Health, Education, and Welfare (USDHEW). (1961). *Handbook for civil defense emergency planning in welfare institutions (draft).* Unpublished manuscript. National Archives.

U.S. Department of Justice. (2011). *Terrorism: National Institute of Justice.* Retrieved from http://www.nij.gov/topics/crime/terrorism/pages/welcome.aspx

U.S. Department of Veterans Affairs. (2015). *National Center for PTSD: Criteria for PTSD.* Retrieved from http://www.ptsd.va.gov/professional/PTSD-overview/dsm5_criteria_ptsd.asp

U.S. Public Health Service (USPHS). (2014). *U.S. Public Health Service Commissioned Corps to help treat Ebola patients in Liberia.* Retrieved from http://www.hhs.gov/about/news/2014/09/16/us-public-health-service-commissioned-corps-help-treat-ebola-patients-in-liberia.html

Vaccarino, V., Goldberg, J., Rooks, C., Shah, A. J., Veledar, E., Faber, T. O., ... Bremner, J. D. (2013). Post-traumatic stress disorder and incidence of coronary heart disease: A twin study. *Journal of the American College of Cardiology, 62*(11), 970–978.

Varcarolis, E., & Halter, M. J. (2014). *Foundations of psychiatric mental health nursing: A clinical approach* (7th ed.). St. Louis, MO: Elsevier-Mosby.

Veenema, T. G. (2013). *Disaster nursing and emergency preparedness for chemical, biological, and radiological terrorism and other hazards* (3rd ed.). New York, NY: Springer Publishing Company.

Wagner, J. M., & Dahnke, M. D. (2015). Nursing ethics and disaster triage: Applying utilitarian ethical theory. *Journal of Emergency Nursing, 41*(4), 300–306.

Wall, E. (2012). Self-care practices and attitudes toward CISD and seeking mental health services among firefighters: A close look at a mid-sized Midwestern urban city. *Master of Social Work Clinical Research Papers, Paper 99.* Retrieved from http://sophia.stkate.edu/msw_papers/99

Watson Institute for International & Public Affairs. (2015). *Iraqi civilians.* Retrieved from http://watson.brown.edu/costsofwar/costs/human/civilians/iraqi

White, J. (2002). The American Psychiatric Nurses Association responds to the September 11 tragedy. *Online Journal of Issues in Nursing, 7*(3), Manuscript 3. Retrieved from www.nursingworld.org/MainMenuCategories/ANAMarketplace/ANAPeriodicals/OJIN/TableofContents/Volume72002/No3Sept2002/APNARespondstoSep11.aspx

thePoint: Everything You Need to Make the Grade!

thePoint® Visit http://thePoint.lww.com/Rector9e for selected readings, study aids for all learning styles, and more!

THE FAMILY AS CLIENT

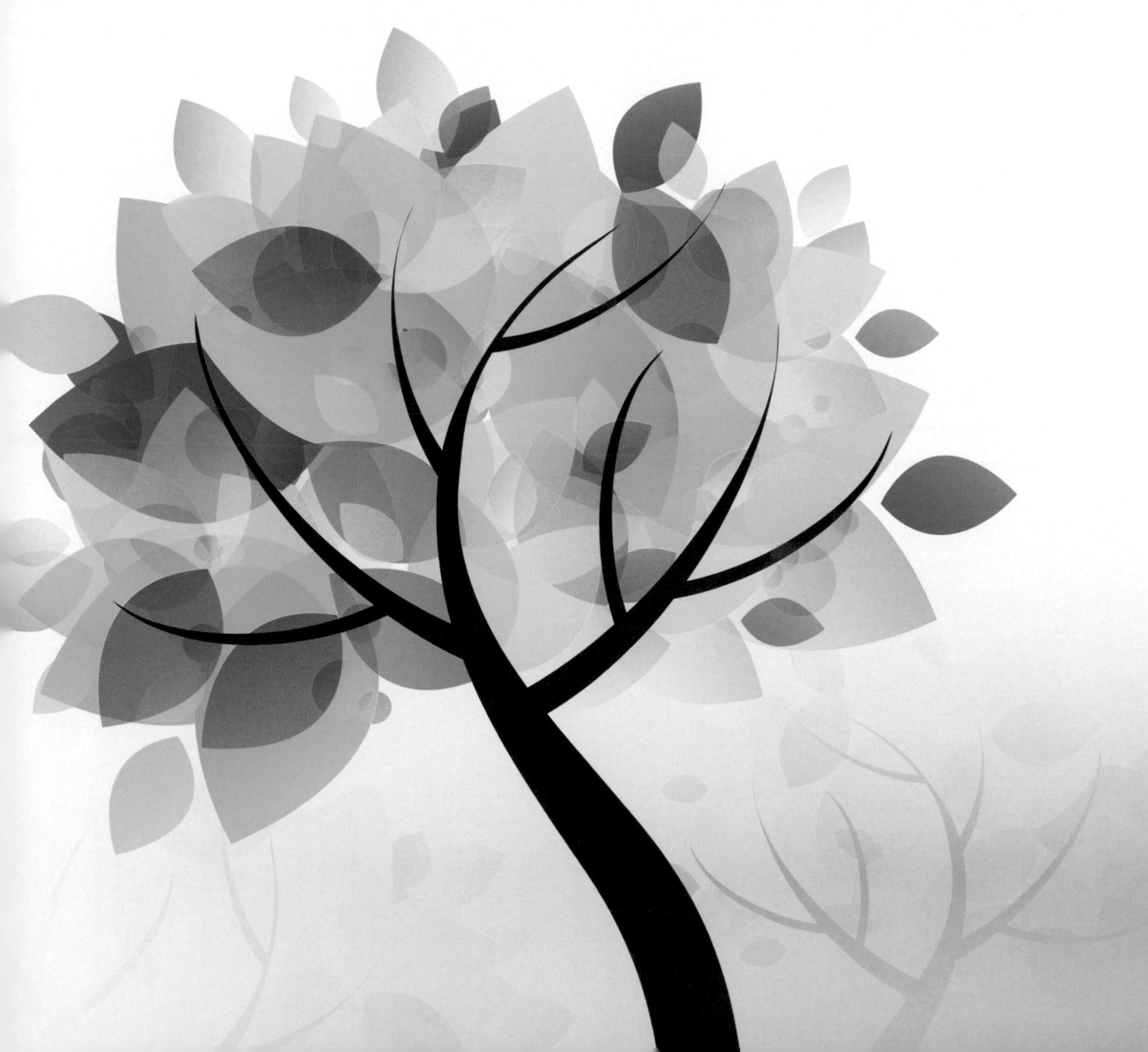

Theoretical Basis for Promoting Family Health

"Family is who they say they are."

—*Wright and Leahey* (2013, p. 55), **Family Nurse Theorists**

KEY TERMS

Family
Family culture
Family functions

Family health
Family life cycle
Family structure

Family system boundaries
Foster families
Gay and lesbian families

Homeless families
Roles

LEARNING OBJECTIVES

Upon mastery of this chapter, you should be able to:

- Define family health nursing.
- Analyze definitions of family.
- Discuss characteristics all families have in common.
- Identify the stages of the family life cycle and the developmental tasks of a family.
- Discuss how a family's culture influences its values, behaviors, and roles.
- Describe the functions of a family.
- Analyze the role of the community health nurse in promoting the health of the family.

Community health nurses are intimately involved with families. The family plays a critical role in the health of its members. Health habits such as preventative care, diet, exercise, and physical activity are developed in the context of family. Health beliefs, genetic influences, and care of the ill family member all take place within the family environment. The community health nurse is in a unique position to influence and promote family health.

Definition of family varies by organization, discipline, and individual. These definitions are certainly changing with recent recognition of same-sex marriage laws. Many family theorists suggest that a family consists of two or more individuals who share a residence or live near one another; possess some common emotional bond; engage in interrelated social positions, roles, and tasks; and share cultural ties and a sense of affection and belonging (Kaakinen, Coehlo, Steele, Tabacco, & Hanson, 2015; Titelman, 2014). There are many definitions of family. One definition that seems the most inclusive and yet the simplest is "family is who they say they are" (Wright & Leahey, 2013, p. 55).

Today's community health nurse needs to understand and work with many types of families, each of which has unique health needs. For example, a young, single mother who is homeless seeks help in caring for her sick infant. A 55-year-old grandfather provides care for his elderly mother, who was recently discharged from the hospital after a stroke. A family from El Salvador needs instruction on the purchase and preparation of food. Why is it important for the community health nurse to understand and respect the unique characteristics, cultures, structures, and functions of each of these families? Do families have characteristics that affect the type of community health nursing intervention? The answer is an unqualified yes. The effectiveness of the community health nurse depends on knowing how to work with all kinds of families.

This chapter explores the nature of families and family health. It draws from various theories to strengthen the student's understanding and appreciation of families as clients. This information will promote the effectiveness of interventions with families at the primary, secondary, and tertiary levels of prevention. See Levels of Prevention Pyramid.

FAMILY HEALTH

Kaakinen et al. (2015) define **family health** as a "dynamic changing state of wellbeing, which includes the biological, psychological, spiritual, sociological, and culture factors of individual members and the whole family system" (p. 5). Family health is concerned with how well the family functions together as a unit. It involves not only the health of the members and how they relate to other members but also how well they relate to and cope with the community, outside the family. In fact, family health, like individual health, ranges along a continuum from wellness to illness. A family may be at one point on that continuum now and at a much different point 6 months from now. Family health refers to the health status of a given family at a given point in time (Kaakinen et al., 2015).

WHAT IS FAMILY HEALTH NURSING?

There are multiple ways that community health nurses can approach families. Nurses can provide care to individuals within the family or to the family as the client (family as context) or to the family as a system. Some nurses view family nursing as part of other specialties such as public health nursing, maternal child nursing, or behavioral health nursing. However, some nurses view family nursing as its own distinct specialty, rich with its own body of literature and research. Each of these approaches with families has their own distinct set of beliefs (Fig. 18–1).

Nurses work with individuals within families every day. Most often, the individual is the recipient of care. While assessing the needs of the individual, the nurse needs to include the family in the assessment, as the family is the pivotal provider of care. This may represent family as context. How does the family assist the individual family member? What are their available resources (physically, emotionally, and spiritually)? Nurses working with families as a system view the family as part of a larger suprasystem that includes many subsystems. The family becomes greater than the sum of all of its parts. A change within the family system affects not only the individual member but all of the family members (Wright & Leahey, 2013). When visualizing a family as a system, it may help to compare it to a mobile. Think of all the pieces suspended freely by a string. If you pull lightly on one piece, all the pieces move, just as a change in one member's health affects the entire family. Can you think of some examples of this in your own family?

Examples of Level of Care

How can this make more sense to us? A nurse receives a referral to visit a new adolescent mother in her home. The baby girl (Rose) is currently 2 weeks old. Her mother (Zoe) is 15 years old. Zoe lives with her mother and three other siblings (13, 11, and 9 years of age). On the referral, Rose is listed as the client and the recipient of care. The nurse assesses Rose's feeding, sleeping, and interaction with her mother. The focus is clearly on the needs of the infant and intervening with any information that may be needed to meet the needs of Rose.

The nurse on the same visit includes information about the family on the assessment from the perspective of the family as context. How would the birth of Rose change the family? Who assists in the care of Rose? Will Zoe remain in school? Who takes care of Rose while she attends school?

The nurse includes information on the assessment looking at the family as a system of care. The nurse would observe Rose and Zoe as members of a family.

LEVELS OF PREVENTION PYRAMID

SITUATION: The family will provide the emotional and material resources necessary for its members' growth and well-being.

GOAL: Using the three levels of prevention, negative health conditions are avoided, promptly diagnosed, and treated, and/or the fullest possible potential is restored.

TERTIARY PREVENTION

Rehabilitation

- After the family suffers a crisis, the members recognize the need for help and accept that help
- Families draw on personal resources to rebuild relationships and heal the family unit

Primary Prevention

Health Promotion and Education

- The family continues using resources that enhance the growth and well-being of individuals and the family as a unit

Health Protection

- Engage in family strengthening practices to protect the family from possible inhibitors to growth and well-being

SECONDARY PREVENTION

Early Diagnosis

- Identification of a family member's personal problems that affect the family as a whole
- Early recognition that problems exist in the relationship among or between family members

Prompt Treatment

- The family seeks out the appropriate resources that brings the family to the highest level of wellness possible

PRIMARY PREVENTION

Health Promotion and Education

- Adults are well prepared for the responsibilities of their union
- Adults enter the relationship with the personal resources necessary to promote the growth and development of their family unit

Health Protection

- Adults are able to provide for basic needs (housing, nutrition, safety)

How are they adjusting to their new roles within the family? How has the birth of Rose changed Zoe's role in the family? Does Zoe's mother interact with her differently? What has changed in the family with the birth of Rose?

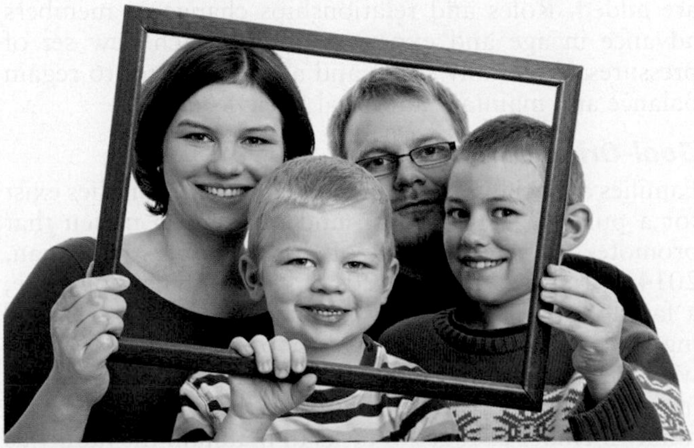

FIGURE 18–1 Community health nurses work with families and individual family members.

It would be important to ask each of the family members their answers to these questions.

DEFINITIONS OF FAMILY

Throughout history, the **family** has been the most basic unit. One of the first steps of the nurse is to define the family. How nurses define a family influences the care that they provide and how they interact with the family. What comes to mind when you hear the word family? How would you define your own family? Is your grandmother a member of your family? Your niece? Your neighbor? A friend? A family pet?

Most of us were raised in families and spent a good portion of our lives within families. Our first experiences with others are from our families. Often, how we interact with others is determined by how we were taught within our family. So we come to our nursing practice with ideas about families based on our own experiences. As the nurse begins working with families, it is important to first reflect on our own definition of a family. Bell (2013) asserts that the way we interact with families actually comes from how we define family so it is important to spend some time looking at this, because it will shape our care.

The United Nations (UN) defines family "as the basic unit of society" (n.d., para. 1). They recognize that there have been many changes in families in the last 50 years due to societal forces such as delayed marriage and child-bearing, smaller family size, increases in divorce rates, and migration (UN, n.d.). In regard to demographic statistics, the UN defines family as "those members of the household who are related, to a specified degree, through blood, adoption, or marriage," acknowledging that the term "related" varies worldwide (2014, para. 3). The U.S. Census Bureau (Vespa, Lewis, & Krider, 2013) views family as people living together and related by birth, adoption, or marriage. Kaakinen et al. (2015) defines family as "two or more individuals who depend on one another for emotional, physical, and economical support. The members of the family are self-defined" (p. 5).

UNIVERSAL CHARACTERISTICS OF FAMILIES

Several observations can be made about families in general. First, each family is unique, with its own distinct set of strengths. As a nurse you want to look first at the family's strengths. When you approach the door of a house to begin your visit with a family, you cannot be sure of what they will be like. You will have to gather information about the family in order to provide the best nursing care possible. Starting with their strengths will only assure your success.

Families share universal characteristics with every other family. These characteristics provide an important key to understanding each family's uniqueness. Five of the most important family characteristics for community health nurses to recognize are as follows:

1. Every family is a small social system.
2. Every family moves through stages in its life cycle.
3. Every family has its own cultural values and rules.
4. Every family has structure.
5. Every family has certain basic functions.

No matter how many families a nurse may visit over the course of a year, each one will have universal features; it is important for PHNs to know each family's unique set of characteristics and their effects on family health. These five universal characteristics of family life, which provide the framework of this chapter, are based on systems theory, sociology, and family development.

Families as Social Systems

Many Americans fall into the habit of viewing families merely as individuals. This may be caused partly by our strong cultural emphasis on individualism. This error also occurs because families are often encountered through the individual members. When a community health nurse sits in a living room talking with a family about their adolescent son who has significant cognitive delays, it is important to keep in mind that all the family members are present by way of their influence. Systems theory offers some insights about how families operate as social systems (Titelman, 2014). Knowing the attributes of living systems or open systems can help strengthen understanding of family structure and function. There are five

attributes of open systems that help explain functions of families: (1) families are interdependent, (2) families maintain boundaries, (3) families exchange energy with their environments, (4) families are adaptive, and (5) families are goal oriented.

Interdependence Among Members

All the members of a family are interdependent; each member's actions affect the other members, and what affects the family system affects each family member. For example, consider the changes a father might make to treat his hypertension. If he cuts back on working overtime, the family's income will be reduced. If he begins to eat different foods, food preparation and eating patterns in the family will be altered. If he starts a new exercise program three evenings a week, this may upset other family routines. Even his ability to carry out his usual roles as husband and father may be affected if, for instance, he has less time to help his children with their homework or share household chores with his wife.

Family Boundaries

Families as systems set and maintain boundaries that can include outside influences (permeable) or not (limiting) (Wright & Leahey, 2013). These boundaries result from shared experiences and expectations and link family members together in a bond that excludes the rest of the world. Also, a greater concentration of energy exists within the family than between the family and its external environment, thereby creating a **family system boundary**.

Energy Exchange

Family boundaries are semipermeable; although they protect and preserve the family unit, they also allow selective linkage with the outside world. To function adequately as open systems, families exchange materials or information with their environment (Friedman, Bowden, & Jones, 2003; Titelman, 2014). This process is called energy exchange. This exchange promotes a healthy ecologic balance between the family system and the environment that is its immediate community.

Adaptive Behavior

Families are adaptive, equilibrium-seeking systems. Families never stay the same. They shift and change in response to internal and external forces (Titelman, 2014). The family composition changes as new members are added. Roles and relationships change as members advance in age and experience. With each new set of pressures, the family shifts and accommodates to regain balance and maintain a normal lifestyle.

Goal-Oriented Behavior

Families as social systems are goal directed. Families exist for a purpose—to establish and maintain a milieu that promotes the development of their members (Titelman, 2014; Wright & Leahey, 2013). To fulfill this purpose, a family must perform basic functions, such as providing love, security, identity, a sense of belonging; assisting with preparation for adult roles in society; and maintaining order and control. In addition to these functions, each family member engages in tasks to maintain the family as a viable unit. See What Do You Think?

What do *you* think?

DEFINITION OF FAMILY

How do you define family? How would you define your own family?

Who do you include as family members? What are your first memories of family?

Family Life Cycle

Many of the characteristics and defined developmental stages of individual growth also apply to families. For example, families change continuously. Families grow and develop as the individuals within them mature and adapt to changes. A family's composition, set of roles, and interpersonal relationships change with time (Friedman et al., 2003; Wright & Leahey, 2013). Families vary with each stage of the family life cycle. See Display 18–1 for some questions to ask yourself about your own family. At what stage are you and your own family?

Consider the following example. The Jordan family, a young married couple, concentrated on learning their new roles of husband and wife and building a mutually satisfying marriage. With the birth of their first child, Ben, the family composition and relationships changed and role transitions occurred. The Jordan family consists of not only a husband and wife but also a father, mother, and son; the family added three new roles. Within the next 4 years, two daughters, Lisa and Tiffany, were born. The introduction of each new member not only increased family size but also significantly reorganized family living. As Duvall and Miller (1985) first pointed out and later Plomin and Daniels (2011) reaffirmed, no two children are born into precisely the same family. The children entered school; Mrs. Jordan went back to work, and soon, Scott was leaving for college. The Jordan family, like every family, is moving through a predictable and sequential pattern of stages known as the **family life cycle**.

PHNs who are knowledgeable about this cycle can provide anticipatory guidance to families. For instance, while teaching prenatal care to the Jordan family, the nurse can help the soon-to-be parents to anticipate the responsibility and costs of raising her child by helping them calculate child care needs. The nurse can assist the family in figuring out the monthly costs of breast-feeding versus buying formula, disposable diapers versus cloth or a diaper service, and the clothing, equipment, and medical costs of infant care. When working with middle-aged parents of an adult son who has had a brain injury, the nurse can discuss what arrangements the parents have made for their son's care after they are older and unable to provide care themselves or after one or both of them die.

Stages of the Family Life Cycle

There are two broad stages in the family life cycle: one of expansion as new members are added and roles and relationships are increased, and one of contraction as family members leave to start lives of their own or age or die (Wright & Leahey, 2013). Within this framework of the expanding–contracting family are more specific phases, such as launching of children and retirement of parents. In some families, expansion and contraction are repeated as various members are added, return home with their children and perhaps a partner, or leave home permanently.

Family Developmental Tasks

To progress through the stages of the life cycle, a family must carry out its basic functions and the developmental tasks associated with those functions. Unlike developmental tasks, which are specific to each age level, family developmental tasks are ongoing throughout the life cycle. All families, for instance, must provide for the physical needs of their members at every stage. The manner and degree to which each function is carried out varies depending on how well members accomplish individual developmental tasks and meet the demand of a particular stage (Rasheed, Rasheed, & Marley, 2011). Physical maintenance, for example, affects the parents' ability to accept responsibility and procure the necessary resources to provide food, clothing, and shelter for their children. At early stages, children are dependent on their parents for meeting these needs; at the school, teenage, and launching stages, children may increasingly contribute to home management and family income. The responsibility for these tasks shifts from just the parents to other family members as well.

Some functions require greater emphasis at certain stages. Socialization, for example, consumes much of a family's time during the early years of child development. These same functions and their associated developmental tasks can be further broken down into actions specific to certain stages. While carrying out its function of maintaining controls, a family sets clearly defined limits for children at the preschool stage: "Do not cross the street"; "You may have dessert only after you finish your meal"; or "Bedtime is at 8 o'clock." During the school stage, control activities may center on allocating responsibilities and division of labor within the family: "Feed the dog"; "Clean your room"; or "Take out the trash." When a family reaches the teenage stage, its control function increasingly focuses on the relationships between family members and outsiders. The family may regulate some activities by setting limits: "Be home by midnight." In areas such as moral conduct, controls may involve family values and therefore be more imperceptible. A family at this stage must recognize the need for young people to assume increasing responsibility for their own behavior and acknowledge its own diminishing control over members who are exploring independence. Duvall and Miller (1985) described these activities as "stage critical" family developmental tasks that must be completed before moving onto the next stage. Others have echoed the concept of critical stages and tasks in family development (Rasheed et al., 2011). Sample community health nursing actions with the family at different stages are presented in Table 18–1.

Table 18-1 Stage Critical Family Developmental Tasks

Stage of Family Life Cycle	Family Position	Stage Critical Family Developmental Tasks	Role of the Community Health Nurse
Forming a partnership	Female partner Male partner	Establishing a mutually satisfying relationship	Interact with family where they are at
Childbearing	Partner–mother Partner–father Infant child(ren)	Adjusting to pregnancy and the promise of parenthood Fitting into the kin network Having and adjusting to infants and encouraging their development Establishing a satisfying home for both parents and infant(s)	Assist them in developing strong relationships
Preschool age	Partner–mother Partner–father Child, siblings	Adapting to the critical needs and interests of preschool children in stimulating, growth-promoting ways Coping with energy depletion and lack of privacy as parents	Assist in preparing for family expansion through education and anticipatory guidance
School age	Partner–mother Partner–father Child, siblings	Fitting into the community of school-age families in constructive ways Encouraging children's educational achievement	Encourage time for each other as adults in a relationship separate from parenting role
Teenage	Partner–mother Partner–father Child, siblings	Balancing freedom with responsibility as teenagers mature and emancipate themselves Establishing outside interests and careers as growing parents	Provide anticipatory guidance for the school-aged children as they grow into adulthood
Launching center	Partner–mother–grandmother Partner–father–grandfather Child, sibling, aunt or uncle	Releasing young adults into work, military service, college, marriage, etc., with appropriate rituals and assistance Maintaining a supportive home base	Provide anticipatory guidance for the contracting family as children leave home
Middle-aged parents	Partner–mother–grandmother Partner–father–grandfather	Rebuilding the relationship Maintaining kin ties with older and younger generations	Prepare adults for grandparenting role
Aging family members	Widow or widower Partner–mother–grandmother Partner–father–grandfather	Adjusting to retirement Coping with bereavement and living alone Closing the family home or adapting it to aging	Assist aging adults with emotional and financial security, as they approach retirement Prepare the aging adults with ways to cope with the losses of old age, including changes in space, work, health, status, and loss of friends and family members

Adapted from Duvall, E. R., & Miller, B. C. (1985). *Marriage and family development.* New York, NY: Harper & Row; and Wright, L. M., & Leahey, M. (2013). *Nurses and families: A guide to family assessment and intervention* (6th ed.). Philadelphia, PA: F. A. Davis.

Family Culture

Family culture is an acquired knowledge that family members use to interpret their experiences and generate their behaviors that in turn influence their actions. The concept of family culture arises from a significant body of literature in the social and behavioral sciences. Culture explains why families behave as they do (McGoldrick, Garcia-Preto, & Carter, 2016; Pender, Murdaugh, & Parsons, 2015). Family culture also gives the community health nurse a basis for assessing family health and designing appropriate interventions. Three aspects of family culture deserve special consideration: (1) family members share certain values that affect family behavior, (2) certain roles are defined for family members, and (3) a family's culture determines its distribution and use of power.

Shared Values and Their Effect on Behavior

Although families share many broad cultural values drawn from the larger society in which they live, they also develop unique characteristics. Every family has its own set of values and rules for operation that can be considered as family (McGoldrick et al., 2016). Some values are explicitly stated: "Family issues and problems must always stay within the family." Such values may give rise to specific operating rules: "Don't tell anyone about our problems." Values such as these may make it difficult for families to ask for help.

Like all cultural values, many family values remain outside the conscious awareness of family members. These values, often not verbalized, become powerful determinants of what the family believes, feels, thinks, and does. Family values include those beliefs transmitted by previous generations, religious influences, immediate social pressures, and the larger society. Values become an integral part of a family's life and are difficult to change. A family that values free expression for every member engages comfortably in loud, noisy debates. Another family that values quietness, order, and control does not tolerate its members raising their voices. One family uses birth control based on beliefs about human life and parental responsibility; another family chooses not to use birth control because the members may feel it is against their religion. How a family views education, health care, lifestyle, courtship, marriage, child rearing, sex roles, or any of the countless other issues requiring choices depends on the cultural values of the family.

Roles

Roles, the assigned or assumed parts that members play during day-to-day family living, are bestowed and defined by the family (Kaakinen et al., 2015). For instance, the father role may be assigned as an authoritative one that includes establishing rules, judging behavior, and administering punishment for violation of rules. In another family, the father role may be defined primarily as that of a breadwinner and supporting the mother's decisions in day-to-day child rearing. If there is an absence of a male parent, a grandfather, uncle, friend, or even the mother may take over the father role. Selection of specific roles to be played in any given family varies depending on the family's structure, needs, and patterns of functioning. In a single-parent family, the parent may need to assume the roles of mother, father, and breadwinner, as well as others.

Families distribute among their members all the responsibilities and tasks necessary to conduct family living. The responsibilities of breadwinner and homemaker, with their accompanying tasks, may belong to husband and wife, respectively, or may be shared if both husband and wife have jobs outside the home. Older children may help younger ones with homework, entertain them, or care for their basic needs. This releases parents for other tasks and increases the responsibility of older children.

Family members may play several roles at the same time. This can be taxing. A woman may play the role of wife to her husband, daughter to her mother, and mother to each of her children. The mother role may involve taking on several additional roles and responsibilities and varies with each child's needs. Parents may care for their children and also have some responsibility for aging parents. This situation characterizes the sandwich generation, and those experiencing this newly coined phenomenon feel the squeeze both in overloaded schedules and financial burden (Parker & Patten, 2013). A single parent often takes on the role of both father and mother but may distribute responsibilities and tasks more widely. A grandmother or a child may assume responsibility for some chores and thereby relieve some of the demands on the single parent. Among families, there is great variation in expectations for each role and in the degree of flexibility in divisions of roles. An example may be specific tasks given to girls versus boys within the family. Girls may be given child care or kitchen responsibilities and boys given yard tasks. Confusion and conflict can develop unless roles are clarified.

Other roles of family may extend beyond the immediate family. There may be extended family members nearby who interact with the family on a regular basis or only on special occasions like birthdays. If both parents are employed, they may have an expansive network of folks within the neighborhood. Friendships are often made with the parents of children's friends, particularly if the children participate in the same activities. Many families enjoy the fellowship of organized religious or cultural groups. This fellowship can be a source of support or comfort, as well as an additional role function for the family members. Family members can also participate in roles outside the family. These may involve local or regional politics, community improvement, volunteerism for nonprofit groups, or other groups outside the home that the community may offer. These diverse role relationships should enrich and energize the participants. However, many people become overcommitted, creating an imbalance of role responsibilities that is draining and causes friction and stress. The community health nurse may work with families to help them achieve a balance of activities that promote family health.

Distribution and Use of Power

Power is the possession of control, authority, or influence over others—assuming patterns in each family. In some families, power is concentrated primarily in one member; in other families, it is distributed on a more egalitarian basis (Perelberg & Miller, 2011). The traditional patriarchal family, in which the father holds absolute authority over the other members, is rare in American

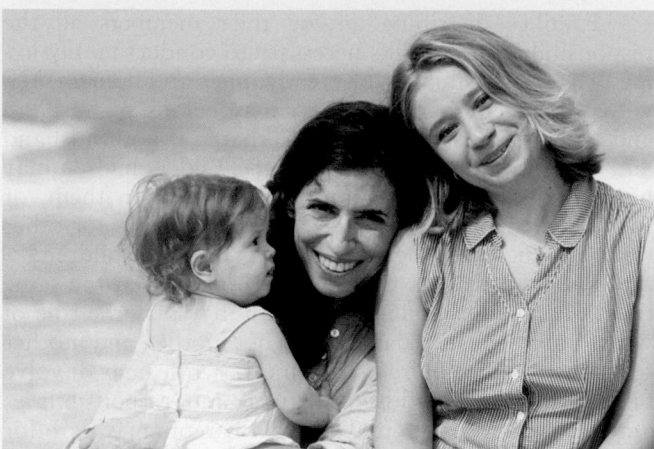

FIGURE 18–2 Families exist in many different forms.

society. However, the pattern of husband as head of the household and dominant member of the family is still frequently seen. The dominant power, whether male or female, holds the majority of the decision-making power, particularly over more important family matters such as employment, finances, and health care. Other areas of decision-making, including choices about vacations, housing, leisure activities, household purchases, and child rearing, may be shared or delegated. With changing societal influences, however, the present trend among American families is toward egalitarian power distribution (Fig. 18–2).

Family Structures

Globally, families—in all varied forms—are the basic social unit (Wright & Leahey, 2013). The meaning of family among the Hmong of northern Laos may include hundreds of people who make up a clan. In Mexico, families remain close, are large, and extend into multiple generations. In Germany and Japan, families are small and tend to the needs of their elders at home. In the United States, where families come from many cultural groups, many variations coexist within communities.

For many people in the United States, the term family used to evoke a picture of a husband, wife, and children living under one roof, with the man as breadwinner and the woman as homemaker. In the past, this nuclear **family structure** was often seen as the norm for everyone. Changes in social values and cultural lifestyles (i.e., women working outside the home) combined with acceptance of alternative lifestyles have changed the definition of family. Today, definitions of a family include unmarried adults living together with or without children, single-parent households, divorced couples combining households with children from previous marriages (the blended family), and gay couples with or without children.

Families come in many shapes and sizes. McGoldrick et al. (2016) find changes in family structure related to societal changes such as increased divorce rates and remarriage rates, changing roles for women, increase in LGBT couples and families, lower birth rates, rise in single-parent families, increase in single-parent adoptions, high rates of unwed childbearing, two-income households, and a greater physical distance among members.

It is a privilege to gain entry into a family's home. This is a uniquely private space belonging to the family. The people who are members of this household interact, care for one another, and bond in ways that may never be fully understood by anyone outside the family. Therefore, being granted entrance into this system gives the community health nurse an opportunity to work with the family that few other professionals experience. Each type of household requires recognition and acceptance by community health nurses, who must help families achieve optimal health.

Family Functions

Families in every culture throughout history have engaged in similar functions: families have produced children, physically cared for their members, protected their health, encouraged their education or training, given emotional support and acceptance, and provided supportive and nurturing care during illness. Some societies have experimented with separation of these functions, allocating activities such as child care, socialization, or social control to a larger group (e.g., government, social systems). In U.S. society, certain social institutions help perform some aspects of traditional **family functions**. Schools, for example, help in child socialization, professionals supervise health care, and religious organizations influence values.

Six functions are typical of American families today and are essential for the maintenance and promotion of family health: (1) providing affection, (2) providing security, (3) instilling identity, (4) promoting affiliation, (5) providing socialization, and (6) establishing controls (Duvall & Miller, 1985; Titelman, 2014; Wright & Leahey, 2013). See Table 18–2 for a list of tasks associated with these functions.

SOCIAL CLASS

As a community health nurse, it is important to include social class of families you are visiting in your assessment. Social class often shapes a family's access and choices to work, educational, and health care opportunities (McGoldrick et al., 2016). Their overall health is often determined by their class position. The biggest predictor of health is your level of wealth (Unnatural Causes, 2008). How healthy we are and how long we live are often related to our social standing. The neighborhoods families choose to live in, and the schools their children attend, are often determined by social class. These decisions/choices have lifelong implications and shape the history of families. See Chapter 25 on social determinants of health and the socioeconomic gradient.

TRADITIONAL FAMILIES

Traditional families are those that are likely most familiar to us. They include the nuclear family—husband, wife, and children living together in the same household. In nuclear families, the workload distribution between the two adults can vary. Both adults may work outside the home; one adult may work outside the home, whereas the other stays at home and assumes primary responsibilities for the household; or partners may alternate, constantly renegotiating work and domestic responsibilities.

Table 18-2 Family Functions	
Functions	**Tasks**
Providing affection	1. Meeting physical needs (food, shelter, clothing, health care) 2. Provides dependability
Providing security and acceptance	1. Provide need fulfillment 2. Offers a safe retreat
Instilling identity and satisfaction	1. Teaching roles 2. Instilling values and goals
Promoting affiliation	1. To give a sense of belonging 2. Provide a connection to a family
Providing socialization	1. Transmit their culture 2. Learn roles within the family
Establishing controls	1. Maintain order 2. Learn right and wrong 3. Teach division of labor

In 2012, according to the U.S. Census Bureau, for the first time, only 48% of American households consist of a married couple with or without children (Vespa et al., 2013). In 2014, 64% of children under the age of 17 years lived with two-parent families (ChildStats.gov, 2015). The percentage of children living in two-parent families continues to decrease.

A nuclear dyad family consists of two adults living together who have no children or who have grown children living outside the home. A single adult family is one in which one adult is living alone by choice or because of separation from a spouse or children or both. Separation may be the result of divorce, death, or distance from children.

Sometimes, in close-knit ethnic communities, families form a kin network, in which several nuclear families live in the same household or near one another and share goods and services. They may own and operate a family business, sharing work and child care responsibilities, income and expenses, and even meals. Variations of this trend are increasing among all groups as children postpone leaving home because of economic conditions, educational plans, or student loans. The number of young adults who continue to live with their parents is on the rise. Nineteen percent of men and ten percent of women between the ages of 25 and 34 years continue to live with their parents (Vespa et al., 2013).

CONTEMPORARY FAMILIES

The traditional nuclear family has been a fundamental part of our cultural heritage shared by many Americans and reinforced by religion, education, and other influential social institutions. Variations from this pattern often were treated as deviant and abnormal. Walsh (2012) describes the continued diversity in types of families and foresees the possibilities of normality and healthy functioning in each of these diverse family types. McGoldrick et al. (2016) fosters the importance of putting a positive spin on the families that make up our world. The nurse is in a unique position to assess families in a strength-based model rather than viewing certain families as deviant. Society has begun to accept contemporary definitions of family.

Divorce

Divorce changes family structures. Half of all marriages now end in divorce (the rate is higher for teen mothers), and the median duration of marriages is approximately 7 years. In the United States, the marriage rate is reported as 6.9 per 1,000 and the divorce rate as 3.6 per 1,000 in 2014 (Centers for Disease Control and Prevention [CDC], 2016). Seventy percent of divorced individuals remarry (McGoldrick et al., 2016). See Table 18–3.

Adjusting to divorce involves a series of transitions and reorganizations for all family members. For children, it may require coping with a new geographic location and a new school, as well as adjusting to changes in the mental and physical health of family members. In addition to the normal growth and developmental changes, children of divorce may face an absent father or mother, interparental conflict, economic distress, parental adjustment, multiple life stressors, and short-term crises.

Blending

Another variation in family composition is the blended family. In this structure, single parents marry and raise the children from each of the previous relationships together. They may be custodial parents who have the children except during planned visits with the noncustodial parent, or they may share custody, so that the children live in the blended arrangement only part time or possibly live in two separate blended homes. The family may include children from the couple, in addition to the children brought into the relationship. Not all divorced adults stay single; most remarry or cohabitate with another adult, who may or may not have children. This new couple may have children from their union, creating an even more complex family. Merged or blended families require considerable adjustment and relearning of roles, tasks, communication patterns, and relationships.

Table 18–3 When Families Divorce

Phase	Emotional Responses	Developmental Issues
1. Stressor leading to marital differences	Reveal the fact that the marriage has major problems	Accepting the fact that the marriage has major problems
2. Decision to divorce	Accepting the inability to resolve marital differences	Accepting one's own contribution to the failed marriage
3. Planning the dissolution of the family system	Negotiating viable arrangements for all members within the system	Cooperating on custody visitation and financial issues Informing and dealing with extended family members and friends
4. Separation	Mourning loss of intact family Working on resolving attachment to spouse	Develop coparental arrangements/relationships Restructure living arrangements Adapt to living apart Realign relationship with extended family and friends Begin to rebuild own social network
5. Divorce	Continue working on emotional recovery by overcoming hurt, anger, or guilt.	Giving up fantasies of reunion Staying connected with extended families Rebuild and strengthen own social network
6. Postdivorce	Separate feelings about ex-spouse from parenting role Prepare self for possibility of changes in custody as child(ren) get older; be open to their needs Risk developing a new intimate relationship	Make flexible and generous visitation arrangements for child(ren) and noncustodial parent and extended family members Deal with possibilities of changing custody arrangements as child(ren) get older Deal with child(ren)'s reaction to parents establishing relationships with new partners

Adapted from McGoldrick, M., Garcia-Preto, N., & Carter, B. (2016). *The expanding family life cycle: Individual, family, and social perspectives* (5th ed.). Upper Saddle River, NJ: Prentice Hall.

Identifiable phases occur in divorce, remarriage, and the blending of families; each phase has its own emotional transitions and developmental issues. We all come to new relationships with our own history from the past.

Because this emerging family pattern has become so prominent in such a short period, it is very possible that the community health nurse is familiar with this pattern or lives in such a family. The Pew Research Center (2011) found that 4 in 10 Americans currently have at least one step-relative, and 3 in 10 have a step or half sibling. Thirteen percent of adults have at least one stepchild. Stepfamilies are less common among those with college educations and higher-income levels. Survey respondents showed higher levels of feeling very obligated to give assistance to biological parents, grown children, and siblings over those with stepparents, stepchildren, or step/half sibling relationships (85% vs. 56%, 78% vs. 62%, and 64% vs. 42%, respectively).

Nursing skills that are needed when working with divorced or blended families include the ability to listen and be empathetic, as well as a nonjudgmental attitude. The nurse can be a rich resource for the family. Support groups for adults and children are excellent resources and provide invaluable services at a time of emotional instability in the family. Peer support groups for children and adolescents and support from within the schools should be used, if available, or started if they do not exist. The community health nurse can have a significant role in community-wide planning if services are needed but unavailable. See Table 18–4.

Single-Parent Family

One of the most common contemporary family structures is the single-parent family mostly headed by a woman. Sometimes single women choose to adopt or have children without being married. Sometimes pregnancy without marriage creates this family unity. In 2013, births to single women remain relatively stable at 41% of all births (ChildStats.gov, 2015). Twenty-four percent of all children live only with their mother, 4% of children live with their father, and 4% live with neither parent. Most of these children live with their grandparents (ChildStats.gov, 2015).

Over time, this form of family has become more accepted by society. It is important for community health nurses to view the strengths of single-parent families. Building on their current strengths can be most helpful in terms of meeting the challenges that they may face. See Population Focus on Families.

Adolescent Parents

Statistics indicate that teenagers are increasingly heads of single-parent families; some of these teen head of households become pregnant in junior high school. The birth rate among teens 15 to 19 years old has continued a steady decline, but teen birth rates in the United States remain the highest among those in developed countries. Specific factors related to teen birth rates are poor performance in school, growing up in a single-parent family,

Table 18-4   Remarriage and Blending Families

Phase	Emotional Responses	Developmental Issues
1. Meeting new people	Allowing for the possibility of developing a new intimate relationship	Dealing with child(ren)'s and ex-family members' reactions to a parent "dating"
2. Entering a new relationship	Completing an "emotional recovery" from past divorce Accepting one's fears about developing a new relationship Working on feeling good about what the future may bring	Recovery from loss of marriage is adequate Discovering what you want from a new relationship Working on openness in a new relationship
3. Planning a new marriage	Accepting one's fears about the ambiguity and complexity of entering a new relationship such as: New roles and responsibilities Boundaries: space, time, and authority Affective issues: guilt, loyalty, conflicts, unresolvable past hurts	Recommitment to marriage and forming a new family unit Dealing with stepchild(ren) as custodial or noncustodial parent Planning for maintenance of coparental relationships with ex-spouses Planning to help child(ren) deal with fears, loyalty conflicts, and memberships in two systems Realignment of relationships with ex-family to include new spouse and child(ren)
4. Remarriage and blending of families	Final resolution of attachment to previous spouse Acceptance of new family unit with different boundaries	Restructuring family boundaries to allow for new spouse of stepparent Realignment of relationships to allow intermingling of systems Expanding relationships to include all new family members Sharing family memories and histories to enrich members' lives

Adapted from McGoldrick, M., Garcia-Preto, N., & Carter, B. (2016). *The expanding family life cycle: Individual, family, and social perspectives* (5th ed.). Upper Saddle River, NJ: Prentice Hall.

having parents with lower levels of education, living in poverty, lack of access to contraception, and being sexually active (Ventura, Hamilton, & Mathews, 2014).

Infants born to teen mothers are at risk for low birth weight, developmental delay, and death before 1 year of age. The infant mortality rate among mothers younger than 15 is twice as high as for women between the ages of 20 and 24 years, and 20% higher among teens between ages 15 and 19 years than from women in their twenties (Ventura et al., 2014). Of all births in 2013 to 15 to 17 year olds, 95% were to unmarried mothers (ChildStats. gov, 2015).

Teen fathers are often left out of the loop for services that communities provide for the teen mother and infant. However, paternal involvement contributes positively to the physical, social, and cognitive development of children. Children with absent fathers are at increased risk for behavioral difficulties and poor academic performance. Longitudinal research found lower birth weights and lower cognitive and behavioral scores at age two and poorer health for children of adolescent fathers when compared with those of adult fathers. Most children of teen fathers live in lower SES households and their mothers frequently do not marry their fathers (Mollborn & Lovegrove, 2011). A father who is emotionally supportive of the mother and provides child care and financial support directly and indirectly affects the well-being of his child.

The implications for the role of the PHN are greatest with the adolescent parent population. For example, nurses work with young teens through schools, clinics, or home-visiting programs to ensure healthy pregnancies and teach parenting skills to the parents and grandparents. Nurses can also ensure that the infant receives immunizations and primary care health services and can provide family planning information to the new parents. SmithBattle, Lorenz, and Leander (2013) suggest that teen mothers respond positively to community health nursing interventions. On a broader scale, community health nurses should collaborate with other professionals to make sure that the community has resources for all levels of prevention, with a focus on primary prevention. By initially approaching the teen parent in the hopes of developing a relationship, positive changes may be set in motion to assist the family in their child-rearing activities (SmithBattle et al., 2013). See Chapter 22.

Cohabitating Couples

Another form of nontraditional families includes couples that form a family alliance outside of a legal marriage. Cohabitating couples may range from young adults living together to an elderly couple sharing their lives outside of marriage to avoid tax penalties or inheritance issues. Cohabitating couples may be heterosexual or gay/lesbian; they may or may not share a sexual relationship. In some instances, these couples have their own biologic

POPULATION-FOCUS ON FAMILIES

How Much Time Do Mothers Need to Spend With Children?

One of the biggest concerns for single mothers is how to best care for their children while at the same time making a living and maintaining a home. Many single mothers feel guilty spending time at work and not having enough time to spend with their young children and adolescents. And early research in this area often touted the need for intensive mothering, spawning the tension between mothers who chose to work versus those choosing to stay home—hence the "Mommy Wars." Many child support structures emphasize the need for mothers of young children to stay home and not work. A study by Milkie, Nomaguchi, and Denny (2015) examined the amount of time mothers spent with their children (ages 0 to 19) on child outcomes of academic performance, as well as emotional and behavioral problems. The data came from two waves of a "nationally representative longitudinal survey of families" (p. 359). The overall findings revealed that none of the measures of maternal time with children were significantly associated with their outcome behaviors. They did find that mother's level of education and family income level were significantly associated with school performance with some subject matter (e.g., reading, math). When compared with children from two-parent homes, those from stepfamilies had greater behavioral problems, and ones from single-mother families had greater emotional problems.

For adolescents, the only differences were behavioral problems for those from single-mother homes. Having time with both parents was beneficial to teens. They noted that the amount of time a mother spends with her 3- to 11-year-old children does not show a significant difference in their outcomes. However, there was some difference noted for adolescents. Time spent in "focused interactions" with adolescents was significantly associated with decreased delinquent behaviors (p. 368). Mother's work hours were negatively associated with their teenager's scores in math. Children and adolescents with a "warmer" mother had better outcomes (p. 369). The researchers noted the limitations of their study, and that mothers often provide engagement with their children in alternative ways (e.g., through proxies [extended family, neighbors, friends], networking with resources [e.g., after-school programs], phone calls) that were not measured in this study. They do encourage mothers to not simply focus time on younger children but to build in quality time with their adolescents.

Do you agree with these findings?

You need more evidence. Where could you find similar research studies that may show differing results?

How could you use this information in your work with single-mother families?

From Milkie, M. A., Nomaguchi, K. M., & Denny, K. E. (2015). Does the amount of time mothers spend with children or adolescents matter? *Journal of Marriage and Family, 77*(2), 355–372.

---

or adopted children. Kuperberg (2014) studied age at "coresidence" and found that a good portion of later marital dissolutions occurred in younger couples with a history of prior cohabitation.

Gay and Lesbian Families

Although the exact number of **gay and lesbian families** is not known, this emerging family type is increasing. It is estimated that there are 600,000 to 4 million children with gay or lesbian parents in the United States (Vespa et al., 2013). Gates (2013) reports there are over 8 million American adults identifying themselves as lesbian, gay, bisexual, and transgender (LGBT), and 3 million of them report having had a child. Six million American children and adults state that they have at least one parent who is LGBT. Almost one half of LGBT women are raising a child and about one fifth of LGBT men. Foster and adopted children are often being raised by LGBT couples, and over 25% of same-sex couples are raising siblings, grandchildren, or other related/nonrelated children. About half of the children living with same-sex couples are non-white (Gates, 2013).

One of the new topic areas established by *Healthy People 2020* is Lesbian, Gay, Bisexual, and Transgender (LGBT) Health, and this speaks to the importance of understanding the discrimination and oppression that LGBT families have faced (Display 18–2). Although

much progress has been made in accepting people with values and beliefs different from those of the mainstream, pervasive homophobia and heterosexism persist (U.S. Department of Health and Human Services, 2016).

Gay and lesbian families have many of the same hopes regarding parenting that any family may have. In addition, they experience the stress that accompanies being stigmatized by much of a society. Lack of acceptance from their families and communities may have negative implications on their own family. Brown (2013) reports that 21% of LGBT participants surveyed have experienced workplace discrimination. Other markers of discrimination (e.g., rejected by family/friend, been a subject of jokes/slurs, threatened or physically attacked, poor service at business, hotel, restaurant) have shown decreases from past year to current year; this indicates that some progress has occurred. But annual family income is lower (39% vs. 38% earning < $30,000; 20% vs. 34% earning < $75,000) for LGBT families than for overall U.S. population.

The nurse can become a valued resource for the family. Through education and anticipatory guidance, the nurse can assist the family to successfully navigate the developmental stages of their children as well as the varied issues faced by families. Research has shown that the psychosocial development of the children of gay or lesbian parents is similar to that of children with

Table 18–5   Questions to Expect from Children About Their Family

Developmental Stage	Concern	Approach
Preschool children	Curious about background of family and meeting other children's parents, or about an absent parent	Answer questions simply and honestly. Talk to your children. Have fun together. Find other families like yours.
School-aged children	Have a better understanding of how their family may be different from other families; may have more questions about family background as they are introduced to other families through peers	Be honest. Talk to your children. Teach your schools. Show unconditional love.
Young and older teens	Know that their family is unique; may become embarrassed by parents. Also may begin to question own sexual orientation	Talk more about your life choices and sexual orientation when asked. Continue to show unconditional love and support.

Adapted from American Academy of Pediatrics. (2015). *Questions to expect*. Retrieved from https://www.healthychildren.org/English/family-life/family-dynamics/types-of-families/Pages/Gay-and-Lesbian-Parents.aspx

heterosexual parents (American Academy of Pediatrics, 2015). The nurse can work with parents to anticipate what questions to expect from their children about their family (Table 18–5).

Older Adults

Elderly individuals are the fastest growing segment of the population. In 2010, 40 million people in the United States were over the age of 65 years or 11% of the total population. This is projected to double by 2030 (AgingStats.gov, 2015). Many older adults live independently well into the eighties and maintain healthy contacts with family and friends. Others feel isolated because of chronic health problems that limit mobility, thereby reducing or eliminating the ability to interact or contribute meaningfully in society (Fig. 18-3).

The community health nurse needs to understand the complex dynamics of such situations and offer support and encouragement as family members work through chronic health problems. Often, a nurse serves an entire community of elders in a senior apartment complex, an assisted living center, or a mobile home community, for whom maintaining wellness is the focus. Keeping physically active, eating healthy meals, receiving appropriate medical care and immunizations, and establishing and

maintaining social contacts are some of the tasks elders should focus on to stay healthy well into old age; these are some of the areas in which the community health nurse can intervene (Touhy & Jett, 2014). See Chapter 24.

Homeless Families

Children make up 39% of the homeless population and 42% of the children are under 6 years of age. Families with young children now account for 40% of the nations' homeless population (National Law Center on Homelessness and Poverty, 2015). On any given night in the United States, 2.5 million children are homeless; this translates into 1 in 30 children. This actually represents an 8% increase from the previous year. Of the adults in homeless families, 29% are working (Bassuk, DeCandia, Beach, & Berman, 2013). You can check your state rates at http://www.homelesschildrenamerica.org/.

Typically, **homeless families** are young single mothers with two children. Ninety-two percent of these women have experienced physical and/or sexual abuse. One in four women is homeless because of violence committed against them. They typically have poorer health than other women and suffer from posttraumatic stress disorder (PTSD) at three times higher rates than other women; one half have a recent history of major depression and one third have a chronic physical condition (National Center on Family Homelessness, 2015).

Homeless families present the PHN with unique challenges. Primarily, the family is in crisis often not being able to provide for its most basic needs. A PHN's knowledge of the resources available in the community is an important first step in providing the family with the help to deal with the crisis and assist in the provision of ongoing shelter, food, health, employment, and schooling needs. See Chapter 28.

Foster Families

Many children are removed from their families because of maltreatment due to abuse, violence, or neglect. In most communities, these children are placed with families known as **foster families** (Gonzalez, 2014). These families take a variety of forms, but all foster families have formal training to accept unrelated children into their homes on

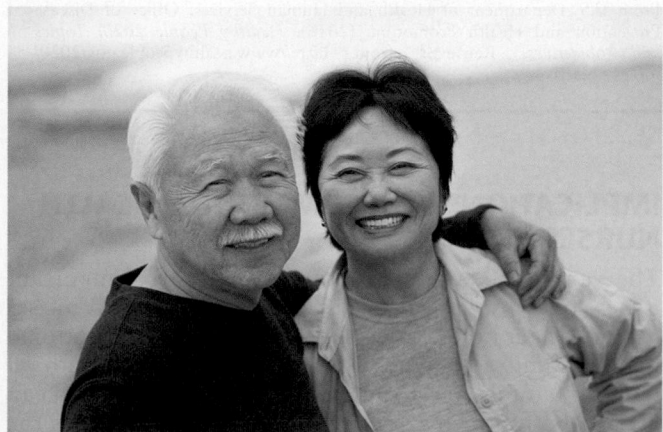

FIGURE 18–3   Older adults constitute a growing population.

DISPLAY 18–2 *HEALTHY PEOPLE 2020* OBJECTIVES

Selected Healthy People Goals and Objectives Related to Family Health

Family Planning

Goal: Improve planning and spacing of pregnancies and prevent unintended pregnancies.

Overview: "Family planning is one of the 10 great public health achievements of the 20th century" (para 2). Family planning services can improve outcomes for families, women, infants, and children.

FP-1   Increase the proportion of adolescents who are connected to a parent or another positive adult caregiver.

FP-5   Reduce the proportion of pregnancies conceived within 18 months of a previous birth.

FP-6   Increase the proportion of females at risk of an unintended pregnancy or their partners who used contraception at most recent sexual intercourse.

FP-8   Reduce pregnancy rates among adolescent females.

FP-9   Increase the proportion of adolescents aged 17 years and under who have never had sexual intercourse.

FP-13   Increase the proportion of adolescents who talked to a parent or guardian about reproductive health topics before they were 18 years old.

Adolescent Health

Goal: Improve the healthy development, health, safety, and well-being of adolescents and young adults.

Overview: Adolescents (ages 10 to 19) and young adults (ages 20 to 24) make up 21% of the population of the United States. The behavioral patterns established during these developmental periods help determine young people's current health status and their risk for developing chronic diseases in adulthood.

AH-3.1 Increase the proportion of adolescents who have an adult in their lives with whom they can talk about serious problems.

AH-3.2 Increase the proportion of parents who attend events and activities in which their adolescents participate.

AH-4   Increase the proportion of adolescents who transition to self-sufficiency from foster care.

AH-4.1 Increase the proportion of adolescents in foster care who exhibit positive early indicators of readiness for transition to adulthood.

Maternal, Infant, and Child Health

Goal: Improve the health and well-being of women, infants, children, and families.

Overview: Improving the well-being of mothers, infants, and children is an important public health goal for the United States. Their well-being determines the health of the next generation and can help predict future public health challenges for families, communities, and the health care system. The objectives of the Maternal, Infant, and Child Health topic area address a wide range of conditions, health behaviors, and health system indicators that affect the health, wellness, and quality of life of women, children, and families.

Morbidity and Mortality

MICH-1   Reduce the rate of fetal and infant deaths.

MICH-8   Reduce low birth weight (LBW) and very low birth weight (VLBW).

Infant Care

MICH-21   Increase the proportion of infants who are breast-fed.

MICH-22   Increase the proportion of employers that have worksite lactation support programs.

Health Services

MICH-30   Increase the proportion of children, including those with special health care needs, who have access to a medical home.

MICH-31   Increase the proportion of children with special health care needs who receive their care in family-centered, comprehensive, coordinated systems.

From U.S. Department of Health and Human Services, Office of Disease Prevention and Health Promotion. (2016). *Healthy People 2020: Topics and objectives*. Retrieved from http://www.healthypeople.gov/2020/topics-objectives

---

a temporary basis, while the children's parents receive the help necessary to reunify the original family. Although this arrangement is not ideal, most foster families provide safe and loving homes for these children in transition. Often, foster children have emotional and physical health problems, and they may never have experienced the positive structure that foster families provide. These problems, which can cause stress for everyone involved, are typically ones that the community health nurse may help to alleviate See Evidence-Based Practice.

IMPLICATIONS FOR COMMUNITY HEALTH NURSES

The variety of family structures raises three important issues for consideration. First, community health nurses can no longer hold to a myth that idealizes the traditional nuclear family. They must be prepared to work with all types of families and to accept them. Unless the PHN can accept the full array of family lifestyles and address the special needs of each, it is questionable that they will be

EVIDENCE-BASED PRACTICE
Parenting Programs for Incarcerated Parents and Their Children

Recognizing the significant public health implications of parents who are in prison and their children was the impetus for a literature review of programs targeting these vulnerable families. Newman, Fowler, and Cashin (2011) cited the intergenerational nature of criminal activity and delinquency as leading to poor choices made by these children during childhood and into their adult years. The risk that these children will themselves develop poor parenting skills and engage in criminal activity is well documented. Families with one or more parents incarcerated are a growing problem in Australia, the United States, and England, with nearly 2 million children in the United States alone having a parent in prison. The authors reviewed the literature on 11 prison programs designed to deliver some level of parenting support using a variety of methods, both short and longer term. These programs were seen to vary in both delivery methods and evaluation; most significantly, few looked at the long-term impact of the programs. Using educationally based approaches covering areas of child development, communication, play skills, child safety, and discipline, they ranged from as few as 5 hours to a program lasting 24 weeks. The potential for improving child–parent relationships through increased contact and facilitation of that contact were seen as essential to both the child's well-being and the recidivism of the parents. The authors stress that addressing this growing public health problem requires assurance that evidence-based approaches are used and evaluation of effectiveness is ongoing.

A more recent study by Whalen and Loper (2014) examines an impact on children when a parent is unable to care for them because of incarceration. The researchers analyzed data from 12 waves of survey data from a U.S. longitudinal study of youth and found that girls who had a household member incarcerated had more family and demographic risk factors present than did those who did not. Using advanced statistical methods, they were able to demonstrate that teen pregnancy could be predicted by the additional variable of household incarceration in addition to basic family and demographic variables. They noted that prevention programs should be developed for at-risk teenage girls who have household members incarcerated along with other family dynamic risk factors.

1. As you will see in Chapter 30, many public health nurses are employed in state and federal prisons; what challenges might they face in providing parenting support to these populations?
2. How could long-term evaluation of these programs be achieved?
3. What challenges from the prison system, the public health care system, schools, and politicians would the public health nurse face in the implementation of programs such as these? What sources of support could be identified?
4. Aside from the literature, what other sources might provide information on parenting support (or lack of) in the prison system?

From Newman, C., Fowler, C., & Cashin, A. (2011). The development of a parenting program for incarcerated mothers in Australia: A review of prison-based parenting programs. *Contemporary Nurse*, 39(1), 2–11; Whalen, M. L., & Loper, A. B. (2014). Teenage pregnancy in adolescents with an incarcerated household member. *Western Journal of Nursing Research*, 36(3), 346–361.

---

able to fully help the family and may even create additional difficulties.

Second, the structure of an individual's family may change several times over a lifetime. A girl may be born into a nuclear family and then become part of a single-parent family when her parents are divorced. As she matures, she may become a single adult living alone and then become a part of a cohabiting couple. Still later, she may marry and have children in a nuclear family. After the death of her husband as a senior citizen, she may have a relationship outside of marriage and choose not to remarry. For the individual, each family form involves changes in roles, interaction patterns, socialization processes, and links with external resources. The community health nurse must learn to address clients' needs throughout these life changes equipping people with the skills needed to deal the inevitability of changing structures.

Finally, each type of family structure creates different issues and problems that, in turn, influence a family's ability to perform basic functions. Gottlieb (2013) recommends a strength-based approach by getting to know families for "what they do best" (p. 1). Wright and Leahey (2013) discuss the need for nurses to identify and develop strengths with families in planning nursing care. This should be a community health nurse's starting point. What are the family strengths? How does the family see their strengths? All families have strengths, although sometimes these are not easily recognized. It is important for the nurse to identify these with the family's collaboration (Display 18–3).

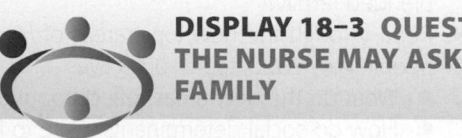

DISPLAY 18–3 QUESTIONS THE NURSE MAY ASK THE FAMILY

1. What are your strengths as a family?
2. If you had to tell me your three most favorite things about your family what would they be?
3. Name one quality about your mother that you really respect. About your father? Your partner? Your child?
4. What is your best memory of your family?

SUMMARY

The family as the unit of service has received increasing emphasis in nursing over the years. Today, family nursing has an important place in nursing practice, particularly in community health nursing. Its significance results from recognizing that the family itself must be a focus of service, that family health and individual health strongly influence each other, and that family health affects community health. A community health nurse's effectiveness in working with families depends on an understanding of family theory and characteristics.

Every family on the globe is unique; its needs and strengths are different from those of every other family. At the same time, each family is alike because of certain shared universal characteristics. Five of these universal characteristics have particular significance for community health nursing: every family is a small social system, has its own cultural values and rules, has structure, has certain basic functions, and moves through stages in its life cycle.

Family patterns influence the role of the community health nurse. The single adolescent parent needs the community health nurse's knowledge of family developmental theory. More complex interaction patterns and living arrangements are created by divorce, remarriage, the blending of families, and the unique relationships these arrangements create. Gay and lesbian families with children may also have special needs calling for a sensitive understanding of society's reaction to their family. Understanding families different needs will help the nurse provide appropriate services.

The chapter ends as it begins with several important points to consider when working with families. The nurse begins where the family is and accepts the family's own definition of who their family is and listens to the family's ideas about the direction of visits and time together. The nurse and the family become partners in providing health care. The nurse should begin the work assessing the family's strengths, which will begin to build a positive relationship between the nurse and the family. This is the essential starting point in the community health nurse's work.

ACTIVITIES TO PROMOTE CRITICAL THINKING

1. Get together with a small group of your peers. Ask each of your peers to define family and then compare each of your definitions. How similar or different are each of the definitions? What in each person's own experience may account for the way they view families?

2. Analyze two families you know well (other than your own) and answer the following questions:
   If the major breadwinner in this family was unable to work or lost his or her job, how would the family most likely respond immediately and in the long term?
   What developmental stage is this family currently in and how does that affect their functioning?
   What are the strengths of the family?
   How could a nurse most effectively intervene in this situation?

3. More LGBT couples are becoming parents. What are some of the characteristics they have in common with other parents? What could be some concerns they might have?

4. Talk with members of a blended family and discuss with each member his or her relationships with stepchildren, stepparents, or siblings. What strengths can they identify in their family? How has this helped them adapt to their blended family?

5. Read through the new topic areas of *Healthy People 2020* that relate to family health at http://www.healthypeople.gov/2020/topics-objectives.
   ● What do the new areas reflect about changes in our society?
   ● How do social determinants relate to family?
   ● *Healthy People 2020* calls for more research in the areas of LGBT parenting issues throughout the life course. What do you think are potential areas of needed research? Back up your position with current research and statistics.

REFERENCES

AgingStats.gov. (2011). *Population*. Retrieved from http://www.agingstats.gov/agingstatsdotnet/Main_Site/Data/2010_Documents/Population.aspx

American Academy of Pediatrics. (2015). *Promoting the wellbeing of children whose parents are gay*. Retrieved from https://www.aap.org/en-us/my-aap/advocacy/Documents/Promoting_the_Well-Being_of_Children_Whose_Parents_Are_Gay.pdf

Bassuk, E. L., DeCandia, C. J., Beach, C. A., & Berman, F. (2014). *America's youngest outcasts: A report card on child homelessness*. Retrieved from http://www.homelesschildrenamerica.org/mediadocs/282.pdf

Bell, J. (2013). Family nursing is more than family centered care. *Journal of Family Nursing, 19*(4), 411–417. doi: 10.1177/1074840713512750.

Brown, A. (2013, November 4). *As Congress considers action again, 21% of LGBT adults say they faced workplace discrimination*. Retrieved from http://www.pewresearch.org/fact-tank/2013/11/04/as-congress-considers-action-again-21-of-lgbt-adults-say-they-faced-workplace-discrimination/

ChildStats.gov. (2015). *America's children: Key national indicators of well-being*. Retrieved from http://www.childstats.gov

Duvall, E. M., & Miller, B. (1985). *Marriage and family development* (6th ed.). Philadelphia, PA: Lippincott Williams & Wilkins.

Friedman, M. M., Bowden, V. R., & Jones, E. G. (2003). *Family nursing: Research, theory, and practice* (5th ed.). Upper Saddle River, NJ: Prentice Hall.

Gates, G. J. (2013). *LGBT parenting in the United States*. Retrieved from http://williamsinstitute.law.ucla.edu/wp-content/uploads/LGBT-Parenting.pdf

Gonzalez, M. J. (2014). Mental health care of families affected by the child welfare system. *Child Welfare, 93*(1), 7–57.

Gottlieb, L. N. (2013). *Strengths based nursing care: Health and healing for person and family*. New York, NY: Springer Publishing Company.

Kaakinen, J. R., Coehlo, D. P., Steele, R., Tabacco, A., & Hanson, S. (2015). *Family health care nursing: Theory, practice and research* (5th ed.). Philadelphia, PA: F. A. Davis Company.

Kuperberg, A. (2014). Age at coresidence, premarital cohabitation, and marriage dissolution: 1985–2009. *Journal of Marriage and Family, 76*(2), 352–369.

McGoldrick, M., Garcia-Preto, N., & Carter, B. (2016). *The expanding family life cycle: Individual, family, and social perspectives* (5th ed.). Upper Saddle River, NJ: Prentice Hall.

Mollborn, S., & Lovegrove, P. J. (2011). How teenage fathers matter for children: Evidence from the ECLS-B. *Journal of Family Issues, 32*(1), 3–30.

National Law Center on Homelessness and Poverty. (2015). *Homelessness in America: Overview of data and causes*. Retrieved from http://www.nlchp.org/documents/Homeless_Stats_Fact_Sheet

Newman, C., Fowler, C., & Cashin, A. (2011). The development of a parenting program for incarcerated mothers in Australia: A review of prison-based parenting programs. *Contemporary Nurse, 39*(1), 2–11.

Parker, K., & Patten, E. (2013, January 30). *The sandwich generation: Rising financial burdens for middle-aged Americans*. Retrieved from http://www.pewsocialtrends.org/2013/01/30/the-sandwich-generation/

Pender, N. J., Murdaugh, C. L., & Parsons, M. A. (2015). *Health promotion in nursing practice* (7th ed.). Boston, MA: Pearson.

Perelberg, R. J., & Miller, A. C. (2011). *Gender and power in families*. London, UK: Karnac Books, Ltd.

Pew Research Center. (2011, January 13). *A portrait of stepfamilies*. Retrieved from http://www.pewsocialtrends.org/2011/01/13/a-portrait-of-stepfamilies/

Plomin, R., & Daniels, D. (2011). Why are children in the same family so different from one another? *International Journal of Epidemiology, 40*(3), 563–582.

Rasheed, J. M., Rasheed, M. N., & Marley, J. A. (2011). *Family therapy: Models and techniques*. Thousand Oaks, CA: Sage Publications, Inc.

SmithBattle, L., Lorenz, R., & Leander, S. (2013). Listening with care: Using narrative methods to cultivate nurses' responsive relationships in a home visiting intervention with teen moms. *Nursing Inquiry 20*(3): 188–198. doi: 1111/j.1440-1800.2012.00606.x.

Titelman, P. (Ed.). (2014). *Differentiation of self: Bowan family systems perspectives*. New York, NY: Routledge.

Touhy, T. A., & Jett, K. F. (2014). *Ebersole and Hess' gerontological nursing & healthy aging* (4th ed.). St. Louis, MO: Elsevier Mosby.

U.S. Department of Health and Human Services, Office of Disease Prevention and Health Promotion. (2016). *Healthy People 2020*. Retrieved from http://www.healthypeople.gov/2020/

United Nations. (2014). *Households and families*. Retrieved from http://unstats.un.org/unsd/demographic/sconcerns/fam/fammethods.htm

United Nations. (n.d.). *Family*. Retrieved from http://www.un.org/en/globalissues/family/

Unnatural Causes. (2008). *Is inequality making us sick?* Retrieved from http://www.unnaturalcauses.org

Ventura, S. J., Hamilton, B. E., & Mathews, T. J. (2014, August 20). National and state pattern of teen births in the United States, 1940–2013. *National Vital Statistics Reports, 63*(4), 1–33. Retrieved from http://www.cdc.gov/nchs/data/nvsr/nvsr63/nvsr63_04.pdf

Vespa, J., Lewis, J. M., & Krider, R. M. (2013). *America's families and living arrangements: 2012 population characteristics*. Retrieved from https://www.census.gov/prod/2013pubs/p20-570.pdf

Walsh, F. (Ed.). (2012). *Normal family processes: Growing diversity and complexity* (4th ed.). New York, NY: Guilford Press.

Wright, L. M., & Leahey, M. (2013). *Nurses and families: A guide to family assessment and intervention* (6th ed.). Philadelphia, PA: F. A. Davis.

CHAPTER 19

Working with Families: Applying the Nursing Process

"If the family were a fruit, it would be an orange, a circle of sections, held together but separable—each segment distinct."

—*Letty Cottin Pogrebin*

KEY TERMS

Community
Conceptual framework
Developmental framework
Eco-map
Family

Family health
Family nursing
Genogram
Home
Interactional framework

Outcome evaluation
Population
Referral
Resource directory
Strengthening

Structural–functional
framework

LEARNING OBJECTIVES

Upon mastery of this chapter, you should be able to:

- Describe the components of the nursing process as they apply to enhancing family health.
- Identify the steps in a successful family health intervention.
- Describe useful activities and actions when intervening on family health visits.
- List at least six specific safety measures the community/public health nurse should take when traveling to a home or making a home visit.
- Describe the effect of family health on individual health.
- Describe individual and group characteristics of a healthy family.
- Identify five family health practice guidelines.
- Describe three conceptual frameworks that can be used to assess a family.
- Describe the 12 major assessment categories for families.
- List the five basic principles the community/public health nurse should follow when assessing family health.
- Discuss the two foci of family health visits: education and health promotion.
- Describe the three types of evaluations that are necessary after family health interventions.

Chapter 18 explored the theoretical basis of family formation and the variety of family structures. Other chapters have stressed that families come in all sizes, consist of members of many ages and biologic relationships, and experience the world filtered through their unique cultures. There are many theoretical approaches and roles to consider when caring for families. This chapter explores the nursing process as it applies to community/public health nurses working with families, the "core unit of service," in the promotion of health and wellness, illness prevention, and overall improved health of the population.

The delivery of care to families occurs in various community settings (i.e., their homes, their work settings, classrooms, clinics and outpatient departments, neighborhood centers, and homeless shelters). Although caring for the family, as a unit of service, is an effective way to treat the population in the communities, a gap often exists between family nursing theory, development, and practice. The problem, in part, is derived from a health care system that tailors services to an individual and not a family and/or a community. This is evident in many third-party payer and reimbursement policies that impose limits to the kinds of services funded, in public health agencies' tendencies to organize services around individuals, and in government requirements that agencies keep statistics for specific diseases or service categories that reflect individual rather than family or aggregate data.

By focusing on the health needs of the core unit of service, the family, public health nurses address the health needs of the communities for the treatment of the population (American Nurses Association [ANA], 2013). Through legal changes, public health nurses are the leaders in using the accessible health care services to prevent illnesses and promote health in families (ANA, 2014; American Public Health Association, 2013; Davis & Gustafson, 2014). Therefore, family health has become the cornerstone for community and population health, making the family the focus of health care and related services.

The family is the basic element of a community and a population. A **family** refers to a group of individuals whose behaviors, actions, health conditions, and interrelationships impact the health of the group and the individuals (Smith, 2013a). A **community** relates to a set of people in families that share a common purpose with a sense of belonging and place (ANA, 2013). A **population** encompasses the total number of persons in families within communities at a specific geographic location (ANA, 2013). Based on the above definitions, providing the family with a positive experience when accessing health services means improved health for the community that leads to a healthier population. With that premise in mind, it is important for families to have equal access to optimal health care, social services, and community resources in a supportive and healthy environment. For example, immunization programs exist for infants and children. Parks, recreational services, organized team sports, and social centers exist for the physical and emotional well-being of families. Pregnant women can attend childbirth education classes and receive medical care throughout the entire pregnancy from their health care providers (Aston et al., 2015; Parthasarathy, Dailey, Young, Lam, & Pies, 2014). Growing families can access parenting classes and support groups for help with developmental crises and in the management of chronic illness (Bahramnezhad, Asgari, Zolfaghari, & Afshar, 2015). Senior centers exist for the older adults in families, and myriad social and recreational activities offer senior discounts. What all these clients have in common is that they are members of families. Maintaining the health of the family is a way to influence the health and wellness of the population.

Think about how your family has influenced you. Did family members impact your choice for a career or the schools you attended? What impact did your family have on your value system, understanding of right or wrong, or your view of health? What role did the family play in the friendships you've formed? How different would your choices for food be if you had grown up with vegetarian parents or parents that annually hunted deer? Clearly, family members influence each other as well as the family as a whole, making it a unique unit of service.

Just as each family is unique, so too are their homes. Some families live in homes that look very much like yours, where you will feel comfortable almost immediately upon entering it. Other families may live in places that may not feel so comfortable to you. Families live in a variety of structures or buildings that define a home (e.g., mobile homes, high-rise inner-city apartments, rural cabins, cardboard boxes, farm labor camps). To a novice public health nurse, it can be daunting to enter a home that is a small and cluttered apartment, a sparsely furnished single room, or a makeshift structure in disrepair. Each home can bring its own set of unique challenges, as well as strengths, to the families you are visiting. These challenges can also influence the way the public health nurse perceives and interacts with the community to promote health, prevent illnesses, and reduce risk.

Family-level problem-solving techniques are needed to deal with important health issues including health promotion, pregnancy and childbirth, acute life-threatening illness, chronic illness, substance abuse, domestic violence, and terminal illness (Aston et al., 2015; Ayala et al., 2014; Bahramnezhad et al., 2015; Dennis, 2014; Kulbok, Thatcher, Park, & Meszaros, 2012; Parthasarathy et al.,

2014; Prichard, Lee, Hutchinson, & Wilson, 2015). The first step is to complete a detailed assessment of the family with emphasis on both internal and external influences (ANA, 2013). This is foundational to the development of a database on which, to formulate a family diagnosis, an essential step before planning, implementation, and evaluation of services can occur. It is important for the novice public health nurse to understand how to execute their practice within the nursing process. With that in mind, this chapter is structured on addressing the *family* health needs through the nursing process: assessing, diagnosing, planning, implementing, and evaluating to enhance family health.

NURSING PROCESS WITH FAMILIES AS CLIENTS

The nursing process (assessing, diagnosing, planning, implementing, and evaluating nursing care) includes steps used to deliver care to clients in acute care settings and in the extensive clinic system. These same steps are used with families and aggregates in community health settings. The difference is the context and client focus (the family) and the consideration of external variables that have not been encountered in other contexts.

For public health nursing, the nursing process is executed with the family at the center of each step, knowing that addressing the health needs of the core unit of service will always transition into the health needs of the community and the population. As shown in Table 19–1, the context and application of each step are tailored to the needs of the population by focusing on the core unit of service (ANA, 2013).

Family assessment refers to a detailed collection of information from the public health nurse's observations about the family and external factors (e.g., family members, extended family, friends, neighbors). This assessment includes verbal and nonverbal cues, what is observed, and what is not observed because certain barriers to health care may be invisible, camouflaged as another issue, or understated (e.g., social bias, cultural prejudices, or geographical constraints). During the family diagnosis process, the public health nurse recognizes patterns, behaviors, and/or seen/unseen routines from the collected information during the assessment. This step involves identifying issues, risks concerns, and problems that can negatively alter the health of the family. During the family planning of care step, targeted outcomes and goals are identified based on the patterns of unhealthy behavior and relationships. A plan of care is created and includes interventions, strategies, and interactions, which involves family resources and external services to promote the health of the family. Implementation of family care plan goes beyond just completing the plan of care to achieve the desired outcomes. The public health nurse collaborates with the family, community resources, and external services to organize and complete the plan of care. The family is educated about the resources and how to use them to address the health problems and promote the **family health**. Also, it is important to be aware of ways to include seen and unseen cultural and social issues in completing the interventions and strategies. Finally, the evaluation step is where the entire process from assessment to implementation is reviewed to determine if (1) the targeted outcomes and goals were achieved, (2) the

	Client = Individual	**Client = Family in Community**
Table 19–1	**The Nursing Process**	
Step 1	Assessment—gather information, subjective and objective, from interviewing client	Assessment—collect detailed health information about families from observations, interactions, and inferences in a systematic and continuous process to understand population's health status
Step 2	Diagnosis—identify problems of concern specific to client and assign action-based categories	Diagnosis and priorities—analyze assessment data to identify patterns of behavior, constraints to health, potential risks, actual risks, and unhealthy routines within and outside family relationships and their interactions
Step 3	Planning—identify interventions and plan of care for client with targeted outcomes and goals	Outcomes identification—in collaboration with the family, determine what the expected outcomes and goals will be for a detailed plan of care Planning—document the plan of care with clearly defined prescriptive interventions and strategies uses resources within the family and community
Step 4	Implementation—execute the interventions for the targeted goals and outcomes with the client	Implementation—work with the family to fulfill the interventions and strategies in the plan of care, which involves, but is not limited to: • Organizing the care • Educating the family about ways to prevent illnesses and promote health • Advising on how to use internal and external resources • Collaborating for health promotion activities
Step 5	Evaluation—review goals and outcomes achieved by the client and determine if further actions are needed	Evaluation—with the family, systematically and continuously review the process in achieving the targeted outcomes with the family and plan for future steps to promote and maintain the health of the family with internal and external services

process was a positive experience for the family, (3) new and current relationships with internal and external resources will maintain and strengthen the efforts for the family health, and (4) the family feels comfortable in participating in their care. With this understanding of the nursing process, the novice public health nurse is ready to prepare to work with families in the community.

Working With Families in Community Settings

Family visits are not limited to the home, and by "thinking outside the box," the nurse has a variety of nonhome settings or public places for visits to accommodate the family's schedules and routines. As long as a family member is comfortable with the nonhome setting, a visit may occur at school or work during a lunch break, in a day care or senior center, in a group home, or myriad after-work or after-school and recreational settings (Dennis, 2014). In general, the nurse must make sure that the family as the client, the school principal, employer, or center director is alright with the visit in a public place, which supports the use of community resources for the family health. This opportunity can be used to strengthen the nurse's relationship with the community and educate the family about community resources, both falling within the steps of the nursing process. The nurse must also remember that families appreciate the individualized effort and respond more positively when nurses are willing to work with family member's schedules (see Perspectives: Voices From the Community).

When making visits in public places, such as worksites or schools, it is important to respect and comply with the family member's wishes (Dennis, 2014). The time and place may have been selected because that individual is able to focus on the visit and feels comfortable to give detailed feedback. The visit may occur during lunch break in a business office on the day that the boss is off or after the lunch crowd disperses in a restaurant so that the individual can take a break. Be mindful of maintaining a confidential atmosphere so that the individual feels safe and not distracted by background noise and/or people. Seek out a place for the visit where other employees or customers cannot overhear your conversation or determine the purpose of the visit. Meeting in the waiting area of a restaurant after lunch may seem ideal, but a table in the back of the restaurant decreases the

risk of distractions, people overhearing the conversation, or people guessing the nature of the visit from the individual's and your body language.

Visiting a family member in the places where he or she spends time during the day can enhance the family assessment. The nurse can assess an individual's ability to function within public places and independent of the home setting. It decreases the potential impact of issues in the home on the individual's response(s) to the questions. The assessment of a child in a day care or an elderly family member in an adult day care will include that individual's ability to manage, participate, and interact in a frequently visited public place. This information can provide insight into problems the family is referring to when you make a home visit. Visiting children during the school hours often give insight into health problems and emotional issues that the parents may be concerned about or unaware of their existence. Such visits can offer the nurse an excellent opportunity to consult with the school's principal, teachers, nurse, counselor, and psychologist. As the public health nurse, you can suggest and coordinate a meeting between the school professionals and the parents while acting as an advocate for the family member(s) and liaison for the school resources during the meeting.

Working With Families Where They Live

Depending on the setting for public health nursing practice, the nurse encounters most family members in their homes and neighborhoods. Some see families in transition, who are living on the streets, in homeless shelters, or with relatives or friends. Regardless of the family's location, the family is the client; the family is the unit of service in public health nursing (Kaakinen, Coehlo, Steele, Tabacco, & Hanson, 2015) (Fig. 19–1).

The Home Visit

It is a privilege to be able to visit families in their homes or private space and work with their neighbors within their community. In this unique setting, you are permitted into the most intimate of spaces that we, as human beings, have. Our homes are our creations, our private spaces; they hold our personal treasures and our memories. A **home** refers to a place that is either a permanent or temporary

PERSPECTIVES
VOICES FROM THE COMMUNITY

I couldn't believe it when she (the community health nurse) said she could visit me during my lunch break. I have been so worried about Ben's hearing and with my new work hours I kept missing her—I got her notes she left in the screen door. She actually drove all the way out to my work to tell me about his hearing test at school and the teacher's classroom changes. I can't afford to lose this job—and she came here!

Mary Anne, 34, Ben's mother

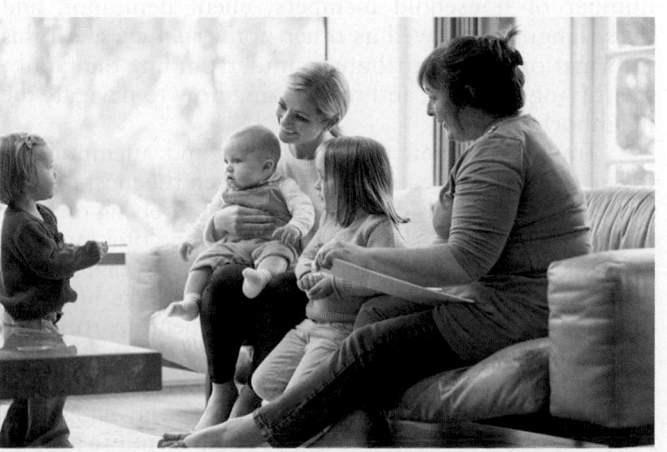

FIGURE 19–1 Home visit with mother and her young children.

residence where an individual eats meals, interacts with others, rests her or his body, and engages in recreational activities (Smith, 2013a). The key to this privilege is trust. Family members must have a certain amount of trust to let a stranger and representative of a governmental agency into their home. Family members are trusting that the visiting stranger is there to help enhance their ability to function as a healthy family with internal and external resources. In the same manner, the nurse must have a certain amount of trust to enter an individual's family home. Once the door is shut behind you, the rules change; you are in the client's world where they are the experts, and you are the guest and may feel like a stranger. Nevertheless, you are trusting that the family welcomes your visit and is ready to work with you for healthier outcomes.

Skills Used During Home Visits

Many skills, in addition to expert nursing skills, are needed when assessing, diagnosing, planning, implementing, and evaluating services in the home to families at a variety of functional levels. Expert interviewing skills and effective communication techniques are essential for effective family intervention (see Chapter 10). It is equally important to enhance these established techniques with your relational skills (e.g., intuition, openness, nurturing, and compassion) (Porr, 2015; SmithBattle, Lorenz, & Leander, 2013). The key to a productive home health visit and effective use of nursing skills is the development of a trusting relationship (Aston et al., 2015). The following paragraphs describe special skills required when making home visits.

Acute Observational Skills

You are preparing for a home visit to a new family in a new environment. You will be using your acute observational skills to assess both the family and the environment, which are equally important for a detailed assessment. Acute observational skills refer to the ability to take note of every detail (physical and nonphysical) that is directly and indirectly related to the family, the environment, the visit, and the entire process. Throughout the visit, you will focus on the family members' concerns and the purpose of the visit while being observant about the neighborhood, travel safety, home environmental conditions, number of household members, client demeanor, and body language, as well as other nonverbal cues. All this information will contribute to understanding the family, identifying patterns, and recognizing how to navigate the neighborhood.

Traveling to new neighborhoods and attempting to locate a family can cause distress to even the most experienced nurse, but this can be decreased by relying on your acute observational skills. Often, the home of a family is difficult to locate because of several reasons that can be addressed by noticing the smallest detail. The house or apartment number is missing, the basement apartment is not numbered, or the residence may be situated behind another house. As you walk through the neighborhood or apartment building, it is useful to notice the layout and the sequence of the addresses, which can help identify a missing address or a house located behind another. Many anomalies in the layout of a building or a neighborhood may make it difficult for the nurse to locate a family. Addresses on referrals may have numbers transposed where 123 Hickory is listed as 132 Hickory. Perhaps there is a North Hickory that is miles away from a South Hickory, or there is a Hickory Boulevard, Drive, Road, Street, Court, Lane, or Way. There is also the chance that the family member has given a fictitious address, for whatever reason, so that the family remains anonymous as long as possible. Again, using your acute observational skills, it may be possible to prepare ahead of the visit by searching for the address or confirming the information with the referral(s) to identify any anomalies. Of course, this search could also provide information about the environmental conditions of the neighborhood.

Observation of Home Environmental Conditions

Conditions in the neighborhood and home environments reveal important information that can guide diagnosing, planning, and intervention with families. While traveling to and arriving at the family home, you have been gathering information about the neighborhood conditions (e.g., cleanliness, street activities, people's interactions/behaviors) and the physical appearance of the apartment or house. This information can provide an assessment of the resources and barriers encountered by the family. It is important to remember that these observations of the external environment may contradict the family's values, resources, and goals. They may have little control over the neighborhood or the building they live in, especially if they are renting. For instance, a young couple with a baby may be able to rent a $775/month apartment, which is only available in a deteriorating low-income neighborhood with dilapidated buildings. You notice that all occupants are renters and that absentee landlords own the building; they may own several buildings, mainly for profit. A manager handles the property and is employed through a management company owned by the landlords. However, the manager does not seem to know any of the landlords. Yet, upon entering the young couple's apartment, you walk into a nicely furnished, uncluttered, and clean home that is opened to you with pride by the family.

In another situation, you have a home visit with an older couple that lives in an upscale suburban neighborhood. They own their own two-story house that has a two-car garage with a well-groomed lawn and several trees. The husband, an older man, who moves very slowly, greets you at the front door. On entering the house, however, you barely can manage to squeeze through a pathway from the front door to the living room, which is made from ceiling-high piles of boxes, newspapers, and furniture. The pathway continues throughout the house and even into a back bedroom with half the bed covered in papers, books, and a few cats. An older woman is reclining in the other half of the bed. After showing you into the bedroom, the husband leaves the bedroom and heads toward the backyard.

There are many environmental conditions in each of these situations that a nurse can observe and use in her or his assessment that will lead to a family diagnosis and a plan of care to assist each family. Most neighborhoods and homes do not present such extremes. However, if you are unprepared for the extremes, they may overwhelm you, and you may become so distracted that you cannot focus wholly on the family and incorporate these important observations into the plan.

Observation of Body Language and Other Nonverbal Cues

You are gathering data as soon as you have knocked on the door or have rung the doorbell, greeted the people in the doorway, and entered the home (see Perspectives: Public Health Nursing Instructor). Your observations are based on how you perceive the sound of the doorbell or doorknocker, the way the door opens, or the manner in which individuals walk toward and open the door. Assessment from these nonverbal cues and body language are observations that will contribute to your initial opinions and perceptions about the family. Being human, you may form opinions or make judgments about the family before the actual beginning of the meeting. Be aware of this possibility so that you can determine the value of these initial opinions and judgments with the information from the family assessment. Also, realize that *all* family members (present or absent) are doing the same with you. Be aware of all household members; acknowledge and greet them. If some are absent, inquire about them. Make this a habit on all visits. Each family member is important and has opinions and health care needs, even if you only see certain members of the family on each visit.

Be observant of family's nonverbal cues such as body language and demeanor because they can provide information that must not be overlooked. Opening statements such as, "You seem anxious today," or "Did I come at a bad time? You seem distracted," will encourage family members to express what is on their minds, which otherwise might not be indicated or addressed. Through their facial expressions, hand gestures, subtle glances, eye movement, and body language, detailed information will be generated to address both direct and indirect concerns of the family. If you are not open to body language while making a visit, you may overlook important cues and continue with *your* agenda instead of the family member's agenda, without realizing that the family is distracted by another, more pressing issue.

On a related note, it is important to be aware of your own body language. Your mannerisms can tell the family a great deal about how you feel being in their home, doing the visit, perceive the family members, and more about you as a person. Fidgeting with car keys during the entire visit or appearing to be rushed can be perceived as nervousness, anxious, or not wanting to be in the current situation—the home visit. Rudeness, unprofessionalism, and not being knowledgeable about the family, the purpose of the visit, and their resources may be a conclusion the family makes from you giving minimal eye contact while continuously looking at your paperwork, chewing gum, or appearing distracted. Your level of discomfort and perhaps "fear" can easily be suggested from the refusal to sit on any of the furniture or a shocked expression at seeing a roach or mouse scampering across the floor. Remember, your behavior will contribute to the family trusting you and your capabilities during the visit and subsequent visits, as well as interventions.

PLANNING THE HOME VISITS TO MEET THE FAMILY HEALTH NEEDS

The greatest barrier to a successful family health visit is lack of planning and preparation. A visit is not successful just because the nurse enters a home or another setting where the family is present. A successful family health visit takes much planning and preparation and requires accurate documentation and follow-up. In addition, safety measures must be followed not only while traveling in the neighborhood, but also in the home.

Components of the Family Health Visit

The structure of family health visits can be divided into five components that follow the nursing process (see Display 19–1). Previsit preparation steps (assessment, diagnosing, and planning) are necessary to ensure that the actual family health visit (implementation) is complete. The documentation and planning for the next visit (evaluation) concludes the responsibilities for one visit and prepares the nurse for the next action needed.

Previsit Preparation

Based on a referral to the agency, public health nurses identify preliminary family diagnoses and design a plan for the initial family health visit. A **referral** is a request for service from another agency or person. This request is formalized by use of a form or information that the originating agency has transferred to the receiving agency. Referrals may be formal, coming from physicians or complementary agencies, or they may be informal, resulting

---

PERSPECTIVES
PUBLIC HEALTH NURSING INSTRUCTOR

How You Knock Helps Families Open the Door

This question may seem trite but, "How do you knock on the door when you visit a family?" Do you use the "I don't want to be here and if they don't hear the knock I can quickly and quietly leave" type of knock that even Superman can't hear? Or do you knock like, "I'm a bill collector and *you better* open this door!" During this knock, the entire family may be running out the back door or through a window! We suggest a knock that is loud enough to be heard, yet friendly and nonthreatening. If necessary, practice "your knock" until you can create this beneficial combination.

With some families, it is helpful to call toward the door as you knock or ring the bell with, "Mrs. Smith, this is Jenny from the Health Department—remember I was coming by today" or, "Ms. Jiminez, it's the student public health nurse, Terry De Leon, and I brought some pamphlets for you" or, "Hello, it's James from the neighborhood clinic, we planned to meet today." Using such a greeting allows the family to know who is at the door and choose to open the door if they want. It will get you into more homes than the "quiet-as-a-mouse" or "bill-collector" knocks.

—Alice K. PHN

DISPLAY 19–1   GUIDELINES FOR MAKING HOME VISITS: 33 STEPS TO SUCCESS

The following guidelines can be followed to evaluate yourself after making a home visit, or it can be an evaluation tool when another nurse (peer or instructor) evaluates you. Rate yourself using the following scale: 0 = does not apply, 1 = unsatisfactory, and 2 = satisfactory.

Rating   *Assessment*

_____ 1. Studies referral, record, or other available data about the family

_____ 2. Gathers community resource information potentially appropriate to the family

_____ 3. Obtains appropriate supplies or educational material in anticipation of family needs

Diagnosis

_____ 4. Identifies reoccurring problems, issues, and/or concerns in both internal and external settings

_____ 5. Detects gaps in the available data and resources

_____ 6. Identifies issues, problems, and/or concerns emphasized by primary client

Planning

_____ 7. Contacts family to set up an appropriate time for the home visit

_____ 8. Ascertains correct address and directions to the family for the home visit

_____ 9. Formulates a written plan for nursing intervention with each family member

_____ 10. Organizes a chart with forms and charting tools based on the focus of the visit

_____ 11. Plans a route to the family's home that is the most direct, being resource efficient

Implementation

_____ 12. Travels the community with safety, locating the family home with ease

_____ 13. Knocks on the door loudly enough to be heard and in a friendly manner

_____ 14. Introduces self to family members in an appropriate manner

_____ 15. Clearly states the reason for the visit

_____ 16. Allows a few moments of socialization before beginning the visit

_____ 17. Smiles; speaks in a pleasant, friendly tone of voice; and maintains eye contact

_____ 18. Uses aseptic technique when providing nursing care

_____ 19 Respects the dignity, privacy, safety, and comfort of family members

_____ 20. Listens attentively to ascertain what family members are saying or implying

_____ 21. Converses with family members during the home visit

_____ 22. Communicates accurate and meaningful information to family members

_____ 23. Responds to family members in a way that encourages them to continue talking

_____ 24. Uses appropriate words of explanation for family member understanding

_____ 25. Utilizes opportunities for incidental teaching

_____ 26. Commends progress made by individual family members

_____ 27. Explains nursing measures before, during, and after each procedure

_____ 28. Shares the results of nursing measures with family members when indicated

_____ 29. Closes the home visit by summarizing the main points of the visit

_____ 30. Makes plans for the next visit, considering family member wishes

Evaluation

_____ 31. Uses information gathered on the home visit to plan care for next visit

_____ 32. Documents home visit in an appropriate and timely manner

_____ 33. Completes a self-evaluation of the home visit

---

from verbal or telephone referrals from friends or relatives who believe that someone needs help. Referrals are the source of new cases for the agencies, and they need timely responses. Some examples include:

- Referrals may come from labor and delivery hospital units, requesting service for low-birth-weight babies and teen mothers.
- Social service agencies might request a home assessment for a child being returned to parents after previous removal from the home.
- A homeless shelter might be seeking services for homeless or transient persons showing signs of uncontrolled diabetes.

- A battered woman's shelter might need services to treat emotional issues of a mother and her children who are running from an abusive husband and father.
- A referral could come via a telephone call from a woman in a city 500 miles away, requesting that a nurse check on an elderly relative who lives alone in the community and has recently exhibited slurred speech and/or has been homebound. Follow-up visits are made to these families based on need and agency protocol.

Nurses must have a physical place to work with access to a telephone, the Internet, and any other supportive resources deemed necessary, such as educational material (pamphlets, brochures, computer, and related Web site addresses to access educational information), charting tools, and any other supplies required for home visits. Nurses also need a **resource directory**, which is a list of resources for the broader community, or a nurse-made directory of resources created over years of working with people in the community. Some agencies issue a nursing bag to their nurses, but if not, many public health nurses become creative and devise their own carryall tote for supplies. The supplies needed depend on the type of visit; some nurses have several totes for different types of visits. Think about what basic supplies you will need to visit a new mother and her infant or an elderly man with hypertension.

Once the nurse is prepared, contact with the family is made. For a home visit, ideally, the referral contains a correct telephone number for the family, a relative, or a neighbor. If the referral or chart does not contain this information, an unannounced visit is scheduled. During this visit, it is important to get a contact number for the family. When calling for the first time, you, the PHN, will:

1. Introduce yourself
2. Explain the reason for the call
3. Give the reason why the family was referred
4. Indicate what the visit consists of
5. Determine when a visit would be convenient for the family and you
6. Get explicit directions to where the family is staying (the referral may have a different address or the family did not mention that they are staying elsewhere)
7. Repeat the date and time of the scheduled visit

It is possible that some people may question the nurse's intention(s) and become defensive or suspicious. For example, a new young mother may think, "Why is this nurse visiting me so close to my time in the hospital? Did I say something or do something wrong with my baby while I was in the hospital?" In this kind of situation, it is very important that the nurse explain that:

- The visit is a follow-up one to see if the move from the hospital to home is okay.
- The visit is an opportunity for her to ask questions because young mothers often have lots of questions about their new babies, especially outside the hospital. It is also a chance for the nurse to show the mother how to handle the baby in the home.
- The visit is a service provided by the agency to all mothers.
- The visit is paid for by taxes, donations, or by the client's health maintenance organization (if applicable). There is no direct cost to the family.

The nurse needs to extract as much as possible from the referral information, allowing him or her to be specific and exact in preparing for the health visit and contacting the family. This will set the stage for a detailed assessment, appropriate family diagnosing and family-oriented care planning. Following logical steps in the previsit preparation will also enhance the nurse's confidence in her or his ability to intuitively recognize patterns and/or trends from the referral information for preliminary diagnoses to guide preliminary care planning.

Making the Visit

Before the day of the scheduled visit, it is useful to call the family you plan to visit and remind them of the meeting and your arrival time. You will want to reiterate why you are visiting and the anticipated length of time needed for the visit. Once you locate the house and meet the family, the following guidelines for initial contact should be used (Aston et al., 2015; SmithBattle et al., 2013; Porr, 2015):

1. Engage the family in a manner to build a supportive and trusting relationship.
   a. Introduce yourself to the family.
   b. Explain the value of the nursing services provided by the agency.
   c. Spend the first few minutes of the visit establishing cordiality and getting acquainted (a mutual discovery or "feeling out" time).
   d. Become acquainted with all family and household members if you are making a home visit.
   e. Encourage each person to speak for himself.
2. Use acute observational skills.
   a. Use your "sixth sense" or intuition as a guide regarding family responses, questions they ask, and your personal safety (trust your feelings).
   b. Be sensitive to verbal and nonverbal cues.
   c. Be accepting and listen carefully.
   d. Be cognizant of possible internal and external stressors and effect on mental status of family.
   e. Be aware of your own personality—balance talking and listening—and be aware of your nonverbal behaviors.
3. Help the family focus on issues and move toward the desired goals.
   a. Be adaptable and flexible (you may be planning a prenatal visit, but the woman delivered her baby the day after you made the appointment, and now there is a newborn).
   b. Be aware that most clients are not extremely ill and have higher levels of wellness than are generally seen in acute care settings.
   c. Be prepared to develop a sustained continuity of care by actively collaborating with the family in addressing their issues.
4. Near the end of the visit, review the important points and emphasize the family strengths.
5. Plan with the family for the next visit.

The length and primary focus of the visit will vary depending on its purpose. A visit shorter than 20 minutes is generally not enough time for a thorough assessment, unless you are dropping off supplies, relaying information about a referral, or stopping by at the family's request, for instance. On the other hand, a visit over 60 minutes should be avoided and, if lengthy assessments are needed, should be conducted over two visits. Families have routines that are important to them, and long visits can negatively impact future ones. Similarly, if the family feels that nothing of value occurred during a visit, they may not continue to make themselves available for future visits. This becomes a balancing act for the family and the nurse, and you may want to work at picking up on nonverbal cues (SmithBattle et al., 2013; Porr, 2015). Long home visits are not a productive way to provide nursing services. Taking up too much of the family time can reflect the nurse's hesitation in trusting the family to understand and/or follow the instructions and feedback. These visits also limit the family's ability to seek out community resources for community-based health care. Remember, the outcome of better health for family members must be demonstrated in order to support and validate the value, as well as justify the cost of public health nursing services (Monsen, et al. 2014) (see Evidence-Based Practice).

Concluding and Documenting the Visit

After planning for the follow-up visit with the family, it is time to say goodbye and end the visit. This is a good time to pack up any paperwork, materials, and supplies used for this visit in your car and get ready for the next home visit on your schedule. By arriving at the next home visit in this manner, you demonstrate your respect for the family's time, ability to be efficient, and professionalism. You are also being "streetwise" when you use the end of the current visit to prepare for the next home visit. It is safer to expose the contents of your car at the end of your time in the current community because the car, with your equipment, is no longer unattended. Getting your supplies, materials, and paperwork together when you arrive at the next home visit gives clues about what is stored in your car's trunk while you are in the family's home and the car is unattended (Jones, 2015; McDonald, Frazer, & Cowley, 2013).

Documentation or charting of each home visit used to be typically completed as soon as the nurse returned to the agency. Today, charting is encouraged at the end of the visit before leaving for the next one on an agency-provided device (laptop, smartphone, or tablet) linked to electronic charting forms and records. You may be able to chart in your own home after the last visit of the day if time is allowed. For the most part, most agencies expect the charting to be completed as soon as practically possible during that workday.

EVIDENCE-BASED PRACTICE

Home Visiting

The Nurse–Family Partnership (NFP) has a long history of providing prenatal and infancy home visits by nurses to first-time at-risk mothers (Eckenrode et al., 2010; U.S. Department of Health & Human Services [USDHHS], 2011). The overall goal of this program is to prevent child abuse and neglect, children's mental health problems, and infant mortality through home visiting during the first 2 years of the child's life. The program has demonstrated positive results in various ethnic and racial groups and in a variety of living contexts through randomized trials (Mejdoubi et al., 2015; USDHHS, 2011). In order to assess other long-term benefits of the program, 19-year-olds ($n = 310$) were recruited from among the 400 families enrolled in the NFP between 1978 and 1980 in a semirural area of New York (Eckenrode et al., 2010). Of the sample, 29% of the mothers had received public health nurse home visits during pregnancy and the child's first 2 years, 25% received home visits during pregnancy, and 45% did not receive either form of home visiting. These young adults completed a telephone interview that assessed high-school graduation, employment, sexual behavior, childbearing, substance use, and criminal behavior. The girls, whose mothers received both pregnancy and infancy visits by the nurse, were less likely to have been arrested or convicted, had fewer children, and had less Medicaid use. With respect to the factors assessed, there were few programmatic effects demonstrated for the boys. The researchers noted that adult patterns of criminal behavior and educational attainment cannot be effectively assessed for 19-year-olds and propose further study of these individuals at 27 years of age. They further suggest examination of the coherence of intervention effects between the mothers and daughters that was not demonstrated with the sons.

Nursing Implications: The NFP has demonstrated that comprehensive home visiting by nurses can have a positive impact on both the mothers and the children. The cost savings in terms of reduced use of public assistance programs, decreased criminal behavior, reduced pregnancy rates, and delayed pregnancy can offset the operating costs of the program. In addition, the academic achievement of these children may ultimately prove beneficial to the long-term economic prospects of these at-risk children and the communities in which they live. Communities considering reducing or eliminating home visiting programs may want to consider retaining them or possibly implementing the NFP program.

Research in other countries and with other populations has confirmed the effectiveness of this PHN home visiting program.

References

Eckenrode, J., Campa, M., Luckey, D. W., Henderson, C. R., Cole, R., Kitzman, H.,...Olds, D. (2010). Long-term effects of prenatal and infancy nurse home visitation on the life course of youths, 19-year follow-up of a randomized trial. *Archives of Pediatrics & Adolescent Medicine, 164*(1), 9–15.

Mejdoubi, J., van den Haijkant, C. M., van Leerdam, F., Heymans, M. W., Crijnen, A. M., & Hirasing, R. A. (2015). The effect of VoorZorg, the Dutch Nurse-Family Partnership, on child maltreatment and development: a randomized controlled trial. *PLoS One, 10*, e0120182. doi: 10.371/journal.pone.0120182.

U.S. Department of Health & Human Services (USDHHS). (2011). *Home visiting evidence of effectiveness: Implementing NFP*. Retrieved from http://homvee.acf.hhs. gov/Implementation/3/Nurse-Family-Partnership-NFP—Program-Model-Overview/14

Agencies use a variety of forms that assist the nurse to document fully and succinctly. Some forms use a checklist format that contains code numbers, letters, or checkmarks on developmental or disease-specific care plans. For example, four pages may be used to document a postpartum visit and newborn assessment: two narrative forms to chart the expectations for the postpartum mother and baby and two forms to chart the head-to-toe assessment of the newborn. These forms contain a place to document parent teaching according to expected parameters and a place for listing other professionals' involvement with the family. The agency may also use similar developmentally focused checklist forms for high-risk infants, high-risk children, adolescents, and older adults. Other forms may focus on chronic illness (e.g., chronic obstructive pulmonary disease, hypertension, diabetes, alcoholism, HIV/AIDS, communicable diseases) that are common in the agency client base.

Focus of Family Health Visits

The focus of family health visits depends on the mission and resources of the agency providing the service and the needs of the families being served. Some agencies provide education, recreational activities such as summer camps, and support groups for families of people with specific health problems such as Alzheimer's disease, asthma, diabetes, or neurologic disorders. Other agencies provide services directed toward those with special social or economic needs, such as immigrant families, people living in poverty, or the homeless (Ballard, Mooney, & Dempsey, 2013; Dennis, 2014; Lynch et al., 2015; Martins et al., 2015; Salem & Ma-Pham, 2015). Home visits may be a part of the service being provided and are best conducted and received in the comfort and privacy of a family's home. In general, family health visits are designed to be educational, to provide anticipatory guidance, and to focus on health promotion or prevention.

Family Education and Anticipatory Guidance

Official agencies, such as county or city health departments, distribute their services based on the broader community's needs. For example, if there is a large population of teen pregnancies and high-risk infants, the health department may contract with hospitals and private health care providers' offices to provide home or clinic visits to all teens and women with high-risk pregnancies and their newborns after delivery (Schaffer, Goodhue, Stennes, & Lanigan, 2012). On these visits, the public health nurse teaches prenatal, postpartum, and newborn care and provides anticipatory guidance (information needed in the future regarding the child and the need for regular infant health care provider visits, immunizations, and safety awareness). Another community may have a significant number of older adults or migrant workers who need to learn how to manage a chronic illness, enhance their nutrition, and practice safety measures to prevent injuries and falls (Ballard et al., 2013; Ramal, Petersen, Ingram, & Champlin, 2012). For a large concentration of active military families at a nearby army base, the PHN needs to collaborate with military personnel in order to gain access to the base and coordinate services that may be requested.

Family Promotion and Illness Prevention

Teaching people how to prevent illness and how to remain healthy is basic to public health nursing (see Chapter 11). Even within the limitations of chronic illnesses, family members can be taught health promotion activities to live as healthfully as possible (Ha, Narendorf, Maria, & Bezette-Flores, 2015; Kulbok et al., 2012; Williford, Fite, Johnson-Motoyama, & Frazer, 2015). Health promotion activities may include screening for hypertension and elevated cholesterol, performing a physical assessment, and teaching about nutrition and safety. Immunizations are another health promotion activity that has been implemented in the United States for years.

Immunizations are *recommended* for all populations, regardless of age, income, culture, or nation of origin. Immunizations are one major step in promoting the family health and preventing illnesses by protecting the health of the individual and the larger community. Although immunizations are a responsibility of all health departments, usually such services are not brought into the home. But, it is the responsibility of the public health nurse to promote family health and prevent illnesses. The public health nurse can provide information about immunizations, teach the importance of following an immunization schedule, and follow up with the family during home visits.

Public health nurses' role and commitment to health promotion are highlighted with the following statements: "The work of public health nurses with individuals and families is informed by the broader context of the community and/or the population. Improvement of population health is accomplished through individual health promotion strategies to increase knowledge; explore health attitudes, beliefs, and values; and facilitate behavior change to optimize personal health" (ANA, 2013, p. 4). This holistic emphasis can also be found in the Patient Protection and Affordable Care Act (ACA). In particular, social determinants of health have been added with the ultimate goal of creating "social and physical environments that promote good health for all" (USDHHS, 2016, para. 3; see Display 19–2). For more on social determinants of health, see Chapters 15 and 25.

Health promotion and/or illness prevention activities can occur during a family health visit, at a family member's home away from home (e.g., work, school, or recreational facility), or at self-help group meetings. Public health nurses provide health promotion services to couples during prenatal classes by teaching about the expected changes during pregnancy and providing anticipatory guidance for safe infant care and postpartum care (Chartier et al., 2015). They may screen older adults at senior centers for hypertension or elevated cholesterol, teach family members who attend support groups such as Alcoholics Anonymous, or provide mental and health assessments for homeless persons.

Personal Safety on the Home Visit

As mentioned earlier, being streetwise is essential when interacting and traveling throughout communities (Jones, 2015). Continuation of personal safety must be considered while maintaining respect for the families, a trusting relationship, and professionalism (Fig. 19–2).

DISPLAY 19-2 *HEALTHY PEOPLE 2020—SELECT TOPICS AND OBJECTIVES*

Topic: Health-Related Quality of Life and Well-Being

Health-related quality of life (HRQoL) is a multidimensional concept that includes domains related to physical, mental, emotional, and social functioning. It goes beyond direct measures of population health, life expectancy, and causes of death. It focuses on the impact health status has on quality of life. A related concept of HRQoL is well-being, which assesses the positive aspects of a person's life, such as positive emotions and life satisfaction.

Source: U.S. Department of Health and Human Services. (2016). *Health-related quality of life & wellbeing.* Retrieved from http://www.healthypeople.gov/2020/topics-objectives/topic/health-related-quality-of-life-well-being

Objective: Social Determinants of Health

Goal: Create social and physical environments that promote good health for all. Emerging Strategies to Address Social Determinants of Health.

Overview: Health starts in our homes, schools, workplaces, neighborhoods, and communities. We know that taking care of ourselves by eating well and staying active, not smoking, getting the recommended immunizations and screening tests, and seeing a health care provider when we are sick all influence our health. Our health is also determined in part by (1) access to social and economic opportunities; (2) the resources and supports available in our homes, neighborhoods, and communities; (3) the quality of our schooling; (4) the safety of our workplaces; (5) the cleanliness of our water, food, and air; and (6) the nature of our social interactions and relationships. The conditions in which we live explain in part why some Americans are healthier than others and why Americans more generally are not as healthy as they could be.

Source: U.S. Department of Health and Human Services. (2016). *Social determinants of health.* Retrieved from http://www.healthypeople.gov/2020/topics-objectives/topic/social-determinants-of-health

Healthy People 2020, Objective: Lesbian, Gay, Bisexual, and Transgender Health

Goal: Improve the health, safety, and well-being of lesbian, gay, bisexual, and transgender (LGBT) individuals.

Overview: LGBT individuals encompass all races and ethnicities, religions, and social classes. Sexual orientation and gender identity questions are not asked on most national or state surveys, making it difficult to estimate the number of LGBT individuals and their health needs. Research suggests that LGBT individuals face health disparities linked to societal stigma, discrimination, and denial of their civil and human rights.

Healthy People 2020, Objective: Genomics

Goal: Improve health and prevent harm through valid and useful genomic tools in clinical and public health practices.

Overview: The new Genomics topic area and objectives for 2020 reflect the increasing scientific evidence supporting the health benefits of using genetic tests and family health history to guide clinical and public health interventions.

Source: U.S. Department of Health and Human Services. (2016). *Healthy people 2020: Topics and objectives.* Retrieved from http://www.healthypeople.gov/2020/topicsobjectives2020/default.aspx

---

Traveling to and in the Neighborhood

When leaving your "base of operation" (e.g., the health department office, neighborhood clinic, homeless shelter, or campus classroom), make sure you have all the necessary supplies, materials, and paperwork for the scheduled home visits. This effort will make your travel to the community and within the neighborhood safe because you know the contents of your car and how to quickly access them. Always keep your "base of operation" (or agency) aware of your plans and how to promptly reach you by leaving an itinerary of your planned travels, the telephone numbers of families you will attempt to visit, and your mobile phone number. Traveling in the community takes a variety of forms and means different things to different people.

If you are traveling in an agency or private car, you need:

- A full gas tank, addresses for families you are visiting, city/county map or GPS, and a mobile phone (helpful to use speed dialing for emergency numbers such as police, fire department, health department, towing and taxi services).

If you are using public transportation, you need:

- Change for each bus trip, a current bus schedule, knowledge of the exit at the bus stop closest to your family's home, knowledge of the bus stop for the return trip to agency or to the next home visit, and a mobile phone (as above).

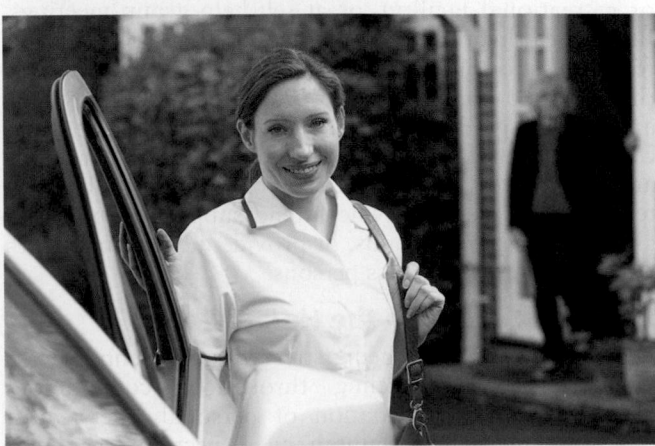

FIGURE 19-2   The public health nurse utilizes appropriate safety measures when making home visits.

You still need to travel safely if you are walking or riding a bicycle to a home visit. Like with all home visits, you will still call ahead to the family and give them an approximate time of your arrival. For some neighborhoods, it is best to ask them to watch out for your arrival. Remember, the families know their neighborhood and may see this as a step toward a trusting relationship. When walking in neighborhoods, be streetwise and walk with direction and purpose. Do not look lost; and if you are, be resourceful in getting help. Use neighborhood shopkeepers as resources for direction and information and as refuge if you feel uncomfortable or threatened. If you need to ask for directions, and you are not near any stores, look for another professional (e.g., a public service employee, police, postal, or utility worker; an apartment manager; or a social worker). If a group of people makes you feel uncomfortable, you want to stay calm. As soon as it is practically possible, cross the street while limiting eye contact with the group, and continue to the home you are intending to visit. Streetwise means to avoid showing fear and/or anxiety while confidently taking measures to remain safe. Always avoid walking through alleys, dark areas, or along buildings that open onto alleys, and stay in the middle of the sidewalk or closer to the street. You may find it helpful to carry a whistle or pepper spray on your key ring.

It is always safest to avoid compromising situations by staying alert and using safe traveling methods whenever you are in public no matter how "safe" the area appears. However, if an individual or group accosts you, immediately try to break free and run to a public place while making loud and lots of noises. Yell "**Fire!**" This response gets more attention than "Help!" Do not argue or challenge a criminal or thief if he or she wants your nursing bag, purse, or wallet. Freely give them up because the contents are not worth your safety; they can always be replaced. Some nurses feel safer after they have attended self-defense classes, which are offered by police departments or through an employee in-service program in some agencies. Nevertheless, the goal in these situations is for you to safely get out of the compromising situation, "not to beat up a perp."

Before venturing into any community, know the neighborhood and what resources are available to you for a safe visit. In some rough inner-city neighborhoods, travel to home visits only in pairs or with a security guard or police escort. Experienced PHNs have found it wise to refuse to visit families living in an isolated area with only one apartment building or with only one block, regardless if it is an inner-city neighborhood or not. Similar issues are found in rural areas known for drug manufacturing and distribution. PHNs understand that it is important to know the safety measures that are used by expert nurses, follow these measures for personal safety, and do not challenge them (Dennis, 2014; Jones, 2015). Safety issues are unique to each community.

Another focus of concern is the perceived risk to self when making a home visit. Feeling and being safe, when traveling to a home visit, can relate to the nurse's perception of a situation, views on risk taking, the traveling conditions (e.g., the time and/or the setting), and coping process (Jones, 2015). What one person sees as a risk, another sees as a challenge or an opportunity. Yet another may see nothing. We each perceive risks differently based on knowledge, experience, and personality.

Arriving at the Home

Make sure you are at the right house. Do not go into the home until you are assured that the family you are intending to visit does live there and is home. For example, you may be planning to visit 16-year-old Jennifer and her 5-day-old infant, Marcus. A 50-year-old man answers the door when you knock. Give your name and ask if Jennifer can come to door because you are here to see her. Do not enter the house even if he invites you in to wait for Jennifer. Smile and let him know that you are comfortable waiting for Jennifer at the door. Remain outside the home and go inside only after you talk to Jennifer at the door. This precaution ensures that the family members you want to visit are really home and that this is the right address.

Friction Between Family Members

During a home visit, two or more family members may begin to argue or physically fight with one another. You want to immediately terminate the visit and inform the family what will take place regarding the home visit. It is highly recommended that you following these steps:

1. Inform the family that the visit is now terminated.
2. Calmly let the family know that such distraction takes away from the purpose of the visit.
3. Inform the family that you will return at another convenient time.
4. Remove yourself from the home.

When two or more family members are physically fighting, never intervene, try to stop the fight, serve as a referee, or assist an adult family member. You may be the next victim. If necessary, call 911 from your mobile phone once you are out of the house. Once you are safe, rely on your acute observation skills to recall the altercation. This data may provide significant information about the family's structure, process, and health. Depending on your assessment and processing of the information, it may be appropriate to discuss the altercation and the friction in the family at a later visit.

Family Members Under the Influence

If the focus of the visit is on two family members and a third member's behavior suggests or indicates drug or alcohol use, you must use your judgment as to the best action to take. Although the agency you work for or the school you attend has guidelines you should follow, it is important for you to assess the situation and proceed accordingly. If the intoxicated person goes to another room and remains quiet/calm, it might be appropriate to continue the visit. You might want to discuss your observations with the two family members. If the intoxicated person remains in the room and interrupts the visit by being abusive or distractive, it is best to terminate the visit. Let the two family members know that you want to reschedule when that family member is not under the influence or is not present. You do not want to put yourself in the middle of a situation that could deteriorate rapidly and compromise your safety.

The Presence of Strangers

In some families, it is common to have extended family members, neighbors, and friends present in the home. Although this is the norm and not distracting to the family, it may be to the nurse because it is a different setting from her or his experience. For example, what would you do if you arrived at a home and you had to weave your way past five teenage boys sitting on the front stoop or steps to the front door? What if you found three men sleeping on the living room floor in the small apartment of a teenage mother and her infant? How would you react to two neighbor children riding their tricycles inside the house during a teaching visit to two young parents who do not seem fazed by the commotion? These situations may not be indicative of danger, but they can make you feel vulnerable and uncomfortable and distract you from the purpose of the visit. Relying on your observation skills, inquire about the people you observe in the periphery of the home visit; ask about their relationship to the family and if they should be included in the visit. The family may suggest that you ignore the other people or say they are transient family members. It may be important to learn who they are, if they have unmet health care needs, or if their presence influences the health of the family you are visiting.

USING THE NURSING PROCESS

The focus of each family visit is different. On the first visit, the public health nurse initiates the nursing process by performing an initial assessment for data that will be later processed for family diagnoses to help the family set their desired goals (see Table 19–1). On subsequent visits, the nurse and the family work collectively on actions and activities to reach the goals. To determine the family's health by using the nursing process in a systematic way, three tools are needed: (1) a conceptual framework on which to base the process, (2) a clearly defined set of data collection categories, and (3) a method of measuring a family's functional level.

Conceptual Frameworks

A **conceptual framework** is a set of concepts integrated into a meaningful explanation that helps the nurse interpret human behavior or situations (Shi & Singh, 2011). Several conceptual frameworks have been used historically to study families (Hill & Hansen, 1960; Reiss, 1981). Three frameworks that are particularly useful in public health nursing are presented here: the interactional, structural–functional, and developmental frameworks (Raingruber, 2014; Shi & Singh, 2011). Although the family remains the core unit of service, steps of the nursing process are centered on the internal interactions, external influences, or a combination of the two.

The **interactional framework** focuses on internal relationships of the family. With this framework, the family is described as a unit of interacting personalities with emphasis on communication, roles, conflict, coping patterns, and decision-making processes (Marlowe, Hodgson, Lamson, White, & Irons, 2014). The family's interactions with the external environment are not emphasized.

The **structural–functional framework** focuses on the family's interaction with the external environment. The family is referred to as a social system in an external environment that results in relationships or interactions with other social systems (e.g., church, school, work, and the health care system). This framework examines the interacting functions between the society and the family. The family social system is built around the family structure, which is used in processing, analyzing, and understanding the function of the family social system in the external environment (Peterson & Bush, 2013).

The **developmental framework** incorporates elements from both interactional and structural–functional frameworks. The family is studied from a life-cycle perspective by examining family members' changing roles and tasks in the members' progression of life-cycle stage within the environment. Internal relationships are studied to understand the development of the family. External environmental influences are examined to recognize how the family structure is created, functions as a social system, and interacts with other social systems. With this framework, the family structure, function, and interaction are viewed in the context of the environment at each stage of family development (Kaakinen et al., 2015).

The concepts of these 3 core frameworks have been combined in various ways to design family assessment, diagnosing process, and intervention models that focus on human–environmental interactions, interactional and structural–functional frameworks, self-care, responses to stressors, and a developmental framework. A combination of the 3 core frameworks is discussed in the Characteristics of Healthy Families section as an initial framework in assessing and diagnosing the family's health by identifying six characteristics. These 3 core frameworks are the basis for various methods of family assessment.

Data Collection Categories

When using a conceptual framework, the public health nurse identifies one or two priority concerns of the family from the previsit preparation for data collection. The conceptual framework gives the nurse a format by which to collect data for specific categories. The amount of data that may be collected about any given family can be voluminous. Considering the nursing process, both the assessment and diagnosing process can be lengthy, time consuming, and ongoing. Often, the most essential data are collected on the first visit. This data may be useful for assessing, diagnosing, care planning, and serving as a guide for subsequent visits in which to obtain additional information.

Certain basic information is needed to determine a family's health status, identify the diagnosis, and design appropriate nursing interventions. Table 19–2 lists the 12 categories, each grouped into one of three data sets: family strengths and self-care capabilities, family stresses and problems, and family resources (Edelman, Kudzma, & Mandle, 2013).

1. *Family demographics* refer to such descriptive variables as a family's composition, socioeconomic status, and members' ages, education, occupation, ethnicity, and religious affiliations.
2. *Physical environment data* describe the internal and external physical environment that consists of the geography, climate, housing, space, social and political structures, food availability and dietary patterns, and any other elements that influence a family's health status.
3. *Psychological and spiritual environment* refers to affective relationships, mutual respect, support, promotion of members' self-esteem and spiritual development, and life satisfaction and goals.
4. *Family structure and roles* include family organization, socialization processes, division of labor, and allocation and use of authority and power.
5. *Family function* refers to a family's ability to carry out appropriate developmental tasks and provide for members' needs.

Table 19-2 Categories of Data Collection for Family Health Assessment

Assessment Categories	Family Strengths and Self-Care Abilities	Family Stresses and Problems	Family Resources
1. Family demographics			
2. Physical environment			
3. Psychological and spiritual environment			
4. Family structure/roles			
5. Family functions			
6. Family values and beliefs			
7. Family communication patterns			
8. Family decision-making patterns			
9. Family problem-solving patterns			
10. Family coping patterns			
11. Family health behavior			
12. Family social and cultural patterns			

6. *Family values and beliefs* deal with raising children, making and spending money, education, religion, work, health, and community involvement. Values and beliefs influence all aspects of family life.
7. *Family communication patterns* include the frequency and quality of communication within a family and between the family and its environment.
8. *Family decision-making patterns* refer to how decisions are made in a family, which includes who makes the decisions and how they are implemented.
9. *Family problem-solving patterns* describe how a family handles problems and involve who deals with the problems, the family's flexible approach to problem solving, and the nature of solutions.
10. *Family coping patterns* encompass how a family handles conflict and life changes; this consists of the nature and quality of family support systems and family perceptions and responses to stressors.
11. *Family health behavior* refers to familial health history, current physical health status of family members, family use of health resources, and family health beliefs.
12. *Family social and cultural patterns* comprise family discipline and limit-setting practices, family initiative/creativity/leadership, family goal setting, family culture, cultural adaptations to present circumstances, and development of meaningful relationships within and outside the family.

FAMILY HEALTH ASSESSMENT

A thorough family health assessment relies on the public health nurse's commitment and determination to learn and understand as possible about the family in order to promote family health. A limited amount of information is given with the referral; however, the assessment allows the nurse to determine the value of that information and any

prior opinions and/or information about the family. Certain assessment tools or guidelines can help the PHN conduct a detailed family assessment and organize data (Fig. 19–3).

Assessment Methods

Assessment methods are used to generate information about selected aspects of family structure and function, and the methods must match the purpose for assessment. The methods may have an informal approach where the nurse relies on her or his acute observational skills for the assessment. In addition, the nurse uses occasional questioning to confirm the observations and determine the next direction to take. A formal approach may include specific questions and assessment tools such as questionnaires, tests, and/or charts/diagrams. The nurse may ask specific questions about each family member, which may include the health data and history of the

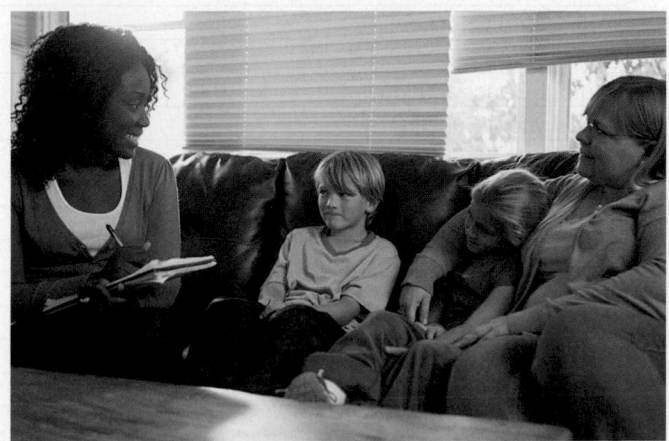

FIGURE 19–3 Family health assessments are foundational to the PHN's work with families.

family. An assessment tool may contain physical data (e.g., height, weight, pulse, temperature, blood pressure) or items related to the family's development. The public health nurse can work with the family in completing tools to gather information on potential health problems that may not be detected by family members. For exam- ple, the use of developmental screening tests for young children can assist in determining if the children were high-risk newborns and the degree to which they have overcome any potential issues. A high-risk infant flow sheet (see Fig. 19–4) is useful in connecting the specific problems with the type of high-risk newborn (e.g., fetal

FLOW SHEET—HIGH-RISK INFANT

Pt's Name _____ Address _____ Phone _____

At Birth: Weight _____   Length _____   Head Circ. _____   APGARS _____

	Date									
Irritability										
Lethargic										
Vomiting										
Diarrhea										
Feedings										
• Amount										
• Frequency										
• Suck										
Seizures/Convulsions										
Stools										
• Color										
• Consistency										
• Frequency										
Urine Output										
Edema										
Eyes Roll										
Temperature										
Pulse										
Respiration										
Weight										
Length										
Femoral Pulses										
Reflexes										
Muscle Tone										
Skin										
• Color										
• Condition										
Auscultate Chest										
Edema										
Output-Concentration										
Respiratory Function										
• Nasal Flaring										
• Grunting										
• Sternal Retracting										
• Tachycardia										
Head Circumference										
Chest Circumference										
Initials										

O - Normal   X - Problem (See Narrative)   C - Counseled for prevention

FIGURE 19–4 High-risk infant flow sheet.

Immunization (Circle & Date)

DTaP 1 2 3 4 _____   PPD _____   MMR _____   Hib _____

Polio 1 2 3 _____   Hep B _____   Varicella _____   PCV _____   RV _____   Flu _____

Instruction	Instruction Date	Pt. Understanding Date	Pamphlets Given Date	Comments	Initials
Review Disease Process					
Temperature Technique					
Feeding & Technique					
Bonding					
General Care					
• Bath					
• Hygiene					
• Formula Preparation					
• Cord Care					
Prevention of Infection					
Environment—Temperature Control					
Position					
Growth & Development					
Safety					
Stimulation					
Immunizations					
Referred to:					
Medical App./Date/M.D.					
S/S of Sick Child					

Initials	Signature

FIGURE 19–4   (*Continued*)

alcohol syndrome newborn, drug-exposed newborn, failure to thrive, birth defect) so that appropriate treatment can be implemented.

The eco-map and the genogram are two assessment tools that are developed and completed by both the family and the nurse. The **eco-map** shows the connections between a family and the other systems in the ecologic environment. Originally designed to help child welfare workers study family needs, the eco-map visually depicts dynamic family–environment interactions (de Cássia Tszesnioski, da Nóbrega, de Lima, & Facundes, 2015). The family or family member is represented by a central circle with smaller satellite circles on the periphery representing people and systems (e.g., school or work) that have significant relationships with the family. Strength of relationships is depicted by the lines to and from the central circle to the satellite circle (see Fig. 19–5). The map is used to discuss and analyze these relationships.

The **genogram** graphically displays family information in a way that provides a quick view of complex family patterns. It is a rich source of hypotheses about a family over a significant period of time, usually three or more generations (Leonidas & Santos, 2015), and is a diagram of the family's genealogy or family relationships.

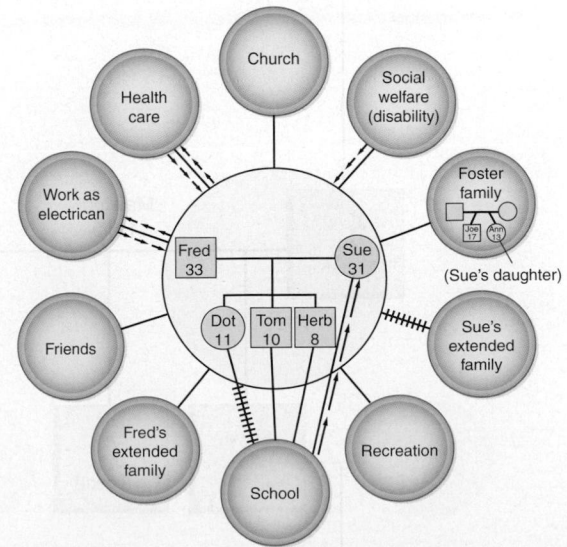

FIGURE 19–5   Eco-map of family's relationship to its environment. Lines indicate types of connections: *solid lines*, strong; *dotted lines*, tenuous; *lines with crossbars*, stressful. *Arrows* signify energy or resource flow, and absence of lines indicates no connection.

The diagram can visually depict significant life events (e.g., birth, death, marriage, divorce, illness), demographic characteristics (e.g., race, religion, social class), occupations, and places of family residence. Again, this tool is completed with the family. It encourages family expression and sheds light on family behavior and problems (see Fig. 19–6). Recognizing the value of this type of assessment, an initiative was launched in 2005 to bring awareness of the familial links between health outcomes and the need to develop prevention strategies based on potential health risks (USDHHS, 2012). Using the downloadable materials provided on the Web site www.hhs.gov/familyhistory/, public health nurses can work with families to create their own family health portrait. The genogram has also been stressed as a useful way to guide clinical and public health interventions (Smith, 2013b).

A detailed family assessment may involve several different instruments to gather data on family structure, function, and development. For consistency and ease of documentation, public health nursing agencies usually develop their own tools, often in the form of questionnaires, checklists, flow sheets, or interview guides (Monsen et al., 2014). The format varies to fit organizational needs. For example, most agencies have changed to computerized information management systems and have adjusted data collection to be technologically compatible. See Chapter 10 for more on electronic health records. Three sample assessment tools are shown in Figures 19–7 to 19–9. Figure 19–7 shows a checklist

format with scores and dates of assessment gathering. It is useful over a span of time for observing family growth or decline, especially for the novice public health nurse, who can document assessment data as rapport with the family is established or as the comfort level with home visits increases.

Figure 19–8 offers an open-ended assessment tool. The open-ended format is brief and lends itself to subjectivity. The goal is to create a document that is informative for all who use it while limiting subjective observations—a difficult task with open-ended tools. Such a tool may be useful in a teen perinatal program or a senior support program, in which a primary nurse makes the home visits and an additional nurse visits occasionally.

Figure 19–9, the self-care assessment guide measures a family member's ability to provide self-care. This assessment tool provides a way to compile the data after gathering the family assessment information. With this method, useful information can be gathered about stressors and self-care practices (e.g., prescription medicines, over-the-counter [OTC] medicines, herbal remedies, nutritional supplements, other complementary therapies). Such assessment tools are useful adjuncts, especially for families coming from various cultural groups. Another assessment method is the use of technology such as videotaping family interactions to provide structured observation and analysis of life-changing events. They are often used in combination with other tools to enhance the breadth of data collection and understanding of the family.

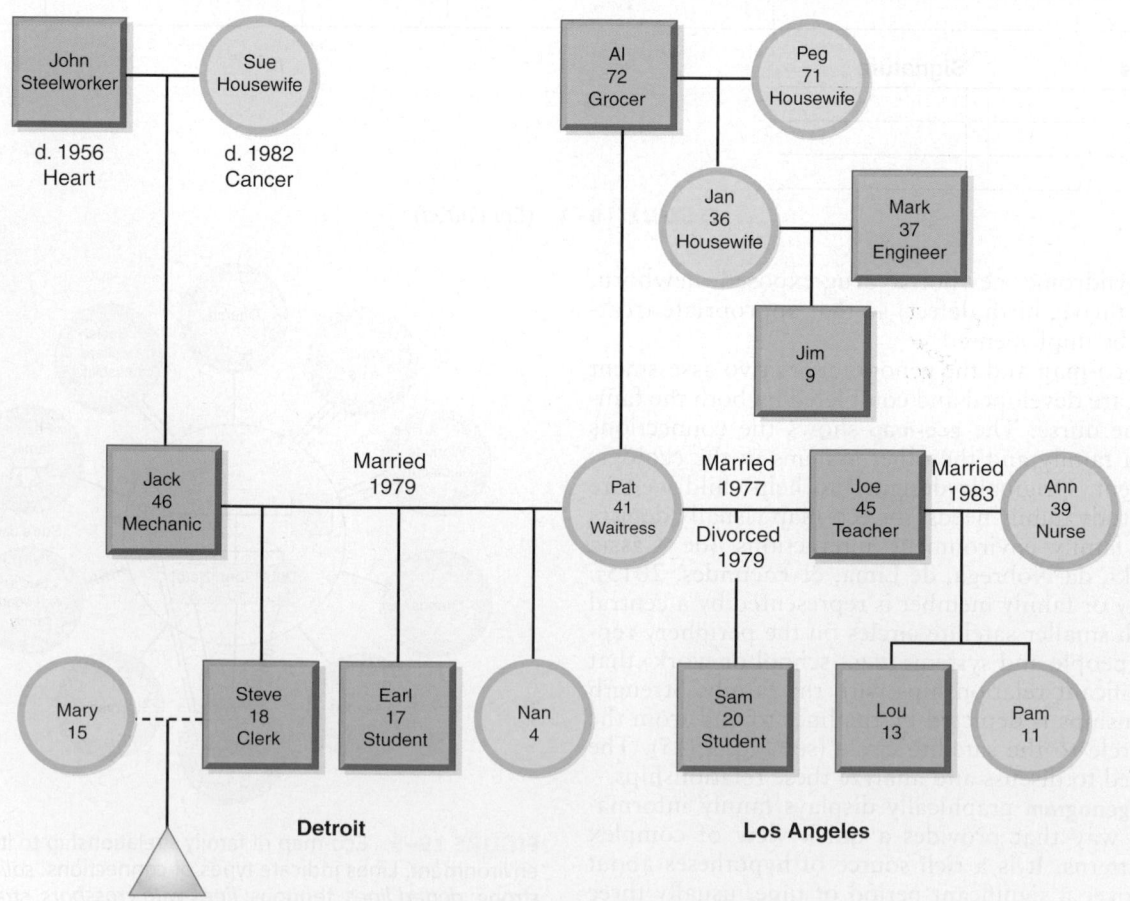

FIGURE 19–6   A genogram depicting three generations of family history. *Square*, male; *circle*, female; *triangle*, infant; *solid line*, married; *broken line*, not married.

Family Assessment

Family Name _____

Family Constellation

Member	Birth Date	Sex	Marital Status	Education	Occupation	Community Involvement

Financial Status _____

Using the following scale, score the family based on your professional observations and judgement:

0 = Never   3 = Frequently
1 = Seldom   4 = Most of the time
2 = Occasionally   N = Not observed

Facilitative Interaction among Members

a. Is there frequent communication among all members?
b. Do conflicts get resolved?
c. Are relationships supportive?
d. Are love and caring shown among members?
e. Do members work collaboratively?

Comments _____
_____

Totals

Enhancement of Individual Development

a. Does family respond appropriately to members' developmental needs?
b. Does it tolerate disagreement?
c. Does it accept members as they are?
d. Does it promote member autonomy?

Comments _____
_____

Totals

(score | date | score | date | score | date | score | date columns)

FIGURE 19–7 Family assessment using questions based on characteristics of healthy families.

	score	date	score	date	score	date	score	date

Effective Structuring of Relationships
  a. Is decision making allocated to appropriate members?
  b. Do member roles meet family needs?
  c. Is there flexible distribution of tasks?
  d. Are controls appropriate for family stage of development?

Comments _____

_____

Totals

Active Coping Effort
  a. Is family aware when there is a need for change?
  b. Is it receptive to new ideas?
  c. Does it actively seek resources?
  d. Does it make good use of resources?
  e. Does it creatively solve problems?

Comments _____

_____

Totals

Healthy Environment and Life-style
  a. Is family life-style health promoting?
  b. Are living conditions safe and hygienic?
  c. Is emotional climate conducive to good health?
  d. Do members practice good health measures?

Comments _____

_____

Totals

Regular Links with Broader Community
  a. Is family involved regularly in the community?
  b. Does it select and use external resources?
  c. Is it aware of external affairs?
  d. Does it attempt to understand external issues?

Comments _____

_____

Totals

FIGURE 19-7 (*Continued*)

Guidelines for Family Health Assessment

A family health assessment can easily result in a lot of data even if the nurse only selects one or two problems to investigate during the home visit. This huge amount of information can challenge even the most experienced of public health nurses. Therefore, here are five guidelines to use when collecting and processing the data for a detailed family health assessment:

1. Focus on the family as a total unit.
2. Ask goal-directed questions.
3. Collect data over time.
4. Combine quantitative and qualitative data.
5. Exercise professional judgment.

You should notice that these guidelines emphasize the family as the core service unit and will strengthen your ability to work collaboratively with the family—promoting a trusting relationship.

Focus on the Family as a Total Unit

Family health is more than the sum of its individual members' health. If you gave a numeric value to the health of each family member and added them up for a total score, the total would not show how healthy that family is. The family is a single entity (a single core unit of service), and it is the family's aggregated behavior that is being assessed (Centers for Disease Control and Prevention, 2012; Rogers, 2012; Wright & Leahey, 2012). Throughout the assessment process, the public health nurse asks, "Is this typical of the family as a whole?" For example, when the nurse is assessing the communication patterns of family members "A" and "B," the nurse is also thinking about

---

FAMILY ASSESSMENT

Family Name _____

Family Constellation

Member names	Occupation	Educational background

_____
_____
_____
_____

Significant change in family life — _____

Coping ability of family — _____

Energy level — _____

Decision-making process within the family — _____

Parenting skills — _____

Support systems of the family — _____

Use of health care (include plans for emergencies) — _____

Financial status — _____

Other impressions — _____

Signature of Nurse _____   Date _____

FIGURE 19–8 Open-ended family assessment.

the other family members. How do these family members communicate? How do they communicate with "A" and "B"? Further observations show good communication among all but one member. After processing the information, the nurse may decide that the family, as a whole, communicates well and supportively even if one family member does not. The nurse will document that one family member's communication behaviors deviated from the family norm, and this difference needs to be considered in the care planning. Remember, one family member can influence the internal functioning of the entire family.

Ask Goal-Directed Questions

Goal-directed questions are the cornerstone of a detailed assessment (Dennis, 2014; Rodriguez & Margolin, 2015). These types of questions significantly contribute to a detective solving a crime, a teacher discerning a student's learning capabilities, or a mechanic repairing that knocking sound in a car engine. Similarly, the nurse asks goal-directed questions when determining a family's level of health, making family diagnoses, and crafting a care plan. As a public health nurse, you must ask questions beyond "How is the family today?" Relevant or goal-directed questions yield relevant data (Rodriguez & Margolin, 2015). The family assessment tool shown in Figure 19–7 provides a sample set of questions to use for a family health assessment. Even if you are hesitant about the wording, these questions can guide your thinking and

observations because they are built on the characteristics of a healthy family. They direct attention to specific aspects of family behavior to facilitate the goal of discovering a family's level of health.

For example, one of your goals is to determine the steps or behaviors a family uses to cope with change—active coping effort. While visiting this family, you watch everyone closely for signs of the family's response(s) to change and the ability to problem-solve any problems resulting from the change. You, the public health nurse, can ask several goal-directed questions. Does this family recognize when a change needs to be made? How does the family react when a change is forced on the family? If a problem arises from the change, such as the baby having diarrhea or constantly crying, will the family be responsible for dealing with the problem? Is there a family member who knows how to solve the problem, and will this person be willing to accept outside assistance? With these questions, the nurse can determine how the family will respond to the problem. The nurse can continue to see how the family will cope with the problem by asking additional questions. Will someone in the family be responsible to seek out resources, such as reading about causes of infant diarrhea or constant crying, using home remedies, or seeking assistance from a public health nurse, a nurse practitioner, or a doctor? Will this person or another family member be comfortable using the identified resources, or will this person try something new to

SELF-CARE ASSESSMENT GUIDE

Name _____ Birth date _____
Address _____ Phone number _____
Names of health care providers visited in past year:

Name	Discipline	Address	Phone number	Times visited past year
1.				
2.				

Surgeries (Include date)

1. _____
2. _____

Major acute illnesses (Include date; indicate whether hospitalization was necessary)

1. _____
2. _____

Chronic illnesses (Include date)

1. _____
2. _____

Age of parents (If deceased, indicate date of death, age at death, and cause of death)

Mother _____ Father _____

Age of grandparents (If deceased, indicate age at death and cause of death)

MGM _____ MGF _____ PGM _____ PGF _____

Natural teeth   Y   N

Dentures or partials   Y   N

Dental care: _____ Brush teeth/Frequency _____
_____ Floss teeth/Frequency _____

Women/men over 50 Sigmoidoscopy/colonoscopy Date _____

Women

Breast self-exam   Y   N   Frequency _____
Mammograms   Y   N   Frequency _____
Pap smears   Y   N   Frequency _____

Men

Testicular self-exam   Y   N   Frequency _____
PSA   Y   N   Date _____ Results _____
TB skin test (Date) _____ Results _____

Immunizations
Td/Tdap _____
Flu vaccine _____
Hepatitis vaccine _____
Zoster _____
Other _____
Weight (At age 25) _____ Current weight _____ Normal weight _____
Height (At age 25) _____ Current height _____
Dietary practices (24-hour dietary recall)
First meal (Time) _____ Contents (Include amount) _____
_____
Second meal (Time) _____ Contents (Include amount) _____
_____
Third meal (Time) _____ Contents (Include amount) _____
_____
Snacks (Include time, contents, and amount) _____
_____
Usual food eaten (not mentioned above) _____
Foods not eaten at all (by preference) _____
Food allergies _____
Medicine allergies _____
Food taboos _____

Religious practices that affect health (prayer, special practices or services) _____
_____

Exercise patterns (Include sample activities, duration, frequency, problems or side effects):
1. _____
2. _____

Medications and therapies

OTC drugs (Include name, length of treatment, frequency of use, side effects):
1. _____
2. _____
3. _____
4. _____

Prescription drugs (Include name, length of treatment, frequency of use, side effects):
1. _____
2. _____
3. _____
4. _____

Folk medicine/home remedies (e.g., postpartum isolation, mustard poultice for chest congestion):
1. _____
2. _____
3. _____
4. _____

Complementary therapies (e.g., biofeedback, imagery, herbalism)
1. _____
2. _____
3. _____
4. _____

Plan for self-care improvement

Overall goal _____
_____

Areas needing modification (e.g., enhancement, moderation, deletion; include short- and long-term goal for each area):
1. _____
STG: _____
LTG: _____
2. _____
STG: _____
LTG: _____

Client role to reach long-term goals
_____

Nurse's role(s) to reach long-term goals (e.g., collaboration, teaching, evaluation)
_____
_____

Others' roles in reaching goals (Include discipline, name, address and phone number)
1. _____
2. _____

Comments
_____
_____
_____
_____

FIGURE 19–9 Self-care assessment guide. (Adapted from Cleveland, L., & Allender, J. A. (1999). Environment: Self-care issues. In L. Cleveland, D. S. Aschenbrenner, S. J. Veneable, & J. A. P. Yensen (Eds), *Nursing management in drug therapy.* Philadelphia, PA: Lippincott Williams & Wilkins, with permission.)

resolve the problem? As the nurse focuses on these behaviors, she or he is asking goal-directed questions aimed at finding out the family's coping skills—one part of assessing the family's total health picture.

Another more open-ended format or approach is to use the assessment categories listed in Figure 19–8. These categories can be instrumental in stimulating nursing questions such as those exploring family support systems. What internal resources or strengths do this family have? What outside person does the family turn to for help and support? How does the family seek out help from the church, the local community center, or any social organization in the community? The open-ended style of this assessment tool allows questions aimed at determining family health within a specific category.

Collect Data Over Time

Assessing the family's health is a timely process, and most likely, information from the first and/or second visits will provide only a partial picture of the family functioning. You want to take your time to accumulate observations, make notes, identify both major and minor issues, and observe the interactions of all family members (Aston et al., 2015; Parthasarathy et al., 2014; Shepherd, 2011). You also want to take your time so that you can develop a trusting and supportive relationship with the family. To assess the family's communication patterns, for instance, the nurse needs to observe the family as a group at mealtime or during some family activity. The family needs to feel comfortable with you, the observing nurse, in the room so that they will respond freely and naturally. Time and patience are needed for such rapport to develop.

We can see the importance of a timely assessment in one nurse's experience. Nurse Jolene Burns was working with the Olson family. They were receiving nursing services for health promotion and discussing ways to discipline their young children. Although Jolene had met with the Olson family twice (first in the clinic and then at home), Mr. Olson had not been present at either visit. A third visit was arranged in the early evening so that Mr. Olson could be present and Jolene could observe the family together. The third visit ended with the Olson family contracting with Jolene for six weekly visits to be held in the late afternoon, when Mr. Olson came home from work. After the fourth visit, she filled out an assessment form to keep as a part of the family record. Jolene's assessment of the Olson family began with the first visit where she made notes on their chart and, guided by questions similar to those in Figure 19–8, kept a brief log. However, it was not until the fourth visit that Jolene felt she had collected enough data to make valid judgments about this family's level of health.

Combine Quantitative With Qualitative Data

Any appraisal of family health relies on both qualitative and quantitative information that is used to create a database for planning care. Qualitative data occurs when the nurse is determining the presence or absence of essential family characteristics. Determining the degree or quantifying if the various signs of health are present or not reflects a quantitative measure. Asking if family members engage in some type of behaviors is qualitative; and, asking how often the family engages in the behaviors is quantitative. What about questions like, "Is this behavior fairly typical of the family" or "Does this behavior occur infrequently?" The first one is qualitative and the second is quantitative.

Figures 19–7 and 19–8 demonstrate ways to measure family health quantitatively. When using the tool in Figure 19–7, the nurse can assess the Beck family's ability to enhance individuality by rating the family's behavior on a scale of 0 (never) to 4 (most of the time). After several observations, the nurse concludes that the family responds appropriately to the members' developmental needs most of the time. So, under the section Enhancement of Individual Development (Fig. 19-7), the nurse scores "a" as 4 and notes the date of the assessment.

A quantitative measure provides a way for the nurse to compare the family's development over several home visits. The nurse can determine if the family's health is progressing or regressing by comparing the present score with previous ones. For instance, you have been working with the Kovacs for 6 months, a total of 12 home visits. After comparing the Kovacs' scores for all assessed areas, you discover a drop in their scores in several areas, suggesting a possible regression in their overall health. Many of their communication patterns, role relationships, and coping skills, in particular, show signs of deterioration. The scored assessment gave a vivid picture of exactly where to target your intervention(s). For this reason, it is useful to conduct periodic assessments when a case is reopened, or every 3 to 6 months if it is kept open for an extended period. The nurse can monitor the progress of high-risk families through early introduction of preventive measures when a trend or regressive behavior is observed. Periodic quantitative assessments also provide a means of evaluating the effectiveness of the planned care and can point to documented signs of growth.

Quantitative data serve another useful purpose. The nurse can compare one family's health status with that of another family as a basis for priority setting and nursing care planning. The difference in the level of health between the Becks and the Kovacs, for example, shows that the Kovacs need considerably more attention right now.

Exercise Professional Judgment

Although nurses seek to validate all their collected data with the use of quantitative measures, a family assessment is still subjective and relies on the nurse's professional judgment or decisions. Assessment tools can guide observations and even quantify the nurse's decisions; but, ultimately, the content of the assessment is driven by the nurse's experiences and intuition (Shepherd, 2011). The nurse may observe that a family makes good use of a community agency, but the decision that using this external resource contributes to the family's health is a subjective one. This determination indicates that effective health care practices depend on sound professional judgment. An assessment tool is only a tool and should be used to guide the care planning. Its value or infallibility should never be overemphasized or interpreted as an absolute and irrevocable statement about a family's health status. These are assessment tools to assist in collecting and organizing the nurse's observations and decisions.

A family health assessment occurs unobtrusively, and any assessment tool is ordinarily not filled out in the family's presence. This documentation occurs at the end of the home visit(s) and is a way to guide the nurse's observations and judgments. Before going into a family's home, the public health nurse may review the questions. She or he may find it helpful to keep the assessment tool in a folder for easy reference during the visit. Depending on the nurse's relationship with the family, notes may be made during or immediately after the encounter. However, the assessment tool is not completed in the presence of the family. Like Jolene, the nurse may choose to keep a short log—an accumulation of notes—until enough data have been collected to complete the assessment form. Occasionally, a family with high self-care capability may be involved in the assessment, such as assisting in developing an eco-map or genogram. This idea should be introduced carefully with the nurse using professional judgment to determine when the family is ready to engage in this kind of self-examination.

THE FAMILY DIAGNOSIS PROCESS

Although the family diagnosing process is critical in moving the data from the family health assessment into care planning, the process is often understated or even omitted when talking about public health nursing. However, it is important to understand how a large amount of information is processed so that the nurse can have objective and realistic family diagnoses. And, this process is an expected standard of practice for public health nurses (ANA, 2013). The family diagnosing process involves the public health nurse using observational skills and clinical reasoning to recognize and understand the patterns in the data from the assessment. This process is key because family diagnosis is the basis for goal setting to reduce family health risks and identify factors that may lead to ongoing risks. In other words, this process is indispensable in planning, implementing, and evaluating the treatment(s) used to address the concerns of the family health.

The diagnosing process involves determining the family's health status based on identified patterns of behavior, barriers preventing the family from being healthy (e.g., potential risks, actual risks, attitudes, beliefs/values, unhealthy routines), and internal and relationships with the external environment (ANA, 2013; Thompson & Adderley, 2015). This process allows the nurse to see what problems take precedence over others and the best action(s) to consider for the desired outcome or goal (McDonald et al., 2013). As indicated earlier, the diagnosing process is lengthy, time consuming, and ongoing. Every interaction with the family provides the nurse with more information that has to be processed and weighed against the known family diagnoses. Using the data from the assessment, the diagnosing process occurs as follows (Odell, 2015; Thompson & Adderley, 2015):

1. Identify the family health problems
   a. Determine what family members are directly and indirectly related to the problem.
   b. Determine what factors from the external environment are related to the problem.
   c. Describe the problem as it impacts the identified family members and external environment.
   d. Indicate the risks that are associated with the description of the problem(s) given in "c."
   e. Prioritize the problems along with their risks with an emphasis on the problems that are overlapping and/or have overlapping risks.
2. Indicate the factors from the family (family unit and family members) and the external environment that are associated with the health problems.
3. Determine the measurements (quantitative and qualitative data) that confirm or verify the health problems.

Sometimes, you, the nurse, will complete this process more than once, especially when there is a lot of data from the assessment, and there may be new information and/or a new understanding of the data. Each review of the data will give a deeper understanding of the problems, their risks, and how to approach them for treatment, as this is an ongoing process with two major goals—improving the health of the family and giving them the tools for health promotion. After prioritizing the problems and measurements, the nurse can begin to craft a plan of care or intervention to move the family toward a state of health. At this point, you have a more detailed understanding of the family, their relationships (internal and external), and a succinct and logical way to promote family health and prevent future illnesses.

PLANNING AND IMPLEMENTING EDUCATION AND HEALTH PROMOTION

Once the public health nurse has recognized the family's patterns of behavior from the assessment, the nurse has also probably identified and/or confirmed the main concerns, problems, and risks (actual and potential). With that information, the PHN is ready to create the care plan with family input and collaboration. At a certain level, care planning has been informally occurring during the assessment and family diagnosing; but at this stage, it becomes formal. The nurse works with the family to determine if the family agrees with the identified problems and the suggested interventions, and each family member is open to discussing the plan of action (de Cássia Tszesnioski et al., 2015; Porr, 2015; SmithBattle et al., 2013). If the family does not agree with the nurse's family assessment and family diagnosing, it is difficult to move forward with a plan of care. The nurse wants to work *with* the family, so the data should be reviewed and family members should be engaged in dialog in order to further understand their concerns and come to an agreement. The goal is to ensure that both the family and the nurse reach a mutual understanding with the best interventions for the family's health being identified and ready to be put into action. This level of communication is important in contributing to a trusting and collaborative relationship, and the family needs to believe in the plan of action or the nurse will be limited in her or his efforts to prevent identified problems and/or risks while promoting the family's health (Aston et al., 2015; Deutsch, Frese, & Sandholzer, 2014).

If the family is not at a level of functioning that enables members to use anticipatory guidance and teaching, the nurse can provide more basic services such as gathering resources and acting as a counselor. Remember, devising a plan of care with certain treatments/interventions and teaching health promotion activities should begin only after family members express an interest and recognize a need. If family members are ready to learn ways to improve their health status, then the nurse determines the best teaching approach to use and tailors interventions to the specific family needs and functional capability (Pereira et al., 2015; Salem & Ma-Pham, 2015; Schaffer et al., 2012). The family's language barriers, previous knowledge and experience, internal and external resources, and availability are important considerations (see Chapter 11).

EVALUATING IMPLEMENTED FAMILY HEALTH PLANS

The final step in the nursing process is evaluation. The evaluation process relates to the appraisal of your work with the family and a determination of what is needed in preparation for the next visit. The evaluation helps you to further individualize services to the family. It is helpful to use a reflective manner in order to informally evaluate the structure–process of the visit. The self-evaluation is often done while completing the other steps of the nursing process, and it becomes a formal evaluation once the outcomes are documented in the client record. A thorough evaluation also assists you in making the most appropriate referrals and contacting key resources to meet family needs.

Types of Evaluation

The evaluation of the family home visit deals with three components—the structure–process, the outcome, and your self-evaluation. Each one provides a different piece of information that can be helpful in determining what made the visit a success and what made it less than successful. Importantly, each can indicate if the outcomes were achieved and how to advance the outcomes to the next level of family health. A question a public health nurse always asks, "Is there something about the structure–process, my level of preparedness, or my behavior that needs to be changed?" Why? The answer to this question, and those like it, can determine the nurse's ability to promote health in the family, the community, and eventually the population.

Structure–Process

Structure–process refers to the organization of the visit and how it proceeded (see Chapter 12, Fig. 12–1). The structure–process of a visit should be analyzed first. Were there aspects of the organization (resources, number of persons present, timing, environment, or presented materials) or the flow of the assessment (use of observational skills, people's attitudes, reliance on standards) that needed to be changed or modified? How could you have arranged these factors differently? Were you organized and prepared for the visit? Were there distractions in the home that influenced the organization of the visit? Ask yourself these questions so that you can plan to adjust your structure–process for the next visit and reduce or avoid disorganizing distractions. For example, if the first visit was made based on limited information from

a referral, you now have additional family data and can be better prepared for the next visit. Perhaps other transportation can be arranged if transportation caused the family to be late for the visit. A visit earlier in the day can prevent the distraction of children returning home from school. If the television was playing loudly during the next visit, you know now to ask the family if they would not mind turning down the volume in the next visit, or turning off the television. You may also ask about choosing a time to visit when they are not watching television. The point is to use the evaluation to modify subsequent visits.

Outcome Evaluation

Evaluating the outcomes of the visit is the second and most important evaluation component because the nurse will want to know if the anticipated outcomes were achieved and what made them possible. This **outcome evaluation** is a formal process that happens with documentation of the home visits. If the outcome is a change in the family's health status based on mutually agreed activities, the agency may determine the effectiveness of this outcome with the Nursing Outcomes Classification (NOC) System and the Nursing Intervention Classification (NIC) System, as well as the Omaha System (see Chapters 12 and 14). Alternatively, there may be agency-driven criteria to rate success and indicate expectations for each client category or visit type. Progression toward an expected outcome may be demonstrated by small changes over time in the family dynamics, which are noted on a visit-by-visit basis. These small changes are viewed cumulatively to determine the success or failure of the family to achieve certain outcomes at the conclusion of agency services. Depending on the conclusions, the decision to terminate services may need to be reevaluated. Possibly, the continuance of service is required, and the terms must be renegotiated. Whatever the decision, the family must be included in the decision-making process.

Self-Evaluation

The third component of evaluation is self-evaluation. What aspect of your performance as a public health nurse facilitated the desired outcome during the home visit? Were you prepared? Did you gather enough data so that you can be prepared to assist the family on the next visit? What would you do differently if you could do the visit over? What went right? What went wrong? What are you going to do on the next visit to make it better? This self-evaluation or reflection can be a useful tool for the public health nurse to recognize her or his strengths and failings with internal measures to improve practice (Edelman et al., 2013).

In some agencies, routine peer evaluations are conducted because sometimes we cannot see our own strengths or weaknesses. An agency staff nurse makes a family visit with the public health nurse and provides feedback based on her or his observations. This is a useful technique to employ outside of planned evaluations of all staff members in the agency. Another perspective might be helpful when working with a family that has not made progress toward the desired outcomes or to a family you have not been able to reach (Porr, 2015).

Consultation with peers can assist you in becoming better prepared or more focused, and it can also improve your interaction with families from different cultures or in difficult situations (Spector, 2013).

Planning for the Next Visit

Planning for the next visit is part of evaluating the family visit. The data collected from the previous visit will guide you to the activities for subsequent visits. You may need to modify goals if the family's situations have changed, making specific outcomes irrelevant. For example, you plan to visit a prenatal family one last time before the second baby is born. Given the information from the last visit, you intend to assess the pregnant mom's rising blood pressure and complaints of backache, as well as go over the baby-sitting arrangements for the 2-year-old child. You arrive for the visit only to discover that the husband and the 2-year-old child are home alone and the husband is about to leave to bring the mother and new baby home from the hospital. The husband asks you about a diaper rash that just appeared on the 2-year-old and how to secure the new car seat into the car. Outcomes for a problem-free pregnancy and healthy birth are no longer relevant; the situation has changed, and now, there are new outcomes to be formulated and addressed with this family.

More frequently, planning for subsequent visits is relatively predictable and is done to ensure that steps toward outcome accomplishment are achieved on the visit. Being totally prepared each time helps assure a successful family visit. Once you have met and gotten to know a family during a visit, the planning can be individualized and tailored to meet the family's needs. This information is not available from a paper referral, which makes planning for that first home visit important. The tone set during the first visit can affect your continued success with the family (see From the Case Files).

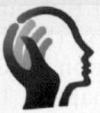 *From the* **Case Files** **I**

A Family Assessment: Meeting Hector's Needs

You are a public health nurse working in Smithville. You have been given a referral for a new client, Hector. Hector is being released from the rehabilitation unit of Metropolis Hospital. Although he lives in Smithville, Metropolis Hospital, 50 miles away, was the only facility willing to accept a Medicaid client with a severe spinal cord injury.

Hector is a 19-year-old Hispanic male who sustained major injury to his spinal cord (T4 injury) in a motorcycle accident. The injury occurred approximately 6 weeks ago. Hector has been diagnosed as paraplegic with some residual limitation of upper body strength and mobility.

Your job is to facilitate Hector's transition from Metropolis Hospital to his home environment. You will be teaching Hector and his family about the following:

1. Nutrition and fluid intake
2. Signs and symptoms warranting follow-up
3. Medication administration
4. Bowel and bladder care
5. Skin care
6. Activities of daily living (ADLs) and self-care with sensory–motor deficits
7. Safety/injury prevention
8. Community resources
9. Rehabilitative services
10. Anticipatory guidance about mood issues (grief, anger, and suicidal ideations), sexual function, fear of abandonment, role change, and social isolation
11. Altered family processes

Following is a synopsis of information obtained during your initial visit with Hector and his family in their home.

Visit One. Hector lives in a migrant labor camp located on the outskirts of Smithville. His family has resided in the camp for 18 years. Those living in the two-bedroom cabin-like home are:

- Hector, your assigned client.
- Hector's uncle Manuel (32 years old). Manuel's job is seasonal; he has been offered a temporary job for a much higher salary, working out of state.
- Hector's brother Efran (16 years old). Efran is considering dropping out of high school in order to assist with the care of his family. His goal is to become an auto mechanic. He is fluent in both Spanish and English.
- Manuel's wife Marisol (29 years old). Marisol was a teacher in Mexico. She is extremely supportive of her family. She is concerned about getting pregnant, but does not believe in the use of birth control.
- Manuel and Marisol's children, Arturo (5 years old) and Anna (6 months old). Arturo begins a Head Start program soon and will be gone for 5 hours each day. Anna is a healthy baby who is being breastfed and is thriving at home.
- Hector's paternal grandmother, Lourdes (74 years old). She has recently arrived from Mexico and plans on assisting in Hector's care. Lourdes has congestive heart failure and arthritis. She is not a legal resident of the United States and is not eligible for medical assistance.

The whereabouts of Hector's mother are unknown. Shortly after Efran was born, she moved from their village in Mexico, remarried, and started another family. She has had no contact with Hector or Efran. Hector's father lives in their home village in Mexico. Although he lived in the migrant camp in Smithville for many years, he recently returned to Mexico, remarried, and

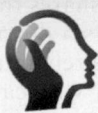

From the Case Files I (Continued)

has two young daughters. He is aware of Hector's injury, but the father has no plans to return to the United States.

Your ability to speak fluent Spanish has enabled you to collect the above information from Hector and Manuel. Manuel has been very involved in Hector's recovery through daily visits to the rehabilitation unit and frequent discussions with Hector's health care providers. Manuel tells you "Hector is like a son to me ... I have a responsibility to my older brother to watch over his son. My brother watched out for me when I was young ... he even left school to work to help support our family." Manuel adds, "We don't have much but we will take care of Hector ... we'll all work together."

You began the visit by explaining your role as home health nurse. You informed the family about the type of services, education, and interventions you are able to provide. You ask Hector and the family to tell you what they have learned from the health care team at the rehabilitation unit and what plans the family have developed to address Hector's medical and psychosocial needs. As you began the visit, you noticed that Hector's grandmother was sitting quietly in the corner of the room rocking Anna. You learned that Efran was working in the fields. Arturo was in school. Manuel, Marisol, and Lourdes were participating in the home visit this morning. The conversation was as follows.

> Nurse: Hector, can you tell me how you feel about being home?
> Hector (looks at Marisol): Okay, I guess.
> Marisol: He's a little scared, I think. He feels like it's going to be too much for us to deal with.
> Nurse (looking at Hector): There's so much happening right now, so much to think about ...
> Hector: Uh-huh.
> (Hector is maintaining eye contact with Manuel and Marisol only; because this is your initial visit to the home, you feel that Hector may be more comfortable in the role of observer.)
> Nurse (looking at Manuel and Marisol): Do you have any questions before we begin?
> Marisol: They gave us a lot of information at the hospital... I'm most afraid about if the phone doesn't work and Hector needs help. What if something happens to Hector and I can't call anyone? That's the only thing I worry about.
> Lourdes: If anything happens to him, I'll be right here with you, "mija." We can do this; we can take care of Hector if we work together.
> Manuel: There is a store with a phone only two blocks away; if you needed to, you can call from there. What I want to know is how we can get Hector into school or something that will help him to be around kids his own age. His English is good enough; he even finished high school. He needs to be ready to make a future for himself.
> Hector (grins and looks at Manuel): Right, uncle that is what I want, too.

You continued the conversation by revisiting Marisol's concerns about access to a telephone in case of an emergency. You

asked specific questions about her concerns and used this as an opportunity to educate the family about circumstances warranting immediate follow-up. Together with the family, you decide that Marisol will develop a list of specific concerns that you will review together at a subsequent visit planned 2 days from today.

Visit One consisted of the following:

I. Assessment
    A. Home environment
        1. Safety
        2. ADLs
    B. Knowledge of disease processes
    C. Fluid volume balance
    D. Nutritional resources of family
        1. Food availability
        2. Food preparation
    E. Insurance and financial status
II. Education
    A. Medications
    B. Warning signs and symptoms and appropriate follow-up procedures
    C. Bowel and bladder care
    D. Hygiene prior to and following patient care

The plan for your visit in 2 days includes the following:

III. Referrals
    A. Community resources
    B. Educational opportunities
    C. Support groups (Spanish speaking)
    D. Peer group opportunities for Hector
IV. Assessment
    A. Continuation of above
V. Education
    A. Continuation of above

Questions

1. What is the social structure of this family (traditional vs. nontraditional)? Be specific about the type of traditional or nontraditional family system that exists in this scenario.
2. Discuss an example of triangulation in this scenario.
3. What essential functions are present within this family system?
4. What developmental stages appear to have been achieved?
5. What steps will you take in order to empower the family to make their own decisions?
6. List the strengths of the family.
7. Prioritize Hector's issues—medical and psychosocial.
8. Prioritize issues facing the other family members.
9. Identify mutual goals for this family:
    *   Immediate
    *   Midrange
    *   Long term
10. What community health nursing interventions will you utilize to achieve these mutual goals?

Referrals

A written or verbal referral (by agency-created form, telephone call, fax, or e-mail) initiates contact with a family. The nurse makes referrals on behalf of the family in addition to responding to a referral to begin the relationship with a family (Fig. 19–10). Families often need access to services beyond the agency's scope, and the nurse's knowledge of other resources can mean the difference between the family having and not having access to additional services. Therefore, nurses must have information available to them about the eligibility requirements and availability of services provided by a multitude of official, voluntary, religious, and neighborhood organizations (Allen, Feinberg, & Mitchell, 2014). Public health nurses need to know how to readily access this information to avoid any delay of the services to the family. This is challenging because there are many organizations that frequently change staff, telephone numbers, Web sites, services, and the populations served. Networking with colleagues on a regular basis helps keep nurses up to date with community services for family referrals (Parthasarathy et al., 2014).

Contacting Resources

At times, public health nurses implement their roles as advocates for families by facilitating easier access to services for the family. Public health nurses know how to access key personnel in agencies and can eliminate some of the red tape involved in obtaining services, as well as provide pointers that may help a family procure needed services. For example, a family may receive faster services by going to an agency early in the morning or in the middle of the week. An agency may process a family faster if all forms are completely filled out and the family member has receipts for the last 3 months' rent and utilities. Also, the nurse can suggest that the family member ask to speak with a certain worker—an informal referral.

When nurses seek informal services for families, a relationship with the director of the agency can help nurses gain services for the family. For example, a family with a personal crisis needs a donation of food and a volunteer to stay with a handicapped child for 3 days while the spouse undergoes surgery. The nurse telephones the religious leader of a neighborhood church, shares the family's requests, clarifies the situation, and gets a donation of food from the church's food pantry. The religious leader also offers the name of a church member who can stay with the child. The family may not have been aware of these services, so the connections provided by the nurse are as important as other public health nursing functions.

EFFECTS OF FAMILY HEALTH ON FAMILY MEMBERS

If a family entails the interrelationships of a group of individuals, then the health of each family member affects the health of others. It is this concerted interlacing of individual health that contributes to the level of the family's health. For example, a woman may be able to successfully cope with the physical and emotional demands of caring for a husband who recently had a stroke. However, caring for a husband can deplete her energies, which leaves her with inadequate reserves to effectively meet her children's needs. The mother's level of health significantly affects the level at which her family functions—how well it is able to solve problems and help all members reach their potential. A healthy family promotes each family member's growth and resistance to illnesses so that the family's health can sustain members during times of crisis such as serious illness, emotional dilemmas, divorce, or death of a family member (Deutsch et al., 2014; Miller, Brody, Yu, & Chen, 2014). On the other hand, a family with underdeveloped coping skills or a limited capacity for problem solving, self-management, or self-care is often unable to promote the potential of its members or assist them in times of need.

Standards and practices for family health influence each member's health. For instance, many adults and children adhere to cultural and family patterns of eating, exercise, and communication. Cultural (see Chapter 5) and family values influence decisions about utilizing preventative health care and adhering to recommendations related to immunizations, regular health assessments, or family planning (Spector, 2013). Family patterns also dictate if family members will participate in their health care as well as follow through and comply with professional advice. A family member influences the family health, and the family, as a unit, can either obstruct or facilitate the health of a family member. Remember, the family is the core unit of service, making it the focus of public health nursing throughout the nursing process.

CHARACTERISTICS OF HEALTHY FAMILIES

How does the community/public health nurse determine family health status? Analysis of how basic functions are met does not give a satisfactory picture of a family's health status. More definitive criteria are needed. Although it is difficult to define a "normal" family, studies have provided some standards that characterize a healthy family (Barker & Chang, 2013; Deutsch et al., 2014; Miller et al., 2014). Over the years, research on families and on family health behavior has produced a growing body of data with which to assess family health.

In looking at families over the years, many similar characteristics have been identified. Some characteristics

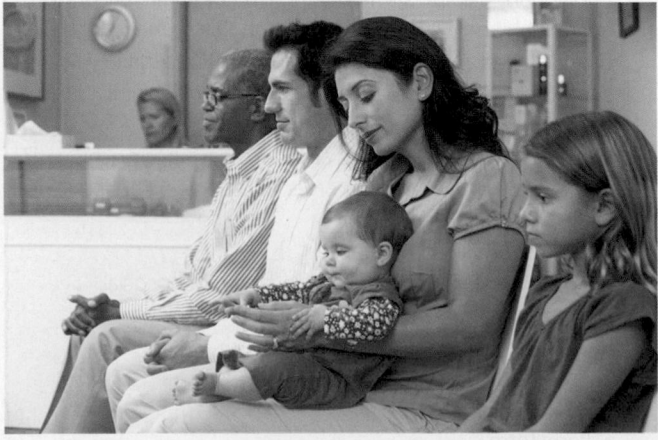

FIGURE 19–10 Referrals are often made to health department clinics or physicians.

are family unity, loyalty and interfamily cooperation, support and security, role flexibility, and constructive relationships with community (Smith, 2013a). Seven major family strengths have been described as important factors for family functioning and coping with crisis— family pride, family support, cohesion, adaptability, communication, religious orientation, and social support (Smith, 2013a). Specific topics have been used to characterize a healthy family (Becvar & Becvar, 2012):

● A legitimate source of authority that is supported and consistent over time
● A stable and consistent system of rules
● Consistent and regular nurturing behaviors
● Effective child-rearing practices
● Stable and well-maintained marriages
● A set of agreed-upon goals toward which the family and individuals work
● Sufficient flexibility to change in the face of both expected and unexpected stressors

The six signs of a healthy family (Parachin, 1997)) have been used to guide and understand family-oriented interventions (Fort et al., 2015). The six signs are maintaining a spiritual foundation, making the family a top priority, asking for and giving respect, communicating and listening, valuing service to others, and expecting and offering acceptance. From this plethora of information about a healthy family, six important characteristics have consistently emerged (Becvar & Becvar, 2012; Kaakinen et al., 2015):

1. A facilitative process of interaction exists among family members.
2. Individual member development is enhanced.
3. Role relationships are structured effectively.
4. Active attempts are made to cope with problems.
5. There is a healthy home environment and lifestyle.
6. Regular links with the broader community are established.

Healthy Communication Among Family Members

Healthy families communicate. Their patterns of communicating are regular, varied, and supportive. Adults talk with and engage adults, children with children, and adults with children (Deutsch et al., 2014; Fort et al., 2015; Miller et al., 2014). These interactions are frequent and assume many forms. Healthy families discuss problems, confront each other when angry, share ideas and concerns, and write or call each other when separated. They communicate through nonverbal means, particularly families from cultural or subcultural groups that are less verbal. There are innumerable ways to convey feelings and thoughts without words (e.g., smiling encouragingly, embracing warmly, frowning disapprovingly, being available, withdrawing for privacy, doing an unsolicited favor, serving refreshments, giving a gift). The family that communicates effectively has family members who are sensitive to one another. They watch for cues and verify messages to ensure understanding. This kind of family recognizes and deals with conflicts as they arise. This family has learned to share and to work collaboratively with each other (Fig. 19–11).

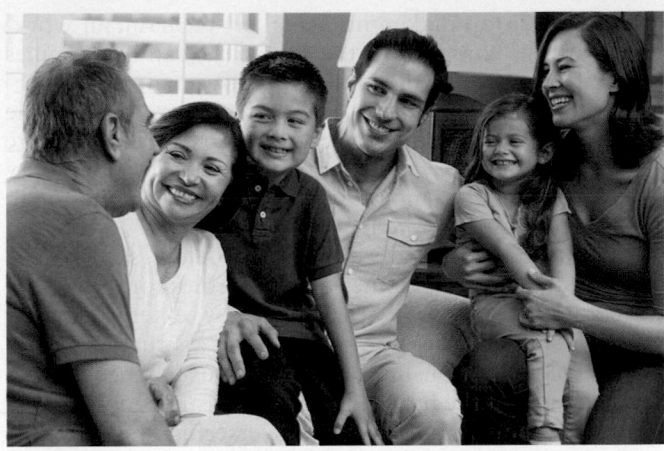

FIGURE 19–11 Good communication promotes healthy families.

Communication is necessary for the functioning of a healthy family. Family members use communication to demonstrate affection and acceptance, to promote identity and fellowship, and to guide behavior through socialization and social ethics. Importantly, effective communication patterns are associated with a family that promotes the health and development of each family member. Healthy families are more likely than unhealthy families to negotiate topics for discussion, use humor, show respect for differences of opinion, and clarify the meaning of one another's communications.

Enhancing Family Members' Development

Healthy families are responsive to the needs of family members and provide the freedom and support necessary to promote each member's growth. If a father in a healthy family loses his job, the family works to support his family role by helping him to use his energy constructively to adjust and find a new job. A healthy family recognizes that a growing child needs a certain level of independence so that the family will increase opportunities for the child to try new things alone. This kind of family can tolerate differences of opinion or lifestyle; each member has the right to be an individual and the family respects this right. A healthy family encourages freedom and autonomy for each of its members because it contributes to the family's stability (Kaakinen et al., 2015).

Patterns of promoting a family member's development vary from family to family, depending on cultural orientation. An Italian American family expresses autonomy differently from a Native American family, but each family promotes freedom and autonomy. This level of family promotion of autonomy leads to increased competence, self-reliance, social skills, intellectual growth, and overall capacity for self-management among family members (Deutsch et al., 2014; Pereira et al., 2015; Whittaker & Cowley, 2012; Wright & Leahey, 2012). See From the Case Files.

Effective Structuring of Family Role Relationships

In healthy families, role relationships are structured to meet the family's changing needs over time (Kaakinen et al., 2014). In the context of a stable society, families establish members' roles and tasks (e.g., breadwinner, primary decision maker, homemaker) to maintain workable patterns throughout the life of the family. Families in rural areas, isolated communities, or religious and subcultural groups are more likely than others to retain role consistency because they face little to no external pressure or need to change. For example, the Amish community in Pennsylvania has maintained marked differentiation in family roles for more than 100 years.

In a technologically advanced society such as the United States, most families establish roles for the changing family needs that are created by external forces. Women entering the workforce create a situation where family roles, relationships, and tasks must change to meet the demands of the family. Husbands assume more homemaking responsibilities such as overseeing child rearing. In some families, children, along with adults, share in the decision making. This equal distribution of power in family decisions may be essential for the survival of a single-parent family. Children may need to assume adult responsibilities in the home so that the parent can work to support the family.

Changing life-cycle stages require alterations in the structure of relationships. The healthy family recognizes the changing developmental needs of family members and adapts parenting roles, family tasks, and controls to fit each stage (Deutsch et al., 2014; Fort et al., 2015; Miller et al., 2014). For example, household chores of increasing complexity and responsibility are assigned as children become capable of handling more responsibility. Rules of conduct are relaxed as members learn to govern their own behavior.

Active Coping Effort

Healthy families actively attempt to overcome life's problems and issues. When faced with change, they assume responsibility for coping and seek to meet the demands of the situation (Becvar & Becvar, 2012; Smith, 2013a). Coping skills are needed to deal with emotional problems stemming from tragedies such as substance abuse/addictions, serious illness, or death. If a family member has a substance abuse problem, all family members may participate in the counseling and treatment opportunities. If a family member is seriously ill, the family may ask for and accept assistance from the extended family and/or public health care workers. In the event of a death in the family, an important step in the healing process is accepting consolation and support from one another, the extended family, and friends or clergy. The healthy family recognizes the need for assistance, accepts help, and pursues opportunities to eliminate or decrease the stressors that affect it (Deutsch et al., 2014; Miller et al., 2014).

More frequently, healthy families cope with less dramatic, day-to-day changes. For instance, one family may cope with the increased cost of food by consuming less meat, eating more vegetables and legumes high in protein, and going out to restaurants less frequently. Healthy families are open to innovation, support new ideas, and find creative and energetic ways to solve problems. One family may try to solve the problem of spending too much on transportation by cutting down on daily travel. The family may even support this change although some family members' jobs are in different areas of town or the family is active in school functions and meetings that occur in the evenings. Responding to a personal need for a healthier lifestyle, another family may solve the same transportation problem by walking, bicycling, or carpooling to school, work, and/or other activities. Active coping may go beyond finding a simple, obvious solution. For example, family members may try to rearrange schedules to avoid frequent trips to regular destinations and plan ahead to avoid last-minute trips to stores. Healthy families actively seek and use a variety of resources to solve problems. These resources may be within the family such as self-care or externally by using community resources. A professional couple faced with the unaffordable expense of daytime babysitting, for instance, arranged their work schedules to share childcare by trading off responsibilities during the first 2 years. Later, they joined a cooperative preschool that provided daily age-appropriate childcare and required the parents to work at the preschool only 1 day a week. In another example, a single parent of five children, who was also a full-time nursing student, was able to finance annually two or three weekend family outings by having everyone in the family participate in collecting and recycling cans and bottles.

Healthy Environment and Lifestyle

Another sign of a healthy family is a healthy home environment and lifestyle (Fig. 19–12). Healthy families create safe and hygienic living conditions for their members. For instance, a healthy family with young children "childproofs" the home by removing potential hazards such as exposed electric outlets and cleaning solvents from the children's reach. A healthy family with an older adult, who is prone to falls, installs night lighting and handrails. A healthy home environment is clean and reduces the spread of disease-causing organisms.

A healthy family lifestyle encourages family members to find balance or harmony in their lives. There is balance between activity and rest so that the family can have sufficient energies for daily living. There is variety in the family diet so that it is both nutritionally sound and appealing. Adequate physical activity helps to maintain a healthy weight while promoting cardiac health. Preventative hygiene habits are taught and followed by

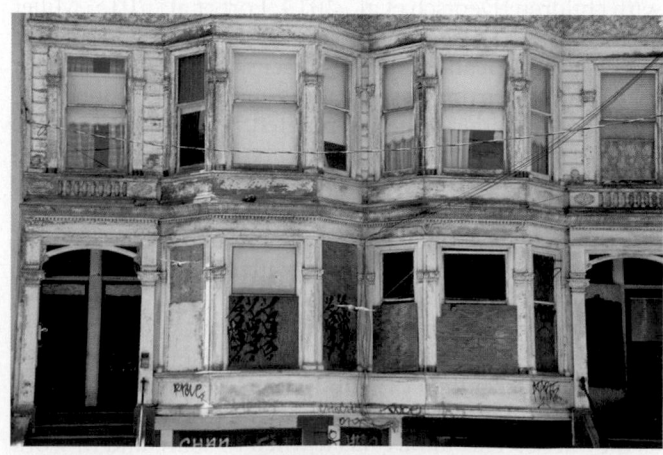

FIGURE 19–12 Families need healthy environments.

family members. Emotional and mental health is encouraged through a support network of caring family members and others. Finally, family members seek out and use health care services and demonstrate adherence to recommended regimens.

The emotional climate of a healthy family is positive and supportive of growth. Contributing to this healthful emotional climate is a strong sense of shared values, often combined with a strong moral ethical orientation (Smith, 2013a). A healthy family demonstrates caring, encourages and accepts expression of feelings, and respects divergent ideas. The home environment makes family members feel welcomed and accepted so that they can express their individuality in simply ways such as their dress or decoration of their room in the home.

Regular Links With the Broader Community

Healthy families maintain dynamic ties with the broader community. They participate regularly in external groups and activities. They may join in local politics, participate in a church bazaar, or promote the school's paper drive to raise money for science equipment. They use external resources suited to family needs. For example, a farming family with teenagers becomes very active in the local 4-H club as a way to promote peer interactions for the adolescents. Another family where the father is out of work joins a job transition support group. A family may be active in a nursing home where a family member resides in order to ensure optimal delivery of nursing home services and maintain that family member's role in the family. Healthy families also know what is going on in the world around them. They show an interest in current events and attempt to understand significant social, economic, and political issues. The families are exposed to a wider range of alternatives and a variety of contacts, which can increase options for finding resources and strengthen coping skills.

Public health nurses need to assess and encourage family's involvement with the broader community as it facilitates a relationship between the family and the community (Davis & Gustafson, 2014; de Cássia Tszesnioski et al., 2015). Importantly, the nurse can promote structural and developmental variations, interaction, coping strategies, and lifestyle for health promotion within the family.

PUBLIC HEALTH NURSING PRACTICE GUIDELINES

The family is often the unit of service in public health nursing (Kaakinen et al., 2015). It is not merely a family-oriented approach in which family concerns that affect the health of an individual are taken into account. A public health nurse asks how the family provides health care to a collection of people. Five principles guide and enhance public health nursing practice:

1. Work with the family collectively.
2. Start at the family's present level of functioning.
3. Adapt nursing interventions to the family's stage of development.
4. Recognize the validity of family structural variations.
5. Emphasize family strengths.

Work With the Family Collectively

Public health nurses focus on the family. They remind themselves that a family is a group of several persons living together and this group or family has a collective personality, collective interests, and a collective set of needs. Viewing a group of people as a unit is similar to the way business organizations are perceived—as a single entity. Many persons may make up the entity, but they function collectively as a single entity with common attributes and activities. For example, you think of a particular corporation as conservative or liberal, not the individual employees. You read and perhaps support the women's group that has taken a stand on family life education, not a specific woman in the group. You believe that it is a government agency that needs to be better organized instead of thinking that it is just one staff member. In each case, the group is viewed collectively. So it is with families. A family has its own personality, interests, and needs.

As much as possible, public health nurses strive to involve all family members during nurse–client interactions (Wright & Leahey, 2012). This approach reinforces the importance of each family member's contributions to the collective functioning of the family. Nurses recognize the importance of encouraging all family members to participate in the work that the nurse and the family jointly agree to do. Like a coach, the nurse rallies family members to work together as a team for their collective benefit. Look at how a nurse works collectively with the Beck family (see Display 19–3).

Start at the Family's Present Level of Functioning

When working with families, public health nurses begin at the present level of functioning and not some arbitrary ideal level. The nurse determines this level of functioning by first conducting a detailed family assessment. As discussed earlier, a family assessment allows the nurse to ascertain the needs and health level of each family member. This assessment will then strengthen the nurse's ability to recognize patterns of behaviors so that she or he can determine collective interests, concerns, problems, risks, and priorities. The accompanying description of the Kovac family illustrates this principle (see Display 19–4).

Adapt Nursing Intervention to the Family's Stage of Development

Every family engages in the same basic functioning. However, every family does not use the same approaches and/or tasks to accomplish these functions. Furthermore, this variation in achieving these functions can and often do vary with each stage of the family's development. A young family, for instance, can meet the family members' affiliation needs by establishing mutually satisfying relationships and meaningful communication patterns. As the family enters later stages of development, bonds change due to some family members becoming part of another family unit (e.g., through marriage or living together) or because of death. Awareness of the family's developmental stage enables the nurse to assess the

---

DISPLAY 19–3 THE BECK FAMILY

A public health nurse had an initial contact with Mr. and Mrs. Beck and their youngest child at the well-baby clinic. The 9-month-old child was over the 95th percentile for weight and at the 40th percentile for height. The nurse also noted that both parents were obese. The nurse asked about the family's eating patterns, the baby in particular, and suggested a home visit to determine whether the Becks were interested in family nursing. The nurse explained the purpose of home visits (to assess all family members, coping patterns, eating patterns, and food purchasing choices) and the importance of including all family members and asked for a time that would be good for the family as a whole. The nurse explained that each person should be involved and committed to the agreed-upon goals; that, like a team of oarsmen, the family has to pull together to accomplish the purpose of the visits. To help the Beck family improve its nutritional status, the nurse might suggest a session of brainstorming to uncover many causes of poor nutrition. More brainstorming might also lead to more solutions and plans for action. On each visit, the nurse views the Becks as a group so that group responses and actions would be expected. Evaluation of outcomes will be based on what the family did collectively. The Becks were interested, and a home visit date was made.

---

appropriateness of the family's level of functioning and to tailor interventions accordingly. Nurses are often adept at family assessment, but they must remember that the assessment is used to determine the problems/risks and implement the interventions needed to move the family to a state of health (Kaakinen et al., 2015; Wright & Leahey, 2012). A nurse's work with the Ravina family illustrates this need (see Display 19–5).

Recognize the Validity of Family Structure Variations

Public health nurses work with families from communities that are rich with diverse cultures and subcultures. For a public health nurse, there is no such thing as a traditional or nontraditional family. Why? The nurse works in communities with varying family structures that reflect these communities. Families can be structured and organized

---

DISPLAY 19–4 THE KOVAC FAMILY

Marcia Kovac brought her baby, Tiffany, to the well-child clinic once but failed to keep further appointments. Concerned that the family might be having other difficulties, Sara Villa, a public health nurse, made a home visit. The mobile home was cluttered and dirty, and the baby was crying in her playpen. Marcia seemed uninterested in the nurse's visit. She listened politely but had little to say. She repeated that everything was okay and that the baby was doing fine, explaining that Tiffany was just fussy because she was teething. As they talked, Marcia's husband Henry, a delivery van driver, stopped by to pick up a sports magazine to read on his lunch hour. The three of them discussed the problems of inflation and how expensive it was to raise a child. Sara reminded the Kovacs that the clinic was free and that they could at least get good health care without extra cost. They agreed without enthusiasm. After Henry left, the nurse spent the remainder of the visit discussing infant care with Marcia, particularly emphasizing regular checkups and immunizations.

The next visit also focused on the baby, but Sara had an uncomfortable feeling that the Kovacs were not really interested in her help. After consulting her supervisor, Sara did what she wished she had done in the first place. She asked to talk with Marcia and Henry together, explained frankly why she had come to their home, and informed them what she could offer in the way of counseling, teaching, support, and referral to other community resources. She then asked them what problems or concerns they had. The Kovacs were more than responsive. They described their financial difficulties and feelings of isolation from family and friends. They were new in the city, and both their families lived some distance away on farms. The neighbors were friendly but not close enough to confide in. They believed they would eventually overcome their problems if they just had "someone to lean on," as they put it.

Now Sara could address the Kovacs' primary needs and concerns for friends and emotional support. The nurse began to address the Kovacs' social needs first by introducing them to a young couples' group that met at the community center. Sara continued to make periodic home visits and shared additional information about community services that the Kovacs might find helpful. She praised Marcia and Henry for following up on immunizations for Tiffany. Over time, Sara saw differences in the family's interest in their relationship with the community and their connection to its services. Sara realized that before she could address the issue of Tiffany's health, she needed to address the emotional health of the parents.

DISPLAY 19–5 THE RAVINA FAMILY

The Ravinas, a couple in their early 70s, recently moved to a retirement complex. They had received nursing visits after Mrs. Ravina's stroke 3 years earlier, but requested service now because Mr. Ravina was feeling "poorly" all the time. He thought that perhaps his diet and lack of activity might be the cause and hoped the nurse might have some helpful suggestions. The couple had eagerly awaited Mr. Ravina's retirement from teaching, with plans to be lazy, travel, visit all their children, and do all those things they never had time to do when they were young. Now, neither of them seemed to have enough energy or the capacity to enjoy their new life. The move from their home of 28 years had been difficult: They were still trying to find space in the tiny apartment for their cherished books and mementos, although they had given many items away.

Ronald Bell, a public health nurse, recognized that the Ravinas were experiencing a situational crisis (leaving their home of 28 years) and a developmental crisis (aging and entering retirement) and may perhaps have some underlying health problems. Many of the Ravinas' expectations for this new life stage were unrealistic; they had not adequately prepared themselves for the adjustments that the loss of their home and retirement would demand. Through discussion, Ronald was able to help the Ravina family understand their situation and express their feelings. He completed physical assessments on the Ravinas and encouraged regular follow-up with their health care provider. He also helped them join a support group of retired persons who were experiencing some of the same difficulties. Because this nurse was able to help the Ravina family through their crisis in a supportive and nonjudgmental manner, he found them receptive later to discussing preparation for the inevitable loss and bereavement that would occur when one of them died. He was adapting his nursing intervention to this family's stage of development.

---

around a single parent, a married couple, an unmarried couple, an older sibling, or a single elderly grandparent. For example, the parents may have full-time careers, a husband may provide childcare as an at-home father, a wife may financially support her family, or the parents may telecommute and work at home. Such variations in structure and organizational patterns lead to individualized patterns of family functioning. Family member roles and tasks may differ from what the nurse is used to or may expect. Public health nurses must learn to understand and accept these variations in family structure and organization in order to address the needs of the families. Therefore, there are two important principles to guide this acceptance and understanding (Miller et al., 2014; Ramal et al., 2012; Salem & Ma-Pham, 2015):

1. *Principle One*—Each family is unique in its combination of structures, composition, roles, and behaviors. As long as a family carries out its functions effectively and demonstrates the characteristics of a healthy family, one must agree that its form, no matter how variant, is valid.
2. *Principle Two*—Families are constantly changing. Throughout the life cycle, a family seldom stays the same for very long. Each of these changes forces a family to adapt to its circumstances.

Let's look at some common ways a family changes in today's society. Marriage or cohabiting (living together) transforms two people into a couple without children. This family structure and the family members' roles may change by adding children, the couple separating, or becoming part of another family that already has children. Consider the young mother with a baby and a husband who has deserted her: the young mother is now forced to assume a single-parent role in order to survive. This change creates varying degrees of stress and demands because she adapts her energies to be a mother and the family's provider.

Although change is a part of the expected life-cycle growth, some changes can be unexpected and have a large effect on the family's structure. As a public health nurse, your responsibility is to help families cope with these changes while you remain nonjudgmental and accepting of the family structure. For example, a nurse personally may find it difficult to work with same sex couples or respect their same sex marriage because this lifestyle conflicts with the nurse's personal set of values. However, the nurse is a professional, and it is her or his responsibility to help promote the collective health of that family. See Chapter 18. All families are unique groups, each with its own set of needs, and they are best served through unbiased care. Consider the nurse's work with James Cutler and Brian Hoag (see Display 19–6).

Empowering Families

Throughout the family visit, the public health nurse realizes that the ultimate goal is to assist the family in becoming independent of services (Deutsch et al., 2014; Miller et al., 2014). This is accomplished through the approach used in conducting the visit and the nurse–client relationship. Your working relationship with the family can be guided by four suggestions:

- The current functioning of the family has worked for the family before meeting you.
- Before doing "something" for a family, consider who did this "something" before you.
- Find family strengths even in the most challenging and compromised family situation.
- Think about your ability to manage, cope, or function as well as the family members if you were in a similar situation.

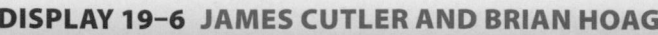

DISPLAY 19–6 JAMES CUTLER AND BRIAN HOAG

James Cutler and Brian Hoag have a 6-year monogamous relationship. A same sex couple, they worked with an attorney to privately adopt a child. The arrangements were completed and their 2-week-old son, Adrian, arrived in their home last week. Helen Jeffers, a public health nurse, receives a referral from the county hospital where Adrian was born. The request is for an assessment of the home situation and parenting skills. At the hospital, the baby tested positive for cocaine with APGAR scores of 6 and 8 and had some initial difficulty sucking. Birth weight was 2,900 g. Discharge weight, at 3 days, was 2,850 g. At her first home visit, Helen finds a neat and orderly two-bedroom condominium that is well equipped with baby supplies. The infant has gained 200 g and is being well cared for by two fatigued parents whose previous contact with infants was limited. James and Brian have many questions and are anxious learners. Helen plans with the couple to make weekly home visits to assess infant growth and development, provide support, and answer questions. She suggests a neighborhood parenting class and finding a reliable babysitter. She also helps James and Brian develop an infant care work schedule. After 6 weeks of intervention, Adrian is thriving. Helen closes the case to home visits, feeling confident that the parents' goal of becoming knowledgeable and confident has been achieved.

Too often, public health nurses focus on a family's weaknesses, looking for and referring to them as *needs* or *problems*. This negative emphasis can be devastating to a family and can undermine any hope of a therapeutic relationship between nurse and family. Many families have strengths that may be overlooked or interpreted as weaknesses by PHNs. It is the nurse's job to recognize the strengths in families and to help families recognize them and understand their potential for self-efficacy (Whittaker & Cowley, 2012). For example, some families create a supportive neighborhood by borrowing needed items (diapers, food, and clothes) from each other, whereas others may pursue more self-reliance by not seeking assistance from outside or infringing on their neighbors' space. Children from large families often learn to physically care for one another, which strengthens their internal relationships. On the other hand, a child from a small family learns to access community resources for care. A large family provides family members with an accepting internal sociomicrocosm, whereas a small family with one or two children learns to interact more with families in the community, enhancing the environment's impact on the family's health. Although family members without a car have to take public transportation or walk to accomplish errands, they are promoting their health by walking while reducing the family expenses. Families need to have their strengths reinforced. Emphasizing a family's strengths fosters a positive self-image, promotes self-confidence and self-efficacy, and often helps a family feel better able to address other problems as they arise.

At times, public health nurses will want to do a simple task for the family such as driving a family member to the clinic or buying a supply of formula or diapers. It might seem like a simple task because "it is on your way" or "there are extra cans of formula or diapers at the agency." But, the nurse should ask, "Will this type of help promote the family's independence and self-efficacy?" A better gift promotes the family's skill of planning ahead to meet the family's transportation needs (make travel arrangements with neighbors or family members, save loose change for the bus, or even walk) or to find ways to use the formula wisely (only fill the bottles with the amount the baby consumes, refrigerate unused formula for later use, or avoid overfeeding the baby). The nurse's gift can be to help the family determine the amount of formula consumed in 24 hours so that the correct quantity is always available. Another gift may be the suggestion to keep a can of powdered formula for emergencies or to completely switch to the powdered formula. These gifts will help the family learn skills to deal with daily situations and crises more effectively.

Finally, you should always look for ways to genuinely praise families for managing in difficult situations. On a home visit, you can empower families by pointing out the positive aspects of their self-care and caregiving, rather than pointing out what they do not do or have (Aston et al., 2015; Pereira et al., 2015).

One helpful communication technique is **strengthening**. This involves verbally listing the positive aspects of an otherwise negative situation in a natural and conversational manner (Aston et al., 2015). For example, a young woman greets you at the door while holding her baby boy. They live in a sparsely furnished one-room apartment, and you notice that the dresser drawer where the baby sleeps is on the floor next to the woman's mattress. She has two baby bottles and a limited assortment of baby clothes. Later during the first visit, you say, "Carlo looks so happy when you cuddle him in your arms, and you are thinking of his safety by letting him sleep in the dresser drawer next to your mattress. I noticed you wash each bottle before making the formula, and you keep him warm in the sleeper and blanket. I think you are managing Carlo's care very well." In this brief scenario, you have positively mentioned bonding, infant health and safety, and proper infant clothing. You have not mentioned the absence of furniture, a full set of bottles, or a variety of clothing. During the rest of the visit, you discuss the services your agency can provide and assess if any of them would be of interest to the young mother. This strengthening technique helps the nurse use a positive approach instead of a negative one that may be viewed by the family as condescending or punitive. The nurse also empowered the young mother to make decisions for her family and to use the nurse as a resource and guide (Wright & Leahey, 2012).

At the least, the public health nurse should be able to say that the family seems to be managing as best as possible if there is nothing else positive to say. This approach does not mean that the nurse should ignore problems. It creates an atmosphere where the assessment can explore all aspects of family functioning, both strengths and weaknesses. Remember, the nurse needs a total picture of the family to know when the family is ready to begin work on problems and to determine adequate nursing care plans. Even as the nurse becomes more aware of a family's unhealthy behaviors, the emphasis should remain on the positive ones. Emphasizing strengths indicates to the family that they are important to the nurse—creating a collaborative relationship.

Family strengths facilitate the ability of the family to meet the needs of the family members and the demands made by systems outside the family unit. Not all behaviors that seem positive are necessarily strengths.

Before the nurse emphasizes a behavior, it should be examined closely to determine if it is actually facilitating family functioning. For instance, a strong work ethic may be viewed a strength when balanced with play and relaxation, but this behavior is a weakness in a family obsessed with working. A public health nurse knows that the amount of free choice, as opposed to compulsive drive, determines if a behavior is either a strength or weakness.

Some behaviors that a nurse may consider as strengths are related to basic family functions, family developmental tasks, and characteristics of family health. For instance, a nurse may wish to note when a family meets family members' needs (physical, emotional, and spiritual needs), shows respect for members' various points of view, or fosters self-discipline in its children. An illustration of this action is in the **family nursing** care of the Stevensons (see Display 19–7).

DISPLAY 19–7   THE STEVENSON FAMILY

The public health nurse, Keith Dow, made an initial home visit after referral by an outpatient physician who was concerned about possible child abuse. Alice Stevenson had brought her baby boy to the emergency room for treatment of a laceration on the forehead. He had fallen off the table while she was changing him, she claimed. A bruise on his arm made the physician suspicious, but Alice explained it was caused by his older brother's rough play. The nurse opened the visit by stating that he was simply following up on the emergency room treatment and wanted to see how the baby was progressing. Keith made no mention of child abuse. He observed the mother and children closely, looking for small things on which to compliment Alice (strengthening) while learning all he could about the family's background. Because the nurse appeared approving rather than suspicious or judgmental, Alice agreed to further visits. During a later visit, Alice admitted to the nurse that she had slapped the baby and her ring cut his forehead. She could not get him to stop crying, no

matter what she did; she just could not endure it any longer, she said. There had been other times when she grabbed him roughly to pull him away from things he wasn't allowed to touch, causing bruises on his arms. Alice told the nurse that she had not planned this baby. When her husband found out she was pregnant, he had left her shortly before the baby was born. Like many abusive parents, Alice had unrealistic expectations of her children's behavior as well as very inadequate self-esteem. Realizing that Alice would be particularly vulnerable to any criticism, the nurse concentrated on her strengths. Keith complimented her on how well she managed her home, dressed the children, maintained her job, and read to her 3-year-old son. It took many visits before Alice trusted the nurse, but in time, they were able to discuss her feelings frankly and work toward improving this family's health. Keith got her to attend a support group for single parents and she began counseling. Emphasizing strengths had provided a bridge for Alice and assisted in bringing her into a helping relationship.

SUMMARY

The family unit remains the focus of service in public health nursing. Family health and the health of each family member strongly influence each other, and family health affects community health. While assessing, diagnosing, planning, implementing, and evaluating are steps used to deliver care to clients in acute care settings and the extensive clinic system, these steps can be used in delivering care to a family as long as the focus is the family. It is family assessment, family diagnosing, family care planning, family health promotion, and family health evaluation.

It is important for the public health nurse to understand healthy family characteristics and to use a variety of tools so that family assessments are thorough.

Healthy families demonstrate six important characteristics: a facilitative process of interaction exists among family members; individual member development is enhanced; role relationships are structured effectively; active attempts are made to cope with problems; there is a healthy home environment and lifestyle; and regular links with the broader community are established.

To systematically assess a family's health, the nurse needs a conceptual framework as a basis for the steps of the nursing process, a clearly defined set of categories for data collection, and a method for measuring the family's level of functioning. The six characteristics of a healthy family provide one assessment framework that public health nurses can use. Assessment tools to aid the nurse in appraising the health of families include the eco-map and the genogram.

There are 12 main categories of family dynamics for which the nurse must collect data: family demographics, physical environment, psychological/spiritual environment, family structure and roles, family functions, family values and beliefs, family communication patterns, family decision-making patterns, family problem-solving patterns, family coping patterns, family health behaviors, and family social and cultural patterns.

Public health nurses enhance their practices with families by observing five principles: work with the family collectively, start at the family's present level of functioning, adapt nursing interventions to the family's stage of development, recognize the validity of family structural variation, and emphasize family strengths.

During assessment, the nurse should focus on the family as a total unit, ask goal-directed questions, collect data over time, combine quantitative with qualitative data, and exercise professional judgment.

Making family health visits is a unique role for nurses and is one of the activities common to most public health nurses. In some agencies, family health visits is the method of choice for most care. In other agencies, a visit is conducted for only the most high-risk families.

When nurses visit families, they must use acute observational skills, good verbal and nonverbal communication, assessment skills, and their intuition to guide them safely in the community and with the families they visit. Some visits are conducted with families in settings other than their homes. Neighborhood clinics, schools, workplaces, or recreational settings may be the preferred or the only locations in which you can gather most of the family members for the visit. Other families may be in transition and living in homeless shelters or with relatives or neighbors. These settings are familiar to the family and provide a unique environment for the nurse in which to visit the family.

Previsit preparation, conduct of the visit, and postvisit documentation are the main components of a family health visit. Each step is important and has value for the success of the next step. Being well prepared for a visit is the first concern (e.g., know the location, have family health status information and needed materials), and the visit should be conducted in an orderly and organized fashion. Time should be allowed for getting acquainted, for the assessment and the nursing diagnosing process, including teaching and anticipatory guidance, and for any other nursing care that may be a part of the visit. The home health visit concludes with a summary of the important parts of the visit and planning for the next visit.

Being safe in a neighborhood is important for all people. Public health nurses spend a great part of the day in the community, and safe travel is important. Use of a personal or agency car, public transportation, or walking to visit families each has its own set of precautions for personal safety. Even in a family's home, personal safety must be a consideration. If family members are arguing or under the influence of drugs or alcohol, the situation may deteriorate rapidly and become unsafe; at this point, it is best to terminate the visit.

During the implementation phase of the family health visit, the nurse may establish a verbal or written contract with the family that permits understanding of the personal roles and responsibilities in the relationship. Empowerment of family members is significant. People who are empowered can help themselves for a lifetime and can make independent decisions about their own health.

Evaluation and preparation for the next visit complete the family health visit cycle. Three types of evaluation can be conducted at the end of a visit: (a) recall of the structure–process assists the nurse in reflecting on the physical aspects of the visit that were positive or negative; (b) discovering these factors can help enhance the positive and eliminate the negative; and (c) evaluating if the outcomes of the visit were achieved through completion of agency documentation. Because the purpose of conducting family health visits is to bring about positive changes in family behaviors, it is necessary to evaluate if both the family and the nurse have achieved the mutual goals. The hardest part of evaluation is self-evaluation where you reflect on your behavior(s) as the PHN and how you conduct home visits. Often, peer evaluation is a helpful way to obtain feedback, because people tend to minimize their own strengths and overlook their weaknesses.

Conducting family health visits involves making referrals to other agencies and services on behalf of the family. One agency cannot provide all the services that a family needs, and PHNs may contact available resources within a community through either written or verbal forms of referral. Public health nurses have unique skills in knowing and locating both official and voluntary services within their community. Such skills come with experience.

ACTIVITIES TO PROMOTE **CRITICAL THINKING**

1. Construct an eco-map of your family or one in your clinical rotation. Ask a peer to do the same, and compare the eco-maps. Assess the balance between your family and the resources in its environment. How does your eco-map compare with that of your peer? What changes are needed in each family system? Are you able to influence the changes that are needed?

2. Draw a genogram of your own family, and ask a peer to discuss it with you. Get input from older family members about illnesses or problems your grandparents or other relatives may have. Make your drawing of the genogram as complete as possible, and then analyze your thoughts and feelings. How did you feel while tracing your family history? Did you learn anything new about your family? Did any family trends or behaviors appear? Did any uncomfortable or suppressed information come to the surface? Do you have any new insights about your family?

3. Assess a family (other than your own) that you know well by completing a family assessment guide. You may use one of the forms in this chapter or an available form from another source. Based on your assessment, recognition of any patterns, or identification of risks (actual or potential), determine as many nursing interventions as you can think of that could be used to promote this family's health as practically as possible.

4. Invite a peer to go on a family health visit with you, and be open to feedback regarding your strengths and weaknesses. How does it make you feel to have someone else on a family health visit with you, knowing they are observing your skills? Offer to do the same for a peer and provide him with feedback. Discuss your experience.

5. Go on several family health visits with an experienced public health nurse and observe the nurse's visiting techniques. Observe how she or he contacts the family; knocks on the door; greets the family; conducts, summarizes, and concludes the visit; and makes plans for the next visit. Discuss the various techniques used and ask questions about your observations to get a better idea of why things are done as they are. Use some of this information on your next home visit.

6. Initiate a small group discussion among your peers about safety on your school campus and in your community. Encourage each person to share the safety habits used. How are these techniques different from safety techniques used when making home visits in the community? If they are different, think about why this is so. Should they be different?

REFERENCES

Allen, D., Feinberg, E., & Mitchell, H. (2014). Bringing life course home: A pilot to reduce pregnancy risk through housing access and family support. *Maternal & Child Health, 18,* 405–412.

American Nurses Association (ANA). (2013). *Public health nursing: Scope and standards of practice* (2nd ed.). Silver Spring, MD: Nursesbooks.org.

American Nurses Association (ANA). (2014). *Health care reform. Health care transformation: The Affordable Care Act and more.* Retrieved from http://www.nursingworld.org/MainMenuCategories/Policy-Advocacy/HealthSystemReform/AffordableCareAct.pdf

American Public Health Association. (2013). *The definition and practice of public health nursing: A statement of the public health nursing section.* Washington, DC: American Public Health Association.

Aston, M., Price, S., Etowa, J., Vukic, A., Young, L., Hart, C.,... Randel, P. (2015). The power of relationships: Exploring how public health nurses support mothers and families during postpartum home visits. *Journal of Family Nursing, 21*(1), 11–34.

Ayala, G. X., Carnethon, M., Arredondo, E., Delamater, A. M., Perreira, K., Van Horn, L.,... Isasi, C. R. (2014). Theoretical foundations of the study of Latino (SOL) youth: Implications for obesity and cardiometabolic risk. *Annals of Epidemiology, 24,* 36–43.

Bahramnezhad, F., Asgari, P., Zolfaghari, M., & Afshar, P. F. (2015). Family-centered education and its clinical outcomes in patients undergoing hemodialysis short running. *Iranian Red Crescent Medical Journal, 17*(6), e20705. doi: 10.5812/ircmj.17(5)2015.20705.

Ballard, J., Mooney, M., & Dempsey, O. (2013). Prevalence of frailty-related risk factors in older adults seen by community nurses. *Journal of Advanced Nursing, 69*(3), 675–684.

Barker, P., & Chang, J. (Eds.). (2013). *Basic family therapy* (6th ed.). Hoboken, NJ: Wiley-Blackwell.

Becvar, D. S., & Becvar, R. J. (2012). *Family therapy: A systematic integration* (8th ed.). New York, NY: Pearson Education.

Centers for Disease Control and Prevention. (2012). *National survey of family growth.* Retrieved from http://www.cdc.gov/nchs/nsfg.htm

Chartier, M. J., Attawar, D., Volk, J. S., Cooper, M., Quddus, F., & McCarthy, J.-A. (2015). Postpartum mental health promotion: Perspectives from mothers and home visitors. *Public Health Nursing, 23*(6), 671–679.

Davis, R. A., & Gustafson, D. T. (2014). Academic-practice partnership in public health nursing: Working with families in a village-based collaboration. *Public Health Nursing, 32*(4), 327–338.

de Cássia Tszesnioski, L., da Nóbrega, K. B. G., de Lima, M. L. L. T., & Facundes, V. L. D. (2015). Building the mental health care network for children and adolescents: Interventions in the territory. *Ciência & Saúde Coletiva, 20*(2), 363–370.

Dennis, T. (2014). Time to tackle domestic violence: Identifying and supporting families. *Community Practitioner, 87*(9), 29–32.

Deutsch, T., Frese, T., & Sandholzer, H. (2014). Factors associated with family-centered involvement in family practice—a cross-sectional multivariate analysis. *Health Communication, 29,* 689–697.

Edelman, C. L., Kudzma, E. E., & Mandle, C. L. (Eds.). (2013). *Health promotion throughout the life span* (8th ed.). St. Louis, MO: Mosby.

Fort, M. P., Castro, M., Peña, L., Hernández, S. H. L., Camacho, G. A., Ramírez-Zea, M., & Martínez, H. (2015). Opportunities for involving men and families in chronic disease management: A qualitative study from Chiapas, Mexico. *BMC Public Health, 15,* 1019.

Ha, Y., Narendorf, S. C., Maria, D. S., & Bezette-Flores, N. (2015). Barriers and facilitators to shelter utilization among homeless young adults. *Evaluation and Program Planning, 53,* 25–33.

Hill, R., & Hansen, D. (1960). The identification of conceptual frameworks utilized in family study. *Marriage and Family Living, 22,* 299–311.

Jones, S. (2015). Implications of case managers' perceptions and attitude on safety of home-delivered care. *British Journal of Community Nursing, 20*(12), 602–607.

Kaakinen, J. R., Coehlo, D. P., Steele, R., Tabacco, A., & Hanson, S. M. H. (2015). *Family health care nursing: Theory, practice, and research* (5th ed.). Philadelphia, PA: F. A. Davis.

Kulbok, P. A., Thatcher, E., Park, E., & Meszaros, P. S. (2012). Evolving public health nursing roles: Focus on community participatory health promotion and prevention. *Online Journal of Issues in Nursing, 17*(2), Manuscript 1. doi: 10.3912/OJIN.Vol17No02Man01.

Leonidas, C., & Santos, M. A. (2015). Family relations in eating disorders: The genogram as instrument of assessment. *Ciência & Saúde Coletiva, 20*(5), 1435–1447.

Lynch, S., Wood, J., Livingood, W., Smotherman, C., Goldhagen, J., & Wood, D. (2015). Feasibility of shelter-based mental health screening for homeless children. *Public Health Reports, 130,* 43–47.

Marlowe, D., Hodgson, J., Lamson, A., White, M., & Irons, T. (2014). Medical family therapy in integrated primary care: An interactional framework. In J. Hodgson, A. Lamson, T. Mendenhall, & D. R. Crane (Eds.), *Medical family therapy: Advanced applications* (pp. 77–94). New York, NY: Springer.

Martins, D. C., Gorman, K. S., Miller, R. J., Murphy, L., Sor, S., Martins, J. C., & Vecchiarelli, M. L. (2015). Assessment of food intake, obesity, and health risk among the homeless in Rhode Island. *Public Health Nursing, 32*(5), 453–461.

McDonald, A., Frazer, K., & Cowley, S. (2013). Caseload management: An approach to making community needs visible. *British Journal of Community Nursing, 18*(3), 140–147.

Miller, G. E., Brody, G. H., Yu, T., & Chen, E. (2014). A family-oriented psychosocial intervention reduces inflammation in low-SES African American youth. *Proceedings of the National Academy of Sciences, 111*(31), 11287–11292.

Monsen, K. A., Chatterjee, S. B., Timm, J. E., Poulsen, J. K., Tchg, D. S., & McNaughton, D. B. (2014). Factors explaining variability in health literacy outcomes of public health nursing clients. *Public Health Nursing, 32*(2), 94–100.

Odell, J. (2015). Clinical decision-making in minor illness. *Nurse Prescribing, 13*(10), 504–507.

Parachin, V. M. (1997, March/April). Six signs of a healthy family. *Vibrant Life, 13,* 5–6.

Parthasarathy, P., Dailey, D. E., Young, M.-E. D., Lam, C., & Pies, C. (2014). Building economic security today: Making the health-wealth connection in Contra Costa County's maternal and child health. *Maternal & Child Health Journal, 18,* 296–404.

Pereira, M. G., Costa, V., Oliveira, D., Ferreira, G., Pedras, S., Sousa, M. R., & Machado, J. C. (2015). Patients' and spouses' contribution toward adherence to self-care behaviors in type 2 diabetes. *Research and Theory for Nursing Practice: An International Journal, 29*(4), 276–296.

Peterson, G. W., & Bush, K. R. (Eds.). (2013). *Handbook of marriage and the family* (3rd ed.). New York, NY: Springer.

Porr, C. J. (2015). Important interactional strategies for everyday public health nursing practice. *Public Health Nursing, 32*(1), 43–49.

Prichard, I., Lee, A., Hutchinson, A. D., & Wilson, C. (2015). Familial risk for lifestyle-related chronic diseases: Can family health history be used as a motivational tool to promote health behavior in young adults? *Health Promotion Journal of Australia, 26,* 122–128.

Raingruber, B. (2014). Health promotion theories. In B. Raingruber (Ed.), *Contemporary health promotion in nursing practice* (pp. 53–94). Sudbury, MA: Jones & Bartlett Learning.

Ramal, E., Petersen, A. B., Ingram, K. M., & Champlin, A. M. (2012). Factors that influence diabetes self-management in Hispanics living in low socioeconomic neighborhoods in San Bernardino, California. *Journal of Immigrant & Minority Health, 14,* 1090–1096.

Reiss, D. (1981). *The family's construction of reality.* Cambridge, MA: Harvard University Press.

Rodriguez, A. J., & Margolin, G. (2015). Military service absences and family members' mental health: A timeline followback assessment. *Journal of Family Psychology, 29*(4), 642–648.

Rogers, J. (2012). Working with families to boost children's continence. *Nursing Times, 108*(50), 16–18.

Salem, B. E., & Ma-Pham, J. (2015). Understanding health needs and perspectives of middle-aged and older women experiencing homelessness. *Public Health Nursing, 32*(6), 634–644.

Schaffer, M. A., Goodhue, A., Stennes, K., & Lanigan, C. (2012). Evaluation of a public health nurse visiting program for pregnant and parenting teens. *Public Health Nursing, 29*(3), 218–231.

Shepherd, M. L. (2011). Behind the scales: Child and family health nurses taking care of women's emotional wellbeing. *Contemporary Nurse, 37*(2), 137–148.

Shi, L., & Singh, D. A. (2011). Conceptual framework of health determinants. In L. Shi & D. A. Singh (Eds.), *The nation's health* (8th ed.; pp. 43–46). Sudbury, MA: Jones & Bartlett Learning.

Smith, C. (2013). A family perspective in community/public health nursing. In F. A. Maurer & C. M. Smith (Eds.), *Community/public health nursing practice: Health for families and populations* (5th ed.; (pp. 322–339). St. Louis, MO: Elsevier Saunders.

Smith, C. (2013). Family case management. In F. A. Maurer & C. M (Eds.), Smith, *Community/public health nursing practice: Health for families and populations* (5th ed.; pp. 340–371). St. Louis, MO: Elsevier Saunders.

SmithBattle, L. S., Lorenz, R., & Leander, S. (2013). Listening with care: Using narrative methods to cultivate nurses' responsive relationships in a home visiting intervention with teen mothers. *Nursing Inquiry, 20*, 199–198.

Spector, R. E. (2013). *Cultural diversity in health and illness* (8th ed.). Upper Saddle River, NJ: Prentice-Hall.

Thompson, C., & Adderley, U. (2015). Diagnostic and treatment decision making in community nurses faced with a patient with possible venous leg ulceration: A signal detection analysis. *International Journal of Nursing Studies, 52*, 325–333.

U.S. Department of Health and Human Services (USDHHS). (2012). *U.S. surgeon general's family health history initiative*. Retrieved from http://www.hhs.gov/familyhistory/

U.S. Department of Health and Human Services (USDHHS). (2016). *Social determinants of health*. Retrieved from http://www.healthy-people.gov/2020/topics-objectives/topic/social-determinants-of-health

Whittaker, K. A., & Cowley, S. (2012). A survey of parental self-efficacy experiences: Maximising potential through health visiting and universal parenting support. *Journal of Clinical Nursing, 21*, 3276–3286.

Williford, A., Fite, P. J., Johnson-Motoyama, M., & Frazer, A. L. (2015). Acculturative dissonance and risks for proactive and reactive aggression among Latino/a adolescents: Implications for culturally relevant prevention and interventions, *Journal of Primary Prevention, 36*, 405–418.

Wright, L., & Leahey, M. (2012). *Nurses and families: A guide to family assessment and intervention* (6th ed.). Philadelphia, PA: F.A. Davis.

thePoint: Everything You Need to Make the Grade!

the**Point**® Visit http://thePoint.lww.com/Allender9e
for selected readings, study aids for all learning styles, and more!

Surgeon General's Family Health History Initiative

Visit http://www.hhs.gov/familyhistory/
for more information about creating a family health portrait as a way to explore and understand the family history.

Violence Affecting Families

"The right things to do are those that keep our violence in abeyance; the wrong things are those that bring it to the fore."

—*Robert J. Sawyer* (1960), Calculating God

KEY TERMS

Adolescent dating violence (ADV)
Battered child syndrome
Child abuse
Child maltreatment
Crisis theory
Cycle of violence
Developmental crisis
Elder abuse
Emotional abuse
Infanticide
Intimate partner violence (IPV)
Mandated reporters
Neglect
Neonaticide
Physical abuse
Sexual abuse
Shaken baby syndrome
Situational crisis
Spectrum of prevention

LEARNING OBJECTIVES

Upon mastery of this chapter, you should be able to:

- Explain the difference between developmental crises and situational crises, and give examples of each within families.
- Discuss strategies to prevent the impact of a situational crisis and a developmental crisis at a primary, secondary, and tertiary level of prevention.
- Discuss the global incidence and prevalence of family violence.
- Describe how the United States has responded to family violence.
- Identify characteristics of abuse against infants, children, and adolescents.
- Describe the "cycle of violence" seen in intimate partner/spousal abuse.
- Explain common types of elder abuse.
- Describe the community health nurse role with families in crises at each level of prevention.
- Use the nursing process to outline nursing actions in developmental and situational crises.

A *family crisis* is a stressful and disruptive event (or series of events) that comes with or without warning and disturbs the equilibrium of the family. A family crisis can also result when usual problem-solving methods fail. All families experience periods of crisis: a toddler is diagnosed with a serious illness; a teenager discovers she is pregnant; a father and sole breadwinner in a family loses his job; a mother's social drinking becomes habitual after her children go off to college; or a family's home is destroyed in a hurricane, earthquake, flood, or fire. If you think back on your family's history, you can probably identify one or more periods of crisis that you and your family members experienced. If so, how directly were you affected? How did the crisis resolve? As a result of the crisis, did any permanent changes occur in your family's dynamics or individual behaviors?

People respond to crises differently. Some people approach crisis as a challenge, an event to be reckoned with, whereas others may feel overwhelmed and defeated or give up. Some individuals seek help if needed and come through the experience unscathed or as survivors, perhaps even stronger than before. Other individuals who are unable to cope with the crisis, or who do not cope well, may suffer severe psychological damage or may inflict their feelings of rage, frustration, or powerlessness onto their children, partners, or elders. This chapter focuses on families that have responded to stressors with violence, neglect, or abuse and those that have experienced stress and loss as a result of violence initiated by others.

Regardless of their responses, families in crisis need help, and community health nurses have a unique opportunity and responsibility to provide that help in a broad variety of situations. For example, in one family, an 8-year-old boy begins doing poorly in school; he wets his pants during class twice in 1 week and starts a small fire in the schoolyard. The school nurse is astute enough to begin an investigation into the family dynamics that may be contributing to these symptoms. In another family, a pregnant woman reschedules her appointment at a community clinic twice and then arrives at the appointment with multiple faded bruises on her face and arms. The clinic nurse uses sensitivity and caring while screening her for intimate partner violence (IPV).

Primary and secondary prevention measures used by community health nurses that help prevent crises include teaching families parenting skills and coping strategies and informing them about community resources. In addition to assessment and education, community health nurses provide tertiary responses with direct assistance during times of crisis. This chapter discusses the knowledge and skills that community health nurses use in their practice of crisis prevention and intervention aimed at promoting improved health for families in the community.

DYNAMICS AND CHARACTERISTICS OF A CRISIS

Researchers have studied the nature of crises and have developed a body of knowledge called stress or **crisis theory**. Initially limited to the field of mental health, crisis theory now influences every field of health care. The theory helps to explain why people respond in certain ways during a crisis and can be predictive of the phases people go through during and after a crisis. These responses and phases are important ideas for the community health nurse to understand before working in prevention or management of crises (Weber, 2011).

How does a crisis occur? Each of us is a dynamic system living within a given environment under circumstances unique to us alone. Our behavior—both consciously and subconsciously—is gauged to maintain a balance within ourselves and in our relations with others. When some internal or external force disrupts our system's balance and alters functioning, a loss of equilibrium occurs. The individual then attempts to restore equilibrium by using whatever resources are available to him or her, in an effort to cope with the situation. Coping refers to those actions and ways of thinking that assist people in dealing with and surviving difficult situations. If individuals cannot readily cope with a stressful event—for example, if one's home is destroyed by fire, or one fails a final examination—the person experiences a crisis (Weber, 2011).

Crises are precipitated by a specific identifiable event that becomes too much for the usual problem-solving skills of those involved. Often, a single distressing event follows a host of previous difficulties and becomes the "straw that breaks the camel's back." For example, a wife who suffers years of spousal abuse finally becomes unable to cope and shoots her husband during a violent attack. Occasionally, tragic events occur suddenly without previous stressors, as when a father is killed in a plane crash or a child drowns in the family swimming pool.

Crises are normal in that all people occasionally feel overwhelmed. A person intervening in a crisis today may well be tomorrow's crisis victim. No individual is immune from sudden overwhelming difficulties. For example, Barbara, a hospice nurse, assists families through crises as part of her job, when suddenly her own spouse is diagnosed with cancer. Her coping skills are strained, as she feels overwhelmed with increased personal demands that require her support and attention.

Often, a crisis is not an event per se, but rather a person's perception of the event. Each person reacts in his own way. A situation that throws one person off course

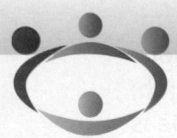

DISPLAY 20–1 TWO FAMILIES' RESPONSE TO CRISIS

The Redondos and the Fosters will be moving to a town in another state, 900 miles away, because of a job change. The Redondos are in crisis over the move. They have never lived in any other town. They will have to leave relatives and lifelong friends who live nearby and a community in which they have been very involved. Mrs. Redondo is the secretary at her family's house of worship. Their teenage daughter, a cheerleader, just started high school. Their son is in kindergarten; Grandma happily watches him in the mornings before school. Everyone is upset because of how the move will affect them. The family is stressed and argues each evening. They don't want to put their house up for sale or even to visit the new community to which they will be moving. Mr. Redondo is second-guessing his decision to move, but his choices were limited as his company is relocating. The Redondos, in crisis, are not exploring alternatives that may allow them to stay in their present community. One possible alternative might be for Mrs. Redondo to work while Mr. Redondo looks for another job. When people perceive that they are in crisis, decision-making and problem-solving become more difficult.

The Fosters, however, are excitedly looking forward to their move. They have two young children who are not yet in school. The move will bring them only 50 miles from old college friends. They hope to realize a significant profit on their house, which they recently remodeled. They can't wait to go "house hunting" in the new town. Everyone is enjoying planning the anticipated move; their two children, aged 3 and 4, have been playing "moving day" with their favorite toys.

Both families are experiencing the same event. The difference is each person's situation and perception of the event. The Redondos' equilibrium is being disrupted. They have not developed previous coping skills and do not see the move as a positive experience. They are at a different time in their family life cycle than are the Fosters. Although the move upsets their equilibrium, too, the Fosters experience it as an exciting event that conjures positive feelings; they are passing these feelings on to their children. They see this move as an opportunity.

---

may merely create an interesting detour for another (see Display 20–1). It is usually the individual's interpretation of the event, rather than the event itself, that is crucial. At other times, a community crisis occurs on a large scale or is so unexpected that the crisis directly involves people who are known by others hundreds of miles away, causing distant friends and relatives shock and sorrow. Examples of such crises are Hurricane Katrina, or an apartment building fire that kills a dozen people, or the terrorist attack in San Bernardino in 2015. Even strangers, knowing no one involved directly, are affected and experience signs and symptoms of stress (Devakumar, Birch, Osrin, Sondorp, & Wells, 2014).

Crises are resolved, either positively or negatively, within a brief period, usually 4 to 8 weeks (Kanel, 2012). People's strong need to regain homeostasis and the intense nature of crises contribute toward making the crisis a temporary condition that will not continue indefinitely. In the family in which the wife shot her abusive husband, as shocking as the event might seem, life returns to a recognizable pattern within a few weeks. Even though family members will feel the change for years, the crisis soon subsides. The husband is hospitalized and recovers from his wound; the wife's case goes to trial, and she is sentenced to 2 years in prison; the children stay with relatives and attend school.

Crisis resolution can be an adaptive process in which growth and improved health occur, or it can be maladaptive, resulting in illness or even death (Weber, 2011). The battered wife reevaluates her life, gets divorced, learns employment skills in jail, and becomes more assertive, with stronger self-esteem; after she is paroled, she returns to her children, now able to support them financially and emotionally. She finds personal growth and health while successfully resolving the crisis. The children settle into their aunt's home with minimal difficulty, start a new school, and visit their mother and father regularly. After release, the mother finds an apartment near her sister's home, so that the children can continue in the same school district. The husband recovers from his wounds, gets counseling, relocates to another town, and sees his children frequently. The crisis situation is resolved at a higher level of wellness for all members than existed before the crisis. In this example, the members are determined to improve their situation by working with skilled health care professionals. By using the resources within the community, this family is healthier after the crisis.

Developmental Crises

Developmental crises are periods of disruption that occur at transition points during normal growth and development (see Display 20–2). When developmental crises occur, people feel threatened by the demands placed on them and have difficulty making the changes necessary to fit the new stage of development (Weber, 2011).

During the process of normal biopsychosocial growth, people go through a succession of life cycle stages, from birth through old age. Each stage differs from the previous one, and transitions from one stage to the next require changes in roles and behavior. Popular and classic authors such as Bridges (1980, 2001), Sheehy (1976, 1992, 1999), and Sheehy and Delbourgo (1996) have called these periods "passages" and "transitions." These transitions are times when developmental or maturational crises occur.

Most family developmental crises have a gradual onset. The change is evolutionary rather than revolutionary. People usually anticipate and even prepare to start

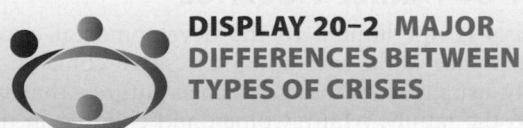

DISPLAY 20-2 MAJOR DIFFERENCES BETWEEN TYPES OF CRISES

Developmental Crisis

Part of normal growth and development that can upset normalcy

Precipitated by a life transition point

Gradual onset

Response to developmental demands and society's expectations

Situational Crisis

Unexpected period of upset in normalcy

Precipitated by a hazardous event

Sudden onset

Externally imposed "accident"

---

school, enter adolescence, leave home, marry, have a baby, retire, or die. Individuals move into and through each transitional period knowing in advance that some kind of change will be required. In many instances, people have already seen others experience these transitions. As a result, developmental crises have a degree of predictability. These developmental crises offer a time for anticipation and adjustment.

Developmental crises arise from both physical and social changes. Each new life stage confronts people with changed relationships, responsibilities, and roles. The transition to parenthood, for example, demands a change in role from caring for oneself and one's mate to include nurturing, caring for, and protecting a completely helpless infant. Relationships with adults, children, and even one's parents also change. Parenthood is an entrance into a previously inexperienced part of the adult world. New parents may fear the unknown. Will this infant develop normally? Can I give adequate care? Parents often feel anxiety about the responsibility of shaping this new person's life, satisfying society's expectations for their child's proper education and training, or bringing children into a world that is in crisis and already overpopulated. Parents may worry about the increased financial burden while struggling with mixed feelings about giving up a large measure of freedom. These transitions put people under considerable stress, which contributes to tension, feelings of helplessness, and resultant crisis. Some people adapt quickly; others cannot cope, probably because earlier developmental crises went unresolved. If people lack a repertoire of adaptive skills, even positive and planned changes can develop into crises (Display 20–3) (Fig. 20–1).

Situational Crises

A **situational crisis** is a stressful, disruptive event arising from external circumstances that occur suddenly, often without warning, to a person, group, aggregate, or community. Typically, the external event requires behavioral changes and coping mechanisms beyond the abilities of the people involved (Weber, 2011).

Such events are not predicted, expected, or planned. The crisis occurs to people because of where they are in time and space. For instance, a baby grabs her mother's hot cup of tea and burns her chest; a college student is raped in the library parking lot; an older adult falls and fractures a hip; a mother with a van full of Little League baseball players is involved in a traffic collision at a busy intersection; or a hurricane devastates a state. These

---

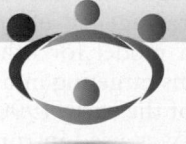

DISPLAY 20-3 A DEVELOPMENTAL CRISIS

Marcia Sand is 39 years old. Married for 22 years, she has been a capable homemaker and mother of four children. Her husband, Lou, a construction worker for the past 20 years, thinks Marcia does a "super job at home." In the past, Marcia's time was filled with cooking, laundry, cleaning, shopping, and meeting the endless demands of the family. Their limited income prompted her to adopt many money-saving strategies. She made most of her own and the children's clothes, did all her own baking, and raised vegetables in her backyard garden. Now, the youngest of the children, Tommy, has just left home to join the Navy. Her husband spends much of his spare time at the local bar with his friends, leaving Marcia alone. With a nearly empty house and little need for cooking, baking, and sewing, Marcia has lost her sense of usefulness. She thinks of taking a job but knows her choices are limited because she has only a high school education. Marcia has not slept well in weeks; she wakes up tired and drags through the day barely able to manage the simplest task. She cries frequently but does not know why. Her hair, always neat and attractive in the past, looks bedraggled, and her shoulders slump. "I just can't seem to get on top of things any more," she complains.

Marcia has entered a developmental crisis that is sometimes called the "empty nest syndrome." She faces a turning point in her life, a time when parenting has seemingly ended. Leaving her satisfying homemaker role, she faces a new life stage filled with unknowns, changes, and a seeming lack of purpose. The transition came about gradually, almost imperceptibly, but now she must deal with it. Yet she feels unable to cope and wishes to turn to someone who would understand and lend her strength. She can be helped, but her crisis could also have been prevented at the precrisis phase. Anticipatory planning could have prevented the dilemma Marcia finds herself in now.

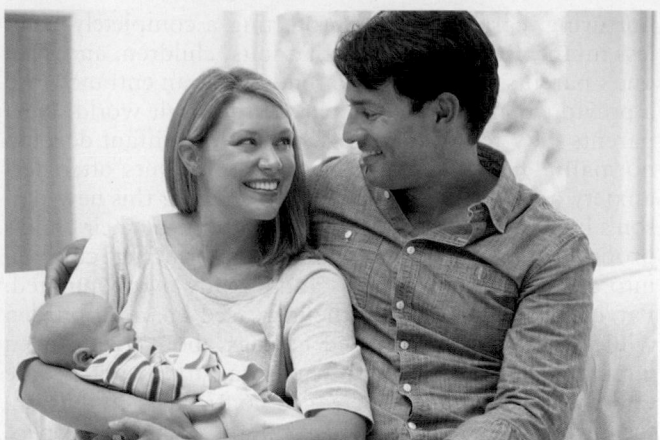

FIGURE 20–1 Young couple with a new baby.

events, which involve loss or the threat of loss, represent life hazards to those affected. Some crisis-precipitating events can be positive, such as a significant job promotion or sudden acquisition of great wealth; however, the change still makes increased demands on individuals who must make major life adjustments. Even positive events involve a modified grieving process, because the individuals involved may be losing or giving up old, familiar, and comfortable situations and facing stressful changes.

Community health nurses see an almost infinite variety of situational crises, including debilitating disease, economic misfortune, unemployment, physical abuse, divorce, unwanted pregnancy, drug and alcohol abuse, sudden death of a loved one, tragic accidents such as a drowning or plane crash, and many others. In each situation, people feel overwhelmed and need help to cope. Skilled intervention can make the difference between a healthy and an unhealthy.

Multiple Crises

Different kinds of crises can overlap in actual experience, compounding the stress felt by the persons involved. For example, a couple may experience a **developmental crisis** (birth) and a situational crisis (birth defect) simultaneously, thus compounding the resulting stress. The developmental crisis of midlife may be complicated by situational crises such as a divorce or job change. With older adults, the developmental crisis of retirement may be compounded by the situational crisis of a fire that destroys the family home. The transition a child faces entering school may occur at the same time the family moves to a new neighborhood and a new infant joins the family. The child must share the parent's attention and affection with a new sibling at a time when all the child's resources are needed to cope with starting school and adjusting to the new neighborhood. Classic research shows that accumulated stresses can lead to ill health (Holmes & Rahe, 1967; Salleh, 2008), and research continues to examine the link between chronic stress and various illnesses (Epel & Lithgow, 2014; Heidt et al., 2014). Those who normally work through one crisis in a healthy way may find that compounding events overwhelm them, causing more stress than they can handle.

HISTORY OF FAMILY VIOLENCE

Family crisis is not limited to the developmental crises people experience or the situational crises that come upon us suddenly, usually from forces—such as nature—that are external to the family. Many women and children in the world also experience the crisis of domestic violence. The terms domestic violence, family violence, and interpersonal violence refer to morbidity and mortality attributable to violence within the home setting, involving action by a family member or intimate partner. Domestic violence involves "a systematic pattern of assaultive and coercive behaviors, including physical, sexual, and psychological attacks and economic coercion, that adults or adolescents use against their intimate partner" (WHO, 2013b, para.1). This type of violence occurs worldwide and is a global public health burden (WHO, 2016a).

Global History

Family violence is not new. For centuries, children were thought of as the property of their parents, and any treatment doled out by the parents was their prerogative. In fact, most countries had animal welfare laws long before child welfare laws were adopted. In addition, the ideology of childhood that emerged in the Western world in the late 1800s assumed that only "abnormal" children needed protection. These children were casualties of an urban–industrial society and were abandoned, dependent, or delinquent—the products of social dislocation such as orphans or refugee children.

In the early 1900s, sensitive leaders concerned with child welfare issues emerged. Several international agencies were created designed to positively affect the health of children. The British Children's Act was passed in 1908, and the first White House Conference on Children was held in 1909. These were early attempts to define a role for the state in the welfare of children. The U.S. conference was the forerunner of the United States Children's Bureau (USCB), and a national voluntary organization, later known as the Child Welfare League of America, was established to complement federal agency efforts (Cheung, 2012). The USCB became a model for other countries, with well-developed programs targeting infant mortality. In one innovative program of the early 1900s, a heated, mobile, child welfare center was used in rural communities and was staffed by a female physician and a public health nurse to improve health care to children.

Other international organizations emerged in the early 1900s, including the International Association for the Promotion of Child Welfare (IAPCW), the League of Red Cross Societies (LRCS), the Save the Children Fund (SCF), and the Save the Children International Union (SCIU). The latter two agencies were immensely successful in raising funds for children in Germany, Austria, France, Hungary, and Serbia. As these organizations began serving the needs of children internationally, they moved from a sentimental depiction of victims to a medical–social–scientific view of children at risk, expanding and uncovering the concepts of child victimization, exploitation, and abuse (Cheung, 2012).

By the mid-1920s, the work of these agencies began to focus on children from non-European countries.

The first conference on children from non-European countries focused on African children in 1931 and included such issues as infant mortality, child labor, education, and child slavery. In 1924, the League of Nations adopted the Declaration of the Rights of the Child, which would influence the League of Nations' successor, the United Nations (UN), in the years to come in the form of the Declaration of the Rights of the Child 1959 and the Convention on the Rights of the Child 1989. The UN continues to hold annual hearings on the Rights of the Child and has addressed global concerns, such as children without parental care, indigenous children, violence against children, children with disabilities, and economic exploitation of children (Office of the United Nations High Commissioner for Human Rights, 2014).

Children are not the only victims of family morbidity and mortality from violence. Historically, women were also treated as property and often suffered physical and psychological damage. Gender-based violence, or violence against women (VAW), has global public health and human rights ramifications (World Health Organization [WHO], 2014). Worldwide, more than 1.3 million people die each year from violence (WHO, 2014). Abuse toward women is often perpetrated by an intimate partner and is not reported. Areas of war and conflict have been known to use sexual violence toward women as a war tactic. Recent global prevalence figures indicate 35% of women worldwide have experienced IPV or non-partner sexual violence in their lifetime (WHO, 2016c). In 2010, the United Nations Entity for Gender Equality and the Empowerment of Women was established and prioritized the prevention of and response to VAW. The first global and regional estimates of VAW was published in 2013, which resulted in clinical and policy guidelines that have been widely disseminated, and 35 countries have participated in programs to build capacity (WHO, 2014). As with children, the rights of women are socially, culturally, and religiously influenced, with change coming slowly.

United States History

The history of treatment of children, women, and elders in the United States began with early immigration to this continent and has been influenced by the cultural and religious practices of early settlers. In addition, necessity, attitudes of the time, and the stress and hardship of life in the colonies and on the frontier influenced how people were treated. Children were born into families to help with the chores of an agricultural society. Families had many children, infant mortality rates were high, and it was not uncommon for half of the children in a family to die before their second birthday. Older people did not retire; they contributed to family survival until they died. There were no special considerations for children, women, or elders. The best a woman could hope for was that the man she married would not abuse her emotionally, physically, sexually, or fiducially (taking advantage of a person's financial resources). Women had limited or no education, resources, or rights, and children had even less. If a woman married "poorly," she would have to live with the consequences. Separation and divorce were either unheard of or were a "death sentence" for the woman and her children, because there was nowhere they could go and no way for the woman to support her family (Cherlin, 2014).

Public Laws and Protection

It took many years for the United States to establish laws that benefited women and children. Nonetheless, the United States began earlier than did many other countries to protect children, women, and elders. The Children's Bureau began to focus on child abuse in the 1960s, supporting development of a child abuse mandatory reporting law in 1962 to be used as a model by the states. The law required health professionals and child care workers to report suspected child abuse to appropriate officials. In 1974, the Child Abuse Prevention and Treatment Act (CAPTA) was passed, becoming Public Law 93-247 (PL 93-247). This law served to reinforce the earlier mandatory reporting law model and was aimed at solving the growing problem of child abuse in the country. PL 93-247 has been amended several times since 1974. The Child Abuse Prevention and Treatment and Adoption Reform Act of 1978 preceded the Family Violence Prevention and Services Act of 1984. Later, all three acts were consolidated into the Child Abuse Prevention, Adoption, and Family Services Act of 1988 (PL 100-294), and most recently, the Act (PL 108-36) was amended and reauthorized as the Keeping Children and Families Safe Act of 2003 (Child Welfare Information Gateway, 2011).

This act supports funding to states in their efforts to prevent violence in families and to identify and treat victims. The funding comes in the form of the CAPTA and state grants that meet eligibility requirements. One aspect of the funding supports the National Child Abuse and Neglect Data System (NCANDS) that tracks reports of child abuse and neglect and all fatalities from child abuse or neglect in the United States. In 2015, NCANDS reported an estimate of 1,520 child deaths caused by injury or neglect (Administration for Children and Families [ACF], 2013b). Information on adoption, out-of-home care for children, preventing and responding to child abuse and neglect, supporting and preserving families, and resources are available via the Child Welfare Information Gateway, a program under the U.S. Department of Health and Human Services (USDHHS), Administration of Children and Families. The Administration on Aging, also under the USDHHS, supports similar programs including the National Center on Elder Abuse (n.d.b) that works to educate and assist families, seniors, and health care and legal providers regarding elder abuse. The Centers for Disease Control and Prevention (CDC, 2013) provide videos and resources on violence prevention.

Healthy People 2020 Goals

The goal for *Healthy People 2020* regarding injury and violence prevention is to "prevent unintentional injuries and violence and reduce their consequences" (USDHHS, 2016a, para. 1). Determinants that affect violence include (1) individual behavior, (2) physical environment, (3) access to services, (4) social environment, and (5) societal-level factors. Through previous tracking and program strategies, new focus areas in violence prevention have been identified. Current *Healthy People 2020* trends identified for youth involve "bullying, dating violence, and sexual violence," whereas the rates and causes of elder abuse were also cited as areas needing more research and strategies for prevention (USDHHS, 2016a, para. 15).

The problem of violence is pervasive, affecting the victim directly and family members and society indirectly. Selected violence and abuse objectives for *Healthy People 2020* include the following:

- Reduce homicides from a baseline of 6.1 deaths per 100,000 population that occurred in 2007 to a target of 5.5 homicides per 100,000 population
- Reduce child maltreatment deaths from 2.3 per 100,000 children under age 18 years for 2008 to a target of 2.1 deaths per 100,000 children in 2020
- Reduce the number of adolescents carrying weapons on school property during the past 30 days from a 2009 baseline of 5.6% of students in grade 9 through 12, to a target of 4.6% (data from Youth Risk Behavior Surveillance System [YRBS], CDC, 2012).

The *Healthy People 2010* final review (CDC, 2011a) demonstrated reductions in several areas and identification of new or modified objectives for 2020. Declines were seen in the following:

- Physical assaults by intimate partners dropped from 3.6 to 2.3 per 1,000 population.
- Rape or attempted rape declined by 66.7% from 1998 to 2009.
- Physical assaults dropped by 47.6% between 1998 and 2009 in the 12 years and older population, whereas physical fighting for 9th to 12th grade students dropped by 13.9%.

The *Healthy People 2020 Leading Health Indicator [LHI] Progress Report for Violence* indicates that the homicide rate has declined 15% from 6.1 deaths per 100,000 people in 2007 to 5.3 per 100,000 population people in 2010, exceeding the HP target of 5.5 per 100,000 (USDHHS, 2014). As of March 2014, progress generally has been positive toward achieving the *Healthy People 2020* targets for the 26 LHIs, with 14 indicators (53.9%) having either met their target or shown improvement (CDC, 2014g).

Social environment and societal-level determinants are expanding in the *Healthy People 2020* tracking to investigate what works in violence prevention. This tracking is multifocused through research, program development, and policy making. Education programs on conflict resolution coping and bullying provide data and strategies to reduce violence among students. Policies and legislation that affect social attitudes and regulations to deter violence, promote community involvement, and create safer communities are also being studied. Investigating individual behaviors, such as risk-taking, drug and alcohol use, or factors influencing individual development, guides further learning of risk, as well as prevention measures.

Myths and Truths About Family Violence

Many myths about family violence need to be dispelled. Strongly held myths by members of society, including community health nurses and other health care providers, may interfere with their ability to help families in crisis get the help they need. Table 20–1 displays some common myths and truths about family violence.

FAMILY VIOLENCE AGAINST CHILDREN

Communicable disease is no longer the leading cause of morbidity and mortality among children. Globally, child maltreatment is a huge problem with a serious impact on victims' physical and mental health, well-being, and development throughout their lives and by extension on the health of societies in general as noted by the WHO and International Society for Prevention of Child Abuse and Neglect in a 2006 press release, yet violence directed at children is preventable. Therefore, ending violence against children would shift resources to aid in prevention of illnesses that affect children worldwide. This continuing morbidity is psychosocial in nature and is associated with behavioral problems that are more difficult to prevent than the diseases known for centuries. The effects of maltreatment of children lead to long-term conditions that include depression, suicide behavior, cardiovascular disease, sexually transmitted disease, and cancers (WHO, 2014).

Child abuse is defined by the federal CAPTA (42 USCA, 5106g) and was amended by the CAPTA Reauthorization Act of 2010 as "at minimum: any recent act or failure to act on the part of a parent or caretaker which results in death, serious physical or emotional harm, sexual abuse or exploitation; or an act or failure to act which presents an imminent risk of serious harm" (Child Welfare Information Gateway, 2012, para. 1). **Child maltreatment** is identified as maltreatment toward a child under age 18 that may include physical, emotional, general neglect, medical or educational neglect, physical punishment or battering, emotional or sexual maltreatment and exploitation, or other exploitation that results in actual or potential harm to the child's health, survival, or dignity in the context of a relationship of responsibility, trust, or power (WHO, 2014).

Child abuse and the associated psychosocial developmental problems are taking a toll globally in human costs and economically in health care services. Worldwide, almost 23% of adults reported physical abuse during their childhood, over 36% reported emotional abuse, and 16.3% reported neglect. Childhood sexual abuse lifetime prevalence rates are 7.6% for boys, but 18% for girls. High rates of all abuse were found in the African region. Victims of child abuse and IPV have a greater health burden, with higher numbers of health care provider visits, hospitalizations, and generally poorer health (WHO, 2014). Identifying and gathering worldwide data about child abuse is difficult because many cases are not investigated and death reports may not be classified as the result of abuse or homicide.

Another concern for children is their role in families that may require very young children to aid the family financially. A child's "chores" may include spending the whole day scrounging around city dumps gathering bits of food, clothing, or other useful or saleable items. Some children are sold for sexual favors, whereas others spend all day working in fields, home businesses, or "sweatshops" for the equivalent of pennies a day. In some societies, female children are not valued and are killed at birth, given away, or sold into slavery for a pittance.

Child abuse in the United States is most often recognized in the categories of neglect, physical abuse, sexual

Table 20–1   Common Myths and Truths About Abuse in Families

Myth	Truth
Violence in families is rare.	Family violence is common and increasing.
Violence occurs most frequently among low-income families.	Family violence occurs across all incomes.
Violence occurs more frequently in some racial and cultural groups.	Family violence occurs across all racial and cultural groups.
Violence in families does not coexist with love.	Love may exist but is unable to be displayed appropriately because of conflicting emotions.
Men who batter women are mentally ill.	The percentage of batterers who are mentally ill is the same as in the general population.
Women who accept battering are mentally ill.	The percentage of battered women who are mentally ill is the same as in the general population; however, they have low self-esteem and a damaged spirit.
Violence occurs only in heterosexual relationships.	Domestic violence has no gender or sexual boundaries; it can occur among all people.
Abused women instigate the battering.	Quite the contrary, they go out of their way not to agitate or confront the abuser.
Abuse occurs when the abuser is under the influence of drugs or alcohol.	It can, but many abusers do not drink or use drugs.
Children should not be taken from their parents.	In some violent families, the safest place for the child is with another family member or a foster home (temporarily or permanently).
Even abusive parents are better for a child than a child living elsewhere.	Children must be protected, and living away from abusive parents may save their lives.
Abused children become abusive adults.	Some may but most can learn how to channel their emotions positively if the cycle of violence is broken.

abuse, and emotional abuse. Often, there is an overlap of maltreatment when a report is made to Child Protective Services (CPS) or the police. The NCANDS reported 3.5 million referrals to CPS departments in 2013, and professionals (e.g., teachers, law enforcement officers, and social services) made 62% of the CPS reports. Infants (birth to 1 year) had the highest victimization rate at 23.1 per 1,000 children in the same age group (ACF, 2013a). Boys were victimized at a higher rate than were girls (2.36 vs. 1.77 per 100,000), whereas 44% of the victims were White, 22% were African American, and 22.4% were Hispanic (ACF, 2013a). Neglect continued as the category of highest occurrence at 79.3%, whereas 18% of children were found to have suffered physical abuse, and sexual abuse was determined as the primary cause in 9.2% of the investigations. Of all child fatalities in the United States, 73.9% were among children 3 years of age or younger (ACF, 2013a). NCANDS estimated 1,560 child fatalities in the United States in 2010 and 1,520 in 2013. The dependence of small children makes them vulnerable to abuse and neglect as shown in both the United States and worldwide child abuse data. Either one or both parents were responsible for almost 80% of all child fatalities (ACF, 2013a).

Nationally, measures have been taken to improve data gathering and information about violence toward children, as well as outcomes for these children. The *National Survey of Child and Adolescent Well-Being* (NSCAW) is a longitudinal study on the well-being of children who have encountered the child welfare system (Office of Planning, Research & Evaluation, 2012). Other important sources of tracking child maltreatment occur in conjunction with *Healthy People 2020*, such as *Youth Risk Behavior Surveillance—United States 2013* (CDC, 2014a; CDC, 2014g; USDHHS, 2016b). The outcomes report describes state-level data and trends, as well as the demographic data of race, age, and ethnicity. Foster care children are also covered in the outcomes report and data. One of the largest investigations ever conducted to assess associations between childhood maltreatment and later-life health and well-being is the Adverse Childhood Experiences Study [ACE]. Study findings suggest certain life experiences are major risk factors leading to illness and death (CDC, 2014b).

Child Neglect

Neglect occurs when the physical, emotional, medical, or educational resources necessary for healthy growth and development are withheld or unavailable. Neglect is obvious to an observer if a very young child is playing unattended outside, is not dressed appropriately for the weather, or has an unkempt appearance. However, neglect is not always so obvious. Parents may refuse to buy eyeglasses for a child who needs them or to access dental care for severely decayed teeth (medical neglect). An 8-year-old may get to school only 3 days a week, possibly without breakfast and no lunch money or packed lunch (educational neglect). A family with three children may live in a sparsely furnished apartment with very little food available and only intermittent heat and multiple people coming and going in the residence, while the children may appear at school unwashed and without coats in winter weather (general neglect). Emotional neglect may be seen when demands placed on a child are excessive or inappropriate for his or her development, or the caretaker berates or verbally humiliates a child frequently and without reason. Thousands of children in the United States experience neglect each day. They are frequently "invisible" victims. At times, sensational stories of severe child neglect are reported in the media and cause public outrage. Examples include 12 children found among piles of garbage in an abandoned apartment building during a drug raid; parents vacationing in Florida while their two daughters, aged 6 and 4, were left unattended at home; or three young children found barely alive, kept in a basement closet. However, most children suffering from neglect do not make newspaper headlines or television reports. They go to school like others, but if a child is fortunate, a school nurse or PHN (or a teacher, neighbor, or counselor) may discover their plight. Because of the invisibility of neglect, its prevalence is hard to estimate. Often, cases of neglect are brought to the attention of the proper authority only during the investigation of other forms of abuse or family issues (Display 20–4) (Fig. 20–2).

Physical Abuse

Physical abuse is intentional harm to a child by another person that results in pain, physical injury, or death. The abuse may include striking, biting, poking, burning, shaking, or throwing the child. Corporal punishment, which involves violence against a child as a form of discipline, was an acceptable form of discipline earlier in our country's history and is still condoned in some subgroups (ACF, 2014). Many parents

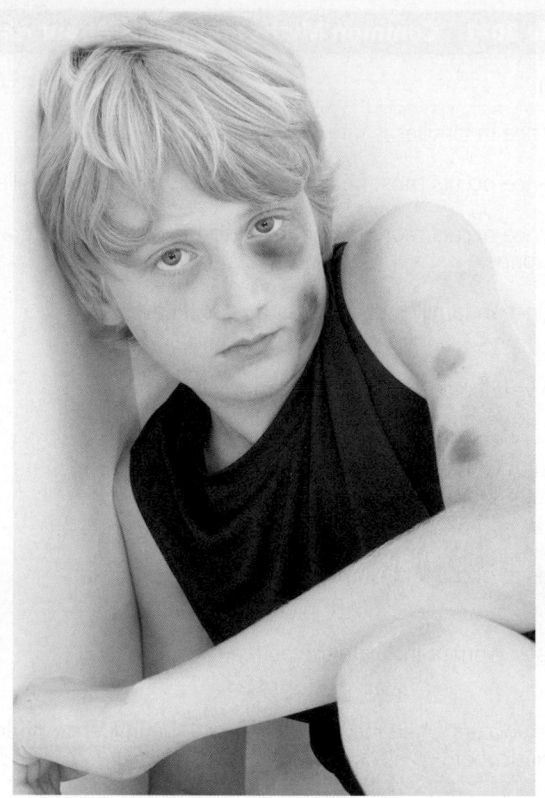

FIGURE 20–2 Young boy with signs of physical abuse.

today were raised in families in which physical punishment was used as a form of discipline. Even today, it is not unusual to see a parent slap the hand of a toddler to get his attention after he has been told not to do something several times or to prevent him from touching something that would hurt him more than a slap on the hand. Most families know where to draw the line. Others—especially if they were raised with "the belt" or "the switch"—see no harm in using the same physical disciplinary practices with their children.

Some parents cannot control the degree of physical punishment they give their child. In one case, a mother repeatedly physically assaulted her young daughter while

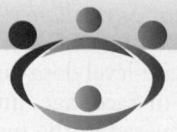

DISPLAY 20–4 SIGNS AND SYMPTOMS OF NEGLECT

Neglect may be suspected if one or more of the following conditions exist:

- The child lacks adequate medical or dental care.
- The child is often sleepy or hungry.
- The child is often dirty, demonstrates poor personal hygiene, or is inadequately dressed for weather conditions.
- There is evidence of poor or inadequate supervision for the child's age.
- The conditions in the home are unsafe or unsanitary.
- The child appears to be malnourished.

- The child is depressed, withdrawn, or apathetic; exhibits antisocial or destructive behavior; shows fearfulness; or suffers from substance abuse or speech, eating, or habit disorders (e.g., biting, rocking, whining).

Adapted from Child Help. (2011). *Speak up be safe prevention education curriculum: Signs and symptoms of child abuse and neglect*. Retrieved from http://www.speakupbesafe.org/parents/warning-signs-of-abuse-and-neglect-for-parents.pdf
New Jersey Department of Children and Families. (n.d.). *Physical and behavioral indicators of child abuse and neglect*. Retrieved from http://www.state.nj.us/dcf/documents/news/publications/Indicators.pdf
Smith, M. A., & Segal, J. (2016). *Child abuse and neglect: Recognizing, preventing, and reporting child abuse*. Retrieved from http://www.helpguide.org/articles/abuse/child-abuse-and-neglect.htm

getting her into the car. The mother's behavior was recorded by the store's parking lot surveillance camera. Intervention and follow-up occurred, including incarceration and counseling for the mother and foster home placement for the child. If physical punishment is administered in anger, while the parent is under the influence of mind-altering substances or out of a sense of frustration, the punishment may cross over to become battering of the child.

C. Henry Kempe identified the **battered child syndrome** in the 1960s as "serious physical abuse" of the child by parents or foster parents (Wolff, 2013, para 4.). This declaration led to a different viewpoint on child abuse as being something that could happen in "average families" and not just those with known psychopathic disorders. Battered child investigations require thorough follow-up and interviews with caretakers, medical personnel, family members, and school personnel. Investigators should be aware that parents often are not able to give credible or even complete explanations for the child's injuries. Severe injuries, like fracture, can be seen on x-rays. Display 20–5 lists behavioral indicators of physical abuse.

Sexual Abuse

Sexual abuse of children includes acts of sexual assault or sexual exploitation of a minor and may consist of a single incident (sexual assault) or many acts over a long period. Sexual abuse is considered to be "exposure of a child to sexual experiences that are inappropriate for his or her level of physical and emotional development, are coercive in nature, and are usually initiated for the purpose of sexual gratification" (Trotman, Young-Anderson, & Deye, in press, p. 1). The abuse usually takes place over some extended time period, and in most cases, the child does not readily disclose the abuse. Sexual assault occurs when there is sexual contact "without consent of the recipient" (Trotman et al., in press, p. 1). It includes rape, gang rape, incest, sodomy, lewd or lascivious acts with a child younger than 14 years of age (in most states), oral copulation, fondling of the child's genitals, penetration of the genital or anal opening by a foreign object, and child molestation. Serious injuries to the child may require trauma care (Abraham, Kondis, & Merritt, 2016). Sexual exploitation of children includes conduct or activities related to pornography that depict minors in sexually explicit situations and promotion of prostitution by minors (U.S. Department of Justice [USDOJ], 2011a). Incest is sexual abuse among family members who are related by blood (e.g., parents, grandparents, older siblings, aunts, and uncles); it constitutes the most hidden form of child abuse. Intrafamilial sexual abuse refers to sexual activity involving family members who are not related by blood (e.g., stepparents, boyfriends). Of the perpetrators who

---

DISPLAY 20–5 SIGNS AND SYMPTOMS OF PHYSICAL ABUSE

Types of Injuries

Types of physical abuse injuries include bruises, burns, bite marks, abrasions, lacerations, head injuries, internal injuries, and fractures.

Behavioral Indicators of Physical Abuse

These behaviors are often exhibited by physically abused children:

- The child is frightened of parents/caretakers or, at the other extreme, is overprotective of parent or caretakers.
- The child is excessively passive, overly compliant, apathetic, withdrawn or fearful, or, at the other extreme, excessively aggressive, destructive, or physically violent.
- The child and/or parent or caretaker attempts to hide injuries; child wears excessive layers of clothing, especially in hot weather; child is frequently absent from school or misses physical education classes if changing into gym clothes is required; child has difficulty sitting or walking.
- The child is frightened of going home.
- The child is clingy and forms indiscriminate attachments.
- The child is apprehensive when other children cry.
- The child is wary of physical contact with adults.
- The child exhibits drastic behavioral changes in and out of parental/caretaker presence.
- The child is hypervigilant.

- The child suffers from seizures or vomiting.
- The adolescent exhibits depression, self-mutilation, suicide attempts, substance abuse, or sleeping and eating disorders.

Other indicators of physical abuse may include the following:

- A statement by the child that the injury was caused by abuse (chronically abused children may deny abuse)
- Knowledge that the child's injury is unusual for the child's specific age group (e.g., any fracture in an infant)
- Knowledge of the child's history of previous or recurrent injuries
- Unexplained injuries (e.g., parent is unable to explain reason for injury; there are discrepancies in explanations; blame is placed on a third party; explanations are inconsistent with medical diagnosis)
- A parent or caretaker who delays seeking or fails to seek medical care for the child's injury

Adapted from Child Help. (2011). *Speak up be safe prevention education curriculum: Signs and symptoms of child abuse and neglect*. Retrieved from http://www.speakupbesafe.org/parents/warning-signs-of-abuse-and-neglect-for-parents.pdf
New Jersey Department of Children and Families. (n.d.). *Physical and behavioral indicators of child abuse and neglect*. Retrieved from http://www.state.nj.us/dcf/documents/news/publications/Indicators.pdf
Smith, M. A., & Segal, J. (2016). *Child abuse and neglect: Recognizing, preventing, and reporting child abuse*. Retrieved from http://www.helpguide.org/articles/abuse/child-abuse-and-neglect.htm

sexually abused their victims, 87.8% were men. The largest relationship category was the parent (91.4%), which reflects the perpetrator could have been a parent to multiple victims. Of the parental relationships, 88.6% were the biological parent, 3.7% the stepparents, and 0.6% were adoptive parents. The age range of the perpetrator was between 6 and 75, with 63.3% being between the ages of 25 and 44, 19.2% between ages of 18 and 24, and 13.1% between ages 45 and 75. Only 2.3% were between ages 6 and 17 (ACF, 2013a). Initial sexual abuse may occur at any age, from infancy through adolescence. However, the largest number of cases involves girls younger than 11 years of age. Regardless of how gentle, trivial, or coincidental the first approach may have seemed, sexual coercion tends to be repeated and to escalate over a period of years. The child may blame himself or herself for tempting or provoking the abuser. Often, the abuser threatens the child or the child's parents in order to assure silence (Trotman et al., in press).

The mother, who is expected to protect the child, may purposely isolate herself from a problem of sexual abuse. Sometimes, the mother is distant, uncommunicative, or so disapproving of sexual matters that the child is afraid to speak up. Sometimes, she is extremely insecure and feels confrontation may cause anger or the loss of her husband or boyfriend, or the mother's economic security may depend on her partner/spouse. The mother may feel threatened or feel that she cannot allow herself to believe or even to suspect that her child is at risk. She may have been a victim herself of child abuse and may not trust her judgment or her right to challenge the man's authority in the home. Some mothers consciously acknowledge that their children are being sexually abused but, for whatever reason, choose to "look the other way." In some cases, families may not permit the child to admit the assault and cooperate with authorities (Trotman et al., in press). Until the victim is old enough to realize that incest or intrafamilial sexual abuse is not a common occurrence, or is strong enough to obtain help outside the family, there is little chance of escape unless the abuse is reported (Townsend & Rheingold, 2013).

Indicators of sexual abuse are seen in various ways, and attention should be given to a history of sexual abuse, sexual behavior indicators, behavioral indicators in younger children and behavioral indicators of sexual abuse in older children and adolescents, and physical symptoms of sexual abuse (see Display 20–6). As mandated reporters, community health nurses should be aware that sexual abuse of a child may surface through a broad range of physical, behavioral, and social symptoms. Some of these indicators, taken separately, may not be symptomatic of sexual abuse and should be examined in the context of other behaviors or situational factors. See Perspectives.

Community health nurses may be part of the Sexual Assault Response Team (SART). This group's responsibilities include obtaining the evidence and providing support to the victim and family after an episode of sexual abuse has been reported. SART members include nurses, physicians, social workers, police, laboratory personnel, lawyers, and district attorney staff (Moylan, Lindhorst, & Tajima, 2015). Care for children who have been

sexually abused varies, as the duration of the molestation, the age, and symptoms of the child will influence their care measures. Besides the physical trauma, children suffer mentally and emotionally. They have an increased risk for posttraumatic stress disorder (PTSD), major depressive disorder, anxiety, loss of self-esteem, thoughts of suicide, and substance abuse or eating disorders. Some victims of child sexual assault and abuse have early sexual intercourse and pregnancy, as well as a higher risk of later sexual victimization (Trotman et al., in press). Parents may also need counseling and support following the investigation and proceedings involving their child's victimization. Family therapy is often beneficial.

The sexual assault nurse examiner's (SANE) role is more explicit in assisting the victim and appropriate family members immediately after the victim presents to the police or to an emergency department setting. The nurse has very specific actions to take to promote trust, obtain needed specimen evidence, and treat the sexual abuse victim. The victim has already been significantly traumatized, and the nurse can be effective in this role only if trust can be established during this critical time after the sexual assault. The SANE is trained to work with victims of all ages, both genders, and under all sexual abuse situations; some specialize in pediatric populations (Trotman et al., in press).

The majority of those committing ongoing sexual abuse and assault against children are relatives, in fact, about 80% of child sexual assaults are committed by someone known to the child (Rape, Abuse, & Incest National Network, 2013). Pedophiles present a danger. A pedophile is an adult whose main sexual interest is a child and tends to be well liked by children. Pedophiles, who most often are men, frequently choose to work in professions or volunteer organizations that allow them easy access to children, where they can develop the trust and respect of children and their parents. The pedophile believes that sex with children is appropriate and often lures children into sexual relationships with love, rewards, promises, and gifts. He may be among a child's family members (e.g., grandfather, father, uncle, cousin) or a trusted community leader the child knows (e.g., next-door neighbor, teacher, coach, or religious leader). Reports of pedophiles among clergy in the Roman Catholic Church have affected the church, its clergy, and its members. The National Sex Offender Public Registry, sponsored through the Department of Justice, is used in all 50 states thereby improving efforts to safeguard all children. This resource provides information regarding the more than 500,000 registered sex offenders throughout the United States (USDOJ, n.d.).

Human trafficking of children on a national and international scale is recognized by the United States in the Trafficking Victims Protection Act (TVPA) of 2000. This federal law defined human trafficking as the recruitment, harboring, transportation, provision, or obtaining of a person for compelled labor or commercial sex or for labor or services through the use of force, fraud, or coercion (ACF, 2015). The law specifically identified any child <18 years who engaged in commercial sex as a victim of trafficking (ACF, 2015). The USDHHS established a National Human Trafficking Resource Center

DISPLAY 20-6 INDICATORS OF SEXUAL ABUSE

I. History of Sexual Abuse

- A child confides to a friend, a classmate, a teacher, a friend's mother, or other trusted adult that she/he has experienced sexual abuse.
- A child may disclose information indirectly by such statements as:
  "I know someone …"
  "What would you do if … ?"
  "I heard something about somebody…"
- The child has torn, stained, or bloody underclothing (among her/his clothing or is wearing it).
- Knowledge that a child's injury/disease (vaginal trauma, sexually transmitted disease) is unusual for the specific age group.
- Unexplained injuries/diseases (parent/caretaker unable to explain reason for injury/disease); there are discrepancies in explanation; blame is placed on a third party; explanations are inconsistent with medical diagnosis.
- A very young girl is pregnant or has a sexually transmitted disease. Pregnancy alone does not constitute sexual abuse, but if there are indications of coercion or significant age disparity between the minor and her partner, this may lead to reasonable suspicion of sexual abuse that must be reported.

II. Sexual Behavioral Indicators of Sexually Abused Children

- Detailed and age-inappropriate understanding of sexual behavior (especially among very young children)
- Sexually explicit language
- Inappropriate, unusual, or aggressive sexual behavior with peers or toys
- Compulsive indiscreet masturbation
- Excessive curiosity about sexual matters or genitalia (self or others)
- Unusually seductive or flirtatious behavior with classmates, teachers, and other adults
- Excessive concern about homosexuality, especially by boys

III. Behavioral Indicators of Sexual Abuse in Younger Children

- Enuresis (wetting pants or bedwetting)
- Fecal soiling
- Eating disturbances such as overeating or undereating
- Fears or phobias
- Overly compulsive behavior
- School problems or significant change in school performance (attitude and grades)
- Age-inappropriate behavior that includes pseudo-maturity or regressive behavior such as bedwetting or thumb sucking
- Inability to concentrate
- Sleeping disturbances (nightmares, fear of falling asleep, fretful sleep pattern, sleeping long hours)
- Drastic behavior changes

- Speech disorders
- Frightened of parents/caretaker or of going home or being at home

IV. Behavioral Indicators of Sexual Abuse in Older Children and Adolescents

- Withdrawal
- Chronic fatigue
- Clinical depression, apathy
- Overly compliant behavior
- Over- or underreaction (hysteria or cavalier attitude) to a genital exam
- Poor hygiene or excessive bathing
- Poor peer relations and social skills; inability to make friends
- Acting out; running away; aggressive, antisocial, or delinquent behavior
- Alcohol or drug abuse
- Prostitution or excessive promiscuity
- School problems, frequent absences, sudden drop in school performance
- Refusal to change clothes for physical education class
- Nonparticipation in sports and social activities
- Fearful of showers or restrooms
- Fearful of home life as demonstrated by arriving at school early and leaving late
- Suddenly fearful of other things (going outside or participating in familiar activities)
- Extraordinary fear of males (in cases of male perpetrator and female victim)
- Self-consciousness of body beyond that expected for age
- Sudden acquisition of money, new clothes, or gifts with no reasonable explanation
- Suicide attempt or other self-destructive behavior
- Crying without provocation
- Setting fires

V. Physical Symptoms of Sexual Abuse

- Sexually transmitted diseases, especially in prepubescent girls
- Genital discharge or infection
- Physical trauma or irritation to the anal/genital area (pain, itching, swelling, bruising, bleeding, lacerations, abrasions), especially if injuries are unexplained or there is an inconsistent explanation
- Pain during urination or defecation
- Difficulty in walking or sitting due to genital or anal pain
- Psychosomatic symptoms (stomach aches, headaches, chronic pain)

Adapted from Child Help. (2011). *Speak up be safe prevention education curriculum: Signs and symptoms of child abuse and neglect*. Retrieved from http://www.speakupbesafe.org/parents/warning-signs-of-abuse-and-neglect-for-parents.pdf
New Jersey Department of Children and Families. (n.d.). *Physical and behavioral indicators of child abuse and neglect*. Retrieved from http://www.state.nj.us/dcf/documents/news/publications/Indicators.pdf
Smith, M. A., & Segal, J. (2016). *Child abuse and neglect: Recognizing, preventing, and reporting child abuse*. Retrieved from http://www.helpguide.org/articles/abuse/child-abuse-and-neglect.htm

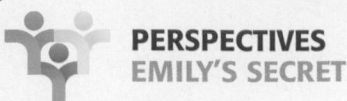

PERSPECTIVES
EMILY'S SECRET

I am a school nurse in a small town. I am assigned to a large school with 1,000 children; this includes every child in town who is in grades K-3, and this is not my only assigned school. I have a busy school nurse office, but I try to be observant to subtle cues. Sadly, sometimes it is so busy that I miss things. Emily, a third grader, had been coming into my office with stomachaches and vague complaints off and on for several months. Thinking back, this usually happened within the last hour of school. After school, she walked to her aunt's house (her mother's sister) and stayed there for a few hours until her mother came to pick her up when she finished working. Emily was a petite child, very quiet, and well behaved, and she usually only responded with a few words in reply to my questions about her ailments. She came in one day with another stomachache and wanted to lie down. I had several children in my office, and when I was free, I asked her what was going on. She shrugged her shoulders and didn't really respond. The final bell rung, and I told her that if she didn't feel well enough to walk home I could call her aunt. She just seemed to really be avoiding having to go to her aunt's house; she wanted me to call her mom at work. The aunt was the emergency contact, so the procedure was to start there. I had a feeling that something was wrong. I had recently attended a workshop on child sexual abuse and remembered that sometimes the hardest thing was to break through the guilt and shame in order for the child to open up to you. I told her that she "could tell me anything, and I wouldn't think that she was bad". She knew I was there to help her, and she began talking. In fact, it was like "verbal vomiting"— the words just came spilling out of her mouth. Her uncle had been "touching her" and she "didn't want to go back there." She began crying and I told her we would call her mom and someone from CPS to help her. I sent someone to get her teacher, a woman with whom she felt comfortable and safe. I stayed with Emily through the lengthy process.

Later, as I thought about the constant stream of children coming into my office everyday, I wondered how many of those kids with subtle, vague complaints might have something they need help with that is as serious as Emily's secret. I try to be even more vigilant and open to their concerns—whatever they may be.

Josie, School Nurse

(2015), which operates a 24-hour crisis line in over 200 languages at 1.888.373.8888.

Emotional Abuse

Emotional abuse of children involves psychological mistreatment or neglect, such as when parents do not provide the normal experiences that produce feelings of being loved, wanted, secure, and worthy (Rodner, 2015), and can be exhibited by insults, belittling, constant humiliation, intimidation, or threats of harm (WHO, 2014). This type of abuse is commonly associated with other types of abuse and may involve verbal abuse, such as name calling, or threatening. A mother may shout at the child, "You're just like your father, a good-for-nothing, lazy bum." A father may say, "You're ugly. You look just like your mother." If the child spills some juice, a parent may scream, "Everything you do is wrong. Can't you do anything right?"

Emotional abuse may also take the form of emotional abandonment. Some parents "shun" their children as a form of punishment. They will not speak to them and do not look at them; they behave as if their child does not exist. This behavior may continue for a day or more, whenever a child displeases the parent. In some cases, the shunning lasts for days.

Verbal threats, although a common discipline practice, are also a form of emotional abuse. Examples of verbal threats include "Take your feet off the furniture or I'll chop your feet off" and "Do that again, and you'll really know what my belt feels like." In the first instance, the child might realize that the parent wouldn't really chop her feet off, but hearing the parent say such a violent thing can be emotionally upsetting. In the second instance, the parent may have beaten the child with a belt in the past, so merely threatening to use the belt again causes emotional trauma. Parental acceptance and rejection have been studied by researchers in the United States and internationally with evidence of empirical cross-cultural generalizations, antecedents, and consequences of undifferentiated rejection. Indifference is an internal psychological feeling or the physical and psychological nonavailability of the parent that is one indicator of emotional abuse (Rodner, 2015).

Emotional abuse alone is rarely reported because it is another "hidden" form of abuse. However, **mandated reporters**, people who have a responsibility for the welfare of children and include public and private school employees; administrators and employees of youth centers and recreation programs; child welfare employees; foster parents; group home and residential facility personnel; social workers; probation workers; health care workers including nurses, doctors, and chiropractors; animal control workers; and personnel working in film development laboratories are required by law to report *suspected* cases of severe emotional neglect or abuse or deprivation in addition to *suspected* neglect and physical or sexual abuse (Child Welfare Information Gateway, 2014). See Display 20–7.

Specific Abusive Situations

The previous information addressed the major types of child abuse in families, yet other patterns of abuse against children need to be discussed. Shaken baby syndrome, Munchausen syndrome by proxy, and maternal filicide defined as a child murdered by the mother are fairly rare, but by the time the symptoms are recognized, it is often too late, with the diagnosis made during subsequent visits to the emergency department or at autopsy.

In addition, Internet crimes against children, child abduction, and crimes against children by babysitters are an increasingly common fear of parents. These types of abuse are occurring more often as children and adolescents have increased time and access to computers and because both parents (or a single parent) must work,

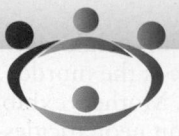

DISPLAY 20-7 SIGNS AND SYMPTOMS OF EMOTIONAL ABUSE OR DEPRIVATION

Emotional abuse should be suspected if the child displays the following behavioral indicators:

- Is withdrawn, depressed, or apathetic
- Is clingy and forms indiscriminate attachments
- "Acts out" and is considered a behavior problem
- Exhibits exaggerated fearfulness
- Is overly rigid in conforming to instructions of teachers, doctors, and other adults
- Suffers from sleep, speech, or eating disorders
- Displays signs of emotional turmoil that include repetitive, rhythmic movements (rocking, whining, picking at scabs)
- Pays inordinate attention to details or exhibits little or no verbal or physical communication with others
- Suffers from enuresis and fecal soiling
- Unwittingly makes comments such as "Mommy always tells me I'm bad"
- Experiences substance abuse problems

Emotional deprivation should be suspected if the child:

- Refuses to eat adequate amounts of food and therefore is very frail
- Is unable to perform normal learned functions for a given age (e.g., walking, talking)
- Displays antisocial behavior (aggression, disruption) or obvious delinquent behavior (drug abuse, vandalism); conversely, the child may be abnormally unresponsive, sad, or withdrawn
- Constantly "seeks out" and "pesters" other adults such as teachers or neighbors for attention and affection
- Displays exaggerated fears

Adapted from Child Help. (2011). *Speak up be safe prevention education curriculum: Signs and symptoms of child abuse and neglect.* Retrieved from http://www.speakupbesafe.org/parents/warning-signs-of-abuse-and-neglect-for-parents.pdf
New Jersey Department of Children and Families. (n.d.). *Physical and behavioral indicators of child abuse and neglect.* Retrieved from http://www.state.nj.us/dcf/documents/news/publications/Indicators.pdf
Smith, M. A., & Segal, J. (2016). *Child abuse and neglect: Recognizing, preventing, and reporting child abuse.* Retrieved from http://www.helpguide.org/articles/abuse/child-abuse-and-neglect.htm

---

while children are spending more time alone or with babysitters. Community concern regarding child abductions by family members or strangers has resulted in the institution of *Amber Alert* systems in many states. School violence is also an area of increasing concern for families and will be addressed.

Shaken Baby Syndrome

Abusive head trauma (AHT) sometimes called **shaken baby syndrome** is the intentional abusive action of violently shaking an infant or toddler, usually a child of 2 years or younger (American Academy of Pediatrics [AAP], 2015). The type of damage that occurs to these infants very seldom occurs through play, as in minor falls or as a result of tossing a baby in the air. The classic medical symptoms associated with infant shaking are bilateral retinal hemorrhage, subdural or subarachnoid hematomas, absence of other external signs of abuse, and symptoms that may include breathing difficulties, seizures, dilated pupils, lethargy, and unconsciousness (Parks, Kegler, Annest, & Mercy, 2012; Parks, Sugerman, Xu, & Coronado, 2012). These injuries occur from a violent, sustained action in which the infant's head, which lacks muscular control, is violently whipped forward and backward, hitting the chest and shoulders. According to experts, an observer would describe the shaking as being "as hard as the shaker was humanly capable of shaking the baby" or "hard enough that it appeared the baby's head would come off." AHT includes violent shaking, but also blunt trauma to the head (Allen, 2014). Within minutes to hours after the injury, the baby begins to show symptoms such as irritability, lethargy, vomiting, breathing problems, seizures, or unconsciousness. A typical explanation given by the parents or caretakers is that the baby was "fine" and then suddenly went into respiratory arrest or began having seizures—both common symptoms of shaken

baby syndrome. Children who survive shaken baby syndrome may require lifelong care if they endure the AHT. Approximately 30 per 100,000 children younger than 1 year of age are injured from AHT, resulting in at least 1,200 seriously injured infants and approximately 80 deaths each year (AAP, 2015).

Munchausen Syndrome by Proxy

The term *Munchausen syndrome* was first used to describe illnesses or symptoms that were provided or simulated by patients themselves and "is a diagnosis applied to parents and other caregivers who intentionally feign, exaggerate, and/or induce illness or injury in a child to get attention from health professionals and others" (Frye & Feldman, 2012, p. 47). Clients with this disorder may intentionally injure him/herself or induce illness in him/herself. *Munchausen syndrome by proxy* is a form of child abuse played out in the medical setting (Gilbert, 2014). In such cases, a parent or caretaker attempts to bring medical attention to self by injuring or inducing illness in his or her child. About 85% to 98% of those perpetrating this are biological mothers of the child, who often form close bonds with health care providers. A majority of these abusers have some type of mental health illness (e.g., borderline personality disorders) or history of abuse in their own childhood (e.g., sexual abuse, child maltreatment, witness to IPV, family mental illness). Although less common than mothers, fathers can also be perpetrators, and often fathers are characterized as emotionally uninvolved or distant from their families and may appear overbearing and demanding to health care providers (Gilbert, 2014). The following scenarios can be typical of these cases:

- The child's parent or caretaker brings the child to the emergency department or calls paramedics repeatedly for alleged problems that have no medical basis.

- The child experiences "seizures" or "respiratory arrest" only when the parent or caretaker is present—never in the presence of a neutral third party or when hospitalized, unless the parent or caretaker reports that the incident occurred in his or her presence alone.
- While the child is hospitalized, the parent or caretaker shuts off intravenous tubes or life-support equipment, causing the child distress, and then turns everything back on and summons help.
- The parent or caretaker induces illness by introducing a mild irritant or poison into the child's body; chronic ingestion of such substances may cause the child's death.
- The child may have many school absences and a complicated medical history according to the child's mother or father who may seem overinvolved or demanding.

Health providers, mental health professionals, and attorneys may be involved in working with such cases, requiring careful attention to the history of the illness/injury, the treatment, documentation, and communication with the parent/caretaker. Allegations of *Munchausen syndrome by proxy* should be investigated by interprofessional teams that may include nurses working with children in community settings such as schools and home health care (Cabral, 2014; Gilbert, 2014; Grace & Jagannathan, 2015). Although the parent may remove the child from care or take the child to another facility or school district if the caregiver's suspicions are aroused, attention to the child's safety is paramount, and a protective order may be considered.

Child Murder by Mother or Father

A rare, yet concerning type of child death is known as *filicide*, defined as child murder by the parent (Debowska, Boduszek, & Dhingra, 2015). The parent or stepparent is frequently the perpetrator when a young child is murdered; maternal filicide is known to occur in all areas of the world. A parent was the perpetrator in the majority of homicides of children under the age of 5, with 33% being killed by their fathers and 30% being killed by their mothers (USDOJ, 2011b). In the United States, the child homicide rate is 7.2 deaths per 100,000 infants under the age of 5. Infants are most likely to be killed by their mother during the first week of life, but thereafter are more likely to be killed by a male (Child Trends Data Bank, 2015). Research indicates five common motives when a parent murders their child. An *altruistic filicide* is defined as a situation when the parent kills a child out of love, in the belief that the child's life or fate is worse than death; the parent may then commit suicide. A second motive that may occur is an *acute psychotic filicide* wherein the mother or father may suffer from delirium or psychosis and murder her or his child as a result of an unstable mental disorder. A third, and the most common, motive is *fatal maltreatment or accidental filicide* is a situation in which the child's death is an unintentional result from repeated abuse or Munchausen syndrome by proxy. *Unwanted child filicide* occurs when the child is unwanted and the parent feels the child is a hindrance. The fifth and most rare motive is a *spouse revenge filicide* when one parent murders the child as revenge toward the other parent, sometimes as a result of adultery (Debowska et al., 2015).

Infanticide is defined as the murder of a child during the first year of life, whereas **neonaticide** is the murder of an infant within the first 24 hours of life. Mothers exhibiting specific risk factors most often commit neonaticides—they are frequently adolescent, unmarried woman with an unwanted pregnancy, and who have received no prenatal care. One consistent feature is often denial about the pregnancy, even as labor begins. The newborn is frequently "disposed of" by "flushing down the toilet, drowning in the toilet or a tub, smashing the head with an object, stabbing....or suffocating" (Malmquist, 2013, p. 402). In the United States, these cases are often handled as homicides, but in other countries, there are specific legal provisions recognizing the physiological changes during birth and the postpartum period that can affect mental capacity and distinguish infanticides from homicides. The United States has provided "safe haven" statutes to encourage desperate mothers to leave their unwanted babies in a safe place, but has not followed suit with other countries regarding alternatives to homicide charges (Malmquist, 2013).

In a recent study, infanticide in the United States was found to be associated with economic stress. Other risk characteristics for maternal filicide include a mother who was (a) socially isolated, (b) poor, (c) acted as a full-time caregiver, and (d) often had a history of domestic violence or relationship problems. Neglectful or abusive mothers were often substance abusers, while the majority of perpetrators exhibited psychosis, depression, or suicidality (Debowska et al., 2015). The rate for infanticide in this country is estimated at 6.0 homicides per 100,000 and is similar to the adult homicide rate (Malmquist, 2013). Measures for prevention and support to mothers include parenting classes, emotional support, providing emergency numbers for support, as well as treating maternal substance abuse. See From the Case Files I for two examples of neonaticide.

Internet Crimes Against Children

Communication technologies provide novel opportunities to pursue, monitor or harass other people (Drebing, Bailer, Anders, Wagner, & Gallas, 2014). Internet crimes are insidious because they come right into the home. Children either unintentionally or intentionally may access an Internet chat room or Web site developed or used by pedophiles. The perpetrator establishes contact, usually passing himself off as a teen or young man who has similar interests, and states affection for and understanding of the youth's "problems." Eventually, the pedophile either sets up a meeting time and place or engages in sexually explicit dialogue with the minor. Many minors find the attention from this stranger inviting or exciting and make plans to meet the person. When this happens, the minor falls victim to this individual, putting the child/adolescent at great risk. This computer-based child abuse risk has led the U.S. Attorney General to authorize a federal awareness and justice program focusing solely on technology-facilitated sexual exploitation and abuse against children, named *Project Safe Childhood* (USDOJ, 2014) (Fig. 20–3).

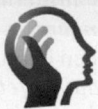

From the Case Files I

Neonaticide

Case #1: A 17-year-old honor student recognized that she was pregnant, but chose not to tell her parents, friends, or her boyfriend. She kept her pregnancy quiet by wearing loose clothing and complaining that she had "gained weight" over Christmas holidays. Home alone, after school, she went into labor while sitting on the toilet. She stretched out on the bathroom floor and labored for several hours with significant blood loss. She delivered her newborn and used scissors to cut the umbilical cord. She was afraid because she had not stopped bleeding. Blood was everywhere, and she got the keys to the car and drove herself to the local hospital. On the way, she felt dizzy and seemed to pass out. Coming to, she continued to drive to the ER. Upon admission, she was treated to control the hemorrhaging. Later, an ER nurse asked about the newborn baby, and the girl said "I left it; it's on the bathroom floor." Police located the dead newborn as described, but no formal charges were ever filed.

Case #2: A 16-year-old girl, having sex with her boyfriend, became pregnant. But, she thought she was just having stomach and GI problems, so she went with her mother to see her pediatrician. He prescribed medication for her symptoms, but she got no relief. Using an over-the-counter pregnancy test, she got a negative result. Her friend encouraged her to go to the walk-in clinic and get another test, but this one was inconclusive and she was now spotting, so she continued to take her birth control pills, thinking she was not pregnant. A few months later, at a family backyard barbeque, she felt like she is getting the "stomach flu" and told her mother she was going to rest in bed. She tried to have a bowel movement, but couldn't. Eventually, she thought she might be in labor and lay down on the floor of the bathroom. To her shock and horror, she gave birth and quickly stabbed the infant and hid it in a trash bin. When the body was discovered, and a court psychiatrist later examined her, she described "watching the birth and the stabbing from a vantage point above her body." Her defense was limited to testimony about whether or not she noticed the baby's fingers moving and trying to counter the pathologist's findings that the lungs had inflated. Her attorney couldn't bring up issues surrounding her pregnancy and *neonaticidal syndrome*. The jury found her guilty of murder, and she was sentenced to prison for a life term.

What are your thoughts about the two cases? Have you seen examples like these in your local or regional newspapers or Web news sources? What preventive programs and policies might be helpful in addressing this issue? Are there EBP population-focused interventions available to address this problem?

Adapted from Malmquist, C. (2013). Infanticide/neonaticide: The outlier situation in the United States. Aggression and Violent Behavior, 18, 399–408.

Community health nurses can assist families to prevent such Internet crimes in various ways by:

- Urging parents to openly discuss with their children the dangers of online "friendships" that seek face-to-face meetings; downloading photos or uploading/posting photos to people they do not really know; giving information that identifies them (name, phone number, school they attend, home address); and responding to e-mails, messages, or tweets that are suggestive or harassing, being aware of phishing and other forms of attempted identity theft
- Establishing parent–child contracts for Internet and smartphone use
- Blocking or only permitting specific phone numbers for smartphone calls and regularly checking for deleted phone calls and texts
- Monitoring the time and Internet sites a child uses (check log of every site accessed on the computer); also the apps on their smartphones
- Keeping the computer in a high-traffic area in the home, affording easy observation of the computer monitor
- Using available parental controls or blocking software
- Installing a firewall, antivirus, and antiadware/spyware programs that increase privacy
- Discouraging downloading of apps, games, and other media that might contain Trojan or worm programs that enable remote access by unauthorized users
- Having access to their child's e-mail and other accounts; randomly checking e-mails and text messages
- Being aware of safeguards in place at their child's school, public areas your child frequents, and homes of their friends (Federal Bureau of Investigation [FBI], n.d.).

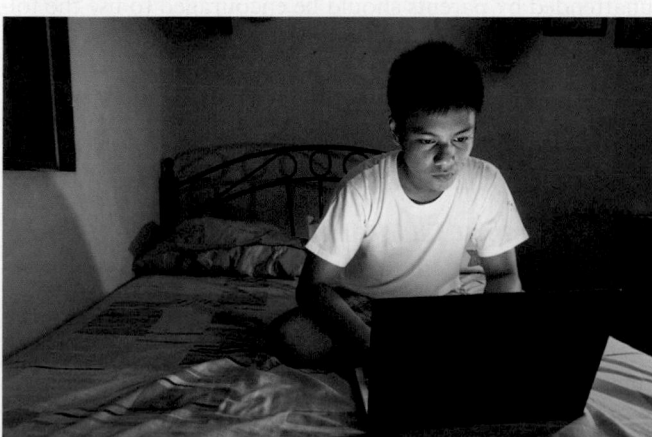

FIGURE 20–3 Children and youth can be victims of Internet crimes.

There is a constant stream of news around cyberbullying and cyberstalking incidents. Cyberstalking has been defined "as the repeated pursuit of an individual using electronic or Internet-capable devices" (Drebing et al., 2014, p. 61). Thirty-three percent of teenagers report that they have been victims of cyberbullying, and 20.8% of kids between the ages of eight and ten report that they have been cyberbullied at least once in their life (Woda, 2015). Effects of cyberbullying can be more far-reaching than those of traditional schoolyard bullying but is often easier to deal with because there is an electronic trail that provides proof to show parents, teachers, and/or even police. As a nurse, make sure families are prepared to identify and appropriately handle cyberbullying, sexting, and threats from online predators. The rule of three is to ignore, save, and report (Woda, 2015).

Furthermore, parents can contact the Cyber Tip Line at (800) 843-5678 or access the Web site (www.cyber-tipline.com) if they suspect that an online predator has contacted their child (National Center for Missing and Exploited Children, 2015).

Child Abduction

Child abduction is a crime that every parent fears, and although stranger abduction happens infrequently, it remains the greatest fear for parents. However, intense media coverage gives the impression that such crimes occur frequently, and this causes great stress among parents and community members. Nationally, the Amber Alert program and the Child Abduction Response Teams (CART) were established to provide a prompt and professional response to child abduction. Amber Alerts are now being sent through the Wireless Emergency Alerts (WEA) program to millions of cell phone users. The goal of the Amber Alert is to provide instant collaboration and partnership in the community to assist in the search and safe recovery of the child (USDOJ, 2013a).

Child abduction by family members or intimate partners, such as a divorced mother, father, stepparent, boyfriend, or grandparents, is more common. Nonetheless, the parent from whom the child was taken may be unaware that the abduction was by a relative or known person and may experience the same type of stress and loss as parents who lose a child by stranger abduction. In some cases, knowing the relative or person who abducted the child causes just as much fear because the abductor may have a history of violence or sexual abuse crimes.

Prevention of child abduction is difficult, and at times, parents who think they have taught their children well may have a false sense of security. Some studies assessed the effects on children of taking a "stranger awareness" class. The class included lessons on avoiding strangers, not talking to strangers, identifying who is a stranger, saying "no" to strangers, and running away and screaming if addressed by a stranger. Yet, researchers found that when the children left the classroom, if an unknown person (a stranger sent in by the researcher) asked the child to help him find a lost puppy or go help them get candy, many of the children responded readily without using any of the actions learned in the stranger awareness class. Parents who watched their children on tapes of these studies could not believe what they saw.

Children are trusting and curious, and they may not consider people who look like their parents as *strangers*.

More encompassing skills programs have been evaluated and found to be effective. *Kidpower Everyday Safety Skills Program* was tested with 128 third-graders using school-based workshops and weekly follow-up exercises, as well as homework assignments and parental involvement (Brenick, Shattuck, Donlan, Duh, & Zurbriggen, 2014). Researchers found that those third-grade students that participated, when compared to students in a control group, had increased safety knowledge at posttest and 3 months after the intervention ended. The children learned about stranger safety, but also boundary setting, help seeking, and maintaining confidence and calmness.

Community health nurses can help parents improve their child's safety by promoting close supervision of young children and practicing behaviors that promote anonymity. Ideas that help improve the child's safety include the following:

- Keeping the child in the seat of a shopping cart and holding the child's hand while in malls or stores
- Keeping a young child in sight at all times when playing outside
- Sharing parental supervision with another mother when children play, so that an adult is always supervising the children
- Not putting the child's name or initials on clothing or backpacks
- Teaching the child a "password" that only the parents and child know to use when a different person is picking them up from a neighborhood activity
- Teaching children to recognize when they feel unsafe and get help
- Making safety plans with children and having them practice getting help
- Helping children understand the different circumstances when it is OK to give out personal information (at school, MD office, lost in a store), and when it is not (stranger they don't know)
- Practicing with children about when to "think first" before they talk to a stranger and to keep walking (Kidpower, 2016, para. 8)

Older children and teens who go outside the home unattended by parents should be encouraged to use the following behaviors that promote safety: staying with groups of other children or teens, having a cell phone, leaving an itinerary with the parents, and not changing their plans without contacting parents. Other measures that can benefit older children and adolescents are attending a self-defense class and carrying a whistle and/or pepper spray.

Crimes Against Children by Babysitters

Crimes against infants and young children by babysitters have been reported in the media (Johnston, 2013). Some parents who have suspected mistreatment of their children by caretakers have used hidden cameras to reveal the problem. Abuse by caretakers is a fear of parents who work and leave their children with others.

The community health nurse can help parents assess day care settings by providing them descriptors for finding good day care providers. Parents who use neighbors as babysitters should get references and should drop by the home or day care setting at various times during the day. They should assess their infants and follow up on any bruises, rashes, burns, conditions, or behaviors they observe that are not normal for their child. With older children, parents need to listen to them and ask about their day and activities. Parents must not ignore signs, such as a child's fear of going to the babysitter or reports of spankings, being shouted at, or other inappropriate treatment. Day care centers and many home day care programs are licensed by the state. Programs for which parent complaints have been filed with licensing agencies are monitored more closely, and the state is mandated to make changes or close the facility if necessary. Parents need to know that their child is safe and cared for when they leave them to pursue their employment or educational activities.

School Violence

An area of growing concern regarding violence against children has been in school settings. Violence in schools may range from bullying, slapping, or punching to weapon use (CDC, 2015g). Random shootings and hostage situations in schools over the past decades have fueled fears about the safety of students and promoted research into how to prevent this type of community violence affecting children. Bullying is defined as "any unwanted aggressive behavior (s) by another youth or group of youths, who are not siblings or current dating partners, involving an observed or perceived power imbalance and is repeated multiple times or is highly likely to be repeated" (CDC, 2015a, p. 1). Bullying can be verbal, social, or physical or happening via Internet, text, or e-mail (cyberbullying). The child that is at high risk to get bullied may have delayed puberty, be gender nonconforming, have unique physical appearance, or be socially rejected and isolated (Simms, Bushman, & Pederson, 2016). Gay, lesbian, bisexual, and transgender youth were more likely than were heterosexual youth to report high levels of bullying (CDC, 2014c). There is evidence that bullying and violence are linked (Simms et al., 2016).

The Youth Risk Behavior Survey collects information about health and prevention issues of adolescents. Included in the survey are questions about violence risks such as fighting, use of illegal drugs, carrying a weapon, and being threatened or injured with a weapon on school property. In 2013, of a national representative sample of youth in grades 9 to 12, 8.1% of the children reported being in a physical fight on school property in the 12 months before the survey, 19.6% reported being bullied on school property and 14.8% reported being bullied electronically, 7.1% reported feeling unsafe at school or on their way to and from school, 5.2% reported carrying a weapon on school property in the 30 days before the survey, and 6.9% reported being threatened or injured with a weapon on school property (CDC, 2015h). School violence has immediate and long-term effects on students demonstrated by an increase in depression, anxiety, psychological problems, and fear (CDC, 2015g). See Chapter 22 for more on school-aged children and adolescents.

The U.S. Department of Education, Department of Health and Human Services, and Department of Justice have collaborated to provide funding, programs, and trainings that improve school safety through the *Safe Schools Healthy Students* initiative. Six areas identified for attention in building safe school climates are

- Creating a safe school environment
- Providing alcohol, drug, and violence prevention and early intervention programs
- Supporting school and community mental health prevention and treatment intervention services
- Providing early childhood psychosocial and emotional development programs
- Addressing education reform
- Designing safe school policies (Safe Schools Healthy Students Initiative, 2016)

Risk factors surrounding youth violence can be categorized as individual risks, relationship risks, and/or community/societal risks. Individual risks for perpetrating youth violence may include a history of violent victimization; a history of early aggressive behaviors, attention deficit, hyperactivity, or learning disorders; an association with delinquent peers; gang involvement; high emotional distress; social rejection; family violence and conflict; or poor behavioral control (CDC, 2012). Low parental involvement, parental substance abuse or criminality, poor supervision, low emotional attachment to the parent, and harsh, lax, or inconsistent forms of discipline increase a child/adolescent's risk for violence (CDC, 2015h). Community and societal risk factors for youth violence are associated with diminished economic opportunities, a high concentration of poverty, transiency, and family disruption, with low levels of community participation (CDC, 2012). Youth development programs address these risk factors in schools and communities, as well as promoting activities that help students in meeting their individual needs. Mentoring has been identified as a beneficial program for at-risk teens when effectively trained and supported mentors are utilized. Social skills, conflict resolution, and programs that support student sports, arts, and extracurricular interests decrease an individual's risk in being involved in violence. School and societal strategies include surveillance, maintenance of facilities, and consistent classroom management techniques, along with adequate student supervision (CDC, 2015e). Parent involvement and education are expanding through programs such as with *Healthy Start* and parent-participation preschools, *Loving Solutions* for elementary age students, and the *Parent Project* for parents of difficult adolescents.

PARTNER/SPOUSAL ABUSE

Adult violence is rooted in childhood violence (Fig. 20–4). A father hits a mother. The mother hits her son. The son hits his sister. The sister hits her little brother. The little brother sets fire to the cat, pulls wings off butterflies, and grows up to be a spouse batterer. Although abused girls may grow up to be abusing mothers, more often they grow up to be abused wives. Researchers may refer to the term domestic violence as punching, grabbing, shoving, slapping, choking, kicking, biting, hitting with a fist or some other object, being beaten, or being threatened with a knife or gun by a spouse or cohabiting partner. The USDOJ (2015, para. 1) defines domestic violence as

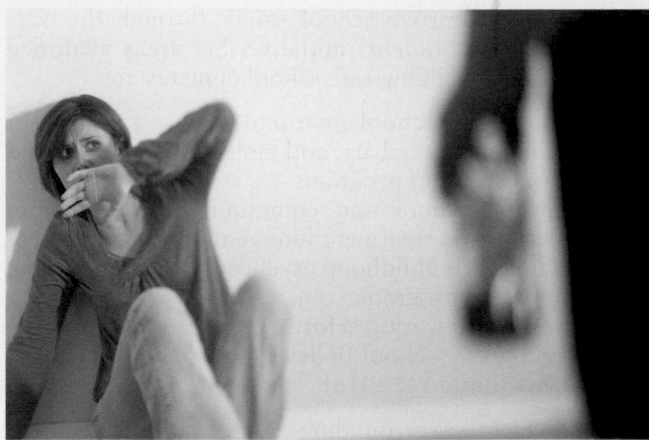

FIGURE 20–4 Domestic violence affects families and not just the immediate victims.

"a pattern of abusive behavior in any relationship that is used by one partner to gain or maintain power and control over another intimate partner"; it may be emotional, economic, physical, psychological, or sexual in nature. See Perspectives: Voices From the Community.

Violence during adolescent relationships sets the stage for problems in future adult relationships (CDC, 2015b). As these minor episodes of violence continue, the victim

---

PERSPECTIVES
VOICES FROM THE COMMUNITY

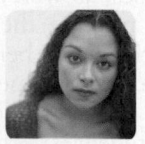

My family was always shouting at each other—it was just the way it was. The hitting—well, that happened, but it wasn't nearly as bad as all that yelling. Now here I am in the same boat all over again—the yelling, the hitting, and I've got this new baby to take care of. I'm just so tired. When the nurse showed up today to check on the baby and me, I swore to myself I wouldn't tell her about the fight we had last night (anyway, it wasn't nearly as bad as the other times). Then she looked at me and asked if I felt safe and that was it ... I said NO before I realized my mouth was even open. I told her that he punched me in the side while I was changing the baby's diaper. She was so kind—she didn't tell me how stupid I was for staying with him, but she did help me look at my options. Because I was holding the baby when he hit me, she said she was required to make a report of child abuse. That was awful news, and I started to cry; but like she said, I could have dropped her or he could have missed me and hit her. I knew he'd be furious when he found out—then I was really in a panic. Well, she told me about a place in town I can stay for a time with the baby, and she helped me make arrangements. I'm so tired and scared, but I know now that I need to keep my baby safe. I still don't know what made me tell the nurse—I guess it was because she asked. I know I'm doing the right thing for my baby and me.

Angie

---

typically feels that she is doing something wrong and attempts to modify her behavior. She also assumes wrongly that once she and her boyfriend are married, these physical assaults will stop automatically or that in time she will be able to "change" him, yet the cycle has already begun.

Cycle of Violence

The **cycle of violence** is a repetitive, cyclic pattern of abuse seen in domestic violence situations. This theory of family violence was first described as a three-phase cycle by Walker (1984), after she studied more than 1,000 battered women and a smaller group of battering men. The cycle includes the tension-building phase, the acute battering incident, and the loving reconciliation (Carrington, 2014). The psychological dynamics of these three phases help explain why women feel so guilty and ashamed of their partner's violence toward them, and why they find it so difficult to leave, even when their lives are in danger (see Display 20–8). Later adaptations of the model included additional phases: tension, buildup, standover, explosion, remorse, buyback, honeymoon, and normality (Carrington, 2014). Some like to begin with the honeymoon phase of the cycle, as this most often reflects the beginning of a relationship and the difficulty many women have in perceiving the explosive, battering phase (Carrington, 2014). Carrington (2014) also sees this cycle as more of a "vortex of violence" that sucks the woman deeper into the violence and giving her the feeling that her former self has been "spun off" the longer she remains in the relationship (p. 456). At first, her choices and security are lost, then her comfort and confidence, until finally hope, trust, and energy vanish. Often, as the cycle of violence continues, the frequency of the cycle increases, with the tension-building phase and the acute battering incident occurring more often and diminishment or elimination of the loving reconciliation phase. Without intervention, this shorter, more violent cycle becomes increasingly risk filled for outcomes that may lead to injury or maiming of a partner, incarceration, or death of a partner.

The Domestic Abuse Intervention Project in Duluth, Minnesota, developed a wheel of violence, identifying power and control at the center and citing eight categories of perpetrator behaviors. This model is a useful tool for visualizing the multidimensional nature of abuse in which threats, coercion, isolation, blaming, intimidation, and use of children, male privilege, and economics convene to control the victim (Fig. 20–5).

Reducing violence and its effects happens strategically at all three levels of prevention. Primary prevention efforts attempt to identify risk factors, reduce risks, and increase social support to prevent violence from occurring. Secondary prevention effort involves developing immediate response to violence that addresses the short-term consequences through emergency response and medical care. Tertiary prevention interventions work to address the long-term effect of trauma through counseling and rehabilitation (CDC, 2013).

Dating Violence

Adolescent dating violence (ADV) includes physical, sexual, emotional, and verbal abuse between teenagers who are or have been in a casual or serious dating relationship. It

DISPLAY 20–8 THE CYCLE OF VIOLENCE

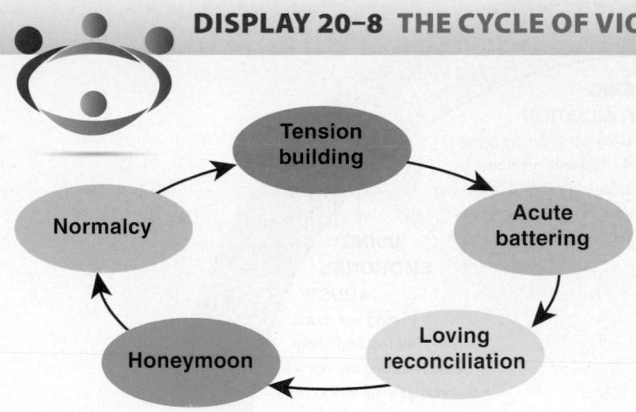

Normalcy/Calm

This is the normal, everyday interaction for the couple. The usual routines are followed and the woman feels she is in a zone of safety. There is no behavior extreme (e.g., anger/violence or honeymoon phase), but this is the time when expectations are advanced and the woman attempts to adapt to them in order to prevent another violent episode.

The Increasing Spiral of Violence

One aspect of the cycle of violence of particular concern is its progressive and spiraling nature. Once violence has begun, every study indicates that it not only continues but, over time, increases in both frequency and severity. As the violence continues, the cycle begins to change. The tension-building phase becomes shorter and more intense, the acute battering incidents become more frequent and severe, and the loving reconciliation phase becomes shorter and less intense. After many years of battering, the man may not apologize at all.

Tension-Building Phase

The woman senses her partner's increasing tension. She may or may not know what is wrong. The partner is "edgy" and lashes out in anger. He challenges her, calls her names, and tells her she is stupid, incompetent, and unconcerned about him. She "tries hard" not to make any "mistakes" that may upset him. She takes the responsibility for making him feel better and begins to set herself up to feel guilt when he eventually explodes in spite of her best efforts to calm and please him. During the increasing tension, the woman is rarely angry even at the most outrageous demands or blame. Rather, she internalizes her appropriate anger at the partner's unfairness and, instead, experiences depression, anxiety, and a sense of helplessness. As the tension in the relationship increases, minor episodes of violence increase, such as pinching, tripping, or slapping. The batterer knows his behavior is inappropriate, and he fears the woman will leave him. This fear of rejection and loss increases his rage at the woman and his need to control her.

Acute Battering Incident: The Explosion

The tension-building phase ends in an explosion of violence. The incident that sets off the man's violence is often trivial or unknown, leaving the woman confused and feeling helpless. The woman may or may not fight back. She may try to escape the violence or call for help. If she cannot escape the beating, she may have a sense of unreality—as if it is a dream. Following the battering, the woman is in a state of physical and psychological shock. She may be passive and withdrawn or hysterical and incoherent. She may not be aware of the seriousness of her injuries and may resist help. The man discounts the episode and also underestimates the woman's injuries. He may not summon medical help even when her injuries are life threatening.

Remorse and Loving Reconciliation

The loving reconciliation phase may begin a few hours to several days following the acute battering incident. Both partners have a profound sense of relief that "it's over." Although the woman is initially angry with her partner, he begins an intense campaign to "win her back." Just as his tension and violence were overdone, his apologies, gifts, and gestures of love may also be excessive. He often promises to "never do this again." Showering her with love and praise helps her repair her shattered self-esteem. It is nearly impossible for her to leave him during this phase as he is meeting her desperate need to see herself as a competent and lovable woman. The woman's feelings of power and romantic ideals are nurtured. She believes this gentle and loving person is her "real" lover. She believes that if only she can find the key, she can stop him from further violent episodes. She believes that no matter how often it has happened before, somehow this episode seems different and it will never happen again.

Honeymoon Phase

This is a continuation of the reconciliation phase after an incident, but it is also commonly the first phase in a new relationship. When we are attracted to someone, we develop feelings and emotions that bond us to the person. The man in this phase wants the woman's trust and devotion and is "kind and loving." Some researchers feel that he is "grooming" her, much like a sexual predator does, to trust him and overlook any subtle signs that might indicate later abuse.

Adapted from Carrington, A. M. (2014). The vortex of violence: Moving beyond the cycle and engaging clients in change. *British Journal of Social Work, 44,* 451–468.
Relationships Australia. (2007). *Safe from violence: A guide for women leaving or separating.* Retrieved from http://www.relationships.org.au/relationship-advice/publications/pdfs/safefromviolence.pdf
Walker, L. E. (1979). *The battered woman.* New York, NY: Harper and Row.

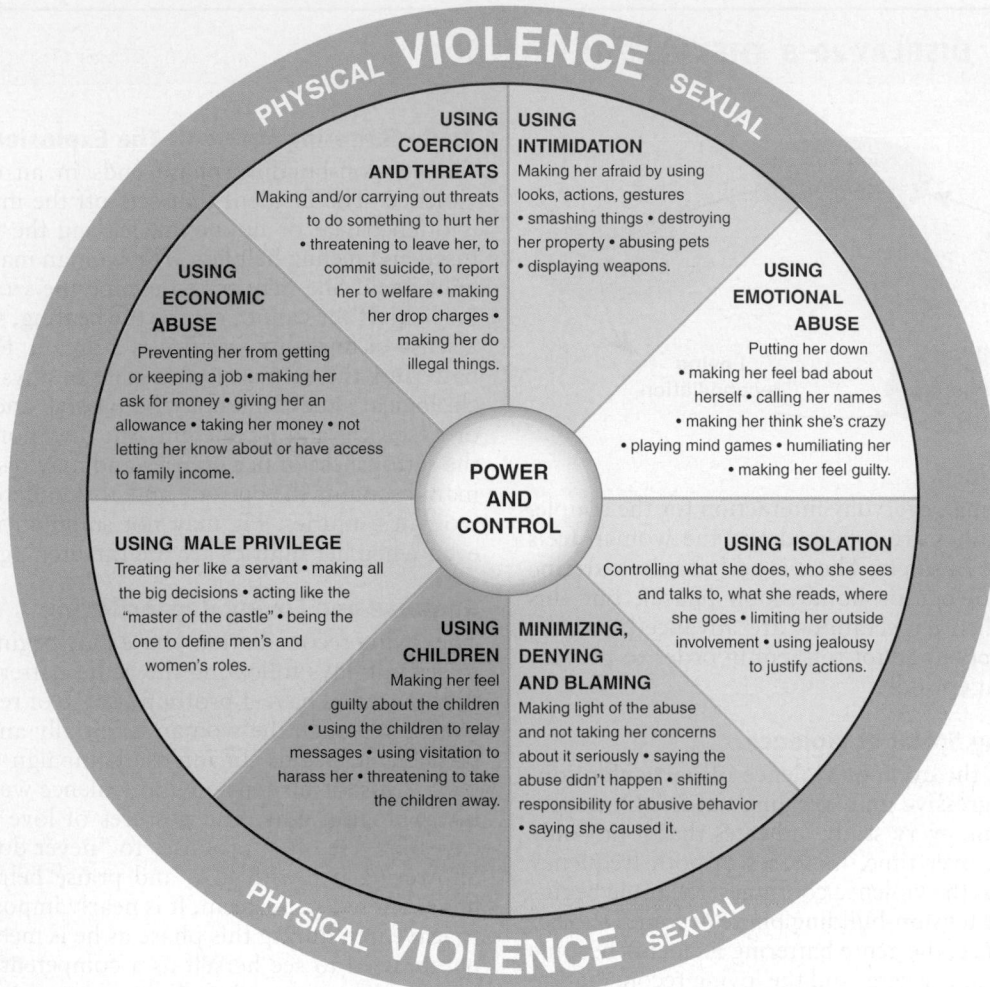

FIGURE 20–5 Wheel of violence.

can be electronic or in person and might occur between a current or former partner (CDC, 2015b). In the United States, ADV was reported by nearly 10% of students in the past 12 months; furthermore, victims of dating violence are at higher risk for dating violence in college (CDC, 2015b). Documented risk factors include poverty, limited education, substance abuse, poor family functioning, child maltreatment, and childhood exposure to IPV (Maas, Fleming, Herrenkohl, & Catalano, 2010; Stewart, Vigod, & Riazantseva, 2016). Research on male aggressors found that those who exhibited physical and psychological dating aggression often had a history of suicide attempts, reports of past physical aggression, and low relationship satisfaction/instability and jealousy (Collibee & Furman, 2016; Kerr & Capaldi, 2011). Teens, male or female, who experience dating violence in adolescence, are more at risk for binge drinking, suicide attempts, doing poorly in school, physical fighting, and sexual activity (CDC, 2015b). Programs through schools and communities, such as *Dating Matters*, are part of a national effort to address harmful beliefs about dating violence and promote healthy and respectful dating relationships (CDC, 2015c). Dating violence in adolescent relationships is a serious and prevalent problem (CDC, 2016). Because of its prevalence, community

health nurses should include screening for dating violence in all encounters with teens.

Intimate Partner Violence

"Intimate partner violence is a pattern of assaultive behavior and coercive behavior that may include physical injury, psychological abuse, sexual assault, progressive isolation, stalking, deprivation, intimidation and reproductive coercion by someone who is, was, or wishes to be involved in an intimate or dating relationship with an adult or adolescent, and is aimed at establishing control of one partner over the other" (American Congress of Obstetricians and Gynecologists, 2012, para. 2). The WHO reported that 30% of women reported being physically abused by an intimate partner at some point in their lives, and 38% of all women who were murdered were murdered by their intimate partner. Approximately, 18.3% of women had experienced sexual violence by an intimate partner (CDC, 2011b; WHO, 2013b). Global prevalence figures indicate that 35% of women worldwide have experienced either IPV or nonpartner sexual violence in their lifetime (WHO, 2013b). The World Health Organization found that approximately 20% of women and 5% to 10% of men had experienced sexual abuse as a child (WHO, 2013a). Because of the nature of **intimate partner violence (IPV)**, the problems are difficult to study and believed to be underreported. Much remains unknown about factors that increase or decrease the likelihood that men will behave violently toward women. Researchers have examined the physical and emotional consequences of partner violence upon women and their children, as well as the impact on their health (Grip, Almqvist, Axberg, & Broberg, 2014; Karakurt, Smith, & Whiting, 2014). There is evidence to support the importance of screening for partner violence and to support plans for interventions for a quicker and healthy recover for women and their children (Garrido, Culhane, Petrenko, & Taussig, 2011; Symes, Maddoux, McFarlane, Nava, & Gilroy, 2014). See Evidence-Based Practice.

Although domestic violence is categorized as physical abuse, sexual abuse, emotional abuse, economic abuse, or psychological abuse, the victim commonly experiences a combination of these abuses or threats of abuse in these areas. Intimidation and threats create an atmosphere of fear for the victim and may include humiliation, isolation, terrorizing, coercing, blaming,

manipulating, stalking, and/or destruction of property or pets valued by the partner. *Stalking* may occur by either partner in a relationship, demonstrated as a "pattern of repeated and unwanted attention, harassment, contact, or any other course of conduct directed at a specific person that would cause a reasonable person to feel fear" (USDOJ, 2016, para. 2). During 1 year, approximately 1.5% of people age 18 or older will be victims of stalking. Divorced or separated women are at greater risk as victims of stalking, whereas harassment occurs equally between men and women (Catalano, 2012). Breiding et al. (2014) note that over 15% of women report a lifetime prevalence of being a victim of stalking behavior, and 9.3% of men. Cyberstalking, a technology-based attack, can also take many forms that can involve harassment, embarrassment, and humiliation of the victim. Approximately 1 million women and 370,000 men have been stalked through technology annually in the United States (Moore, 2014).

IPV is a leading cause of morbidity and mortality in women worldwide, as well as a public health and human rights issue (WHO, 2012b). In the United States, IPV

EVIDENCE-BASED PRACTICE

Generational Transmission of Intimate Partner Violence

About one quarter of women will experience domestic violence or IPV during their lifetime, and research has linked child exposure to IPV and later adult domestic violence behavior. Some posit that children adopt behaviors that have been role modeled by parents; however, most children who have witnessed IPV do not abuse their partners in adulthood. Others found that abused children, compared to IPV-exposed children, have a similar or even higher risk of becoming perpetrators of IPV as adults. Research has also indicated that there may be an even greater effect for those children who are both abused and who witness interparental violence. Eriksson and Mazerolle (2015) wanted to know if examining gender role–specific behavior would give a clearer indication of generational transmission. They inspected effects of experiencing domestic violence and child abuse among a group of 303 males who had been arrested on drug-related charges. Further, they examined the differences between childhood observations of mothers abusing fathers and fathers abusing mothers or bidirectional abuse on later IPV behavior in adulthood. Tools and interviews helped determine if participants had themselves been a perpetrator of IPV, if they had experienced physical abuse in their childhood, and if they had observed parental violence (and if father and/or mother was the perpetrator). The Beliefs About Wife Beating scale, along with demographic information, also provided data. Ethnicity was fairly evenly split (46.5% White, 53.5% non-White), and the majority had completed high school (63.4%). Over 44.2% had initiated alcohol use early, and almost half had tried hard drugs (49.8%) or been involved in IPV (43.6%). Almost one in five had experienced child abuse and over 40%

had observed IPV, most commonly father-only violence (24.4%). Almost one third had attitudes that indicated justification for wife beating.

Using bivariate analysis, they found that having attitudes that justified wife beating and childhood observation of parental IPV were significantly associated (p = 0.043), but child abuse was not. Having attitudes justifying wife beating was not a mediating variable between childhood observation of IPV and adult perpetration of IPV, but attitudes did have a "direct effect on IPV perpetration" (p. 956). With logistic regression, they determined that those who witnessed parental IPV in childhood were significantly more likely to perpetrate IPV as adults (B = 1.76, p = 0.001 for bidirectional IPV; B = 1.02, p = 0.001 for father-only IPV) and those who both witnessed IPV and were abused as children were even more likely to be adult domestic abusers (B = 1.53, p = 0.001). No significant association was found for observation of mother-only IPV and later adult IPV perpetration. Thus, the researchers concluded that there could be a gender-specific connection to male IPV perpetration (e.g., male children who observe their fathers beating their mothers are more likely to do the same as adults).

Given this evidence and after examining other research on this topic, what interventions might you consider when working with families dealing with domestic violence?

From Eriksson, L., & Mazerolle, P. (2015). A cycle of violence? Examining family-of-origin violence, attitudes, and intimate partner violence perpetration. *Journal of Interpersonal Violence, 30*(6), 945–964.

affects more than 34.2 million women each year with 23 million being raped during their lifetime. Almost 80% of victims experienced the first rape or IPV before age 25, and 40% before the age of 18. Approximately 19.3% of women and 1.7% of men have been raped during their lifetime (Breiding et al., 2014; CDC, 2011b). Health care providers have a responsibility and opportunity to assess and initiate a safety plan when these patients are seen in the emergency room. A compendium of assessment tools for IPV can be found on the CDC Web site.

Violence During Pregnancy

IPV during pregnancy increases a woman's vulnerability to her and her fetus. A form of physical violence during pregnancy is when abusive partners target a woman's abdomen, not only hurting the women but also potentially jeopardizing the pregnancy (WHO, 2011). Abuse during pregnancy results in higher rates of intrauterine growth retardation and preterm labor that can lead to low birth weight and neonatal risks. One international study of domestic violence during pregnancy found a prevalence rate of 43.4% (Coutinho et al., 2015). Approximately 4% of women with a recent live birth in a 30-state area reported some

form of IPV in the 12 months prior to becoming pregnant (Child Health USA, 2013). Abuse during pregnancy has been linked with maternal health problems such as smoking, alcohol and substance abuse, delay in prenatal care, stress, physical injuries, headaches, and lack of attachment to the infant (WHO, 2011). Among pregnant women in the United States, homicide is the second most prevalent cause of traumatic death (McMahon & Armstrong, 2012). One finding in a U.S. 11-city review found pregnancy significantly increased a woman's risk of IPV homicide, as men who abused their partner during pregnancy were particularly more dangerous and, therefore, more likely to commit homicide (WHO, 2011). *Femicide*, the killing of women because they are women, happens globally with 35% of all murders of women reportedly committed by an intimate partner (WHO, 2012a). See Chapter 21 for more on maternal child health issues.

Abuse is more likely to be reported by pregnant adolescents than pregnant adults and by women with unplanned pregnancies compared with other pregnant women (WHO, 2011). Unemployment, low levels of education, and an immigrant partner were noted as predictive factors in one study (Coutinho et al., 2015).

DISPLAY 20–9 DOMESTIC VIOLENCE SCREENING TOOL

Although some research notes that screening and educational interventions/providing resources on domestic or IPV do not lead to increased knowledge and behavior change (Klevens, Sadowski, Kee, & Garcia, 2015), this type of screening remains part of the Women's Preventive Services Guidelines (Health Resources & Services Administration, n.d.).

Frame the Questions by Stating:

"Because abuse and violence are common in the lives of women, I have begun to ask about it with all women (or all pregnant women). I don't know if this is a problem for you, but I would like to ask you some questions, talk about ways to reduce your risk of being hurt, and give you some information and phone numbers that might be helpful to you."

Universal Questions

	Yes	No
1. Do you feel safe in your current relationships? Comments: _____	___	___
2. Have you ever been physically abused (pushed, shoved, hit, punched, bitten, burned, etc.)? Comments: _____	___	___
3. Have you ever been emotionally abused (neglected, called names, controlled, threatened, had your activities or decisions hindered, been	___	___

denied resources to meet your physical or financial needs)?
Comments: _____

4. Have you ever been sexually abused (forced to have an unwanted sexual act)? ___ ___
Comments: _____

5. Have your children ever been threatened or abused?
Comments: _____

6. Do you want to talk to someone ___ ___ about receiving help?
Comments: _____

Resources

National Domestic Violence Hotline:
1-800-799-SAFE (7233)
Local Battered Women's Shelter _____
Local Department of Women's Health Services _____
Other resources _____

Adapted from Basile, K. C., Hertz, M. F., & Back, S. E. (2007). *Intimate partner violence and sexual violence victimization assessment instruments for use in healthcare settings: Version 1*. Atlanta, GA: Centers for Disease Control & Prevention.
Health Resources & Services Administration. (n.d.). *Women's preventive services guidelines: Affordable Care Act expands prevention coverage for women's health and wellbeing.* Retrieved from http://www.hrsa.gov/womensguidelines/
Klevens, J., Sadowski, L. S., Kee, R., & Garcia, D. (2015). Does screening or providing information on resources for intimate partner violence increase women's knowledge? Findings from a randomized controlled trial. *Journal of Women's Health Issues and Care, 4*(2), 81.
U.S. Department of Health & Human Services. (2013). *Health providers' role in screening and counseling for interpersonal and domestic violence.* Retrieved from http://www.womenshealth.gov/publications/our-publications/fact-sheet/screening-counseling-fact-sheet.html#moreInfo

The pregnant women in that study reported the pregnancies as planned, but not monitored closely. Teen pregnancy is linked to various types of violence, and several studies found that teens are at increased risk of abuse during pregnancy (National Campaign to Prevent Teen Pregnancy, 2014). IPV rates for adolescents seeking prenatal care range from 16% to 37% (Kulkarni, Lewis, & Rhodes, 2011). Pregnant teens that have been abused also associate with other adverse health behaviors such as smoking and alcohol and substance abuse. Once born, the infant of an abused teen or adult is at risk for child abuse.

Studies indicate that the prenatal care visit is one of the few times when women are seen by the helping professions. This visit is an important opportunity to identify women who are abused and therefore at risk for homicide. It is imperative that nurses conduct an assessment for danger and lethality, so that the women can be aware of their own level of risk and take safety precautions as needed. A series of questions requiring a "yes" or "no" response and inquiries about occurrences of abuse, escalation of abuse, frequency, severity, weapons, drugs or alcohol use by the perpetrator, and safety of other children should be incorporated into prenatal home visit assessments. This is especially important with women who have not followed through with prenatal care, thereby allowing health care professionals to monitor the progress of their pregnancies (Display 20–9).

Batterer Characteristics

Although men who batter come from all walks of life educationally, culturally, and socioeconomically, perpetrators have some common characteristics. The following attributes represent personal characteristics often seen in batterers:

- Low income
- Low self-esteem
- Low academic achievement
- Involvement in aggressive or delinquent behavior as youth
- Heavy alcohol and drug use
- Depression
- Anger and hostility
- Personality disorders
- Prior history of being physically abusive
- Having few friends and being isolated from other people
- Unemployment
- Emotional dependence and insecurity
- Belief in strict gender roles (e.g., male dominance and aggression in relationships)
- Desire for power and control in relationships
- Being a victim of physical or psychological abuse—this is consistently one of the strongest predictors of perpetration (CDC, 2015f, para. 4).

Relationship, community, and societal factors have also been identified that affect a perpetrator's risk for battering. Identified relationship factors include marital fights and tension, divorce and separations, money problems, and problematic and difficult family relationships, as well as the male's need for dominance and control in the relationship. Societal factors associated with increased risk are strict role stereotyping about the roles the husband and wife should follow in a relationship. Aspects identified within a community that lead to increased risks for IPV may be a lack of resources in the community, a failure or unwillingness of others to intervene or contact authorities when they are aware of the abuse, and factors associated with poverty, such as overcrowding and unemployment (CDC, 2015f).

Victim Characteristics

Studies have also revealed risk factors associated with victims. Increasing the victim's abilities to manage and improve their behaviors and understanding of relationship patterns and abuse allows victims to change their risk of being a victim. Individual risk factors for IPV victims include:

- A prior history of IPV
- Being female
- Young age, especially if pregnant
- From low-income household
- Witnessing or experiencing violence as a child
- Lower education level
- Unemployment
- Single parent with children or separated/divorced/previously widowed
- For men, having a different ethnicity from their partner
- For women, having a greater education level than their partner
- For women, being American Indian/Alaska Native or African American
- For women, being disabled
- For women, having a verbally abusive, jealous, or possessive partner
- Veterans and active-duty military
- Some research indicates higher levels of IPV (especially emotional victimization) in same-sex couples (Hart & Klein, 2013)

Marked differences between partner's incomes, levels of education, or job status place a victim more at risk for IPV. Community characteristics are similar to those of the perpetrator, revealing that those communities with fewer available resources, in areas of poverty, and having a lack of sanctions against violent behaviors increase one's risk; there is some indication that rates of IPV are higher in rural versus urban areas. Traditional gender roles, such as a belief that men work and women are submissive and should stay home, are societal risk factors associated with higher IPV risk (Hart & Klein, 2013).

Effects of Violence on Children

Twenty to fifty percent of children around the world suffer from abuse (Finkelhor, 2013). The consequences of exposure to violence and abuse hinder children's health and development and can have lifelong impact, negatively affecting health and increasing the risks of further victimization and becoming a perpetrator of violence (WHO, 2013a). Sexual assault in children can result in PTSD, suicidal thoughts, depression, and later risk of substance abuse and nonviolent or violent criminal behavior (Trotman et al., in press). Children who are exposed to family violence are more at risk for abuse and for violence later in their life as either a perpetrator or a victim. Although domestic violence may not be directed at a child, that child may become a victim as a bystander or when trying to protect a parent. Effects of family violence are often seen in emotional, cognitive, physical, and/or behavioral manifestations of the child. Children who have been exposed to violence are more likely to use drugs and alcohol, experience depression anxiety and/or posttraumatic stress syndrome, do poorly in school, or exhibit delinquency/participate in criminal activity. More immediate child reactions include high levels of activity, anxiety, and aggression, as well as problems with sleep/nightmares, concentration, and separation anxiety (National Child Traumatic Stress Network, n.d.).

Most often, wife abuse and child abuse occur together. Literature reviews consistently suggest that a positive correlation exists between children's witnessing IPV and some aspects of impaired child development. Young children are particularly vulnerable to the effects of violence, as they lack the ability to understand the trauma and are likely to exhibit somatic complaints (e.g., headaches, eating or sleep problems) and/or behavior regression, such as clinging, whining, or becoming nonverbal (National Child Traumatic Stress Network, n.d.). Meanwhile, school-age children and adolescents are more likely to either act out with delinquent behaviors or withdraw. It is more common for girls to become withdrawn and an important reason for health care providers to include an assessment for family violence concerns. Children in families with domestic violence are at risk for depression, negative mental health effects, and consequences that last far into their adult lives. These maladjustments may be behavioral (aggression and conduct problems), emotional (withdrawal, anxiousness, fearfulness), social, cognitive (learning disabilities), and/or physical. Researchers have linked physical alterations in the child's brain (e.g., cerebral cortex, limbic system, corpus callosum, hypothalamus) with PTSD following child exposure to domestic violence (Tsavoussis, Stawicki, Stoicea, & Papadimos, 2014). For some children, high cortisol and other hormonal responses may lead to chronic levels of arousal, aggression, anxiety, depression, eating disorders, and other problems (e.g., self-harm, general irritability). In others, during adulthood, attempts to adjust to new stressors may lead to down-regulation of receptors and the ability to only respond minimally to stress hormones. Providers who work with children need to listen in a sincere, nonjudgmental manner and provide ongoing support when assisting the child and family with resources, such as counseling, education, or community violence prevention programs (Fig. 20–6).

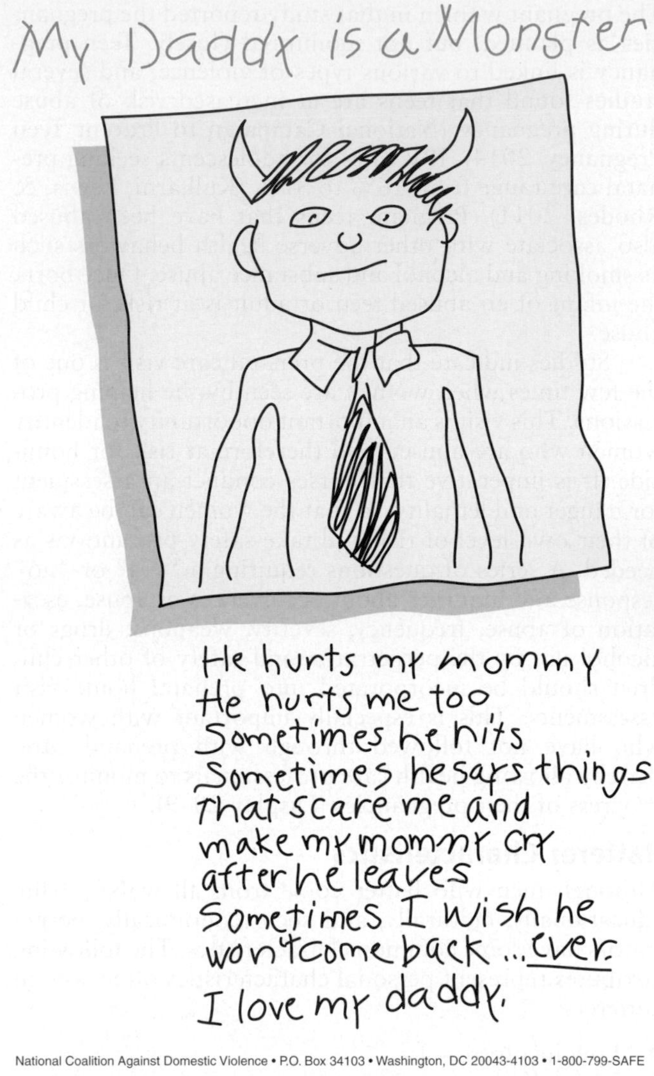

MISTREATMENT OF ELDERS

"Elder mistreatment (i.e., abuse and neglect) is defined as intentional actions that cause harm or create a serious risk of harm (whether or not harm is intended) to a vulnerable elder by a caregiver or other person who stands in a trust relationship to the elder. This includes failure by a caregiver to satisfy the elder's basic needs or to protect the elder from harm" (National Center on

National Coalition Against Domestic Violence • P.O. Box 34103 • Washington, DC 20043-4103 • 1-800-799-SAFE

FIGURE 20–6 Poster of "My Daddy Is a Monster."

Elder Abuse, Elder Abuse [NCEA], 2013b, para 3). The mistreatment or exploitation of older adults may involve physical, sexual, or emotional or psychological abuse; neglect; abandonment; financial or material exploitation; or self-neglect or any combination of these mistreatments (NCEA, n.d.a; Falk et al., 2012). Of the population ages 60 or older, 1 out of every 10 who live at home suffers abuse, neglect, or exploitation. Abuse against elders is not new, but research on elder abuse is new. Until recently, the reasons for elder abuse were extrapolated from the literature on abuse in younger populations. The Elder Justice Roadmap (USDOJ, 2013b) provides specific recommendations for five top priorities and delineates action items for direct service, education, policy, and research.

As longevity increases, and the number of elderly individuals in the population increase, so does the incidence of elder abuse (Administration on Aging, 2015). Forms of physical abuse were found to include rough handling during caregiving, pinching, hitting, and slapping. Emotional abuse, which can take many forms, included being shouted at or threatened and having needed care withheld. More rarely, elders are sexually abused, which may include rape. Some elders are neglected by those they depend on to meet their caregiving needs. Elders with dementia and those requiring assistance for all activities of daily living (ADLs) are more at risk because of caregiver stress or burnout, which increases an elder's risk for abuse and neglect. With neglect, the elder may appear unwashed and unkempt or may suffer from malnutrition and dehydration or even pressure sores. Elders who are dependent on others for their care often do not report abuse for fear of being abandoned. They feel powerless and at a loss about how to change a bad situation. They often fear reprisal from the perpetrator if they tell others about the abuse.

Older adults are frequently exploited in a variety of ways. Family members may take their Social Security retirement money, savings, or investments and use these funds on themselves. Criminals often approach elders with get-rich-quick schemes, sham investment opportunities, or overpriced home repairs or as collectors for illegitimate charities, thereby preying on the trusting nature of older adults. See Chapter 24 for more on older adults.

Perpetrator and Victim Characteristics

The incidence and prevalence of **elder abuse** is very difficult to estimate as every 1 in 24 cases are not reported, but estimates are often about 1 in 10 elderly experiencing some type of abuse (National Center on Elder Abuse [NCEA], n.d.b). Adult protective services show an increased trend in reporting, and information is becoming more available.

Approximately two thirds of elder abuse victims are women, often about half of individuals suffering from dementia (USDOJ, 2013b). Ninety percent of abusers are family members, most often the elder's adult children, spouses, and partners. Family members who feel burdened by their caregiver responsibilities and who abuse drugs or alcohol or have a mental or emotional illness abuse at higher rates than those who do not (NCEA, 2013b).

The dominant underlying factors that contribute to abuse of an elder by a family member are social isolation and pathology on the part of the perpetrator. Research has identified emotional or financial dependence on the victim, alcohol use, and isolation or few external contacts as major contributing factors. Abuse happens more frequently to elderly individuals with dementia, and individuals with mental illness are often perpetrators (Rosen, 2014).

Some characteristics of older people appear to increase their risk of abuse. These risks include dementia and poor health, increased age, disability, and lesbian, gay, bisexual, and transgender (LGBT) lifestyle and being a resident of an assisted living facility (NCEA, 2013a). Newly diagnosed cognitive impairment correlates with occurrences of abuse. If violence or threats of violence by the elder toward the caregiver accompany dementia, this contributes to the elder's risk for abuse. The failing health of an elder may also contribute to self-neglect or diminished ability for self-defense or escape from maltreatment. Finally, if the abuser and victim live together, the close proximity can bring up unresolved family conflicts or create new conflicts and tension (NCEA, 2013b). Abuse

in an elder often leads to a downward spiral in their life with a loss of independence, increased health complications, and greater risk of mortality especially in most vulnerable populations (Dong & Simon, 2014).

Risk Factors

Regardless of the type of abuse an elder suffers or the motivation of the abuser, two factors are common to all elder abuse situations. The first factor is the *invisibility* of elders in general and abused elders specifically. Reasons for invisibility among the elderly are multifaceted. Older people usually have less contact with the community. They are no longer in the workforce or in public on a regular basis, which keeps their problems hidden longer. In addition, older adults are reticent to admit to being abused or neglected. Because the abuser is most often a family member, the elder desires to protect the abuser; without this abusing family member, the elder may be entirely alone. On the other hand, the elder may fear reprisal from the abuser for coming forward with a self-report of abuse or telling someone about the home situation. Cultural and societal values also contribute to keeping "family matters" private, while shame and embarrassment make it difficult for many elders to tell others of the abuse (New York City Elder Abuse Center, 2013).

The second risk factor is the *vulnerability* of older adults. Vulnerability refers to a cluster of risk factors that include age, sex, race and ethnicity, socioeconomic status, cognitive impairment, depression, functional ability, social network, and social participation (Dong & Simon, 2014). Many elders who are frail are dependent on others for some aspect of their day-to-day survival. At first, they may need to rely on others for transportation, shopping, and housekeeping. Later, they may need help with financial affairs, cooking, and laundry. In time, the elder may need help managing medications, bathing, and eating. The degree to which an elder needs assistance is often kept hidden from others because the elder fears being removed from his present living situation and being placed in a more restrictive environment. Additionally, vulnerability in elders is increased when any of the following characteristics are present: (1) impairment and isolation, (2) poverty and pathologic caregivers, (3) learned helplessness and living in a violent subculture, and (4) living in deteriorating housing and crime-ridden neighborhoods.

Prevention of Elder Abuse

Awareness of elder abuse and education about the types of abuse via media campaigns has improved community recognition of the problem. Increasing attention is now directed at the unique care needs of elders, including resources for the elderly, and the need for caregiver respite has also received increased attention and services. Training for caregivers as well as health care and social service providers that focus on recognizing stress and initiating measures for intervening has developed new understanding of effective interventions (e.g., use of physical therapists, occupational therapists, and geropsychiatrists). Statutory requirements for reporting abuse and providing crisis hotlines for reporting elder abuse are also integral aspects of a community's response to the problem of elder abuse

(Falk et al., 2012). World Elder Abuse Awareness Day has been designated as an annual observance on June 15th to promote public awareness and prevention education regarding elder abuse (NCEA, 2015).

OTHER FORMS OF FAMILY VIOLENCE

Three other forms of violence that directly affect families are suicide, homicide, and rape. These three forms of violence demonstrate the ultimate extreme of violence to the victim and are the most traumatic to the surviving family members.

Suicide

Suicide is taking action that causes one's own death. In the United States, suicide is the 10th leading cause of death. Not all suicide attempts are successful, approximately 1.3 million adults (aged 18 or older) attempted suicide in 2013 (CDC, 2015d). These attempts to cause or actually cause self-harm are known as *parasuicidal acts*. In 2013, 494,169 individuals were treated in emergency departments for self-inflicted injuries (CDC, 2015d). Gender has an influence on suicide rates and fatalities—men are four times more likely than women to die and represent 77.9% of all suicides (CDC, 2015d). The *Healthy People 2010* goal was to reduce suicides to not more than 6 per 100,000 people, yet in 2013, there were 41,149 suicides, a rate of 12.6 per 100,000. Suicide is the leading cause of death among persons aged 10 to 14.

Worldwide, 75% of suicides occur in low- and middle-income countries with a global mortality rate of 11.4 per 100,000 people. The estimate for suicide attempts is up to 20 times more frequent than the fatality rate. Older men have traditionally had the highest suicide rate, 57% higher in men than in women, although there is a noted increase in younger and older people in higher-income countries (WHO, 2016b). The association between mental health disorders and suicide is well established in high-income countries, particularly depression and alcohol use disorders; many suicides happen impulsively in moments of crisis. Rates are high in vulnerable groups such as refugees, migrants, prisoners, and LGBT populations (WHO, 2014).

It is important to be aware of warning signs of potential suicide when working with people in crisis. The strongest risk for suicide is a previous suicide attempt (WHO, 2014). Warning signs fall into three categories: what the person talks about, types of behaviors, and mood. The more warning signs the greater the risk (American Foundation for Suicide Prevention [AFSP], 2016). An individual may talk about not having a reason to live, feeling trapped, or suicide. Threats or comments that indicate a plan or giving personal items away are potential indicators of a person contemplating suicide. Isolation, sleeping too much, acting recklessly, and increased use of alcohol or drugs are high-risk behaviors for suicide. Moods that may reflect increased risk are depression, irritability, rage, humiliation, and anxiety. Access to guns increases one's risk regardless of age, gender, or ethnicity because firearms are the most utilized method of suicide. Health providers and others may find *IS PATH WARM*, a mnemonic from the American Association of Suicidology

helpful when looking at possible warning signs for suicide (AAS, 2014). These signs are:

I—ideation
S—substance abuse
P—purposelessness
A—anxiety
T—trapped
H—hopelessness
W—withdrawal
A—anger
R—recklessness
M—mood change

Completed suicides are carried out in a variety of ways, some more violent than others. Women usually choose less violent methods, such as overdosing on medications. Men choose more violent forms of suicide, such as hanging, use of firearms, or vehicle crashes. Deaths from suicide are underreported because of a tendency to group them as accidental deaths or deaths from undetermined causes. See Chapter 27 for more on behavioral health in the community.

Community awareness campaigns and education programs are needed to help a person recognize the risks and the importance of initiating prevention for someone who is suicidal. Crisis hotlines with 24-hour access are a vital resource for a distraught individual, friend, or loved one to contact and find help during a crisis and to learn about local resources to contact. Appropriate and consistent treatment, most often a combination of antidepressants and psychotherapy approach, is needed for those suffering from depression because individuals with a major depressive disorder have approximately a 20 times higher risk for suicide than the general population (AAS, 2014). The surviving loved ones require attention to their grief and bereavement. Support groups often provide benefits, allowing the bereaved to share their intense feelings of guilt and learn how to deal with any sense of a stigma, embarrassment, or shame felt by the survivors.

Homicide

Homicide is any non–war-related action taken to cause the death of another person. Violence has historically been associated with crime and is generally categorized by the method or age group affected. In 2012 globally, intentional homicide took the lives of half a million people (United Nations Office on Drugs & Crime, 2016). In 2013, 12,253 murders were committed and 89.3% involved males. In incidents of murder in which the victim relationship was known, 55.9% were killed by someone they knew, 24.9 % of victims were killed by family members, and the relationship was unknown in 45.5 % of murder and manslaughter incidents in 2013 (FBI, 2014). Young adults ages 18 to 24 had the highest homicide rate of any age group from 2002 to 2011 with a rate of 11.9 per 100,000 in 2011 (Bureau of Justice Statistics [BJS], 2013).

The homicide rate in the United States has declined by nearly half, from 9.3 to 4.7 per 100,000 in 1992 and 2011, respectively (BJS, 2013), which is below the *Healthy People 2020* objective of 5.5 per 100,000 (USDHHS, 2016a). Many homicide casualties are victims of domestic abuse as the cycle of violence escalates; a partner may be killed during a violent episode or by a recruited third party. Homicide in young infants and children is most often perpetrated by a parent, a stepparent, or a caregiver. Conflict between adolescent males may escalate if weapons or guns are available, resulting in homicide.

Evidence suggests that violence can be prevented by measures aimed at individuals, families, relationship, community, and society. The Community Guide provides evidence-based recommendations for each level of prevention (CDC, 2015e). Although biologic and personal factors may influence one's predisposition to violence, an interaction between one's family, community, cultural, and other factors combine to create violence (WHO, 2014). The WHO cites four key steps in developing a public health approach to violence. These steps include

- Uncovering as much knowledge as possible about all aspects of violence
- Investigating why it occurs
- Exploring means of violence prevention
- Taking action, which includes disseminating information and evaluating programs' effectiveness (WHO, 2014)

Prevention methods include education programs for preschool, school-aged children, and adolescents to decrease bullying and improve social skills; parent education courses and parent resources such as advice lines, support groups, or a crisis nursery; and community measures that improve firearm safety and reduce firearm injuries.

Rape

Rape is an act of aggression in which the perpetrator is motivated by a desire to dominate, control, and degrade the victim. Once considered an act of sexuality, it is now believed to be a combination of domination and sexuality or defined as a "sexual expression of aggression." The National Violence Against Women Survey (NVAWS) working with the CDC and National Institute of Justice reports that 302,091 women and 92,748 men are raped each year in the United States. Furthermore, the survey estimates that one in five women and one in 71 men have been a rape victim at some time during their life, with 42.2% of all rapes occurring before the age of 18 and 12.3% of the rapes occurring before age 12 of female rape victims (CDC, 2014f). Female rape victims reported intimate partners (51.1%), family members (12.5%), and acquaintances (40.8%) as perpetrators (CDC, 2014e).

The violence of rape creates physical and psychological harm for the victim and those close to them. Health problems for the victim may include head, pelvic, back, or facial pain; depression; suicidal ideation; eating disorders; gastrointestinal disorders; or substance abuse (Breiding et al., 2014). Fear, anxiety, or shame may become debilitating for the victim. Counseling and professional care are necessary for the rape victim from the time the rape is reported through any legal process that may result.

Community measures useful in preventing rape include Rape Prevention and Education (RPE) program for adolescents and college students, date rape education, hotlines staffed to provide help for victims of rape or VAW, and having trained professionals, such as SART members, on hand (CDC, 2014d). SART members are trained to understand the psychological and physical assessment needs of the victim, as well as the legal requirements for an investigation and court proceeding (Moylan et al., 2015). Rape crisis centers and state sexual assault coalitions work together with law enforcement, health care providers, and community-based organizations (CBOs) to provide community education and care and support to victims.

LEVELS OF PREVENTION: CRISIS INTERVENTION AND FAMILY VIOLENCE

Family violence is a family crisis and needs intervention. Community health nurses are in a unique position to prevent, identify, and intervene during crisis situations. Because community health nurses encounter people in their own settings, a more accurate assessment with direct observation, discussion, and intervention can occur. The community health nurse's assessment skills, familiarity with the community, and access to resources enhance his ability to help families in crisis. By using the three levels of prevention, the nurse can begin to assist families in a variety of ways to counter problems arising from domestic violence.

Primary Prevention

The cycle of violence within the family can be interrupted. Even when partners, spouses, or parents have been brought up in violent homes by abusive parents, they can learn to rechannel and control their emotions and behaviors and use more appropriate coping strategies. Primary prevention is the most effective level of intervention in terms of promoting clients' health and containing costs. Primary prevention reflects a fundamental human concern for well-being and includes planned activities undertaken by the nurse to prevent an unwanted event from occurring, to protect current health and healthy functioning, and to promote improved states of health for all members of a community. For the community health nurse, any activity that fosters healthful practices will counteract unhealthful influences, thereby empowering an individual or family help prevent a crisis. Health promotion must take into account the physical, psychological, sociocultural, and spiritual needs of the individual and family.

Opportunities for families to improve relationships with their partner or spouse and children may begin with learning social problem-solving skills. Both partners benefit by participating in these learning sessions/opportunities. Assertiveness skills for women provide a foundation on which additional empowerment can build. Many people have not learned positive problem-solving skills that are socially acceptable, while women may have learned passivity and submissiveness in response to their own childhood parenting or from an abusive upbringing.

Healthy self-esteem improves education and occupational success. If poverty is a factor related to the violence, adequate educational preparation and having a successful employee role may eliminate this stressor. Violence occurs across all socioeconomic levels; however, if a family is so impoverished that its basic needs cannot be met, stress can lead vulnerable family members to seek illegal ways to solve their financial problems. Living in neighborhoods where criminal activity is common often leads to increased violence and risk of abuse.

Parenting, one of life's most difficult roles, influences children in their coping strategies, decision-making, and sense of self-confidence. Parenting classes are an important resource to assist parents, particularly parents who are at high risk, such as teens, people with no exposure to children in their upbringing, and people raised in violent and abusive families. Parenting classes offer an opportunity for parents to share information and the stresses of parenting, while learning new strategies for managing their children's behaviors and appropriate physical, emotional, and developmental expectations for their children's ages.

Community health nurses often make home visits to families based on referrals from hospital perinatal departments. During the mother's postpartum stay, a nurse may have noted some inappropriate parenting behaviors or that the parents may meet high-risk parameters set by the hospital, such as being age 17 or younger, being a single parent, or having a history of substance abuse. On the first few visits to the family, the nurse can assess parenting skills and need for further teaching. If a parenting class is recommended, the course should cover age-appropriate content, such as safety, breast-feeding, formula preparation, food progression, anticipatory guidance for growth and development, discipline techniques including behavior modification and time-out, well-baby care, and immunizations. Additional benefits for the parents are the social support they receive from participating with other parents and having the opportunity to share needs and concerns about child rearing.

Home visiting has been formalized into public health nursing model programs around the country, based on two decades of work by David Olds and others. This evidenced-based program has shown that nurse follow-up and interventions during the pregnancy and for the first 2 years of the child's life was effective in preventing child abuse, decreasing the mother's reliance on government assistance, having mothers with longer spacing between their children and fewer subsequent pregnancies, and improving health habits, such as less smoking by mothers (Eckenrode et al., 2010; USDHHS, 2011). In these programs, a nurse visits the mother and child on a regular basis over 1 to 3 years, teaching and role modeling parenting techniques, providing needed support, and initiating necessary referrals. Home visitation by nurses is a means of reducing all-cause mortality among mothers and in first-born children preventable-cause mortality (Olds et al., 2014; Miller, 2015).

The interrelatedness between families and communities cannot be overlooked or underestimated. Neighborhoods need to be enfranchised, developed, and attentive to the needs for health and safety for all community members. Empowered families and communities can take back their neighborhoods from criminals, and their empowerment acts as a source of growth for other families.

Secondary Prevention

Early diagnosis and prompt treatment of the effects of family crisis or violence is the focus at a secondary level of prevention. Secondary prevention seeks to reduce the intensity and duration of a crisis and to promote adaptive behavior. By creating a positive relationship with family members and seeing them in their homes, the community health nurse can often uncover and intervene in a crisis or stop abusive situations.

People in crisis need help. Often, they desperately want help. The crisis, or violence, and its associated disequilibrium, has a twofold effect on the individuals involved: it renders them temporarily helpless and unable to cope on their own, and it makes them especially receptive to outside influence. Community health nurses can implement crisis resolution models to assist clients at the secondary level. The following process has been used successfully in the mental health field by those working on crisis hot lines, in mental health centers, or in emergency departments (James & Gilliland, 2013). These steps are as follows:

1. Establish rapport.
2. Assess the individual and the problem for lethality.
3. Identify major problems and intervene.
4. Deal with feelings.
5. Explore alternatives and coping mechanisms.
6. Develop an action plan.
7. Follow up, including anticipatory planning for coping with future crises.

People in crisis will seek and generally receive some kind of help, but the nature of that help may act in favor of or against a healthy outcome from which the participants can grow and evolve. A client's desire for assistance gives the helping professional a prime opportunity to intervene; this opportunity also presents a challenge to make the intervention as effective as possible (Fig. 20–7). Behaviors found to be helpful in these interventions include the following:

- *Respect confidentiality.* Discussions must occur in private, without other family members present or in within the proximity for hearing. Confidentiality is essential to build trust and ensure the client's safety.
- *Believe and validate the client's experiences.* Listen to and believe the client. Acknowledge the client's feelings, and validate that many others have had similar experiences.
- *Acknowledge any injustice.* In the case of violence, acknowledge that no one deserves to be abused.
- *Respect clients' autonomy.* Respect their right to make life decisions, particularly regarding whether to involve the police. Validate and respect clients' choices. They are the experts in their lives.
- *Help the client plan for future safety.* What past strategies have been successful for self-protection? Does the client

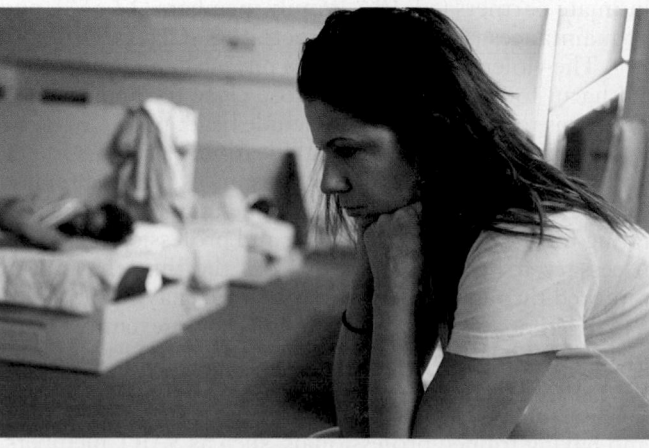

FIGURE 20–7 PHN client in a homeless shelter.

have a safe place to escape to if necessary? If children are involved, what plans are available to protect them? Help clients to recognize danger in their lives.

- *Promote access to community services.* Know the resources in your community. Is there a shelter for battered or homeless clients? A domestic violence hotline? A rape crisis center? Give clients the appropriate phone numbers (James & Gilliland, 2013).

The Quality and Safety Education for Nurses Project [QSEN] provides a guide for preparing future nurses to improve the quality and safety of the health care system in which they work (QSEN Institute, 2014). Knowledge, skills, and attitudes are delineated for the domain of safety. Although framed specifically for acute care settings the domain of safety identifies factors that create a culture of safety such as communication and reporting systems (i.e., mandatory reporting). Effective use of strategies to assess and reduce harm is important when working with families in crisis. Valuing safety, vigilance, monitoring, and reporting are skills necessary for community health nursing practice.

One goal of crisis intervention should be to help clients reestablish a sense of safety and security while allowing them to ventilate their feelings and have those feelings validated. This process helps reestablish equilibrium at as healthy a level as possible and can result in client change and growth. Minimally, the goal is to resolve the immediate crisis and restore clients to their precrisis level of functioning. Ultimately, however, intervention seeks to improve their functioning to a healthier, more mature level that will enable them to cope with and prevent future crises. As discussed earlier, crises tend to be self-limited; intervention time generally lasts from 4 to 8 weeks, with resolution (one way or another) within 2 or 3 months (James & Gilliland, 2013). The urgency of the situation represents a window of opportunity that invites prompt, focused attention by the client and nurse in working together to achieve intervention goals.

Special programs for children who live in homes where crises and violence are chronic include Head Start programs for prekindergarten children who meet certain socioeconomic characteristics. These programs are designed to give children social and academic stimulation, thereby increasing their skills for when they enter kindergarten. Other programs for social skills development may include a Special Friends program designed explicitly for children who have survived abusive situations, or primary intervention programs (PIP), in which the child works with a trained, supportive, and caring adult.

Abuse survivors and those living in homes with domestic violence experience multiple developmental and psychological problems. Children who are experiencing academic and social failure should receive ongoing services as needed through their elementary, middle, and high school grades. Early identification and intervention with conduct-disordered youth ensure that appropriate resources are obtained and, hopefully, that behavior outbursts and violence will be eliminated. School nurses are important interprofessional team members in providing assessments and programs for these youth.

Intervention at the secondary level for adults who experience abuse focuses on women and their children. Shelters for women and children are available in most communities and offer a variety of services, including counseling, classes in self-esteem building and assertiveness training, referrals to or programs for job training, and even money/budgeting and time management classes. Some shelters offer programs that last up to 2 years with progressive independence and employment skill development while the women and their children live in a protected home environment with their addresses kept confidential from abusers.

Depending on the situation that brings the woman to a shelter, the perpetrator may or may not be incarcerated or on probation. If arrested during the most recent violent episode, the abuser may be released, on parole, or incarcerated. Even while incarcerated, the abuser may be able to take part in an anger management class, psychological counseling, substance abuse treatment, Alcoholics Anonymous (AA) meetings, or Narcotics Anonymous (NA) meetings. Visits between the abuser and the children are supervised, if that is part of a court order.

At times, the nurse may be responding to a referral regarding suspected abuse; at other times, an abusive or neglectful situation may be uncovered on a home visit made for another reason. In any case, the community health nurse has an important role in reporting suspected abuse and encouraging the child, partner/spouse, or elder to go to the appropriate facility to seek care and to file required documentation about the abuse (see From the Case Files II).

Reporting Abuse

All states have reporting laws for suspected abuse, although states differ on aspects of the timeline for reporting, who to notify, and the sequence of events. The following steps represent one state's guidelines for reporting suspected child abuse (Child Welfare Information Gateway, 2014):

1. All mandated reporters must report known or suspected abuse.
2. Immediately, or as soon as reasonably possible, a local child protective agency (police department after normal working hours) must be contacted and given a verbal report. During this verbal report, mandated reporters must give their name—which is kept confidential and may be revealed only in court or if the reporter waives confidentiality (others can give information anonymously)—the name and age of the child, the present location of the child, the nature and characteristics of the injury, and any other facts that led the reporter to suspect abuse or that would be helpful to the investigator.
3. Within 2 working days, a written report must be completed by the mandated reporter and filed. If a mandated reporter fails to report known or suspected instances of child abuse, they may be subject to criminal liability, punishable by up to 6 months in jail or a fine of $1,000.

Similar steps are required for nurses when reporting elder abuse. Cases of maltreatment and neglect among elders are reported to a local area agency on aging, Adult Protective Services, or to the police, and a screening/documentation form is used to gather and record pertinent information. Guidelines for filing the report and agency notification are specific within each state.

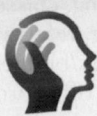

From the Case Files **II**

Community Health Nursing and a Potential Family in Crisis

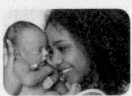

You are a community health nurse working for Smithville Health Department. You are following up on a referral from a community clinic's family planning clinic. The referral was made for a 19-year-old woman, Sandy, who presented in clinic and exhibited inappropriate behaviors with her 6-month-old daughter. In their referral, staff stated that they observed the mother shouting at the child, accusing her of "being spoiled rotten." They added that the mother appeared quite anxious and seemed to have difficulty waiting the 15 minutes for her examination. Although the behaviors described in this referral were insufficient to warrant a report to social services, the staff felt that this young mother would benefit from intervention on the part of the nurse.

You prepare for this home visit by reviewing the medical records of both Sandy and her child to determine whether the family has had previous involvement with social service agencies such as CPS. You find that the maternal grandparents made a referral to Child Welfare on behalf of Sandy when she was 15. They were concerned about the relationship between Sandy and her stepfather. The report cited suspected sexual involvement between the two. An investigation occurred but was inconclusive, and the charges were never pursued.

You also discuss the case with family planning and immunization clinic staff, because the family receives services at both clinics. The staff advises you that they are familiar with Sandy and her husband Nick. They state that their only interaction with Nick was during a family planning clinic 2 months ago. They report that Sandy appeared anxious and in a hurry on that day, stating, "I really need to hurry, Nick is waiting in the car and he gets impatient." Shortly after that, the staff tells you, Nick came running into the clinic shouting, "What the hell is taking you people so long?" He reportedly glared at Sandy, and the two quickly exited the clinic.

You phone the client and advise her that you are a nurse with the local health department. You inform her that nurses often visit new mothers to assist them in finding resources. You add that as a community health nurse, you will be available to talk with her about her child's growth and development.

The client expresses interest in the visit and states, "I want you to show me some things about feeding her and stuff. I need help figuring out what to do at night, she still isn't sleeping much and it's driving me crazy." You advise the client that you will be happy to discuss those issues with her and that you will bring information that you will review with her. You add that you noted in her medical record that the father of the baby is living in the home and assure her that she may involve other family members, including the father of the baby, in the home visit. You jointly decide that the visit will occur the following day at 10:30 AM and that the father of the baby will be present if his work schedule allows.

On the day of the visit, as you walk up the stairs toward the apartment, you notice someone looking at you through the curtains. As you near the apartment door, the curtains close. Your repeated knocking on the door is met with no response. You call the client's name but there is no answer.

1. Would this scenario provoke anxiety for you? How would you deal with your reaction?
2. How is this different from a scenario in the acute care setting in which a supervisor would be readily available?
3. Given this scenario, what actions will you take?
4. If you had been working in the family planning clinic on the day that Nick came in, what, if anything, would you have done differently?
5. As young parents, Nick and Sandy are part of an aggregate that has unique risk factors for parenting. List as many of these risk factors as you can think of and brainstorm about possible community health nursing interventions for each.
6. What methods would you suggest the clinic staff utilize to detect signs and symptoms of physical, sexual, or emotional abuse among this aggregate?

In cases of partner/spousal abuse, adults who are mentally competent cannot be removed involuntarily from the abusive situation. The community health nurse can encourage the victim to leave the perpetrator for the victim's safety until the perpetrator gets professional help and can give information regarding community resources, such as a shelter for women and children. If the adult has a life-threatening injury or illness, medical follow-up must be encouraged; however, the victim may still be reluctant to seek help. At times, another family member or neighbor who witnesses the abusive event calls 911; when the police and paramedics arrive, the victim may have support to seek care and needed protection. A PHN completes a domestic violence screening/documentation form as a part of the official health records for the client.

Tools

Assessment of suspected abuse cannot be overemphasized. The community health nurse may be the only person entering the home of a family in crisis where abuse is occurring. Asking the right questions, being a careful observer, and following the correct reporting process and recording procedures may mean the difference between life and death for a victim of violence.

Displays 20–10, 20–11, and 20–12 consist of three sample tools that the community health nurse and other advocates can use in their role as a mandated reporter. These forms include a Suspected Child Abuse Report, a two-page Medical Report of Suspected Child Abuse, and a Domestic Violence Screening/Documentation Form.

(*Text continues on page 719*)

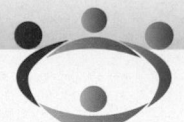

DISPLAY 20–10 SUSPECTED CHILD ABUSE REPORT

SUSPECTED CHILD ABUSE REPORT

To Be Completed by Reporting Party
Pursuant to Penal Code Section 11166

A. CASE IDENTIFICATION

TO BE COMPLETED BY INVESTIGATING CPA

VICTIM NAME: _____

REPORT NO./CASE NAME: _____

DATE OF REPORT: _____

B. REPORTING PARTY

NAME/TITLE

ADDRESS

| PHONE ( ) | DATE OF REPORT | SIGNATURE |

C. REPORT SENT TO

☐ POLICE DEPARTMENT ☐ SHERIFF'S OFFICE ☐ COUNTY WELFARE ☐ COUNTY PROBATION

| AGENCY | ADDRESS |

| OFFICIAL CONTACTED | PHONE ( ) | DATE/TIME |

D. INVOLVED PARTIES

VICTIM

| NAME (LAST, FIRST, MIDDLE) | ADDRESS | BIRTHDATE | SEX | RACE |

| PRESENT LOCATION OF CHILD | | PHONE ( ) |

SIBLINGS

NAME	BIRTHDATE	SEX	RACE	NAME	BIRTHDATE	SEX	RACE
1.				4.			
2.				5.			
3.				6.			

PARENTS

| NAME (LAST, FIRST, MIDDLE) | BIRTHDATE | SEX | RACE | NAME (LAST, FIRST, MIDDLE) | BIRTHDATE | SEX | RACE |

| ADDRESS | | ADDRESS |

| HOME PHONE ( ) | BUSINESS PHONE ( ) | HOME PHONE ( ) | BUSINESS PHONE ( ) |

E. INCIDENT INFORMATION

IF NECESSARY, ATTACH EXTRA SHEET OR OTHER FORM AND CHECK THIS BOX. ☐

| 1. DATE/TIME OF INCIDENT | PLACE OF INCIDENT | *(CHECK ONE)* ☐ OCCURRED ☐ OBSERVED |

IF CHILD WAS IN OUT-OF-HOME CARE AT TIME OF INCIDENT, CHECK TYPE OF CARE:

☐ FAMILY DAY CARE ☐ CHILD CARE CENTER ☐ FOSTER FAMILY HOME ☐ SMALL FAMILY HOME ☐ GROUP HOME OR INSTITUTION

2. TYPE OF ABUSE: *(CHECK ONE OR MORE)* ☐ PHYSICAL ☐ MENTAL ☐ SEXUAL ASSAULT ☐ NEGLECT ☐ OTHER

3. NARRATIVE DESCRIPTION:

4. SUMMARIZE WHAT THE ABUSED CHILD OR PERSON ACCOMPANYING THE CHILD SAID HAPPENED:

5. EXPLAIN KNOWN HISTORY OF SIMILAR INCIDENT(S) FOR THIS CHILD:

SS 8572 (Rev. 1/93)

INSTRUCTIONS AND DISTRIBUTION ON REVERSE

<u>**DO NOT**</u> submit a copy of this form to the Department of Justice (DOJ). A CPA is required under Penal Code Section 11169 to submit to DOJ a Child Abuse Investigation Report Form SS-8583 if (1) an active investigation has been conducted and (2) the incident is <u>**not**</u> unfounded.

Police or Sheriff-WHITE Copy; County Welfare or Probation-BLUE Copy; District Attorney-GREEN Copy; Reporting Party-YELLOW Copy

DISPLAY 20–11 MEDICAL REPORT: SUSPECTED CHILD ABUSE

DOJ 900   84 89220

MEDICAL REPORT—SUSPECTED CHILD ABUSE

HOSPITAL

INSTRUCTIONS: ALL PROFESSIONAL MEDICAL PERSONNEL ARE REQUIRED BY SECTION 11166 OF THE PENAL CODE TO COMPLETE THIS FORM IN CONJUNCTION WITH THE SS 8572 SUSPECTED CHILD ABUSE REPORT WHERE CHILD ABUSE, AS DEFINED BY SECTION 11165 OF THE PENAL CODE, IS SUSPECTED. THE REPORTS, DOJ 900 AND SS 8572, MUST BE SUBMITTED TO A POLICE OR SHERIFF'S DEPARTMENT, OR A COUNTY PROBATION OR WELFARE DEPARTMENT WITHIN 36 HOURS. PROFESSIONAL MEDICAL PERSONNEL MEANS ANY PHYSICIAN AND SURGEON, PSYCHIATRIST, PSYCHOLOGIST, DENTIST, RESIDENT, INTERN, PODIATRIST, CHIROPRACTOR, LICENSED NURSE, DENTAL HYGIENIST OR ANY OTHER PERSON WHO IS CURRENTLY LICENSED UNDER DIVISION 2 (COMMENCING WITH SECTION 500) OF THE BUSINESS AND PROFESSIONS CODE. EACH PART OF THE FORM MUST BE COMPLETED UNLESS INAPPLICABLE. IN FILLING OUT THIS FORM, NO CIVIL LIABILITY ATTACHES AND NO CONFIDENTIALITY IS BREACHED.

I. GENERAL INFORMATION Print or type

PATIENT'S NAME

HOSPITAL ID NO.

ADDRESS	CITY	COUNTY	STATE	PHONE

AGE	BIRTHDATE	RACE	SEX	DATE AND TIME OF ARRIVAL	MODE OF TRANSPORTATION	DATE AND TIME OF DISCHARGE

ACCOMPANIED TO HOSPITAL BY: NAME	ADDRESS	CITY	STATE	RELATIONSHIP

PHONE REPORT MADE TO	ID NO.	DEPARTMENT	PHONE	RESPONDING OFFICER/AGENCY

NAME OF: ☐ FATHER ☐ STEPFATHER	ADDRESS	CITY	COUNTY	HOME PHONE	BUS. PHONE	AGE/DOB

NAME OF: ☐ MOTHER ☐ STEPMOTHER	ADDRESS	CITY	COUNTY	HOME PHONE	BUS. PHONE	AGE/DOB

SIBLINGS: LAST NAME, FIRST	DOB	LAST NAME, FIRST	DOB	LAST NAME, FIRST	DOB

II. MEDICAL EXAMINATION

A. History   1. EXPLANATION OF INJURIES BY PARENT OR PERSON ACCOMPANYING CHILD (LOCATION, DATE, TIME AND CIRCUMSTANCES)

2. PATIENT'S STATEMENT EXPLAINING INJURY (PARAPHRASE)

3. PATIENT'S EMOTIONAL REACTION TO EXAMINATION (SUBMISSIVE, COMPLIANT, ETC.)

4. PREVIOUS HISTORY OF CHILD ABUSE (IF KNOWN)

B. Sexual Assault   Perform exam only if necessary.

1. ACTS COMMITTED: NOTE—COITUS, FELLATIO, CUNNILINGUS, SODOMY

2. DURING ASSAULT
☐ VAGINAL PENETRATION (HOW)

☐ ANAL PENETRATION (HOW)

EJACULATION: ☐ VAGINAL ☐ ORAL ☐ ANAL ☐ OTHER:

☐ CONDOM USED ☐ VOMITED ☐ LOSS OF CONSCIOUSNESS ☐ OTHER:

3. AFTER ASSAULT:
☐ WIPED/WASHED ☐ BATHED ☐ DOUCHED ☐ VOMITED ☐ CHANGED CLOTHES ☐ BRUSHED TEETH ☐ DEFECATED ☐ OTHER:

C. Physical Examination	DATE AND TIME OF EXAM	DATE AND TIME OF ASSAULT	BP	PULSE	RESP	TEMP

HEIGHT	WEIGHT	HEAD CIRCUM	LAST TETANUS	KNOWN ALLERGIES	CURRENT MEDICATION

DIAGNOSTIC DATA

Check if indicated and incorporate results in written examination at left

☐ X-rays (skull, chest, longbone, full skeletal)

☐ Bleeding, coagulation, tourniquet, tests

☐ Funduscopic

☐ Other

DISPLAY 20-11 MEDICAL REPORT: SUSPECTED CHILD ABUSE (Continued)

DOJ 900

DATE	HOSPITAL ID NO.	HOSPITAL

PHYSICAL EXAMINATION (CONTINUED) LOCATE AND DESCRIBE IN DETAIL ANY INJURIES OR FINDINGS: TRAUMA, BRUISES, ERYTHEMA, EXCORIATIONS, LACERATIONS, WOUNDS. TRACE OUTLINE USED AND INDICATE LOCATION OF WOUNDS/LACERATIONS USING 'X' FOR SUPERFICIAL, 'O' FOR DEEP. SHADE FOR BRUISES OR BURNS. BESIDE EACH INJURY INDICATED NOTE COLOR, SIZE, PATTERN, TEXTURE, AND SENSATION. WRITE OVER UNUSED OUTLINES. DESCRIBE IN DETAIL SHAPE OF ARM OR OTHER BRUISES WHICH MAY INDICATE FORCE.

D. PELVIC A PELVIC EXAMINATION SHOULD NOT BE PERFORMED UNLESS THE PARENT, GUARDIAN OR MINOR CONSENT OR UNLESS NECESSARY AS PART OF TREATMENT. SEE DEPARTMENT OF HEALTH REGULATIONS TITLE 22, DIVISION 2, VICTIMS OF SEXUAL ASSAULT. SAME INSTRUCTIONS AS GENERAL PHYSICAL. IN ADDITION, NOTE PUBIC HAIR COMBINGS WHERE INDICATED, DRIED SECRETIONS AND RECENT INJURIES TO HYMEN. TRACE AND OUTLINE AS ABOVE.

V. SPECIMENS

STAINS/FOREIGN MATERIALS
(WHEN INDICATED)

LOOSE HAIR	____	FINGERNAIL SCRAPINGS	____
BLOOD	____	DIRT OR GRAVEL	____
THREADS	____	VEGETATION	____
GRASS	____	CLOTHING	____
DRIED SECRETIONS	____		

	SLIDES	SWABS
VAGINAL	____	____
RECTAL	____	____
ORAL	____	____
ASPIRATES/WASHINGS	____	____
BITE MARKS	____	____
OTHER	____	____

III. DIAGNOSTIC IMPRESSION OF TRAUMA AND INJURIES

IV. TREATMENT/DISPOSITION OF PATIENT

A. ☐ GC CULTURE ☐ VDRL ☐ PREGNANCY TEST ☐ POST COITAL ESTROGEN ☐ VD PROPHYLAXIS ☐ OTHER:

MOTILE SPERM: ☐ PRESENCE ☐ ABSENCE ☐ NOT TAKEN ☐ FAMILY ASSESSMENT BY: ☐ NOT ORDERED

B. ORDERS:

PATIENT'S SAMPLES TIME OF COLLECTION AT MD DISCRETION

BLOOD	____
HAIR FROM HEAD	____
SALIVA	____
HAIR FROM PUBIC AREA	____

C. DISPOSITION: ☐ ADMIT TRANSFERRED TO:

☐ RELEASED ACCOMPANIED BY: NAME   ADDRESS   RELATIONSHIP

D. FOLLOW-UP WITHIN:

☐ MEDICAL
____ HRS ____ DAYS

☐ SOCIAL SERVICES
____ HRS ____ DAYS

☐ PRIVATE MD
____ HRS ____ DAYS

☐ OTHER
____ HRS ____ DAYS

I HAVE RECEIVED THE INDICATED ITEMS AS EVIDENCE AND A COPY OF THIS REPORT.

OFFICER: ID NO.:   DATE:

NURSE   SIGNATURE OF EXAMINATION PHYSICIAN

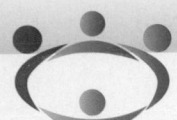

DISPLAY 20–12 DOMESTIC VIOLENCE SCREENING/DOCUMENTATION FORM

DV SCREEN
- ☐ Screened
    - ☐ Yes
    - ☐ No
    - ☐ Probable/Suspected DV
- ☐ Not Screened

<u>Routinely Screen at Each Visit</u>
"Because violence is so common in women's lives, I've begun to ask about it routinely."

<u>Ask Direct Questions</u>
"I'm concerned that your injuries/symptoms may have been caused by someone hurting you. Is this what happened to you?"
            -OR-
"Has your intimate partner or ex-partner ever physically hurt you? Have they ever *threatened* to hurt you or someone close to you?"

<u>Assess Patient Safety</u>

- ☐ Yes ☐ No Is patient afraid to go home?
- ☐ Yes ☐ No Has physical violence increased in severity over past years?
- ☐ Yes ☐ No Have threats of homicide been made?
- ☐ Yes ☐ No Have threats of suicide been made?
- ☐ Yes ☐ No Is alcohol or substance abuse also a problem?
- ☐ Yes ☐ No Is there a gun in the house?
- ☐ Yes ☐ No Is patient afraid of their partner?
- ☐ Yes ☐ No Was safety plan discussed?

<u>Referrals</u>
- ☐ hotline number given
- ☐ legal referral made
- ☐ shelter number given
- ☐ in-house referral made
- ☐ discharge instructions given

Date _____ Patient ID#_____
Patient Name _____
Provider Name _____
Patient Pregnant? Yes ____ No ____

Describe frequency and severity of present and past abuse (use direct quotes as much as possible)

_____
_____
_____
_____
_____
_____

Describe location and extent of injury

_____
_____
_____
_____
_____
_____

<u>Indicate where injury was observed</u>

☐ Yes ☐ No Photographs taken?
☐ Yes ☐ No Consent to be photographed?
(Attach Photographs) + Appropriate Form

Tertiary Prevention

Tertiary prevention focuses on the rehabilitation of the family from the violence and crisis they have sustained. The family may never again have the same connections because partners may separate—by choice, motivated by fear or hatred; by court order, if the perpetrator is incarcerated; or by death. If the family chooses to stay together, long-term intervention for all family members is needed to establish a climate more conducive to family normalcy. Many of the services discussed as part of the secondary level of prevention are continued into the tertiary prevention phase to promote healing and to restore and promote family growth.

If incarceration is a part of tertiary prevention, the effects of having one family member living in this environment must be factored into the services and support provided by the community health nurse to the family as a whole (see Chapter 30 for information on working in correctional facilities). Even if the partner/spouse has separated from the perpetrator emotionally and/or legally, the perpetrator usually has legal rights to see the children. This may mean that other family members, usually from the abuser's side of the family, can bring the children to the prison to visit their parent. Just making arrangements for these visits can cause stress to the visitors. The community health nurse needs to be aware of the complicated dynamics and emotional stress such difficult situations can produce for all family members. The victim-perpetrator relationship is as complex as the forces that created the violence and abuse.

FAMILIES FACING VIOLENCE FROM OUTSIDE THE FAMILY

The concern of violence coming into the family from outside the home, often beyond the family's control, is a relatively new phenomenon in the United States. There has always been some degree of violence that affects families in their homes, such as burglaries, or at times murder, or abduction. Increasingly, however, home invasion, a form of forced entry to terrorize family members, is a violent crime perpetrated most frequently by strangers. Other forms of violence of which families are more aware include the potential for terrorist activities through planned community violence (such as the 9/11 attacks or the Sandy Hook school shooting) and biologic, chemical, or radioactive actions (see Chapter 17). Communities have developed resources such as the National Organization for Victim Assistance (NOVA) and crisis response teams (CRT), to assist individuals and groups experiencing a disaster or violent event (e.g., child murder or school shootings).

Home invasion is an increasing new form of terror. It occurs mainly in large cities, although rural areas are not immune. *Home invasion* is the purposeful and sudden entry into a home by force while the family is home and awake. The effectiveness of this form of terror relies on surprise. Motivation may be material or thrill; household belongings are frequently stolen while family members are incapacitated by being bound, blindfolded, and/or gagged. In some cases, family members are killed. Often, the perpetrators are under the influence of drugs or alcohol, and at times, the violence may be gang related.

Violence, terrorism, and war profoundly affect individuals, families, and society (Devakumar et al., 2014). Lethal violence can create a climate of fear and uncertainty. Intentional homicide victimizes the family and the community of the victim (United Nations Office on Drugs and Crime, 2016). Fear of violence can create psychological and physiologic stress reactions similar to the sensations that occur when one actually experiences the violence. These fears should not be ignored. It is important to understand the impact of violence on the health of individuals, families, and the community (Joyce, Najera-Aguiree, Brown, & Sievers, 2014).

So many forces in the social, cultural, and physical environment conspire against an individual's desire to change behavior. Poverty, associated with overcrowding, lack of institutional relationships and low levels of community participation, and sanctions provide a catalyst for community violence. Historically, society has depended on the criminal justice system to respond to community violence with emphasis on deterrence and incarceration, which has limited prevention capacity. Community correctional facilities provide a form of rehabilitation in some states, to facilitate transitioning of prisoners back to community after incarceration.

To put primary prevention into practice an integrated multifaceted approach is required. The **Spectrum of Prevention** offers a systematic framework for developing effective and sustainable primary prevention programs (Cohen, Chavez, & Chehimi, 2010). The *Spectrum* identifies multiple levels for community intervention: (1) strengthening individual knowledge and skills, (2) promoting community education, (3) educating providers, (4) fostering coalitions and networks, (5) changing organizational practices, and (6) influencing policy and legislation. When used together, these levels are complementary and create synergy that results in greater effectiveness (Cohen et al., 2010).

Nurses may work at each level of the *Spectrum*, by educating individuals and high-risk target populations, working on coalitions to foster increased awareness and use of screening tools by health care providers, and working with multisector partnerships to foster change in workplace, organizational, and community policy. Nurses may work with extended family members of the victims or families who have reported such a happening in their neighborhood and are now fearful of a reoccurrence. See Chapters 11 and 12. The role of the nurse includes four steps discussed in the generic approach to crisis intervention (see discussion in "Generic Approach").

METHODS OF CRISIS INTERVENTION

Crisis intervention in community health nursing uses either a generic or individual approach, or both (Fig. 20–8). For the majority of crisis encounters, the generic approach is more appropriate. Family violence is a major situational crisis in which community health nurses intervene. However, many other situational and developmental crises affect families, and these families are benefited by the skills of the community health nurse. Newly recognized crises include community violence coming into the home and the potential of terrorism at home.

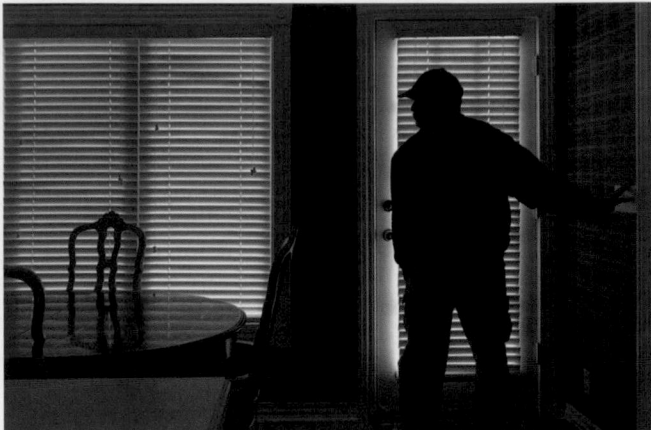

FIGURE 20–8 Crime is a type of community violence that can affect families.

Generic Approach

The generic approach creates interventions to fit a particular type of crisis, focusing on the nature and course of the crisis rather than on the psychodynamic of each client (James & Gilliland, 2013). Crisis intervention using the generic approach is tailored to a specific kind of crisis, situational or developmental, and comprises four important elements: (1) use of adaptive behavior and coping strategies, (2) support of the individual/family, (3) preparation for the practical and emotional future, and (4) anticipatory guidance.

As an example, the generic approach is used with families experiencing child abuse. The child may be in foster care while the family receives needed services and rebuilds itself. The nurse encourages the parents to discuss and analyze their feelings, teaches stress reduction techniques and positive coping skills, and creates a supportive, caring atmosphere, especially through self-help groups such as Parents Anonymous. The nurse can help individual family members strengthen their self-esteem by encouraging positive interpersonal relationships. The community health nurse also teaches needed parenting skills, providing anticipatory guidance, so that parents are prepared to raise their children with consistent and age-appropriate discipline techniques.

The generic approach does not require advanced professional psychotherapy skills. More importantly, this approach works well with families, groups, and even communities in crisis. The community health nurse may work with a group of cancer clients, abused elders, adolescents struggling with developmental crisis, or an entire community recovering from a natural or man-made disaster. The generic approach allows the nurse to intervene with any group of people who have a crisis in common. This approach also offers a broad base of support because the crisis group members can provide resources for one another beyond those brought by the nurse.

Individual Approach

The individual approach is used for clients who do not respond to the generic approach or who need special therapy. Individual crisis intervention should not be confused with individual psychotherapy, which tends to focus on a client's developmental past. In contrast, crisis intervention directs treatment toward the immediate state of disequilibrium, identifying its causes and developing coping mechanisms. Family members or significant others are included during the process of crisis resolution. An entire group may need this type of intervention. If this approach is needed, clients should be referred to a professional with specialized training.

ROLE OF THE COMMUNITY HEALTH NURSE IN CARING FOR FAMILIES IN CRISIS

Crisis intervention in community health assumes that clients have resources. If their potential for managing stressful events can be tapped, people in crisis will need

Table 20–2	Levels of Prevention to Promote Crisis Resolution	
Phase	**Goals**	**Interventions**
Primary prevention		
Precrisis	Health promotion	Anticipatory guidance
	Disease prevention	Reduce factors that increase vulnerability
	Education	Reduce hazards in some events (safety and multiplicity of stressors)
		Reinforce positive coping strategies
		Mobilize social support and other resources
Secondary prevention		
Crisis	Reduction of stress load	Assist with reaction to the event and functioning
	Cure or restoration of function	Allow behavior: dependence, grief
		Set goals with client
		Refer to resources
Tertiary prevention		
Postcrisis	Rehabilitation and maintenance	Promote adaptation to a changed level of wellness
		Promote interdependence
		Reinforce newly learned behaviors, lifestyle changes, coping strategies
		Explore application of learned behaviors to new situations
		Identification and use of additional resources

minimal direct assistance. In accordance with the self-care concept, crisis intervention seeks to identify and build on client strengths. James and Gilliland (2013) outlined a series of four steps for intervention during crisis: assessment, planning, intervention, and resolution. Interventions to promote crisis resolution are presented using the three levels of prevention in Table 20–2.

Assessment and Nursing Diagnosis

Initially, the nurse must assess the nature of the crisis and the client's response to it. How severe is the problem, and what risks are the clients facing? Are other people also at risk? Assessment must be rapid but thorough and focused on specific areas.

First, the nurse concentrates on the immediate problem during the assessment. Why have clients asked for help right now? How do they define the problem? What precipitated the crisis? When did it occur? Was it a sudden accidental or situational event, or a slower developmental one?

Next, the nurse focuses on the clients' perceptions of the event. What does the crisis mean to them, and how do they think it will affect their future? Are they viewing the situation realistically? When a crisis occurs to a family or group, some members see the situation differently from others. During intervention, all family members should be encouraged to express themselves, to talk about the crisis, and to share their feelings about its meaning. Acceptance of the wide range of feelings is important.

Determine who is available to offer support to the individual or family. Consider family, friends, clergy, other professionals, community members, and agencies. Who are the clients close to, and whom do they trust? One advantage of group intervention is that the members provide some of this support for one another. In subsequent sessions, the quality of support should be evaluated. Sometimes, a well-meaning individual can worsen the situation or deter clients from facing and coping with reality.

Finally, the nurse assesses the clients' coping abilities. Have they had similar kinds of experiences in the past? What techniques have they tried in this situation, and if they did not work, why not? Clients should be encouraged to think of other stress-relieving techniques, perhaps ones they have used in the past, and to try them.

The nurse gathers all of these data and mentally begins to form nursing diagnoses. As a plan of care is developed for the client, these nursing diagnoses are formalized in writing. Standardized nursing diagnoses are available for reference, or the agency where the nurse works may have a preferred format for nursing diagnoses. These nursing diagnoses are effective tools for the nurse to begin planning interventions. When the violence problem is more community centered the Omaha System of documentation and information management may be useful as a nomenclature as it comprehensively includes the family and community as clients or modifiers. The system consists of three relational, reliable, and valid components used together: the Problem Classification Scheme, Intervention Scheme, and the Problem Rating Scale for Outcomes (Martin & Monsen, 2015). The Problem Classification Scheme includes neighborhood/workplace safety in the environmental domain. The benefits of using the Omaha system enables interdisciplinary problem identification and functioning with intervention targets that reflect communication with health team members across multiple settings, using electronic health records (Bowles, 2011; Bowles et al., 2013; Martin & Monsen, 2015).

Planning Therapeutic Interventions

Several factors influence clients' reaction to crises. Nurses should try to determine what factors are affecting clients before making intervention plans. The major balancing factors—clients' perceptions of the event, situational supports, human resources, and clients' coping skills—have been assessed in the first step (James & Gilliland, 2013). While continuing to explore these, the nurse now also considers the clients' age, past experiences with similar types of situations, sociocultural and religious influences, general health status, and the actual assets and liabilities of the situation. This assessment helps clarify the situation and gives the nurse an opportunity to further encourage the clients' participation in the resolution process. If clients are defensive, resistant, and rigid, they are not processing clearly and can complete only simple tasks. It will take time before these clients can begin to solve problems related to the effects of the crisis on themselves and the loss they are experiencing, but the nurse will want to encourage them to reach this level.

A therapeutic plan is based on multiple factors:

- The kind of crisis (situational or developmental, acute or chronically recurring)
- The effect the crisis is having on clients' lives (can they still work, go to school, and keep house, or are they secured within their home for an indefinite period, not knowing whether other family members have survived a major natural or man-made crisis?)
- Where they are in coming to resolution of the crisis
- The ways in which significant others are affected and respond
- Their level of preparation for such a crisis
- The clients' strengths and available resources

Using this problem-solving process, the nurse and clients develop a plan. They review the event that precipitated the crisis, obvious symptoms, and the disruption in the clients' lives. The plan may focus on several areas. For instance, clients may need to grasp intellectually the meaning of the crisis, to engage in greater expression of feelings, or work both on the intellectual and emotional aspects. Part of the plan may be directed toward finding appropriate and safe shelter, counseling, or physical care. Another part may focus on helping clients identify and use more effective coping techniques or locate supportive agencies and resources. The plan may also include development of realistic goals for the future.

Implementation

During implementation, communication between the nurse and clients is important. Discussions about what is happening, reviewing the family's plan and rationale for this approach, and making appropriate changes are necessary parts of this communication. Assigning definite activities at the end of each session will help clients try out different solutions and evaluate various coping behaviors (Gambrill, 2013). Using the following guidelines is helpful during implementation:

1. *Demonstrate acceptance of clients.* A crisis often shatters the ego. Clients need to feel the support of a positive, caring person who does not judge their feelings or behavior. Some negative expressions, such as anger, withdrawal, and denial, are normal aspects of the crisis phase. Accept them as normal.
2. *Help clients confront crisis.* Clients need to face and discuss the situation. Expressing their feelings reduces tension and improves reality perception. Recounting what has actually occurred may be painful, but it helps clients confront the crisis. Do not assume that once clients have told about the event, no further recounting is necessary. Each time the story is told, the client comes closer to dealing realistically with the crisis.
3. *Help clients find facts.* Distorted ideas and unknown factors of the situation create additional tension and may lead to maladaptive responses. For instance, it would help inexperienced parents to know that children younger than 2 years of age cannot deliberately misbehave. Facts about childhood development and parenting training may be important for preventing crisis.
4. *Help clients express feelings openly.* Suppressed feelings can be harmful. For instance, a widow may feel guilty that she is glad her husband is gone. Expression of such feelings helps reduce tension and gives clients an opportunity to deal with them.
5. *Do not offer false reassurance.* Clients need to face reality, not avoid it. A statement such as "Don't worry, it will all work out" is demeaning and meaningless. Instead, make positive statements about faith in the clients' ability to cope: "It is a very difficult situation, but I believe you will be able to deal with it."
6. *Discourage clients from blaming others.* Clients often blame others as a way to avoid reality and the responsibility for problem-solving. Withhold judgment when clients blame others, but point out other causal factors and avenues for dealing with the situation.
7. *Help clients seek out coping mechanisms.* Explore and test old and new techniques to reduce stress and anxiety. Ask questions. What are the things that need to be done? What do clients think they can do? This assistance gives clients more adaptive energy to work toward resolution.
8. *Encourage clients to accept help.* Denial in the early phases of crisis cuts off help. Encouraging clients to acknowledge the problem is a first step toward acceptance of help. Often, clients fear the loss of their independence and the invasion of their privacy. A client may say, "We ought to be able to handle this problem." At this point, the community health nurse can reassure clients that people in a crisis of this sort almost always need help. Preparing people to accept help enables them to make the best use of what others have to offer.
9. *Promote development of new positive relationships.* Clients who have lost significant others through unintentional or intentional death, divorce, incarceration, or an act of perpetrated violence should be encouraged to find new connections, purpose, and people to fill the void and provide needed supports and satisfactions.

Evaluation of Crisis Resolution and Anticipatory Planning

In the final step, clients and the nurse evaluate, stabilize, and plan for the future. Evaluating the outcome of the intervention might address the following:

- Are the clients using effective coping skills and exhibiting appropriate behavior?
- Are adequate resources and support persons available?
- Is the diagnosed problem solved?
- Have the desired results been accomplished?

Analysis of these outcomes will provide a greater understanding for coping with future crises.

To stabilize the change that has occurred, identify and reinforce all of the positive coping mechanisms and behaviors. Discuss why they are effective, and explore ways to use them in future stressful situations. Summarize the crisis experience, emphasizing the clients' successes with coping, reconfirm their progress, and reinforce their self-confidence. It is especially important to point to the evidence that the client has reached their pre crisis level, or an even higher level of functioning.

Clients' plans for the future should include setting realistic goals and means to implement them. Review with clients how their handling of the present crisis can help them cope with, minimize, or preferably prevent future crises.

SUMMARY

Crisis is a temporary state of severe disequilibrium for persons who face a threatening situation. A crisis is a state that individuals can neither avoid nor solve with their usual coping abilities and occurs when some force disrupts normal functioning, thereby causing a loss of balance or normalcy in life. Crises create tension; subsequently, efforts are made to solve the problem and reduce the tension. If such efforts meet with failure, people feel upset, redefine the situation, and try other solutions, and if failure continues, the person eventually reaches the breaking point.

Two main types of crisis are developmental and situational. Developmental crises are disruptions that occur during transitional periods in normal growth and development. These transitions usually have a gradual onset and are often predictable. Situational crises are precipitated by an unexpected external event and occur suddenly, sometimes without warning.

Family violence constitutes a unique crisis for the victim and the entire family and is becoming disturbingly prevalent in the world. Historically, family violence is not new. Only in the last half century of our nation's history have laws and societal concerns been raised about the treatment of spouse/partners, children, and seniors. Although advances in human rights have been made, abuses against women and children remain socially and culturally accepted in some countries, and attitudes have been slow to change.

Child abuse occurs among children of all ages, from infancy through the teen years, and may be physical, emotional, and/or sexual. Neglect and sexual exploitation are additional forms of child abuse. Neglect may be described as general neglect or specific, such as medical or educational neglect. Child abuse, such as shaken baby syndrome or Munchausen syndrome by proxy, is sometimes identified only on autopsy. Teen dating violence, violence during pregnancy, and VAW in general constitutes partner/spousal abuse. Finally, a most unsettling form of violence—elder abuse, neglect, and exploitation—is occurring more frequently than previously suspected.

New and unexpected forms of violence are becoming a reality in our unsettled world. Within communities, violence comes into the home in the form of Internet crimes against children, child abductions, and home invasions. Globally, terrorist groups threaten attacks on civilians in the United States and abroad. For people in the Unites States, this form of terror is a new reality. Preparation against and survival of such attacks is a new concern for most Americans, and the community health nurse has an important role to play (see Chapter 17). Community violence creates fear and uncertainty and impacts individuals and families that may live, work, play, and pray in close proximity.

Community health nurses use three levels of prevention when working with families. Primary prevention focuses on providing people with the skills and resources to prevent violent situations. Secondary prevention involves immediate intervention at the time of the violent episode. This secondary level includes providing different services for each family member, such as medical attention, emotional support, and police involvement. Tertiary prevention offers family rebuilding services and helps the family establish equilibrium with a structure that may be different, but healthier. The *Spectrum of Prevention* offers a multidimensional approach to building community capacity to address issues of violence.

People in crisis need and often seek help. Crisis intervention builds on these two phenomena to achieve its primary goal—reestablishment of equilibrium. The two major methods of crisis intervention are the generic and the individual approaches. The generic approach is used with groups of people involved in the same type of crisis, such as rape victims, mothers who have lost children because of drunken driving, or a family experiencing child abuse. The individual approach is used if clients do not respond to the generic approach or need additional therapy. Crisis intervention begins with assessment of the situation, followed by planning a therapeutic intervention. The nurse then implements and carries out the intervention, building on the strengths and self-care ability of clients. Crisis intervention concludes with resolution and anticipatory planning to avert possible future crises.

Regardless of the method of intervention the community health nurse uses, the steps of the nursing process provide a framework within which to intervene. Assessing the family's assets and liabilities, their willingness to change, and the nature of the violence helps the nurse form a nursing diagnosis. With this diagnosis, the nurse can begin to plan appropriate interventions and implement plans in concert with the family. Evaluation of the intervention techniques provides the nurse with new data to assist with ongoing assessment of the family's progress and additional anticipatory guidance needs.

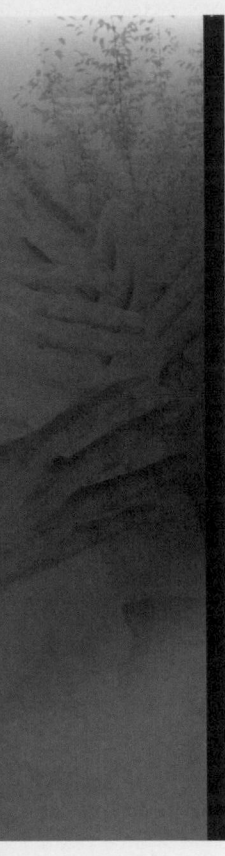

ACTIVITIES TO PROMOTE **CRITICAL THINKING**

1. What are the major differences between a developmental and a situational crisis? Give examples of each from personal experiences.
2. Describe a developmental crisis experienced by a family. What was this family's response? Describe some actions a PHN might have taken (alone or within an interdisciplinary team) to help the family cope with the crisis.
3. Search news sources (e.g., news programs, Internet news) for examples of developmental or situational crises occurring to families. Analyze the situations and anticipate what the role of a community health nurse would be during the crises selected.
4. Family violence is a significant public health problem. Assume that a battered wife becomes a community health nurse's client, and the nurse suspects there may be more women with this problem in the community. Describe how the nurse might provide assistance using the crisis intervention steps. Then discuss how a three-level preventive program might be instituted in the community.
5. Talk with a PHN or social worker that has experience in child abuse cases. What are the most frustrating aspects of their job and why? Do they feel that the system can protect children from their abusers and why or why not? If possible, discuss cases (no names) dealing with physical, emotional, and sexual abuse, as well as neglect. How can nurses be more attuned to signs and symptoms of abuse?
6. With a group of fellow students, explore the child abuse and domestic violence statistics for your city, county, and state. Compare these with national statistics. Research available programs at each level to address these problems. If possible, volunteer at a battered women's shelter to learn more about this problem.
7. Research statistics and evidence-based practice related to Veteran's health and domestic violence. Does this population (e.g., active military, returning veterans) have higher rates of spousal abuse than the general population? Does the Veterans Administration offer any special programs to address this issue (e.g., for the serviceman, spouse)?

REFERENCES

Abraham, M., Kondis, J., & Merritt, D. F. (2016). Case series: Vaginal rupture injuries following sexual assault in children and adolescents. *Journal of Pediatric and Adolescent Gynecology, 29*(3), e49–e52. doi: 10.1016/j.jpag.2015.12.009.

Administration for Children and Families (ACF). (2013a). *Child maltreatment 2013.* Retrieved from https://www.acf.hhs.gov/sites/default/files/cb/cm2013.pdf

Administration for Children and Families (ACF). (2013b). *National survey of child and adolescent well-being (NSCAW).* Retrieved from http://www.acf.hhs.gov/sites/default/files/cb/cm2013.pdf#page=6

Administration for Children and Families (ACF). (2014). *Human Rights Council—Child rights connect.* Retrieved from http://www.childrightsconnect.org/connect-with-the-un-2/human-rights-council/

Administration for Children and Families (ACF). (2015). *Child victims of human trafficking.* Retrieved from http://www.acf.hhs.gov/program/endtrafficking

Administration on Aging. (2015). *What is elder abuse?* Retrieved from www.aoa.gov/AoA_programs/elder_rights/EA_prevention/whatisEA.aspx

Allen, K. A. (2014). The neonatal nurse's role in preventing abusive head trauma. *Advances in Neonatal Care, 14*(5), 336–342.

American Academy of Pediatrics (AAP). (2015). *Abusive head trauma (shaken baby syndrome).* Retrieved from https://www.aap.org/en-us/about-the-aap/aap-press-room/aap-press-room-media-center/Pages/Abusive-Head-Trauma-Fact-Sheet.aspx

American Association of Suicidology (AAS). (2014). *Warning signs.* Retrieved from http://www.suicidology.org/resources/warning-signs

American Congress of Obstetricians and Gynecologists. (2012). *Intimate partner violence.* Retrieved from http://www.acog.org/Resources-And-Publications/Committee-Opinions/Committee-on-Health-Care-for-Underserved-Women/Intimate-Partner-Violence

American Foundation for Suicide Prevention (AFSP). (2016). *Suicide warning signs.* Retrieved from http://afsp.org/about-suicide/risk-factors-and-warning-signs/

Bowles, K. H. (2011, July). Achieving meaningful use with standardized data. *Online Journal of Nursing Informatics, 15*(2), 1–2.

Bowles, K. H., Potashnik, S., Ratcliffe, S. J., Rosenberg, M., Shih, N., Topaz, M., ... Naylor, M. D. (2013). Conducting research using the electronic health record across multi-hospital systems. *The Journal of Nursing Administration, 43*(6), 355–360.

Breiding, M. J., Smith, S. G., Basile, K. C., Walters, M. L., Chen, J., & Merrick, M. T. (2014). Prevalence and characteristics of sexual violence, stalking, and intimate partner violence victimization: National intimate partner and sexual violence survey. USA, 2011. *Morbidity and Mortality Weekly Report, 63*(SS08), 1–18. Retrieved from http://www.cdc.gov/mmwr/preview/mmwrhtml/ss6308a1.htm?s_cid=ss6308a1_e

Brenick, A., Shattuck, J., Donlan, A., Duh, S., & Zurbriggen, E. L. (2014). Empowering children with safety skills: An evaluation of the Kidpower Everyday Safety-Skills Program. *Children and Youth Services Review, 44*, 152–162.

Bridges, W. (1980). *Transitions: Making sense of life's changes* (2nd ed.). Cambridge, MA: Perseus Publishing.

Bridges, W. (2001). *The way of transition: Embracing life's most difficult moments.* Cambridge, MA: Perseus Publishing.

Bureau of Justice Statistics (BJS). (2013). *Homicide in the U.S. known to law enforcement, 2011.* Retrieved from http://www.bjs.gov/index.cfm?ty=pbdetail&iid=4863

Cabral, R. (2014). Identifying cases of fabricated, exaggerated or induced illness. *British Journal of School Nursing, 9*(2), 78–82.

Carrington, A. M. (2014). The vortex of violence: Moving beyond the cycle and engaging clients in change. *British Journal of Social Work, 44*, 451–468.

Catalano, S. (2012). *Stalking victims in the United States—revised.* Retrieved from http://www.bjs.gov/index.cfm?ty=pbdetail&iid=1211

Centers for Disease Control and Prevention (CDC). (2011a). *Healthy people 2010 final review.* Retrieved from http://www.cdc.gov/nchs/data/hpdata2010/hp2010_final_review.pdf

Centers for Disease Control and Prevention (CDC). (2011b). *The national intimate partner and sexual violence survey: 2010 summary* report. Retrieved from http://www.cdc.gov/violenceprevention/intimatepartnerviolence

Centers for Disease Control and Prevention (CDC). (2012). *CDC releases 2013 Youth Risk Behavioral Survey (YRBS) results*. Retrieved from http://www.cdc.gov/Features/YRBS

Centers for Disease Control and Prevention (CDC). (2013). *Help stop violence before it happens*. Retrieved from http://vetoviolence.cdc.gov

Centers for Disease Control and Prevention (CDC). (2014a). *Adolescent health: Healthy People 2020*. Retrieved from http://www.healthy-people.gov/2020/topics-objectives/topic/Adolescent-Health

Centers for Disease Control and Prevention (CDC). (2014b). *Adverse Child Experiences (ACE) study*. Retrieved from http://www.cdc.gov/violenceprevention/acestudy/

Centers for Disease Control and Prevention (CDC). (2014c). *LGBT youth*. Retrieved from http://www.cdc.gov/lgbthealth/youth.htm

Centers for Disease Control and Prevention (CDC). (2014d). *Rape Prevention and Education (RPE) program*. Retrieved from http://www.cdc.gov/violenceprevention/rpe/

Centers for Disease Control and Prevention (CDC). (2014e). *Sexual violence: Facts at a glance*. Retrieved from http://www.cdc.gov/violenceprevention/pdf/sv-datasheet-a.pdf

Centers for Disease Control and Prevention (CDC). (2014f). *Youth risk behavior surveillance, United States, 2013*. Retrieved from http://www.cdc.gov/mmwr/pdf/ss/ss6304.pdf

Centers for Disease Control and Prevention (CDC). (2014g). *Understanding sexual violence. Fact sheet 2014*. Retrieved from http://www.cdc.gov/violenceprevention/pdf/sv-factsheet.pdf

Centers for Disease Control and Prevention (CDC). (2015a). *Bullying research: Featured topic*. Retrieved from http://www.cdc.gov/ViolencePrevention/index.html

Centers for Disease Control and Prevention (CDC). (2015b). *Dating Matters® initiative*. Retrieved from http://www.cdc.gov/violenceprevention/datingmatters/index.html

Centers for Disease Control and Prevention (CDC). (2015c). *Dating Matters® initiative funded programs*. Retrieved from http://www.cdc.gov/violenceprevention/datingmatters

Centers for Disease Control and Prevention (CDC). (2015d). *Suicide facts at a glance 2015*. Retrieved from http://www.cdc.gov/violenceprevention/pdf/suicide-datasheet-a.pdf

Centers for Disease Control and Prevention (CDC). (2015e). *The community guide: Guide to community preventive services: Violence*. Retrieved from www.thecommunityguide.org

Centers for Disease Control and Prevention (CDC). (2015f). *Teen dating violence*. Retrieved from http://www.cdc.gov/ViolencePrevention/intimatepartnerviolence/teen_dating_violence.html

Centers for Disease Control and Prevention (CDC). (2015g). *Understanding school violence: Fact sheet*. Retrieved from http://www.cdc.gov/violenceprevention/youthviolence/school violence

Centers for Disease Control and Prevention (CDC). (2015h). *Youth violence: Risk and protective factors*. Retrieved from http://www.cdc.gov/violenceprevention/youthviolence/riskprotectivefactors.html

Centers for Disease Control and Prevention (CDC). (2016). *Teen dating violence*. Retrieved from http://www.cdc.gov/Features/datingviolence

Cherlin, A. J. (2014). *Labor's love lost: The rise and fall of the working-class family in America*. New York, NY: Russell Sage Foundation.

Cheung, M. (2012). *Child sexual abuse: Best practices for interviewing and treatment*. Chicago, IL: Lyceum Books.

Child Health USA. (2013). *Intimate partner violence and pregnancy*. Retrieved from http://mchb.hrsa.gov/chusa13/perinatal-risk-factors-behaviors/p/intimate-partner-violence-pregnancy.html

Child Trends Data Bank. (2015). *Infant homicide: Child trends*. Retrieved from http://www.childtrends.org/?indicators=infant-homicide

Child Welfare Information Gateway. (2011). *About CAPTA: A legislative history*. Retrieved from https://www.childwelfare.gov/pubPDFs/about.pdf

Child Welfare Information Gateway. (2012). *Definitions of child abuse and neglect in federal law*. Retrieved from https://www.childwelfare.gov/topics/can/defining/federal/

Child Welfare Information Gateway. (2014). *Mandatory reporters of child abuse and neglect*. Washington, DC: U.S. Department of Health and Human Services, Children's Bureau. Retrieved from https://www.childwelfare.gov/topics/systemwide/laws-policies/statutes/manda/

Cohen, L., Chavez, V., & Chehimi, S. (2010). *Prevention is primary: Strategies for community well-being*. San Francisco, CA: Jossey-Bass.

Collibee, C., & Furman, W. (2016). Chronic and acute relational risk factors for dating aggression in adolescence and young adulthood. *Journal of Youth and Adolescence, 45*(4), 763–776.

Coutinho, E., Almeida, F., Duarte, J., Chaves, C., Nelas, P., & Amaral, O. (2015). Factors related to domestic violence in pregnant women. *Procedia—Social and Behavioral Sciences, 171*, 1280–1287.

Debowska, A., Boduszek, D., & Dhingra, K. (2015). Victim, perpetrator, and offense characteristics in filicide and filicide-suicide. *Aggression and Violent Behavior, 21*, 113–124.

Devakumar, D., Birch, M., Osrin, D., Sondorp, E., & Wells, J. C. K. (2014). The intergenerational effects of war on the health of children. *BMC Medicine, 12*, 57. doi: 10.1186/1741-7015-12-57.

Dong, X., & Simon, M. (2014). Vulnerability risk index profile for elder abuse in a community-dwelling population. *American Geriatrics Society, 62*(1), 10–15.

Drebing, H., Bailer, J., Anders, A., Wagner, H., & Gallas, C. (2014). Cyberstalking in a larger sample of social network users: Prevalence, characteristics, and impact upon victims. *Cyberpsychology, Behavior, and Social Networking, 17*(2), 61–67.

Eckenrode, J., Campa, M., Luckey, D. W., Henderson, C. R. Cole, R., Kitzman, H., ... Olds, D. (2010). Long-term effects of prenatal and infancy nurse home visitation on the life course of youths: 19-year follow-up of a randomized trial. *Archives of Pediatrics and Adolescent Medicine, 164*(1), 9–15.

Epel, E. S., & Lithgow, G. J. (2014). Stress biology and aging mechanisms: Toward understanding the deep connection between adaptation to stress and longevity. *Journals of Gerontology. Series A, Biological Sciences and Medical Sciences, 69*(Suppl. 1), s10–s16.

Eriksson, L., & Mazerolle, P. (2015). A cycle of violence? Examining family-of-origin violence, attitudes, and intimate partner violence perpetration. *Journal of Interpersonal Violence, 30*(6), 945–964.

Falk, L., Baigis, J., & Kopac, C. (2012). Elder mistreatment and the elder justice act. *Online Journal of Issues in Nursing, 17*(3). doi: 10.3912/OJIN.Vol17No03PPT01.

Federal Bureau of Investigation (FBI). (2014). *Crime in the United States, 2013: Expanded homicide data*. Retrieved from https://www.fbi.gov/about-us/cjis/ucr/crime-in-the-u.s/2013/crime-in-the-u.s.-2013/offenses-known-to-law-enforcement/expanded-homicide/expandhomicidemain_final.pdf

Federal Bureau of Investigation (FBI). (n.d.). *A parent's guide to Internet safety*. Retrieved from https://www.fbi.gov/stats-services/publications/parent-guide/parentsguide.pdf

Finkelhor, D. (2013). *Promoting research to prevent child maltreatment*. Washington, DC: Crimes Against Children Research Center. Optimus Study. Retrieved from http://www.who.int/violence_injury_prevention/violence/child/ispscan_report_june2013.pdf

Frye, E., & Feldman, M. (2012). Factitious disorder by proxy in educational settings: A review. *Educational Psychology Review. 24*, 47–61. doi: 10.1007/s10648-011-9180-9.

Gambrill, E. (2013). *Social work practice: A critical thinker's guide* (3rd ed.). New York, NY: Oxford University Press.

Garrido, E. R., Culhane, S. E., Petrenko, C. L., & Taussig, H. N. (2011). Psychosocial consequences of intimate partner violence (IPV) exposure in maltreated adolescents: Assessing more than IPV Occurrence. *Journal of Family Violence, 26*, 511–518.

Gilbert, J. (2014). Munchausen syndrome by proxy and the implications for childbirth educators. *International Journal of Childbirth Education, 29*(3), 73–79.

Grace, E., & Jagannathan, N. (2015). Munchausen syndrome by proxy: A form of child abuse. *International Journal of Child & Adolescent Health, 8*(3), 259–263.

Grip, K. K., Almqvist, K., Axberg, U., & Broberg, A. G. (2014). Perceived quality of life and health complaints in children exposed to intimate partner violence. *Journal of Family Violence, 2*, 681–692. doi: 10.1007/s10896-014-9622-5.

Hart, B. J., & Klein, A. R. (2013). *Practical implications of current intimate partner violence research for victim advocates and service providers*. Retrieved from https://www.ncjrs.gov/pdffiles1/nij/grants/244348.pdf

Health Resources & Services Administration. (n.d.). *Women's preventive services guidelines: Affordable Care Act expands prevention coverage for women's health and wellbeing*. Retrieved from http://www.hrsa.gov/womensguidelines/

Heidt, T., Sager, H. B., Courties, G., Dutta, P., Iwamoto, Y., Zaltsman, A., ... Nahrendorf, M. (2014). Chronic variable stress activates hematopoietic stem cells. *Nature Medicine, 20*, 754–758.

Holmes, T., & Rahe, R. (1967). The social readjustment rating scale. *Journal of Psychosomatic Research, 11,* 213–217.

James, R. K., & Gilliland, B. E. (2013). *Crisis intervention strategies* (7th ed.). Belmont, CA: Brooks/Cole, Cengage Learning.

Johnston, J. E. (2013). Babysitters from hell: Childcare providers who kill kids. *Psychology Today.* Retrieved from https://www.psychology-today.com/blog/the-human-equation/201312/babysitters-hell-0

Joyce, B. L., Najera-Aguire, S., Brown, N., & Sievers, V. (2014). The impact of violence on nursing students in Mexico: A lived experience. *International Journal of Health, Wellness, and Society, 3*(3), 57–65.

Kanel, K. (2012). *A guide to crisis intervention* (5th ed.). Stamford, CT: Cengage Learning.

Karakurt, G., Smith, D., & Whiting, J. (2014). Impact of intimate partner violence on women's mental health. *Journal of Family Violence, 29,* 693–702. doi: 10.1007/s10896-014-9633-2.

Kerr, D. C., & Capaldi, D. M. (2011). Young men's intimate partner violence and relationship functioning: Long-term outcomes associated with suicide attempt and aggression in adolescence. *Psychological Medicine, 41*(4), 759–769.

Kidpower. (2016). *Protecting children from stranger abduction/kidnapping.* Retrieved from https://www.kidpower.org/library/article/safety-tips-kidnapping/

Klevens, J., Sadowski, L. S., Kee, R., & Garcia, D. (2015). Does screening or providing information on resources for intimate partner violence increase women's knowledge? Findings from a randomized controlled trial. *Journal of Women's Health Issues and Care, 4*(2), 81.

Kulkarni, S. J., Lewis, C. M., & Rhodes, D. M. (2011). Clinical challenges in addressing intimate partner violence with pregnant and parenting adolescents. *Journal of Family Violence, 26,* 565–574. doi: 10.1007/s10896-011-9393-1.

Maas, C. D., Fleming, C. B., Herrenkohl, T. I., & Catalano, R. F. (2010). Childhood predictors of teen dating violence. *Violence and Victims, 25*(2), 131–147.

Malmquist, C. P. (2013). Infanticide/neonaticide: The outlier situation in the United States. *Aggression and Violent Behavior, 18,* 399–408.

Martin, K., & Monsen, K. (2015). *The Omaha System: Solving the clinical data-information puzzle.* Retrieved from http://www.omahasystem.org/overview.html

McMahon, S., & Armstrong, D. Y. (2012). Intimate partner violence during pregnancy: Best practices for social workers. *Health and Social Work, 37*(1), 9–17.

Miller, T. R. (2015). Projected outcomes of nurse-family partnership home visitation during 1996–2013, USA. *Prevention Science, 16*(6), 765–777. doi: 10.1007/s11121-015-0572-9.

Moore, A. (2014). *Cyberstalking and women: Facts and statistics.* Retrieved from http://womensissues.about.com/od/violenceagainstwomen/a/CyberstalkingFS.htm

Moylan, C. A., Lindhorst, T., & Tajima, E. A. (2015). Sexual Assault Response Teams (SARTs): Mapping a research agenda that incorporates an organizational perspective. *Violence Against Women, 21*(4), 516–534.

National Campaign to Prevent Teen Pregnancy. (2014). *Teen pregnancy and violence.* Retrieved from https://thenationalcampaign.org/sites/default/files/resource-primary-download/violence.pdf

National Center for Missing and Exploited Children. (2015). *Cyber tipline.* Retrieved from http://www.cybertipline.com

National Center on Elder Abuse (NCEA). (2013a). *Mistreatment of lesbian, gay, bisexual and transgender (LGBT) elders: Research brief.* Retrieved from http://www.ncea.aoa.gov/Resources/Publication/docs/NCEA-LGBT-ResearchBrief-508.pdf

National Center on Elder Abuse (NCEA). (2013b). *Statistics/data.* Retrieved from http://www.ncea.aoa.gov/Library/Data/index.aspx on January 9, 2016.

National Center on Elder Abuse (NCEA). (2015). *World elder abuse awareness day.* Retrieved from http://www.ncea.aoa.gov on January 10, 2016.

National Center on Elder Abuse (NCEA). (n.d.a). *Elder abuse: The size of the problem.* Retrieved from http://www.ncea.aoa.gov/library/data/

National Center on Elder Abuse (NCEA). (n.d.b). *Home.* Retrieved from http://www.ncea.aoa.gov

National Child Traumatic Stress Network. (n.d.). *Children and domestic violence.* Retrieved from http://www.nctsn.org/content/children-and-domestic-violence

National Human Trafficking Resource Center. (2015). *Human trafficking.* Retrieved from https://traffickingresourcecenter.org

New York City Elder Abuse Center. (2013). *Podcast: A conversation with Ashton Applewhite on ageism and elder justice.* Retrieved from http://nyceac.com/elder-justice-dispatch-nyceac-podcast-a-conversation-with-ashton-applewhite-on-ageism-elder-justice/

Office of Planning, Research & Evaluation. (2012). *National survey of child and adolescent well-being (NSCAW).* Retrieved from http://www.acf.hhs.gov/programs/opre/research/project/national-survey-of-child-and-adolesce

Office of the United Nations High Commissioner for Human Rights. (2014). *Committee on the rights of the child.* Retrieved from http://www.ohchr.org/english/bodies/crc/discussion.htm

Olds, D. L., Kitzman, H., Knudtson, M. D., Anson, E., Smith, J. A., & Cole, R. (2014). Effect of home visiting by nurses on maternal and child mortality. *JAMA Pediatrics, 168*(9), 1–12.

Parks, S. E., Kegler, S. R., Annest, J. L., & Mercy, J. A. (2012a). Characteristics of fatal abusive head trauma among children in the USA: 2003–2007: An application of the CDC operational case definition to national vital statistics data. *Injury Prevention, 18,* 193–199.

Parks, S. E., Sugerman, D., Xu, L., & Coronado, V. (2012b). Characteristics of non-fatal abusive health trauma among children in the USA, 2003–2008: Application of the CDC operational case definition to national hospital inpatient data. *Injury Prevention, 18,* 392–398.

QSEN Institute. (2014). *Quality and safety competencies.* Retrieved from http://qsen.org/competencies/pre-lecensure-ksas/

Rape, Abuse, & Incest National Network. (2013). *The offenders.* Retrieved from https://rainn.org/get-information/statistics/sexual-assault-offenders

Rodner, R. (2015). *Introduction to interpersonal acceptance-rejection theory: Methods, evidence and implications.* Retrieved from http://csiar.uconn.edu/introduction to partheory

Rosen, A. (2014). Where mental health and elder abuse intersect. *Journal of the American Society on Aging, 38*(3), 75–79.

Safe Schools Healthy Students Initiative. (2016). *About the Safe Schools Healthy Students (SS/HS) initiative: A comprehensive approach to youth violence prevention.* Retrieved from http://www.samhsa.gov/safe-schools-healthy-students/about

Salleh, M. R. (2008). Life event, stress and illness. *Malaysian Journal of Medical Sciences, 15*(4), 9–18.

Sheehy, G. (1976). *Passages: Predictable crises of adult life.* New York, NY: Dutton.

Sheehy, G. (1992). *The silent passage.* New York, NY: Ballantine.

Sheehy, G. (1999). *Understanding men's passages: Discovering the new map of men's lives.* New York, NY: Ballantine Books.

Sheehy, G., & Delbourgo, J. (1996). *New passages: Mapping your life across time.* New York, NY: Ballantine Books.

Simms, L., Bushman, S., & Pedersen, S. (2016). *Bullying: How to prevent it and help children who are victims.* Retrieved from http://center4research.org/violence-risky-behavior/z-other-violence/b

Stewart, D. E., Vigod, S., & Riazantseva, E. (2016). New developments in intimate partner violence and management of its mental health sequelae. *Current Psychiatry Reports, 18*(4). doi: 10.1007/s11920-015-0644-3.

Symes, L., Maddoux, J., McFarlane, J., Nava, A., & Gilroy, H. (2014). Physical and sexual intimate partner violence, women's health and children's behavioural functioning: Entry analysis of a seven-year prospective study. *Journal of Clinical Nursing, 23,* 2909–2918. doi: 10.1111/jocn.12542.

Townsend, C., & Rheingold, A. (2013). *Estimating a child sexual abuse prevalence rate: A review of child sexual abuse prevalence studies.* Charleston, SC: Darkness to Light. Retrieved from http://www.d2l.org/site/c.4dICIJOkGc

Trotman, G. E., Young-Anderson, C., & Deye, K. P. (2015). *Acute sexual assault in the pediatric and adolescent population. Journal of Child and Adolescent Gynecology.* doi: 10.1016/j.jpag.2015.05.001.

Tsavoussis, A., Stawicki, S. P. A., Stoicea, N., & Papadimos, T. J. (2014). Child-witnessed domestic violence and its adverse effects on brain development: A call for societal self-examination and awareness. *Frontiers in Public Health, 2,* 178. doi: 10.3389/fpubh.2014.00178.

U.S. Department of Justice (USDOJ). (2015). *Domestic violence.* Retrieved from http://www.justice.gov/ovw/domestic-violence

U.S. Department of Justice (USDOJ). (2016). *Stalking.* Retrieved from http://www.justice.gov/ovw/stalking

U.S. Department of Health and Human Services (USDHHS). (2011). *Home visiting evidence of effectiveness: Implementing NFP*. Retrieved from http://homvee.acf.hhs.gov/Implementation/3/Nurse-Family-Partnership-NFP—Program-Model-Overview/14

U.S. Department of Health and Human Services (USDHHS). (2014). *Healthy People 2020 leading health indicators: Injury and violence*. Retrieved from http://www.healthypeople.gov/sites/default/files/HP2020_LHI_Injury_Viol.pdf

U.S. Department of Health and Human Services (USDHHS). (2016a). *2020 topics & objectives: Injury and violence prevention*. Retrieved from https://www.healthypeople.gov/2020/topics-objectives/topic/injury-and-violence-prevention/objectives

U.S. Department of Health and Human Services (USDHHS). (2016b). *Adolescent health*. Retrieved from http://www.healthypeople.gov/2020/topics-objectives/topic/Adolescent-Health

U.S. Department of Justice (USDOJ). (2011a). *Child abuse and mistreatment*. Retrieved from http://www.nij.gov/topics/crime/child-abuse/Pages/welcome.aspx

U.S. Department of Justice (USDOJ). (2011b). *Homicide trends in the United States 1980–2008*. Retrieved from http://bjs.gov/content/pub/pdf/htus8008.pdf

U.S. Department of Justice (USDOJ). (2013a). *Amber Alert: America's missing: Broadcast emergency response*. Retrieved from http://www.amberalert.gov/ on January 1, 2016

U.S. Department of Justice (USDOJ). (2013b). *The elder justice roadmap*. Retrieved from http://ncea.aoa.gov/Library/Gov_Report/docs/EJRP_Roadmap.pdf

U.S. Department of Justice (USDOJ). (2014). *Project safe childhood fact sheet*. Retrieved from http://www.justice.gov/psc/project-safe-childhood-fact-sheet

U.S. Department of Justice (USDOJ). (n.d.). *About NSOPW*. Retrieved from https://www.nsopw.gov/en/Home/About

United Nations Office on Drugs and Crime. (2016). *Global study on homicide*. Retrieved from https://www.unodc.org/documents/gsh/pdfs/2014_GLOBAL_HOMICIDE_BOOK_web.pdf

Walker, L. E. A. (1984). *The battered woman syndrome*. New York, NY: Springer Publishing.

Weber, J. G. (2011). *Individual and family stress and crises*. Thousand Oaks, CA: Sage Publications, Inc.

Woda, T. (2015, January). Cyberbullying: Children as victims and predators. *USA Today Magazine*.

Wolff, L. (2013, March 6). *The battered child syndrome: 50 years later*. Retrieved from http://www.huffingtonpost.com/larry-wolff/battered-child-syndrome_b_2406348.html

World Health Organization (WHO). (2011). *Intimate partner violence during pregnancy*. Retrieved from http://whqlibdoc.who.int/hq/2011/WHO_RHR-11.35

World Health Organization (WHO). (2012a). *Femicide*. Retrieved from http://apps.who.int/iris/bitstream/10665/77421/1/WHO_RHR_12.38_eng.pdf

World Health Organization (WHO). (2012b). *Intimate partner violence*. Retrieved from http://apps.who.int/iris/bitstream/10665/77432/1/WHO_RHR_12.36_eng.pdf

World Health Organization (WHO). (2013a). *Summary report*. Retrieved from http://www.who.int/violence_injury_prevention/violence/child/ispscan_report_june2013.pdf

World Health Organization (WHO). (2013b). *Violence against women: A global picture health response*. Retrieved from http://www.who.int/mediacentre/news/releases/2013/violence_against_women_20130620/en

World Health Organization (WHO). (2014). *Global status report on violence prevention*. Retrieved from http://www.who.int/violence_injury_prevention/violence/status_report/2014/report/Narrative.pdf?ua=1

World Health Organization (WHO). (2016a). *Global health observatory data*. Retrieved from http://www.who.int/gho/mental_health/suicide_rates_text/en/ on January 16, 2016

World Health Organization (WHO). (2016b). *Suicide fact sheet*. Retrieved from http://www.who.int/mediacentre/factsheets/fs398/en/

World Health Organization (WHO). (2016c). *Violence against women*. Retrieved from http://www.who.int/mediacentre/factsheets/fs239/en

thePoint: Everything You Need to Make the Grade!

thePoint® Visit http://thePoint.lww.com/Rector9e for selected readings, study aids for all learning styles, and more!

PROMOTING AND PROTECTING THE HEALTH OF AGGREGATES WITH DEVELOPMENTAL NEEDS

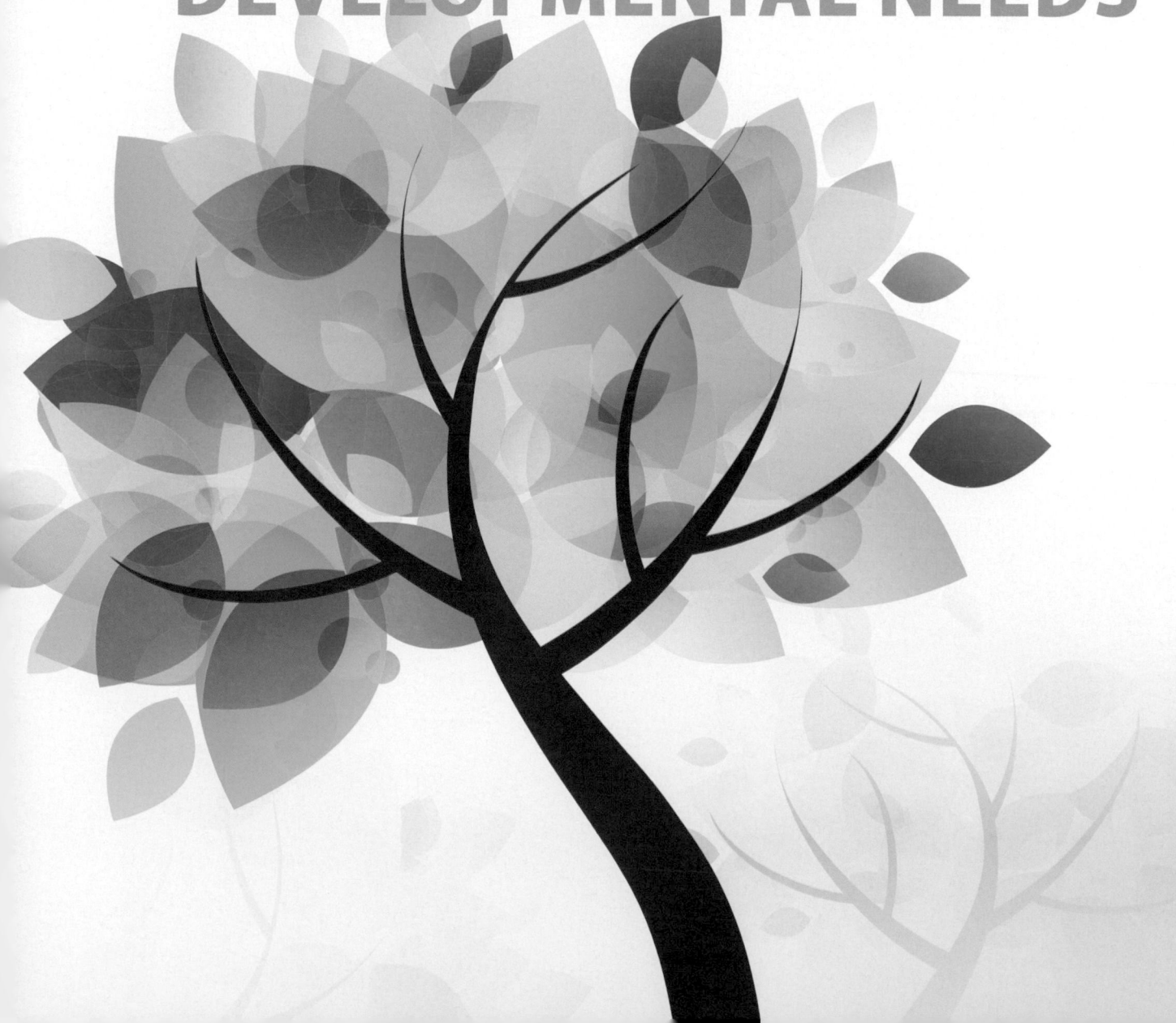

Maternal–Child Health: Working with Perinatal, Infant, Toddler, and Preschool Clients

"Be gentle with the young."

—*Juvenal* (55–127 AD)

KEY TERMS

Alcohol-related birth defects
Alcohol-related
  neurodevelopmental
  disorder
Child abuse
Environmental tobacco
  smoke (ETS)

Fetal alcohol effects
Fetal alcohol spectrum
  disorders
Fetal alcohol syndrome
Gestational diabetes mellitus
  (GDM)
Head Start

High-risk families
Infant
Low birth weight (LBW)
Population health
Preconception care
Preschooler
Shaken baby syndrome

Smokeless tobacco products
Sudden infant death
  syndrome (SIDS)
Toddler
Very low birth weight (VLBW)

LEARNING OBJECTIVES

Upon mastery of this chapter, you should be able to:

- Identify major health problems and concerns for childbearing women, infant, toddler, and preschool populations globally and in the United States.
- Identify the *Healthy People 2020* goals established for the maternal–child population.
- Discuss major risk factors and special complications for childbearing families.
- Describe the important considerations in developing effective health promotion programs to fit the needs of diverse maternal–child populations.
- Describe various roles of a public and community health nurse in serving the maternal–child population.
- Describe a variety of programs that promote and protect health and prevent illness and injury of infant, toddler, and preschool populations.
- State the recommended immunization schedule for infants and children and give the rationale for the timing of each immunization.
- Give examples of methods and interventions the public and community health nurse might use in working with infants, toddlers, and preschool populations to help promote their health.

Maternal and child populations have always been priorities for public health and public and community health nursing (P/CHN). These populations consist of childbearing women, including pregnant adolescents, and infants and children through adolescence. In this chapter, the focus is on childbearing women, including adolescents and infants through age 4. Often, more than half of P/CHN practice in official public health agencies involves primary prevention work with mothers, such as family planning, **preconception care**, provision of prenatal care, and monitoring infant health. Why should maternal–infant populations require this amount of attention from P/CHN? Despite advanced technology and availability of excellent perinatal services in the United States, we often have less than optimal birth outcomes—for instance, 318,847 low-birth-weight (LBW) and 381,321 preterm infants were born in 2014 (Centers for Disease Control and Prevention [CDC], 2016j). Also, certain segments of the maternal and infant populations, such as adolescent mothers and those who are economically disadvantaged or women and children of color, remain at high risk for disparities in regard to maternal deaths and complications and child risk and illness. Although some women receive excellent prenatal care and benefit from diagnostic and technological resources, many others are without access to prenatal care.

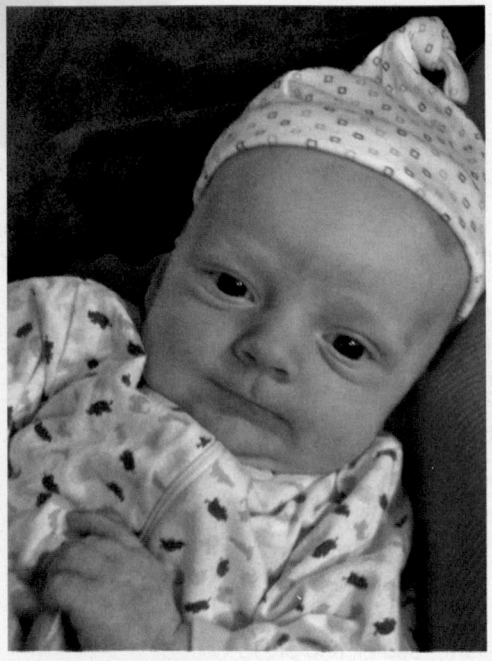

Child Health USA (U.S. Department of Health and Human Services, Health Resources and Services Administration, Maternal and Child Health Bureau, 2014) reports that adequate prenatal care is associated with adequate health insurance. In 2012, 88% of privately insured women and 83% of Medicaid insured women received adequate prenatal care (four or more provider visits during pregnancy). Seventy-two percent of those who were uninsured were least likely to receive adequate prenatal care. This correlates to health inequity characteristics such as race and ethnicity, poverty, and low maternal education levels (less than high school education).

Historically, the health of U.S. women and children has largely fallen under the umbrella of Title V, of the Social Security Act, enacted in 1935. (For more on the Social Security Act, see Chapter 6.) Funding for state Maternal and Child Health and Crippled Children programs was part of this original legislation, as was some provision for child welfare services. Title V is "the longest-standing public health legislation in American history" and came to fruition after other legislation established a National Birth Registry; provided *Infant Care*, the first educational pamphlet; established the Children's Bureau; and enacted the first Child Labor Law of 1916 (Maternal Child Health Bureau [MCHB], n.d.b, para. 4). For an illustration of MCHB functions and programs, see Display 21–1.

In 1909, formal prenatal care was first provided in Boston by the Instructive District Nursing Association and spread across the country to outpatient clinics (MCHB, n.d.b). Since the inception of Title V, many programs have been developed with the goal of improving the health of women of childbearing age, as well as infants and children. Research areas have included prenatal and pregnancy, child development and parenting, improving health care systems and delivery of care, as well as obesity, nutrition, medical homes, school services and outcomes, and behavioral health (MCHB, n.d.c). Healthy Start grants were first awarded in 1991 to 15 agencies, with the goal of reducing rates of infant mortality, LBWs, premature births, and maternal deaths (MCHB, n.d.a). Evaluation of Healthy Start programs reveals that almost all programs provide home visitation to prenatal clients, and most continued these visits to infants and toddlers. Health education, smoking cessation counseling, services for perinatal depression, and involvement of male partners are hallmarks of most programs.

In 2016, $345 million in grants were awarded to expand the Maternal, Infant, and Early Childhood Home Visiting Program (Federal Home Visiting Program). This program provides PHN visits, assistance from social workers, early childhood educators, and other professionals to expectant families, much like the program designed by David Olds (Health Resources & Services Administration [HRSA], 2016). Early improvements in six benchmark areas were noted:

- Maternal and newborn health
- Child injuries, child maltreatment, and ED visits
- School readiness and achievement
- Crime or domestic violence

DISPLAY 21–1 TYPES OF SERVICES OFFERED THROUGH FEDERAL MATERNAL–CHILD HEALTH FUNDING

Direct Health Care Services (Gap Filling)

Examples: Basic Health Services and Health Services for Children with Special Health Care Needs (CSHCN)

Enabling Services

Examples: Transportation, Translation, Outreach, Respite Care, Health Education, Family Support Services, Purchase of Health Insurance, Case Management, Coordination with Medicaid, WIC, and Education

Population-Based Services

Examples: Newborn Screening, Lead Screening, Immunization, Sudden Infant Death Syndrome Counseling, Oral Health, and Injury Prevention

Infrastructure Building Services

Examples: Needs Assessment, Evaluation, Planning, Policy Development, Coordination, Quality Assurance, Standards Development, Monitoring, Training, Applied Research, Systems of Care, and Information Systems

U.S. Department of Health and Human Services. (2008). *State MCH-Medicaid Coordination: A Review of Title V and Title XIX Interagency Agreements* (2nd ed.). Retrieved from http://mchb.hrsa.gov/pdfs/statemch-medicaid.pdf

- Family economic self-sufficiency
- Service coordination/referrals for other community resources/support (MCHB, 2016, p. 4).

This chapter addresses major areas of concern regarding population health for maternal–infant clients. It also explores the global needs of and related services available to the youngest and thus most vulnerable of society's members. Health services that are commonly available in the United States for pregnant and postpartum women, infants, toddlers, and the preschool population are examined, and the role of the public and community health nurse in providing those services is explored.

HEALTH STATUS AND NEEDS OF PREGNANT WOMEN AND INFANTS

Public and community health nurses constitute a key group of health professionals involved in both program planning and the actual delivery of services to mothers and babies in the community. In the public health sector, these nurses are the largest group of professionals practicing public health. A solid understanding of vital statistics and other data regarding mothers and infants is important to determine the appropriateness and the effectiveness of programs and services. A review of some global and national vital statistics provides insight into the major problems facing maternal and child populations.

Global Overview

One of the major indicators of **population health** is maternal health, which is often measured by the maternal mortality rate (MMR). The MMR is a measure of obstetric risk and is determined by dividing the number of maternal deaths by the number of live births per 100,000. Most maternal deaths are the result of direct causes (complications of pregnancy, labor, and delivery), hypertensive disorders, intervention omissions or incorrect treatment, the chain of events resulting from any one of these, and unsafe abortions. In 2015, more than 50% of maternal deaths occurred in sub-Saharan Africa and about 33% in South Asia. In these developing countries, the MMR is 239 per 100,000 live births. This compares to developed countries, such as Canada, Australia, New Zealand, Japan, and most European countries where the MMR is around 12 per 100,000 live births—a very wide disparity (World Health Organization [WHO], 2016b). The U.S. MMR was 17.8 per 100,000 women in 2011 and 15.9 in 2012 (CDC, 2016k). Ireland and Greece's MMR is <4, making them very good places for expectant mothers. Although the MMR has decreased since 1990 by 44%, the worldwide goal is to eliminate maternal mortality by 2030 (WHO, 2015c). This goal is achievable because most maternal mortality can be prevented. For an example of a country that has implemented successful policies to eliminate maternal–child inequities, see Evidence-Based Practice: Reducing Child Mortality in Bangladesh.

Infant Mortality

Another critical population health indicator is the infant mortality rate (IMR). Globally, 6.3 million children under 5 years died in 2013; 44% of these deaths took place in the neonatal period and are primarily caused by preterm birth, birth asphyxia, and infection. More than half of the deaths for children under 5 years are preventable and the interventions are affordable (WHO, 2015c). In the United States, the IMR was 6.14 infant deaths under age one per 1,000 live births in 2010, a decrease from 6.86 in 2005 (MacDorman, Mathews, Mohangoo & Zeitlin, 2014). For non-Hispanic Blacks, the rate is 2.3 times higher than for the non-Hispanic White population at 12.67 versus 5.52 (HRSA, 2013). Among American Indian and Alaska Natives, the IMR is also higher at 8.42 and 7.29, whereas Asian/Pacific Islanders have a much lower overall rate of 4.51, but some variability exists with Native Hawaiians having higher rates. See Figure 21–1 for U.S. infant mortality rate ethnic comparison data. WHO estimated in 2015 that 800,000 million infants worldwide would be saved if there were more infants exclusively breast-fed for the first 6 months of life. Currently, breast-feeding practice worldwide is at 35% (WHO, 2015b).

HIV/AIDS

There are 36.9 million individuals living with human immunodeficiency virus (HIV). Almost 70% of all cases are found in sub-Saharan Africa (WHO, 2016a). Most children with acquired immunodeficiency syndrome (AIDS) are children of HIV-positive mothers (WHO, 2015a). Mother-to-child transmission (MTCT) of HIV can be almost fully prevented with antiretroviral

EVIDENCE-BASED PRACTICE

Reducing Child Mortality in Bangladesh

Child mortality rates have declined significantly in Bangladesh over the last decade. In 2000, Bangladesh experienced a 53% reduction in the under-five mortality rate (88 per 1,000) compared to 41 per 1,000 in 2012. Additionally, the neonatal mortality rate was decreased by 40% from 40.7 per 1,000 in 2000 to 24.4 per 1,000 in 2012. Routine childhood immunizations, oral rehydration therapy, and supplementation of vitamin A are interventions that have significantly influenced this reduction in child mortality rates. It is estimated that 98% of the children aged 12 to 23 months have access to routine immunizations. Completed immunization rates are at 93% among these children. Furthermore, the government of Bangladesh implemented a nutrition plan in its National Health Strategy. This included utilizing community health workers to improve access to health care, improvements in the quality of health care, and increases in the number of health facilities that have demonstrated improved rates. Although these improvements are dramatic, additional improvements in sustainable trends and equity are essential (Baruah et al., 2013).

Baruah, S., Haines, S., Hewitt, S., Holly, L., Jensen, P., Johnson, R., ... Olayemi, D. (2013). *Lives on the line: An agenda for ending preventable child deaths.* London, UK: Save the Children.

treatment for mother and infant (WHO, 2015a). To reduce MTCT, women must seek prenatal care early enough in their pregnancies for the antiretroviral drug to be effective. Antiretroviral therapy was provided to an estimated 14.9 million persons in 2014, and approximately 823,000 of them were children (WHO, 2015a).

National Overview

In the United States, 3.9 million women gave birth in 2013, 1% more for the first time since 2007 (Martin, Hamilton, Osterman, Curtin, & Matthews, 2015). The general fertility rate declined to a total of 62.5 births per 1,000 women ages 15 to 44 years. Birth rates declined for non-Hispanic White and Hispanic populations and remained unchanged for African American women. Just over 40% of births were to unmarried women (Martin et al., 2015). When unmarried women rely on a single income, financial resources are more limited, and many of these women raise their children at poverty or near poverty income levels, which impacts their health and their children's health over the life course of both.

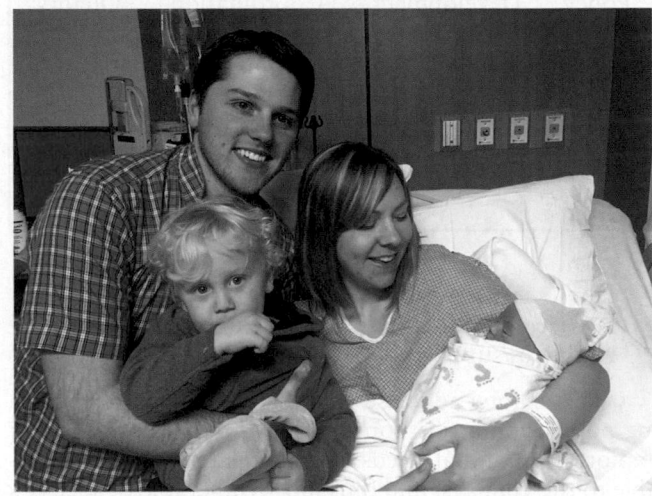

Support for mothers and children helps ensure healthier families. (Author's private photo with permission from Christian and Samantha Nelson.)

Birth Weight and Preterm Birth

Birth weight is one of the most important predictors of infant mortality. **Low-birth-weight (LBW)** babies are those weighing <2,500 g (or <5.5 pounds) at birth; **very-low-birth-weight (VLBW)** babies weigh <1,500 g (or <3 pounds 4 ounces) at birth. In the last 25 years, the rate of preterm births has increased by 33% with the majority of these births occurring late preterm (34 to 36 weeks' gestation) (Shapiro-Mendoza & Lackritz, 2012). Presently, preterm birth rates have been slowly declining. Preterm birth rates for 2013 were 11.39% and declined for non-Hispanic White, African Americans, and Hispanics; overall LBW rates were unchanged at 8.02% down from the 2006 high of 8.32% (Martin et al., 2015). Statistics for VLBW are 1.5% overall but 3.0% for African Americans

FIGURE 21–1 U.S. infant mortality rates, by race and Hispanic ethnicity of mother: comparisons for 2000, 2005, and 2010. (From MacDorman, M. F., & Mathews, T. J. (2014). QuickStats: Infant mortality rates, by race and Hispanic ethnicity of mother— United States, 2000, 2005, and 2010. *Morbidity & Mortality Weekly Report (MMWR), 63*(1), 25. Retrieved from http://www.cdc.gov/mmwr/preview/mmwrhtml/mm6301a9.htm)

(Figure 21–1: Bar chart — Deaths per 1,000 live births, comparing 2000, 2005, and 2010 across Total, White non-Hispanic, Black non-Hispanic, and Hispanic groups.)

(Martin et al., 2011). These numbers represent a significant disparity for African Americans.

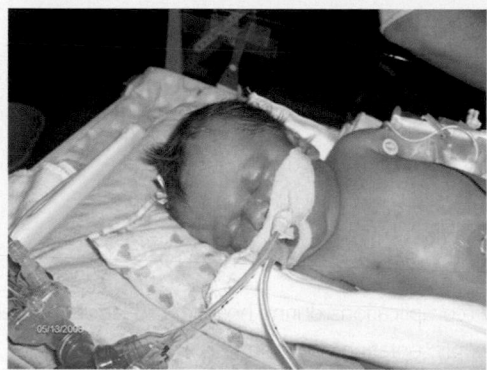

Infant in NICU. (Author's private photo with permission from Danielle Rector.)

Infant complications of preterm birth include hearing and vision problems; acute respiratory, gastrointestinal, and immunologic problems; and central nervous system (CNS), motor, cognitive, behavioral, and socioemotional disorders. A variety of growth concerns as well as acute and chronic health and developmental problems often occur, and the families of these infants are burdened with additional economic and emotional costs. In a study of preterm infants from birth to age two, those with feeding difficulties and at risk for feeding difficulties had significant neurodevelopmental problems such as impaired cognition, language, motor, and socioemotional skills that led to increased parental stress, poorer maternal mental health, or family stressors than those preterm infants that did not have feeding difficulties. Maternal mortality, LBW, and VLBW births are three areas requiring attention by health care providers and the public health system. Public and community health nurses can contribute to reducing these rates and societal costs by outreach, surveillance, health teaching, counseling, and referral (Save the Children, 2015).

In addition to infant deaths and LBW, the effects of pregnancy and childbirth on women are other important indicators of health and reflect discrepancies in access to reproductive health care. The United States is not ranked among the top 10 countries in maternal–child health in the *2015 Mother's Index*. It is ranked 33rd out of the more developed countries. The U.S. ranking is largely due to poorer scores on the indices of maternal and child health. Eastern European countries, such as Slovakia, the Czech Republic, Belarus, Croatia, and the developing countries such as Peru and Ethiopia, rank higher than the United States (Save the Children, 2015).

In the United States, the MMR is higher than in other developed countries, mostly because of the disparities found among women of color. The MMR for Blacks (42.8 per 100,000 live births) is four times greater than that for Whites (12.5), and the gap has continued to widen since 1986 when the MMR surveillance was initiated (CDC, 2016k). Pregnancy-related death risk increases with age and with lack of prenatal care for women of every race, but the risk of pregnancy-related death for U.S. Black women is three to four times greater

than for White women. Even though maternal deaths are low, most maternal deaths are preventable.

One of the maternal–child objectives for *Healthy People 2020* is to improve the proportion of infants who are breast-fed. Breast-feeding is beneficial to both mother and infant, and currently, 79.2% of mothers reported ever breast-feeding. Only 49.4% of U.S. infants were breast-fed for the recommended 6-month period, and 18.8% were breast-fed exclusively for this 6-month period. These proportions do not reach the *Healthy People 2020* targets of 81.9% for "ever breast-feeding," and 60.6% for "breast-feeding for the first 6 months" (CDC, 2014a). An evidence-based quality improvement project that promoted mother-to-infant skin-to-skin contact in the delivery room showed significant improvement in exclusive breast-feeding (Brown, Kaiser, & Nailon, 2014). It is estimated that if 90% of U.S. families would comply with the recommended American Academy of Pediatrics guidelines regarding exclusive breast-feeding, $3.7 billion in direct and indirect pediatric health costs and $10.1 billion in premature death related to pediatric disease would be saved (Bartick, 2011). See Table 21–1 for *Healthy People 2020* maternal, infant, and child health objectives.

Adolescent Mothers

In 1991, after a steady 5-year upward trend, the United States reached a 20-year high in the number of children born to teen mothers (aged 15 to 19 years). That trend then declined with 2013 marking a 57% decline in teen birth rates (Ventura, Hamilton, & Matthews, 2014). In 2013, there were 26.5 births per 1,000 women age 15 to 19 years (Martin et al., 2015). The drop in teen birth rates translates into an estimated 4 million fewer births to teenagers from 1992 through 2012. The decrease in teen birth rate can be attributed to several behavioral changes, such as decreased sexual activity, increase use of contraception at first sex and at most recent sex, and the increased use of contraception methods (Ventura et al., 2014). Although the United States has seen a decrease in teen births, the country continues to have much higher teen birth rates compared to other developed countries, including Canada and the United Kingdom (United Nations Statistics Division, 2015). See Chapter 22 for more on adolescent pregnancy.

The *Healthy People 2020* (USDHHS, 2016) document encompasses specific goals and objectives for the maternal–child population, based on the previous achievements in the same or similar areas. After years of working toward improving maternal–child health, the United States has made limited progress. One objective, however, has been met; 70% of infants are now sleeping on their backs, up from a 35% baseline. The rate for sudden infant death syndrome (SIDS) had dropped by over 50% since 1994. This can be attributed to the national public health education campaign known as "Back to Sleep" (Eunice Kennedy Shriver National Institute of Child Development and Health, 2016).

Risk Factors for Pregnant Women and Infants

Most pregnant women in the United States are healthy; they have normal pregnancies and produce healthy babies. Many factors contribute to the health problems of those mothers

Table 21–1 *Healthy People 2020:* **Summary of Objectives for Maternal, Infant, and Child Health**

Goal: Improve the health and well-being of women, infants, children, and families

Number	Objective

Morbidity and Mortality

MICH-1	Reduce the rate of fetal and infant deaths
MICH-2	Reduce the 1-year mortality rate for infants with Down's syndrome
MICH-3	Reduce the rate of child deaths
MICH-4	Reduce the rate of adolescent and young adult deaths
MICH-5	Reduce the rate of maternal mortality
MICH-6	Reduce maternal illness and complications because of pregnancy (complications during hospitalized labor and delivery)
MICH-7	Reduce cesarean births among low-risk (full-term, singleton, vertex presentation) women
MICH-8	Reduce low birth weight (LBW) and very low birth weight (VLBW)
MICH-9	Reduce preterm births

Pregnancy Health and Behaviors

MICH-10	Increase the proportion of pregnant women who receive early and adequate prenatal care
MICH-11	Increase abstinence from alcohol, cigarettes, and illicit drugs among pregnant women
MICH-12	Increase the proportion of pregnant women who attend a series of prepared childbirth classes (Archived)
MICH-13	Increase the proportion of mothers who achieve a recommended weight gain during their pregnancies (Developmental)

Preconception Health and Behaviors

MICH-14	Increase the proportion of women of childbearing potential with intake of at least 400 mcg of folic acid from fortified foods or dietary supplements
MICH-15	Reduce the proportion of women of childbearing potential who have low red blood cell folate concentrations
MICH-16	Increase the proportion of women delivering a live birth who received preconception care services and practiced key recommended preconception health behaviors
MICH-17	Reduce the proportion of persons aged 18–44 years who have impaired fecundity (physical barrier preventing pregnancy or carrying pregnancy to term)

Postpartum Health and Behavior

MICH-18	Reduce postpartum relapse of smoking among women who quit smoking during pregnancy
MICH-19	Increase the proportion of women giving birth who attend a postpartum care visit with a health worker (Developmental)

Infant Care

MICH-20	Increase the proportion of infants who are put to sleep on their backs
MICH-21	Increase the proportion of infants who are breast-fed
MICH-22	Increase the proportion of employers that have worksite lactation support programs
MICH-23	Reduce the proportion of breast-fed newborns who receive formula supplementation within the first 2 days of life
MICH-24	Increase the proportion of live births that occur in facilities that provide recommended care for lactating mothers and their babies

Disability and Other Impairments

MICH-25	Reduce the occurrence of fetal alcohol syndrome (FAS)
MICH-26	Reduce the proportion of children diagnosed with a disorder through newborn blood spot screening who experience developmental delay requiring special education services
MICH-27	Reduce the proportion of children with cerebral palsy born as LBW infants (<2,500 g)
MICH-28	Reduce occurrence of neural tube defects
MICH-29	Increase the proportion of young children with autism spectrum disorder (ASD) and other developmental delays who are screened, evaluated, and enrolled in special services in a timely manner

(continued)

Table 21–1 *Healthy People 2020:* **Summary of Objectives for Maternal, Infant, and Child Health (***Continued***)**	
Number	**Objective**
Health Services	
MICH-30	Increase the proportion of children, including those with special health care needs, who have access to a medical home
MICH-31	Increase the proportion of children with special health care needs who receive their care in family-centered, comprehensive, and coordinated systems
MICH-32	Increase appropriate newborn blood spot screening and follow-up testing
MICH-33	Increase the proportion of VLBW infants born at level III hospitals or subspecialty perinatal centers

Source: USDHHS. (2016). *Healthy People 2020: Maternal, infant, and child health objectives.* Retrieved from https://www.healthypeople.gov/2020/topics-objectives/topic/maternal-infant-and-child-health/objectives

and babies who figure in the statistics on infant mortality and LBW. The factors associated with LBW and infant mortality can be grouped into three categories (CDC, 2014e):

1. Lifestyle: Smoking, secondhand smoke exposure, inadequate nutrition, alcohol consumption, substance abuse, late prenatal care, environmental toxins, stress, violence, and lack of social support
2. Sociodemographic: Maternal age below 15 and above 35, low educational level, poverty, domestic violence, and unmarried status
3. Medical and gestational history: Primiparity, multiple gestation, short interpregnancy intervals, premature rupture of the membranes, uterine abnormality, febrile illness during pregnancy, spontaneous abortion, genetic factors, gestation-induced hypertension, less than ideal weight gain during pregnancy, and diabetes

It is in the area of lifestyle choices that nurses can have the most significant impact on pregnancy outcomes such as LBW, preterm birth, and infant mortality. Programs that provide access and funding to PHNs are available through federal, state, and local funding.

Substance Use and Abuse

Another area of concern is substance use and abuse among the childbearing population. The range of adverse consequences associated with the use of tobacco, alcohol, and illicit drugs during pregnancy is wide and includes preterm birth, LBW, and fetal alcohol syndrome (FAS) (described later in this chapter). This puts these women and their unborn children in double jeopardy; not only are they at risk from the consequences of alcohol or drug use, but also they do not receive the preventive prenatal care that can eliminate or reduce other obstetric complications. This is most often related to the pregnant woman's concerns about legal ramifications of substance use while pregnant if they do seek care. In a study conducted in the Netherlands, nurse home visitor intervention had significant effects on the cessation and reduction of smoking in pregnant women compared to regular care (Mejdoubi et al., 2014).

Substance abuse during pregnancy is a problem with staggering social and medical implications, such as preterm births, LBW, miscarriage, placental abruption, developmental delays, and child behavior and learning problems later in life (American Pregnancy Association, 2016). The precise rate of substance abuse among pregnant women is difficult to determine. In a large study

($n = 27,874$) of substance abuse and pregnancy, 26.3% of the women reported previous use and 2.6% current use. Adverse outcomes of these pregnancies included LBW, preterm birth, babies born small for gestational age (SGA), and admissions to neonatal intensive care units (NICUs). The investigators also noted that many substance-using women also used tobacco and alcohol while pregnant (Hayatbakhsh et al., 2012). In a large Danish population study, it was found that among opiate-exposed newborns compared to nonexposed newborns there was greater prevalence of preterm birth, LBW at term, and being SGA. In addition, there were twice the number of congenital birth defects (Nørgaard, Nielsson, & Heide-Jørgensen, 2015).

In the United States, almost 90% of substance-abusing women are of reproductive age and are most commonly reported to abuse cocaine, methamphetamines, heroin and opioids, alcohol, marijuana, and tobacco. Also, the use of several substances—or polysubstance abuse—is fairly common in this population (Hayatbakhsh et al., 2012). The use of stimulants such as cocaine and methamphetamines during pregnancy is associated with impaired fetal growth, neonatal seizures, and congenital anomalies. Neonatal withdrawal is characterized by abnormal functions of the gastrointestinal tract, the CNS, and the respiratory system. Poor feeding, abnormal sleep patterns, long-term learning disabilities, and delayed language development may be observable results of maternal drug use.

The United States has seen an increased incidence of neonatal abstinence syndrome (NAS) as a result of heroin or opioid use in pregnancy. It is estimated that from 2009 to 2012, the incidence increased from 3.4 to 5.8 per 1,000 births. Geographically, this increase has been seen in the Southeast states of Kentucky, Tennessee, Mississippi, and Alabama and the South Central states of Texas, Oklahoma, Arkansas, and Louisiana (Patrick, Davis, Lehmann, & Cooper, 2015). NAS occurs as a result of the sudden discontinuation of fetal exposure to substances such as heroin or other opioids during pregnancy. Withdrawal symptoms experienced by these infants include irritability, excessive/high-pitched crying, tremors, and gastrointestinal problems such as diarrhea. In the event nonpharmacologic care does not alleviate these symptoms, morphine is the most commonly used pharmacologic treatment for NAS. The long-term effects of NAS are not known and are currently being studied (Kocherlakota, 2014).

A lifestyle choice that includes the use of drugs during pregnancy, and subsequent maternal addiction, has placed millions of children at risk. These children are seen in NICUs, foster care, special education programs in the public schools, and later in the juvenile court system. Family structure patterns are altered because grandparents may find themselves primary caregivers for their grandchildren. A woman who is an illicit intravenous drug user may lose her inhibitions and engage in high-risk sexual behaviors introducing other public health problems; these include acquisition of sexually transmitted infections (STIs), including HIV, and possible spread of the infection to the fetus or others (CDC, 2015h). The primary, secondary, and tertiary prevention interventions of the PHN cannot be underestimated when drug use takes such a high toll on every aspect of society.

Alcohol Use

Another societal problem is the use and addiction to alcohol. It is difficult to establish accurate statistics on the number of women who drink during pregnancy, but results from the 2011 to 2013 Behavioral Risk Factor Surveillance System (BRFSS) indicate that roughly 1 in 10 pregnant women drank alcohol within the past 30 days, compared to 53.6% of nonpregnant women. Prevalence of binge drinking was 18.2% for nonpregnant women, and 3.1% for pregnant women, with a 4.6 times greater rate for unmarried pregnant women (Tan, Denny, Cheal, Sniezek, & Kanny, 2015).

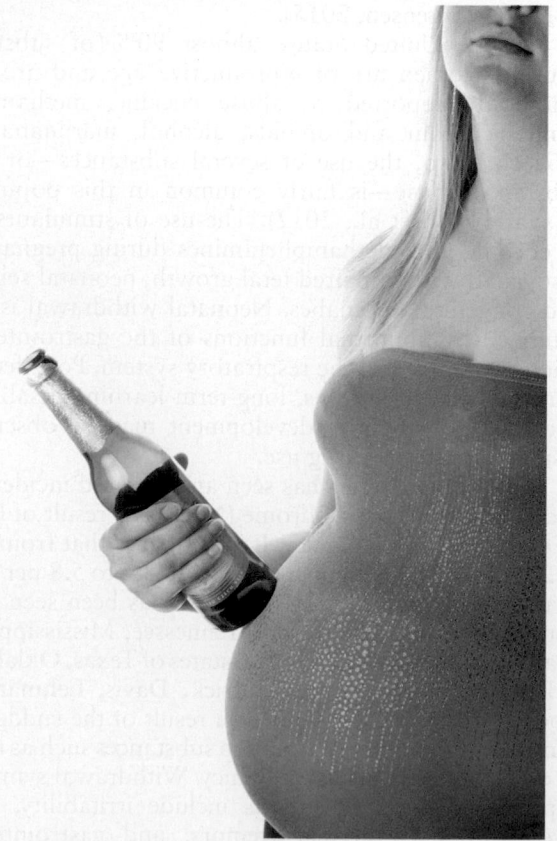

Alcohol use during pregnancy can cause serious problems for the fetus.

Alcohol use can cause devastating effects in the fetus, even when limited to early pregnancy and in the absence of addiction, and can lead to an array of neurocognitive and behavioral disorders, sometimes with structural anomalies, now described as **fetal alcohol spectrum disorders** (FASD). For example, regular intake of alcohol during pregnancy, especially in the first trimester, can cause the most recognizable form of the disorder: **fetal alcohol syndrome**, which is characterized by structural abnormalities of the head and face (e.g., microcephaly and flattening of the maxillary area), intrauterine growth retardation, decreased birth weight and length, developmental delays related to CNS abnormalities that can cause intellectual impairment, hyperactivity, altered sleep patterns, feeding problems, perceptual difficulties, impaired concentration, mood problems, and language dysfunction (NCBDDD, 2015b). FASD is estimated to occur at a rate of 0.2 to 1.5 per 1,000 live births in selected areas of the United States (NCBDDD, 2015a). Among the Native American population, alcohol abuse is a major public health problem, and FASD rates are as high as 8.97 per 1,000. PHNs working collaboratively with FASD specialists among this population have been effective in preventing FASD and in helping children born with FAS (Beckett, 2011). This completely preventable leading cause of birth defects imposes major costs for educational and health care systems.

What was once termed **fetal alcohol effects** (FAEs) syndrome, characterized as causing some but not all of the symptoms of FASD, is now separated into the more descriptive categories of **alcohol-related birth defects** (ARBDs), indicating problems with hearing, bones, heart, and kidneys, and **alcohol-related neurodevelopmental disorder** (ARND), represented by mental or functional problems, including cognitive and/or behavioral abnormalities (NCBDDD, 2015b). Recent research has helped to better classify the fetal effects of alcohol and may continue to lead to more specific classifications. These conditions occur in children whose mothers have used varying amounts of alcohol while pregnant, and physical signs are often much more subtle than in cases of FAS. However, those with FASD may have one or more of the following behaviors or characteristics (NCBDDD, 2015b):

- Small size for gestational age or small stature in relation to peers
- Facial abnormalities (e.g., smooth philtrum)
- Poor coordination
- Hyperactivity, attention problems, and learning disabilities
- Difficulties in school, especially with math
- Developmental disabilities (e.g., speech and language delays)
- Intellectual disability or low IQ
- Vision and hearing problems; problems with heart, kidneys, and bones
- Poor reasoning and judgment skills
- Sleep and sucking disturbances in infancy (para. 5)

It is important to provide evidence-based primary prevention before pregnancy and to reach women before a lifestyle of drinking becomes such a part of their lives that they are unable or unwilling to abstain during pregnancy. For example, the Pregnancy Risk Assessment Monitoring System (PRAMS) is a surveillance system developed by the CDC and state health departments to collect population-based information on maternal preconception, prenatal, pregnancy, and postpartum behaviors and experiences. Recent data collection revealed that prior to conception, 23% of women used tobacco and 12.8% continued to smoke while pregnant (CDC, 2013b). Children are also at risk based on maternal alcohol use during child-rearing, especially for adolescent mothers age 15 to 19 years.

Working with women of childbearing age to improve their general health behaviors and promote better preparation for pregnancy is essential. For those pregnant women and mothers already using substances, maternal drug and alcohol treatment programs that focus on supportive parent–child attachment, enhancement of parenting and child-rearing capabilities, and encouragement of the use of support systems that can improve child health and cognitive development are needed. In-home family skills training and parenting education programs that are evidence based and promote PHN and client rapport can be effective methods of working with substance-abusing mothers and their at-risk children; however, more studies are recommended. In a systematic review of home visitation with alcohol- and drug-using mothers, there was no significance in reduction of substance abuse among mothers entering drug and alcohol rehabilitation programs for those receiving home visitation. However, individual studies showed significance of home visitation in reducing these mothers' involvement with Child Protective Services indicating a positive effect on parenting and childcare practices even if it did not effectively diminish the addictive behavior (Turnbull & Osborn, 2012).

Tobacco Use

Tobacco use has increased dramatically among women, especially since the women's movement of the 1970s, inevitably affecting maternal and newborn health. The nicotine in tobacco is a major addictive substance, and smoking is an addiction that many people find difficult to stop. Although the risk factors of smoking are well documented, many pregnant women continue to smoke. Smoking during pregnancy is one of the most studied risk factors in obstetric assessment. Women, who may have started smoking as adolescents, often continue to smoke in response to life stressors. From a population and community health nurse perspective, one study found that a higher level of smoking in one's neighborhood environment increased smoking during pregnancy for Latina women (Chesnokova, French, Weibe, Camenga, & Yun, 2015). The use of e-cigarettes, or vaping, is considered to be a health danger for pregnant women and developing fetuses. This nicotine delivery system poses threats to the baby. Also, the exhaled aerosol that is advertised to be "water vapor" actually contains nicotine and other chemicals such as metals, nitrosamines, and volatile organic compounds (CDC, 2016h).

Passive smoking or **environmental tobacco smoke (ETS)**—exposure to tobacco smoke from other people smoking in one's environment—also puts a person at risk for smoking-related disease. The Surgeon General has outlined major conclusions related to ETS based on years of research findings. One conclusion is that there is no risk-free level of secondhand smoke. Related to children and ETS, there is an increased risk of SIDS, more acute respiratory infection, ear disease, worse asthma, and risk for poor lung growth (CDC, 2013b). If a pregnant woman lives with a smoker, she and her fetus can be negatively affected by the other person's addiction. The use of **smokeless tobacco products**, such as snuff and chewing tobacco, has led to an increase in oral cancers related to tobacco exposure. Maternal smokeless tobacco use among some women has been associated with lower birth weight by an average of 78 g, controlling for other factors, and a mean of 331 g for pregnant women who smoke (England et al., 2012). An initial health history of a pregnant woman should always include the assessment of tobacco use, smoking status, and exposure to smoke in the personal environment.

Public and community health nurses and other health care professionals must be involved in the control of tobacco products on many levels, especially in health policy development, community outreach, education, and advocacy. It is very common to see smoking incentives and advertisements in poorer neighborhoods and communities of color. It is also important to have skills in smoking risk assessment, cessation options, and symptom management interventions for smoking withdrawal. Nurses should serve as positive nonsmoking role models and to be active in research implementation using clinical guidelines and evidenced-based practices. In the case of tobacco control, health policy development has made important strides at the grassroots level (see Chapter 13). A top priority of health care policy development is to reduce access of youth to tobacco products by restricting tobacco product advertising and promotion. Some significant policy steps that have been taken to discourage young people from smoking include imposing substantial cigarette excise taxes; requiring that public places, such as malls, restaurants, and even bars, be smoke-free; monitoring tobacco retailers for illegal sales to minors; and keeping cigarettes in locked cases. Most smokers become addicted to tobacco use in their early teens. If fewer adolescents begin smoking (primary prevention), there will be fewer women of childbearing age who smoke in the future (CDC, 2015e).

The community health nurse must not only advise clients to quit smoking but also offer supportive and empathetic approaches to stress reduction during smoking cessation, including methods or interventions that can help other symptom management that is associated with smoking cessation. For example, the PHN may counsel clients individually, refer for behavioral therapy, provide self-help manuals, or recommend nicotine replacement therapy or medication. Other approaches, such as support groups, can be helpful. Any permanent reduction in the number of cigarettes smoked, amount of secondhand smoke inhaled, or amount of smokeless tobacco products used is helpful in improving the health of the mother and her fetus. Particular attention should be paid to adolescent mothers (15 to 19 years), as their rates of smoking are much higher than for adolescents of similar age who are not mothers (Substance Abuse & Mental Health Services Administration, 2014).

Nurses can be positive role models for health and demonstrate health promotion strategies to clients by their own behavior—if a nurse has struggled with smoking cessation, her admission of failures or explanation of successful strategies offers an opportunity to enhance credibility with clients as they recognize that the nurse struggles with some of the same health issues.

Intimate Partner Violence

Intimate partner violence (IPV) is any coercive action taken by someone against an intimate partner (New York City Department of Health and Mental Hygiene, 2012). Pregnancy is a vulnerable period for women and can increase their risk for IPV. IPV can range from physical abuse to woman and fetus (e.g., blows to the belly) to psychological coerciveness. It is estimated that between 4% and 8% of pregnant women from all walks of life experience IPV per year (New York City Department of Health and Mental Hygiene, 2012). Reasons for increased IPV during pregnancy can be an unintended pregnancy, increased stress related to supporting a child, and jealousy. Victims of IPV have high levels of stress that may lead to or prevent cessation of smoking and substance use such as alcohol and drugs. These women may also avoid prenatal care services for a variety of reasons such as injuries, control by their partners, and a lack of resources such as transportation or money for mass transit. Pregnant women who experience psychological IPV have a 1.5- to 2-fold increase in the risk of postpartum depression (Beydoun, Beydoun, Kaufman, & Zonderman, 2012). IPV can also have effects on the newborn and infant. In a study of low-income women who had experienced IPV, posttraumatic effects were found to influence the infant as indicated by regulatory issues and socioemotional problems (Ahifs-Dunn & Huth-Bock, 2014).

Sexually Transmitted Infections

The Centers for Disease Control and Prevention (CDC) estimates the prevalence of all STI cases in the general population to be 110 million, with an annual incidence of 20 million, and health care costs of $16 billion. The CDC (2013a) has recommended STI screening of all pregnant women at the initial prenatal visit for *Chlamydia*, hepatitis, HIV, and syphilis. Further, they recommend screening high-risk pregnant women for gonorrhea.

STIs can pass from mother to baby. Syphilis can cross the placenta and infect the fetus, as can HIV—which can also be passed to the infant through breast-feeding (CDC, 2016l). Between 2012 and 2014, the rate of congenital syphilis rose 38% to 11.6 cases per 100,000 live births (Bowen, Su, Torrone, Kidd, & Weinstock, 2015). Other STIs (e.g., gonorrhea, hepatitis B, *Chlamydia*, genital herpes) can infect the baby as it passes through the birth canal during delivery. LBW, stillbirth, conjunctivitis, blindness, deafness, neurologic damage, chronic liver disease, and cirrhosis, along with neonatal sepsis and pneumonia, are possible infant complications of maternal STIs. Mothers may have premature rupture of membranes and resultant infection or may have a premature onset of labor. Some STIs can lead to cervical and other cancers, pelvic inflammatory disease, infertility, chronic hepatitis, and many other health problems (CDC, 2016m). Vaginosis during pregnancy has been linked to premature labor. However, a Cochrane systematic review determined that giving antibiotics to all pregnant women to "eradicate all vaginosis" did not significantly reduce the overall incidence of preterm births and that more evidence is needed (Brocklehurst, Gordon, Heatley, & Milan, 2013, para. 3).

A pregnant woman who discovers she has an STI often feels ashamed, betrayed, embarrassed, and angry. Those who are asymptomatic may not realize they are infected or deny the existence of the disease and fail to carry out the treatment plan after diagnosis. Although educating the pregnant client about the effects of STIs is critical, providing information alone is not enough. The community health nurse has a pivotal role in enhancing the empowerment of women so they can act on the information they receive. The PHN engages with the pregnant clients and helps them understand that they have control over their bodies. Usually, STIs are first discovered in pregnancy during routine prenatal screening, which places the clinic nurse and the nurse who may make home visits in the position to take an affirmative approach to treatment and follow-up.

HIV and AIDS

The HIV epidemic is the great tragedy of the final two decades of the 20th century, but great strides are being made in the 21st century. As a result of early detection and antiviral therapy, there has been a substantial decline in the number of infants born with HIV since the height of the epidemic. A large-scale study conducted from 2005 to 2008 examining the association between mother and child HIV transmission in 15 jurisdictions of the United States found that of the 8,054 births of HIV-infected mothers, 179 infants (2.2%) were diagnosed with HIV. It was concluded that there was an increased risk of having an HIV-infected infant among those mothers that received late testing/prenatal care or no prenatal antiretroviral therapy (Whitmore et al., 2012). An HIV-positive woman who is pregnant or who has delivered a baby requires special nursing management of the pregnancy and of the family after the birth of the newborn. There are many teaching opportunities for the PHN during a high-risk pregnancy, such as helping the client identify, change, or curtail high-risk behaviors and promoting adherence to prenatal and HIV care. Success in changing behaviors often requires an interdisciplinary approach of health care, social, emotional, and financial resources (Bungay, Massaro, & Gilbert, 2014 CDC, 2015f).

In the United States and other developed nations, HIV-infected women are advised not to breast-feed their infants because there is a chance that the infants will become infected with HIV from breast milk (Mofenson et al., 2013). The community health nurse focuses teaching on providing a safe, available, and low-cost form of infant formula. In developing countries, the lack of clean water still makes formula feeding dangerous, and breast-feeding is usually recommended. The infection rate for HIV from breast-feeding and the mortality rate from formula made with impure water are about the same, resulting in a dilemma for women and health care providers in developing countries.

Poor Nutrition, Weight Gain, and Oral Health

Nutrition is very important to the unborn child, and mothers' choices, even before conception, can affect the baby's health and development. It is at about 3 weeks' gestation—often before the woman recognizes that she is pregnant—the infant's neural tube is forming. Hormones and nutrients set gene switches that affect later life.

Research has demonstrated a positive correlation between weight gain during pregnancy and normal birth weight in the babies. In 2009, the Institute of Medicine (IOM) released new guidelines for weight gain during pregnancy based on body mass indices (BMIs). Weight gain between 25 and 35 pounds during pregnancy is recommended for women with BMIs ranging from 18.5 to 24.9, and the recommendation is 28 to 40 pounds for underweight women with a BMI under 18.5, whereas overweight women with a BMI between 25 and 29 should gain 15 to 25 pounds, and obese women with a BMI over 30.0 should hold their weight gain to between 11 and 20 pounds (IOM, 2009). The American College of Obstetricians and Gynecologists (ACOG) reaffirmed in 2015 that the 2009 IOM gestational weight gain guidelines are important for clinicians to use. It is recommended that clinicians determine a woman's BMI at the initial prenatal visit and discuss weight gain, diet, and exercise goals initially and throughout the pregnancy (ACOG, 2013b).

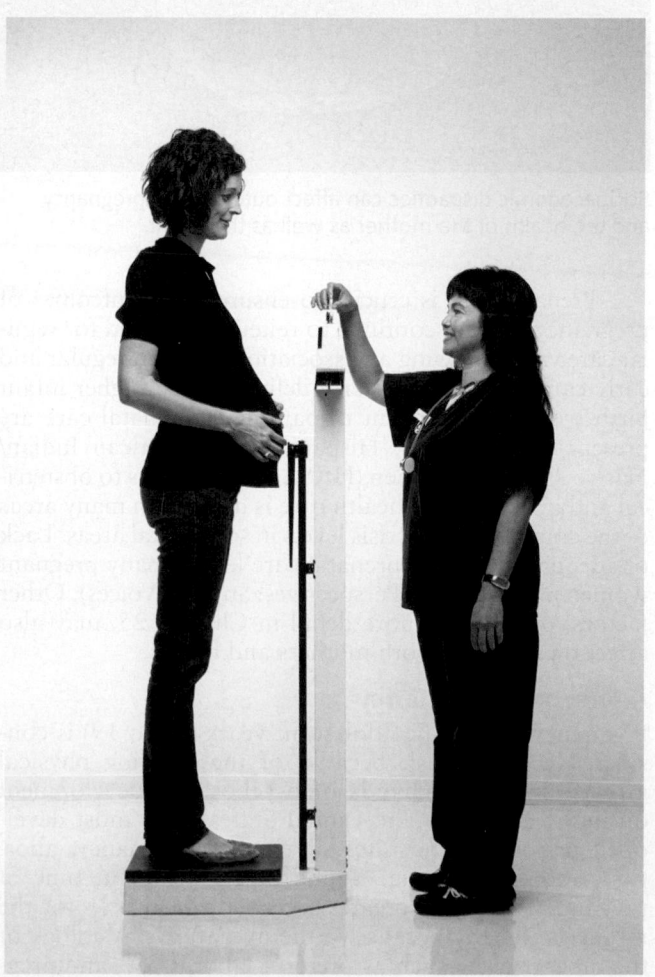

Weight gain during pregnancy should be monitored regularly.

Obesity currently affects about 36% of all American women (National Institute of Diabetes and Digestive and Kidney Diseases, 2012). Approximately 20% of UK women weighed at their first prenatal visit were determined to be obese (Midwives Information & Resource Service, 2016). Studies have shown that about 48% of pregnant women in the United States gain more than the recommended amount of weight (CDC, 2016n). Gestational diabetes poses the greatest risk to obese pregnant women and increases the risk for preterm birth (CDC, 2014e). Obese women often have nutritional deficiencies, such as anemia, and low levels of B12 and folic acid and need to be guided toward eating less processed foods, more lean meats, and more fruits and vegetables (University of Rochester Medical Center, 2011). PHNs who work with morbidly obese pregnant women can help them most by emphasizing good nutrition and by encouraging them to maintain their prepregnant weight without drastically reducing caloric intake. This can be accomplished primarily by a marked decrease in consumption of "empty calories" from junk food and replacing with increased intake of fruits, vegetables, and low-fat sources of calcium. Pregnancy is never a time for dieting. Following nutritional guidelines ensures the proper number of servings and portion sizes. Nutritional counseling can have an additional benefit in that it may ultimately decrease the risk of obesity or eating disorders in the client's children. For women who are prone to gaining too much weight, nutrition-rich, low-calorie foods are recommended.

Exercise during pregnancy is essential and can moderate maternal weight gain and improve overall fitness that is desirable for the labor and delivery process. After assessment, the PHN can determine whether the unwanted weight gain is related to the consumption of additional calories, to limited activity, or to fluid retention. Each cause must be managed differently. Underweight women have twice as many LBW babies as women whose weight is within normal range. Low maternal weight gain is associated with LBW infants who have higher incidences of growth problems, developmental delays, CNS disorders, and mental retardation (Han, et al., 2011). Nutritional teaching is part of the PHN's role when working with a pregnant woman who has difficulty gaining the recommended weight during pregnancy. Finding ways to add calories to foods and increasing the woman's desire to eat are effective methods to improve maternal weight gain. Insufficient caloric intake in pregnant adolescents (who themselves are still growing) is an additional concern for their future health and health of the infant over the life course.

Oral health during pregnancy is also very important to assess (Oral Health Care During Pregnancy Expert Workgroup, 2012). Periodontal infection may affect around 40% of women of childbearing age and is especially common among disadvantaged and ethnic or racial minorities who may not have adequate access to dental health care. Maternal periodontal disease has been linked to preterm birth, LBW, preeclampsia, and early fetal loss; however, recent studies have not shown the reduction of preterm birth or LBW among those infants whose mothers received periodontal therapy in pregnancy. Therefore, additional research in this area is needed. Although the research is conflicting, it is evident that dental health procedures have generally been found to be effective and safe for pregnant women, especially during the second trimester (ACOG, 2013a). Sugar-free gums that contain xylitol and chlorhexidine may be helpful in reducing the maternal–child transmission of caries-causing bacteria (Nayak, Nayak, & Khandelwal, 2014). Not only dental health is important during pregnancy but poor dental hygiene and disease have been linked to health conditions, such as cardiovascular disease and diabetes. High maternal levels of the bacteria that cause cavities have been associated with a greater chance of subsequent dental caries in the infant (ACOG, 2013a).

Public and community health nurses should teach women of childbearing age the importance of regular dental health checkups and proper dental hygiene, along with making referrals for dental treatment when needed. Because there is frequently a shortage of dental providers to see vulnerable or low-income women, the nurse sometimes has to advocate for pregnant women who have major oral health treatment problems, such as gingivitis or dental caries or infections. Dental health should be a part of general primary preventive education for all childbearing-age women and a major teaching and screening element of prenatal care.

Socioeconomic Status and Social Inequality

As noted earlier, poverty plays a role in pregnancy and birth outcomes. Social and economic disparities are factors in preterm birth in both developed and developing nations and reflect some of the social determinants of health. These relationships may be more indirect, as poorer women often lack health insurance, have less access to quality prenatal care services, have poorer nutrition, and are exposed to more situational and psychological stressors. In the United Kingdom, a retrospective study with a very large sample ($n = 59,487$) was done that focused on the poorly understood factors that delay seeking antenatal care and engagement in that care. Findings indicated that higher parity, pregnancy during the teenage years, higher parity, non-White ethnic background, unemployment, unmarried, poor social support, and smoking were significantly associated with late access to antenatal services and poor fetal outcomes (Kapaya et al., 2015). Prenatal stress is difficult to research because of the multiple variables that can affect prenatal stress. In vitro fertilization (IVF) is a relatively new area to consider for pregnancy stress. Differences in stress based on method of pregnancy (IVF and spontaneous pregnancy) indicate that the sources of prenatal stress differ based on pregnancy method and that nurses should be aware of the pregnancy method in their assessment interview when discussing stress (Shih et al., 2015). Other stressors should also be assessed (e.g., unintended pregnancy; nutrition; chronic stress and daily hassles; levels of social support; mental health issues, such as depression or anxiety, work stressors, racism, or discrimination; and any significant life events, such as death or other significant losses).

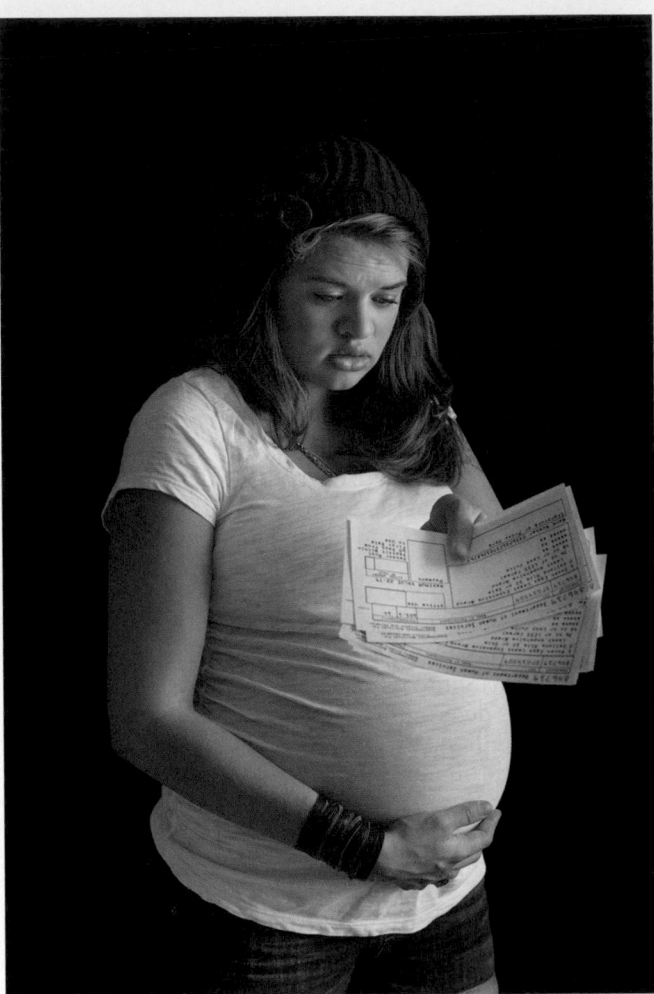

Socioeconomic disparities can affect outcomes of pregnancy and the health of the mother as well as the infant.

Prenatal care is crucial to ensure good outcomes of pregnancy. Studies continue to reiterate the need for regular care visits, showing an association between regular and early care and fewer preterm deliveries and higher infant birth weights. Significant disparities in prenatal care are present among Black, Hispanic, and American Indian/Native American women (HRSA, n.d.). Access to obstetrical and gynecological health care is difficult in many areas of the country. It is at crisis levels in some rural areas. Lack of adequate access to prenatal care leaves many pregnant women in danger (see Perspectives: Student Voices). Other factors, outlined in more detail in Chapter 25, may also affect the health of both mothers and babies.

Adolescent Pregnancy

Pregnancy during the adolescent years (13 to 19) is considered a health risk because of the ongoing physical growth and the demands of psychosocial development during these years. The United States leads most developed nations in the rates of teenage pregnancy, abortion, and childbearing. Young maternal age at time of pregnancy and birth creates several medical risks for the mother and baby because of the immature physiology of the mother-to-be such as preterm labor, LBW, and pregnancy complications. There are also many social risks

PERSPECTIVES STUDENT VOICE

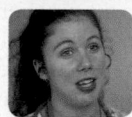

I began working as a nurse's aide at our local hospital when I started nursing school. I learned firsthand the dangers of childbirth and the long-term consequences that can result. One night, a single young female reported to the emergency room in labor and was admitted to the labor and delivery department and seen by the nurse midwife who had provided prenatal care for the mother in the clinic. The young mother-to-be was very excited. Her contractions continued, and she did not progress with the labor process, so she was to be started on oxytocin (Pitocin) to increase the effectiveness of her labor. The nurse midwife checked on her patient frequently, but problems began after the first 8 hours of labor. As the dosage was increased, the fetus reacted with bradycardia, and the nurse midwife did not notify the physician. The Pitocin dosage was decreased and then the heart rate stabilized; this process continued for three cycles. The nurse midwife signed off her 12-hour shift and handed care of the patient over to the nurse midwife coming on shift. Again, whenever the Pitocin dosage was increased to the point of becoming effective, the fetus would respond with bradycardia. Report was given, and the physician in charge was still not notified. The first two times, the fetus recovered. The third time, the fetus did not recover; instead, the bradycardia increased. By this time, the mother had been in labor for over 24 hours, and the fetus was in irreversible distress. The physician was notified of an emergency and reported to the bedside within 5 minutes. An emergency cesarean section was performed, and the Apgar scores at delivery were 0 at 1 minute, 0 at 5 minutes, 0 at 10 minutes, and 3 at 15 minutes. The infant was severely neurologically damaged. I found out later that the infant was diagnosed with severe cerebral palsy and will never walk, talk, or feed normally. She cannot swallow and will require suctioning, gastrostomy tube feeding, and total care throughout her lifetime. She is also cortically blind. The hospital and physician were sued. The nurses and the nurse midwives in the labor and delivery room were found negligent in not reporting to the physician when the patient's labor failed to progress. The nurse midwives from both shifts were found negligent for failure to recognize fetal distress and summon the physician. A multimillion-dollar award was given, and the nurses and nurse midwives employed by the hospital were fired. It is sad to think that this tragedy could have been avoided with prudent nurse–patient advocacy, reporting, and appropriate documentation—the things our nursing instructors are always drumming into our heads. I know that as a new graduate, I am now in a position of responsibility to make decisions to notify the physician or not. I have decided that the choice should always be to notify the physician. Even though it may seem inconvenient, it really should be done. I will never forget this case and its long-reaching consequences for the child and family, as well as for the nursing staff and nurse midwives.

Lyndsay, Student Nurse

such as high school dropout rates, lifetime poverty for mother and children, high rates of incarceration of the teen's child in later years, and poor school performance. Infants born to Black adolescents are more likely to be LBW babies than are infants of White teens. Infants born to very young adolescents (aged 10 to 14 years) are at very high risk for neonatal mortality. Adolescent mothers have increased psychological risks, such as isolation, powerlessness, depressive disorders, and increased somatic complaints. Developmental and maturational processes are disrupted or compromised. There is also a high prevalence of psychological distress that impacts the mental health of the teen parent and their offspring, with not enough community mental health resources in many communities (Smithbattle & Freed, 2015). It is important for PHNs to assess each pregnant adolescent's situation in order to promote the best outcomes based on available evidence and community resources including family support and living situation, relationship with the father of the baby and other supportive friends, school plans, and the ability to care for her own health and that of her infant, as well as her hopes, goals, strengths, and weaknesses, in order to effectively plan interventions (Nurse-Family Partnership, 2011).

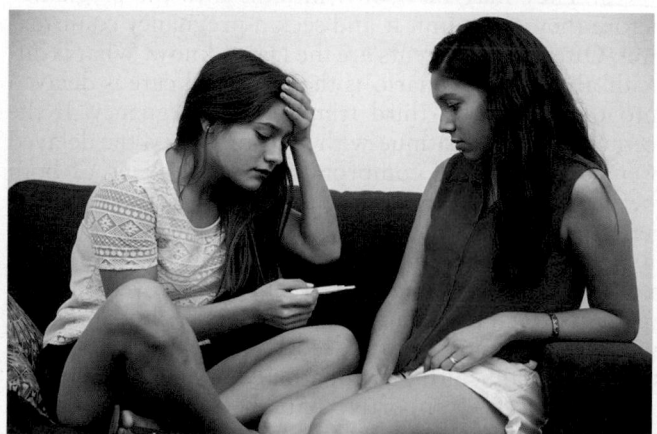

Adolescent pregnancy poses risks for both mother and baby.

The markers for successful pregnancy outcomes and future life events are complex and dependent on the expectant mother's health behavior, social determinants, and living environment. The mother's educational attainment, marital experiences, subsequent fertility behavior, labor force experience, occupational attainment, and experiences with poverty and public assistance are all directly related to the adolescent pregnancy and are often negatively affected (Pinzon, Jones, Committee on Adolescence, & Committee on Early Childhood, 2012). The issues of adolescent parenting are complex. They encompass many areas, including emotional, physical, and social issues, and the life experiences of adolescent mothers are often characterized as unequal to those of their peers who delayed childbirth (Ruedinger & Cox, 2012). Pregnant adolescents are less likely to receive early and continuous prenatal care, and they are more likely to use alcohol and to smoke during their pregnancies. Moreover, their diets are often lacking in essential vitamins and minerals.

The P/CHN has a unique challenge when developing plans of care and implementing them with pregnant teens. Part of the challenge is the developmental needs of the adolescent mother herself and preparation for becoming a mother. Teaching and counseling related to pregnancy-related changes and prenatal self-management, preparation for labor and delivery, breast-feeding, and infant care and development are some of the most immediate learning needs Development of a trusting relationship helped teens to continue breast-feeding. Emotional support is provided by relationships that engender love and appreciation, and instrumental support is more concrete (e.g., a ride to the clinic, help with homework, or money to buy food). Informational support is the provision of information or advice. Another issue with pregnant adolescents is the problem of repeated pregnancies. Public and community health nurses can provide interventions that may help postpone subsequent pregnancies such as counseling, referral, and intensive case management (Nurse-Family Partnership, 2011).

Emotional Needs

Teenagers who become pregnant deal with this change in their life in a variety of ways. Some have such a strong denial system that they deny the pregnancy, even to themselves. They may be 3 or 4 months into the pregnancy before they can admit it and seek a pregnancy confirmation. Often, their parents are the last to know. What is difficult about this scenario is that prenatal care is delayed into the second or third trimester of pregnancy. If the teen chooses to continue with the pregnancy, the delayed prenatal care could compromise the well-being of both the young mother and the fetus. Teenagers also take longer to develop their competence and identity as mothers in many cases. The major life transition of "becoming a mother" can take longer or create more developmental and situational risk. Early interventions for both prenatal and parenting support are needed to build resilience and strong mental health (Smithbattle & Freed, 2015).

Caring and supportive parents, community health nurses, and school nurses can be instrumental in guiding an adolescent through this difficult time. Adolescent parents have difficult choices to make, including decisions about continuing with the pregnancy, keeping the baby, or finding adoptive parents. Some may choose abortion. These choices are difficult, may be strongly influenced by peer opinions and social pressure, and are fraught with emotion. Adolescents and supportive parents, in consultation with professionals, can explore all options. This may be the time that the nurse first begins to work with the teen, perhaps at school or in a school-based clinic. First contact may also occur in a clinic or physician's office or on a home visit resulting from a referral from a health care provider. Home visiting programs for adolescent mothers have been effective in improving prenatal care, parenting scores, and school continuation rates (Peacock, Konrad, Watson, Nickel, & Muhajarine, 2013). The nurse can offer educational services, emotional support, and referrals for services as needed. Because postpartum depression is not uncommon, and adolescents are at increased risk, it may be important for P/CHN contact to continue periodically for 1 to 2 years postpartum. The goal of any pregnancy is positive maternal–infant outcomes, including a positive relationship. For some adolescent mothers, positive relationships are more difficult to achieve than for older mothers. Positive relationships and self-esteem have an impact on the quality of mothering and positive responses to infant distress. In classic home visitation studies conducted by Olds et al. (2007), by Nurse–Family Partnership (2011), and by Koniack-Griffin, Anderson, Verzemnieks, and Brecht (2000) and Koniack-Griffin et al. (2002) and (2003), intensive intervention programs improved parenting outcomes, including self-esteem and self-confidence. A recent systematic review confirmed that home visiting programs were effective in improving child development, reducing child abuse, and overall improving the lives of at-risk children and their families (Peacock et al., 2013).

Public health nurses who have special training in the evidenced-based home visitation models for high-risk maternal–child populations can provide each participant with services that promote the overall health of the mother and maternal–infant bonding. Results of studies, like those for the Nurse–Family Partnership, can further guide nurses in their work with pregnant adolescents and their children (Olds et al., 2013).

Physical Needs

Pregnant teens have myriad physical needs that can be addressed by routine prenatal care and education, but there is a need for continuity if such endeavors are to be successful. Routine prenatal care is one of the most important needs, and adolescents may require assistance in recognizing the value of health professionals monitoring the pregnancy. Some may feel embarrassed and uncomfortable with male health care providers and refuse to keep appointments or may want to be accompanied by the baby's father or a girlfriend. Whatever it takes to get the teen to prenatal appointments should be encouraged, including making arrangements for transportation (e.g., procuring bus tokens, calling a taxi, or arranging for a friend or social worker to drive the teen to her appointments). Where feasible, specialty-focused clinics for pregnant and parenting teens may be most effective. School-based clinics have shown promise in providing easily accessible prenatal care. One study found a 14.2% increase in school attendance with a program targeted to pregnant teens, the Prenatal at School Program (Griswold et al., 2012). The pregnant adolescent needs education regarding changes in her emotional state and her body, the growth and development of the fetus, dietary requirements, and rest and relaxation needs. She also needs anticipatory guidance for caregiving and parenting. Teaching can take place as part of each prenatal appointment, in specific classes at school for pregnant teens, in the health department clinic, or during home visits. In each setting, the PHN can modify the teaching methods to the setting and the individual needs of the adolescent. Studies show that home visits and motherhood classes are effective in promoting better outcomes for adolescents and their infants (Schaffer, Goodhue, Stennes, & Lanigan, 2012). Changing adolescent behavior during pregnancy can be challenging, and P/CHNs must keep in mind the developmental differences between early, middle, and late adolescents with regard to intentions and health habits. The P/CHN may focus on one important and seemingly less complex issue of nutrition during pregnancy. However, it is a more difficult task to change the eating habits of teens than it is to change those of adults. In their stage of development, adolescents usually are more concerned with body image than with fetal growth and development. Fad diets, peer pressure, and personal control are all issues with which the pregnant adolescent is struggling. If a teen has been raised in poverty, a multiplicity of other issues can affect her motivation to make dietary changes during pregnancy. Adolescents are more often concerned with present needs and respond better to relaxed, informal group approaches to education that involve topics of their choosing and do not resemble the school setting. Pregnancy diaries, creative activities (crafts, drawing, making snacks), small group activities and games, videos with discussions, social media and computer-assisted interventions, and visits to local community resources (hospital delivery rooms, social services, lactation counselors) are more appealing than classroom lectures. Programs that offer empowerment and group prenatal care are helpful. Also, teaching and support groups may be helpful in promoting healthy prenatal behaviors and preparing for motherhood (National Clearinghouse on Families & Youth, n.d.).

Social Needs

Peer support and acceptance is an expected part of adolescent development but can also influence the stress level of the teen. There may be changes in acceptance by social groups or in types of activities (e.g., surfboarding, mountain climbing) based on the pregnancy. The group may participate in behaviors that the pregnant adolescent should not participate in, such as smoking, drinking, or taking illicit drugs. This causes conflict for a pregnant teen who has a strong need to be accepted by her peer group and who also knows that she has a responsibility to her unborn child. Peer support almost universally changes once an adolescent girl finds herself pregnant. This can lead to conflict and isolation. The PHN can facilitate help for the adolescent client to problem solve her dilemma by providing a social support system among the attendees at prenatal classes. The nurse can also convince the teen's parents or other adults in her life to offer her more support. Often, a developmental crisis such as an adolescent pregnancy can help cement the mother–daughter relationship. It takes time and work on the part of the parents and the teen. The adolescent will need the support of her parents after the baby is born,

and strengthening the relationship during pregnancy is an important start. Another social outlet and an important resource is school. The teen should be encouraged to continue her studies, with the goal of graduation. This helps her chances for self-sufficiency, employment, and stable housing, as well as a sense of self-worth (Family and Youth Services Bureau, n.d.). Teen pregnancy and education are discussed more thoroughly in Chapter 22.

Maternal Developmental Disability

For couples that are developmentally disabled, having a child puts increased stress on a system that is already burdened. Parenting requires attending to not just the child's physical care but socialization and developmental stimulation, well-child and illness health care, emotional nurturing, and age-appropriate supervision. Depending on the social support, and coping skills of the developmentally delayed parent, the stress and need for emotional control and positive decision making can be monumental. Evidence from a large cohort study in Britain found that, for 4- to 6-year-olds, there was "no association of parental IQ with conduct or emotional problems" in the children; however, for children age 7 into adolescence, "strong evidence was observed" between lower parental IQ and child "conduct, emotional, and attention problems" (Whitley, Gale, Deary, Kivimaki, & Batty, 2011, p. 1032). Confounding variables included the environment of the home, parental affect, and child IQ. Even though there may not be strong evidence for these problems, children are still at risk for understimulation and environmental insecurity. Parent training/childcare skills programs, peer-to-peer support groups, community agencies, and careful home monitoring can reduce the risk of child abuse and neglect and promote more effective parenting (Promising Practices Network, 2012).

Much of the pediatric literature discusses the needs of developmentally disabled infants and children and the roles of nurses and health care professionals in assisting the families of these children. Developmentally disabled adults, however, are not often represented in studies of parenting, so there is limited information about their experiences and success as parents. Sometimes bizarre behaviors can occur because the parent does not understand basic concepts regarding normal child development. As with nondevelopmentally delayed parents, more responsive and involved developmentally disabled parents have better parenting outcomes. Periodic developmental screening, infant stimulation and home visitation programs, and special health care instruction have demonstrated some evidence-based results (Promising Practices Network, 2012), but there is a great need for more research. How does the PHN work with developmentally disabled parents effectively? Most importantly, nursing support must enhance the natural resilience of the family. Extended family support systems, along with community agencies and religious organizations that provide services for mentally disabled adults and children, can improve the outcomes for these families. The success of family support depends on immediate and continuing health promotion visits by multidisciplinary providers. The goal is to establish safe parenting routines that will serve as a foundation for parenting skills needed when the infant begins to walk and explore—a time when the infant's safety is more in jeopardy. A list of helpful resources is available from Connecticut Department of Developmental Services (2014).

The establishment of a trusting relationship between the nurse and the family is of foremost importance. Teaching by demonstration with many visual aids and prompts, along with games and creative approaches to engage and sustain attention, can challenge the nurse's creativity. Modeling of appropriate parenting behavior needs to occur on each visit. Supervision and monitoring of family functioning must continue until the child reaches adulthood. As part of the transition to other systems of care, PHNs often advocate for families with maternal developmental disability regarding the plan of care, interpreting it for other professionals and multiple disciplines. Many agencies employing nurses cannot provide the intensive follow-up that such a family requires. It is then necessary to make referrals to organizations that can provide support, such as the American Association of Retarded Citizens (AARC) or Exceptional Parents Unlimited. The nurse may stay involved as a consultant to the paraprofessionals or make periodic home visits at times of developmental or situational crisis.

Complications of Childbearing

Some maternal deaths are not preventable (e.g., amniotic fluid embolism). Morbidity is also a factor, and although some major risk factors among pregnant women and infants have been discussed, several common medical complications of childbearing bear mentioning. The effects of hypertensive disease in pregnancy, gestational diabetes, postpartum depression, and grief in families who have lost a child are important areas in which the P/CHN can intervene effectively.

Hypertensive Disease in Pregnancy

Blood pressure measurements in all people show daily variation, regardless of physical and mental activities. Hypertension in pregnancy may be chronic or related specifically to pregnancy. In a 13-year study (1995–2008) reviewing primary and secondary chronic hypertension in pregnancy, the prevalence almost doubled during the study period (0.90% to 1.52%), and this was shown to contribute to adverse maternal outcomes of renal failure, pulmonary edema, preeclampsia, and in-hospital mortality (Bateman et al., 2012).

Preeclampsia results in new-onset high blood pressure and protein in the urine, along with nondependent edema, and can result in eclampsia (characterized by convulsions and/or coma), pulmonary edema, liver rupture, renal failure, disseminated intravascular coagulopathy (DIC), and cortical blindness, as well as maternal death. The effects from pregnancy-induced hypertension on infants are often serious because placental health is associated with fetal growth (Skjaerven, Klungsoyr, Morken, Rich-Edwards, & Wilcox, 2015). Although protein in the urine has been a consistent marker, it may take a while to show up in lab tests and is no longer required in order for a health care provider to diagnose preeclampsia (ACOG, 2013c). Various biomarkers are helpful in predicting preeclampsia early in pregnancy (e.g., placental protein-13, PAP-A), and others (homocysteine, asymmetric dimethylarginine [ADMA], leptin) found during the first trimester can be indicative of third trimester onset (Masoura et al., 2012). A prospective study of 252 women found that in the 49 who developed preeclampsia, ADMA and homocysteine levels began to rise 1 month prior to onset, indicating that careful monitoring of these biomarkers may help identify pregnant women at risk of developing this condition (Lopez-Alarcón et al., 2015). It occurs in about 6% to 8% of pregnancies and the goal is to prevent maternal cardiac or cerebrovascular complications and preserving the fetal circulation until the baby can safely be delivered; some risk to mother is still present in the immediate postpartum period (Kattah & Garovic, 2013). Various methods are employed to attempt to prevent and control hypertension during pregnancy, namely, careful and constant monitoring of blood pressure, use of blood pressure medications if needed, frequent prenatal visits with monitoring of lab tests, a diet rich in fresh fruits and vegetables, lower sodium food choices, adequate fluid intake, weight gain limitations, rest, and regular exercise. Intermittent fetal monitoring may be required. These remain the most common preventive suggestions that PHNs, in collaboration with the clients' primary health care providers, can give to their pregnant clients. A calm environment, periods of rest, and the pregnant woman either elevating her feet or reclining in a left sidelying position are also recommended. Additional assessment data may guide the nurse to focus teaching on stress reduction techniques and modification or elimination of smoking. Public and community health nurses can provide frequent monitoring of blood pressure and other symptoms and encourage the client to be vigilant in keeping prenatal appointments. However, medication or even hospitalization may be necessary. The PHN can offer support and understanding while continuing to be a resource for the client as the pregnancy progresses and the infant is born.

Gestational Diabetes

Gestational diabetes mellitus (GDM) occurs in pregnant women who have never had a problem with high blood glucose but do during pregnancy. The average onset for GDM is around the 24th week of pregnancy (American Diabetes Association, 2016). GDM is estimated to occur in about 2% to 10% of pregnancies and is estimated to cost $1.3 billion (Dall et al., 2014). For the mother with GDM, there is a higher risk of hypertension, preeclampsia, urinary tract infections, cesarean section, and future risk of type 2 diabetes. As far as pathophysiology, GDM is similar to type 2 diabetes, and more than one third of women with GDM eventually develop type 2 diabetes during their lifetimes. Although type 2 diabetes prevalence is higher in some racial and ethnic groups, for GDM, the effects of poorer pregnancy outcomes are spread out across ethnic and racial groups with similar rates of complications of pregnancy-induced hypertension and preterm birth (Mocarski & Savitz, 2012). Because growth and maturation of the fetus are closely associated with the delivery of maternal nutrients, particularly glucose, maintenance of appropriate glucose levels is essential to the health of the fetus. Daily self-monitoring of blood glucose levels is recommended. Women should be encouraged to monitor blood glucose levels regularly 6 weeks postpartum and periodically throughout their life (CDC, 2012a).

The infant is at increased risk for fetal death because GDM has been associated with macrosomia, or large-for-gestational-age (LGA) babies, birth injuries such as broken shoulders, breathing problems, and abnormally high blood sugars at birth (Rosenstein et al., 2012). The public and community health nurse can help in the control of GDM by encouraging early prenatal care, adequate nutrition, rest and exercise, and adherence to the particular dietary, activity, and blood glucose monitoring regimen suggested by the woman's health care provider. Those P/CHNs working with pregnant women should provide education on early warning signs for GDM and the importance of regular prenatal care, reminder about getting the glucose tolerance test around the 24th week of pregnancy, and follow-up.

Postpartum Depression

Although most people recognize the common fleeting mood swings immediately after childbirth known as "baby blues," high-profile cases like Andrea Yates, who suffered from postpartum psychosis and drowned her five small children, are rare (1 or 2 per 1,000 births) but nonetheless tragic (Criminal Justice, n.d.). Actresses Brooke Shields and Hayden Panettiere, among others, have discussed their postpartum depression and treatment with antidepressant medications, making this condition more visible and less stigmatizing (Davis, 2016).

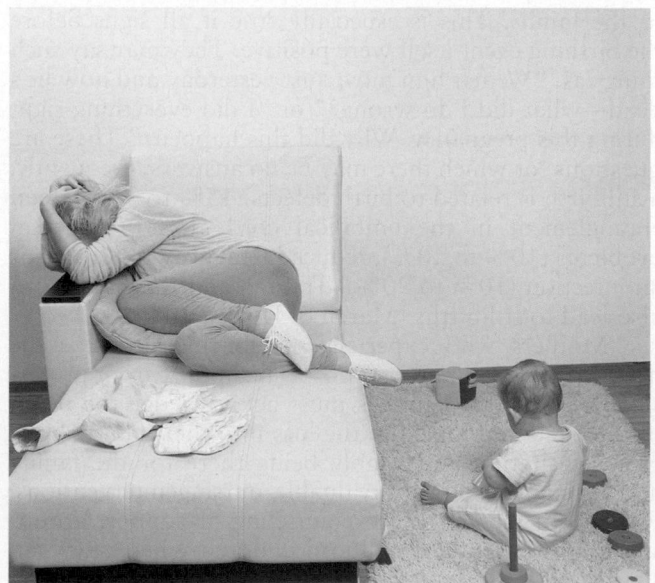

PHNs need to watch for signs of postpartum depression among their clients and offer assistance.

According to a national survey, approximately 11% of nonpregnant and 8% of postpartum women experienced depression from 2005 to 2009 (Ko, Farr, Dietz, & Robbins, 2012). Also, depression and posttraumatic stress disorder (PTSD) have been found in both mothers

and fathers subsequent to a healthy birth following a prior perinatal loss (Christiansen, Elklit, & Olff, 2013). Meta-analyses have indicated that risks for postpartum depression include a family history of psychiatric illness, poor social support, stressful life events, anxiety during pregnancy, the personality traits of neuroticism, and more recently perfectionism (Gelabert et al., 2012). Depression can affect anyone, even women without a history of prior depression. Perinatal depressive symptoms may not indicate major clinical depression. Nevertheless, symptoms may cause considerable psychological distress, such as irritability and restlessness; feeling hopeless, sad, and overwhelmed; having little energy or motivation and crying unexpectedly; sleeping and eating too little or too much; problems with cognition (memory, decision making, focus); loss of pleasure or interest in usually pleasant activities; and withdrawal from family and friends.

The value of confidantes to new mothers is evident, and mothers should be encouraged to ask for help from family and friends or to talk with other new mothers or join support groups. Group and individual therapy are helpful, as is medication. PHNs can encourage new mothers with depressive symptoms to sleep while baby is sleeping, be realistic and not try to be the perfect homemaker, ask for help from her partner with feedings during the night and with household chores, get out of the house periodically, and spend quality time with her partner. They can also refer them for a mental health evaluation.

There are several nonpharmacological interventions the nurse can initiate in addition to the ones mentioned above. First, caffeine can lead to sleep disturbance, and alcohol is a depressant that has been implicated in depression. A simple yet helpful suggestion is the elimination of both. Getting adequate sleep is important because sleep deprivation exacerbates psychiatric symptoms. Napping when the baby naps, resting when possible throughout the day, and going to bed early (albeit with the knowledge that sleep may be interrupted two or more times to feed the infant) will provide more hours of rest and sleep. Exercise is helpful and raises levels of endorphins. Anxiety symptoms often coexist with depression. Relaxation techniques that reduce anxiety can be helpful, including listening to relaxing music, doing yoga, or performing a simple exercise routine. Having a daily routine and setting realistic goals are also helpful (Griffin, 2016). Participation in a support group allows women to identify with others who may be experiencing similar difficulties. Through discussion, women provide each other with both emotional and practical support.

A final area of assistance is client education. A woman with postpartum depression is more likely to manage her depression successfully if she is aware of the symptoms of depression; the need for a support system; the importance of adequate rest, sleep, and nutrition; and the possibility of supportive psychological or pharmacologic therapy. The critical nature of postpartum depressive symptoms and the potential negative ramifications for mothers and their children are evident. Depression during pregnancy can result in lower birth weight or premature infants. Moreover, postpartum depression can affect parenting and infant stimulation that can lead to delays in infant language development and emotional bonding, lower activity levels, and behavior and sleep problems. Untreated depression can lead to substance abuse, inadequate prenatal care and nutrition, poor pregnancy outcomes, family disruption, and inadequate mother–infant bonding. However, the safety of antidepressants in pregnant and breast-feeding women is not clear. Even though psychotropic medications have been shown to cross the placental barrier and have been found both in amniotic fluid and breast milk, the ACOG encourages routine depression screenings and recommends that the use of antidepressants be individualized (ACOG, 2015). Further research supports the importance of prenatal health care providers collaborating with psychiatric health care providers to determine the best treatment for pregnant and lactating women (Chaudron, 2013). Women on any medications should be educated and advised to discuss with their providers if they become pregnant.

Community health nurses can intervene by initiating primary preventive mental health and coping measures that promote mental health throughout pregnancy and the postpartum period. Helping pregnant women to appreciate themselves and their strengths, embrace their new body changes, and positively anticipate their new role is primary preventive intervention for good mental health and promotion of attachment to their infant. If women are assessed to be at risk, mental health resources can be identified, and then, positive mental health outcomes may be fostered by supporting their self-esteem, optimizing the quality of their primary intimate relationships, anticipatory guidance on issues that may arise during pregnancy and the postpartum period, and reducing day-to-day stressors. At times, the nurse's efforts alone are not sufficient, and a referral to community mental health services for early detection and treatment is essential for the women and their children.

Fetal or Infant Death

An infrequent role for nurses in maternal–child health is that of grief counselor, but this may be a role for the advanced practice nurse in certain settings or communities. A couple may experience a miscarriage or ectopic pregnancy, stillbirth, or the death of an infant from **sudden infant death syndrome (SIDS)**, which is "the unexpected, sudden death of a child under age 1, with onset of the fatal episode apparently occurring during sleep, that remains unexplained after a thorough investigation, including performance of a complete autopsy and review of the circumstances of death and the clinical history" (Trachtenberg, Haas, Kinney, Stanley, & Krous, 2012, p. 630). The exact cause of SIDS is not certain, but it may be associated with brainstem control of heart and lung functions (Illinois Department of Public Health, n.d.). It is more common in boys and most often occurs in infants between 1 and 4 months of age (Safe to Sleep, 2015). Increased rates of SIDS are associated with side/stomach sleeping position, exposure to cigarette smoke, premature birth, cosleeping, having a sibling that died of SIDS, and soft bedding in the crib. SIDS is the leading cause of

death for infants from 1 to 12 months of age; about 2,500 infants die annually from SIDS. Since 1990, the SIDS rate has dropped, but the rates for Black and American Indian/Alaska Native infants are disproportionately higher (Illinois Department of Public Health, n.d.). A study by Trachtenberg et al. (2012) examined changed in San Diego after the Back to Sleep campaign was initiated. Infant deaths while in prone position dropped from 84% in 1991–1993 to 48.5% in 1996–2008. However, bed sharing increased from 19.2% to 37.9% overall, and for infants ≤2 months, it is more than doubled (29% to 63.8%). Researchers noted that 99% of SIDS infants had a minimum of one risk factor and only 5% had no extrinsic risk factors.

In each situation of loss, the PHN has an important supportive role. People respond to grief in a variety of ways: some express deep sadness, shock, or disbelief; some weep and are unable to talk; and others talk incessantly about regrets or guilt. Even if a miscarriage occurs early in a pregnancy, the bonding between the mother and fetus has begun, and expressions of grief may be as intense as with the loss of an infant or child. Women often have feelings of abandonment, bereavement, and guilt, thinking that they did something wrong. When parents are unable to identify the exact cause of their fetal loss, they have a more difficult time letting go of grief and anxiety. Increased anxiety levels are also found, sometimes more frequently than depression. Psychological counseling has been associated with greater decreases over time in levels of worry, grief, and self-blame (Bhat & Byatt, 2016). For couples that have delivered a stillborn baby, the shock is compounded by the experience of carrying the pregnancy to full term, along with the anticipation of an imminent delivery and the expectation of an addition to the family. This is especially true if all signs before the birthing event itself were positive. They may say such things as, "We felt him move just yesterday and now he's dead—what did I do wrong?" or "I did everything right during this pregnancy. Why did this happen?" These are questions for which there may be no answers. Frequently, a stillbirth is related to birth defects (15% to 20%), fetal entanglement in the umbilical cord (15%), placental problems (10% to 20%), reduced fetal growth (20%), or an infection (10% to 20%). Trauma and *Rh* disease can also lead to stillbirths (March of Dimes, 2015).

Mothers who experience stillbirths recognize the need for spiritual and psychosocial support from professional caregivers. Families must acknowledge the death of the child and integrate the loss into their family lives. Home visitation and simply being there for the family and listening well are invaluable nursing interventions. Referral to mental health counseling or support groups specific to parents of stillborn children where they can share their feelings may be very helpful (March of Dimes, 2015). Providing continuity and support to the family for months after the death of an infant gives the P/CHN an opportunity to assess the family for signs of unresolved grief. Grieving families may find comfort, support, and helpful information from support groups and resources such as Compassionate Friends or First Candle. When a family experiences loss of an infant after the baby has been brought home from the hospital, grief and guilt are compounded by the loss of an anticipated future and the disrupted continuity in family life. An infant may die of SIDS, a congenital anomaly, an infection, or an accident. There are constant reminders of the infant's presence in the home from memories, photos, videos, and accumulated possessions. This death disrupts family homeostasis and the psychological and physiologic equilibrium of the family. In many cases, the police are involved and an autopsy is required, contributing to the anguish of the grieving family. This promotes both guilt and loss of self-esteem and can even threaten the marriage.

INFANTS, TODDLERS, AND PRESCHOOLERS

Healthy children are a vital resource to ensure the future well-being of nations. They are the parents, workers, citizens, leaders, and decision makers of tomorrow, and their health and safety depend on today's decisions and actions. Their futures lie in the hands of those people responsible for their well-being, including the PHN, whose dominant responsibility is to the community and populations, such as dependent children.

The well-being of children has been a subject of great public health concern globally and in the United States. Its importance has been emphasized through development of numerous laws and services, yet the needs of many children continue to go unmet. Young children (up to age 4) are totally dependent on their caregivers. This contributes to their vulnerability during these years. Many young children often go to bed hungry; some infants and toddlers do not receive even the most basic immunizations before they reach school age. Accidents and injuries are a leading cause of death; preventable communicable diseases increase mortality among the very young.

Whereas the United States provides leadership in many arenas, its failure to protect and promote the health of its youngest citizens represents a significant population health breakdown. However, in many other nations—mostly less-developed countries—child health and well-being are in even greater jeopardy.

Global History of Children's Health Care

Only recently in the history of the world have children been considered valuable assets, even in countries where there are now well-developed programs of infant health promotion and protection, infant and child day care services, and strict educational expectations for all children. In some countries today, however, female infants and children or those born with congenital anomalies are not valued. Countries, such as India and China, provide inequitable care for male and female children. Gender-selective abortions or infanticide also occur. Some birth, growth, and developmental rituals are harsh and would be considered illegal if judged by Western standards. Cultural practices that are fostered by political forces prevent many countries from improving the health of infants and young children (Save the Children, 2015). For these reasons, there are great differences globally in child health care systems. The health of children in one country can affect that of children in other countries, including the United States. Major natural disasters place whole populations at risk, especially the very young and the very old.

National Perspective on Infants, Toddlers, and Preschoolers

The **infant** (birth to 1 year), **toddler** (ages 1 and 2 years), and **preschooler** populations (ages 3 and 4 years) are generally healthy years. Most U.S. children have a usual source of health care (96.9%), and their parents report them to be in excellent or very good health (Bloom, Cohen, & Freeman, 2011; CDC, 2016f). Growth and development of infants and young children should be monitored regularly. Pediatricians and P/CHNs often provide anticipatory guidance for parents so that they better understand what to expect as their child grows and can plan for safety issues that may arise. See "Internet Resources" posted on thePoint (http://thepoint.lww.com/Rector) for growth charts and educational resources.

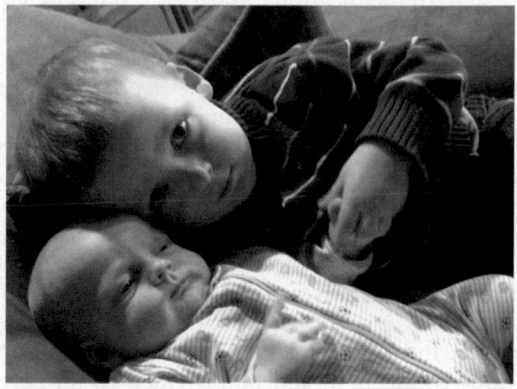

Author's private photo with permission from Deanna Rector.

The IMR in 2013 was 5.96 per 1,000 live births. The mortality rate for children ages 1 to 4 years is 25.5 per 100,000. Major causes of death include congenital malformations or deformities, as well as chromosomal abnormalities. The mortality rate for children ages 5 to 14 years is 13.0 per 100,000. Major causes are unintentional injuries (motor vehicle crashes, falls, drowning, fires, and burns), cancer, and suicide (CDC, 2016g; Xu, Murphy, Kochanek, & Bastian, 2016). Some variation in mortality rates continues among racial/ethnic groups.

Accidents and Injuries

Toddlers and preschoolers are at risk for many types of accidents and unintentional injuries, such as those caused by unsafe toys, falls, burns or scalding, drowning, motor vehicle crashes, and poisonings. These unintentional injuries are the leading cause of mortality and morbidity for children from age birth to 19 years (CDC, 2015a). Male children have higher rates of death from injuries than females; it is almost twice the rate. Causes of injury deaths vary across age groups. For those children under age one, about 66% are caused by suffocation. Between ages 1 and 4, drowning is the leading cause. In 15- to 19-year-olds, being a passenger in a motor vehicle crash was the most frequent cause of injury death. American Indian/Alaska Native children had the highest death rates from injury, and Asian/Pacific Islander children had the lowest. The loss of children's lives resulting from all injuries combined represents a staggering number of productive life years lost to society. Childhood unintentional injuries lead to almost 12,175 deaths annually (CDC, 2015a).

The *National Action Plan for Child Injury Prevention* addresses child safety and provides an agenda for injury prevention (CDC, 2012b). It brings together 60 partners in implementing injury prevention activities and providing a blueprint for collecting/interpreting data and surveillance and plans to promote research and enhance communication/education/training on injury prevention. Improving the outcomes of childhood injuries by working with health care and health systems and supporting strong policies to prevent injuries are further goals. Risks for childhood injuries that increase child vulnerability include "poverty, crowding, young maternal age, single parent households, and low maternal educational status" (USDHHS, CDC, & National Center for Injury Prevention & Control, 2012, p. 9). Using a public health model, the three levels of prevention are utilized to prevent injuries from occurring (e.g., safety latches on cabinets containing cleaning supplies or medications), minimize injuries (e.g., child safety seats), and improve emergency response and care after injury occurs (e.g., paramedica, trauma care). For instance, to prevent infant suffocation and SIDS, infants should go to sleep on their backs, in a crib or child-friendly bed without soft bedding or pillows, and parents should be cautioned about risk factors for SIDS and the potential dangers of sleeping with their babies. Information about the SIDS prevention campaign *Back to Sleep* should be provided to all parents of infants, and education should begin with hospital nurses and continue with PHNs in the community.

Burn injuries can affect children of all ages. Bath water that is too hot can also cause serious scalding injuries. Cigarette lighters and matches are fascinating to young children. Toddlers or preschoolers may be able to start a flame, injuring or killing themselves or others. The sound of a smoke alarm may frighten young children, and it is important for P/CHNs to instruct parents not only to teach their young children about fire prevention but also to be aware of the sound of the alarm and know what actions to take when they hear it, such as the *Stop Drop and Roll* program taught in Head Start and other preschool programs (National Fire Protection Association, n.d.). The PHN should also take every opportunity on home visits and in other health education settings to ask or observe if parents have a functional smoke detector in their home. Most community fire departments will install and test smoke detectors for free. Preventing the sources of injury or death from burns may be accomplished by eliminating opportunity and source. Through child supervision, safe storage of matches and lighters, and keeping children away from stoves and electrical outlets, burns and fires can be prevented.

Drowning is another category of unintentional injury in children. Brief lapses in supervision can have disastrous consequences. Young children are at risk for drowning wherever water occurs in depths exceeding a few inches—such as in toilet bowls, bathtubs, mop buckets or cans filled with rainwater, puddles, ponds, spas, and swimming pools. Lakes, rivers, streams, and irrigation ditches or canals are other water hazards. Infants, toddlers, and preschool-aged children are especially vulnerable because they are not aware of water dangers and they explore without fear. Poor children, especially children of color, are at higher risk for drowning because of lack of access to swimming lessons. The PHN can work with community groups and recreation centers to promote swimming for children. Parents need to provide a drown-free environment. Guidelines include the following (American Academy of Pediatrics, 2016; Government of Alberta, 2015):

- Bathe young children in shallow water.
- Never leave young children unattended during a bath.
- Keep toilet lids down and bathroom doors closed—preferably secured with childproof safety handles.
- Never leave full mop buckets unattended.
- Eliminate water collection sites around the home by turning over or removing empty buckets, containers, flowerpots, and other items that can collect rainwater.
- Fence swimming pool areas and install childproof locks or alarm devices that sound when the water is disturbed.
- Promote water safety measures, including teaching young children to swim.
- Be aware of the dangers of open pool drains and suction outlets than can lead to drain entrapment and hair entanglement and ensure that drain covers and safety vacuum-release systems are installed.
- Vigilant supervision of young children at play to prevent involvements with neighborhood water sources.

Supervising children in or around bathtubs, spas, pools, or other water receptacles is critical and requires close (arm's length) distances. Parents of young children should be encouraged to get CPR training. The real dangers of accidental drowning are related in From the Case Files I.

Injuries and deaths from motor vehicle crashes continue to be a major safety problem in the United States. Although 88.5% of United States families use safety belts (Pickrell & Li, 2016), some families do not use infant safety seats or child booster seats consistently, even though for decades the law has required their use. Many families have them and use them regularly but do not install them properly, placing the child at as much risk as if there were no restraint. Greenwall (2015, para. 3) reports that 59% of child car seats and 20% of child booster seats were "misused" (e.g., not properly installing seat or restraining child). The most current recommendations for safety seat use are categorized by age. For children birth up to age 2 years, a rear-facing seat should be used (placed in car's back seat); the child should continue in rear-facing seat until reaching the height or weight limit of the seat placed in the back seat; age 2 to at least 5 years, child should use forward-facing car seat until reaching upper weight and height limit for the seat; age 5 years and up, keep child in back seat with a seat belt–buckled booster seat until they reach height limit of 57 inches and can use a car seat belt alone; seat belts are considered to be properly fitting when the lap belt portion lays across the upper thighs (not stomach area) and the seat belt lays across the chest and not the neck (CDC, 2016g). There is much opportunity in this area for the

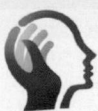

From the Case Files I

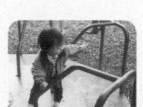

Mop Bucket Drowning

I am a Head Start nurse, and one of my assigned centers is located within a farm-labor camp. There are many large, hardworking families in the camp. Older siblings often watch over young children and help with household chores. Most families keep their cinder block homes tidy and clean, and floors are constantly being mopped (no one has carpeting—it is a bare-minimum type of accommodation). One day, several children were absent from school, and when I made home visits to determine the cause of the absences, I discovered that one of the Garcia family's children, a toddler named Miguel, had unexpectedly died. Because many of the absent children were cousins, parents had kept them home while attending to the family. I knew the Garcia

family well, and when I stopped by to check on them, they told me that Miguel had fallen into a large mop bucket the older sister had been using to clean the kitchen floor. She had gone outside for just a minute to separate the 5-year-old twins who were fighting, and when she returned, she found Miguel head first in the bucket. She tried to revive him but could not. The parents were working, trying to earn extra money for an elderly grandmother who needed surgery, and only learned of the tragedy when they returned home at the end of a long day. It was a very sad situation, and it reminded me of how even an everyday item can become deadly. Safety and prevention of unintentional injuries, especially with curious toddlers and preschoolers, is extremely important to teach all families.

Myra, Head Start Nurse

community health nurse to educate the public and ensure that parents have the information and skills to secure their children properly when traveling by car. Safety seat clinics, where installations are checked and corrected, can

help to promote the proper use of age-appropriate child restraints. See Evidence-Based Practice: Getting Families to Use Child Booster Seats for an example of effective interventions.

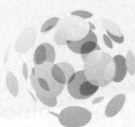

EVIDENCE-BASED PRACTICE

Getting Families to Use Child Booster Seats

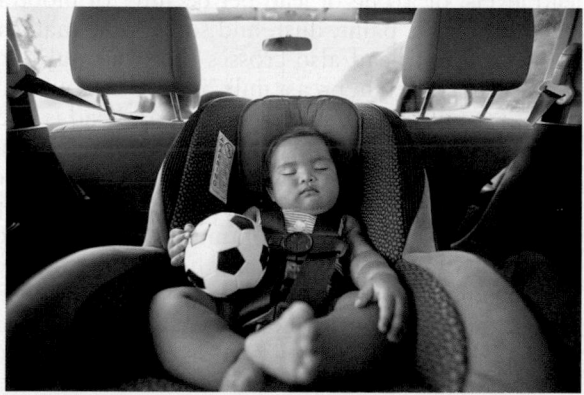

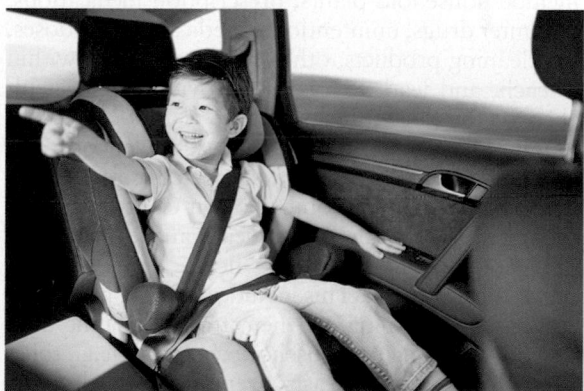

Many health departments, law enforcement, and social service agencies educate parents about the laws and benefits related to the use of child safety seats. Still, not every family consistently uses them. Education and awareness are essential to increase the use of child safety seats.

The Strike Out Child Passenger Injury (Strike Out) intervention program provided booster seat education for children ages 4 to 7 years at instructional baseball programs in four states. Twenty communities participated in the nonrandomized, controlled trial. The study tested the effectiveness of the education program before and after baseball season in increasing proper restraint use among participating children.

Findings revealed that the intervention program did increase the use of child restraint use in three of the four participating states (Alabama +15.5%, Arkansas +16.1%, and Illinois +11.0%). The study reinforces the importance that unique interventions can positively influence child safety use. It is essential for PHN/community health nurses to use evidence and a variety of approaches to combat public health problems.

Source: Aitken, M. E., Miller, B. K., Anderson, B. L., Swearingen, C. J., Monroe, K. W., Daniels, D.,... Mullins, S. H. (2013). Promoting use of booster seats in rural areas through community sports programs. *The Journal of Rural Health, 29*(s1), s70–s78.

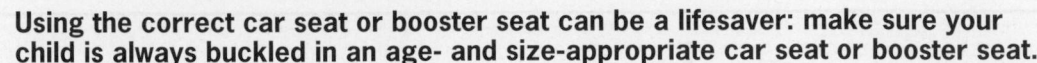

Using the correct car seat or booster seat can be a lifesaver: make sure your child is always buckled in an age- and size-appropriate car seat or booster seat.

Birth 1   2   3   4   5   6   7   8   9   10   11   12+

Age by Years*

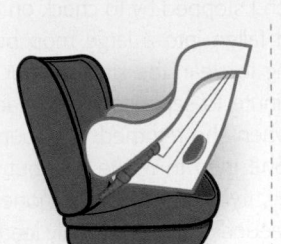 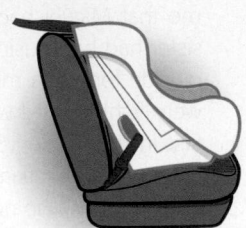 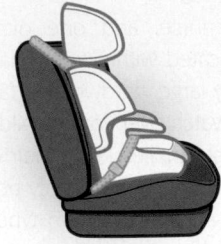 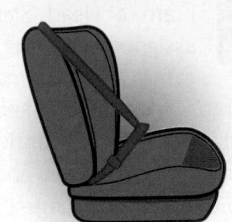

REAR-FACING CAR SEAT

Birth up to Age 2*
Buckle children in a rear-facing seat until age 2 or when they reach the upper weight or height limit of that seat.

FORWARD-FACING CAR SEAT

Age 2 up to at least age 5*
When children outgrow their rear-facing seat, they should be buckled in a forward-facing car seat until at least age 5 or when they reach the upper weight or height limit of that seat.

BOOSTER SEAT

Age 5 up until seat belts fit properly*
Once children outgrow their forward-facing seat, they should be buckled in a booster seat until seat belts fit properly. The recommended height for proper seat belt fit is 57 inches tall.

SEAT BELT

Once seat belts fit properly without a booster seat
Children no longer need to use a booster seat once seat belts fit them properly. Seat belts fit properly when the lap belt lays across the upper thighs (not the stomach) and the shoulder belt lays across the chest (not the neck).

Keep children ages 12 and under in the back seat. Never place a rear-facing car seat in front of an active air bag.

*Recommended age ranges for each seat type vary to account for differences in child growth and height/weight limits of car seats and booster seats. Use the car seat or booster seat owner's manual to check installation and the seat height/weight limits, and proper seat use.

Child safety seat recommendations: American Academy of Pediatrics.
Graphic design: adapted from National Highway Traffic Safety Administration.
www.cdc.gov/motorvehiclesafety/cps

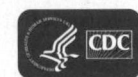

Poisoning is a constant safety concern for young children, and toddlers are most often at risk. Sources of poisoning include household plants, prescription medications, over-the-counter drugs, unintentional medication overdoses, household cleaning products, other chemicals stored within a child's reach, and lead. PHNs can provide parents with the number for the Poison Help Hotline (1-800-222-1222) and encourage them to post it next to each telephone and call immediately in the event of a suspected poisoning or overdose (American Association of Poison Control Centers [AAPCC], n.d.b). They can also educate and demonstrate for parents how to childproof the home by eliminating major sources of poisoning. This includes keeping plants out of a child's reach or eliminating them from the home until the child is older, locking up household chemicals (e.g., toilet bowl cleaner, bleach, mouthwash, oven and drain cleaners, pesticides, gasoline, paint thinner, hair products) and storing them out of a child's sight and reach, using childproof medication containers, and storing all medicines in a locked box with a key that is kept out of reach (AAPCC, n.d.a). Alcoholic beverages should also be kept out of reach, as should tobacco products. Outside hazards, such as wild mushrooms and poisonous plants, flowers, and berries, must also be considered (AAPCC, n.d.b). It is also important to eliminate sources of lead in and around the home.

Lead Poisoning

Lead poisoning historically resulted in encephalopathy and death. Today, morbidity from lead poisoning is subtle and most often affects the child's CNS with long-term changes in behavior and IQ. The CDC estimates that 250,000 children between the ages of 1 and 5 years have elevated blood lead levels, or 10 µg of lead per deciliter of blood (CDC, 2016i). Lead in paint, dust, and soil can be inadvertently consumed, and lead also crosses the placental barrier. It can be transferred in breast milk and is also found in some infant formulas (Schnur & John, 2014). Lead is one cause of childhood poisoning. There is no safe level of lead, and the elimination of elevated blood lead levels in children is a U.S. health goal. The primary sources of lead exposure in preschool-aged children continue to be lead-based paint and lead-contaminated soil and house dust. The critical age of exposure (or peak level) is thought to be between ages 18 and 36 months. Levels generally begin to decline after age 3 years. Children who live in poverty and play in substandard housing areas remain at risk for direct exposure to significant sources of lead. Lead safety and housing code enforcement, along with periodic monitoring to detect new lead hazards, can help prevent future lead exposures. Public and community health nurses, working together with environmental health sanitarians, should promote opportunities for blood lead screening, especially if it is suspected that children in certain homes, apartments, or neighborhoods are at risk for lead poisoning. Children have also been exposed to lead in some toys, candies, cosmetics, traditional medicines, and eating or drinking utensils imported from other countries. Many of these have been tested and revealed to have high levels of lead. Education and public awareness campaigns can help prevent this type of lead poisoning. Cost–benefit analysis has estimated a return of between $17 and $221 for every dollar spent in lead paint hazard control (Schnur & John, 2014). One example is Rochester, NY; the city passed a comprehensive rental housing-based lead law in 2005. Researchers subsequently evaluated its effects by reviewing city inspections of housing and health department data on child blood lead levels and discussed the new law with landlords. They noted reduced lead hazards in housing and decreased blood lead levels in children (Korfmacher, Ayoob, & Morley, 2012). PHNs can alert clients to the dangers of lead and its sources and work as an advocate for policies to reduce this danger for infants and children. See Chapter 9 for more on lead poisoning and water contaminated with lead.

Child Maltreatment

Child maltreatment is a major public health concern for the United States. It is any type of abuse directed at a child under 18 years old. Child maltreatment can be physical, emotional, and sexual abuse and child neglect (e.g., withholding feeding or medical care). Neglect is more an act or acts of omission in which a child's basic needs are not met. Children under age 4 years are at the greatest risk for severe abuse and neglect (CDC, 2014d). In 2012, approximately 686,000 children were found by child protective workers to be abused or neglected, and 1,740 died of neglect or abuse (CDC, 2014d). In 2014, over 702,000 children were documented victims of **child abuse** and neglect and over 1,500 children died from abuse or neglect (CDC, 2016d). Exposure of infants to drugs in utero is considered by many states as a form of neglect. In recent years, there has been an increase in reported cases of physical and sexual abuse in day care centers, nursery schools, children's organizations, and churches. Evidence suggests there are multiple long-term complications that occur because of child maltreatment. These complications include mental disorders, substance use, suicide attempts, STIs, and risky sexual behavior (Norman et al., 2012). It is believed that many more children also suffer from forms of abuse and neglect, but thousands of cases are not reported and not reflected in the statistics. The problem is often difficult to detect and is underreported (CDC, 2014d). One example of an often-overlooked form of abuse is shaken baby syndrome. **Shaken baby syndrome**, suspected in infants or toddlers who exhibit traumatic brain injuries caused by violent shaking or impact, is characterized by a triad of symptoms: retinal hemorrhage, subdural hemorrhage, and/or subdural hemorrhage with few signs of external trauma (Ramya, 2014). The soft brain tissues are injured as they move violently against the rough cranial bones as the infant is shaken or thrown against a hard object.

Failure to thrive (FTT) is characterized by slowing growth rate in height and weight, as well as head circumference among infants and toddlers. If an infant's growth rate is consistently below third to fifth percentiles, drops more than two percentiles, or is lower than the 80th percentile of median weight for height, a diagnosis of FTT may be made. Problems with growth may be due to many behavioral or physiological etiologies for infants but can also be related to child neglect or abnormal maternal–infant bonding. Child neglect differs from child abuse in that the action of the parent or guardian is more one of omission with neglect rather than commission as in the case of an injury related to abuse. Risk factors that point to child neglect as the basis for FTT include those most often cited for abuse and neglect, along with specific concerns about parents intentionally withholding food, being resistant to recommended interventions, and having rigid beliefs about nutrition and health regimens that may jeopardize the infant. The exact incidence of FTT is difficult to determine and no accurate estimates are available. The PHN can take a careful nutritional history and determine the mother's knowledge of basic infant needs, as well as checking for developmental milestones. A psychosocial history is also helpful (e.g., income/poverty level, cultural beliefs, social support networks, domestic abuse, substance abuse, mental health disorders), with careful attention to maternal bonding and feeding practices. Growth problems in the first 2 months of life may result in cognitive, language/speech, and fine motor deficits in childhood, and early intervention programs that involve home visitation have been effective in attenuating the long-term effects of FTT (Sirotnak, Chiesa, Windle, & Pataki, 2015).

Child maltreatment is seldom the result of any single factor but rather a combination of a chaotic environment, stressful situations, and parents who have difficulty coping with problems and stress (USDHHS, Administration for Children & Families, 2016). Risk factors for child maltreatment are found in four general areas (CDC, 2016d):

- Parent or caregiver behaviors
- Family/community characteristics
- Child factors
- Environment

Parental behaviors may include personality characteristics that include an external locus of control and poor self-esteem, along with problems with impulse control and antisocial behavior. Witnessing violence during one's own childhood may influence the use of violence as a form of parental discipline. Depression and anxiety may also play a role, and parents who had a childhood history of abuse or neglect may maltreat their children. Substance abuse is often a factor in child abuse and neglect cases. Alcohol and drug abuse often lead to neglect, as parents use money meant for household expenses on substances. Little knowledge of normal age-appropriate child development can result in unrealistic expectations. Holding negative attitudes toward their children, viewing them as property, exhibiting harsh parenting styles and verbal aggression, not knowing how to handle children's behaviors, and being easily frustrated are parental characteristics that have also been associated with risk of child maltreatment. Young parental age is also a factor, although this may be because it is also associated with poverty, lower levels of social support, and higher levels of stress. Cohabitation or sharing child supervision with a nonbiological parent can also increase the risk of child maltreatment under certain conditions (American Psychological Association, 2016; CDC, 2016d; USDHHS, 2016).

Family characteristics that include disorganization, IPV and marital conflict, financial stress and unemployment, and social isolation may lead to increased risk of child maltreatment. Children living with single parents (most often mothers) are at higher risk of physical and sexual abuse, as well as neglect; they are also more likely to live in poverty. Single parents have the sole caretaker burden and experience more stress than parents who have joint responsibilities. In a national study, children from single parent homes where a cohabiting partner is present have 10 times higher rates of abuse than children living with both biological parents; they also have 8 times higher rates of neglect. Neglect, including emotional neglect, often occurs in children living with single parents. The lowest rates of abuse and neglect were found for children living with both biological parents. Families in which child neglect occurs often are characterized by greater numbers of children or report a larger number of people living in the household. The household is frequently more chaotic, with constantly changing players—for example, mothers and children living on and off with grandmothers, aunts, boyfriends, or others. Families at high risk for child abuse may be those that are either chronically troubled or temporarily experiencing increased stressed. Disadvantaged communities and neighborhood violence can also increased risk factors for child abuse (American Psychological Association, 2016; CDC, 2016d; National Parents Organization, 2016).

Child characteristics often involve younger age (≤4) in cases of physical abuse and neglect, because of the greater need for continual care by the parent/caregiver. Maltreatment rates vary by gender (there are more girls than boys, mostly because of higher incidence of sexual abuse) and race/ethnicity (Black children have significantly higher rates than White or Hispanic). Children who are premature or LBW may be at greater risk of maltreatment because of the greater parental stress engendered by more demands on the caregiver. Children with difficult temperaments or behavior problems, or whose parents perceive them to have problems, including disabled children, could be at greater risk for abuse or neglect because of the greater caregiving demands and few community respite resources (Sedlak et al., 2010).

The environment can play a part, along with parental, family, and child factors, in determining risk for child abuse and neglect. Parents who maltreat their children have reported more loneliness, greater isolation, and lower levels of social support. Social isolation may indicate a lack of positive role models to help them better understand parenting and the consequences of child maltreatment. Unemployment, poverty, and neighborhood factors such as crime, violence, and substance use play a part in the stress placed on families. Strong, significant relationships have been found between unemployment, poverty, and child maltreatment, especially child neglect. The availability of affordable, quality, licensed day care facilities is recognized as one long-term solution for the prevention of child abuse. When their young children are safely cared for, two parents or a single parent can work and provide more resources for the family, thereby decreasing the stress that may precipitate abuse. Although poverty and lower parental education level are often linked with child abuse and neglect, no socioeconomic level is immune. Parent training programs can help teach parents to cope with fussy infants and difficult toddlers, and child sexual abuse prevention programs may also be helpful. However, P/CHN home visitation programs, like the Nurse–Family Partnership, have been researched and found to be very effective (American Psychological Association, 2016; CDC, 2016e; Krugman, Lane, & Walsh, 2007; National Bureau of Economic Research, 2016). Also, mandated reporters need to take the initiative to report suspected abuse. Only 54% of mandated reporters working in schools, compared to 77% of health agency staff and 87% of law enforcement staff, reported abuse in the last national study of child maltreatment (Sedlak et al., 2010). About 20% of schools forbid staff from making direct Child Protective Services reports. School nurses and other community health nurses can lobby for safer reporting policies and educate school staff on how to report suspected abuse.

A child with high self-esteem and an optimistic and creative nature and who is independent and uses humor is better able to cope with the adversity of child maltreatment. Other protective factors include positive mentors and role models (e.g., teachers, clergy, neighbors, peers), as well as social supports (e.g., safe schools/neighborhoods, regular health care). A parent who listens to the child's concerns, provides consistent monitoring/expectations/rules, and allows for safe ways for the child to exert independence promotes good child health and development. When families can provide for themselves, have a socially supportive network of neighbors/friends/family, and are able to cope with stressors involved in daily life, their children are at decreased risk of abuse (American Psychological Association, 2016; CDC, 2016d; USDHHS, 2016). See Display 21–2. See also Chapters 20, 22, and 30 for more on child abuse and neglect.

Communicable Diseases

Infants, toddlers, and preschool-aged children experience a high frequency of acute illnesses, more so than any other age group. Acute conditions commonly seen from birth

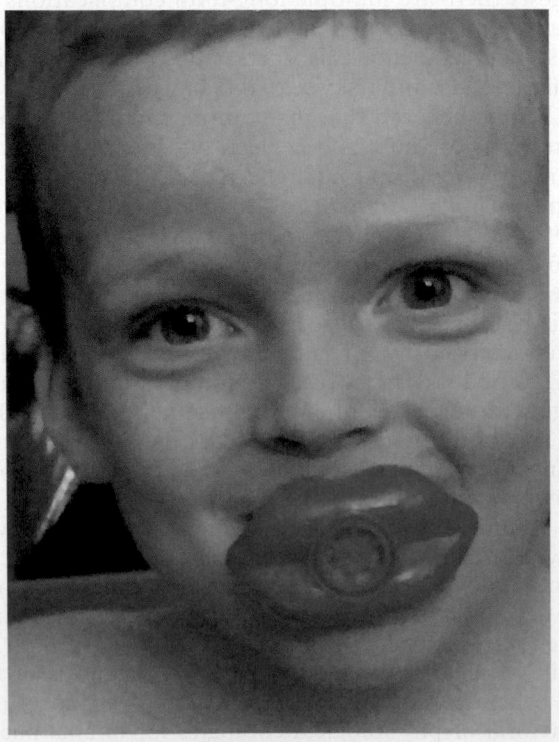

Infants, toddlers, and preschoolers are constantly putting things in their mouth and sharing items with others. (Author's photo used with permission from Deanna Rector.)

DISPLAY 21-2   REPORTS OF AN EMERGENCY FOSTER HOME

The following are examples of the various situations from which abused and neglected children come, as reported by a couple who had an emergency foster home for the county department of social services. The examples represent children placed with them over a 2-year period in which they cared for 256 children.

- Two-week-old Jose was taken to their home because the parents (under the influence of drugs) were found swinging Jose upside down in circles in an infant carrier as they walked along a downtown street at 3 AM. After being returned to his parents, he returned to foster care 1 month later after being found abandoned in an infant carrier at the county fair.
- Andre, Otis, and Selma, ages 8, 5, and 4, went to the foster home when the social services agency discovered they had been living with their father in an abandoned car for 2 years. They stayed for 3 weeks while the social worker found suitable housing for this family and counseling for the father.
- Victoria, 5 years old, a loving and passive child, arrived wearing a diaper and appeared developmentally delayed. She had a history of being physically and sexually abused. Her family was very dysfunctional, and it took the social worker several weeks to sort out relatives and their intentions before placing Victoria in a long-term foster home.
- Ronald and Randall, 6-year-old twin boys who were forced to "sexually please their mother" for several years, came to the emergency foster home before being placed with relatives while their

mother underwent psychiatric treatment. The boys began counseling during their stay in the emergency foster home.
- Antoinette, age 7, had severe asthma and was very withdrawn. She came to the emergency foster home because her mother (and the mother's boyfriend) refused to care for her. The child came with every photograph of herself and personal mementos because the mother wanted no reminders of the child. The social worker located a grandmother who would be the child's guardian.
- Thirteen-year-old Robert came home from school one day and found his mother and all their furniture gone. After a few weeks of Robert living in the basement of the apartment building, someone alerted the social services agency, and he was placed in the emergency foster home for 2 months. His mother finally called social services after 6 weeks, saying Robert was too difficult for her to handle, but she may want to see him again someday. Robert was eventually placed in a group home for boys.
- Quyn, a 17-year-old Laotian girl, came into foster care after being referred by the school nurse because of wounds observed on her wrists and ankles. Quyn reported being strapped to a chair for 12 or more hours at a time by her father because she was not following the old ways and was shaming the family by being seen in public with a boy, and without a chaperone. Several meetings were held between the parents, a Southeast Asian community leader, and the social worker to resolve this situation so that Quyn could go home safely.

---

to age 5 include fever, respiratory infections (including ear infections, colds, influenza), conjunctivitis (pink eye), and gastrointestinal problems. Communicable diseases are prevalent in these age groups, as very young children are building an immune system and are just beginning to come in contact with a greater number of people outside their families (Benaroch, 2015).

Acute respiratory illnesses (ARIs) are common in children under age five. PHNs need to emphasize that over-the-counter cough and cold medications should not be used for children under age 2. The U.S. Food and Drug Administration (FDA) questioned their safety and effectiveness at a hearing in October 2007, and manufacturers removed medication targeted to infants and toddlers; they also changed labels all cold and cough medications to read that they should not be used in children under age 4 (Hampton, Nguyen, Edwards, & Budnitz, 2013). This was in response to emergency room visits and deaths linked to their toxic effects. In 2011, the FDA formally recommended that the drugs not be used in children under age 2 as they had "serious and potentially life-threatening side effects" (FDA, 2011, para. 1). Evidence has found a reduction in emergency department (ED) visits related to cough and cold medication adverse drug events for infants and toddlers under 2 and children 2 to 3 years

of age (Hampton et al., 2013). However, parents may be uninformed about this and may use old bottles or try to give smaller doses of adult medications to their infants and toddlers. Public and community health nurses should inform parents of the dangers and suggest safer interventions (Stockwell et al., 2014).

Bronchiolitis is the most common type of lower respiratory infection among infants and starts with a runny nose, fever, and cough. It is a common cause of hospitalization in this age group; about 2% of children with respiratory syncytial virus (RSV), the most common cause of bronchiolitis, are hospitalized every year. The majority of hospitalizations for bronchiolitis are for infants 6 months and younger. RSV is the cause in 70% of cases and can rise to 100% during winter epidemics. Although wheezing, tachypnea, and chest retractions can be frightening to parents, most healthy infants survive (95%). However, P/CHNs working with at-risk infants need to work with parents and pediatricians to ensure that palivizumab (monoclonal antibody) or RSV immunoglobulin is given to preterm infants or those born closer to term but exposed to environmental pollution or to other children. An effective RSV vaccine has not yet been found, but palivizumab (Synagis) can be used to help prevent the most severe cases of RSV in high-risk infants (e.g., premature, congenital heart problems) and is given monthly by injection during RSV season (Benaroch, 2015; CDC, 2015d; Mersch & Nettleman, 2011).

As with older children and adults, air pollution increases the susceptibility of bronchitis and other respiratory illnesses among infants and children under age 5. Preschool-aged children are a target population for respiratory illness monitoring. A study of gene–environment interactions found an incidence rate of 53 episodes of bronchitis over 1,000 child months, indicating an "air pollution-induced pathogenesis" of inflammatory bronchitis (Ghosh et al., 2016). Public and community health nurses can inform families who live in areas where air pollution is significant to take the necessary precautions (see Chapter 9).

Vaccine-Preventable Diseases

Vaccines are one of the greatest achievements of public health. The number of childhood vaccines increased from 5 in 1961 to 16 in 2011 (Hinman, Orenstein, & Schuchat, 2011). Since 1980, there has been a 99% or greater decrease in deaths because of the vaccine-preventable diseases of mumps, pertussis, tetanus, and diphtheria and 80% or greater decline in deaths associated with vaccines instituted since 1980: hepatitis A and B, *Haemophilus influenzae* type B (HiB), and varicella. Smallpox has been eradicated worldwide, and the viruses for polio, rubella, and measles are no longer endemic in the United States. The decline in the number of cases of measles, mumps, rubella, pertussis, and tetanus has been dramatic (99.9%, 95.9%, 99.9%, 92.2%, and 92.9%, respectively), and cases of varicella have declined 88%. Intensive immunization campaigns have been successful in preventing infectious diseases and improving public health by reducing death and suffering from several microbial threats (Nabel, 2013). It is estimated that the childhood series of vaccines (DTP, polio, MMR, Hib, hepatitis B, and varicella) saves almost $10 billion in direct costs, $33 billion in indirect costs, 14 million infections, and 33,000 premature deaths for each fully vaccinated U.S. birth cohort (Schuchat, 2011). Newborns immature immune systems and lack of exposure to antigens, along with somewhat porous physical barriers to microbes, put them at high risk of infection. By the age of 4 to 6 months, however, a brisker antibody response to vaccines becomes possible. Successful infant and childhood immunization programs have been responsible for high vaccine coverage and the subsequent decline in morbidity and mortality from these preventable diseases.

The CDC's Advisory Committee on Immunization Practices develops policies and guidelines, based on review of current scientific research. The committee provides suggestions for available immunizations for the 17 vaccine-preventable diseases through the Vaccines for Children Program, a federal program providing uninsured and low-income families with vaccines at no charge through their primary care providers and local health department clinics. The National Immunization Survey provides surveillance for this program, with recent findings revealing that vaccination coverage rates for children aged 19 to 35 months was met or near *Healthy People 2020* objectives (Hill, Elam-Evans, Yankey, Singleton, & Kolasa, 2015).

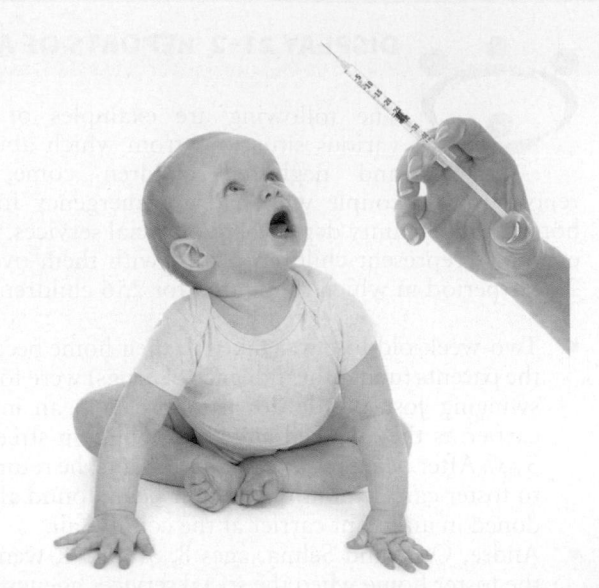

State-level immunization registries help track vaccine coverage at all age levels. Because day care centers and schools require proof of immunization, vaccination rates have improved over the last two decades. The 2009 HITECH Act proposed adoption of electronic health records (EHRs) and Immunization Information Systems (IIS) are a logical extension of that law. State and federal immunization databases help public health agencies track of immunization levels and provide data for further education, planning, and services (Hedden, Jessop, & Field, 2012). The financing of immunizations for infants and children has significantly improved as a result of two major initiatives. The Vaccines for Children Program and the Child Health Insurance Program (CHIP) cover children on Medicaid, uninsured children, and American Indian/Alaska Native children. In addition, underinsured children who receive immunizations at federally qualified health centers and rural health clinics are covered. Additional state programs and funds help provide free or low-cost vaccines for children who are not covered by the other programs. There are several ways for PHNs to help all families obtain free or low-cost immunizations and contribute to maintaining adequate levels of community immunity to communicable disease (see Chapters 8, 10 and 12).

Even if financial barriers are removed, there are other barriers. Transportation is a significant problem for some parents, especially in rural areas and for families in urban areas who have several children and need to take public transportation. All 50 states provide for medical exceptions to mandatory vaccination, and 47 allow religious exemptions; 18 permit philosophical or personal exemptions (National Conference of State Legislatures, 2016). Despite public health announcements in the media, some mothers remain unaware of the disabling consequences of diseases such as polio and do not realize the importance of fully vaccinating their children. Also, as more vaccines become available and the deadly diseases they prevent become a distant memory in the public's mind, more concerns about the safety of vaccines emerge. There has not been any link established between thimerosal, a vaccine preservative, and autism (Colaizzo, 2016). The use of thimerosal has been reduced or completely curtailed; single-dose packaging does not require the ethyl mercury preservative (Hinman et al., 2011). Numerous Web sites have emerged that advise against childhood immunization and provide graphic horror stories about the handful of severe reactions to vaccination. Media coverage and online Web sites about vaccine adverse events also contribute to decreased compliance on the part of parents in getting their children immunized. Public and community health nurses and other health professionals are encouraged to provide parents of very young children with meaningful stories of preventable deaths because of vaccines and to educate parents about scientifically based Web sites and resources rather than relying solely on dispassionate facts and figures.

At the start of the 21st century, some resurgence of pertussis, varicella, and mumps was noted, and changes were made to vaccination recommendations. Pertussis immunity was found to wane with age, and a reformulated vaccine was recommended for adolescents and adults (Tdap) so that pertussis was not inadvertently spread among infants who had not yet received their full vaccine series (Hinman et al., 2011). A two-dose varicella series is now recommended over the single-dose vaccine; measles outbreaks were found in populations where parents had refused MMR vaccination and received personal belief exemptions (Faulkner et al., 2015; Hinman et al., 2011; Kutty et al., 2015; Lopez, Schmid, & Bialek, 2015). Greater education and improved education and policies are needed to overcome this concern (see Chapters 10 and 13).

Worldwide, vaccine coverage has increased because of effects of manufacturers and philanthropists (e.g., Bill & Melinda Gates Foundation). The WHO has specific disease eradication and vaccine promotion programs around the world (see Chapter 16).

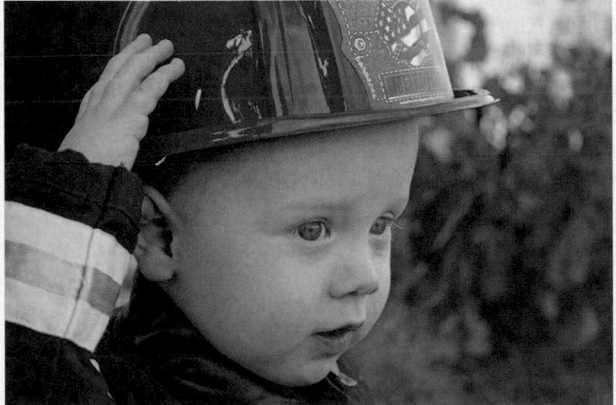

Dress up and playtime are important for toddler and preschooler development. (Author's photo used with permission from Samantha Nelson.)

Chronic Diseases

Infants and young children can be afflicted with chronic diseases that affect their quality of life. For instance, the most common chronic disease among the 6 to 11 age group is *dental caries* (CDC, 2014c). Some children begin to show signs and symptoms of cavities by the age of 10 months, and decay can begin to develop as soon as teeth erupt. Enamel defects, and subsequent caries, are more prevalent in children living in poverty and in preterm or LBW infants. One study examining the association of household socioeconomic status (SES) and food security with children's oral health outcomes found that in children aged 5 to 17 those with lower SES and those low to very low food security had significantly higher dental caries (Chi, Masterson, Carle, Mancl, & Coldwell, 2014). Dental sealants are helpful in preventing further cavities (CDC, 2014c, 2015g).

Asthma symptoms may begin in infants and toddlers. Asthma is considered by some to be the most common chronic disease of childhood, with 8.6% (6.3 million) of children younger than age 18 years diagnosed with asthma (CDC, 2016a). Inner-city, low-income, and minority children are disproportionately affected, and asthma hospitalizations are common. Otitis media in infancy and early childhood has been shown to exert an effect on the developing immune system and increases the risk for asthma and eczema (MacIntyre & Heinrich, 2012). Public and community health nurses can assist families in finding appropriate health care providers and encourage proper administration of asthma medications and treatments. They can also teach families to reduce the presence of asthma triggers in their homes (see Chapters 9 and 22 for more information on environmental triggers, asthma, and other chronic diseases of childhood and adolescence).

Autism is a developmental spectrum disorder that is often first noticed in toddlers. Parents become aware that the child's communication and interaction with others are different and that the child may also display obsessive and narrow interests. Autism spectrum disorder (ASD) is a complex developmental disorder and spectrum of ASD indicates that symptoms for each child varies and may range from mild to severe (CDC, 2016b). A child's communication skills and interaction with others are most often affected, along with obsessive behavior and narrowed interests. Behaviors associated with autism include:

- Language problems (no language, delay in language, repetitive use of language)
- Motor mannerisms (often repetitive rocking, hand flapping, object twirling)
- Fixation on objects (restricted interests)
- No spontaneous play or make-believe play; no interest in peers (problems making friends)
- Little or no eye contact (may also resist hugging)

Boys are four times more likely than girls to develop autism. An average of 41% of children with ASD also have intellectual disabilities (NCBDDD, 2012). What causes autism is unclear—some genetic links have been found, but environment may also be a factor. There is a higher risk of subsequent children having autism in a family with one autistic child or a parent with ASD (CDC, 2016b; National Institute of Neurological Disorders and Stroke [NINDS], 2015). It is often associated with other disorders (e.g., congenital rubella syndrome, Down syndrome, fragile X syndrome, tuberous sclerosis), but the exact causes are not fully understood (CDC, 2014b; NINDS, 2015). The CDC is conducting multistate research, the Study to Explore Early Development (SEED), to get a clearer picture of the number of children with ASD, "discover the risk factors and causes, and raise awareness of the signs and symptoms" (NCBDDD, n.d., para. 6). Families may need to be referred to early educational intervention programs and social service agencies for assistance. Parents need to be vigilant with daycares and preschools about their child's environmental sensitivities. It is important for PHNs to educate parents that parenting practices are *not* a cause of autism and that multiple, large-scale research studies on childhood immunizations have shown that there is no relationship between immunizations and autism (CDC, 2016b; National Vaccine Information Center, 2016; NINDS, 2015).

Sickle cell disease, an inherited blood disorder, affects thousands of children in the United States, most often those of African or Hispanic Caribbean ancestry. The characteristic chronic and severe anemia are common in young children with this condition, and it can affect memory, learning, and behavior. Children can also exhibit jaundice, gallstones, and joint pain. When both parents have the genetic mutation, the newborn will be afflicted with the disease. Those with the sickle cell trait have no symptoms of the disease but can pass it on to their offspring. In many states, routine newborn screening for sickle cell anemia is offered. Because sickle cell anemia can lead to splenic sequestration (or pooling of blood in the spleen), many children either have nonfunctioning spleens or have had them surgically removed. Risk of infection is always a concern when this occurs before age five (University of Chicago Medical Center, 2016). Public and community health nurses working with populations at risk for this disease can educate and refer families for diagnosis and treatment.

The incidence of *food allergies* is increasing in the population. Infants with close family members who have atopic diseases are at risk for development of allergies. Prolonged breast-feeding for 1 year is recommended for these infants or the use of hypoallergenic infant formula. The National Institute of Allergy and Infectious Diseases (2012) does not recommend a delay in the introduction of the most allergic foods (milk, eggs, and peanuts) for infants past the usual 4 to 6 month of age as this will not prevent a child from developing an allergy. Fortunately, once allergies are diagnosed, they can be managed through dietary changes and by avoidance of allergy-producing foods. Parents need to be educated, so that they can consistently read food labels and alert family members to the young child's allergy so that inappropriate foods are avoided.

Other chronic illnesses can have a profound effect on child and family. *Muscular dystrophy* (MD) and *cystic fibrosis* (CF) are two diseases that not only affect quality of life but also severely shorten the child's life. MD is a constellation of genetic disorders characterized by progressive atrophy and weakening of skeletal muscles. The onset of some forms of MD begins in infancy or early childhood, and MD is more common in boys (1 in than 3,300 male births). Girls are usually carriers, but a few may be "manifesting carriers" that have milder symptoms of muscle weakness (Muscular Dystrophy Association, 2016, para. 16). *Duchenne MD* usually begins before age 6 and progresses rapidly until most boys are wheelchair bound and require a ventilator (NINDS, 2016). Genetic testing can determine who is a carrier of the gene and can aid in confirming the clinical diagnosis.

CF is a genetic disease that usually begins in infancy—about 1,000 new CF cases are diagnosed annually and 75% are diagnosed before a child reaches age two. CF is characterized by a persistent cough or wheeze, shortness of breath, poor weight gain despite a good appetite, and a salty taste to the skin. Sticky, thick mucus builds up in the lungs and digestive tract. Respiratory infections become increasingly more frequent as the child ages. It is the major cause of severe chronic lung disease in children. Chest physiotherapy to help mobilize secretions is performed daily, usually by the parents. Sometimes, a vibrating inflatable vest is used that loosens mucus. Aerosolized antibiotic treatments and mucus-thinning medications help to improve lung function and reduce respiratory infections. Mucus also affects the pancreas and prevents release of digestive enzymes needed to digest food and absorb nutrients. Pancreatic enzyme supplements help with nutrient absorption (Cystic Fibrosis Foundation, n.d.; PubMed Health, 2014). Community health nurses reinforce these techniques and teach the family to avoid exposure to respiratory infections and to initiate prescribed antibiotic prophylaxis promptly. As much as feasible, the young child should be involved in his own care, offered valid choices, and encouraged to participate in decision-making. The family needs genetic counseling and emotional support as members work through feelings of anticipatory grief.

Antecedents for a number of chronic diseases that develop in adolescence and adulthood may be found in infancy and early childhood. Recent research has noted that genetics may account for 30% to 40% of risk, but environment (e.g., diet) may be responsible for 60% to 70% of risk of *diabetes*. Further, there is some evidence that suggests that exclusive, long-term breast-feeding may result in less risk of type 1 diabetes (Patelarou et al., 2012). More epidemiologists are beginning to recognize the importance of a life course approach and the effects of social determinants relative to chronic disease and early death and the societal costs of disadvantaged fetal and child health and development (Roberts & Bell, 2015). Among other variables, diet and nutrition play an important role in later health, and more research about these health connections are being released every year.

Poor Nutrition and Dental Hygiene

Other health problems found in the birth to preschool-aged group include nutritional problems (underfeeding or overfeeding, overeating, and inappropriate food choices) and poor dental health. Nutritional and dental health needs are great during this period of rapid growth. Many factors contribute to early nutritional and dental problems.

A Healthy Start is foundational to well-being later in life. Nutrition is basic in strengthening this foundation. Bonding between mother and infant and overall maternal health are predictors of infant weight gain. Both nutrition and bonding can be accomplished by breast-feeding. Some of the benefits of breast-feeding include (American Academy of Pediatrics, 2012):

- *Convenience*: Milk is always at the perfect temperature, and no preparation is needed; the infant can instantly begin feeding when hungry.
- *Cost*: No formula or bottles to buy; costs are limited to healthful diet for the mother, breast pads, nursing bras, and (possibly) a breast pump.

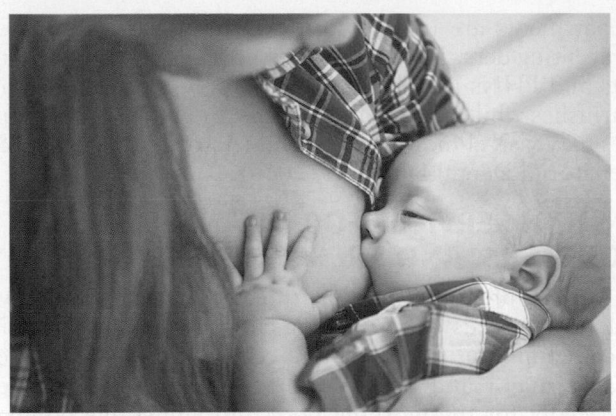

Breast-feeding has many benefits for both infant and mother.

- *Nutrition*: Breast milk is species specific; the proteins are easily digested, and fats are well absorbed; it is the most complete form of nutrition for human infants.
- *Anti-infective and antiallergic properties*: Breast milk contains immunoglobulins, enzymes, and leukocytes that protect against pathogens, and it decreases the incidence of allergy by eliminating exposure to potential antigens. Babies exclusively breast-fed for 6 or more months have fewer respiratory illnesses, ear infections, and cases of diarrhea. The chance of hospitalization for respiratory infection is reduced by 72% for infants that are breast-fed for more than 4 months.
- *Infant growth*: Breast-fed babies usually gain weight at a more moderate rate and are leaner than bottle-fed babies; rapid weight gain in infancy has been associated with later chronic diseases.
- *Long-term health effects*: Breast-feeding exclusively for at least 6 months is associated with reduced risk of overweight in later life, and breast-fed infants have slightly higher IQ scores and less change of developing atopic dermatitis, asthma, and inflammatory bowel disease. Incidence of type 1 diabetes is reduced by 30% and type 2 diabetes is reduced 40%, among infants receiving only breast milk for a minimum of 3 months.
- *Benefits for mothers*: Breast-feeding burns extra calories, helps to reduce postpartum bleeding, and delays ovulation and menstruation; it also lowers the risk of later ovarian and breast cancers. Studies show that the longer the period of lactation, the lower chance she has of developing hyperlipidemia, hypertension, cardiovascular disease, and diabetes.

The benefits of breast-feeding are well established and include protection against respiratory infections and diarrhea, long-term increased cognitive development through adolescence, and some improvement in blood pressure and total cholesterol. A systematic review found that breast-feeding had a positive effect on cognition and was associated with improved results on intelligence tests (Horta, Loret de Mola, & Victora, 2015). Several systematic reviews have found that the longer a mother breast-feeds her infant, the greater the protection against later obesity for the child (Yan, Liu, Zhu, Huang, & Wang, 2014). Public and community health nurses can encourage pregnant women to consider the benefits of breast-feeding their infants and provide education and interventions to assist them with the most common barriers: concern about

insufficient supply of breast milk, problems with the baby latching onto the breast, painful nipples, and scheduling problems. Women often choose to breast-feed their babies when they fully understand the health effects for their infants and themselves and when they receive positive influence from family and friends. The community health nurse can join with labor and delivery nurses and lactation consultants in promoting breast-feeding among mothers in the community. Nurses can lobby local hospitals to educate new mothers about the benefits of breast-feeding and stop the routine distribution of free samples of infant formula.

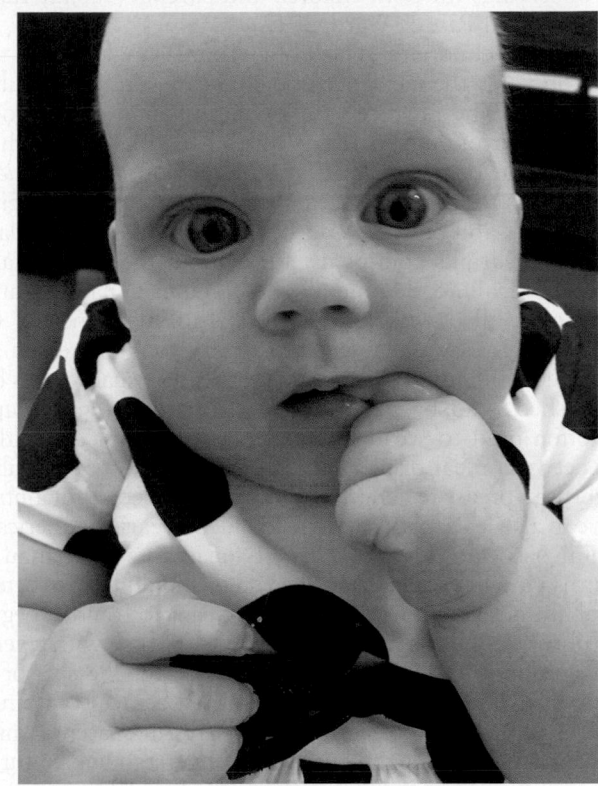

Breast-feeding gives infants a healthy head start. (Author's photo used with permission from Deanna Rector.)

Child and adolescent obesity prevalence in 2009 to 2010 was 16.9%, with 9.7% of infants and toddlers characterized as overweight. A significant trend in obesity prevalence was found for males between the ages of 2 and 19 over the previous 12-year period; this was not the case for females (Ogden, Carroll, Kit, & Flegal, 2012). In 2011 to 2012, there was a higher prevalence of obesity among Hispanic children and adolescents (22.4%) and non-Hispanic Blacks (20.2%) than among non-Hispanic Whites (14.1%) (CDC, 2015c). Another large study of 4-year-olds found prenatal and early childhood risk factors to be more prevalent among Black and Hispanic populations (e.g., maternal depression, rapid infant weight gain, higher sugar-sweetened beverage intake, and higher intake of fast foods). There were also lower rates of breast-feeding among those populations (Perrin et al., 2014).

Childhood obesity can be connected to the rise in type 2 diabetes (Copeland et al., 2013). Although overfeeding can lead to problems, poor infant growth is also problematic. The pattern of growth may also be important, such as growth problems in infancy along with overweight in later childhood. The most common sources of energy and nutrients for infants and toddlers are breast milk, formula, and milk. Fortified foods (e.g., grain-based foods with added vitamin A, folate, and iron) become increasingly more significant in toddler diets. In general, most nutrition recommendations include providing for a wide variety of foods for children. Public and community health nurses can encourage parents to continue to introduce new healthy foods to their toddlers and not give up or give in too soon. Home visiting programs that promote fruit and vegetable consumption in preschoolers have been shown to be effective in increasing the number of servings for both children and parents (Tabak, Tate, Stevens, Siega-Riz, & Ward, 2012).

Young children's diets, often unreasonably high in sugar, increase the incidence of dental caries in this population group. The practice of allowing infants to feed from the bottle beyond 15 to 16 months, or to fall asleep with a bottle, can lead to *baby bottle tooth decay* or *nursing caries*. Baby bottle tooth decay occurs when others persist in giving toddlers and preschool-aged children milk, juice, sodas, or sugared drinks continually throughout the day (Çolak, Dülgergil, Dalli, & Hamidi, 2013). Frequent snacking and sippy cups filled with juice or sugary drinks can lead to cavities. It is recommended that sugary foods be eaten at mealtimes and not as snacks and that regular snack times be established. Also, between ages 6 and 12 months, sippy cups are often used to wean infants from the breast or bottle, but between-meal drinks should consist of water or milk. Nighttime breast-feeding beyond what is needed for nutrition can also lead to increased risk of dental caries (American Dental Association, 2016). Parents of infants older than 6 months who have several erupted teeth should be instructed to rub the infant's gums with a damp, clean cloth and to begin toothbrushing, using a soft pediatric toothbrush with a very small amount of fluoride toothpaste—about the size of a grain of rice. The first dental exam should be made within 6 months of the first tooth eruption. Addressing parental misconceptions about dental health and understanding cultural beliefs and practices related to dental health and hygiene are important (American Dental Association, 2016).

Fluoride supplementation may be needed by 6 months of age if local water supplies are not fluoridated. Generally, breast-feeding infants do not require supplemental fluoride, and liquid or chewable fluoride supplements should not be given with formula or milk because absorption will be decreased (Çolak et al., 2013). As children reach the toddler years, they are able to brush their own teeth. Toothpaste should be used sparingly, and adults should continue to supervise tooth brushing. Children of this age can get overzealous with the amount of toothpaste they use and it should not be ingested. The American Academy of Pediatric Dentistry (2013) recommends an initial dental visit no later than 12 months of age. Medicaid benefits among states have varying dental benefits. Oral checks by health care providers should be a part of the well-child checks, especially in the younger years.

Dental caries is a preventable condition that can be addressed with proper nutrition and hygiene. The younger the age when dental caries first appear, the greater the risk for future tooth decay that increases the risks of chronic health conditions due the inflammatory response. Untreated dental caries can also lead to serious infections. Pain can interfere with learning at school. Many health departments are using fluoride varnishes as a means of preventing dental caries in young children. Dental hygienists and PHNs may be trained to apply the sealants and varnishes while making home visits, or children and families may visit clinics for treatment (Association of State & Territorial Dental Directors, 2015).

HEALTH SERVICES FOR INFANTS, TODDLERS, AND PRESCHOOLERS

A variety of programs that directly or indirectly serve the health needs of very young children may be found in most communities. Public and community health nurses play a major and vital role in delivering these services especially for the working poor and vulnerable populations. In public and community health, programs fall into three categories, which approximate the three priorities of PHN practice: prevention, protection, and promotion.

Preventive Health Programs

Neighborhood community centers found in urban and rural settings provide families with parenting education, health and safety education, immunizations, various screening programs, and family planning services. In some areas, nurse-run clinics are established at local schools or community centers to assist in outreach services to the community. Public and community health nurses, in collaboration with an interdisciplinary team, are often the primary care providers in these programs. The major goals are to keep communities healthy by focusing on primary and secondary prevention services. Three examples of preventive health programs for infants and young children are immunization programs, parent training programs, and quality day care health services.

Immunization Programs

Health departments, community clinics, and private health care providers continue to offer immunizations against the major childhood infectious diseases—measles, mumps, rubella, varicella, polio, diphtheria, tetanus, pertussis, hepatitis A and B, and Hib—some of which can cause permanent disability and even death. Pneumococcal, meningococcal, and influenza vaccines are also recommended, as is the vaccine for rotavirus (CDC, 2016c). Many of these diseases no longer plague infants and children, and newer vaccines offer an even greater promise of health. The current immunization schedule is available in Chapter 22.

Although the threat of these diseases has been substantially reduced, vigilance is still essential. Low immunization levels in many areas of the United States, particularly among the poor and medically underserved, and increased disease rates signal the need for constant surveillance, outreach programs, and innovative educational efforts. PHNs can help young families find low-cost vaccinations by using the Vaccines.gov Web site (http://www.vaccines.gov/getting/where/). Whenever infants and young children come in contact with public health and other community clinics, it is always important to check immunizations and provide the necessary vaccines. Public and community health nurses are deeply involved in preventive activities that promote immunizations. One important intervention is to provide each parent with immunization record that they can keep so that they have a record of their children's immunizations. This is very important until a national immunization registry is implemented. Health departments and day care centers often work collaboratively to provide vaccinations. A compulsory immunization law, varying in its application from state to state, has enabled public health personnel to carry out these preventive services (Groom et al., 2015).

Parent Training Programs

Parent education and training programs have been useful in providing parents with the tools needed to deal with the stresses and challenges of parenting effectively. A meta-analysis of 77 program evaluations revealed that effective programs consist of teaching parents to use time-out rather than corporal punishment as a means of discipline, promoting consistency in discipline, encouraging emotional communication skills and positive parent–child interaction, and requiring that parents practice these skills during classroom sessions. An effective training program for parents of preschool children is the Incredible Years Parent Training Program. Parent participants report decreased levels of stress and positive changes in their children after participating in this program (Moreland, Felton, Hanson, Jackson, & Dumas, 2016).

Some health and social service agencies offer this program for high-risk families of young children, and some evaluation studies have found this program to improve behavior and reduce symptoms of attention deficit hyperactivity disorder (ADHD) in preschool-aged children (Trillingsgaard, Trillingsgaard, & Webster-Stratton, 2014).

Quality Day Care and Preschool Programs

In 2011, nonrelative child providers cared for approximately 51% of children (birth to 4 years) of working mothers (Federal Interagency Forum on Child and Family Statistics, 2015). About 24% spent time in center-based child care. A study examining the effects of home environment and childcare facilities impact on the development of children's language, communication, and early literacy found quality childcare centers combined with a stimulating home environment resulted in better cognitive and language development (Pinto, Pessanha, & Aguiar, 2013).

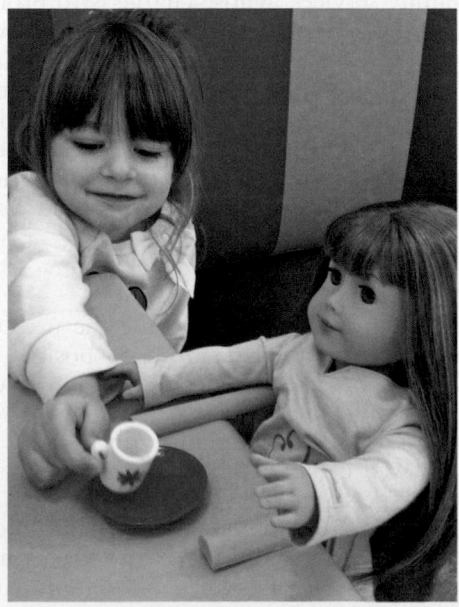

Author's private photo with permission from Danielle Rector.

Although safe, affordable child care is important, the long-term benefits of early childhood education are numerous. These benefits include higher rates of high school completion, college attendance, and full-time employment and lower rates of felony arrests, convictions, and incarcerations (Goodwin & Miller, 2013). **Head Start**, a federally funded program that offers early childhood education to low-income children between ages 3 and 5, has consistently demonstrated significant improvements in preschoolers' social, emotional, and cognitive development, and those attending Head Start do better on several developmental and educational measures. Head Start children are also more likely to receive dental and health screenings, to have up-to-date immunization coverage, to have better school attendance, and to be less likely to be held back in school. The benefits of Head Start extend to families because more Head Start parents read more frequently to their children than do parents of children not enrolled in the program. Because parents of preschoolers in Head Start must demonstrate parent involvement in the program, they are more likely to demonstrate upward mobility and positive growth (Cooper & Lanza, 2014; Lee, 2016; Nix et al., 2016). Many states provide preschool programs, and Head Start has been criticized for uneven effectiveness in learning outcomes (Whitehurst, 2013). However, the quality of day care and preschool programs varies considerably; licensing laws can regulate only minimum safety and health standards. In addition, numerous childcare operations are too small to require licensing, leaving quality and compliance unevaluated. Community and public health nurses can influence the quality of day care and preschool programs through active childcare consultation efforts that focus on health educational efforts for staff, monitoring of health and safety standards, and working to improve the state's or community's role in passing stronger licensing laws. They can also work with parents and communities providing referral to regulatory agencies and teaching about what characteristics to look for in a quality childcare center.

Health Protection Programs

Health protection programs for infants and young children are designed to protect them from illness and injury. Ultimately, these programs may even protect their lives.

Safety and Injury Protection

Accident and injury control programs serve a critical role in protecting the lives of children. Efforts to prevent motor vehicle crashes, a major cause of death, may include driver education programs, better highway construction, improved motor vehicle design and safety features, and continuing research into the causes of various types of crashes. Injury prevention and reduction have been addressed through strategies such as state laws requiring the use of safety restraints (e.g., seat belts, child safety seats), availability of front and side driver and passenger airbags, substitution of other modes of travel (air, rail, or bus), lower speed limits, stricter enforcement of drunk-driving laws, safer automobile design, and helmets for motorcyclists, bicycle riders, and skaters.

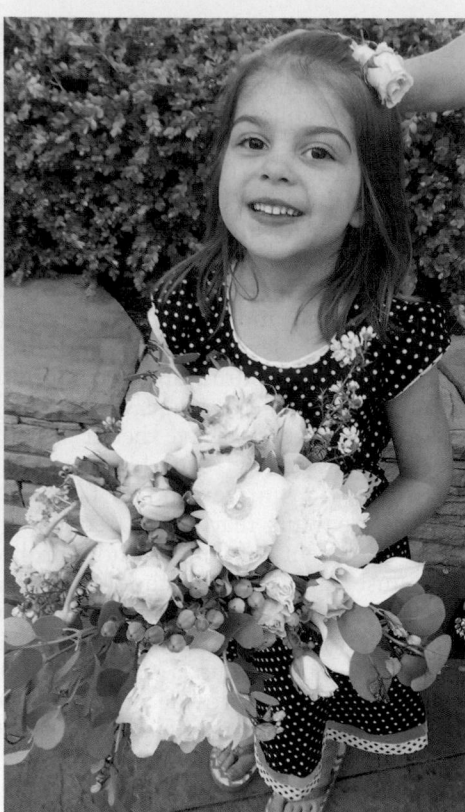

A preschooler helps the bride with her bouquet. Author photo used with permission of Tobey Roos.

For infants, toddlers, and preschool-aged children to be safe when traveling in vehicles, they must be restrained in an approved infant carrier, child restraint seat, or booster seat. These must be positioned and secured as described by the manufacturer; used at all times, even for the shortest distances; placed in the back seat, never in the front seat; and installed in the appropriate position (facing rear or front) based on the weight or age of the infant or young child. Hospital-based and community programs provide training, education, and child safety seat checks improving child safety and safety seat use (Brown, Finch, Hatfield, & Bilston, 2011; McDonald et al., 2016).

Lead poisoning prevention programs can be found in most state and local health departments. The Lead Contamination Control Act of 1988 provided for CDC funding and programs to eliminate childhood lead poisoning (CDC, 2015b). The CDC provides technical assistance, training, and surveillance at a national level. PHNs can help with targeted screening and case management and provide education to clients and communities about lead poisoning at the local level. They also work with environmental health personnel and epidemiologists to reach out to neighborhoods and communities at risk for testing. See more on this in Chapter 9.

Protection From Child Abuse and Neglect

Services to protect children from abuse are not as well developed or effective as safety and injury prevention programs, an observation accounted for by a variety of factors. Most child abuse occurs in the home, so only the most blatant situations become evident to outsiders.

Public and community health nurses and providers who see injured children may find parents' explanations plausible and may not suspect or want to believe that abuse might be responsible. Avoidance of legal involvement keeps others from reporting suspected cases. In order to protect children, this attitude must change among professionals who work with children and other community members. With reporting and intervening in child abuse, nurses practice a form of professional coercion to protect children from threats to their health.

For many years, states have had mandatory reporting laws. Enacted in 1974, the Child Abuse Prevention and Treatment Act (CAPTA) supplies funding to states to aid in preventing and investigating child abuse and neglect. Over the years, numerous amendments have expanded the definition of child abuse and the persons who are required to report. People mandated to report suspected child abuse include all those who work with children: day care providers, teachers, social workers, nurses, doctors, clergy, coaches, and so forth. In addition, animal humane workers and commercial photograph developers are mandated reporters. Procedures for reporting categories of child abuse have also been clarified, and 1990 updates included services for homeless children and families. Today, professionals and the public are more aware of the problem, and there has been an increase in reporting. In 1974, the National Center for Child Abuse and Neglect was established as a result of the CAPTA. The center collects and analyzes information on child abuse and neglect, serves as an information clearinghouse, publishes educational materials on the subject, offers technical assistance, and conducts research into the problem. The Adoption and Safe Families Act, enacted in 1997, gives further direction in working with families and promotes the safety of children while recognizing the child's need for a permanent home (U.S. Department of Health and Human Services, 2016).

In addition, these acts spurred all of the states to pass mandatory reporting laws and design procedures for investigation of suspected cases of child abuse and neglect. All states have some form of child protective services or family services, whose charge is to protect children and strengthen families. They often work with law enforcement and the judicial system, but health professionals and educators are also important team members. The basic dilemma facing those who work in this area is maintaining the family unit, if possible while at the same time keeping children safe. Most professionals adopt the *levels of prevention* model to describe child abuse and neglect prevention efforts.

Primary Prevention

Primary prevention measures include the use of public service announcements that promote positive parenting, family support groups, and public awareness campaigns about child maltreatment and how to report it, along with establishing community education to enhance the general well-being of children and their families. Educational-type services are designed to enrich the lives of families, to improve the skills of family functioning, and to prevent the stress and problems that might lead to dysfunction and abuse or neglect. The Safe Environment for Every Kid (SEEK) program has been effective in helping to prevent child maltreatment (Dubowitz, Lane, Semiatin, & Magder, 2012; Dubowitz et al., 2011).

Primary prevention also focuses on parent preparation during the prenatal period; practices that encourage parent–child bonding during labor, delivery, the postpartum period, and early infancy; and provision of information regarding support services for families with newborns. This is often the ultimate outcome sought by home visitation programs carried out or managed by PHNs. It is also helpful to provide parents of children of all ages with information regarding child-rearing strategies, anticipatory guidance for developmental milestones and tasks, and community resources. Child sexual abuse prevention curricula, such as *Good Touch/Bad Touch*, teach children skills to avoid victimization, promote discussion with children, and encourage them to tell an adult.

Secondary Prevention

Services are designed to identify and assist families who may have risk factors for impaired parenting to prevent abuse or neglect. **High-risk families** are those families that exhibit the symptoms (risk factors) of potentially abusive or neglectful behavior or that are under the types of stress associated with abuse or neglect. These can include families living in poverty, substance abuse or mental health problems, parents who were abused when they were children, and parents or children with developmental disabilities. Early intervention with high-risk families can improve emotional and functional coping and help prevent further problems. High school parent education programs for pregnant adolescents, home visitation programs targeted to at-risk families, and respite care for families with special needs children are all examples of secondary prevention actions. Family resource centers in schools or community centers located in low-income neighborhoods can offer resource and referral services to families who may be dealing with multiple sources of stress. Evidenced-based home visitation programs, such as the Nurse–Family Partnership, Early Head Start, and Healthy Families America, provide parental support and education and promote healthier family functioning and have resulted in decreased rates of child abuse and neglect (Kopko, n.d.).

Tertiary Prevention

Intervention and treatment services are designed to assist a family in which abuse or neglect has already occurred, so that further abuse or neglect may be prevented and the consequences of abuse or neglect may be minimized. Often, families are referred to mental health counselors to improve family communication and functioning. Some families may require crisis respite when they feel they cannot manage the stresses of child care. Role models, through the use of parent mentor programs, provide support and nonjudgmental coaching to parents who have sometimes been the victims of abuse themselves (Child Welfare Information Gateway, n.d.).

The public health nurse and school nurse have major roles in all levels of prevention of child maltreatment. In addition, the nurse is in a unique position to detect early signs of neglect and abuse. The nurse must establish rapport with families and assist with appropriate interventions and referrals at the secondary and tertiary levels of prevention. The advanced practice nurse may also work with families of abused and neglected children as part of an interdisciplinary approach with teachers, the department of social services, the judicial system, foster families, and other health care providers if needed. The effectiveness of local programs depends, in large measure, on the willingness of health professionals to increase their awareness and work as a team to detect, report, develop, and evaluate interventions for the perpetrators and victims of abuse and neglect. Ongoing education of health care providers is recommended to increase awareness of changing child abuse patterns, new reporting laws, and resources available to families.

Health Promotion Programs

Early childhood development and intervention programs are designed to have positive effects on the outcomes of children's cognitive and social development. Some health promotion programs have considered children's physical health, and fewer have focused on parent–child interaction and child social development. All are considered important health promotion programs from birth through preschool years.

Infant Brain Development Research and Parent–Child Interactions

New research into the normal brain development of infants and toddlers has revealed that brain maturation in the first few years of life is very rapid: the brain grows to 80% of adult size by age 3, and the myelination pattern of an 18- to 24-month-old child is similar to that of an adult (Zero to Three, 2016). The prefrontal cortex of 4-year-olds is already functional and becomes more organized throughout later adolescence. Early environment exerts a lasting influence on brain development, even in the womb. Appropriate early environment and stimulation promotes healthy development.

Because brain development is thought to be "activity dependent," and *pruning* or selection of only the most active neural circuits occurs in early childhood, parents are encouraged to provide appropriate nutrition, avoid potentially harmful substances, and provide appropriate stimulation for their infants, toddlers, and preschoolers (Zero to Three, 2016). During the first 2 years, when rapid myelination is taking place, 50% of total calories should come from fat, but after age 2, 1% or 2% milk should be the norm. Harmful substances, such as tobacco (cigarettes), chemicals, and radiation, should be avoided during pregnancy, as should contact with people who have infectious diseases. Meaningful parent–child interactions should be established early; they include holding, rocking, comforting, touching, talking, and singing. When parents talk to infants and read to young children, children later demonstrate more advanced language and literacy skills. Providing a caring and supportive environment, with opportunities to learn and explore, is supportive of healthy brain development and promotes secure infant attachment (Zero to Three, 2016). Young children who do not have early exposure to this type of environment—for example, those who are in institutional care—exhibit delays in cognitive and social development, as well as attachment disorders (van IJzendoorn et al., 2011). Important parental behaviors that promote social development include gazing into an infant's eyes, paying attention to and interacting with toddlers, and listening to and answering preschoolers' questions. Providing infants and young children with secure, learning-rich environments where they can use their senses to discover new things helps them to maximize their potential. Emotional comfort and a secure environment ensure that young children will better deal with their feelings. Public and community health nurses can provide information to parents on the most current research results about brain development as well as tangible suggestions such as low-cost brain-stimulating toys and community resources to encourage quality parent–child interactions that promote appropriate physical growth and cognitive and social development.

Developmental Screening

With the emphasis on infant and early childhood development, PHNs often routinely carry out developmental screenings. Tools such as the Ages and Stages Questionnaire (ASQ-3), Ages and Stages Social Emotional Questionnaire (ASQ: SE), Parents' Evaluation of Developmental Status (PEDS), the Child Developmental Inventory, the Denver II, and the Bayley Infant Neurodevelopmental Screening (BINS) are often used by PHNs and other child development professionals as they make routine home and childcare center visits to follow at-risk infants, children, and families. They may also access families during outreach interventions at special events such as community health fairs. Those working with high-risk or medically vulnerable infant programs periodically screen their clients to determine gaps in development and provide suggestions to parents that promote advancement (Oregon Health Plan, 2015).

Developmental screening tools are also helpful in educating parents about normal child development and can provide a means of anticipatory guidance on developmental milestones and future safety issues. *Bright Futures*, an important resource for nurses and parents, provides tools to help families determine appropriate developmental milestones and expected behaviors, along with suggestions about when to seek help from professionals. A variety of screening tools available to nurses and other health professionals, ranging from parent report instruments to those that involve direct assessment of behaviors and skills, can examine overall physical and cognitive development or screen for such things as temperament, behavior, autism, and speech and language problems. It is important for the PHN to use tools that have reported validity and reliability. Early identification of problems can lead to interventions such as enrollment in early intervention programs and help children with school readiness. These early intervention programs are available in most communities or through the public school system. Early identification is essential, but unfortunately, many children with developmental disabilities are not recognized before age 10 (Boyle et al., 2011).

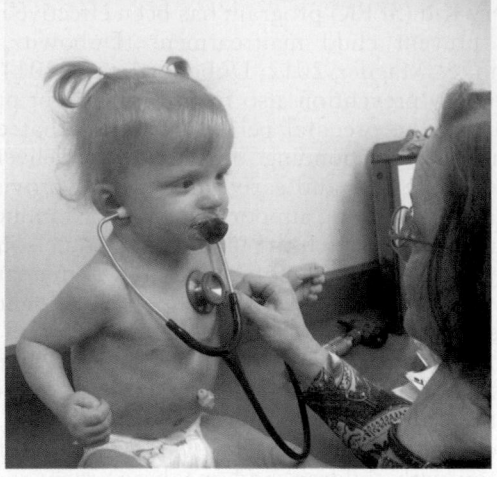

Private author's photo used with permission of Tamara Harris and Lisa Sharp, APRN, BC.

Programs for Children with Special Needs

Many children have special needs. They may have a congenital or acquired developmental disability, birth defect, or a chronic emotional, mental, or physical disease. The CDC conducts a periodic randomized national survey on CSHCN, with the most recent data available for analysis being 2009 to 2010 (CDC, 2015d). About 1 in every 33 U.S. infants are born with a birth defect each year (CDC, 2014b, 2015d). Some children suffer injuries after birth (see From the Case Files II). Autism and other mental or behavioral disorders develop after infancy and may require special services. Educational, health, and social or recreational services should be available for all children.

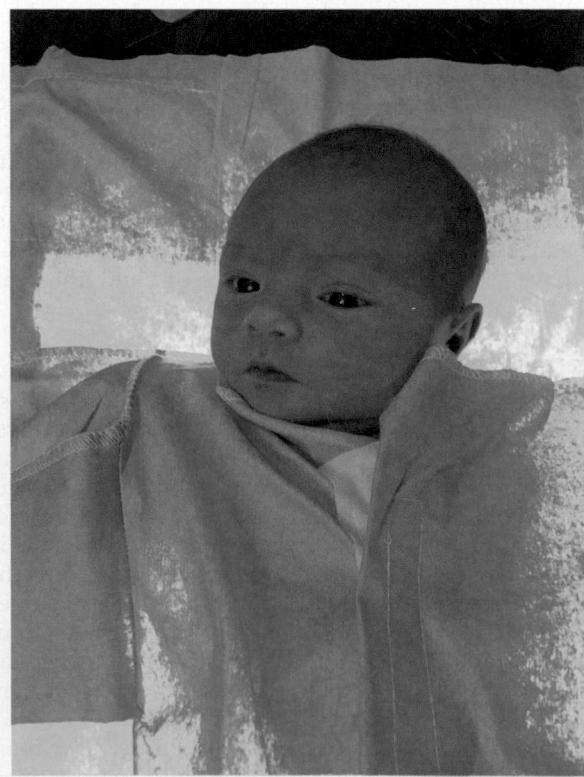

Infant using bili-blanket. Author's private photo with permission from Samantha Nelson.

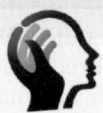

From the Case Files II

A Case of Kernicterus

A young mother was hospitalized for the birth of her second daughter, a beautiful little girl born without incident. The infant was taken to the mother for feeding and care by the nursing staff, and the mother noticed that her daughter was not very active. The infant had difficulty latching on for breast-feeding. The mother told her obstetrical nurse that the infant seemed very different from her first child. The infant was irritable, but the nurse reassured the mother that the baby was fine and "not all babies are alike." Still, the new mother was concerned.

By the second day, the mother noticed that the baby was not very alert and did not want to feed. She also noticed that the baby's color was "yellowish," and the mother notified the nurse. Again, the nurse reassured the mother that this was "normal" for infants of Asian descent. The baby still was not feeding well, and there was yellowish-orange color stool in the baby's diaper. The mother notified the nurse and asked the nurse to call the doctor. The nurse refused and told the mother that she was "overreacting." The nurse again reassured the mother that the baby was "fine" and no action was taken. The mother felt that the nurse was not listening to her concerns. The baby continued to be irritable, and the nurse said that the baby just needed to breast-feed and was insistent that the new mother was "not breast-feeding properly." The new mother was instructed not to give the baby water or additional fluids, so that the baby would breast-feed. No additional fluids were offered. The young mother was not satisfied with the nursing care and was offended that the nurse would not listen to her. A referral was made to the breast-feeding specialist at the hospital to help the new mother feed her infant. There were no phone calls documented to the physician nor was there documentation of the "yellowish-orange" stool. (The young mother kept the diaper for further proof of her concerns, though.) There was no documentation of irritability, inability to breast-feed, lethargy, or jaundiced appearance of the skin. The physician discharging the infant did not receive any information regarding irritability or yellowish stool. The nursing emphasis postpartum was on breast-feeding, and the nurses documented that the young mother had an "uncooperative attitude."

The young mother and infant were discharged home on the second postpartum day. No blood work was done for the "yellowish" color of the baby's skin, even though the yellowish tone to lower extremities and abdomen was documented in the nurse's notes and on the discharge summary. No referrals were made to Home Health or Public Health for follow-up.

Within 48 hours of discharge, the young mother brought her lethargic baby to the hospital's emergency room. On day 4 of life, the infant's bilirubin was 46. The infant was severely neurologically damaged, and the brain damage that resulted was irreversible. She was diagnosed with severe cerebral palsy, secondary to kernicterus (excessive bilirubin). The child will never be able to walk or talk. She will be fed through a gastrostomy tube for the rest of her life. She has normal intelligence, but it is locked into a dysfunctional body. The patient and family were devastated.

The physician and hospital (nurses) were sued. The nurses on duty could not defend their actions with their charting or lack thereof. The attorneys for the hospital, representing the physician and nurses, could not defend the actions of their clients. A multimillion-dollar settlement was granted, and the nurses were fired. Unfortunately, this is not an isolated case. The irreversible brain damage that occurs as a result of untreated hyperbilirubinemia should not occur in the 21st century. This was a no-win situation that could have been avoided with proper nursing intervention. Hyperbilirubinemia should always be in the forefront of newborn assessment during the first few days of life.

The nurses involved in this case were not acting as the patient's advocate. The young mother tried to tell the nurses, and the nurses should have listened to their patient. The physician should have been notified immediately when signs and symptoms were first noted. Incorrect assumptions were made because of the nationality of the patient, an indication of lack of cultural competence. Home health nursing or public health nursing care should have been arranged for infant follow-up after discharge, but these interventions did not happen.

Linda O., Certified Life Care Planner, Nurse Consultant

Federal law mandates early identification and intervention services for those with a variety of developmental disabilities. Developmental delays are characterized by slower development in one or more areas. The Individuals with Disabilities Education Act (IDEA) provides early intervention services, usually at home, for those from birth to age 2 who have developmental delays in physical, cognitive, communication, social/emotional, and adaptive development. Intervention services are also available to children with a mental or physical

problem that is likely to result in a developmental delay. Newborns can receive infant stimulation services at home or in some schools specially designed to meet the needs of the very young. These programs are offered on a part-time basis for 1 to 2 hours, two to three times a week. Special education preschools are available for young children from ages 3 to 5. By preschool age, children may advance to half-day programs. Additional services can be provided to assist the families in getting children to the programs. Door-to-door bus service in specially equipped small buses or vans safely transports young children who arrive at school in wheelchairs or with other assistive devices (Child Welfare Information Gateway, 2013).

Availability of health services for children with special needs varies with the size of the community. In small rural communities, children and their parents may have to travel long distances to receive specialized services, and in inner-city neighborhoods, lack of money for transportation can make even nearby services equally inaccessible. Accessibility is also influenced by lack of knowledge, attitudes, and prejudices. Another area of concern for special needs children is quality day care for their child. Research has shown that including special needs children in early childcare programs provides a positive experience for those children along with their normal developing peers (Extension, 2015). Public health nurses must recognize the power of these immobilizing factors and be able to deal with them effectively to make positive changes. See Chapter 25 for more on barriers to health care.

Most communities offer additional social and recreational programs for children with special needs. For example, American Lung Association affiliate offices sponsor camping programs for children with asthma or other lung diseases. Often, these are camps for school-aged children that may last up to 1 week and be located in mountain or beach areas, but they may also be day camps, with parents in attendance for preschoolers. Nationwide programs, such as the Special Olympics, offer recreational competition for children with special needs in a variety of sports, such as bowling, track and field, skiing, and swimming. The PHN best serves families as a resource for such programs. Some parents are not aware of the rights or services available for their special needs children. Nurses can advocate for parents and help establish services in communities where needed services are lacking.

Nutritional Programs

Adequate nutrition must begin before birth. One of the most productive health promotion programs is the Special Supplemental Food Program for Women, Infants, and Children (WIC). In addition to supporting women and young children with nutritious foods and achieving the initial goals of decreasing the rates of preterm and LBW babies, increasing the length of pregnancy, and reducing the incidence of infant and child iron deficiency anemia, WIC also improves pregnant women's nutritional status. WIC is not an entitlement program, but rather, Congress sets funding and eligibility requirements yearly (U.S. Department of Agriculture, 2016).

WIC provides information to parents about eating healthfully and promoting healthy rates of growth. Parents become more aware of the need to reduce consumption of saturated fat, salt, sugar, and overprocessed foods. The P/CHN, through nutrition education, reinforcement of positive practices, and referral, plays a significant role in promoting the health of infants and young children (see Levels of Prevention Pyramid). For more information about WIC, see Chapter 22.

ROLE OF THE PUBLIC AND COMMUNITY HEALTH NURSE

Public and community health nurses face the challenge of continually assessing each population's current health problems as well as determining available and needed services. PHN interventions with maternal, infant, toddler, and preschool populations are focused on health promotion, health protection, and early intervention. They may include work in family planning or high-risk clinics, telephone information services and hotlines, outreach interventions, childcare consultation, or home visitation programs. The nurse uses educational and health coaching interventions when teaching family planning, nutrition, safety precautions, and appropriate health seeking or childcare skills. Such interventions involve providing information and encouraging client groups (parents and young children) to participate in their own health care. Other interventions include strategies in which the nurse uses a greater degree of persuasion or positive manipulation, such as conducting voluntary immunization programs, working in a lead screening program, encouraging smoking cessation during pregnancy, preventing communicable diseases, and encouraging appropriate use of child safety devices such as car seats. Finally, the nurse may use interventions that motivate people into adherence with laws that require certain immunizations or mandate reporting of suspected child abuse and environmental health standards violations, such as sanitation issues. PHN home visiting programs are effective in addressing needs of high-risk and hard to reach families (Avellar & Supplee, 2013). See Chapter 6 for new programs available through health care reform.

The PHN acts as an advocate and a resource for childbearing women and couples and families of young children. The PHN may be called upon to provide information to young mothers about infant temperament, sleep schedules, colic, parenting, discipline, toilet training, television or video choices, and nutrition and feeding. The nurse should be aware of federal, state, and local laws that preserve and protect the rights of children and families. Knowledge about educational, medical, social, and recreational services needed by young families is helpful. The nurse works to secure these services in the

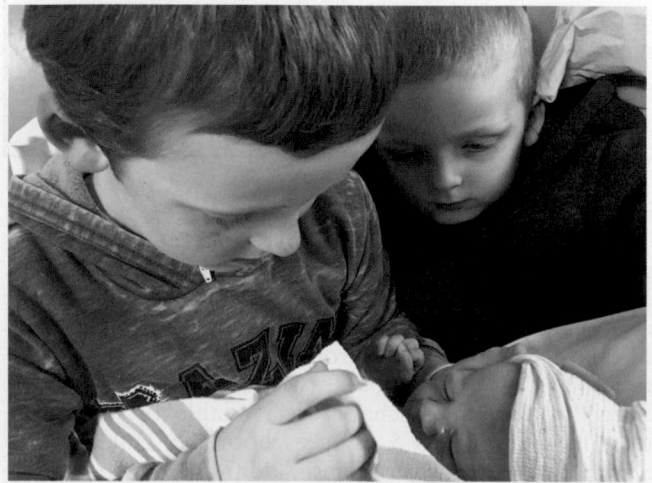

Public health nurses' role with young families is very important. (Author's photo used with permission of Deanna Rector.)

LEVELS OF PREVENTION PYRAMID

SITUATION: Desire for a healthy, full-term infant

GOAL: Using the three levels of prevention, negative health conditions are avoided, promptly diagnosed, and treated, and/or the fullest possible potential is restored.

TERTIARY PREVENTION

Rehabilitation	Primary Prevention	
	Health Promotion and Education	*Health Protection*
• The parents and significant others begin to bond with the newborn. • Parents get to know the newborn and establish a successful breast- or bottle-feeding routine. • The infant returns home in an age-appropriate infant car seat, which is used properly when traveling. • The infant's birth is celebrated according to cultural and religious preferences. • Parents resume sexual intercourse using a family planning method of their choice. • The parents enjoy the new life they have created.	• Educate about benefits of early postpartum care. • Set goals with client to make and keep appointments for postpartum and newborn visits to health care providers.	• Educate to avoid exposure to people with infectious diseases. • Educate and follow up to assure that infant immunization schedule begins on time and continues through childhood.

SECONDARY PREVENTION

Early Diagnosis	Prompt Treatment
• The mother starts prenatal care early in the first trimester and continues care at regular intervals throughout the pregnancy.	• The mother does not use alcohol, tobacco, or other mood-altering substances during the pregnancy. • The mother takes a daily prenatal vitamin with folic acid. • Parents avoid exposure to people with infectious disease. • The mother has adequate nutrition, rest, sleep, and exercise. • The mother begins supportive services if eligible (WIC, Temporary Assistance for Needy Families). • Family and significant others continue to be supportive. • The parents attend labor preparation, infant care, and parenting classes. • Name(s) is selected for the infant. • Delivery method and location are selected. • The home is prepared for the infant, e.g., adequate infant furnishings and supplies are acquired within the parents' budget. • Preparations and plans are made regarding breast- or bottle-feeding. • A pediatrician or pediatric nurse practitioner is selected. • An infant car seat is acquired and properly installed. • Plans are made to get to the chosen health care facility when in labor.

PRIMARY PREVENTION

Health Promotion and Education	Health Protection
• The pregnancy is planned. • Pregnancies are spaced 2 years (or more) apart. • Mother has a positive attitude going into the pregnancy. • A health care provider is chosen. • There are financial resources to meet the expanding family's needs. • Family and significant others are supportive. • Mother's weight is as close to ideal as possible before conception.	• Parents do not use alcohol, tobacco, or other mood-altering substances when planning to conceive. • The mother begins a vitamin regimen containing folic acid before the pregnancy.

community. Ensuring that families have the resources to provide a safe and healthy environment for their children can take many forms. The nurse may lobby to change existing laws, initiate the effort needed to establish programs and services in the community, and teach families about infant safety or the importance of immunizations.

The PHN also has skills of community and neighborhood assessment. These skills are vital to health departments and community-based organizations and primary care centers for development of programs needed for women and children (Stewart-Brown & Schrader-McMillan, 2011).

SUMMARY

Maternal–child health clients are an important population group to PHNs because their physical and emotional health is vital to the future of society. The United States does not fare well in comparison to other developed nations on maternal–child health indicators. Most developed countries have universal home visiting programs by nurses for new mothers and families, especially for the first-born child and those at high risk.

Problems of substance abuse, sexually transmitted diseases, and teen pregnancy can lead to less than optimal outcomes for newborns. Complications of pregnancy and childbirth, such as hypertension, gestational diabetes, postpartum depression, and fetal or infant death, offer opportunities for community health nurses to provide education, outreach, monitoring, and support.

IMRs in the United States are higher than those in many other countries around the world. Toddler and young child mortality and morbidity are often related to unintentional injuries. Worldwide, toddlers and preschoolers are at risk for accidents (falls, drowning, burns, and poisoning); acute illnesses, particularly respiratory illnesses; and nutritional, dental, and emotional ailments. Violence against children and deaths from homicide elicit valid concerns. These problems create major challenges for the PHN who seeks to prevent illness and injury among children and to promote and protect their health. The public health intervention of outreach is one community intervention that can lead to prevention.

Health services for children span three categories: preventive, health protecting, and health promoting. The PHN plays a vital role in each. Preventive services include immunization programs, along with quality day care and preschool. Health protection services include accident and injury prevention and control, as well as services to protect children from child abuse. Health promotion services include infant development through effective parent–child interaction, developmental screening, and services to children with special needs.

The role of PHNs includes providing interventions to serve young children's health needs (e.g., educational interventions for parents on nutrition and healthy habits). Other interventions involve encouraging age-appropriate immunizations or cessation of smoking during pregnancy, and community health nurses may employ persuasive tactics, coaching, and motivational strategies to move clients toward more positive health behaviors.

ACTIVITIES TO PROMOTE **CRITICAL THINKING**

1. What specific objectives has your local health department developed for mothers and infants to help achieve the goals listed in the *Healthy People 2020* document? How do your county's statistics compare with those of others in your state on (1) infant mortality rates (collectively and by specific ethnic groups), (2) incidence of LBW and VLBW infants, and (3) incidence of birth defects?
2. Locate some national Web sites that give you current information about progress toward meeting some of the *Healthy People 2020* goals with mothers, infants, toddlers, and preschool-aged children. Are we making progress? What can a PHN do locally to promote meeting these goals? What needs to be done on the regional, state, or national level?
3. Describe three different maternal–child populations in your county. What are their most pressing health needs? Do any existing services target these populations? How well, in your judgment, are clients' needs being met? Interview a city or county PHN and other public health professionals to help you find answers.

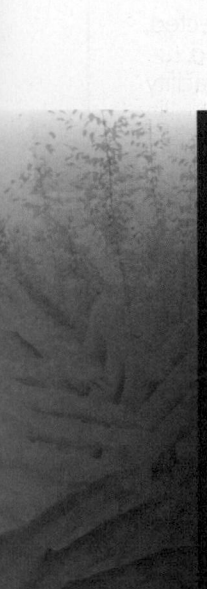

4. Sonia, an 18-year-old woman, is single and 14 weeks pregnant. Her first prenatal visit was made at the urging of her aunt, who uses the health department women's clinic. Sonia reluctantly admitted to the clinic nurse that the pregnancy was unplanned. She consumes alcohol two to three times a week—frequently as much as six 12-ounce cans of beer and 16 ounces of wine—and she smokes one pack of cigarettes a day. She has tried a variety of street drugs in the last 3 months but does not use any on a regular basis. The clinic nurse believed that Sonia might not return for regular prenatal care and made a referral to the PHN for follow-up home visits to assess Sonia's home environment and educate about prenatal care and preparation for the infant. You have been assigned to the case. How would you approach Sonia and make her feel comfortable with you? Design a plan of care to address Sonia's needs. What specific services and programs might you recommend? What barriers might exist? How would the prenatal and postpartum teaching delivered to Sonia differ from care needed by other single teens?

5. What is the major cause of death among infants, toddlers, and preschool-aged children? What community-wide interventions could be initiated to prevent these deaths? Select one intervention for each age group, and describe how you and a group of community health professionals might develop this preventive measure.

6. Describe one health promotion program that you as a PHN could initiate and carry out to improve the health of children in a day care center or preschool program.

7. Look at the pertussis, MMR, and maternal–child health vital statistics in your county or community. What do these statistics tell you about your community's health? What other related statistics are important to gather to determine if your community is a positive and healthy place for childbearing women and young children?

8. Go to the **Centers for Disease Control and Prevention** (CDC) Web site (www.cdc.gov) and look up the current childhood immunization schedule for children ages 0 to 4 years. How would you determine how to modify the schedule for a 30-month-old who is missing his last set of immunizations?

REFERENCES

Ahifs-Dunn, S. M., & Huth-Bocks, A. C. (2014). Intimate partner violence and infant development: The moderating effects of maternal trauma symptoms. *Infant Mental Health Journal, 35*(4), 322–335. doi: 1002/imhj2145S.

American Academy of Pediatric Dentistry. (2013). Guideline on periodicity of examination, preventive dental services, anticipatory guidance/counseling, and oral treatment for infants, children, and adolescents. *Pediatric Dentistry, 35*(5), E148.

American Academy of Pediatrics. (2012). *Executive summary: Breastfeeding and the use of human milk.* Retrieved from https://www2.aap.org/breastfeeding/files/pdf/Breastfeeding2012ExecSum.pdf

American Academy of Pediatrics. (2016). *Prevention of drowning.* Retrieved from http://pediatrics.aappublications.org/content/126/1/178

American Association of Poison Control Centers (AAPCC). (n.d.a). *Prevention.* Retrieved from http://www.aapcc.org/prevention/

American Association of Poison Control Centers (AAPCC). (n.d.b). *Working with AAPCC.* Retrieved from http://www.aapcc.org/working-aapcc/

American College of Obstetricians and Gynecologists (ACOG). (2013a, August). *Committee opinion: Oral health care during pregnancy and through the lifespan.* Retrieved from http://www.acog.org/Resources-And-Publications/Committee-Opinions/Committee-on-Health-Care-for-Underserved-Women/Oral-Health-Care-During-Pregnancy-and-Through-the-Lifespan

American College of Obstetricians and Gynecologists (ACOG). (2013b, January). *Committee opinion: Weight gain during pregnancy.* Retrieved from http://www.acog.org/Resources-And-Publications/Committee-Opinions/Committee-on-Obstetric-Practice/Weight-Gain-During-Pregnancy

American College of Obstetricians and Gynecologists (ACOG). (2013c). *Hypertension in pregnancy.* Retrieved from http://www.acog.org/Resources-And-Publications/Task-Force-and-Work-Group-Reports/Hypertension-in-Pregnancy

American College of Obstetricians and Gynecologists (ACOG). (2015, July 27). *ACOG statement on depression screening.* Retrieved from http://www.acog.org/About-ACOG/News-Room/Statements/2015/ACOG-Statement-on-Depression-Screening

American Dental Association. (2016). *Statement on early childhood caries.* Retrieved from http://www.ada.org/en/about-the-ada/ada-positions-policies-and-statements/statement-on-early-childhood-caries

American Diabetes Association. (2016). *Gestational diabetes.* Retrieved from http://www.diabetes.org/diabetes-basics/gestational/

American Pregnancy Association. (2016). *Using illegal drugs during pregnancy.* Retrieved from http://americanpregnancy.org/pregnancy-health/illegal-drugs-during-pregnancy/

American Psychological Association. (2016). *Understanding and preventing child abuse and neglect.* Retrieved from http://www.apa.org/pi/families/resources/understanding-child-abuse.aspx

Association of State & Territorial Dental Directors. (2015, March). *Best practice approaches for state and community oral health programs.* Retrieved from http://www.astdd.org/docs/bpar-selants-update-03-2015.pdf

Avellar, S. A., & Supplee, L. H. (2013). Effectiveness of home visiting in improving child health and reducing child maltreatment. *Pediatrics, 132*(Suppl 2), s90–s99.

Bartick, M. (2011). Breastfeeding and the US economy. *Breastfeeding Medicine, 6*(5), 313–318.

Bateman, B. T., Bansil, P., Hernandez-Diaz, S., Myhre, J. M., Callaghan, W. M., & Kuklina, E. V. (2012). Prevalence, trends, and outcomes of chronic hypertension: A nationwide sample of delivery admissions. *American Journal of Obstetrics and Gynecology, 206*(2), 134.e1–134.e8.

Beckett, C. D. (2011). Fetal alcohol spectrum disorders: A Native American journey to prevention. *Family and Community Health, 34*(30), 242–245.

Benaroch, R. (2015). *Childhood illness: The facts.* Retrieved from http://www.webmd.com/children/ss/slideshow-childhood-illnesses-to-know

Beydoun, H., Beydoun, M., Kaufman, J., & Zonderman, A. (2012). Intimate partner violence against adult women and its association with major depressive disorder, depressive symptoms and postpartum depression: A systematic review and meta-analysis. *Social Science & Medicine, 75*(6), 959–975.

Bhat, A., & Byatt, N. (2016). Infertility and perinatal loss: When the bough breaks. *Current Psychiatry Reports, 18*(3), 1–11.

Bloom, B., Cohen, R. A., & Freeman, G. (2011). Summary health statistics for U.S. children: National Health Interview Survey, 2010. *Vital Health Statistics, 10*(250). Retrieved from http://www.cdc.gov/nchs/data/series/sr_10/sr10_250.pdf

Bowen, V., Su, J., Torrone, E., Kidd, S., & Weinstock, H. (2015). Increase in incidence of congenital syphilis—United States, 2013–2014. *Morbidity & Mortality Weekly Report (MMWR), 64*(44), 1241–1245.

Boyle, C. A., Boulet, S., Schieve, L., Cohen, R. A., Blumberg, S. J., Yeargin-Allsopp, M., ... Kogan, M. D. (2011). Trends in the prevalence of developmental disabilities in U.S. children, 1997–2008. *Pediatrics, 127*(6), 1034–1042. doi: 10.1542/peds.2010-2989.

Brocklehurst, P., Gordon, A., Heatley, E., & Milan, S. J. (2013, January 31). *Antibiotics for treating bacterial vaginosis in pregnancy.* Retrieved from http://www.cochrane.org/CD000262/PREG_antibiotics-for-treating-bacterial-vaginosis-in-pregnancy

Brown, J., Finch, C. F., Hatfield, J., & Bilston, L. E. (2011). Child restraint fitting stations reduce incorrect restraint use among child occupants. *Accident Analysis & Prevention, 43*(3), 1128–1133.

Brown, P. A., Kaiser, K. L., & Nailon, R. F. (2014). Integrating quality improvement and translational research models to increase exclusive breastfeeding. *Journal of Obstetric, Gynecological, and Neonatal Nursing, 43*(5), 545–553. doi: 10.1111/1552-6909.12482.

Bungay, V., Massaro, C. L., & Gilbert, M. (2014). Examining the scope of public health nursing practice in sexually transmitted infection prevention and management: What do nurses do? *Journal of Clinical Nursing, 23*(21/22), 3274–3285.

Centers for Disease Control and Prevention (CDC). (2012a). *Diabetes and pregnancy.* Retrieved from http://www.cdc.gov/Features/DiabetesPregnancy/

Centers for Disease Control and Prevention (CDC). (2012b). *National action plan for childhood injury prevention.* Retrieved from https://www.cdc.gov/safechild/pdf/national_action_plan_for_child_injury_prevention-a.pdf

Centers for Disease Control and Prevention (CDC). (2013a). *CDC fact sheet: Incidence, prevalence, and cost of sexually transmitted infections in the United States.* Retrieved from https://www.cdc.gov/std/stats/sti-estimates-fact-sheet-feb-2013.pdf

Centers for Disease Control and Prevention (CDC). (2013b). *PRAMS and smoking.* Retrieved from http://www.cdc.gov/prams/TobaccoandPRAMS.htm

Centers for Disease Control and Prevention (CDC). (2014a). *Breastfeeding report card: United States, 2014.* Retrieved from http://www.cdc.gov/breastfeeding/pdf/2014breastfeedingreportcard.pdf

Centers for Disease Control and Prevention (CDC). (2014b). *Facts about birth defects.* Retrieved from http://www.cdc.gov/ncbddd/birthdefects/facts.html

Centers for Disease Control and Prevention (CDC). (2014c). *Hygiene related diseases: Dental caries (tooth decay).* Retrieved from http://www.cdc.gov/healthywater/hygiene/disease/dental_caries.html

Centers for Disease Control and Prevention (CDC). (2014d). *Understanding child maltreatment.* Retrieved from http://www.cdc.gov/violenceprevention/pdf/CM-FactSheet-a.pdf

Centers for Disease Control and Prevention (CDC). (2014e). *Premature births and the environment.* Retrieved from http://ephtracking.cdc.gov/showRbPrematureBirthEnv.action#exposure

Centers for Disease Control and Prevention (CDC). (2015a). *CDC Childhood injury report.* Retrieved from http://www.cdc.gov/safechild/child_injury_data.html

Centers for Disease Control and Prevention (CDC). (2015b). *CDC's lead poisoning prevention program.* Retrieved from http://www.cdc.gov/nceh/lead/about/program.htm

Centers for Disease Control and Prevention (CDC). (2015c). *Childhood obesity facts.* Retrieved from http://www.cdc.gov/obesity/data/childhood.html

Centers for Disease Control and Prevention (CDC). (2015d). *State and local area integrated telephone survey (SLAITS): National survey of children with special health care needs.* Retrieved from http://www.cdc.gov/nchs/slaits/cshcn.htm#09-10

Centers for Disease Control and Prevention (CDC). (2015e). *Highlights: Minors' access to tobacco.* Retrieved from http://www.cdc.gov/tobacco/data_statistics/sgr/2000/highlights/minor/index.htm

Centers for Disease Control and Prevention (CDC). (2015f). *HIV and substance use in the United States.* Retrieved from http://www.cdc.gov/hiv/risk/substanceuse.html

Centers for Disease Control and Prevention (CDC). (2015g). *School-based dental sealant programs.* Retrieved from http://www.cdc.gov/oralhealth/dental_sealant_program/

Centers for Disease Control and Prevention (CDC). (2015h). *STDs during pregnancy statistics.* Retrieved from http://www.cdc.gov/std/pregnancy/stats.htm

Centers for Disease Control and Prevention (CDC). (2016a). *Asthma.* Retrieved from http://www.cdc.gov/nchs/fastats/asthma.htm

Centers for Disease Control and Prevention (CDC). (2016b). *Autism spectrum disorder (ASD).* Retrieved from http://www.cdc.gov/ncbddd/autism/research.html

Centers for Disease Control and Prevention (CDC). (2016c). *Birth-18 years & "catch-up" immunization schedules.* Retrieved from http://www.cdc.gov/vaccines/schedules/hcp/child-adolescent.html#chgs

Centers for Disease Control and Prevention (CDC). (2016d). *Child abuse and neglect: Risk and protective factors.* Retrieved from http://www.cdc.gov/violenceprevention/childmaltreatment/riskprotectivefactors.html

Centers for Disease Control and Prevention (CDC). (2016e). *Child abuse prevention.* Retrieved from http://www.cdc.gov/features/healthychildren/

Centers for Disease Control and Prevention (CDC). (2016f). *Child health.* Retrieved from http://www.cdc.gov/nchs/fastats/child-health.htm

Centers for Disease Control and Prevention (CDC). (2016g). *Child passenger safety: Get the facts.* Retrieved from http://www.cdc.gov/motorvehiclesafety/child_passenger_safety/cps-factsheet.html

Centers for Disease Control and Prevention (CDC). (2016h). *Dual use of tobacco products.* Retrieved from http://www.cdc.gov/tobacco/campaign/tips/diseases/dual-tobacco-use.html

Centers for Disease Control and Prevention (CDC). (2016i). *Lead.* Retrieved from http://www.cdc.gov/nceh/lead/

Centers for Disease Control and Prevention (CDC). (2016j). *National Center for Health Statistics: Birth weight and gestation.* Retrieved from http://www.cdc.gov/nchs/fastats/birthweight.htm

Centers for Disease Control and Prevention (CDC). (2016k). *Pregnancy mortality surveillance system.* Retrieved from http://www.cdc.gov/reproductivehealth/maternalinfanthealth/pmss.html

Centers for Disease Control and Prevention (CDC). (2016l). *STDs & pregnancy: CDC fact sheet.* Retrieved from http://www.cdc.gov/std/pregnancy/STDFact-Pregnancy.htm

Centers for Disease Control and Prevention (CDC). (2016m). *STDs during pregnancy. Fact sheet.* Retrieved from http://www.cdc.gov/std/pregnancy/stdfact-pregnancy.htm

Centers for Disease Control and Prevention (CDC). (2016n). *Weight gain during pregnancy.* Retrieved from http://www.cdc.gov/reproductivehealth/maternalinfanthealth/pregnancy-weight-gain.htm

Chaudron, L. H. (2013). Complex challenges in treating depression during pregnancy. *American Journal of Psychiatry, 170,* 12–20.

Chesnokova, A., French, B., Weibe, D., Camenga, D. R., & Yun, K. (2015). Association between neighborhood-level smoking and individual smoking risk: Maternal smoking among Latina women in Pennsylvania. *Public Health Reports, 130*(6), 672–683.

Chi, D. L., Masterson, E. E., Carle, A. C., Mancl, L. A., & Coldwell, S. E. (2014). Socioeconomic status, food security, and dental caries in US children: Mediation analyses of data from the National Health and Nutrition Examination Survey, 2007–2008. *American Journal of Public Health, 104*(5), 860–864.

Child Welfare Information Gateway. (2013). *Addressing the needs of young children in child welfare: Part C—early intervention services.* Retrieved from https://www.childwelfare.gov/pubPDFs/partc.pdf

Child Welfare Information Gateway. (n.d.). *Framework for prevention of child maltreatment.* Retrieved from https://www.childwelfare.gov/topics/preventing/overview/framework/

Christiansen, D. M., Elklit, A., & Olff, M. (2013). Parents bereaved by infant death: PTSD symptoms up to 18 years after the loss. *General Hospital Psychiatry, 35*(6), 605–611.

Colaizzo, G. R. (2016). Misinformed parents, unvaccinated children and the fabricated vaccine-autism scare. *Paediatrics and Health, 4*(1), 1.

Çolak, H., Dülgergil, C. T., Dalli, M., & Hamidi, M. M. (2013). Early childhood caries update: A review of causes, diagnoses, and treatments. *Journal of Natural Science, Biology, & Medicine, 4*(1), 29–38.

Connecticut Department of Developmental Services. (2014). *Parents with intellectual disability—resource guide.* Retrieved from http://www.ct.gov/dds/lib/dds/pwid/pwid_resource_guide.pdf

Cooper, B. R., & Lanza, S. T. (2014). Who benefits most from Head Start? Using latent class moderation to examine differential treatment effects. *Child Development, 85*(6), 2317–2338.

Copeland, K. C., Silverstein, J., Moore, K. R., Prazar, G. E., Raymer, T., Shiffman, R. N., ... Flinn, S. K. (2013). Management of newly diagnosed type 2 diabetes mellitus (T2DM) in children and adolescents. *Pediatrics, 131*(2), 364–382.

Criminal Justice. (n.d.). *Postpartum depression, psychosis, and infanticide.* Retrieved from http://criminal-justice.iresearchnet.com/crime/domestic-violence/postpartum-depression-psychosis-and-infanticide/

Cystic Fibrosis Foundation. (n.d). *About Cystic Fibrosis.* Retrieved from https://www.cff.org/What-is-CF/About-Cystic-Fibrosis/

Dall, T. M., Yang, W., Halder, P., Pang, B., Massoudi, M., Wintfeld, N., ... Hogan, P. F. (2014). The economic burden of elevated blood glucose levels in 2012: Diagnosed and undiagnosed diabetes, gestational diabetes mellitus, and prediabetes. *Diabetes Care, 37*(12), 3172–3179.

Davis, A. (2016). *Pregnancy 101: 11 celebrities who battled postpartum depression.* Retrieved from http://www.health.com/health/gallery/0,,20448173,00.html/view-all

Dubowitz, H., Lane, W. G., Semiatin, J. N., & Magder, L. S. (2012). The SEEK model of pediatric primary care: Can child maltreatment be prevented in a low-risk population? *Academic Pediatrics, 12*(4), 259–268.

Dubowitz, H., Lane, W. G., Semiatin, J. N., Magder, L. S., Veneplally, M., & Jans, M. (2011). The safe environment for every kid model: Impact on pediatric primary care professionals. *Pediatrics, 127*(4), e962–e970.

England, L. J., Kim, S. Y., Shapiro-Mendoza, C. K., Wilson, H. G., Kendrick, J. S., Satten, G. A., ... Callaghan, W. M. (2012). Maternal smokeless tobacco use in Alaska Native women and singleton infant birth size. *Acta Obstetricia et Gynecologica Scandinavica, 91*(1), 93–103. PMID: 21902677

Eunice Kennedy Shriver National Institute of Child Development and Health. (2016). *Back to Sleep public education campaign.* Retrieved from http://www.nichd.nih.gov/sids/

Extension. (2015, September 8). *What is inclusive childcare?* Retrieved from http://articles.extension.org/pages/61602/what-is-inclusive-child-care

Family and Youth Services Bureau. (n.d.). *Working with pregnant and parenting teens: Overview.* Retrieved from https://www.acf.hhs.gov/sites/default/files/assets/pregnant-parenting-teens-tips.pdf

Faulkner, A., Skoff, T., Martin, S., Cassiday, P., Tondella, M. L., & Liang, J. (2015). *Pertussis.* Retrieved from http://www.cdc.gov/vaccines/pubs/surv-manual/chpt10-pertussis.html

Federal Interagency Forum on Child and Family Statistics. (2015). *America's children: Key national indicators of well-being, 2015.* Washington, DC: U.S. Government Printing Office.

Gelabert, E., Subira, S., Garcia-Esteve, L., Navarro, P., Plaza, A., Cuyas, E., ... Martin-Santos, R. (2012). Perfectionism dimensions in major postpartum depression. *Journal of Affective Disorders, 136*(1–2), 17–25.

Ghosh, R., Rossner, P., Honkova, K., Dostal, M., Sram, R. J., & Hertz-Picciotto, I. (2016). Air pollution and childhood bronchitis: Interaction with xenobiotic, immune regulatory and DNA repair genes. *Environment International, 87,* 94–100.

Goodwin, B., & Miller, K. (2013, May). Teaching self-regulation has long-term benefits. *Educational Leadership, 70*(8)80–82.

Government of Alberta. (2015). *Child safety: Preventing drowning.* Retrieved from https://myhealth.alberta.ca/Health/Pages/conditions.aspx?hwid=ue5148spec

Greenwall, N. K. (2015, June). *National child restraint use special study. Traffic Safety Facts Research Note (Report No. DOT HS 812 157).* Washington, DC: National Highway Traffic Safety Administration. Retrieved from http://www-nrd.nhtsa.dot.gov/Pubs/812157.pdf

Griffin, R. M. (2016). *Depression health center: 10 natural depression treatments.* Retrieved from http://www.webmd.com/depression/features/natural-treatments

Griswold, C. H., Nasso, J. T., Swider, S., Ellison, B. R., Griswold, D. L., & Brooks, M. (2012). The prenatal care at school program. *Journal of School Nursing, 29*(3):196–203. doi: 10.1177/1059840512466111.

Groom, H., Hopkins, D. P., Pabst, L. J., Morgan, J. M., Patel, M., Calonge, N., et al. (2015). Immunization information systems to increase vaccination rates: A community guide systematic review. *Journal of Public Health Management and Practice, 21*(3), 227–248.

Hampton, L. M., Nguyen, D. B., Edwards, J. R., & Budnitz, D. S. (2013). Cough and cold medication adverse events after market withdrawal and labeling revision. *Pediatrics, 132*(6), 1047–1054.

Han, Z., Lutsiv, O., Mulla, S., Rosen, A., Beyene, J., & McDonald, S. D. (2011). Low gestational weight gain and the risk of preterm birth and low birth weight: A systematic review and meta analyses. *Acta Obstetricia et Gynecologica Scandinavica, 90*(9), 935–954.

Hayatbakhsh, M. R., Fenady, V. J., Gibbons, K. S., Kingsbury, A. M., Hurrion, E., Mamun, A. A., et al. (2012). Birth outcomes associated with cannabis use before and during pregnancy. *Pediatric Research, 71*(2), 215–219.

Health Resources & Services Administration (HRSA). (2013). *Child health USA, 2012.* Retrieved from http://mchb.hrsa.gov/publications/pdfs/childhealth2012.pdf

Health Resources & Services Administration (HRSA). (2016, April 1). *HRSA awards $345 million to support families through voluntary home visiting program.* Retrieved from http://www.hrsa.gov/about/news/pressreleases/160401homevisiting.html

Health Resources & Services Administration (HRSA). (n.d.). *Prenatal—first trimester care access.* Retrieved from http://www.hrsa.gov/quality/toolbox/measures/prenatalfirsttrimester/

Hedden, E. M., Jessop, A. B., & Field, R. I. (2012). Childhood immunization information system exchange with payers: State and federal policies. *Journal of Managed Care Medicine, 15*(3), 11–18.

Hill, H. A., Elam-Evans, L. D., Yankey, D., Singleton, J. A., & Kolasa, M. (2015). National, state and selected local area vaccination among children aged 19–35 months—United States, 2014. *Morbidity and Mortality Weekly Report (MMWR), 64*(33), 889–896.

Hinman, A. R., Orenstein, W. A., & Schuchat, A. (2011). Vaccine-preventable diseases, immunizations, and MMWR—1961–2011. *Morbidity and Mortality Weekly Report (MMWR), 60*(4), 49–57.

Horta, B. L., Loret de Mola, C., & Victora, C. G. (2015). Breastfeeding and intelligence: A systematic review and meta-analysis. *Acta Paediatrica, 104*(467), 14–19.

Illinois Department of Public Health. (n.d.). *Sudden infant death syndrome and infant mortality.* Retrieved from http://www.idph.state.il.us/sids/sids_factsheet.htm

Institute of Medicine (IOM). (2009). *Weight gain during pregnancy: Reexamining the guidelines.* Retrieved from http://www.iom.edu/Reports/2009/Weight-Gain-During-Pregnancy-Reexamining-the-Guidelines.aspx

Kapaya, H., Mercer, E., Boffey, F., Jones, G., Mitchell, C., & Anumba, D. (2015). Deprivation and poor psychosocial support are key determinants of late antenatal presentation and poor fetal outcomes: A combined retrospective and prospective study. *BMC Pregnancy Childbirth, 15*(1): 309 doi: 10.1186/s12884-015-0753-3.

Kattah, A. G., & Garovic, V. D. (2013). The management of hypertension in pregnancy. *Advances in Chronic Kidney Disease, 20*(3), 229–239.

Ko, J. Y., Farr, S. L., Dietz, P. M., & Robbins, C. L. (2012). Depression and treatment among US pregnant and nonpregnant women of reproductive age, 2005–2009. *Journal of Women's Health, 21*(8), 830–836.

Kocherlakota, P. (2014). Neonatal abstinence syndrome. *Pediatrics, 134*(2), e547–e561.

Koniack-Griffin, D., Anderson, N. L. R., Brecht, M. L., Verzemnieks, I., Lesser, J., & Kim, S. (2002). Public health nursing care for adolescent mothers: Impact on infant health and selected maternal outcomes at 1 year post-birth. *Journal of Adolescent Health, 30,* 44–54.

Koniack-Griffin, D., Anderson, N. L. R., Verzemnieks, I., & Brecht, M. L. (2000). A public health nursing early intervention program for adolescent mothers: Outcomes from pregnancy through 6 weeks postpartum. *Nursing Research, 49,* 130–138.

Koniack-Griffin, D., Verzemnieks, I. L., Anderson, N. L. R., Brecht, M. L., Lesser, J., Kim, S., et al. (2003). Nurse visitation for adolescent mothers: Two-year infant health and maternal outcomes. *Nursing Research, 52*(2), 127–136.

Kopko, K. (n.d.). *Nurse-family partnership program demonstrates results.* Retrieved from http://www.human.cornell.edu/hd/outreach-extension/loader.cfm?csModule=security/getfile&PageID=43498

Korfmacher, K. S., Ayoob, M., & Morley, R. (2012). Rochester's lead law: Evaluation of a local environmental health policy innovation. *Environmental Health Perspectives, 120*(2), 309–315.

Krugman, S. D., Lane, W. G., & Walsh, C. M. (2007). Update on child abuse prevention. *Current Opinions in Pediatrics, 19*(6), 711–718.

Kutty, P., Rota, J., Bellini, W., Redd, S. B., Barksey, A., & Wallace, G. (2015). *Measles*. Retrieved from http://www.cdc.gov/vaccines/pubs/surv-manual/chpt07-measles.html

Lee, K. (2016). Impact of Head Start's entry age and enrollment duration on children's health. *Social Work, 61*(2), 137–145.

Lopez, A., Schmid, S., & Bialek, S. (2015). *Varicella*. Retrieved from http://www.cdc.gov/vaccines/pubs/surv-manual/chpt17-varicella.html

Lopez-Alarcón, M., Montalvo-Velarde, I., Vital-Reyes, V. S., Hinojosa-Cruz, J. C., Leaños-Miranda, A., & Martinez-Basila, A. (2015). Serial determinations of asymmetric dimethylarginine and homocysteine during pregnancy to predict pre-eclampsia: A longitudinal study. *British Journal of Obstetrics and Gynaecology, 122*(12), 1586–1592.

MacDorman, M., Mathews, T., Mohangoo, A., & Zeitlin, J. (2014). International comparisons of infant mortality and related factors: United States and Europe, 2010. *National Vital Statistics Reports, 63*(5), 1–6. Retrieved from http://www.cdc.gov/nchs/data/nvsr/nvsr63/nvsr63_05.pdf

MacIntyre, E. A., & Heinrich, J. (2012). Otitis media in infancy and the development of asthma and atopic disease. *Current Asthma & Allergy Reports, 12*(6), 547–550.

March of Dimes. (2015). *Loss and grief: Stillbirth*. Retrieved from http://www.marchofdimes.com/baby/loss_stillbirth.html

Martin J. A., Hamilton B. E., Osterman M. J. K., Curtin, S. C., & Matthews, T. J. (2015). Births: Final data for 2013. *National Vital Statistics Reports, 64*(1). Hyattsville, MD: National Center for Health Statistics.

Martin, J. A., Hamilton, B. E., Ventura, S. J., Osterman, M. J., Kirmeyer, S., Mathews, T. J., et al. (2011). Births: Final data for 2009. *National Vital Statistics Reports, 60*(1). Retrieved from http://www.cdc.gov/nchs/data/nvsr/nvsr60/nvsr60_01.pdf

Masoura, S., Kalogiannidis, I. A., Goutsioulis, A., Koiou, E., Athanasiadis, A., & Vavatsi, N. (2012). Biomarkers in pre-eclampsia: A novel approach to early detection of the disease. *Journal of Obstetrics & Gynecology, 32*(7), 609–616.

Maternal Child Health Bureau (MCHB). (2016). *The Maternal, Infant, and Early Childhood Home Visiting Program: Partnering with parents to help children succeed*. Retrieved from http://mchb.hrsa.gov/programs/homevisiting/programbrief.pdf

Maternal Child Health Bureau (MCHB). (n.d.a). *Healthy Start*. Retrieved from http://mchb.hrsa.gov/programs/healthystart/

Maternal Child Health Bureau (MCHB). (n.d.b). *Historical timeline*. Retrieved from http://www.mchb.hrsa.gov/timeline/

Maternal Child Health Bureau (MCHB). (n.d.c). *Overview of funded projects*. Retrieved from http://mchb.hrsa.gov/research/about-projects.asp

McDonald, E. M., Mack, K., Shields, W. C., Lee, R. P., & Gielen, A. C. (2016). Primary care opportunities to prevent unintentional home injuries: A focus on children and older adults. *American Journal of Lifestyle Medicine*, Epub ahead of print. pii: 1559827616629924.

Mejdoubi, J., van den Heijkant, S. M., van Leerdam, F. M., Crone, M., Crijnen, A., & HiraSing, R. A. (2014). Effects of nurse home visitation on cigarette smoking, pregnancy outcomes and breastfeeding: A randomized controlled trial. *Midwifery, 30*(6): 688–695.

Mersch, J., & Nettleman, M. D. (2011). *Respiratory syncytial virus (RSV)*. Retrieved from http://www.medicinenet.com/respiratory_syncytial_virus/page4.htm

Midwives Information & Resource Service. (2016, March 3). *Over 20% of pregnant women are obese, statistics show*. Retrieved from https://www.midirs.org/over-20-of-pregnant-women-are-obese-statistics-show/

Mocarski, M., & Savitz, D. A. (2012). Ethnic differences in the association between gestational diabetes and pregnancy outcome. *Maternal and Child Health Journal, 16*(2), 364–373.

Mofenson, L. M., Flynn, P. M., Aldrovandi, G. M., Chadwick, E. G., Chakraborty, R., Cooper, E. R., et al. (2013). Infant feeding and transmission of human immunodeficiency virus in the United States. *Pediatrics, 131*(2), 391–396.

Moreland, A. D., Felton, J. W., Hanson, R. F., Jackson, C., & Dumas, J. E. (2016). The relation between parenting stress, locus of control and child outcomes: Predictors of change in a parenting intervention. *Journal of Child and Family Studies, 25*(6) 1–9.

Muscular Dystrophy Association. (2016). *Duchenne muscular dystrophy (DMD)*. Retrieved from https://www.mda.org/disease/duchenne-muscular-dystrophy/causes-inheritance

Nabel, G. J. (2013). Designing tomorrow's vaccines. *New England Journal of Medicine, 368*(6), 551–560.

National Bureau of Economic Research. (2016). *Poverty and mistreatment of children go hand in hand*. Retrieved from http://www.nber.org/digest/jan00/w7343.html

National Center on Birth Defects & Developmental Disabilities (NCBDDD). (2012). *How many children have autism?* Retrieved from http://www.cdc.gov/ncbddd/features/counting-autism.html

National Center on Birth Defects & Developmental Disabilities (NCBDDD). (2015a). *Fetal alcohol spectrum disorders (FASD): Data & statistics*. Retrieved from http://www.cdc.gov/ncbddd/fasd/data.html

National Center on Birth Defects & Developmental Disabilities (NCBDDD). (2015b). *Fetal alcohol spectrum disorders (FASD): Facts about FASDs*. Retrieved from http://www.cdc.gov/ncbddd/fasd/facts.html

National Center on Birth Defects & Developmental Disabilities (NCBDDD). (n.d.). *CDC's study to explore early development*. Retrieved from http://www.cdc.gov/ncbddd/autism/documents/SEED_10yrs.pdf

National Clearinghouse on Families & Youth. (n.d.). *YES! Youth empowerment strategies for all working with pregnant and parenting youth*. Retrieved from http://ncfy.acf.hhs.gov/publications/youth-empowerment-strategies/pregnant-parenting

National Conference of State Legislatures. (2016). *States with religious and philosophical exemptions from school immunization requirements*. Retrieved from http://www.ncsl.org/research/health/school-immunization-exemption-state-laws.aspx

National Fire Protection Association. (n.d). *Know when to stop, drop, and roll*. Retrieved from http://www.nfpa.org/public-education/resources/education-programs/learn-not-to-burn/learn-not-to-burn-grade-1/know-when-to-stop-drop-and-roll

National Institute of Allergy and Infectious Diseases. (2012). *Food allergy: An overview*. Retrieved from http://www.niaid.nih.gov/topics/foodAllergy/Documents/foodallergy.pdf

National Institute of Diabetes and Digestive and Kidney Diseases. (2012). *Overweight and obesity statistics*. Retrieved from http://www.niddk.nih.gov/health-information/health-statistics/Pages/overweight-obesity-statistics.aspx

National Institute of Neurological Disorders and Stroke (NINDS). (2015). *NINDS learning disabilities information page*. Retrieved from http://www.ninds.nih.gov/disorders/learningdisabilities/learningdisabilities.htm

National Institute of Neurological Disorders and Stroke (NINDS). (2016). *Muscular dystrophy: Hope through research*. Retrieved from: http://www.ninds.nih.gov/disorders/md/detail_md.htm

National Parents Organization. (2016). *New study: Child abuse down, but kids in single parent families far more likely to be abused*. Retrieved from https://nationalparentsorganization.org/blog/6210-new-study-child-abu-6210

National Vaccine Information Center. (2016). *Autism*. Retrieved from http://www.nvic.org/vaccines-and-diseases/Autism.aspx

Nayak, P. A., Nayak, U. A., & Khandelwal, V. (2014). The effect of xylitol on dental caries and oral flora. *Clinical, Cosmetic and Investigational Dentistry, 6*, 89–94. http://doi.org/10.2147/CCIDE.S55761

New York City Department of Health and Mental Hygiene. (2012). *Intimate partner violence*. Retrieved from http://www.nyc.gov/html/doh/html/epi/domviol.shtml

Nix, R. L., Bierman, K. L., Heinrichs, B. S., Gest, S. D., Welsh, J. A., & Domitrovich, C. E. (2016). The randomized controlled trial of Head Start REDI: Sustained effects on developmental trajectories of social-emotional functioning. *Journal of Consulting and Clinical Psychology, 84*(4), 310–322.

Nørgaard, M., Nielsson, M. S., & Heide-Jørgensen, U. (2015). Birth and neonatal outcomes following opioid use in pregnancy: A Danish population study. *Substance Abuse, 9*(Suppl 2), 5–11.

Norman, R. E., Byambaa, M., De, R., Butchart, A., Scott, J., & Vos, T. (2012). The long-term health consequences of child physical abuse, emotional abuse, and neglect: A systematic review and meta-analysis. *PLoS Med, 9*(11), e1001349.

Ogden, C. L., Carroll, M. D., Kit, B., & Flegal, K. (2012). Prevalence of obesity & trends in body mass index among US children & adolescents, 1999–2010. *JAMA, 307*(5), 483–490.

Olds, D. L., Holmberg, J. R., Donelan-McCall, N., Luckey, D. W., Knudtson, M. D., & Robinson, J. (2013). Effects of home visits by paraprofessionals and by nurses on children: Follow-up of a randomized trial at ages 6 and 9 years. *JAMA Pediatrics, 168*(2), E1–E8.

Olds, D., Kitzman, H., Hanks, C., Cole, R., Anson, E., Sidora-Arcoleo, K., … Bondy, J. (2007). Effects of nurse home-visiting on maternal and child functioning: Age 9 follow-up of a randomized trial. *Pediatrics, 120*(4), E832–E845.

Oral Health Care During Pregnancy Expert Workgroup. (2012). *Oral health care during pregnancy: A national consensus statement.* Washington, DC: National Maternal and Child Oral Health Center Resource.

Oregon Health Plan. (2015, November). *Developmental screening for young children guidance document.* Retrieved from https://www.oregon.gov/oha/analytics/CCOData/Developmental%20Screening%20Guidance%20Document%20-%20Nov%202015.pdf

Patelarou, E., Girvalaki, C., Brokalaki, H., Patelarou, A., Androulaki, Z., & Vardavas, C. (2012). Current evidence on the associations of breastfeeding, infant formula, and cow's milk introduction with type 1 diabetes mellitus: A systematic review. *Nutrition Reviews, 70*(9), 509–519.

Patrick, S. W., Davis, M. M., Lehmann, C. U., & Cooper, W. O. (2015). Increasing incidence and geographic distribution of neonatal abstinence syndrome: United States 2009-2012. *Journal of Perinatology, 35*(8), 650–655.

Peacock, S., Konrad, S., Watson, E., Nickel, D., & Muhajarine, N. (2013). Effectiveness of home visiting programs on child outcomes: A systematic review. *BMC Public Health, 13*(1), 1.

Perrin, E. M., Rothman, R. L., Sanders, L. M., Skinner, A. C., Eden, S. K., Shintani, A., … Yin, H. S. (2014, April). Racial and ethnic differences associated with feeding- and activity-related behaviors in infants. *Pediatrics, 133*(4), e857–e867.

Pickrell, T. M., & Li, R. (2016, February). Seat belt use in 2015—Overall results. *Traffic Safety Facts (Report No. DOT HS 812 243).* Washington, DC: National Highway Traffic Safety Administration. Retrieved from http://www-nrd.nhtsa.dot.gov/Pubs/812243.pdf

Pinto, A. I., Pessanha, M., & Aguiar, C. (2013). Effects of home environment and center-based child care quality on children's language, communication, and literacy outcomes. *Early Childhood Research Quarterly, 28*(1), 94–101.

Pinzon, J. L., Jones, V. F., Committee on Adolescence, & Committee on Early Childhood. (2012). Care of adolescent parents and their children. *Pediatrics, 130*(6), e1743–e1756.

Promising Practices Network. (2012). *Infant health and development programs.* Retrieved from http://www.promisingpractices.net/program.asp?programid=136

Nurse-Family Partnership. (2011). *Proven effective through extensive research.* Retrieved from http://www.nursefamilypartnership.org/proven-results

Pub Med Health. (2014). *Cystic fibrosis.* Retrieved from http://www.ncbi.nlm.nih.gov/pubmedhealth/PMH0063023/

Ramya, A. P. M. K. (2014). Shaken Baby Syndrome. *Narayana Nursing Journal, 3*(4), 22–25.

Roberts, J. & Bell, R. (2015). *Social inequalities the leading causes of early death: A life course approach.* Retrieved from http://www.instituteofhealthequity.org/projects/social-inequalities-in-the-leadingcauses-of-early-death-a-life-course-approach

Rosenstein, M. G., Cheng, Y. W., Snowden, J. M., Nicholson, J. M., Doss, A. E., & Caughey, A. B. (2012). The risk of stillbirth and infant death stratified by gestational age in women with gestational diabetes. *American Journal of Obstetrics and Gynecology, 206*(4), 309,e1–e7.

Ruedinger, E., & Cox, J. E. (2012). Adolescent childbearing: Consequences and interventions. *Current Opinion in Pediatrics, 24*(4), 446–452.

Safe to Sleep. (2015). *Fast facts about SIDS.* Retrieved from https://www.nichd.nih.gov/sts/about/SIDS/Pages/fastfacts.aspx

Save the Children. (2015). *State of the world's mothers: 2015.* Retrieved from http://www.savethechildren.org/site/c.8rKLIXMGIpI4E/b.8585863/k.9

Schaffer, M. A., Goodhue, A., Stennes, K., & Lanigan, C. (2012). Evaluation of a public health nurse visiting program for pregnant and parenting teens. *Public Health Nursing, 29*(3), 218–231.

Schnur, J., & John, R. M. (2014). Childhood lead poisoning and the new Centers for Disease Control and Prevention guidelines for lead exposure. *Journal of the American Association of Nurse Practitioners, 26*(5), 238–247.

Schuchat, A. (2011). Human vaccines and their importance to public health. *Procedia in Vaccinology, 5,* 120–126.

Sedlak, A. J., Mettenburg, J., Basena, M., Petta, I., McPherson, K., Greene, A., et al. (2010). *Fourth national incidence study of child abuse and neglect (NIS-4): Report to Congress.* Retrieved from http://www.acf.hhs.gov/sites/default/files/opre/nis4_report_congress_full_pdf_jan2010.pdf

Shapiro-Mendoza, C. K., & Lackritz, E. M. (2012, June). Epidemiology of late and moderate preterm birth. *Seminars in Fetal and Neonatal Medicine, 17*(3), 120–125.

Shih, F. F., Chen, C. H., Ciao, C. Y., Li, C. R., Kup, F. C., & Lai, T. J. (2015). Comparison of pregnancy stress between in vitro fertilization/embryo transfer and spontaneous pregnancy in women during early pregnancy. *Journal of Nursing Research, 23*(4), 280–289. doi: 10.1097/jnr.0000000000000089.

Sirotnak, A. P., Chiesa, A., Windle, M. L., & Pataki, C. (2015, November 4). *Failure to thrive.* Retrieved from http://emedicine.medscape.com/article/915575-overview#showall

Skjaerven, R., Klungsoyr, K., Morken, N. H., Rich-Edwards, J., & Wilcox, A. J. (2015). [77-OR]: Preeclampsia and maternal mortality, the importance of size of the fetus. *Pregnancy Hypertension: An International Journal of Women's Cardiovascular Health, 5*(1), 41.

Smithbattle, L., & Freed, P. (2015). Teen mother's mental health. *MCN: The American Journal of Maternal Child Health Nursing, 41*(1), 31–36.

Stewart-Brown, S. L., & Schrader-McMillan, A. (2011). Parenting for mental health: What does the evidence say we need to do? *Health Promotion International, 26*(Suppl 1), i10–i28.

Stockwell, M. S., Catallozzi, M., Larson, E., Rodriguez, C., Subramony, A., Andres Martinez, R, … Meyer, D. (2014). Effect of a URI-related educational intervention in Early Head Start on ED visits. *Pediatrics, 133*(5), e1233–e1240.

Substance Abuse & Mental Health Services Administration. (2014). *Results from the 2013 national survey on drug use and health: Summary of national findings (NSDUH Series H-48, HHS Pub No. [SMA] 14-4863).* Rockville, MD: U.S. Department of Health and Human Services. Retrieved from http://www.samhsa.gov/data/sites/default/files/NSDUHresultsPDFWHTML2013/Web/NSDUHresults2013.pdf

Tabak, R. G., Tate, D. F., Stevens, J., Siega-Riz, A. M., & Ward, D. S. (2012). Family ties to health program: A randomized intervention to improve vegetable intake in children. *Journal of Nutrition Education and Behavior, 44*(2), 166–171.

Tan, C. H., Denny, D. H., Cheal, N. E., Sniezek, J. E., & Kanny, D. (2015). Alcohol use and binge drinking among women of childbearing age—United States, 2011-2013. *Morbidity & Mortality Weekly Report (MMWR), 64*(37), 1042–1046.

Trachtenberg, F. L., Haas, E. A., Kinney, H. C., Stanley, C., & Krous, H. F. (2012). Risk factor changes for sudden infant death syndrome after initiation of back-to-sleep campaign. *Pediatrics, 129*(4), 630–638.

Trillingsgaard, T., Trillingsgaard, A., & Webster-Stratton, C. (2014). Assessing the effectiveness of the "Incredible Years® parent training" to parents of young children with ADHD symptoms—a preliminary report. *Scandinavian Journal of Psychology, 55*(6), 538–545.

Turnbull, C., & Osborn, D. A. (2012). Home visits during pregnancy and after birth for women with an alcohol or drug problem. *Cochrane Database Syst Rev, 1*(1), CD004456. PMID 22258956

U.S. Department of Agriculture. (2016). *Women, Infants and Children (WIC): About WIC.* Retrieved from http://www.fns.usda.gov/wic/aboutwic/

U.S. Department of Health and Human Services, Centers for Disease Control and Prevention, & National Center for Injury Prevention and Control. (2012). *National action plan for childhood injury prevention.* Retrieved from http://www.cdc.gov/safechild/pdf/national_action_plan_for_child_injury_prevention.pdf

U.S. Department of Health and Human Services, Health Resources and Services Administration, Maternal and Child Health Bureau. (2014). *Child Health USA 2014.* Rockville, MD: U.S. Department of Health and Human Services, 2014.

U.S. Department of Health and Human Services (USDHHS). (2016). *Healthy People 2020.* Retrieved from http://www.healthypeople.gov/2020/default.aspx

U.S. Department of Health and Human Services (USDHHS), Administration for Children and Families. (2016). *Child maltreatment.* Retrieved from http://www.acf.hhs.gov/programs/cb/resource/child-maltreatment-2014

U.S. Food & Drug Administration (FDA). (2011). *Public health advisory: FDA recommends that over-the-counter (OTC) cough and cold products not be used for infants and children under 2 years of age*. Retrieved from http://www.fda.gov/drugs/drugsafety/postmarketdrugsafetyinformationforpatientsandproviders/drugsafetyinformationforheathcareprofessionals/publichealthadvisories/ucm051137.htm

United Nations Statistics Division. (2015). *Demographic yearbook 2013*. New York, NY: United Nations Statistics Division. Retrieved from http://unstats.un.org/unsd/demographic/products/dyb/dyb2013/Table10.pdf

University of Chicago Medical Center. (2016). *Sickle cell disease*. Retrieved from http://www.uchicagokidshospital.org/specialties/anemias/sickle-cell/

University of Rochester Medical Center. (2011, December 21). *Myths and truths of obesity and pregnancy*. Retrieved from https://www.urmc.rochester.edu/news/story/3371/myths-and-truths-of-obesity-and-pregnancy.aspx

Van IJzendoorn, M. H., Palacios, J., Sonuga-Barke, E., Gunnar, M., Vorria, P., McCall, R. B., ... Juffer, F. (2011). Children in institutional care: Delayed development and resilience. *Monographs of the Society for Research in Child Development, 76*(4), 8–30.

Ventura, S. J., Hamilton, B. E., & Matthews, T. J. (2014). National and state patterns of teen births in the United States, 1940-2013. *National Vital Statistics System, 63*(4), 1–34.

Whitehurst, G. J. (2013, January 16). *Can we be hard-headed about preschool? A look at Head Start*. Retrieved from http://www.brookings.edu/research/papers/2013/01/16-preschool-whitehurst

Whitley, E., Gale, C., Deary, I., Kivimaki, M., & Batty, D. (2011). Association of maternal and paternal IQ with offspring conduct, emotional, and attention problem scores: Transgenerational evidence from the 1958 British Birth Cohort Study. *Archives of General Psychiatry, 68*(10), 1032–1038.

Whitmore, S. K., Taylor, A. W., Espinoza, L., Shouse, R. L., Lampe, M. A., & Nesheim, S. (2012). Correlates of mother-to-child transmission of HIV in the United States and Puerto Rico. *Pediatrics, 129*(1), e74–e81.

World Health Organization (WHO). (2015a). *HIV/AIDS*. Retrieved from http://www.who.int/mediacentre/factsheets/fs360/en/

World Health Organization (WHO). (2015b). *10 facts on breastfeeding*. Retrieved from http://www.who.int/features/factfiles/features/en/

World Health Organization (WHO). (2015c). *Trends in maternal mortality 1990-2015*. Retrieved from http://www.who.int/reproductivehealth/publications/monitoring/m

World Health Organization (WHO). (2016a). *Global health observatory (GHO) data: HIV/AIDS*. Retrieved from http://www.who.int/gho/hiv/en/

World Health Organization (WHO). (2016b). *Media centre: Maternal mortality*. Retrieved from http://www.who.int/mediacentre/factsheets/fs348/en/

Xu, J., Murphy, S. L., Kochanek, K. D., & Bastian, B. A. (2016, February 16). Deaths: Final data for 2013. *National Vital Statistics Report, 64*(2). Retrieved from http://www.cdc.gov/nchs/data/nvsr/nvsr64/nvsr64_02.pdf

Yan, J., Liu, L., Zhu, Y., Huang, G., & Wang, P. P. (2014). The association between breastfeeding and childhood obesity: A meta-analysis. *BMC Public Health, 14*, 1267. Retrieved from http://bmcpublichealth.biomedcentral.com/articles/10.1186/1471-2458-14-1267

Zero to Three. (2016). *Frequently asked questions about brain development*. Retrieved from http://www.zerotothree.org/site/PageServer?pagename=ter_key_brainFAQ

School-Age Children and Adolescents

"Youth isn't always all it's touted to be."

—**Lawana Blackwell,** The Dowry of Miss Lydia Clark, 1999

KEY TERMS

Anorexia nervosa
At risk of overweight
Attention deficit hyperactivity
   disorder (ADHD)

Autism spectrum disorder
   (ASD)
Binge eating
Bulimia

Eating disorders
Food insufficiency
Learning disability
Overweight

Pediculicide
Pediculosis

LEARNING OBJECTIVES

Upon mastery of this chapter, you should be able to:

- Identify major health problems and concerns for U.S. school-age children and adolescent populations.
- Explain how health status can influence academic achievement.
- State the recommended immunization schedule for school-age children and adolescents.
- Examine the trends in mortality and injury among school-age children and adolescents and identify the most important areas needing intervention.
- Discuss *Healthy People 2020* objectives affecting adolescents and the barriers that may be involved in attaining these objectives.
- Describe types of programs and services that promote health and prevent illness and injury of school-age children and adolescent populations.

According to Erick Erickson's developmental framework, the school-age and adolescent years are a time of task mastery and development of competence and self-identity. During these years, children grow physically, as well as emotionally and socially. They move from the total control of parents and families during infant and toddler years to deriving more and more influence from outside the home—from school, teachers, peers, and other groups (Adler-Tapia, 2012).

The challenges of childhood and adolescence include developmental issues, school concerns, behavioral and learning problems, emotional and mental health issues, and the risk behaviors characteristic of teenage years. This chapter explores the health needs of school-age children and adolescents and describes various services that address those needs, along with the community health nurse's role in assisting families with children.

SCHOOL—CHILD'S WORK

In the United States in 2011, about 55 million school-age children and adolescents (5 to 18 years old) attended more than 132,000 public, private, and charter schools (National Center for Education Statistics [NCES], 2014, Table 105.30; National Clearinghouse for Educational Facilities, 2012). In 2014, the U.S. population aged 0 to 17 was composed of 51.9% White/non-Hispanic, 13.8% Black/non-Hispanic, 4.8% Asian/non-Hispanic, 24.4% Hispanic, and 5.2% all other groups (Federal Interagency Forum on Child and Family Statistics [FCFS], 2015a).

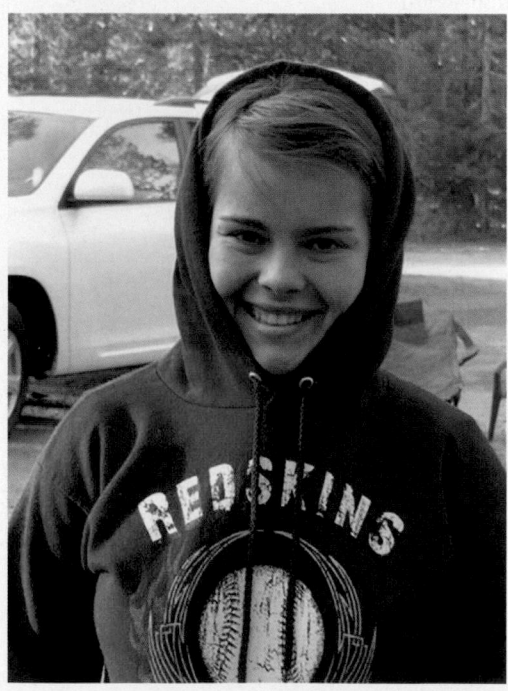

High school is a critical time in an adolescent's life. (Author's private photo with permission from Merysa Schultz.)

Children and adolescents spend most of their waking hours in school. Their academic success can predict future education, employment, and income. The quality of their educational experiences (e.g., teacher–child interactions) can influence learning (Gifford, Evans, Berlin, & Bai, 2011; Quan-McGimpsey, 2011). These children are the parents, workers, leaders, and decision makers of tomorrow, and their future success depends in good measure on achievement of their educational goals today. Child health has been linked to school success—healthy children are found to be more motivated and prepared to learn (Centers for Disease Control and Prevention [CDC], 2014b; London & Castrechini, 2011), and coordinated school health programs are linked to academic achievement (Ickovics et al., 2014). This is well known to school nurses and public health nurses (PHNs) working in schools.

HEALTH PROBLEMS OF SCHOOL-AGE CHILDREN

The well-being of children has been a subject of great concern in the United States since the days of Lillian Wald. For many years, international organizations, including the World Health Organization (WHO), the United Nations International Children's Education Fund (UNICEF), and U.S. governmental agencies, nonprofit groups, and charitable foundations, have focused their resources on improving the health and well-being of children (U.S. Department of Health and Human Services [USDHHS], 2015a). Nonetheless, the needs of millions of children in the United States and worldwide remain unmet. The *Healthy People 2020* document has four objectives for early (birth to age 8) and middle childhood (aged 6 to 12):

- Increase the proportion of children who are ready for school in all five domains of healthy development (physical and social–emotional development, approaches to learning, language, and cognitive development).
- Increase the proportion of parents who use positive parenting and communicate with their health care professionals about positive parenting.
- Decrease the proportion of children who have poor quality of sleep.
- Increase the proportion of elementary, middle, and senior high schools that require health education (USDHHS, 2015b).

Even in the wealthiest nations, many children face complex and often chronic health problems that cause them to miss school days or participate only marginally in the classroom. Because childhood is a critical period during which certain behaviors or health conditions are known to lead to more serious adult illnesses, it is vital for community health nurses and school nurses to screen children and identify problems early (Haines et al., 2011; Ruggieri & Bass, 2015). The chronic health problems of children younger than age 18 are often characterized by severity (e.g., persistence of symptoms and impact on social functioning) and duration (usually longer than 3 to 12 months) and often include

- Diabetes
- Asthma
- Autism spectrum disorder (ASD)
- Cystic fibrosis
- Spina bifida
- Neuromuscular disorders
- Juvenile rheumatoid arthritis
- Seizure disorders
- Hemophilia
- Congenital heart disease
- Attention deficit hyperactivity disorder (ADHD)
- Nutritional problems—anemia or obesity/overweight
- Cerebral palsy
- Mental illnesses (Perrin, Andersen, & Van Cleave, 2014)

Other conditions may also be defined as chronic, such as allergies, ear infections, and sinusitis, as well as hearing or speech disorders. Some chronic conditions may affect a child socially and emotionally, as well as physically. School attendance and relationships with family and peers may be affected.

Chronic Diseases

Stomachaches, headaches, colds, and flu are frequent complaints of school-age children, but it is not uncommon for this same age group to be afflicted with some type of chronic disease. Common chronic problems include hay fever, sinusitis, dermatitis, tonsillitis, asthma, and hearing difficulties. Chronic health problems such as these can affect a child's ability to learn and/or his or her physical and social development. Other more serious conditions, such as diabetes, sickle cell anemia, or seizure disorders, have definite effects on academic achievement and educational attainment (Champaloux & Young, 2015).

The growth in the number of chronic health conditions in children and adolescents has been astounding. Since 1960, when <2% reported a condition that interfered with daily activities, the incidence rose by 400% in 2010 when 8% reported severe health conditions. Most of the increase has centered on four broad areas: asthma, mental health conditions, obesity, and neurodevelopmental disorders. Rates of asthma and obesity have begun to slow at the start of the 21st century. Growth, in some cases, has been thought to be because of an interaction of genetic susceptibility and exposures or environmental triggers, along with changes in diet and exercise as well as use of electronic devices (e.g., computers, televisions, video games). Some of the conditions, such as ASD and **attention deficit hyperactivity disorder (ADHD)**, are thought to be increasing because of better public awareness and diagnosis rather than actual increases in prevalence. Gender differences in chronic health conditions have been found, with males having 50% higher rates. Racial/ethnic

differences have also been noted, as Black children have higher rates than White children, despite income level. Puerto Rican children's rate of asthma is 140% higher than that of White children. These differences are also found with obesity: Black children and Hispanic children had reported rates of 24% and 21%, respectively, in 2009–2010. For ADHD, White and Black children have the largest share of prevalence compared to Hispanics (Perrin et al., 2014).

A large study of almost 100,000 children and adolescents born to immigrant or U.S.-born parents found lower prevalence of behavioral problems and depression in immigrant children, and autism prevalence for immigrant Asian children of only 0.3%, whereas the rate for native-born White and Hispanic children was between 1.3% and 1.4%. Interestingly, immigrant children had lower rates of asthma, ADHD, learning disabilities, speech/hearing and sleep problems, and total number of chronic health conditions than native-born children. The risk rose as their mother's years in this country increased over time (Singh, Yu, & Kogan, 2013).

The numbers of children with chronic conditions are increasing, and more children with significant health problems are present in schools (National Association of School Nurses, 2012). In the school setting, some children require specialized physical health care procedures, such as catheterization, suctioning, or ventilator care. The U.S. Supreme Court ruled that even complex nursing services (i.e., ventilator care) must be provided by schools, even though school nurses are not always present in each school building every day (New York State United Teachers, 2012). The Individuals with Disabilities Education Act (IDEA) and Section 504 of the Rehabilitation Act of 1973 mandate that services must be provided for children identified as *disabled*. Many conditions may be characterized as disabling under these two laws, including autism, deafness or hearing impairment, blindness or vision impairment, emotional disturbances, mental retardation, specific learning disabilities (LD), speech or language impairments, or other health impairments (e.g., ADHD, asthma). Once they have been characterized as disabled, children may qualify for special educational services. Children with chronic health conditions that can affect learning (e.g., diabetes, seizure disorders) may receive medications or other related services while in school, to maintain their health and promote their ability to learn.

Chronic diseases of childhood and adolescence affect the entire family and can lead to developmental and social issues for children, as well as missed school days and eventual school failure (CDC, 2014b; Reuben & Pastor, 2013). In a large study of over 22,700 students with chronic health conditions in grades 2 through 11, researchers found that seizure and neurodevelopmental disorders (e.g., autism, ADHD) were associated with poor school performance. Diabetes and cardiovascular disorders were not independently associated with low school performance, and asthma had a weak association before adjustments were made for absenteeism. The adjusted odds ratio for any chronic health condition and below average performance for math was 1.25 when compared to students without chronic health conditions (Crump et al., 2013).

Many children with chronic health conditions take multiple medications at home and at school. One study that examined parents' mediation administration for children with seizure disorders and sickle cell disease included 52 home visits and 280 medications administered at home. Researchers found 61 medication errors, and 31 errors with the potential for harm or injury, as well as 9 causing actual injury (Walsh et al., 2011). Problems in communication with the physician, pharmacy, and spouse led to failure to fill new prescriptions, failure to change dosage, and problems with medication preparation, all leading to inaccurate medication administration. Also, 95% of parents didn't use support tools like reminders or alarms to remind them to give medications on time. Home visits and consultations by PHNs and school nurses could be helpful to parents and children or youth with chronic health conditions. See Chapter 30 for more on school nursing.

Asthma

Asthma is one of the most common chronic diseases of childhood. In 2013, it was estimated that 13% of children younger than age 18 have at some time been diagnosed with asthma. Childhood asthma rates steadily increased between 1997 and 2011; however, during 2012–2013, the prevalence of diagnosed asthma slightly decreased. Black, non-Hispanic children exhibited the highest asthma attack rates at 13%, compared with 8% for White, non-Hispanic children and 7% for children of Mexican heritage. Overall, about 5% of all children reported an episode within the past year (FCFS, 2015b).

Although reasons for increased cases of asthma over the past two decades are somewhat unclear, experts speculate that better recognition and diagnosis of the disease, overcrowded conditions, and exposure to air pollution (indoor or outdoor), allergens, and irritants in the environment are probable culprits and may trigger asthma attacks. Many schools have high levels of allergens and irritants. Children and adolescents with asthma may have attacks triggered by infections, exposure to cigarette smoke, stress, strenuous exercise, or weather changes (e.g., cold, wind, rain; Sleath et al., 2011; Sweet, Polivka, Chaudry, & Bouton, 2014).

Pediatric asthma is among the respiratory system ailments (including pneumonia and acute bronchitis) that were the top cause of hospital stays for children in 2012 (Witt, Weiss, & Elixhauser, 2014). Treatment for chronic asthma usually includes cromolyn sodium, leukotriene modifiers, inhaled and oral corticosteroids or long-acting beta agonists, and anti-IgE therapy, but acute symptoms may involve inhaled $beta_2$ agonists and sometimes anticholinergics (National Heart, Lung, and Blood Institute, 2014). Parent and child education, along with adherence to oral corticosteroid regimens, can help decrease the number of emergency room visits and hospitalizations because of asthma attacks (Sweet et al., 2014).

Teaching families to reduce allergens in their homes by controlling dust mites, vacuuming frequently, preventing animal dander and the entry of pollen into the home, and avoiding mold and mold spores may help minimize asthma symptoms for many children. In addition, families should be educated on the danger of indoor environments with mold and mold spores and the use of household items or products (e.g., furniture, flooring, and paints) made from volatile organic compounds (VOCs) (Asthma and Allergy Foundation of America [AAFA], 2015). School nurses and PHNs often work with students, families, and physicians to develop an asthma action plan to control, prevent, or minimize the untoward effects of acute asthma episodes. The goal is to control asthma symptoms and minimize school absences resulting from asthma (Basch, 2011a). Asthma triggers are noted, and school staff members are taught to assist the child in avoiding these triggers. Peak flow meters can be used to determine early signs of asthma problems and to facilitate early interventions; asthma action plans and holding chambers/spacers are used. Although only one third of schools have a full-time school nurse (viewed as vital to the success of an asthma control program), 80% allowed students to self-administer their inhalable asthma medications (Robert Wood Johnson Foundation, 2013).

Monitoring asthma medications and teaching proper methods of inhaler use are also vital school nursing or PHN functions. Although the link between asthma and academic achievement is not definitive, some evidence exists that school nurse case management of asthmatic children can lead to fewer absences and contribute to better overall asthma control (Healthy Schools Campaign, 2014).

Autism

Autism spectrum disorder (ASD) is a complex developmental disorder often originally noticed within the first few years of life. The spectrum of ASD indicates that symptoms for each child varies and may range from mild to severe (CDC, 2014a). A child's communication skills and interaction with others are most often affected, along with obsessive behavior and narrowed interests. Behaviors associated with autism include

- Language problems (no language, delay in language, repetitive use of language)
- Motor mannerisms (often repetitive rocking, hand flapping, object twirling)
- Fixation on objects (restricted interests)
- No spontaneous play or make-believe play; no interest in peers (problems making friends)
- Little or no eye contact (may also resist hugging)

Autism prevalence has been estimated at approximately 1 out of every 68 children (CDC, 2014a). The yearly expense for care of an autistic child is approximately $17,000 greater than the cost of a child without ASD (CDC, 2014a). When autism involves intellectual disabilities, the lifetime cost may be as high as $2.4 million/individual and $1.4 million if no intellectual disability is involved (Autism Society of America [ASA], 2014). Autism is not a new disorder—descriptions of autistic behavior have been identified in 18th century writings. Currently, early detection and intervention therapies focusing on speech, coordination, and interaction skills can help to improve development. Boys are five times more likely than girls to have the disorder (CDC,

2014a). Because autism is a "spectrum disorder" that presents differently among individuals, behaviors and severity can vary widely (ASA, 2014).

The cause of autism is not clear—some genetic links have been found, but environment may also be a factor. There is a higher risk of subsequent children having autism in a family with one autistic child or a parent with ASD (CDC, 2014a; National Institute of Neurological Disorders and Stroke [NINDS], 2012). It is often associated with other disorders (e.g., congenital rubella syndrome, Down syndrome, fragile X syndrome, tuberous sclerosis), but the exact causes are not fully understood (CDC, 2014a; NINDS, 2012).

PHNs may come in contact with families dealing with autism through work in well-child or immunization clinics. It is important to educate parents that parenting practices are now known *not* to be a cause of autism and that multiple, large-scale research studies on childhood immunizations have shown no relationship between immunization and autism (CDC, 2014a; NINDS, 2012; National Vaccine Information Center, 2012). The CDC is conducting a multiyear study to identify risk factors for autism, the Study to Explore Early Development (SEED), in an effort to better understand the causes of autism. It is also important to assist families in accessing services for their children, as early intervention is most helpful.

Diabetes

Diabetes is another common chronic illness in children, with type 1 being the leading cause of diabetes in all children (National Diabetes Education Program, n.d.). About 50% of children diagnosed with type 1 diabetes mellitus (T1DM) are diagnosed before age 10, but most children with type 2 diabetes (T2DM) are diagnosed after age 10, with a mean of 13.5 years (Jesitus & Kim, 2015). Redondo and colleagues (2014) found that newly diagnosed autoimmune T1DM children who were obese had higher levels of proinflammatory adiposity-induced biomarkers than those who were lean, adding that this may contribute to diabetic complications and cardiovascular disease (CVD). Both type 1 (T1DM) and type 2 diabetes (T2DM) are found in school-age children, with T2DM rising almost exponentially in this age group, leading some scientists to call this a major public health crisis. T2DM in children and adolescents, virtually nonexistent before 1999, now comprises about half of new cases in many communities (Reinehr, 2014) and 8% to 45% of all new T2DM diagnoses in the United States (Caple & March, 2015). This epidemic is thought to stem from increasing rates of childhood obesity, sedentary lifestyle, and the predisposition of certain ethnic groups (e.g., American Indian, Mexican American) to the disease. Some research has shown a connection between a secreted protein, pigment epithelium-derived factor (PEDF), and childhood obesity with insulin resistance in obese children, both with and without type 2 diabetes, leading researchers to put a greater emphasis on obesity as a risk factor (Tryggestad, Wang, Zhang, Thompson, & Short, 2015). A family history of T2DM may also play a role; in over 74% of cases, the child or adolescent has a first- or second-degree relative with

T2DM (Reinehr, 2014). A longitudinal study of 699 10- to 17-year-olds with recent-onset T2DM, the Treatment Options for Type 2 Diabetes in Adolescents and Youth (TODAY) study, concluded that the disease progression for children and youth is different than for adults and that it progresses more rapidly than originally expected. Early results revealed that 50% of participants required insulin within only a few years of diagnosis and, by the end of the 4-year study, almost one third had hypertension, 17% had early signs of kidney disease, and 13% demonstrated signs of visual problems. Early and aggressive treatment is recommended, as 50% of participants responded to metformin therapy and were able to maintain glycemic control over the time period of the study (TODAY Study Group, 2012).

Another recent national study with shocking results found an increase in the prevalence of prediabetes/diabetes from a rate of 9% in 1999 to 23% in 2008 (May, Kuklina, & Yoon, 2012). This study included youth aged 12 to 19 years, and researchers found that those who were more overweight or obese had greater increased prevalence of CVD risk factors (e.g., hypertension, higher LDL cholesterol). Approximately 37% of those of normal weight, 49% of those considered overweight, and 61% of obese adolescents had at least one CVD risk factor. Other considerations include "chronic and toxic levels of stress… that lead to a number of chronic physical conditions," and, with the rise in obesity and metabolic disorder among children and adolescents, screening for CVD risk factors (e.g., cholesterol, hypertension) needs to be more routine and widespread (Halfon, Verhoef, & Kuo, 2012, p. 51).

A more recent category of diabetes, double diabetes, is found when a child or adolescent presents features of both T1DM and T2DM. For instance, when a child with T2DM develops antibodies to β cells or when an adolescent with T1DM becomes overweight or obese, they may be characterized as having double diabetes (Cleland, Fisher, Colhoun, Sattar, & Petrie, 2013; Pozzilli, Guglielmi, Caprio, & Buzzetti, 2011; Robinson & Estell, 2012).

Research continues on the pathophysiology of the disease and prevention strategies (e.g., lifestyle changes, causes of autoimmunity), as well as refining methods of diagnosis and treatment (e.g., insulin pumps, continuous glucose monitoring, closed loop systems). Even though carbohydrate counting has not shown definitive results, it is still largely used (Cameron & Wherrett, 2015). Large-scale studies of T1DM youth under age 18 have shown racial/ethnic disparities in both methods of treatment and outcomes (Willi et al., 2015).

Younger children with T1DM, especially those who use insulin pumps, may need careful monitoring, something that is not always possible for the school nurse, who is often assigned to several school sites and may not be present when problems arise. Also, it is important for PHNs and others working with children and youth who have diabetes to consider their psychosocial needs, as well as their physical needs (see Evidence-Based Practice). A multidisciplinary team approach to care is needed, coordinating family, school staff, and physician collaboration. See Chapter 30 for more on the school nurse's role with school-age children with diabetes.

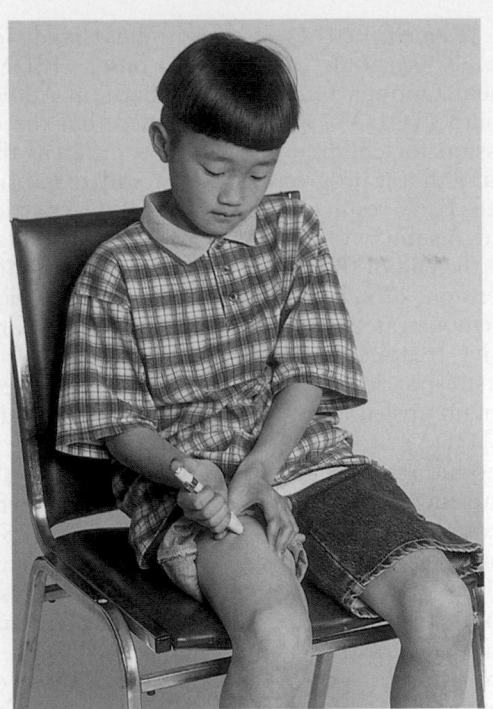

PHNs and school nurses work with diabetic school-age children to assure proper glucose monitoring and insulin administration.

Children and adolescents with diabetes may be reluctant to comply with their medical regimen, but strict adherence has proved to reduce later microvascular complications. Intensive treatment control in a study of adolescent diabetics reduced clinical neuropathy by 60%, retinopathy by 53%, and microalbuminuria by 54%, as well as HbA1c levels; at a 17-year follow-up, cardiovascular events were 50% lower and clinical neuropathy 60% lower in those adhering to stricter control. Although vascular complications in childhood and adolescence are rarely clinically evident, intensive treatment is beneficial for long-term outcomes (Donaghue et al., 2014). Testing blood glucose levels and taking insulin at school can be frustrating and cause children to feel singled out or different from their peers. Adolescents with T1DM or T2DM have higher rates of depression than those without diabetes (Hood et al., 2014). Also, other researchers noted that, among adolescents with diabetic duration of 2 to 5 years, early microvascular complications are not uncommon (Cho et al., 2011), and puberty is noted to accelerate diabetes complications in a recent review of research (Cho, Craig, & Donaghue, 2014). It is important for school nurses and PHNs to understand each child's unique concerns and to alert teachers and school personnel to the signs and symptoms (as well as treatment) of hypoglycemia.

In addition to the obvious emergency health-related concerns for diabetic children, other studies have demonstrated mild cognitive impairments and somewhat reduced intellectual functions in children with T1DM that may affect school achievement (Cato et al., 2014; Schwartz, Axelrad, & Anderson, 2014). A comparative study of children between ages 4 and 10, with and without diabetes, found slower growth of white and gray brain matter and differences in white and gray matter regions of the brain in those children with diabetes. Researchers concluded

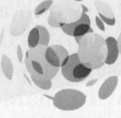

EVIDENCE-BASED PRACTICE

Children and adolescents with diabetes (both T1DM and T2DM) are faced with additional challenges. They are required to pay stricter attention to their health and management of their chronic condition. In addition, there are emotional costs. Nurses Sparapani, Jacob, and Nascimento (2015) wanted to better understand the emotional impact of children with diabetes. They conducted a small qualitative study with nineteen 7- to 12-year-olds with T1DM to determine feelings, thoughts, and self-management of diabetes. In an effort to better engage the children, they used puppets that the children created to help them convey their thoughts and feelings. When asked, "What is it like to be a child with T1DM?" their responses were grouped into four main themes: (a) conflicting desires, (b) insecurity, (c) fear, and (d) pain.

They expressed worry about control of their diabetes, dietary restrictions, and hypoglycemic reactions. They expressed frustration about not being able to eat sweets. One girl said, "I think if there were no sugar in the world, the world would be a better place" (p. 18). When having to monitor blood sugar and administer insulin, most children noted fear of needles and skin pricks, and some asked their parents to do this for them. Children noted the need for control of their diabetes, with one girl stating, "if you have a lot of sugar, you can amputate a leg, an arm, and even, you can die" (p. 18). Other children could not fully explain their disease and were ashamed of talking about it with others. Some mentioned problems in relationships with other children, because of their diet restrictions and need for self-care. One girl, testing her blood sugar in class, relayed "I am ashamed of the others who keep looking at me" (p. 19).

In addition to the usual developmental stressors of childhood, these children had additional conflicts: on the one hand, they want to be children like their peers and do what they wanted, but, on the other hand, they must adhere to the restrictions imposed upon them by having T1DM. Children in this study reported problems relating to peers, and some assistance may be needed with that. One child participant noted that a hypoglycemic episode was used to gain access to "sweets" (p. 20); because this propensity for sweet things is a common childhood occurrence, this should be kept in mind. Adults (e.g., parents, caretakers, nurses) need to be aware of children's physical needs and offer assistance, but they also must consider their emotional and psychosocial needs.

Sparapani, V. D., Jacob, E., & Nacimento, L. C. (2015). What is it like to be a child with type 1 diabetes mellitus? *Pediatric Nursing*, 41(1), 17–22.

that chronically higher levels of glucose could be harmful to brain development (Mauras et al., 2015). Moreover, the youth's own perception of obesity and overweight has been found to correlate with lower academic performance (Florin, Shults, & Stettler, 2011). Boogerd and colleagues (2015) found more psychosocial problems among children with T1DM than among a group of healthy children, although in 40% of their sample, neither parents nor children (ages 4 to 16) reported any psychosocial problems. Alerting teachers to these concerns may help them better understand the academic complications of this disease and ensure their support.

It is imperative to teach children and families that proper diet, oral antidiabetic medications or insulin administration, physical activity, and blood glucose testing are

vital strategies to keep blood glucose levels as close to normal as possible. The prevention of T2DM through education and improvement in exercise, nutrition, and lifestyle can be one of the most important areas of focus for health professionals who work with the school-age population—including PHNs who may come into contact with them during immunization or child health clinics. Health education and health promotion to decrease childhood obesity and sedentary lifestyles may help stem the tide of T2DM in children and adolescents (see Levels of Prevention Pyramid).

Juvenile Rheumatoid Arthritis

Juvenile rheumatoid arthritis is a painful autoimmune disorder characterized by persistent joint swelling and stiffness with periods of remission and flare-up. It is

---

LEVELS OF PREVENTION PYRAMID

SITUATION: The public health nurse and children with type 2 diabetes (T2DM)

GOAL: By using the three levels of prevention, negative health conditions are avoided, promptly diagnosed and treated, and/or the fullest possible potential is restored.

TERTIARY PREVENTION

Rehabilitation	Primary Prevention	
	Health Promotion and Education	*Health Protection*
• Monitor the child's health • Work closely with the child, family, physician, and teacher to ensure proper follow-up • Be alert to monitor for any possible complications (e.g., medication side effects)	• Continue to promote a healthy lifestyle that includes appropriate food choices and daily physical activity within the limitations of T2DM	• Educate the teachers on safety precautions for children in their classroom diagnosed with T2DM • Monitor children taking medications for T2DM (e.g., over- or underdosage and adverse reactions)

SECONDARY PREVENTION

Early Diagnosis	Prompt Treatment
• Teach older children to calculate their body mass index (BMI) • Monitor BMI scores • Yearly screenings for height and weight (calipers are useful) • Complete health histories on at-risk children	• Initiate referrals for health care provider follow-up in collaboration with parents of students at risk for T2DM • Initiate referrals to health care providers in collaboration with parents of students with signs and symptoms of T2DM

PRIMARY PREVENTION

Health Promotion and Education	Health Protection
• Educate to promote good nutrition and a physically active lifestyle • Provide classroom contact in the early primary grades to encourage children to make good food choices • Limit passive activities and increase sports and physical activity • Teach older children how to make better food choices at fast-food restaurants	• Advocate for policies that limit access to sugary beverages and snacks at school, and programs that raise awareness and family involvement in better nutrition and promote physical activity for families.

often diagnosed between the ages of 6 months and 16 years. It is treated with nonsteroidal anti-inflammatory drugs (NSAIDs), disease-modifying antirheumatic drugs (DMARDs), such as methotrexate, and sometimes corticosteroids or newer biologic response modifiers (Pub Med Health, 2011). Exercise is often an important component of therapy, and an adapted physical education program may be developed for these children. Long-term sequelae may result, such as slow rate of growth or uneven growth of arm or leg, as well as pericarditis and joint destruction. Many adolescents with this disorder require additional support and counseling (Pub Med Health, 2011). Once again, the school nurse or PHN can serve as a liaison between the health care and education communities and advocate for any necessary accommodations.

Seizure Disorders

Seizure disorders are not uncommon in the school-age population. Epilepsy is a disorder of the brain in which neurons sometimes transmit abnormal signals. Epilepsy is considered to be one of the most common disabling neurologic conditions, and it is most common in the very young and in elderly populations. Over 300,000 children under age 15 and more than 570,000 older adults have epilepsy; more than 90,000 children may have treatment-resistant seizures (Epilepsy Foundation, n.d.). Lifetime prevalence of seizure disorders/epilepsy is estimated at 10.2 per 1,000, and prevalence is higher in low-income families, as well as for male, older children. Those with seizure disorders have an increased risk for developmental (ASD, delays), mental health (e.g., anxiety, depression, ADHD, conduct disorders), and physical comorbidities (e.g., headaches) and were over 2.5 times more likely to repeat a grade (Russ, Larson, & Halfon, 2012). Although sudden unexplained death can occur in children with epilepsy, it is considered quite rare and is much more common among adults with epilepsy (Arts, 2012). More commonly, childhood deaths are due to the underlying conditions causing the seizures, and some are due to accidents that happen while the child is seizing (e.g., drowning, falls).

Although there are some instances of intractable or drug-resistant epilepsy, many children diagnosed with seizure disorders/epilepsy can have their seizures controlled with medications such as Tegretol, Dilantin, Depakote, Neurontin, Topamax, and Lamictal (WebMD, 2012). Vagus nerve stimulators are used in some cases after other treatments have failed (Elliott et al., 2011; Wilfong, 2015). Rectal diazepam is commonly prescribed for younger children and those with developmental disabilities, yet nurses are not always available to make an appropriate nursing assessment of the child before the drug is given to stop a seizure (Wong-Kisiel, 2013). Often, school secretaries or health aides are trained to give the emergency medication—highlighting the conflict between education laws and nurse practice acts (see more on this in Chapter 30). Treatment of epilepsy has been greatly enhanced by the use of newer anti-epilepsy drugs (AEDs) specific to the pediatric population and, in some cases, by a diet rich in proteins and fats and low in carbohydrates—a *ketogenic diet* (Epilepsy Foundation, n.d.).

It is important to monitor medication compliance and teach school staff about first-aid measures for seizure victims. When teachers are anxious about having a child with epilepsy in the classroom, educational programs for them and other school staff members can be provided. Community health nurses or school nurses can help allay fears and promote appropriate and timely care.

Family dynamics are also a consideration, as behavior problems can arise (Rodenburg, Wagner, Austin, Kerr, & Dunn, 2011; Sprague-McRae & Rosenblum, 2013). Children and adolescents with seizure disorders may feel embarrassed or be the victims of teasing or bullying. They may exhibit signs of school avoidance, or they may have problems learning. Seizure activity, along with the side effects of antiepileptic medications, may lead to problems with memory and learning, as well as changes in behavior (Epilepsy Foundation, n.d.). Moreover, seizures can affect short-term memory or language functions (Epilepsy Foundation, n.d.). It is important for school nurses to work with children with epilepsy and to teach all students about the disease process and the need for empathy and understanding.

Childhood Cancers

In 2013, cancer was the leading cause of death from disease among U.S. children between infancy and age 14 years. Leukemias and brain, central nervous system, and neuroblastoma cancers are the most common types of childhood cancers (National Cancer Institute [NCI], 2015). Childhood cancers, especially leukemias, now have better outcomes than ever before. Five-year survival rates for childhood cancers increased from 60% in the 1970s to 86% in recent years, generally as a result of treatment advances and participation in clinical trials (NCI, 2015). More children are surviving childhood cancers, and concern has shifted to later complications of treatment rather than about cancer recurrence. Survivors are at greater risk of gastrointestinal, auditory, and cardiovascular complications (Goldsby et al., 2011; Whelan et al., 2011). Also, children who have been treated with chemotherapy and/or radiation may develop a second primary cancer, and the risk of leukemia may be increased (NCI, 2014). White children, more than children from any other racial/ethnic group, are more likely to develop a childhood cancer (NCI, 2014).

The cause of most childhood cancers remains unknown; however, acquired immune deficiency syndrome (AIDS), high levels of ionizing radiation, Down syndrome, and other genetic syndromes (e.g., Gorlin syndrome) have been linked to a higher risk for some childhood cancers. Pesticide exposure may be a factor, but research findings have not been decisive. Parental smoking may be linked to an increased cancer risk, but evidence for this is also inconclusive (NCI, 2014).

Because many children return to school after initial hospitalization and treatment for cancer, school nurses or PHNs can help make this transition easier by educating classmates about cancer (e.g., it is not contagious), helping the children make necessary adjustments, and vigilantly protecting any immunocompromised students from communicable diseases (American Cancer Society, n.d.; Hakim, 2015).

Behavioral and Learning Problems

Other childhood health problems, less easy to detect and measure but often just as debilitating, are those of emotional, behavioral, and intellectual development. Although these problems are not new, awareness and concern have increased as the rates of occurrence for other life-threatening childhood diseases have diminished. Emotional or behavior problems and LD are prevalent in childhood. Of the 5.7 million school-age children with disabilities in the United States, 42% have LDs (National Center for Learning Disabilities [NCLD], 2014). One classic study of national data found a lifetime prevalence of LD at 9.7% (Altarac & Saroha, 2007). In a national survey, 6.4 million of 4- to 17-year-olds reported being diagnosed with ADHD. Parent report of ADHD was 22%, with rates increasing 3% annually from 1997 to 2006 and approximately 5% from 2003 to 2011. Approximately 5.6% of girls and 13.2% of boys reported having a diagnosis of ADHD. LDs, along with ADHD, were reported in 4% of children; and this was more commonly found in the older age group of 12 to 17 years (NCLD, 2014)

Learning Disabilities

Children and adults who have average or above-average intelligence and who demonstrate significant difficulties in one or more areas of learning (e.g., reading, writing, mathematics, attention, coordination) may have a **learning disability**. Thinking and organization skills can also be affected. LD may occur in one area or be overlapping—they are often lifelong conditions (NINDS, 2015). LDs, or learning disorders, are often recognized as the child progresses in school, and special education services may be needed. Causes of LD and emotional behavioral problems appear to have genetic, environmental, and cultural influences. Approximately 8% to 10% of students have an LD, formally defined as a "neurologically based processing disorder" (Silver, 2011, para 5). About two thirds of learning disabled students receiving special education services are male (NCLD, 2014). The number of children with LD in the lowest economic group is greater than that in the highest economic group (NCLD, 2014). Additionally, children and adolescents with LD are more likely to have health and safety concerns than those without LD (American Academy of Pediatrics, 2015).

Children with LDs can be helped through special education services. In fact, about 41% of children receiving special education services have an LD (NCLD, 2014). Students must first be carefully diagnosed through psychoeducational testing (IQ testing, achievement tests, and measures of processing abilities); then, special education or resource teachers can build on the child or adolescent's strengths while working to compensate for weaknesses (NINDS, 2015). Some LDs are apparent in early school years, whereas others do not present problems until early adolescence. Battles over homework, poor grades, acting out in school, or frequent child complaints about school, teachers, or schoolwork are often harbingers of LDs. Common signs of LDs are (LD Online, 2014; Silver, 2011):

- Reading problems
- Writing problems (fine-motor control and handwriting; problems with spelling, grammar, punctuation, capitalization; difficulty controlling flow of thoughts)

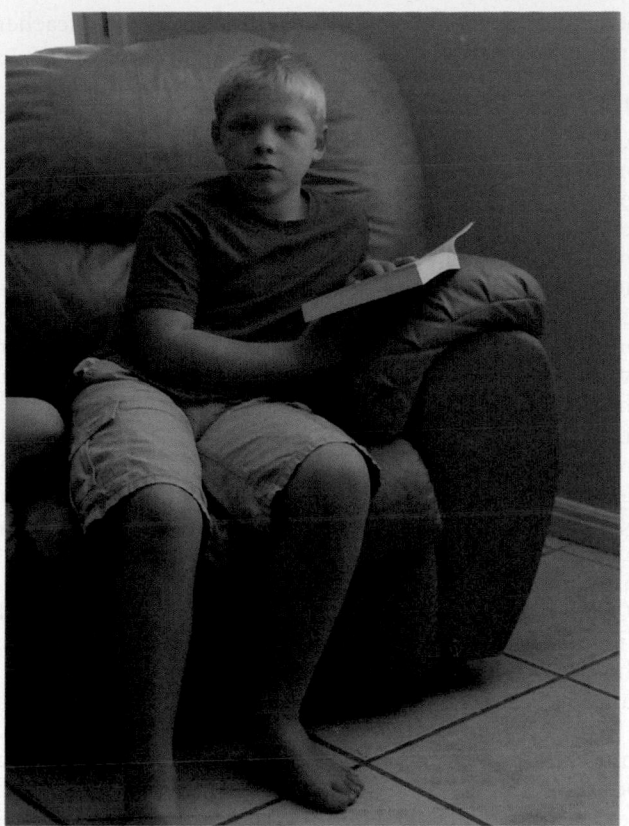

Reading is an important to education and may be problematic for children with learning disabilities. (Author's private photo with permission of Danielle Rector.)

- Math problems (problems learning and understanding concepts, missing steps or sequencing of problems, and placement of numbers in columns)
- Language problems (cannot quickly process what is heard, problems with multiple instructions, difficulty organizing thoughts and speaking in classroom situations)
- Motor problems (problems with fine-motor planning activities, such as tying, cutting, coloring, and gross motor planning, such as jumping and running; trouble with visual–motor activities, such as hitting or catching a ball)
- Sequencing (getting letters or numbers out of order); organization (messy binders)
- Memory (difficulty retaining what was learned); abstraction (confused, or not understanding what was said)

If LDs are not dealt with in childhood and adolescence, they can lead to later, more serious, problems related to employment, relationships, and quality of life in adulthood. Approximately 55% of adults (18 to 64 years) with LD, compared with 76% of those without LD, reported that they were employed. Children can receive services in schools, based on IDEA and Section 504; provisions of the Americans with Disabilities Act (ADA) provide protections for adults with LD (NCLD, 2014). The PHN and school nurse can assist individuals and families in recognizing LDs and locating necessary resources. Some students with significant LDs may qualify for special education services, and school nurses can be helpful in facilitating this process along with teachers and learning specialists.

Attention Deficit Hyperactivity Disorder

ADHD, a common childhood disorder, is a cluster of problems related to hyperactivity, impulsivity, and inattention. Its estimated prevalence has ranged from 3% to 5%, representing about 2 million children (National Institute of Mental Health (NIMH), n.d.a). As mentioned earlier, there is an overall 9.5% lifetime prevalence of ADHD, with one study indicating 9% lifetime prevalence for 13- to 18-year-olds, and 1.8% for severe ADHD (Merikangas et al., 2010). Another study found the rate of ADHD diagnosis increased from 7% to 9% from 1998 to 2009, with the largest increase among low-income and poor children, and higher prevalence among non-Hispanic White children (Akinbami, Liu, Pastor, & Reuben, 2011). The National Resource Center on ADHD (CHADD) states that the rate of ADHD diagnosis increased to 10.2% between the years 2012 and 2014 (CHADD, 2015a). Along with the increase in ADHD diagnosis, there has been a rise in prescriptions to treat this disorder; there has also been a rise in ADHD stimulant medication abuse by adolescents. It is estimated that 5% to 10% of high school students misuse the stimulants and poison control centers calls rose over a 7-year period by 76%—a rate much higher than for overall substance abuse calls. ADHD prescription estimates over the same time period showed increases of 133% for amphetamines, 52% for methylphenidates, and 80% for combined medications (Clemow & Walker, 2014). Clemow and Walker (2014) indicate that 5% to 35% of college students use ADHD medications to enhance studying and improve attention problems, although they had no medical justification for use. Although research has shown medications to be effective in controlling behavioral issues, and with less success improve academic achievement, medication titration is a trial-and-error proposition (Hale et al., 2011). Boys are often recognized as having ADHD in early elementary grades, because they most often exhibit hyperactivity symptoms. Girls, on the other hand, are at increased risk for not receiving appropriate services because they often do not exhibit the hyperactivity component and may not be appropriately diagnosed and treated for ADHD.

Although a number of parents believe that sugar, food-coloring agents, or other food additives may worsen ADHD symptoms in their children, research shows no behavioral or learning differences in double-blind studies using sugar and sugar substitutes. And additive-free or non-Western diets are difficult to achieve (Millichap & Yee, 2012). Some research shows that prenatal exposure to nicotine and psychosocial adversity are associated with ADHD (CDC, 2015a). Symptoms of ADHD may be related to such diverse causes as lead poisoning and traumatic brain injuries, but new research focuses on evidence of decreased blood flow in the prefrontal regions of the brain, and the inherited tendencies for problems with dopamine receptors and transporter genes, and research noting that some of the same genes found in childhood ADHD may also be found in adult ADHD (Franke et al., 2012; Thapar, Cooper, Jefferies, & Stergiakouli, 2012).

Some researchers are developing functional and structural imaging techniques to identify adolescent ADHD (Iannaccone et al., 2015). These findings support a neurobiological basis for the condition. Some evidence indicates that children with ADHD who are medicated properly later show peak cortical thickness in the frontal areas of the brain consistent with control subjects without ADHD, indicating that medication can restore brain development to a more normal rate, rather than the 3-year delay seen in previous studies (NIMH, n.d.a). Some classic family and twin studies reveal a higher heritability factor for ADHD and its symptoms of inattention and hyperactivity than for other psychiatric disorders, and researchers consider ADHD a heritable, familial disorder (Bezdjian, Baker, & Tuvblad, 2011) In families that have children with ADHD, about 25% of close relatives also had ADHD (NIMH, n.d.a).

Not all behaviors related to ADHD, such as hyperactivity, may truly be ADHD. Health and psychological professionals must take a careful history and note if sudden family changes may have recently occurred (e.g., divorce, death, family crises) that may cause children to behave erratically. Untreated chronic middle ear infections, undetected temporal lobe seizures, and anxiety or depression can also be the source of some behavior problems that mimic ADHD, as can other brain disorders (NIMH, n.d.a). Although some health professionals believe that many of the symptoms found in people with ADHD are part of the normal spectrum of human behavior, others note that people with ADHD have functional impairment in academic, social, or occupational areas resulting from their problem behaviors. Noted differences have even been reported in the results of electroencephalograms between children with and without ADHD, possibly because of cortical hypoarousal in children with ADHD (Nazari, Wallois, Aarabi, & Berquin, 2011). Over time, nursing researchers have documented data from children and adolescents who described their difficulties, as well as mother's parenting experiences (Paidipati & Deatrick, 2015). This disorder can be very disruptive for children and families, and additional support and counseling are often needed.

At each stage of development, those with ADHD are presented with distinct challenges. For example, children in elementary school are often involved in conflicts with peers and have problems organizing tasks. They may be more prone to accidents and may have more school-related problems, such as grade retention and suspension or expulsion. They often have problems with grooming and handwriting, and they exhibit difficulty sleeping and making friends. As adolescents, 80% still exhibit symptoms of inattentiveness, hyperactivity, and impulsiveness. Compared with non-ADHD teens, they may have more conflict with their parents, poorer social skills, and ongoing problems at school. They may face more difficulty driving and are more prone to injury while driving, biking, or walking than their peers. They are also more likely to use tobacco and alcohol, spend less time with their families, and more often experience negative moods. As young adults, they are less likely to be enrolled in college, more likely to have begun sexual activity at an earlier age and to have been treated for a sexually transmitted infection (STI), and more likely to experience lower job performance ratings than their peers. In adulthood, they tend to have more marital and occupational problems. They often have less formal education and lower levels of savings. Poor social skills may also continue to be an issue (NIMH, n.d.a). About 60% of adults with ADHD were first diagnosed as children. Adult ADHD is thought to affect 4.4% of U.S. adults, and it often goes undiagnosed and untreated; only 10% to 25% of those having adult ADHD have been diagnosed and are receiving treatment. Almost 95% of them continue to have attention deficit problems, but about one third report symptoms of hyperactivity (Anxiety and Depression Association of America (ADAA), n.d.).

ADHD is sometimes found with associated disorders, such as communication or language disorders and LDs. About half of ADHD children and adolescents have learning or other mental disorders. Common comorbid conditions are bipolar, depressive, and anxiety disorders, Tourette's syndrome, as well as conduct disorders and oppositional defiant disorder (NIMH, n.d.). Childress and Berry (2012) note that ADHD is associated with higher risk of psychiatric disorders (e.g., conduct, mood, substance abuse disorders). Differentiating between ADHD and bipolar condition can be difficult in early childhood, as bipolar disorder in children can present as a chronic mood problem, with some symptoms related to depression, irritability, and elation (CHADD, 2015b). There is a growing body of evidence showing the use of stimulant medications to treat ADHD may reduce the risk of developing later psychiatric comorbidities (including substance abuse disorder). A meta-analysis of studies on adults with ADHD found that those who took stimulant medication had normalization of ADHD structural abnormalities (e.g., reduced gray matter volume), as did those with increasing age, indicating some preliminary evidence of benefits to use of stimulant medications and the improvement in brain structure over time (Nakao, Radua, Rubia, & Mataix-Cols, 2011). However, a longitudinal study over an 8-year period found that adolescents with ADHD are at higher risk of using cigarettes and abusing substances; the authors concluded that ADHD, not treatment medications, was the major influence (Stovell, 2013). Although the medications are helpful, they can also be abused.

Collaboration among the child's family, school, and physician is needed to diagnose ADHD and to plan appropriate interventions and educational accommodations. Although parents have a wealth of knowledge about the child, teacher confirmation of ADHD-related behaviors is very important. School nurses and PHNs can assist parents in recognizing the symptoms of ADHD and in obtaining appropriate treatment and follow-up.

A multimodal treatment approach is recognized as most effective. This includes medication, usually methylphenidate (Ritalin, Metadate, or Concerta), dextroamphetamine (Dexedrine or Dextrostat), or combined dextroamphetamine and amphetamine (Adderall), school accommodations for learning problems, and social skills training for the child with ADHD (NIMH, n.d.a). Family and individual counseling, parent support groups, and training in behavior management techniques, as well as

family education about the condition, are also essential features of this treatment method. Not all children and adolescents respond to medication and a good number do not fully comply with their medication regimen; medication dosage must be carefully monitored and adjusted (Charach & Fernandez, 2013). The main goal of medical treatment for school-age children is academic improvement. If this does not occur, medication may need to be changed or discontinued. Parental response, severity of ADHD symptoms in children, and types of treatment plans are all important factors in the success of interventions for ADHD children and families. School nurses and community health nurses can work closely with school staff, parents, and physicians in determining the efficacy of treatment regimens.

Parents often voice concern about giving their children a stimulant medication to treat ADHD, and some families pursue alternative treatments (Charach, Yeung, Volpe, Goodale, & Dosreis, 2014). Families may use some type of complementary and alternative medicine (e.g., acupuncture, nutritional supplements, diet), and they may not discuss this fact with health care providers. Neurofeedback has produced some promising results, and newer equipment and techniques are even more efficient (Koberda et al., 2014). Nonstimulant medications, such as clonidine, atomoxetine (Strattera), and guanfacine hydrochloride (Intuniv), have been used in children and adolescents (DeSousa & Kalra, 2012).

Parental resistance to treatment may result from side effects (e.g., problems with sleep, appetite, greater anxiety) or stem from fears about later abuse of substances. However, Cormier (2012) indicates that most parents eventually reach a point where medication administration is felt to be both beneficial to the child's function and a less disruptive family life. As adolescents, those with ADHD may experiment with alcohol and other substances earlier than non-ADHD teens do, whereas concurrent hyperactivity has been shown to predict low self-esteem, leading to social withdrawal and abuse of substances (CHADD, 2015c). One large-scale Finnish study found that symptoms of inattentiveness and hyperactivity in childhood were more predictive of alcohol use disorders and illicit drug use in later adolescence than an ADHD diagnosis (Sihvola et al., 2011). Some pediatricians are recommending supplementation with omega-3 fish oils when parents refuse medication, as there has been some evidence that this may be beneficial in reducing symptoms (Millichap & Yee, 2012).

Behavioral and Emotional Problems

The lifetime prevalence of any mental disorder among 13- to 18-year-olds is 46.3% (Merikangas et al., 2010; NIMH, n.d.b). It is estimated that 5.4% of children between the ages of 6 and 17 have ever been diagnosed with a behavioral or conduct problem (Ghandour, Kogan, Blumberg, Jones, & Perrin, 2012). About 10% of children and adolescents have been diagnosed at some point with anxiety or depression. Around 20% of school-age children display behaviors consistent with oppositional defiant disorder (e.g., hostile, stubborn, disobedient, belligerent, defiant), and 2.1% of children have been diagnosed with conduct disorder characterized by a persistent violation of norms/rules and others' rights (American Academy of Child & Adolescent Psychiatry [AACAP], 2011a). Early symptoms of conduct disorder (CD) in 3-year-old preschool children (e.g., fighting, stealing, property destruction) have been shown to be predictive of later conduct disorder at age 6, with an effect stronger for boys than girls (Rolon-Arroyo, Arnold, & Harvey, 2014). Symptoms of conduct disorder, sometimes thought to be a more severe form of antisocial behavior than oppositional defiant disorder, is often characterized by behaviors that may include destruction of property, fire setting, cruelty to animals or people, and/or bullying and threatening behavior. Schizophrenia in childhood affects 1 in 40,000 children under age 12, and adult schizophrenia, which affects 1 in 100 people, usually begins in young adulthood (age 18 for males, age 25 for females). Bipolar disorder, most often found in adults, is also found in children and adolescents. Early identification of children and adolescents at risk for developing bipolar disorder may be accomplished through the use of behavior checklists and other psychometric tools that reveal higher scores related to aggression, delinquent behavior, and attention problems or withdrawal and anxiety/depression (Axelson et al., 2015). It is important to find referral sources for these children and their families, and this may be difficult in more rural or outlying areas.

School-age problem behaviors stem from many causes, some of them genetic and others environmental. Corporal punishment may be a risk factor for antisocial behavior, and several studies have noted a link between corporal punishment and restricted development of cognitive ability, as well as increased externalizing behaviors and receptive vocabulary scores (Gershoff, Lansford, Sexton, Davis-Kean, & Sameroff, 2012; MacKenzie, Nicklas, Waldfogel, & Brooks-Gunn, 2013). For children who already live in difficult situations, repeated spanking and harsh parenting measures only amplify the cumulative risk (MacKenzie, Nicklas, Brooks-Gunn, & Waldfogel, 2014). Physical punishment (e.g., slapping, spanking, pinching, pulling ears) is thought to both trigger and maintain child behavior problems, and decreasing this parental behavior could be associated with better child mental health and lower levels of behavior problems (Scott, 2012). Despite decades of research highlighting its deleterious effects, 55.2% of mothers and 43.2% of fathers of children age 3 were found to use spanking as a disciplinary measure in an urban birth cohort study (MacKenzie, Nicklas, Waldfogel, & Brooks-Gunn, 2012). Researchers found that 5-year-old children whose mothers spanked them frequently at age 3 were more likely to have externalizing behavior and decreased verbal expression at age 5. The effects of corporal punishment and the use of parental psychological aggression were shown to continue to affect children into adulthood, even after positive parenting was incorporated. These adults had higher levels of anxiety and poorer self-esteem (Taillieu & Brownridge, 2013).

Children are barometers of their environment. The current rate of divorce in the United States is double what it was in the 1950s. Over the last 30 years, the percentage of children living with two married parents decreased from close to 80% to 64% in 2014; about 4%

of children lived with two unmarried parents. Four percent of children did not live with either parent, and 56% of those children lived with grandparents. The majority of children living with one parent live with their mother. Children of divorce are more likely to exhibit behavior problems, with children who are products of highly contentious divorces most at risk (FCFS, 2015d). School nurses can be alert to early symptoms and refer parents to marital counseling or suggest family therapists. Some schools also offer support groups for children of divorce.

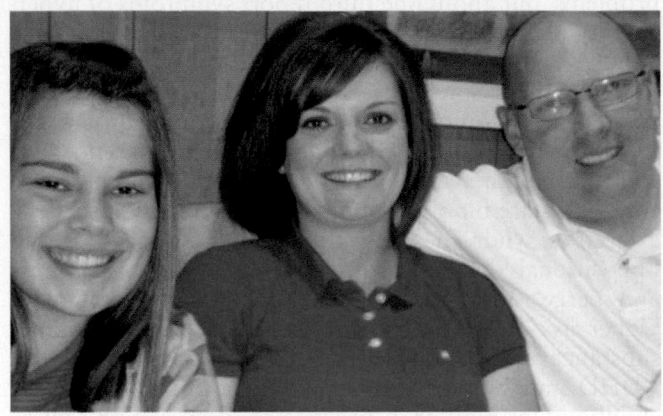

Fewer children now live in two-parent homes. (Author's private photo with permissions of Merysa Schultz, Deanna Rector, Jon Rector.)

School refusal, where a child develops a pattern of refusing to go to school or remain in school for the entire school day, is found in 2% to 5% of school-age children and differs from truancy. Unlike truancy, school refusal is commonly associated with symptoms of emotional distress—usually anxiety or depression—but may also be associated with oppositional defiant disorder, ADHD, or other disruptive behavior disorders. Often, the children complain of headaches, stomachaches, or other physical ailments, but some are motivated to miss school to gain parental attention (ADAA, n.d.). School refusal (formerly called school phobia) is most commonly found in children between ages 5 and 6 or ages 10 and 11. Transitional periods, such as school entry or moving to middle school or high school, are often the most difficult. Rates are generally reported by parents to be higher for girls and younger children (ADAA, n.d.). Children usually present to the school nurse or PHN with headaches and/or abdominal pains. They may throw tantrums, cry, or exhibit panic and fear to their parents in an attempt to stay home from school. Sometimes, children are afraid of something in the school environment (e.g., bullies, teachers, test taking), or they may have a type of separation anxiety. Family enmeshment or detachment, or high levels of family conflict, may contribute to school refusal problems, as well as parental anxiety disorders like agoraphobia and panic disorder (Maynard et al., 2015). The best interventions include early return to school, with parental involvement in school, systematic desensitization (graded exposure to the classroom), relaxation training, and counseling being the most effective (ADAA, n.d.). Family therapy and cognitive–behavioral therapy is often used (Maynard et al., 2015). Occasionally, antidepressant medications are used as well. PHNs and school nurses can serve as a liaison with the child, family, school, and health care/mental health care providers to promote a positive outcome.

Disabled Children

Children with disabilities accounted for almost 6% of the total school-age population in 2010. Cognitive and self-care difficulties were the two most common disabilities reported, followed by vision, ambulatory, and hearing problems (Brault, 2011). Between 2012 and 2013, almost 6.4 million students were classified as disabled, or 13% of school-age students; this was down slightly from 2003 to 2004 (13.7%). The most commonly cited disabilities are specific LD, speech or language disability, intellectual disability, emotional disturbance, and other health impairments (NCES, 2015). The prevalence of developmental disabilities in children aged 3 to 17 increased from 12.84% to 15.04% between 1997 and 2008. Hispanic children had the lowest prevalence, and boys had higher overall prevalence than girls. Rates for autism and ADHD, along with other developmental delays, increased; hearing loss declined (Boyle, Boulet, Schieve, & Cohen, 2011; CDC, 2015e).

Many children with perceived disabilities or problems are referred for assessment and possible placement in special education programs each year. School nurses often serve as a liaison between parents, physicians, and educators and are part of the team developing an individualized education plan (IEP) for children who qualify for special education services. Most children receive special services in a regular classroom because *full inclusion* or *mainstreaming* legislation mandates that fewer children be segregated into special classes or separate schools. See Chapter 26 for more on clients with disabilities and Chapter 30 for more on school nursing.

Problems Associated with Economic Status

After reaching a low point (16.2%) in 2000, childhood poverty in the United States rose to 22 % in 2013 (FCFS, 2015d). This increase in poverty did not vary by parents' place of birth, employment status, or educational level, leading many to speculate that this jump in the poverty rate reflects overall economic conditions. According to the Children's Defense Fund (CDF, 2014), 1 in 5 Black and 1 in 7 Hispanic children live in extreme poverty, as does 1 in 18 White children. About 1 in 3 children of color lives in poverty, along with 1 in 10 White children. Overall, children make up 24% of the U.S. population, but they represent 34% of all those in poverty (Addy & Wight, 2012; CDF, 2014). Although the United States ranked number one among industrialized nations in gross domestic product (GDP), health expenditures, defense expenditures, and military technology, it ranked 17th in reading scores and 30th in infant mortality. It ranked last because of high rates of relative child poverty and adolescent birth mothers (aged 15 to 19) and was also last in protecting children against gun violence (CDF, 2014). It is in society's best economic interest to care for its children, because they will become the taxpayers of tomorrow. Historically, experts posited that single-parent families (usually without an adult man present), welfare

reform, and economic trends that kept less well-educated populations from entering all but the most menial jobs combined to produce a powerful synergistic effect on children and adolescents.

Poverty has profound and lasting effects on children, as research has consistently shown over many years. A classic study found that more than 20% of low-income children between the ages of 6 and 17 have some type of mental health problem (Chau & Douglas-Hall, 2007). A large, often cited, birth cohort study found that family poverty predicted increased rates of depression and anxiety in adolescents and young adults and that an increased frequency of child poverty exposure, or repeated exposures, was associated with poorer mental health and reduced levels of cognitive development (Najman et al., 2010). Childhood poverty, leading to high levels of chronic stress and allostatic load, is inversely associated with adult working memory levels (Evans & Fuller-Rowell, 2013). Evans and Fuller-Rowell (2013) indicate, however, that a child with enhanced self-regulatory skills may be somewhat protected from the adverse effects of poverty. Children living in poverty have poorer health and are more likely to suffer from a chronic health condition (e.g., asthma, anemia), as well as injuries and accidents (CDF, 2014). As adolescents, they more often experience depression and mental health problems and engage in more health risk behaviors (e.g., smoking, early sexual activity), and more externalizing/adolescent delinquent behaviors (Child Trends Databank, 2015a).

As adults, these children will be more likely to have lower occupational status and lower wages. Poor children and adolescents are at higher risk for negative cognitive outcomes and learning problems, resulting in fewer school days, lower math and reading scores, more grade failures, and earlier high school dropout (Child Trends Databank, 2015a). Parental education level and employment status play large roles in childhood poverty. For children with parents having less than a high school diploma, 85% live in low-income families; and 73% of children with one parent who works less than full time annually live in poverty (Addy & Wight, 2012).

The social, emotional, and behavioral problems of some poor children may be the end result of disproportionate exposure to environmental toxins, parental substance abuse, maternal depression, trauma and abuse, divorce, violent crime, low-quality child care, inadequate nutrition, and decreased cognitive stimulation and exposure to vocabulary in early childhood and infancy (Child Trends Databank, 2015a).

The relationship between lower socioeconomic status (SES) and poor health persists throughout childhood and adolescence into adulthood (Doubeni et al., 2012), and childhood SES is strongly associated with morbidity and mortality during adulthood (Cheng, Goodman, & Committee on Pediatric Research, 2015). A population-based cohort study found that lower childhood SES was significantly related to obesity and higher systolic blood pressure in women, and some association was found for men and smoking. These outcomes are cardiovascular risk factors, and even when social inequalities level off with age, early poverty may affect cardiovascular health through these risk factors (Schumann et al., 2011). A study by Levine, Cole, Weir, and Crimmins (2015) examined childhood SES, traumas, and health, as well as adult traumas and SES, and found that childhood traumas were associated with an increase in "inflammatory transcription" in later adulthood (p. 16). Childhood traumas also potentiated the effect of low SES in adulthood on elevated "inflammatory gene expression" (p. 16); researchers thought that early childhood traumas may affect the stress response throughout life and affect health outcomes in later adult life, especially for those who have lower SES. Another study, looking at childhood SES and affect on adult health over time, found racial/ethnic differences among men in their study with White men most affected by adult low SES (Hargrove & Brown, 2015).

Some specific physical health problems are related to poverty (e.g., lead poisoning, iron deficiency anemia, increased susceptibility to illness). Children living in poorer neighborhoods are exposed to higher levels of community violence and may be more prone to seeing the world as a hostile and dangerous place; they are often also exposed to higher levels of family violence and are more at risk of subsequent mental health issues (Child Trends DataBank, 2015b). Longitudinal research, along with a series of preliminary studies, on the many stresses of childhood poverty (e.g., crowded homes/classrooms, inadequate child care, low SES, family/peer problems) found that levels of the stress hormone cortisol influenced results on school readiness testing and affected cognitive functioning (e.g., impulse/emotional control, planning, attention): that, in turn, affects school success (Blair, 2012). For more affluent children, other stressors (e.g., divorce, learning disabilities, harsh parenting) can affect stress levels and outcomes. Continuing periods of high stress can lead to either high levels of cortisol or immediately high dropping to very low levels that blunt children's responses to new challenges. Those with blunted responses or very high cortisol responses were found to have lower executive function and more problems with writing, math, and reading, as well as poor self-control in class. The reverse was found for those with more characteristic patterns of cortisol response (elevated with stressful event and then normalized afterward). Children were tested in Head Start and again in kindergarten. Parenting style was also examined, and lower SES parents were more prone to harsher forms of discipline that demanded obedience. Their children had lower executive functioning and either high or blunted cortisol levels. Parents using a more sensitive approach, who interacted with children during play and allowed more exploration, had children with better executive function and normal cortisol response. Researchers saw this as evidence that parenting style was an important part of child stress response. They noted that psychological stress in childhood "can substantially shape the course of their cognitive, social, and emotional development … and impair specific learning abilities in children, potentially setting them back in many domains of life" (p. 67).

The negative impact of childhood poverty on learning and later income along with health continues to be well documented. Schickedanz, Dreyer, and Halfon (2015) state "poverty is the most pervasive of risks for America's children" (p. 1111). It is important to put in place programs and safeguards to reduce child poverty and its long-term negative effects (Anthony, King, & Austin, 2011; Schickedanz et al., 2015). Many school-age children suffer from the effects of poverty-related hunger. It is difficult to concentrate and learn properly if meals are often skipped or if food consistently does not provide enough nourishment (American Psychological Association, [APA] n.d.). **Food insufficiency** is defined as not having enough food to eat, whereas food insecurity is characterized by "reduced quality, variety, or desirability" of one's diet, but there may be no real indication of a reduction of food intake (U.S. Department of Agriculture [USDA], 2011, para. 5). About 15.4% of U.S. households reported some degree of food insecurity in 2014, representing 48.1 million people. Variation among states occurs, with North Dakota reporting 8.4% and Mississippi 22%. In December 2014, more than 46.2 million Americans participated in the Supplemental Nutrition Assistance Program (SNAP, or food stamps); this represents a decrease of approximately 0.5 million over the previous year (Food Research & Action Center [FRAC], 2015). About 30% of those who are eligible use any of the largest federal food assistance programs, such as food stamps, free or reduced school lunches, and women, infants, and children (WIC). Thus, children go hungry because many eligible families do not use these services. In 2013, about 14.6% of Americans surveyed reported a hardship providing food for their families (FRAC, 2015). Those children who participate in school lunch and breakfast programs suffer fewer of the side effects of hunger that affect learning; however, not all schools participate in these programs. For more on poverty, see Chapter 25.

Welfare Reform

Welfare reforms enacted in 1996 (i.e., the Personal Responsibility and Work Opportunity Reconciliation Act [PRWORA]) have been successful in moving many families from welfare to work. With a combination of welfare time limits, increasing work requirements/sanctions, and reducing financial disincentives for work, welfare reform and work success programs were projected to lead to greater employment. Although the number of families receiving cash assistance (Temporary Assistance for Needy Families [TANF]) decreased between 2001 and 2008, the number increased between 2008 and 2010 as the recession spread nationally. The majority of TANF adult recipients are single mothers with young children and Hispanic children represented the greatest number of recipient children in 2011 (Folk, 2014).

A study of Wisconsin welfare leavers found that those who left before the recession had less difficulty finding jobs and child care, whereas those exiting the welfare system during the recession had lower employment rates and more difficulty with child care because of sporadic employment (Kwon & Meyer, 2011). More than 1 million single mothers are now thought to be in the "no work, no welfare" group—with no jobs and no government support. Although welfare reform was found to reduce the probability of high school dropout by 15%

for adolescents from disadvantaged families, it also decreased the probability of college enrollment for adult women eligible for welfare by 20% (Dhaval, Corman, & Reichman, 2012). As part of welfare reform, the mission of case workers changed from eligibility verification/payments to service delivery/promoting client self-sufficiency; the decline in social worker caseloads by over half has been linked to a drop in service to qualifying families, rather than a reduction in the numbers of poor families (Godfrey & Yoshikawa, 2011). Also, employment and earnings success are often tied to client–caseworker interaction and personalized client attention, with great variation among states and counties (Godfrey & Yoshikawa, 2011).

The SNAP, formerly the Food Stamp Program, is one of the largest programs offered by federal Food and Nutrition Services. In 2013, the number of children receiving SNAP benefits rose to 20.5 million. This increase in SNAP recipients coincided with the U.S. Great Recession of 2007–2009. Positive health benefits for children are linked with SNAP. These positive outcomes include improved birth outcomes and improved adult health and self-sufficiency (Child Trends Databank, 2015c). Although children living in immigrant families are more likely to live in poverty than their counterparts with native-born parents, immigrant families are less likely to receive SNAP benefits. This disparity is thought to be the result of additional challenges faced by foreign-born parents such as language and cultural barriers (Hanson, Koball, Fortuny, & Chaudry, 2014). Some affected by welfare reform decreased their food stamp participation while turning more to the special supplemental food program for WIC, or the National School Lunch/Breakfast Program, as a source of essential food items for their children. Safety-net programs—specifically, WIC and the Food Stamp Program—have been shown to reduce the risk of nutrition-related problems (e.g., anemia, nutritional deficiency, failure to thrive). They have also been associated with a reduction in the risk of child abuse and neglect (Slack et al., 2011). Some studies indicate that about half of the families who leave welfare for work actually have fewer economic resources than they had while on welfare. Research regarding PRWORA and the ensuing SNAP and TANF programs suggests that increased evaluation is needed regarding the effectiveness at reducing poverty and the overall effect for children's health (Pimpare, 2013).

Although almost 22% of children live below the federal poverty level ($23,624 or less for family of four in 2013), economists note that families need about twice the income of the federal poverty level to survive (Child Trends DataBank, 2015a; Coverage for All, 2012). These families are characterized as low income, and more than 16 million children live in these circumstances. Millions more children live in moderate-income families that have inadequate child care, limited health insurance, limited access to higher education, and poor housing. Almost 20% of children live in distressing situations and are at risk of being homeless. In 2013, about 10% of children living in low-income families did not have health insurance and approximately 9% of children living below the poverty line had no health insurance (Miller, 2011). Public

insurance now covers the majority of poor (81%) and low-income (68%) children. Abdus, Hudson, Hill, and Seldon (2014) indicate, however, that although Medicaid and Children's Health Insurance Program (CHIP) offer insurance coverage for low-income children, insurance premiums are associated with increased numbers of uninsured children. See Chapters 6 and 25 for more on insurance and vulnerable populations.

Injuries

The loss of children's lives that results from all injuries combined suggests a staggering loss to society in the number of years of productive life lost. An injury is damage to the body, either unintentional or intentional, but use of the word accident is considered incorrect, as injuries may be prevented through environmental, individual behavioral, legislative, and institutional policy changes. In the United States, unintentional injuries are the leading cause of death and disability for children between the ages of 1 and 19 years. Approximately 36% of all childhood and adolescent deaths result from unintended injuries. One out of nine children under the age of 19 years in the United States will be seen in the emergency room for unintentional injuries, with the resulting annual cost of medical treatment estimated at $11.5 billion (CDC, 2012a; Child Trends Databank, 2015e). The total lifetime cost for injured children between the ages 0 and 14 years is approximately $80 billion. The causes of death vary between age groups. Motor vehicle–related injuries remain the leading cause of death for children age 5 to 19 years and ranks second for children 0 to 4 years of age. Other common causes of death include suffocation, drowning, and poisoning (Child Trends Databank, 2015e).

Injuries are responsible for approximately 75% of deaths during adolescence. The death rate for adolescents (15 to 19 years) dropped to 45 per 100,000 in 2013 from 49 per 100,000 in 2011. During 2013, approximately 60% of adolescent deaths were a result of motor vehicle accidents or were firearms related (FCFS, 2015a, 2015c). For children aged 5 to 14, the death rate in 2012 and 2013 was 13 per 100,000, with the death rate dropping by 58% since 1980 (FCFS, 2015c). Black, non-Hispanic children had the highest death rates at 40/100,000 (ages 1 to 4) and 18/100,000 (ages 5 to 14). As the leading cause of childhood death, unintentional injury and injury death rates were 8 (1 to 4 years) and 4 (5 to 14 years) per 100,000 overall. For the 5- to 14-year-olds, this was followed by cancer (2), homicide (1), and birth defects (1). Injury death rates have dropped over the past two decades (FCFS, 2015c).

For all racial and ethnic groups, death rates were higher for infants and late adolescents and dropped during the middle years. Homicide rates were highest for black children in all age groups (Sumner et al., 2015). Injuries not resulting in death often cause permanent disabilities or emotional and physical consequences for children and their families.

Each year, about 4 million children and adolescents are injured at school, and over 1 million sports- or recreation-related injuries occur in 0- to 19-year-olds (CDC, 2013c). Nonfatal injuries among adolescents most often involve being struck by or against an object or person, but for younger children, the cause is most often a fall (FCFS, 2015c).

A large-scale study examining the risk factors for passenger deaths in fatal motor vehicle crashes found that in more than 21% of cases of child passenger fatalities, alcohol was a factor. Quinlan, Shults, and Rudd (2014) indicate that alcohol-impaired driving continues to be a safety threat to child passengers. Although the overall fatality rate associated with young drivers (age 15 to 20 years) has steadily decreased since 2004, 9% of all drivers involved in a fatal accident are within this age group (National Center for Statistics and Analysis, 2015b). Suicide was the second leading cause of death of 15- to 19-year-olds during 2011 and homicide ranked third. Firearms were involved in 42% of teen suicides and 87% of teen homicides (Child Trends Databank, 2015d).

Another, more recent danger for adolescents is use of cell phones while driving. Although not only a concern among adolescents, among the general population, cell phone usage while driving leads to distractions and has been estimated to lead to a three times greater risk of crashing (Fitch et al., 2013). In 2014, it was estimated that cell phone use was involved in 26% of all car accidents. Approximately 10% of drivers under the age of 20 involved in a motor vehicle accident report being distracted at the time of the crash (National Highway Traffic Safety Administration, n.d.). The use of cell phones can lead to injury in younger populations, as many school-age children now have them. It is estimated that approximately 78% of teens (age 12 to 17 years) now have cell phones (Madden, Lenhart, Duggan, Cortesi, & Gasser, 2013). An interesting pair of longitudinal studies (first with 13,000 and later with 28,745 children) examined exposure to cell phones prenatally and postnatally; researchers found that behavior problems at age 7 were associated with cell phone exposure before birth and cell phone use in early childhood (Divan, Kheifets, Obel, & Olsen, 2012). In comparing American drivers to those in European countries, the prevalence of talking on a cell phone while driving was found to be 68% in the United States, much higher than 21% in the United Kingdom. Texting or emailing while driving was 31% in the United States and only 15% in Spain (Naumann & Dellinger, 2013). Legislation in many states has banned the use of cell phones (talking and/or texting) while driving. A study by Ferdinand, Menachemi, Sen, Blackburn, and Morissey (2014) found 31 states passed texting-while-driving laws, with 7 of the states banning only young drivers. Researchers found that where laws were primarily enforced (officer can stop driver for any reason), rather than secondarily enforced (officer must have another reason to stop driver in order to cite for texting), mortality reduction was improved. Also, broader texting bans were helpful in reaching the younger, more at-risk populations and that handheld bans were the most effective method of targeting the adult population. The research regarding cell phone use and distracted driving legislation continues and Qiao and Bell (2015) also indicate that legislation specific to texting while driving is effective at decreasing high school student text use.

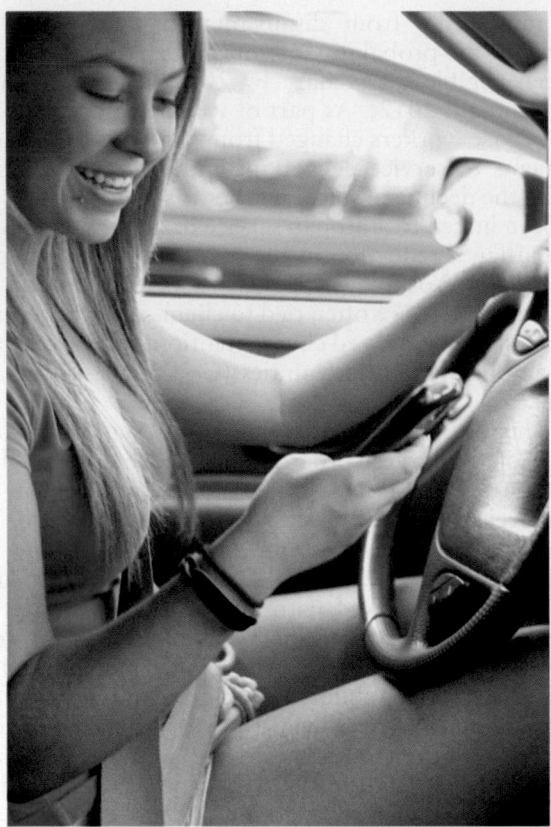

Cell phone use while driving is dangerous, especially for inexperienced adolescent drivers.

For children and adolescents, aged 6 to 19, unintentional strangulation deaths from the "choking game" are often misreported (Mechling, Ahern, & McGuiness, 2013). This behavior involves self-strangulation or strangulation by a friend through the use of hands or a noose, causing a brief euphoric high because of cerebral hypoxia. Most of the victims are male (estimated at almost 87%), and the average age is estimated at 13.3 years. Survivors may have serious neurological impairments, concussions/broken bones, or eye hemorrhages (Mechling et al., 2013). Most parents were unaware of this potentially fatal activity until a child's death occurred, but warning signs, such as bloodshot eyes; disorientation after being alone; belts, scarves, and ropes tied to doorknobs or bedroom furniture; and marks on the neck, should lead parents to suspect this dangerous activity (Mechling et al., 2013). Although difficult to track because of misreporting, the game continues to be of concern among the adolescent population and has recently shown resurgence on social media (Ruryk, 2015)).

PHNs can promote injury prevention and control through education, promotion of safety engineering and environmental protection strategies, and legislative advocacy. PHNs can advance the prevention of unintentional injuries and deaths by working with families to initiate consistent use of seat belts and child safety seats in vehicles and the use of helmets and other protective gear for children riding bikes and skateboarding (see From the Case Files I). Where water is a natural hazard, wearing life jackets while boating and swimming can help decrease accidental drowning. Promotion of smoke and carbon

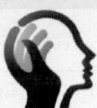

From the Case Files I

The use of restraints (seatbelts, infant car seats, child booster seats) has been shown to be an effective population-level intervention that reduces fatalities and serious injuries (National Center for Statistics and Analysis, 2015a,b). I was part of a group of pediatric nurses, epidemiologists, health educators, and physicians from a large mid-Western medical center who worked with 20 elementary schools to evaluate the most effective way to provide information on booster seat use in kindergarten children. Because we understood that most children use a seat belt and not a car or booster seat, increasing their chances of injury, we wanted to address this issue even though our state did not have any specific regulation about booster seats at that time. Our group designed three interventions: (1) a group receiving information only, (2) a group receiving a 1-hour class for parents offered at the school, or (3) a classroom presentation for children about proper booster seat use with a follow-up letter to parents about the presentation. Three to six months later, telephone follow-up was made. Parents in all three groups did not report the 70% goal of knowledge that booster seat use could protect their children in an automobile crash. The group with the greatest improvement in booster seat use was the one receiving a parent presentation and a booster seat. It was difficult to determine the best educational approach, because the demographics of the three groups were too different (language spoken, immigrant status, reading level), but we believed that the gift of a booster seat, along with personal contact and interaction, was most effective. Involving both parents and children was thought to be a better way to go in future research. The use of written educational material alone did not increase use of booster seats. Written information alone is often not effective—a good thing to keep in mind when you drop off pamphlets to clients and don't spend time going over them and answering questions.

—Julie, RN

Adapted from Philbrook, J., Kiragu, A., Geppert, J., Graham, P., Richardson, L., & Kriel, R. (2009). Pediatric injury prevention: Methods of booster seat education. Pediatric Nursing, 35(4), 215–220.

monoxide detectors, poison prevention, and sudden infant death syndrome (SIDS) education can help to further decrease injury death rates. Teaching parents about presetting hot water heaters to lower than 130°F, recognizing the hazards of infant walkers, storing matches and lighters safely, and using pool fencing can help to prevent common unintentional injuries (Safe Kids Worldwide, 2015). Advocacy for stricter seat belt and child safety seat enforcement, as well as programs to provide child safety seats and bicycle helmets, has been shown to positively affect mortality and injury rates (National Center for Statistics and Analysis, 2015a).

Community health nurses can work with their local health departments and community action groups to provide seats and helmets to families who cannot afford them, organize clinics to educate about proper installation and use, and encourage local police to enforce seat belt and safety seat laws.

Communicable Diseases

The mortality rates of school-age children 5 to 14 years old are comparatively low and have decreased substantially over the last century, a reduction that can be attributed to the effective prevention and control of the acute infectious diseases of childhood, a significant achievement in the last century. Although mortality rates are low in this country, worldwide mortality because of communicable diseases is 6 million deaths annually; morbidity because of communicable diseases among school children worldwide is also high. Tuberculosis (TB), HIV, and malaria are common, as is pneumonia because of upper respiratory infections and parasitic infections (World Bank, 2011). Among school children, the incidence rates of measles, rubella (German measles), pertussis (whooping cough), infectious parotitis (mumps), and varicella (chickenpox) have dropped considerably because of widespread immunization efforts (see Fig. 22–1 for childhood immunization schedule).

Over the past several decades, the incidence of vaccine-preventable diseases has generally decreased, although in recent years, multiple measles outbreaks were reported. In 2014, the largest number of measles cases was reported since 2000. The 667 cases involved persons from 27 different states (CDC, 2015g). A total of 159 cases of measles were reported to the CDC between January and April 2015 in the United States. Of these cases, 96% were import associated and 80% were either unvaccinated or persons with unknown vaccination status. The reported cases of mumps, hepatitis A, and meningococcal disease decreased in the under age 5 population between 2007 and 2009 (Maternal and Child Health Bureau, 2011). Some of these communicable illnesses carry potentially serious complications, such as birth defects from rubella and nerve deafness from mumps. Cases of pertussis increased by 15% between 2013 and 2014. This increase included children from all ages, with infants exceeding all other groups. The majority of pertussis-related deaths occurred in infants (CDC, 2015i).

Vigorous campaigns have been undertaken by health departments to get children immunized. Along with the standard diphtheria, tetanus, and pertussis vaccine, an immunization for mumps, measles, and rubella (MMR) has been available for more than 25 years, and newer vaccines for *Haemophilus influenzae* type b (Hib), hepatitis A and B, and varicella have been developed and are now included in the childhood immunization schedule. Meningococcal, pneumococcal, and rotavirus vaccines have also been added, along with yearly influenza vaccines for all children younger than age 5 (Barclay, 2012). Human papillomavirus (HPV) for girls aged 11 and above was recommended in 2009, and in 2011, the Advisory Committee on Immunization Practices recommended routine use for 11- and 12-year-old males. It recommended

Recommended immunization schedule for persons aged 0 through 18 years – United States, 2016.
(FOR THOSE WHO FALL BEHIND OR START LATE, SEE THE CATCH-UP SCHEDULE [FIGURE 2]).
These recommendations must be read with the footnotes that follow. For those who fall behind or start late, provide catch-up vaccination at the earliest opportunity as indicated by the green bars in Figure 1.
To determine minimum intervals between doses, see the catch-up schedule (Figure 2). School entry and adolescent vaccine age groups are shaded.

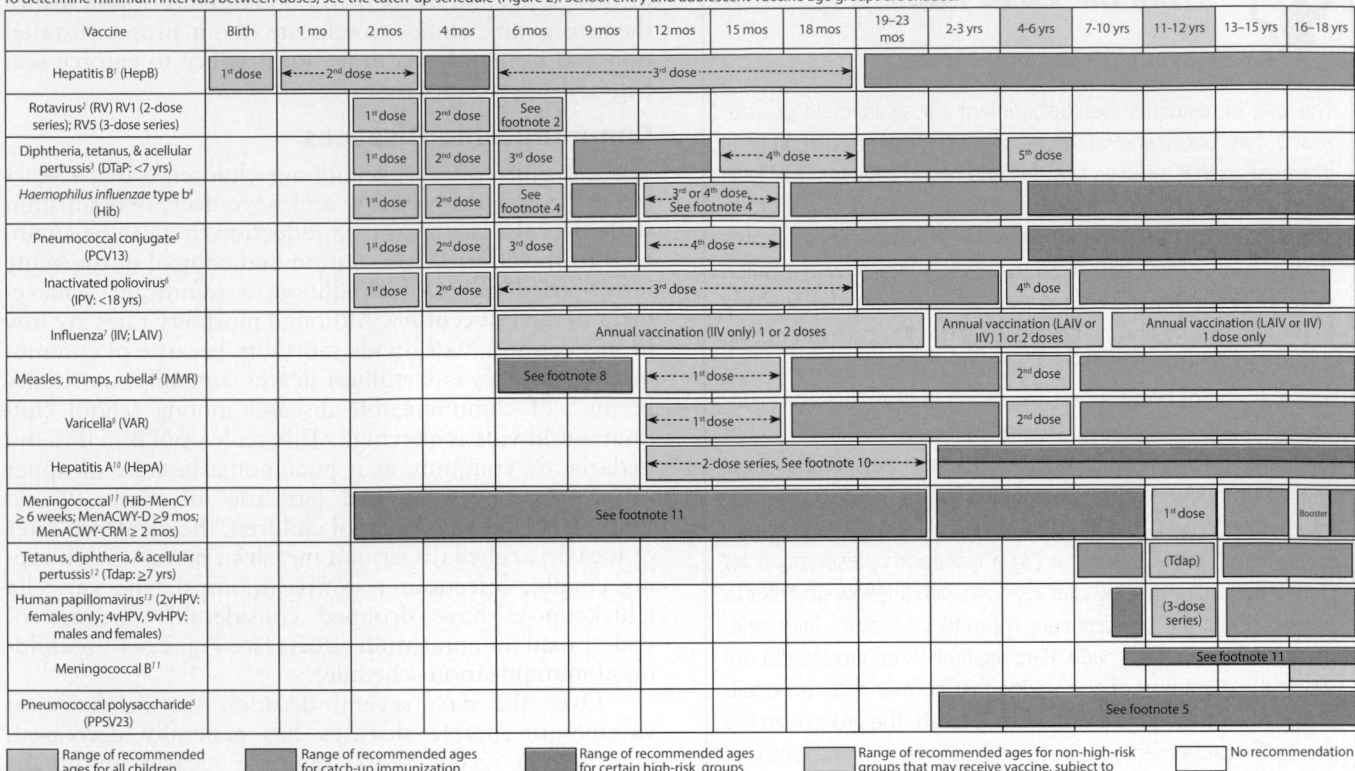

FIGURE 22–1 Childhood immunization schedule, 2015. (Retrieved from http://www.cdc.gov/vaccines/schedules/downloads/child/0-18yrs-child-combined-schedule.pdf.)

that previously unvaccinated 13- to 26-year-olds also receive the vaccine, noting that males up to age 21 may be safely vaccinated (Petrosky et al., 2015).

As increasing numbers of school-age children must show proof of required vaccinations before they are allowed to enroll in school, the percentages of children in this age group who are immunized against specific diseases may continue to rise. But more parents of young children are choosing not to immunize their children, invoking religious or personal belief exceptions. This practice has led to outbreaks of vaccine-preventable diseases including the 2014–2015 measles outbreak in a recreational theme park (CDC, 2015g; Reinberg, 2011). However, immunization compliance for adolescents has often been problematic because of lack of sufficient insurance coverage and poor systems for tracking and recall, as well as fewer well-child visits to health care providers among this age group. This has improved in recent years, though. Results from a 2013 national immunization survey revealed that 70.4% of children between ages 19 and 35 months have received the full vaccine series. Results, however, also indicate continuing disparities between vulnerable populations; for example, non-Hispanic black children were less likely to receive the full immunization

series than non-Hispanic white children. Strategies shown to improve vaccination rates include the Vaccine for Children (VFC) Program, cost reduction, home visits, and linking vaccination opportunities with WIC visits. Among adolescents, vaccination rates increased for the Tdap and meningococcal conjugate vaccine. Lower rates were documented for the HPV vaccine and recommendations made for clinicians to administer all of the age-appropriate vaccines in a single visit (USDHHS, 2015b). Diekema (2012) suggests that efforts to improve immunization rates should focus on eliminating socioeconomic barriers, strengthening school-entry requirements, addressing vaccine misinformation, and using effective communication to influence the vaccine-hesitant. See Figure 22–2, adolescent immunization schedule.

With the marked rise in community-acquired methicillin-resistant *Staphylococcus aureus* (CA-MRSA), PHNs and school nurses must be alert when skin infections or other conditions do not resolve quickly in children and adolescents (CDC, 2013b). Sports teams, for instance, may spread this infection, along with others like molluscum contagiosum, as participants come into close contact. Referral to an infectious disease specialist may need to be considered (Fritz et al., 2012).

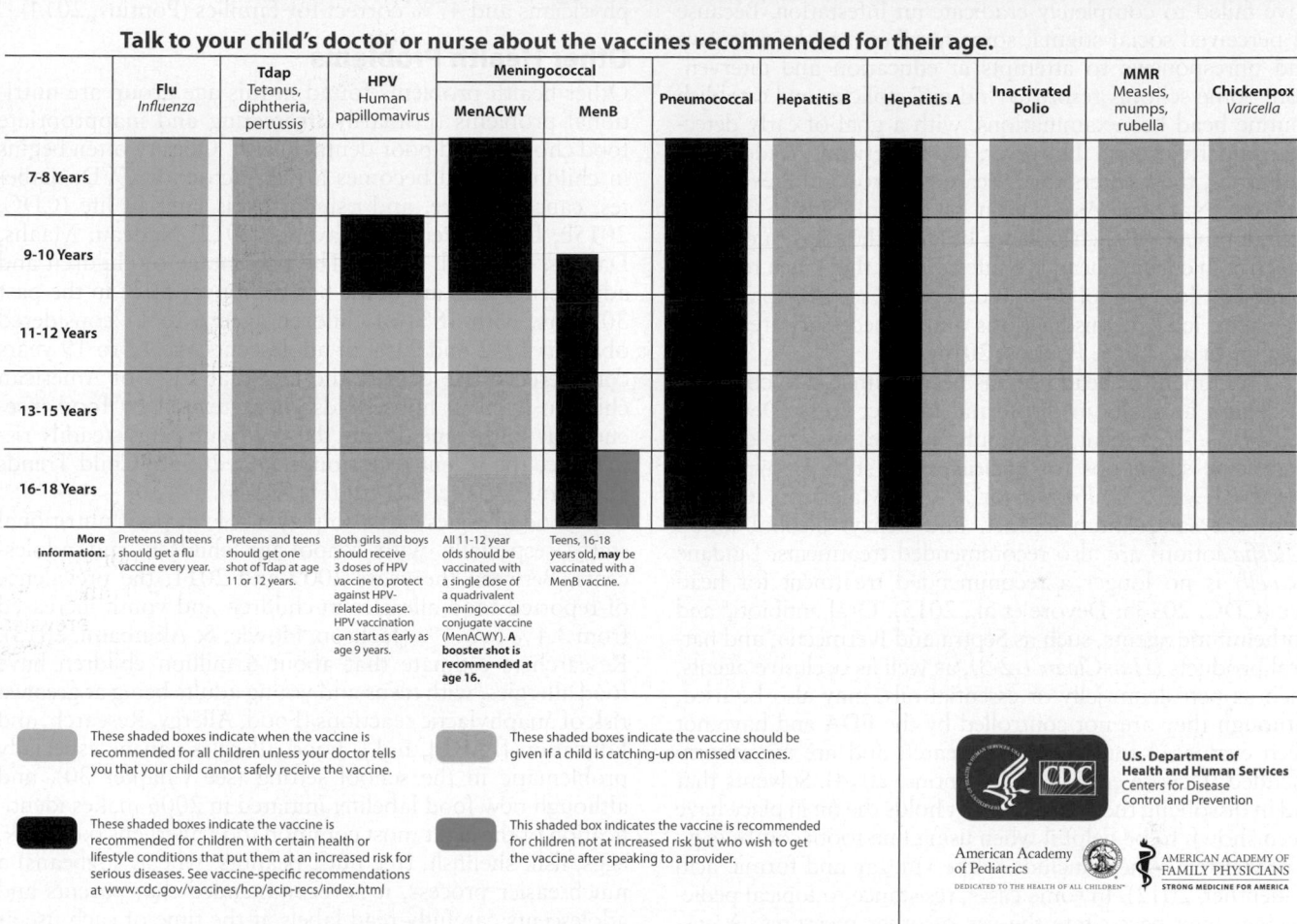

FIGURE 22–2 Adolescent immunization schedule, 2015. (Retrieved from http://www.cdc.gov/vaccines/who/teens/downloads/parent-version-schedule-7-18yrs.pdf.)

Head Lice

Pediculosis (head lice) is a frustrating and common problem for many preschool and school-age children, and the incidence has been increasing with approximately 6 to 12 million 3- to 11-year-olds infected annually (CDC, 2013a). Preschoolers and elementary-age children and their caretakers and family members are at highest risk for head lice. Close crowded conditions can also be a risk factor (CDC, 2013a). An infestation of *Pediculus humanus* var. *capitis*, the parasite that lives and feeds on the human scalp, can be an embarrassing nuisance to families of any socioeconomic level. These very tiny, wingless insects need blood to survive and can cause itching and skin irritation. They do not transmit disease, but secondary bacterial infections can occur from children scratching their scalps (CDC, 2013a; Pontius, 2014). They are most often found behind the ears, toward the nape of the neck, where hair is usually thickest, but their pearly white eggs (nits) are distributed all over the head. They are attached to the hair shaft with a glue-like substance and can be detected by careful examination of the scalp. Nits typically hatch within 8 to 9 days, and the immature

louse passes through three developmental stages before reaching adulthood during the next 9 to 12 days. Viable nits are closer than one-quarter inch from the scalp, and those further away are not viable. Adult head lice, similar in size to a sesame seed, may be whitish, gray, or brown colored and may live for about 30 days. Without treatment, the cycle repeats every 3 weeks. Complete eradication generally requires that all viable nits be removed along with lice; family and close contacts should be checked for head lice and, if found, treated at the same time (Devore, Schutze, & Council on School Health & Committee on Infectious Diseases, 2015; Pontius, 2014).

Head lice are most often transmitted by direct contact (head-to-head) or may occasionally be passed from infected to uninfected children through shared items such as combs and brushes, hats, scarves, sheets, and towels (items called *fomites*). However, this is thought to rarely be the case. Most infestations begin in the community, not in schools. Children who play closely together and share beds give head lice the opportunity to crawl from one person's head to another's. Contrary to some popular myths, lice do not fly or jump, and they cannot be contracted from animals—they live only on humans. They do not survive long off the human head, generally 1 or 2 days (CDC, 2015a; Devore et al., 2015; Pontius, 2014). Schools may have recurring outbreaks of head lice that can be traced back to particular families who have failed to completely eradicate an infestation. Because of perceived social stigma, some families may be defensive and unresponsive to attempts at education and intervention. Some schools resort to "no-nit" policies and establish routine head lice examinations, with a goal of early detection and treatment. However, the American Academy of Pediatrics, the Centers for Disease Control and Prevention, and the National Association of School Nurses call for abandonment of such policies because they have not been effective in curbing head lice infestations, they often result in significant lost school days and negative social impact, and they may lead to misdiagnosis and unnecessary treatment (Devore et al., 2015; Pontius, 2014).

Treatment of head lice has been estimated to cost over $1 billion annually in direct and indirect costs (Devore et al., 2015). Treatment commonly includes over-the-counter insecticide shampoos (or **pediculicides**), such as pyrethrin-based *RID*, *R&C*, *Pronto*, or *A-200*. Malathion (*Ovide*), from chrysanthemum extract, and benzyl alcohol lotion (*Ulesfia* lotion) are also recommended treatments. Lindane (*Kwell*) is no longer a recommended treatment for head lice (CDC, 2013a; Devore et al., 2015). Oral antibiotic and anthelmintic agents, such as Septra and Ivermectin, and natural products (*HairClean 1-2-3*), as well as occlusive agents, such as petroleum jelly or essential oils, may also be used, although they are not controlled by the FDA and have not been evaluated for safety by research and are not recommended (Devore et al., 2015; Pontius, 2014). Solvents that aid in dissolving the "cement" that holds the nit in place have been shown to be helpful when using fine-tooth combs (e.g., LiceMeister)—these include white vinegar and formic acid (Guenther, 2012). In some cases, resistance to topical pediculicides may necessitate the use of other measures. A custom machine, blasting hot air for 30 minutes (*AirAllé*), has shown some promising results but is expensive and requires training for operators. Frustrated families, having repeated problems with head lice infestations, have tried such unusual remedies as kerosene, acetone, bleach, vodka, and other extreme measures to try to kill lice and nits without success. Such flammable agents are not appropriate treatment for head lice (Devore et al., 2015; Pontius, 2014).

School nurses and PHNs also need to educate families about reducing reinfestations by careful application of pediculicides, retreating in 2 weeks if necessary, and cleaning of any fomites (e.g., combs, hats, towels, sheets, clothing, upholstered furniture) and removal of any viable nits. Drying sheets, blankets, and towels on high heat and washing all hats and clothing are effective measures. It is not necessary to use fumigant sprays, as they can be toxic (CDC, 2013a). It is difficult, however, to prevent children—who are social creatures—from coming into close contact with one another and becoming reinfected. In some larger cities, entrepreneurs have started nit removal businesses (e.g., Nit Pickers, Hair Fairies) to assist parents with this tedious task, but most experts in the field feel that this is an unnecessary expense (Pontius, 2014). Some resistance to pediculicides has been found, but most treatment failures have been found to be because of initial misdiagnosis, noncompliance or inappropriate application of

treatments, new lice infestation after treatment, and using products that do not kill eggs (no ovicidal ingredients). When checked by an entomologist, head lice samples sent for identification were found to be only 11% accurate for physicians and 47% correct for families (Pontius, 2014).

Other Health Problems

Other health problems found in this age group are nutritional problems (primarily overeating and inappropriate food choices) and poor dental health. Obesity often begins in childhood and becomes a risk factor for CVD, diabetes, cancer, stroke, and osteoarthritis later in life (CDC, 2015b; Dixon, Pena, & Taveras, 2012; Nadeau, Maahs, Daniels, & Eckel, 2011). The percentage of children and adolescents who are obese has risen over 50% in the past 30 years, with 18% of children aged 6 to 11 considered obese in 2012 and 21% of adolescents age 12 to 19 years considered obese despite the fact that 21% of American children lived in households characterized by food insecurity at some time during the year with rates steadily rising since the recent recession (CDC, 2015b; Child Trends Databank. 2014c, 2014d) (Fig. 22–3).

Food allergies can also play a role in poor nutritional status, especially with school-age children and adolescents. Between the years 2009 and 2011, the prevalence of reported food allergies in children and youth increased from 3.4% to 5.1% (Jackson, Howie, & Akinbami, 2013). Researchers estimate that about 6 million children have food allergies, with teens and young adults being at greatest risk of anaphylactic reactions (Food, Allergy, Research, and Education [FARE], n.d.). Food allergies can be especially problematic in the school setting (see Chapter 30), and although new food labeling initiated in 2006 makes identification of the eight most common food allergens (i.e., milk, eggs, fish, shellfish, tree nuts, peanuts, wheat, soybeans) a much easier process, it is recommended that parents and adolescents carefully read labels at the time of each use as ingredients can change without warning (FARE, n.d.).

Dental caries is another common problem among school-age children. Approximately 17% of U.S. schoolchildren (5 to 19 years) have untreated cavities. In 2013, 83% of children age 2 to 17 visited a dentist during the year (CDC, 2015d).

Childhood Obesity

About one third of U.S. children are classified as overweight or at risk of becoming overweight (CDC, 2015b; Gurnani, Birken, & Hamilton, 2015). The CDC uses the term **overweight**, rather than obese, in defining children who have a BMI at or above the 95th percentile. Children with a BMI between the 85th and 94th percentile are defined as **at risk of overweight** (National Heart, Lung, and Blood Institute, 2013). (See Display 22–1 for an explanation and examples.) The obesity rate has tripled for children and adolescents, and about 17% of children aged 2 to 19 are obese. Although there has been a decrease in obesity in 2- to 5-year-old children, the rate has remained constant for adolescents through 2012 (Ogden, Carroll, Kit, & Flegal, 2014). In New York, the drop in early childhood obesity was thought to be related to home food consumption changes at the prompting of media messages and school/child care policy changes that also reinforced behavioral change (Farley & Dowell, 2014). Obese

Catch-up immunization schedule for persons aged 4 months through 18 years who start late or who are more than 1 month behind —United States, 2016.
The figure below provides catch-up schedules and minimum intervals between doses for children whose vaccinations have been delayed. A vaccine series does not need to be restarted, regardless of the time that has elapsed between doses. Use the section appropriate for the child's age. Always use this table in conjunction with Figure 1 and the footnotes that follow.

Vaccine	Minimum Age for Dose 1	Minimum Interval Between Doses			
		Dose 1 to Dose 2	Dose 2 to Dose 3	Dose 3 to Dose 4	Dose 4 to Dose 5
Children age 4 months through 6 years					
Hepatitis B[1]	Birth	4 weeks	8 weeks *and* at least 16 weeks after first dose. Minimum age for the final dose is 24 weeks.		
Rotavirus[2]	6 weeks	4 weeks	4 weeks[2]		
Diphtheria, tetanus, and acellular pertussis[3]	6 weeks	4 weeks	4 weeks	6 months	6 months[3]
Haemophilus influenzae type b[4]	6 weeks	4 weeks if first dose was administered before the 1st birthday. 8 weeks (as final dose) if first dose was administered at age 12 through 14 months. No further doses needed if first dose was administered at age 15 months or older.	4 weeks[4] if current age is younger than 12 months **and** first dose was administered at younger than age 7 months, **and** at least 1 previous dose was PRP-T (ActHib, Pentacel) or unknown. 8 weeks *and* age 12 through 59 months (as final dose)[4] • if current age is younger than 12 months **and** first dose was administered at age 7 through 11 months (wait until at least 12 months old); OR • if current age is 12 through 59 months **and** first dose was administered before the 1st birthday, **and** second dose administered at younger than 15 months; OR • if both doses were PRP-OMP (PedvaxHIB; Comvax) **and** were administered before the 1st birthday (wait until at least 12 months old). No further doses needed if previous dose was administered at age 15 months or older.	8 weeks (as final dose) This dose only necessary for children aged 12 through 59 months who received 3 doses before the 1st birthday.	
Pneumococcal[5]	6 weeks	4 weeks if first dose administered before the 1st birthday. 8 weeks (as final dose for healthy children) if first dose was administered at the 1st birthday or after. No further doses needed for healthy children if first dose administered at age 24 months or older.	4 weeks if current age is younger than 12 months and previous dose given at <7months old. 8 weeks (as final dose for healthy children) if previous dose given between 7-11 months (wait until at least 12 months old); OR if current age is 12 months or older and at least 1 dose was given before age 12 months. No further doses needed for healthy children if previous dose administered at age 24 months or older.	8 weeks (as final dose) This dose only necessary for children aged 12 through 59 months who received 3 doses before age 12 months or for children at high risk who received 3 doses at any age.	
Inactivated poliovirus[6]	6 weeks	4 weeks[6]	4 weeks[6]	6 months[6] (minimum age 4 years for final dose).	
Measles, mumps, rubella[8]	12 months	4 weeks			
Varicella[9]	12 months	3 months			
Hepatitis A[10]	12 months	6 months			
Meningococcal[11] (Hib-MenCY ≥ 6 weeks; MenACWY-D ≥9 mos; MenACWY-CRM ≥ 2 mos)	6 weeks	8 weeks[11]	See footnote 11	See footnote 11	
Children and adolescents age 7 through 18 years					
Meningococcal[11] (Hib-MenCY ≥ 6 weeks; MenACWY-D ≥9 mos; MenACWY-CRM ≥ 2 mos)	Not Applicable (N/A)	8 weeks[11]			
Tetanus, diphtheria; tetanus, diphtheria, and acellular pertussis[12]	7 years[12]	4 weeks	4 weeks if first dose of DTaP/DT was administered before the 1st birthday. 6 months (as final dose) if first dose of DTaP/DT or Tdap/Td was administered at or after the 1st birthday.	6 months if first dose of DTaP/DT was administered before the 1st birthday.	
Human papillomavirus[13]	9 years	Routine dosing intervals are recommended.[13]			
Hepatitis A[10]	N/A	6 months			
Hepatitis B[1]	N/A	4 weeks	8 weeks **and** at least 16 weeks after first dose.		
Inactivated poliovirus[6]	N/A	4 weeks	4 weeks[6]	6 months[6]	
Measles, mumps, rubella[8]	N/A	4 weeks			
Varicella[9]	N/A	3 months if younger than age 13 years. 4 weeks if age 13 years or older.			

For further guidance on the use of the vaccines mentioned below, see: http://www.cdc.gov/vaccines/hcp/acip-recs/index.html. For vaccine recommendations for persons 19 years of age and older, see the Adult Immunization Schedule.

Additional information
- For contraindications and precautions to use of a vaccine and for additional information regarding that vaccine, vaccination providers should consult the relevant ACIP statement available online at http://www.cdc.gov/vaccines/hcp/acip-recs/index.html.
- For purposes of calculating intervals between doses, 4 weeks = 28 days. Intervals of 4 months or greater are determined by calendar months.
- Vaccine doses administered 4 days or less before the minimum interval are considered valid. Doses of any vaccine administered ≥5 days earlier than the minimum interval or minimum age should not be counted as valid doses and should be repeated as age-appropriate. The repeat dose should be spaced after the invalid dose by the recommended minimum interval. For further details, see *MMWR, General Recommendations on Immunization and Reports* / Vol. 60 / No. 2; Table 1. *Recommended and minimum ages and intervals between vaccine doses* available online at http://www.cdc.gov/mmwr/pdf/rr/rr6002.pdf.
- Information on travel vaccine requirements and recommendations is available at http://wwwnc.cdc.gov/travel/destinations/list.
- For vaccination of persons with primary and secondary immunodeficiencies, see Table 13, *"Vaccination of persons with primary and secondary immunodeficiencies,"* in *General Recommendations on Immunization* (ACIP), available at http://www.cdc.gov/mmwr/pdf/rr/rr6002.pdf.; and American Academy of Pediatrics. "Immunization in Special Clinical Circumstances," in Kimberlin DW, Brady MT, Jackson MA, Long SS eds. *Red Book: 2015 report of the Committee on Infectious Diseases. 30th ed.* Elk Grove Village, IL: American Academy of Pediatrics.

1. **Hepatitis B (HepB) vaccine. (Minimum age: birth)**
Routine vaccination:
At birth:
- Administer monovalent HepB vaccine to all newborns before hospital discharge.
- For infants born to hepatitis B surface antigen (HBsAg)-positive mothers, administer HepB vaccine and 0.5 mL of hepatitis B immune globulin (HBIG) within 12 hours of birth. These infants should be tested for HBsAg and antibody to HBsAg (anti-HBs) at age 9 through 18 months (preferably at the next well-child visit) or 1 to 2 months after completion of the HepB series if the series was delayed; CDC recently recommended testing occur at age 9 through 12 months; see http://www.cdc.gov/mmwr/preview/mmwrhtml/mm6439a6.htm.
- If mother's HBsAg status is unknown, within 12 hours of birth administer HepB vaccine regardless of birth weight. For infants weighing less than 2,000 grams, administer HBIG in addition to HepB vaccine within 12 hours of birth. Determine mother's HBsAg status as soon as possible and, if mother is HBsAg-positive, also administer HBIG for infants weighing 2,000 grams or more as soon as possible, but no later than age 7 days.

Doses following the birth dose:
- The second dose should be administered at age 1 or 2 months. Monovalent HepB vaccine should be used for doses administered before age 6 weeks.
- Infants who did not receive a birth dose should receive 3 doses of a HepB-containing vaccine on a schedule of 0, 1 to 2 months, and 6 months starting as soon as feasible. See Figure 2.
- Administer the second dose 1 to 2 months after the **first** dose (minimum interval of 4 weeks), administer the third dose at least 8 weeks after the second dose AND at least 16 weeks after the first dose. The final (third or fourth) dose in the HepB vaccine series should be administered **no earlier than age 24 weeks**.
- Administration of a total of 4 doses of HepB vaccine is permitted when a combination vaccine containing HepB is administered after the birth dose.

Catch-up vaccination:
- Unvaccinated persons should complete a 3-dose series.
- A 2-dose series (doses separated by at least 4 months) of adult formulation Recombivax HB is licensed for use in children aged 11 through 15 years.
- For other catch-up guidance, see Figure 2.

2. **Rotavirus (RV) vaccines. (Minimum age: 6 weeks for both RV1 [Rotarix] and RV5 [RotaTeq])**
Routine vaccination:
Administer a series of RV vaccine to all infants as follows:
   1. If Rotarix is used, administer a 2-dose series at 2 and 4 months of age.
   2. If RotaTeq is used, administer a 3-dose series at ages 2, 4, and 6 months.
   3. If any dose in the series was RotaTeq or vaccine product is unknown for any dose in the series, a total of 3 doses of RV vaccine should be administered.

Catch-up vaccination:
- The maximum age for the first dose in the series is 14 weeks, 6 days; vaccination should not be initiated for infants aged 15 weeks, 0 days or older.
- The maximum age for the final dose in the series is 8 months, 0 days.
- For other catch-up guidance, see Figure 2.

3. **Diphtheria and tetanus toxoids and acellular pertussis (DTaP) vaccine. (Minimum age: 6 weeks. Exception: DTaP-IPV [Kinrix]: 4 years)**
Routine vaccination:
- Administer a 5-dose series of DTaP vaccine at ages 2, 4, 6, 15 through 18 months, and 4 through 6 years. The fourth dose may be administered as early as age 12 months, provided at least 6 months have elapsed since the third dose.
- Inadvertent administration of 4th DTaP dose early: If the fourth dose of DTaP was administered at least 4 months, but less than 6 months, after the third dose of DTaP, it need not be repeated.

Catch-up vaccination:
- The fifth dose of DTaP vaccine is not necessary if the fourth dose was administered at age 4 years or older.
- For other catch-up guidance, see Figure 2.

4. ***Haemophilus influenzae* type b (Hib) conjugate vaccine. (Minimum age: 6 weeks for PRP-T [ACTHIB, DTaP-IPV/Hib (Pentacel) and Hib-MenCY (MenHibrix)], PRP-OMP [PedvaxHIB or COMVAX], 12 months for PRP-T [Hiberix])**
Routine vaccination:
- Administer a 2- or 3-dose Hib vaccine primary series and a booster dose (dose 3 or 4 depending on vaccine used in primary series) at age 12 through 15 months to complete a full Hib vaccine series.
- The primary series with ActHIB, MenHibrix, or Pentacel consists of 3 doses and should be administered at 2, 4, and 6 months of age.
- The primary series with PedvaxHib or COMVAX consists of 2 doses and should be administered at 2 and 4 months of age; a dose at age 6 months is not indicated.
- One booster dose (dose 3 or 4 depending on vaccine used in primary series) of any Hib vaccine should be administered at age 12 through 15 months. An exception is Hiberix vaccine. Hiberix should only be used for the booster (final) dose in children aged 12 months through 4 years who have received at least 1 prior dose of Hib-containing vaccine.
- For recommendations on the use of MenHibrix in patients at increased risk for meningococcal disease, please refer to the meningococcal vaccine footnotes and also to *MMWR* February 28, 2014 / 63(RR01);1-13, available at http://www.cdc.gov/mmwr/PDF/rr/rr6301.pdf.

Catch-up vaccination:
- If dose 1 was administered at ages 12 through 14 months, administer a second (final) dose at least 8 weeks after dose 1, regardless of Hib vaccine used in the primary series.
- If both doses were PRP-OMP (PedvaxHIB or COMVAX), and were administered before the first birthday, the third (and final) dose should be administered at age 12 through 59 months and at least 8 weeks after the second dose.
- If the first dose was administered at age 7 through 11 months, administer the second dose at least 4 weeks later and a third (and final) dose at age 12 through 15 months or 8 weeks after second dose, whichever is later.
- If first dose is administered before the first birthday and second dose administered at younger than 15 months, a third (and final) dose should be administered 8 weeks later.
- For unvaccinated children aged 15 months or older, administer only 1 dose.
- For other catch-up guidance, see Figure 2. For catch-up guidance related to MenHibrix, please see the meningococcal vaccine footnotes and also *MMWR* February 28, 2014 / 63(RR01);1-13, available at http://www.cdc.gov/mmwr/PDF/rr/rr6301.pdf.

FIGURE 22–3 Catch-up schedule for immunizations, 2016. (Retrieved from http://www.cdc.gov/vaccines/schedules/downloads/child/0-18yrs-child-combined-schedule.pdf.)

4. ***Haemophilus influenzae*** **type b (Hib) conjugate vaccine (cont'd)**

Vaccination of persons with high-risk conditions:
- Children aged 12 through 59 months who are at increased risk for Hib disease, including chemotherapy recipients and those with anatomic or functional asplenia (including sickle cell disease), human immunodeficiency virus (HIV) infection, immunoglobulin deficiency, or early component complement deficiency, who have received either no doses or only 1 dose of Hib vaccine before 12 months of age, should receive 2 additional doses of Hib vaccine 8 weeks apart; children who received 2 or more doses of Hib vaccine before 12 months of age should receive 1 additional dose.
- For patients younger than 5 years of age undergoing chemotherapy or radiation treatment who received a Hib vaccine dose(s) within 14 days of starting therapy or during therapy, repeat the dose(s) at least 3 months following therapy completion.
- Recipients of hematopoietic stem cell transplant (HSCT) should be revaccinated with a 3-dose regimen of Hib vaccine starting 6 to 12 months after successful transplant, regardless of vaccination history; doses should be administered at least 4 weeks apart.
- A single dose of any Hib-containing vaccine should be administered to unimmunized* children and adolescents 15 months of age and older undergoing an elective splenectomy; if possible, vaccine should be administered at least 14 days before procedure.
- Hib vaccine is not routinely recommended for patients 5 years or older. However, 1 dose of Hib vaccine should be administered to unimmunized* persons aged 5 years or older who have anatomic or functional asplenia (including sickle cell disease) and unvaccinated persons 5 through 18 years of age with HIV infection.

** Patients who have not received a primary series and booster dose or at least 1 dose of Hib vaccine after 14 months of age are considered unimmunized.*

5. **Pneumococcal vaccines. (Minimum age: 6 weeks for PCV13, 2 years for PPSV23)**

Routine vaccination with PCV13:
- Administer a 4-dose series of PCV13 vaccine at ages 2, 4, and 6 months and at age 12 through 15 months.
- For children aged 14 through 59 months who have received an age-appropriate series of 7-valent PCV (PCV7), administer a single supplemental dose of 13-valent PCV (PCV13).

Catch-up vaccination with PCV13:
- Administer 1 dose of PCV13 to all healthy children aged 24 through 59 months who are not completely vaccinated for their age.
- For other catch-up guidance, see Figure 2.

Vaccination of persons with high-risk conditions with PCV13 and PPSV23:
- All recommended PCV13 doses should be administered prior to PPSV23 vaccination if possible.
- For children 2 through 5 years of age with any of the following conditions: chronic heart disease (particularly cyanotic congenital heart disease and cardiac failure); chronic lung disease (including asthma if treated with high-dose oral corticosteroid therapy); diabetes mellitus; cerebrospinal fluid leak; cochlear implant; sickle cell disease and other hemoglobinopathies; anatomic or functional asplenia; HIV infection; chronic renal failure; nephrotic syndrome; diseases associated with treatment with immunosuppressive drugs or radiation therapy, including malignant neoplasms, leukemias, lymphomas, and Hodgkin disease; solid organ transplantation; or congenital immunodeficiency:
  1. If neither PCV13 nor PPSV23 has been received previously, administer 1 dose of PCV13 now and 1 dose of PPSV23 at least 8 weeks later.
  2. If PCV13 has been received previously but PPSV23 has not, administer 1 dose of PPSV23 at least 8 weeks after the most recent dose of PCV13.
  3. If PPSV23 has been received but PCV13 has not, administer 1 dose of PCV13 at least 8 weeks after the most recent dose of PPSV23.
- For children aged 6 through 18 years with chronic heart disease (particularly cyanotic congenital heart disease and cardiac failure), chronic lung disease (including asthma if treated with high-dose oral corticosteroid therapy), diabetes mellitus, alcoholism, or chronic liver disease, who have not received PPSV23, administer 1 dose of PPSV23. If PCV13 has been received previously, then PPSV23 should be administered at least 8 weeks after any prior PCV13 dose.
- A single revaccination with PPSV23 should be administered 5 years after the first dose to children with sickle cell disease or other hemoglobinopathies; anatomic or functional asplenia; congenital or acquired immunodeficiencies; HIV infection; chronic renal failure; nephrotic syndrome; diseases associated with treatment with immunosuppressive drugs or radiation therapy, including malignant neoplasms, leukemias, lymphomas, and Hodgkin disease; generalized malignancy; solid organ transplantation; or multiple myeloma.

6. **Inactivated poliovirus vaccine (IPV). (Minimum age: 6 weeks)**

Routine vaccination:
- Administer a 4-dose series of IPV at ages 2, 4, 6 through 18 months, and 4 through 6 years. The final dose in the series should be administered on or after the fourth birthday and at least 6 months after the previous dose.

Catch-up vaccination::
- In the first 6 months of life, minimum age and minimum intervals are only recommended if the person is at risk of imminent exposure to circulating poliovirus (i.e., travel to a polio-endemic region or during an outbreak).
- If 4 or more doses are administered before age 4 years, an additional dose should be administered at age 4 through 6 years and at least 6 months after the previous dose.
- A fourth dose is not necessary if the third dose was administered at age 4 years or older and at least 6 months after the previous dose.
- If both OPV and IPV were administered as part of a series, a total of 4 doses should be administered, regardless of the child's current age. If only OPV were administered, and all doses were given prior to 4 years of age, one dose of IPV should be given at 4 years or older, at least 4 weeks after the last OPV dose.
- IPV is not routinely recommended for U.S. residents aged 18 years or older.
- For other catch-up guidance, see Figure 2.

7. **Influenza vaccines. (Minimum age: 6 months for inactivated influenza vaccine [IIV], 2 years for live, attenuated influenza vaccine [LAIV])**

Routine vaccination:
- Administer influenza vaccine annually to all children beginning at age 6 months. For most healthy, nonpregnant persons aged 2 through 49 years, either LAIV or IIV may be used. However, LAIV should NOT be administered to some persons, including 1) persons who have experienced severe allergic reactions to LAIV, any of its components, or to a previous dose of any other influenza vaccine; 2) children 2 through 17 years receiving aspirin or aspirin-containing products; 3) persons who are allergic to eggs; 4) pregnant women; 5) immunosuppressed persons; 6) children 2 through 4 years of age with asthma or who had wheezing in the past 12 months; or 7) persons who have taken influenza antiviral medications in the previous 48 hours. For all other contraindications and precautions to use of LAIV, see *MMWR* August 7, 2015 / 64(30):818-25 available at http://www.cdc.gov/mmwr/pdf/wk/mm6430.pdf.

For children aged 6 months through 8 years:
- For the 2015-16 season, administer 2 doses (separated by at least 4 weeks) to children who are receiving influenza vaccine for the first time. Some children in this age group who have been vaccinated previously will also need 2 doses. For additional guidance, follow dosing guidelines in the 2015-16 ACIP influenza vaccine recommendations, *MMWR* August 7, 2015 / 64(30):818-25, available at http://www.cdc.gov/mmwr/pdf/wk/mm6430.pdf.
- For the 2016-17 season, follow dosing guidelines in the 2016 ACIP influenza vaccine recommendations.

For persons aged 9 years and older:
- Administer 1 dose.

8. **Measles, mumps, and rubella (MMR) vaccine. (Minimum age: 12 months for routine vaccination)**

Routine vaccination:
- Administer a 2-dose series of MMR vaccine at ages 12 through 15 months and 4 through 6 years. The second dose may be administered before age 4 years, provided at least 4 weeks have elapsed since the first dose.
- Administer 1 dose of MMR vaccine to infants aged 6 through 11 months before departure from the United States for international travel. These children should be revaccinated with 2 doses of MMR vaccine, the first at age 12 through 15 months (12 months if the child remains in an area where disease risk is high), and the second dose at least 4 weeks later.
- Administer 2 doses of MMR vaccine to children aged 12 months and older before departure from the United States for international travel. The first dose should be administered on or after age 12 months and the second dose at least 4 weeks later.

Catch-up vaccination:
- Ensure that all school-aged children and adolescents have had 2 doses of MMR vaccine; the minimum interval between the 2 doses is 4 weeks

9. **Varicella (VAR) vaccine. (Minimum age: 12 months)**

Routine vaccination:
- Administer a 2-dose series of VAR vaccine at ages 12 through 15 months and 4 through 6 years. The second dose may be administered before age 4 years, provided at least 3 months have elapsed since the first dose. If the second dose was administered at least 4 weeks after the first dose, it can be accepted as valid.

Catch-up vaccination:
- Ensure that all persons aged 7 through 18 years without evidence of immunity (see *MMWR* 2007 / 56 [No. RR-4], available at http://www.cdc.gov/mmwr/pdf/rr/rr5604.pdf) have 2 doses of varicella vaccine. For children aged 7 through 12 years, the recommended minimum interval between doses is 3 months (if the second dose was administered at least 4 weeks after the first dose, it can be accepted as valid); for persons aged 13 years and older, the minimum interval between doses is 4 weeks.

10. **Hepatitis A (HepA) vaccine. (Minimum age: 12 months)**

Routine vaccination:
- Initiate the 2-dose HepA vaccine series at 12 through 23 months; separate the 2 doses by 6 to 18 months. Children who have received 1 dose of HepA vaccine before age 24 months should receive a second dose 6 to 18 months after the first dose.
- For any person aged 2 years and older who has not already received the HepA vaccine series, 2 doses of HepA vaccine separated by 6 to 18 months may be administered if immunity against hepatitis A virus infection is desired.

Catch-up vaccination:
- The minimum interval between the 2 doses is 6 months.

Special populations:

10. **Hepatitis A (HepA) vaccine. (cont'd)**
- Administer 2 doses of HepA vaccine at least 6 months apart to previously unvaccinated persons who live in areas where vaccination programs target older children, or who are at increased risk for infection. This includes persons traveling to or working in countries that have high or intermediate endemicity of infection; men having sex with men; users of injection and non-injection illicit drugs; persons who work with HAV-infected primates or with HAV in a research laboratory; persons with clotting-factor disorders; persons with chronic liver disease; and persons who anticipate close personal contact (e.g., household or regular babysitting) with an international adoptee during the first 60 days after arrival in the United States from a country with high or intermediate endemicity. The first dose should be administered as soon as the adoption is planned, ideally 2 or more weeks before the arrival of the adoptee.

11. **Meningococcal vaccines. (Minimum age: 6 weeks for Hib-MenCY [MenHibrix], 9 months for MenACWY-D [Menactra], 2 months for MenACWY-CRM [Menveo], 10 years for serogroup B meningococcal [MenB] vaccines: MenB-4C [Bexsero] and MenB-FHbp [Trumenba])**

Routine vaccination:
- Administer a single dose of Menactra or Menveo vaccine at age 11 through 12 years, with a booster dose at age 16 years. Adolescents aged 11 through 18 years with human immunodeficiency virus (HIV) infection should receive a 2-dose primary series of
- Menactra or Menveo with at least 8 weeks between doses. For children aged 2 months through 18 years with high-risk conditions, see below.

Catch-up vaccination:
- Administer Menactra or Menveo vaccine at age 13 through 18 years if not previously vaccinated.
- If the first dose is administered at age 13 through 15 years, a booster dose should be administered at age 16 through 18 years with a minimum interval of at least 8 weeks between doses.
- If the first dose is administered at age 16 years or older, a booster dose is not needed.
- For other catch-up guidance, see Figure 2.

Clinical discretion:
- Young adults aged 16 through 23 years (preferred age range is 16 through 18 years) may be vaccinated with either a 2-dose series of Bexsero or a 3-dose series of Trumenba vaccine to provide short-term protection against most strains of serogroup B meningococcal disease. The two MenB vaccines are not interchangeable; the same vaccine product must be used for all doses.

Vaccination of persons with high-risk conditions and other persons at increased risk of disease:

Children with anatomic or functional asplenia (including sickle cell disease):

Meningococcal conjugate ACWY vaccines:
1. Menveo
   - *Children who initiate vaccination at 8 weeks:* Administer doses at 2, 4, 6, and 12 months of age.
   - *Unvaccinated children who initiate vaccination at 7 through 23 months:* Administer 2 doses, with the second dose at least 12 weeks after the first dose AND after the first birthday.
   - *Children 24 months and older who have not received a complete series:* Administer 2 primary doses at least 8 weeks apart.
2. MenHibrix
   - *Children who initiate vaccination at 6 weeks:* Administer doses at 2, 4, 6, and 12 through 15 months of age.
   - If the first dose of MenHibrix is given at or after 12 months of age, a total of 2 doses should be given at least 8 weeks apart to ensure protection against serogroups C and Y meningococcal disease.
3. Menactra
   - *Children 24 months and older who have not received a complete series:* Administer 2 primary doses at least 8 weeks apart. If Menactra is administered to a child with asplenia (including sickle cell disease), do not administer Menactra until 2 years of age and at least 4 weeks after the completion of all PCV13 doses.

Meningococcal B vaccines:
1. Bexsero or Trumenba
   - *Persons 10 years or older who have not received a complete series.* Administer a 2-dose series of Bexsero, at least 1 month apart. Or a 3-dose series of Trumenba, with the second dose at least 2 months after the first and the third dose at least 6 months after the first. The two MenB vaccines are not interchangeable; the same vaccine product must be used for all doses.

Children with persistent complement component deficiency (includes persons with inherited or chronic deficiencies in C3, C5-9, properidin, factor D, factor H, or taking eculizumab (Soliris®):

Meningococcal conjugate ACWY vaccines:
1. Menveo
   - *Children who initiate vaccination at 8 weeks:* Administer doses at 2, 4, 6, and 12 months of age.
   - *Unvaccinated children who initiate vaccination at 7 through 23 months:* Administer 2 doses, with the second dose at least 12 weeks after the first dose AND after the first birthday.
   - *Children 24 months and older who have not received a complete series:* Administer 2 primary doses at least 8 weeks apart.
2. MenHibrix
   - *Children who initiate vaccination 6 weeks:* Administer doses at 2, 4, 6, and 12 through 15 months of age.
   - If the first dose of MenHibrix is given at or after 12 months of age, a total of 2 doses should be given at least 8 weeks apart to ensure protection against serogroups C and Y meningococcal disease.
3. Menactra
   - *Children 9 through 23 months:* Administer 2 primary doses at least 12 weeks apart.
   - *Children 24 months and older who have not received a complete series:* Administer 2 primary doses at least 8 weeks apart.

Meningococcal B vaccines:
1. Bexsero or Trumenba
   - *Persons 10 years or older who have not received a complete series.* Administer a 2-dose series of Bexsero, at least 1 month apart. Or a 3-dose series of Trumenba, with the second dose at least 2 months after the first and the third dose at least 6 months after the first. The two MenB vaccines are not interchangeable; the same vaccine product must be used for all doses.

For children who travel to or reside in countries in which meningococcal disease is hyperendemic or epidemic, including countries in the African meningitis belt or the Hajj
- administer an age-appropriate formulation and series of Menactra or Menveo for protection against serogroups A and W meningococcal disease. Prior receipt of MenHibrix is not sufficient for children traveling to the meningitis belt or the Hajj because it does not contain serogroups A or W.

For children at risk during a community outbreak attributable to a vaccine serogroup
- administer or complete an age- and formulation-appropriate series of MenHibrix, Menactra, or Menveo, Bexsero or Trumenba.

For booster doses among persons with high-risk conditions, refer to *MMWR* 2013 / 62(RR02);1-22, available at http://www.cdc.gov/mmwr/preview/mmwrhtml/rr6202a1.htm.

For other catch-up recommendations for these persons, and complete information on use of meningococcal vaccines, including guidance related to vaccination of persons at increased risk of infection, see *MMWR* March 22, 2013 / 62(RR02);1-22, and *MMWR* October 23, 2015 / 64(41); 1171-1176 available at http://www.cdc.gov/mmwr/pdf/rr/rr6202.pdf, and http://www.cdc.gov/mmwr/pdf/wk/mm6441.pdf.

12. **Tetanus and diphtheria toxoids and acellular pertussis (Tdap) vaccine. (Minimum age: 10 years for both Boostrix and Adacel)**

Routine vaccination:
- Administer 1 dose of Tdap vaccine to all adolescents aged 11 through 12 years.
- Tdap may be administered regardless of the interval since the last tetanus and diphtheria toxoid-containing vaccine.
- Administer 1 dose of Tdap vaccine to pregnant adolescents during each pregnancy (preferred during 27 through 36 weeks gestation) regardless of time since prior Td or Tdap vaccination.

Catch-up vaccination:
- Persons aged 7 years and older who are not fully immunized with DTaP vaccine should receive Tdap vaccine as 1 (preferably the first) dose in the catch-up series; if additional doses are needed, use Td vaccine. For children 7 through 10 years who receive a dose of Tdap as part of the catch-up series, an adolescent Tdap vaccine dose at age 11 through 12 years should NOT be administered. Td should be administered instead 10 years after the Tdap dose.
- Persons aged 11 through 18 years who have not received Tdap vaccine should receive a dose followed by tetanus and diphtheria toxoids (Td) booster doses every 10 years thereafter.
- Inadvertent doses of DTaP vaccine:
  - If administered inadvertently to a child aged 7 through 10 years may count as part of the catch-up series. This dose may count as the adolescent Tdap dose, or the child can later receive a Tdap booster dose at age 11 through 12 years.
  - If administered inadvertently to an adolescent aged 11 through 18 years, the dose should be counted as the adolescent Tdap booster.
- For other catch-up guidance, see Figure 2.

13. **Human papillomavirus (HPV) vaccines. (Minimum age: 9 years for 2vHPV [Cervarix], 4vHPV [Gardasil] and 9vHPV [Gardasil 9])**

Routine vaccination:
- Administer a 3-dose series of HPV vaccine on a schedule of 0, 1-2, and 6 months to all adolescents aged 11 through 12 years. 9vHPV, 4vHPV or 2vHPV may be used for females, and only 9vHPV or 4vHPV may be used for males.
- The vaccine series may be started at age 9 years.
- Administer the second dose 1 to 2 months after the first dose (minimum interval of 4 weeks); administer the third dose 16 weeks after the second dose (minimum interval of 12 weeks) and 24 weeks after the first dose.
- Administer HPV vaccine beginning at age 9 years to children and youth with any history of sexual abuse or assault who have not initiated or completed the 3-dose series.

Catch-up vaccination:
- Administer the vaccine series to females (2vHPV or 4vHPV or 9vHPV) and males (4vHPV or 9vHPV) at age 13 through 18 years if not previously vaccinated.
- Use recommended routine dosing intervals (see Routine vaccination above) for vaccine series catch-up.

FIGURE 22–3 *(continued)*

children are more likely to become obese adults. A classic Surgeon General's report states that there is a 70% chance of adult overweight or obesity if an adolescent is overweight; if at least one parent is overweight, the risk jumps to 80% (2007). Results of a recent Youth Risk Behavior Survey (YRBS) indicated that almost 78% of high school students surveyed ate fewer than five servings of fruits and vegetables the day before, and almost 30% drank soda at least once a day (CDC, 2013c).

The poor eating habits that develop during childhood are generally thought to persist into adulthood, contributing to the leading causes of death and disability—CVD,

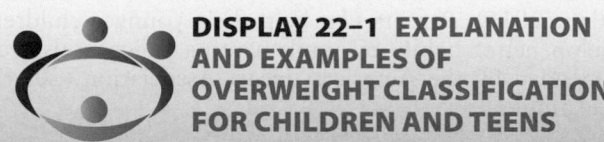

DISPLAY 22–1 EXPLANATION AND EXAMPLES OF OVERWEIGHT CLASSIFICATION FOR CHILDREN AND TEENS

BMI is used as a screening tool to identify weight problems in children and teens. The criteria are different from those used for adults, as body fat differs between boys and girls and the amount of body fat changes with age. BMI-for-age growth charts for boys and girls are available at http://www.cdc.gov/growthcharts.

Weight Status Category	Percentile Range
Underweight	Less than the 5th percentile
Healthy weight	5th percentile to less than the 85th percentile
At risk of overweight	85th to less than the 95th percentile
Overweight	Equal to or greater than the 95th percentile

Source: Centers for Disease Control and Prevention. (2015). *About child & teen BMI.* Retrieved from http://www.cdc.gov/healthyweight/assessing/bmi/childrens_bmi/about_childrens_bmi.html

cancer, and diabetes. Treating hypertension and high cholesterol, stopping tobacco use, controlling diabetes, reducing obesity, and improving physical activity are all helpful in reducing CVD. Evidence of early atherosclerosis and fatty streaks has been found in autopsy studies of children as young as 6 years, and many now acknowledge the need to prevent cumulative cardiac risk factors, per a classic study by Masia et al. (2009). Childhood cancer survivors were examined and found to have evidence of stiffness in carotid arteries and increased risk for CVD and early arteriosclerosis (Dengel et al., 2014). Another study found that obese 7- to 14-year-olds had "early subclinical arthrosclerosis when compared to their normal weight peers" (Alpsoy et al., 2014, p. 141). Childhood obesity is also associated with metabolic syndrome, insulin resistance, as well as CVD and hypertension (Saha, Sarkar, & Chatterjee, 2011). Preventive measures and early management of cardiovascular risk factors are now considered more effective forms of treatment than just clinical treatment of the disease complications after the fact. Aside from its relationship with inactivity, television viewing and other sedentary behaviors have been associated with higher intake of fats, sweet and salty snacks, and carbonated drinks, as well as lower intakes of fruits and vegetables in a systematic review of studies with children, adolescents, and adults (Pearson & Biddle, 2011). Watching television while eating meals has been shown to lead to increased frequency of poor food choices, and food is the most heavily advertised product on children's television. Highly sweetened products (e.g., sweetened beverages and sugar-rich cereals), as well as fast food, are the most frequently advertised foods. American children and adolescents watch more than 3 to 4 hours of television daily, and

increased television watching has been associated with less exercise, increased overweight, lower grades, and less time spent reading (AACAP, 2011b). A review of international research on food marketing to children through the use of television and the Internet found prevalent food advertising promoting "energy dense, nutrient poor foods" and that "even short-term exposure results in children increasing their food consumption" (Boyland & Whalen, 2015, p. 331). In a study examining causes of weight loss failures, bulletin board, chat room, and pool responses over a 10-year period on an interactive weight loss Web site for preteens and teens were analyzed. Researchers found that many of the participants showed symptoms of substance abuse addiction (per DSM-IV criteria) when they discussed their "relationship with highly pleasurable foods" (Pretlow, 2011, p. 295).

As children move from elementary to middle school, their food choices change dramatically. Fad diets and peer pressure become more of an issue. Media fast-food promotion, targeted to middle and high school students, is common. Diets most often include fast-food French fries and hamburgers, pizza, and sweetened carbonated beverages. The average adolescent diet consists of excess fat and added sugars and often is lacking in micronutrients, such as calcium, iron, and zinc, as well as many vitamins and folic acid. Deficits in micronutrients can compromise development; some people advocate multiple food fortification to improve nutritional status and reduce anemia, but unequivocal evidence is lacking (Best et al., 2011). A study by Bruening et al. (2014) suggests an association between adolescent friends, sugar-sweetened drinks, and fast-food restaurant visits, noting that nutrition education efforts could be improved by taking into consideration the influence of friends. They recommend that parents, schools, and communities work with youth to find other venues for friend groups that will not expose adolescents to unhealthy foods. This is also a time when school-based nutrition education programs can have an influence. During the 2014–2015 school year, under the direction of the Healthy, Hunger-Free Kids Act of 2010, new school meal standards were outlined. In addition, all schools are now required to sell "Smart Snacks" in vending machines, a la carte, and in school stores (CDC, 2015c; Food & Nutrition Service, 2014; USDA, 2015). Some school-based programs also include physical activity, but one longitudinal study of over 200 children concluded that physical activity was not the cause of obesity, but rather, it was the result; they questioned if this might be the reason why most efforts to reduce childhood obesity through increased physical activity have not been very successful (Metcalf et al., 2011) (see Using the Nursing Process).

For many years, research studies have examined childhood obesity and its causes. A link between weight gain in early infancy and later risk of obesity may exist (Young, Johnson, & Krebs, 2012). In a retrospective cohort study, 18-month-olds who were obese or overweight were two times more likely to be obese between the ages of 4 and 6. Those that were obese at 18 months of age were over three times more likely to be obese when they were between age 4 and 6 (Wheeler, 2013). In another long-term study following children from age 5 to age 15, intake of sweetened beverages (not fruit juice or milk) was associated with greater adiposity and higher body fat percentages and waist circumference at age 15 (Brown, Halverson, Cohen, Lazorick, & Skelton, 2015). Some studies show that children who are lacking in sleep duration may have higher BMIs (odds ratio 2.15), and other studies have shown that having an obese mother is significantly associated with childhood overweight or obesity (Fatima, Doi, & Mamun, 2015; Rosas et al., 2011; Young et al., 2012). A longitudinal study of 13,170 UK children between the ages of 7 and 11 found that both sugar-sweetened and artificially sweetened beverages were associated with increases in body fat percent-

ages and BMI (Laverty, Magee, Monteiro, Saxena, & Millett, 2015). Parents can help their younger children develop better habits by implementing suggestions recommended by the American Heart Association (2014), for example:

- Serve a variety of fruits and vegetables. Limit juice to 4 to 6 oz. per day.
- Keep fat intake between 25% and 35% of total daily calories (aged 4 to 18).
- Provide foods low in saturated fat, trans fat, cholesterol, added sugar, and salt.

USING THE NURSING PROCESS

James Lopez is entering third grade. His teacher comes to you, the school nurse, because she is concerned about his poor performance in school. He frequently comes to school late and often puts his head on his desk and appears to be falling asleep. You notice that James has gained a significant amount of weight over the summer. His face is much fuller now than in his second grade picture.

Assessment (Initial Visits)

You call James' mother and make an appointment for a home visit.

You do a health history, noting family history of diabetes, current eating, activity, and sleeping patterns for James and the family, and determine whether he has a regular physician and insurance or Medicaid.

You assess his vital signs, height and weight, hearing, and vision.

You talk more with his teacher about his activity on the playground and any signs of excessive thirst, hunger, or general fatigue.

Nursing Diagnoses

After a home visit, a meeting with James' teacher, and two observations and interviews with James, you decide on the following nursing diagnoses:

1. Nutrition: More than Body Requirements related to James' eating as a way of coping and his sedentary lifestyle.
2. Altered Family Process related to mother's recent change from being a stay-at-home single mom to attending truck driving school (necessitating absences of several days at a time, with James cared for by a married teenage sister and her husband).

Findings, Plan, and Implementation

James has been eating large quantities of snack food and fast-food meals for the last 3 months, since his mother started her training. He has also quit participating in soccer and baseball, because his mother can no longer provide transportation. His bicycle was recently stolen, and he spends a lot of time playing video and computer games. James misses his mother when she is away and says that he "stays up late watching television" and has "trouble getting up for school" when he is at his sister's house.

You plan to work with the family to refer James to his physician to rule out diabetes. A family meeting is scheduled so that you can provide some health education on childhood obesity and inactivity. You discuss some possible interventions that the family can put into place:

- Decrease reliance on fast-food meals.
- Have a regular evening mealtime and encourage less snacking.
- Provide fresh fruit and vegetable snacks and decrease purchases of high-calorie, high-fat snack foods.
- Decrease sedentary activity (e.g., video and computer games, television viewing) and increase physical activity (e.g., team sports, walking, bicycling, active outdoor games).
- Establish a reasonable bedtime and consistently enforce it.
- Offer referral for family counseling so that James can discuss his feelings in a safe environment.
- With the family's input, seek ways for James and his mother to keep in better contact and for his sister to gain a greater understanding of good parenting practices.
- Meet with the teacher, the family, and James to discuss ways to help with his school performance.
- Continue to monitor James' progress with monthly height and weight checks, personal interviews, home visits, and teacher conferences.

Evaluation

The physician reported that James does not have diabetes; however, if he continues to gain weight and remains inactive, he is at a higher risk for type 2 diabetes. Evaluation of nursing diagnoses 1 and 2 includes the following goals:

- The family will report less reliance on fast food and more meals cooked at home.
- The family will report more purchases of fresh fruits and vegetables and fewer purchases of high-calorie, high-fat snacks.
- James will report more physical exercise (by the use of a calendar) and fewer hours spent in sedentary activity (corroborated by family).
- James will exhibit less tardiness and fewer signs of sleep deprivation at school, and his school performance will improve.
- James and his family will complete sessions with a family counselor.
- James' weight will remain stable or will decrease as his height increases over time.

- Encourage kids to eat only enough calories to maintain healthy weight.
- Help kids be physically active at least 60 minutes each day.
- Serve whole-grain/high-fiber cereals and breads.
- Serve low-fat and fat-free dairy products (two to three cups of milk daily).
- Serve fish more often, but avoid fried fish.
- Keep introducing a variety of healthy foods, but don't overfeed your child.

One European study found that children and adolescents who had higher consumption of dairy products (e.g., yogurt, milk) had lower levels of body fat and were at less risk of CVD and showed evidence of better cardiorespiratory fitness (Moreno, Bel-Serrat, Santaliestra-Pasias, & Bueno, 2015).

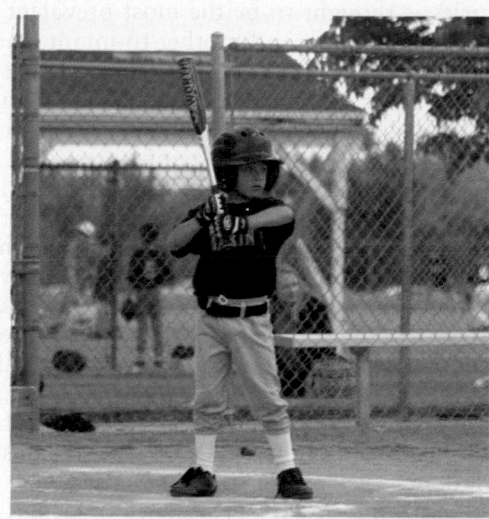

Physical activity is important for health and in childhood obesity prevention. Author's private photo with permission of Holly Raphael.

Inadequate Nutrition

Poor nutritional status of schoolchildren is a global issue but also a problem in this country. Undernutrition can also have serious consequences, including effects on the cognitive development and academic performance of children and chronic health (Weitzman & Zhou, 2012). Irritability, lack of energy, and difficulty concentrating are only some of the problems that arise from skipped meals or consistently inadequate nutrition. Infection and illness that lead to loss of school days can affect academic progress and interfere with the acquisition of basic skills, such as reading and mathematics. Food insecurity has been associated with child development problems, psychological and social issues, and poor general health (Weitzman & Zhou, 2012).

About 14.0% of U.S. households reported some degree of food insecurity in 2014, representing 48.1 million people. Approximately 19.2% of households with children were food insecure, and of those headed by single women with children, 35.3% reported food insecurity (Coleman-Jensen, Rabbitt, Gregory, & Singh, 2015). Reviews of research studies done over the past 15 years have shown mixed results with the association of food insecurity and childhood obesity (Eisenmann, Gundersen, Lohman, Garasky, & Stewart, 2011; Larson, & Story, 2011). A national study by Kaur, Lamb, and Ogden (2015) suggests that there is an association between food insecurity and obesity in school-age children (6 to 11 years) but not between preschoolers, age 2 to 5 years. These results provide additional validation for healthy school meal programs. There is some indication that there is a significant relationship between food insecurity and increased BMI in young adult females, and a growing consensus that both problems warrant further research (Gooding, Walls, & Richmond, 2011).

Longitudinal research has found that long-term childhood exposure to poverty is related to young adult overweight and obesity for White, Black, and Hispanic young women (Hernandez & Pressler, 2014). A Canadian study found that parents and caregivers viewed their low-income status as a contributing factor for poor nutrition in their children and cited dependence on nutrient-poor, energy-dense food because it was longer lasting than more nutritious fresh foods and easier to obtain (Bhawra, Cooke, Hanning, Wilk, & Gonneville, 2015). Research findings of Holben and Taylor (2015) confirm the relationship between food insecurity and central obesity.

Undernutrition is frequently associated with poverty and hunger, but social pressure to be thin can also spark purposeful undernutrition. Because prepubertal children often exhibit a period of adiposity before a growth spurt, they are at risk for developing **eating disorders**. Along with childhood obesity, prevention of eating disorders is also a high priority in this age group. Some sources find pediatric eating disorders to be more prevalent than T2DM, and minority groups, boys, and younger children have higher rates. The lifetime prevalence for anorexia nervosa is 0.5% to 2%, and for bulimia, it is 0.9% to 3%, with mortality rates of 5% to 6% and around 2%, respectively (Campbell & Peebles, 2014). A landmark 5-year study of the frequency of reading magazine articles about dieting and weight loss found that girls who frequently read these magazines were two times more likely to engage in unhealthful weight-control measures (e.g., skipping meals, smoking more cigarettes, fasting) than those who did not read magazine articles about dieting and weight loss. Extreme weight-control measures (e.g., laxative use, vomiting) were found three times more often in high-frequency readers versus nonreaders (van den Berg, Neumark-Sztainer, Hannan, & Haines, 2007). The Youth Risk Behavior Survey (SYRBS) found that almost 14% of high school students reported not eating for 24 hours or more in order to keep from gaining or lose weight; vomiting and laxatives were used by 4% (CDC, 2013c). A study by Holm-Denoma, Hankin, and Young (2014) suggests that for boys, the association between depression and eating disorders was greater between third and sixth grades and then stabilized. However, eating disorder symptoms and depressive symptoms became more manifest in females between sixth and ninth grade. They recommend that eating disorder prevention programs begin before age 12 and depressive symptom interventions target males by third grade and females by sixth grade.

Although there has been some concern about the possibility that obesity prevention measures may lead to eating disorders, no real evidence of that has surfaced, and experts feel that both problems can be effectively addressed through evidence-based interventions. Suggestions include stressing family meals and physical activities, promoting a positive body image, avoiding weight talk, and decreasing media focus. More specific suggestions include:

- Foods to *encourage* (fruits, vegetables) versus foods to *limit* (high-fat/high-sugar/low nutritional value) rather than *good* or *bad* foods
- A focus on dietary restraint/portion size rather than dieting or deprivation
- More research on the continuum of mindless eating to obsessive preoccupation with food intake and on helping individuals more effectively use internal cues for hunger or satiety
- Simultaneous promotion of healthy eating behaviors while protecting positive body images in children (Campbell & Peebles, 2014)

It is important to talk with overweight children and adolescents about their experiences of being mistreated because of their problems with weight and to encourage families to not just talk about weight but to do more together to promote healthy eating and increased physical activity. Also, early detection of eating disorder is important, as this problem can irreversibly affect growth and development and early intervention and treatment show better outcomes (Campbell & Peebles, 2014). School nurses and PHNs should be aware of signs and symptoms of this disorder, noting that T1DM children may be at higher risk, and watch for unexplained weight loss, stunting of normal growth patterns, concerns about body image, delayed puberty, and abnormal or restrictive eating (e.g., newly committed vegetarians, food rituals, swallowing disorders, textural aversions). They can provide families with necessary information to promote healthful eating and exercise, as well as provide guidance for parental and child support (Hertz, Jones, Barrios, David-Ferdon, & Holt, 2015). Some school districts include BMI screening programs as part of healthy lifestyle promotion (Ruggieri & Bass, 2015), and school nurses are encouraged to provide educational programs that promote healthy eating and help students see through advertising efforts that promote an unrealistic body image (Funari, 2013).

Inactivity

An association between poor eating habits and physical inactivity has been found in numerous research studies (Nesbit, Kolobe, Sisson, & Ghement, 2014). More television watching, fewer family meals eaten together at home, and living in an unsafe neighborhood were shown to be associated with overweight (Nesbit et al., 2014). The YRBS revealed that 66.7% of children surveyed who were enrolled in physical education classes did not attend class on a daily basis. In addition, fewer than 19% of respondents stated that they were physically active for 60 minutes daily. Almost 33% watched three or more hours of television daily and just below 25% used a computer (other than for schoolwork) or played a video game on a daily basis (CDC, 2013c).

In a study of adolescent girls and their families, researchers found that parents' modeling of physical activity, television viewing, fruit and vegetable consumption, and use of soft drinks were significantly associated with the teens' behaviors, indicating that improvements in parent behaviors can affect adolescents (Bauer, Neumark-Sztainer, Fulkerson, Hannan, & Story, 2011). School nurses and PHNs can work with families to increase their levels of physical activity and to encourage limited television viewing for school-age children. They can also advocate for increased physical education in the school setting and for increased safe recreational opportunities in all neighborhoods.

Dental Health

Dental caries is thought to be the most prevalent childhood infectious disease, and mother-to-infant transmission of the bacteria most commonly involved in tooth decay occurs before primary teeth are visible (Caple & Schub, 2015). Caries affect 37% of children between the ages of 2 and 8, with 14% having untreated cavities in primary (baby) teeth. About 21% of children (6 to 11 years of age) have dental caries in their permanent teeth and 6% have untreated caries. Hispanic children have the highest rates of decay in both primary and permanent teeth (CDC, 2015d). In a classic study, comparing African refugee children with U.S. children, the rate of dental caries for refugee children was half that of U.S. children (Cote et al., 2004). Poor children report twice the rate of untreated dental caries than do children from higher-income families (CDC, 2012b). Those children with high or very high food insecurity were found to have significantly higher prevalence of dental caries than those children living in food-secure households (two times the rate) (Chi, Masterson, Carle, Mancl, & Coldwell, 2014).

The prevalence of dental caries in school-age children has decreased significantly since the early 1970s because of community fluoridation projects and the use of fluoride toothpaste (FCFS, n.d., Table HC4.C). Fluoridated drinking water, the availability of school-provided fluoride rinse or gel, and dental sealant programs are cost-effective, proven methods of reducing dental caries in school-age children (National Institute of Dental & Craniofacial Research, 2015).

The peak incidence of dental caries is found among school-age children and adolescents, although the effects of decay are observed in adulthood as caries activity recurs or various restorations fracture or wear out and must be replaced. In 2013, 88% of children age 2 to 17 years visited a dentist in the past year, but for children living in poverty, only about 82.3% did, and approximately 56% of uninsured children saw a dentist. Over time, these rates have improved with coverage through the State Children's Health Insurance Program (SCHIP) and preventive programs such as community water fluoridation and the expansion of sealant programs. The number of children between 5 and 19 years with untreated dental caries has decreased from 24% in 1994 to 17% in 2011–2012 (FCFS, 2015e). Yet, access to dental care is still problematic. Barriers to dental care are more prevalent among the poor (Caple & Schub, 2015).

Financial barriers and lack of education lead to poor dental health values and adversely affect the appropriate use of early dental services and conscientious personal oral health care. School-based dental sealant program research was reviewed and found to be effective in managing cavities in this age group (CDC, 2015j). Prescription fluoride supplements should be used when drinking water is deficient in fluoride and children are at high risk of developing cavities. Some interventions have shown promise in reducing caries transmission and improving tooth-brushing habits. Motivational interviewing with parent post–dental examination of their children, along with a brief instructional DVD were employed in a large-scale study, and at 6-month follow-up, researchers found that participating caregivers were more apt to check children's teeth and ensure nightly brushing. This continued at the 2-year follow-up (Ismail, Ondersma, Jedele, Little, & Lepkowski, 2011). Second through fifth grade students' motivations for brushing teeth were examined in focus group research. Cues to motivate brushing included wanting to have good teeth, relatives with dentures, social media that instructed them on the link between oral health and CVD or smoking, and cancer (Walker, Steinfort, & Keyler, 2015). Albert, Barracks, Bruzelius, and Ward (2014) found that a Web-based educational program significantly increased knowledge of caries transmission and plans to prevent maternal caries transmission between pre- and posttest in a largely college-educated group of participants. PHNs and other community health nurses working with school-age children and families can promote good dental health through education and advocacy, as well as through collaboration to provide adequate dental services to uninsured children and promotion of fluoridation and sealant programs.

ADOLESCENT HEALTH

Adolescence is a time of self-discovery, movement toward self-reliance, increasing opportunities, and pivotal choices that can affect the remainder of an individual's life. Adolescence generally begins with puberty and encompasses the ages between 10 and 24; it consists of early adolescence (aged 10 to 14), middle adolescence (15 to 17), and late adolescence (18 to mid-20s). Adult society largely segregates adolescents and often has ambiguous expectations for them (Park, Scott, Adams, Brindis, & Irwin, 2014). Adolescents are part of a subculture, one with its own language, dress, social mores, and values. The tasks of adolescence remain fairly constant: adolescents must become autonomous, come to grips with their emerging sexuality and the skills necessary to attract a mate, and acquire skills and education that can prepare them for adult roles, all while resolving identity issues and developing values and beliefs (Park et al., 2014). The search for and expression of developing identity, along with the strong drive for social acceptance, are evident in the personal home pages and blogs of adolescents on social networking Internet sites such as Twitter and Facebook (Spies-Shapiro & Margolin, 2014).

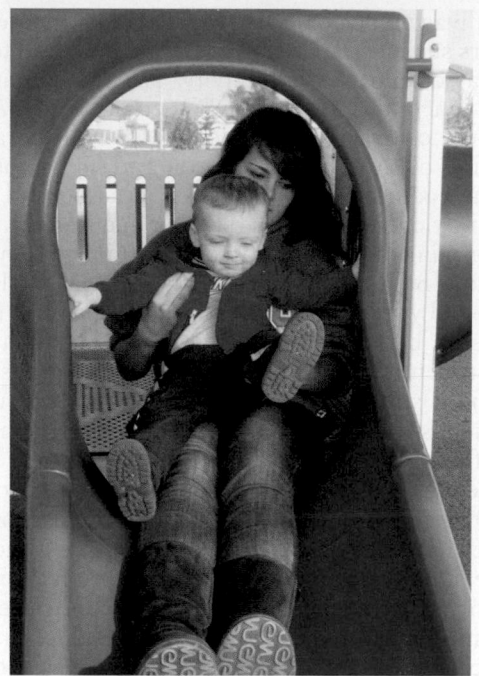

Common first jobs for adolescents include babysitting and yard work. (Author's private photo with permissions of Merysa Schultz and Deanna Rector.)

Adolescents are generally healthy, but parents and teens may differ in their perceptions of the adolescent's health. Adolescents from lower-income brackets frequently report poorer health than those from higher-income groups. As with other population groups, socioeconomic level and health are inversely related for adolescents. Adolescents also exhibit inverse relationships between income level and school achievement, most likely because of a lack of successful strategies for academic success (Office of Disease Prevention and Health Promotion, 2014a; Oyserman, Johnson, & James, 2011). Parental long-term unemployment is also negatively associated with adolescent self-reported health status and depressive symptoms and psychosomatic complaints. These, along with poor health behaviors related to lack of physical activity and drug use or smoking, contribute to self-perceived poor or fair health (Nichols, Mitchell, & Lindner, 2013). Social stressors and strained relations with peers and parents are also related to health complaints, including psychosomatic complaints (Child Trends Databank, 2014e; van Geelan, Rydelius, & Haagquist, 2015). Common complaints of adolescents include sleep deprivation, fatigue, chronic insomnia, acne, and concerns about weight and body image (van Geelan et al., 2015). As children become adolescents, their sleep patterns change—they move from early risers/sleepers to staying up later and sleeping in later or catching up on sleep over weekends. This transition becomes more apparent through high school. Scientists believe that these changes in circadian and homeostatic sleep regulation support this delayed sleep phase, and there are concerns about consistent lack of sleep (Orzech, Acebo, Seifer, Barker, & Carskadon, 2014). A national survey of adolescents revealed that 68.9% reported getting insufficient sleep and this was associated with higher odds of several risk behaviors such as use of cigarettes, alcohol, and tobacco, as well as current sexual activity, physical fighting, and physical inactivity (McKnight-Eily et al., 2011). Another U.S. survey of over 14,000 adolescents corroborated the association of short sleep duration and high cholesterol, with "each additional hour of sleep … associated with … significantly decreased odds of being diagnosed with high cholesterol in young adulthood" for females (Gangwisch, Malaspina, Babiss & Opler, 2010, p. 956; IglayReger et al., 2014). Lytle, Pasch, and Farbakhsh (2011) found a relationship between sleep duration and BMI in middle school students but did not find the same results among high school students. They noted that waking up later on weekends was related to lower body fat and healthier weight for girls, but not for boys, and warned "inadequate sleep is a risk factor for early adolescent obesity" (p. 324). Sleep deprivation, along with television viewing time, has been related to increased BMI and blood pressure, and a poor body weight perception (being overweight or underweight) has predicted problem behaviors in both male and female adolescents (Nesbit et al., 2014). Many schools have instituted later start times in order to correlate with youth circadian rhythms. Recent studies confirm the support for delaying adolescent school start times and indicate benefits of improved duration of sleep, decreased daytime sleepiness, and reductions in depression and caffeine use (Minges & Redecker, 2016). One study suggests that the benefit of delayed start times past 8:01 AM is not significant. Based on research findings, Paksarian, Rudolph, He, and Merikangas (2015) recommend that modest delays in start times may be beneficial but other factors, such as travel time to school, should be considered. Further research in this area is suggested.

In the past, routine health care visits by adolescents were not commonplace. However, newer recommended vaccines and better awareness of the health needs of adolescents have led to improvement, but concerns remain. In 2012, 88.1% of 10- to 17-year-olds had a physician visit within the past year, and 73.8% had a well-child checkup (Park et al., 2014). This shows an increase in visits compared to data from an earlier national survey when 38% of adolescents had a visit for preventive care within the last year, but only 40% spent time alone with their health care provider (Irwin, Adams, Park, & Newacheck, 2009). Sadly, only 10% had all areas of recommended anticipatory guidance addressed (e.g., healthy diet, seat belt/helmet use, smoking/secondhand smoke), and teens from low-income or uninsured families were at greater risk of not having any preventive health care visits. Most health care visits for adolescents were for female reproductive health care, and birth control was a common prescription written at outpatient visits. An update to the 2009 review indicates that the majority of health indicators have changed very little for adolescents over the past decade (Park et al., 2014). However, encouraging trends among adolescents and youth include a decrease in unintentional injury, tobacco use, and assault rates. Increases were also noted in exercise trends. Additionally, the number of adolescents having health care insurance has increased with the advent of the Affordable Care Act, Medicaid Expansions, and CHIP (Park et al., 2014).

Although hospitalization rates for adolescents are low, the leading cause of hospitalization in 15- to 24-year-olds is pregnancy related. Trauma and mental disorders were the next two causes of hospitalization, and trauma-related disorders are the leading reason for emergency room visits. Almost 17% of adolescents have some special health care need; this prevalence has changed little (Park et al., 2014).

Health literacy during adolescence is an important consideration. Teens are frequent users of mass media (Internet, television, radio, text messaging), and specific health-related educational interventions can be targeted to them by using these media. One study found that 56% of high school students in an online sample had heard of MedlinePlus, and 52% had "adequate levels of health literacy" as measured by an online test (Ghaddar, Valerio, Garcia, & Hansen, 2012, p. 28). PHNs can help young people find reliable sources of information, as well as work with families to ensure proper monitoring of Internet use. Sexual predators, pornography, and cyberbullying are among the Internet dangers encountered by adolescents (Spies-Shapiro & Margolin, 2014).

During the period that roughly encompasses the teen years, adolescents encounter many complex changes, physically, emotionally, cognitively, and socially (Park et al., 2014). Rapid and major developmental adjustments create a variety of stresses with concomitant problems that have an impact on health. Recent advanced neuroimaging techniques have demonstrated marked changes in the adolescent brain, especially related to white and gray matter and the prefrontal cortex (Krongold, Cooper, & Bray, 2015). The uneven changes in brain development may help explain the risk-taking behaviors and higher incidence of unintentional injuries found in this population (Steinberg, 2015).

Unintentional injuries were the leading cause of death in the 10- to 19-year-old age group. Most deaths in this adolescent/young adult age group are due to preventable causes. The overall injury death rate in 2009 for adolescents 10 to 14 years of age was 17.9 per 100,000 and for 15- to 19-year-olds, it was 69.7, indicating a dramatic rise as teens gain more freedom and begin to drive (Kochanek, Kirmeyer, Martin, Strobino, & Guyer, 2012). In 2013, nearly 75% of adolescent deaths were related to injury with unintentional injuries responsible for approximately 50% of these adolescent deaths. Motor vehicle and firearm-related deaths accounted for approximately 60% of adolescent injury deaths (FCFS, 2015a). The death rate from motor vehicle–related injuries for this age group peaked during the 1970s and 1980s and then declined throughout the next two decades, although motor vehicle–related injuries remain the number one cause of injury mortality for this age group (Park et al., 2014). Gender differences are also apparent: girls are much less likely than boys to engage in behaviors that put them at risk for injuries, resulting in twice the rate of unintentional injury death rate for male than female adolescents. This gender difference has persisted over three decades and is greater than age or ethnic differences in both unintentional and violence-related injury deaths (FCFS, 2015a; Sorenson, 2011) (see Fig. 22–4).

Unintentional injuries also cause the greatest level of morbidity, and the largest cause is transportation (drivers

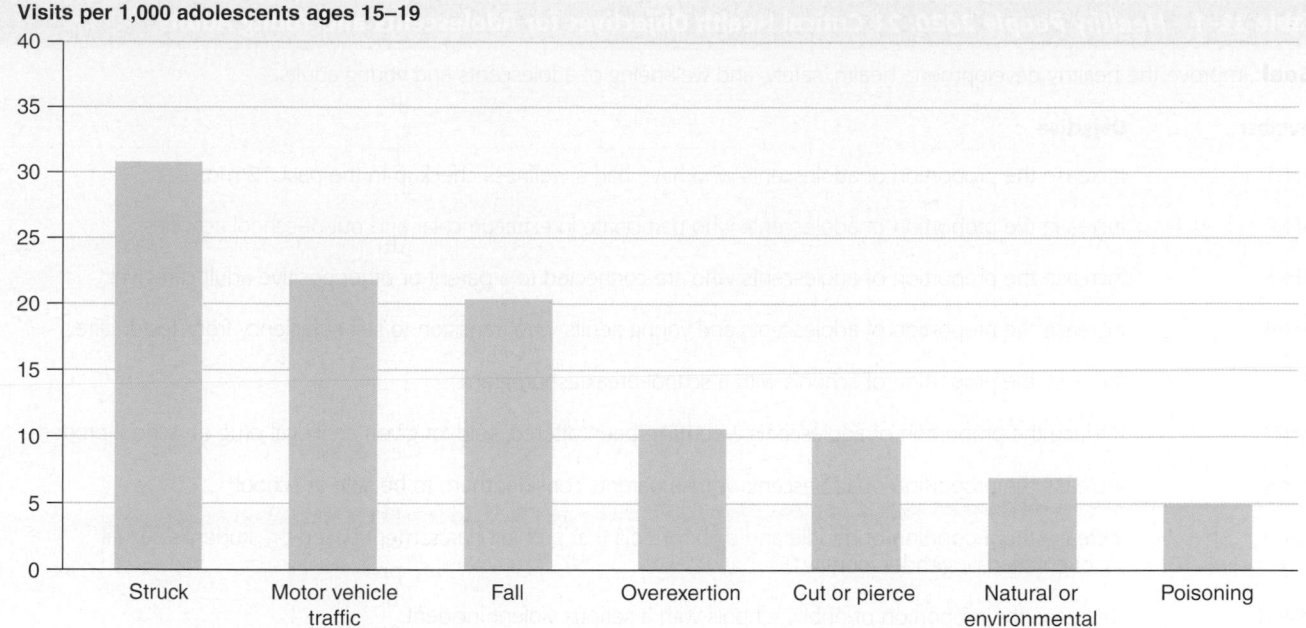

FIGURE 22–4   Death rates among adolescents aged 15 to 19 by all causes and all injury causes and selected mechanisms of injury, 1980–2009. (From http://www.childstats.gov/americaschildren/phenviro8.asp.)

and passengers, bicyclists, pedestrians). Other causes include crime, drowning, poisoning, fires, sports, and recreation, reckless driving, and work-related injuries (Steinberg, 2015). Almost 2.6 million sports- and recreation-related injuries (aged 0 to 19) are treated annually in EDs. The causes of most injuries requiring treatment include bicycling, playground activities, football, basketball, and soccer. Football and girl's soccer have the highest injury rates among youth sports (0.47 and 0.36 per 1,000 exposures), and the incidence of traumatic brain injury (TBI)/concussion ED visits has risen 60% over the last decade (CDC, 2015f).

Health Objectives for Adolescents

Healthy People 2020 objectives are focused on improving the health of all Americans. Goals and objectives for adolescent health have been developed. Because much of the mortality and morbidity in this age group stems from risk-taking behaviors, many objectives addressing alcohol-related unintentional injuries, violent behaviors, and suicide and mental health issues, as well as more responsible reproductive health behaviors, are included throughout the document under Substance Abuse, Mental Health, etc. (Jiang, Kolbe, Seo, Kay, & Brindis, 2011; see Table 22–1). The 2014 review of these critical objectives found overall mortality trends varied, with decreases for 15- to 19-year teens since 2007. Trends in injury mortality for ages 10 to 24 years decreased with the exception of motor vehicle accidents associated with alcohol-impaired young drivers. Adolescent use of seat belts improved. The objectives related to violence and mental health objectives have shown mixed results. Overall, homicide rates show little change for the adolescent age group. Black, non-Hispanic and Hispanic male homicide rates have decreased, although the current rate for this population is six to seven times greater than the general

rate. Suicide rates and reported attempted suicides are not significantly improved, and only modest increases are found in other objectives related to mood and treatment. Binge drinking and marijuana use remain the same, and physical activity reports are improving. Tobacco use has gone down considerably; unfortunately, this rate increases fourfold between the teen years and young adulthood. Obesity and overweight rates remain at about 17%. The adolescent pregnancy rate has decreased and related objectives are on pace to reach targets (e.g., never having sex, used a condom with last sexual contact). *Chlamydia* infection rates have increased but may be an artifact of more sensitive testing and improved reporting (Park et al., 2014). Analysis of the *21 Critical National Health Objectives* for *Healthy People 2010* relating to adolescents and young adults revealed that only 2 targets had been met (i.e., rode with a driver who had drunk alcohol, physical fighting), but progress had been made toward 12 of the objectives. Jiang and colleagues (2011) reported that no progress was made on four objectives and two objectives actually showed worse results (i.e., rates of *Chlamydia* infection and overweight). But significant progress was made in decreasing adolescents' use of alcohol or illicit drugs (Office of Disease Prevention and Health Promotion, 2014b).

Because adolescents have less contact with the health care system than children, many conditions may go undetected. Also, a shift occurs from a childhood preponderance of physical conditions to more social behavioral problems in adolescence. Risk behaviors become much more evident, along with their attendant outcomes: unsafe sexual activity, substance use, violence, and motor vehicle–related issues. Also, the transition from high school into early adulthood is often difficult and those individuals with mental health issues often have worse

Table 22–1 *Healthy People 2020:* 21 Critical Health Objectives for Adolescents and Young Adults

Goal: Improve the healthy development, health, safety, and well-being of adolescents and young adults.

Number	Objective
AH-1	Increase the proportion of adolescents who have had a wellness checkup in the past 12 mo.
AH-2	Increase the proportion of adolescents who participate in extracurricular and out-of-school activities.
AH-3	Increase the proportion of adolescents who are connected to a parent or other positive adult caregiver.
AH-4	Increase the proportion of adolescents and young adults who transition to self-sufficiency from foster care.
AH-5	Increase the proportion of schools with a school breakfast program.
AH-7	Reduce the proportion of adolescents who have been offered, sold, or given an illegal drug on school property.
AH-8	Increase the proportion of adolescents whose parents consider them to be safe at school.
AH-9	Increase the proportion of middle and high schools that prohibit harassment based on student's sexual orientation or gender identity.
AH-10	Decrease the proportion of public schools with a serious violent incident.
AH-11	Reduce adolescent and young adult perpetration of, as well as victimization by, crimes.

From U.S. Department of Health and Human Services (USDHHS). (2014). *Adolescent health*. Retrieved from http://healthypeople.gov/2020/topicsobjectives2020/objectiveslist.aspx?topicId=2

outcomes than those with physical conditions (Park, Adams, & Irwin, 2011).

Emotional Problems and Suicide

The adolescent years are a time of rapid growth and change. Hormonal influences may cause a teen to be emotional and unpredictable at times (Chulani & Gordon, 2014). The influence of peers increases, and peer pressure may influence behavior. Teens test family rules and generally search for their own identity and individuality apart from the family. Most parents and teens ride out this period with love and understanding and no long-term negative effects. For some children, however, a real or perceived lack of emotional support can lead to temporary or permanent emotional problems. Additionally, increased risk behaviors such as suicide, risky sexual behavior, and mental health disorders are associated with child and adolescent maltreatment (Chulani & Gordon, 2014; National Institute of Justice, 2011; Norman, et al., 2012). Gender differences in types and trajectories of emotional and behavioral problems have also been noted, with more females developing adolescent-onset depression and males demonstrating more conduct problems at an earlier age of onset (Zimmer-Gembeck & Skinner, 2015).

Depression, schizophrenia, and eating disorders may first appear during adolescence. About 50% of mental health conditions begin before age 14, and 75% by age 21. It is estimated that approximately 20% of adolescents have mental health disorders with depression being the most commonly reported diagnosis. Prevalence rates of depression vary (Fig. 22–5). About 29% of high school students report feelings of sadness or hopelessness every day for longer than 2 weeks. Of those reporting symptoms, 36% are female and 22% are male. Anxiety disorders such as OCD, posttraumatic stress disorder, social anxiety disorders, and phobias are reported by approximately 10% of students between ages 12 and 17 years (Murphey, Barry, Vaughn, Guzman, & Terzian, 2013). Researchers have concluded that 26% to 30% of adolescents display symptoms of emotional distress, and about 9% have moderate to severe symptoms (Child Trends Databank, 2014a). Adolescent brain maturation may explain susceptibility to depression during this period of development (Ahmed, Bittencourt-Hewitt, & Sebastian, 2015).

Many adolescents are reluctant to seek help for emotional problems, or help may not be readily available to them. Most mental health disorders are treatable; however, it is estimated that approximately 60% to 90% do not receive treatment. Barriers to treatment may include social stigma and missed opportunities for identification and prevention (Murphey et al., 2013). Survey results have found that 12.7% of youth aged 12 to 17 have been given some type of mental health services, but the usual disparities apply (e.g., ethnicity, income level, rural vs. urban locale). Treatment for serious mental health problems may include hospitalization or placement in a group home. The most common reasons for youths to receive mental health treatment during 2012 include depression (50.7%), home-based problems (29.1%), rule breaking (24.2%), suicidal ideation or suicide attempts (23.8%), and fear/anxiety (22.7%) (Substance Abuse and Mental Health Services Administration [SAMHSA], 2013). Mental health disorders experienced during adolescence may persist into adulthood. It is critical to identify negative adolescent mental health behaviors, provide access to services, and educate teens about healthy physical and mental health skills. School-based programs to

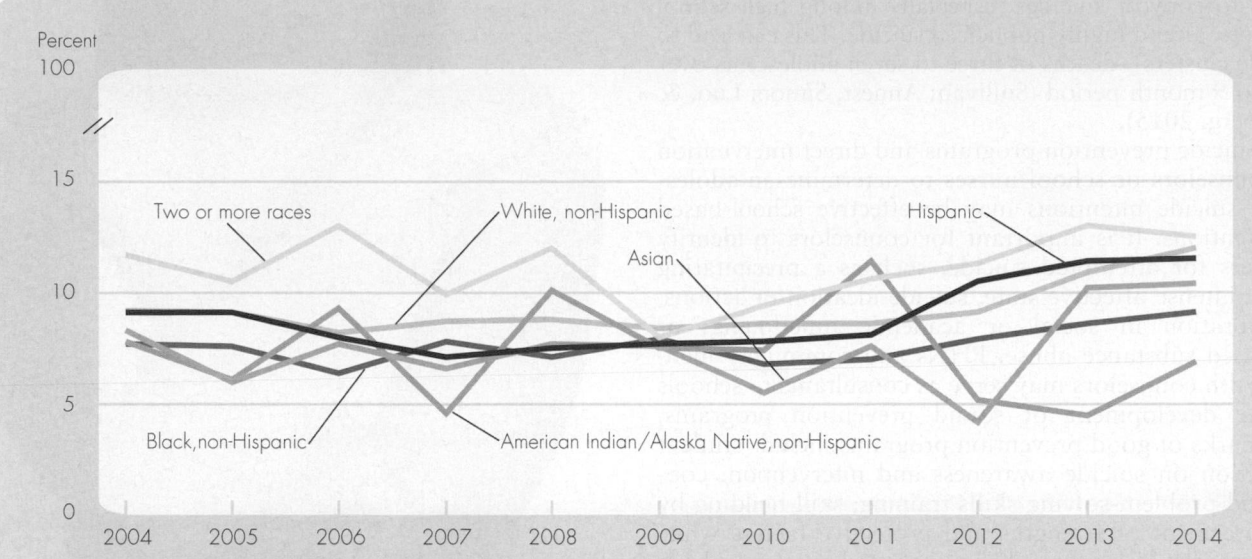

NOTE: MDE is defined as a period of at least two weeks when a person experienced a depressed mood or loss of interest or pleasure in daily activities plus at least four additional symptoms of depression (such as problems with sleep, eating, energy, concentration, and feelings of self-worth) as described in the fourth edition of the *Diagnostic and Statistical Manual of Mental Disorders (DSM-IV)*. The 1997 Office of Management and Budget standards were used to collect race and ethnicity data. Persons could select one or more of five racial groups: White, Black or African American, American Indian or Alaska Native, Native Hawaiian or Other Pacific Islander, or Asian. Respondents could choose more than one race. Those reporting more than one race were classified as "Two or more races." Data on Hispanic origin are collected separately. Persons of Hispanic origin may be of any race.

SOURCE: Substance Abuse and Mental Health Services Administration, National Survey on Drug Use and Health.

FIGURE 22-5 Percentage of youth ages 12 to 17 who had at least one major depressive episode (MDE) in the past year by race and Hispanic origin, 2004–2014. (Retrieved from http://www.childstats.gov/americaschildren/health_fig.asp.)

educate adolescents about depression and suicide prevention have been useful (Melnyk et al., 2015; Murphey et al., 2013). For some, more universal approaches are viewed as more effective in preventing a wider range of social and emotional problems (Durlak, Weissberg, Dymnicki, Taylor, & Schellinger, 2011). PHNs and school nurses often participate in the development or administration of these types of programs.

Suicide is the third leading cause of death in 10- to 14-year-olds and the second leading cause in 15- to 24-year-olds. In 2013, suicide accounted for 11.3% of child and adolescent deaths. This is an increase from 10.7% in 2012 (Osterman, Kochanek, MacDorman, Strobino, & Guyer, 2015). Overall, male suicide rates are four times higher than female rates and comprise 77.9% of all suicides (CDC, 2016). A classic study found that a psychiatric diagnosis is noted in 90% of suicide victims, with depression reported in over 50% of all cases (National Alliance for Mental Illness [NAMI], 2011). Untreated depression is often a factor in adolescent suicide and should be screened for and evaluated (Pelkonen, Karlsson, & Marttunen, 2011). Although questions have been raised and the FDA issued a black box warning that adolescents beginning treatment may be at increased for suicidal ideation, selective serotonin reuptake inhibitors (SSRIs) are among the more commonly prescribed antidepressant medications and are not considered to increase suicide risk (Cousins & Goodyer, 2015). In 2013, almost 17% of high school students reported that they seriously considered suicide in the previous 12 months (up from 13.8% in 2009), and 8%

made at least one suicide attempt. Almost 2.7% made an attempt that required medical attention. Suicide rates for adolescent female versus male students are higher (10.6% vs. 5.4%; Child Trends Databank, 2015d). As adolescents grow older, they are more at risk for suicide: the rate increases from 1.5 per 100,000 for ages 10 to 14 to 8.2 for ages 15 to 19. It is 12.8 for older adolescents (20 to 24), and about 2 million adolescents attempt suicide each year (NAMI, 2011).

Male adolescents are more likely to die as a result of suicide; females are more likely to report suicide attempts. It is important to question a teen about a history of depression or feelings of hopelessness, as well as the quality and quantity of her social support systems and the availability of means to follow through on suicide threats; it is also helpful to have intensive therapy visits early on and discussions about safety planning (Pelkonen et al., 2011). School and discipline problems, family discord, and depression, as well as drug and alcohol abuse, can increase the risk of suicide (Adrian, Miller, McCauley, & Stoep, 2015). Recent stressful events and preoccupation with suicide, as well as substance use, are also important to note. Being bullied, a history of sexual or physical abuse, aggressive conduct disorders, and personality disorders are risk factors for adolescent suicide attempts (Murphey et al., 2013). Major depressive disorder is most commonly associated with lifetime prevalence of adolescent suicidal ideation, plans, and attempts. This is followed by "specific phobia, oppositional defiant disorder, IED, substance abuse, and conduct disorder" (Nock, et al., 2013, p. 303). *Suicide contagion* refers to copycat suicides, especially among high school students, after a highly publicized suicide. This can lead to suicide clusters—deaths of three to seven adolescents over a 3- to 9-month period (Sullivan, Annest, Simon, Luo, & Dahlberg, 2015).

Suicide prevention programs and direct intervention by counselors or school nurses to determine an adolescent's suicide intentions may be effective school-based interventions. It is important for counselors to identify markers for attempted suicide, such as a precipitating event, intense affective state, suicide ideation or actions, deterioration in social or academic functioning, or increased substance abuse. PHNs and community mental health counselors may serve as consultants to schools in the development of sound prevention programs. Hallmarks of good prevention programs include student education on suicide awareness and intervention; coping and problem-solving skills training; skill building by reinforcement of strengths and protective factors while dealing with risk-taking behaviors; and teaching about the association between suicide and mental health (especially depression). Suicide screening is often thought to be effective in reducing suicidal ideation (Gray & Dihigo, 2015). Youth suicide has been of great concern over the past several decades. Communities across the nation have been urged to implement effective school-based suicide prevention programs. Although many programs have been implemented, many have not been based on evidence or have not shown a positive impact. The "Surviving the Teens" program is designed to help all adolescents and specifically identify teens exhibiting help-seeking behaviors. This evidence-based program teaches adolescents to communicate emotional health issues and seek help when experiencing suicidal ideation. It also teaches teens how to help friends experiencing depression or suicidal ideation. The program demonstrated a decrease in suicidal ideation reports and increased help seeking by youth over a 3-month period (Strunk, Sorter, Ossege, & King, 2014). Another study examined the effect of the 12-month "COPE Healthy Lifestyles TEEN Program" on adolescent obesity and depressive symptoms. Study results demonstrated improved outcomes for both long-term physical and mental health among participating teens (Melnyk et al., 2015). Skills training programs that target a broader range of problems (e.g., depression, anxiety, negative self-perceptions) have been effective in teaching adolescents how to monitor feelings, identify triggers, and avoid and reframe negative thoughts. Relaxation skills training, learning how to seek out help from others, and promoting healthier responses to stress have also been successful in impacting internalizing behaviors (Terzian, Hamilton, & Ericson, 2011). Brown and Green (2014) indicate that research gaps in the literature continue; however, follow-up screening and the expansion of services and research within new populations and settings are needed (Fig. 22–6).

A behavior that can sometimes accidentally result in suicide is *self-injury* or *cutting*. Adolescents with this abnormal behavior who overdose, head bang, cut, burn, brand, mark, or otherwise dangerously harm themselves are attempting to find relief from profound psychological pain. The physical injury distracts them from these pain-

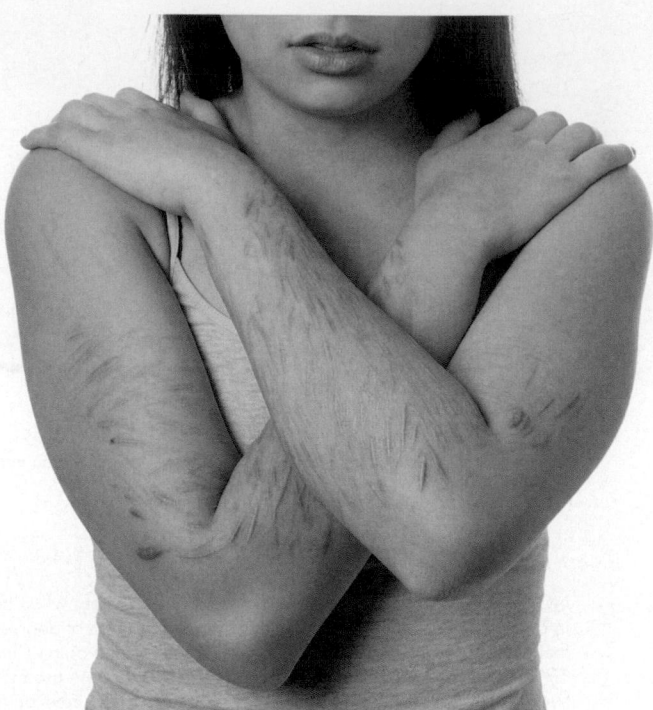

FIGURE 22–6 A young woman with evidence of "cutting" self-injury.

ful emotions, possibly giving them a feeling of control or providing a means of feeling emotions when they are cut off from them. Scars often remain long after the behavior has stopped (AACAP, 2013). A large study of almost 2,000 adolescents found an 8% rate of self-harm and a reduction in frequency of self-injury with age (7% no longer self-harmed as young adults). Adolescent self-harming behaviors were associated with use of marijuana, alcohol, and cigarettes, as well as higher rates of depression and anxiety symptoms and antisocial behavior (Moran et al., 2012). One smaller longitudinal study found that over the 2.5 years, data were collected, 18% of 11- to 14-year-olds engaged in nonsuicidal self-injury, with 14% reported as new cases (Hankin & Abela, 2011). This behavior most often begins in early adolescence or late childhood. It can continue into adulthood. It is more common in girls and in those with a family history of suicide, self-injury, or maternal depression. Isolation, neglect, or abuse may predispose an adolescent to this behavior. Depression, poor quality of relationships, excessive seeking of reassurance, and eating disorders are commonly associated with self-injury. PHNs and school nurses can provide education to adolescents and families about this condition and can work with schools to promote prevention strategies, such as early detection and referral to mental health providers.

Violence

The total costs of youth violence (e.g., quality of life, medical costs, lost productivity) are more than $158 billion each year (Hammond & Arias, 2011). The Youth Risk Behavior Surveillance, United States, 2013, indicated that 17.9% of 9th through 12th grade students carried a weapon at least one day within 30 days of the survey and 5.2% of students had carried a weapon such as a gun, knife, or club one day prior to the survey. In 2013, 7.1% of students did not go to school on at least one day prior to the survey because of safety concerns (Kann et al., 2014).

Homicide is the third leading cause of death for adolescents and youth (aged 15 to 24), it is more common in males than females, and in 87% of adolescent cases, it involved the use of a firearm. In 2013, the homicide rate was the lowest it has been since before 1970 at 6.7 deaths per 100,000 (Child Trends Databank, 2015d). The homicide rate among African American male adolescents is 45.0 per 100,000, and for Hispanic males, it is 11.7; it is only 2.2 among White males, indicating a wide disparity (Child Trends Databank, 2015d). Almost 1,580 homicides of school-age youth occurred in the 2008–2009 school year, but only 17 of these occurred on school grounds (Robers, Zhang, & Truman, 2012). In 2011, there were 11 homicides of school-age youth at school (National Center for Injury Prevention and Control, 2015).

Delinquency is thought to peak during middle adolescence—around age 16. The National Institute of Justice (2014) indicates that 40% to 60 % of juvenile offenders no longer participate in or offend by early adulthood. Children assault and kill other children at school and on the streets. Eight percent of high school students reported being injured or threatened with a weapon, such as a gun, knife, or club, on school grounds. Four percent of students (aged 12 to 18) reported victimization during the 6 months prior to the survey, and public school students had twice the rate of those in private schools (Robers et al., 2012).

Gangs are often associated with teen violence. U.S. gangs are now found in communities across the country, with a rise in gang membership to more than 1 million members. Authorities believe that gangs are responsible for up to 85% of crimes and are the primary distributor of most illegal drugs. In 2011, 18% of adolescents (12 to 18 years) indicated that there were gangs present at school. The 2012 National Youth Gang Survey reported an increase in the number of gangs, gang membership, and gang-related homicides (Egley, Howell, & Harris, 2014). Although youth gangs may not effectively manage drug distribution as well as more established, older gangs, they are involved in various forms of violence that often includes intergang conflict (Egley & Howell, 2011). Public schools reported gang activity at 16% in 2009–2010, down from 20% 2 years earlier; but 20% of students reported gang presence at their schools with more high school students than sixth graders noting gangs being present (Robers et al., 2012). Although gang members may engage in violence and intimidation, other instances of school violence have captured greater media attention. Incidents of high school shootings, such as the one at Columbine High School, have raised concerns among parents and teachers. These high-profile events are rare, but they bring attention to the need for change. School violence has been linked to bullying and the overall school environment and should be addressed quickly. However, the incidence of homicides on school property has actually decreased over the past 15 years (Virginia Youth Violence Project, n.d.). Multiple successful antigang programs have been implemented in communities including Homeboy Industries, Boys Town and SOS Villages, and Open Door Youth Gang Alternatives

in an effort to prevent gang activity (National Crime Prevention Council, 2012).

Bullying can result in depression, social anxiety, internalizing and psychosomatic symptoms, loneliness, and poor school performance (Hertz et al., 2015). Daily or weekly bullying incidents were reported by 23% of public schools during the 2009–2010 school year, and 28% of students reported bullying at school; cyberbullying was reported by 6% of students (Robers et al., 2012). The percentage of young adolescents who do not feel safe at school decreased slightly over the past 5 years. In 2013, 17.9% of adolescents reported carrying a weapon to school during the past month (5.5% carried a gun), and more than 24.7% were involved in physical fights in the last year (8.1% on school property). Males were more likely to be involved in carrying weapons and fighting (Kann et al., 2014). Another form of violence found among adolescents and young adults is dating violence (or date rape), and females can also be the perpetrators of this although it is more common among males (Kann et al., 2014).

Cultural and environmental influences on youth include the violence to which children and adolescents are exposed. Increased aggressive behavior among children and teens has been attributed to violence in the environment, the home (spousal and child abuse), and the community, as well as to what children see on television and in movies. The effects of family violence (domestic violence, child maltreatment) can lead to internalizing and externalizing behaviors among youth (Child Trends Databank, 2015b). Personally experiencing violence and witnessing it as a child are risk factors for adolescent behaviors such as school dropout, running away from home, attempting suicide, and delinquency (Child Welfare Information Gateway, 2013). Violence is an increasing threat as students move from elementary school into middle and high school. Ninth grade students reported the highest rate of physical fights in a study of high school students (Robers et al., 2012). However, adolescents who are better connected to school are less likely to engage in violent behaviors. A longitudinal study of early adolescents found links between poor school engagement and delinquency, as well as depression and substance use (Li & Lerner, 2011). School climate is important in reducing the levels of violence in this age group, as is adequate parental support (Sumner et al., 2015). Family cohesion can also be a mediating factor for delinquency as a consequence of childhood effects of violence (Barr et al., 2012; Child Trends Databank, 2015b).

In 1994, with the implementation of the Gun-Free School Act and the Safe and Drug-Free Schools and Communities Act, juvenile crime rate peaked and then decreased over the next decade. During this time, zero-tolerance policies were implemented in schools in an effort to decrease weapon bearing at schools (Kang-Brown, Trone, Fratello, & Daftery-Kapur, 2013). In 2009–2010, 39% of public schools took serious disciplinary action against youth accused of specific offenses (Robers et al., 2012). Many schools now have metal detectors and security guards, and some schools conduct random searches of students' lockers in an effort to prevent violence. In 2008, the American Psychological Association Zero Tolerance Task Force examined 20 years of research studies and found little evidence of effectiveness and some indication that these policies actually may be worse than ineffective. They noted that these policies actually lead to increased violent and disruptive behavior and higher dropout rates. The task force found that a disproportionate number of Black and Hispanic students were expelled or suspended from school and that zero-tolerance policies do not consider children's lapses in judgment as a normal aspect of development. They recommended adaptations to zero-tolerance policies to make them more flexible and individualized to students, school sites, and situations. Students with disabilities are also disproportionately affected and this type of school discipline is seen as reactive, rather than proactive, and punitive, rather than corrective (Kang-Brown et al., 2013). Research over the past two decades validated concerns regarding the effectiveness of zero-tolerance policies in schools and a more positive approach to discipline has been recommended (Kang-Brown et al. 2013). In 2014, the Obama Administration recommended that zero-tolerance policies be discontinued in schools (Hefling, 2014).

Community efforts, youth development and violence prevention programs, and parenting education have been used to address youth violence, and a multimodal approach is often most effective (Allison, Edmonds, Wilson, Pope, & Farrell, 2011; Child Trends Databank, 2015b). Because family cohesion has been found to be a moderating influence for adolescents who witness community violence, programs that improve parenting practices and promote family cohesion are needed (Barr et al., 2012). Focusing on high-risk youth to improve parenting, peer relationships, academic achievement, and social cognition may be an effective means of preventing adolescent conduct disorder and delinquency (Child Trends Databank, 2015b).

Substance Abuse

Substance abuse among young people was almost unknown before 1950, and rare before 1960, but exploded in the mid-1960s. By 1981, 66% of high school students had ever tried an illicit drug and this dropped to 47% by 2008 (Johnston, O'Malley, Bachman, & Schulenberg, 2009). With the exception of a decrease in tobacco use, substance abuse among adolescents has changed very little over the past decade (Park et al., 2014). Adolescent drug experimentation and use pose serious physical and psychological threats. A national survey of high school students found that nearly 4 out of 10 teens reported drinking alcohol within 30 days before the survey and approximately 2 of 10 students reported binge drinking within the previous 2 weeks. In 2011, 50% of adolescents reported using an illicit drug by their senior year in high school. Forty-six percent of those students report using marijuana at least once. Prescription drug abuse is reported by 22% of 12th grade students and approximately 8% reported ever using inhalants like glue or aerosols (Murphey et al., 2013).

Why do adolescents turn to alcohol or illicit drugs? Substance abuse is one of the greatest threats to adolescent health. There are many influences associated with adolescent substance use including influence and monitoring by parents and guardians, family structure, history of physical abuse and maltreatment, adult example and parental substance use, and teen peer influence. Some research indicates that friend and peer influence becomes an even stronger predictor of substance abuse as a teen ages (Ewing et al., 2015). Depression has also been linked to alcohol and substance use (Fig. 22–7). Increased emphasis on family values is noted to be a

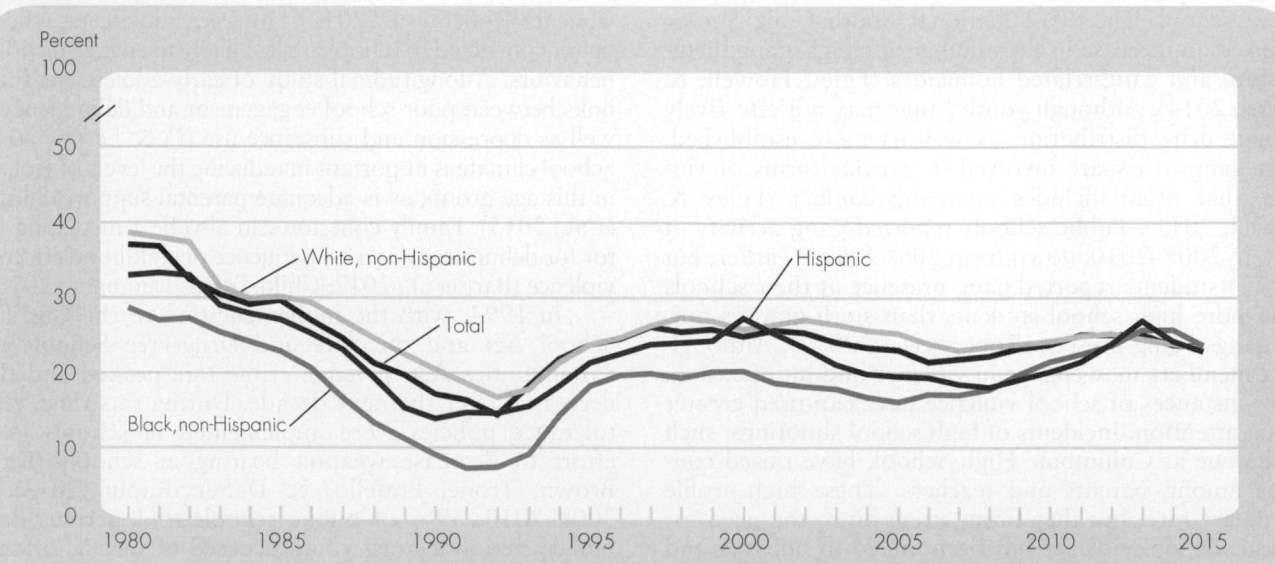

NOTE: Use of "any illicit drug" includes any use of marijuana, LSD, other hallucinogens, crack, other cocaine, or heroin, or any use of other prescription narcotics, amphetamines, barbiturates, or tranquilizers not under a doctor's orders. Persons of Hispanic origin may be of any race. Data on race and Hispanic origin are collected separately.

SOURCE: National Institute on Drug Abuse, Monitoring the Future Survey.

FIGURE 22–7 Percentage of 12th grade students who reported using any illicit drugs in the past 30 days by race and Hispanic origin, 1980–2015. (Retrieved from http://www.childstats. gov/americaschildren/beh_fig.asp.)

protective factor for alcohol use. This includes not only the parenting style of the adolescent's parents but also the parenting influences of the teen's friend's parents (Ewing, et al., 2015; Shikaya, Christakis, & Fowler, 2012).

Alcohol is the most frequently used substance for U.S. adolescents—it is often their first drug of choice. In one large study, the reasons cited by adolescents for trying alcohol included such things as "to find out what effect it would have," "to have more fun at a party," and "because it was exciting." Teens drinking for the last two reasons were more likely to engage in risky drinking, and those with symptoms of depression were three times more likely to binge drink (Kuntsche & Muller, 2012, p. 34). The teen brain is very susceptible to the damaging effects of alcohol and a number of social, physical, and academic are associated with its use. Early drinkers more often report damaged family relationships, academic problems, problems with concentration and memory, use of other substances, and delinquent behavior in middle and high school. Analysis of national survey data found that adolescents who begin first alcohol use before the age of 13 had significantly more involvement in violent behaviors and suicide attempts than those who delayed the initiation of alcohol (Murphey et al., 2013). Early use of alcohol was found to be a marker for later alcohol and drug dependence (SAMHSA, 2014), and age of alcohol initiation for Whites was earlier than for Blacks and Hispanics and more quickly progressed to alcohol dependence in a recent national survey (Alvanzo et al., 2011). It is important to stress education and prevention in late childhood to delay the initiation of alcohol use.

More than $1.7 billion was spent on alcohol advertising in 2009, and some feel that this influences adolescent drinking (Moreno, 2011; Murphey, Barry, Vaughn, Guzman, & Terzian, 2012). A study regarding brand-specific alcohol advertising and underage alcohol consumption by teens indicates that exposure via advertising was a significant predictor of consumption by the adolescent (Ross et al., 2015). Ross et al. (2015) recommend that decreased exposure of alcohol brands may be beneficial in decreasing underage consumption of alcohol. Binge drinking is generally defined as having five or more drinks at one time—usually within a couple of hours—and it often increases as adolescents get older (Murphey et al., 2012). Binge drinking has been associated with poor academic achievement and other risk behaviors (e.g., sexual activity, smoking, using illicit drugs, riding with a driver who had been drinking, attempting suicide), and the more adolescents binge drink, the more they engage in risk behaviors (Park et al., 2014). Adolescent binge drinking was associated and parental alcoholism was influential in later adult substance use disorders (Murphey et al., 2012).

Family drinking and perceived family norms related to drinking have been found to affect adolescents' perceptions of the benefits of drinking. This perception, in turn, predicts their drinking behavior (Murphey et al., 2012). Parenting practices (e.g., monitoring, discipline, enforcing rules related to alcohol use) have also been found to have an influence on adolescent drinking behavior (Ewing et al., 2015). Factors prevalent during adolescence, such as divorce, parental trust, social class

and relationships, along with depressive symptoms and poor impulse control and self-esteem, were associated with excessive alcohol use in adults (SAMHSA, 2014).

Adolescents who are engaged emotionally and connected to school generally have better outcomes; lower levels of engagement were linked to substance use and delinquency in one longitudinal study (Li & Lerner, 2011). Positive parenting practices such as open communication, monitoring adolescent activities, and teaching methods of self-control have also been associated with a reduction in adolescent alcohol use (Murphey et al., 2012). Family mealtimes have been shown to promote family cohesion and problem- and emotion-focused coping by encouraging parents to help their children feel part of the family and allowing them valuable time to coach them in effective methods for dealing with daily stresses and problems. The benefits of family mealtime include improved self-esteem, improved mental health, decreased alcohol and substance abuse, and decreased depression (Harrison et al., 2015). To promote the health and welfare of adolescent children, it is vital to stress to families with young children the continued importance of family meals throughout adolescence (Fig. 22–8).

Marijuana is the most commonly used illicit drug among 14- to 17-year-olds—46% of high school seniors reported ever using marijuana. Use of marijuana by early adolescents has remained constant, but middle to late adolescent use has slightly increased since 2009 (Murphey et al., 2013). This is an important finding, because early marijuana use (before age 15) has been associated with a much greater likelihood of adult cocaine and heroin use and drug dependency (Office of National Drug Control Policy, 2012). Marijuana use has negative health effects, including anxiety, panic attacks, increased heart rate, frequent respiratory infections, impaired memory and learning, and tolerance. Regular marijuana smokers often have respiratory complications similar to those of tobacco smokers—cough, phlegm, respiratory infections, and airway obstruction (Office of National Drug Control Policy, 2012).

Inhalant abuse is very common and frequently used by young teens. Inhalant use begins in early adolescence—more 12- and 13-year-olds reported using inhalants than

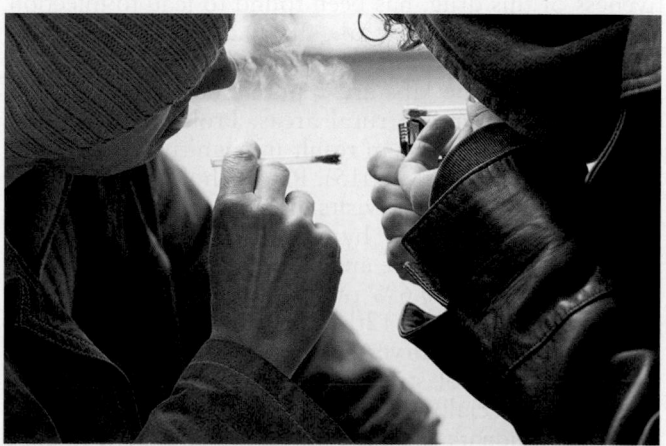

FIGURE 22–8 Marijuana use is common among adolescents.

any other illicit drug. The most commonly reported inhalants used were shoe polish, glue or toluene, spray paints, and lighter fluid or gasoline (Johnston, O'Malley, Miech, Bachman, & Schulenberg, 2015). Other inhalants commonly used include amyl nitrite "poppers"; locker room deodorizers or "rush"; cleaning fluid, degreasers, or correction fluid; halothane, ether, or other anesthetics; lacquer thinner or other paint solvents; butane or propane gases; nitrous oxide or "whippets"; and other aerosol sprays (Center for Behavioral Health Statistics and Quality, 2015). Inhalant abuse can result in severe nervous system damage or death. Control of legal products, such as spray paint, lighter fluid, household solvents, gasoline, and glue, is difficult, making this problem almost impossible to monitor adequately.

Other drugs that are used by adolescents and young adults include "club drugs" such as MDMA (Ecstasy), a synthetic drug with amphetamine and hallucinogenic properties, and its purer form "Molly" often glamorized by singers and musicians; Rohypnol (the date rape drug that is often mixed with alcohol to produce sedative hypnotic effects); ketamine (a rapid-acting anesthetic); lysergic acid diethylamide (LSD), a hallucinogen originally popularized in the 1960s; and gamma-hydroxybutyrate (GHB, a drug that is touted as a synthetic steroid in fitness clubs and that has been associated with sexual assaults). Fentanyl use has been noted in several areas of the country, along with its derivative, acetyl fentanyl, and overdoses have occurred leading to deaths. Rates of use for ketamine, Rohypnol, and GHB have declined over the past few years, but psilocybin or "magic mushrooms" are still widely used. Ecstasy use has generally declined but may become popular again among younger adolescents. Over-the-counter cold and cough medications containing the cough suppressant dextromethorphan are sometimes used to produce a "high," and between 2% and 4.1% of adolescents are reported to have used them (Johnston et al., 2015; Templeton, 2013). Visits to the ED and deaths have occurred from the use of many of these drugs.

Cocaine use has remained steady in recent years, after peaking in the late 1990s. Heroin use fell below peak levels reached in 2001 but continues to remain steady. Smoking or snorting of heroin, which is popular among adolescents and young adults because they mistakenly believe it precludes the strong physical addictiveness of this drug, has been found to lead to injection drug abuse (Johnston et al., 2015). Methamphetamine may be smoked, along with marijuana, or injected. Methamphetamine labs are a public health hazard and can often be found in rural areas. Prolonged exposure to methamphetamine can result in cognitive deficits and psychosis (Chen et al., 2015). PHNs should be aware of this when making home visits in outlying areas.

Another drug used by adolescents is anabolic steroids. The illicit use of anabolic steroids is difficult to monitor; however, 0.6% of 8th graders, 0.8% of 10th graders, and 1.5% of 12th graders reported using steroids in a national survey (Johnston et al., 2015). A survey of high school students noted that use was higher in males, especially those participating in sports, and 49% of students believed that athletic performance could be improved with steroid use; 38% thought that use improved appearance (Lorang, Callahan, Cummins, Achar, & Brown, 2011). Some coaches have, at times, turned a blind eye to steroid abuse, but educational campaigns to fight the rising level of abuse in adolescents have led to decreases in use since peak levels were reached in 2000. Adverse effects of illicit steroid use include irritability, increased risk-taking behavior, extreme mood swings, paranoia, jealousy, and euphoria, as well as psychiatric conditions that may be intensified or induced. Because steroids are often readily available through Internet pharmacies, policymakers, health educators, and parents must make adolescents aware of the dangers, such as altered serotonin levels and increased aggression (U.S. Food and Drug Administration [FDA], 2013). A recent study regarding parental communication with adolescent athletes indicates that discussions should emphasize "protective" health and the social consequences of misusing steroids (Dodge & Clark, 2015).

Adolescents are becoming more involved with prescription drugs, often found in their parents' medicine cabinets, purchased on the Internet, or bought from friends at school (McCabe et al., 2012). Medications are often mixed with alcohol, and adolescents often mistakenly believe prescription medications are safer than street drugs when used to produce a high. Ritalin, prescribed to students with ADHD, may be given or sold to others, but the most commonly used medications are OxyContin, Vicodin, tranquilizers, and sedatives. In 2014, 3.3% of high school seniors tried OxyContin, and 4.8% of high school seniors used Vicodin (Johnston et al., 2015). Although the prevalence rates have decreased, the trend is concerning because of society's nonchalant, casual attitude toward prescription medications and their easy access. Early onset (before age 13) of nonmedical use of prescription medications is a predictor of later prescription drug abuse and drug dependence (Swartz & Bilbo, 2013). A large national survey found the number of adolescents admitting to nonmedical use of prescription drugs remained about the same between 2012 and 2014. Although the most common nonmedical use of a substance was pain medications, sedatives, stimulants, and tranquilizers were also frequently abused. Approximately 655,000 teens between ages 12 and 17 years abused psychotherapeutic drugs during 2014 (Center for Behavioral Health Statistics and Quality, 2015).

Tobacco products are also easily acquired, often from parents. About $10 billion is spent annually on marketing tobacco products (Koch, 2012). Approximately one in three high school seniors report ever trying a cigarette. In 1997, 25% of 12th graders reported to regular smoking; however, this percentage has been steadily declining, and in 2014, it reached an all-time low of 7% of high school students reporting to daily, regularly smoking (Office of Adolescent Health, 2015). Males almost exclusively use smokeless tobacco products (e.g., snuff, chew), and 8.4% of 12th graders reported using smokeless tobacco during 2014. Electronic cigarettes (e-cigarettes) are becoming increasingly used in the adolescent population. Between the years 2010 and 2014, the number of adolescents reporting that they had used e-cigarettes in the past 30 days increased from 1.5% to 17.2%. Of concern is the unknown long-term effect of e-cigarettes

POPULATION-FOCUS
SUBSTANCE ABUSE PREVENTION FOR ADOLESCENTS

School nursing runs in my family. In the 1980s, when my mother was a school nurse in a small, rural school district located in an agriculturally dependent county, there was only one high school in the small town of about 10,000 people. School personnel were aware of some "keg parties" after football games, and the occasional alcohol-related fight on school property between some of the rougher students, but they were not fully aware of the substance abuse problems. The school psychologist conducted an anonymous survey and found, much to the surprise of teachers and administrators, that most of the teens involved in alcohol and drug abuse were the athletes and cheerleaders. They had assumed that the lower-income, trouble-making kids were much more involved, but this was not necessarily the case. My mother worked with the psychologist to implement health education classes in the high school and eventually the middle school and elementary schools to address this issue and health promotion in general.

I am a school nurse at a more suburban, larger school district serving over 30,000 students with four high schools, a charter high school and a continuation high school. Each high school has a full-time school nurse, and the middle schools have one most of the week. We utilize evidence-based practice as school nurses, and there are many resources available to us. We are aware of national surveys on substance use among adolescents and have conducted some ourselves (e.g., YRBS) in order to better understand our students' needs. Although alcohol is still a concern, drug use has increased since my mom's school nursing experience. A national survey found that almost 1 in 10 adolescents use some type of illicit drugs (Center for Behavioral Health Statistics and Quality, 2015), and 7.4% are currently using marijuana; this is similar to statistics in 2005. The next concern is illicit use of psychotropic drugs (i.e., prescription-type pain relievers, stimulants, sedatives, and tranquilizers), and 2.6% of 12- to 17-year-olds are currently using these (1.9% use pain relievers, 0.7% use stimulants, 0.2% use sedatives, and 0.4% use tranquilizers). When you consider that 2.5% of the population (over the age 12) use psychotropic prescription drugs either nonmedically or illicitly, you have a clearer picture of the problem.

The district school nurses met with our advisory board, parent groups, school administration, and eventually the school board to discuss the problem and address potential interventions. We discussed our population demographics, our various cultural and ethnic influences, and our community statistics. After examining the best research-based methods, we found that school-based interventions can be effective if they include the following components (Griffin & Botvin, 2010; Lowe, Acevedo, Griffin, & Botvin, et al., 2013):

- Social Resistance Skills—Increasing students' awareness of the social influences around them that encourage substance use and then given them specific skills sets to more effectively withstand media and peer pressures to drink and use drugs or tobacco.
- Normative Education—There is a need to correct teens' misperceptions that "everybody is doing it" and become part of the crowd. Information from national, state, and local surveys are used to demonstrate actual prevalence rates, and data from current research are presented that show substance abuse is not socially acceptable and is a danger.
- Competence Enhancement—Life skills such as problem-solving and decision-making are taught, as well as cognitive skills for resistance of adverse influences (peers, media). Skills are also taught to improve self-esteem and self-control, along with coping strategies to reduce anxiety and relieve stress (e.g., relaxation). Students are also taught assertiveness and social skills. All of these are helpful to the development of adolescents in their everyday experiences, even when not facing pressures to drug experimentation.

Family-focused prevention programs often provide skills to parents (e.g., parenting, helping children develop social resistance skills, monitoring/rule setting). Some programs included children and their families (e.g., improve communication, family functioning, develop family rules on substance abuse/enforcement). These family bonding interventions have been found to be most effective. Community-based prevention programs usually not only include both school-based and family-based intervention components but also encompass mass media campaigns and policy/legislative initiatives, along with other community activities and improvements (e.g., teen-focused recreation). These have also shown promise when they are comprehensive and well coordinated and have broad support of stakeholders (Griffin & Botvin, 2010).

Some programs have shown great promise in addressing nonmedical prescription drug use, along with other substances. *Life Skills Training* was found to be the only school program that, when delivered without family and community interventions or other methods, significantly reduced use of nonmedical prescription drugs in 12th grade comparative to the control group. It was considered the most cost-effective program. When a family-based program, *Strengthening Families*, was added for 6th graders, the results doubled (Crowley, Jones, Coffman, & Greenberg, 2014).

Our school district decided to purchase the Life Skills Training program for elementary, middle, and high school students. They also plan to institute a family-based prevention program for upper elementary students and their parents within the next few years.

(continued)

POPULATION-FOCUS
SUBSTANCE ABUSE PREVENTION FOR ADOLESCENTS (Continued)

I hope we can eventually encourage a more community-based approach to population health for our children and adolescents. I feel that with the resources we have today, we can really make a difference in the lives of our students and their families. I know my mother is proud of the work I am doing, and I hope my daughter considers carrying on the family tradition!

Holly, Age 30, School Nurse

Center for Behavioral Health Statistics and Quality. (2015). *Behavioral health trends in the United States: Results from the 2014 National Survey on Drug Use and Health* (HHS Publication No. SMA 15-4927, NSDUH Series H-50). Retrieved from http://www.samhsa.gov/data/

Crowley, D. M., Jones, D. E., Coffman, D. L., & Greenberg, M. T. (2014). Can we build an efficient response to the prescription drug abuse epidemic? Assessing the cost effectiveness of universal prevention in the PROSPER trial. *Preventive Medicine, 62,* 71–77.

Griffin, K. W., & Botvin, G. J. (2010). Evidence-based interventions for preventing substance use disorders in adolescents. *Child & Adolescent Psychiatric Clinics of North America, 19*(3), 505–526.

Lowe, S. R., Acevedo, B. P., Griffin, K. W., & Botvin, G. J. (2013). Longitudinal relationships between self-management skills and substance use in an urban sample of predominately minority adolescents. *Journal of Drug Issues, 43*(1), 103–118.

and the possibility that adolescents using e-cigarettes may later use tobacco (Johnston et al., 2015).

Social disapproval and heightened perception of health risks are thought to help contribute to the downward trend of smoking and smokeless tobacco use, along with price increases and advertising bans (Johnston et al., 2015). But tobacco marketing continues to be problematic, as the tobacco industry has joined with convenience stores to more prominently display tobacco products, and even though state and federal taxes comprise about half the cost of a pack of cigarettes, states have not always sufficiently invested these funds in adolescent tobacco prevention (Koch, 2012). One longitudinal study found that adolescents who had low academic aspirations, perceived themselves to be unconventional, and had internalizing behaviors (e.g., depressive symptoms) were less likely to participate in smoking cessation programs. Parental smoking also was a negative influence, and other research demonstrated less effective quit attempts for adolescents with at least one smoking parent (Kong, Carmenga, & Krishnan-Sarin, 2012). Motivational interviewing techniques may be an effective intervention for smoking cessation. This strategy has been shown to be effective when used during in-person counseling and with telephone counseling (Boccio et al., in press; Lindson-Hawley, Thompson, & Begh, 2015). In addition, parental disapproval was related to a greater number of attempts at abstinence for boys but not for girls (Kong et al., 2012).

Primary health care providers do not always question adolescents about smoking, drinking, and use of other substances. Some evidence highlights the effectiveness of brief interventions by health care providers in encouraging smoking cessation and improvement in other risk behaviors. Research recommends that health care professional counseling be provided as a preventive measure to adolescent tobacco users (Schauer, Agaku, King, & Malarcher, 2014). But the long-term effectiveness of this type of intervention was not demonstrated in a Finnish cohort study (Saari, Kentala, & Mattila, 2012). PHNs and community health nurses can provide information to teens about smoking cessation programs and promote primary prevention by educating children and adolescents to choose not to smoke or engage in other health risk behaviors. They can also encourage physicians and parents to question and monitor adolescents about smoking and the use of tobacco products.

Teen Sexuality and Pregnancy

Teenage pregnancies, sexually transmitted diseases (STDs), and HIV/AIDS are public health concerns associated with the sexual activity of adolescents. In the 2013 YRBS, 46.8% of high school students reported ever having sexual intercourse, and 59.1% used a condom during their last sexual intercourse. Almost 15% reported having had sexual intercourse with four or more persons, and 19.0% used birth control pills to prevent pregnancy (Kann et al., 2014). In 2013, teens (aged 15 to 19) experienced 274,641 pregnancies and those under age 14 had 3,108 pregnancies (Ventura, Hamilton, & Matthews, 2014). Although early sexual debut has been associated with delinquency, as well as with other negative outcomes, a recent study by Butera, Lanza, and Coffman (2014) suggests that more research is needed regarding this effect. Research findings posit that early sex and delinquency may have a common cause (such as family structure and maternal education) and that interventions for early sex prevention "may not be an effective intervention target for reducing rates of adolescent delinquency" (Butera et al., 2014, p. 405). Early puberty has also been related to greater sexual activity and higher rates of delinquency in a large study of 9- to 13-year-olds (Negriff, Susman, & Trickett, 2011).

The United States leads most developed nations in rates of teenage pregnancy, abortion, and childbearing. The teen birth rate in this country declined to its lowest level in 70 years from 1991 to 2009; yet the U.S. rate was six to nine times higher than that of "developed countries with the lowest birth rates" (Pazol et al., 2011, p. 419). Despite a slight increase in 2006–2007, since 1991, pregnancy and birth rates for 15- to 19-year-old girls have declined by 37%. In 2013, the rate was 26.6 births per 1,000 females. The rate for Hispanic adolescent girls was 46.3 per 1,000; for non-Hispanic Blacks, the rate was 43.9 per 1,000. For non-Hispanic Whites, the rate was 20.5 per 1,000. There is a wide discrepancy between states, with rates varying from 13.84 to 47.5, and southern and southwestern states having higher numbers of teen pregnancies and births (Ventura et al., 2014). Some research has indicated that shared social norms about adolescent pregnancy may vary among racial/ethnic groups, and this may account for a larger amount of influence than religious or socioeconomic factors (Mollborn, Domingue, & Boardman, 2011). An examination of state-level characteristics found that those states with higher rates in 1991 and sharper increases through 2007 were more likely to have higher rates of unemployment, unmarried births, violent crime, and a higher proportion of Hispanic and Black residents than lower birth rate states. They were also less likely to have public funding for abortion (Terzian & Moore, 2012). The downward trend for teen birth rates is thought to be associated with a drop in the percentage of students who had sexual intercourse and those having sex without contraception. The use of two forms of birth control (i.e., condoms together with birth control pills or Depo-Provera) increased from 5% to 9% in the decade preceding 2009 (Pazol et al., 2011). The rate of teenage abortion was 17.8 per 1,000 in 2008, the lowest since abortions became legal. This declining trend continued in 2010, when the rate was 14.7 per 1,000. The highest rate was in 1988 at 43.5 (Kost & Henshaw, 2014). The rate of adolescent fatherhood also declined; between 1991 and 2010, it dropped from 25 to 16 per 1,000 males. Almost half of male teens state they would be very upset if they were responsible for a pregnancy (Guttmacher Institute, 2014).

Teenage pregnancy is associated with increased health risks to both the mother and the child. These risks include increased risk of illness and death, increased risk of mother's death from violence, and increased developmental concerns of the child. In addition, young mothers are more likely to live in poverty and to be delayed in their own education (Medline Plus, 2015). Young mothers are more likely to smoke tobacco and are at high risk of bearing infants with low birth weights. They are also less likely to receive adequate prenatal care or to gain the recommended weight during pregnancy. Adolescent mothers are at a greater risk than mothers over age 20 to experience a complication of pregnancy (e.g., anemia, hypertension, premature labor), and the risk increases for those under age 15 (Wallace & Harville, 2013). Compared with women giving birth at age 30, teen mothers can expect 2 years less education and they are 10% to 12% less likely to finish high school; they are also less likely to attend college (Basch, 2011b). Adolescent girls living with a single parent or not living with either parent have higher teen birth rates than those who live with both parents (Wildsmith, Manlove, Jekielek, Moore, & Mincieli, 2012). The children of adolescent mothers are more likely to exhibit disorganized attachment with the mother, suffer abuse, and show developmental delays. Their mothers also face social, physical, and mental health challenges (Crugnolaa, Ierardia, Gazzottia, & Albizzatib, 2014). Teenage mothers who choose to end their pregnancies by abortion may additionally encounter other physical and psychosocial complications (SmithBattle & Fried, 2016).

By 19 years of age, 71% of males and females have had sexual intercourse. Approximately 16% of teens have had sex by age 15 (Guttmacher Institute, 2014). As such, it would behoove U.S. society to provide effective sexuality education. There is often debate about the virtues of comprehensive versus abstinence-only educational programs. Despite the contentiousness about the subject, in 2006, 87% of private and public schools in the United States required health education, most of it at the high school level. Most adolescents (age 15 to 19) received education about STIs (93%) and abstinence (84%), but about 33% were not instructed about contraception. Many sexually active teens have no instruction on contraception before their first sexual experience (33% girls, 46% boys; Fields, 2012; Guttmacher Institute, 2012). Teaching about contraception has not been shown to increase the risk of adolescent sexual activity or STIs, but it may decrease the risk of pregnancy. Analysis of data from a national survey found that sex education, of any type, when compared to no education was associated with delayed sexual intercourse for both adolescent males and females. When education included instruction in birth control, along with abstinence, adolescents were more likely to use contraception (birth control pills or condom) at first sexual intercourse and less likely to have a much older partner (Lindberg & Maddow-Zimet, 2012). Besides formal education through schools, adolescents note that peers, the media, and parents are also sources of information on sexual health. Between 70% and 79% of teens report talking with a parent about sex, although girls more often talk with parents about how to say no to sex or use birth control (Guttmacher Institute, 2012, 2014) (Fig. 22–9).

Pregnancy prevention programs can be effective in reducing teen pregnancy and birth rates, as well as in reducing the number of second births to teenage mothers. A prospective cohort study found that increased levels of sexuality education within schools was associated with decreased teen birth rates, although the reverse was

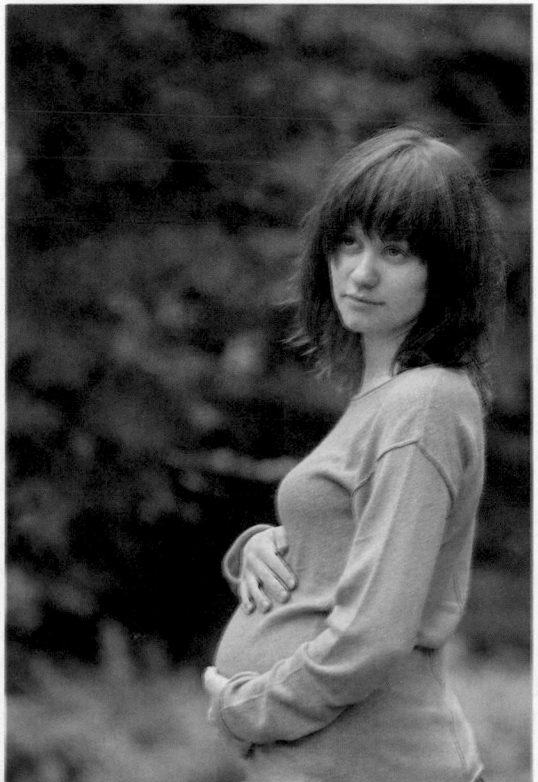

FIGURE 22–9 Pregnancy prevention programs can be helpful in decreasing rates of adolescent pregnancy.

found in some states with higher religiosity and political conservatism (Cavazos-Rehg et al., 2012). Another study comparing the curriculum effectiveness of the comprehensive teen pregnancy prevention (TPP) intervention and the abstinence-only TPP taught in schools indicates that the comprehensive TPP program is slightly more effective than the abstinence intervention. Results were based on adolescent attitudes and perceptions, knowledge-based questions, and behavioral outcomes. Study recommendations include the "need to focus on improving attitudes about sexual activity, especially related to male and female sexuality, peer norms, and refusal skills" (Oman, Merritt, Fluhr, & Williams, 2015, p. 892). Positive youth development (PYD) programs have been found to promote adolescent sexual and reproductive health by focusing on social and cognitive competence, prosocial bonding, future orientation, and self-determination. These programs focus on overall youth development, not just sexuality, and emphasize positive, personal strengths of all adolescents (Geldhof et al., 2014).

Primary care providers often miss opportunities to provide counseling on prevention of pregnancy, HIV, and STDs, as well as other risk factors for unintentional injury (Ozer et al., 2011). Nurses can provide information and counseling on birth control and emergency contraception to adolescent clients and collaborate with schools to promote effective pregnancy prevention programs. It is important for PHNs to provide education and health counseling on these subjects. A recent study by Borawski et al. (2015) demonstrated the importance of nursing collaboration in high school sexual education and counseling, stating "those taught by school nurses reported significant and sustained changes (up to 12 months after intervention) in attitudes, beliefs, and efficacy" (p. 189).

Sexually Transmitted Infections

STI and HIV infections are epidemic among adolescents worldwide (World Health Organization, 2016). More than 20 diseases can be transmitted sexually; only the most common are reportable. Each year, about half of the STI cases occur among the 15- to 24-year-old age group, even though they represent only 25% of the population of sexually active individuals. These diseases include syphilis, gonorrhea, *Chlamydia*, HPV, and herpes simplex virus. Approximately 30 of the 100 known types of HPV strains are sexually transmitted; some of these are related to cervical cancer, and others lead to genital warts. Gardasil, a vaccine effective against some forms of HPV-related disease, can be administered in three doses to 11- to 12-year-old females and now to males as well (Dunne et al., 2011; Guttmacher Institute, 2014).

Chlamydia, gonorrhea, and syphilis are other STDs/STIs found in the adolescent population. Of the 19 million new cases of STIs annually, about half are among adolescents (15 to 24 years old), and 21% of 13- to 24-year-olds in reporting states had a new HIV infection in 2011 (Guttmacher Institute, 2014). In the adolescent population, STIs are more common among those engaging in sexual risk behaviors. In 2013, 46% of high school students reported ever having sexual intercourse and 34% were active within the previous 3 months. Almost 15% had sex with four or more

partners, and 59% used a condom with their last sexual contact (Child Trends Databank, 2014b). *Chlamydia* is the most common STI; adolescent girls 15 to 19 years of age had the second highest reported cases of *Chlamydia* and gonorrhea. Adolescent males had a lower prevalence of both *Chlamydia* and gonorrhea (CDC, 2015k).

About one in four adolescent females (aged 15 to 19) have an STI; and the rate for African American girls is 4.9 times the rate for white females (CDC, 2015k). Compared with adults, adolescents (10 to 19 years) and young adults (20 to 24 years) are at increased risk for acquiring STIs. Reasons for this may include a greater likelihood of multiple sex partners, unprotected intercourse, and selection of higher-risk partners, as well as immature biology making them more vulnerable to infection and earlier sexual initiation. Barriers to improvement include lack of health insurance and transportation, concerns about confidentiality, and lack of quality STI prevention services or clinics targeted to younger age groups (CDC, 2015k). Adolescent girls also have a physiologically amplified susceptibility to *Chlamydia* infection because of increased cervical ectopy (CDC, 2014d). Serious complications from STIs include pelvic inflammatory disease (PID), sterility, increased risk of cancers of the reproductive system, and, with syphilis, blindness, mental illness, and death. There are also complications for the unborn children of those infected with STIs. In one study on follow-up for adolescents with STIs diagnosed in EDs, a large number did not receive appropriate treatment. Of those who did, 25% did not realize they had an STI, which put them at risk of avoiding reinfection and nontreatment of sexual partners (Reed & Huppert, 2011).

Even though death rates from HIV/AIDS have dramatically fallen, new HIV infections reported annually do not reflect the same steep decline. It is estimated that as many as 50% of youth with HIV are not aware of their infection (CDC, 2015m). Adolescents and young adults (aged 13 to 24) comprised 26% of all new cases of HIV infection in 2010 and black youth accounted for 57% of the new cases. New medications are thought to be the cause of the declining death rate, whereas new cases are increasing within adolescent and young adult populations. Females, males having sex with other males, injection drug users, and racial minorities have higher rates of STI/HIV during adolescence Also, those experiencing childhood sexual abuse are more at risk for HIV/AIDS risk behaviors as adolescents (CDC, 2015k, 2015m).

As noted earlier, sex education is effective at both delaying the onset of sexual activity and increasing the use of contraception in adolescents who are already sexually active. It is also effective in increasing safer sex practices, knowledge of birth control method efficacy, and overall sexual knowledge when that content is taught (Borawski et al., 2015). Prevention strategies, identified by systematic review of research, found the best strategies to reduce sexual risk behaviors included targeting behaviors that are most easily amenable to change (e.g., condom use, decreased number of sexual partners, abstinence), tailoring programs to the target population (e.g., subgroups such as African American females, gay/bisexual males), using theory as a guide in development of programs (e.g., modeling discussions with partners about condom use, skill building by role-playing situations, increasing self-efficacy), and addressing a broader content than just STI/HIV prevention education (e.g., problem-solving, social skills, gender pride, capacity building). Evidence-based interventions are the most effective (CDC, 2015m). See Chapter 30 for the school nurse's role with STI/HIV.

Acne

About 80% of individuals between the ages of 11 and 30 have acne. Most of these are adolescents, although pediatric acne (ages 7 to 11) cases are growing (Mancini, Baldwin, Eichenfield, Friedlander, & Yan, 2011). The precise cause of acne is not fully understood. It is generally related to several factors. Genetics plays a part (there is often a family history of acne), and hormonal influences are also at play (especially an increase in male hormones), and greasy cosmetics may plug cells of follicles, producing a plug (National Institute of Arthritis and Musculoskeletal and Skin Diseases [NIAMSD], 2014). Acne generally begins during puberty (10 to 12 years of age) with the increase in circulating male hormones that stimulate sebaceous glands in the skin. The excess sebum (oil) causes irritation in the pores and results in a buildup of cells, leading to whiteheads. Open pores are known as blackheads. A red and inflamed pustule can develop or, in serious cases of acne, cysts or nodules can form. Untreated, this can lead to pitting and scarring.

It is now known that greasy foods and chocolate do not cause acne but may be aggravating factors (along with stress, environmental irritants, and certain cosmetics) in susceptible adolescents. Abrasive scrubbing of the skin; pressure from backpacks, tight collars, or sports helmets; and picking or squeezing blemishes may make acne worse (NIAMSD, 2014). Common treatment regimens include skin cleansers, peelers, and medications to decrease sebaceous gland activity. Topical retinoids are the first-line drugs of choice because of their anti-inflammatory properties. Benzoyl peroxide is used to kill bacteria on the skin and in the pores. It may be sold over the counter (OTC) or by prescription. Other OTC medications include salicylic acid and resorcinol. Retin A (a topical vitamin A ointment), glycolic acid, and alpha hydroxy acids help to peel the impacted cells from the pores. Antibiotics (oral or topical), such as tetracycline (Ala-Tet) or doxycycline (Adoxa), may be prescribed to help control bacteria on the skin. Isotretinoin (Accutane) reduces the size and activity of sebaceous glands but can cause liver or kidney dysfunction. Because of an extremely high risk of birth defects, female adolescents taking Accutane are prescribed oral contraceptives; these may also be prescribed for girls not taking this drug who have hormonally influenced acne (NIAMSD, 2014; Ramanathan & Hebert, 2011). Sun sensitivity is another side effect of this medication. Corticosteroids may be injected directly into the comedones. Dapsone gel (Aczone) can be applied twice daily to the face, and some adolescents choose to try complementary therapies such as tea tree oil, aloe vera, or witch hazel, as well as biofeedback and hypnosis (Ramanathan & Hebert, 2011).

The best preventive measures are keeping the skin clean, eating a balanced diet that includes fresh fruits and vegetables, drinking lots of water, and getting adequate sleep. It is important for male adolescents to shave carefully and for all teens with acne to avoid touching their faces or picking at their blemishes. They may want to use skin and hair products that are noncomedogenic. Adolescents with severe acne may need to be referred to dermatologists who specialize in this skin disorder.

Poor Nutrition and Eating Disorders

Poor nutrition and obesity are not uncommon among adolescents, whose diets often consist of snacks with limited nutritional value interspersed among unhealthful meals. Increased fast-food consumption has been tied to poor diets and the increase in obesity in the United States (Brown et al., 2015). The eating behavior of adolescents is influenced by many things, among them psychosocial factors, family and peers, availability of fast food, and mass media marketing (Brown et al., 2015). Girls are more at risk for problems with nutrition for several reasons: they tend to diet inappropriately, to have more finicky eating habits, and to be less physically active than teenage boys. Boys typically eat large quantities of food, which increases the likelihood of obtaining adequate nutrients, and they also tend to be more physically active than girls. The quality of an adolescent's diet has implications for later health, as evidenced by a study of fruit and vegetable consumption among 13- to 17-year-olds. The beneficial effects of vegetable and fruit intake on inflammatory and oxidative stress markers were already evident in these adolescents, indicating a good basis for future health (Kann et al., 2014). Habitual unhealthy snacking is of concern among the adolescent population. A study by De Vet, Stok, De Wit, and De Ridder (2015) shows promising results for adolescent snacking and suggests that self-regulation strategies may be helpful in curbing an adolescent's habitual unhealthy eating.

Issues with body image and control are at the heart of anorexia nervosa and bulimia nervosa, common problems for adolescent girls. Eating disorders are considered psychiatric conditions, but there is a continuum of altered eating that does not fall within the diagnostic guidelines of an eating disorder (American Dietetic Association, 2011). **Anorexia nervosa** is an eating disorder with an emotional etiology that is characterized by body image disturbance (i.e., girls see themselves as fat although they may be extremely thin), an intense fear of becoming fat or gaining weight, and refusal to maintain adequate body weight (i.e., BMI of 18 or greater). **Bulimia** is an eating disorder characterized by recurrent episodes of binge eating with repeated compensatory mechanisms to prevent weight gain, such as vomiting (purging type) and fasting or exercise (nonpurging type). Lifetime prevalence of anorexia nervosa is 0.3%, and bulimia is 0.9% (Swanson, Crow, LeGrange, Swendsen, & Merikangas, 2011).

Binge eating, also a recognized eating disorder, involves recurrent episodes of binge eating without fasting, self-induced vomiting, or other compensatory measures, and lifetime prevalence of this disorder is 1.6% (Swanson et al., 2011). Self-esteem, depressive symptoms, and emotional eating are very sensitive predictors of binge eating, and 34% of adolescents have reported secretive eating (Knatz, Maginot, Story, Neumark-Sztainer, &

Boutelle, 2011). Low levels of support from peers can also be linked to binge eating, and binge eating is associated with an increased risk of becoming overweight or obese (Knatz et al., 2011). There is evidence of later onset of eating disorders in males versus females, with a peak in prevalence before age 25 (Michison & Mond, 2015).

These diseases have emotional causes that are often associated with role impairment and other psychiatric conditions, along with suicidality, and pose complex challenges to treatment (Swanson et al., 2011). A review of current research on eating disorders notes how environmental factors (e.g., nutrition, stress) may lead to epigenetic changes that affect the risk of developing an eating disorder (Campbell, Mill, Uher, & Schmidt, 2011). There is some evidence of mother and peer attitudes and behaviors increasing the risk of later escalations of symptoms among adolescents. The transition from adolescence into young adulthood is an important one as "eating disorder risk factors and symptoms increase over time" (Linville, Stice, Gau, & O'Neill, 2011, p. 749). Nutrition education, psychological counseling, and cognitive–behavioral techniques that teach clients how to control stimuli, substitute alternative behaviors, and use positive visualization are all part of treatment; development of a support network is also important. Family and individually based treatments are most often used for severe cases of adolescent eating disorders and have been studied most often. Self-concept is often distorted and self-esteem is low; therefore, activities are initiated to improve the adolescents' feelings about themselves and to bolster their coping mechanisms. Medications (e.g., antidepressants) have been used to treat some adolescents with eating disorders, but there is little evidence of their effectiveness (Lock, 2010).

The key to prevention with girls may be tied to perceptions of their appearance and education about the risks of dieting. One classic study indicated that adolescent girls who were severe dieters were 18 times more likely to develop an eating disorder than those who did not diet. Even moderate dieters were at risk; they were five times more likely to develop an eating disorder. Psychiatric morbidity was also a factor; it increased risk sevenfold. Exercise is seen as a more viable alternative than extreme dieting for adolescents who want to control their weight. Adolescents who use unhealthy and extreme weight-control behaviors (e.g., binge eating, fasting, skipped meals) continue these behaviors into adulthood. This is more common for females, but one third of males reported these behaviors in a recent study (National Association of Anorexia Nervosa and Eating Disorders, 2015; Pedersen, 2011).

HEALTH SERVICES FOR SCHOOL-AGE CHILDREN AND ADOLESCENTS

A number of programs serve the health needs of school-age children and adolescents. Community health nurses play a major and vital role in delivering these services. Such programs fall into three categories that approximate the three practice priorities of community health nursing practice: illness prevention, health protection, and health promotion.

Preventive Health Programs

Among programs to prevent physical illness and other health problems among adolescents are immunizations and TB testing, as well as school- and community-based education and support programs. Private and public counseling programs and other social services are also geared to promote health and prevent illness.

Immunizations and Tuberculosis Testing

PHNs are deeply involved in each of the preventive activities of immunizations and tuberculosis testing. Health departments and schools often work collaboratively to provide immunization services. Compulsory immunization laws are helpful in carrying out these preventive services, but recent survey results reveal that not all adolescents are fully covered. A national immunization survey revealed mixed results for achievement of *Healthy People 2020* goals for adolescent vaccination (80% coverage). Whereas there were significant increases in vaccination rates for hepatitis B, varicella, tetanus/diphtheria/acellular pertussis (Tdap), and meningococcal conjugate vaccine, HPV lagged behind at 57% for females and 35% for males (Schneyer, Yang, & Bocchini, 2015). It is important for adolescents, as well as adults, to get a single dose of Tdap to protect themselves and infants who may be around them from whooping cough. Although pertussis in adolescents or adults often manifests as an upper respiratory infection with a chronic cough, for infants who have not yet been fully immunized, it can lead to serious complications. It is now recommended that all pregnant women receive a Tdap dose with each pregnancy, including adolescents who may have more recently received an update (Schneyer et al., 2015).

In the recent past, adolescents were only given "catch-up" vaccinations (those missed in childhood), except for a tetanus/diphtheria booster. Now, recommended immunizations include Tdap, meningococcal vaccine (MCV4), pneumococcal polysaccharide vaccine (PPV), both hepatitis A and B, influenza vaccine, and HPV vaccine for both boys and girls—along with any missed vaccines, for example, polio and varicella (see Figs. 22–2 and 22–3). Often, school nurses and community health nurses work with nurse volunteers to provide immunization clinics at elementary and middle schools; these are convenient for adolescents and their parents. School-based clinics are also great places to catch adolescents who need updated immunizations. There is some evidence that adolescent vaccinations are becoming more available at retail pharmacies—much like flu shots for older adults (Goad, Taitel, Fensterheim, & Cannon, 2013; Skiles, Cai, English, & Ford, 2011). Researchers note, however, that higher levels of medical and dental health needs are met when children and adolescents have a *medical home* (or regular source of primary care). But only 56.9% of 1- to 17-year-olds did in 2007, and adolescents were less likely than younger children to have a medical home (Strickland, Jones, Ghandour, Kogan, & Newacheck, 2011). Another study, using national data from 2007 to 2008 survey and telephone follow-up, noted 58% of children overall had a medical home, but only 53.4% of those ages 12 to 17 (Aysola, Bitton, Zaslavsky, & Ayanian, 2013).

Although immunization clinics may improve rates of compliance, it is recommended that 11- and 12-year-olds be scheduled for routine health care visits to their physicians, so that immunizations can be administered, checked, and updated. Adolescents who have not had chickenpox and have not received prior vaccination should be given the varicella virus vaccine. Routine visits give the health care provider an opportunity to discuss risk behaviors and health concerns with adolescents and to intervene early as problems arise.

In addition to immunizations required for school entry, many states or local school districts now require TB skin tests for school-age children and adolescents. Children have a much higher risk of disease progression than do adults. Annual testing is often recommended for children and adolescents from high-risk populations (CDC, 2014d). Annual testing is often recommended for children and adolescents from high-risk populations. Targeted TB skin testing identifies adolescents and children at risk for latent TB who could benefit from treatment to prevent progression of the disease. See Chapter 8 for more on TB skin testing. The following questions should be asked to determine risk:

- Was the child born outside the United States? If so, where? (Children born in Asia, Africa, Latin America, and Eastern Europe require TB skin testing.)
- Has the child traveled outside the United States? If so, where and with whom? (If child stayed with friends/family in Latin America, Asia, Africa, or Eastern Europe for 1 week or more, TB skin testing should be done.)
- Has the child been exposed to anyone with TB? Who? Did contact person have active or latent TB? When was child exposed and what was the nature of contact? (Notify the local health department if the child had contact with a person having TB.)
- Does the child have close contact with a person who had a positive TB skin test? (Other questions may relate to contact with persons who have HIV, have been in jail or shelters, or are injection drug users; or if the child ingested raw milk/products? Does the child live in a household with members who were born or traveled outside the United States?)
- Positive skin tests for children and adolescents have three cutoff points (CDC, 2014c):
  - Induration ≥5 mm (if child has close contact with known or suspected TB, if child or adolescent is suspected of having TB disease, if child or adolescent's immune system is suppressed).
  - Induration ≥10 mm (if child or adolescent is at an increased risk of disseminated disease or if child or adolescent has been exposed to cases of TB disease).
  - Induration ≥15 mm (if child is 4 years old or older and has no known risk factors).

Education and Social Services

The health education of school-age children and adolescents includes a wide variety of approaches and can range from the basics of handwashing for elementary school students (Lecky et al., 2011) to hearing conservation for students who like to listen to loud music (Blood & Blood, 2011).

Parental support services are commonly available through many public and private agencies, including churches. These services can have long-range effects on the health of school-age children, because emotionally healthy parents and stable families offer a healthful environment and support system for children and can facilitate their progress in school. In most states, community health nurses provide teaching and counseling services to parents in their homes and in groups. School nurses, school mental health counselors, and school psychologists also organize parent support groups in local schools. This is particularly important during periods of transition (e.g., from elementary to middle school, from middle to high school). Discussing parenting concerns and increasing parents' understanding of normal child growth and development help to allay fears and prevent problems. Through such efforts, family violence and abuse can be averted. Reduction in rates of divorce and the attendant consequences may also be a benefit of strengthening family resilience.

Family planning programs, often stationed strategically in inner cities, near schools, or in school-based clinics, provide birth control information and counseling to young people. In some communities, the school-based clinic dispenses condoms. In many states, adolescents have the right to consent for sexual and reproductive health care without parental permission. It is important that health care providers be aware of local and regional options for counseling (Society for Adolescent Health and Medicine, 2014). PHNs, in collaboration with an interdisciplinary team, are usually the primary care providers in these programs. Their major goals are to prevent teenage pregnancy, educate teens about reproduction and contraception, and encourage responsible sexual behavior. Teaching parents about adolescent sexuality is important, as parents can influence their child's sexual behavior (Dittus et al., 2015). A review of studies examining caregiver-targeted interventions that address adolescent risk/protective behaviors noted that personal contact targeting parents and other caregivers leads to effective improvements in adolescent health (Burrus et al., 2012; Dittus et al., 2015). Other forms of contact were not as effective (e.g., Internet), but person-to-person interventions were the most effective.

Providing STI services and HIV/AIDS education can be a daunting task. Many young people with STIs are often afraid or embarrassed to seek help, and others who have been exposed to the HIV virus may not know that they are infected. Gay and bisexual young men are particularly at risk, as are youth who have been sexually abused. Furthermore, community health professionals receive very little training in these areas and may be uncomfortable and judgmental in their approaches. Quality services that are easily accessible, provide anonymity for clients, are age appropriate or targeted to adolescents, and are staffed with health care providers who exhibit nonjudgmental attitudes are better able to attract young people who need help (Borawski et al., 2015). Some argue that drastic changes in the provision of services to young people are needed to effect change, as adolescents often feel more comfortable when services are targeted to them rather than the general population.

Vulnerable groups, particularly minority youth, inner-city residents, incarcerated youth, and LGBT adolescents, may be best reached at targeted sites (e.g., STD clinics, HIV testing sites in clinics and health departments, family planning clinics, private health care providers, schools, juvenile rehabilitation facilities, employers). PHNs are available in most of these settings; they are usually the professionals who deal most directly with these clients. An open, matter-of-fact, yet respectful, demeanor is helpful in reaching adolescents and establishing rapport and trust with them. This is especially helpful when dealing with sexual issues. Youth asset development programs, mentioned in Chapter 11, have been shown to reduce health risk behaviors, including sexual risk-taking (CDC, 2015k). Improved public awareness and education, screening of high-risk groups, appropriate treatment of infected people, and identification and treatment of sexual partners can reduce the threat of STIs (Fig. 22–10).

PHNs should educate parents about the effects of smoking in the home and its relationship to adolescent smoking. A national survey on tobacco use among youth found that smoking at home was associated with current smoking across all of adolescence, whereas smoking decreased as adolescents moved from early to middle stages in relationship to peer smoking influences (Villanti, Boulay, & Juon, 2011). Media campaigns for tobacco use prevention have been successful, as have some school-based education programs. In 2014, the U.S. Federal Drug Administration (FDA) launched the first national antitobacco campaign targeting youth (U. S. Food and Drug Administration, FDA, 2014). Targeted smoking cessation messages from peers that emphasized benefits of quitting were the most effective for adolescents in one evaluative study (Latimer et al., 2012). Social marketing campaigns to decrease alcohol, drug, and tobacco use have also shown some effectiveness among adolescents (Jones, 2014). It is essential that PHNs work with law enforcement officials, school district administrators, and other community agencies to ensure compliance with local regulations and prevent or delay the use of tobacco products. Information on smoking cessation and resources to help prevent tobacco use by children and adolescents is available through the Foundation for a Smokefree America.

Health Protection Programs

Safety and Injury Prevention

Accident- and injury-control programs serve a critical role in protecting the lives of school-age children and adolescents. They are cost-effective: seat belt laws, child safety seats, and helmet laws have saved millions of dollars in medical care. Efforts to prevent motor vehicle accidents, a major cause of death, include driver education programs, better highway construction, improved motor vehicle design and safety features, and continuing research into what causes various types of crashes. Injury prevention and reduction have been addressed through strategies such as state laws requiring the use of safety restraints, installation of driver and front passenger airbags, substitution of other modes of travel (air, rail, or bus), lower speed limits, stricter enforcement of drunk driving laws, graduated drivers licenses (GDLs) for teenagers, safer automobile design, and helmets for motorcyclists, bicycle riders, and skaters. Although adolescents may have negative attitudes toward GDLs and learner supervision requirements, these have been effective in reducing deaths and injuries (Brookland & Begg, 2011).

In developing interventions, community health nurses need to recognize that adolescents are prone to risk-taking/novelty-seeking behaviors as a result of their cognitive, physical, and psychosocial developmental stage (Johnson & Jones, 2011). Students Against Drunk Driving (SADD) and Friday Night Live activities can promote more responsible driving habits among teens. Communities can also work with law enforcement officials to ensure compliance with mandatory seat belt laws and to promote safe speeds and appropriate driving behaviors near schools.

Safety programs also seek to protect school-age children and adolescents from the hazards of poisonings, ingestion of prescription or OTC drugs, product-related accidents (unsafe toys, bicycles, skateboards, skates, playground equipment, and furniture), and recreational accidents, including drowning and sports-related injuries. Safety services assume various forms. Poison control centers in many localities offer information and emergency assistance. Whereas the federal Consumer Product Safety Commission monitors the safety of products, education programs in schools or through local fire or police departments teach school-age children about bicycle and water safety, fire dangers, and hazards related to poisoning. Generally, the community health nurse can educate families to recognize potentially hazardous situations and encourage efforts to eliminate them. Working with school nurses and school district officials to reduce playground hazards can contribute to the reduction of school-related injuries.

Environmental hazards and other dangers await school-age children and adolescents in the workforce. There were approximately 18.1 million workers under age 24 in 2013, and 357 workers under age 24 died from

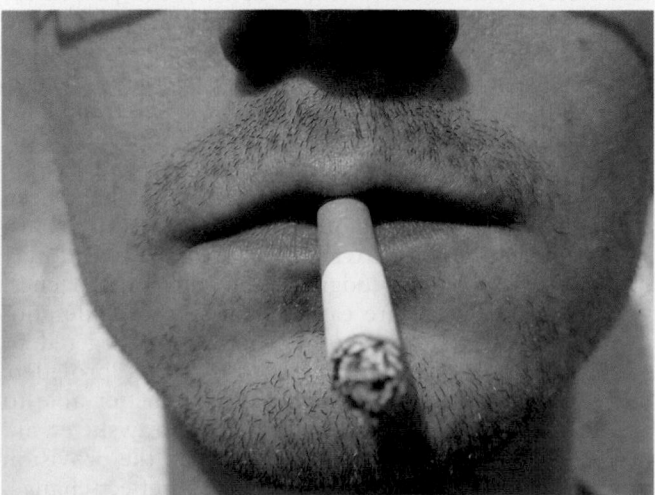

FIGURE 22–10 Children and adolescents can be influenced by adults' smoking in the home.

a work-related injury in 2012. Hospitals treated almost 800,000 work-related injuries that occurred to adolescent workers between 1998 and 2007, almost twice the rate for workers over age 25. One *Healthy People 2020* objective seeks to reduce the number of ED-treated occupational injuries among 15- to 19-year-olds (CDC, 2015l). Because teens often work in restaurants where floors can be slippery and kitchen equipment can be hazardous, they have a higher frequency of workplace injuries. The federal government notes that fatal occupational injuries among adolescents are most often in the service sector (32%), construction (28%), wholesale/retail trade (10%), and agriculture (10%). The highest death rates in mining, agriculture, and construction were among younger workers (Estes, Jackson, & Castillo, 2010). Public health nurses can join with occupational health nurses and school nurses to teach parents and children about the dangers and risks inherent in the workplace, and they can work with local employers to ensure safe working conditions and reasonable hours of employment that do not interfere with school. One study noted that 17- and 18-year-old students working an average of 14.7 hours weekly who experienced lack of adequate sleep, psychological distress, and higher physical work had greater levels of fatigue (Laberge et al., 2011).

Infectious Diseases

Programs that protect school-age children and adolescents against infectious diseases encompass such efforts as closing swimming pools that have unsafe bacteria counts, conducting immunization campaigns in conjunction with influenza or measles outbreaks, and working with hospital pediatric units to reduce the incidence and threat of iatrogenic disease. Prevention of community-acquired MRSA is a new challenge for public schools, and PHNs may work with school nurses or others to provide educational programs covering a variety of infectious diseases. Epidemiologic investigations, especially with school sports teams, may be necessary to determine the cause of outbreaks (Fritz et al., 2012).

Child Protective Services

In 1974, the National Center for Child Abuse and Neglect was established as a result of the Child Abuse Prevention and Treatment Act. The center collects and analyzes information on child abuse and neglect, serves as an information clearinghouse, publishes educational materials on the subject, offers technical assistance, and conducts research into the problem (Administration on Children and Families [ACF], 2015a).

In 2013, an estimated 3.5 million referrals were made alleging child abuse and/or neglect of approximately 6.4 million children. Over 60% of these referrals were screened and almost 3.2 million cases had Child Protective Services (CPS) responses. Over 679,000 cases of child abuse or neglect were substantiated (ACF, 2015b). Most victims suffered from neglect (79.5%), approximately 18% were physically abused, and 9% were sexually abused. There were 2.04 deaths per 100,000 children, and 73.9% of children were under age 3. More than 70% of deaths were attributed to neglect or a combination of neglect and another form of maltreatment. Nearly 50% of deaths were attributed to physical abuse or a combination of physical abuse and another form of maltreatment. Most perpetrators of child abuse and maltreatment—more than 80%—were biological parents. Fathers or male caretakers are most often perceived to be perpetrators for physical abuse fatalities; mothers are more often thought to be associated with deaths stemming from neglect (Child Welfare Information Gateway, 2015). Consequences for affected children include lower self-esteem, depression, suicide, self-abuse, substance abuse, eating disorders, less empathy for others, antisocial behavior, delinquency, aggression, violence, low academic achievement, and sexual maladjustment. Long-term emotional, social, cognitive, and physical consequences are well documented and often follow abused children into adolescence and adulthood—posttraumatic stress disorder, poor attachment and problems with trust, difficulties with language development and abstract reasoning, high-risk health behaviors, and abusive or violent behavior (Child Welfare Information Gateway, 2013). These findings were first noted in a large-scale, landmark research study, the Adverse Childhood Experiences study (Felitti et al., 1998).

Neglectful families are generally profiled as having high levels of problems among adults, reports of stressful life events, and a higher incidence of maternal depression, and these families often live at or below the poverty level. Children and adolescents who are raised in blended homes (where one parent is not their biologic parent) are at greater risk of physical or sexual abuse (Friedman & Billick, 2015). Adolescents who run away, act out at school, commit illegal acts, or engage in high-risk behaviors (e.g., drug abuse, sexual promiscuity) may be exhibiting externalizing behaviors in response to years of abuse and neglect (Child Welfare Information Gateway, 2013; Felitti et al., 1998). Young adults who have been arrested for general or violent offenses and those who use illicit drugs are more likely to have been abused or neglected in adolescence (Sumner et al., 2015).

The average lifetime cost per child nonfatal victim of maltreatment is estimated in 2010 at $210,012, and for each child death, it is $1,272,900 including the loss of productivity (Fang, Brown, Florence, & Mercy, 2012). Services to protect children from abuse are not as well-developed or as effective as safety and injury protection programs, for a variety of reasons. Most child abuse occurs in the home, so only the most blatant situations become evident to outsiders. Child social workers are also often unable to assess recurrent risk of child maltreatment. A wish to avoid legal involvement keeps others from reporting suspected cases, although this attitude is changing among professionals who work with children and other community members (Sumner et al., 2015). Teachers (17.5%), legal and law enforcement personnel (17.5%), social services staff (11.5%), and medical personnel (9%) were the highest reporters of child abuse in 2013; others reporting maltreatment include friends, neighbors, relatives (18.6%), and anonymous reporters (19.8%; Child Welfare Information Gateway, 2015).

In some areas, PHNs are working together with social workers, mental health workers, and substance abuse counselors as part of a team that provides services to families. Improved training of mandated reporters, such as teachers and physicians, has led to better reporting of abuse; as professionals and the public become more aware of the problem, an increase in reporting has occurred. Child abuse prevention education programs can be found in many public health departments and through some school districts as a primary preventive intervention. Primary prevention of child maltreatment can also occur through home visiting programs utilizing PHNs. These visits can also help to connect high-risk families to the community and promote better child outcomes (Miller, 2015).

Families often have many time constraints that can lead to difficulties in providing adequate social support and sufficient opportunities for teaching children socialization skills and appropriate methods of coping with stress. Family stressors can cause parental conflict and lead to disruptions in parent–child relationships. Outcomes for children are worse when these situations occur early in childhood and continue for longer periods of time. Programs that target at-risk families, especially adolescent mothers and young couples prone to partner violence or harsh parenting practices, may help to prevent later child abuse. PHNs, school nurses, and other nurses working in the community setting must be vigilant for signs of family stress, harsh parenting practices, family violence, and other risk factors for child abuse and neglect and provide resources and respite as needed (Miller, 2015; Sumner et al., 2015). Home visiting programs such as the Nurse Family Partnership Program are showing promising and far-reaching effects for families at risk for child maltreatment. Projected outcomes include decreases in infant deaths, child maltreatment, violent crimes, and youth substance abuse (Miller, 2015).

Child death review teams are found at state and local levels and, through their work, improvements in interagency collaboration, procurement of more comprehensive data sets, and identification of gaps in CPS have led to better services for families and prosecution of abusers, along with improvements in child protective and other community supportive services (Keleher & Arledge, 2011).

Oral Hygiene and Dental Care

School-based programs that provide fluoride rinses and dental sealants and promote toothbrushing and nutrition education for dental health can be found in most areas of the country. Fluoridation of community water supplies is considered the most effective, safe, and low-cost means of protecting the dental health of children and adolescents. Fluoridation of drinking water, school-provided fluoride rinse or gel, and dental sealant programs are cost-effective and can reduce dental caries (CDC, 2015j; FCFS, 2015e).

Fluoride makes teeth less susceptible to decay by increasing the resistance of tooth enamel to the bacterially produced acid in the mouth. Since 1945, public water supplies have been fluoridated at relatively low cost to communities. Water fluoridation has been ranked as one of the 10 greatest public health achievements of the 20th century (Division of Oral Health, 2012).

Some individuals and groups oppose fluoridation because of possible adverse effects (including fluorosis, which can cause mottling of tooth enamel). Research results have been mixed, although most studies have supported the low risk of water fluoridation and the benefits of decreased caries. In the United States, because of children's potential for multiple exposures to fluoride through drinking water, processed foods and beverages, toothpaste, gels, and rinses, physicians may prescribe lower doses of fluoride supplements or deem that they are not needed (American Academy of Pediatrics, n.d.). Although most dental care is focused on children, adolescents remain in need of dental health services. In addition to regular dental care, good nutrition, and proper oral hygiene, PHNs can promote public water fluoridation as an important program for protecting children's dental health. Nurses can also recommend that parents talk with their primary health care provider and dentist about fluoride varnish or supplements (CDC, 2015h).

Health Promotion Programs: Nutrition and Exercise

Nutrition and weight-control programs form another important set of health promotion services. Children need to learn sound dietary habits early in life to establish healthy lifelong patterns. Being overweight during childhood or adolescence may persist into adulthood and may increase the risk for some chronic diseases later in life (Dixon et al., 2012; Nadeau et al., 2011). Some school programs teach and provide good nutrition and encourage eating patterns that prevent obesity (USDA, 2015). A number of weight-control programs for overweight children and adolescents are available through schools, health departments, community health centers, health maintenance organizations, and private groups.

Children and adolescents are particularly vulnerable to media and peer pressures with regard to their food choices. Because of increased rates of childhood obesity and a greater awareness of the need for better nutrition in adolescence, legislative support to limit soft drink sales at public schools is growing. Parents and children are becoming more aware of the need to cut consumption of saturated fat, salt, sugar, and overprocessed foods and increase fruit and vegetable consumption in order to feel and look better. The community health nurse, through nutrition education and reinforcement of positive practices, plays a significant role in promoting the health of children.

SUMMARY

Physical health and illness, developmental issues, schooling, behaviors, and emotional and mental problems are major concerns for all Americans and especially for U.S. school-age and adolescent populations. Children and adolescents are important population groups to community health nurses, because their physical and emotional health can affect not only their academic achievement but also the future of society. This population particularly needs the guidance and direction that can be provided by community health nurses. Among the health problems that affect learning and achievement in school-age children are chronic diseases, such as asthma, autism, and diabetes; behavioral and learning problems, such as ADHD and learning and other disabilities; poverty; injuries; communicable diseases, such as measles and mumps; and dietary problems involving inadequate nutrition, obesity, inactivity, and poor dental health.

One nationwide measure to prevent communicable diseases is the federally and state-mandated immunization program for school-age children and adolescents. Among vaccines given on schedule throughout childhood are those that prevent polio, smallpox, diphtheria, tetanus, typhoid, and many other diseases, so that these diseases will not be passed from one person to another in epidemic proportion.

Mortality rates for children and adolescents have decreased dramatically since the early 1900s, but morbidity rates remain high. Children and adolescents are vulnerable to many illnesses, injuries, and emotional problems, often as a result of a complex and stressful environment. Violence against children and deaths because of homicide occur in the United States at alarming rates. Unintentional injuries, suicide, and homicide are the leading threats to life and health for adolescents. Other health problems include alcohol and drug abuse, unplanned pregnancies, STIs and HIV/AIDS, and poor nutrition. All of these problems create major challenges for the community health nurse who seeks to prevent illness and injury among children and adolescents and to promote their health.

Among the objectives for children and adolescents proposed by *Healthy People 2020*, some key goals are reduction of alcohol-related unintentional injuries; declines in violent behaviors, suicide, and mental health issues; and more responsible reproductive health behaviors. Barriers to achieving these goals vary. Some include economic inequities; lack of sufficient immunization, educational, and community-supported health programs; and the presence of risk behaviors typical among developing youth. Community health nurses play a large role in promoting the health of young people, their families, and communities through education programs and by developing strategies to support healthy growth and development and prevent risky behaviors that lead to injury, teen pregnancy, and sometimes death.

Health services for children and adolescents span three categories: prevention, health protection, and health promotion. The community health nurse plays a vital role in each. Preventive services may include immunization programs, parental support services, family planning programs, services for those with STIs, and alcohol and drug abuse prevention programs. Health protection services often include accident and injury control, programs to reduce environmental hazards and control infectious diseases, and services to protect children and adolescents from child abuse and neglect. Health promotion services may include programs in nutrition and weight control, along with HIV/AIDS prevention, and smoking, alcohol, and drug abuse education. PHNs are integral to the health and well-being of children and adolescents, through their work with families, schools, and other community agencies.

ACTIVITIES TO PROMOTE CRITICAL THINKING

1. You are a community health nurse assigned to work at a school. You learn that more than 20% of the students in this school district are receiving Ritalin, Adderall, or some other medication for treating ADHD. What issues should you consider in determining whether these medications are being appropriately prescribed?

2. What is the major cause of death among younger school-age children? Adolescents? What community-wide interventions could be initiated to prevent these deaths? Select one intervention for children and one for adolescents and describe how you and a group of community health professionals might develop effective preventive measures.

3. A 14-year-old girl from a middle-class family and a 14-year-old girl from a poor family both come to the health department clinic where you work. The girls have similar symptoms that suggest gonorrhea. Would your assessment and intervention be the same for the two girls? What are your values and attitudes toward people with infections that are sexually transmitted? Does social class, race, age, or sex make any difference in how you feel about them? What is one action the community health nurse can take to prevent such infections in this population group?

4. Discuss possible methods of doing nutritional assessments in school-age children and adolescents. What programs could be instituted to encourage healthier diets and increased exercise? What other factors might need to be considered? How could you, as a community health nurse, work with schools and parents to increase physical activity and improve nutrition for school-age children and adolescents?

5. A new elementary school to which you have been assigned has repeated outbreaks of head lice and very limited access to health care. Search the Web for research into the causes for recurrent head lice infestations and effective over-the-counter treatment products. Are "no-nit" policies effective? Why or why not? Discuss possible education programs you might implement or other innovative methods of treatment and control you might be able to institute.

6. Your school district allows personal exemptions for vaccination (i.e., parents can refuse to get mandatory vaccinations for their children based upon personal, not solely religious, beliefs). You have been informed by the public health department that there is a measles epidemic in your county. What actions will you need to take in regard to these unvaccinated children and their families? What are your feelings and attitudes about personal exemptions?

REFERENCES

Abdus, S., Hudson, J., Hill, S. C., & Seldon, T. M. (2014). Children's health insurance program premiums adversely affect enrollment, especially among lower-income children. *Health Affairs, 33*(8), 1353–1360.

Addy, S., & Wight, V. R. (2012). *Basic facts about low-income children, 2010: Children under age 18*. Retrieved from http://www.nccp.org/publications/pub_1049.html

Adler-Tapia, R. (2012). *Child psychotherapy: Integrating developmental theory into clinical practice*. New York, NY: Springer Publishing Co.

Administration on Children and Families. (2015a). *Child abuse & neglect*. Retrieved from http://www.acf.hhs.gov/programs/cb/focus-areas/child-abuse-neglect

Administration on Children and Families. (2015b). *Child maltreatment 2013*. Retrieved from http://www.acf.hhs.gov/sites/default/files/cb/cm2013.pdf#page=15

Adrian, M., Miller, A. B., McCauley, E., & Stoep, A. V. (2015). Suicidal ideation in early to middle adolescence: Sex specific trajectories and predictors. *Journal of Child Psychology and Psychiatry* Advance online publication. doi: 10.1111/jcpp.12484.

Ahmed, S. P., Bittencourt-Hewitt, A., & Sebastian, C. L. (2015). Neurocognitive bases of emotion regulation development in adolescence. *Developmental Cognitive Neuroscience, 15*, 11–25.

Akinbami, L. J., Liu, X., Pastor, P. N., & Reuben, C. A. (2011). Attention deficit hyperactivity disorder among children aged 5–17 years in the United States, 1998–2009. *NCHS Data Brief, 70*. Retrieved from http://www.toxicpsychiatry.com/storage/ADHD%20NCHS%20stats%20age%205-17%20years%20US%2098-2009%20Akinbami%20et%20al.pdf

Albert, D., Barracks, S., Bruzelius, E., & Ward, A. (2014). Impact of a web-based intervention on maternal caries transmission and prevention knowledge, and oral health attitudes. *Maternal and Child Health Journal, 18*(7), 1765–1771.

Allison, K. W., Edmonds, T., Wilson, K., Pope, M., & Farrell, A. D. (2011). Connecting youth violence prevention, positive youth development, and community mobilization. *American Journal of Community Psychology, 48*(1–2), 8–20.

Alpsoy, S., Akyuz, A., Akkoyun, D. C., Nalbantoglu, B., Topcu, B., & Mustafa, M. (2014). Effect of obesity on endothelial function and subclinical atherosclerosis in children. *European Journal of General Medicine, 11*(3), 141–147.

Altarac, M., & Saroha, E. (2007). Lifetime prevalence of learning disability among US children. *Pediatrics, 119*(Suppl. 1), s77–s83.

Alvanzo, A., Storr, C., La Flair, L., Green, K., Wagner, F., & Crum, R. (2011). Race/ethnicity and sex differences in progression from drinking initiation to the development of alcohol dependence. *Drug and Alcohol Dependence, 118*(2–3), 375–382.

American Academy of Child & Adolescent Psychiatry (AACAP). (2011a). *Children with oppositional defiant disorder*. Retrieved from http://www.aacap.org/page.ww?section=Facts%20for%20Families&name=Children%20With%20Oppositional%20Defiant%20Disorder

American Academy of Child & Adolescent Psychiatry (AACAP). (2011b). *Children and watching TV*. Retrieved from http://www.aacap.org/cs/root/facts_for_families/children_and_watching_tv

American Academy of Child & Adolescent Psychiatry. (2013). *Self-injury in adolescents*. Retrieved from http://www.aacap.org/AACAP/Families_and_Youth/Facts_for_Families/FFF-Guide/Self-Injury-In-Adolescents-073.aspx

American Academy of Pediatrics. (2015). *Health and safety of children with ADHD*. Retrieved from https://www.healthychildren.org/English/health-issues/conditions/adhd/Pages/Health-and-Safety-of-Children-with-ADHD.aspx

American Academy of Pediatrics. (n.d.). *Children's oral health*. Retrieved from https://www2.aap.org/oralhealth/pact/ch6_sect3b.cfm

American Cancer Society. (n.d.). *Children diagnosed with cancer: Returning to school.* Retrieved from http://www.cancer.org/treatment/childrenandcancer/whenyourchildhascancer/

American Dietetic Association. (2011). Position of the American Dietetic Association: Nutrition intervention in the treatment of eating disorders. *Journal of the American Dietetic Association, 111,* 1236–1241.

American Heart Association. (2014). *Dietary Recommendations for healthy children.* Retrieved from http://www.heart.org/HEARTORG/GettingHealthy/HealthierKids/HowtoMakeaHealthyHome/Dietary-Recommendations-for-HealthyChildren_UCM_303886_Article.jsp#.Vm4ukUorKM8

American Psychological Association. (n.d.). *Effects of poverty, hunger, and homelessness on children and youth.* Retrieved from http://www.apa.org/pi/families/poverty.aspx

American Psychological Association Zero Tolerance Task Force. (2008). Are zero tolerance policies effective in the schools? An evidentiary review and recommendations. *American Psychologist, 63*(9), 852–862.

Anthony, E., King, B., & Austin, M. J. (2011). Reducing child poverty by promoting child well-being: Identifying best practices in a time of great need. *Children and Youth Services Review, 33,* 1999–2009.

Anxiety and Depression Association of America (ADAA). (n.d.). *School refusal.* Retrieved from http://www.adaa.org/living-with-anxiety/children/school-refusal

Arts, W. F. (2012). Risk and causes of death in children with a seizure disorder. *Developmental Medicine & Child Neurology, 54,* 582–587.

Asthma and Allergy Foundation of America (AAFA). (2015). *Asthma overview.* Retrieved from http://www.aafa.org/page/asthma.aspx

Autism Society of America (ASA). (2014). *About autism: Facts and statistics.* Retrieved from http://www.autism-society.org/what-is/facts-and-statistics/

Aysola, J., Bitton, A., Zaslavsky, A. M., & Ayanian, J. Z. (2013). Quality and equity of primary care with patient-centered medical homes: Results from a national survey. *Medical Care, 51*(1), 68–77.

Axelson, D., Goldstein, B., Goldstein, T., Monk, K., Yu, H., Hickey, M. B., Sakolsky, D.,...Birmaher, B. (2015). Diagnostic precursors to bipolar disorder in offspring of parents with bipolar disorder: A longitudinal study. *American Journal of Psychiatry, 172*(7), 638–646. Retrieved from http://dx.doi.org/10.1176/appi.ajp.2014.14010035

Barclay, L. (2012). *AAP updates childhood and adolescent immunization schedules.* Retrieved from http://www.medscape.com/viewarticle/757879

Barr, S. C., Hanson, R., Begle, A. M., Kilpatrick, D. G., Saunders, B., Resnick, H., & Amstadter, A. (2012). Examining the moderating role of family cohesion on the relationship between witnessed community violence and delinquency in a national sample of adolescents. *Journal of Interpersonal Violence, 27*(2) 239–262. doi: 10.1177/0886260511416477.

Basch, C. E. (2011a). Asthma and the achievement gap among urban minority youth. *Journal of School Health, 81*(10), 606–613.

Basch, C. E. (2011b). Teen pregnancy and the achievement gap among urban minority youth. *Journal of School Health, 81*(10), 614–618.

Bauer, K., Neumark-Sztainer, D., Fulkerson, J., Hannan, P., & Story, M. (2011). Familial correlates of adolescent girls' physical activity, television use, dietary intake, weight, and body composition. *International Journal of Behavioral Nutrition and Activity, 8,* 25. Retrieved from http://www.ijbnpa.org/content/8/1/25

Best, C., Neufingerl, N., Del Rosso, J., Transler, C., van den Briel, T., & Osendarp, S. (2011). Can multi-micronutrient food fortification improve the micronutrient status, growth, health, and cognition of schoolchildren? A systematic review. *Nutrition Reviews, 69*(4), 186–204.

Bezdjian, S., Baker, L. A., & Tuvblad, C. (2011). Genetic and environmental influences on impulsivity: A meta-analysis of twin, family and adoption studies. *Clinical Psychology Review, 31*(7), 1209–1223.

Bhawra, J., Cooke, M. J., Hanning, R., Wilk, P., & Gonneville, S. L. (2015). Community perspectives on food insecurity and obesity: Focus groups with caregivers of metis and off-reserve first nations children. *International Journal for Equity in Health, 16*(14), 96.

Blair, C. (2012). Treating a toxin to learning. *Scientific American Mind, 23,* 64–67.

Blood, I. M., & Blood, G. W. (2011). Podcasts, Google, and YouTube—oh my! An innovative online course for university students on preventing hearing loss. *Perspectives on Public Health Issues Related to Hearing and Balance, 1*(1), 4–12.

Boccio, M., Sanna, R. S., Adams, S. R., Goler, N. C., Brown, S. D., Neugebauer, R. S., ... Schmittdiel, J. A. (in press). Telephone-based coaching: A comparison of tobacco cessation programs in an integrated health care system. *American Journal of Health Promotion.* doi: http://dx.doi.org/10.4278/ajhp.140821-QUAN-424.

Boogerd, E. A., Damhuis, A., van Alfen-vander Velden, J., Steeghs, M., Nopordam, C., Verhaak, C., & Vermaes, I. (2015). Assessment of psychosocial problems in children with type 1 diabetes and their families: The added value of using standardized questionnaires in addition to clinical estimations of nurses and pediatricians. *Journal of Clinical Nursing, 24*(15/16), 2143–2151.

Borawski, E. A., Tufts, K. A., Trapl, E. S., Hayman, L. L., Yoder, L. D., & Lovegreen, L. D. (2015). Effectiveness of health education teachers and school nurses teaching sexually transmitted infections/human immunodeficiency virus prevention knowledge and skills in high school. *Journal of School Health, 85*(3), 189–196. doi: 10.1111/josh.12234.

Boyland, E. J., & Whalen, R. (2015). Food advertising to children and its effects on diet: Review of prevalence and impact data. *Pediatric Diabetes, 16*(5), 331–337.

Boyle, C. A., Boulet, S., Schieve, L., & Cohen, R. (2011). Trends in the prevalence of developmental disabilities in US children 1997–2008. *Pediatrics, 127*(6), 1034–1042.

Brault, M. W. (2011). *School-aged children with disabilities in U.S. metropolitan statistical areas: 2010.* Retrieved from http://www.census.gov/prod/2011pubs/acsbr10-12.pdf

Brookland, R., & Begg, D. (2011). Adolescent, and their parents, attitudes towards graduated driver licensing and subsequent risky driving and crashes in young adulthood. *Journal of Safety Research, 42*(2), 109–115.

Brown, G. K., & Green, K. L. (2014). A review of evidence-based follow-up care for suicide prevention: Where do we go from here? *American Journal of Preventive Medicine, 47*(3), S209–S215.

Brown, C. L., Halverson, E. E., Cohen, G. M., Lazorick, S., & Skelton, J. A. (2015). Addressing childhood obesity: Opportunities for prevention. *Pediatric Clinics of North America, 62,* 1241–1261.

Bruening, M., MacLehose, R., Eisenberg, M. E., Nanney, M. S., Story, M., & Neumark-Sztainer, D. (2014). Associations between sugar-sweetened beverage consumption and fast-food restaurant frequency among adolescents and their friends. *Journal of Nutrition Education and Behavior, 46*(4), 277–285.

Burrus, B, Leeks, K, Sipe, T, Dolina, S, Soler, R, Elder, R, ... Community Preventative Services Task Force. (2012). Person-to-person interventions targeted to parents and other caregivers to improve adolescent health: A community guide systematic review. *American Journal of Preventive Medicine, 42*(3), 316–326.

Butera, N. M., Lanza, S. T., & Coffman, D. L. (2014). A framework for estimating causal effects in latent class analysis: Is there a causal link between early sex and subsequent profiles of delinquency? *Prevention Science, 15*(3), 397–407. doi: 10.1007/s11121-013-0417-3.

Cameron, F. J., & Wherrett, D. K. (2015). Care of diabetes in children and adolescents: Controversies, changes, and consensus. *Lancet, 385,* 2096–2106.

Campbell, I. C., Mill, J., Uher, R., & Schmidt, U. (2011). Eating disorders, gene-environment interactions and epigenetics. *Neuroscience and Biobehavioral Reviews, 35*(3), 784–793.

Campbell, K. & Peebles, R. (2014). Eating disorders in children and adolescents: State of the art review. *Pediatrics, 134*(3), 582–592.

Caple, C., & March, P. (2015). *Diabetes mellitus, type 2: Prevention in children and adolescents.* Evidence-Based Care Sheet. Glendale, CA: CINHAL Information Systems.

Caple, C., & Schub, T. (2015). *Dental caries in children and adolescents.* Evidence-Based Care Sheet. Glendale, CA: CINHAL Information Systems.

Cato, M. A., Mauras, N., Ambrosino, J., Bondurant, A., Conrad, A. L., Kollman, C., ... Hershey, T. (2014). Cognitive functioning in young children with type 1 diabetes. *Journal of the International Neuropsychological Society, 20,* 238–247.

Cavazos-Rehg, P., Krauss, M., Spitznagel, E., Iguchi, M., Schootman, M., Cottler, L., ... Bierut, L. J. (2012). Associations between sexuality education in schools and adolescent birthrates. *Archives of Pediatrics and Adolescent Medicine, 166*(2), 134–140.

Center for Behavioral Health Statistics and Quality. (2015). *Behavioral health trends in the United States: Results from the 2014 national survey on drug use and health.* Retrieved from http://www.samhsa.gov/data/sites/default/files/NSDUH-FRR1-2014/NSDUH-FRR1-2014.pdf

Centers for Disease Control and Prevention (CDC). (2012a). *Protect the ones you love: Child injuries are preventable*. Retrieved from http://www.cdc.gov/safechild/

Centers for Disease Control and Prevention (CDC). (2012b). *Oral health disparities as determined by selected Healthy People 2020 oral health objectives for the United States, 2009–2010*. Retrieved from http://www.cdc.gov/nchs/data/databriefs/db104.htm.

Centers for Disease Control and Prevention (CDC). (2013a). *Head lice*. Retrieved from http://www.cdc.gov/parasites/lice/head/epi.html

Centers for Disease Control and Prevention (CDC). (2013b). *Methcillin-resistant Staphylococcus aureus (MRSA infections): Information and advice about MRSA for school and daycare officials*. Retrieved from http://www.cdc.gov/mrsa/community/schools/

Centers for Disease Control and Prevention (CDC). (2013c). *Youth risk behavior surveillance system*. Retrieved from http://www.cdc.gov/HealthyYouth/yrbs/

Centers for Disease Control and Prevention (CDC). (2014a). *Community report on autism: 2014*. Retrieved from http://www.cdc.gov/ncbddd/autism/states/comm_report_autism_2014.pdf

Centers for Disease Control and Prevention (CDC). (2014b). *Health and academic achievement*. Retrieved from http://www.cdc.gov/healthyyouth/health_and_academics/pdf/health-academic-achievement.pdf

Centers for Disease Control and Prevention (CDC). (2014c). *Tuberculosis: Testing & diagnosis*. Retrieved from http://www.cdc.gov/tb/topic/testing/

Centers for Disease Control and Prevention (CDC). (2014d). *Tuberculosis (TB): Children*. Retrieved from http://www.cdc.gov/tb/topic/populations/tbinchildren/default.htm

Centers for Disease Control and Prevention (CDC). (2015a). *Attention-deficit/hyperactivity disorder (ADHD)*. Retrieved from http://www.cdc.gov/ncbddd/adhd/data.html

Centers for Disease Control and Prevention (CDC). (2015b). *Childhood obesity facts*. Retrieved from http://www.cdc.gov/healthyschools/obesity/facts.htm

Centers for Disease Control and Prevention (CDC). (2015c). *Competitive meals in schools*. Retrieved from http://www.cdc.gov/healthyschools/nutrition/standards.htm

Centers for Disease Control and Prevention (CDC). (2015d). *Dental caries and sealant prevalence in children and adolescents in the United States, 2011–2012*. Retrieved from http://www.cdc.gov/nchs/data/databriefs/db191.htm#how

Centers for Disease Control and Prevention (CDC). (2015e). *Developmental disabilities*. Retrieved from http://www.cdc.gov/ncbddd/developmentaldisabilities/about.html

Centers for Disease Control and Prevention (CDC). (2015f). *Heads up*. Retrieved from http://www.cdc.gov/headsup/index.html

Centers for Disease Control and Prevention (CDC). (2015g). *Measles cases and outbreaks*. Retrieved from http://www.cdc.gov/measles/cases-outbreaks.html

Centers for Disease Control and Prevention (CDC). (2015h). *Oral and dental health*. Retrieved from http://www.cdc.gov/nchs/fastats/dental.htm

Centers for Disease Control and Prevention (CDC). (2015i). *Pertussis outbreak trends*. Retrieved from http://www.cdc.gov/pertussis/outbreaks/trends.html

Centers for Disease Control and Prevention (CDC). (2015j). *School-based dental sealant programs*. Retrieved from http://www.cdc.gov/oralhealth/dental_sealant_program/

Centers for Disease Control and Prevention (CDC). (2015k). *2014 sexually transmitted diseases surveillance*. Retrieved from http://www.cdc.gov/std/stats14/default.htm

Centers for Disease Control and Prevention (CDC). (2015l). *Young worker safety and health*. Retrieved from http://www.cdc.gov/niosh/topics/youth/

Centers for Disease Control and Prevention (CDC). (2015m). *HIV among youth*. Retrieved from http://www.cdc.gov/hiv/group/age/youth/

Centers for Disease Control & Prevention (CDC). (2016). *National suicide statistics*. Retrieved from http://www.cdc.gov/violenceprevention/suicide/statistics/

Champaloux, S. W., & Young, D. R. (2015). Childhood chronic health conditions and educational attainment: A social ecological approach. *Journal of Adolescent Health, 56*(1), 98–105.

Charach, A., & Fernandez, R. (2013). Enhancing ADHD medication adherence: Challenges and opportunities. *Current Psychiatry Report, 15*(371), 1–8. doi: 10.1007/s11920-013-0371-6.

Charach, A., Yeung, E., Volpe, T., Goodale, T., & Dosreis, S. (2014). Exploring stimulant treatment in ADHD: Narratives of young adolescents and their parents. *BMC Psychiatry, 12*(14), 110. doi: 10.1186/1471-244X-14-110.

Chen, C., Lin, S., Chen, Y., Huang, M., Chen, T., Ree, S., & Wang, L. (2015). Persistence of psychotic symptoms as an indicator of cognitive impairment in methamphetamine users. *Drug and Alcohol Dependence, 148*, 158–164.

Cheng, T. L., Goodman, E., & Committee on Pediatric Research. (2015). Race, ethnicity, and socioeconomic status in research on child health. *Pediatrics, 135*(1), e225-e237.

Chi, D. L., Masterson, E. E., Carle, A. C., Mancl, L. A., & Coldwell, S. E. (2014). Socioeconomic status, food security, and dental caries in US children: Mediation analyses of data from the National Health and Nutrition Examination Survey, 2007–2008. *American Journal of Public Health, 104*(5), 860–864.

Child Trends Databank. (2014a). *Adolescents who felt sad or hopeless*. Retrieved from http://www.childtrends.org/?indicators=adolescents-who-felt-sad-or-hopeless

Child Trends Databank. (2014b). *Condom use*. Retrieved from http://www.childtrends.org/?indicators=condom-use

Child Trends Databank. (2014c). *Food insecurity*. Retrieved from http://www.childtrends.org/?indicators=food-insecurity

Child Trends Databank. (2014d). *Overweight children and youth*. Retrieved from http://www.childtrends.org/?indicators=overweight-children-and-youth

Child Trends Databank. (2014e). *Profiles of adolescents who are not in good health*. Retrieved from http://www.childtrends.org/?research-briefs=profiles-of-adolescents-who-are-not-in-good-health&rbp=1

Child Trends Databank. (2015a). *Children in poverty*. Retrieved from http://www.childtrends.org/?indicators=children-in-poverty

Child Trends Databank. (2015b). *Identifying the determinants of violence (Research Brief Publication # 2015-10)*. Retrieved from http://www.childtrends.org/?research-briefs=preventing-violence&rbp=1

Child Trends Databank. (2015c). *Recipient of SNAP benefits (food stamps)*. Retrieved from http://www.childtrends.org/www.childtrends.org/?indicators=food-stamp-receipt

Child Trends Databank. (2015d). *Teen homicide, suicide, and firearm deaths*. Retrieved from http://www.childtrends.org/?indicators=teen-homicide-suicide-and-firearm-deaths

Child Trends Databank. (2015e). *Unintentional injuries*. Retrieved from http://www.childtrends.org/?indicators=unintentional-injuries

Child Welfare Information Gateway. (2013). *Long-term consequences of child abuse and neglect*. Retrieved from https://www.childwelfare.gov/pubpdfs/long_term_consequences.pdf

Child Welfare Information Gateway. (2015). *Child maltreatment 2013. Summary of key findings*. Retrieved from https://www.childwelfare.gov/pubPDFs/canstats.pdf

Children's Defense Fund (CDF). (2014). *The state of America's children, 2014*. Retrieved from http://www.childrensdefense.org/library/state-of-americas-children/

Childress, A. C., & Berry, S. A. (2012). Pharmacotherapy of attention-deficit hyperactivity disorder in adolescents. *Drugs, 72*(3), 309–325.

Cho, Y. H., Craig, M. E., & Donaghue, K. C. (2014). Puberty as an accelerator of diabetes complications. *Pediatric Diabetes, 15*(1), 18–26.

Cho, Y. H., Craig, M. E., Hing, S., Gallegos, P. H., Poon, M., Chan, A., & Donaghue, K. C. (2011). Microvascular complications assessment in adolescents with 2- to 5-year duration of type 1 diabetes from 1990 to 2006. *Pediatric Diabetes, 12*, 682–689.

Chulani, V., & Gordon, L. P. (2014). Adolescent growth and development. *Primary Care: Clinics in Office Practice, 41*(3), 465–487.

Cleland, S. J., Fisher, B. M., Colhoun, H. M., Sattar, N., & Petrie, J. R. (2013). Insulin resistance in type 1 diabetes: What is "double diabetes" and what are the risks? *Diabetologia, 56*(7), 1462–1470.

Clemow, D. B., & Walker, D. J. (2014). The potential for misuse and abuse of medications in ADHD: A review. *Postgraduate Medicine, 126*(5), 64–81.

Coleman-Jensen, A., Rabbitt, M. P., Gregory, C., & Singh, A. (2015). *Household food insecurity in the United States 2014*. Retrieved from http://www.ers.usda.gov/media/1896841/err194.pdf

Cormier, E. (2012). How parents make decisions to use medication to treat their child's ADHD: A grounded theory study. *Journal of the American Psychiatric Nurses Association, 18*(6), 345–356.

Cote, S., Geltman, P., Nunn, M., Lituri, K., Henshaw, M., & Garcia, R. (2004). Dental caries of refugee children compared with U.S. children. *Pediatrics, 114*(6), E733–E740.

Coverage for All. (2012). *2012 federal poverty level*. Retrieved from http://coverageforall.org/pdf/FHCE_FedPovertyLevel.pdf

Cousins, L., & Goodyer, I. (2015). Antidepressants and the adolescent brain. *Journal of Psychopharmacology, 29(5),* 545–555. doi: 10.1177/0269881115573542.

Crugnolaa, C. R., Ierardia, E., Gazzottia, S., & Albizzatib, A. (2014). Motherhood in adolescent mothers: Maternal attachment, mother–infant styles of interaction and emotion regulation at three months. *Infant Behavior and Development, 37(1),* 44–56.

Crump, C., Rivera, D. London, R., Landau, M., Erlendson, B., & Rodriguez, E. (2013). Chronic health conditions and school performance among children and youth. *Annals of Epidemiology, 23(4),* 179–184.

Dengel, D. R., Kelly, A. S., Zhang, L., Hodges, J. S., Baker, K. S., & Steinberger, J. (2014). Signs of early sub-clinical atherosclerosis in childhood cancer survivors. *Pediatric Blood & Cancer, 61(3),* 532–537.

DeSousa, A., & Kalra, G. (2012). Drug therapy of attention deficient hyperactivity disorder: Current trends. *Mens Sana Monographs, 10(1),* 45–69.

De Vet, E., Stok, F. M., De Wit, J., & De Ridder, D. (2015). The habitual nature of unhealthy snacking: How powerful are habits in adolescence? *Appetite, 95,* 182–187.

Devore, C. D., Schutze, G. E., & Council on School Health & Committee on Infectious Diseases. (2015, April). Head lice. *Pediatrics.* doi: 10.1542/peds.2015-0746.

Dhaval, M. D., Corman, H., & Reichman, N. E. (2012). Effects of welfare reform on education acquisition of adult women. *Journal of Labor Research.* doi: 10.1007/s12122-012-9130-4.

Diekema, D. S. (2012). Improving childhood vaccination rates. *New England Journal of Medicine, 366(5),* 391–393.

Dittus, P. J., Michael, S. L., Becasen, J. S., Gloppen, K. M., McCarthy, K., & Guilamo-Ramos, V. (2015). Parental monitoring and its associations with adolescent sexual risk behavior: A meta-analysis. *Pediatrics, 136(6),* 1587–1599.

Divan, H. A., Kheifets, L., Obel, C., & Olsen, J. A. (2012). Cell phone use and behavioural problems in young children. *Journal of Epidemiology & Community Health, 66(6),* 524–529.

Division of Oral Health. (2012). *Community water fluoridation.* Retrieved from http://www.cdc.gov/fluoridation/

Dixon, B., Pena, M., & Taveras, E. (2012). Lifecourse approach to racial/ethnic disparities in childhood obesity. *Advances in Nutrition: An International Review Journal, 3,* 73–82.

Dodge, T., & Clark, P. (2015). Influence of parent–adolescent communication about anabolic steroids on adolescent athletes' willingness to try performance-enhancing substances. *Substance Use & Misuse, 50(10),* 1307–1315. doi: 10.3109/10826084.2014.998239.

Donaghue, K. C., Wadwa, R. P., Dimeglio, L. A., Wong, T. Y., Chiarelli, F., Marcovecchio, M. L., ... Craig, M. E. A. (2014). ISPAD clinical practice consensus guidelines 2014 compendium: Microvascular and macrovascular complications in children and adolescents. *Pediatric Diabetes, 15*(Suppl. 20), 257–269.

Doubeni, C. A., Schootman, M., Major, J. M., Torres-Stone, R. A., Laiyemo, A. O., Park, Y., ... Schatzkin, A. (2012). Health status, neighborhood socioeconomic context, and premature mortality in the United States: The National Institutes of Health–AARP Diet and Health Study. *American Journal of Public Health, 102(4),* 680–688.

Douglas-Hall, A., & Chau, M. (2008, October). Basic facts about low-income children, birth to age 18. Fact Sheet. *National Center for Children in Poverty.* Retrieved from http://www.nccp.org/publications/pdf/text_845.pdf

Dunne, E. F., Markowitz, L. E., Chesson, H., Curtis, C. R., Saraiya, M., Gee, J., D., & Unger, E. R. (2011, December 23). Recommendations on the use of quadrivalent human papillomavirus vaccine in males—Advisory Committee on Immunization Practices (ACIP), 2011. *Morbidity & Mortality Weekly Report (MMWR), 60(50),* 1705–1708.

Durlak, J. A., Weissberg, R. P., Dymnicki, A. B., Taylor, R., & Schellinger, K. (2011). The impact of enhancing students' social and emotional learning: A meta-analysis of school-based universal interventions. *Child Development, 82(1),* 405–432.

Egley, A., & Howell, J. (2011, June). *Highlights of the 2009 National Youth Gang Survey.* Washington, DC: U.S. Department of Justice.

Egley, A., Howell, J. C., & Harris, M. (2014, December). *Highlights of the 2012 National Youth Gang Survey.* U. S. Department of Justice. Retrieved from http://www.ojjdp.gov/pubs/248025.pdf.

Eisenmann, J. C., Gundersen, C., Lohman, B., Garasky, S., & Stewart, S. (2011). Is food insecurity related to overweight and obesity in children and adolescents? A summary of studies, 1995–2009. *Obesity Reviews, 12(5),* e73–e83.

Elliott, R., Rodgers, S. D., Bassani, L., Morsi, A., Geller, E. B., Carlson, C., ... Doyle, W. K. (2011). Vagus nerve stimulation for children with treatment-resistant epilepsy: A consecutive series of 141 cases. *Journal of Neurosurgery: Pediatrics, 7(5),* 491–500.

Epilepsy Foundation. (n.d.). *About epilepsy.* Retrieved from http://www.epilepsyfoundation.org/aboutepilepsy/

Estes, C., Jackson, L., & Castillo, D. (2010). Occupational injuries and deaths among young workers—United States, 1998–2007. *Morbidity & Mortality Weekly, 59(15),* 449–455.

Evans, G. W., & Fuller-Rowell, T. E. (2013). Childhood poverty, chronic stress, and young adult working memory: The protective role of self-regulatory capacity. *Developmental Science 16(5),* 688–696. doi: 10.1111/desc.12082.

Ewing, B. A., Osilla, K. C., Pedersen, E. R., Hunter, S. B., Miles, J. N., & D'Amico, E. J. (2015). Longitudinal family effects on substance use among an at-risk adolescent sample. *Addictive Behaviors, 41,* 185–191.

Fang, X., Brown, D., Florence, C., & Mercy, J. (2012). The economic burden of child maltreatment in the United States and implications for prevention. *Child Abuse and Neglect, 36(2),* 156–165.

Farley, T. A., & Dowell, D. (2014). Preventing childhood obesity: What are we doing right? *American Journal of Public Health, 104(9),* 1579–1583.

Fatima, Y., Doi, S. A., & Mamun, A. A. (2015). Longitudinal impact of sleep on overweight and obesity in children and adolescents: A systematic review and bias-adjusted meta-analysis. *Obesity Review, 16(2),* 137–149.

Federal Interagency Forum on Child and Family Statistics (FCFS). (2015a). *Adolescent injury and mortality.* Retrieved from http://www.childstats.gov/americaschildren/phys8.asp

Federal Interagency Forum on Child and Family Statistics (FCFS). (2015b). *America's children: Key national indicators of wellbeing, 2015: Asthma.* Retrieved from http://www.childstats.gov/americaschildren/health8.asp.

Federal Interagency Forum on Child and Family Statistics (FCFS). (2015c). *America's children: Key national indicators of wellbeing, 2015: Child injury and mortality.* Retrieved from http://www.childstats.gov/americaschildren/phys7.asp

Federal Interagency Forum on Child and Family Statistics (FCFS). (2015d). *America's children: Key national indicators of wellbeing, 2015: Child poverty.* Retrieved from http://www.childstats.gov/americaschildren/family1.asp

Federal Interagency Forum on Child and Family Statistics (FCFS). (2015e). *America's children: Key national indicators of wellbeing, 2015: Oral health.* Retrieved from http://www.childstats.gov/americaschildren/care4.asp

Federal Interagency Forum on Child and Family Statistics (FCFS). (n.d.). *Oral health: Percentage of children ages 5–17 with untreated dental caries.* Retrieved from http://www.childstats.gov/americaschildren/tables.asp

Felitti, V. J., Anda, R. F., Nordenberg, D., Williamson, D. F., Spitz, A. M., Edwards, V., ... & Marks, J. S. (1998). Relationship of childhood abuse and household dysfunction to many of the leading causes of death in adults: The adverse childhood experiences (ACE) study. *American Journal of Preventive Medicine, 14(4),* 245–258.

Ferdinand, A. O., Menachemi, N., Sen, B., Blackburn, J. L., & Morissey, M. (2014). Impact of texting laws on motor vehicular fatalities in the United States. *American Journal of Public Health, 104(8),* 1370–1377.

Fields, J. (2012). Sexuality education in the United States: Shared cultural ideas across a political divide. *Sociology Compass, 6(1),* 1–14.

Fitch, G. A., Soccolich, S. A., Guo, F., McClafferty, J., Fang, Y., Olson, R. L., ... Dingus, T. A. (2013). *The impact of hand-held and hands-free cell phone use on driving performance and safety-critical event risk (Report No. DOT HS 811 757).* Washington, DC: National Highway Traffic Safety Administration. Retrieved from http://www.distraction.gov/downloads/pdfs/the-impact-of-hand-held-and-hands-free-cell-phone-use-on-driving-performance-and-safety-critical-event-risk.pdf

Florin, T. A., Shults, J., & Stettler, N. (2011). Perception of overweight is associated with poor academic performance in US adolescents. *Journal of School Health, 81(11),* 663–670.

Folk, G. (2014). *Temporary Assistance for Needy Families (TANF): Size and characteristics of the cash assistance caseload.* Retrieved from https://www.fas.org/sgp/crs/misc/R43187.pdf

Food, Allergy, Research, and Education (FARE). (n.d.). *Food allergy facts and statistics for the U.S.* Retrieved from http://www.foodallergy.org/document.doc?id=194

Food and Nutrition Service. (2014). *Healthier school day*. Retrieved from http://www.fns.usda.gov/healthierschoolday

Food Research & Action Center (FRAC). (2015). *SNAP/food stamp participation*. Retrieved from http://frac.org/federal-foodnutrition-programs/snapfood-stamps/

Franke, B., Faraone, S. V., Asherson, P., Buitelaar, J., Bau, C. H. D., Ramos-Quiroga, J. A., Mick, E., ... Reif, A. (2012). The genetics of attention deficit/hyperactivity disorder in adults, a review. *Molecular Psychiatry, 17*(10), 960–987.

Friedman, E., & Billick, S. B. (2015). Unintentional child neglect: Literature review and observational study. *Psychiatric Quarterly, 86*(2), 253–259. doi: 10.1007/s11126-014-9328-0.

Fritz, S. A., Long M., Gaebelein, C. J., Martin, M. S., Hogan, P. G., & Yetter, J. (2012). Practices and procedures to prevent the transmission of skin and soft tissue infections in high school athletes. *Journal of School Nurses, 28*(5), 389–396.

Funari, M. (2013). Detecting symptoms, early intervention, and preventative education: Eating disorders & the school-age child. *NASN School Nurse, 28*(3), 162–166.

Gangwisch, J., Malaspina, D., Babiss, L., Opler, M. (2010). Short sleep duration as a risk factor for hypercholesterolemia: Analyses of the National Longitudinal Study of Adolescent Health. *Sleep, 33*(7), 956–961.

Geldhof, G. J., Bowers, E. P., Mueller, M. K., Napolitano, C. M., Callina, K. S., & Lerner, R. M. (2014). Longitudinal analysis of a very short measure of positive youth development. *Journal of Youth and Adolescence, 43*(6), 933–949.

Gershoff, E., Lansford, J., Sexton, H., Davis-Kean, P., & Sameroff, A. (2012). Longitudinal links between spanking and children's externalizing behaviors in a national sample of White, Black, Hispanic, and Asian American families. *Child Development, 83*, 838–843. doi: 10.1111/j.1467-8624,2911.01732.x.

Ghaddar, S., Valerio, M., Garcia, C., & Hansen, L. (2012). Adolescent health literacy: The importance of credible sources for online health information. *Journal of School Health, 82*(1), 28–36.

Ghandour, R., Kogan, M., Blumberg, S., Jones, J., & Perrin, J. (2012). Mental health conditions among school-aged children: Geographic and sociodemographic patterns in prevalence and treatment. *Journal of Developmental and Behavioral Pediatric, 33*(1), 42–54.

Gifford, B., Evans, K., Berlin, L., & Bai, Y. (2011). *America's promise alliance: 10 indicators of academic achievement and youth success*. Retrieved from http://files.eric.ed.gov/fulltext/ED540104.pdf

Goad, J. A., Taitel, M. S., Fensterheim, L. E., & Cannon, A. E. (2013). Vaccinations administered during off-clinic hours at a national community pharmacy: Implications for increasing patient access and convenience. *Annals of Family Medicine, 11*(5), 429–436.

Godfrey, E. B., & Yoshikawa, H. (2011). Caseworker-recipient interaction: Welfare office differences, economic trajectories, and child outcomes. *Child Development, 83*(1), 382–398.

Goldsby, R., Chen, Y., Raber, S., Li, L., Diefenbach, K., Shnorhavorian, M., ... Diller, L. (2011). Survivors of childhood cancer have increased risk of gastrointestinal complications later in life. *Gastroenterology, 140*(5), 1464–1471.

Gooding, H. C., Walls, C., & Richmond, T. (2012). Food insecurity and increased BMI in young adult women. *Obesity (Silver Spring), 20*(9), 1896–1991.

Gray, B. P., & Dihigo, S. K. (2015). Suicide risk assessment in high-risk adolescents. *Nurse Practitioner, 40*(9), 30–37. doi: 10.1097 /01.NPR.0000470353.93213.61.

Guenther, L. (2012). *Pediculosis*. Retrieved from http://www.emedicine.com/med/topic1769.htm

Gurnani, M., Birken, C., & Hamilton, J. (2015). Childhood obesity: Causes, consequences, and management. *Pediatric Clinics of North America, 62*(4), 821–840.

Guttmacher Institute. (2014, May). *American teens' sexual and reproductive health*. Retrieved from http://www.guttmacher.org/pubs/FB-ATSRH.html

Guttmacher Institute. (2012, February). *Facts on American teens' sources of information about sex*. Retrieved from http://www.guttmacher.org/pubs/FB-Teen-Sex-Ed.html

Haines, J., Ziyadeh, N., Franko, D., McDonald, J., Mond, J., & Austin, S. B. (2011). Screening high school students for eating disorders: Validity of brief behavioral and attitudinal measures. *Journal of School Health, 81*(9), 530–535.

Hakim, H. (2015). *Protecting children with weakened immune systems from measles*. Retrieved from http://www.cancer.net/blog/2015-02/protecting-children-weakened-immune-systems-measles

Hale, J., Reddy, L., Semrud-Clikeman, M., Hain, L., Whitaker, J., Morley, J., ... Jones, N. (2011). Executive impairment determines ADHD medication responses: Implications for academic achievement. *Journal of Learning Disabilities, 44*(2), 196–212.

Halfon, N., Verhoef, P. A., & Kuo, A. A. (2012). Childhood antecedents to adult cardiovascular disease. *Pediatrics in Review, 33*(2), 51–61.

Hammond, W. R., & Arias, I. (2011). Broadening the approach to youth violence prevention through public health. *Journal of Prevention and Intervention in the Community, 39*(2), 167–175.

Hankin, B. L., & Abela, J. R. (2011). Nonsuicidal self-injury in adolescence: Prospective rates and risk factors in a 2 1/2 year longitudinal study. *Psychiatry Research, 186*(1), 65–70.

Hanson, D., Koball, H., Fortuny, K., & Chaudry, A. (2014). *Low-income immigrant families' access to SNAP and TANF*. Retrieved from http://www.urban.org/sites/default/files/alfresco/publication-pdfs/2000013-Low-Income-Immigrants-Families-Access-to-SNAP-and-TANF.pdf

Hargrove, T. W., & Brown, T. H. (2015). A life course approach to inequality: Examining racial/ethnic differences in the relationship between early life socioeconomic conditions and adult health among men. *Ethnicity & Disease, 25*(3), 313–320.

Harrison, M. E., Norris, M. L., Obeid, N., Fu, M., Weinstangel, H., & Sampson, H. (2015). Systematic review of the effects of family meal frequency on psychosocial outcomes in youth. *Canadian Family Physician, 61*(2), e96–e106.

Healthy Schools Campaign. (2014). *Research shows full-time school nurses improve student health and learning*. Retrieved from http://www.healthyschoolscampaign.org/blog/research-shows-full-time-school-nurses-improve-student-health-and-learning

Hefling, K. (2014, January 8). *Obama administration recommends ending "zero-tolerance" policies in schools. Associated Press*. Retrieved from http://www.pbs.org/newshour/rundown/obama-administration-recommends-ending-zero-tolerance-policies-in-schools/

Hernandez, D. C., & Pressler, E. (2014). Accumulation of childhood poverty on young adult overweight or obese status: Race/ethnicity and gender disparities. *Journal of Epidemiology & Community Health, 68*(5), 478–484.

Hertz, M. F., Jones, S. E., Barrios, L., David-Ferdon, C., & Holt, M. (2015). Association between bullying victimization and health risk behaviors among high school students in the United States. *Journal of School Health, 85*, 833–842.

Holben, D., & Taylor, C. A. (2015). Food insecurity and its association with central obesity and other markers of metabolic syndrome among persons aged 12 to 18 years in the United States. *Journal of the American Osteopathic Association, 115*(9), 536–543.

Holm-Denoma, J. M., Hankin, B. L., & Young, J. F. (2014). Developmental trends of eating disorder symptoms and comorbid internalizing symptoms in children and adolescents. *Eating Behaviors, 15*(2), 275–279.

Hood, K. K., Beavers, D. P., Yi-Frazier, J., Bell, R., Dabela, D., Mckeown, R. E., & Lawrence, J. M. (2014). Psychosocial burden and glycemic control during the first 6 years of diabetes: Results from the SEARCH for diabetes in youth study. *Journal of Adolescent Health, 55*(4), 498–504.

Iannaccone, R., Hauser, T. U., Ball, J., Brandeis, D., Walitza, S., & Brem, S. (2015). Classifying adolescent attention-deficit/hyperactivity disorder (ADHD) based on functional and structural imaging. *European Child & Adolescent Psychiatry, 24*(10), 1279–1289.

Ickovics, J. R., Carroll-Scott, A., Peters, S. M., Schwartz, M., Gilstad-Hayden, K., & McCaslin, C. (2014). Health and academic achievement: Cumulative effects of health assets on standardized test scores among urban youth in the United States. *Journal of School Health, 84*(1), 40–48.

IglayReger, H. B., Peterson, M. D., Liu, D., Parker, C. A., Woolford, S. J., Gafka, B. J., ... Gordon, P. (2014). Sleep duration predicts cardiometabolic risk in obese adolescents. *Journal of Pediatrics, 164*(5), 1085.e1–1090.e1.

Irwin, C., Adams, S., Park, M. J., & Newacheck, P. (2009). Preventive care for adolescents: Few get visits and fewer get services. *Pediatrics, 123*(4), e565–e572.

Ismail, A. I., Ondersma, S., Jedele, J. M., Little, R. J., & Lepkowski, J. M. (2011). Evaluation of a brief tailored motivational intervention to prevent early childhood caries. *Community Dentistry & Oral Epidemiology, 39*(5), 433–448.

Jackson, K. D., Howie, L. D., & Akinbami, L. J. (2013). *Trends in allergic conditions among children: United States, 1997–2011 (NCHS Data Brief, no. 121).* Hyattsville, MD: National Center for Health Statistics. Retrieved from http://www.cdc.gov/nchs/data/databriefs/db121.pdf

Jesitus, J., & Kim, J. (2015, April 1). Prediabetes or T2D? *Contemporary Pediatrics.* Retrieved from http://contemporary-pediatrics.modernmedicine.com/contemporary-pediatrics/news/prediabetes-or-t2d?page=full

Jiang, N., Kolbe, L., Seo, D. C., Kay, N. S., & Brindis, C. (2011). Health of adolescents and young adults: Trends in achieving the 21 critical national health objectives by 2010. *Journal of Adolescent Health, 49*(2), 124–132.

Johnson, S. B., & Jones, V. C. (2011). Adolescent development and risk of injury: Using developmental science to improve interventions. *Injury Prevention, 17*, 50–54.

Johnston, L. D., O'Malley, P. M., & Bachman, J. G., Schulenberg, J. E. (2009). *Monitoring the future: National results on adolescent drug use. Overview of key findings, 2008 (NIH Publication No. 09-7401).* Bethesda, MD: National Institute on Drug Abuse.

Johnston, L. D., O'Malley, P. M., Miech, R. A., Bachman, J. G., & Schulenberg, J. E. (2015). *Monitoring the future national survey results on drug use: 1975-2014: Overview, key findings on adolescent drug use.* Ann Arbor, MI: Institute for Social Research, University of Michigan.

Jones, S. (2014). Using social marketing to create communities for our children and adolescents that do not model and encourage drinking. *Health & Place, 30*, 260–269. doi: 10.1016/j.healthplace.2014.10.004.

Kang-Brown, J., Trone, J., Fratello, J., & Daftery-Kapur, T. (2013). *A generation later: What we've learned about zero tolerance in schools.* Retrieved from http://www.vera.org/sites/default/files/resources/downloads/zero-tolerance-in-schools-policy-brief.pdf

Kann, L., Kinchen, S., Shanklin, S. L., Flint, K. H., Hawkins, J., Harris, W. A., ... Zaza, S. (2014). Youth risk behavior surveillance—United States, 2013. *Morbidity and Mortality Weekly Report, 63*(4), 1–168. Retrieved from http://www.cdc.gov/mmwr/pdf/ss/ss6304.pdf

Kaur, J., Lamb, M. M., & Ogden, C. L. (2015). The Association between Food Insecurity and Obesity in Children—the National Health and Nutrition Examination Survey. *Journal of the Academy of Nutrition and Dietetics, 15*, 751–758.

Keleher, N., & Arledge, D. N. (2011). Role of child death review team in a small rural county in California. *Injury Prevention, 17*, i19–i22.

Knatz, S., Maginot, T., Story, M., Neumark-Sztainer, D., & Boutelle, K. (2011). Prevalence rates and psychological predictors of secretive eating in overweight and obese adolescents. *Childhood Obesity, 7*(1), 30–35.

Koberda, J. L., Koberda, P., Moses, A., Winslow, J., Bienkiewicz, A., & Koberda, L. (2014). Z-score LORETA neurofeedback as a potential therapy for ADHD. *Biofeedback, 42*(2), 74–81.

Koch, W. (2012, March 13). Teen tobacco "epidemic" shocks Surgeon General. *USA Today.* Retrieved from http://yourlife.usatoday.com/health/story/2012-03-08/Teen-tobacco-epidemic-shocks-surgeon-general/53404520/1

Kochanek, K., Kirmeyer, S., Martin, J., Strobino, D., & Guyer, B. (2012). Annual summary of vital statistics: 2009. *Pediatrics, 129*(2), 338–351.

Kong, G., Carmenga, D., & Krishnan-Sarin, S. (2012). Parental influence on adolescent smoking cessation: Is there a gender difference? *Addictive Behaviors, 37*(2), 211–216.

Kost, K., & Henshaw, S. (2014, May). *U.S. teenage pregnancies, births and abortions, 2010: National trends by age, race and ethnicity.* Washington, DC: Guttmacher Institute.

Krongold, M., Cooper, C., & Bray, S. (2015). Modular development of cortical gray matter across childhood and adolescence. *Cerebral Cortex Advance Access,* 1–12. doi: 10.1093/cercor/bhv307.

Kuntsche, E., & Muller, S. (2012). Why do young people start drinking? Motives for first-time alcohol consumption and links to risky drinking in early adolescence. *European Addiction Research, 18*(1), 34–39.

Kwon, H. C., & Meyer, D. R. (2011). How do economic downturns affect welfare leavers? A comparison of two cohorts. *Children and Youth Services Review, 33*, 588–597.

Laberge, L., Ledoux, E., Auclair, J., Thuilier, C., Gaudreault, M. Gaudreault, M., ... Perron, M. (2011). Risk factors for work-related fatigue in students with school-year employment. *Journal of Adolescent Health, 48*(3), 289–294.

Larson, N., & Story, M. (2011). Food insecurity and weight status among U.S. children and families. *American Journal of Preventive Medicine, 40*(2), 166–173.

Latimer, A., Kerishnan-Sarin, S., Cavallo, D., Duhig, A., Salovey, P., & O'Malley, S. (2012). Targeted smoking cessation messages for adolescents. *Journal of Adolescent Health, 50*(1), 47–53.

Laverty, A. A., Magee, L., Monteiro, C. A., Saxena, S., & Millett, C. (2015). Sugar and artificially sweetened beverage consumption and adiposity changes: National longitudinal study. *International Journal of Behavioral Nutrition and Physical Activity, 12*, 137.

LD Online. (2014). *Common signs of learning disabilities.* Retrieved from http://www.ldonline.org/ldbasics/signs

Lecky, D., McNulty, C., Adriaenssens, N., Herotova, T., Holt, J., Touboul, P., ... e-Bug Working Group. (2011). What are school children in Europe being taught about hygiene and antibiotic use? *Journal of Antimicrobial Chemotherapy, 66*(Suppl. 5), v13–v21.

Levine, M. E., Cole, S. W., Weir, D. R., & Crimmins, E. M. (2015). Childhood and later life stressors and increased inflammatory gene expression at older ages. *Social Science & Medicine, 130*, 16–22.

Li, Y., & Lerner, R. M. (2011). Trajectories of school engagement during adolescence: Implications for grades, depression, delinquency, and substance use. *Developmental Psychology, 47*(1), 233–247.

Lindberg, L. D., & Maddow-Zimet, I. (2012). Consequences of sex education on teen and young adult sexual behaviors and outcomes. *Journal of Adolescent Health.* doi: 10.1016/j.jadohealth.2011.12.028.

Lindson-Hawley, N., Thompson, T. P., & Begh, R. (2015). Motivational interviewing for smoking cessation. *Cochrane Database Systemic Review, 3*, CD006936. doi: 10.1002/14651858.CD006936.pub3.

Linville, D., Stice, E., Gau, J., & O'Neill, M. (2011). Predictive effects of mother and peer influences on increases in adolescent eating disorder risk factors and symptoms: A 3-year longitudinal study. *International Journal of Eating Disorders, 44*(8), 745–751.

Lock, J. (2010). Treatment of adolescent eating disorders: Progress and challenges. *Minerva Psichiatr, 51*(3), 207–216.

London, R. & Castrechini, S. (2011). A longitudinal examination of the link between youth physical fitness and academic achievement. *Journal of School Health, 81*(7), 400–408.

Lorang, M., Callahan, B., Cummins, K., Achar, S., & Brown, S. (2011). Anabolic androgenic steroid use in teens: Prevalence, demographics, and perception of effects. *Journal of Child and Adolescent Substance Abuse, 20*(4), 358–369.

Lytle, L., Pasch, K., & Farbakhsh, K. (2011). The relationship between sleep and weight in a sample of adolescents. *Behavior and Psychology, 19*(2), 324–331.

MacKenzie, M. J., Nicklas, E., Waldfogel, J., & Brooks-Gunn, J. (2012). Corporal punishment and child behavioral and cognitive outcomes through 5 years-of-age: Evidence from a contemporary urban birth cohort study. *Infant and Child Development, 21*(1), 3–33.

MacKenzie, M. J., Nicklas, E., Waldfogel, J., & Brooks-Gunn, J. (2013). Spanking and child development across the first decade of life. *Pediatrics, 132*(5), e1118-e1125.

MacKenzie, M. J., Nicklas, E., Brooks-Gunn, J., & Waldfogel, J. (2014). Repeated exposure to high-frequency spanking and child externalizing behavior across the first decade: A moderating role for cumulative risk. *Child Abuse & Neglect, 38*(12), 1895–1901.

Madden, M., Lenhart, A., Duggan, M., Cortesi, S., & Gasser, U. (2013). *Teens and technology.* Retrieved from http://www.pewinternet.org/files/old-media/Files/Reports/2013/PIP_TeensandTechnology2013.pdf

Mancini, A. J., Baldwin, H. E., Eichenfield, L., Friedlander, S., & Yan, A. (2011). Acne life cycle: The spectrum of pediatric disease. *Seminars in Cutaneous Medicine and Surgery, 30*(3 Suppl.), s2–s5.

Maternal and Child Health Bureau. (2011). *Vaccine-preventable diseases.* Retrieved from http://mchb.hrsa.gov/chusa11/hstat/hsc/pages/209vpd.html

Mauras, N., Mazaikam P., Buckingham, B., Weinzimer, S., White, N., Tsalikian, E., ... Marzelli, M. (2015). Longitudinal assessment of neuroanatomical and cognitive differences in young children with type 1 diabetes: Association with hyperglycemia. *Diabetes, 54*(5), 1770–1779.

May, A. L., Kuklina, E. V., & Yoon, P. W. (2012). Prevalence of cardiovascular disease risk factors among US adolescents, 1999–2008. *Pediatrics, 29*(6), 1035–1041. doi: 10.1542/peds.2011-1082.

Maynard, B. R., Brendel, K. E., Bulanda, J. J., Heyne, D., Thompson, A. & Pigott, T. D. (2015). Psychosocial interventions for school refusal behavior with elementary and secondary school students: A systematic review. *Campbell Systematic Reviews, 12*. doi: 10.4073/csr.2015.12.

McCabe, S. E., West, B., Teter, C., Cranford, J., Ross-Durow, P., & Boyd, C. (2012). Adolescent nonmedical users of prescription opioids: Brief screening and substance use disorders. *Addictive Behaviors, 37*(5), 651–56.

McKnight-Eily, L., Eaton, D., Lowry, R. Croft, J., Presley-Cantrell, L., & Perry, G. (2011). Relationships between hours of sleep and health-risk behaviors of US adolescent students. *Preventive Medicine, 53*(4–5), 271–273.

Mechling, B., Ahern, M. A., & McGuiness, T. M. (2013). The choking game: A risky behavior for youth. *Journal of Psychosocial Nursing and Mental Health Services, 51*(12), 15–20.

Medline Plus. (2015). Teenage pregnancy. Retrieved from https://medlineplus.gov/teenagepregnancy.html

Melnyk, B., Jacobson, D., Kelly, S. A., Belyea, M. J., Shaibi, G. Q., Small, L., O'Haver, J. A., & Marsiglia, F. (2015). Twelve-month effects of the COPE Healthy Lifestyles TEEN Program on overweight and depressive symptoms in high school adolescents. *Journal of School Health, 85*(12), 861–870.

Merikangas, K. R., He, J. P., Brody, D., Fisher, P. W., Bourden, K., & Koretz, D. S. (2010). Prevalence and treatment of mental disorders among U.S. children in the 2001–2004 NHANES. *Pediatrics, 125*(1), 75–81.

Metcalf, B. S., Hosking, J., Jeffery, A. N., Voss, L. D., Henley, W., & Wilkin, T. J. (2011). Fatness leads to inactivity, but inactivity does not lead to fatness: A longitudinal study in children (EarlyBird 45). *Archives of Disease in Childhood, 96*(10), 942–947.

Michison, D., & Mond, J. (2015). Epidemiology of eating disorders, eating disordered behavior, and body image disturbance in males: A narrative review. *Journal of Eating Disorders, 3*(20). doi: 10.1186/s40337-015-0058-y.

Miller, P. M. (2011). A critical analysis of the research on student homelessness. *Review of Educational Research, 81*(3), 308–337.

Miller, T. R. (2015). Projected outcomes of Nurse-Family Partnership Home visitation during 1996–2013, USA. *Prevention Science, 16*(6), 765–777. doi: 10.1007/s11121-015-0572-9.

Millichap, J. G., & Yee, M. W. (2012). The diet factor in attention-deficit/hyperactivity disorder. *Pediatrics, 129*(2), 330–337.

Minges, K. E. & Redecker, N. S. (2016). Delayed school start times and adolescent sleep: A systematic review of the experimental evidence. *Sleep Medicine Reviews, 28*, 82–91. doi: 10.1016/j.smrv.2015.06.002.

Mollborn, S., Domingue, B. W., & Boardman, J. D. (2011, November). *Racial, socioeconomic, and religious influences on school-level teen pregnancy norms and behaviors: Working paper*. Boulder, CO: Institute of Behavioral Science, University of Colorado.

Moran, P., Coffey, C., Romaniuk H., Olsson, C., Borschmann, R., Carlin, J., & Patton, G. (2012). The natural history of self-harm from adolescence to young adulthood: A population-based cohort study. *The Lancet, 379*(9812), 21–27.

Moreno, L. A., Bel-Serrat, S., Santaliestra-Pasias, A., & Bueno, G. (2015). Dairy products, yogurt consumption, and cardiometabolic risk in children and adolescents. *Nutrition Review, 73*(Suppl.1), 8–14.

Moreno, M. A. (2011). Advice for parents: Media influence on adolescent alcohol use. *Archives of Pediatric & Adolescent Medicine, 165*(7), 680.

Murphey, D., Barry, M., Vaughn, B., Guzman, L., & Terzian, M., (2012, November). *Adolescent health highlights: Alcohol use*. Retrieved from http://www.childtrends.org/wp-content/uploads/2013/05/Child_Trends-2012_11_01_AHH_AlcoholUse.pdf

Murphey, D., Barry, M., Vaughn, B., Guzman, L., & Terzian, M., (2013, September). *Adolescent health highlights: Illicit drug use*. Retrieved from http://www.childtrends.org/wp-content/uploads/2013/09/Illicit-drug-use-Highlight-9.13.pdf

Nadeau, K., Maahs, D., Daniels, S., & Eckel, R. (2011). Childhood obesity and cardiovascular disease: Links and prevention strategies. *Nature Reviews Cardiology, 8*, 513–525.

Najman, J. M., Hayatbakhsh, M., Clavarino, A., Bor, W., O'Callaghan, M., & Williams, G. (2010). Family poverty over the early life course and recurrent adolescent and young adult anxiety and depression: A longitudinal study. *American Journal of Public Health, 100*(9), 1719–1723.

Nakao, T., Radua, J., Rubia, K., & Mataix-Cols, D. (2011). Gray matter volume abnormalities in ADHD: Voxel-based meta-analysis exploring the effects of age and stimulant medication. *American Journal of Psychiatry, 168*(11), 1154–1163.

National Alliance for Mental Illness (NAMI). (2011). *Suicide in youth*. Retrieved from http://www.nami.org/Template.cfm?Section=By_Illness&template=/ContentManagement/ContentDisplay.cfm&ContentID=10210

National Association of Anorexia Nervosa and Eating Disorders. (2015). *About eating disorders*. Retrieved from http://www.anad.org/get-information/about-eating-disorders/

National Association of School Nurses. (2012). *Chronic health conditions managed by school nurses: Position statement*. Retrieved from https://www.nasn.org/PolicyAdvocacy/PositionPapersandReports/NASNPositionStatementsFullView/tabid/462/ArticleId/17/Chronic-Health-Conditions-Managed-by-School-Nurses-Revised-January-2012

National Cancer Institute (NCI). (2014). *Fact sheet: Childhood cancers*. Retrieved from http://www.cancer.gov/types/childhood-cancers/child-adolescent-cancers-fact-sheet

National Cancer Institute (NCI). (2015). *A snapshot of pediatric cancers*. Retrieved from http://www.cancer.gov/research/progress/snapshots/pediatric

National Center for Education Statistics (NCES). (2014). *Digest of education statistics*: 2013. Retrieved from https://nces.ed.gov/programs/digest/d13/tables/dt13_105.30.asp?referrer=report

National Center for Education Statistics (NCES). (2015). *The condition of education, chapter 2, section: Elementary/secondary enrollment: Children and youth with disabilities*. Retrieved from http://nces.ed.gov/programs/coe/pdf/coe_cgg.pdf

National Center for Injury Prevention and Control. (2015). *Understanding school violence*. Retrieved from http://www.cdc.gov/violenceprevention/pdf/school_violence_fact_sheet-a.pdf

National Center for Learning Disabilities (NCLD). (2014). *The state of learning disabilities*. Retrieved from http://www.fmptic.org/download/2011_state_of_ld_final.pdf

National Center for Statistics and Analysis. (2015). *Occupant protection: 2013 data (Traffic Safety Facts DOT HS 812 153)*. Washington, DC: National Highway Traffic Safety Administration. Retrieved from http://www-nrd.nhtsa.dot.gov/Pubs/812153.pdf

National Center for Statistics and Analysis. (2015). *Young drivers: 2013 data (Traffic Safety Facts DOT HS 812 200)*. Washington, DC: National Highway Traffic Safety Administration. Retrieved from http://www-nrd.nhtsa.dot.gov/Pubs/812200.pdf

National Clearinghouse for Educational Facilities. (2012). *How many schools are there in the U.S.?* Retrieved from http://www.ncef.org/ds/statistics.cfm#

National Crime Prevention Council. (2012). *Keeping kids cool & confident and out of gangs*. Arlington, VA: Author.

National Diabetes Education Program. (n.d.). *The facts about diabetes: A leading cause of death in the U.S.* Retrieved from http://ndep.nih.gov/diabetes-facts/index.aspx

National Heart, Lung, and Blood Institute. (2013). *Calculate body mass index*. Retrieved from http://www.nhlbi.nih.gov/health/educational/wecan/healthy-weight-basics/body-mass-index.htm

National Heart, Lung, and Blood Institute. (2014). *How is asthma treated and controlled?* Retrieved from http://www.nhlbi.nih.gov/health/health-topics/topics/asthma/treatment

National Highway Traffic Safety Administration. (n.d.). *Distracted driving: Facts and statistics*. Retrieved from http://www.distraction.gov/stats-research-laws/facts-and-statistics.html

National Institute of Arthritis and Musculoskeletal and Skin Diseases (NIAMSD). (2014). *What is acne?* Retrieved from http://www.niams.nih.gov/health_info/Acne/acne_ff.asp#c

National Institute of Dental & Craniofacial Research. (2015). *Data and statistics*. Retrieved from http://www.nidcr.nih.gov/DataStatistics/

National Institute of Justice. (2011). *Impact of child abuse and maltreatment on delinquency, arrest, and victimization*. Retrieved from http://www.nij.gov/topics/crime/child-abuse/pages/impact-on-arrest-victimization.aspx.

National Institute of Justice. (2014). From juvenile delinquency to young adult offending. Retrieved from http://www.nij.gov/topics/crime/Pages/delinquency-to-adult-offending.aspx

National Institute of Mental Health (NIMH). (n.d.a). *NIMH pages about attention deficit hyperactivity disorder (ADHD)*. Retrieved from http://www.nimh.nih.gov/topics/topic-page-adhd.shtml

National Institute of Mental Health (NIMH). (n.d.b). *Statistics: Any disorder among children*. Retrieved from http://www.nimh.nih.gov/topics/topic-page-adhd.shtml

National Institute of Neurological Disorders and Stroke (NINDS). (2012). *Autism fact sheet*. Retrieved from http://www.ninds.nih.gov/disorders/autism/detail_autism.htm?css=print

National Institute of Neurological Disorders and Stroke (NINDS). (2015). *NINDS learning disabilities information page*. Retrieved from http://www.ninds.nih.gov/disorders/learningdisabilities/learningdisabilities.htm

National Resource Center on ADHD (CHADD). (2015a). *Data and statistics: General prevalence*. Retrieved from http://www.chadd.org/Understanding-ADHD/About-ADHD/Data-and-Statistics/General-Prevalence.aspx

National Resource Center on ADHD (CHADD). (2015b). *Pediatric bipolar disorder: Bipolar disorder and ADHD*. Retrieved from http://www.chadd.org/Understanding-ADHD/For-Parents-Caregivers/Coexisting-Conditions-in-Children/Pediatric-Bipolar-Disorder.aspx

National Resource Center on ADHD (CHADD). (2015c). *Substance abuse and ADHD*. Retrieved from http://www.chadd.org/Understanding-ADHD/For-Parents-Caregivers/Coexisting-Conditions-in-Children/Substance-Abuse-and-ADHD.aspx

National Vaccine Information Center. (2012). *Introduction to autism information*. Retrieved from http://www.nvic.org/vaccines-and-diseases/Autism.aspx

Naumann, R., & Dellinger, A. (2013). Mobile device use while driving: United States and seven European countries, 2011. *Morbidity & Mortality Weekly Report, 62*(10), 177–182.

Nazari, M. A., Wallois, F., Aarabi, A., & Berquin, P. (2011). Dynamic changes in quantitative electroencephalogram during continuous performance test in children with attention-deficit/hyperactivity disorder. *International Journal of Psychophysiology, 81*(3), 230–236.

Negriff, S., Susman, E., & Trickett, P. (2011). The developmental pathway from pubertal timing to delinquency and sexual activity from early to late adolescence. *Journal of Youth and Adolescence, 40*(10), 1343–1356.

Nesbit, K. C., Kolobe, T. H., Sisson, S. B., & Ghement, I. R. (2014). A model of environmental correlates of adolescent obesity in the United States. *Journal of Adolescent Health, 55*, 394–401.

New York State United Teachers. (2012, April 24). *Fact sheet 12-14: Supreme Court rules on nursing services under the IDEA*. Retrieved from http://www.nysut.org/resources/all-listing/2012/april/fact-sheet-12-14--supreme-court-rules-on-nursing-services-under-the-idea

Nichols, A., Mitchell, J., & Lindner, S. (2013). *Consequences of long-term unemployment*. Retrieved from http://www.urban.org/sites/default/files/alfresco/publication-pdfs/412887-Consequences-of-Long-Term-Unemployment.PDF

Nock, M. K., Green, J. G., Hwang, I., McLaughlin, K. A., Sampson, N. A., Zaslavsky, A. M., & Kessler, R. C. (2013). Prevalence, correlates, and treatment of lifetime suicidal behavior among adolescents: Results from the national comorbidity survey replication adolescent supplement. *JAMA Psychiatry, 70*(3), 300–310. doi: 10.1001/2013.jamapsychiatry.55.

Norman, R. E., Byambaa, M., De, R., Butchart, A., Scott, J., and Vos, T. (2012). The long-term health consequences of child physical abuse, emotional abuse, and neglect: A systematic review and meta-analysis. *PLoS Med, 9*(11), e1001349. doi: 10.1371/journal.pmed.1001349.

Office of Adolescent Health. (2015). *Trends in adolescent tobacco use*. Retrieved from http://www.hhs.gov/ash/oah/adolescent-health-topics/substance-abuse/tobacco/trends.html

Office of Disease Prevention and Health Promotion. (2014a). *Healthy People 2020: Adolescent health*. Retrieved from http://www.healthypeople.gov/2020/topics-objectives/topic/Adolescent-Health

Office of Disease Prevention and Health Promotion. (2014b). *Healthy People 2020 leading health indicators: Progress update*. Retrieved from https://www.healthypeople.gov/sites/default/files/LHI-Progress-Report-ExecSum_0.pdf

Office of National Drug Control Policy. (2012). *Marijuana: Know the facts*. Retrieved from http://www.whitehouse.gov/sites/default/files/page/files/marijuana_fact_sheet_3-28-12.pdf

Ogden, C. L., Carroll, M. D., Kit, B. K., & Flegal, K. M. (2014). Prevalence of childhood and adult obesity in the United States, 2011–2012. *The Journal of the America Medical Association, 311*(8), 806–814. doi: 10.1001/jama.2014.732.

Oman, R. F., Merritt, B. T., Fluhr, J., & Williams, J. M. (2015). Comparing school-based teen pregnancy prevention programming: Mixed outcomes in an at-risk state. *Journal of School Health, 85*(12), 886–893.

Orzech, K. M., Acebo, C., Seifer, R., Barker, D., & Carskadon, M. (2014). Sleep patterns are associated with common illness in adolescents. *Journal of Sleep Research, 23*, 133–142.

Osterman, M. J. K., Kochanek, K. D., MacDorman, M. F., Strobino, D. M., & Guyer, B. (2015). Annual summary of vital statistics: 2012–2013. *Pediatrics, 135*(6), 1115–1125.

Oyserman, D., Johnson, E., & James, L. (2011). Seeing the destination but not the path: Effects of socioeconomic disadvantage on school-focused possible self content and linked behavioral strategies. *Self and Identity, 10*(4), 474–492.

Ozer, E. M., Adams, S., Orrell-Valente, J. K., Wiobbelsman, C., Lustig, J. L., Millstein, S., … Irwin, C. (2011). Does delivering preventive services in primary care reduce adolescent risky behavior? *Journal of Adolescent Health, 49*(5), 476–482.

Paidipati, C. P., & Deatrick, J. A. (2015). The role of family phenomena in children and adolescents with attention deficit disorder. *Journal of Child and Adolescent Psychiatry, 28*, 3–13.

Paksarian, D., Rudolph, K. E., He, J., & Merikangas, K. R. (2015). School start time and adolescent sleep patterns: Results from the US National Comorbidity Survey—adolescent supplement. *American Journal of Public Health, 105*(7), 1351–1357.

Park, M., Adams, S., & Irwin, C. (2011). Health care services and the transition to young adulthood: Challenges and opportunities. *Academic Pediatrics, 11*(2), 115–122.

Park, M. J., Scott, J. T., Adams, S. H., Brindis, C. D., & Irwin, C. E. (2014). Adolescent and young adult health in the United States in the past decade: Little improvement and young adults remain worse off than adolescents. *Journal of Adolescent Health, 55*, 3–16.

Pazol, K., Warner, L., Gavin, L., Callaghan, W. M., Spitz, M., Anderson, J., … Kann, L. (2011). Vital signs: Teen pregnancy—United States, 1991–2009. *Morbidity and Mortality Weekly Report, 60*(13), 414–420.

Pearson, N., & Biddle, S. (2011). Sedentary behavior and dietary intake in children, adolescents, and adults. *American Journal of Preventive Medicine, 41*(2), 178–188.

Pedersen, T. (2011, June 26). *Teens' unhealthy eating behaviors continue into adulthood*. Retrieved from http://psychcentral.com/news/2011/06/26/teen-unhealthy-eating-behaviors-continue-into-adulthood/27252.html

Pelkonen, M., Karlsson, L., & Marttunen, M. (2011). Adolescent suicide: Epidemiology, psychological theories, risk factors, and prevention. *Current Pediatric Reviews, 7*(1), 52–67.

Perrin, J. M., Andersen, L. E., & Van Cleave, J. (2014). Changing epidemiology of children's health: The rise in chronic conditions among infants, children, and youth can be met with continued health system innovations. *Health Affairs, 33*(12): 2099–2105.

Petrosky, E., Bocchini, J. A., Jr., Hariri, S., Chesson, H., Curtis, C. R., Saraiya, M., … Markowitz, L. E. (2015). Use of 9-valent human papillomavirus (HPV) vaccine: Updated HPV vaccination recommendations of the Advisory Committee on Immunization Practices. *Morbidity and Mortality Weekly Report, 64*(11), 300–304.

Pimpare, S. (2013). Welfare reform at 15 and the state of policy analysis. *Social Work, 58*(1), 53–62.

Pontius, D. J. (2014). Demystifying pediculosis: School nurses taking the lead. *Pediatric Nursing, 40*(5), 226–235.

Pozzilli, P., Guglielmi, C., Caprio, S., & Buzzetti, R. (2011). Obesity, autoimmunity, and double diabetes in youth. *Diabetes Care, 34*(Suppl. 2), s166–s170.

Pretlow, R. A. (2011). Addiction to highly pleasurable food as a cause of the childhood obesity epidemic: A qualitative Internet study. *Eating Disorders, 19*(4), 295–307.

Pub Med Health. (2011). *Juvenile rheumatoid arthritis*. Retrieved from http://www.ncbi.nlm.nih.gov/pubmedhealth/PMH0001487/

Qiao, N., & Bell, T. (2015) State all-driver distracted driving laws and high school students' texting while driving behavior. *Traffic Injury Prevention, 4*, 1–4.

Quan-McGimpsey, S. (2011). Early education teachers' conceptualizations and strategies for managing closeness in childcare: The personal domain. *Journal of Early Childhood Research, 9*(3), 232–246.

Quinlan, K., Shults, R. A., & Rudd, R. A. (2014). Child passenger deaths involving alcohol-impaired drivers. *Pediatrics, 133*(6), 966–972. doi: 10.1542/peds.2013-2318.

Ramanathan, S., & Hebert, A. A. (2011). Management of acne vulgaris. *Journal of Pediatric Health Care, 25*(5), 332–337.

Redondo, M. J., Rodriguez, L. M., Haymond, M. W., Hampe, C. S., Smith, E. O., Balasubramanyan, A., & Devaraj, S. (2014). Serum adiposity-induced biomarkers in obese and lean children with recently diagnosed autoimmune type 1 diabetes. *Pediatric Diabetes, 15*(8), 543–549.

Reed, J. L., & Huppert, J. S. (2011). Adolescent sexually transmitted infections: A community epidemic. *Journal of Prevention and Intervention in the Community, 39*(3), 243–255.

Reinberg, S. (2011). Unvaccinated kids behind largest U.S. measles outbreak in years: Study. *U.S. News & World Report.* Retrieved from http://health.usnews.com/health-news/family-health/childrens-health/articles/2011/10/20/unvaccinated-kids-behind-largest-us-measles-outbreak-in-years-study

Reinehr, T. (2014). Type 2 diabetes mellitus in children and adolescents. *World Journal of Diabetes, 4*(6), 270–281.

Reuben, C. A., & Pastor, P. N. (2013). The effect of special health-care needs and health status on school functioning. *Disability and Health Journal, 6,* 325–332.

Robers, S., Zhang, J., & Truman, J. (2012). *Indicators of school crime and safety: 2011.* Washington, DC: National Center for Education Statistics.

Robert Wood Johnson Foundation. (2013). *School nurse shortage may imperil some children, RWJF scholars warn.* Retrieved from http://www.rwjf.org/en/library/articles-and-news/2013/12/School-Nurse-Shortage-May-Imperil-Some-Children.html

Robinson, M., & Estell, K. (2012). Defining double diabetes in youth: Nutrition intervention and treatment guidelines. *Topics in Clinical Nutrition, 27*(3): 277–290.

Rodenburg, R., Wagner, J., Austin, J., Kerr, M., & Dunn, D. (2011). Psychosocial issues for children with epilepsy. *Epilepsy and Behavior, 22*(1), 47–54.

Rolon-Arroyo, B., Arnold, D. H., & Harvey, E. A. (2014). The predictive utility of conduct disorder symptoms in preschool children: A 3-year follow-up study. *Child Psychiatry & Human Development, 45*(3), 329–337.

Rosas, L. G., Guendelman, S., Harley, K., Fernald, L. C. H., Neufeld, L., Mejia, F., & Eskenazi, B. (2011). Factors associated with overweight and obesity among children of Mexican descent: Results of a binational study. *Journal of Immigrant & Minority Health, 13,* 169–180.

Ross, C. S., Maple, E., Siegel, M., DeJong, W., Naimi, T. S., Padon, A. A., … Jernigan, D. H. (2015). The relationship between population-level exposure to alcohol advertising on television and brand-specific consumption among underage youth in the US. *Alcohol and Alcoholism, 50*(3), 358–364.

Ruggieri, D. G., & Bass, S. B. (2015). A comprehensive review of school-based body mass index screening programs and their implications for school health: Do the controversies accurately reflect the research? *Journal of School Health, 85*(1), 61–72.

Ruryk, J. (2015, May 7). *Social media fads fuel risky behavior.* Retrieved from http://www.cbc.ca/news/trending/social-media-fads-fuel-risky-behaviour-1.3065082

Russ, S. A., Larson, K., & Halfon, N. (2012). A national profile of childhood epilepsy and seizure disorder. *Pediatrics, 129*(2), 256–264.

Saari, A. J., Kentala, J., & Mattila, K. (2012). Long-term effectiveness of adolescent brief tobacco intervention: A follow-up study. *BMC Research Notes, 5,* 101. Retrieved from http://www.biomedcentral.com/content/pdf/1756-0500-5-101.pdf

Safe Kids Worldwide. (2015). *Safe kids worldwide safety tips.* Retrieved from http://www.safekids.org/safetytips

Saha, A. K., Sarkar, N., & Chatterjee, T. (2011). Health consequences of childhood obesity. *Indian Journal of Pediatrics, 78*(11), 1349–1355.

Schauer, G. L., Agaku, I. T., King, B. A., & Malarcher, A. M. (2014). Health care provider advice for adolescent tobacco use: Results from the 2011 National Youth Tobacco Survey. *Pediatrics, 143*(3), 446–455.

Schickedanz, A., Dreyer, B. P., & Halfon, N. (2015). Childhood poverty understanding and preventing the adverse impacts of a most-prevalent risk to pediatric health and well-being. *Pediatric Clinics of North America, 62,* 1111–1135. doi: http://dx.doi.org/10.1016/j.pcl.2015.05.008.

Schneyer, R. J., Yang, C., & Bocchini, J. A. (2015). Immunizing adolescents: A selected review of recent literature and US recommendations. *Current Opinion in Pediatrics, 27*(3), 405–417. doi: 10.1097/MOP.0000000000000228.

Schumann, B., Kluttig, A., Tiller, D., Werdan, K., Haerting, J., & Greiser, K. (2011). Association of childhood and adult socioeconomic indicators with cardiovascular risk factors and its modifica-

tion by age: The CARLA Study, 2002–2006. *BMC Public Health, 11,* 289.

Schwartz, D. D., Axelrad, M. E., & Anderson, B. J. (2014). A psychosocial risk index for glycemic control in children and adolescents with type 1 diabetes. *Pediatric Diabetes, 15*(3), 190–197.

Scott, S. (2012). Parenting quality and children's mental health: Biological mechanisms and psychological interventions. *Current Opinion in Psychiatry, 25*(4), 301–306.

Shikaya, H. B., Christakis, N A., & Fowler, J. H. (2012). Parental influence on substance use in adolescent social networks. *Archives of Pediatric & Adolescent Medicine, 166*(12), 1132–1129.

Sihvola, E., Rose, R., Dick, D., Korhonen, T., Pulkkinen, L., Raevuori, A., … Kaprio, J. (2011). Prospective relationships of ADHD symptoms with developing substance use in a population-derived sample. *Psychological Medicine, 41,* 2615–2623.

Silver, L. (2011). *Doctor to doctor: Information learning disabilities for pediatricians and other physicians.* Retrieved from http://www.ldaamerica.org/aboutld/professionals/doctor_to_doctor.asp

Singh, G. K., Yu, S. M., & Kogan, M. D. (2013). Health, chronic conditions, and behavioral risk disparities among U.S. immigrant children and adolescents. *Public Health Reports, 128*(6), 463–479.

Skiles, M. P., Cai, J., English, A., & Ford, C. A. (2011). Retail pharmacies and adolescent vaccination: An exploration of current issues. *Journal of Adolescent Health, 48*(6), 630–632.

Slack, K. S., Berger, L., DuMont, K., Yang, M. Y., Kim, B., Erhard-Eietzel, S., & Holl, J. (2011). Risk and protective factors for child neglect during early childhood: A cross-study comparison. *Children and Youth Services Review, 33*(8), 1354–1363.

Sleath, B., Carpenter, D., Saynor, R., Ayala, G., Williams, D., Davis, S., … Yeatts, K. (2011). Child and caregiver involvement and shared decision-making during asthma pediatric visits. *Journal of Asthma, 48*(10), 1022–1031.

SmithBattle, L. & Fried, P. (2016). Teen mothers' mental health. *American Journal of Maternal/Child Nursing, 41*(1), 31–36. doi: 10.1097/NMC.0000000000000198.

Society for Adolescent Health and Medicine. (2014). Sexual and reproductive health care: A position paper of the Society for Adolescent Health and Medicine. *Journal of Adolescent Health, 54,* 491–496.

Sorenson, S. B. (2011). Gender disparities in injury mortality: Consistent, persistent, and larger than you'd think. *American Journal of Public Health, 101*(Suppl. 1), s353–s358.

Spies-Shapiro, L. A., & Margolin, G. (2014). Growing up wired: Social networking sites and adolescent psychosocial development. *Clinical and Child Family Psychology Review, 17*(1), 1–18. doi: 10.1007/s10567-013-0135-1.

Sprague-McRae, J. M., & Rosenblum, R. K. (2013). Chronic neurological conditions in the classroom: A school nurse curriculum for sustaining a healthy learner. *Pediatric Nursing, 39*(6), 276–282.

Steinberg, L. (2015). How to improve the health of American adolescents. *Perspectives on Psychological Science, 10*(6), 711–715. doi: 10.1177/1745691615598510.

Stovell, K. (Ed.) (2013). Researchers look at links between ADHD, stimulant medications and SUDs. *Alcoholism Drug Abuse Weekly, 25*(7), 1–4.

Strickland, B. B., Jones, J., Ghandour, R., Kogan, M., & Newacheck, P. (2011). The medical home: Health care access and impact for children and youth in the United States. *Pediatrics, 127*(4), 604–611.

Strunk, C. M., Sorter, M. T., Ossege, J., & King, K. A. (2014). Emotionally troubled teens' help-seeking behaviors: An evaluation of Surviving the TEENS® suicide prevention and depression awareness program. *Journal of School Nursing, 30*(5), 366–375.

Substance Abuse and Mental Health Services Administration (SAMHSA). (2013). *Results from the 2012 National Survey on Drug Use and Health: Mental health findings (NSDUH Series H-47, HHS Publication No. [SMA] 13-4805).* Retrieved from http://archive.samhsa.gov/data/NSDUH/2k12MH_FindingsandDetTables/2K12MHF/NSDUHmhfr2012.htm#sec4-2

Substance Abuse and Mental Health Services Administration (SAMHSA). (2014). *The TEDS report: Age of substance use initiation among treatment admissions aged 18 to 30.* Retrieved from http://www.samhsa.gov/data/sites/default/files/WebFiles_TEDS_SR142_AgeatInit_07-10-14/TEDS-SR142-AgeatInit-2014.htm

Sullivan, E. M., Annest, J. L., Simon, T. R., Luo, F., & Dahlberg, L. L. (2015). Suicide trends among persons aged 10–24 years—United States, 1994–2012. *Morbidity and Mortality Weekly Report, 64*(8), 201–205.

Sumner, S. A., Mercy, J. A., Dahlberg, L. L., Hillis, S. D., Klevens, J., & Houry, D. (2015). Violence in the United States: Status, challenges, and opportunities. *Journal of the American Medical Association, 314*(5), 478–488.

Swanson, S. A., Crow, S., LeGrange, D., Swendsen, J., & Merikangas, K. (2011). Prevalence and correlates of eating disorders in adolescents. *Archives of General Psychiatry, 68*(7), 714–723.

Swartz, J. M., & Bilbo, S. D. (2013). Adolescent morphine exposure affects long-term microglial function and later-life relapse liability in a model of addiction. *The Journal of Neuroscience, 33*(3), 961–971. doi: 10.1523/JNEUROSCI.2516-12.2013.

Sweet, L. L., Polivka, B. J., Chlaudry, R. V., & Bouton, P. (2014). The impact of an urban home-based intervention program on asthma outcomes in children. *Public Health Nursing, 31*(30), 243–252.

Taillieu, T. L., & Brownridge, D. A. (2013). Aggressive parental discipline experienced in childhood and internalizing problems in early adulthood. *Journal of Family Violence, 28*, 445–458.

Templeton, D. (2013, September 9). Music scene's Molly is not a friend to drug users. *Pittsburgh Post-Gazette*. Retrieved from http://www.post-gazette.com/news/health/2013/09/09/Music-scene-s-Molly-is-not-a-friend-to-drug-users/stories/201309090185

Terzian, M., Hamilton, K., & Ericson, S. (2011). *What works to prevent or reduce internalizing problems or socio-emotional difficulties in adolescence*. Washington, DC: Child Trends.

Terzian, M., & Moore, K. A. (2012). *Examining state-level patterns in teen childbearing: 1991 to 2009*. Washington, DC: Child Trends.

Thapar, A., Cooper, M., Jeffries, R., & Stergiakouli, E. (2012). What causes attention deficit hyperactivity disorder? *Archives of Disease in Childhood, 97*(3), 260–265.

TODAY Study Group. (2012). A clinical trial to maintain glycemic control in youth with type 2 diabetes. *New England Journal of Medicine, 366*, 2247–2256.

Tryggestad, J. B., Wang, J. J., Zhang, S. X., Thompson, D. M., & Short, K. R. (2015). Elevated plasma pigment epithelium-derived factor in children with type 2 diabetes mellitus is attributable to obesity. *Pediatric Diabetes, 16*(8), 600–605.

U.S. Department of Agriculture (USDA). (2011). *Food security in the United States: Definitions of hunger and food security*. Retrieved from http://www.ers.usda.gov/briefing/foodsecurity/labels.htm

U.S. Department of Agriculture (USDA). (2015). *Nutrition standards for school meals*. Retrieved from http://www.fns.usda.gov/school-meals/nutrition-standards-school-meals

U.S. Department of Health and Human Services (USDHHS). (2015a). *Child health USA 2014*. Retrieved from http://mchb.hrsa.gov/chusa14/

U.S. Department of Health and Human Services (USDHHS). (2015b). *Early and middle childhood: Healthy People 2020*. Retrieved from http://www.healthypeople.gov/2020/topics-objectives/topic/early-and-middle-childhood/objectives

U.S. Food and Drug Administration (FDA). (2013). *Teens and steroids: A dangerous combo*. Retrieved from http://www.fda.gov/downloads/ForConsumers/ConsumerUpdates/UCM373284.pdf

U.S. Food and Drug Administration (FDA). (2014). *FDA News Release: FDA launches its first national public education campaign to prevent, reduce youth tobacco use*. Retrieved from http://www.fda.gov/NewsEvents/Newsroom/PressAnnouncements/ucm384049.htm

van den Berg, P., Neumark-Sztainer, D., Hannan, P., & Haines, J. (2007). Is dieting advice from magazines helpful or harmful? Five-year associations with weight-control behaviors and psychological outcomes in adolescents. *Pediatrics, 119*(1), E30–E37.

van Geelan, S. M., Rydelius, P., & Haagquist, C. (2015). Somatic symptoms and psychological concerns in a general adolescent population: Exploring the relevance of DSM-5 somatic symptom disorder. *Journal of Psychosomatic Research, 79*(4), 251–258.

Ventura, S. J., Hamilton, B. E., & Matthews, T. J. (2014). National and state patterns of teen births in the United States, 1940–2013. *National Vital Statistics Reports, 63*(4), 1–33.

Villanti, A., Boulay, M., & Juon, H. S. (2011). Peer, parent and media influences on adolescent smoking by developmental stage. *Addictive Behaviors, 36*(1–2), 133–136.

Virginia Youth Violence Project. (n.d.). *School violence myths*. Retrieved from http://youthviolence.edschool.virginia.edu/violence-in-schools/survey-hoax.html

Walker, K. K., Steinfort, E. L., & Keyler, M. J. (2015). Cues to action as motivators for children's brushing. *Health Communication, 30*(9), 911–921.

Wallace, M. E., & Harville, E. W. (2013). Predictors of healthy birth outcome in adolescents: A positive deviance approach. *Journal of Pediatric and Adolescent Gynecology, 25*(5), 314–321.

Walsh, K. E., Mazor, K. M., Stille, C. J., Torres, I., Wagner, J. L., Moretti, J., … Gurwitz, J. H. (2011). Medication errors in the homes of children with chronic conditions. *Archives of Disease in Childhood, 96*(6), 581–586.

WebMD. (2012). *Drugs for children with epilepsy*. Retrieved from http://www.webmd.com/epilepsy/medicines-for-children-with-epilepsy

Weitzman, M., & Zhou, S. (2012). Commentary on household hardships, public programs, and their associations with the health and development of very young children: Insights from Children's HealthWatch. *Journal for Applied Research on Children, 3*(1), article 13.

Wheeler, J. J. (2013). Risk of obesity at 4 to 6 years of age among overweight or obese 18-month-olds. *Canadian Family Physician, 59*(4), e202–e208.

Whelan, K., Stratton, K., Kawashima, T., Leisenring, W., Hayashi, S., Waterbor, J., … Martens, A. C. (2011). Auditory complications in childhood cancer survivors: A report from the childhood cancer survivor study. *Pediatric Blood and Cancer, 57*(1), 126–134.

Wildsmith, E., Manlove, J., Jekielek, S., Moore, K. A., & Mincieli, L. (2012). Teenage childbearing among youth born to teenage mothers. *Youth & Society, 44*(2), 258–283.

Wilfong, A. (2015). *Patient information: Treatment of seizures in children (Beyond the basics)*. Retrieved from http://www.uptodate.com/contents/treatment-of-seizures-in-children-beyond-the-basics#H3

Willi, S. M., Miller, K. M., DiMeglio, L. A., Klingensmith, G. J., Simmons, J. H., Tamboriane, W. V., … Lipman, T. H. (2015). Racial-ethnic disparities in management and outcomes among children with type 1 diabetes. *Pediatrics, 135*(3), 424–434.

Witt, W. P., Weiss, A. J., & Elixhauser, A. (2014). *Statistical brief #187: Overview of hospital stays for children in the United States, 2012*. Retrieved from https://www.hcup-us.ahrq.gov/reports/statbriefs/sb187-Hospital-Stays-Children-2012.jsp

Wong-Kisiel, L. (2013). *Six questions to help decide whether your child should have acute rescue medications for breakthrough seizures in the community*. Retrieved from http://www.epilepsy.com/article/2013/4/six-questions-help-decide-whether-your-child-should-have-acute-rescue-medications

World Bank. (2011). *Health, nutrition, and population*. Retrieved from http://web.worldbank.org/WBSITE/EXTERNAL/TOPICS/EXTSOCIALPROTECTION/EXTDISABILITY/0,,contentMDK:20208203~menuPK:418901~pagePK:148956~piPK:216618~theSitePK:282699,00.html

World Health Organization. (2016). *Sexually transmitted infections among adolescents: The need for adequate health services*. Retrieved from http://www.who.int/maternal_child_adolescent/documents/9241562889/en/

Young, B. E., Johnson, S. L., & Krebs, N. F. (2012). Biological determinants linking infant weight gain and child obesity: Current knowledge and future directions. *Advances in Nutrition: An International Review Journal, 3*, 675–686.

Zimmer-Gembeck, M. J., & Skinner, E. A. (2015). Adolescent vulnerability and the distress of rejection: Associations of adjustment problems and gender with control, emotions, and coping. *Journal of Adolescence, 45*, 149–159.

thePoint: Everything You Need to Make the Grade!

Adult Women and Men

"Male and female represent the two sides of the great radical dualism. But in fact, they are perpetually passing into one another. Fluid hardens to solid, and solid rushes to fluid. There is no wholly masculine man, no purely feminine woman."

—*Margaret Fuller* (1810–1850), Woman in the Nineteenth Century, 1845

KEY TERMS

Adult
Anorexia nervosa
Binge eating
Bioidentical hormone therapy
Bisexual
Bulimia nervosa
Cancer

Cardiovascular disease
Chronic fatigue and immune dysfunction syndrome/ myalgic encephalomyelitis
Chronic lower respiratory disease
Diabetes mellitus
Erectile dysfunction

Genitourinary syndrome of menopause (GSM)
Health disparities
Health literacy
Hormone replacement therapy (HRT)
Life expectancy
Menopause

Obesity
Osteoporosis
Prostate
Substance use
Transgender
Unintentional injuries

LEARNING OBJECTIVES

Upon mastery of this chapter, you should be able to:

- Identify key demographic characteristics of women and men throughout the adult life span.
- Provide a health profile of adult women and men living in the United States.
- Discuss the major chronic illnesses found in adult women and men in the United States.
- Compare and contrast the manifestations of chronic illnesses in adult women and men.
- Identify primary, secondary, and tertiary health promotion activities designed to improve the health of women and men.
- Describe the role of the community health nurse in promoting the health of adult women and men across the life span.

The term *adult* has many different meanings in society. To children, an adult is anyone in authority, including a 14-year-old babysitter. As people age, they tend to redefine the term upward. It is not unusual, for example, to hear an elderly person describe a couple in their mid-30s as "kids." The U.S. Criminal Justice System distinguishes between adults and juveniles for purposes of delimiting types of crimes and possibilities for punishment, and labor legislation provides different protections for children than for adult workers. Even hospitals and health care systems vary somewhat as to the ages at which they distinguish pediatric and geriatric clients from middle-aged adults.

How would you characterize an adult? Does your definition rest solely on age or is it influenced by other factors, such as marital status, employment status, financial independence, amount of responsibility for self and others, and so on? For the purposes of this chapter, an **adult** is defined as anyone 18 years of age or older. Obviously, there are tremendous differences in health profiles and health care needs as people age. As adults enter their middle years (35 to 65), they experience many normal physiologic changes. However, some changes are the result of disease, environment, or lifestyle and can be modified through behavior change (Fig. 23–1).

Throughout history, the health care needs of women and men have differed more often than shown similarities. Many health promotion and health protection programs are designed specifically for women or for men. Mammography screening programs and prenatal clinics are designed with women's health in mind. Teaching testicular self-examination (TSE) and prostate cancer screening are health promotion programs for men. Programs in many areas, such as cardiac rehabilitation, stress management, and dating violence prevention, may have had one gender in mind at one time but are now established as programs for both genders. Nevertheless, morbidity and mortality statistics, historical development of research foci, and workforce changes require that health care needs of women and men be examined separately. This chapter focuses on the health of women and men across the adult life span. A physical profile of middle-aged adults is organized by body systems and can be found in Display 23–1.

DEMOGRAPHICS OF ADULT WOMEN AND MEN

Examining mortality statistics provides key information to understanding changes in the health and well-being of a population. In 2012, a total of 2,543,279 people died

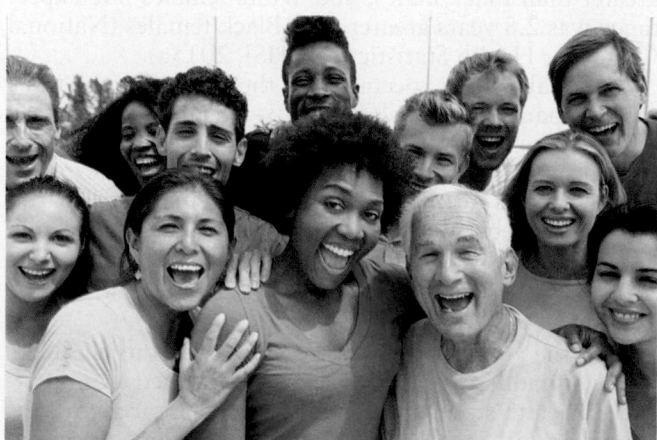

FIGURE 23–1 Health care needs for men and women of varying ages are often different.

in the United States. The age-adjusted death rate was 732.8 per 100,000 for all ages (Murphy, Kochanek, Xu, & Heron, 2015). Causes of death varied by age, gender, and ethnicity, but the 10 leading causes of death for all people in rank order included the following:

1.	Diseases of the heart (heart disease)	599,711
2.	Malignant neoplasms (cancer)	582,623
3.	Chronic lower respiratory diseases (CLRDs)	143,489
4.	Cerebrovascular diseases (stroke)	128,546
5.	Accidents (unintentional injuries)	127,729
6.	Alzheimer's disease	83,637
7.	Diabetes mellitus (diabetes)	73,932
8.	Influenza and pneumonia	50,636
9.	Nephritis, nephritic syndrome, and nephrosis (kidney disease)	45,622
10.	Intentional self-harm (suicide)	40,600

Diseases of the heart and malignant neoplasms accounted for 46.5% of deaths in 2012, and these diseases are the top two causes of death for both women and men. Differences include the following:

- Cerebrovascular diseases (stroke) were the third leading cause of death for women.
- Unintentional injuries (accidents) were the third leading cause of death in men (Murphy et al., 2015).

In 2012, deaths because of four causes increased significantly: intentional self-harm (suicide) by 2.7%, unintentional harm (accidents) by 1.1%, malignant neoplasms (cancer) by 1.0%, and diseases of the heart (heart disease) by 0.5%. Deaths from influenza and pneumonia and Alzheimer's disease decreased significantly, 5.9% and 1.6%, respectively (Heron, 2015).

Since the beginning of the 21st century, the major causes of death have remained fairly consistent. This was a major shift from the turn of the 20th century, when communicable

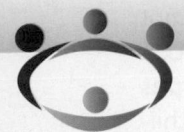

DISPLAY 23–1 PHYSICAL PROFILE OF MIDDLE-AGED ADULTS BY BODY SYSTEM

Body System	Physical Characteristic
Skeletal system	Intervertebral disks flatten over time.
Integumentary system	Decreased secretions by sebaceous glands lead to drier skin.
	Sweat glands diminish in size and number.
	Skin loses elasticity and is more prone to wrinkles.
	Hair bulbs lose melanin usually resulting in gray hair by age 50.
Muscular system	Muscle fibers decrease by approximately 10%.
	Lean body mass is replaced by adipose tissue.
	Decreased grip strength occurs at this age.
Endocrine and reproductive system	Menses stops.
	Synthesis of estrogen decreases.
	Tissues of the reproductive system (e.g., cervix and uterus) gradually atrophy.
	Uterine changes make pregnancy less likely.
	Intercourse may be more painful because of diminishing natural lubrications.
	Less frequent erections
	Testosterone levels decline gradually.
Neurologic system	Nerve impulses are conducted 5% slower.
	Cognition is unaffected, although there is a gradual loss of neurons.
	Eyesight is poorer because of loss of elasticity in the lens.
	Auditory discrimination of certain tones and consonants gradually decreases.
Cardiovascular system	By age 50, the heart's efficiency may be only 80%.
	Elasticity of heart and blood vessels decreases.
	Cardiac output decreases.
Respiratory system	Elasticity of lungs decreases.
	Breathing capacity decreases to 75% because of diminished strength of chest wall muscles.
Urinary system	Decreased glomerular filtration rate appears in women.
	Loss of bladder tone and tissue atrophy may lead to incontinence or possibly prolapse.
	In men, an enlarged prostate may result in nocturia or dribbling.

diseases, such as tuberculosis and pneumonia, were leading causes of death. The shift from communicable to chronic illness can be attributed to the significant advances in public health, prevention, technology, pharmacotherapy, and biomedical research. See Chapters 1 and 7.

LIFE EXPECTANCY

Life expectancy is the average number of years that an individual member of a specific cohort (usually a single birth year) is projected to live. It is another standard measurement used to compare the health status of various populations, typically calculated from age-specific death rates. Health statistics often report life expectancy figures at birth, at 65 and 75 years of age (see Table 23–1).

In the United States, life expectancy has increased consistently over time. Between 1990 and 2013, life expectancy at birth increased 4.6 years for men and 2.4 years for women. The gap between men and women narrowed from 6.8 years in 1990 to 4.8 years in 2013. There are, however, differences in the life expectancy

between Whites and Blacks for both genders. In 2013, life expectancy at birth for White males was 4.4 years greater than Black males, and White females' life expectancy was 2.8 years greater than Black females (National Center for Health Statistics [NCHS], 2015a).

Globally, life expectancy in the United States trails that of many countries (Table 23–2). Japan reports the highest life expectancy for males and females. In all countries, disparities exist between male and female life expectancy, some as much as 6.7 years. The smallest disparity can be found between women and men living in Iceland, at 2.7 years (NCHS, 2015a).

HEALTH DISPARITIES

One of the goals of *Healthy People 2020* is to eliminate **health disparities**. A health disparity is defined as a difference in health status that occurs by gender, race/ethnicity, education or income, disability, geographic location, or sexual orientation (U.S. Department of Health and Human Services [USDHHS], 2015). Disparities in health

Table 23–1   Life Expectancy at Birth and 65 Years of Age According to Sex: United States, Selected Years, 1900–2013

Year	At Birth			At 65 Years		
	Both Sexes	Male	Female	Both Sexes	Male	Female
1900	47.3	46.3	48.3	—	—	—
1950	68.2	65.6	71.1	13.9	12.8	15.0
1960	69.7	66.6	73.1	14.4	12.9	15.9
1970	70.8	67.1	74.7	15.2	13.1	17.1
1980	73.7	70.0	77.4	16.5	14.2	18.4
1990	75.4	71.8	78.8	17.3	15.2	19.1
2000	76.8	74.1	79.3	17.7	16.1	19.1
2010	78.7	76.2	81.0	91.1	17.7	20.3
2013	78.8	76.4	81.2	19.3	17.9	20.5

—, data not available.
Extracted from National Center for Health Statistics (NCHS). (2015). *Health, United States 2014*. Retrieved from http://www.cdc.gov/nchs/data/hus/hus14.pdf

occur when one segment of the population has a higher incidence of disease or mortality rate than another or when survival rates are less for one group than another (Meyer, Yoon, & Kaufmann, 2013). Often, persons with the greatest health burden have the least access to health care services, adequate health care providers, information, communication technologies, and supporting social services. Interdisciplinary, collaborative, public, and private approaches as well as public–private partnerships are needed to develop strategies to address the health

Table 23–2   Life Expectancy at Birth for Selected Countries by Sex, 2012

	Female	Male	Disparity
Japan	86.4	79.9	6.5
France	85.4	78.7	6.7
Switzerland	84.9	80.6	4.3
Spain	85.5	79.5	6.0
Australia	84.3	79.9	4.4
Iceland	84.3	81.6	2.7
Germany	83.3	78.6	4.7
Greece	83.4	78.0	5.4
Korea	84.6	77.9	6.7
United States	80.4	75.4	5.0

Extracted from National Center for Health Statistics (NCHS). (2015a). *Health, United States 2014*. Retrieved from http://www.cdc.gov/nchs/data/hus/hus14.pdf

disparity goal of *Healthy People 2020*. Chapter 25 discusses health disparities in more detail.

HEALTH LITERACY

Health literacy is defined as the degree to which individuals have the capacity to obtain, process, and understand basic health information and services needed to make appropriate health-related decisions. The ability to read and understand health information is key to managing health problems. Low health literacy contributes to health disparities and has been documented as an increasing problem among certain racial and ethnic groups, non–English-speaking populations, and persons over 65 years of age in the United States (American Medical Association, 1999; Beauchamp et al., 2015; Weiss, 2014). See Chapters 1 and 11 for additional information on health literacy.

MAJOR HEALTH PROBLEMS OF ADULTS

Morbidity and mortality among adults vary substantially by age, gender, and race/ethnicity. Several leading causes of death are presented in this section. Heart disease is the first leading cause of death in adults and is presented along with stroke. Malignant neoplasms, chronic lower respiratory diseases (CLRDs), unintentional injuries, and diabetes mellitus are among the top 10 leading causes of death and are discussed separately. Other selected major causes of death are covered in detail in other chapters: suicide (Chapter 27), Alzheimer's disease (Chapter 24), and homicide (Chapters 17 and 20).

Coronary Heart Disease and Stroke

Over the last three decades, cardiovascular mortality in the United States has declined by about 50%. These gains are attributed to increased use of evidence-based medical therapies for secondary prevention and reduction in risk factors associated with lifestyle and environment. Despite these gains, 31.3% of all deaths in the United States are still due to cardiovascular disease (CVD). Currently, an estimated 85.6 million adults (>1 in 3) are living with one or more types of CVD and over half of these individuals are 60 years of age or older. It is estimated that every 34 seconds, an American will have a coronary event and every 60 seconds, someone dies from a heart-related disease. By 2030, researchers predict that 43.9% of the population will have some form of CVD (Centers for Disease Control and Prevention [CDC], 2015a; Mozaffarian et al., 2015; Patel, Winkel, Ali, Narayan, & Mehta, 2015) (Fig. 23–2).

CVD and stroke are responsible for 15% of total national health expenditures. Annually, this represents $320.1 billion for direct and indirect costs. The direct costs ($195.6 billion) include expenditures for physicians and other health care professionals, hospital services, prescribed medications, and home health care, but not the cost of nursing home care. The indirect costs ($124.5 billion) include lost productivity attributed to premature CVD and stroke morality (CDC, 2015a; Mozaffarian et al., 2015).

Through ongoing research, we now know that CVD affects more women than men, but there are also race/ethnicity disparities in heart disease that we are still discovering. For example, Black and Hispanic/Latino women are at a higher risk of death from heart disease, yet they are less likely to recognize their risks. The overall death rate in 2009 from CVD was 236.1 per 100,000 persons, but death rates among Black females and males in the same year were higher than the general population, (267.9 and 387.0, respectively). In addition, Blacks are twice as likely to have a first stroke and much more likely to die from one compared to Whites (Graham, 2014; Singh, Hu, Wheeler, & Hall, 2015).

Just like the general population, CVD is the leading cause of death among Hispanics/Latinos living in the United States. However, most studies on prevalence and incidence of CVD in Hispanics/Latinos have primarily included Mexicans. Recent estimates indicate that the prevalence of CVD is 33.4% for Mexican males and 30.7% for Mexican females. This is lower than the overall prevalence among Whites (36.6% males and 32.4% females) and Blacks (44.4% males and 48.9% females),

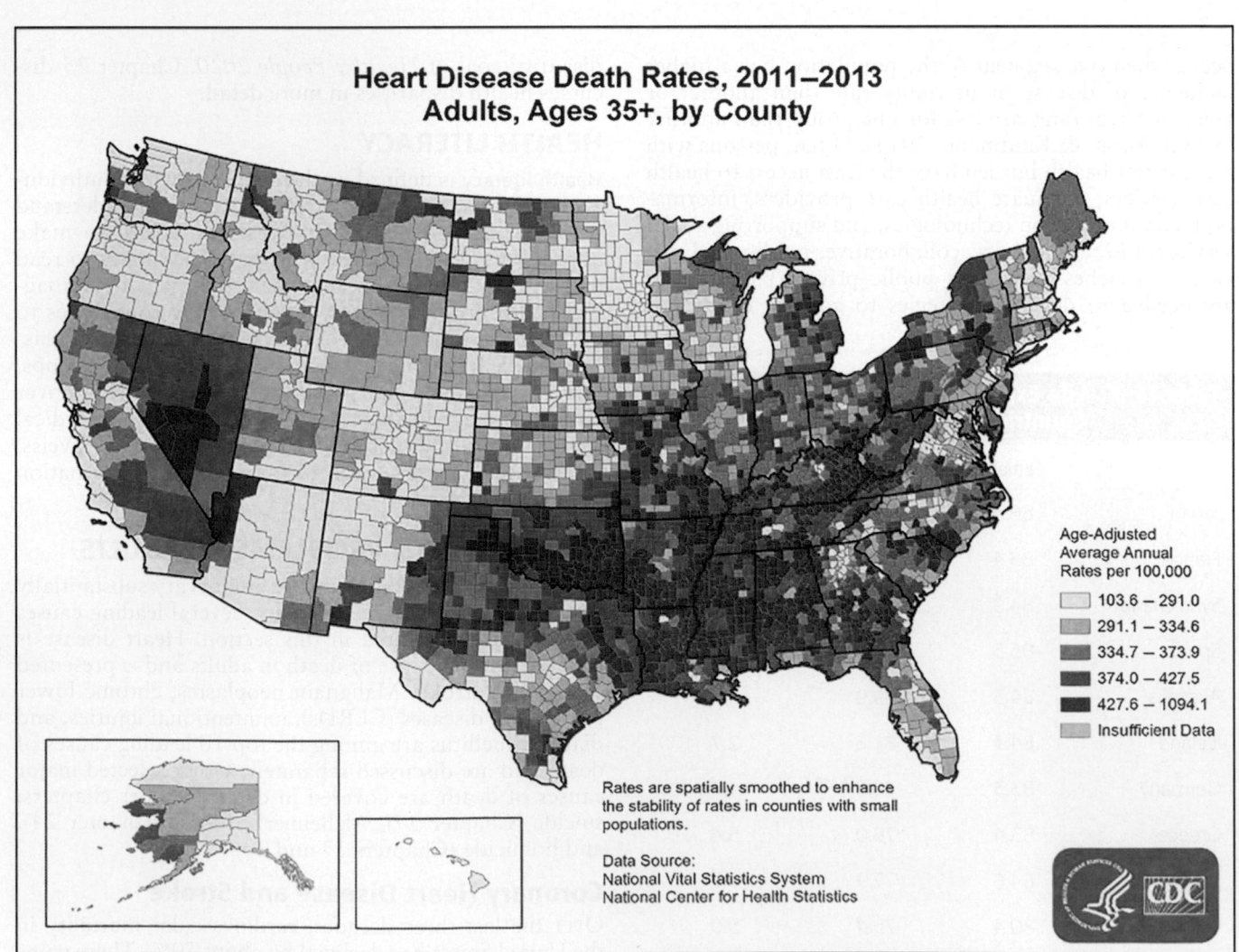

Heart Disease Death Rates, 2011–2013
Adults, Ages 35+, by County

Age-Adjusted
Average Annual
Rates per 100,000

- 103.6 – 291.0
- 291.1 – 334.6
- 334.7 – 373.9
- 374.0 – 427.5
- 427.6 – 1094.1
- Insufficient Data

Rates are spatially smoothed to enhance
the stability of rates in counties with small
populations.

Data Source:
National Vital Statistics System
National Center for Health Statistics

FIGURE 23–2 Heart disease death rates, 2011 to 2013 adults ages 35+ by county. (Retrieved from http://www.cdc.gov/dhdsp/maps/national_maps/hd_all.htm)

but the lack of data from other Hispanic/Latino groups (Puerto Ricans, Central and South Americans) does not allow for an accurate prevalence rate of CVD among this population (Graham, 2014; Rodriguez et al., 2014).

Asian Americans are a rapidly growing racial/ethnic group in the United States, but understanding CVD among this population is distorted by the aggregation of subgroups (Asian Indians, Chinese, Filipinos, Japanese, Koreans, and Vietnamese) in epidemiological reports. Limited data suggest that some subgroups may be at higher risk for CVD compared to others (de Souza & Anand, 2014). Based on available data, it appears that CVD causes more deaths for Asian Americans than all forms of cancer combined. The estimated prevalence of coronary heart disease (CHD) in Asian and Pacific Islanders is 4.3% compared to 6.4% of the total U.S. population (American Heart Association [AHA], 2013a; Graham, 2014; Jose et al., 2014).

Unfortunately, in the United States, racial/ethnic minority populations encounter more barriers to CVD diagnosis and care, receive lower-quality treatment, and experience worse health outcomes. Such disparities are linked to complex factors such as income and education, genetic and physiological factors, access to care, and communication barriers. To tackle inequalities in CVD morbidity and mortality, actions that focus on the social determinants of health are needed. This includes development and implementation of health and social policy interventions that improve access to and quality of health care services and a reduction in poverty and unemployment (Graham, 2014; Singh, Siapush, Azuline, & Williams, 2015).

Risk factors contributing to CVD can be separated into two categories: personal and hereditary. Personal risk factors include gender, age, race/ethnicity, cholesterol levels, diabetes, obesity, physical inactivity, high blood pressure (BP), and cigarette smoking. The most modifiable of these factors are cholesterol, high BP, cigarette smoking, obesity, and physical inactivity. Heredity obviously cannot be changed. About half of all Americans (47%) have at least one of the three key risk factors for heart disease: high BP, high cholesterol, and cigarette smoking. The likelihood of heart disease or stroke multiplies with the increasing number of risk factors present (CDC, 2015b; Patel et al., 2015) (Table 23–3).

Stroke ranks fourth among all causes of death in the United States and is a leading cause of serious physical and cognitive long-term disability in adults. Approximately 795,000 Americans experience a new or recurrent stroke each year—610,000 of these are first attacks and 185,000 are recurrent attacks. On average, someone in the United States has a stroke every 40 seconds. Disparities exist among people who are at risk for having a stroke. For example, women have a higher lifetime risk of having stroke as compared to men, with approximately 55,000 more women than men experiencing a stroke each year. Risk of having a first stroke is nearly twice as high for Blacks than Whites, and Blacks are more likely to die following a stroke as compared to their White counterparts. The risk for stroke among Hispanics/Latinos falls between that of Whites and Blacks. In the southeastern United States (the "Stroke Belt"), stroke death rates are higher than in any other part of the country (see Fig. 23–3). Strokes cost the United States about $34 billion each year. This total includes the cost of health care services, medications, and missed days of work (CDC, 2015c; Mozaffarian et al., 2015).

Cancer

Cancer is a major chronic illness and the second leading cause of death in the United States (Murphy, Xu, & Kochanek, 2013). The National Cancer Institute's (NCI) Surveillance, Epidemiology, and End Stage Program (SEER) estimated that in 2012, there were approximately 13.7 million Americans living with cancer. It is estimated that in 2015, 1,658,370 new cancer cases will be diagnosed and, of these cases, 589,430 persons are expected to die. Approximately 78% of all cancers are diagnosed in persons 55 years of age and older, and as individuals age, they are more likely to develop cancer. Among ethnic groups, Blacks are more likely to develop and die from cancer. Over their lifetime, men living in the United States are more likely to

---

Table 23–3   Primary Risk Factors for Coronary Heart Disease and Symptoms of Heart Attack in Adults

Risks	Symptoms
• Age	• Pain: chest, neck, jaw, arm, shoulders, upper part of abdomen, or back
• Gender	• Chest: pressure, squeezing, or fullness
• Heredity (includes race/ethnicity)	• Shortness of breath
• Cigarette smoking	• Cold sweat
• Sedentary lifestyle	• Nausea and vomiting
• Excess body weight	• Light-headedness or sudden dizziness
• Hypertension	• Feeling unusually tired without cause
• Diabetes mellitus, HbA1C	
• Hyperlipidemia	
• Stress	

Risks adapted from Goff, D. C., Jr., Loyd-Jones, D. M., Bennett, G., Coady, S., D'Agostino, R. B., Sr., Gibbons, R., Greenland, P., ... Wilson, P. F. (2014). 2013 ACC/AHA guideline on the assessment of cardiovascular risk: A report of the American College of Cardiology/American Heart Association task force on practice guidelines. *Circulation, 129*(25 suppl), S49–S73.
Symptoms adapted from American Heart Association. (2015). *Warning signs of a heart attack.* Retrieved from http://www.heart.org/HEARTORG/Conditions/HeartAttack/WarningSignsofaHeartAttack/Warning-Signs-of-a-Heart-Attack_UCM_002039_Article.jsp#.VkIgMcud8io
National Heart, Lung, and Blood Institute. (2015). *What are the symptoms of a heart attack?* Retrieved from http://www.nhlbi.nih.gov/health/health-topics/topics/heartattack/signs

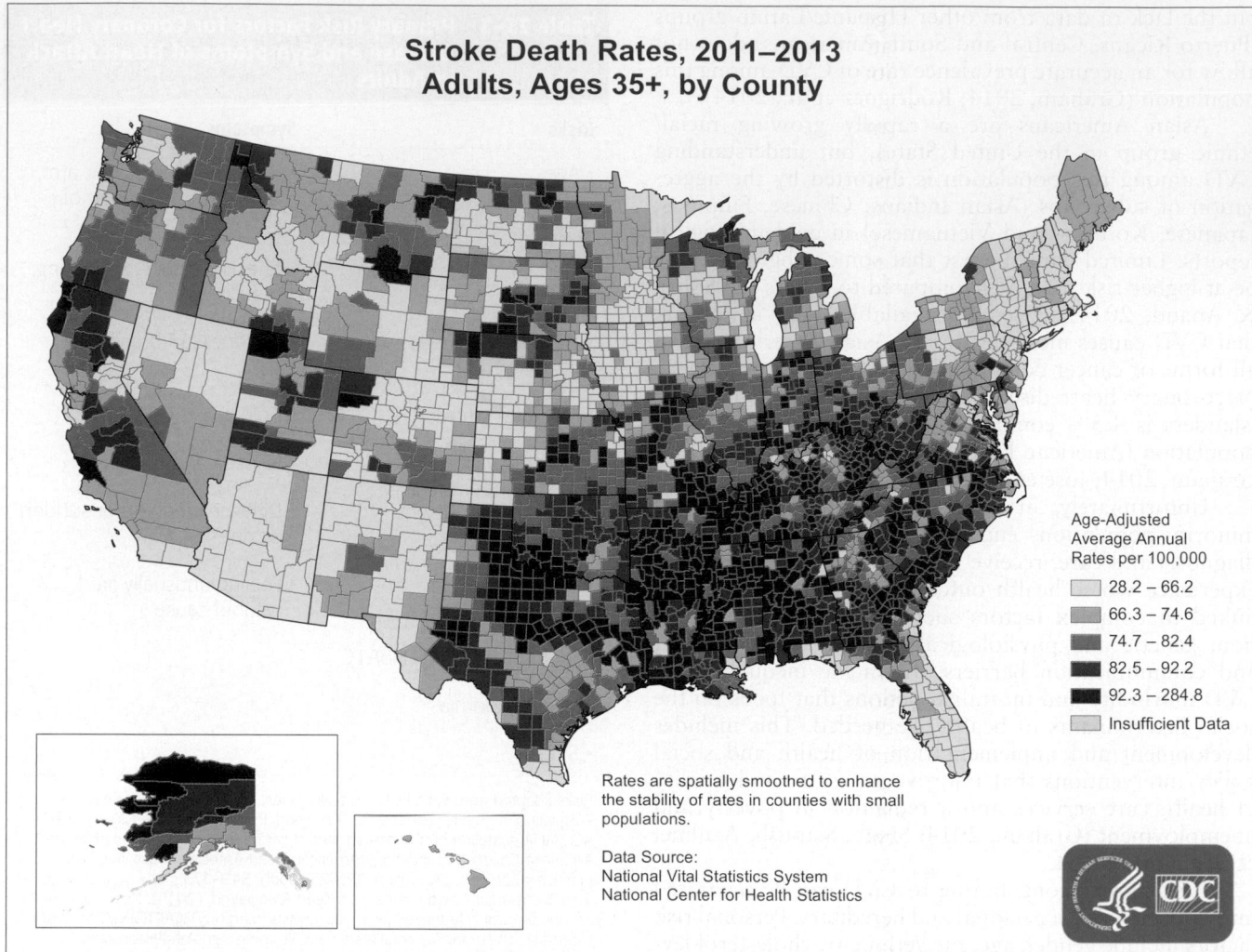

Stroke Death Rates, 2011–2013
Adults, Ages 35+, by County

Age-Adjusted
Average Annual
Rates per 100,000

- 28.2 – 66.2
- 66.3 – 74.6
- 74.7 – 82.4
- 82.5 – 92.2
- 92.3 – 284.8
- Insufficient Data

Rates are spatially smoothed to enhance
the stability of rates in counties with small
populations.

Data Source:
National Vital Statistics System
National Center for Health Statistics

FIGURE 23–3 Stroke death rates, 2011 to 2013 adults ages 35+ by county. (Retrieved from http://www.cdc.gov/dhdsp/maps/national_maps/stroke_all.htm)

EVIDENCE-BASED PRACTICE
Landmark Research on Cardiovascular Disease

The hallmark Framingham Heart Study identified major risk characteristics associated with the development of CVD and the effects of related factors such as blood triglycerides, gender, and psychosocial issues. The study began in 1948 under the direction of National Heart Institute, now known as the National Heart, Lung, and Blood Institute (NHLBI). At that time, the death rates from CVD were rising, but little was known about the general causes of heart disease and stroke. The Framingham Heart Study researchers recruited 2,336 men and 2,873 women between the ages of 30 and 62 in an effort to identify common factors or characteristics that contribute to CVD. All participants lived in the town of Framingham, Massachusetts. Every 2 years, these individuals were scheduled for an extensive medical history, physical examination, and laboratory tests. In 1971, the study enrolled 5,124 of the original participants'

adult children and their spouses (offspring cohort) (NHLBI, 2015).

In an effort to reflect the changing demographics that occurred in the town of Framingham since the original cohort was enrolled, researchers implemented a new study in 1994. This study included individuals of Black, Hispanic/Latino, Asian, Indian, Pacific Islander, and Native American origin (Omni cohort). In 2002, a third generation (the children of the offspring cohort) was recruited and a second group of Omni participants was enrolled in 2003. Over the last several years, investigators expanded their research into the role of genetics and CVD. Between 1950 and 2015, a total of 3,093 research articles have been published in peer-reviewed medical journals. Fortunately, findings from the Framingham Heart Study will continue to make important scientific contributions about the causes and treatment of CVD and related health issues (NHLBI, 2015).

develop cancer than women. The Agency for Healthcare Research and Quality (AHRQ) estimated the total expenditures for cancer in 2011 at $88.7 billion (American Cancer Society [ACS], 2015a; SEER, 2015).

Cancer is caused by internal and external factors. External factors include tobacco and alcohol use, chemicals, radiation, infectious organisms, and poor lifestyle choices. Internal factors are inherited gene mutations, hormones, immune conditions, and gene mutations that occur from metabolism. These factors can occur in isolation or together to initiate illness. However, only a small percentage of cancers are hereditary. The ACS estimates that in 2015, cancer deaths caused by tobacco use will reach 171,000 and one third of cancer cases will be related to overweight or obesity, physical inactivity, and/or poor nutrition. Screenings can reduce the cancer mortality rate, especially malignancies associated with the breast, colon, rectum, cervix, and lung (ACS, 2015a).

Lung cancer is the number one cause of cancer deaths among adults. An estimated 158,040 or 27% of all cancer deaths in 2015 will be attributed to lung cancer (ACS, 2015a). Overall, death rates have been declining for both men (since 1991) and women (since 2003). Cigarette smoking is the predominant risk factor for lung cancer. Quantity of cigarettes smoked and the number of years a person smoked both increase an individual's risk of developing lung cancer. Other risk factors include occupational or environmental exposure to secondhand smoke, radon, asbestos, genetic susceptibility (disease at an early age), and a history of tuberculosis. Current efforts to reduce mortality by early detection have been unsuccessful. Early detection of lung cancer by chest x-ray, analysis of cells in sputum, and fiberoptic examination of the bronchial passages has shown limited effectiveness in reducing lung cancer deaths. However, low-dose spiral computed tomography (CT) scans and molecular markers in sputum have produced more promising results in detecting lung cancers at an earlier stage of the disease (ACS, 2015a; U.S. Preventive Services Task Force, 2014a).

Colon and rectal cancers are the third most common cancers in adults. Among adults, an estimated 93,090 cases of colon and 39,610 cases of rectal cancers are expected to occur in 2015 and result in 49,700 deaths. The risk of developing colorectal cancer increases with age, and 90% of all cases are diagnosed in individuals 50 years of age or older. There are several modifiable factors associated with the increased risk of colorectal cancer. These factors include obesity, physical inactivity, a diet high in red or processed meat, alcohol consumption, long-term smoking, and low intake of whole grains, fruits, and vegetables. Other risk factors include certain inherited genetic mutations, personal or family history of polyps or colorectal cancer, and personal history of chronic inflammatory bowel disease. Screening for colon and rectal cancer should begin at age 50 for men and women who are at average risk (ACS, 2015a; see Display 23–2).

Chronic Lower Respiratory Diseases

Chronic lower respiratory disease (CLRD) comprises three major conditions: chronic bronchitis, emphysema, and asthma. CLRD is the third leading cause of death in the United States. The term chronic obstructive pulmonary disease (COPD) includes emphysema and chronic bronchitis. COPD is a major cause of disability, and over 11 million adults in the United States (aged 18 and over) are estimated to have the disease. However, approximately 24 million adults in the United States demonstrate evidence of impaired lung function, which could indicate an underdiagnosis of COPD (American Lung Association

---

DISPLAY 23–2 SCREENINGS AND CHECKUP SCHEDULE FOR WOMEN AND MEN

	When?	Ages 20–39	Ages 40–49	Age 50+
Physical Exam: Performed to review overall health status. Have a thorough physical examination and discuss health-related concerns and topics.	Every 3 years	X		
	Every 2 years		X	
	Every year			X
Blood Pressure: High blood pressure can have no symptoms but can cause permanent damage to body organs and systems.	Every year	X	X	X
Blood Tests and Urinalysis: Screens for various illnesses and diseases, such as cholesterol, kidney, or thyroid disorders, before problems or symptoms occur.	Every 3 years	X		
	Every 2 years		X	
	Every year			X
Electrocardiogram (EKG): EKG screens for heart abnormalities.	Baseline–age 30	X		
	Every 2 years		X	
	Every year			X
Immunizations				
Tetanus and diphtheria booster (plus 1-time booster of pertussis—Tdap)	Every 10 years	X	X	X
Flu vaccine	Every year	X	X	X

(continued)

DISPLAY 23–2 SCREENINGS AND CHECKUP SCHEDULE FOR WOMEN AND MEN
(Continued)

Pneumonia vaccine: Administered earlier if there is a history of diabetes, sickle cell, HIV/AIDS, pulmonary, cardiovascular, or liver disease	Age 65			X
Zoster vaccine	Age 60			X
HPV: Discuss with your health care provider.		X		
Rectal Exam: Screens for hemorrhoids, lower rectal problems, colon, and prostate cancer	Every year	X	X	X
Prostate-Specific Antigen (PSA) Blood Test: PSA is produced by the prostate. Levels increase when there is an infection, enlargement, or cancer. Testing should be done in collaboration with your health care provider.	Every year			X
Clinical Breast Exam (Women): Breast exam by health care provider	As recommended by health care provider			
Mammography (Women): Screening should begin at age 50 unless recommended sooner by health care provider.	Every 2 years			X
Pelvic Exam: A pelvic exam is performed to evaluate the size and position of the vagina, cervix, uterus, fallopian tubes, and ovaries.	Every year beginning at age 21 (unless sexually active at an earlier age)	X	X	X
Pap Test: A Pap test is performed to look for changes in the cells of the cervix, such as dysplasia or cancer.	Every 3 years	X	X	X
Self-Exams: *Testicles* are examined to find lumps. *Skin* is checked to look for signs of changing moles, freckles, or early skin cancer. *Oral* to look for cancerous lesions in the mouth.	Monthly	X	X	X
Fecal Occult Blood Test: Screens the stool for microscopic amounts of blood that can be the first indication of polyps or colon cancer	Every year			X
Colon Rectal Health: A flexible endoscope is used to examine the rectum, sigmoid, and descending colon for cancer at its earliest stages. The exam also detects polyps that can progress to cancer if not found early. Or, colonoscopy every 10 years starting at age 50	Every 5 years			X
Lung: Current or former smokers ages 55–74 in good health with at least 30 pack-year history should consider having a low-dose helical CT scan.	Discuss with health care provider			X
Hepatitis C: Get screened once if born between 1945 and 1965, ever injected drugs, or received a blood transfusion before 1992.	Discuss with health care provider			
TB Test: Should be done on occasion of exposure or suggestive symptoms at the direction of the health care provider. Some occupations may require more frequent testing for public health indications.	Every 5 years	X	X	X

Adapted from American Cancer Society. (2015). *Cancer facts and figures* 2015. Retrieved from http://www.cancer.org/acs/groups/content/@editorial/documents/document/acspc-044552.pdf
Agency for Healthcare Research and Quality. (2014a). *Men: Stay healthy at any age.* Retrieved from http://www.ahrq.gov/sites/default/files/publications/files/healthy-men.pdf
Agency for Healthcare Research and Quality. (2014b). *Women: Stay healthy at any age.* Retrieved from http://www.ahrq.gov/sites/default/files/publications/files/healthy-women.pdf
Men's Health Network. (n.d.a). *Get it checked. Checkup and screening guidelines for men.* Retrieved from http://www.menshealthnetwork.org/library/getitcheckedpostermen.pdf
Men's Health Network. (n.d.b). *Get it checked. Checkup and screening guidelines for women.* Retrieved from http://www.menshealthnetwork.org/library/getitcheckedposterwomen.pdf

[ALA], 2015a; Guarascio, Ray, Finch, & Self, 2013). By 2020, the annual cost of medical care for adults living with COPD will be more than $49 billion. Medicare and Medicaid pay for the majority of national health care costs related to this disease, 51% and 25%, respectively. On average, total costs incurred by COPD patients are approximately $6,000 higher than non-COPD patients (CDC, 2014a; Ford et al., 2015).

Cigarette smoking is the major risk factor for developing COPD, accounting for 85% to 90% of cases. Pipe, cigar, and other types of tobacco smoke also can cause COPD, especially if the smoke is inhaled. The remaining COPD cases are attributable to environmental exposures and genetic factors (ALA, 2015b). Since 2000, the number of women dying from COPD has surpassed the number of men. This rise is probably related to the increase in smoking among women after World War II and the difference in how cigarette smoke is metabolized by women as compared to men. Women are also more vulnerable to lung damage from cigarette smoke and other pollutants because their lungs are smaller, and research has found that estrogen plays a role in worsening the disease (ALA, 2013a).

People of all ages can develop chronic bronchitis, but it occurs more frequently in people who are 45 years of age or older. Many adults who develop chronic bronchitis are smokers and women are more than twice as likely as men to be diagnosed with the disease. Contact with dust, chemical fumes, and vapors from certain jobs also increase the risk for developing chronic bronchitis. Examples include jobs in coal mining, textile manufacturing, grain handling, and livestock farming; work in nail salons has also been associated with respiratory and neurological effects (ALA, 2013b; CDC, 2014e; Halldin, Doney, & Hnizdo, 2015).

The exact cause of asthma is unknown, but research indicates that both genetic and environmental factors contribute to its cause. In the United States, approximately 18.9 million adults have been diagnosed with asthma. Among adults, the prevalence rate is highest among 18- to 24-year-olds (10.3%) and lowest among adults 65 years of age or older (8.1%). The prevalence of asthma is higher in women (10.7%) than men (6.5%), respectively. When compared with White adults (8.7%), higher rates of asthma occur in multiracial (15.1%) and Black (10.8%) adults. Approximately one in three adults miss at least 1 day of work because of asthma (ALA, 2015c; CDC, 2013a).

Unintentional Injuries

Unintentional injuries refer to any injury that results from unintended exposure to physical agents, including heat, mechanical energy, chemicals, or electricity. They are the fifth leading cause of death overall and the leading cause of death for persons 44 years of age and younger. The top three causes of unintentional injuries include motor vehicle crashes, poisoning, and falls. Approximately 193,000 Americans die from injury each year—one person every 3 minutes. However, millions of other people are injured every year and survive. These individuals are often left to face lifelong mental, physical, and financial problems (CDC, 2015d, 2015e) (Fig. 23–4).

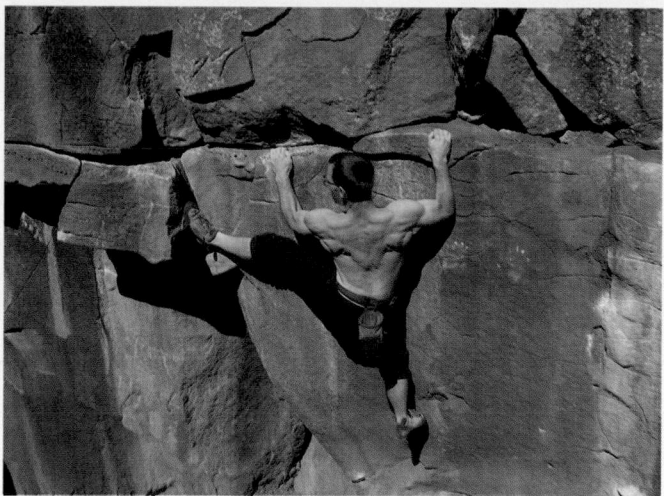

FIGURE 23–4 Unintentional injuries are the leading cause of death for those aged 44 years and younger.

In 2013, 3 million people were hospitalized due to injuries and 27 million were treated in emergency departments. The costs associated with fatal injuries were $214 billion, whereas nonfatal injury costs were over $457 billion. Males account for the majority of fatal injury costs (78%, $166.7 billion), as well as nonfatal injury costs (63%, $287.5 billion; CDC, 2015d, 2015e; Florence, Simon, Haegerich, Luo, & Zhou, 2015).

Mortality from unintentional injuries in the United States based on age includes the following:

- Unintentional poisoning is the leading cause of death among persons 25 to 64 years of age and younger.
- Motor vehicle accident is the leading cause of death among persons 15 to 24 years of age and second among persons 25 years of age and older.
- Firearm suicide is the third leading cause of death among persons 35 years of age and older.
- Firearm homicide is the third leading cause among persons 25 to 34 years of age.
- Unintentional falls are the leading cause of death among persons 65 years of age and older (CDC, 2015f).

Drugs, both pharmaceutical and illicit, cause the vast majority of poisoning deaths in the United States. From 2000 to 2013, the age-adjusted drug-poisoning death rate more than doubled, from 6.2 to 13.8 per 100,000. Of the 43,982 deaths because of drug poisoning in 2013, 81% were unintentional, 12% were suicides, and 6% were of undetermined intent. Opioid analgesic pain relievers are involved in a substantial number of drug-poisoning deaths. These include natural and semisynthetic opioid analgesics such hydrocodone, morphine, and oxycodone. Synthetic opioid analgesics that contribute to drug-poisoning mortality are fentanyl and methadone (NCHS, 2015b). See Chapter 27 for more on substance use.

In 2012, there were 22,912 motor vehicle–related fatalities and over 2.5 million emergency department visits for motor vehicle crash–related injuries. Approximately 7.5% of the persons who came to the emergency department were admitted to the hospital because of their injuries.

The average lifetime medical cost per treated and released patient was $3,362, whereas a hospitalized patient's average lifetime cost was $56,674. The lifetime cost of work loss because of motor vehicle crash injuries was $9.4 billion for treated and released patients and $23.5 billion for hospitalized patients (Bergen et al., 2014).

Despite increasing traffic on highways, motor vehicle crash injuries have declined almost 25% between 2004 and 2013. This decline is due to improvement in vehicle and road designs, seat belt laws, ignition interlocks to prevent alcohol-impaired driving, publicized sobriety checkpoints, and graduated driver licensing systems for teens (Dischinger, Ryb, Kufera, & Ho, 2013; National Highway Traffic Safety Association, 2014).

A *disabling injury* is one that results in restriction of normal activities of daily living (ADLs) beyond the day on which the injury occurred. Disabling injuries occur disproportionately among the young and the elderly. Seat belts, helmets, smoke detectors, and poison control centers save billions of dollars in direct and indirect medical costs. These primary and secondary prevention strategies save lives and money. See Chapter 26 for more on those living with disabilities and chronic illness.

An *unsafe condition* is any environmental factor, either social or physical, that increases the likelihood of an unintentional injury. An icy walkway is an example of an unsafe condition; although it poses a hazard, it does not cause an injury but makes it more likely that an injury will occur. *Injury prevention* and *injury control* refer to any effort to prevent injuries or lessen their severity. These efforts often focus on assessment of the environment for unsafe conditions, such as loaded guns in the home or asbestos in school buildings and workplaces (Li & Baker, 2014).

Diabetes Mellitus

Diabetes mellitus is the seventh leading cause of death in the United States. According to the CDC, over 29 million Americans have type 1 or type 2 diabetes (CDC, 2015g; see Fig. 23–3). Diabetes affects 12.3% of Americans 20 years of age and older and 25.9% of Americans 65 years of age and older. Among individuals 20 years of age and older with diabetes (diagnosed and undiagnosed), 13.4 million (11.2%) are women and 15.5 million (13.6%) are men (see Table 23–4). After adjusting for population age differences, minorities continue to have higher rates of diabetes. Among individuals 20 years of age or older, 7.1% of Whites, 8.4% of Asian Americans, 12.8% of Hispanics, 13.2% of Blacks, and 15.9% of Native Americans were diagnosed with diabetes between 2010 and 2012. In 2012, there were 1.7 million new cases of diabetes diagnosed in people 20 years of age and older (CDC, 2015g; CDC, 2015h) (Fig. 23–5).

Diabetes is a major chronic health condition that puts individuals at risk for other serious health conditions including heart disease, stroke, hypertension (HTN), blindness, kidney disease, and nervous system disease (i.e., neuropathy, which is a loss of sensation or pain in the feet or hands). Because diabetes can affect any part of the body, damage to other body systems can be minimized by good blood glucose control (assessed by hemoglobin A1c [HbA1c]). In 2012, the estimated direct

Table 23–4	Diagnosed and Undiagnosed Diabetes Among People Ages 20 Years or Older, United States, 2012	
Group	**Number or Percentage Who Have Diabetes**
Ages 20 y or older	28.9 million, or 12.3%, of all people in this age group
Ages 65 y or older	11.2 million, or 25.9%, of all people in this age group
Men	15.5 million, or 13.6%, of all men ages 20 y or older
Women	13.4 million, or 11.2%, of all women ages 20 y or older

Extracted from Centers for Disease Control and Prevention (CDC). (2015). *National diabetes statistics report: Estimates of diabetes and its burden in the United States; 2014.* Atlanta, GA: U.S. Department of Health and Human Services; 2014. Retrieved from http://www.cdc.gov/diabetes/pubs/statsreport14/national-diabetes-report-web.pdf

and indirect costs for individuals diagnosed with diabetes totaled $245 billion. Direct costs represented medical care, and indirect costs were for disability, work loss, and premature mortality. After adjusting for population age and gender differences, people diagnosed with diabetes had expenditures that were 2.3 times greater than individuals who did not have diabetes (CDC, 2015g).

Obesity

Obesity is defined as having a body mass index (BMI) of 30 or greater and is recognized as a national health threat and a major public health challenge. Individuals who have a BMI of 40 or greater or are more than 100 pounds overweight are considered to have extreme or severe obesity. In 2011 to 2012, based on data from the

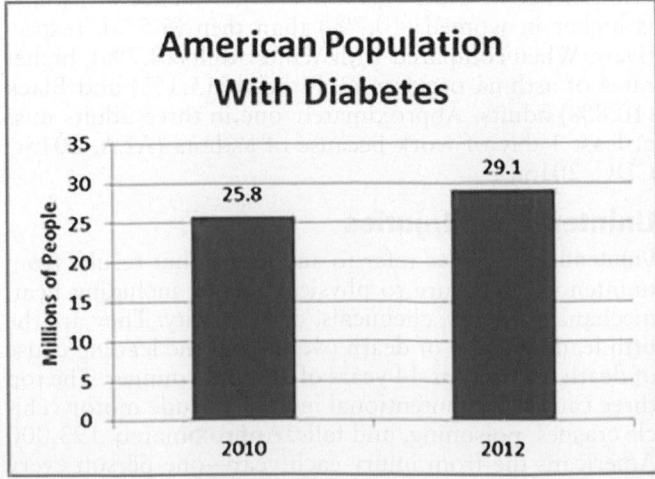

FIGURE 23–5 Rising prevalence of diabetes in the United States. (Adapted from American Diabetes Association. (2014). *National diabetes statistics report, 2014.* Retrieved from http://www.diabetes.org/diabetes-basics/statistics/?loc=db-slabnav)

National Health and Nutrition Examination Survey, the age-adjusted prevalence of obesity in the United States indicated that among adults 34.9% were obese and 6.4% extremely obese (National Institute of Diabetes and Digestive & Kidney Diseases [NIDDKD], 2012). Based on the National Health Survey from 2012, more men than women were overweight, obesity was greatest among Native Americans (41%), Blacks (36%), and 32% of Hispanics/Latinos (Blackwell, Lucas, & Clarke, 2014; Ogden, Carroll, Kit, & Flegal, 2014). Obesity is a major risk factor for CVD, along with certain types of cancer, type 2 diabetes, obstructive sleep apnea, and premature death (CDC, 2015k). One of the *Healthy People 2020* objectives is to decrease the proportion of adults who are obese by 10% (USDHHS, 2015).

Over the past 20 years, there has been a dramatic increase in obesity in the United States. Currently, every state in the country has a prevalence of obesity >20%, 45 states have a prevalence ≥25%, and 3 states exceed 35% (i.e., Arkansas, West Virginia, and Mississippi). Arkansas has the highest prevalence of obesity at 39.5%, and Colorado the lowest at 21.3% (Robert Wood Johnson Foundation, 2015). Recent medical care costs related to obesity in the United States are estimated to be $147 billion (CDC, 2015l). This high prevalence and cost of this disease underscore the need for additional measures to educate persons regarding healthier lifestyle choices, increasing physical activity, and decreasing caloric intake.

Bariatric surgery is a clinically and cost-effective intervention for moderately to severely obese individuals; however, this is a very serious decision. There are four types of bariatric produces: adjustable gastric band, Roux-en-Y gastric bypass, biliopancreatic diversion with a double-duodenal switch, and vertical sleeve gastrectomy. Careful consideration must be given; for example, the individual has been unsuccessful in losing weight, the person is knowledgeable regarding risks and benefits of the surgery, the person is aware of how life may change following surgery, and a commitment by the person of engaging in healthy eating following the surgery to maintain weight loss, to name a few. The average cost of a bariatric procedure is $20,000 to $25,000, and about $1.5 billion is spent annually (NIDDKD, 2011). However, research supports the notion that bariatric surgery is a cost-effective procedure when obesity is viewed as a chronic disease (Wang & Furnback, 2013).

Substance Use

According to the Substance Abuse and Mental Health Services Administration (SAMHSA), a **substance use** disorder occurs when the recurrent use of alcohol and/or drugs causes clinically and functionally significant impairment such as health problems, disability, and failure to meet major responsibilities at work, school, or home. It is a serious and continuing problem among adult women and men living in the United States (Center for Behavioral Health Statistics and Quality, 2015).

In 2014, 139.7 million Americans aged 12 or older reported current use of alcohol, 60.9 million reported binge alcohol use in the past month, and 16.3 million reported heavy alcohol use in the past month. In the United States, a standard drink contains 0.6 ounces of alcohol:

12 ounces of beer, 8 ounces of malt liquor, 5 ounces of wine, or 1.5 ounces of 80-proof distilled spirits. Definitions for the different levels of drinking include the following:

- Moderate drinking—According to the *Dietary Guidelines for Americans*, moderate drinking is up to one drink per day for women and up to two drinks per day for men.
- Binge drinking—SAMHSA defines binge drinking as drinking five or more alcoholic drinks on the same occasion on at least 1 day in the past 30 days. The National Institute on Alcohol Abuse and Alcoholism defines binge drinking as a pattern of drinking that produces blood alcohol concentrations of >0.08 g/dL. This usually occurs after four drinks for women and five drinks for men over a 2-hour period.
- Heavy drinking—SAMHSA defines heavy drinking as drinking five or more drinks on the same occasion for each of five or more days in the past 30 days (CDC, 2014b; Center for Behavioral Health Statistics and Quality, 2015).

In 2014, males 18 years of age and older were more likely than women to have had at least 1 day of heavy drinking in the past year. From 2004 to 2013, the percentage of women who had at least one heavy drinking day in the past year increased from 11.2% to 14.5%. Among men, the percentage that had at least one heavy day of drinking decreased from 31.6% in 1997 to 27.8% in 2006 but then increased to 32.4% in 2009. Since 2009, there has been no change in the drinking rate among men. Based on race/ethnicity, White adults (30.6%) were more likely to have had at least one heavy day of drinking in the past year followed by Hispanic/Latinos (21.7%) and Black adults (16.4%) (USDHHS, CDC, & NCHS, 2015).

Alcohol consumption is very common in our society, but excessive use can harm an individual's health. Between 2006 and 2010, excessive alcohol use accounted for 1 in 10 deaths among adults 20 to 64 years of age, and it is currently the third leading lifestyle-related cause of death in the United States (CDC, 2014c; Kanny et al., 2015). In 2013, alcohol-impaired driving fatalities accounted for 10,076 deaths. This represents 30.8% of overall driving fatalities during that year (National Institute on Alcohol Abuse and Alcoholism, 2015). In 2010, excessive use of alcohol cost the United States over $249 million or about $2.05 per drink ($807 per person). Government-sponsored health programs paid for $100.7 billion (40.4%) of these costs (Sacks, Gonzales, Bouchery, Tomedi, & Brewer, 2015).

Tobacco use is a major public health problem and the leading cause of preventable diseases and deaths in the United States. More than 10 times as many U.S. citizens have died prematurely from cigarette smoking than have died in all the wars fought by the United States during its history (USDHHS, 2014a). Because of the significance of the problem, 18 of the *Healthy People 2020* objectives are related to tobacco use.

Among adults 18 years of age or older, 18 out of every 100 adults (42.1 million or 17.8%) currently smoke cigarettes and young adults 18 to 24 years of age are more likely to smoke than people 65 years of age or older. When examining cigarette smoking based on gender, men are more likely to smoke cigarettes (20.5%)

than women (15.3%). The prevalence of smoking based on race/ethnicity indicates that American Indians and Alaska Natives (26.1%) smoke more cigarettes than Whites (19.4%), Blacks (18.3%), and Hispanics/Latinos (12.1%). In the United States, the rate of cigarette smoking is lowest among Asians, at 9.5% (CDC, 2015i).

Despite significant declines in cigarette smoking among adults in the United States over the past five decades, the use of other tobacco products such as cigars and smokeless tobacco has been unchanged. Additionally, the prevalence and use of emerging products such as electronic cigarettes (e-cigarettes) and water pipes/hookahs have rapidly increased. During 2012–2013, an estimated 21.3% of adults in the United States used any tobacco product every day or some days. The prevalence of every day or some day use was cigarettes (18%), cigars/cigarillos/filtered cigars (2%), regular pipes (0.3%), water pipes/hookah (0.5%), and e-cigarettes (1.9%), and 2.5% used smokeless tobacco (Agaku et al., 2014).

In the United States, smoking is responsible for 87% of lung cancer deaths, 32% of CHD deaths, and 79% of COPD cases. Changes in the design and composition of cigarettes have increased the risk of developing adenocarcinoma of the lung, the most common type of lung cancer. Between 1959 and 2010, lung cancer risks for smokers rose dramatically. Among female smokers, the risk increased 10-fold, and it doubled for male smokers (USDHHS, 2014a). Smoking-related illness in the United States costs more than $300 billion each year. This includes approximately $170 billion for direct medical care for adults and more than $156 billion in lost productivity (CDC, 2015j). To reduce tobacco-related disease and deaths in the United States, population-level interventions such as mass antitobacco campaigns, comprehensive smoke-free laws, regulation of tobacco products, and increased access to smoking cessation programs are critical (CDC, 2014d).

The health and well-being of millions of Americans is impacted by *illicit drug use*. Illicit drug use refers to use and misuse of illegal and controlled drugs. In 2014, an estimated 27 million persons (ages 12 and older) used an illicit drug in the past 30 days. This represents about 1 in 10 Americans or 10.2% of the population. The most common illicit drugs used in the United States are marijuana (22.2 million people) and nonmedical use of prescription pain relievers (4.3 million). The percentage of persons 12 years of age and older in the United States who were current illicit drug users in 2014 was higher that than the percentages from 2002 to 2013. This increase may be reflective of a rise in illicit drug use among adults aged 26 and older (Center for Behavioral Health Statistics and Quality, 2015).

Prescription drug misuse or abuse is the intentional or unintentional use of medication without a prescription, in a way other than prescribed, or for the experience or feeling the drug elicits. The illegal use of prescription drugs is one of the fastest-growing forms of drug abuse and is a major public health concern. Although many medications can be abused, the following three classes are most common:

- Opioids—usually prescribed to treat pain
- Central nervous system (CNS) depressants—used to treat anxiety and sleep disorders
- Stimulants—most often prescribed to treat attention deficit hyperactivity disorder (ADHD; National Institute on Drug Abuse [NIDA], 2014)

Overall, males are more likely than females to abuse prescription drugs in all age groups, except the youngest (12 to 17 years of age). Prescription drug abuse is highest (11.8%) among young adults 15 to 18 years of age. However, it is important to note that illicit drug use is increasing among the baby boomers (persons between the ages of 50 and 69). This is because illicit drug use was historically higher in this generation as compared to those of previous generations (NIDA, 2015; SAMHSA, 2015a).

Nonmedical use of prescription pain relievers varies by race/ethnicity: Asians (1.8%), Blacks (3.6%), Whites (4.3%), Hispanics/Latinos (4.5%), and American Indians/Alaska Natives (6.9%). The highest rates of nonmedical use of prescription pain relievers were found to be among individuals of two or more races (8.1%) (SAMHSA, 2015b). A recent study estimated the number of emergency department visits for nonmedical use of prescription drugs, over-the-counter drugs, or other pharmaceuticals to be over 1.2 million. Overall, medical emergencies related to nonmedical use of pharmaceuticals increased 132% between the years 2004 and 2011 (USDHHS, SAMHSA, & Center for Behavioral Health Statistics and Quality, 2013). This health issue is covered in greater detail in Chapter 27.

WOMEN'S HEALTH

Women have not been the focus of medical attention throughout the centuries. Health benefits achieved by women were incidental compared to men. Advances in women's health are very recent and primarily an advantage for women living in Western countries, where the women's or feminist movement has made major inroads (Fig. 23–6).

Overview of Factors Influencing Women's Health

Women's rights in the United States started in the second half of the 19th century and over time addressed issues directly or indirectly impacting the health of women:

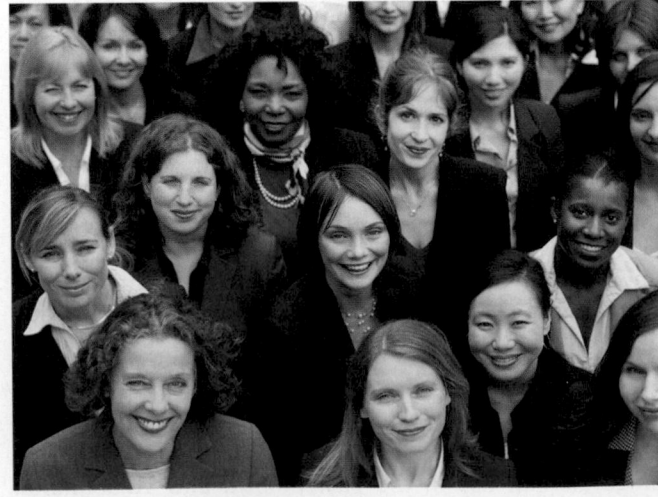

FIGURE 23–6 Women's health has not historically been the focus of health care research.

voting rights, labor laws, reproductive rights, and violence against women (Fried, 2013; International Women's Day, 2015). This section of the chapter examines women's health concerns over the adult life span and the major causes of acute and chronic illness and death and the issues, trends, and policies that have and currently affect women.

Women's health is still overlooked in much of the world. Only in the past few decades has the health of women been a formidable issue in the United States, coming not so coincidently with the modern women's feminist movement that began in the 1960s. The landmark 1963 publication *The Feminine Mystique* helped launch the modern women's movement by critically examining the role of women in American society (Foster, 2015; Friedan, 2013). The Boston Women's Health Book Collective's *Our Bodies, Ourselves* (initial release 1973) represented the first book to explore women's health issues, exclusively written by and for women. In addition, this publication served as a model for women who wanted to learn about themselves, communicate their findings with doctors, and challenge the medical establishment to change and improve the care that women received (Our Bodies Ourselves, 2015). To further expand the dialogue regarding women's health, consumer activists created the National Women's Health Network in 1975, primarily to shape health policy and support consumer health decisions (National Women's Health Network, 2015). These historical occurrences likely contributed to more female researchers and women as participants in research. Feminists paved the way for women to have their voices heard on many health, social, and political issues. Women sought out higher-education opportunities in greater numbers and entered workplaces once solely occupied by men, especially during and after World War II. These positive changes escalated women toward greater equality, and with equality came the freedom—and pressure—for women to compete with men in their social and work settings. Issues related to women's health were discovered as a result of research that now more regularly includes women. The importance of women's research was reaffirmed in the National Institute of Health's (NIH) Revitalization Act of 1993, Subtitle B—clinical research equity regarding women and minorities to "identify projects for research on women's health that should be conducted or supported by the national research institutes; identify multidisciplinary research relating to research on women that should be so conducted or supported ..." (NIH, 1993, section 486).

Women's Health Research

In response to changing priorities, researchers have designed and implemented major studies that focus exclusively on women. Five significant studies have and continue to provide important health information about women:

- The *Women's Health Initiative* (WHI), a major 15-year research program addressing the most common causes of death, disability, and poor quality of life in postmenopausal women—CVD, cancer, and osteoporosis
- The *Women's Health Study* (WHS) that evaluated the effects of vitamin E and low-dose aspirin therapy in

primary prevention of CVD and cancer in apparently healthy women
- The *Nurses' Health Study I* involved with investigating risk factors for cancer and CVD, and the *Nurses' Health Study II* that researched diet and lifestyle risk factors in a population younger than the original Nurses' Health Study cohort
- The *Nurses' Health Study III* that is investigating women's health issues related to lifestyle fertility/ pregnancy, environment, and nursing exposures

The *WHI* addressed CVD, cancer, and osteoporosis and was one of the largest prevention studies of its kind in the United States, starting in 1991 and spanning 15 years. The three major components of the WHI were a randomized controlled clinical trial of promising but unproven approaches to prevention, an observational study to identify predictors of disease, and a study of community approaches to developing healthful behaviors. This study was sponsored by the NIH and the NHLBI involving 161,808 women ages 50 to 79 and was considered to be one of the most far-reaching clinical trials for women's health ever undertaken. Enrolled women participated in a follow-up phase of this study until 2010. To date, more than 616 publications have been associated with findings from this study, which address coronary artery calcium, breast cancer risk, colorectal cancer, venous thrombosis, peripheral arterial disease risk, risk of CHD, dementia and cognitive function, and the effects of estrogen alone in reducing the risk of CHD (Database of Genotypes and Phenotypes, n.d.).

The *WHS* was a randomized, double-blind, placebo-controlled clinical trial sponsored by the NHBLI and the NCI. It was the first large clinical trial to study the use of low-dose aspirin to prevent heart attack and stroke in women 45 years of age and older. This study began in 1991 and continued through March 2009 for additional observation and follow-up of the original 28,345 participants. Current findings indicate that low-dose aspirin does not prevent first heart attacks or death from cardiovascular causes in women; however, stroke was found to be 17% lower in the aspirin group. More than 110 professional articles are associated with this investigation. Recent publications address the association of dietary fat intake with risk of atrial fibrillation in women and the novel protein glycan biomarker and future CVD events (WHS, 2015).

The *Nurses' Health Studies* (three separate phases) represent the longest running study related to women's health in the world, investigating factors that influence the health of women. The *Nurses' Health Study I*, a prospective study that began in 1976, enrolled 122,000 registered nurses ages 30 to 55 from 11 states that responded to 170,000 mailed questionnaires. Every 2 years, participants received a follow-up questionnaire with questions about diseases and health-related topics including smoking, hormone use, and menopausal status. Later in the study, questions regarding diet and nutrition and quality of life were added. The *Nurses' Health Study II* represented women who started using oral contraceptives in adolescence, a population with long-term exposure during early reproductive years. Participants were between

25 and 42 years of age, and 116,686 women were enrolled and followed forward in time. Every 2 years, participants received a follow-up questionnaire and were surveyed about diseases and health-related topics including smoking, hormone use, pregnancy history, and menopausal status. Women also received nutrition and quality-of-life assessments later in the study. The *Nurses' Health Study III* began recruitment in 2010 and will continue until 100,000 nurses (registered and licensed practical, 22 to 45 years of age) are enrolled. Also, nurses from Canada are participants and the study aims to be more representative of the diverse backgrounds of nurses. This investigation is supported by major nursing organizations. Overall, as of 2015, outcomes from phases I and II have spawned 1,200 professional publications (Harvard School of Public Health & Brigham and Women's Hospital, 2013; Nurses' Health Study, n.d.)

Women's Health Promotion Across the Life Span

What health care needs do women have that are different from those of men? Is there a need to look at health promotion throughout the life cycle of adult women? How is the health of an 18-year-old different from that of a 50-year-old woman? Most of us would have no trouble agreeing that women have different health care needs that must be considered and that these concerns vary with age. Knowing what the needs are is essential to knowing how to help women promote their health.

Healthy People 2020 Goals for Women

As a nation, we have been focusing on improving the health of all citizens through the *Healthy People* initiatives, commencing with the 1979 Surgeon General's report, *Healthy People: The Surgeon General's Report on Health Promotion and Disease Prevention*, providing measurable population objectives. *Healthy People 2000* set a standard for change and improvement in objectives that were met or exceeded in some areas and were far from being reached in others. In that initiative, objectives in 14 areas focused specifically on women's health. *Healthy People 2010* focused on two overarching goals: increasing the quality of life and eliminating health disparities, containing 25 objectives relating to women. *Healthy People 2020* reaffirmed the goals of *2010* and added two additional goals: quality of life, healthy development, along with healthy behaviors across the life span and creating social and physical environments that promote good health (USDHHS, 2015). In the nation's fourth generation of health planning, 27 objectives pertain to the health of women (Display 23–3). As the community health nurse works with women at various stages in the life cycle, the objectives in *Healthy People 2020* can give structure to program planning and services offered to women in the community at the primary, secondary, and tertiary levels of prevention.

Young Adult Women (18 to 35 Years)

Women in the earlier years of adulthood have different tasks to accomplish and issues to address than do women in later adulthood, and the transition from adolescence to adulthood can be stressful. There are major developmental tasks that young women need to accomplish such as forming an identity and the development of intimacy. Behaviors associated with young adulthood include attracting and choosing a significant other for the long term and establishing a home. Young women during this stage also prepare and choose a life's work that is personally satisfying, plan for children by using a variety of parenting models (childbirth, adoption, foster parenting),

---

What do *you* think?

A woman's dressing style that included a tightly laced corset was popular from the late 1700s throughout the late 1800s in Germany, England, and the United States. In 1793, this practice was brought into question by S. T. von Soemmerring, an anatomist. He identified compression of rib cages and internal organs as contributing to digestive problems, fainting, and shortness of breath. For the next century, dress reformers advocated looser lacing and clothes that allowed for a more natural movement. However, these reformers belonged to the "radical fringe" of the feminist movement, and the tiniest waists, regardless of their impact on health, continued to be in vogue as both middle-class and upper-class women sought the "hourglass" figure. More recently, hiatal hernias caused by overly tight girdles and corsets have been termed "Soemmerring's syndrome" in tribute to the first physician to warn of the dangers, more than 200 years ago.

In 2015, thanks to social media and our fascination with celebrities and social media personalities, waist trainers (a newer version of the traditional corset) have become popular. Even though some women have fainted from having worn them for extended periods, and despite the fact that there is no evidence to show that they truly reduce fat at the waistline, there is still the allure of a tiny waist even over a century after Soemmerring's findings.

Do you know someone who has tried a waist trainer? What was their reason for using it? What was their experience like? As a PHN, how would you approach this subject with them?

Adapted from Fee, E., Brown, T. M., Lazarus, J., & Theerman, P. (2002). The effects of the corset. *American Journal of Public Health*, 92, 1085. Retrieved from http://www.ncbi.nlm.nih.gov/pmc/articles/PMC3222278/pdf/0921085.pdf
Thapoung, K. (2015, September 25). Celebrities swear by it, but is waist training actually healthy? *Marie Claire*. Retrieved from http://www.marieclaire.com/health-fitness/a13489/celebrities-swear-by-it-but-is-waist-training-actually-healthy/

DISPLAY 23–3 *HEALTHY PEOPLE 2020* OBJECTIVES FOR WOMEN

1. Reduce the breast cancer death rate, from 22.9 deaths per 100,000 women to 20.6 deaths per 100,000.
2. Reduce the death rate from cancer of the uterine cervix, from 2.4 deaths per 100,000 to 2.2 deaths per 100,000 women.
3. Reduce invasive uterine cervical cancer from 7.9 new cases per 100,000 females to 7.1 new cases per 100,000 females.
4. Reduce late-stage female breast cancer from 43.2 new cases per 100, 000 females to 41.0 new cases per 100,000 females.
5. Increase the proportion of women who receive a cervical cancer screening based on the most recent guidelines from 84.5% of women aged 21 to 65 years to 93% of women aged 21 to 65 years.
6. Increase the proportion of women who receive a breast cancer screening based on the most recent guidelines from 73.7% of females aged 50 to 74 years to 81.1% of females aged 50 to 74 years.
7. Increase the proportion of pregnancies that are intended, from 51% to 56%.
8. Reduce the proportion of females experiencing pregnancy despite use of a reversible contraceptive method from 12.4% to 9.9%.
9. Reduce the proportion of pregnancies conceived within 18 months of a previous birth from 35.3% to 31.7%.
10. Increase the proportion of females or their partners at risk of unintended pregnancy who used contraception at most recent sexual intercourse from 83% to 91.3%.
11. Reduce pregnancy rates among adolescent females aged 15 to 17 years from 40.2 pregnancies per 1,000 to 36.2 pregnancies per 1,000.
12. Increase the proportion of females in need of publically supported contraceptive services and supplies who receive those services and supplies from 53.8% to 64.5%.
13. Increase the proportion of women with a family history of breast and/or ovarian cancer who receive genetic counseling from 23.3% to 25.6%.
14. Reduce the rate of maternal mortality from 12.7% to 11.4%.
15. Reduce maternal illness and complications because of pregnancy (complications during hospitalized labor and delivery) from 31.1% to 28%.
16. Reduce cesarean births among low-risk (full-term, singleton, vertex presentation) women from 26.5% to 23.9%.
17. Increase the proportion of pregnant women who receive early and adequate prenatal care form 70.8% to 77.9%.
18. Increase abstinence from alcohol, cigarettes, and illicit drugs among pregnant women from 89.4% to 98.3%.
19. (Developmental) Increase the proportion of pregnant women who attend a series of prepared childbirth classes.
20. (Developmental) Increase the proportion of mothers who achieve a recommended weight gain during their pregnancies.
21. Increase the proportion of women of childbearing potential with intake of at least 400 µg of folic acid from fortified foods or dietary supplements from 23.8% to 26.2%.
22. Reduce the proportion of women of childbearing potential who have low red blood cell folate concentrations from 24.5% to 22.1%.
23. Increase the proportion of women delivering a live birth who received preconception care services and practiced key recommended preconception health behaviors (took multivitamins/folic acid every day in the month prior to pregnancy) from 30.1% to 33.1%.
24. (Developmental) Reduce postpartum relapse of smoking among women who quit smoking during pregnancy.
25. (Developmental) Increase the proportion of women giving birth who attended a postpartum care visit with a health worker.
26. Reduce iron deficiency among young children and females of childbearing age (12 to 49 years) from 10.4% to 9.4%.
27. Reduce iron deficiency among pregnant females from 16.1% to 14.5%.

Adapted from U.S. Department of Health and Human Services (USDHHS). (2015). *Healthy people 2020*. Retrieved from http://www.healthypeople.gov/2020/default.aspx

and develop a personal philosophy that encompasses meaningful and comforting spiritual beliefs that are consistent with day-to-day living (Hutteman, Hennecke, Orth, Reitz, & Specht, 2014; Lane, 2015) (Fig. 23–7).

Women in this age group tend to be healthy. Unfortunately, during this period, many women engage in health risk behaviors such as physical inactivity, eating poorly, participating in unprotected sexual intercourse, and smoking. Some, if not all, of these behaviors may have been established in adolescence and represent modifiable

behaviors. If not addressed, these behaviors can contribute significantly to the leading causes of morbidity and mortality: diseases of the heart and vascular systems, cancers, chronic respiratory diseases, and diabetes (USDHHS, Health Resources and Services Administration, Maternal and Child Health Bureau, 2013); the majority of health concerns for many of these women are related to eating disorders, reproductive health and sexually transmitted infections (STIs), physical activity, mental health and mood disorders, and substance use.

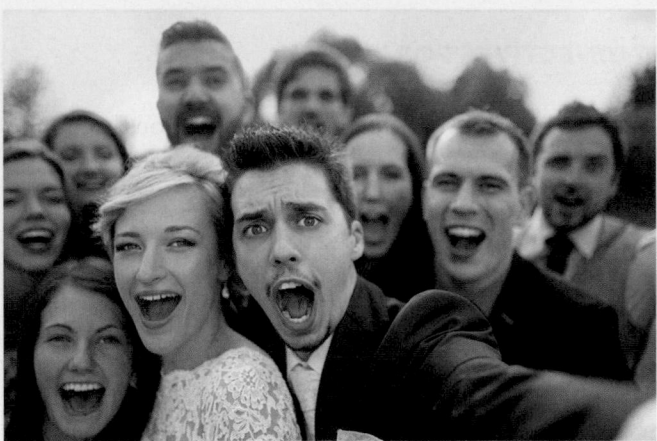

FIGURE 23–7 Choosing a significant other is a developmental task of young adulthood.

Eating Disorders

Eating disorders are complex, chronic illnesses primarily affecting young women. There is no single cause of these disorders; however, several things may contribute: culture, personal characteristics, emotional disorders, stressful events, biology, and families. The three most common are anorexia nervosa, bulimia nervosa, and binge eating. **Anorexia nervosa** is an eating disorder that is marked by weight loss, emaciation, a disturbance in body image, and a fear of weight gain. Persons affected lose weight either by excessive dieting or by purging themselves of ingested calories. This illness is typically found in industrialized nations and usually begins in the teen years. Young women are 10 to 20 times more likely than young men to suffer from this disorder. The young woman claims to feel fat even when she is emaciated. Refusal to maintain body weight can be life threatening because of electrolyte disturbances, anemia, and secondary cardiac arrhythmias. Affected women need to understand that low body weight can cause the body to stop producing estrogen, which leads to amenorrhea (absent menstrual periods). Low estrogen levels contribute to losses in bone density. If anorexia nervosa is suspected, the client must be referred to a health care provider for follow-up as soon as possible (Bulik, 2014; Chelvanayagam & Newell, 2015; National Institute of Mental Health, n.d.; Office on Women's Health, 2012a).

A related disorder, **bulimia nervosa**, is marked by recurrent episodes of binge eating, self-induced vomiting and diarrhea, misuse of laxatives or diuretics, excessive exercise, strict dieting or fasting, and an exaggerated concern about body shape or weight in self-evaluation. Females in cultures where emphasis is placed on a certain ideal of beauty, individuals who have been sexually abused or come from families with a history of eating disorders, and individuals with low self-esteem and a history of not being "in control" or with communication and emotional difficulties are at greater risk. The community health nurse should refer a woman suspected of practicing bulimic behaviors to an appropriate health care provider (National Eating Disorders Collaboration, 2015a; Office on Women's Health, 2012b).

Binge eating is an eating disorder characterized by repeated episodes of uncontrolled eating. It is the newest clinically recognized eating disorder. The onset is usually in late adolescence and the early 20s and starts following significant weight loss from dieting. However, many binge eaters are obese because they usually do not induce vomiting and diarrhea or engage in excessive exercise. Typically, individuals with this disorder eat quickly, eat until they are uncomfortably full, eat when they are not hungry, eat large amounts of food alone, have difficulty expressing their feelings, have difficulty controlling impulses and stress, and feel depressed about overeating. This disorder also puts these women at increased risk for type 2 diabetes, high cholesterol, osteoarthritis, kidney disease or renal failure, heart disease, and high BP (National Eating Disorders Collaboration, 2015b; Office on Women's Health, 2012c).

Overall, eating disorders are not gender specific; females are commonly affected; however, millions of men and boys battle all forms of this illness. Because of the complexities of these disorders, there are differences of opinion in the literature among the experts regarding this topic (National Eating Disorders Association, n.d.). The community health nurse can play a vital role in identifying affected persons and refer these individuals to appropriate health care providers, mental health counselors, and self-help groups. A screening tool that may be helpful in this effort is the Malnutrition Universal Screening Tool, a five-step instrument to identify adults who are malnourished, at risk of malnutrition (undernutrition), or obesity (British Association for Parental and Enteral Nutrition, 2015).

Reproductive Health

By age 25, at least 50% of childbearing women have given birth once. Women (also men) need to be as healthy as possible to have positive pregnancy outcomes. Based on published research and input of experts from the CDC/ATSDR Preconception Care Work Group and the Select Panel on Preconception Care, the CDC (2015m) has made 10 recommendations for preconception care and health care. Four goals of preconception care are to improve knowledge and attitudes, assure that all women of childbearing age in the United States receive preconception care services, reduce risks through interventions, and reduce disparities in adverse pregnancy outcomes. The recommendations for preconception care address (Fig. 23–8):

- Consumer awareness
- Individual responsibility
- Preventive visits
- Interventions for identified risks
- Interconception care
- Prepregnancy checkups
- Health insurance coverage for women with low incomes
- Public health programs and strategies
- Monitoring improvements
- Research (CDC, 2015m)

Although preconception care is addressed in *Healthy People 2020*, many of the preconception objectives are

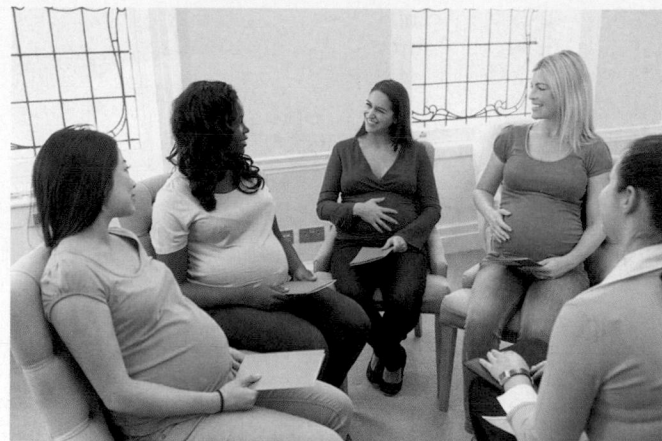

FIGURE 23–8 A group of pregnant women at a support group class.

related to family planning and maternal health (see Display 23–3). Community health nurses have been at the forefront of maternal and child health care for decades, and they must continue to strive to incorporate components of preconception care into their practices. Nurses must advocate for clients to influence public policy, which has the potential to improve access to care for many women and improve pregnancy outcomes (CDC, 2015m).

Sexual health and STIs are important health concerns for young women. Sexual activity typically commences in adolescence and continues throughout the life span. STIs are epidemic in the United States, especially among young adults (see Chapter 8). Many of the common infections are asymptomatic, but not always. The two most common STIs affecting women are Chlamydia and gonorrhea. Approximately 1.4 million cases of Chlamydia occurred in the United States in 2014, and this STI is the most reported nationally notifiable disease. Females 20 to 24 years of age have the second highest rate, preceded by 15- to 19-year-old adolescents. The rate of gonorrhea is lower than Chlamydia, but in 2014, there were 350,062 cases reported, making it the second most nationally reported notifiable disease in the United States. The current prevalence is 110.7 cases per 100,000 persons. Historically, gonorrhea rates for men were higher than women, and in 2014, this continued, with 120.1 cases per 100,000 for men and 101.3 per 100,000 for women. Both Chlamydia and gonorrhea are underdiagnosed, which can have deleterious consequences for women. If treatment is delayed, women can develop pelvic inflammatory disease, chronic pelvic pain, ectopic pregnancy, and infertility (CDC, 2015n, 2015o). See Chapter 8 for more information on communicable diseases.

Community health nurses working with adult women need to provide factual information to increase women's knowledge of STI risk. This information should be a part of frank discussions regarding condom use, sexual partners (male and female), type of sexual activity (oral, anal, vaginal), life-threatening consequences of an undiagnosed STI, and undesirable pregnancy outcomes. Outside of abstinence, condom use is the first line of prevention against STIs. See Evidence-Based Practice.

EVIDENCE-BASED PRACTICE

Bridging Financial Gaps

A survey was conducted using a 15-item instrument (multiple choice and completion questions; English and Spanish versions) at 21 metropolitan sexually transmitted disease (STD) clinics in the United States from August to December in 2013. The aim was to assess the characteristics of STD clinic patients, their reasons for seeking care at the clinics, and the patients' ability to access health care at other providers. The survey was distributed to 100 males and 100 females at each clinic while they were waiting for service. Time to complete the survey was 5 minutes. The overall response rate was 86.6%, and 4,364 individuals completed the survey. Of the patients who declined to complete the survey, 86 cited language barrier as the reason. Researchers noted the most frequently reported reasons for persons using the clinics were a perceived health problem or STD symptoms (18.9%), STD screening (33.8%), and HIV testing (13.6%). However, the main reasons why patients selected the STD clinic included walk-in or same-day appointments (49.5%), low cost of care (23.9%), or availability of expert STD care (8.3%). Of note, if the STD clinics were not available, 20.9% of patients would have delayed seeking care (waiting to see what would happen) and 50.2% would have sought care at an emergency room or urgent care provider.

STI are a major burden on the already overtaxed public health system. More than 19 million new STI cases are diagnosed annually and over $15.6 billion are spent to diagnose and treat STIs and their complications in the United States. When interacting with clients who are sexually active, nurses need to consider incorporating brief educational interventions about STIs into client care; nurses cannot assume that persons are knowledgeable. The more informed individuals are about STI transmission and prevention, the more likely they are to protect themselves. By increasing knowledge and prevention strategies, the costs related to STI treatment can be reduced.

Hoover, K. W., Parsell, B. W., Leichliter, J. S., Habel, M. A., Tao, G., Pearson, W. S., & Gift, T. L. (2015). Continuing need for sexually transmitted disease clinics after the Affordable Care Act. *American Journal of Public Health, 105*(Suppl 5), S690–S695. doi: 10.2105/AJPH.2015.302839.

American Sexual Health Association. (2015). *Statistics.* Retrieved from http://www.ashasexualhealth.org/stdsstis/statistics/

Adult Women (35 to 65 Years)

Women in the adult age group of 35 to 65 years have established themselves into patterns of living that have served them well or ill. During this period, the results of years of choices may present themselves in the form of chronic illnesses. Nevertheless, many women in this age group have time to change health habits to possibly reverse encroaching chronic illnesses. For other women, lifestyle choices and undetected diseases have shortened their life spans, and large numbers of women in this age group are dying prematurely.

Menopause and Hormone Replacement Therapy

Menopause is a time that marks the permanent cessation of menstrual activity (last menstrual period). The average age is 51 years (range = 45 to 55); however, it can occur as early as age 40. Perimenopause, or the time period that leads up to the last menstrual cycle, is characterized by cycle changes and irregularity. Menstrual flow may be light or heavy, and spotting may occur, depending on varying estrogen and progesterone levels. This perimenopausal period may last 10 years, and women may see their health care providers more frequently because of irregular bleeding that could be due to more serious causes (American College of Obstetricians and Gynecologists [ACOG], 2011). Natural menopause is defined as cessation of menstrual periods for 12 consecutive months, with no other apparent cause. Because of the sudden loss of estrogen with surgical removal of the ovaries, some women have an early, *surgical menopause*. Because estrogen levels do not simply decline evenly over time, but rather have peaks and valleys, blood tests are not effective in the diagnosis (Bostock-Cox, 2015). Menopause symptoms differ among women and may last from months to years. They range from hardly noticeable in some women to very severe in others. Symptoms include nervousness or anxiety, hot flashes (flushes), chills, excessive sweating (often at night), excitability, fatigue, mood disorders (apathy, mental depression, crying episodes), insomnia, palpitations, vertigo, headache, numbness, tingling, myalgia, urinary disturbances, and vaginal dryness (National Institute on Aging, 2015; Shaheen, Mahmood, & Kadri, 2015). Some women experience problems with sexual functions (e.g., infrequent sexual relations, decreased libido), and one study of almost 500 women who had wither a natural menopause or a surgical menopause found an association between problems with sexual functioning and the intensity of menopausal symptoms like hot flashes and sweating, especially for those experiencing surgical menopause (Topatan & Yildiz, 2012). The *Study of Women's Health Across the Nation* (SWAN) revealed that hot flashes and some of the other menopausal symptoms may last longer than the 7 years previously thought; in fact, they may last up to 14 years and Australian researchers noted that a small percentage of women (about 7%) may experience them well into their 60s (Freeman, Sammel, & Sanders, 2014; Harvard Health, 2015) (Fig. 23–9).

Genitourinary syndrome of menopause (GSM) describes a group of symptoms related to decreased estrogen and other steroids involved in changes to the female genitourinary

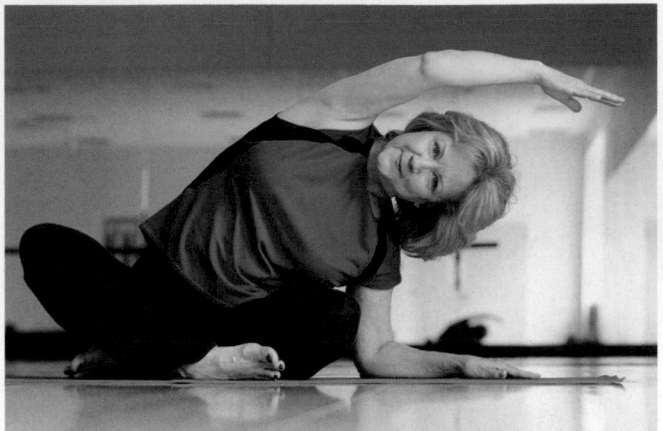

FIGURE 23–9 Menopause is another transitional period in a woman's life, and healthy diet and exercise are important.

system. These symptoms include genital dryness, irritation, or burning, sexual symptoms that include inadequate lubrication and painful or impaired sexual functioning, and symptoms of urinary frequency, urgency, painful urination, and frequent urinary tract infections (Portman & Gass, 2014). Sleep problems are common among menopausal women, and researchers noted more restless sleep, decreased quality of sleep, and more instances of waking during the night among postmenopausal women, compared to premenopausal women (Lampio et al., 2014). Many women complain of weight gain, especially in the abdominal area, during perimenopause. Davis et al. (2012) found that all weight gain can't be blamed on the menopausal transition period, but there are indications that the hormonal changes accompanying menopause are correlated with both an increased level of body fat and increased levels abdominal fat. Those women who received **hormone replacement therapy (HRT)** generally had an overall fat mass reduction and increased insulin sensitivity, along with lower rates of type 2 diabetes. Lifestyle interventions (e.g., healthy diet, exercise programs) have also shown promise in addressing changes in body weight during menopause (Jull et al., 2014).

Other research on menopausal symptoms and outcomes includes topics such as hot flashes and dizziness during menopause, iron changes during menopause and associated insulin resistance, and earlier age of menopause being associated with cumulative lead exposures, as well as the effects of premature menopause and later life cognitive functioning and later age of natural menopause and increased cardiovascular death rates (Eum, Weisskopf, Nie, Hu, & Korrick, 2014; Kim, Nan, Kong, & Harlow, 2012; Owada & Suzuki, 2014; Ryan et al., 2014; Tom, Cooper, Wallace, & Guralnik, 2012).

How do women really feel about menopause? Anthropologists at the University of Hawaii conducted a qualitative study of a multiethnic sample of 185 women who were pre-, peri-, and postmenopausal. The most common theme among premenopausal women was anxiety over the expected changes that would occur during menopause. They feared the stories that they had heard from others about this stage of life, such as the "hormonal rages, personality changes," depression, osteoporosis, divorce, and sexual or physical dysfunctions (Morrison et al., 2014, p. 535). For perimenopausal women, they were transitioning from negative to more positive thoughts about the experience. The benefits of no longer having periods or worrying about getting pregnant, and liberation from an intense focus on family concerns to being more able to take care of themselves, seemed less frightening than the stories they had heard from other women of the "raging menopausal maniacs." For postmenopausal women, there was more of a focus on developing a "postmenstrual identity" as a wiser, more optimistic woman who has gone through a natural body change.

A quantitative study of over 1,000 baby boomer females from a national sample examined adaptation to menopause and resulted in a two-factor model. Women who had positive responses to menopausal effects about the end of menstruation/loss of fertility were generally less educated, but more financially secure, and older than those who had more positive viewpoints toward physical attractiveness and health concerns related to menopause (Strauss, 2011).

The Endocrine Society recommendations include menopause diagnosis; discussions about menopausal symptoms, osteoporosis, cancer screening, and assessment for CVD; along with a determination of the need for hormonal therapy (usually estrogen for those having had a hysterectomy and estrogen/progesterone for those who have not). In some cases, SSRIs or other medications are indicated, and vaginal lubricants or hormone creams are used (Stuenkel et al., 2014). Bethany Hays (2011), an OB/GYN physician and contributor to a functional medicine textbook, considers that menopause is not a hormone deficit disorder, as many believe, but a period of necessary normal hormonal adjustment. She describes the hormonal balancing act between adrenaline, insulin, and cortisol, along with estrogen, progesterone, and testosterone, and notes that dysregulation of the hyopothalamus because of estrogen changes leads to hot flashes. Estrogen and testosterone are involved in decreased libido and atrophic vaginitis, and she cautions health care providers to use hormone therapy carefully. She prefers delivery of hormones by transdermal patches or vaginal creams and urges physicians to pay careful attention to a woman's signs and symptoms and to regularly utilize lab tests in order to "normalize hormone levels across the board" (p. 43).

Based on the severity of symptoms and to address long-term body changes such as bone loss and the risk for CVD, HRT may be recommended. Treatment typically involves the use of estrogen alone, estrogen plus progesterone, or estrogen plus progestin (a synthetic hormone with effects similar to progesterone). However, there still remains controversy regarding use of HRT as evidenced by the following: in 2002, researchers found an increased rate of breast cancer, ovarian cancer, heart disease, and stroke among healthy women in the *WHI* study who were taking combined estrogen and progestin HRT. The initial reaction to this information was a dramatic decline in prescribing by physicians, which included both combined HRT and estrogen alone. The debate over the risk versus benefit of long-term HRT is ongoing; however, there is strong agreement that HRT should not be used for the primary or secondary prevention of CVD. However, it is clear that menopausal women should discuss the risks of HRT with their primary care provider (deVilliers et al., 2013; LaCroix et al., 2011; Mosca et al., 2011; NCI, 2011; Stuenkel et al., 2014). Some providers voice concern about the changes in treatment options for menopausal women, and the lack of physician training on this issue, as well as not providing hormone therapy for the "20% to 30% of those who experience distressing symptoms without adequate relief" (Manson & Kaunitz, 2016; Rubenstein, 2014, p. 218). In place of HRT, some women choose to use **bioidentical hormone therapy**—chemically similar hormones derived from plants—that may (e.g., micronized estradiol and progesterone) or may not be approved (e.g., Triest, Biest, pregnenolone) by the Food and Drug Administration (FDA). Both the FDA and the Endocrine Society have determined that the term bioidentical hormone therapy is not scientifically based and is used mainly for marketing purposes (ACOG, 2012). Researchers examined the differences in menopausal symptom relief between those women taking bioidentical hormones that have been prepared by a compounding pharmacist (BCH) and other women using conventional HRT (Iftikhar, Shuster, Johnson, Jenkins, & Wahner-Roedler, 2014). About 59% of BCH preparations also included androgens, and both groups of women reported similar menopausal symptoms at baseline. Both groups reported relief of symptoms, but those using BCH therapy had better relief of sexual symptoms of menopause; researchers thought this might have been related to the inclusion of androgens like testosterone. The greatest concern involved lack of knowledge in the BCH group. Women in the study thought BCH compounds were safer than HRT; however, BCH risk is similar to that of HRT (Iftikhar et al., 2014). A systematic review of the use of soy isoflavones for relieving the vaginal dryness of menopause was inconclusive, although some relief was indicated (Ghazanfarpour, Sadeghi, & Roudsari, 2016). Jacob (2016) reports a 79% drop in HRT use from 2002 to 2010, after the *WHI* study results were publicized and notes that between 50% and 80% of women now use some type of nonhormonal therapy to deal with menopausal symptoms. Cognitive behavioral therapy, hypnosis, and the SSRI paroxetine have been shown to decrease both the frequency and irritation of night sweats and hot flashes. Short-term HRT can relieve the vasomotor symptoms (e.g., hot flashes) and presents a low risk to women who do not have breast cancer and CVD risks. A smartphone/tablet app, *MenoPro*, helps women and health care providers evaluate all available recommended options. Risk calculators for osteoporosis/fracture, breast cancer, and CVD, as well as information of various medications, are also available on the app.

Osteoporosis

A gradual loss in bone density is known as **osteoporosis**. Typically, bone density peaks about age 25, and over time, bones become fragile and easily facture. It is estimated that one out of five women in the United States has *osteoporosis*. Therefore, it is important for women to build strong bone early. Bone density is influenced by many factors such as heredity, race/ethnicity, physical activity, and nutrition. It is important for women of all ages to maintain a healthy diet and engage in physical activity. There are several classes of medications that can be used to treat osteoporosis: bisphosphonates (helps build bone mass), selective estrogen receptor modulators (slows rate of bone loss), calcitonin (slows rate of bone loss), and teriparatide (helps build up new bone). Every woman 65 years of age or older should be screened for osteoporosis (Office on Women's Health, 2012d). See Chapter 24 for more on osteoporosis in older women.

Heart Disease

Heart disease, or CVD, is the number one killer of women, causing the death of 292,188 females in 2009 (CDC, 2013b). Racial disparity exists, with CVD-related death rates for Black women at 204.5 per 100,000 compared to 150.5 per 100,000 for White women. The most common heart problem, CHD, is underdiagnosed, undertreated, and underresearched in women. In addition, women have a higher mortality rate after heart attack and poorer outcomes than do men, and this may be related to delayed diagnosis and treatment. Risk factors for heart disease in women are age, family history, race/ethnicity, physical inactivity, obesity, diabetes mellitus, high BP, high cholesterol, and cigarette smoking (Boudi, 2015; CDC, 2013b; Kochanek, Xu, Murphy, Miniño, & Kung, 2011; Mosca et al., 2011).

Family history, race/ethnicity, and advancing age cannot be changed, but women can make lifestyle changes to alter other risk factors. The remaining risk factors are issues that the community health nurse can discuss with female clients in this age group. Community health nurses can help raise awareness regarding heart disease when working with women at the individual, family, or aggregate levels. Some important facts that can be shared are as follows:

- More than 1 million Americans have a heart attack yearly, and about half of them are women (Rajan, 2015).
- According to a recent survey, 36% of women were not aware that heart disease was the leading cause of death in women (CDC, 2013b).
- Almost two thirds of women who suddenly die from heart disease have had no previous symptoms (CDC, 2013b).
- Heart disease is sometimes thought of as a "man's disease," but about the same number of women and men die each year of heart disease (CDC, 2013b).
- Women have atypical heart symptoms or less acute chest pain, which may delay them from seeking care (CDC, 2013b).
- Hormone therapy does not reduce coronary events (deVilliers et al., 2013).
- Nine out of 10 women have at least one risk factor for heart disease (Heart Foundation, 2015).
- One in 3 female deaths are from CVD, compared with 1 in 31 from breast cancer (Heart Foundation, 2015).

An excellent lay resource is "*Go Red for Women*," a public awareness program of the American Heart Association to help improve knowledge (AHA, 2015).

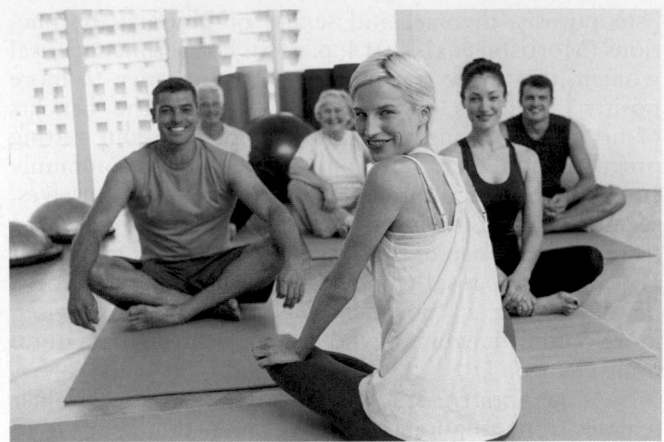

FIGURE 23–10 Regular exercise is an important part of health promotion.

Also, *Well-Integrated Screening and Evaluation for Women across the Nation* (WISEWOMAN), a CDC program that helps women with little or no health insurance reduce their risk for heart disease, stroke, and other chronic diseases (located in 21 sites across 19 states), can be helpful. The program assists women ages 40 to 64 in improving their diet, physical activity, and other behaviors. This program also provides cholesterol tests and other screening (CDC, 2013b; Mosca et al., 2011) (Fig. 23–10).

Regular exercise is an important part of health promotion.

Cancer

Cancer is the second leading cause of death for women, estimated to kill 24,480 females in the United States in 2015. Genetic mutations play a role in cancer; but only a small percentage of cancers are hereditary. Thus, the vast majority of cancers are random, and most cancers (78%) occur in persons 55 years of age and older. The lifetime risk of a woman getting cancer is a little more than one in three. To help address this disparity, community health nurses can provide more opportunities for education and screening for this population. Screening has reduced the deaths for cancers of the breast, colon, rectum, and cervix (ACS, 2015a).

Breast cancer is the most common cancer among women; however, more women die of lung cancer. In 2015, it is estimated that 40,290 deaths related to breast cancer will occur (ACS, 2015a). Overall, the death rates from breast cancer have declined since 1990, and the biggest decline was among women under 50 years of age. This can be attributed to early detection and improvements in treatment. The sooner breast cancer is discovered, the more successfully it is treated. By obtaining regular clinical breast exams and mammograms, eating a diet low in fat and high in fruits and vegetables, breast-feeding (if possible), and avoiding prolonged use of menopausal HRT, a woman is doing what she can to promote breast health. Although breast self-examination (BSE) continues to be taught in many communities, it is no longer considered to be a routine screening recommendation. However, it is important that women be aware of any overt changes in their breasts, especially changes

Table 23–5 Breast Cancer Death Rates Among All Women: 2008 to 2012

(Age-Adjusted Rates per 100,000)

Women	Rate
All races	21.9
Black	30.2
White	21.3
American Indian/Alaska Native	15.0
Hispanic	14.5
Asian/Pacific Islander	11.4

Extracted from Surveillance, Epidemiology, and End Stage Program (SEER). (n.d.). *SEER stat fact sheets: Female breast cancer.* Retrieved from http://seer.cancer.gov/statfacts/html/breast.html

related to size, shape, symmetry, and nipple discharge. Knowledge of and engaging in BSE can heighten awareness of breast changes for many women. The community health nurse has many resources available to provide information and to teach women in their homes, small groups in clinics, or in various other community settings to enhance knowledge of breast health (ACS, 2015b). See Chapters 11 and 12. See Table 23–5.

Screening for breast cancer is important as it leads to early detection when tumors are likely to be smaller and confined to the breast. Early detection is associated with better prognosis for survival. In April of 2015, the U.S. Preventive Services Task Force released its breast cancer screening draft recommendations for public comment. These recommendations are based on the current scientific evidence so that women can make the best choices regarding their breast health in concert with health care providers. These recommendations are biennial mammography screening for women 50 to 75 years; evidence is insufficient to assess the benefits and harms of screening mammography in women 75 years and older; current evidence is insufficient to assess the additional benefits and harms of clinical breast examination (CBE) beyond screening mammography in women 40 years or older; BSE is not recommended; and biennial mammography screening before the age of 50 years should be an individual decision and the patient's context (risk for disease) should be taken into account. Women who have a first-degree relative with breast cancer (mother, sister), have a breast cancer gene (BRCA 1 or BRCA 2), or have had previous breast cancer are at a higher risk for developing the disease than other women in the general population. Therefore, these individuals need to consult their physicians regarding timelines for screenings (ACS, 2015b; NCI: SEER, n.d.).

Papanicolaou (Pap) smears have improved early detection and prevention of cervical cancer dramatically. Both the incidence and the death rates for cervical cancer have declined in recent decades because of treatment of preinvasive cervical lesions. The major

risk factors for this disease are infection with certain types of the human papillomavirus (HPV), unprotected intercourse at an early age, and multiple sex partners. In 2015, it is estimated that 12,900 new cases of invasive cervical cancer will be diagnosed in the United States, contributing to 4,100 deaths among women from this disease. The 5-year survival rate for this cancer, if prompt treatment is initiated, is 68% for all stages and 91% for local infiltration, making it one of the most successfully treated cancers. Community health nurses can continue to improve screening and early diagnosis through education and advocating for low-cost screening, which will allow many at-risk elderly, low-income, and rural women access to regular Pap screenings. In addition, making women aware of the HPV vaccines Gardasil (given between the ages of 9 to 26 years), Gardasil 9 (works against nine different viruses, given between the ages of 9 and 26 years), and Cervarix (effective against two different viruses, given between the ages of 9 to 25 years) may reduce the incidence of cervical cancer in upcoming decades. Of note, both Gardasil vaccines are approved for use in males (ACS, 2015a; NCI, 2015).

Ovarian cancer contributes to more deaths than any other cancer of the female reproductive system and accounts for 5% of cancer deaths among women. Examining 2007 to 2011 data, death rates have steadily declined by 2% each year since 2007. In 2015, a total of 21,290 cases were anticipated and 14,180 deaths were expected. The primary risk factor for this disease is heredity, or a strong family history of breast or ovarian cancer. The 5-year survival rate is 45% compared to cervical (70%) and breast (89%) cancers. Women at high risk should receive a pelvic exam, a transvaginal ultrasound, and a blood test for the tumor marker CA 125. An ongoing clinical trial in the United Kingdom is examining the efficacy of screening, using the serial values of CA 125 to estimate risk and referring women with high risk for ultrasound examination to improve survival. Therefore, public health nurses need to continue to stress the importance of early detection (ACS, 2015a; Hartge, 2011).

Chronic Fatigue and Immune Dysfunction Syndrome/Myalgic Encephalomyelitis

Chronic fatigue and immune dysfunction syndrome (CFIDS) also known as **myalgic encephalomyelitis (ME)** is characterized by persistent and debilitating fatigue and additional nonspecific symptoms such as sore throat, headache, painful muscles, joint pain, difficulty thinking, and loss of short-term memory. It is estimated that ME affects between 836,000 and 2.8 million persons in the United States and the majority are women. Rest does not relieve the fatigue. Symptoms may wax and wane and are difficult to validate objectively, but they are subjectively debilitating. Symptoms can last for months or years. Because the cause is unknown, there is no specific treatment and no prevention suggestions. Treatment is focused on supportive care for the associated pain, depression, and insomnia. The ME/CFS Initiative provides support and information for women and is one of seven organizations that contributed to the newly released paper, *Impact of Chronic Overlapping Pain Conditions on Public Health* *and the Urgent Need for Safe and Effective Treatment*, a report that raises awareness of chronic pain conditions that disproportionately impact women. The community health nurse can assess activity level and degree of fatigue, emotional response to the illness, and coping ability. Emotionally supportive family members and health care providers are helpful. Referring women to mental health counseling or a local support group is useful for many women and within the role of the community health nurse (CDC, 2015p; Chronic Pain Research Alliance, 2015; Institute of Medicine, 2015; Solve ME/CFS Initiative, 2015).

MEN'S HEALTH

Gender is among the numerous factors that influence health. More male neonates die at birth, and men are more likely to die earlier from a chronic illness than women. This is evidenced by the difference in life expectancy between men and women in the United States; women survive an average of 5 years longer than men (Mathews, MacDorman, & Thoma, 2015; Xu, Kochanek, Murphy, & Arias, 2014) (Fig. 23–11).

Overview of Factors Influencing Men's Health

The concept of masculinity is an influencing factor in men's health. Men are socialized to be independent and conceal their vulnerability. Therefore, even when they are aware of personal physical or mental health problems, they are less likely to access the health care system. How the male identity is maintained can include activities that are hazardous to their health, and the result is a high death rate from unintentional injuries among young men. Examples of these activities include working in dangerous jobs, engaging in behaviors that lead to increased risk of homicide or car crashes, excessive alcohol consumption, smoking, substance use, and unsafe sex practices (Gough, 2013; Levant & Wimer, 2014; Lutfiyya, Cannon, & Lipsky, 2014).

Factors that contribute to the deteriorating state of men's health include a lack of quality health education programs for men, health care services that are only

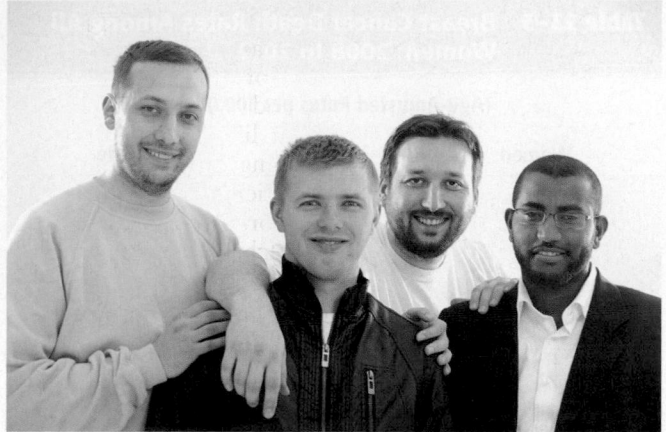

FIGURE 23–11 Men have different health care needs at various stages of life.

accessed half as much by men when compared to women, and a lack of male gender-specific research (Lipsky, Cannon, & Lutfiyya, 2014). Considering all of these factors, the PHN must determine the health care needs of men at various stages and how nurses can best meet these needs throughout the adult life span.

Men's Health Promotion Across the Adult Life Span

In the early years of young adulthood (between 18 and 35 years), men continue to grow and mature. Adult men aged 35 to 65 years have reached maturity, the peak of their physical and intellectual development, and their greatest earning power. What specific needs do men in these age groups have? Are their needs being met through provided services?

Healthy People 2020 Goals for Men

Although *Healthy People 2020* includes 27 health objectives specifically for women and 7 for men, many apply to both women and men of all ages. The 7 men's objectives focus on prostate health, reproductive health, and disease prevention among men, especially men who have sex with men (MSM) (see Display 23–4).

DISPLAY 23–4 *HEALTHY PEOPLE 2020* OBJECTIVES FOR MEN

1. Reduce the number of prostate cancer death rates from 23.5 deaths per 100,000 to 21.2 deaths per 100,000
2. (Developmental) Increase the proportion of men who have discussed with their health care provider whether or not to have a prostate-specific antigen (PSA) test to screen for prostate cancer
3. Increase the proportion of sexually active males aged 15 to 44 years who received reproductive health services by 10%, from 14.9% to 16.4%
4. Reduce the number of new AIDS cases among adolescents and adult MSM by 10%, from 16,749 new cases to 15,074 new cases
5. Increase the proportion of adolescents and adults who have been tested for HIV in the last 12 months among (developmental) MSM
6. (Developmental) Decrease the proportion of MSM who reported unprotected anal sex in the past 12 months
7. Increase the proportion of sexually active unmarried males 15 to 44 years of age who used a condom at last intercourse by 10%, from 60.7% to 55.2%

Adapted from U.S. Department of Health and Human Services (USDHHS). (2015). *Healthy people 2020: Topics and objectives*. Retrieved from https://www.healthypeople.gov/2020/topics-objectives

Young Adult Men (18 to 35 Years)

The young adult male has many tasks to accomplish. These tasks include the acquisition of training or education that will lead to a personally and financially rewarding career, selecting a compatible lifetime companion and establishing a life together, finding comfort with and meaning to existence through practicing and internalizing a belief and value system that works for him, actively planning for having (or not having) children, and participating in the betterment of the greater community. Young men may choose work that involves physical labor, office work, or a variety of other endeavors, including active duty military. They may also be veterans of military service (Fig. 23–12).

Depending on his attitudes and practices before a man enters young adulthood, he may or may not be enticed to experiment or continue with the use of tobacco, alcohol, or illicit drugs. Experimentation or usage of these substances can occur in college, the military, or working at a full-time job. Young men also engage in behaviors or take risks without thinking about the consequences. They respond to challenges such as drag racing, exceeding speed limits, and binge drinking. This is an important age group for the PHN to reach with health information because decisions made in these formative years affect how young men live the rest of their lives. The nurse can meet with young adult men in work settings, college campuses, military bases, health clubs and bars, and at single-adult groups sponsored by religious communities and other organizations.

Another issue to address during the early years is the young man's attitudes and beliefs toward sex and sexual experimentation. Young men may question their sexuality as they mature, and during this stage, some men come to the realization that they are homosexual. **Gay** is a commonly accepted term for a homosexual—a person who has sexual interest in or sexual intercourse exclusively with members of his or her own gender. Some men who have sex with men, women, or both often do not consider themselves to be gay or **bisexual**. They are categorized as MSM. When taking a sexual history, community health nurses must ask men if they have sex with women, men, or both, and they should be aware of issues affecting the lesbian, gay, bisexual, and transgender (LGBT) population.

Transgender, another term associated with sexuality, is used to describe individuals who experience and/or express their gender differently from what people might expect. These individuals express characteristics that do not correspond with the person's apparent or presumed gender. An example is when a presumed male chooses to put on makeup and clothes that a female would traditionally wear. Some transgender individuals define themselves as *female to male* or *male to female* and may take hormones and/or undergo medical procedures to enhance or make permanent their gender selection, including gender reassignment surgery. Others prefer to simply be called *male* or *female*—the gender they present to others, whether or not they have undergone permanent gender reassignment.

Sexual experimentation, whether heterosexual or homosexual, can place young men at risk for diseases that affect long-term health or are life threatening. Men who are sexually active can reduce the possibility of being infected with an STI by limiting the number of sexual partners and using condoms consistently and correctly. Condoms also serve as a form of birth control for men. *Monogamy*, having sex with only one partner and abstinence can further reduce or eliminate the chance of contracting an STI. Public health nurses can serve as a resource for young men and can help them obtain free or low-cost condoms and treatment for STIs.

Human Immunodeficiency Virus and Men

Despite advances in the prevention and treatment of human immunodeficiency virus (HIV), the disease continues to disproportionately impact men in the United States. At the end of 2012, there were 42 jurisdictions in the United States with numerically stable HIV estimates. Within these jurisdictions, the CDC estimated 914,826 persons aged 13 and older were living with HIV. The percentage or persons living with the disease ranged from 110 cases per 100,000 in Iowa to 3,936 cases per 100,000 in Washington, DC. Because the percentage of persons diagnosed with HIV varies by geographic region, it is important that prevention, testing, and treatment interventions be tailored for each area's distinctive milieu (CDC, 2015q; Hall et al., 2015).

In 2012, men accounted for 75% of all diagnoses of HIV infection among adults and adolescents, and 69% of those males were men who had sex with men (MSM). The rate of HIV infection among men was 540.7 per 100,000 persons compared to 167.0 in women. Most new infections occurred in adult males aged 25 to 34 years, except among Black men for whom 38% of all new infections occurred in the youngest age group, 13 to 24 years. When examining trends in the disease based on race/ethnicity, the burden of the disease is highest among men of color. The rate of new HIV infections among Black men is 6.5 times higher than White men and 2 times higher than Hispanic/Latino men (CDC, 2015r; Singh, Hu, Wheeler, & Hall, 2014).

Alcohol and illicit drug use are known to decrease social inhibitions and increase the risk for HIV transmission through risky sexual behaviors (e.g., lack of condom

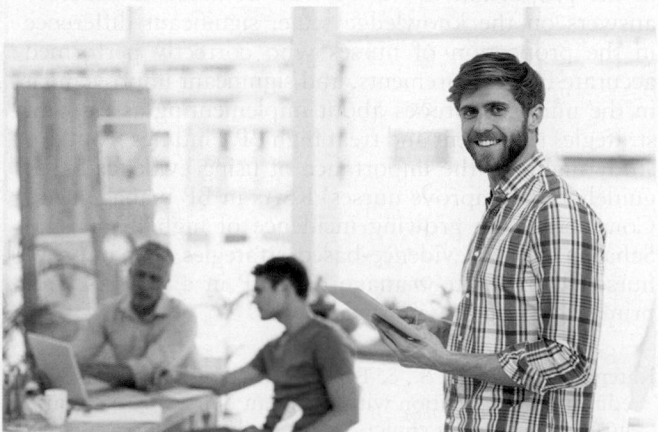

FIGURE 23–12 Choosing a career path is one developmental task for young adult males.

use) and the sharing of needles or other injection equipment. Community health nurses must be able to talk openly and nonjudgmentally with men about their use of substances and their sexual relationships. These conversations can be challenging, but they have to occur if the number of HIV infections is to be reduced (CDC, 2015s; USDHHS, 2014b).

Testicular Cancer

The risk for testicular cancer is a health problem that young men should be aware of even before early adulthood. The disease occurs most often in men between 20 and 34 years of age. Only a few risk factors have been identified that increase a young man's chance of developing testicular cancer. These include a personal history of an undescended testicle, family history of testicular cancer, race/ethnicity (White), age, and tall stature (ACS, 2015c; Ghazarian, Trabert, Devesas, & McGlynn, 2015). It is a rare form of cancer and is not on the list of objectives for men in *Healthy People 2020*. However, if detected early, this cancer is highly curable. According to the American Cancer Society, it may be beneficial to the overall health of a young man to know how to perform a testicular self-exam (TSE), although clinical guidelines

no longer recommend this (ACS, 2015c; U.S. Preventive Services Task Force, 2014b). Teaching men how to do this exam appropriately is a role for nurses working in community settings such as schools and clinics (see Display 23–5).

The choices a young adult man makes during these years establish healthy eating, work, rest, and exercise habits that will benefit him for a lifetime. A man should follow the dietary food guidelines that are recommended by U.S. Department of Agriculture (2016) when considering personal likes and dislikes. He and his family will benefit if he is able to balance work and home, doing his best in both settings. Establishing a pattern of rest that allows his body to recover and refresh from a day full of meaningful activities will help him look forward to each day. He should establish an exercise routine that meets his personal needs, fits his skills and talents, and includes some physical activities that involve his family. These choices provide him with the knowledge that he is doing everything he can to keep himself healthy and to prevent the two major killers of men—heart disease and cancer. However, there are additional considerations. Typically, young adult clients have few interactions with health care providers in any given year. It is often assumed that young

---

EVIDENCE-BASED PRACTICE

The Global Community

HTN has become a significant cardiovascular disorder in sub-Saharan Africa and it is estimated that by 2025, 41.7% of males and 38.7% of females in this part of the world will develop HTN. To prepare nurses and physicians working with hypertensive patients, the World Health Organization (WHO) developed comprehensive HTN guidelines for low- and middle-income countries.

Little is known about the capacity of Ugandan nurses to address early detection, risk assessment, and patient education on diet, physical activity, and other lifestyle changes for hypertensive patients. Based on the WHO HTN guidelines, a nurse-led pilot project aimed at enhancing nurses' knowledge, attitude, and skills in early detection, risk assessment, and patient education was implemented at Mulago Hospital's medical outpatient clinic.

To evaluate outcomes of the project, a one-group pre-/poststudy using convenience sampling was designed and implemented. The education intervention was conducted over 3 months and consisted of 22 hours of didactic classroom sessions that focused on improving the nurses' knowledge, skills, and attitudes (KSA) related to HTN management. To enhance self-directed learning, a CD-ROM on HTN management was given to each nurse. The participants were also involved in clinic sessions that focused on using the WHO risk prediction charts, accurate BP measuring techniques, motivational interviewing for patient education on lifestyle changes, and implementation

of the WHO HTN guidelines. The nurses' KSAs were measured using pre-/postintervention instruments. The measures included a researcher-developed knowledge scale, a technique skills checklist that assessed accurate BP measurement skills, and an adapted version of the *Respondents' Attitude to Assessment Strategies for Prevention of High Blood Pressure* survey.

Seven nurses working in the outpatient clinic participated in the study. All participants were female and ranged in age from 37 to 53 years. Mean years of nursing experience were 2.8 ± 4.1 and 71% received nursing education in Uganda. The study found that after the educational intervention, there was significant difference in the proportion of nurses who obtained satisfactory answers on the knowledge scale, significant difference in the proportion of nurses who correctly performed accurate BP measurements, and significant improvement in the nurses' attitudes about implementing assessment strategies to prevent and treat high BP. Findings from this study highlight the importance of using evidence-based guidelines to improve nurses' KSAs in BP management. Considering the growing incidence of high BP in sub-Saharan Africa, evidence-based strategies that improve nurses' capacity to manage high BP in a low resource primary care setting is crucial.

Katende, G., Groves, S., & Becker, K. (2014). Hypertension education intervention with Ugandan Nurses working in hospital outpatient clinic: A pilot study. *Nursing Research and Practice, 2014*. doi: 10.1155/2014/710702.

DISPLAY 23–5 PERFORMING TESTICULAR SELF-EXAMINATION (TSE)

- TSE should be performed monthly.
- TSE should be done right after a hot shower or bath. The scrotum is most relaxed then, which makes it easier to examine the testicles.
- Examine one testicle at a time. Use both hands to gently roll each testicle (with slight pressure) between your fingers. Place your thumbs over the top of your testicle, with the index and middle fingers of each hand behind the testicle, and then roll it between your fingers.
- The epididymis, which feels soft, rope-like, and slightly tender to pressure, is located at the top of the back part of each testicle. This is a normal lump.

- One testicle (usually the right one) is slightly larger than the other; this is normal.
- When examining each testicle, feel for any lumps or bumps along the front or sides. Lumps may be as small as a piece of rice or a pea.
- If there are any swellings, lumps, or changes in the size or color of a testicle, or if there is any pain or achy area in your groin, let your doctor know right away.
- Lumps or swelling may not be cancer, but a physician should be consulted.

Adapted from American Cancer Society. (2015). *Testicular self-exam.* Retrieved from http://www.cancer.org/cancer/testicularcancer/moreinformation/doihavetesticularcancer/do-i-have-testicular-cancer-self-exam

---

adult males in this age range are not at risk for physical or psychological disease. This is a myth. It is important for people in this age group to have regular health check-ups, be assessed for early signs of disease, and engage in health promotion activities (Fig. 23–13).

Adult Men (35 to 65 Years)

Men in the developmental stage between 35 and 65 years of age are often faced with caring for their own families and children, as well as aging parents and in-laws. The physical, economic, and emotional demands can be great: older adults may have extended care needs while, simultaneously, the family must bear the economic burdens of putting children through college. Meanwhile, men are adjusting to the reality that their career path is probably set and many of their life choices have been made.

The term "midlife" is applied to the first half of this age period, 35 to 49 years. It is a time when many men focus on a reappraisal of values, priorities, and personal relationships. As the term "midlife crisis" implies, this can be one of the more difficult stages of life. It can be an emotional time of doubt and anxiety when a man becomes uncomfortable with the idea that his life is half over. He may believe that he has not accomplished enough, or he may struggle to find new meaning or purpose in his life. Men may experience boredom with their personal life, job, or partners, and a desire to make changes in these areas may occur (Lachman, 2015; Robinson & Wright, 2013).

The later years in this stage, ages 50 to 64, involve preparation for retirement. In anticipation of retirement, these years are marked by expanded social relationships and pursuit of new hobbies to fill increased leisure time, along with anticipating finishing a career and accumulation of the best retirement benefits. The decisions made during these years will play out over the rest of a man's life and could alter how a spouse or long-term partner lives out their years. Health problems that were left undiagnosed when the man was younger begin to emerge. Peers may be suffering and succumbing to diseases, and a man begins to adjust to the potential loss of loved ones, particularly a spouse or long-term companion (Cahill, Giandrea, & Quinn, 2013; Wang & Shi, 2014).

Successful navigation of this stage can be fulfilling but may require a man to enhance his self-care skills. This includes having a positive attitude toward aging, one that examines the benefits of maturity, finds a balance between work and home, and maintains a healthy lifestyle by eating balanced meals and obtaining regular exercise. The community health nurse can provide anticipatory guidance to men approaching this stage and provide them with information on ways to manage life more effectively.

Reproductive Health

During this stage, especially when a man has decided that his family is complete, he may choose a permanent form of birth control. For men, permanent birth control can be obtained through a surgical procedure called *vasectomy*. A vasectomy entails removal of all or a segment of the vas deferens, so that sperm cannot be released. The procedure is routinely conducted on an outpatient basis, is minimally invasive, and takes about 30 minutes. Vasectomies

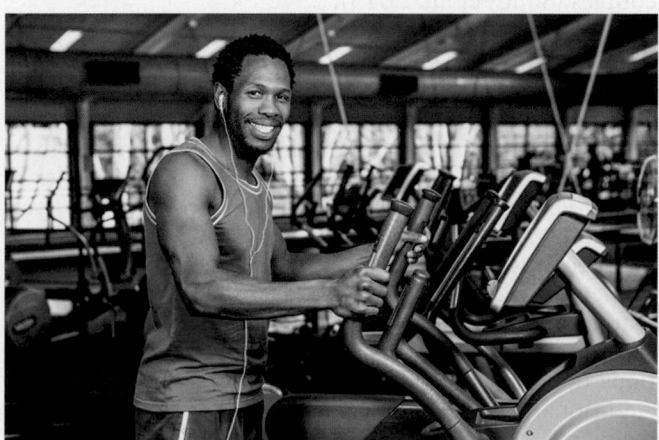

FIGURE 23–13 Adult men are encouraged to maintain good health through eating a healthy diet and getting regular exercise.

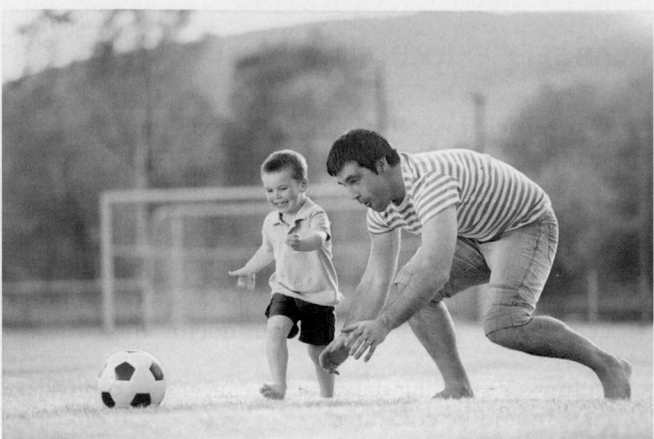

FIGURE 23–14 Reproductive health is also an important consideration for men.

are considered permanent; however, with the advent of microsurgical techniques, vasectomy reversals are now possible (Rayala & Viera, 2013) (Fig. 23–14).

Compared to tubal ligation (a surgical form of contraception for women), vasectomy is equally effective in preventing pregnancy. But, vasectomy is simpler, faster, safer, and less expensive. When compared to the expense of a tubal ligation, a vasectomy is about one fourth of the cost. Despite its advantages, vasectomy has low utilization as a form of contraception. In the United States, only 5.7% of all couples that use some form of contraception rely on a vasectomy (Sharlip et al., 2012). Among married couples, the prevalence of vasectomy as a form of birth control is higher, at 13.1% (Anderson et al., 2012). Reasons for low use of vasectomy include lack of knowledge, misconceptions, lack of access, provider bias, and patient preferences (Shih, Zhang, Bukowski, & Chen, 2014). Men who select vasectomy are largely a homogenous group of older White, well-educated men of high economic status who have children (Eeckhaut, 2015; Sharma et al., 2013).

Erection problems are common among men of all ages but especially in men as they age. **Erectile dysfunction** (ED), sometimes called *impotence*, is the repeated inability to get or keep an erection firm enough for sexual intercourse. The word impotence may also be used to describe other problems that interfere with sexual intercourse, such as lack of sexual desire and problems with ejaculation or orgasm. Using the term *erectile dysfunction* makes it clear that these other issues are not involved (Corona, Rastrelli, Maseroli, Forti, & Maggi, 2013; Mola, 2015).

Because an erection requires a specific sequence of events, ED can occur when any of the associate events are disrupted. The sequence includes nerve impulses in the brain, spinal column, and areas around the penis, as well as response in muscles, fibrous tissues, veins, and arteries in and near the corpora cavernosa. Damages to nerves, arteries, smooth muscles, and fibrous tissues, often as a result of disease, are the most common causes of ED. Comorbidities such as diabetes, kidney disease, chronic alcoholism, multiple sclerosis, atherosclerosis, vascular disease, and neurologic disorders are primary health risk factors for ED (Besiroglu, Otunctemur, & Ozbeck, 2015; McMahon, 2014).

Lifestyle choices that contribute to heart disease and vascular problems also increase the risk of ED. Smoking, being overweight, and lack of exercise are possible causes of ED. Surgery (especially radical prostate and bladder surgery for cancer) can injure nerves and arteries near the penis, causing ED. Injury to the penis, spinal cord, prostate, bladder, and pelvis can lead to ED by harming nerves, smooth muscles, arteries, and fibrous tissues of the corpora cavernosa. In addition, many common medicines—antihypertensives, antihistamines, antidepressants, tranquilizers, appetite suppressants, and cimetidine—can produce ED as a side effect (Maiorino, Bellastella, & Esposito, 2015; Meldrum et al., 2012).

In diagnosing ED, the medical history should include whether or not erections occur at other times. If an erection can be achieved with masturbation or upon awakening, the problem is probably not physical and is related to stress or an emotional problem. Treatment for ED usually proceeds from least to most invasive. For some men, making a few healthy lifestyle changes may solve the problem. Smoking cessation, weight loss, and increased physical activity may help some men regain sexual function. Cutting back on any drugs with harmful side effects is considered next. For example, drugs for high BP work in different ways. If a particular drug is causing problems with erection, a different class of BP medicine might work just as well. Psychotherapy and behavior modifications in some men should also be considered (Maiorino et al., 2015; McMahon, 2014).

Drugs for treating ED can be taken orally, injected directly into the penis, or inserted into the urethra at the tip of the penis. In March 1998, the U.S. FDA approved sildenafil citrate (Viagra), the first pill to treat ED. Since then, vardenafil hydrochloride (Levitra [oral], Staxyn [sublingual]), tadalafil (Cialis), and avanafil (Stendra) have also been approved. The aforementioned medications all belong to a class of drugs called phosphodiesterase (PDE) type 5 inhibitors. These medications are currently the first line of therapy for treating ED. The drugs work by relaxing smooth muscles in the penis during sexual stimulation and allow increased blood flow. They can be taken as needed before sexual activity, up to once a day. Low-dose daily dosing rather than "on-demand" dosing has been found to be beneficial for some couples (Smith et al., 2013).

Heart Disease and Men

Cardiovascular disease is a term that refers to the broadest category of diseases that affect the heart and blood vessels. About one in three adult men have some form of CVD and it is the leading cause of death among males in most racial/ethnic groups. Despite a decline in the overall death rate from CVD, the burden of disease among men remains high. In 2009, CVD caused 386,436 deaths in men, a rate of 236.1 deaths per 100,000. It was estimated in 2010 that 74.9% of all coronary artery bypass surgeries and 67.1% of percutaneous coronary interventions (angioplasty) procedures were performed on men. Additionally, in 2011, 68.7% of all heart transplant recipients were male (AHA, 2013b; CDC, 2015t).

Approximately 70% to 89% of sudden cardiac events occur in men, and 50% of these men have no previous symptoms of disease. The average age for a first heart attack among men is 66 years. About 8.5% of White men, 7.9% of Black men, and 6.3% of Mexican American men have some coronary disease. The rate of a first cardiovascular event rises from 3 per 1,000 men at 35 to 44 years of age to 74 per 1,000 men at 85 to 94 years of age. It is interesting to note, if all forms of major CVD were eliminated, life expectancy among all persons would increase by almost 7 years (CDC, 2015t; Mozaffarian et al., 2015).

Major risk factors for heart disease in men include HTN, hyperlipidemia (high LDL), tobacco use, diabetes, obesity/overweight, lack of physical activity, excessive alcohol consumption, stress, and low daily fruit and vegetable consumption. When working with adult men, the community health nurse should educate men about the importance of modifying factors that increase their risk of developing CVD (Campos-Outcalt, 2014). PHNs should discuss the signs and symptoms of a heart attack and how to access emergency medical treatment with adult males.

Prostate Health

Prostate health is another concern that may occur later in this life stage. The **prostate** is a doughnut-shaped gland located at the bottom of the bladder, about halfway between the rectum and the base of the penis. The prostate encircles the urethra. The walnut-sized gland produces most of the fluid in semen. Men can experience infection (prostatitis), prostate enlargement (benign prostatic hyperplasia [BPH]), and prostate cancer (ACS, 2015d).

BPH is very common among men. The primary risk factor for developing BPH is age. Nearly 50% of men over 50 years of age report symptoms that are related to prostate gland enlargement.

Symptoms of BPH are caused by an obstruction of the urethra and gradual loss of bladder function, which results in incomplete emptying of the bladder. The most commonly reported symptoms of BPH involve lower urinary tract symptoms (LUTS), such as hesitant, interrupted, or weak urinary stream, urgency or leaking of urine, and more frequent urination, especially at night. Men often report the symptoms of BPH before the physician diagnoses it through a digital rectal examination (DRE). Treatment for BPH can include medication or surgery to reduce the size of the prostate (McVary et al., n.d.).

Prostate cancer is the most frequently diagnosed cancer in men and the second leading cause of cancer death. According to the ACS, 1 man in 7 will get prostate cancer during his lifetime and 1 man in 38 will die from the disease. However, most prostate cancers grow slowly and do not cause any health problems in men who have them. More than 2.9 million men in the United States who have been diagnosed with prostate cancer at some time in their lives are still alive today. Prior to age 40, prostate cancer is very rare, but the chance of having prostate cancer rises rapidly after age 50. About 6 cases in 10 are diagnosed in men 65 years of age and older. Age is the strongest risk factor for prostate cancer, but family history and ethnicity also need to be considered. Prostate cancer occurs more often in Black men than in men of other races and occurs less often in Asian and Hispanic/Latino men. The reasons for these racial and ethnic differences are not clear. Starting at age 50, all men should talk to their health care provider about the pros and cons of screening for prostate cancer. This discussion should start at age 45 if a man is Black or has a father or brother who had prostate cancer before age 65. Men with two or more close relatives who had prostate cancer before age 65 should talk with their health care provider about screening for prostate cancer at age 40 (ACS, 2015d; CDC, 2015u). The effectiveness of the screening test, prostate-specific antigen (PSA), has been brought into question, and the U.S. Preventive Services Task Force (2015) has outlined a framework for further study and review.

Treatment for prostate cancer depends on the man's age, overall health status, and stage of disease. Treatment options include surgery to remove all or part of the prostate (prostatectomy), radiation, and hormone therapy. Surgery, radiation, and hormone therapy all have the potential to disrupt sexual desire and performance, temporarily or permanently. Urinary dysfunction and incontinence are common side effects that occur after surgery or radiation. Rather than immediate treatment, watchful waiting or active surveillance is an option that may be appropriate for older men with limited life expectancy and/or less aggressive tumors (Filson, Marks, & Litwin, 2015). A community health nurse can reinforce or clarify information shared with the man by his health care provider, discuss his treatment options with him and his family, and provide the support they may need if prostate cancer is diagnosed.

ROLE OF THE COMMUNITY HEALTH NURSE

The community health nurse works with adults in all age groups using the three levels of prevention—primary, secondary, and tertiary—as a guide. Interventions are conducted at the individual, family, group, and aggregate levels to make progress toward the *Healthy People 2020* objectives (see Levels of Prevention Pyramid).

Client teaching by the community health nurse is a major factor in preventing and managing chronic diseases. The challenge to the nurse is to be prepared to discuss issues, backed up with knowledge of and access to the appropriate community resources, to meet client needs. What the nurse can accomplish can be quite dramatic in terms of reducing days in the hospital because of chronic disease, improving quality of life for the chronically ill person, and preventing a combination of unhealthy habits from becoming causative factors in new cases of chronic disease. See Chapter 26 for more on chronic diseases and disabilities. A nursing care plan matrix can guide the community health nurse in discussing areas of health promotion and protection with the client. An example of a nursing care plan matrix for young adults can be found in Display 23–6.

Primary Prevention

Primary prevention activities focus on education to promote a healthy lifestyle. Much of the community health nurse's time is spent in the educator role. When working with individuals, the PHN should encourage routine health examinations, healthy eating habits, adequate sleep, moderate drinking, and no smoking. Among aggregates, the community health nurse focuses on community needs for services and programs that will keep that population healthy, such as providing flu clinics, teaching sexual responsibility, and preventing STIs.

LEVELS OF PREVENTION PYRAMID

SITUATION: Breast cancer

GOAL: Using the three levels of prevention, negative health conditions are avoided or promptly diagnosed and treated, and the fullest potential is restored.

TERTIARY PREVENTION

Rehabilitation	Primary Prevention	
	Health Promotion and Education	*Health Protection*
• Recovery at home with return to activities of daily living within 2 weeks	• Maintains periodic follow-up with health care provider, follow-up mammogram at 6 and 12 months, and as recommended by health care provider • Education regarding risk for other cancers (cervical, ovarian, uterine, etc.)	• Practice breast self-examination (BSE) and receive mammograms as recommended; receives screening for ovarian cancer—transvaginal ultrasonography and blood test for tumor marker CA 125

SECONDARY PREVENTION

Early Diagnosis	Prompt Treatment
• Identification of lump in left breast, appointment made with health care provider for evaluation • Receives mammogram and sonogram	• Needle aspiration of lump followed by cytologic studies • Lumpectomy with removal of two suspicious lymph nodes • Low-dose radiation

PRIMARY PREVENTION

Health Promotion and Education	Health Protection
• Education regarding for BSE and mammograms, as needed • Education regarding environmental exposure and breast cancer (smoking, alcohol, chemicals) • Education regarding low-fat diet and maintaining a body mass index <29	• Avoidance of environmental exposures that may contribute to cancer • Performs BSE and obtains mammogram when appropriate

The community health nurse may collaborate with community leaders and other stakeholders in designing programs, work with committees to secure funding, or approach the state legislature to lobby for needed changes to state laws and policies governing the health of adults. At other times, the nurse works with small groups of adults who could benefit from making healthy choices in diet, relaxation, and physical activity. Likewise, it is not unusual for the PHN to work with an individual to promote healthy living. An example of available resources on smoking cessation to those working with the veteran population is shared in Population-Focus.

Secondary Prevention

Secondary prevention focuses on screening for early detection and prompt treatment of diseases. Throughout the life span, screening tests can help adults identify disease early (see Display 23–2). A significant amount of the community health nurse's time is spent in assessing the need for planning, implementing, or evaluating programs that focus on the early detection of diseases. This is followed with teaching to prevent further damage from the disease in progress or to prevent the spread of the disease, if it is communicable. Examples of secondary prevention programs include establishing mammography clinics, teaching breast and TSE, and screenings—BP, blood glucose, BMI, and cholesterol. Wherever adults gather in groups, this is a good place to provide both primary and secondary health care and prevention services (AHRQ, 2014a, 2014b).

Tertiary Prevention

The tertiary level of prevention focuses on rehabilitation and preventing further damage to an already compromised system. Many adults with whom a community health nurse works have chronic diseases, conditions

DISPLAY 23–6 NURSING CARE PLAN MATRIX FOR HEALTH PROMOTION, YOUNG ADULTS: 18 TO 35

Community health nurses can use this matrix to individualize teaching, services, and/or care to young adult clients. Use the questions to stimulate the development of an individualized approach that is client focused and client driven with the community health nurse acting as the catalyst. In any or all of these areas, the community health nurse may (1) discuss issues and commend the client for positive attitudes and behaviors (e.g., when the client is making healthful decisions, such as condom use for his/her health and the health of significant others), (2) discuss the issues and guide the client to resources that will enhance more positive behaviors and decisions (e.g., flu shot clinic or healthy lifestyle program for adults), or (3) discuss the issues and inform the client that immediate changes must be made to protect the health of self or others and inform/utilize the appropriate resources as soon as possible (e.g., follow-up for symptoms related to suspected STI).

1. *Life partner*. Ascertain whether the client is looking for a life partner or is choosing to live a single life. Discuss how the single life is satisfying for the client and ways to make it richer.

   Discuss settings in which client can meet others (male or female, based on sexual preference) with similar interests, philosophy, and outlook, such as work settings, school settings, faith communities, recreational communities, and the like.

   Discuss what the client is looking for in a potential life partner, expectations for the relationship, what the client contributes, how the client compromises and resolves conflict, and other issues. If in a relationship, what is good, what needs improving, and how to initiate change.

2. *Life's work*. How is the client preparing for his/her life's work (education, formal training, on the job training)? Will the life's work provide resources for client's life plans? Will the work choice provide long-term satisfaction? Is the work choice a "stepping stone" to another work role? How will/does he/she handle work and rearing children? What needs changing or can be improved in the work/children arrangement?

3. *Planning for children*. What knowledge does he/she have about family planning? What methods fit best with his/her philosophy, religious beliefs, and lifestyle? What are the long-term effects of the choices? How many children is the client planning to rear? Has he/she thought through the ramifications of this number? If choosing not to have (or unable to have) children, how will he/she deal with this? Does he/she want alternative suggestions for raising a child (adoption, foster parenting) or information about interacting with children (volunteering)?

4. *Maintaining physical and mental health*. In this area, the community health nurse needs to explore all areas of health promotion and protection. This will include discussions regarding primary and secondary prevention. Primary prevention discussions could include:
   - Diet and nutrition
   - Physical and leisure activities
   - Safe sex practices
   - Periodic health examinations
   - Personal safety—seat belts, protective helmets, dating violence, etc.
   - Immunizations
   - Regular use of sunscreen
   - Stress reduction activities

   Secondary prevention discussions could include:
   - Breast self-examination
   - Testicular self-examination
   - Smoking cessation
   - Pelvic exams and Pap smears
   - Counseling and support at times of stress

5. *Developing a life's philosophy*. Discuss client's personal life satisfaction, which may include religiosity and spirituality, living in congruence with cultural/ethnic/family beliefs and expectations, and coming to a comfortable level of satisfaction with life choices, having few regrets.

POPULATION-FOCUS
PUBLIC HEALTH AND THE VETERAN POPULATION

The Clinical Public Health group in the Veterans Health Administration provides expertise and leadership that is focused on preventing illness and promoting quality of life for the veteran population through sound policy and practice. The mission is accomplished through education and outreach, policy development, clinical demonstration projects, population-based surveillance, performance measurement and improvement, clinical guidelines, and research. Current focus areas for the veteran population include HIV, hepatitis C, influenza, health care–associated infections, and smoking and tobacco use. The veteran population is disproportionately affected by smoking-related illnesses. Many veterans began smoking in the military and this remains a significant public health challenge in VA clinics. The U.S. Department of Veterans Affairs Public Health Web site "Quit Tobacco" was developed specifically for the veteran population to provide evidence-based information and helpful resources for veterans interested in improving their health by quitting the use of tobacco. The Web site is resource rich and can be accessed by any veteran or health care professional at http://www.publichealth.va.gov/smoking/quit/index.asp. One particularly meaningful resource for the veteran population is a 27-minute video episode of *The American Veteran Show* that presents the story of several veterans' experiences in a VA tobacco cessation clinic led by a VA nurse practitioner.

Bryan, Associate Director for Patient Services, VA Clinic

resulting from another disease, or long-standing injuries with resulting disability. Ideally, negative health conditions can be prevented. If not, the next best thing is for them to be diagnosed early, without damage to an individual's health. But if negative health conditions have not been treated or brought under control, then the individual is at a tertiary level of prevention. At this level of prevention, the nurse focuses on maintaining quality of life.

Depending on the client's age, tertiary prevention can be simple or very complex. A 19-year-old man who breaks his leg while skiing needs information about using crutches safely, a reminder to eat protein foods for bone healing, and an appointment to return to his health care provider if he experiences various symptoms and to get the cast removed. He generally needs no additional help from others. Tertiary prevention in this case is uncomplicated. On the other hand, a 62-year-old woman who is 70 pounds overweight with out-of-control blood glucose levels, symptoms of congestive heart failure, and difficulty walking more than 20 feet has much to accomplish in order to feel healthy.

Can the nurse help the woman lose weight? Will weight loss bring her diabetes under control and alleviate congestive heart failure symptoms? With some weight reduction, will she be able to walk more easily? Or, will the woman feel better with physical therapy and a different medication regimen? Is there a quicker, safer, and better approach? On assessment, the nurse discovers that the woman has been as much as 80 pounds overweight for 40 years. Will this information alter the nurse's approach to helping this woman? What additional information does the nurse need?

Caring for people at the tertiary level of prevention can become quite complicated because many body systems may be involved. In addition, all people function within many social systems, which may include family expectations, roles people have within the family, expected behaviors, community system knowledge and involvement, personal expectations, motivation, and support. Working at the tertiary level involves all of the nurse's skills in addition to community resources and a client who can be or wants to be motivated.

SUMMARY

The 20th century saw a shift in the leading causes of death, from communicable to noncommunicable diseases. Currently, the five leading causes of death in adults are diseases of the heart, malignant neoplasms, CLRDs, cerebrovascular diseases, and unintentional injuries—none of which are communicable. The health care needs of adults are of great concern. Many needs are the same for both women and men, but the important differences were addressed in this chapter.

Adults have health care needs that change as they age. Diet and exercise, obesity, substance use, safety, and healthy lifestyle choices are issues that adults must consider throughout their lives. Heart disease and cancers remain important concerns for both men and women, and health decisions made as a young adult can have a major impact on persons as they age.

Chronic illness is an issue of increasing concern for both men and women as life expectancies increase. Community health nurses should use the three levels of prevention to promote health across the life span. Primary prevention activities focus on education to promote a healthy lifestyle. Secondary prevention focuses on screening for early detection and prompt treatment of diseases. The community health nurse's role at this stage is to assess needs; to plan, implement, or evaluate programs that focus on the early detection of diseases; and to educate clients to prevent further damage from or spread of disease. The tertiary level of prevention focuses on rehabilitation and prevention of further damage to an already compromised system. At this level of prevention, the nurse focuses on maintaining quality of life.

ACTIVITIES TO PROMOTE **CRITICAL THINKING**

1. Using the newspaper or online news sources, select three articles that relate to a preventable chronic disease. For each article, summarize the content, identify the likely cause, and describe how the disease may have been prevented.
2. You are asked to offer a weight control program for 12 young adults who are residents in an apartment complex that has monthly programs related to health and wellness. The ages of the intended participants range from 20 to 30. What steps would you take to develop a successful program? What would be important to emphasize with this age group? What resources (e.g., smartphone apps, online information) might be useful to them in adhering to a healthy diet and exercise program?

3. Using nursing and other health care databases, research a chronic disease associated with men or women aged 35 to 65. In a small group discussion with your classmates, identify selected concerns and discuss both personal responsibility and societal responsibility regarding management of this health problem.

4. Access the Web site for the Nurses' Health Study 3 at (http://www.nhs3.org/). If you were to join the study what would be the benefits to you personally and to your nursing practice? Would you encourage other nurses to participate? What strategies might you use to encourage participation? What research findings from this study may have personal benefits to you or members of your family?

5. Arrange to have a discussion with a nurse leader in the Veteran's Administration (VA) health care system to gain a better understanding of the role they play in improving the health of veteran populations.

   ● When completing health histories or screening veterans for health-related issues, what are important things to look for and/or ask about? What health issues are prevalent in the veteran population? How does diversity within the veteran population relate to prevalence of critical issues?

   ● Think about how nursing assessment, planning, intervention, and evaluation can be applied to address functioning across all dimensions when working with veterans attempting to reintegrate into their community. How might you be able to impact community responsiveness to the veteran culture and needs of returning veterans?

6. Visit a local veteran's organization (e.g., VFW, American Legion) in your community and discuss the resources available in the community. Explore veteran online resources (www.va.gov) and review the history and programs available.

   ● What are family health considerations for veterans? Do these differ from the general population? What community resources are available for family health needs and concerns? Are there any access challenges for veterans and their families for the services they need?

   ● What resources are available to the veteran population to address health-related issues? How well do those resources provide culturally competent, evidence- based care for this population? What resources are needed that might not be available in the community? What options do veterans have for accessing needed resources?

   ● What are the mechanisms through which coordination of services occurs for veterans in the community? Are there formal structures that facilitate coordination across agencies? Are there particular issues or segments of the veteran population that are "falling through the cracks" or are underserved?

REFERENCES

Agaku, I. T., King, B. A., Husten, C. G., Bunnell, R., Ambrose, B. K., Hu, S. S., ... Day, H. R. (2014). Tobacco product use among adults—United States, 2012–2013. *Morbidity and Mortality Weekly Report, 63*(25), 542–547. Retrieved from http://www.cdc.gov/mmwr/preview/mmwrhtml/mm6325a3.htm

Agency for Healthcare Research and Quality (AHRQ). (2014a). *Men: Stay healthy at any age.* Retrieved from http://www.ahrq.gov/sites/default/files/publications/files/healthy-men.pdf

Agency for Healthcare Research and Quality (AHRQ). (2014b). *Women: Stay healthy at any age.* Retrieved from http://www.ahrq.gov/sites/default/files/publications/files/healthy-women.pdf

American Cancer Society (ACS). (2015a). *Cancer facts and figures 2015.* Retrieved from http://www.cancer.org/acs/groups/content/@editorial/documents/document/acspc-044552.pdf

American Cancer Society (ACS). (2015b). *Breast cancer prevention and early detection.* Retrieved from http://www.cancer.org/acs/groups/cid/documents/webcontent/003165-pdf.pdf

American Cancer Society (ACS). (2015c). *Testicular cancer.* Retrieved from http://www.cancer.org/cancer/testicularcancer/detailedguide/testicular-cancer-detailed-guide-toc

American Cancer Society (ACS). (2015d). *Prostate cancer.* Retrieved from http://www.cancer.org/cancer/prostatecancer/

American College of Obstetricians and Gynecologists (ACOG). (2011). *FAQ: Perimenopausal bleeding and bleeding after menopause.* Retrieved from http://www.acog.org/~/media/For%20Patients/faq162.pdf

American College of Obstetricians and Gynecologists (ACOG). (2012). *Committee opinion: Compounded bioidentical menopausal hormone therapy.* Retrieved from http://www.acog.org/Resources-And-Publications/Committee-Opinions/Committee-on-Gynecologic-Practice/Compounded-Bioidentical-Menopausal-Hormone-Therapy

American Heart Association (AHA). (2013a). *Asian & Pacific Islanders and cardiovascular disease.* Retrieved from https://www.heart.org/idc/groups/heart-public/@wcm/@sop/@smd/documents/downloadable/ucm_319570.pdf

American Heart Association (AHA). (2013b). *Statistical fact sheet 2013 update: Men and cardiovascular disease.* Retrieved from https://www.heart.org/idc/groups/heart-public/@wcm/@sop/@smd/documents/downloadable/ucm_319573.pdf

American Heart Association (AHA). (2015). *Go red for women.* Retrieved from https://www.goredforwomen.org

American Lung Association (ALA). (2013a). *Taking her breath away. The rise of COPD in women.* Retrieved from http://www.lung.org/assets/documents/research/rise-of-copd-in-women-full.pdf

American Lung Association (ALA). (2013b). *Trends in COPD (chronic bronchitis and emphysema): Morbidity and mortality.* Retrieved from http://www.lung.org/assets/documents/research/copd-trend-report.pdf

American Lung Association (ALA). (2015a). *Lung health and diseases: How serious is COPD?* Retrieved from http://www.lung.org/lung-health-and-diseases/lung-disease-lookup/copd/learn-about-copd/how-serious-is-copd.html

American Lung Association (ALA). (2015b). *Lung health and diseases: What causes COPD.* Retrieved from http://www.lung.org/lung-health-and-diseases/lung-disease-lookup/copd/symptoms-causes-risk-factors/what-causes-copd.html

American Lung Association (ALA). (2015c). *Lung health and diseases: Asthma.* Retrieved from http://www.lung.org/lung-health-and-diseases/lung-disease-lookup/asthma/

American Medical Association Ad Hoc Committee on Health Literacy for the Council on Scientific Affairs. (1999). Health literacy: Report of the council on scientific affairs. *Journal of the American Medical Association, 281,* 552–557.

Anderson, J. E., Jamieson, D. J., Warner, L., Kissin, D. M., Nangia, A. K., & Macaluso M. (2012). Contraceptive sterilization among married adults: Nation data on who chooses vasectomy and tubal ligation. *Contraception, 85*(6), 552–557. doi: 10.1016/j.contraception.2011.10.009.

Beauchamp, A., Buchbinder, R., Dodson, S., Batterham, R. W., Elsworth, G. R., McPhee, C., ... Osborne, R. H. (2015). Distribution of health literacy strengths and weaknesses across socio-demographic groups: A cross-sectional survey using the Health Literacy Questionnaire (HLQ). *BMC Public Health, 15*(678), 1–13. doi: 10.1186/s12889-015-2056-z.

Bergen, G., Peterson, C., Ederer, D., Florence, C., Haileyesus, T., Kresnow, J., & Xu, L. (2014). Vital signs: Health burden and medical costs of nonfatal injuries to motor vehicle occupants—United States, 2012. *Morbidity and Mortality Weekly Report, 63*(40), 894–900. Retrieved from http://www.cdc.gov/mmwr/preview/mmwrhtml/mm6340a4.htm

Besiroglu, H., Otunctemur, A., & Ozbeck, E. (2015). The relationship between metabolic syndrome, its components, and erectile dysfunction: A systematic review and a meta analysis of observational studies. *Journal of Sexual Medicine, 12*(6), 1309–1318. doi:10.111/jsm.12885

Blackwell, D. L., Lucas, J. W., & Clarke, T. C. (2014). Summary health statistics for U.S. adults: National Health Interview Survey, 2012. *National Center for Health Statistics. Vital Health Statistics, 10*(260), 1–161. Retrieved from http://www.cdc.gov/nchs/data/series/sr_10/sr10_260.pdf

Bostock-Cox, B. (2015). Focus on women's health: The menopause. *Practice Nurse, 45*(5), 10–14.

Boudi, F. B. (2015, November 22), Risk factors for coronary artery disease. *Medscape.* Retrieved from http://emedicine.medscape.com/article/164163-overview

British Association for Parental and Enteral Nutrition. (2015). *Malnutrition universal screening tool.* Retrieved from http://www.bapen.org.uk/screening-for-malnutrition/must/introducing-must

Bulik, C. (2014). *9 Eating disorders myths busted.* Retrieved from http://www.nimh.nih.gov/news/science-news/2014/9-eating-disorders-myths-busted.shtml

Cahill, K. E., Giandrea, M. D., & Quinn, J. F. (2015). Retirement patterns and the macroeconomy, 1992–2010: The prevalence and determinants of bridge jobs, phased retirement, and reentry among three recent cohorts of older adults. *The Gerontologist, 55*(3), 384–403. doi: 10.1093/geront/gnt146.

Campos-Outcalt, D. (2014). The new cardiovascular disease prevention guidelines: What do you need to know. *The Journal of Family Practice, 63*(2), 89–93. Retrieved from http://www.jfponline.com/specialty-focus/cardiovascular/article/the-new-cardiovascular-disease-prevention-guidelines-what-you-need-to-know/d2536cc91ae97a71ff807cced7765a61.html

Center for Behavioral Health Statistics and Quality. (2015). *Behavioral health trends in the United States: Results from the 2014 National Survey on Drug Use and Health (HHS Publication No. SMA 15-4927, NSDUN Series H-50).* Retrieved from http://www.samhsa.gov/data/sites/default/files/NSDUH-FRR1-2014/NSDUH-FRR1-2014.pdf

Centers for Disease Control and Prevention (CDC). (2013a). *Asthma facts. CDC's national asthma program grantees.* Retrieved from http://www.cdc.gov/asthma/pdfs/asthma_facts_program_grantees.pdf

Centers for Disease Control and Prevention (CDC). (2013b). *Women and heart disease fact sheet.* Retrieved from http://www.cdc.gov/dhdsp/data_statistics/fact_sheets/docs/fs_women_heart.pdf

Centers for Disease Control and Prevention (CDC). (2014a). *Increase expected in medical cares costs for COPD.* Retrieved from http://www.cdc.gov/features/ds-copd-costs/

Centers for Disease Control and Prevention (CDC). (2014b). *Fact sheet—Alcohol use and your health.* Retrieved from http://www.cdc.gov/alcohol/fact-sheets/alcohol-use.htm

Centers for Disease Control and Prevention (CDC). (2014c). *Alcohol and public health: Data, trends and maps.* Retrieved from http://www.cdc.gov/alcohol/data-stats.htm

Centers for Disease Control and Prevention (CDC). (2014d). *Best practices for comprehensive tobacco control programs—2014.* Retrieved from http://www.cdc.gov/tobacco/stateandcommunity/best_practices/pdfs/2014/comprehensive.pdf

Centers for Disease Control and Prevention (CDC). (2014e). *Nail technicians' health and workplace exposure control.* Retrieved from http://www.cdc.gov/niosh/topics/manicure/

Centers for Disease Control and Prevention (CDC). (2015a). *Heart disease fact sheet.* Retrieved from http://www.cdc.gov/dhdsp/data_statistics/fact_sheets/fs_heart_disease.htm

Centers for Disease Control and Prevention (CDC). (2015b). *Heart disease risk factors.* Retrieved from http://www.cdc.gov/heartdisease/risk_factors.htm

Centers for Disease Control and Prevention (CDC). (2015c). *Stroke in the United States.* Retrieved from http://www.cdc.gov/stroke/facts.htm

Centers for Disease Control and Prevention (CDC). (2015d). *Injury prevention and control: Data & statistics. Key injury and violence data.* Retrieved from http://www.cdc.gov/injury/wisqars/overview/key_data.html

Centers for Disease Control and Prevention (CDC). (2015e). *Injury prevention and control: Data & statistics. Costs of injuries and violence in the United States.* Retrieved from http://www.cdc.gov/injury/wisqars/overview/cost_of_injury.html

Centers for Disease Control and Prevention (CDC). (2015f). *10 Leading causes of injury deaths by age group highlighting unintentional injury deaths, United States—2013.* Retrieved from http://www.cdc.gov/injury/images/lc-charts/leading_causes_of_injury_deaths_highlighting_unintentional_injury_2013-a.gif

Centers for Disease Control and Prevention (CDC). (2015g). *National diabetes statistics report: Estimates of diabetes and its burden in the United States, 2014.* Atlanta, GA: U.S. Department of Health and Human Services; 2014. Retrieved from http://www.cdc.gov/diabetes/pubs/statsreport14/national-diabetes-report-web.pdf

Centers for Disease Control and Prevention (CDC). (2015h). *Diabetes report card 2014.* Atlanta, GA: Centers for Disease Control and Prevention, U.S. Department of Health and Human Services. Retrieved from http://www.cdc.gov/diabetes/pdfs/library/diabetes-reportcard2014.pdf

Centers for Disease Control and Prevention (CDC). (2015i). *Current cigarette smoking among adults in the United States.* Retrieved from http://www.cdc.gov/tobacco/data_statistics/fact_sheets/adult_data/cig_smoking/

Centers for Disease Control and Prevention (CDC). (2015j). *Economic facts about U.S. tobacco production and use.* Retrieved from http://www.cdc.gov/tobacco/data_statistics/fact_sheets/economics/econ_facts/

Centers for Disease Control and Prevention (CDC). (2015k). *Adult obesity causes and consequences.* Retrieved from http://www.cdc.gov/obesity/adult/causes.html

Centers for Disease Control and Prevention (CDC). (2015l). *Adult obesity facts.* Retrieved from http://www.cdc.gov/obesity/data/adult.html

Centers for Disease Control and Prevention (CDC). (2015m). *Preconception health and health care.* Retrieved from http://www.cdc.gov/preconception/index.html

Centers for Disease Control and Prevention (CDC). (2015n). *Chlamydia.* Retrieved from http://www.cdc.gov/std/stats14/chlamydia.htm

Centers for Disease Control and Prevention (CDC). (2015o). *Gonorrhea.* Retrieved form http://www.cdc.gov/std/stats14/gonorrhea.htm

Centers for Disease Control and Prevention (CDC). (2015p). *Chronic fatigue syndrome.* Retrieved from http://www.cdc.gov/cfs/index.html

Centers for Disease Control and Prevention (CDC). (2015q). *HIV Surveillance Report, 2013, vol. 25.* Retrieved from http://www.cdc.gov/hiv/pdf/library/reports/surveillance/cdc-hiv-surveillance-report-vol-25.pdf

Centers for Disease Control and Prevention (CDC). (2015r). *HIV among men in the United States.* Retrieved from http://www.cdc.gov/hiv/group/gender/men/index.html

Centers for Disease Control and Prevention (CDC). (2015s). *HIV risk and prevention.* Retrieved from http://www.cdc.gov/hiv/risk/

Centers for Disease Control and Prevention (CDC). (2015t). *Men and heart disease fact sheet.* Retrieved from http://www.cdc.gov/dhdsp/data_statistics/fact_sheets/fs_men_heart.htm

Centers for Disease Control and Prevention (CDC). (2015u). *Should I get screened for prostate cancer?* Retrieved from http://www.cdc.gov/cancer/prostate/basic_info/get-screened.htm

Chelvanayagam, S., & Newell, C. (2015). Differentiating between eating disorders and gastrointestinal problems. *Gastrointestinal Nursing, 13*(7), 56–62. doi: 10.12968/gasn.2015.13.7.56.

Chronic Pain Research Alliance. (2015). *Advancing Research—Changing Lives.* Retrieved from http://www.chronicpainresearch.org/site/index

Corona, G., Rastrelli, G., Maseroli, E., Forti, G., & Maggi, M. (2013). Sexual function of the ageing male. *Best Practice & Research Clinical Endocrinology & Metabolism, 27*(4), 581–601. doi: 10.1016/j.beem.2013.05.007.

Database of Genotypes and Phenotypes. (n.d.). *Women's health initiative clinical trial and observational study SHARe.* Retrieved from http://www.ncbi.nlm.nih.gov/projects/gap/cgi-bin/study.cgi?study_id=phs000200.v1.p1

Davis, S. R., Castelo-Branco, C., Chedraui, P., Lumsden, M. A., Nappi, R. E., Shah, D., & Villaseca, P. (2012). Understanding weight gain at menopause. *Climacteric, 15*(5), 419–429.

de Souza, R. J., & Anand, S. S. (2014). Cardiovascular disease in Asian Americans: Unmasking the heterogeneity. *Journal of the American College of Cardiology, 64*(23), 2495–2497. doi: 10.1016/j.jacc.2014.09.050.

deVilliers, T. J., Gass, M. L., Haines, C. J., Hall, J. E., Lobo, R. A., Pierroz, D. D., & Rees, M. (2013). Global consensus statement on menopausal hormone therapy. *Climacteric, 16*, 203–204.

Dischinger, P. C., Ryb, G. E., Kufera, J. A., & Ho, S. M. (2013). Declining statewide trends in motor vehicle crashes and injury related hospital admissions. *Annals of Advances in Automotive Medicine, 57*, 247–256. Retrieved from http://www.ncbi.nlm.nih.gov/pmc/articles/PMC3861824/pdf/ffile058.pdf

Eeckhaut, M. C. (2015). Marital status and female and male contraceptive sterilization in the United States. *Fertility and Sterility, 103*(6), 1509–1515. doi: 10.1016/j.fertnstert.2015.02.036.

Eum, K. D., Weisskopf, M. G., Nie, L. H., Hu, H., & Korrick, S. A. (2014). Cumulative lead exposure and age at menopause in the Nurses' Health Study cohort. *Environmental Perspectives, 122*(3), 229–236.

Filson, C. P., Marks, L. S., & Litwin, M. S. (2015) Expectant management for men with early stage prostate cancer. *CA: A Cancer Journal for Clinicians, 65*(4), 264–282. doi: 10.3322/caac.21278.

Florence, C., Simon, T., Haegerich, T., Luo, F., & Zhou, C. (2015). Estimated lifetime medical and work loss costs of fatal injuries—United States, 2013. *Morbidity and Mortality Weekly, 64*(38), 1074–1077. Retrieved from http://www.cdc.gov/mmwr/preview/mmwrhtml/mm6438a4.htm

Ford, E. S., Murphy, L. B., Khavjou, O., Giles, W. H., Hole, J. B., & Croft, J. B. (2015). Total and state-specific medical and absenteeism costs of COPD among adults aged ≥ 18 years in the United States for 2010 and projections through 2020. *Chest, 147*(1), 311–345. doi: 10.1378/chest.14-0972.

Foster, J. E. (2015). Women of a certain age: "Second wave" feminists reflect back on 50 years of struggle in the United States. *Women's Studies International Forum, 50*, 68–79. doi: 10.1016/j.wsif.2015.03.005.

Freeman, E. W., Sammel, M. D., & Sanders, R. J. (2014). Risk of long-term hot flashes after natural menopause: Evidence from the Penn Ovarian Aging Study cohort. *Menopause, 21*(9), 924–932.

Fried, M. G. (2013). Reproductive rights activism in the post-Roe era. *American Journal of Public Health, 103*, 10–14. doi: 10.2105/AJPH.2012.301125.

Friedan, B. (2013). *The feminine mystique* (50th anniversary ed.). New York, NY: W. W. Norton and Company.

Ghazanfarpour, M., Sadeghi, R., & Roudsari, R. L. (2016). The application of soy isoflavones for subjective symptoms and objective signs of vaginal atrophy in menopause: A systematic review of randomized controlled trials. *Journal of Obstetrics & Gynaecology, 36*(2), 160–171.

Ghazarian, A. A., Trabert, B., Devesas, S. S., & McGlynn, K. A. (2015). Recent trends in the incidence of testicular germ cell tumors in the United States. *Andrology, 3*(1), 13–18. doi: 10.111/andr.288.

Gough, B. (2013). The psychology of men's health: Maximizing masculine capital. *Health Psychology, 32*(1), 1–4. doi: 10.1037/a0030424.

Graham, G. (2014). Population-based approaches to understanding disparities in cardiovascular disease risk in the United States. *International Journal of General Medicine, 7*, 393–400. doi: 10.2147/IJGM.S65528.

Guarascio, A. J., Ray, S. M., Finch, C. K., & Self, T. H. (2013). The clinical and economic burden of chronic obstructive pulmonary disease in the USA. *ClinicoEconomics and Outcomes Research, 5*, 235–245. doi: doi.org./10.2147/CEOR.S34321.

Hall, H. I., An, Q., Tang, T., Song, R., Chen, M. Green, T., & Kang, J. (2015). Prevalence of diagnosed and undiagnosed HIV infection—United States, 2008–2012. *Morbidity and Mortality Weekly Report, 63*(24), 657–662. Retrieved from http://www.cdc.gov/mmwr/preview/mmwrhtml/mm6424a2.htm?s_cid=mm6424a2_e

Halldin, C. N., Doney, B. C., & Hnizdo, E. (2015). Changes in prevalence of chronic obstructive pulmonary disease and asthma in the US population and associated risk factors. *Chronic Respiratory Disease, 12*(1), 47–60. doi: 10.1177/1479972314562409.

Hartge, P. (2011). Reducing cancer death rates through screening. *Cancer, 17*, 449–450. doi: 10.1002/cncr.25622.

Harvard Health. (2015, May). *Harvard women's health watch: Menopause symptoms can last longer than you expect.* Retrieved from http://www.health.harvard.edu/womens-health/menopause-symptoms-can-last-longer-than-you-expect

Harvard School of Public Health & Brigham and Women's Hospital. (2013). *Nurses Health Study 3: A historic study, a nursing tradition.* Retrieved from http://www.nhs3.org/index.php/our-story

Hays, B. (2011). Giving menopause its proper place. *Integrative Medicine, 19*(4), 40–43.

Heart Foundation. (2015). *Heart disease: Scope and impact.* Retrieved from http://www.theheartfoundation.org/heart-disease-facts/heart-disease-statistics/

Heron, M. (2015). Deaths: Leading causes for 2012. *National Vital Statistics Report, 64*(10). Retrieved from http://www.cdc.gov/nchs/data/nvsr/nvsr63/nvsr63_09.pdf

Hutteman, R., Hennecke, M., Orth, U., Reitz, A. K., & Specht, J. (2014). Developmental tasks as a framework to study personality development in adulthood and old age. *European Journal of Personality, 28*, 267–278. doi: 10.1002/per.1959.

Iftikhar, S., Shuster, L. T., Johnson, R. E., Jenkins, S. M., & Wahner-Roedler, D. L. (2011). Use of bioidentical compounded hormones for menopausal concerns: Cross-sectional survey in an academic menopause center. *Journal of Women's Health, 20*(4), 559–565.

Institute of Medicine. (2015). *Beyond Myalgic Encephalomyelitis/Chronic Fatigue Syndrome, redefining an illness, report guide for clinicians.* Retrieved from http://iom.nationalacademies.org/~/media/Files/Report%20Files/2015/MECFS/MECFScliniciansguide.pdf

International Women's Day. (2015). *About International Women's Day (March 8).* http://www.internationalwomensday.com/about.asp#.Vkpaer9wKmU

Jacob, J. A. (2016). Can nonhormonal treatments dial down the heat during menopause? *Journal of the American Medical Association. 315*(1), 14–16.

Jose, P. O., Frank, A. T. H., Kapphahn, K. I., Goldstein, B. A., Eggleston, K., Hastings, K. G., … Palaniappan, L. P. (2014). Cardiovascular disease mortality in Asian Americans. *Journal of the American College of Cardiology, 64*(23), 2486–2494. doi: 10.1016/j.jacc.2014.08.048.

Jull, J., Stackey, D., Beach, S., Dumas, A., Strychar, I. Ufholz, L. A., … Prud'homme, D. (2014). Lifestyle interventions targeting body weight changes during the menopause transition: A systematic review. *Journal of Obesity, 2014*, 824318.

Kanny, D., Brewer, R. D., Mesnick, J. B., Paulozzi, L. J., Naimi, T. S., & Lu, H. (2015). Vital signs: Alcohol poisoning deaths—United States, 2010–2012. *Morbidity and Mortality Weekly Report, 63*(53), 1238–1242. Retrieved from http://www.cdc.gov/mmwr/preview/mmwrhtml/mm6353a2.htm

Kim, C., Nan, B., Kong, S., & Harlow, S. (2012). Changes in iron measures over menopause and associations with insulin resistance. *Journal of Women's Health, 21*(8), 872–877.

Kochanek, K. D., Xu, J., Murphy, S. L., Miniño, A. M., & Kung, H. (2011). Deaths: Preliminary data for 2009. *National Vital Statistics Report, 59*(4), 1–51. Retrieved from http://www.cdc.gov/nchs/data/nvsr/nvsr59/nvsr59_04.pdf

Lachman, M. E. (2015). Mind the gap in the middle: A call to study midlife. *Research in Human Development, 12*(3–4), 327–334. doi: 10.11080/15427609.2015.1068948.

LaCroix, A. Z., Chlebowski, R. T., Manson, J. E., Aragaki A. K., Johnson, K. C., Martin, L., … Wactawski-Wende, J. (2011). Heath outcomes after stopping conjugated equine estrogens among postmenopausal women with prior hysterectomy: A randomized clinical trial. *Journal of the American Medical Association, 305,* 1305–1314. doi: 10.1001/jama.2011.382.

Lampio, L., Polo-Kantola, P., Polo, O., Kauko, T., Aittokallio, J., & Saaresranta, T. (2014). Sleep in midlife women: Effects of menopause, vasomotor symptoms, and depressive symptoms. *Menopause, 21*(11), 1217–1224.

Lane, J. A. (2015). Counseling emerging adults in transition: Practical applications of attachment and social support research. *The Professional Counselor, 5*(1), 30–42. doi: 10.15241/jal.5.1.30.

Levant, R. F., & Wimer, D. J. (2014). Masculinity constructs as protective buffers and risk factors for men's health. *American Journal of Men's Health, 8*(2), 110–120. doi: 10.177/1557988313494408.

Li, G., & Baker, S. P. (Eds.) (2014). *Injury research: Theories, methods and approaches.* New York, NY: Springer Publishing.

Lipsky, M. S., Cannon, M., & Lutfiyya, M. N. (2014). Gender and health disparities: The case of male gender. *Disease-A-Month, 60*(4), 138–144. doi: 10.1016/j.disamonth2014.001.

Lutfiyya, M. N., Cannon, M., & Lipsky, M. S. (2014). An argument for male gender as a root cause or fundamental social determinant of health. *Disease-A-Month, 60*(4), 145–149. doi: 10.1016/j.disamonth.2014.02.002

Maiorino, M. I., Bellastella, G., & Esposito, K. (2015). Lifestyle modifications and erectile dysfunction: What can be expected? *Asian Journal of Andrology, 17*(1), 5–10. doi: 10.4103/1008-682X.137687.

Manson, J., & Kaunitz, A. M. (2016). Menopause management—Getting clinical care back on track. *New England Journal of Medicine, 374*(9), 803–806.

Mathews, T. J., MacDorman, M. F., & Thoma, M. E. (2015). Infant mortality statistics from the 2013 period linked birth/infant death data set. *National Vital Statistics Reports, 64*(9). Retrieved from http://www.cdc.gov/nchs/data/nvsr/nvsr64/nvsr64_09.pdf

McMahon, C. G. (2014). Erectile dysfunction. *Internal Medicine Journal, 44*(1), 18–26. doi: 10.111/imj.12325.

McVary, K. T., Roehrborn, C. G., Avins, A.L., Barry, M. J., Bruskewitz, R. C., Donnell, R. F., ... Wei, J. T. (n.d.). *American Urological Association (AUA) guideline: Management of benign prostatic hypertrophy.* Retrieved from https://www.auanet.org/education/guidelines/benign-prostatic-hyperplasia.cfm

Meldrum, D. R., Gambone, J. G., Morris, M. A., Esposito, E., Giugliano, D., & Ignarro, L. J. (2012). Lifestyle and metabolic approaches to maximizing erectile and vascular health. *International Journal of Impotence Research, 24*(2), 61–68. doi: 10.1038.ijir.2011.51.

Meyer, P. A., Yoon, P. W., & Kaufmann, R. B. (2013). Introduction: CDC health disparities and inequalities report—United States, 2013. *Morbidity and Mortality Weekly Supplement, 62*(3). Retrieved from http://www.cdc.gov/mmwr/pdf/other/su6203.pdf

Mola, J. R. (2015). Erectile dysfunction in the older adult male. *Urologic Nursing, 35*(2), 87–93. doi: 10.7257/1-53-816X.2015.35.2.87.

Morrison, L. A., Brown, D. E., Sievert, L. L., Reza, A., Rahberg, N., Mills, P., & Goodloe, A. (2014). Voices from the Hilo Women's Health Study: Talking story about menopause. *Health Care for Women International, 35,* 529–548.

Mosca, L., Benjamin, E. J., Berra, K., Bezanson, J. L., Dolor, R. J., Lloyd-Jones, D. M., ... Wenger, N. K. (2011). Effectiveness-based guidelines for the prevention of cardiovascular disease in women—2011 update: A guideline from the American Heart Association. *Circulation, 123,* 1243–1262. doi: 10.1161/CIR.0b013e31820fa.

Mozaffarian, D. Benjamin, E. J., Go, A. S., Arnett, D. K., Blaha, M. J., Cushman, M., de Ferranti, S., ... Turner, M. B. (2015). Heart disease and stroke statistics—2015 update. *Circulation, 131,* e29–e322. doi: 10.1161/CIR.0000000000000152.

Murphy, S. L., Kochanek, M. A., Xu, J., & Heron, M. (2015). Deaths: Final data 2012. *National Vital Statistics, 63*(9). Retrieved from http://www.cdc.gov/nchs/data/nvsr/nvsr63/nvsr63_09.pdf

Murphy, S. L., Xu, J., & Kochanek, K. D. (2013). Deaths: Final data for 2010. *National Vital Statistics Reports, 61*(4), 1–118. Retrieved from http://www.cdc.gov/nchs/data/nvsr/nvsr61/nvsr61_04.pdf

National Cancer Institute (NCI). (2011). *Menopausal hormone therapy and cancer.* Retrieved from http://www.cancer.gov/about-cancer/causes-prevention/risk/hormones/mht-fact-sheet

National Cancer Institute (NCI). (2015). *Human papillomavirus (HPV) vaccines.* Retrieved from http://www.cancer.gov/about-cancer/causes-prevention/risk/infectious-agents/hpv-vaccine-fact-sheet#q5

National Center for Health Statistics (NCHS). (2015a). *Health, United States 2014.* Retrieved from http://www.cdc.gov/nchs/data/hus/hus14.pdf

National Center for Health Statistics (NCHS). (2015b). *NCHS data on drug poisoning deaths.* Retrieved from http://www.cdc.gov/nchs/data/factsheets/factsheet_drug_poisoning.pdf

National Eating Disorders Association. (n.d.). *Learn.* Retrieved from http://www.nationaleatingdisorders.org/learn

National Eating Disorders Collaboration. (2015a). *What is bulimia nervosa?* Retrieved from http://www.nedc.com.au/bulimia-nervosa

National Eating Disorders Collaboration. (2015b). *What is binge eating disorder?* Retrieved from http://www.nedc.com.au/binge-eating-disorder

National Heart, Lung and Blood Institute (NHLBI). (2015). *The Framingham Heart Study.* Retrieved from https://www.framinghamheartstudy.org

National Highway Traffic Safety Administration. (2014). *U.S. Department of Transportation announces decline in traffic fatalities in 2013.* Retrieved from http://www.nhtsa.gov/About+NHTSA/Press+Releases/2014/traffic-deaths-decline-in-2013

National Institute of Diabetes and Digestive and Kidney Diseases (NIDDKD). (2011). *Bariatric surgery for severe obesity.* Retrieved from http://www.niddk.nih.gov/health-information/health-topics/weight-control/bariatric-surgery-severe-obesity/Pages/bariatric-surgery-for-severe-obesity.aspx

National Institute of Diabetes and Digestive and Kidney Diseases (NIDDKD). (2012). *Overweight and obesity statistics.* Retrieved from http://www.niddk.nih.gov/health-information/health-statistics/Pages/overweight-obesity-statistics.aspx

National Institute of Mental Health. (n.d.). *Eating disorders.* Retrieved from https://www.nimh.nih.gov/health/topics/eating-disorders/index.shtml

National Institute on Aging. (2015). *Menopause.* Retrieved from https://www.nia.nih.gov/health/publication/menopause

National Institute on Alcohol Abuse and Alcoholism. (2015). *Alcohol facts and statistics.* Retrieved from http://www.niaaa.nih.gov/alcohol-health/overview-alcohol-/alcohol-facts-and-statistics

National Institute on Drug Abuse (NIDA). (2014). *Prescription drug abuse.* Retrieved from http://www.drugabuse.gov/publications/research-reports/prescription-drugs/what-are-some-commonly-abused-prescription-drugs

National Institute on Drug Abuse (NIDA). (2015). *DrugFacts: Nationwide trends.* Retrieved from http://www.drugabuse.gov/publications/drugfacts/nationwide-trends

National Institutes of Health (NIH). (1993). *National Institutes of Health Revitalization Act of 1993, Subtitle B—Clinical research equity involving women and minorities.* Retrieved from http://orwh.od.nih.gov/about/pdf/NIH-Revitalization-Act-1993.pdf

National Women's Health Network. (2015). *About the National Women's Health Network.* Retrieved from https://www.nwhn.org/about-us/

Nurses' Health Study. (n.d.). *Publications.* Retrieved from http://www.channing.harvard.edu/nhs/?page_id=154

Office on Women's Health. (2012a). *Anorexia nervosa fact sheet.* Retrieved from http://www.womenshealth.gov/publications/our-publications/fact-sheet/anorexia-nervosa.html

Office on Women's Health. (2012b). *Bulimia nervosa fact sheet.* Retrieved from http://www.womenshealth.gov/publications/our-publications/fact-sheet/bulimia-nervosa.html

Office on Women's Health. (2012c). *Binge eating disorder fact sheet.* Retrieved from http://womenshealth.gov/publications/our-publications/fact-sheet/binge-eating-disorder.html

Office on Women's Health. (2012d). *Osteoporosis fact sheet.* Retrieved from http://womenshealth.gov/publications/our-publications/fact-sheet/osteoporosis.html

Ogden, C. L., Carroll, M. D., Kit, B. K., & Flegal, K. M. (2014). Prevalence of childhood and adult obesity in the United States, 2011–2012. *Journal of the American Medical Association, 311,* 806–814. doi: 10.1001/jama.2014.732.

Our Bodies Ourselves. (2015). *History.* Retrieved from http://www.ourbodiesourselves.org/history/

Owada, S., & Suzuki, M. (2014). The relationship between vasomotor symptoms and menopause-associated dizziness. *Acta Otolaryngologia, 134*(2), 146–150.

Patel, S. A., Winkel, M., Ali, M. K., Narayan, K. M. V., & Mehta, N. K. (2015). Cardiovascular mortality associated with 5 leading risk factors: National and state preventable fractions estimated from survey data. *Annals of Internal Medicine, 163,* 245–253. doi: 10.7326/M14-1753.

Portman, D. J., & Gass, M. (2014). Genitourinary syndrome of menopause: New terminology for vulvovaginal atrophy from the International Society for the Study of Women's Sexual Health and the North American Menopause Society. *Menopause, 21*(10), 1063–1068.

Rajan, S. P. (2015). Review and investigation on future research directions of mobile based telecare system for cardiac surveillance. *Journal of Applied Research and Technology, 13*(4), 454–460.

Rayala, B. Z. & Viera, A. (2013). Common questions about vasectomy. *American Family Physician, 88*(11), 757–761. Retrieved from http://www.aafp.org/afp/2013/1201/p757.pdf

Robert Wood Johnson Foundation. (2015). *Adult obesity in the United States.* Retrieved from http://stateofobesity.org/adult-obesity/

Robinson, O. C., & Wright, G. R. (2013). The prevalence, types and perceived outcomes of crisis episodes in early adulthood and midlife: A structures retrospective-autobiographical study. *International Journal of Behavioral Development, 37*(5), 407–416. doi: 10.177/01665025413492464.

Rodriguez, C. J., Allison, M., Daviglus, M. L., Isasi, C. R., Keller C., Leira, E. D., ... Sims, M. (2014). Status of cardiovascular disease and stroke in Hispanics/Latinos in the United States: A science advisory from the American Heart Association. *Circulation, 130*(7), 593–625. doi: 10.1161/CIR.0000000000000071.

Rubenstein, H. (2014). Defining what is normal at menopause: How women's and clinician's different understandings may lead to a lack of provision for those in most need. *Human Fertility, 17*(3), 218–222.

Ryan, J., Scali, J., Carrière, I., Amiva, H., Rouaud, O., Berr, C., ... Ancelin, M. L. (2014). Impact of premature menopause on cognitive function in later life. *BJOG: An International Journal of Obstetrics & Gynaecology, 121*(13), 1729–1739.

Sacks, J. J., Gonzales, K. R., Bouchery, E. E., Tomedi, L. E., & Brewer, R. D. (2015). 2010 National and state costs of excessive alcohol consumption. *American Journal of Preventive Medicine, 49*(5), e73–e79. doi: 10.1016/j.amepre.2015.05.031.

Shaheen, S., Mahmood, A., & Kadri, F. (2015). Menopause and HRT: Clinical pattern and awareness. *The Professional Medical Journal, 22,* 904–909. Retrieved from http://www.theprofesional.com/article/vol.%2022%20no.%2007/prof-2772.pdf

Sharlip, I. D., Belker, A. M., Honig, S., Labrecque, M., Marmar, J. L., Ross, L. S., ... Sokal, D. C. (2012). *Vasectomy: American Urological Association guidelines.* Retrieved from https://www.auanet.org/common/pdf/education/clinical-guidance/Vasectomy.pdf

Sharma, V., Le, B. V., Sheth, K. R., Zargaroff, S., Dupree, J. M., Cashy, J., & Brannigan, R. E. (2013). Vasectomy demographics and postvasectomy desire for future children: Results from a contemporary national survey. *Fertility and Sterility, 99*(7), 1880–1885. doi: 10.1016/j.fertnstert.2013.02.032.

Shih, G., Zhang, Y., Bukowski, K., & Chen, A. (2014). Bringing men to the table: Sterilization can be for him or her. *Clinical Obstetrics and Gynecology, 57*(4), 731–740. doi: 10.1097/GRF 0000000000000060.

Singh, S., Hu, X., Wheeler, W., & Hall, H. I. (2014). HIV diagnoses among men who have sex with men and women—United States and 6 dependent areas, 2008–2011. *American Journal of Public Health, 104*(9), 1700–1706. doi: 10.2105/AJPH.2014.301990.

Singh, G. K., Siapush, M., Azuline, R. E., & Williams, S. D. (2015). Widening socioeconomic and racial disparities in cardiovascular disease mortality in the United States, 1969–2013. *International Journal of MCH and AIDS, 3*(2), 106–118. Retrieved from http://mchandaids.com/wp-content/uploads/2015/04/IJMA_20150415_02_Widening-SES-Race-and-Trends-in-CVD-Mortality.pdf

Smith, W. B., McCaslin, I. R., Gokce, A., Mandava, S. H., Tros, L., & Hellstrom, W. J. (2013). PDE5 inhibitors: Consideration for preference and long-term adherence. *The International Journal of Clinical Practice, 67*(8), 768–780. doi: 10.111/ijcp.12074.

Solve ME/CFS Initiative. (2015). *What is ME/CFS?* Retrieved from http://solvecfs.org/what-is-mecfs/

Strauss, J. R. (2011). Contextual influences on women's health concerns and attitudes toward menopause. *Health & Social Work, 36*(2), 121–127.

Stuenkel, C. A., Davis, S. R., Gompel, A., Lumsden, M. A., Murad, M. H., Pinkerton, J. V., & Santen, R. J. (2015). Treatment of symptoms of the menopause: An Endocrine Society Clinical Practice Guide. *Journal of Clinical Endocrinology & Metabolism, 100*(11). doi: http://dx.doi.org/10.1210/jc.2015-2236.

Substance Abuse and Mental Health Services Administration (SAMHSA). (2015a). *Specific populations and prescription drug misuse and abuse.* Retrieved from http://www.samhsa.gov/prescription-drug-misuse-abuse/specific-populations

Substance Abuse and Mental Health Services Administration (SAMHSA). (2015b). *Nonmedical use of prescription pain relievers by race and ethnicity.* Retrieved from http://www.samhsa.gov/data/sites/default/files/report_1972/Spotlight-1972.pdf

Surveillance, Epidemiology, and End Stage Program (SEER). (2015). *SEER stat fact sheets: All cancer sites.* Retrieved from http://seer.cancer.gov/statfacts/html/all.html

Surveillance, Epidemiology, and End Stage Program (SEER). (n.d.). *SEER stat fact sheets: Female breast cancer.* Retrieved from http://seer.cancer.gov/statfacts/html/breast.html

Tom, S. E., Cooper, R., Wallace, R. B., & Guralnik, J. M. (2012). Type and timing of menopauses and later life mortality among women in the Iowa established populations for the Epidemiological Study of the Elderly cohort. *Journal of Women's Health, 21*(1), 10–16.

Topatan, S., & Yildiz, H. (2012). Symptoms experienced by women who enter into natural and surgical menopause and their relation to sexual functions. *Health Care for Women International, 33*(6), 525–539.

U.S. Department of Agriculture. (2016). MyPlate. Retrieved from https://www.choosemyplate.gov/MyPlate

U.S. Department of Health and Human Services (USDHHS). (2014a). *The Health consequences of smoking: 50 years of progress. A report of the Surgeon General.* Retrieved from http://www.surgeongeneral.gov/library/reports/50-years-of-progress/full-report.pdf

U.S. Department of Health and Human Services (USDHHS). (2014b). *Who is at risk for HIV?* Retrieved from https://www.aids.gov/hiv-aids-basics/prevention/reduce-your-risk/who-is-at-risk-for-hiv/

U.S. Department of Health and Human Services (USDHHS). (2015). *Healthy people 2020: Disparities.* Retrieved from http://www.healthypeople.gov/2020/about/foundation-health-measures/Disparities

U.S. Department of Health and Human Services (USDHHS), Centers for Disease Control and Prevention (CDC), & National Center for Health Statistics (NCHS). (2015). *Alcohol consumption early release of selected estimates based on data from the National Health Interview Survey, 2014, 58–62.* Retrieved from http://www.cdc.gov/nchs/data/nhis/earlyrelease/earlyrelease 201506_09.pdf

U.S. Department of Health and Human Services (USDHHS) & Health Resources and Services Administration, Maternal and Child Health Bureau. (2013). *Women's health USA 2013.* Retrieved from http://www.mchb.hrsa.gov/whusa13/

U.S. Department of Health and Human Services (USDHHS), Substance Abuse and Mental Health Services Administration (SAMHSA), & Center of Behavioral Health Statistics and Quality. (2013). *Drug abuse warning network, 2011: National estimates of drug related emergency department visits.* Retrieved from http://www.samhsa.gov/data/sites/default/files/DAWN2k11ED/DAWN2k11ED/DAWN2k11ED.pdf

U.S. Preventive Services Task Force. (2014a). *Talking with patients about screening for lung cancer.* Retrieved from http://www.uspreventiveservicestaskforce.org/Page/Name/tools-and-resources-for-better-preventive-care

U.S. Preventive Services Task Force. (2014b). *Final recommendation statement: Testicular cancer, screening.* Retrieved from http://www.uspreventiveservicestaskforce.org/Page/Document/RecommendationStatementFinal/testicular-cancer-screening

U.S. Preventive Services Task Force. (2015). *Draft research plan: Prostate cancer, screening.* Retrieved from http://www.uspreventiveservicestaskforce.org/Page/Document/draft-research-plan/prostate-cancer-screening1

Wang, C. M., & Furnback, W. (2013). Modeling the long-term outcomes of bariatric surgery: A review of cost-effective studies. *Best*

Practice & Research Clinical Gastroenterology, 27, 987–995. doi: 10.1016/j.bpg.2013.08.022.

Wang, M., & Shi, J. (2014). Psychological research in retirement. *Annual Review of Psychology, 65,* 209–233. doi: 1146/annurev-psych-010213-115131.

Weiss, B. D. (2014). How to bridge the health literacy gap. *Family Practice Management, 21*(1), 14–18. Retrieved from http://www.aafp.org/fpm/2014/0100/p14.html

Women's Health Study (WHS). (2015). *A randomized trial of low-dose aspirin and vitamin E in the primary prevention of cardiovascular disease and cancer.* Retrieved from http://clinicaltrials.gov/show/NCT00000479

Xu, J. Q., Kochanek, K. D., Murphy, S. L., & Arias, E. (2014). Mortality in the United States, 2012. *National Center for Health Statistics Data Brief, 168.* Retrieved from http://www.cdc.gov/nchs/data/databriefs/db168.pdf

thePoint: Everything You Need to Make the Grade!

thePoint® Visit http://thePoint.lww.com/Allender9e
for selected readings, study aids for all learning styles, and more!

Older Adults: Aging in Place

"We are always the same age inside."

—*Gertrude Stein* (1874–1946), Poet and Novelist

KEY TERMS

Ageism
Aging in place
Alzheimer's disease (AD)
Arthritis
Assisted living
Case management
Centenarians

Continuing care retirement
  communities (CCRCs)
Custodial care
Elder abuse
Geriatrics
Gerontology
Hospice

Long-term care
Nursing home
Obesity
Oldest old
Osteoporosis
Palliative care
Polypharmacy

Respite care
Senility
Skilled nursing facilities
Supercentenarians

LEARNING OBJECTIVES

Upon mastery of this chapter, you should be able to:

- Describe the global and national health status of older adults.
- Identify and refute at least three common misconceptions about older adults.
- Describe characteristics of healthy older adults.
- Provide an example of primary, secondary, and tertiary prevention practices in the older adult population.
- Identify four chronic conditions most commonly found in the older adult population.
- Identify four types of elder abuse.
- Discuss four primary criteria for effective programs for older adults.
- Describe various types of living arrangements and care options as older adults age in place.
- Describe the difference between hospice and palliative care.
- Describe the future of an aging America and the role of the community health nurse.

Older Americans constitute a large and rapidly growing population group. If you aren't already part of it, you will be in the future. Perhaps your parents and grandparents are in that group now. Improved medical care, advances in public health standards, and focus on prevention have contributed to dramatic increases in life expectancy in the United States. A child born in 2013 could expect to live 78.8 years, about 30 years longer than a child born in 1900 (Administration on Aging, 2014). A second reason for the huge growth in the number of older adults began in 2011 as the baby boomers (people born after World War II between the years of 1946 and 1964) reached age 65.

- Between 2003 and 2013, the population aged 60 and over increased 30.7% from 48.1 to 62.8 million (Administration on Aging, 2014).
- Older adults represent 14.1% of the U.S. population, about one in every seven Americans (Administration on Aging, 2014).
- The result is that in the time period between 2011 and 2029, when the last of the baby boomers turns 65, there will be an era of unprecedented growth in the older population.

The number of older adults is projected to more than double to 98 million by 2060 (Administration on Aging, 2014). Looking forward to the changing health needs of the nation, *Healthy People 2020*, the road map for health in the United States, lists four overarching goals:

1. Attain high-quality, longer lives free of preventable disease, disability, injury, and premature death.
2. Achieve health equity, eliminate disparities, and improve the health of all groups.
3. Create social and physical environments that promote good health for all.
4. Promote quality of life, healthy development, and healthy behaviors across all life stages (U.S. Department of Health and Human Services, 2016).

The future older population is expected to be better educated than the current one. The increased levels of education will most likely accompany better health, higher incomes, more wealth, and consequently a higher standard of living in retirement. As people retire at younger ages and in better health, they will require programs and services that support preventive health measures. The programs provide opportunities for continued well-being and enhanced quality of life and contribute to overall longevity. This group's potential for longevity could result in impending poor retirement planning and dwindling finances, increased living costs, increasing chronic disease and disability, diminishing functional capacity, and ongoing losses (Holland, 2014; National Institute on Aging, 2015c).

Health care costs in the United States continue to rise:

- The cost of providing health care for an American 65 years and older is three to five times greater than the cost for someone younger (CDC, 2013c).
- The total national health expenditures (NHEs): $2.9 trillion (CDC, 2015e).
- Total NHEs as a percent of gross domestic product: 17.4% (CDC, 2015e).
- Annual per capita NHEs: $9,255, up from $147 in 1960 (CDC, 2015e; Kaiser Family Foundation, 2013).

Of the total health expenditures:

- 32.1% are spent for hospital care.
- 5.3% for nursing home facilities and continuing care retirement communities.
- 20.1% for physician and clinical services.
- 9.3% for prescription drugs (Kaiser Family Foundation, 2013).

The growth of the aging population presents opportunities for public health nurses to work with communities to strengthen and expand programs and services targeted to seniors, to advocate for the needs of the aging population with government agencies and other organizations, and to assure access to quality health care services that address their unique and complex problems (United Nations, 2015).

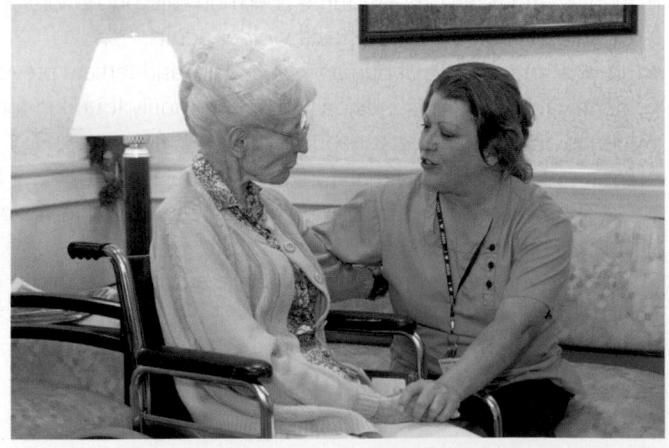

This chapter first examines the characteristics of the aging population in the United States and the global challenge of an aging society. Some myths and misconceptions about older adults are described, and ageism is discussed. Next, the primary, secondary, and tertiary health needs of older adults are explored. Diseases common among older adults are reviewed. Several types of elder abuse are described along with factors that contribute to the abuse of seniors. Finally, population-based health services and nursing interventions applied to the health of the aging population are discussed in light of cost containment and comprehensive care.

GERIATRICS AND GERONTOLOGY

Geriatrics is the medical specialty that deals with the health and social care of the older adult. A geriatrician is a medical doctor with specialized training in geriatrics. Geriatrics includes the physiology of aging, diagnosis and treatment of diseases affecting the aged and resulting from the aging process, and the complex psychosocial issues associated with the aging population. Geriatrics, like other medical specialties with the exception of palliative care, focuses on abnormal conditions and the treatment and cure of those conditions. In the past, geriatric nursing focused primarily on the sick aged. As the nursing profession has grown, its scope has broadened. Many nurses choose to be involved with community-based nursing, focusing on prevention and improved health behaviors for the growing aging population.

Gerontology refers to the study of all aspects of the aging process, including economic, social, clinical, and psychological factors, and their effects on the older adult and on society. Gerontology is a broad, multidisciplinary practice, and gerontological nursing concentrates on promoting the health and maximum functioning of older adults.

PHNs work with many types of older people. In one instance, the nurse may work to promote and maintain the health of a vigorous 80-year-old man who lives alone in his home. As another example, the nurse may give postsurgical care at home to a 69-year-old woman teaching her husband how to care for her and helping them contact community resources for assistance with shopping, meals, housekeeping, and transportation services. Perhaps, nursing intervention focuses on teaching nutrition and maintaining a healthful lifestyle for an extended family that includes a 73-year-old grandmother. The nurse may also lead a bereavement support group for senior citizens whose spouses have recently died. The possibilities are limitless and ever expanding.

A PHN works with older adults at the individual, family, and group levels. However, a community health perspective must also concern itself with the aggregate of older adults. There are many groups of seniors with whom the nurse may choose to work, such as those who attend an adult day care center, belong to a retirement community, live in a nursing home, or use Meals on Wheels. Other groups include residents of a senior citizens' apartment building, retired business and professional women, older post–cataract surgery patients at risk for glaucoma, the older poor, Alzheimer's disease (AD) sufferers, and the homeless. Work with clients can also involve political advocacy.

HEALTH STATUS OF OLDER ADULTS

The growth in the number of older adults in the United States is due to two factors—longer life spans and aging baby boomers These two factors will combine to double the population of Americans aged 65 years or older

during the next 25 years to about 72 million. By 2030, older adults will account for roughly 20% of the U.S. population (CDC, 2013c).

The proportion of individuals aged 65 and older is projected to increase from 12.4% in 2000 to 20.23% by the year 2050 (HelpGuide, 2015d). People are living longer as a result of improved health care, eradication and control of many communicable diseases, use of antibiotics and other medicines, healthier dietary practices, safer global water supplies, regular exercise, and accessibility to a better quality of life including education and social services. Increased life expectancy reflects, in part, the success of public health interventions, but public health programs must now respond to new challenges including the growing burden of chronic illness, injuries, and disabilities; increasing concerns about future caregiving; and rapidly rising health care costs.

The rising number of older adults increases demands on the public health system and on medical and social services and health care delivery. Currently, 50 million older adults have some type of disability (Healthy People. gov, 2015a). Chronic diseases that affect older adults disproportionately contribute to disability, diminish quality of life, and increase health care costs:

- Of those, over 65, 59% report arthritis as the leading cause of disability (CDC, 2013a).
- Diabetes and AD affect one in four and one in nine, respectively, of those aged 65 and older and are expected to have even greater effects on the U.S. health care system in the next few decades (Alzheimer's Association, 2014; CDC, 2013c).

Two key challenges that are new to the public health arena, although they have long been the target of health care and aging services professions, are preventing and treating cognitive decline and addressing end-of-life issues. Meeting these challenges, along with the increasing number of individuals with chronic conditions, is critical to ensuring that the aging population can look forward to their later years. As more and more Americans reach age 65, society is increasingly challenged to help them grow old with dignity and comfort.

Global Demographics

The unprecedented growth in older adults is not limited to the United States but is happening worldwide. In 2010, an estimated 524 million people were aged 65 or older— 8% of the world's population. By 2050, this number is expected to nearly triple to about 1.5 billion, representing 16% of the world's population (National Institute on Aging, 2015b). Life expectancy at birth around the world now is 67. Life expectancy has increased in developing countries since 1950, although the amount of increase varies (Central Intelligence Agency [CIA], 2015). The high percentages of older adults are in part the result of a longer life span, but they also reflect low birth rates in many countries (National Institute on Aging, 2015b).

Although more developed countries have the oldest population profiles, the vast majority of older people—and the most rapidly aging populations—are in less developed countries. Between 2010 and 2050, the number of older people in less developed countries is projected to increase more than 250%, compared with a 71% increase in developed countries (National Institute on Aging, 2015b). In most of the world, the population of those over 85 years of age is the fastest growing segment of the population and is projected to increase 151% between 2005 and 2030 (National Institute on Aging, 2015b). Because of this demographic shift along with altered societal expectations, changes in attitudes and social policies worldwide are needed; many countries have few or no social programs, pensions, or health care services available for their older adult populations.

National Demographics

As a result of demographic transitions including declining infant and childhood mortality, lower fertility rates, and improvements in adult health, the shape of the global age distribution is changing. The age distribution in developed countries, such as the United States, represents a larger proportion of older to younger populations. By 2025, the United States is expected to have 80% more older adults than in 2000, but working-age adults will grow by only 15% (Ortman, Velkoff, & Hogan, 2014).

There are disparities in life expectancy among various subgroups in the population. Life expectancy is highest for White Americans and lowest for Black Americans, who have the highest death rates of any of America's racial and ethnic groups. Although life expectancies have been increasing for all Americans in general, a variety of factors have caused those figures to level off in recent years. These factors include unhealthy lifestyles and societal problems, such as deaths caused by firearms, substance abuse, and human immunodeficiency virus in older adults.

The Hispanic, Black, and Asian populations have been expanding and are projected to grow substantially through 2025 (Healthy People.gov, 2015b). Although the older population is not expected to become majority–minority in the next four decades, it is projected to be 42% minority in 2050, up from 20% in 2010 (Healthy People.gov, 2015b). Thirty-three percent are projected to be minority in 2050, up from 15% in 2010.

The health status of racial and ethnic minorities of all ages lags far behind that of nonminority populations. For a variety of reasons, older adults may experience the effects of health disparities more dramatically than any other population group. In an effort to help address these health disparities, the Racial and Ethnic Approaches to Community Health (REACH, 2015) program supports community-based coalitions in the design, implementation, and evaluation of innovative strategies to reduce or eliminate health disparities among racial and ethnic minorities. Methods utilized include "capacity building, targeted actions, community/system change, widespread risk/protective behavior change, and health disparity reduction" (p. 2). An example of one of these programs, along with other public health nursing research targeted to the older adult population, is highlighted in Evidence-Based Practice. The goal of REACH is to achieve health equity, eliminate disparities, and improve the health of all groups (CDC, 2015r).

Current research has shown that although many efforts—such as aspirin use for high-risk adults, tobacco use screening and brief intervention, colorectal cancer screening for adults over age 50, and immunization for pneumococcal disease for those aged 65 and older—can be very effective, they are not always implemented or consistently utilized. Nevertheless, older people are healthier than ever before. Increasing numbers of capable older adult people are living independently. Hearty older adults—people older than 65 years of age who maintain a level of wellness and activity, well above present expectations for that age—are increasing in number. Many continue to work and stay involved in community programs and activities. Some have become valuable volunteers, helping others in such community activities as hospice and literacy programs for adults, serving as foster grandparents, working in libraries and homeless shelters, or providing services such as Meals on Wheels. Research has shown a connection between positive health effect and community involvement/participation, volunteering, and other forms of social capital.

Not only are more people living into old age but also, once they get there, they are living longer. In 2010, slightly more than 14% of the older population will be 85 and older. By 2050, that proportion is expected to triple (U.S. Census Bureau, 2015). Because of this expansion, subcategories of the over-65 age group are being used. **Oldest old** refers to people who are 85 and above (Segen's Medical Dictionary, 2015); it is the fastest growing age group in the United States and worldwide. Those 100 years old or older are called **centenarians**. A new category for those who have lived 110 years is called **supercentenarians** (Gerontology Research Group, 2015).

Growth in the number of older adults will significantly affect health care resources, housing options for older adults, and national longevity statistics. As the number of older people increases, so, too, will their need for assistance with activities of daily living (ADLs) and other services. Many people will be involved with the care of a family member who needs assistance in attending to ADLs such as dressing, eating, toileting, and bathing; and researchers are seeking effective methods of providing respite to caregivers and reducing costs. In the United States, approximately 80% of older adults have one chronic condition and half of older adults have two chronic conditions. It is estimated that health care costs for chronic disease treatment account for more than 75% of national health expenditures (Kaiser Family Foundation, 2013). Approximately 7 of 10 deaths are from chronic conditions such as heart disease, cancer, and respiratory deaths (CDC, 2015j). Death is only part of the picture of the burden of chronic disease among older Americans. These conditions can cause years of pain, disability, and loss of function and independence before resulting in death. In addition to chronic conditions that require ongoing monitoring and management, the PHN should anticipate the needs of many older adults who will face the loss of a spouse, helpmate, or companion and who may experience loneliness, social isolation, and depression.

Many older adults live in poverty; over 4.2 million older adults (9.5%) were below federal the poverty level in 2013. This poverty rate is statistically different from the poverty rate of 9.1%, only a year earlier in 2012

EVIDENCE-BASED PRACTICE

These are only a few examples of research that may benefit your elderly clients.

A Racial and Ethnic Approaches to Community Health (REACH) study conducted in 16 disadvantaged black communities looked at 5-year trends in self-reported vegetable and fruit consumption and compared results with trends among other black populations and white populations in 14 states. Participatory interventions were used with the REACH participants to improve their consumption of vegetables and fruits. After interventions, there was a 7.4% increase in consumption in the REACH participants and no change among the comparison groups. Researchers estimated that the disparity between the 16 disadvantaged REACH communities and the comparison groups decreased 33% over the course of the study.

Liao, Y., Siegel, P., Zhou, H., Grimm, K., Njai, R., Kent, C., & Giles, W. (2015). Reduced disparity in vegetable consumption in 16 disadvantaged Black communities: A successful 5-year community-based participatory intervention. *Journal of Racial & Ethnic Health Disparities, 2*(2), 211–218.

Improving the health status of immigrant populations has not always been an easy task. Two nurse researchers examined health care utilization and management of hypertension in a group of elderly Korean immigrants recruited from a senior center and a church. Baseline blood pressures were taken and participants completed a health care utilization questionnaire. Findings noted 87% of participants had regular health exams and were aware of their hypertension diagnoses as well as were taking their prescribed antihypertensive medications. About 63% of the elderly Korean participants had hypertension, but not all hypertension was managed effectively. Most had health insurance (95.7%), a much higher number than other elderly ethnic groups (e.g., 29.2% Hispanics, 14.8% Asian/Pacific Islanders). This may help explain higher rates of health care exams and medication compliance in this group. Also, the senior center offered regular blood pressure checks, had assigned meal coordinators for this specific population, and offered social support for this specific group of older adults. This is an example of community agencies and community health nurses targeting programs and interventions to specific populations.

Sin, M. K., & Hirsch, A. (2013). Health care utilization and hypertension management in community-based elderly Korean immigrants. *Journal of Immigrant & Minority Health, 15*, 1090–1095.

Assisted living facilities are not always well regulated, making their elderly residents more vulnerable. Two gerontology nurse researchers examined neglect and neglect-related outcomes in these facilities based on complaint investigations. They specifically examined elder neglect (medical, personal, environmental), the frequency of neglect-related outcomes (health services, physical psychosocial), and the degree to which practices of the facilities (inadequate staffing, hiring, and business practices) and staff insufficiencies (qualifications, education, attitudes) were associated with neglect. They looked at citations that were issued during routine inspections of facilities and the narrative reports done for investigation of complaints. A total of 165 facilities were included, mostly in urban areas, with a total of 616 complaints. Citations were given for inappropriate care, hiring, staffing, and business practices and inadequacies in staff education, attitude of staff, and staff qualifications. For neglect outcomes, injuries were the most common and some deaths occurred. Psychosocial outcomes were found in 23.6% of facilities; more than half of facilities had elderly patients relocated because of neglect. When comparing citations and types of neglect, all were statistically significant except for inappropriate business practices. Staff attitudes and inappropriate staffing were associated with a higher number of citations and all three types of neglect. Personal neglect was found to be the most common type in this study, and <10% of facilities had no reports involving neglect. Neglect often resulted in infections, injuries, and death and increases health care costs. Failure to complete background checks on staff, overcrowding, and improper financial transactions were noted as inappropriate institutional practices. Public health nurses need to participate in research on assisted living facilities and not succumb to the preconceived ideas that these are private-pay, well-run places for older adults needing assistance. National databases are needed to help families determine best placements for their loved ones, and public health nurse surveyors could be helpful in this endeavor. This vulnerable population needs PHN services; they remain members of the communities served by PHNs and deserve protection.

Phillips, L. R., & Ziminski, C. (2012). The public health nursing role in elder neglect in assisted living facilities. *Public Health Nursing, 29*(6), 499–509.

(Administration on Aging, 2014). However, in 2013, the Supplemental Poverty Measure (SPM) from the U.S. Census Bureau adjusted for regional costs of living and nondiscretionary expenses and revealed another calculation of poverty level for older adults at 14.8% (over 5% points higher than the official 9.5% rate). This increase is mainly due to adding in medical out-of-pocket expenses that were not included in the original poverty level calculations (Administration on Aging, 2014).

The education level of the older population is rising. Between 1970 and 2014, the percentage of older persons who had completed high school increased from 28% to 84%. In 2014, about 26% had a bachelor's degree or higher. Considerable racial/ethnic differences were found in the proportion completing high school (i.e., 88% of non-Hispanic Whites, 76% of Asians, 74% of African Americans, 76% of American Indian/Alaska Natives, 54% of Hispanics). Only 30% of older Whites, and 9%

of older African Americans, had high school diplomas in 1970 (Administration on Aging, 2014). With higher levels of education should come broader health consumerism and improved quality of life.

DISPELLING AGEISM

Ageism is a term that describes negative stereotyping of older adults and discrimination because of older age. In America, ageism is a major problem (Ageism Hurts.org, 2015). These stereotypes often arise from negative personal experiences, myths shared over time, and a general lack of current information. Unfortunately, health concerns and symptoms in older adults are often overlooked or dismissed as part of the normal aging process. By becoming more aware of myths and realities, PHNs can better improve the health and quality of life of the growing population of older adults. Ageism can interfere with effective practice and prevent the kind of comprehensive and interdisciplinary services and care that aging persons need and deserve. Ageism has an impact on both society and culture, even though most individuals are not aware of it. Ageism objectifies older adults and can create needless fear, waste, illness, and misery. "Ageism is to old age as racism is to skin color and sexism is to gender.... In its worst form, ageism leads to elder abuse, mistreatment, and neglect" (Robnett & Chop, 2015, p. 22). Most people know little about aging and may have negative stereotypes about older adults. PHNs must guard against ageism in their practice by dispelling common myths and misconceptions.

The Myth of Senility

Myth: It is normal for older adults to become more confused and childlike and forgetful and to lose contact with reality as they age. They become "senile."

Reality: Senility is an obsolete term used to describe deterioration in the mental functions of some older people. The word implies that with growing old come symptoms of forgetfulness, confusion, and changes in behavior and personality. This term is stereotypical, implying that older people are mentally deficient. Memory loss is *not* an inevitable part of the aging process (Alzheimer's Association, 2015b). The brain is capable of producing new brain cells at any age, so significant memory loss is *not* an inevitable result of aging. But, just as it is with muscle strength, you have to use it or lose it. Lifestyle, health habits, and daily activities have a huge impact on the health of the brain. At any age, there are many ways you can improve your cognitive skills, prevent memory loss, and protect your gray matter (HelpGuide, 2015b).

Certainly, Alzheimer's and arteriosclerosis cause memory loss and altered behavior in the older adult, but many older adults have similar symptoms as a result of anxiety, loss, depression, or grief or simply from side effects of medications or changes in their routines. These reactions need to be diagnosed by health care providers and differentiated from disease processes. A recent review of the available literature on the relationship between exercise and cognition indicates that social engagement and physical activity may help maintain cognitive functioning in older adults (Bherer, Erickson, & Liu-Ambrose, 2013; HelpGuide, 2015b). Age-related memory loss can be the result of several physiological factors.

First, the hippocampus, a region of the brain involved in the formation and retrieval of memories, often deteriorates with age. Second, growth factors—hormones and proteins that protect and repair brain cells and stimulate neural growth—decline with age. Third, older people often experience decreased blood flow to the brain. This can impair memory and lead to changes in cognitive skills (Pavlopoulos et al., 2013). Intelligence, learning ability, and other intellectual and cognitive skills do not decline with age. Cognitive deficits are often caused by reversible factors (Gutchess, 2014). Sometimes, even what looks like significant memory loss can be caused by treatable conditions and reversible external factors such as medication side effects, depression, vitamin B_{12} deficiency, thyroid problems, alcohol abuse, or dehydration (HelpGuide, 2015b). Generally, older people are capable of making their own decisions; they want and need the freedom to make choices and to be as independent as their limitations will allow.

The Myth of the Rocking Chair

Myth: As age increases, older adults withdraw, become inactive, and cease being productive.

Reality: Whereas some older adults do become disengaged, many remain active for as long as possible. Diminished capabilities and personal preferences affect the level of activity. As age advances, older adults do not necessarily become inactive and sit in rocking chairs on the porch. The average American retires at age 63. Prior to the 1990s, the average age of retirement had been declining. Now, it is moving upward. A recent trend has been for retirees to return to work; in 2012, almost 27% of 65- to 74-year-olds were working and this number is expected to rise to 31.9% by 2022 (Pew Research Center, 2014).

Labor force participation rates of those over 60 (not retired) have been increasing over the past decade for men and women age 62 to 64 (4% increase for men and 12% increase for women). The Center for Retirement Research at Boston College found that older workers who are more productive remain in the workplace for a longer period than do those who are less productive (Burtless, 2013). Millions of Americans older than age 65 choose to work full- or part-time, and many others, who are not included in labor statistics, work but do not report their earnings. An example is the grandmother who chooses to give up full-time employment in an unsatisfying job to babysit for three preschool grandchildren and is paid in cash by her two children. The grandmother gets to spend time with growing grandchildren and supplement her retirement income, the parents feel comfortable that their mother is caring for their children, and the grandchildren are experiencing the joy of being with their grandparent. In another situation, active retired older adults assist with their two children's businesses. The mother types legal documents for the son's law practice during busy times, and the father helps out on Saturdays at the daughter's pool supply store. Everyone wins in these situations.

Meaningful activity remains important to seniors. Healthy older people usually do not disengage or withdraw and isolate themselves from society; rather, they are active and involved. Remaining active—through a daily routine, purposeful behavior, and a positive view of life—produces the best psychological climate.

The Myth of Homogeneity

Myth: As older adults age, they lose their individual differences and become progressively more alike.

Reality: As a person ages, his/her personality remains fairly constant. Not only are individual differences retained, these differences become even more pronounced with age. Generally, an older adult becomes more like the person he or she was in youth (i.e., a talkative teenager, e.g., becoming a talkative older person or a stubborn youngster carrying the trait of stubbornness into old age). Except for changes in physical appearance and experiencing more physical problems, being "old"

feels no different from how we feel now or when we were young. In reality, an old person is a young person who has just lived longer. Not all elderly drive slowly or are cantankerous or politically conservative (Storlie, 2015).

The aging process is quite distinct among older people, and they age at widely disparate rates. Some people still play golf, drive a car, and participate in social and community activities at age 85; others are frail and cannot move about well, needing assistance with their ADLs. Some prefer to equate "real age" with biological age, not chronological age; this depends on how well an individual promotes self-care, both physically and mentally. Exercise, nutrition, vitamins, seat belt use, and other factors are thought to play a role in healthy aging. Physical, social, and mental health parameters; life experiences; and genetic traits all combine to make aging an individualized process (see Levels of Prevention Pyramid).

LEVELS OF PREVENTION PYRAMID

SITUATION: Making a healthy transition into a satisfying old age

GOAL: Using the three levels of prevention: health promotion improves overall health and well-being and prevents or delays chronic diseases, whereas secondary prevention ensures prompt early diagnosis and treatment of conditions, and tertiary prevention aids in rehabilitation and continuing health promotion, preventing or delaying chronic diseases, to promptly diagnose and treat conditions, until the fullest possible potential is restored

TERTIARY PREVENTION

Rehabilitation	Primary Prevention	
	Health Promotion and Education	*Health Protection*
• Adapt to changed roles with spouse and significant others. • Maintain health while assessing increasing dependency needs, including alternative housing, modifications in transportation, and changing health care needs.	• Periodically review and update will, insurances, and other important documents as needed. • Keep beneficiaries or executors aware of changes in and location of documents and personal wishes regarding end-of-life care and funeral/burial arrangements.	

SECONDARY PREVENTION

Early Diagnosis	Prompt Treatment
• Follow the U.S. Task Force Recommendations for regular screening of potential health problems. • Reflect on past successes and contributions to the workforce.	• Allow time for adaptation to this life transition. • Organize new free time into satisfying and enriching activities.

PRIMARY PREVENTION

Health Promotion and Education	Health Protection
• Early preparation—emotionally and financially. • Plan ahead for changes in health status and potential need for long-term care. • Complete documents, such as a will and a living will.	• Regularly assess health status. • Follow the U.S. Task Force Recommendations for immunizations. • Implement a health-promoting regimen that includes diet and exercise. • Assess living environment for safety hazards.

The Myth of Inability

Myth: Older adults are forgetful, are unable to learn new things, and are set in their old ways of doing things.

Reality: Learning is a lifetime ability that continues into old age. Although older adults may experience some difficulty with short-term (or working) memory as they get older, their long-term memory generally remains sound. People at any age can learn new information and skills. Research indicates that older people can learn new skills and improve old ones, including cognitive training and exercise interventions, as well as how to use a computer and the Internet (Bherer, 2015; Rose et al., 2015). Learning occurs best in a self-paced, supportive environment. Studies have demonstrated that exercising the brain improves memory (HelpGuide, 2015g). Older adults have spent a lifetime adapting to change, with varying measures of success. People older than 65 years grew up during a time when having an automobile was a luxury, and many did not have a microwave oven, computer, or utilize social media until they were in middle adulthood. Older adults learned to adapt to these changes, and they are becoming increasingly computer literate today. The ability to change does not depend on age but rather on personality traits acquired throughout life or, sometimes, because of socioeconomic difficulties. For example, elders living on fixed incomes may be faced with inflationary costs. This may cause them to vote against a school levy that would increase taxes, although they otherwise would be very supportive of schools because they value education.

MEETING THE HEALTH NEEDS OF OLDER ADULTS

No one knows conclusively all of the variables that influence healthy aging, but it is known that a lifetime of healthy habits and circumstances, a strong social support system, and a positive emotional outlook all significantly influence the resources people bring to their later years. Most people recognize a healthy older person when they meet one. See From the Case Files I for an example of healthy aging.

What is healthy old age? As was mentioned earlier, the vast majority (94%) of our older adults, even those with chronic diseases or other disabilities, are living outside institutions and are relatively independent. Their ability to function is a key indicator of health and wellness and is an important factor in understanding healthy aging. Good health in the older adult means maintaining the maximum possible degree of physical, mental, and social vigor. It means being able to adapt, to continue to handle stress, and to be active and involved in life and living. In short, healthy aging means being able to function, even when disabled, with a minimum of help from others.

Wellness among the older population varies considerably. It is influenced by many factors, including personality traits, life experiences, current physical health, and current societal supports and personal health behaviors including smoking, obesity, and excessive alcohol use. One way to measure healthy aging on a large scale is the degree to which states have met or exceeded targets on the *Healthy People 2020* older adult health indicators. The National Report Card on Healthy Aging tracks 15 indicators of older adult health, 8 of which are identified

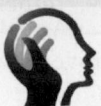

From the **Case Files** I

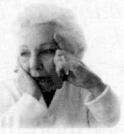

I am a PHN and live next door to Minerva Blackstone, affectionately called Minnie by her friends. Minnie is a lively 87-year-old woman who enjoys life. Every day, except in bad weather, she walks a half mile to visit her granddaughter Karen. There, she works on the quilt she is making for Karen. In addition, twice a week, Minnie takes the city bus to the senior citizens' center to join her friends in an exercise class. Although her eyesight has somewhat diminished, Minnie enjoys reading in the evening or crocheting while she watches television. Mysteries and comedies are her favorite kinds of stories.

Minnie is a happy person but is not content unless she is up on the latest political developments. She always has opinions on current events and expresses them with vigorous shakes of her curly white hair at her monthly group meeting on women and politics. She has a good appetite and generally sleeps well. Minor arthritis does not hamper her activities, nor does the hypertension that she controls by taking her medication with conscientious regularity. Minnie is enjoying a healthy, successful old age.

Carole Stokes, District PHN

in *Healthy People 2020*, the national health agenda of the U.S. Department of Health and Human Services. These 15 indicators are grouped into four areas: Health Status, Health Behaviors, Preventive Care and Screening, and Injuries. In addition, the report assigns a "met" or "not met" score to states on the basis of their attainment of *Healthy People 2020* targets (CDC, 2013c, 2015j; *Healthy People 2020*, 2015c). As of 2013, goals for mammograms, colorectal screening, and taking blood pressure medications have been met. Also, rates of smoking have dropped for older adults, as have rates for obesity and those not engaging in leisure time physical activity within the last month (CDC, 2013c). In addition, the report assigns a "met" or "not met" score to states on the basis of their attainment of *Healthy People 2020* targets (CDC, 2013c). The United States has met six of the *Healthy People 2020* targets in this report (p. ii to iii):

- Having no leisure time physical activity in past month (31.4% vs. goal of 32.6% reporting leisure physical activity)
- Obesity (24.5% vs. goal of 30.6% reported that they are obese)
- Current smoking (8.4% vs. goal of 12% reported that they are currently smoking)
- Taking medications as directed for high blood pressure (94.1% vs. goal of 77.4%)
- Having mammograms within past 2 years (81.9% vs. goal of 70%)
- Screenings for colorectal cancer (72.2% vs. goal of 70%)

However, every state has considerable work to do on other indicators for older adults.

- Flu vaccine in past year—no states met the 2020 target of 90% (total was 66.9%)
- Ever had pneumonia vaccine—no states met the 2020 target of 90% (total was 68.1%)

Other actions that can increase healthy aging include addressing health disparities among older adults, encouraging people to plan for end-of-life care and communicate their wishes through advance directives, improving oral health and increasing physical activity among seniors by promoting environmental changes, increasing adult immunization levels, and preventing falls. Some older adults demonstrate maximum adaptability, resourcefulness, optimism, and activity. Others, often those from whom we tend to draw our stereotypes, have disengaged and present a picture of dependence and resignation. Most older adults fall somewhere in between these two extremes. Although the level of wellness varies among older adults, that level can be raised. The goals in community health nursing are to maximize the wellness potential of older adult clients and to support their highest level of functional ability enabling them to remain independent. Nurses must analyze and build on an older person's strengths rather than focus on the difficulties or deficits. The goal for an aging population is to enable older people to thrive and have the highest quality of life for as long as possible, not merely to survive (Altarum Institute, 2012).

Effective nursing among any population requires familiarity with that group's health problems and needs. Aging, in and of itself, is not a health problem. Rather, aging is a normal, irreversible physiologic process. Its pace, however, can sometimes be slowed, as researchers are discovering, and many of the problems associated with aging can be prevented. The aging process is subtle, gradual, and lifelong. One can see remarkable differences among individuals in the rate of aging. Even in a single individual, various systems of the body age at different rates. Therefore, chronologic age cannot readily be a reliable indicator of health needs. Methods for calculating your "real" or biological age can give you a better picture of your body's true state of health (see http://www.biological-age.com/about.html for a calculator you can use for yourself and your clients).

However, the proportion of people with health problems increases with age, and as a group, older adults are more likely than younger ones to suffer from multiple, chronic, and often disabling conditions requiring ongoing care and management.

LEVELS OF PREVENTION

Older adults, like any age group, have certain basic needs: physiologic and safety needs, as well as the needs for love and belonging, self-esteem, and self-actualization. Their physical, emotional, and social needs are complex and interrelated. The following sections discuss these needs according to primary, secondary, and tertiary prevention activities.

Primary Prevention

As discussed previously in this text, primary prevention activities involve those actions that keep one healthy. Such primary prevention activities as health education, follow-through of sound personal health practices (e.g., flossing, seat belt use, exercise), recommended routine screenings, and maintenance of an appropriate immunization schedule ensure that older adults are doing all that they can to maintain their health. The list in Display 24–1 includes strategies for successful aging. It provides primary

---

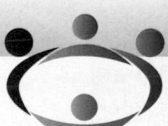

DISPLAY 24–1 STRATEGIES FOR SUCCESSFUL AGING

- Do at least 30 minutes of sustained, rhythmic, vigorous exercise four to five times a week.
- Use complementary/alternative therapies (e.g., meditation, yoga, Tai Chi).
- Eat "like a bushman" (a healthy diet of fruits, whole grains, vegetables, and lean meat).
- Get as much sleep and rest as needed.
- Maintain a sense of humor and deflect anger.
- Set goals and accept challenges that force you to be as alive and creative as possible.
- Do cognitively challenging activities for at least 6 hours each week (e.g., crossword puzzles, playing cards, reading).
- Don't depend on anyone else for your well-being.
- Be necessary and responsible; live outside yourself (give to others, become involved).
- Don't slow down. Stick with the mainstream. Avoid the shadows. Stay together. Maintain energy flow in a purposeful direction; aging need not be characterized by losses. Maintain contacts with family and friends, and stay active through work, recreation, and community. Find meaning in your life.
- Get regular checkups. Maintain good dental health.
- Don't smoke—it's never too late to quit.
- Practice safety habits at home to prevent falls and fractures. Always wear seat belts when traveling by car.
- Avoid overexposure to the sun and the cold.
- If you drink, moderation is the key—when you drink, let someone else drive.
- Keep personal and financial records in order to simplify budgeting and investing—plan long-term housing and financial needs.
- Keep a positive attitude toward life—do things that make you happy.

Adapted from Shapira, E. Z. (2011). *A new wrinkle: What I learned from older people who never acted their age*. Bloomington, IN: iUniverse; Harmell, A. L., Jeste, D., & Depp, C. (2014). Strategies for successful aging: A research update. *Current Psychiatry Reports*, 16(10), 476.

prevention activities the PHN can use when working with older adults, either individually or in groups.

Nutrition and Oral Health Needs

People who have maintained sound dietary habits throughout their life have little need to change in old age. The USDA replaced the food pyramid with MyPlate as a visual to guide the food intake of Americans (U.S. Department of Agriculture, 2015). Tufts University has modified MyPlate for older adults (see Fig. 24–1). The modifications include an emphasis on drinking plenty of fluids such as water and/or fat-free milk and high-fiber intake, as well as adding multivitamins to the diet. Also emphasized is the importance of regular exercise with icons depicting common activities that include daily errands and household chores (Tufts University, 2015).

Many older adults have not established such habits but may be required to do so because of disease processes such as diabetes or cardiovascular disease. It is generally believed that older people need to maintain their optimal weight by eating a diet that is low in fats, moderate in carbohydrates, and high in proteins with a daily calorie count of 1,200 to 1,600. Foods with "empty calories," such as salty snacks, candy, fatty foods, and alcohol, should be limited; they meet hunger needs by satisfying appetite only, while providing little nutrition. Cereals and whole grains, dried beans, and nuts can provide fiber needed by seniors, and eating colorful fruits and vegetables (rather than fruit juice) also contributes to fiber and may help to prevent macular degeneration. Another important thing to remind older adults to do is to drink adequate amounts of liquids, especially water. Eight glasses a day are recommended, and many older adults have a diminished feeling of thirst and can easily become dehydrated if they do not purposefully plan their fluid intake. Older adults need less vitamin A but more calcium and vitamin D (for healthy bones), more folic acid, and more vitamins B_6 and B_{12} (for cognitive health) than younger adults. Many communities offer meals to seniors, either at senior centers or by way of Meals on Wheels, through grants provided by the Older Adult Nutrition Program (Administration on Aging, 2015).

Major advances in the field of oral health including community water fluoridation, advanced dental technology, better oral hygiene, and more frequent use of dental services have had a substantial impact on the number of older adults who retain their natural teeth. Before the time of widespread fluoride use, it was common for people to lose most or all of their teeth by midlife. The percentage of older adults who have lost all their natural teeth has declined to 18%, surpassing the *Healthy People 2020* target of no more than 20% (CDC, 2015k). Severe tooth loss in older adults compromises the quality of their nutrition. Most people can keep their natural teeth for a lifetime with preventive oral health (CDC, 2015l). The percentage of adults ages 65 and over with a dental visit in the past year was 60.6% (CDC, 2015k). Oral health is integral to general health and well-being throughout one's life. A good deal of research has demonstrated the connection between oral health and general health due to chronic inflammation that releases cytokines and C-reactive protein causing endothelial damage and cholesterol plaque attachment in cardiovascular disease and stroke. Poor oral

health has also been associated with peripheral vascular disease, diabetes, and risk for death caused by pneumonia in nursing homes (Igari, Kudo, Toyofuku, Inoue, & Iwai, 2014). Even those with dentures must be vigilant in maintaining oral health, as they are still at risk from inflammatory processes leading to diseases like pneumonia. The oral health of older adults, however, is often neglected. Many older adults especially those who are disadvantaged and with limited incomes have decreased nutritional and fluid intake, changes in gums and increased periodontal disease, as well as a higher incidence of dry mouth. Saliva contains minerals for rebuilding of tooth enamel as well as antimicrobial components (Carpenter, 2013; CDC, 2015i; National Institute on Aging, 2015b). Fluid intake and oral hygiene are appropriate topics for anticipatory guidance from PHNs working with older adults.

Oral health and hygiene needs do not decrease with age. Eating, chewing, and swallowing should be an uncomplicated and natural process. Eating should remain a pleasurable social experience, preferably taking place in the company of others. PHNs can assist older adults with meal management by following the suggestions outlined in Display 24–2 and Figure 24–1.

In addition to maintaining a healthy diet, older adults are cautioned to limit the use of alcohol, avoid tobacco, drink fluoridated water or use fluoride toothpaste, practice good oral hygiene, and have regular dental checkups (CDC, 2015k). They should also avoid the habitual use of laxatives, instead adding more fiber and bulk to their diet with fresh fruits and vegetables. Also, inadequate fluid intake can contribute to bowel and bladder problems. Following a diet that includes eight or more 8-ounce glasses of fluid daily assists the gastrointestinal and genitourinary systems in their functions. Increased physical activity and exercise helps maintain regularity of bowel function in older adults.

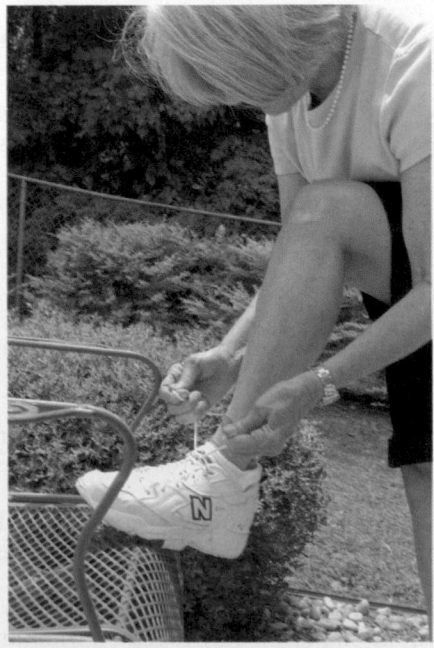

Physical activity, drinking plenty of water, and adding fiber and bulk to their diet with fresh fruits and vegetables are healthy ways seniors can assure good bowel patterns.

DISPLAY 24–2 MEAL MANAGEMENT CONSIDERATIONS

- Complete a safety check with the older adult to assess the ability to operate stoves and microwave ovens. Include the elder's ability to reach and put things on and off stove burners.
- Arrange kitchen shelves so that commonly used items can be reached from an easy standing level.
- Suggest use of turntables and long-handled "grabbers" while discouraging use of step stools or ladders.
- Assess the elder's typical meal for quality and availability—can be accomplished for all meals by doing a 24-hour dietary recall—begin with the most recent meal and work backward.
- To ensure that elders eat an appropriate number of times a day, suggest that they "eat by the clock" or with a certain TV show.
- Help older adults build support system for sharing grocery shopping, cooking, and meals.

- Suggest they bake once a week for an activity or shop with another elder.
- Suggest buying convenience foods, making sure they have nutritional value, such as frozen vegetables or dinners.
- Consider community resources to assist with shopping, transportation, or meal preparation as needed. Keeping a continuous shopping list helps elders to remember needed grocery items and provides a reference if someone offers to assist with shopping.
- Help older adults consider increasing socialization by eating together with friends—rotating among three to four friends each week or eating out with friends and selecting restaurants that are physically and financially accessible.

MyPlate for Older Adults

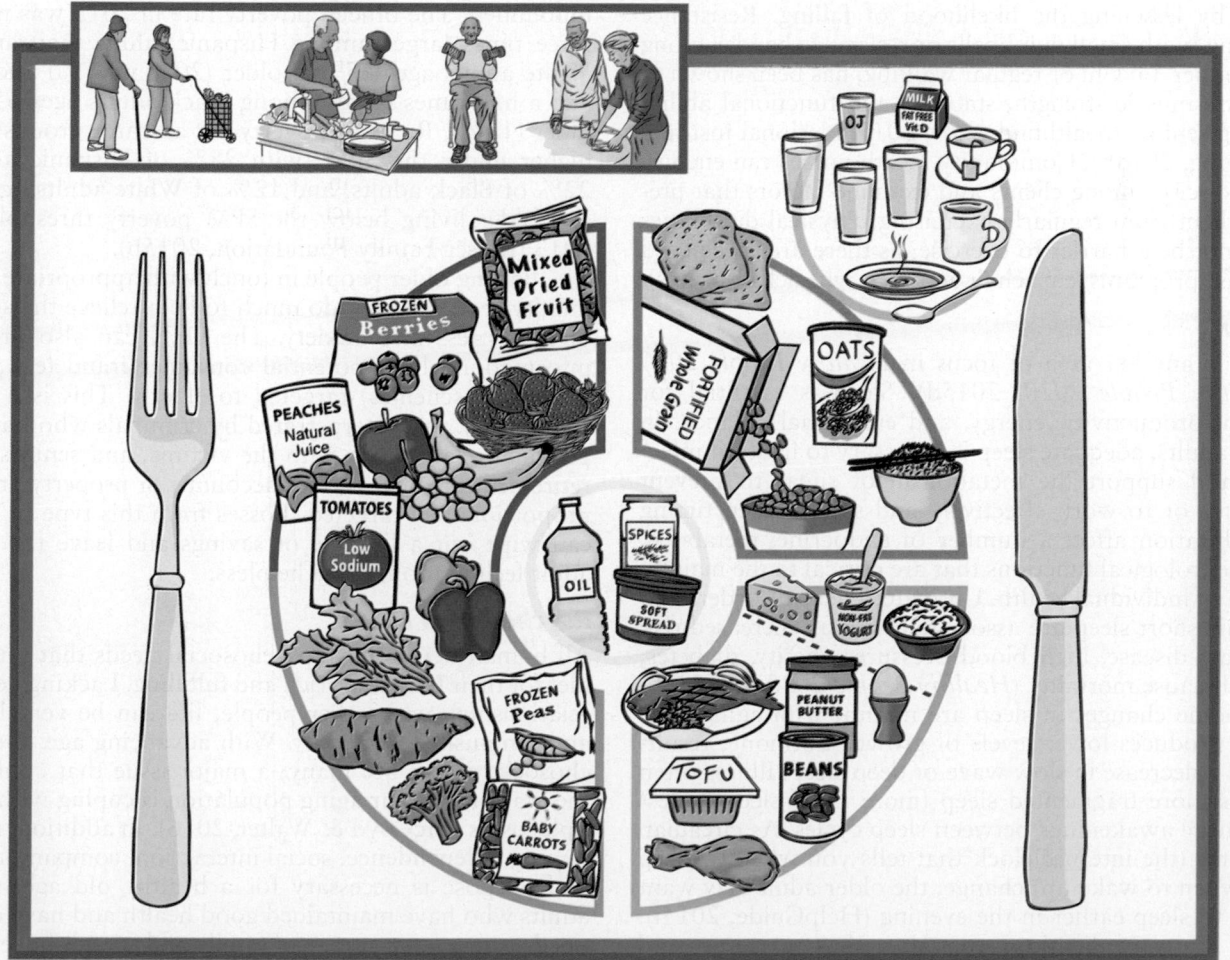

2011© TUFTS UNIVERSITY

FIGURE 24–1   MyPlate for older adults. (Copyright (Tufts University, 2011). Used with permission.)

Exercise Needs

Older adults need to exercise; in fact, they thrive when exercise is incorporated into their daily routine (National Institute on Aging, 2015b). Research demonstrates that exercise and increased physical activity have multiple benefits for the older adult including arthritis relief, restoration of balance and reduction of falls, strengthening of bone, proper weight maintenance, improved glucose control, and overall mortality (Beherer, Erickson, & Liu-Ambrose, 2013; Kokkinos, 2012; Reiner, Niermann, Jekauc, & Woll, 2013; Taylor, 2014). It also contributes to a healthy state of mind, improved sleep, and reduces the risk of heart disease (CDC, 2014). Aging does not and should not involve passivity; instead, physical activity and movement contribute to the quality of intellectual and physical performance in old age. Exercise, such as a daily walk, can keep muscles in good tone, enhance circulation, and promote mental health and adequate sleep (Healthy People 2020, 2015d; National Institute on Aging, 2015b). Exercise may occur in connection with such activities as homemaking chores, gardening, hobbies, or recreation and sports. Often, such physical outlets are enjoyed in the company of other people, meeting social and emotional needs as well as physical ones. Even among the very old, an exercise routine that includes activities to improve strength, flexibility, and coordination may indirectly, but effectively, decrease the incidence of osteoporotic fractures by lessening the likelihood of falling. Resistance training (with small dumbbells or resistance bands), along with either Tai Chi or regular walking, has been shown to increase muscle strength, stability, and functional ability among seniors (healthfinder.gov, 2015; National Institute on Aging, 2015b). Community health nurses can encourage exercise among clients and examine factors that prevent them from regularly exercising. Physical disabilities need not be a barrier to exercise, as there are specialized exercise programs (e.g., chair aerobics, wheelchair fitness).

Sleep

Sleep is another area of focus in *Healthy People 2020* (*Healthy People 2020*, 2015d). Sleep is essential for health, productivity, energy, and emotional balance. In older adults, adequate sleep is necessary to fight off infection and support the metabolism of sugar to prevent diabetes or to work effectively and safely. Sleep timing and duration affect a number of endocrine, metabolic, and neurological functions that are critical to the maintenance of individual health. Untreated, sleep disorders and chronic short sleep are associated with an increased risk of heart disease, high blood pressure, obesity, diabetes, and all-cause mortality (*Healthy People 2020*, 2015d).

Some changes in sleep are natural with aging. The body produces lower levels of growth hormone, resulting in a decrease in slow wave or deep sleep. Illness often means more fragmented sleep (more rapid sleep cycles) and more awakenings between sleep cycles. As circadian rhythms (the internal clock that tells you when to sleep and when to wake up) change, the older adult may want to go to sleep earlier in the evening (HelpGuide, 2015i). Also, many medications can alter sleep patterns, and snoring, which may worsen with age, is a common cause of sleep disturbance (National Sleep Foundation, n.d.).

Economic Security Needs, Poverty

Economic security is another major need for older adults. Worrying about finances is often one of the most debilitating factors of old age. Fearing the potential cost of major illness and not wanting to be a burden on family or friends, many older people conserve their limited finances by establishing frugal eating patterns, using health resources sparingly, not taking their medications or only taking medications in partial doses, reducing costs for home heating and cooling, and, in general, spending little on themselves. People sometimes have to choose between food, housing, and medications. Another factor that is driving up the cost of health care for the aging population is that many clients wait until they are more seriously ill before seeking health care. In waiting for conditions to improve or go away, they often miss out on important preventive health measures and community-based programs that can maximize function and help the client maintain health at a higher level (U.S. Preventive Services Task Force [USPSTF], 2015). Too often, the fear—let alone the reality—of financial difficulties prevents older adults from leading full and active lives (Wallace, 2014–2015).

For older adults today who have lived many years past retirement and perhaps have not planned for sufficient financial security to maintain them throughout these additional, unexpected years, the fears are not unfounded. The official poverty rate in 2013 was nearly three times larger among Hispanic adults than among White adults ages 65 and older (20% vs. 7%) and two and a half times larger among Black adults ages 65 and older (18%). Rates of poverty for all three groups were higher under the SPM, with 28% of Hispanic adults, 22% of Black adults, and 12% of White adults ages 65 and older living below the SPM poverty thresholds in 2013 (Kaiser Family Foundation, 2015b).

Putting older people in touch with appropriate community resources can do much to help relieve the source of that stress and anxiety. The PHN can also provide information about potential consumer fraud (e.g., telemarketing schemes) targeted to elderly. This is a form of financial abuse perpetrated by criminals who have no personal relationship with the victims, and seniors with retirement income, savings accounts, or property are disproportionately targeted. Losses from this type of fraud can wipe out a lifetime of savings and leave the older adult feeling foolish and helpless.

Psychosocial Needs

All human beings have psychosocial needs that must be met for their lives to be rich and fulfilling. Lacking healthy relationships with other people, life can be very lonely and diminished in quality. With advancing age, the psychosocial issues are many; a major issue that confronts the majority of our aging population is coping with multiple losses (McCoyd & Walter, 2016). In addition, maintaining independence, social interaction, companionship, and purpose is necessary for a healthy old age. Older adults who have maintained good health and have developed a supportive system of family and friends have more fulfilled lives. Programs such as Friendly Visitors, where volunteers regularly meet with isolated seniors either in their homes or long-term care facilities, can be an effective method of increasing social support for those who have no family members nearby.

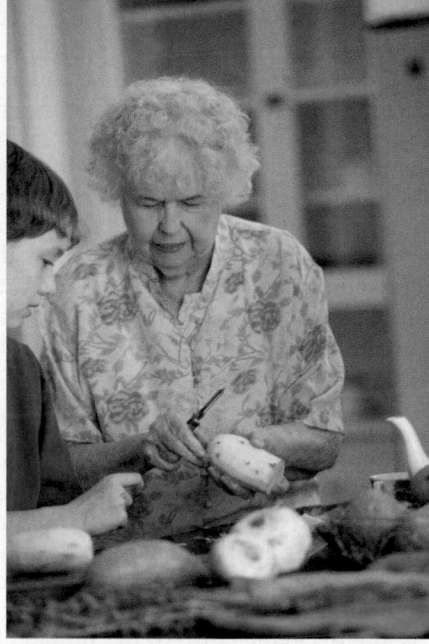

A supportive system of family and friends helps older adults meet their psychosocial needs.

Spiritual Needs

Holistic nursing is a hallmark of community and public health nursing. This means a focus on body, mind, and spirit. The word spirit comes from the Latin meaning "breath" and refers to the core of an individual, the part that gives meaning to life (New World Encyclopedia, 2015). Spirituality is far more encompassing than religion, though we often see the two used interchangeably. Many people think that spirituality and religion are the same; religion and spirituality may exist together; however, a spiritual component exists in all people, but not everyone is religious (Center on Aging Studies Without Walls, n.d.). Religion is generally recognized to be the practical expression of spirituality, or the organization, rituals, and practice of one's beliefs. Religion includes specific beliefs and practices, whereas spirituality is far broader.

Religion and associated activities are common among older adults. Older adults may turn to spirituality and religion when they meet difficult life-changing events and experience personal losses. Their reaction to these events and losses may cause distress and temporary or chronic psychological conditions (Noronha, 2015). Many older persons report that religion helps them cope or adapt with losses or difficulties. While other sources of well-being decline, religion may become more important over time. At the time when religious support is most needed, older persons are often less able to access it because of failing health, immobility, or lack of transportation.

Individuals within different cultures have varying philosophies and practices of spirituality, but derive

similar positive outcomes. For many, old age may be a time of life review. These years become a time of redefining self without the association of lifelong friends, spouses, or work that helped define the self during decades of adult life. This may be a time of reevaluation of what gives meaning and satisfaction in life.

Faith-based nursing is one of the community nursing roles that epitomizes this holistic approach of caring for their clients, many of whom are older adults (see Chapter 31). Faith community nursing, or parish nursing, began in the mid-1980s as a way for nurses working with church congregations to integrate healing and faith (Pappas-Rogich, 2012). Ebersole and Hess' gerontological nursing text (Touhy & Jett, 2014) elucidates, nurses can support the spiritual dimension of older clients in times of difficulty by developing the following skills:

- Listening
- Being aware of signs of mental health problems and urge professional help
- Sharing concern and observations
- Providing privacy
- Reassuring the value of the person
- Allowing decisions to be made
- Accepting without judgment
- Helping express religious, spiritual, or social needs
- Recognizing cultural differences
- Keeping separate values and spiritual beliefs that are different
- Referring to professionals when needs are beyond listener's ability to help
- Using humor as appropriate

Coping with Multiple Losses and Suicide

Older adults may experience multiple losses, including loss of income and prestige from a career once practiced or the economic stability of an enjoyable job, loss of space due to replacement of a larger residence by a much smaller home or apartment, and reductions in health and vitality that may result in limited movement or pain as a daily concern or may necessitate another move to a more dependent living environment. Repetitive losses occur as significant others, relatives, friends, and acquaintances die. There are no right or wrong ways to grieve, but there are healthy ways to cope with the pain. Assisting older adults to handle with these losses is an important role of the public health nurse. To do this, PHNs need to be aware of some of the facts about grief.

First, it is not true that ignoring pain will help it go away faster. In the long run, ignoring pain will only make it worse. It is necessary to face grief and deal with it in order to experience real healing; and feeling sad, or frightened, or lonely is a normal reaction to loss. Second, crying does not mean you are weak. Crying is a normal response to loss, but this does not mean that someone who does not cry does not feel the loss. It may just be shown in a different way. Third, there is no set time for grieving. It will differ from person to person (HelpGuide, 2015d). For about 15% of the bereaved population, grief becomes an endless "loop of suffering"; this is described as prolonged grief disorder, and it requires specialized psychological counseling techniques much like posttraumatic stress disorder (Maercker & Lalor, 2012; Schumer, 2009, p. 2). The most important tip for assisting older adults in coping with grief and loss is making sure they have the support of other people. Wherever it comes from, connecting with others helps the healing process.

As Kübler-Ross (1969) stated in her classic work, there are five stages of grief: denial, anger, bargaining, depression, and finally acceptance. Inadequate coping with the compounding losses can make an older person believe that life holds no meaning. Depression may be a difficult problem for older adults. Social and emotional withdrawal can often occur, as can suicide. Although older populations have a much lower rate of suicide attempts than younger age groups do, the rate of completed suicide is high.

- In 2013, the highest suicide rate was among people 45 to 64 years old (19.1 per 100,000). The second highest rate (18.6 per 100,000) occurred in those 85 years and older.
- For many years, the suicide rate has been about four times higher among men than among women. In 2013, men had a suicide rate of 20.2 per 100,000, and women had a rate of 5.5 per 100,000.
- Of those who died by suicide in 2013, 77.9% were male and 22.1% were female.
- In 2013, Whites had the highest U.S. suicide rate (14.2) and American Indians and Alaska Natives had the second highest rate at 11.7 (American Foundation for Suicide Prevention, 2015).

Because most persons who commit suicide have visited their primary care provider in the last month of their lives, recognition and treatment of depression in health care settings is a promising way to prevent suicide in this age group (Raue, Ghesquiere, & Bruce, 2014).

Mortality after bereavement is high and can sometimes be prevented through nursing intervention. The experience of loss and the mourning process among elders have been examined in many studies. It has been found that the ability to mourn prior states of one's self and the past is crucial to successful aging. Life review can be liberating and can provide energy for current living, including planning for the future. Although men and women experience similar levels of depression during early bereavement, it is often more difficult for men to seek and receive social support. Depression has been found to increase the risk of death for those who have lost a spouse, independent of age or bereavement. The death of a spouse has effects upon the health of the surviving spouse, and depression can exacerbate these effects. In addition to preventing early deaths after the loss of a spouse, the greater goal for the nurse in promoting successful aging can be accomplished when the nurse recognizes the significance of accepting all the losses of aging. The loss of a spouse is much more frequent for women than for men. With this knowledge, a woman who was in a more passive, dependent role may become more anxious when her spouse dies. For couples that were especially close, the wife may be more inclined to experience significant depression (Vitelli, 2015).

Maintaining Independence

Older people need independence, and those who stay independent are happier. As much as possible, they need to make their own decisions and manage their own lives. Even those with activity limitations because of disability can still exercise decision-making options about many, if not most, aspects of their daily living. Unfortunately, because many older adults have chronic diseases, it can be more difficult for them to maintain their independence.

The number of disabled U.S. adults is increasing; 47.5 million U.S. adults report a disability. More than one third of these are aging baby boomers. Arthritis is the most common cause of disability. The number of people reporting a disability increases with age, with women having a higher prevalence of disability than men at all ages. Given the size of the baby boomer generation, the number of adults with disabilities is likely to increase dramatically as they enter into higher-risk age groups over the next 20 years (CDC, 2013c).

The need for autonomy—to be able to assert oneself as a separate individual—is important for all people. Independence helps to meet the need for self-respect and dignity. They need to have their ideas and suggestions heard and acted upon, and they ought to be addressed by their preferred names in a respectful tone of voice. Respect for the older adult is not a strong value in American society, but it is highly valued in Asian, Italian, Hispanic, and Native American cultures. Older people represent a rich resource of wisdom, experience, and patience that is often unacknowledged in the United States.

Interaction, Companionship, and Purpose

Older people need companionship and social interaction, particularly if they live alone. The company of other people and the companionship of a household pet offer avenues for expression along with response and it adds meaning to life. As people age, their social networks weaken, and PHNs and others can help to improve their psychosocial health by working at individual, family, and community levels. The problem is of greatest significance for women, who outnumber men considerably in the later years and who more frequently live alone.

It is also important for older adults without companions to discover and develop a friendship with someone who can be considered a *confidante*, someone in whom the older adult can confide, share reflections on the past, and trust. It could be a close friend, a sibling, a son or daughter, or an acquaintance. This person is usually seen daily or is engaged on the telephone each week. In particular, mothers and daughters form confidante bonds. Many women consider a sibling a confidante, especially if that person lives close by; this is especially true for childless and single women.

Meaningful activity is another need of the older adult that adds purpose to life. Some kind of active role in community life is essential for mental health, satisfaction, and self-esteem. These activities can range from involvement in hobbies, such as gardening or crafts, to volunteer work or even full-time employment. Examples include the federally supported Foster Grandparents and Senior Companions programs, which engage millions of Americans in service. These older adults work part-time offering companionship and guidance to handicapped children, the terminally ill, and other people in need (Corporation for National & Community Service, n.d.).

Additional volunteering opportunities abound. Internationally, many older professionals join the Peace Corps, which was initiated in the early 1960s. In this program, people of all ages work for 2-year periods in global communities that are in need of services to improve personal health, education, environment, and the larger community (Peace Corps, 2015). On the national level, the AmeriCorps program is similar but with a 10-month commitment volunteering with local and national nonprofit and government agencies. Retired people can volunteer to help others, donating their skills at a time in their lives when they are in transition from employment to retirement or to fill active retirement years (AmeriCorps, 2015). Through the Corporation for National and Community Service, older adults can volunteer in the Retired and Senior Volunteer Program (RSVP) or the Foster Grandparent Program. The Senior Companion Program and Senior Corps program engage seniors in a bevy of activities designed to improve people's lives and the environment (Senior Corps, 2015). Environmental Alliance for Senior Involvement (EASI) is a nonprofit coalition of aging, volunteer, and environmental organizations that began in 1991 (Environmental Alliance for Senior Involvement, 2015). It sponsors various environmentally focused programs, such as assisting the Hawk Mountain Sanctuary to protect birds of prey or monitoring streams and other waterways for cleanliness.

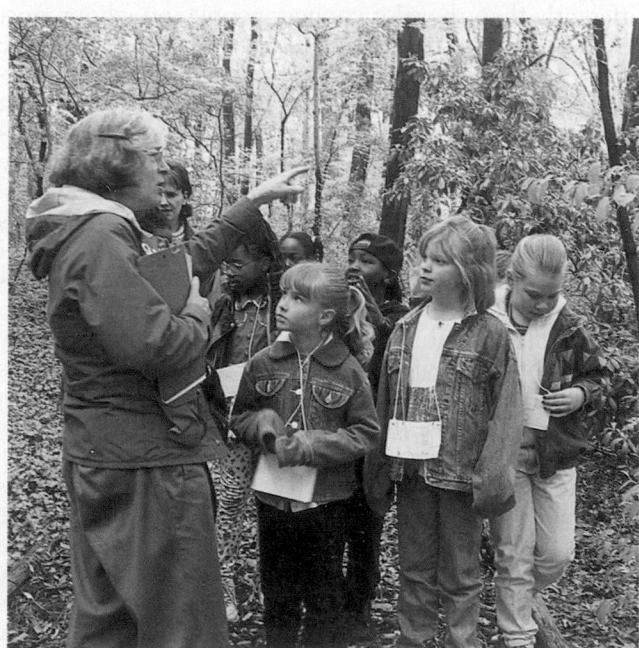

Volunteering can be a rewarding experience for older adults.

Many older adults choose not to engage in long-term volunteering, and other programs are more appropriate for them. Elderhostel, Inc., the not-for-profit world leader in lifelong learning since 1975, is the creator of Road Scholar educational adventures providing high-quality, affordable, educational adventures for adults who desire lifelong learning. It is the nation's first and the world's largest education and travel organization for older adults, offering more than 7,000 learning adventures in all 50 states and more than 150 countries (Road Scholar, 2015). Their theme-based, short-term (3 days to 3 weeks) educational programs are infused with a spirit of camaraderie and adventure. The success of this program is based on recognizing that learning is a lifelong process that is rewarding at any age—and it is learning without any test or term papers! Elderhostel is inspired by the youth hostels and folk schools of Europe but guided by the needs and interests of older citizens.

Safety Needs

People of all ages have safety needs, and safety issues are a major concern for older adults and the PHNs who work with them. Several areas of focus are discussed here: personal health and safety, home safety, and community safety.

Personal health and safety includes three major areas: immunizations, prevention of falls, and drug safety.

Immunizations

Older adults are at increased risk for many vaccine-preventable diseases. Preventable illnesses cause substantial morbidity and mortality in older patients, who tend to have more medical comorbidities and are at higher risk for complications. Acute respiratory infections, including pneumonia and influenza, are the eighth leading cause of death in the United States, accounting for 56,000 deaths annually. On average, influenza leads to more than 200,000 hospitalizations and 36,000 deaths each year (Greenberg, 2012; CDC, 2015p).

Each year in the United States, about 9 out of 10 flu-related deaths and more than 6 out of 10 flu-related hospital stays occur in people over the age of 65. Nonetheless, vaccination rates in the United States do not meet targets. In the United States, the majority of deaths from influenza occur among those over 65, yet only 65% of older adults were immunized against the flu; this is short of the *Healthy People 2010 and 2020* targets of 90%. Only 60.6% of Americans 65 and older were immunized against pneumococcal pneumonia (Greenberg, 2012). The CDC recommends that all adults over 50 receive three immunizations, one each for influenza, pneumonia, and shingles (CDC, 2015m). While influenza does kill an estimated 36,000 people per year, in older adults, it is the exacerbating effect on other conditions (e.g., pneumonia, congestive heart failure, or chronic obstructive pulmonary disease [COPD]) that makes flu of great concern in older adults (National Foundation for Infectious Diseases, 2015). Racial and ethnic disparities exist among older adults receiving influenza vaccines; therefore, it is important to include outreach efforts, such as culturally targeting communication, reaching out to those providers serving this population, and offering vaccination clinics in underserved sections of the community.

Pneumococcal vaccine coverage rates have also increased steadily from 38.4% in 1995 to 66.8% in 2009, but improvement is still needed. In 2012, only 60% were vaccinated, even further from reaching the *Healthy People 2020* goal of 90% vaccine coverage for those aged 65 and older (Alliance for Aging Research, 2015). However, incidence rates for pneumonia have been generally decreasing since 2000, largely because of more people being vaccinated. Similar to flu vaccination, certain racial and ethnic groups remain substantially below those of the general population. Attempts to improve immunization coverage involve changing provider knowledge, attitudes, and behavior through reminders and standing orders, so that "missed opportunities" when seeing clients are prevented. One simple method is to ask clients about their beliefs and fears related to immunizations and then to address them directly and honestly. Additional opportunities for vaccinating people exist beyond the primary care setting, as PHNs are well aware. People can be reached during emergency department visits, during screening procedures such as colonoscopies, at neighborhood and senior centers, at religious facilities, and in other settings where elders may gather. Regardless of the site, a method for tracking and communicating vaccinations is needed so that vaccination information may be documented and shared with the elder's primary care provider. Clinicians often fail to document immunizations for adult patients. Immunizations protect more than the at-risk population; they protect society as a whole. People of any age with a chronic illness, such as heart disease, diabetes, or chronic respiratory disease, and people older than 65 years of age should be encouraged to receive an annual flu vaccine and the pneumonia vaccine every 5 years (CDC, 2015l).

Shingles is caused by the varicella–zoster virus (VZV); this is the same virus that causes chickenpox. Anyone who has had chickenpox can develop shingles because VZV remains in the nerve cells of the body after the chickenpox infection clears, and VZV can reappear years later causing shingles. Shingles is a painful localized skin rash often with blisters. The disease most commonly occurs in people 50 years old or older, people who have medical conditions that keep the immune system from working properly, or people who receive immunosuppressive drugs (CDC, 2015m). The CDC recommends Zostavax for use in people 60 years old and older to prevent shingles. This is a one-time vaccination. There is no maximum age for getting the shingles vaccine (CDC, 2015n). In 2012, only 20% of people age 65 and older received this vaccine; this is below the *Healthy People 2020* target of 30%. The incidence of shingles was on the rise until the vaccine was developed in 2006; since 2008, it has generally been on the decline (Alliance for Aging Research, 2015).

Fall Prevention

Every year, about one third of U.S. adults age 65 and over experience a fall. Falls are the most common cause of hospitalization due to nonfatal trauma (more than 734,000) and over 21,700 deaths are attributed to falls yearly. The total costs related to fall injuries was $34 billion in 2013. Even minor falls can seriously impact the lives of seniors, limiting their social activity and leading to isolation and dependency (National Council on Aging, n.d.a). Environmental hazards (e.g., lack of nonslip surfaces and handrails) and host conditions (e.g., poor vision, problems with balance) are often the causative factors in falls. Fall prevention includes asking older adults about their concerns related to fall risk, discussing their current health conditions (e.g., vision problems, medications that cause dizziness), asking about current vision and recent eye exams (e.g., is current eyeglass prescription being used, do bifocals cause problems when using stairs), noticing if they have difficulty getting out of chairs or are unsteady while walking (e.g., do they need someone to assist them, do they hold onto furniture, could they benefit from a consultation with a physical therapist to improve strength, balance, and gait), and asking whether they check with their physician and pharmacist regularly about the medications they take (e.g., are there drug interactions and side effects that cause dizziness or visual issues, do they take sleep medications that may affect balance) and whether their home is an obstacle course (e.g., make sure paths are free from clutter; do they need a consultation with occupational therapist to ensure good lighting, stair handrails on both sides, grab bars in shower and next to toilets, or use of shower chair). The use of a home safety checklist can give the nurse a baseline of information from which to begin teaching and providing interventions to ensure continued safety for many independent seniors who choose to remain in their homes (National Council on Aging, n.d.b). See Display 24–3 for guidelines to assess the senior client's environment.

Medications

Medications are often prescribed to control the effects of chronic conditions, and older adults' bodies can react differently than those of younger people (on whom most new drugs are tested). A significant safety issue for the older adult arises from the use of prescription and over-the-counter (OTC) drugs. Problems can arise from a single difficulty or a combination of issues such as (1) number of medications taken daily, (2) absorption rate of medications, (3) drug interactions, and (4) side effects.

Older adults often have multiple chronic diseases for which they take prescription medications. It is not unusual for older people to be taking 4 to 6 medications daily and fill 13 prescriptions or more each year. Although older adults constitute only 13% of the population, they account for approximately one third of all medications prescribed in the United States (National Institute on Drug Abuse, 2014). In addition, many older adults take OTC medications and/or dietary supplements.

Older adults often receive multiple prescriptions from multiple providers and sometimes from multiple pharmacies. This puts them in danger of receiving double doses of the same or similar medications. **Polypharmacy** involves the use of multiple medications (more than is medically necessary). Almost 50% of older adults take at least one medication that is not medically necessary (Maher, Hanlon, & Hajjar, 2014). This can happen, for instance, when one health care provider prescribes a brand-name medication and a second one writes a prescription for the same medication but in generic form. Often, the person has no idea that they are taking two doses of the same medication Also, common medications like acetaminophen can be found in a variety of OTC and prescription medications (e.g., cold remedies, arthritis

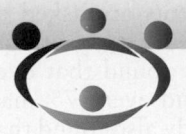

DISPLAY 24-3 GUIDELINES FOR ASSESSING THE SAFETY OF THE ENVIRONMENT

Illumination and Color Contrast

- Is the lighting adequate but not glare producing?
- Are the light switches easy to reach and manipulate?
- Can lights be turned on before entering rooms?
- Are night-lights used in appropriate places?
- Are there working flashlights close by (bedroom, kitchen, bath, living room)?
- Is color contrast adequate between objects such as a chair and floor?

Hazards

- Are there throw rugs, highly polished floors, or other hazardous floor coverings?
- If area rugs are used, do they have a nonslip backing and are the edges tacked to the floor?
- Are there cords, clutter, or other obstacles in pathways?
- Is there a pet that is likely to be running underfoot?

Furniture

- Are chairs the right height and depth for the person?
- Do the chairs have armrests?
- Are tables stable and of the appropriate height?
- Is small furniture placed well away from pathways?

Stairways

- Is lighting adequate?
- Are there light switches at the top and bottom of the stairs?
- Are there securely fastened handrails on both sides of the stairway?
- Are all the steps even?
- Are the treads nonskid?
- Should colored tape be used to mark the edges of the steps, particularly the top and bottom steps?

Bathroom

- Are grab bars placed appropriately for the tub and toilet?
- Does the tub have skid-proof strips or a rubber mat in the bottom?
- Has the person considered using a tub seat?
- Is the height of the toilet seat appropriate?
- Has the person considered using an elevated toilet seat?
- Does the color of the toilet seat contrast with surrounding colors?
- Is toilet paper within easy reach?

Temperature

- Is the temperature of the room(s) comfortable?
- Can the person read the markings on the thermostat and adjust it appropriately?
- During cold months, is the room temperature high enough to prevent hypothermia?
- During hot weather, is the room temperature cool enough to prevent hyperthermia?

Overall Safety

- How does the person obtain objects from hard-to-reach places?
- How does the person change overhead light bulbs?
- Are doorways wide enough to accommodate assistive devices?
- Do door thresholds create hazardous conditions?
- Are telephones easily accessible, especially for emergency calls?
- Would it be helpful to use a cordless portable phone or a cellular phone?
- Would it be helpful to have some emergency call system available?
- Does the person wear sturdy shoes with nonskid soles?
- Are smoke alarms present and operational?
- Is there a carbon monoxide detector (if the house has gas appliances)?
- Does the person keep a list of emergency numbers by the phone?
- Does the person have an emergency exit plan in the event of fire?

Bedroom

- Is the height of the bed appropriate?
- Is the mattress firm at the edges to provide enough support for sitting?
- If the bed has wheels, are they locked securely?
- Would side rails be a help or a hazard?
- When side rails are in the down position, are they completely out of the way?
- Is the pathway between the bedroom and bathroom clear of objects and adequately illuminated, particularly at night?
- Would a bedside commode be useful, especially at night?
- Does the person have sufficient physical and cognitive ability to turn on a light before getting out of bed?
- Is furniture positioned to allow safe use of assistive devices for ambulation?
- Is a telephone situated near the bed?

Kitchen

- Are storage areas used to the best advantage (e.g., are objects that are most frequently used in the most accessible places)?
- Are appliance cords kept out of the way?
- Are nonslip mats used in front of the sink?
- Are the markings on stoves and other appliances clearly visible?
- Does the person know how to use the microwave oven and other appliances safely?

Assistive Devices

- What assistive devices are used?
- Is a call light available, and does the person know how to use it?
- Would the person benefit from any assistive devices that are not being used?
- Are assistive devices being used safely and properly, or do they present additional hazards?

Adapted from Miller, C. A. (2015). *Nursing for wellness in older adults* (7th ed.). Philadelphia, PA: Wolters Kluwer.

topical ointments), and inadvertent overdosing can be a real problem.

Absorption time is usually slower in older adults, and distribution changes as drugs may stay in the body longer because of a higher percentage of fat stores, along with reduced liver and kidney function that affect clearance time. Most adverse drug events (ADEs) are due to drug interactions. The greater number of medications taken, the more likely there will be side effects. Polypharmacy is linked to adverse clinical outcomes such as drug interactions, ADEs, diminished functional capacity, multiple geriatric syndromes (e.g., cognitive impairment, falls, urinary incontinence), and it also leads to increased health care costs (Maher et al., 2014). Multiple medications or complicated drug regimens for many older people can lead to unexpected and dangerous drug interactions or drug–disease interactions; sometimes, medications are prescribed for symptoms that may actually be a side effect of an original medication.

Medication side effects or drug interactions can lead to falls and further disability. Older adults need education about the drugs they take and their possible effects. They also need proper supervision of their overall medication intake, including complementary and alternative therapies (e.g., herbal treatments) and OTC drugs (Public Citizen's Health Research Group [PCHRG], 2015). It is also important for all seniors to keep a list of their current medications and doses, and to have this available in the event of an emergency. However, many hospitals and providers prefer the "brown bag method" of determining accurate medication information; patients are asked to bring everything they take with them. One study of hospital discharges among elderly patients found that over 41% were taking 5 to 8 medications and over 37% had 9 or more prescriptions. This earlier study also found that 58.6% took at least one prescribed medication that was unnecessary (Hajjar et al., 2005). This is an area in which the community health nurse can intervene very effectively (see Display 24–4).

The consequences of polypharmacy are enormous. Approximately 30% of hospital admissions of older adults are drug related. Each year, in hospitals alone, there are 28,000 cases of life-threatening heart toxicity from adverse reactions to digoxin, the most commonly used form of digitalis (i.e., drug that regulates the speed and strength of heartbeats) in older adults. Because as many as 40% or more of these people are using this drug unnecessarily, many of these injuries are preventable (PCHRG, 2015). Each year, 41,000 older adults are hospitalized—and 3,300 of these people die—from ulcers caused by NSAIDs (i.e., nonsteroidal anti-inflammatory drugs, usually for treatment of arthritis). Each year, 32,000 older adults suffer from hip fractures attributable to drug-induced falls, resulting in more than 1,500 deaths. A long-term care study showed that polypharmacy was a risk factor for falls. In another study, the main categories of drugs responsible for the falls leading to hip fractures were sleeping pills and minor tranquilizers (30%),

---

DISPLAY 24–4 PROMOTING POLYPHARMACY SAFETY IN THE OLDER ADULT THROUGH MEDICATION REVIEW

- Ask the client to bring all of his or her medications for you to examine.
- List all medications, along with dosage and time taken.
- Note the pharmacy or pharmacies where each prescription originates. Has more than one physician prescribed medications for the client?
- Ask about medical conditions and diseases for which he or she takes medications. Does the client have a clear understanding of each medication and its benefits and potential side effects?
- Ask the client for which condition or disease each medication is prescribed. Does the client understand the basic disease process and how the prescribed medication works?
- Are there duplicate medications (e.g., contain the same active ingredient, both a generic and a proprietary form)?
- Ask if they feel that they are taking any medications that may no longer be needed.
- Ask if they are concerned about the number of medications they are taking.
- What are the most common side effects of each medication?
- Is the dosage prescribed within the recommended range?

- Is the client experiencing any symptoms of potential drug interactions (e.g., nausea, headaches, dizziness)?
- Is one medication being used to treat possible side effects of another medication?
- Ask if the client takes all medications as prescribed. Are any doses or medications skipped?
- Does the client use a daily or weekly pill box? Does the client have some system of checking off when medications have been taken each day?
- Is the client taking any medications that were prescribed for someone else?
- Is the client taking any OTC medications, nutritional supplements, or herbal remedies? For what purpose or condition? For what length of time has each been used?

Adapted from Hanlon, J., & Schmader, K. (2010). What types of inappropriate prescribing predict adverse drug reactions in older adults? *Annals of Pharmacotherapy, 44*(6), 1110–1111; Heuberger, R. A., & Caudell, K. (2011). Polypharmacy and nutritional status in older adults. *Drugs & Aging, 28*(4), 315–323; Loya, A. M., Gonzalez-Stuart, A., & Rivera, J. O. (2009). Prevalence of polypharmacy, polyherbacy, nutritional supplement use, and potential product interactions among older adults living on the United States–Mexico border. *Drugs & Aging, 26*(5), 428–436; Reeve, E., Shakib, S., Hendrix, I., Roberts, M. S., & Wiese, M. D. (2013). Development and validation of the patients' attitudes towards deprescribing (PATD) questionnaire. *International Journal of Clinical Pharmacy, 35*, 51–56.

antipsychotic drugs (52%), and antidepressants (17%). All of these categories of drugs are often prescribed unnecessarily, especially in older adults (PCHRG, 2015). Two million older Americans are addicted, or at risk of addiction, to minor tranquilizers or sleeping pills because they have used them daily for at least 1 year, even though there is no acceptable evidence that the tranquilizers are effective for more than 4 months (PCHRG, 2015).

Safety in the Community

Safety can involve many things, such as pedestrian and driving issues, crime and fear of crime against older adults, and environmental factors such as sun exposure, pollution, heat, and cold.

Because of age-related changes in vision, hearing, mobility, and the effects of polypharmacy, older adults are at risk in the community as pedestrians and as drivers. Automobile crashes and pedestrian injuries can be life-threatening events when elders are involved. As pedestrians, older adults must be increasingly vigilant to traffic patterns, sidewalk irregularities, and the possibility of being a victim of street crime. Often out of necessity and pride, elders drive longer than their abilities permit. As people age, they are more prone to lapses in memory and attention, problems with depth perception and gauging distance of cars in traffic, reduced manual dexterity and reaction time, and impairment of other skills critical to driving safety (Governor's Highway Safety Association, 2015; HelpGuide, 2015g). Older adults are more likely to receive traffic citations and be involved in an automobile accident than younger people. Fatal car crashes rise sharply after a person turns 70 (CDC, 2015b, 2015h, 2015i; PCHRG, 2015). In 2012, more than 5,560 older adults were killed and more than 214,000 were injured in motor vehicle crashes. This amounts to 15 older adults killed and 586 injured in crashes, on average, every day (CDC, 2013a, 2015i).

Although many older adults are fearful of being victims of crime, rates of nonfatal violent crime and property crime against the elderly are lower than in all younger age groups. See Display 24–5 for actions PHN can take to assist elders with a fear of crime.

The ratio of property crime to violent crime is higher among the elderly (13 to 1) than for younger ages (2 to 1 for 25 to 49, and 5 to 1 for 50 to 64). Also, there is more identity theft among those age 65 and older (5%) than for those 16 to 24 (3.8%). The incidents of identity theft are higher in the age groups 25 to 49 and 50 to 64 (7.9% and 7.8%, respectively). Over 59% of elderly report being victimized in or near their homes (Morgan & Mason, 2014).

Environmental factors can affect health and safety of elders when outside their homes. Sun exposure, pollution, and heat and cold can have negative effects on older adults. Like infants and children, they are vulnerable to climatic changes, and preventive measures should be taken. Sunblock should be used when gardening or reading and walking outdoors for longer than 10 minutes, even on days when the sky is overcast. Hot and cold weather can negatively impact older adults. Even in their homes, the elderly need to be aware of the temperature. In warm weather, they may not realize that they are thirsty

---

DISPLAY 24–5 REDUCING THE FEAR OF CRIME

- Allow elder adults time to discuss their fears of crime.
- Facilitate a realistic self-assessment of their ability to avoid crime and to defend themselves.
- Teach basic safety and security techniques.
- Correct the elder's sensory losses if possible, such as by getting a hearing aid or glasses.
- Correct a physical disability if possible, such as by treating the pain of arthritis or obtaining physical therapy.
- Facilitate access to safe, reliable, and affordable transportation.
- Identify family members, friends, neighbors, or caregivers who can support efforts to leave the home on a more regular basis.
- Encourage an elder to make a daily telephone or e-mail contact with at least one supportive person.
- Encourage the elder to get to know his or her neighbors.
- Encourage elders to travel and conduct community activities and errands together.
- Encourage participation in local senior centers and other community-based programs.
- Refer to alternative housing options available for older adults.
- Provide information on local services that assist and support crime victims.

---

or feel that they are hot. They may not want to run their air conditioning (or their heaters in cold weather) in an effort to reduce their expenses (UC Davis Health System, 2015). Teaching geographically and seasonally appropriate safety precautions is the responsibility of PHNs providing services to older adults in the community.

Secondary Prevention

Secondary prevention focuses on early detection of disease and prompt intervention (see Chapter 1). Much of the PHN's time is spent in educating the community on preventive measures and positive health behaviors. This includes encouraging individuals to obtain routine screening for diseases such as hypertension, diabetes, or cancer, which, if identified early, can be treated successfully. Many nurses, working in collaboration with community agencies, are in positions to establish screening programs based on the desires and demographics of the community and agency focus, making them accessible to the population being served.

Older adults need to be encouraged to follow the routine health screening schedule prescribed by their clinic or health care provider. The preventive screening services described in Table 24–1 was developed by the U.S. Preventive Services Task Force and is presented here as a guide. An immunization schedule for adults is found

Table 24–1 Preventive Services Recommended for Older Adults

Screening	Men	Women	Grade
Abdominal aortic aneurysm	65–75 years, who have ever smoked		B
Alcohol misuse	Over age 18	Over age 18	B
Aspirin/prevention of cardiovascular disease	Ages 45–79 When benefit (CVD) outweighs potential harm (GI bleed)	Ages 45–79 When benefit (CVD) outweighs potential harm (GI bleed)	A
Mammography		Ages 50–74, screen every 2 years	B
Cervical cancer/Pap		Older than 65, do not screen	D
Colorectal cancer	Ages 50–75, screen annually with high-sensitivity fecal occult blood testing (FOBT); screening colonoscopy every 10 years	Ages 50–75, screen annually with high-sensitivity FOBT; screening colonoscopy every 10 years	A
Type 2 diabetes	Asymptomatic adults with sustained B/P >135/80	Asymptomatic adults with sustained B/P greater than >135/80	B
Hypertension	All adults	All adults	A
Lipid disorders	Age 35+	Age 45+	A
Lung cancer	Asymptomatic, age 55–80, 30-pack-a-year history, current smoker or quit within last 15 years	Asymptomatic, age 55–80, 30-pack-a-year history, current smoker or quit within last 15 years	B
Obesity	All adults	All adults	B
Osteoporosis		Age ≥65, no fractures or secondary causes	B
Tobacco use	All adults	All adults	A

Source: U.S. Preventive Services Task Force (USPSTF). (2014). *The guide to clinical preventive services*. Washington, DC: Agency for Healthcare Quality & Research (AHRQ).

in Table 24–2. Resources that can be utilized by the PHN working with older clients are listed in Display 24–6.

Diseases and Conditions Common in Old Age

Alzheimer's Disease

Alzheimer's disease (AD) is the most common form of dementia in older adults, first described in 1907 by Dr. Alois Alzheimer. He depicted the symptoms that are now known as AD. Although much is still unknown about this devastating disease, we do know that:

- It's the only cause of death among America's top ten that cannot be prevented, cured, or slowed.
- Almost two thirds of Americans who have an Alzheimer's diagnosis are women.
- One in three seniors dies of Alzheimer's or dementia.
- Alzheimer's disease is the sixth leading cause of death in America.
- Only 45% of those with Alzheimer's disease or their caregivers report being told of their diagnosis. More than 90% of those with the four most common kinds of cancers report being told of their diagnosis.
- In 2015, Alzheimer's and other dementias will cost the nation $226 billion. By 2040, they could cost as much as $1.1 trillion (CDC, 2015b).

- The number of people who develop this disease doubles every 5 years as people live beyond age 65 (CDC, 2015b).
- Every 67 seconds, another person develops AD, and this will change to every 33 seconds by the year 2050 (Alzheimer's Association, 2015a).
- Age is the greatest risk factor for AD. Most individuals with AD are over age 65 (Alzheimer's Association, 2015c).
- One of three people age 85 or older has the disease (CDC, 2015a).
- AD increased 66% in the years between 2000 and 2008. It is the only major disease that increased during that time frame. Because of this growth, *Healthy People 2020* designated dementias, including AD, as one of the new focus areas (*Healthy People 2020, 2015a*).
- By 2050, this number is projected to rise to 14 million, a nearly threefold increase (CDC, 2015b).
- Among adults from the ages of 65 to 86, AD is the fifth leading cause of deaths.
- In 2013, an estimated 5 million Americans aged 65 years or older had Alzheimer's disease. This number may triple to as high as 13.8 million people by 2050 (CDC, 2015b).

Table 24-2 Recommended Immunizations for Older Adults

Recommended immunization schedule for adults aged 19 years or older, by vaccine and age group[1]

VACCINE ▼ AGE GROUP ►	19–21 years	22–26 years	27–49 years	50–59 years	60–64 years	≥ 65 years
Influenza[*,2]	1 dose annually					
Tetanus, diphtheria, pertussis (Td/Tdap)[*,3]	Substitute Tdap for Td once, then Td booster every 10 years					
Varicella[*,4]	2 doses					
Human papillomavirus (HPV) Female[*,5]	3 doses					
Human papillomavirus (HPV) Male[*,5]	3 doses					
Zoster[6]					1 dose	
Measles, mumps, rubella (MMR)[*,7]	1 or 2 doses depending on indication					
Pneumococcal 13-valent conjugate (PCV13)[*,8]	1 dose					
Pneumococcal 23-valent polysaccharide (PPSV23)[8]			1 or 2 doses depending on indication			1 dose
Hepatitis A[*,9]	2 or 3 doses depending on vaccine					
Hepatitis B[*,10]	3 doses					
Meningococcal 4-valent conjugate (MenACWY) or polysaccharide (MPSV4)[*,11]	1 or more doses depending on indication					
Meningococcal B (MenB)[11]	2 or 3 doses depending on vaccine					
Haemophilus influenzae type b (Hib)[*,12]	1 or 3 doses depending on indication					

*Covered by the Vaccine Injury Compensation Program

Recommended for all persons who meet the age requirement, lack documentation of vaccination, or lack evidence of past infection; zoster vaccine is recommended regardless of past episode of zoster

Recommended for persons with a risk factor (medical, occupational, lifestyle, or other indication)

No recommendation

Report all clinically significant postvaccination reactions to the Vaccine Adverse Event Reporting System (VAERS). Reporting forms and instructions on filing a VAERS report are available at www.vaers.hhs.gov or by telephone, 800-822-7967.

Information on how to file a Vaccine Injury Compensation Program claim is available at www.hrsa.gov/vaccinecompensation or by telephone, 800-338-2382. To file a claim for vaccine injury, contact the U.S. Court of Federal Claims, 717 Madison Place, N.W., Washington, D.C. 20005; telephone, 202-357-6400.

Additional information about the vaccines in this schedule, extent of available data, and contraindications for vaccination is also available at www.cdc.gov/vaccines or from the CDC-INFO Contact Center at 800-CDC-INFO (800-232-4636) in English and Spanish, 8:00 a.m. - 8:00 p.m. Eastern Time, Monday - Friday, excluding holidays.

Use of trade names and commercial sources is for identification only and does not imply endorsement by the U.S. Department of Health and Human Services.

The recommendations in this schedule were approved by the Centers for Disease Control and Prevention's (CDC) Advisory Committee on Immunization Practices (ACIP), the American Academy of Family Physicians (AAFP), the America College of Physicians (ACP), the American College of Obstetricians and Gynecologists (ACOG) and the American College of Nurse-Midwives (ACNM).

From Centers for Disease Control and Prevention (CDC). (2015m). *Recommended adult immunization schedule, by vaccine and age group.* Retrieved from http://www.cdc.gov/vaccines/schedules/hcp/imz/adult.html

---

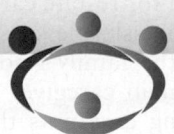

DISPLAY 24-6 PROGRAMS AND SERVICES FOR OLDER ADULTS

Resources for Community Health Nurses to Utilize with Clients

- Communication services (phones, emergency access to health care)
- Dental care services
- Dietary guidance and food services (such as Meals on Wheels, commodity programs, or group meal services)
- Escort and protective services
- Exercise and fitness programs
- Financial aid and counseling
- Friendly visiting and companions
- Health education
- Hearing tests and hearing aid assistance
- Home health services (including skilled nursing and home health aide services)
- Home maintenance assistance (housekeeping, chores, and repairs)
- Legal aid and counseling
- Library services (including tapes and large-print books)
- Medical supplies or equipment
- Medication supervision
- Podiatry services
- Recreational and education programs (community centers, Elderhostel)
- Routine care from selected health care practitioners
- Safe, affordable, and ability-appropriate housing
- Senior citizens' discounts (food, drugs, transportation, banks, retail stores, and recreation)
- Social assistance services offered in conjunction with health maintenance
- Speech or physical therapy
- Spiritual ministries
- Transportation services
- Vision care (prescribing and providing eyeglasses, diagnosis and treatment of glaucoma and cataracts)
- Volunteer and employment opportunities (Vista, RSVP)

Adapted from U.S. Preventive Services Task Force (USPSTF). (2014). *The guide to clinical preventive services.* Washington, DC: Agency for Healthcare Quality & Research (AHRQ).

The occurrence of AD is not a normal development in the aging process. Alzheimer's disease has no survivors. It destroys brain cells and causes memory changes, erratic behaviors, and loss of body functions. It slowly and painfully takes away a person's identity and ability to connect with others, think, eat, talk, walk, and find his or her way home (Alzheimer's Association, 2015b).

As the disease progresses, these changes become so severe that they interfere with the individual's daily functioning, resulting in total dependence on others for care and eventually in death. On average, a person with Alzheimer's lives 4 to 8 years after diagnosis but can live as long as 20 years, depending on other factors (Alzheimer's Association, 2015d). Although AD is the sixth leading cause of death among all Americans and the fifth leading cause of death for 65- to 85-year-olds (CDC, 2015b), those most often diagnosed with AD are generally over age 65 (late-onset AD). However, it is possible for the disease to occur in people between the ages of 30 and 60, but early-onset AD is usually considered an inherited form of the disease; another risk factor for Alzheimer's (Alzheimer's Association, 2015c).

There is a simple way to describe the difference between the normal forgetfulness of aging and AD. From time to time, we all forget where we have put our keys, but people with early-stage AD may notice that they tend to forget things more often—especially recent activities or events, or names of familiar things or people (Alzheimer's Association, 2015d). Although these symptoms are bothersome, they are usually not serious enough to cause alarm. As the disease advances, the symptoms become serious enough to cause people with AD or their family members to recognize that things are not right and that help is needed. In the middle stages of AD, people eventually forget how to do simple tasks like brushing their teeth or combing their hair, and they begin to no longer be able to think clearly. They eventually have problems speaking, understanding, reading or writing, or recognizing people they have known for years. People who suffer from AD may become anxious or aggressive and may wander away from home, thus requiring the need for total care.

There is no single test to identify AD (Alzheimer's Association, 2015b). It is recommended that health care providers offer a comprehensive exam including a complete health history; physical exam; lab tests; neurologic, functional, and mental status assessments; along with possible brain scans. A comprehensive assessment is needed because many conditions, including some that are treatable or reversible (e.g., thyroid disease, depression, brain tumors, drug reactions), may cause dementia-like symptoms. Physicians are now able to accurately diagnose 80% to 90% of people who show symptoms, but the only definitive diagnosis of AD is done at autopsy by the examination of brain tissue (National Institute on Aging, 2015a). Probable causes of AD are many. Promising leads involve the role of neurotransmitters, proteins, metabolism, environmental toxins, and genes. Research has shown links between some genes and AD, with three gene variants identified for early-onset AD and one that boosts risk for late-onset type.

- In 2015, the direct costs to American society of caring for those with Alzheimer's will total an estimated $226 billion, with half of the costs borne by Medicare.

- Nearly one in every five Medicare dollars is spent on people with Alzheimer's and other dementias. In 2050, it will be one in every three dollars.
- Average per-person Medicare spending for those with Alzheimer's and other dementias is three times higher than average per-person spending across all other seniors. Medicaid payments are 19 times higher.
- Unless something is done, in 2050, Alzheimer's will cost over $1.1 trillion (in 2015 dollars). Costs to Medicare will increase over 400% to $589 billion.
- In 2014, 15.7 million family and friends provided 17.9 billion hours of unpaid care to those with Alzheimer's and other dementias—care valued at $217.7 billion.
- Nearly 60% of Alzheimer's and dementia caregivers rate the emotional stress of caregiving as high or very high; about 40% suffer from depression (Alzheimer's Association, 2015a, para. 12 to 24).

Several medications have been approved for use with Alzheimer's patients. Medications called cholinesterase inhibitors are prescribed for mild to moderate AD. However, these drugs only delay the progression of symptoms for a limited time. At best, available medications "turn back the clock somewhat" with the disease worsening at a slower rate, or the drugs control some of the client's behaviors that jeopardize safety, thereby promoting caregiver management.

How does this disease impact the role of the PHN? Often, the person with AD is cared for at home until very late in the disease course. Perhaps more than any other disease, AD is responsible for enormous caregiver burden. In fact, because of the physical and emotional toll of caregiving, Alzheimer's and dementia caregivers had $9.7 billion in additional health care costs of their own in 2014 (Alzheimer's Association, 2015a).

The intense care given to these clients can be a constant drain on the emotional and physical reserves of their families, which highlights the need for respite care. The client exhibits depression, agitation, sleeplessness, and anxiety, which can greatly upset the family's normal routine. In many situations, the main caregiver is an aged spouse. The stress of providing care puts the caregiver's health at risk, as well. In 1992, Congress created the Alzheimer's Disease Supportive Program to encourage states to provide support for persons and families with Alzheimer's. The intensity of caregiving is aptly described in a book written for AD family members: *The 36-Hour Day* (Mace & Rabins, 2006). Another good book is *The Theft of Memory: Losing my Father, One Day at a Time by* award winning author Jonathan Kozol. This is the personal story of his experience with his father, a brilliant neurologist who suffered from Alzheimer's (Kozol, 2015). Another good resource is Braff and Olenik's (2003) *Staying Connected While Letting Go: The Paradox of Alzheimer's Caregiving* (see What Do You Think?).

Because so many older adults afflicted with AD reside at home with their family members providing care to them, it is important for the PHN to monitor and assess the levels of stress on family members. The nurse can intervene as necessary and provide caregivers with methods to cope and adapt as needed, making applicable referrals. The nurse can assist with planning

What do *you* think?

Have you heard of the *Best Friends* approach to Alzheimer's care? This method has changed the caregiving approach to AD and is changing the lives of caregivers, families, and clients. It improves the quality of life not only for clients with AD but also for those providing care. *Best Friends* is a groundbreaking and uplifting method for the care of people with AD. It builds on the essential elements of friendship: respect, empathy, support, trust, and humor. These are the building blocks of a care model that is both effective and flexible enough to adapt to each person's remaining strengths and abilities. The *Best Friends* approach does not just prevent catastrophic episodes; it makes every day consistently reassuring, enjoyable, and secure.

From Bell, V. & Troxel, D. (2011). *An overview of the Best Friends™ approach to Alzheimer's care.* Baltimore, MD: Health Professions Press. (*Best Friends™* is a trademark of Health Professions Press, Inc.).

and preparing the caregiver for what lies ahead. Most communities have resources for clients and their families. They may provide family and caregiver support groups, respite care, counseling, and legal or financial consultation. These services are available through local agencies, such as the Area Agency on Aging, but there are also government-sponsored national resources that offer information, referral services, and educational materials (e.g., Alzheimer's Association) all of which can be accessed by the PHN, the home health/hospice nurse, or the families in need. Some may find online support groups helpful. The nurse needs to know what resources are available in order to guide families to them (see Using the Nursing Process).

Arthritis

Arthritis encompasses more than 100 diseases and conditions that affect joints, surrounding tissues, and other connective tissues and is the leading cause of disability for adults in the United States (CDC, 2015c). Types of arthritis include osteoarthritis (OA), rheumatoid arthritis (RA), gout, and fibromyalgia. OA is the most common form of arthritis affecting both young and old, with two thirds of sufferers younger than age 65 (National Institute of Arthritis and Musculoskeletal and Skin Diseases [NIAMS], 2014a). However, the incidence increases with age. For those aged 18 to 44, 7.6% report physician-diagnosed arthritis. For those 45 to 64, the incidence rises to 29.8%, and for those 65 and older, 50% report physician-diagnosed arthritis. By 2030, it is estimated that 25% of the total adult population will have physician-diagnosed OA (CDC, 2013a; NIAMS, 2015). With OA, the number of cartilage cells diminishes, cartilage becomes ulcerated and thinned, subchondral bone is exposed, and bony surfaces rub together resulting in joint destruction (NIAMS, 2014b). This disease is no longer considered to be only a normal consequence of aging. Risk factors include obesity, repetitive mechanical overuse of a joint, and heredity (CDC, 2015a). For those underweight or of normal weight, 16.4% have arthritis. Among those who are overweight, 21.4% have arthritis, and this increases to 66% for those who are obese (CDC, 2013a). Classic symptoms include aching, stiffness, and limited motion of the involved joint. Discomfort increases with overuse and during damp weather. Acetaminophen is the first drug of choice; however, clients often find a combination of medications and daily routines that helps them the most. The nurse can best assist these clients by assessing the safety of a particular regimen and suggesting treatment changes as new research becomes available, including new medications, surgical options for joint replacement, and dietary changes, such as vitamins and foods high in essential fatty acids (NIAMS, 2015). Arthritis limits ADLs and quality of life and is a costly disability. Forty-two percent of those with arthritis report activity limitations. In 2003, arthritis-related costs totaled $218 billion. This included $81 billion for medical costs and $47 billion in lost earnings (CDC, 2013a).

RA is a progressive chronic condition that begins during young adulthood and becomes disabling as the disease continues, attacking tissues of the joints and causing systemic damage in the later years (NIAMS, 2014b). It affects diarthrodial (synovial line) joints. This form of arthritis is an autoimmune disease that causes inflammation, deformity, and crippling. RA is treated with anti-inflammatory agents, corticosteroids, antimalarial agents, gold salts, and immunosuppressive drugs. Joint discomfort is often relieved by gentle massage, heat, and range-of-motion exercises (NIAMS, 2014a).

The PHN needs to be aware of the major differences between these two prevalent forms of arthritis. Recommended treatments, including physical therapy, diet, and medication, change as more evidence-based research is conducted on arthritis (NIAMS, 2014a). It is helpful to keep up-to-date on treatments, as these conditions are treated in the community and affect a large portion of the midlife and older populations that a PHN may carry in his or her caseload.

Cancer

Cancers, which are characterized by the uncontrolled growth and spread of abnormal cells, steadily increase in incidence in aging adults. Cancer causes 13% (7.6 million) of deaths worldwide. Age is a fundamental risk factor of cancer with the incidence of cancer rising dramatically with age (World Health Organization [WHO], 2012). The leading types of cancers are breast, prostate, lung, and colorectal cancers (CDC, 2012a). One popular theory is that as the body ages, the immune system declines, losing its ability to serve as a buffer against abnormal cancer cells that have been forming in the body throughout life. Tobacco use is a major risk factor for cancer. Harmful alcohol use, poor diet, and physical inactivity are other main risk factors (CDC, 2013b).

It is particularly important for the CHN to be aware of the increased incidence of cancer in older clients because older people often underreport symptoms that may be early signs of cancer. It is vital for PHNs, through assessments at clinics, on home visits, or during participation in screening programs, to encourage

USING THE NURSING PROCESS WHEN WORKING WITH OLDER ADULTS

Assessment

Mr. and Mrs. Boxwell are in their late 70s and have lived modestly on a fixed income since Mr. Boxwell's retirement. However, their budget has been strained this year as they have had $300 to $400 a month in out-of-pocket expenses for prescription medications. Mrs. Boxwell confessed to you (the community health nurse visiting them after receiving a referral from the coordinator of the senior center they attend) that at times, they will skip medication doses to "make ends meet" in some months. They both take drugs for high blood pressure; also, Mrs. Boxwell is diabetic and Mr. Boxwell has heart failure. They live in a small, older home, and their older model car is seldom driven as they report "the traffic is getting worse" and they have "come close to having a car crash two times" while they were driving in the past 3 months. They are receptive to your suggestions and are trying to stay healthy and independent.

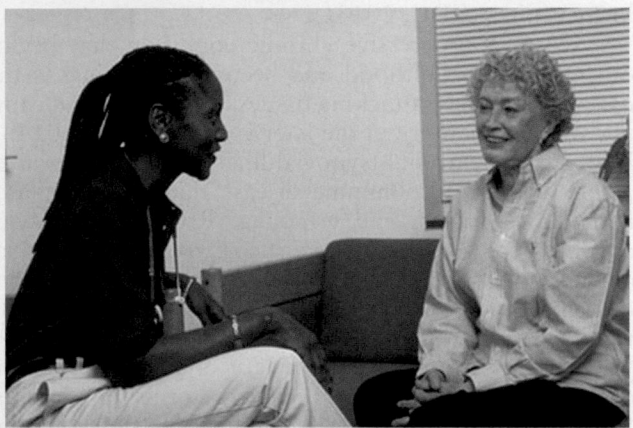

Nursing Diagnoses

1. The clients are at risk for an alteration in their health status due to insufficient finances to purchase needed medications for chronic diseases.
2. The clients are at risk for altered safety when driving related to chronic health problems, diminished driving skills, and a history of near automobile crashes.

Plan and Implementation

- **DIAGNOSIS 1**

The community health nurse will explore the clients' eligibility for Medicare Part D and Medicaid. It is possible these clients are eligible, yet unaware of these programs.

The community health nurse will consult with the clients' primary health care provider and ask for a change in prescriptions from brand names to generic. Also, ordering some medications in larger doses that come in scored tablets may be less expensive, and the client can safely break the larger pills in half. Mrs. Boxwell will check with her present distributor of diabetic supplies about getting larger quantities, generic brands of syringes, alcohol pads, etc.

- **DIAGNOSIS 2**

Mr. Boxwell will look into selling the car and exploring the bus schedule and other senior shuttle services that can be used to travel to the doctor and grocery store. Mr. and Mrs. Boxwell's daughter spends a day with them monthly and takes them wherever they want to go, as long as it is "a fun outing," and they will look into coordinating errands with her.

Evaluation

The couple is eligible for Medicare Part D, and this will help defray the out-of-pocket costs for medications. They have reduced medication costs as much as possible and report not missing any prescribed medications.

They sold their car and are negotiating the bus in good weather and using a taxi in the winter or when it is raining (they figured they save $1,000 a year in auto insurance, auto maintenance, and gasoline, whereas the bus and taxi cost them about $22 a month).

Because the couple is receptive to the help you have provided, you initiate a discussion regarding their long-term plans for housing needs as they get older. They are not opposed to a senior housing option and have been talking about it with their daughter. They are going to talk with a realtor about selling their house, explore some senior apartments with their daughter on her monthly visits, and review their budget.

---

clients to report untoward symptoms in order to promote early detection, which gives clients their best chance of survival (American Cancer Society, 2014). Adherence to the health care practitioner's recommended schedule for health screening should be encouraged. In addition, being aware of and educating clients about the American Cancer Society's *Signs and Symptoms of Cancer* can possibly save their lives (see Display 24–7).

Cardiovascular Disease

Following arthritis and hearing impairment, hypertension is the third most frequent chronic condition for people older than age 65. About 66% of those between 65 and 75 have been diagnosed with hypertension, as have about 75% of those 75 years and older heart disease (CDC,

2015j). Hypertension increases with age and affects men more frequently than women; it is more prevalent in minorities. For example, hypertension in White adult males is 61%, whereas the prevalence in Black males is 71% and it is 69% in Hispanic males. Among females, the prevalence of hypertension in White women is 47%; in Black females it is 51%, and in Hispanic females, the prevalence is 65%. Older adults have difficulty managing ADLs if antihypertensive medications lower their blood pressure too dramatically. Hypotension leads to problems of safety, including a higher risk of falls; blood pressure should be monitored by the PHN, and the client should be taught to also self-monitor. Both hypertension and hypotension can have significant detrimental effects on the health of older adults (CDC, 2015j).

DISPLAY 24-7 SIGNS AND SYMPTOMS OF CANCER

There are some general signs and symptoms of cancer that can be helpful to PHNs when working with clients:

- Unexplained weight loss
- Pain
- Fever
- Fatigue
- Skin changes (hyperpigmentation, erythema, jaundice, itching, and excess hair growth)

Other common signs and symptoms of more specific types of cancers:

- Change in bowel habits or bladder function
- White patches inside mouth or white spots on the tongue
- Sores that do not heal
- Indigestion or trouble swallowing
- Unusual bleeding or discharge
- Thickening or lump in breast or other parts of the body
- Recent change in wart or mole; any new skin changes
- Nagging cough or hoarseness

Source: American Cancer Society. (2014). *Signs and symptoms of cancer*. Retrieved from http://www.cancer.org/cancer/cancerbasics/signs-and-symptoms-of-cancer

Heart disease is the leading cause of death for both men and women in the United States (Centers for Disease Control and Prevention [CDC], 2015f). Risk factors in the aging population associated with cardiovascular disease (CVD) include tobacco use or exposure to tobacco smoke, inappropriate nutritional patterns, diabetes, high cholesterol, and lack of exercise. There are also regional differences in the pattern of deaths from heart disease: The southeastern coastal plains (Appalachia) and lower Mississippi River Valley (southern parts of Georgia and Alabama) have the highest death rates. Blacks and Whites generally have higher rates of heart disease death than do Hispanics or Asians and other races/ethnicities (CDC, 2015g). See Chapter 29 for more information on this and on the "Stroke Belt."

Disease prevention is an important role for the PHN. Based on the knowledge of the prevalence of hypertension in older adults, the nurse can provide primary prevention by teaching community groups and individuals about this condition and ways to prevent its occurrence and can provide secondary prevention by screening seniors on a regular basis.

Depression and Suicide

Depression is not a normal part of growing older, yet it is one of the most common, and most treatable, of all the mental disorders in older adults (CDC, 2015d). It is a major health concern in this population and can be life threatening if unrecognized and untreated. Research has shown that medical costs are much higher for older adults who have medical conditions in addition to depression (National Institute of Mental Health, 2015). Biological, psychological, and social changes place older adults at high risk for the development and recurrence of depression. It is frequently related to multiple losses, such as retirement, a health change, or the death of a significant other. Depression is reported to be more common in women than in men. However, as mentioned earlier in this chapter, depression in men is more severe, resulting in suicide at a higher rate than among women. Higher levels of perceived social support are related to lower instances of depression among all people, and women especially seem to make these supportive connections throughout life more effectively than do men. The nurturing, reassurance, and support women get from intimate relationships with other women are not often as highly developed in men, and for this reason, men display more symptoms of depression after a loss.

The nurse needs to keep in mind the many potential causes of depression. Medical conditions, such as stroke, cancer, vitamin B_{12} deficiency, diabetes, chronic pain with dependence on prescription painkillers, or insomnia, may lead to depressive symptoms. Many prescription drugs can trigger or exacerbate depression. These include blood pressure medications, sleeping pills, calcium channel blockers, ulcer medications, and painkillers. Dementia and depression can be confused. Never assume that loss of mental sharpness is just a sign of old age. It may be difficult to differentiate whether an older adult is suffering from grief, depression, or dementia (National Institute of Mental Health, 2015). As mentioned earlier, older populations may have a lower rate of suicide attempts than younger age groups do, but the rate of completed suicide is high.

PHNs can help elders prevent the overwhelming signs and symptoms of depression related to losses by working with community groups. Through senior centers, adult housing units, senior day care centers, or men's and women's groups at religious centers, the PHN can meet with seniors to offer support, teach strategies to improve the quality and quantity of support systems, invite mental health speakers to discuss the topic of depression prevention, and generally assess the holistic health status of the elders in that setting. The increased years added to life through the advances of the past few decades in medications and treatment should lead to healthy and happy later life for seniors, filled with activities that bring joy and contentment. Years lost to depression are a wasted resource that may be prevented through early intervention and treatment.

Diabetes

According to the American Diabetes Association (2015b), 9.3% of all Americans have diabetes mellitus (DM). For those age 65 or older, the percentage jumps to 25.9%, or 11.2 million people. In 2012, $245 billion was attributable to diagnosed diabetes, including $176 billion in direct costs and $69 billion in indirect costs (disability, work loss, premature mortality). Diabetes mellitus (DM) affects the health of older people and limits their ability to perform activities.

The prevalence of diabetes varies by race:

- 17.5% of American Indians/Alaska Natives
- 16.3% of American Indians/Native Americans
- 13.2% of Hispanics
- 12.9% of non-Hispanic Blacks
- 9.1% of Asian Americans
- 7.6% of non-Hispanic Whites 18 and older (Food and Drug Administration [FDA], 2015)

The number of people with DM has increased sixfold since 1958, and 95% of these have type 2 diabetes. Type 2 diabetes can often be prevented with adherence to proper diet and regular exercise with the addition of oral medications, when needed. More Americans than ever suffer from various forms of DM, and the resulting rates of death and serious complications, such as adult blindness, kidney disease, and foot or leg amputations, are especially high for older adults and racial/ethnic minority populations (American Diabetes Association, 2015a, 2015b). In the past, DM was not always managed effectively; fear and misinformation about the disease may hinder today's elders from getting an early diagnosis or from participating in effective teaching and instruction on how to manage their diabetes.

Being diagnosed with DM can cause depression or anger, and the PHN must tailor educational programs to meet individual client needs. The plan should be comprehensive, with special emphasis placed on the areas in which each client needs information. For example, a spouse may be concerned about preparing meals that meet her husband's needs, whereas the husband may be more concerned with how the disease will affect his long days on the golf course or sexual functioning. In contrast, a single older woman may worry whether she can see well enough to draw up her insulin or can afford to pay for diabetic supplies and special foods. All newly diagnosed diabetics need a comprehensive overview of the disease process followed by an individualized approach for ongoing control and management of the disease.

Self-care behaviors (e.g., appropriate diet, glucose monitoring, medication management, foot care) are not often consistently practiced, yet they are necessary to promote good health and fewer complications (American Diabetes Association, 2015a). PHNs are ideally situated to meet group and individual needs. They have the resources and skills to plan and implement diabetic education classes for groups of elders, in addition to making home visits to address specific learning deficits that impact an individual's ability to manage his or her diabetes properly. The group setting allows elders to share their experiences, learn from each other, and benefit from the support of the group. Home visits permit the nurse to focus on an assessment of the client, home, family support, diabetic supplies and technique, and overall health management.

Obesity

The CDC defines **obesity** as a body mass index (BMI) of 30 or greater (2012c). Worldwide obesity has more than doubled since 1980, overtaking underweight as a cause of death. In 2014, over 600 million adults worldwide were obese (WHO, 2015). In the United States, more than one third of older adults aged 65 and older were classified as obese in 2007–2010. By 2050, the number of obese U.S. older adults is expected to more than double, rising from 40.2 to 88.5 million (WHO, 2015). Both aging and obesity contribute to increased use of health care services. Consequently, an increase in the proportion of older adults who are obese may compound health care spending.

Obesity prevalence is higher in:

- Both women and men who are 65 to 75 than those who are older than 75
  - Men age 65 to 74: 36.4%
  - Men age 75 and over: 27.4%
  - Women age 65 to 74: 44.2%
  - Women age 75 and over
  - Women age 75 and over (CDC, 2015j)

Obesity prevalence among women aged 65 to 74 was higher than in women aged 75 and older in all racial and ethnic groups except for non-Hispanic Black women. The overall prevalence of obesity among older adults and the racial and ethnic patterns are similar to estimates previously reported for the entire adult population (CDC, 2012b). Among older men, there were no differences between racial and ethnic groups in obesity prevalence. However, among older women, non-Hispanic Black women had higher obesity prevalence than older, non-Hispanic White women. Although these same patterns have been shown among middle-aged women, the values are significantly lower among the oldest adults, those aged 75 and over (CDC, 2012b). Socioeconomic disparities in obesity prevalence, as measured by educational attainment and observed in women aged 20 and over, were also found among those aged 65 to 74, but the relationship diminished and even disappeared in those aged 75 and over. Among all women, there was a significant trend in lower obesity prevalence among those with the highest education. This was also true for women aged 65 to 74, but among women aged 75 and over, no difference was observed in obesity prevalence by educational attainment (CDC, 2012b).

Osteoporosis

Osteoporosis is a disease of bone in which the amount of bone is decreased and the strength is reduced. Osteoporosis is a generalized, persistent, and disabling disease that can overshadow every facet of an older adult's overall functional level and independence. It causes acute and chronic pain, subsequent fractures, decreased physical activity, limited mobility, changes in body image, role changes, a reduction in ability to perform ADLs, and depression.

Researchers estimate that one in five women in the United States has osteoporosis and that half of the women over 50 will have a fracture of the hip, wrist, or vertebrae; it is considered a major public health threat for approximately 44 million U.S. adults over age 50 (International Osteoporosis Foundation, n.d.). In osteoporosis, calcium leaches from the bone mass and results in small holes forming in the bones. These empty spaces within the bone increase susceptibility to fractures of hip, wrist, or vertebra. The risk of osteoporosis increases with age. As the disease progresses, other characteristics appear, such as compression of the vertebrae that result in loss of height and the hunched back deformity known as dowager's hump.

Proper diet and exercise throughout life are now recognized as the most effective measure to maintain bone health. There is growing evidence that calcium and vitamin D supplementation can help lower rates of fractures and reduce bone loss in the elderly. Higher protein intake may also help prevent bone loss (International Osteoporosis Foundation, n.d.). There are many FDA-approved drugs to treat osteoporosis that can be prescribed by a primary care provider. Therefore, identification of risk factors and regular screenings are essential to prevent the progression of this debilitating disease (National Center for Biotechnology Information, 2015). See Chapter 23 for more on medications.

PHNs can focus their teaching on primary prevention and ensure that people eat diets rich in vitamin D and calcium, and include calcium supplements as needed. Not smoking, maintaining a healthy weight, participating in weight-bearing activities, and receiving ongoing bone density screenings are all positive health behaviors that can contribute to strong bones throughout life. The value of hormone replacement therapy (HRT) in women—its benefits and possible long-term side effects—must be considered on the advice of the primary care provider, whose judgment should be based on the latest research findings along with the individual woman's needs.

Tertiary Prevention

Tertiary prevention involves follow-up and rehabilitation after a disease or condition has occurred or been diagnosed and initial treatment has begun. Chronic diseases that are common among older adults, such as heart failure, stroke, diabetes, cognitive impairment, or arthritis, cannot always be prevented but can frequently be postponed into the later years of life through a lifetime of positive health behaviors. However, when they occur, the debilitating symptoms and damaging effects can be controlled through healthy choices encouraged by the PHN and recommended by the primary care practitioner.

Although many older adults are considered generally healthy, 80% have at least one chronic condition and 50% have at least two (CDC, 2013c). A small proportion suffer more disabling forms of disease, such as COPD, cerebral vascular accidents (CVAs), cancer, or DM, with some requiring extensive care and ongoing medical management. The most common health problems of older people in the community are arthritis, reduced vision, hearing loss, heart disease, peripheral vascular disease, and hypertension. Heart disease and cancer pose their greatest risks as people age, as do other chronic diseases and conditions, such as stroke, chronic lower respiratory diseases, Alzheimer's disease, and diabetes. Influenza and pneumonia also continue to contribute to older adult deaths among older adults, despite the availability of effective vaccines (CDC, 2013c).

The tragedy of these leading killers is that they are often preventable. Although the risk for disease and disability clearly increases with advancing age, poor health is not always an inevitable consequence of aging. Even though many older adults experience relatively good health, almost all may expect to be chronically ill for an extended amount of time at the end of their lives. Chapter 26 expands on clients with disabilities and chronic illnesses and the role of the PHN working with these populations in the community.

HEALTH COSTS FOR OLDER ADULTS: MEDICARE AND MEDICAID

As the number of older adults grows, so do costs for health care:

- NHEs grew 3.6% to $2.9 trillion in 2013, or $9,255 per person, and accounted for 17.4% of gross domestic product (GDP).
- Medicare spending grew 3.4% to $585.7 billion in 2013, or 20% of total NHE.
- Medicaid spending grew 6.1% to $449.4 billion in 2013, or 15% of total NHE (Centers for Medicare & Medicaid Services, 2015).

Despite the expenditures, it is a myth that Medicare or Medicaid covers all health care costs for older adults. In actuality, an older adult spends a great deal out of pocket for health care. Individuals and their families cover 52% of long-term care costs out of pocket. The cost of paid long-term care is only the tip of the iceberg. Approximately 75% of long-term care services and support are provided on an unpaid basis by family members. This is often done at a heavy physical and financial cost, including lost opportunities for employment, health insurance, and retirement savings. Services for older adults are very expensive. Some examples of average costs in the United States for health care services are:

- $17,904 annually for adult day care services
- $44,616 annually for homemaker services
- $45,760 annually for a home health aide
- $43,200 annually for care in an assisted living facility
- $80,300 annually for a semiprivate room in a nursing home (Genworth, 2015)

Most **long-term care** isn't generally provided solely for the purpose of medical care but rather help with basic personal tasks of everyday life, or ADLs. Medicare doesn't cover custodial care, if that's the only care needed, and most nursing home care is custodial care. Therefore, most nursing home stays do not qualify for Medicare coverage. The average cost per year of a private room in a nursing home is $94,170, rising 3.6% annually. In many areas, it costs much more (John Hancock, 2013). Medicaid is the primary payer for long-term services (Kaiser Family Foundation, 2015a).

Medicare

Although Medicare does cover many services for older adults, there can be significant out-of-pocket costs. Some examples follow (Medicare.gov, 2015a).

NOT covered by Medicare:
- Long-term care (also called custodial care)
- Most dental care and dentures
- Eye examinations related to prescribing glasses
- Cosmetic surgery
- Acupuncture

- Hearing aids and exams for fitting them
- Routine foot care (Medicare.gov, 2015b)

Part A (hospital insurance) covers:
- Inpatient care in hospitals (such as critical access hospitals, inpatient rehabilitation facilities, long-term care hospitals)
- Inpatient care in a skilled nursing facility (limitations apply)
- Hospice care services
- Home health services
- Religious nonmedical health care institution

Services NOT covered by Part A:
- Custodial care (or long-term care).
- If beneficiaries are hospitalized, they pay a $1,288 deductible. If their stay lasts longer than 60 days, they are billed $322 per day for days 61 through 90 and $644 beyond that (Medicare.gov, 2016).

Hospitalizations and rehospitalizations are a significant expense for the Medicare program. A major theme of health care reform was the prevention of hospitalizations by providing more supportive care at home, care that is generally covered by the Medicaid programs.

Part B (supplementary medical insurance for physician visits):
- Beneficiaries pay 20% of the Medicare-approved amount for any visits to their doctor.
- Medicare premiums for medical insurance (part B) are $1,380 per person per year for most beneficiaries and are higher for those with incomes above $80,000 (Medicare.gov, 2015b).

Part C (Medigap—private health plans)
Part D (prescription drug benefits):

The Part D national base beneficiary premium for prescription drug coverage is $388 per person annually. A beneficiary's actual costs depend on the plan that is selected.

For more on Medicare, see Chapter 6.

Medicaid

Although the majority of people enrolled in Medicaid are children and families, most Medicaid spending goes for services provided to people aged 65 and over, and people with disabilities (Kaiser Family Foundation, 2015a).

For seniors, one of the most significant gaps in Medicare coverage is the cost of **custodial care** or help with ADLs like bathing, dressing, eating, getting into or out of a chair, or using the bathroom. Contrary to what many people believe, Medicare does not cover this kind of care, either in a nursing home or in the beneficiary's own home. Funding for this type of care is generally covered by Medicaid waiver programs and through the use of Older Americans Act funds.

It is another myth that Medicaid is a program for the poor whereas Medicare is for those who are financially secure. In FY 2010, 14% of all Medicaid beneficiaries—9.6 million—were "dual eligible" seniors and younger persons with disabilities who are covered by Medicare as well. One of every five Medicare beneficiaries is a dual eligible client. Dual eligible beneficiaries are very poor and many have high health and long-term care needs. Medicaid assists them with their Medicare premiums and cost sharing and covers full Medicaid benefits for a large majority of them—most importantly, long-term services and supports, which Medicare does not cover (Kaiser Family Foundation, 2015b).

Medicare and Medicaid are integral programs that provide quality health care for older adults across the country. Further cuts to these programs will affect the livelihood of many individuals. Given recent economic problems, increased spending in these programs is not feasible, nor sustainable. Our only chance to continue to help older adults live healthier and happier lives is to create innovations in Medicare and Medicaid that result in savings to both programs and increased efficiency and quality in the care that these programs provide.

If seniors' health and long-term services and support needs are not met, their condition ultimately can deteriorate to the point where they need to be hospitalized or admitted to a skilled nursing facility where cost of care is markedly higher.

ELDER ABUSE

Elder abuse is a problem that is underrecognized and underreported, and it has devastating consequences. Unfortunately, we simply do not know for certain how many people are suffering from elder abuse and neglect, at there are few reliable national measures of "elder" abuse. This is partially because there is no uniform reporting system for elder abuse in the United States. Additionally, the available national incidence and prevalence data from administrative records are unreliable because states have different definitions of elder and different reporting mechanisms (National Institute of Justice, 2015a). The complexity of defining elder abuse, and the debate over the classification of types of mistreatment compounds the task of evaluating the magnitude of the problem. **Elder abuse** or mistreatment (i.e., abuse and neglect) is defined as intentional actions that cause harm or create a serious risk of harm (whether or not harm is intended) to a vulnerable elder by a caregiver or other person who stands in a trust relationship to the elder. This includes failure by a caregiver to satisfy the elder's basic needs or to protect the elder from harm (National Center on Elder Abuse, n.d.a).

Signs of elder abuse may be missed by professionals working with older Americans because of lack of training on detecting abuse. The elderly may be reluctant to report abuse themselves because of fear of retaliation, because of lack of physical and/or cognitive ability to report, or because they don't want to get the abuser (90% of whom are family members) in trouble. Below is a sampling of findings about the incidence and prevalence of elder abuse and neglect:

- Major recent studies found that 7.6% to 10% of participants experienced abuse in the year prior to data collection. Also, for 1 in 10 adults who reported that they experienced abuse, financial abuse was included in the report.
- An increasing trend in reporting of elder abuse is seen when examining available data from state Adult Protective Services (APS) agencies.

- Even though there are APS agencies in all 50 states (programs differ by state), and most states have mandatory reporting laws for elder abuse, a large number of cases of neglect, elder abuse, and financial mistreatment are still undetected each year.
- In one study, it was estimated that the involvement of authorities is only found in 1 in 14 cases of elder abuse. A study on elder abuse prevalence in the state of New York found that there are 24 unknown cases for every case known to APS.
- Major financial exploitation is self-reported at a much higher rate (41 per 1,000) than neglect or physical, emotional, and sexual abuse (National Center on Elder Abuse, n.d.b).

The National Institute of Justice conducted a large survey of older adults. They found that 1.6% of the respondents reported physical abuse, but only 31% had reported the incident. When other forms of abuse were included, 11% of those surveyed had some kind of mistreatment in the previous year, with over 5.2% reporting financial abuse, 5.1% citing emotional mistreatment, and 5.1% experienced potential neglect (National Institute of Justice, 2015a). Older adults are at increased risk for abuse due to social isolation, mental impairment, and dependence on others.

Physical abuse, neglect, emotional or psychological abuse, verbal abuse and threats, financial abuse and exploitation, sexual abuse, and abandonment are considered forms of elder abuse (National Center on Elder Abuse, n.d.a).

In some states, self-neglect is also considered a form of mistreatment. This occurs when an older adult neglects to take care of his or herself in a way that leads to illness or injury. Self-neglect includes such behaviors as failing to take medications, refusal to seek medical attention for a serious illness, leaving a burner on the stove on and unattended, poor hygiene, dressing inappropriately for the weather, or confusion. Self-neglect is the form of abuse most commonly reported to APS (National Center on Elder Abuse, n.d.b).

It is notable that financial abuse often accompanies one of the other forms of abuse. The financial abuse of seniors is a growing problem, often called the "crime of the 21st century." It is one of the most sinister forms of abuse. A senior can be financially stable and living independently one day, and become destitute and forced to live in a facility the next as a result of abuse. Sadly, most elder abuse occurs in the elder's own home, and the abuser is usually a family member. In states reporting in a survey of APS agencies, almost half of all cases investigated were substantiated. Most victims of elder abuse are White (77.1%), and the majority of victims are reported to be over age 80 and female (American Psychological Association, 2012). The most common perpetrators of elder abuse are spouses or partners of elders, often in a relationship with long-term domestic violence. Family members account for 76% of reported mistreatment. Abusers, particularly adult children, are often dependent on the victim for financial assistance, housing, or because of personal problems such as mental illness, alcohol, or drug abuse (National Institute of Justice,

2015a). The most common types of financial mistreatment were having someone steal or spend their money, sell or take their property, or forge their signature. The risk of financial mistreatment was higher for individuals who engaged in fewer social or other activities outside of the home (e.g., participating in social activities away from home, getting together with people who do not live in the home, going to the movies), had low self-control, were male and identified as a racial minority (National Institute of Justice, 2015b).

An elder person in immediate danger should be removed from his or her environment; however, elder abuse does not often come to the attention of PHNs or other providers of services to older adults. It is estimated that five occurrences of neglect, abuse, exploitation, or self-neglect go unreported for every case that is reported. Therefore, nurses working in the community with older adults must be vigilant for signs of elder abuse and knowledgeable about reporting laws.

Various state, local, and county agencies investigate and enforce elder abuse laws. The first agency to respond to a report of elder abuse in most states is APS. In some states, certain professionals are required or encouraged to report elder abuse; there are generally doctors and nurses, psychologists, police officers, social workers, and employees of banks and other financial institutions. The National Institute of Justice (2013, para. 1) has identified four areas that are potential markers for identifying elder abuse:

- Physical condition and quality of care (e.g., unreported injuries, malnourishment)
- Facility/housing characteristics (e.g., unchanged linens, strong odors)
- Inconsistencies in statements/records (e.g., statements given vs. what you see)
- Staff/family member behaviors (e.g., evasiveness, lack of knowledge or concern)

APPROACHES TO OLDER ADULT CARE

In general, nursing service to seniors can be divided into two approaches: geriatrics and gerontology. In addition, healthy older adults can be effectively cared for in the community through case management approaches, which focus on all three types of services: primary, secondary, and tertiary. The ultimate goal of community-based case management for the aging population is to enhance the quality of care by decreasing fragmentation, maximizing resources, and providing the highest quality of care possible.

Case Management and Needs Assessment

Case management involves assessing needs, planning and organizing services, and monitoring responses to care throughout the length of the caregiving process, condition, or illness. This concept, which has been practiced by PHNs for many years, focuses primarily on the health needs of clients. Social workers use case management to address their clients' social needs, including their financial problems. Some HMOs provide a coordinated system of services for their enrolled clients. However, many communities provide no such advocate for their older residents, and a more comprehensive, community-wide system approach needs to be developed in order to serve the entire older adult population. Such a system might be based in an agency specifically designed to serve as case manager or agent to assess clients' needs and assemble existing agencies and services to meet those needs.

Various techniques or tools are available to assess the needs of older adults:

- The Older Americans Resources and Services Information System (OARS), developed by Duke University Center for the Study of Aging and Human Development (2014), utilizes two sections of one tool—OARS Multidimensional Functional Assessment Questionnaire (OMFAQ)—to determine levels of functioning in five areas (mental health, physical health, economic resources, social resources, and ability to perform ADLs), along with the extent and intensity of utilization, as well as perceived need, of services. Administration time is about 45 minutes, and this tool is commonly used in research and to determine effectiveness of services, as well as assessment of functional status.
- The Barthel Index assesses functional independence and is often used to determine the levels of disability or dependence of stroke victims with respect to ADLs (Mahoney & Barthel, 1965).
- The Modified Rankin Scale (MRS) is another common tool used for this purpose (Bonita & Beaglehole, 1988; Sulter, Steen, & De Keyser, 1999).
- The Katz Index of ADLs is based on an evaluation of the functional independence or dependence of clients with respect to bathing, dressing, toileting, and related tasks (Katz, 1963).
- The Instrumental Activities of Daily Living Scale looks at an older adult's ability to perform such activities as using the telephone, shopping, doing laundry, and handling finances (Graf, 2013).
- Other tools sometimes used with clients include the Stanford 7-day Physical Activity Recall (PAR) questionnaire (Sallis, Buono, Roby, Micale, & Nelson, 1993) and the Physical Activity Scale for the Elderly (PASE) (Washburn, Smith, Jette, & Janney, 1993). All of these tools measure physical activity and functioning.

A frequently overlooked area of assessment is the client's spiritual needs. Religious dedication and spiritual concern often increase in later years. Limited ability or lack of transportation may prevent older people from attending religious services or engaging in spiritually enhancing activities. Self-health ratings, including clients' reports on their spiritual needs, provide another useful assessment technique.

HEALTH SERVICES FOR OLDER ADULT POPULATIONS

How well are the needs of older adults being met? To answer this question, other questions must be raised. Do health programs for older adults encompass the full range of needed services? Are programs both physically and financially accessible? Do they encourage clients to function independently? Do they treat senior citizens with respect and preserve their dignity? Do they recognize older adults' needs for companionship, economic security, and social status? If appropriate, do they promote meaningful activities instead of overworked games or activities such as bingo, shuffleboard, and ceramics? Are health care services and other social services provided based on evidence and research?

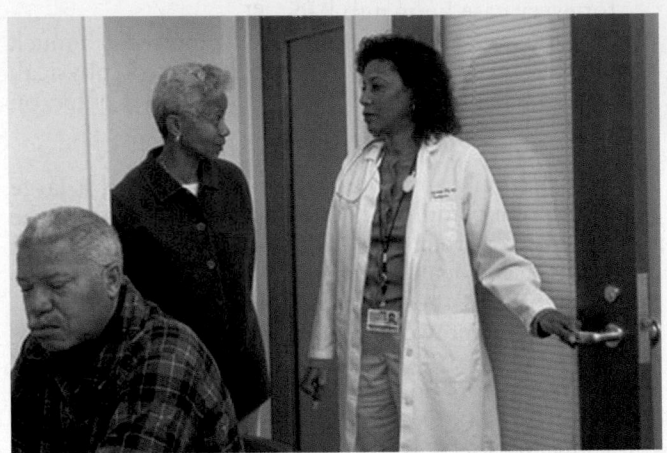

Effective services for older adults should be comprehensive, coordinated, and accessible and demonstrate evidence-based quality.

Criteria for Effective Service

Several criteria help to define the characteristics of an effective community health service delivery system. Four, in particular, deserve attention. In order to be effective, it should be *comprehensive*. Many communities provide some programs, such as limited health screening or selected activities, but do not offer a full range of services to more adequately meet the needs of their senior citizens. Gaps and duplication in programs most often result from poor or nonexistent community-wide planning. Furthermore, such planning should be based on thorough assessment of the needs of the population in that community. A comprehensive set of services should provide the following:

1. Adequate financial support
2. Adult day care programs
3. Access to high-quality health care services (prevention, early diagnosis and treatment, rehabilitation)
4. Health education (including preparation for retirement)
5. In-home services
6. Recreation and activity programs that promote socialization
7. Specialized transportation services

A second criterion for a community service delivery system is *coordination*. Often, older people go from one agency to the next. After visiting one place for food stamps, they go to another for answers to Medicare questions, another for congregate dining, and still another for health screenings. Such a patchwork of services reflects a system organized for the convenience of providers rather than consumers. It encourages misuse and discourages effective use. Instead, there should be coordinated, community-wide assessment and planning. Communities must consider alternatives that can meet many needs in one location, such as multiservice agencies and interdisciplinary collaborative programs.

A coordinated information and referral system provides another link. Most communities need this type of information network, which contains a directory of all resources and services for the older adult and includes the name and telephone number of a contact person with each listing. Such a network is available in many communities and should be developed in those without one. A simplified information and referral system that includes one number (i.e., an "800 number") that can connect seniors with available resources and services is particularly helpful to older people. In most communities, coordination is not present, or it is not done with any regularity or thoroughness. Many agencies in a given community do not coordinate services but instead deliver their own services in a patchwork and uncoordinated fashion. Collaboration among those who provide services to seniors can provide vital information for planning and implementing needed programs.

A third criterion is *accessibility*. Too often, services for seniors are inconveniently located or are prohibitively expensive. Some communities are considering multiservice community centers to bring programs and services for elderly closer to home. The Program of All-Inclusive Care of the Elderly (PACE) is one example of this (National PACE Association, 2015). Comprehensive services are offered to eligible nursing home patients, including personal, health care, and housing services (e.g., adult day care, meals, social workers, nurses, primary care physicians, dentists, podiatrists, optometrists, prescriptions, medical specialists, and acute and nursing home care). More convenient, and perhaps, specialized transportation services and more in-home services, such as home health aides, homemakers, and Meals on Wheels, may further solve accessibility problems for many older adults. Federal, state, and private funding sources can be tapped to ease the burden on the economically pressured population.

Finally, an effective community service system for older people should promote *quality* programs. This means that services should truly address the needs and concerns of a community's senior citizens and be based on scientific evidence. In evaluation of the quality regarding the needs of today's elders and in anticipation of the larger numbers to come, many options are becoming available. A range of housing types, from luxurious retirement communities with all amenities for the active and healthier senior to secure and more modestly priced or low-income apartments for independent senior living, are being built in most communities.

The concept of **continuing care retirement communities (CCRCs)**, sometimes referred to as total life centers, allows seniors to "age in place," with flexible accommodations designed to meet their health and housing needs as these needs change over time (American Association of Retired Persons [AARP], 2015a). CCRCs are the most expensive long-term care solution available to seniors; however,

they provide all levels of living, from total independence to the most dependent, and are designed to meet the continuous living needs of older aging adults. Residents entering CCRCs sign a long-term contract that provides for housing, services, and nursing care, usually all in one location. Many seniors enter into CCRC contracts while they are healthy and active, knowing they will be able to stay in the same community and receive nursing care should this become necessary. Seniors who invest in a CCRC have adequately planned for housing and care for the remainder of their life and have the financial means to support it. Entrance fees can range from $3,000 to $5,000 to 1,000,000 and monthly fees from $3,000 to $5,000 (AARP, 2015b). Others may choose to remain in their own home because they do not desire living arrangements that include only older adults or because they have not planned adequately for the expense. Nevertheless, demand is increasing for this type of housing option.

Although only 1.4 million people in the United States live in **skilled nursing facilities**, such organizations remain the most visible type of health service for older adults (CDC, 2015q). These facilities provide skilled nursing care along with personal care that is considered nonskilled or custodial care, such as bathing, dressing, feeding, and assisting with mobility and recreation. Currently, approximately 2 million people are receiving nursing home care.

Some struggle to maintain the appearance of doing well in order to maintain their independence. Often, they fear that their children or others will make decisions for them that include leaving their homes. Home, whatever form it takes, is where these people believe they are the happiest.

There is increased emphasis on providing needed services for elders at home. This trend started several years ago when it became evident that people improved more quickly and at lower cost when they were cared for as outpatients in their own homes. Today's emphasis on cost control gives added support for providing services at home. Given the increase in longevity, the potential for cost savings appears significant if care for dependent older people can be maintained at home. Doing so encourages functional independence as well as emotional well-being, but needs must be assessed. What are the needs of this specific population group in terms of nutrition, exercise, economic security, independence, social interaction, meaningful activities, and preparation for death? Planning for quality community services depends on having adequate, accurate, and current data. Periodic needs assessment is a necessity to ensure updated information, and initiate and promote quality services.

Services for Older Adults by Level of Care Required

The majority of older adults want to remain in their own homes for the remainder of their lives and be as independent and in control of their lives as possible (HelpGuide, 2015i). Partners for Livable Communities (2015) outline a blueprint for developing livable communities where peoplecan live in their own communities and grow old with all the services necessary. **Aging in place** is a term used for seniors who choose to remain in their own homes.

To successfully remain at home, older adults need transportation, a home that can be modified if moving up and down stairs becomes problematic, a yard that can be maintained, personal care if needed, a way to safely take medications, live in a safe neighborhood, and have family or friends who can assist when needed (HelpGuide, 2015f).

Maintaining functional independence should be the primary goal of services for the older population. Assessment of needs, ability to function and the use of tools, such as the previously cited OARS, the Instrumental Activities of Daily Living Scale, or other tools, form the basis for determining appropriate services. Although many of the well seniors can assess their own health status, some are reluctant to seek needed help. Therefore, outreach programs serve an important function in many communities, as they locate people in need of health or social assistance and refer them to appropriate resources.

Health screening is another important program for early detection and treatment of health problems among older adults. Conditions that are easily screened include hypertension, glaucoma, hearing disorders, cancers, diabetes, anemia, depression, mild cognitive impairment, and nutritional deficiencies. At the same time, assessment of clients' socialization, housing, and economic needs, along with proper referrals, can prevent further problems from developing that would compromise their health status. Health maintenance programs may be offered through a single agency, such as an HMO, or they may be coordinated by a case management agency with referrals to other providers. These programs should cover a wide range of services needed by the senior population, such as those listed in Display 24–6.

At times, seniors who remain in their own homes or apartments need home care services brought to them. Other seniors live with family members and go to an adult day care center during the day. The third category of living arrangements includes those that are short term. It may be a rehabilitation hospital for recovery and physical therapy related to a hip fracture, or respite care, which gives the usual caregiver a much-needed rest from 24-hour-a-day caregiving and helps prevent "burnout." Families of terminally ill clients and those with severe dementia cared for at home often use respite services.

Adult Day Care

Day care services offer a place where older adults can go during the day for social activities, nutrition, nursing care, and physical or speech therapies. They can be publicly or privately funded, nonprofit or for-profit. The average price for adult day care is $64.00 per day, and Medicare does not cover this service (HelpGuide, 2015a).

Home Care Services

Home care provides services such as skilled nursing care, psychiatric nursing, physical and speech therapies, homemaker services, social work services, and dietetic counseling (see Chapter 32). These services are useful for families who are caring for an older person, especially if the caregivers work and no one is at home or available during the day. One disadvantage to those remaining in their homes is that services for dependent older adults in the community are often fragmented, inadequate, and inaccessible, and at times, operate with little or no quality control.

Independent Living

This is a general term for any housing arrangement designed exclusively for seniors. Types of independent living facilities include subsidized senior housing, retirement communities, and senior apartments restricted to those who are older (usually 55+) (HelpGuide, 2015h). These facilities provide minor assistance with ADLs and maintenance for the housing facility.

The *Village Concept* is a relatively new solution for independent living in which older adults live in their own homes in a village, giving them access to services such as transportation and grocery shopping or helping with household chores provided by the village. This means that the older adult is not dependent on family or friends. This option requires a membership fee, often more than $500 a year, based on services needed (AARP Public Policy Institute, n.d.).

The dependent older adult needs someone in the community to assess their particular needs; assemble, coordinate, and monitor the appropriate resources and services; and serve as their advocate. Some communities have ombudsmen to serve in this role. But PHNs can easily fill the role of case manager for clients. This case management approach tailors services to the long-term needs of clients and enables them to function longer outside of institutions.

Assisted Living

Assisted living or assisted living facilities (residences) provide supervision or assistance with ADLs, coordination of services by outside health care providers, and monitoring of resident activities to help to ensure their health, safety, and well-being. Assistance may include the administration or supervision of medication or personal care services provided by trained staff. It is less costly than care in a nursing home (Medline Plus, 2015).

Assisted living as it exists today emerged in the 1990s as an alternative on the continuum of care for older adults. Usually, it includes seniors for whom independent living is no longer appropriate, but who do not need the 24-hour medical care provided by a nursing home. Assisted living is a philosophy of care and services promoting independence and dignity. Other names for assisted living are residential care, board and care, congregate care, sheltered housing, adult congregate living care, adult living facilities, supported care, enhanced care, adult homes, retirement residences, adult foster care, and community-based retirement facilities. There is no nationally recognized definition of assisted living. Regulation and licensing of these facilities occur at the state level, and each has its own definition of the term it uses to describe assisted living. More than two thirds of the states use the licensure term "assisted living." Other licensure terms used for this type of care include residential care home, assisted care living facilities, and personal care homes. Because the term assisted living has not been defined in some states, it is often a marketing term used by a variety of senior living communities, licensed or unlicensed. The difference in licensing is usually based on the size of the facility or the services it can offer.

Services that are provided include help with ADLs, health care management and monitoring, housekeeping and laundry, transportation, security, recreation, and either reminders or help with medications. Although skilled nursing care is not provided, assisted living is an expensive option ranging in cost from <$10,000 to over $50,000 a year with an average rate of $1,800.00 per month (Genworth, 2015). Medicare does not cover the costs of assisted living; therefore, almost all of the expenses must be paid for out of pocket (HelpGuide, 2015c). Medicare only pays for medical care, not housing costs. Medicaid may help pay some assisted living costs and limited custodial home care but not generally for housing costs related to personal care homes. Those facilities focusing on the care of people with AD are physically designed with clients' safety and individual needs considered, and are staffed with trained paraprofessionals.

Nursing homes/long-term care/skilled nursing facilities include those services that provide care for people at different stages of dependence for extended periods of time. New choices are now available and provide housing for larger numbers of older adults than do nursing homes. The average nursing home cost is over $90,000 for a private room, and Medicare only covers limited stays in long-term care. For 100 days following a hospital stay, Medicare covers a nursing or rehabilitation center. Medicare does not, however, pay for custodial care (care that includes help with ADLs but not skilled nursing care). Medicaid will pay for nursing home care for those with limited assets (HelpGuide, 2015c, 2015e).

Medicare and Medicaid generally pay only for care in skilled nursing facilities. Medicaid may pay for care in intermediate care facilities but only after the client meets income and asset tests that leave them essentially indigent. Medicaid coverage of assisted living services is available in a few states that can grant Medicaid waivers. The average length of time a senior remains in an assisted living residence is about 28.3 months (National Center for Assisted Living, 2015). Because of licensing restrictions, when someone becomes bedridden or needs additional assistance or skilled nursing care, they generally must move from assisted care into another facility.

Nursing home reform was legislated in the late 1980s, putting increased demands on facilities to provide competent resident assessment, timely care plans, quality improvement, and protection of resident rights (Omnibus Budget Reconciliation Act, 1987). This increased complexity of services has resulted in increased costs in these facilities. Staffing needs increase as care becomes more complex and the resident population grows. Licensed personnel must be knowledgeable decision-makers, managers of unskilled staff, staff educators, and role models, as well as efficient and effective administrators in an essentially autonomous practice setting. And, as the population grows, the need for greater numbers of both licensed and attendant staff becomes more evident. Because many of these jobs offer low pay and are without substantial benefits or a career ladder, it is projected that it will remain difficult to staff for rising demand.

In the past, nursing homes had stigmas attached to them. Many people saw them as places that enforced dehumanizing and impersonal regulations, such as segregation of sexes, strict social policies, and sometimes overuse of chemical and physical restraints. Media attention to such conditions, together with current licensing regulations, should make these types of practices the rare exception. In addition, as competition comes from facilities offering lower levels of care (e.g., assisted living centers), residents in nursing homes who are receiving minimal care may be able to find other types of housing.

Even in institutions in which the quality of care is outstanding, costs are so high that family resources are soon depleted if not planned for long in advance of the need. Although Medicaid pays for skilled nursing costs if the client meets low-income and asset requirements, and Medicare pays for a limited period of care, clients and families pay more than half of the total costs. Life savings that older parents had hoped to leave to their children may be quickly consumed, forcing them into indigence.

END OF LIFE: ADVANCE DIRECTIVES, HOSPICE, AND PALLIATIVE CARE

A final need of older adults is preparing for a dignified death. In her classic work, *On Death and Dying*, Elisabeth Kübler-Ross (1969) described death as the final stage of growth and one that deserves the same measure of quality as other stages of life. Although death is a natural part of life, many older people fear death as an experience of pain, humiliation, discomfort, or financial concern for loved ones. Sometimes, very aggressive and heroic medical treatments are offered to those near the end of their lives, often at the urging of family members. Planning for a dignified death is an important issue for many older people, and PHNs can facilitate conversations among family members and provide necessary information and resources.

Advance Directives

Living wills and advance health care directives (AHCDs), sometimes referred to as *advance directives*, are legal documents that instruct others about end-of-life choices should an individual be unable to make decisions independently. The forms for advance directives are available for every state online through CaringInfo.org (National Hospice and Palliative Care Organization, n.d.). An AHCD only becomes effective under the circumstances specified in the document. This document allows for appointment of a health care agent who will have the legal authority to make health care decisions on behalf of the patient and for specific written instructions for future health care in the event of any situation in which the patient can no longer speak for himself or herself. Examples include:

- The use of dialysis and breathing machines
- Use of resuscitation if breathing or heartbeat stops
- Tube feeding
- Organ or tissue donation

Having such documents prepared and making them known to significant others can ensure that wishes will be honored. These documents can provide clear directions for families and health care professionals and are gaining more recognition and importance as a result of increasing ethical dilemmas and challenges brought on by advances in technology (American Medical Association, 2015). Advance directives can be revoked or replaced at any time, as long as the individual in question is capable of making his or her own decisions. It is recommended that these documents be reviewed every 2 years or so, or in the event of a change in health status, and revised to ensure that they continue to accurately reflect an individual's wishes.

Hospice

Hospice is an option that takes a multidisciplinary approach to end-of-life care and needs. Hospice is more a concept of care than a specific place, although some hospice organizations provide individuals with a place to die with dignity if they have no home or choose not to die at home. Hospice is an option for people with a "projected" life expectancy of 6 months or less and often involves palliative care (pain and symptom relief) as opposed to ongoing curative measures. Staff is on call 24 hours a day, 7 days a week. In 2011, $1.65 million patients received services from hospice, and 44.6% of deaths occurred under hospice care. Over 39% of hospice patients were over age 85, and 66.4% of all hospice care is given in the patient's own home (National Hospice and Palliative Care Organization, 2015). The Medicare hospice benefit, enacted by Congress in 1982, is the predominant source of payment for hospice. The number of hospice programs nationwide continues to increase—from the first program that opened in 1974 to approximately 5,300 programs today. The majority of hospices are independent, freestanding agencies, whereas the remaining agencies are either part of a hospital system, home health agency, or nursing home. Hospices may range in size from small, all-volunteer agencies that care for fewer than 50 patients per year to large, national corporate chains, employing nurses and other staff members that care for thousands of patients each day (National Hospice and Palliative Care Organization, 2015).

Hospice enables many clients to live their end days to the fullest, with purpose, dignity, grace, and support;

in fact, one recent large-scale study found that hospice patients survived 29 days longer than nonhospice patients (National Hospice and Palliative Care Organization, 2015). Hospice care focuses on all aspects of an individual's life and well-being: physical, social, emotional, and spiritual. Individuals are permitted to go on and off hospice care as needed or if they change their mind and decide to return to curative treatment. Some community health nursing agencies offer hospice programs staffed by their nurses. It is a service that has been well received by older adults, meets important needs, and is growing in use (eldercare.gov, 2015). See Chapter 32 for more on hospice and palliative care in the community.

Palliative Care

Palliative care consists of comfort and symptom management and does not provide a cure. For most chronic ongoing health conditions—such as diabetes, high blood pressure, congestive heart failure, arthritis, and COPD—there are no cures, only symptom relief. Relative to the senior population, which suffers from more chronic conditions than the rest of the population, palliative care should not be viewed as synonymous with hospice or end-of-life care. Rather, palliative care should be viewed as any care primarily intended to relieve the burden of physical and emotional suffering that often accompanies the illnesses associated with aging. Palliative care should be a major focus of care throughout the aging process, regardless of whether death is imminent within 6 months (National Hospice and Palliative Care Organization, 2015). Many seniors are now "preplanning"

POPULATION-FOCUS ON ADVANCE DIRECTIVES

Advance-directives are a very personal and individual matter. Whenever you or I go into the hospital or surgery center for a procedure, we are usually asked by an admitting nurse or clerk if we have an advance-directive (no matter our age or health status). How many people actually answer in the affirmative? Autonomy is a hallmark of ethical thought. We believe that people should be able to choose for themselves and have their choices respected; hence, the right to leave the hospital against medical advice (AMA). Therefore, we wait for patients to express their preference about advance directives (or the choice to have none).

Have you ever considered this from a population perspective? When someone does not choose a plan for end-of-life care, the option by default generally becomes full medical treatment and lifesaving measures to delay death, despite the futility of the pending outcome. Often, this causes needless suffering and is costly in terms of manpower and resources. But, do individuals truly understand their options? Can we offer better explanations of the alternatives? Behavioral economists explain that people are not always good at systematically looking at best evidence in order to make decisions. We rely on what others think or on rules of thumb because we are often faced with "decision fatigue." We are programmed to avoid loss and seek immediate rewards. Taking this

into consideration, and the knowledge that terminal patients want comfort and quality of life at the end of life, researchers gave participants three options: (1) advance directives for comfort-oriented care (where life might be shorter), (2) advance directives for a longer life (where there might be more pain and suffering), and (3) no directives. Because of the way choices were structured, twice as many people chose the option with comfort as the goal over the other two choices. They termed this "choice architecture," as this reframing of the choices to draw attention to outcomes helps to "nudge" people toward their definitive goals (Hostetter & Klein, 2013, June–July, para.17).

The argument could be made that evidence supports advance directives for comfort-oriented care, but is it ethical to influence behavior in this way? The elderly are a growing population, and the lack of advance directives does lead to more economic burden on the healthcare system. Population-focused initiatives are needed to educate the elderly about advance directives and the potential outcomes of the choices they make. Can you think of creative ways of addressing this issue on a population level?

Hostetter, M., & Klein, S. (2013, June–July), In focus: using behavioral economics to advance population health and improve the quality of health care services. *Matters Quality*. Retrieved from http://www.commonwealthfund.org/publications/newsletters/quality-matters/2013/june-july/in-focus

their funerals. This option is gaining momentum in the senior population and allows individuals to make arrangements with a funeral home of their choice, selecting interment or cremation, a memorial service or a celebration of life gathering, music to be played, and other personal details. All options are chosen by the senior rather than leaving these choices and decisions solely to their family members. Other older adults may place less emphasis on the rituals, as was demonstrated by one older adult who left these choices to her children by telling them, "Surprise me!"

CARE FOR THE CAREGIVER

The burden of caregiving is receiving more attention in recent years because it is such a demanding and costly role. An increasing number of older people are cared for in their home by a spouse or other family member on an unpaid basis. Almost 75% of persons receiving care at home rely exclusively on informal caregivers, usually women between the ages of 45 and 64. The demands of caregiving exact a toll on the caregiver, who not only may miss important screening and health care visits for self but also often give up a social life. Caregiving has been associated with increased levels of depression and anxiety, as well as increased use of psychoactive medications, poorer levels of self-reported health, compromised immune function, and increased mortality. For example, there are nearly 15 million Alzheimer's and dementia caregivers providing 17 billion hours of unpaid care valued at $202 billion (AARP, 2015b). These caregivers suffer not only emotionally but also physically. Because of the toll of caregiving on their own health, caregivers for those with AD and dementia had $7.9 billion in additional health care costs. More than 60% of family caregivers report high levels of stress because of the prolonged duration of caregiving and 33% report symptoms of depression (National Alliance for Caregiving and the AARP Public Policy Institute, 2015). Their own decline in health compromises their ability to be a caregiver unless they get some relief (see Chapter 32).

Respite care is a service that is receiving increasing attention. It provides time off for caregivers, including family members, who care for someone who is ill, injured, or frail. Respite care can take place in an adult day center, in the home of the person being cared for, or even in a residential setting such as an assisted living facility or nursing home. Although there are different approaches to respite care, all have the same basic objective: to provide caregivers with planned temporary, intermittent, substitute care, allowing for relief from the daily responsibilities of caring for the care recipient (AARP, 2015b). Respite care is sometimes available through agencies that provide volunteers to relieve caregivers; neighbors, churches, or volunteer organizations may be potential sources of assistance. Some skilled nursing facilities provide an extra room to give temporary institutional housing for the older adults while caregivers take a break over a weekend, for instance. Clients may also need a change from the constant interaction with their caregivers. Long-term care insurance may cover some costs of respite care. The 2000 Older Americans Act Amendments provided funding for states to work through the National Family Caregiver Support Program (NFCSP) to address respite care specifically on the local level (CDC, 2015o).

THE COMMUNITY HEALTH NURSE IN AN AGING AMERICA

PHNs can make a significant contribution to the health of older adults. Because these nurses are in the community and already have contact with many seniors, they are in a prime position to begin needs assessments and mutual planning for the health of this group. Case management is often a critical aspect of the nurse's role because the PHN must know what resources are available and when and how to make referrals for these older clients (see From the Case Files II).

Older adults are changing dramatically. The numbers and types of home care services, for example, are mushrooming. Many entrepreneurs, including nurses, who recognize the potential of this growing market, have begun offering goods and services targeted to older adults. PHNs must keep abreast of new developments, programs, regulations, and social and economic forces, along with their potential impacts on the provision of health services.

More importantly, PHNs need to be proactive, designing interventions that maximize nursing's resources and provide the greatest benefit to clients. For example, nurses might develop an older adult case management program that consists of a community-wide assessment, information, and referral service. Such a program might contract with existing agencies to serve as a clearinghouse for the older adult and to channel clients to appropriate services. Financing of such a program might be based on tax dollars (if it is a public agency), grants, or some innovative fee-for-service reimbursement system.

Many of the older population's health problems can be prevented and their health promoted. Changing to a healthier lifestyle is one of the most important preventive measures the nurse can emphasize. Education and support are two keys to the success of these changes.

The role of the PHN as a teacher is an important one. Educating older adults about their health conditions, safety, and use of medications is another important way to prevent problems. Influenza and pneumonia can be prevented through regular health maintenance, which includes immunizations. Other problems associated with environmental conditions and the aging process, such as arthritis, diabetes, and some cancers, can be diagnosed and treated early, thereby minimizing their deleterious effect on functional independence.

Many types of accidents that frequently happen to older adults are preventable. PHNs can make a difference through their work with individuals, families, and aggregates in promoting and teaching safety measures to prevent such accidents. As discussed earlier, falls are a leading cause of injury and death for the older adult and result from a combination of internal factors (e.g., diseases, effects of medicines) and external factors (e.g., lighting, area rugs, lack of handrails) that are preventable or controllable. Nurses can make a difference in the lives of older clients by using available materials and their own resources when teaching about safety.

PHNs face a serious challenge in addressing the needs of the growing and aging population. At the same time, nursing can be at the forefront of developing innovative health services for seniors, rising to meet the opportunity and the challenge.

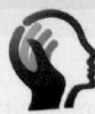

From the Case Files II

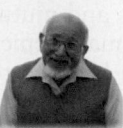

Johnny Jessup is 94 years old and lives with his wife, age 86, in a small mobile home on some acreage in a rural area of our county. He had mastoiditis as a child and lost a good deal of hearing. His vision is good, though, and he only wears glasses for reading. He was diagnosed with prostate cancer 20 years ago and still suffers from the radiation treatments he had at that time. He wears a protective "diaper" because he is often bowel incontinent. He is generally in good health, with no hypertension or evidence of heart disease. He spends most of his days outside, watering his berries, flowers, and fruit trees. He worked as a farmer and laborer—always outside—and he enjoys being in the sun and away from the television that his wife, Maude, likes to watch. He has difficulty hearing it, and when he turns up the volume, it "hurts her ears" and they argue over that. They have one son who lives in the same town, but he works long hours at his job. They speak by phone every other day, and he comes by to visit when he can. Their three grandsons are all away at college and they rarely see them.

As a young man, Johnny liked to dance, and he occasionally will go to the local senior center dances. Maude does not like to dance and will not accompany him there. Sometimes, this is a source of stress. Johnny likes to drink an "occasional cold beer," but he never drinks "hard liquor." He quit smoking 25 years ago, but he had been a heavy smoker from the age of 20. His appetite has usually been good, but he sometimes has difficulty eating fresh fruit or nuts because of his bowel problems. Maude has recently been having memory lapses and some difficulty remembering to turn off the stove and close the refrigerator door. She has trouble with a number of daily tasks. She likes to have someone bring them fast food as a treat every week, and they now require assistance with errands and most housekeeping tasks.

Recently, Johnny noticed that he was having more difficulty doing his outside chores. He seems more "weak" and "tired" and he has recently had quite a bit of "nausea and vomiting." Maude and Johnny's son took them for an appointment with his urologist, and it was determined that his prostate-specific antigen (PSA) was elevated.

You are a district PHN and have recently been assigned to the Jessup family to assess their functional limitations and provide them with information on resources they might need over the next few months. How would you begin your visit? How can you best determine their functional and physical limitations? What other assessments could be helpful (social, spiritual, mental/cognitive, etc.)? What resources and services might be helpful to them?

PERSPECTIVES
VOICES FROM THE COMMUNITY

Continuing Care Centers—A Solution for Aging Adults

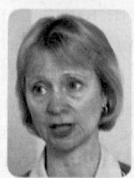

I am really sold on continuing care retirement communities! We have one in our area that is a big hit with our middle- and upper-income folks. The Otterbein Lebanon Retirement Community is a model continuing care center and is one of five Otterbein homes located in Ohio. With housing options for 1,200 residents on a 1,500-acre campus in rural southeastern Ohio, older adults can choose housing options that include freestanding two- and three-bedroom homes, one-bedroom cottages, or apartment-style one- or two-bedroom or one-room studio units, where they live independently.

They are licensed for 296 beds, including assisted living options from one-room studio apartments (with limited facilities for meal preparation) to semiprivate rooms in which nurses oversee medication and staff is available to assist with personal care. If caregiving needs become greater, additional services are available. Both skilled nursing services and a freestanding 30-bed Alzheimer's living unit exist for the frailest older adults. This is a real advantage for my clients who want to remain in the same place, even as their physical condition may worsen.

Regardless of the living arrangement, the residents are free to come and go as they wish and all have access to congregate dining in their large and attractive restaurant-style dining room.

The retirement community is expanding. One hundred and ten patio homes were built in 1999–2000 with additional expansion planned.

The Otterbein Lebanon Retirement Community also provides a health clinic, adult day care, and the other usual services found in a community: a bank, post office, ice cream parlor, a small convenience store, hairdresser, library, a church (with a 70-member choir, a bell choir, and men's and women's clubs), a thrift shop, and an arts and crafts shop open to the public. Because of the popularity of this Otterbein Lebanon Community, there is a waiting list for some independent living areas.

Many of the assisted living and skilled nursing beds are occupied by residents who moved into the independent living areas 10 to 15 years ago while they were in their 70s or 80s. Their ages now range from the late 80s to older than 100, and care needs have increased. This is wonderful because, in this type of setting, frail people do not have to leave their community to get the care they need, and longtime friends are nearby to care for them or offer companionship. It is not unusual to see many of the independent seniors volunteering to help feed the frail patients in the skilled nursing care units. In fact, residents volunteer more than 85,000 hours a year to the Otterbein Lebanon Retirement Community. They know that when they need the care, a senior friend will be there for them.

Judy, PHN

SUMMARY

The number of older adults (age 65 and older) is increasing and becoming a larger percentage of the total U.S. population. Women commonly outlive men by a number of years, making women a larger part of this older population. With improved medicines and medical technology, many people are now living well into the 80s and 90s, and in relatively good health. This extended life expectancy is good news; however, it has also created a myriad of new health needs and concerns, not only for the older population but also for health care facilities and professionals who deliver services to older adults.

Healthy longevity is the goal for the aging population and is a focus of *Healthy People 2020*. This means being able to function as independently as possible; maintaining as much physical, mental, and social vigor as possible; and adapting to life's changes while coping with the stresses and losses and still being able to engage in meaningful activity.

To promote and maintain health and prevent illness, older people need to be educated about their own health care needs. In particular, they should understand the potential hazards of drug interactions if they are taking multiple medications. They also need good nutrition and adequate exercise; they need to be as independent and self-reliant as possible; they need coping skills to face the possibility of financial insecurity and the loss of a spouse or other loved ones; they need social interaction, companionship, and meaningful activities; and they need to resolve anxieties regarding their own eventual death.

The most common health problems of older adults are chronic and often progressive conditions such as arthritis, vision and hearing loss, heart disease, hypertension, and diabetes, all of which can become disabling conditions. Other major causes of death or disability include cancer, CVAs, AD, along with accidents and injuries resulting from falls, fires, or automobile crashes. Older adults also often suffer adverse side effects from polypharmacy (multiple medications prescribed for various chronic conditions), making this a danger. Many of these health problems, along with accidents and injuries, associated with old age are preventable to some extent, and early diagnosis and treatment of some conditions can minimize their adverse effects.

Too frequently, older adults suffer from the emotional side effects of aging, such as feelings of distress and anxiety regarding their future, loneliness and social isolation when loved ones or friends die, and even depression, feeling that life is over and they have no purpose or meaningful function in life. However, older people can also enter this phase of life determined to keep physically and mentally healthy, interacting with others and making viable contributions to others and society.

Many programs are available to older adults, both for those who are healthy and active, along with those needing some level of dependent or semidependent care. Programs for hearty older people include health maintenance programs that cover a wide range of health services, wellness programs, health screening, outreach programs, social assistance programs, and information about volunteering and educational opportunities in the community. A variety of living arrangements and care options are available from which to choose and can be tailored to the older person's desires and needs. These include continuing care centers, which offer a full range of living arrangements—from totally independent living to skilled nursing services—all within one community. There are also facilities that provide skilled nursing and custodial care, assisted living, home care, day care, respite care, and hospice.

The community health perspective includes a case management approach that offers a centralized system for assessing the needs of older people and then matching those needs with the appropriate services. The PHN should also seek to serve the entire older population by assessing the needs of the population, examining the available services, and analyzing their effectiveness. The effectiveness of programs can be measured according to four important criteria (targeted to the specific needs of the population): comprehensiveness, effective coordination, accessibility, and quality.

The PHN can make significant contributions to the health of the older population as a whole by being aware of new developments and programs that become available, new regulations, and innovative social and economic forces and their impacts on the provision of health services. More importantly, the nurse can design interventions that maximize nursing resources and provide the greatest benefit to the older adult population.

ACTIVITIES TO PROMOTE **CRITICAL THINKING**

1. On the Internet, search for and download instructions for filling out your own advance directive. Complete the form for your state and discuss your wishes with someone who is likely to be involved in your health care.

2. Picture an older adult you know well or know a great deal about. Make a list of characteristics that describe this person. How many of these characteristics fit your picture of most senior citizens? What are your biases (ageisms) about them?

3. If you were Minnie Blackstone's community health nurse (see From the Case Files I), what interventions would you consider using to maintain and promote her health? Why?

4. As part of your regular community health nursing workload, you visit a senior day care center one afternoon each week. You take the blood pressures of several people who are taking antihypertensive medications and do some nutrition counseling. The center accommodates 60 senior clients, and you would like to serve the health needs of the aggregate population. List five potential health needs of this group. What actions might you consider taking at an aggregate level? With whom would you consult as you plan programs at the center?

5. Assume that you have been asked by your local health department to determine the needs of the older adult population in your community. How would you begin conducting a needs assessment? What data might you want to collect? How would you find out what services are already being offered and whether they are adequate?

6. Visit a continuing care center in your community. Assess the housing options, services, and health care provisions. Would you live here when you are older? How would you feel about a family member living here? What would you change if you could?

7. Search the Internet for examples of innovative programs for elders in the community at the primary, secondary, and tertiary levels of care. Determine whether such programs could work in your own community.

8. Discuss with a group of your classmates how you may be able to assist older adults with their spiritual health. What are important considerations to keep in mind? Pair with another student and practice how you would open a conversation about this with an elderly client.

9. In From the Case Files II, how would you address the subject of advance directives? Where could you locate information specific to your state? Who else should you include in this conversation? Why is it important to have current advance directives in place?

REFERENCES

AARP Public Policy Institute. (n.d.). *The village: A growing option for aging in place.* Retrieved from http://assets.aarp.org/rgcenter/ppi/liv-com/fs177-village.pdf

Administration on Aging. (2014). *A profile of older Americans: 2014.* Retrieved from http://www.aoa.acl.gov/Aging_Statistics/Profile/Index.aspx

Administration on Aging. (2015). *Elderly nutrition program.* Retrieved from http://www.acl.gov/NewsRoom/Publications/docs/Elderly_Nutrition_Programs_1.pdf

Ageism Hurts. (2015). *What is ageism.* Retrieved from http://ageismhurts.org/what-is-ageism

Alliance for Aging Research. (2015). *Our best shot: Expanding prevention through vaccination in older adults.* Retrieved from http://agingresearch.org/backend/app/webroot/files/Pressroom/136/Our%20Best%20Shot%20%20Expanding%20Prevention%20through%20Vaccination%20in%20Older%20Adults%20October%202015.PDF

Altarum Institute. (2012, September). *Recommendations to promote health and wellbeing among aging populations.* Retrieved from http://healthyamericans.org/assets/files/Prevention%20Recommendations%20for%20Aging%20Populations2.pdf

Alzheimer's Association. (2014). *2014 Alzheimer's disease facts and figures.* Retrieved from https://www.alz.org/downloads/facts_figures_2014.pdf

Alzheimer's Association. (2015a). *2015 Alzheimer's disease facts and figures.* Retrieved from http://www.alz.org/facts/overview.asp

Alzheimer's Association. (2015b). *Alzheimer's myths.* Retrieved from http://www.alz.org/alzheimers_disease_myths_about_alzheimers.asp

Alzheimer's Association. (2015c). *Risk factors.* Retrieved from http://www.alz.org/alzheimers_disease_causes_risk_factors.asp?WT.mc_id=risk_factors_02&gclid=CPyM2-aoxKkCFQsj7AodlA1Vkw

Alzheimer's Association. (2015d). *Stages of Alzheimer's.* Retrieved from http://www.alz.org/alzheimers_disease_stages_of_alzheimers.asp

American Association of Retired People (AARP). (2015a). *About continuing care retirement communities.* Retrieved from http://www.aarp.org/relationships/caregiving-resource-center/info-09-2010/ho_continuing_care_retirement_communities.html

American Association of Retired People (AARP). (2015b). *The cost of caregiving.* Retrieved from http://www.aarp.org/relationships/caregiving/info-01-2010/ginzler_impact_of_caregiving.html

American Cancer Society. (2014). *Cancer treatment & survivorship: Facts & figures.* Retrieved from http://www.cancer.org/acs/groups/content/@research/documents/document/acspc-042801.pdf

American Diabetes Association. (2015a). *Diabetes complications.* Retrieved from http://www.diabetes.org/living-with-diabetes/complications/

American Diabetes Association. (2015b). *FAST FACTS: Data and statistics about diabetes.* Retrieved from http://professional.diabetes.org/admin/UserFiles/0%20-%20Sean/Documents/Fast_Facts_3-2015.pdf

American Foundation for Suicide Prevention. (2015). *Understanding suicide: Facts and figures.* Retrieved from https://www.afsp.org/understanding-suicide/facts-and-figures

American Medical Association. (2015). *Advance care directives.* Retrieved from http://www.ama-assn.org/ama/pub/physician-resources/medical-ethics/about-ethics-group/ethics-resource-center/end-of-life-care/advance-care-directives.page?

American Psychological Association. (2012). *Elder abuse: In search of solutions*. Retrieved from http://www.apa.org/pi/aging/resources/guides/elder-abuse.aspx

AmeriCorps. (2015). *AmeriCorps*. Retrieved from http://www.nationalservice.gov/programs/americorps

Bherer, L. (2015). Cognitive plasticity in older adults: Effects of cognitive training and physical exercise. *Annals of the New York Academy of Sciences, 1337*, 1–6.

Bherer, L., Erickson, K. L., & Liu-Ambrose, T. (2013). A review of the effects of physical activity and exercise on cognitive and brain functions in older adults. *Journal of Aging Research, 2013*, 657508. doi: 10.1155/2013/657508.

Bonita R., & Beaglehole R. (1988). Modification of Rankin Scale: Recovery of motor function after stroke. *Stroke, 19*(12), 1497–1500.

Braff, S., & Olenik, M. R. (2003). *Staying connected while letting go: The paradox of Alzheimer's caregiving*. New York, NY: M. Evans & Co.

Burtless, G. (2013). *The impact of population aging and delayed retirement on workforce productivity*. Retrieved from http://crr.bc.edu/wp-content/uploads/2013/05/wp_2013-111.pdf

Carpenter, G. H. (2013). The secretion, components, and properties of saliva. *Annual Review of Food Science Technology, 4*, 267–276.

Center on Aging Studies Without Walls. (n.d.). *Spirituality and aging*. Retrieved from http://cas.umkc.edu/casww/sa/spirituality.htm

Centers for Disease Control and Prevention (CDC). (2012a). *2012 top ten cancers*. Retrieved from https://nccd.cdc.gov/uscs/toptencancers.aspx

Centers for Disease Control and Prevention (CDC). (2012b). *Prevalence of obesity among older adults in the United States, 2007–2010*. Retrieved from http://www.cdc.gov/nchs/fastats/obesity-overweight.htm

Centers for Disease Control and Prevention (CDC). (2012c). *Defining adult overweight and obesity*. Retrieved from http://www.cdc.gov/obesity/adult/defining.html

Centers for Disease Control and Prevention (CDC). (2013a). *Arthritis-related statistics*. Retrieved from http://www.cdc.gov/arthritis/data_statistics/arthritis_related_stats.htm

Centers for Disease Control and Prevention (CDC). (2013b). *Cancer prevention and control*. Retrieved from http://www.cdc.gov/cancer/dcpc/prevention/other.htm

Centers for Disease Control and Prevention (CDC). (2013c). *The state of aging in America 2013*. Retrieved from http://www.cdc.gov/mmwr/preview/mmwrhtml/mm5206a2.htm

Centers for Disease Control and Prevention (CDC). (2014). *Physical activity*. Retrieved from http://www.cdc.gov/physicalactivity/growingstronger/index.html

Centers for Disease Control and Prevention (CDC). (2015a). *Addressing the nation's most common cause of disability: At a glance 2015*. Retrieved from http://www.cdc.gov/chronicdisease/resources/publications/aag/arthritis.htm

Centers for Disease Control and Prevention (CDC). (2015b). *Alzheimer's disease*. Retrieved from http://www.cdc.gov/aging/agingis.htm

Centers for Disease Control and Prevention (CDC). (2015c). *Arthritis: Addressing the nation's most common cause of disability: At a glance 2015*. Retrieved from http://www.cdc.gov/chronicdisease/resources/publications/aag/arthritis.htm

Centers for Disease Control and Prevention (CDC). (2015d). *Depression is not a normal part of growing older*. Retrieved from http://www.cdc.gov/aging/mentalhealth/depression.htm

Centers for Disease Control and Prevention (CDC). (2015e). *Health expenditures*. Retrieved from http://www.cdc.gov/nchs/fastats/health-expenditures.htm

Centers for Disease Control and Prevention (CDC). (2015f). *Heart disease*. Retrieved from http://www.cdc.gov/heartdisease/statistics.html

Centers for Disease Control and Prevention (CDC). (2015g). *Heart disease facts and statistics*. Retrieved from http://www.cdc.gov/heartdisease/statistics.htm

Centers for Disease Control and Prevention (CDC). (2015h). *Older adult drivers*. Retrieved from http://www.cdc.gov/motorvehiclesafety/older_adult_drivers/

Centers for Disease Control and Prevention (CDC). (2015i). *Older adult drivers data & statistics*. Retrieved from http://www.cdc.gov/Motorvehiclesafety/Older_Adult_Drivers/data.html

Centers for Disease Control and Prevention (CDC). (2015j). *Older persons' health*. Retrieved from http://www.cdc.gov/nchs/fastats/older-american-health.htm

Centers for Disease Control and Prevention (CDC). (2015k). *Oral and dental health*. Retrieved from http://www.cdc.gov/nchs/fastats/dental.htm

Centers for Disease Control and Prevention (CDC). (2015l). *The oral health of older Americans*. Retrieved from http://www.cdc.gov/nchs/data/ahcd/agingtrends/03oral.pdf

Centers for Disease Control and Prevention (CDC). (2015m). *Recommended adult immunization schedule, by vaccine and age group*. Retrieved from http://www.cdc.gov/vaccines/schedules/hcp/imz/adult.html

Centers for Disease Control and Prevention (CDC). (2015n). *Shingles vaccination: What you need to know*. Retrieved from http://www.cdc.gov/vaccines/vpd-vac/shingles/vacc-need-know.htm

Centers for Disease Control and Prevention (CDC). (2015o). *Caregiving*. Retrieved from http://www.cdc.gov/aging/caregiving/index.html

Centers for Disease Control and Prevention (CDC). (2015p). *Estimating seasonal influenza-associated deaths in the United States: CDC study confirms variability of flu*. Retrieved from http://www.cdc.gov/flu/about/disease/us_flu-related_deaths.htm

Centers for Disease Control and Prevention (CDC). (2015q). *Nursing home care*. Retrieved from http://www.cdc.gov/nchs/fastats/nursing-home-care.htm

Centers for Disease Control and Prevention (CDC). (2015r). *Racial and ethnic approaches to community health (REACH)*. Retrieved from www.cdc.gov/nccdphp/dch/programs/reach

Centers for Medicare & Medicaid Services. (2015). *NHE fact sheet*. Retrieved from https://www.cms.gov/research-statistics-data-and-systems/statistics-trends-and-reports/nationalhealthexpenddata/nhe-fact-sheet.html

Central Intelligence Agency. (2015). *The world factbook*. Retrieved from https://www.cia.gov/library/publications/the-world-factbook/geos/xx.html

Corporation for National & Community Service. (n.d.). *Foster grandparents*. Retrieved from http://www.nationalservice.gov/programs/senior-corps/foster-grandparents

Duke University. (2014). *Older Americans resources and services (OARS): The methods and its uses*. Center for the Study of Aging and Human Development. Retrieved from http://centerforaging.duke.edu/services/141

Eldercare.gov. (2015). *Hospice care*. Retrieved from http://www.eldercare.gov/Eldercare.NET/Public/Resources/Factsheets/Hospice_Care.aspx

Environmental Alliance for Senior Involvement. (2015). *Volunteer opportunities for the elderly*. Retrieved from www.easi.org/

Food and Drug Administration (FDA). (2015). *Fighting diabetes' deadly impact on minorities*. Retrieved from http://www.fda.gov/ForConsumers/ConsumerUpdates/ucm389919.htm

Genworth. (2015). *Compare long term care costs across the United States*. Retrieved from https://www.genworth.com/corporate/about-genworth/industry-expertise/cost-of-care.html

Gerontology Research Group. (2015). *Supercentenarians*. Retrieved from http://www.grg.org/calment.html

Governor's Highway Safety Association. (2015). *Mature driver laws*. Retrieved from http://www.ghsa.org/html/stateinfo/laws/older-driver_laws.html

Graf, C. (2013). The Lawton instrumental activities of daily living (IADL) scale. *Try this: Best practices in nursing care to older adults*, Issue no. 23. Retrieved from http://consultgerirn.org/uploads/File/trythis/try_this_23.pdf

Greenberg, S. A. (2012). *Try this: Best practices in nursing care to older adults immunizations for older adults*. Retrieved from http://consultgerirn.org/uploads/File/trythis/try_this_21.pdf

Gutchess, A. (2014). Plasticity of the aging brain: New directions in cognitive neuroscience. *Science, 346*(6209), 579–582.

Hajjar, E. R., Hanlon, J.T., Sloan, R. J., Lindblad, C. I., Pieper, C. F., Ruby, C. M., ... Schmader, K. E. (2005). Unnecessary drug use in frail older people at hospital discharge. *Journal of the American Geriatric Association, 53*(9), 1518–1523.

Healthfinder.gov. (2015). *Lower your risk of falling*. Retrieved from http://healthfinder.gov/prevention/ViewTopic.aspx?topicID=17&cnt=1&areaID=5

Healthy People 2020. (2015a). *Dementias, including Alzheimer's disease*. Retrieved from http://www.healthypeople.gov/2020/topicsobjectives2020/overview.aspx?topicid=7

Healthy People 2020. (2015b). *Find evidence-based information and recommendations related to older adults.* Retrieved from http://www.healthypeople.gov/2020/topics-objectives/topic/older-adults/ebrs

Healthy People 2020. (2015c). *Sleep health.* Retrieved from http://www.healthypeople.gov/2020/topicsobjectives2020/overview.aspx?topicid=38

Healthy People 2020. (2015d). *Healthy People 2020 leading health indicators: Progress update.* Retrieved from http://www.healthy-people.gov/2020/leading-health-indicators/Healthy-People-2020-Leading-Health-Indicators%3A-Progress-Update

HelpGuide. (2015a). *Adult day care.* Retrieved from http://www.help-guide.org/articles/caregiving/adult-day-care-services.htm

HelpGuide. (2015b). *Age-related memory loss.* Retrieved from http://www.helpguide.org/articles/memory/age-related-memory-loss.htm

HelpGuide. (2015c). *Assisted living facilities.* Retrieved from http://www.helpguide.org/articles/senior-housing/assisted-living-facilities.htm

HelpGuide. (2015d). *Coping with grief and loss.* Retrieved from http://www.helpguide.org/home-pages/grief-loss.htm

HelpGuide. (2015e). *A guide to nursing homes.* Retrieved from http://www.helpguide.org/articles/senior-housing/guide-to-nursing-homes.htm

HelpGuide. (2015f). *Home care services for seniors: Services to help you stay at home.* Retrieved from http://www.helpguide.org/articles/senior-housing/home-care-services-for-seniors.htm

HelpGuide. (2015g). *How to improve your memory.* Retrieved from http://www.helpguide.org/articles/memory/how-to-improve-your-memory.htm

HelpGuide. (2015h). *Senior housing.* Retrieved from http://www.help-guide.org/home-pages/senior-housing.htm

HelpGuide. (2015i). *Sleep.* Retrieved from http://www.helpguide.org/home-pages/sleep.htm

Holland, K. (2014). *Older Americans are ill-prepared for hefty health-care costs: Study.* Retrieved from http://www.cnbc.com/2014/10/14/older-americans-are-ill-prepared-for-hefty-health-care-costs-study.html

Igari, K., Kudo, T., Toyofuku, T., Inoue, Y., & Iwai, T. (2014). Association between periodontitis and the development of systemic diseases. *Oral Biology and Dentistry, 2,* 4. http://dx.doi.org/10.7243/2053-5775-2-4

International Osteoporosis Foundation. (n.d.). *Facts and statistics.* Retrieved from http://www.iofbonehealth.org/facts-statistics

John Hancock. (2013, July 30). *John Hancock national study finds long-term care costs continue to climb across all provider options.* Retrieved from http://www.johnhancock.com/about/news_details.php?fn=jul3013-text&yr=2013

Kaiser Family Foundation. (2013). *Trends in U.S. health spending.* Retrieved from http://kff.org/health-costs/

Kaiser Family Foundation. (2015a). *Medicaid moving forward.* Retrieved from http://kff.org/health-reform/issue-brief/medicaid-moving-forward/

Kaiser Family Foundation. (2015b). *Poverty among seniors: An updated analysis of national and state level poverty rates under the official and supplemental poverty measures.* Retrieved from http://kff.org/medicare/issue-brief/poverty-among-seniors-an-updated-analysis-of-national-and-state-level-poverty-rates-under-the-official-and-supplemental-poverty-measures/

Katz, S. (1963). Studies of illness in the aged. The index of ADL: A standardized measure of biological and psychosocial function. *Journal of the American Medical Association, 185,* 914–919.

Kokkinos, P. (2012). Physical activity, health benefits, and mortality risk. *International Scholarly Research Notices, 2012,* Article ID 718789, 14 pages. doi: 10.5402/2012/718789.

Kozol, J. (2015). *The theft of memory: Losing my father, one day at a time.* New York, NY: Crown Publishers.

Kübler-Ross, E. (1969). *On death and dying.* Touchstone, NY: Scribner.

Mace, N. L., & Rabins, P. V. (2006). *The 36-hour day: A family guide to caring for people with Alzheimer disease, other dementias, and memory loss in later life.* Baltimore, MD: The Johns Hopkins University Press.

Maercker, A., & Lalor, J. (2012). Diagnostic and clinical considerations in prolonged grief disorder. *Dialogues in Clinical Neurosciences, 14*(2), 167–176.

Maher, R. L., Hanlon, J. T., & Hajjar, E. R. (2014). Clinical consequences of polypharmacy in the elderly. *Expert Opinion on Drug Safety, 13*(1).

Mahoney, F., & Barthel, D. (1965). Functional evaluation: The Barthel Index. *Maryland State Medical Journal, 14,* 56–61.

McCoyd, J. L. M., & Walter, C. A. (2016). *Grief and loss across the lifespan: A biopsychosocial perspective* (2nd ed.). New York, NY: Springer Publishing Co.

Medicare.gov. (2015a). *Medicare benefits.* Retrieved from http://www.medicare.gov/navigation/medicare-basics/medicare-benefits/medicare-benefits-overview.aspx

Medicare.gov. (2015b). *What's not covered by part A & part B?* Retrieved from https://www.medicare.gov/what-medicare-covers/not-covered/item-and-services-not-covered-by-part-a-and-b.html

Medicare.gov. (2016). *Your Medicare coverage.* Retrieved from https://www.medicare.gov/coverage/hospital-care-inpatient.html

Medline Plus. (2015). *Assisted living.* Retrieved from https://www.nlm.nih.gov/medlineplus/assistedliving.html

Morgan, R. E., & Mason, B. J. (2014). *Special report: Crimes against the elderly, 2003–2013.* Retrieved from http://www.bjs.gov/content/pub/pdf/cae0313.pdf

National Alliance for Caregiving and the AARP Public Policy Institute. (2015). *Caregiving in the U.S. 2015.* Retrieved from http://www.caregiving.org/caregiving2015/

National Center for Assisted Living. (2015). *Assisted living: Resident profile.* Retrieved from http://www.ahcancal.org/ncal/resources/Pages/ResidentProfile.aspx

National Center for Biotechnology Information. (2015). *Osteoporosis.* Retrieved from http://www.ncbi.nlm.nih.gov/pubmedhealth/PMH0001400/

National Center on Elder Abuse. (n.d.a). *Frequently asked questions.* Retrieved from http://ncea.acl.gov/faq/index.aspx

National Center on Elder Abuse. (n.d.b). *Statistics/data.* Retrieved from http://www.ncea.aoa.gov/Library/Data/index.aspx

National Council on Aging. (n.d.a). *Falls prevention facts.* Retrieved from https://www.ncoa.org/news/resources-for-reporters/get-the-facts/falls-prevention-facts/

National Council on Aging. (n.d.b). *Six steps to protect your older loved one from a fall.* Retrieved from https://www.ncoa.org/healthy-aging/falls-prevention/preventing-falls-tips-for-older-adults-and-caregivers/6-steps-to-protect-your-older-loved-one-from-a-fall/

National Foundation for Infectious Diseases. (2015). *Influenza.* Retrieved from http://www.nfid.org/influenza/

National Hospice and Palliative Care Organization. (2015). *Choosing a hospice.* Retrieved from http://wiww.nhpco.org

National Hospice and Palliative Care Organization. (n.d.). *Download your state's advance directives.* Retrieved from http://www.caring-info.org/i4a/pages/index.cfm?pageid=3289

National Institute of Arthritis and Musculoskeletal and Skin Diseases (NIAMS). (2014a). *Living with arthritis: Health information basics for you and your family.* Retrieved from http://www.niams.nih.gov/Health_Info/Arthritis/default.asp

National Institute of Arthritis and Musculoskeletal and Skin Diseases (NIAMS). (2014b). *Rheumatoid arthritis.* Retrieved from http://www.niams.nih.gov/Health_Info/Rheumatic_Disease/default.asp

National Institute of Arthritis and Musculoskeletal and Skin Diseases (NIAMS). (2015). *Arthritis.* Retrieved from http://www.niams.nih.gov/Health_Info/Arthritis/default.asp

National Institute of Justice. (2013). *Identifying elder abuse.* Retrieved from http://www.nij.gov/topics/crime/elder-abuse/pages/identifying.aspx

National Institute of Justice. (2015a). *Extent of elder abuse victimization.* Retrieved from http://www.nij.gov/topics/crime/elder-abuse/Pages/extent.aspx

National Institute of Justice. (2015b). *Financial exploitation of the elderly.* Retrieved from http://www.nij.gov/topics/crime/elder-abuse/pages/financial-exploitation.aspx

National Institute of Mental Health. (2015). *Depression.* Retrieved from http://www.nimh.nih.gov/health/publications/depression/index.shtml

National Institute on Aging. (2015a). *About Alzheimer's disease: Diagnosis.* Retrieved from https://www.nia.nih.gov/alzheimers/topics/diagnosis

National Institute on Aging. (2015b). *Exercise & physical activity: Your everyday guide from the National Institute on Aging.* Retrieved from https://www.nia.nih.gov/health/publication/exercise-physical-activity/introduction

National Institute on Aging. (2015c). *Why population aging matters: A global perspective.* Retrieved from https://www.nia.nih.

gov/publication/why-population-aging-matters-global-perspective/trend-3-rising-numbers-oldest-old

National Institute on Drug Abuse. (2014). *Prescription drug abuse.* Retrieved from http://www.drugabuse.gov/publications/research-reports/prescription-drugs/trends-in-prescription-drug-abuse/older-adults

National PACE Association. (2015). *Is PACE for you?* Retrieved from http://www.npaonline.org/pace-you

National Sleep Foundation. (n.d.). *Aging and sleep.* Retrieved from https://sleepfoundation.org/sleep-topics/aging-and-sleep

New World Encyclopedia. (2015). *Spirit.* Retrieved from http://www.newworldencyclopedia.org/entry/Spirit

Noronha, K. J. (2015). Impact of religion and spirituality on older adulthood. *Journal of Religion, Spirituality & Aging, 27*(1), 16–33.

Omnibus Budget Reconciliation Act. (1987). *Federal nursing home reform act from the Omnibus Budget Reconciliation Act of 1987.* Retrieved from www.ncmust.com/doclib/OBRA87summary.pdf

Ortman, J., Velkoff, V., & Hogan, H. (2014). The older population in the United States, current population reports, P25-1140. *U.S. Census Bureau.* Retrieved from https://www.census.gov/prod/2014pubs/p25-1140.pdf

Pappas-Rogich, M. (2012). Faith community nurses: Protecting our elders through immunizations. *Journal of Christian Nursing, 29*(4), 232–237.

Partners for Livable Communities. (2015). *The aging in place initiative.* Retrieved from www.livable.org/livability-resources/16-aging?start=21

Pavlopoulos, E., Jones, S., Kosmidis, S., Close, M., Kim, C., Kovalerchik, O., ... Kandel, E. R. (2013). Molecular mechanism for age-related memory loss: The histone-binding protein RbAp48. *Science Translational Medicine, 5*(200), 200ra115.

Peace Corps. (2015). *Volunteer programs.* Retrieved from http://www.peacecorps.gov/volunteer/

Pew Research Center. (2014). *Number of older Americans in the workforce is on the rise.* Retrieved from http://www.pewresearch.org/fact-tank/2014/01/07/number-of-older-americans-in-the-workforce-is-on-the-rise/

Public Citizen's Health Research Group (PCHRG). (2015). *Drug-induced diseases.* Retrieved from http://www.worstpills.org/public/page.cfm?op_id=5

Racial and Ethnic Approaches to Community Health (REACH). (2015). *About REACH.* Retrieved from http://www.cdc.gov/reach/about.htm

Raue, P. J., Ghesquiere, A. R., & Bruce, M. L. (2014). Suicide risk in primary care: Identification and management in older adults. *Current Psychiatry Reports, 16*(9), 466–478.

Reiner, M., Niermann, C., Jekauc, D., & Woll, A. (2013). Long-term health benefits of physical activity: A systematic review of longitudinal studies. *BMC Public Health, 13*, 813. doi: 10.1186/1471-2458-13-813.

Road Scholar. (2015). *Explore the world with Road Scholar.* Retrieved from http://www.roadscholar.org/

Robnett, R. H., & Chop, W. C. (2015). *Gerontology for the health care professional* (3rd ed.). Burlington, MA: Jones and Bartlett Learning.

Rose, N. S., Rendell, P. G., Hering, A., Kliegel M., Bidelman, G. M., & Craik, F. (2015). Cognitive and neural plasticity in older adults' prospective memory following training with the Virtual Week computer game. *Frontiers in Human Neuroscience, 9*, 592. doi: 10.3389/fnhum.2015.00592.

Sallis, J. F., Buono, M. J., Roby, J. J., Micale, F. G., & Nelson, J. A. (1993). Seven-day recall and other physical activity self-reports in children and adolescents. *Medicine & Science in Sports & Exercise, 25*(1), 99–108.

Schumer, F. (2009, September 28). After a death, the pain that doesn't go away. *New York Times.* Retrieved from http://www.nytimes.com/2009/09/29/health/29grief.html?pagewanted=all&_r=0

Segen's Medical Dictionary. (2015). *Oldest old.* Retrieved from http://medical-dictionary.thefreedictionary.com/oldest+old

Senior Corps. (2015). *12 great reasons to become a senior volunteer.* Retrieved from http://www.seniorcorps.org

Storlie, T. A. (2015). *Person-centered communication with older adults: The professional provider's guide.* Boston, MA: Elsevier/Academic Press.

Sulter, G., Steen, C., & De Keyser, J. (1999). Use of the Barthel index and modified Rankin scale in acute stroke trials. *Stroke, 30*(8), 1538–1541.

Taylor, D. (2014). Physical activity is medicine for older adults. *Postgraduate Medical Journal, 90*, 26–32.

Touhy, T. A., & Jett, K. F. (2014). *Ebersole and Hess' gerontological nursing & healthy aging* (4th ed.). St. Louis, MO: Elsevier Mosby.

Tufts University. (2015). *MyPlate for older adults.* Retrieved from http://now.tufts.edu/news-releases/tufts-university-nutrition-scientists-unveil-

UC Davis Health System. (2015). *Elderly need special care in hot weather.* Retrieved from http://www.ucdmc.ucdavis.edu/welcome/features/20080723_healthtip_heat/index.html

U.S. Census Bureau. (2015). *The next four decades: The older population in the United States: 2010 to 2050.* Retrieved from http://www.census.gov/prod/2010pubs/p25-1138.pdf

U.S. Department of Agriculture. (2015). *MyPlate.* Retrieved from http://www.choosemyplate.gov/

U.S. Department of Health and Human Services (USDHHS). (2016). *Healthy people 2020: About healthy people.* Retrieved from http://healthypeople.gov/2020/about/default.aspx

U.S. Preventive Services Task Force. (2015). *Information for health professionals.* Retrieved from http://www.uspreventiveservicestask-force.org/Page/Name/tools-and-resources-for-better-preventive-care

United Nations. (2015). *The 2015 revision of world population prospects.* Retrieved from http://www.un.org/en/development/desa/population/events/other/10/index.shtml

Vitelli, R. (2015, March 16). Grief, loneliness, and losing a spouse: Learning to live with grief and loneliness after the death of a spouse. *Psychology Today.* Retrieved from https://www.psychologytoday.com/blog/media-spotlight/201503/grief-loneliness-and-losing-spouse

Wallace, S. P. (2014–2015, Winter). Equity and social determinants of health among older adults. *Generations, 4*, 6–11.

Washburn, R. A., Smith, K. W., Jette, A. M., & Janney, C. A. (1993). The Physical Activity Scale for the Elderly (PASE): Development and evaluation. *Journal of Clinical Epidemiology, 46*(2), 153–162.

World Health Organization (WHO). (2012). *Key facts about cancer.* Retrieved from http://www.who.int/cancer/about/facts/en/

World Health Organization (WHO). (2015). *Obesity and overweight.* Retrieved from http://www.who.int/mediacentre/factsheets/fs311/en/

UNIT 7

PROMOTING AND PROTECTING THE HEALTH OF VULNERABLE POPULATIONS

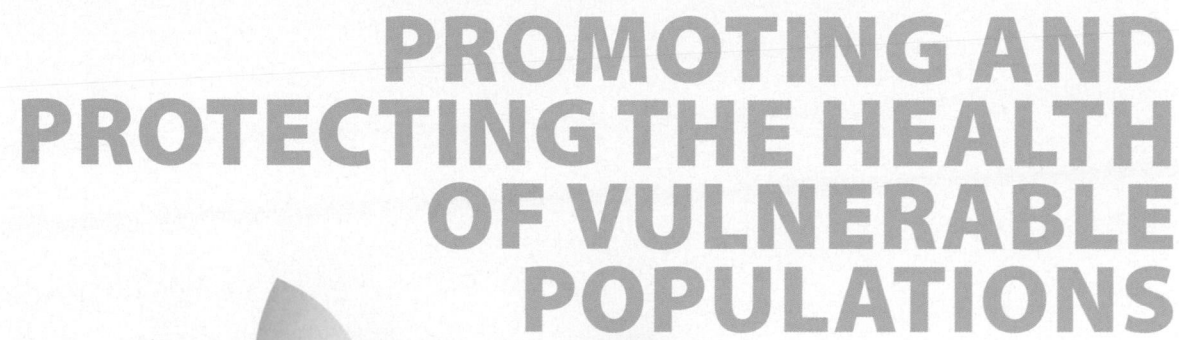

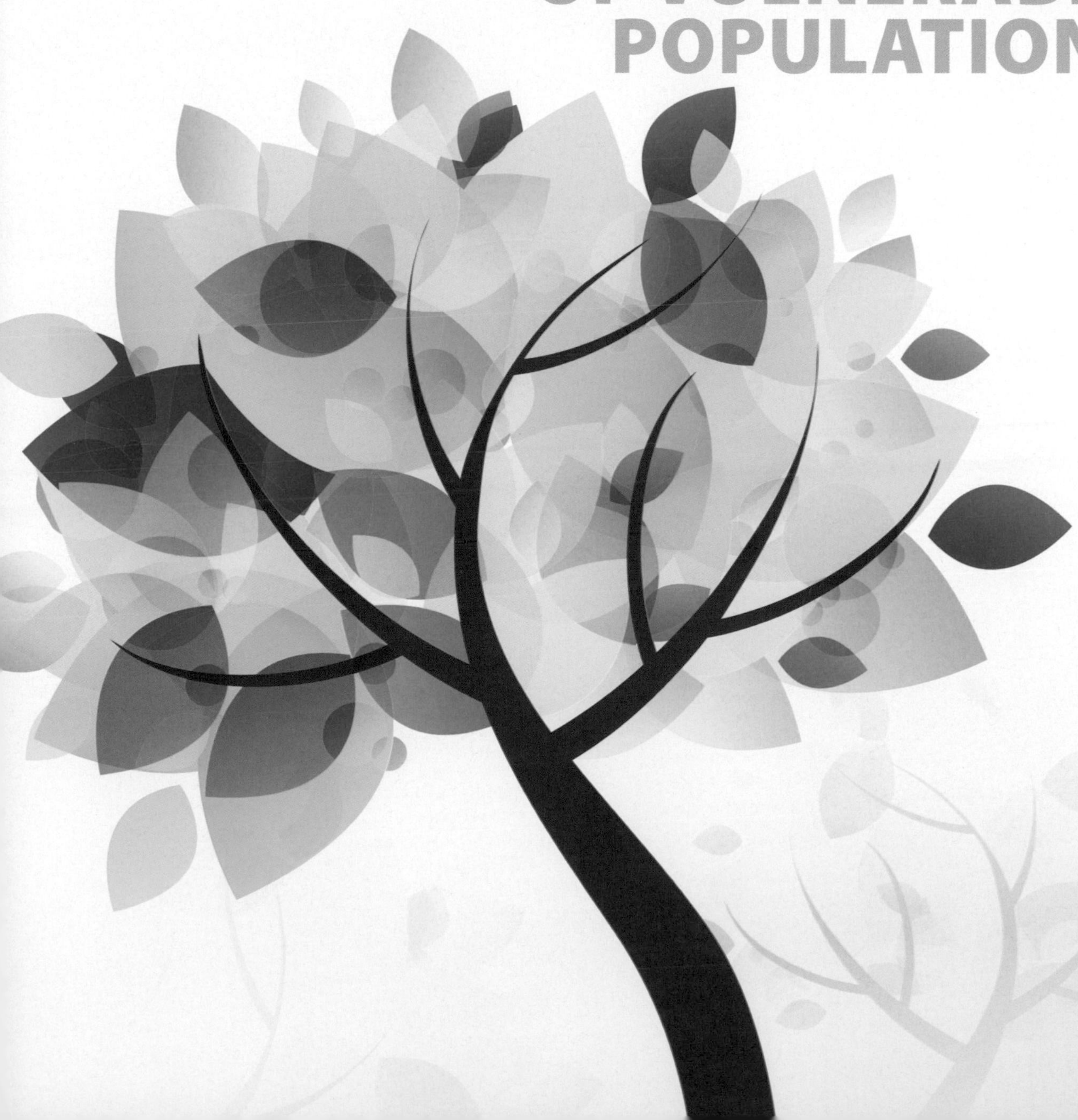

Working with Vulnerable People

"How far you go in life depends on your being tender with the young, compassionate with the aged, sympathetic with the striving, and tolerant of the weak and the strong—because someday you will have been all of these."

—*George Washington Carver* (1860–1943), **Botanist and Scientist**

KEY TERMS

Differential vulnerability
  hypothesis
Empowerment strategies
Environmental resources

Health disparities
Human capital
Racial/ethnic disparities
Racism

Relative risk
Social capital
Social determinants of health
Socioeconomic gradient

Socioeconomic resources
Vulnerability
Vulnerable populations

LEARNING OBJECTIVES

Upon mastery of this chapter, you should be able to:

- Describe the term "vulnerable populations."
- Describe and explain a conceptual model of vulnerability.
- Discuss the effects of vulnerability and relative risk.
- Differentiate between the concepts of social capital and human capital.
- Identify the key premise of the differential vulnerability hypothesis.
- List three of the most common factors related to vulnerability.
- Explain the socioeconomic gradient in health.
- Describe three types of health disparities.
- Describe four PHN roles or behaviors that help promote client empowerment.

Vulnerability is susceptibility to poor health. The public health nurse (PHN) caseload often consists largely of vulnerable populations. Often, **vulnerable populations** are subpopulations, such as ethnic or racial minorities, the uninsured, those with HIV/AIDS, children, the elderly, the poor, and those who are homeless (Shi & Stevens, 2011; Stremikis, Berensohn, Shih, & Riley, 2011). These subpopulations often have higher morbidity and mortality rates, less access to health care (and disparities in outcomes of health care), shorter life expectancy, and an overall diminished quality of life than does the population in general (Agency for Healthcare Research and Quality [AHRQ], 2015; Shi & Stevens, 2011).

In this chapter, we examine popular models and theories of vulnerability, important concepts, and contributing factors. We also briefly discuss health disparities that are more common among vulnerable members of society and the role of PHNs working with these groups. This chapter provides an overview of this subject and lays the foundation for other chapters in this section.

THE CONCEPT OF VULNERABLE POPULATIONS

Models and Theories of Vulnerability

Flaskerud and Winslow (1998) developed a popular conceptual framework of vulnerability that contains three related concepts: resource availability, relative risk, and health status (de Chesnay & Anderson, 2016). The authors posited that a lack of resources (e.g., socioeconomic and environmental) increases a population's exposure to risk factors and reduces individuals' ability to avoid illness. A community's health status can be observed by noting disease prevalence along with morbidity and mortality rates. Within this framework, the more risk a population faces, the greater the effect on their health status (e.g., higher morbidity and mortality rates). A feedback loop exists from health status to resource availability as higher morbidity and mortality further deplete community resources (Fig. 25–1). The central point of the model demonstrates the importance of nursing research and practice, along with ethical and policy analysis, in affecting resources, relative risk, and health status. This can occur by direct interaction with one or more of these three factors (e.g., reducing risk factors through education) or indirectly through intervention at the junction of two factors (e.g., working to minimize morbidity related to a specific risk factor such as encouraging the consistent use of statins for hypercholesterolemia).

To further define model components, Flaskerud and Winslow explained that **socioeconomic resources** include human capital (e.g., jobs, income, housing, education), social connectedness or integration (e.g., social networks or ties; social support or the lack of it, characterized by marginalization), and social status (e.g., position, power, role). **Environmental resources** deal mostly with access to health care and the quality of that care. The authors noted the differential access to health care among the poor, different ethnic and racial groups, and other underserved populations. Limited access or lack of access to care can arise from many sources, including crime-ridden neighborhoods, insufficient transportation systems, lack of adequate numbers and types of providers, limited choices of health care plans, or no health insurance. **Relative risk** refers to exposure to risk factors identified by a substantial body of research as lifestyle, behaviors and choices (e.g., diet, exercise, use of tobacco, alcohol and other drugs, sexual behaviors), use of health screening services (e.g., mammogram, colonoscopy), and stressful events (e.g., crime, violence, abuse, firearm use). The authors noted, for instance, that in populations of single-parent female-headed homes in poverty with little or no access to social programs, violence and homicide are more prevalent. Flaskerud and Winslow provided evidence of the link between poor health status and socioeconomic resource availability through the loss of income, jobs, and health insurance. In the case of environmental resources, high morbidity in an already underserved population will only exacerbate access problems. See Figure 25–1 for Flaskerud and Winslow's Vulnerable Populations Conceptual Model.

This conceptual model has generated a large body of research. Selected studies are displayed in Display 25–1. Adaptations of the model and extensions to newer conceptual frameworks include a framework to develop advocacy and promote empowerment in African American grandmothers caring for their grandchildren (Carr, 2011),

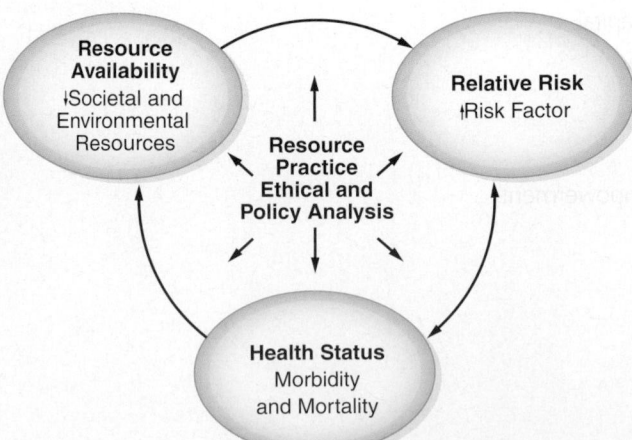

FIGURE 25–1 Vulnerable populations conceptual model. (Adapted from Flaskerud, J. H., & Winslow, B. J. (1998). Conceptualizing vulnerable populations health-related research. *Nursing Research,* 47(2), 69–78.)

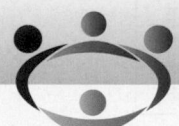

DISPLAY 25-1 SELECTED STUDIES USING FLASKERUD AND WINSLOW'S VULNERABLE POPULATIONS CONCEPTUAL MODEL

Author(s) (Year)	Vulnerable Population	Focus of Study
Flaskerud and Nyamathi (2000)	Low-income Latina women	HIV education, counseling, and testing
Missildine et al. (2009)	Special medical needs evacuees during Hurricane Gustav	Nursing interventions
Cloutier-Fisher and Kobayashi (2009)	Socially isolated populations in Canada	Public health planning
Scott (2009)	African American men	Health promotion intervention
Copeland (2007)	Family members of violent mentally ill	Conceptualizing family members as vulnerable population
Sumner, Wong, Schetter, Myers, and Rodreguez (2011)	Low-income pregnant and postpartum Latinas	Predicting posttraumatic stress disorder symptoms
Springer, Black, Martz, Deckys, and Soelberg (2010)	Somali Bantu refugees in Idaho	Cultural assessment
Strehlow and Gongwa (2005)	Vulnerable populations in academic nursing center for homeless	Administrative perspectives of vulnerable populations
Salem et al. (2013)	Homeless adults	Frailty
Flynn, Budd, and Modelsk (2008)	Pregnant adolescents	Enhancing utilization of resources
Gonzalez-Guarda, Peragallo, Vasquez, Urrutia, and Mitrani (2009)	Hispanic women	Relationship among resource availability, intimate partner violence, and depression
Albarran and Nyamathi (2011)	HIV and Mexican migrant workers in the United States	Review of literature
Kueny, Berg, Chowdhury, and Anderson (2011)	Children in homes of Latino families	Assessment of cultural and environmental barriers to making asthma-focused changes
Rawlett (2011)	Medically underserved, rural populations	Vulnerability
Palmer et al. (2014)	Older adults	Risk reduction of vulnerability to nursing home placement

a model for risk reduction among older adults vulnerable to nursing home placement (Palmer et al., 2014), living with spinal cord injury (Fyffe, Botticello, & Myaskovsky, 2011), and developing a Caregiver Empowerment Model for family members caring for aging parents (Jones, Winslow, Lee, Burns, & Esther-Zhang, 2011).

Gelberg, Andersen, and Leake (2000) advanced another classic model, the Behavioral Model for Vulnerable Populations, looking at population characteristics (predisposing and enabling factors and needs) as an explanation for health behaviors and eventual health outcomes (Burg & Oyama, 2016). Predisposing factors included demographic variables (e.g., gender, age, marital status), social variables (e.g., education, employment, ethnicity, social networks), and health beliefs (e.g., values and attitudes toward health and health care services, knowledge of disease). Social structures (e.g., acculturation and immigration), sexual orientation, and childhood characteristics (e.g., mobility, living conditions, history of substance abuse, criminal behavior, victimization, or

mental illness) were also considered predisposing factors. Enabling factors included personal and family resources, as well as community resources (e.g., income, insurance, social support, region, health services resources, public benefits, transportation, telephone, crime rates, social services resources). Perceived health needs and population health conditions also were considered, as were health behaviors including diet, exercise, tobacco use, self-care, and adherence to care. The use of health services (e.g., ambulatory and inpatient care, long-term care, alternative health care) and personal health practices (e.g., hygiene, unsafe sexual behaviors, food sources) combined with the other factors to produce outcomes such as perceived and evaluated health and general satisfaction with health care services. The model has been used in research with homeless adults (Stein, Andersen, Robertson, & Gelberg, 2012) and in examining barriers to interconceptual care (Hogan et al., 2012), with mixed results. See Figure 25–2 Interrelated Pathways Linking Education to Health.

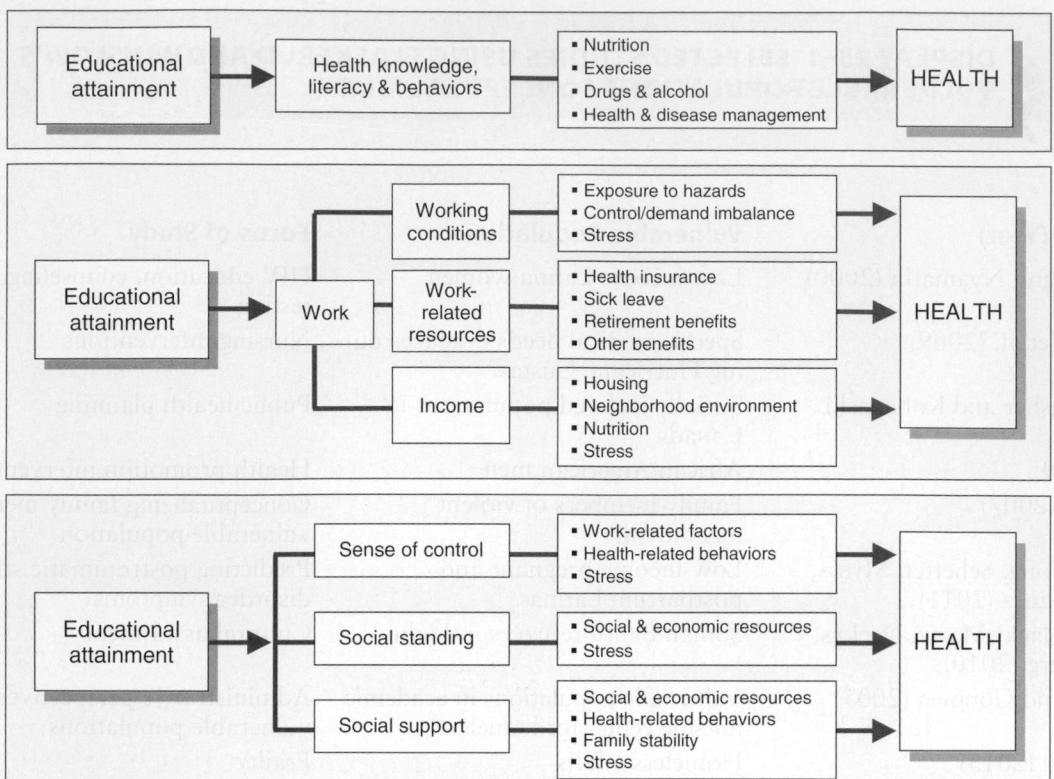

FIGURE 25–2 Interrelated pathways linking education to health. (From Braveman, P., Ergerter, S., & Williams, D. R. (2011). The social determinants of health: Coming of age. *Annual Review of Public Health, 32*, 381–398, 386, used with permission.)

LuAnn Aday (2001) advanced the well-known Framework for Studying Vulnerable Populations that includes both macro- and microperspectives (Burg & Oyama, 2016). Aday described the effects of policies on both communities and individuals, including social and economic policies, community-oriented health policies, as well as medical care and public health policies. She noted that community resources (e.g., strong neighborhoods, close ties between citizens) have a direct effect on individual resources (e.g., social status, social ties, human capital). For instance, a community with a high proportion of children, adolescents, and elderly and a majority of single female-headed households will likely also be characterized by lower education levels, higher unemployment, and lower income levels along with a subsequently higher relative risk of poor health status. When strong social networks are present and housing is adequate, the relative risk of poor psychological, social, or physical health decreases.

Aday subscribed to a **differential vulnerability hypothesis** that "negative or stressful events (such as unemployment, divorce, or death of a loved one) hurt some people more than others" (2001, p. 4). Even though we all are subjected to stressful events (nursing school, for instance), Aday cited research showing that low socioeconomic status (SES) groups, for example, are more adversely affected by stressful or negative events than are those with higher SES. Chronic stressors manifested by the lack of material resources and social marginalization experienced in childhood and early adolescence can lead to real physical changes and are the basis of vul-

nerability to poor health in adulthood. The relationship between lower SES and poor health persists throughout childhood and adolescence into adulthood (Cheng, Goodman, & Committee on Pediatric Research, 2015; Doubeni et al., 2012). Childhood traumas are associated with an increase in "inflammatory transcription" in later adulthood (Levine, Cole, Weir, & Crimmins, 2015, p. 16). Childhood traumas also potentiated the effect of low SES in adulthood on elevated "inflammatory gene expression" (p. 16); researchers believe that early childhood traumas may affect the stress response throughout life and influence health outcomes in later adult life, especially for those who have lower SES. The expression and interaction of these developmental genes with physical and social environments can produce long-term poor health outcomes. In other words, early chronic stressors can induce physiological changes that lead to later negative health outcomes.

Like Flaskerud and Winslow, Aday noted that social status (e.g., age, gender, race, ethnicity) affects social capital and human capital. **Social capital** consists of marital status, family structure, social ties and networks, and membership in voluntary organizations, such as a church or clubs. Aday linked **human capital** to investments in individuals' capabilities and skills (e.g., education, job training) and noted that human capital encompasses jobs, income, housing, and education. Aday described research showing that better health status is associated with higher education levels and noted that the personal and political power of individuals and communities differentially affect their efforts to gain access to adequate schools, housing, and employment. "The social status and social capital resources of individuals and groups in a community influence the level of investments that are likely to be made in the schools, jobs, housing, and associated earning potential of the families and individuals living within it" (2001, p. 8).

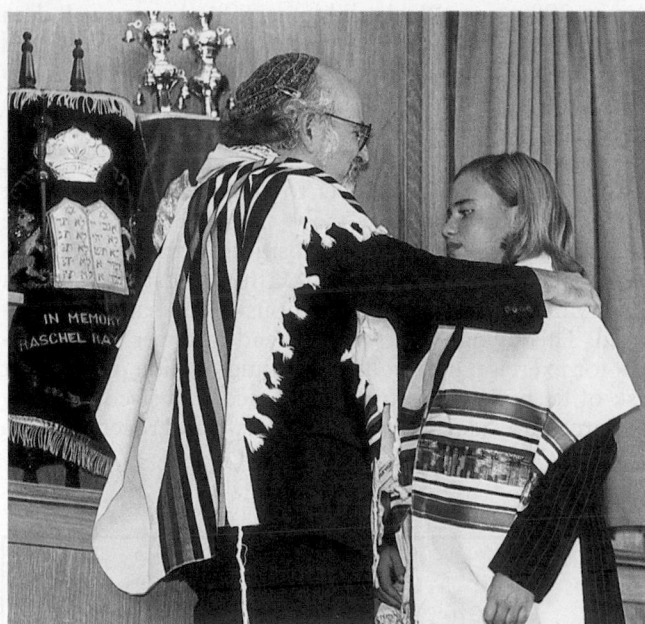

Social capital can include social ties and networks afforded by religious affiliations.

The importance of social capital is sometimes missed, as it can be subtle and less obvious than the lack of money or jobs. But the presence of friends and family or someone to rely on in case of an emergency can be invaluable in assisting individuals through many of life's difficulties. Social support, or a close confidante, can promote social and psychological health and help counteract the effects of stressful events. In our mobile society, many people live great distances from family members and have difficulty establishing new friendships. Those who live alone or who are socially isolated are at greatest risk of vulnerability, increased morbidity and mortality, and decreased overall health (Lubben, Gironda, Sabbath, Kong, & Johnson, 2015); thus, PHNs should be aware of this and strive to provide additional support and resources.

A general model of vulnerability helps to explain individual and community risk factors that lead to vulnerability, as well as problems with access to care and quality of care received that impact health outcomes on both an individual and community level as described in a seminal article by Shi, Stevens, Lebrun, Faed, and Tsai (2008). Vulnerable populations often experience clusters of risk factors, and these are viewed as cumulative. The specific combinations of risks (e.g., low income, low education) are more detrimental to health outcomes, as is the greater number of risk factors that accumulate over time.

Most nursing students are familiar with Maslow's Hierarchy of Needs (Maslow, 1987), with physiological needs (e.g., water, food, air) as the base of a pyramid, and the needs for safety, belonging, esteem, and self-actualization building from the basic needs. Chronic poverty, environments of crime and violence, or disenfranchisement, racism, and discrimination (vulnerability) can keep people from meeting the higher needs (Bates, 2016). **Racism** is largely defined as believing that race is the primary factor of our capacities and traits as humans and that any racial differences result in feelings of either superiority or inferiority.

Who Is Considered Vulnerable?

In her classic book, Aday (2001) included the following factors and populations in the description of who is considered vulnerable:

- Income and education
- Age and gender
- Race and ethnicity
- Chronic illness and disability
- HIV/AIDS
- Mental illness and disability
- Alcohol and substance abuse
- Familial abuse
- Homelessness
- Suicide and homicide risk
- High-risk mothers and infants
- Immigrants and refugees

Other authors considered the uninsured and underinsured as vulnerable populations because of their difficulties with health care access and the potential for poor health outcomes, as well as victims of bullying and crime, children in foster care, those in the gay/lesbian community, veterans and returning military personnel, and victims/survivors of torture and terrorism (Gitterman, 2014; Shi & Stevens, 2011). Although many segments of the population may be considered vulnerable at some point in their lives, some population segments are more often identified as vulnerable because of their long-term situations (de Chesnay & Anderson, 2016). The very young and the very old have particular risk factors that increase their chances of poor health, as well as unique issues with access to health care. An extensive body of research substantiates the reality of higher morbidity and mortality rates for racial and ethnic minorities than for the White population, thus demonstrating **racial/ethnic disparities** in health (Cantu, Hayward, Hummer, & Chiu, 2013; Dubowitz, Basurto-Davila, & Lurie, 2011; Institute of Medicine [IOM], 2003; Neumayer & Plümper, 2015).

Prevalence of Vulnerable Populations and Causative Factors

Because many of the previously listed conditions and categories have overlapping populations, it is difficult to access accurate data and statistics for each group or category. For example, someone with little education and low income may also be a member of a racial or ethnic minority and may have inadequate housing along with a chronic illness and high-risk births. Rates of low birth weight and infant mortality, along with teenage pregnancy and inadequate prenatal care for mothers, are indicators of substantial problems in that particular area. For example, racial and ethnic differences have been found in studies of perinatal outcomes among mothers with gestational diabetes (Nguyen et al., 2012) and in birth outcomes studies in New York City (Almeida, Mulready-Ward, Bettegowda, & Ahluwalia, 2014).

Root causes of vulnerability, such as low SES, lack of insurance coverage, racism, and discrimination, have been widely researched. Which cause or causes are considered most important? The exact weight of the interaction of these causes has been difficult to ascertain. The current approach to understanding the complex interrelationships among the causes and factors related to vulnerability is to examine multiple determinants of health (Freudenberg & Olden, 2010; Krewski et al., 2014); this chapter focuses on the social determinants of health. See From the Case Files.

Poverty

If only one indicator is measured—poverty—it is evident that vulnerability touches a large segment of the American population, as well as the global one. An estimated 896 million people worldwide lived on or below $1.90 a day in 2012 (World Bank, 2015). Data indicated that in 2014, about 46.7 million people in the United States (14.8%)

lived in poverty (Center for Poverty Research, University of California, & Davis, n.d.). For 2015, the poverty thresholds were $11,670 for a single individual, $15,730 for a family of two, and $23,850 for a family of four (U.S. Department of Health and Human Services [USDHHS], 2014). In 2013, about 15.6 million (22%) of all American children under 18 years of age were in families living in poverty. However, there are racial/ethnic disparities as 39% were Black children, 36% American Indian and Alaskan Native, 32% Hispanic, 13% White, and 13% Asian. The percentage of children living in poverty increased 4% from 2008 to 2013 (Institute of Education Sciences & National Center for Education Statistics, n.d.).

How does poverty make one vulnerable to poor health outcomes? The answer to this question is complex and is being addressed by many investigators to provide a complete answer. One supposition is that having less money means being less able to afford most aspects of a quality life, including adequate housing in a safe neighborhood. This living situation may lead to fewer opportunities for exercise, especially if walking outside puts one at risk of becoming a victim of violence. Fewer community resources are usually available, such as grocery stores,

---

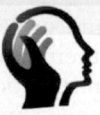 ### From the Case Files I

Natalie and the Social Determinants of Health

My mother's high school friend, Natalie, had her first baby at age 16. He was 10 weeks early, and weighed a little over 2 lb. Her family was poor and mostly ate meals with a lot of fried meat and potatoes. They rarely bought fresh fruits and vegetables, and she worked at a nearby fast-food restaurant for minimum wage and no health insurance was available. She didn't know about family planning services, so she and her boyfriend had unprotected sex and she got pregnant. At that time, "no smoking" ordinances were not common, and even though she was not a smoker at the time, she was exposed to secondhand smoke at home and at work. Her older siblings had problems with substance abuse and her father was often violent with her mother. My mother helped her buy a pregnancy test at the local pharmacy, and she tried to find an obstetrician, but the closest one was 50 mi away. She had no car, and there was no bus service available. She didn't know about prenatal vitamins but wanted to have a healthy baby, so she "ate for two," especially when she could have free burgers and fries at work. It was difficult for her to exercise after dropping out of school, because the rural roads where she lived had no sidewalks; also, there were no parks or recreation facilities. She ended up with terribly severe headaches and saw bright stars in her visual field. She had to be rushed by taxi to the regional hospital, and they diagnosed her with preeclampsia; her son was born prematurely. He had to be on a ventilator in the NICU and had some cognitive deficits

that caused him a lot of later problems in school. He dropped out at the beginning of high school and then got into problems with substance abuse and the legal system. He is about 8 years older than me, and I hear about him from my mom. Natalie later developed respiratory problems and is now disabled, living on a fixed income from Social Security. She never married, but had two more children. I am now in nursing school and learning about vulnerable populations and social determinants of health in my public health nursing course. I talk with my mother every weekend by phone, and I asked her about her friend, Natalie. I now feel that I could begin to understand all of the things that were stacked against her in life. My mother finished high school and married my father, whose family owned a large farming interest in our county. She had a very different life than her friend, Natalie. She uses a treadmill every day at home and tries to cook healthy meals. My mom and dad have a good relationship, and my family lives a comfortable life. I have seen a real-life example of vulnerability and how social differences (e.g., poverty, education, social support) can affect health and social outcomes. I hope to learn more about how to change things for people who are more vulnerable, like my mother's friend, Natalie.

Brynn, Senior Nursing Student

Adapted from County of Los Angeles Public Health. (2013). Social determinants of health: How social and economic factors affect health. Retrieved from http://publichealth.lacounty.gov/epi/docs/SocialD_Final_Web.pdf

quality schools, recreation facilities, and health care providers. Lower income level is associated with lower levels of education and often results in a person having to work at jobs where he or she is exposed to higher risks (e.g., mining), or the need to work at more than one job in order to make ends meet, and often without health insurance coverage (Centers for Disease Control & Prevention [CDC], 2015a). Because of the lack of free time, one may be less likely to shop for fresh fruits and vegetables and to cook healthy meals, with a consequent reliance on fast foods. Inadequate childcare, lower social class, and stigmatization can cause ongoing psychological stress. There may be less control over transportation and work schedules, along with a greater degree of stress on the job and at home. Chronic stress takes a toll on one's body as it can lead to health problems through neuroendocrine and immune pathways (Heffner, 2011). The resulting consequences of chronic stress may lead to rapid aging and damaged health through such behaviors as smoking and excess drinking (see Perspectives: Student Voices). Neighborhood characteristics (e.g., high levels of poverty/physical disorder, low levels of safety) have been linked to significantly higher serum cortisol levels in European American (White) children, but not for African American children. Researchers thought that this reflected an adaptive mechanism for coping with stress, as the differences disappeared as both groups of children approached puberty. They noted that disruption in cortisol levels has negative effects on mental and physical health (Dulin-Keita, Casazza, Fernandez, Goran, & Gower, 2012).

Research has shown that those groups with the lowest income and with the least education were consistently less healthy than were those with the most income and most education (World Health Organization, 2016a). Lower SES can affect health outcomes throughout life (Cheng et al., 2015). As one example, poor prenatal nutrition can lead to learning and memory problems in childhood, as well as type 2 diabetes and cardiovascular disease in later life (de Souza, Fernandes, & Tavares do Carmo, 2011; Finney-Brown, 2012; Martin-Gronert & Ozanne, 2010). Another example is the risk posed by environmental lead to exposure the intellectual development of children. Studies have shown reduced IQ scores for children with lead poisoning and the potential influence of exposure to lead on health and SES of affected populations (Jakubowski, 2011). Poverty and race/ethnicity are often intertwined, but SES is considered a consistent and robust variable related to health and death (Krieger et al., 2014; Montez & Berkman, 2014; Montez & Zajacova, 2013; Neumayer & Plümper, 2015).

If we examine just one aspect of poverty—access to healthy food—research has found that race and environment play a significant role. Neighborhood disparities in access to fruits, vegetables, and other healthy foods have

 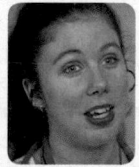

PERSPECTIVES STUDENT VOICE

A Nursing Student's View of the Aftermath of Hurricane Katrina

I was beginning my last year of nursing school when Hurricanes Katrina and Rita hit the Gulf Coast of Louisiana and Mississippi. Like most people, I was fixated on the television coverage of this natural disaster. A lot of the round-the-clock coverage focused on New Orleans, and much of that city seemed to be under water. People in flooded areas were stranded on housetops, while families could be seen walking on highways to get to Red Cross shelters. A horrifying image that I recall clearly was one of yellow school buses, mostly underwater, that were a key part of the city's disaster plan and were supposed to be used to assist those without personal means of transportation to move to higher ground.

It was like watching a very bad dream. We have had disasters in this country, but I did not expect to witness the lack of organization and preparation that seemed to abound with Katrina. I couldn't understand why masses of people didn't leave the area before the storms hit and why it took so long for the federal government to respond to the needs of American citizens. Those people who tried to leave found themselves delayed by the slowly moving parking lots that had once been interstate freeways. Even with personal transportation, evacuation was difficult!

What seemed very clear after Katrina was that there are large numbers of poor and vulnerable people in this country; I had not been previously aware of this. Did you know that most of those who died were poor and Black? This doesn't seem right. Didn't we abolish segregation and advance civil rights? In our community health nursing class, we discussed vulnerable populations and read some articles about this disaster. We talked about health disparities. I had never really thought about that before, but it rings true to me now. Some groups of people have higher numbers of deaths and more problems with certain diseases than do other groups. We do have different levels of health care for different groups, and some people can only access the health care system by coming to the ED.

I now have a better understanding of how things happened with Katrina. When you have little money, no reliable transportation, no extended support systems, and inadequate information about an impending disaster, you are vulnerable and at the mercy of government systems that often cannot respond quickly. I often wonder how I would fare if something happened suddenly, and I couldn't access cash from my bank account, or my car was low on gas, and I hadn't bought groceries in a couple of weeks. Would I be able to survive a natural disaster like an earthquake? I have family close by and many friends, some in nursing school, who could help me. That makes me less vulnerable, but I still should do a better job of being prepared.

Brooke, Nursing Student

been documented in a large-scale nationwide study and in studies in various parts of the United States (Carroll-Scott et al., 2013; Dubowitz et al., 2011; Hilmers, Hilmers, & Dave, 2012). Other researchers have noted the association of greater access to supermarkets (and limited access to convenience stores) with healthier diets and lower rates of obesity. They conducted a later study, finding that convenience stores and fast-food restaurant workers were concentrated in the South and Midwest where obesity prevalence is higher than in the Northeast and West (Michimi & Wimberly, 2010, 2015). The researchers concluded that the food environment landscapes at the metropolitan area level help explain the patterns of obesity.

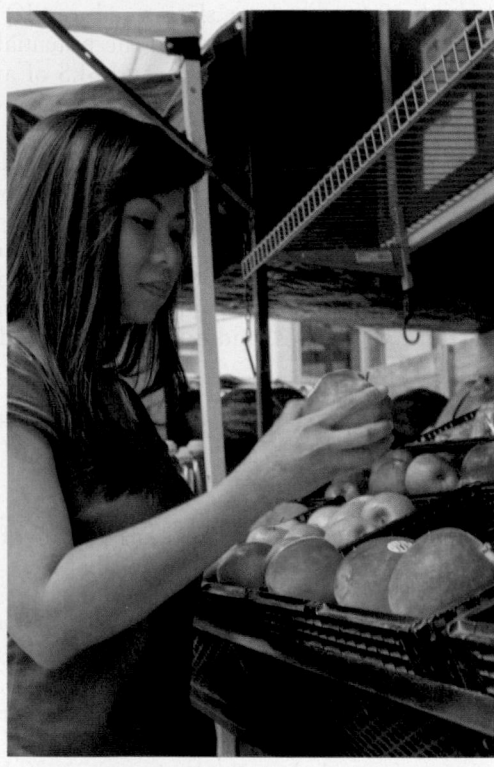

Income and race/ethnicity influence access to healthy food.

Another risk factor for the poor is the finding that the highest amount of pollution is most often found in neighborhoods where there is more poverty, lower education levels, and higher rates of unemployment (CDC, 2015a). Others noted an association between SES and poorer respiratory health, often due to living conditions, such as ambient air pollution and smoking (Hajat, Vardoulakis, Heaviside, & Eggen, 2014; Kanervisto et al., 2011), and because of a higher smoking prevalence among those with lower SES (Hiscock, Bauld, Amos, Fidler, & Munafo, 2012). Also, research has shown that lower SES groups are as likely as higher ones to attempt smoking cessation but are less likely to be successful in their efforts (Hiscock, Dobbie, & Bauld, 2015). The lower success in quitting smoking is being examined to find more effective evidence-based treatment for low-income populations (Evans et al., 2015).

At the population level, increases in total income and reductions in poverty levels are "strongly associated with subsequent improvements in population health" (Aday, 2005, p. 190). This is proven out in an examination of maternal mortality outcomes in Cambodia over the past 15 years. Maternal mortality declined from 472 per 100,000 live births in 2000 to 2005 to 206 in the period 2006 to 2010. Factors that contributed to this were noted to be reduction in poverty associated with economic growth and the country's increased stability and peace, as well as improved education levels (particularly for girls), greater access to health information and services, more births at facilities or with birth attendants, expanded midwifery education, and provision of antenatal care, along with free health care (Liljestrand & Sambath, 2012). Income affects health, and poor health can affect the income of an individual as well as that of a nation (see Chapter 6).

Uninsured and Underinsured

If the uninsured is also classified as a vulnerable population, even more Americans join the ranks, because the majority of those without health insurance are working adults who are not eligible for Medicaid or Medicare. The percentage of uninsured in 2013, was estimated at 16.7%. In 2015, 10.7% of people in the United States were without health insurance (Kaiser Family Foundation, 2015). The percentage of uninsured in 2013 was estimated at 16.7. The decline in the percentage of uninsured is attributable in great part to the Patient Protection and Affordable Care Act (ACA), signed into law by President Barack Obama on March 23, 2010. This law requires most U.S. citizens and legal residents to have health insurance coverage, along with many other provisions (Knickman & Kovner, 2015). See Chapter 6 for more on the ACA. Although the improvement in health insurance coverage is encouraging, disparities in access to health care continue. In 2014, 31 million people were underinsured in the United States, which was unchanged from 2010. In 2003, 1% of privately insured adults had a deductible of $3,000 or more, but that increased to 11% in 2014 (Collins, Rasmussen, Beutel, & Doty, 2015). Also, most health care experts feel that there will still be disparities in quality, access, and outcomes for those who are more vulnerable (Stremikis et al., 2011).

How does having inadequate or no health insurance lead to poor health outcomes? As explained in Chapter 6, those with few or no resources in this area do not utilize early screenings and preventive measures, and they delay getting treatment in an effort to save money. Those without health insurance receive care only for the problem at hand and not always for underlying causes. They do not get regular physical examinations and may be inadequately immunized against common diseases. Thus, they are at risk for poorer general health. Also, when examination and subsequent treatment are delayed, diseases, such as cancer or cardiovascular illness, may result in earlier death.

Race and Ethnicity

The United States is a multiracial, multiethnic country. About one third of the population belongs to a racial or ethnic minority group, and this proportion will continue to increase as minorities are projected to constitute more than half of all children by 2023 (U.S. Census Bureau, 2008, 2011). Hispanics represent the largest minority group (16% of the total population, up from 13% in 2000 census), and they are also the fastest growing group with a lifetime average number of children per woman of 2.53, compared to 1.71 for White women (Ennis, Rios-Vargas, & Albert, 2011; Pew Research Center, 2015).

Blacks and Hispanics report higher levels of metabolic and vascular diseases, as well as cognitive impairment (Apridonidze, Shaqra, Ktaich, Liu, & Bella, 2011). In 2010, Blacks represented 12% of the population, but they have accounted for 44% of new HIV infections; Blacks have the "most severe burden of HIV of all racial/ethnic groups" (CDC, 2015b, para. 2). Preterm births are more prevalent among Blacks, and infant mortality rates for Blacks have been consistently more than twice the rate for Whites (Office of Disease Prevention and Health Promotion, 2015a). Life expectancy for all minority races has been consistently lower than that of Whites since 1901. Life expectancy for Blacks was only 33.7 years in 1901, whereas for Whites, it was 49.4 years. The gap narrowed, but the racial/ethnic disparity still exists. In 2010, the life expectancy at birth for the White population was 78.7 years, for the Black population was 75.1 years, and for the Hispanic population was 81.4 years (Arias, 2014).

Why does simply being a member of a racial/ethnic minority group make someone vulnerable? The reasons are complex and are beginning to be understood. Williams and Mohammed (2013) found in a review of the scientific research that racism affects the health of minority racial populations in multiple ways. The authors found that institutional racism in policies and procedures reduced access to housing, neighborhood and educational quality, employment opportunities, and other societal resources. A second type of racism is cultural racism that affects economic status and health by creating a policy environment adverse to equal policies. A third finding from the review indicated that experiences of racial discrimination are a type of psychosocial stressor that can increase health risks.

Recent immigrants have healthier exercise and dietary patterns than do those born inside the United States. For Asian Americans, one study found that native language retention was associated with lower rates of obesity in first- and second-generation participants when compared with those who become fully acculturated (Wang, Quong, Kanaya, & Fernandez, 2011). Others note the generational link between minority group membership and low educational attainment (e.g., father's education level) and the tie between education and health (Cutler & Lleras-Muney, 2010). A majority of Hispanics and Blacks have spent a lifetime at a lower level of educational attainment and continue to lag behind in most areas. One bright spot is that 2012 college enrollments for Hispanics rose to 49%, above those for Whites at 47% (Krogstad & Fry, 2014).

VULNERABILITY AND INEQUALITY IN HEALTH CARE

Social Determinants of Health

The World Health Organization has defined the social determinants of health as "the conditions in which people are born, grow, live, work, and age," including the health system (World Health Organization, 2016b, para. 1). Commonly acknowledged factors, such as social norms or attitudes (e.g., discrimination, racism), exposure to crime, violence, and social disorder; and concentrated poverty, are associated with health outcomes and are recognized as **social determinants of health** (CDC, 2015a; USDHHS, n.d.). The unequal distribution of these factors among certain groups is thought to contribute to **health disparities** that are persistent and pervasive. The IOM report *For the Public's Health: The Role of Measurement in Action and Accountability* called for addressing the underlying factors, not only the data on morbidity/mortality (2010). When we address health disparities, we must consider these social determinants and work on all levels—individual, aggregate, community, and population—to reduce them. For instance, a safe and nourishing diet is needed to be healthy. Safe and accessible drinking water is also required, as are adequate housing, a supportive environment, and appropriate levels of exercise. The distribution of health care providers (e.g., nurses, physicians, dentists) across the United States leaves many areas and populations underserved. Political resources and social structures can also influence health, and health policies are needed to address multiple inequities and disadvantages that are associated with poorer health (Boyce & Olster, 2011; Embrett & Randall, 2014). You can check your own county's health ranking at http://www.countyhealthrankings.org/.

Social determinants of health are related to both morbidity and mortality. Quantified deaths that could be attributed to social factors in the United States were recently reported. The authors found that in 2000, about 245,000 deaths were attributable to low education, 176,000 to racial segregation, 162,000 to low social support, 133,000 to individual-level poverty, 119,000 to income inequality, and 39,000 to area-level poverty (Galea, Tracy, Hoggatt, DiMaggio, & Karpati, 2011). Moreover, it is estimated that only 10% to 15% of the increase in length of life in Western nations can be attributed to improved medical care, according to Raphael's classic treatise (2003).

In an effort to improve the health of disadvantaged groups, early public health efforts addressed determinants of health such as sanitation and poverty, along with living conditions and other environmental issues, as noted in Chapters 2 and 7. The present need to address underlying social conditions to improve health status is borne out by current research on race and socioeconomic class (Williams & Mohammed, 2013). It is now widely acknowledged that to truly have an impact on the health of the population, there is a need to improve social conditions (Bharmal, Derose, Felician, & Weden, 2015; Braveman & Gottlieb, 2014; CDC, 2016; County of Los Angeles Public Health, 2013; IOM, 2003). Political action and participatory action research are vital tools in reducing the effects of these conditions, as are methods of community empowerment (Commission on Determinants of Health Knowledge Networks, Lee, & Sadana, 2011; Sadana & Blas, 2013; see Chapters 4 and 13). See Figure 25–3 *Healthy People 2020* and Social Determinants of Health.

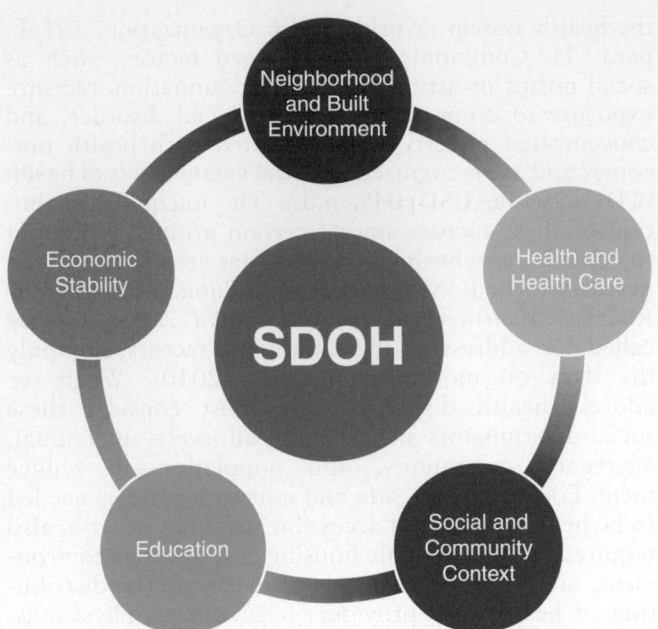

FIGURE 25–3 *Healthy People 2020* and Social Determinants of Health. (From U.S. Department of Health and Human Services. (2016). *Social determinants of health*. Retrieved from http://www.healthypeople.gov/2020/topics-objectives/topic/social-determinants-of-health)

Socioeconomic Gradient of Health

A series of large-scale, longitudinal studies in England, the now classic Whitehall studies, divided British civil servants into socioeconomic groups based upon their occupational status (e.g., executives to unskilled workers). What the investigators discovered was an improvement in mortality and morbidity rates as the level of occupation and pay increased. Those at the lowest levels had the poorest health, but as they moved up the salary scale and occupational level, their health improved. What makes this so interesting is that all of the workers had basic health insurance coverage and free medical care—no real problems with access to health care existed. Although less pronounced, even when the researchers adjusted for diet, exercise, and smoking, the gradient persisted (Marmot, Ryff, Bumpass, Shipley, & Marks, 1997; Marmot & Wilkinson, 2006). The investigators of one study found higher prevalence of heart disease for all participants at the lower end of the social stratus. The researchers also found death rates for diabetic participants to be about 200% higher in the lowest social group when compared to the highest (Chaturvedi, 1998). A U.S. study, following up on children of Framingham study subjects, found the association between lower socioeconomic position and coronary heart disease; a later study found higher odds of smoking, excess consumption of alcohol, and obesity that "may contribute to adult cardiometabolic disease" by the predisposition of these unhealthy behaviors (Loucks et al., 2009; Non et al., 2016, para. 5).

This inverse relationship between social class or income and health has been termed the **socioeconomic gradient** (Blazquez, Cottini, & Herrarte, 2014). It has been found in populations around the world, although not always unfailingly, and has been related to poor health outcomes regarding cardiovascular disease among the Greek population (Naska, Katsoulis, Trichopoulos, & Trichopoulou, 2011); cancer incidence, mortality, and survival in Western countries (Merletti, Galassi, & Spadea, 2011); injury rates, such as blunt and penetrating injuries (Zarzaur, Croce, Fabian, Fischer, & Magnotti, 2010); increased burden of chronic illness among Argentine citizens, especially those in urban areas (Fleischer, Roux, Alazraqui, Spinelli, & De Maio, 2011); and outcomes of adult asthma and rhinitis (Trupin et al., 2013).

The socioeconomic gradient has also been noted in behaviors, such as smoking, that are highest among those who are from the working class and who have low income and low educational levels (Hiscock et al., 2012; Yarnell et al., 2012). The gradient is also apparent in studies of hospital deaths. A large English study found a socioeconomic gradient with a 29.5% difference for in-hospital mortality (Wu, Jen, Bottle, Liaw, Ayulin, & Majeed, 2011). Other studies found higher rates of in-hospital mortality in U.S. pediatric patients and Iranian acute coronary syndrome patients (Abbasi et al., 2015; Colvin et al., 2013). Low birth weights and breast-feeding also demonstrate a socioeconomic gradient. Lower levels of education and income are associated with higher rates of low birth weight, whereas those at the higher levels of occupation and income are more likely to breast-feed their infants than are those at the lower levels (Madden, 2014; Yang, Platt, Dahhou, & Kramer, 2014).

Health Disparities

Health disparities are differences in the quantity of disease, burden of disease, and other adverse health conditions present in different groups (Braveman & Gottlieb, 2014). Health disparities may be unavoidable, such as health-damaging behaviors that are chosen by an individual despite health education and counseling efforts, but most are thought to be due to inequities that can be corrected (Sadana & Blas, 2013). A long-held belief about health inequities, adopted by the World Health Organization, is that health differences that are avoidable and unnecessary are patently unfair and unjust (Whitehead & Dahlgren, 2006). Health disparities can be objectively viewed as a disproportionate burden of morbidity, disability, and mortality found in a specific portion of the population in contrast to another.

The topic of social determinants of health was added to *Healthy People 2020* (Office of Disease Prevention and Health Promotion, 2015b). The *2014 National Healthcare Quality and Disparities Report* revealed that disparities persist, but several racial disparities in rates of childhood immunizations and adverse events associated with procedures have been eliminated (AHRQ, 2015). Reported disparities exist in the areas of quality of health care, access to care, levels and types of care, and care settings; they exist within subpopulations (e.g., elderly, women, children, rural residents, disabled) and across clinical conditions. Thus, to continue the work on eliminating health disparities, one goal for *Healthy People 2020* is to "achieve health equity, eliminate disparities, and improve the health of all groups" (USDHHS, 2016, para. 5).

Poor access to quality care and overt discrimination are examples of disparities. Discrimination can occur during service delivery if health care providers are biased against a specific group or hold stereotypical beliefs about that group. Providers may also not be confident about providing care for a racial or ethnic group with whom they are unfamiliar. Language may be a problem, as can cultural values and norms that are unfamiliar to providers. Patients can also react to providers in a way that promotes disparities; patients may not trust the information given to them and may not follow it as explained, leading to inadequate care (AHRQ, 2014b; Barkauskas, Pohl, Tanner, Onifade, & Pilon, 2011; Kaiser Family Foundation, 2012).

Access to Care

The IOM (2003) report *Unequal Treatment: Confronting Racial and Ethnic Disparities in Health Care* noted a large body of research highlighting the higher morbidity and mortality rates among all racial and ethnic minority groups when compared with Whites. This report drew attention to an issue that continues today and remains relevant. Differences in health care access were also explained, be it in the form of inadequate or no health insurance, problems getting health care, the quality of care, fewer choices in where to go for care, or the lack of a regular health care provider. For instance, because there are fewer numbers of health care providers in minority neighborhoods, finding a primary care provider is more difficult for those living in these areas. Often, sufficient transportation is not available, or clinic hours may be unrealistic for individuals working long hours (AHRQ, 2014b; Benatar, Garrett, Howell, & Palmer, 2012; IOM, 2003).

Residential segregation, although illegal, still exists and can play a role in health disparities. Many vulnerable populations, especially racial and ethnic minority groups and low-income populations, find health care at safety-net hospitals and community clinics where they are at the mercy of balanced budgets and vast bureaucratic systems (AHRQ, 2015; IOM, 2003). However, more recent data showed that the ACA is improving access for uninsured individuals to safety-net clinics in states with expanded Medicaid coverage (Angier et al., 2015). Other geographic factors can affect access to health care services. For example, a classic study by O'Mahony et al. (2008) found that only 25% of pharmacies in non-White neighborhoods, compared with 72% in predominately White neighborhoods, stocked sufficient opioid drugs to meet the needs of palliative care patients in different New York neighborhoods. Disparities were also found in hospice care among 8,211 older women dying from ovarian cancer; researchers found that a larger percentage of Black women, and those receiving fee-for-service Medicare, as well as those in the lowest income bracket, never received any type of hospice care (Fairfield et al., 2012). This lack of access to proper medication and care represents a disparity in health care.

Health care access is also problematic for other vulnerable groups. For example, services and resources for the mentally ill and substance abusers are often fragmented and inadequate, as are those for abusing families and homeless persons. Refugees and immigrants may have difficulty finding affordable and easily accessible health care, largely because of their lack of health insurance and the need to find care at free clinics or emergency rooms (Edberg, Cleary, & Vyas, 2011). When vulnerable individuals cannot get appropriate health care or treatment for illness or disease, for whatever reason, they are more likely to have health deficits.

Quality of Care

Quality of care should result in an "increased likelihood of desired health outcomes" and should be "consistent with current professional knowledge" (IOM, 2003, p. 31). Care quality can include areas such as patient safety issues, timeliness and effectiveness of patient care, and patient centeredness. Inequalities in the quality of care persistent (AHRQ, 2015). Research indicates that racial and ethnic minority clients feel more comfortable and satisfied with care from a health care provider who comes from the same racial and/or ethnic group (AHRQ, 2014b). However, a shortage of ethnically diverse health care providers exists. Despite racial and ethnic minorities constituting 37% of the U.S. population, only 19% of registered nurses (RNs) are from minority racial and ethnic groups (American Association of Colleges of Nursing, 2015).

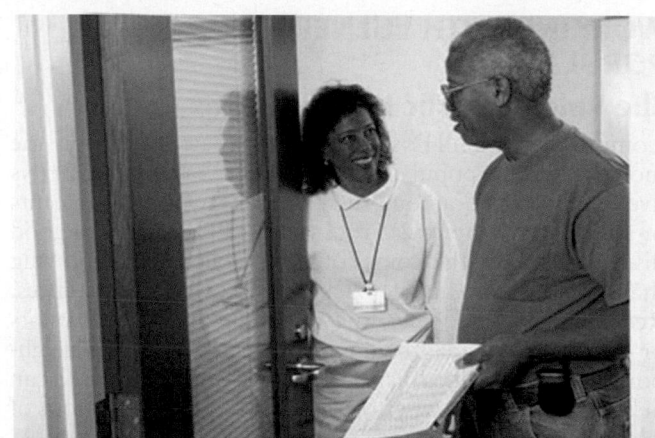

Racial and ethnic minority clients often prefer health care providers from the same racial and ethnic background.

Lack of access to quality health care services is common among racial and ethnic minority groups. Significant disparities in the quality of care were found in a study of over 2.3 million racial and ethnic minority patients receiving care in 4,450 hospitals for myocardial infarction, heart failure, and/or pneumonia, thought to be due to receiving care in hospitals that were lower performing in quality care (Hasnain-Wynia et al., 2010). More recent research looked at 17 quality performance measures among patients with over 12 million hospitalizations for three conditions (i.e., myocardial infarction, pneumonia, heart failure) over a 6-year period beginning after the Centers for Medicare and Medicaid Services instituted their Hospital Inpatient Quality Reporting System (Trivedi et al., 2014). Performance rates increased for all racial/ethnic groups, and the performance gap between White and Black patients over the course of the study dropped to 3.8% from 12.3% initially. For Hispanics, the performance improved to 1.1% from a high of 5.6%. Researchers also examined between hospital differences, a concern in the previous study, and found "greater improvement among hospitals that disproportionately serve minority patients" noting that when quality care is a focus, everyone benefits (Trivedi et al., 2014, p. 2306). A smaller 3-year study of more than 400 clinic patients with diabetes found improvements for hemoglobin A1c levels and no significant differences related to race or gender. Lee, Palacio, Alexandraki, Stewart, and Mooradian (2011) posited that having a medical home was the critical factor in decreasing health disparities for this population.

Communication can be a factor in poor quality of care. Marginalized vulnerable populations, such as substance abusers, at-risk mothers and infants, abusing families, suicide- and homicide-prone individuals, and the mentally ill or disabled, may feel they are treated as "second-class citizens," and cultural barriers and misunderstandings can lead to a discontinuation of recommended regimens. Poor health outcomes may result as effectiveness of health care for vulnerable populations is not often considered or even well defined (AHRQ, 2014b; Sadana & Blas, 2013).

WORKING WITH VULNERABLE POPULATIONS

The Role of Public Health Nurses

Community and PHNs often focus their efforts on the most vulnerable populations. In Lillian Wald's time, PHNs lived and worked among their clients, living in tenements or slums (see Chapter 2). Today, most PHNs travel a good distance to reach the homes of vulnerable clients, knowing that they can leave and go back to their own circumstances. Recognizing that demeaning or dehumanizing behaviors or language that may be directed toward clients or neighborhoods exemplifies disrespect and is often fear based can help us all to focus our efforts (see Fig. 25–2 Dimensions of Meaning). See Perspectives: One PHN's Opinion.

Effective Caring

One nursing goal for clients is to help them develop their capabilities to make choices and be in charge of their lives. Achieving this goal can be challenging for nurses when working with the most vulnerable clients because they are often the most disenfranchised and fearful of others. PHNs often must tailor interventions to vulnerable clients' specific needs, and these clients often require periods of intense support (Monsen, Radosevich, Kerr, & Fulkerson, 2011). One nurse described vulnerable individuals as being behind a locked door: "the door is shut and you can't get back in" (Zerwekh, 2000, p. 50). Opening that door is the first step to working effectively with these clients. Engagement and development of rapport are essential. See Figure 25–4.

Because vulnerability often equates with feelings of powerlessness, the actions of PHNs can either promote engagement or destroy chances for rapport. **Empowerment strategies** can be used by PHNs in their work with clients, once trust and rapport have been established. An often-cited Canadian study found three phases of PHN–client

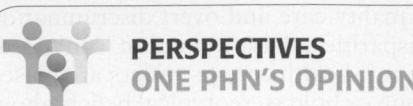

PERSPECTIVES
ONE PHN'S OPINION

All of us, at some level, have some apprehension of the disenfranchised, whether it's because we worry that we could be in that place or because we feel that there may be some potential for harm to us. I love working with my clients and have adapted a more realistic perspective of the vulnerable and disenfranchised. I try to picture myself in their shoes. What would I do if I had all of those things working against me that they are forced to deal with on a daily basis? I have tried to reframe what some people see as their weaknesses and view them as strengths. For instance, the ability to "not sweat the small stuff" and ignore less important things that they can do little about could be a good quality for many of us hardworking mothers to embrace. I see working with vulnerable clients as an important component of students' clinical experiences, and as their preceptor, I encourage them to become engaged with my vulnerable families. I strongly feel that it is necessary so that they can better understand client circumstances and needs. It also helps them to be competent nurses, no matter where they work. My clients are admitted into the hospital and use the emergency department and outpatient clinics. They may need assistance and encouragement in following through with health care interventions, and I want students working with me to understand how to be most effective in providing quality outcomes for them. Helping vulnerable clients is part of our rich nursing heritage, exemplified by Lillian Wald and many others. We are part of a long chain of caring, safety-net nurses who work with some of the most vulnerable among us.

Jamie, PHN

What is the PHN's role with vulnerable populations, and how can nurses learn to be most effective when working with vulnerable groups?

engagement: getting past the fear, working to build trust, and seeking mutual ground (Jack, DiCenso, & Lohfeld, 2005). The personal values, experiences, characteristics, and actions of both nurses and clients influenced the speed at which this process took place and the eventual level of connection. Helping clients identify their fears and clearly defining the PHN role with the client and family were also important. Building and preserving relationships with clients is a central focus of PHN home visits. An Australian nurse, Margaret McAllister (2010), cites three important phases: joining, building, and extending. Joining involves getting to know your client—their strengths and weaknesses and their vulnerabilities and needs. It also includes building trust and rapport and helping them to feel accepted, engaged, and ready. The building phase involves working with individual clients to improve their social connections, build their strengths, and work toward their goals. Building self-efficacy, motivation, and health literacy are essential in this stage, as are helping them with coping skills and giving encouragement as they build resilience. Extending strategies include helping clients to use new strategies and apply them in other situations. Phone calls and other methods of checking in with clients are

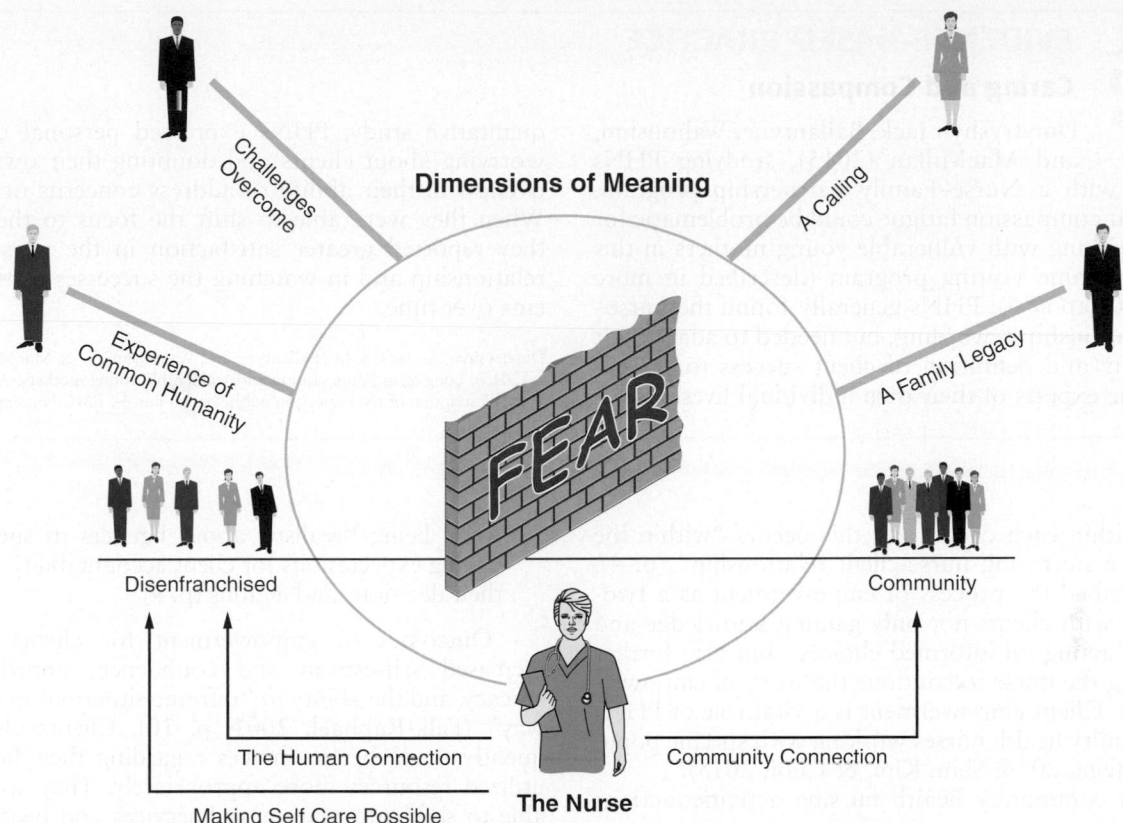

FIGURE 25–4 Breaking through the wall. Fearless caring with separated and often frightened clients has 10 themes that can be organized into three meta-themes: the human connection, the community connection, and making self-care possible. The nurse goes around the separating wall of fear. (Adapted from Zerwekh, J. (2000). Caring on the ragged edge: Nursing persons who are disenfranchised. *Advances in Nursing Science, 22*(4), 47–61.)

used to help them change behaviors and access services. Negotiation and teamwork approaches are helpful in this stage. Keeping a focus on solutions rather than problems helps build client strengths. Six principles of solution-focused nursing, built upon mental health nursing concepts, are helpful (McAllister, 2010).

1. The person, not the problem, is your focus.
2. Strengths, not just problems, can be found and further developed. Begin with an emphasis on strengths, as this can build client hope and self-confidence.
3. Resilience is equally as important as vulnerability.
4. Move beyond an individual focus to examine unjust societal and cultural forces, and actively work toward to alter these.
5. Nurses are not only concerned with illness care but with helping clients adapt/grow.
6. A proactive, not reactive, approach is needed that involves the three stages of client involvement (i.e., joining, building, extending).

These solution-focused nursing principles of client empowerment are exemplified in a study directed by the American Academy of Nursing. In examining the commonalities of nurse-designed models of health care, the authors of this study found four common elements: health defined holistically; individual-, family-, and community-centric approaches to care that put the people and their concerns

ahead of provider-defined priorities; relationship-based care that enabled individual/family/community engagement and partnerships that were time-consuming to develop, but crucial for building action and behavior change; and interventions incorporated ongoing group and public health approaches to improve health of vulnerable and underserved populations (Mason, Jones, Roy, Sullivan, & Wood, 2015).

Working with disadvantaged populations can be challenging and exhausting. Often, novice community health nurses feel overwhelmed and suffer "compassion fatigue" when confronted with the crushing realities that their vulnerable, disenfranchised clients face on a daily basis. Feelings of guilt sometimes surface when nurses contrast their own life experiences with those of their clients. To be effective in working with vulnerable populations, it is often more helpful to donate money and items on a group level rather than an individual level and to work for substantial changes in community attitudes and policies. Also, it is vital to remain grounded to continue to have the necessary energy and compassion. See Evidence-Based Practice.

Empowerment

In Chapter 13, the author discussed the concept of empowerment and applied it to the PHN's role when working with communities. In Falk-Raphael's classic article (2001), empowerment is defined as "an active, internal process of growth" that is reached by actualizing the full potential

EVIDENCE-BASED PRACTICE

Caring and Compassion

Dmytryshyn Jack, Ballantyne, Wahoushm, and MacMillan (2015), studying PHNs working with a Nurse–Family Partnership program, found that compassion fatigue could be problematic for nurses working with vulnerable young mothers in this long-term home visiting program (described in more detail in Chapter 4). PHNs generally found the nurse–client relationship rewarding, but needed to adapt their philosophy and definition of client success to see clients as the experts of their own individual lives. In this qualitative study, PHNs expressed personal costs of worrying about clients and doubting their own effectiveness in their ability to address concerns of clients. When they were able to shift the focus to the client, they reported greater satisfaction in the nurse–client relationship and in watching the successes of their clients over time.

Dmytryshyn, A., Jack, S. M., Ballantyne, M., Wahoushm O., & MacMillan, H. L. (2015). Long-term home visiting with vulnerable young mothers: An interpretive description of the impact on public health nurses. *BMC Nursing*, 14, 12.

---

inherent within each client, and this occurs "within the context of a nurturing nurse-client relationship" (p. 4). PHNs described the process of empowerment as a two-way street, with clients not only gaining knowledge and skills and "acting on informed choices" but also further empowering the nurse to continue the work of empowerment (p. 6). Client empowerment is a vital role of PHNs and community health nurses working with specific populations (Ortega, 2016; Shin, Kim, & Choi, 2015).

Which community health nursing activities/actions are most effective in promoting empowerment among nurses' vulnerable clients? In Falk-Raphael's (2001) well-known qualitative study of PHNs and their clients, several themes were noted as components of the PHN role:

- *Having a client-centered approach*, denoted by flexibility in dealing with clients, for example, "meeting them where they are," "communicating at their level," and "backing off and following client's agenda" (p. 6)
- *Developing a trusting relationship* based on mutual respect and dignity, for example, clients as active partners with the PHN assuming more or less responsibility as needed; being empathetic, nonjudgmental, and "creating a safe environment" (p. 7)
- *Employing advocacy*, both at an individual level as well as political advocacy, for example, using their role and power as a professional to cut through bureaucratic red tape, connecting clients with available community resources, supporting clients in reaching their health goals, making their expertise available, and being a client resource as someone who is open and "available" (p. 8)
- *Being a teacher and role model*, using a variety of strategies and providing opportunities for clients to safely practice new skills. For example, using strategies such as teaching classes, providing individual coaching, providing positive reinforcement and support, demonstrating skills such as assertiveness, and encouraging community action/participation are helpful
- *Capacity building* through encouraging and supporting of clients' work toward attaining health goals, for example, "reflective listening and an empathetic approach" focusing on strengths, not limitations; facilitating client "self-exploration" and providing encouragement for them to "act on their choices"

while being "realistic about barriers to success"; or having expectations for client accountability regarding their decisions and actions (p. 9)

Outcomes of empowerment for clients included increased self-esteem and confidence, improved self-efficacy, and the ability to "reframe situations in a positive way" (Falk-Raphael, 2001, p. 10). Clients also subsequently made better choices regarding their health and utilized resources more appropriately. They were better able to seek information and services and became more politically active. Clients' focus became more proactive than reactive, and they felt that they could communicate more effectively to define boundaries or express feelings. Consequently, clients were also better able to collaborate with their health care providers, becoming more trusting partners in care by demonstrating ownership for their actions and their health. Some clients noted a newfound ability to see their communities in a more holistic way and looked for ways to change things for the better. A large part of PHN practice is to work with the vulnerable and encourage them to become more self-reliant and responsible for their health (Cawley, 2012). Both the client and the PHN undergo a "transformation" when empowerment strategies are employed (Dowling, Cooney, & Casey, 2011, p. 476). Literature on client empowerment was searched and interviews conducted with key informants (e.g., health researchers, patients, patient care representatives, primary care clinicians) in research conducted to produce a conceptual map of patient empowerment (Bravo et al., 2015). Some indicators of patient empowerment included self-efficacy and a sense of personal control over their health as well as the care they receive, along with health literacy, and feeling respected. These led to a more active role in decision-making and management of care, eventually leading to better health outcomes.

Making a Difference

External support, along with temperament and other individual factors, has been associated with coping with stress and adverse situations. The support can be from family members, neighbors, friends, teachers, or others. PHNs can provide external support at both the individual and population levels (see Perspectives: Voices from the Community). For example, research has shown the

PERSPECTIVES
VOICES FROM THE COMMUNITY

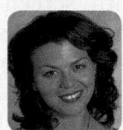

A View of Katrina's Aftermath: Nurse Volunteer

I had never been a Red Cross volunteer before, but Katrina touched my heart, and I signed up. Suddenly, I was headed to New Orleans to help in a shelter. The sheer number of people streaming into the shelter astounded me— people who had lost everything. Some of these people had waited on housetops to be rescued. Others had walked for hours to reach the shelter. A common theme among them was their vulnerability. Many were members of vulnerable populations even before Katrina struck.

At first, most were relieved to be safe and dry. However, that changed as they realized what they had lost and how uncertain their futures were. Many of the older people and those with chronic illnesses had significant health problems that worsened while they were residents of the shelter. Although they were provided with food, it was sometimes difficult for them to get the exact food they needed for their special diets. Some of them did not have all of their medications, and it took some time to complete health histories and secure necessary prescriptions. The weather was very muggy and hot, and there was little privacy. Even though the governor had called out the National Guard, people had to protect their few belongings, as theft was rampant. Toilet and bathing facilities were inadequate, space was limited, and fights often broke out between people who had been

pushed to the limits of their composure. People had to show identification to apply for emergency loans or to receive other assistance. Some of them had lost all documents in the flooding or had lost things on the way to the shelter. Standing in line was physically difficult for many people, but lines were long and standing was necessary in order to get assistance.

Many people were displaced, and a good number of them were separated from their families and friends, with no idea whether they were dead or alive. It was difficult to reconnect people, as individuals were evacuated to diverse locations. Communication was often a problem until phone lines and cell towers were back up and running.

I was there to help and to listen and provide care, but sometimes I felt frustrated and ineffective. I wanted to advocate for people and improve on systems of care, but this was almost impossible in such an erratic and crisis-driven system. Better systems need to be in place before the next disaster strikes, especially for the most vulnerable. All in all, it was a rewarding experience, and I was able to make a difference for some people on an individual basis. But there were so many who needed significant and long-term assistance!

Helena, RN, PHN, Red Cross Volunteer

Adapted from Saunders, J. M. (2007). Vulnerable populations in an American Red Cross shelter after hurricane Katrina. *Perspectives in Psychiatric Care, 43*(1), 30–37.

effectiveness of social support provided by nurses in promoting consistent program participation and positive social and health outcomes among low-income pregnant women and their children, not only in America but around the world (Coalition for Evidence-Based Policy, 2015; Mejdoubi et al., 2013; Mejdoubi et al., 2015; Nurse-Family Partnership, 2011a, 2011b, 2011c, Olds et al., 2010; USDHHS, 2011; 2015). PHNs can assist vulnerable individuals in several ways.

Through work with individual clients, PHNs can expand their own empowerment strategies to serve the community. Being aware of the community's pulse is vital and can be accomplished not only through home visits but also by attending community-level meetings and through the development of partnerships organized around specific health issues or community problems. Early detection of problems at the community level can lead to the development of programs and services to provide early intervention and avert costly tertiary care or to actively meet the needs of specific groups, such as low-income elderly and new parents (Breitenstein et al., 2012; Cawley, 2012; Marek, Stetzer, Adams, Popejoy, & Rantz, 2012; Rantz et al., 2011).

Using Evidence to Reduce Vulnerability

Community health nurses can assist vulnerable populations, communities, individuals, and families to reduce their vulnerability by using evidence from research, expert opinion, and best practices (see Chapter 4 on Evidence-Based

Practice). Often, evidence is embedded in policies, procedures, and clinical guidelines. Thus, the first place to locate evidence for practice is in the specific agency documentation for nursing practice. Sometimes, a community need is discovered that requires creative thinking and evidence-based interventions. See Population Focus—Reaching Out to the Underserved Poor in Rural Communities.

Many areas for improvement of the lives of vulnerable populations lie in areas related to prevention and health promotion, as described above. Primary prevention is readily available in the form of immunizations for children, adolescents, and adults. Nursing activities to promote increasing immunization levels among vulnerable people will result in greater economic and social returns for the whole community. Similar is the involvement of nurses in smoking prevention and smoking cessation activities. Also, some vulnerable subpopulations require additional insight and experience. See Perspectives: Picking up on Clues.

In addition to immunizations, smoking cessation, and other preventive interventions, the following topics are highlighted as evidence-based concepts shown to improve the health status of vulnerable populations: health literacy, access to nursing services, and policy.

Improving Health Literacy

People living in low-income communities often have low educational levels that are related to low literacy and low health literacy levels. An estimated 80 million Americans have limited health literacy. Because clients have difficulty

POPULATION-FOCUS
REACHING OUT TO THE UNDERSERVED POOR IN RURAL COMMUNITIES

Community Preventive Health Collaborative (CPHC) is a program developed by nursing faculty from a university in California's southern central valley. The program was designed to address the serious burden of chronic diseases including obesity, diabetes, heart disease, and hypertension in the large, agricultural county by expanding the reach of the health care workforce through the participation of nursing students and utilizing evidence-based practice interventions. Students enroll in an elective CPHC service-learning course in order to provide health education and health screening tests for blood pressure, blood sugar, total cholesterol, and body mass index.

Rural community residents face many struggles including poverty and lack of access to health care. Long and laborious work schedules, cultural values and priorities, and limited finances may influence when and how often health services are sought out. Chronic diseases may go on for a long period of time without detection. Therefore, services that can reach at-risk populations at no cost to the client are greatly needed in rural communities.

When CPHC began providing services in the rural areas of the county, the population of interest was agricultural workers. An agricultural company in our region partnered with us to provide the services. Clinics were held in a variety of locations including outdoors at an operations plant, indoors in an employee break room, and at a community health center. The process began with a health history interview that examined social factors such as diet and exercise, smoking and other substance use, and clients' health insurance status. Student nurses were able to provide health education and brochures to clients in an effort to encourage healthy lifestyle modification. Then screening tests were performed, and if elevations were found, the client was educated about his or her risks and a referral was given. The client was encouraged to seek follow-up care from a primary care provider. If the client did not already have a primary care provider, students provided information about the employer's clinic and a list of community clinics in the area. Some clients consented for follow-up contact from student nurses and received phone calls one month after their health screening to provide additional information and resources and to determine if a primary care visit had been made.

Since 2011, CPHC has provided health screenings to over 4,000 individuals. The program continues to benefit the community by reaching out to medically underserved regions and provides health promotion and preventive health services to community members that most likely would not have received these services if it weren't for student nurses. CPHC provides services at community locations such as senior centers, community centers, and health fairs and at swap meets in our region. Most recently, CPHC has implemented referrals to PHN home visiting services. Student nurses who are currently in their community health nursing rotation now accept the referrals and visit clients in their homes to provide continuity of service. They offer in-depth health teaching related to their diagnosed health conditions and work with clients to link them with community resources (e.g., available nutrition or exercise classes).

Not only do community members benefit from the services provided by student nurses, it also greatly enhances the student nurses' experience as they reach out to medically underserved communities with health promotion and preventive health strategies. Students shared what the experiences meant to them; here are a few examples:

- *CPHC program was beneficial to my perspective as a health professional. I am now able to appreciate the role of the PHN through community outreach, health promotion, advocacy, and empowering individuals through awareness.*
- *CPHC has really enabled me to interact with the public, especially the underserved community. I have gained knowledge on barriers to healthcare that populations encounter.*
- *CPHC has helped me to have an open mind regarding barriers that prevent clients from achieving optimal health outcomes.*

Nurses in the community setting are able to conduct a community assessment and develop strategies and evidence-based interventions that address problems in order to improve health outcomes at the community level. CPHC is an example of nurses and nursing students joining with the community to offer evidence-based care to those who are most vulnerable to poorer health outcomes.

Judy H. Pedro, MSN, RN, APHN-BC
Community Health Nursing Faculty

---

obtaining, processing, and understanding health information, it is not surprising that low health literacy is associated with poorer health outcomes and poorer use of health care services (Berkman, Sheridan, Donahue, Halpern, & Crotty, 2011; IOM, 2014). Limited skills in health literacy can negatively impact client health behaviors, as well as decisions related to health, and health outcomes (Ferguson & Pawlack, 2011). A systematic review found that low health literacy was associated with more emergency care use, higher hospitalization rates, fewer instances of influenza vaccine and mammography, poorer ability to read labels and interpret health messages, and greater inability to demonstrate appropriate medication administration, as well as higher mortality and poorer overall health status among senior citizens (AHRQ, 2014a). In addition, low literacy or illiteracy is a contributing factor to unemployment and underemployment within vulnerable groups, thus increasing risk for low income and poverty.

PERSPECTIVES
PICKING UP ON CLUES

I have been a PHN for many years and been fortunate enough to work with various populations. I remember a case when I learned that although experience is a valuable asset, sometimes this contributes to assessment miscues. I had an established relationship with a socioeconomically disadvantaged postpartum client, who was experiencing anxiety, feelings of being overwhelmed, and insomnia. The interventions that I had successfully used for so many other moms in similar situations with postpartum depression had failed with this client. It was not until I inquired about a picture of my client, Nancy, in her military uniform that she shared with me that she had served for a few years in the Middle East. She further stated that she did not like to discuss her past, she regretted not being physically able to continue her military career, and she just wanted to "get some sleep." Long story short, we were able to get Nancy into a Veteran's Administration (VA) residential treatment program for substance abuse and medical treatment for traumatic brain injury (TBI). I learned through this encounter that experience coupled with a patient-centered assessment, minus my internal preconceptions, results in the best outcomes for patients. Nancy had more than the usual stressors affecting her, and I was glad that I was finally able to pick up on those clues and address her needs more completely.

Tessa, PHN

The implications of health literacy for public health are as important as those for acute care settings (IOM, 2014). See Chapter 10 for more on health literacy.

Assisting vulnerable groups and communities to improve health literacy is one approach for reducing vulnerability and improving health outcomes. Many cities have literacy programs that use volunteers to provide tutoring. This is an excellent way for nurses to give back to the community. Literacy training contributes to health literacy by improving reading, writing, and comprehension skills. A crucial aspect of improving health literacy is improvements in public schools so that more students graduate with adequate skills for higher education and employment. In addition, it is estimated that tens of millions of U.S. adults are unable to read complex texts, which includes many health-related materials (Roundtable on Health Literacy et al., 2015).

Some research shows that low-literacy clients may learn better with the use of multiple methods for teaching, such as pictures, small group classes, and audiovisual materials (Horowitz, Clovis, Wang, & Kleinman, 2013; Wolf et al., 2009). Written material should be carefully reviewed for reading level before it is given to clients. Many tools, such as Fry Readability Graph and Gunning-FOG formula, are available for testing reading levels of written material (Medline Plus, 2015). The CDC has developed the Clear Communication Index that provides a set of evidence-based criteria for developing and assessing public communication material for diverse populations (Baur & Prue, 2014). See Chapter 11.

A special challenge for nurses is preparing or locating material for clients who do not speak English. Health care agency resources need to be devoted to meeting the needs of clients who have no or few skills in English. This area of need is usually beyond the ability of the individual nurse, but the need can be made known to agency administration. A number of health literacy resources are available from the American Medical Association (Coleman, 2011).

Improving Access to Nursing Services

Results from over three decades of research have demonstrated that home visiting by RNs is effective in improving outcomes for low-income women and children. David Olds and his research team, including Harriet Kitzman, an RN, have conducted much of the work done to demonstrate these dramatic results. Studies show that home visiting to low-income women and their children results in fewer cases of child abuse and neglect, longer spacing between pregnancies, avoidance of substance abuse and criminal behavior, and less dependence on government assistance. For the children of low-income, unmarried women, the children had fewer arrests and convictions, smoked and drank alcohol less, and had fewer sexual partners than did the children who did not have nurse home visits (Olds et al., 1997). More recently, the Olds team found that families who were visited in their homes by PHNs demonstrated lasting positive effects (Eckenrode et al., 2010; Olds et al., 2010) and a promising means of reducing mortality among mothers and children (Olds et al., 2014), as well as reducing intimate partner violence (Mejdoubi et al., 2013).

Other research demonstrating the benefits of PHN interventions and nurse home visiting includes studies on managing clients with HIV (Haley et al., 2014), new mothers released from the hospital (Paul et al., 2011),

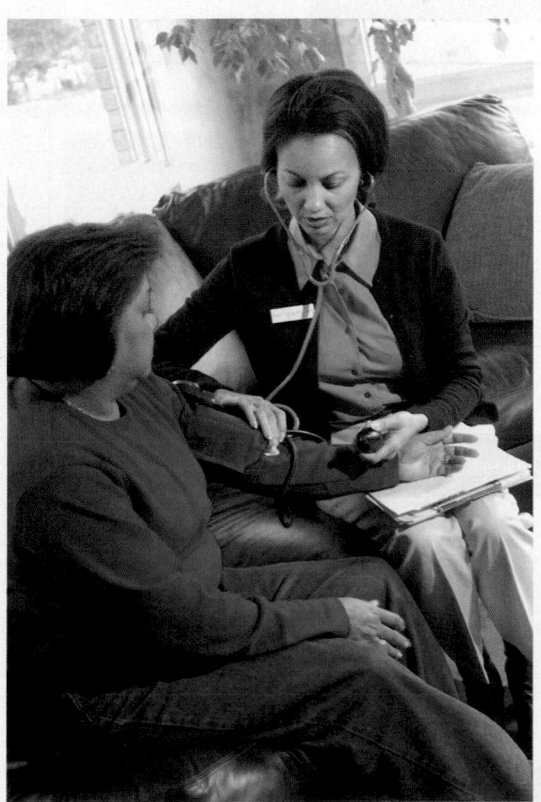

Home visiting has been shown to have positive outcomes for a variety of vulnerable populations.

and transitional care programs for the elderly (Ornstein, Smith, Foer, Lopez-Cantor, & Soriano, 2011). See Chapter 4 for more on this line of research.

Home visiting can be provided from almost any setting that provides services to communities. The usual settings are local health departments, home health care agencies, community-based hospice agencies, and visiting nurse associations. In addition, school nurses, ambulatory nurses, parish or faith-based nurses, and nurses have recently provided limited home visiting services to clients or families seen in a variety of settings, including outpatient clinics, Head Start programs, places of worship, and health centers. Expanding home visiting to all vulnerable groups holds promise for improving the health of many individuals and communities.

School-based clinics have improved access and outcomes for preventive care like immunizations, chronic disease management (e.g., diabetes, asthma, obesity), and adolescent reproductive health services and have been associated with improved academic achievement (Keeton, Soleimanpour, & Brindis, 2012). These clinics are included in health care reform funding, largely because of their proven track record for accessibility and quality. Nurse-managed clinics have also increased access to care for communities, and they may be able to access funding through the ACA (Hansen-Turton, 2012; Holt, Zabler, & Baisch, 2014). See Chapters 30 and 31. Improving access to nursing care in the community has been shown to have benefits for population and individual health.

Improving Health and Public Policy

Policies to reduce vulnerability for individuals, families, and communities have been shown to be effective at all levels: local, state, and national. Policy based on evidence is an important component of reducing vulnerability for communities and individuals. This section of the chapter addresses health and public policy, including policy in schools, cities, counties, and health care settings. Policy includes social, economic, environmental, and health aspects. See Chapter 13 for an expansive discussion of policy.

Small changes in policy can make a big difference in outcomes for vulnerable communities. For example, policies to provide healthy foods in school vending machines provide healthier choices for all students, not just those considered vulnerable. Mandatory activity time for all school children contributes to preventing obesity and enhancing learning in all children as well as those who are most vulnerable because of low income and ethnicity (Beets, Tilley, Kim, & Webster, 2011; Cradock et al., 2011).

Communities that lack safe places for physical activities need to have attention directed to the appropriate governing bodies, such as the city council or the department of recreation. Community residents can be effective in bringing about change that improves a total community (Gortmaker et al., 2011). One model that addresses both individual and social determinants of health in a straightforward manner is the County Health Rankings Model (see Fig. 25–5).

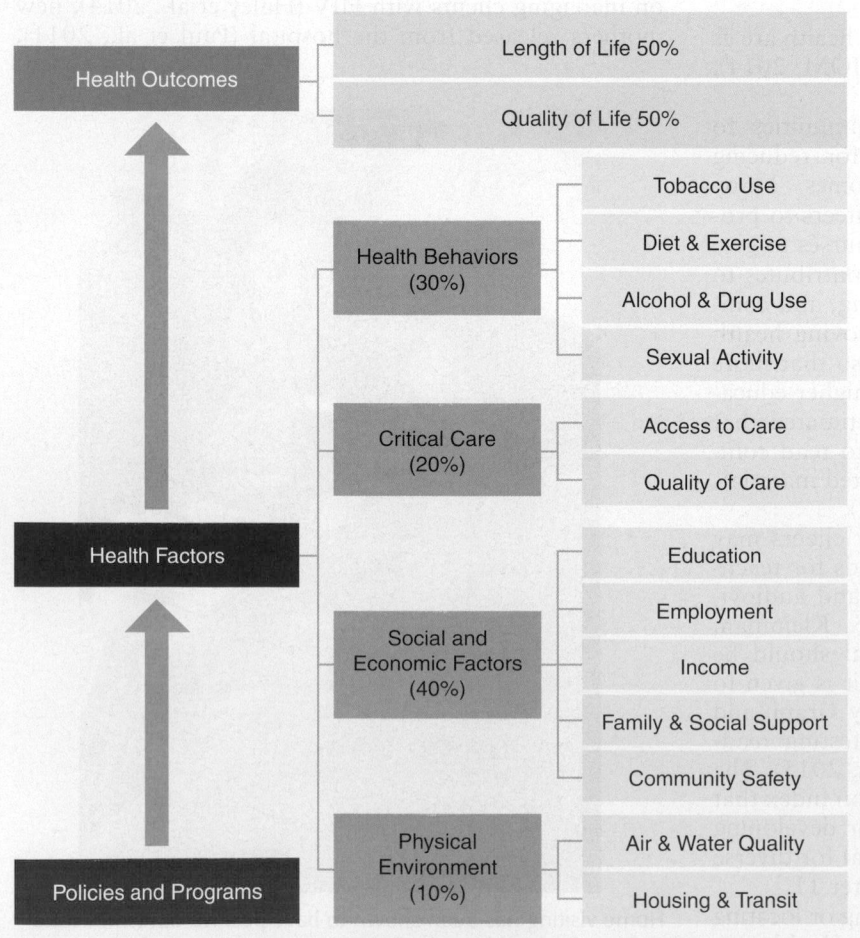

FIGURE 25–5 County Health Rankings Model. (From County of Los Angeles Public Health. (2013). *Social determinants of health: How social and economic factors affect health.* Retrieved from http://publichealth.lacounty.gov/epi/docs/SocialD_Final_Web.pdf, used with permission.)

SUMMARY

Vulnerable populations are at risk for poor health outcomes. Various models or theoretical frameworks examine personal and environmental resources and risks relative to vulnerability. Vulnerability is associated with increased risk for morbidity and mortality. Poverty, age, gender, and race or ethnicity are leading factors that make aggregates vulnerable, as can being uninsured or underinsured, a single parent, and those with little or no education. Vulnerable groups can include chronically ill or disabled, high-risk mothers and infants, those with HIV/AIDS, and the mentally ill or disabled. Alcohol and substance abusers, those prone to suicide and homicide, the homeless, abusing families, and immigrants or refugees can also be characterized as vulnerable.

It is difficult to calculate the exact numbers of Americans who are members of vulnerable groups largely because of the overlap in populations, but it involves a significant proportion of the total population. As an example of overlap in populations, low-income status is often associated with underinsurance or race and ethnicity and may also be related to homelessness and high-risk births.

Social determinants of health are strongly associated with health outcomes. Examples of social determinants of health are social norms or attitudes, such as discrimination and racism; exposure to crime, violence, and social disorder; and concentrated poverty. The socioeconomic gradient, an inverse relationship between social class/income and health, has been repeatedly demonstrated in research conducted around the world.

Health disparities are defined as differences in access to quality health care and in health outcomes and are usually characterized as avoidable and unfair. One of the goals of *Healthy People 2020* is to achieve health equity, eliminate disparities, and improve the health of all groups. Many disparities occur along income/class or racial/ethnic lines. A good deal of research is under way to determine more specifically the causes and consequences of health disparities.

Community health nurses often work with vulnerable populations, and nurses must learn to break through barriers of fear—their own and that of their clients. To be effective, PHNs must establish a sense of trust and rapport with their clients by finding common ground. Connecting with clients and connecting clients to the community and available resources are key factors in successful PHN–client relationships. Coaching and mentoring clients to solve their own problems and make necessary changes are also effective behaviors of PHNs.

Empowerment strategies with individual clients can help them to meet their full potential while also providing empowerment to the nurses working with them. Flexible, client-centered approaches, based on trust and mutual respect, have been found to be most effective. A nonjudgmental attitude and openness with clients lay the foundation for development of effective relationships. Community health nurses who work at empowering clients are advocates at the individual level as well as the political level. The nurse is a resource to clients without being paternalistic. Nurses provide a safe place for clients to try out skills and demonstrate new, healthier behaviors. PHNs build capacity through active, reflective, empathetic listening and serve as role models and teachers. Empowered clients have greater self-confidence and are better able to collaborate with health care providers. Often, empowered clients become more engaged with their communities and neighborhoods.

Community health nurses can provide individual support as well as support and leadership for vulnerable communities. Political action can involve not only health policy issues but also political activism on the part of underserved populations to improve housing, education, and employment. Action at the community or population level is an effective and efficient way to have the "biggest bang for the buck" when improving the health of vulnerable populations.

ACTIVITIES TO PROMOTE **CRITICAL THINKING**

1. Identify at least four vulnerable groups within your community. Using the Flaskerud and Winslow (1998) model depicted in this chapter, determine the health status for each of these groups. Describe the relative risk for each group.
   a. Find available community resources for each of the identified groups. Where are the resources located? How easily accessible are they? What outreach services do they provide for the vulnerable population they serve? Describe some socioeconomic resources. What areas are most deficient?
2. Pick a client from your community health nursing clinical assignment. In a respectful way, discuss your apprehensions about working in the community (e.g., very different from hospital setting) and ask about any concerns your client may have experienced in permitting you access to her or his home. Outline ways in which you could build upon this mutual sharing to achieve mutual trust and rapport.
3. Discuss how you might apply the principles of solution-focused nursing with either one of your community health nursing clinical clients/families or with someone with whom you have a relationship (acquaintance or family member who may fall within the definition of vulnerable). How might you discern a difference in their responses to your conversations and interactions with them? What behaviors would you expect to change?
4. Talk to two expert PHNs and discuss the concept of empowerment with them. What strategies have they used with clients? Ask each to share an example in which they feel that they made a real difference in the lives of their clients. Note any similarities with the roles and behaviors of PHNs and client empowerment described in this chapter.
5. Check with the health department about any interagency groups or committees that may be addressing the needs of vulnerable populations in your community. What issues are most important to this group? Who are the members? Note the agencies represented. Are there any community members present? If possible, attend a meeting or access minutes of a recent meeting and determine the types of issues being discussed. Is there a sense of community involvement and participation?
6. With a group of students, each of you search for a current evidence-based article on vulnerable populations based on ideas from this chapter. Discuss the main points of each article and how they may relate to vulnerable populations (e.g., health disparities, socioeconomic gradient), as well as individual clients you may be seeing in your clinical rotations (e.g., empowerment, health literacy). Based upon the research findings, what interventions might be most helpful? Are they feasible in your area? With your specific populations?

REFERENCES

Abbasi, S. H., De Leon, A. P., Kassaian, S. E., Karimi, A., Sundin, O, Jalali, A., ... & Macassa, G. (2015). Introducing the Tehran Heart Center's premature coronary atherosclerosis cohort: THC-PAC study. *International Journal of Preventive Medicine, 6*, 36.

Aday, L. A. (2001). *At risk in America: The health and health care needs of vulnerable populations in the United States* (2nd ed.). San Francisco, CA: Jossey-Bass.

Aday, L. A. (Ed.). (2005). *Reinventing public health: Policies and practices for a healthy nation.* San Francisco, CA: Jossey-Bass.

Agency for Healthcare Research and Quality (AHRQ). (2014a). *Health literacy interventions and outcomes, update.* Retrieved from http://archive.ahrq.gov/research/findings/evidence-based-reports/er199-abstract.html#Report

Agency for Healthcare Research and Quality (AHRQ). (2014b). *Improving cultural competence to reduce health disparities for priority population.* Retrieved from http://effectivehealthcare.ahrq.gov/index.cfm/search-for-guides-reviews-and-reports/?pageaction=displayproduct&productid=1934

Agency for Healthcare Research and Quality (AHRQ). (2015). *2014 National healthcare quality and disparities report (AHRQ Pub. No. 15–0007).* Rockville, MD: Author.

Albarran, C. R., & Nyamathi, A. (2011). HIV and Mexican migrant workers in the United States: A review applying the vulnerable populations conceptual model. *Journal of the Association of Nurses in AIDS Care, 22*(3), 173–185.

Almeida, J., Mulready-Ward, C., Bettegowda, V., & Ahluwalia, I. (2014). Racial/ethnic and nativity differences in birth outcomes among mothers in New York City: The role of social ties and social support. *Maternal & Child Health Journal, 18*(1), 90–100.

American Association of Colleges of Nursing. (2015). *Fact sheet: Enhancing diversity in the nursing workforce.* Retrieved from http://www.aacn.nche.edu/media-relations/diversityFS.pdf

Angier, H., Hoopes, M., Gold, R., Bailey, S. R., Cottrell, E. K., Heintzman, J., ... DeVoe, J. E. (2015). An early look at rates of uninsured safety net clinic visits after the Affordable Care Act. *Annals of Family Medicine, 13*(1), 10–16. doi: 10.1370/afm.1741.

Apridonidze, T., Shaqra, H., Ktaich, N., Liu, J., & Bella, J. (2011). Relation of components of the metabolic syndrome to left ventricular geometry in Hispanic and non-Hispanic Black adults. *American Journal of Cardiovascular Disease, 1*(1), 84–91.

Arias, E. (2014). United States life tables, 2010. *National Vital Statistics Reports, 63*(7), 1–63.

Barkauskas, V. H., Pohl, J. M., Tanner, C., Onifade, T. J., & Pilon, B. (2011). Quality of care in nurse-managed health centers. *Nursing Administration Quarterly, 35*(1), 34–43.

Bates, B. (2016). *Learning theories simplified and how to apply them to teaching.* Thousand Oaks, CA: Sage.

Baur, C., & Prue, C. (2014). The CDC clear communication index is a new evidence-based tool to prepare and review health information. *Health Promotion Practice, 15*(5), 629–637. doi: 10.1177/1524839914538969.

Beets, M. W., Tilley, F., Kim, Y., & Webster, C. (2011). Nutritional policies and standards for snacks served in after-school programmes: A review. *Public Health Nutrition, 1*, 1–9.

Benatar, S., Garrett, A. B., Howell, E., & Palmer, A. (2012). Midwifery care at a freestanding birth center: A safe and effective alternative to conventional maternity care. *Health Services Research, 48*(5), 1750–1768.

Berkman, N. D., Sheridan, S. L., Donahue, K. E., Halpern, D. J., & Crotty, K. (2011). Low health literacy and health outcomes: An updated systematic review. *Annuals of Internal Medicine, 155*(2), 97–107.

Bharmal, N., Derose, K. P., Felician, M., & Weden, M. M. (2015). *Working paper: Understanding the upstream social determinants of health.* Santa Monica, CA: RAND Health.

Blazquez, M., Cottini, E., & Herrarte, A. (2014). The socioeconomic gradient in health: How important is material deprivation? *The Journal of Economic Inequality, 12*(2), 239–264.

Boyce, C. A., & Olster, D. H. (2011). Strengthening the public research agenda for social determinants of health. *American Journal of Preventive Medicine, 40*(Suppl. 1), s86–s88.

Braveman, P., & Gottlieb, L. (2014). The social determinants of health: It's time to consider the causes of the causes. *Public Health Reports, 129*(Suppl. 2), 19–31.

Bravo, P., Edwards, A., Barr, P. J., Scholl, I., Elwyn, G., McAllister, M.; & Cochrane Healthcare Quality Research Group. (2015). Conceptualizing patient empowerment: A mixed methods study. *BMC Health Services, 15*, 252.

Breitenstein, S. M., Gross, D., Fogg, L., Ridge, A., Garvey, C., Julion W., & Tucker, S. (2012). The Chicago Parent Program: Comparing 1-year outcomes for African American and Latino parents of young children. *Research in Nursing & Health, 35*(5), 475–489.

Burg, M. A., & Oyama, O. (2016). *The behavioral health specialist in primary care: Skills for integrated practice.* New York, NY: Springer Publishing Co.

Cantu, P. A., Hayward, M. D., Hummer, R. A., & Chiu, C. T. (2013). New estimates of racial/ethnic differences in life expectancy with chronic morbidity and functional loss: Evidence from the National Health Interview Survey. *Journal of Cross-Cultural Gerontology, 28*, 283–297.

Carr, G. F. (2011). Empowerment: A framework to develop advocacy in African American grandmothers providing care for their grandchildren. *International Scholarly Research Network (ISRN) Nursing.* doi: 10.5402/2011/531717.

Carroll-Scott, A., Gilstad-Hayden, K., Rosenthal, L., Peters, S. M., McCaslin, C., Joyce, R., & Ickovics, J. R. (2013). Disentangling neighborhood contextual associations with child body mass index, diet, and physical activity: The role of built, socioeconomic, and social environments. *Social Science & Medicine, 95*, 106–114.

Cawley, T. (2012). How can the empowerment role of public health nurses (PHNs) be fostered? A review of an exploratory research study conducted in Ireland. In J. Maddock (Ed.), Current evidence, public health, social, and behavioral health. Retrieved from http://cdn.intechopen.com/pdfs-wm/36948.pdf

Center for Poverty Research, University of California, Davis. (n.d.). *How many people are poor?* Retrieved from poverty.ucdavis.edu/faq/how-many-people-are-poor

Centers for Disease Control and Prevention (CDC). (2015a). *CDC health disparities and inequalities report, United States, 2013.* Retrieved from http://www.cdc.gov/mmwr/pdf/other/su6203.pdf

Centers for Disease Control and Prevention (CDC). (2015b). *HIV among African Americans.* Retrieved from http://www.cdc.gov/hiv/group/racialethnic/africanamericans/

Centers for Disease Control and Prevention (CDC). (2016). *Social determinants of health.* Retrieved from http://www.healthypeople.gov/2020/topics-objectives/topic/social-determinants-of-health

Chaturvedi, N. (1998). Socioeconomic gradient in morbidity and mortality in people with diabetes: Cohort study findings from the Whitehall study and the WHO multinational study of vascular disease in diabetes. *British Medical Journal, 316*(7125), 100–105.

Cheng, T. L., Goodman, E., & Committee on Pediatric Research. (2015). Race, ethnicity, and socioeconomic status in research on child health. *Pediatrics, 135*(1), e225–e237.

Cloutier-Fisher, D., & Kobayashi, K. (2009). Examining social isolation by gender and geography: Conceptual and operational challenges using population health data in Canada. *Gender, Place, and Culture, 16*(2), 181–199.

Coalition for Evidence-Based Policy. (2015). *Social programs that work: Nurse-Family Partnership—top tier.* Retrieved from http://evidencebasedprograms.org/1366-2/nurse-family-partnership

Coleman, C. (2011). Teaching health care professionals about health literacy: A review of the literature. *Nursing Outlook, 59*, 70–78.

Collins, S. R., Rasmussen, P. W., Beutel, S., & Doty, M. M. (2015). *The problem of underinsured and how rising deductibles will make it worse—findings from the Commonwealth Fund biennial health insurance survey, 2014.* Retrieved from www.commonwealthfund.org/publications/issue-briefs/2015/may/problem-of-underinsurance

Colvin, J. D., Zaniletti, I., Fieldston, E. S., Gottlieb, L. M., Raphael, J. L., Hall, M., ... Shah, S. S. (2013). Socioeconomic status and in-hospital pediatric mortality. *Pediatrics, 131*(1), e182–e190.

Commission on Determinants of Health Knowledge Networks; Lee, J. H., & Sadana, R. (Eds.). (2011). *Improving equity in health by addressing social determinants.* Retrieved from https://www.cugh.org/sites/default/files/Improving%20Equity%20in%20Health%20by%20Addressing%20Social%20Determinants.pdf

Copeland, D. (2007). Conceptualizing family members of violent mentally ill individuals as a vulnerable population. *Issues in Mental Health Nursing, 28*(9), 943–975.

County of Los Angeles Public Health. (2013). *Social determinants of health: How social and economic factors affect health.* Retrieved from http://publichealth.lacounty.gov/epi/docs/SocialD_Final_Web.pdf

Cradock, A. L., McHugh, A., Mont-Ferguson, H., Grant, L., Barrett, J. L., Want, Y. C., & Gortmaker, S. L. (2011). Effect of school district policy change on consumption of sugar-sweetened beverages among high school students, Boston, Massachusetts, 2004–2006. *Preventing Chronic Disease, 8*(4), A74.

Cutler, D., & Lleras-Muney, A. (2010). Understanding differences in health behaviors by education. *Journal of Health Economics, 29*(1), 1–28.

De Chesnay, M., & Anderson, B. A. (Eds.). (2016). *Caring for the vulnerable: Perspectives in nursing theory, practice, and research* (4th ed.). Burlington, MA: Jones & Bartlett Learning.

de Souza, A. S., Fernandes, F. S., & Tavares do Carmo, M. D. (2011). Effects of maternal malnutrition and postnatal nutritional rehabilitation on brain fatty acids, learning, and memory. *Nutrition Reviews, 69*(3), 132–144.

Doubeni, C. A., Schootman, M., Major, J. M., Torres-Stone, R. A., Laiyemo, A. O., Park, Y., ... Schatzkin, A. (2012). Health status, neighborhood socioeconomic context, and premature mortality in the United States: The National Institutes of Health–AARP Diet and Health Study. *American Journal of Public Health, 102*(4), 680–688.

Dowling, M., Cooney, A., & Casey, D. (2011). A concept analysis of empowerment in chronic illness from the perspective of the nurse and the client living with chronic obstructive pulmonary disease. *Nursing and Healthcare of Chronic Illness, 3*(4), 476–487.

Dubowitz, T., Basurto-Davila, R., & Lurie, N. (2011). Racial/ethnic differences in US health behaviors: A decomposition analysis. *American Journal of Health Behavior, 35*(3), 290–304.

Dulin-Keita, A., Casazza, K., Fernandez, J. R., Goran, M. I., & Gower, B. (2012). Do neighborhoods matter? Neighborhood disorder and long-term trends in serum cortisol levels. *Journal of Epidemiology & Community Health, 66*(1), 2429.

Eckenrode, J., Campa, M., Luckey, D. W., Henderson, C. R., Jr., Cole, R., Kitzman, H., ... Olds, D. (2010). Long-term effects of prenatal and infancy nurse home visitation on the life course of youths: 19-year follow-up of a randomized trial. *Archives of Pediatrics & Adolescent Medicine, 164*(1), 9–15.

Edberg, M., Cleary, S., & Vyas, A. (2011). A trajectory model for understanding and assessing health disparities in immigrant/refugee communities. *Journal of Immigrant and Minority Health, 13*(3), 576–584.

Embrett, M. G., & Randall, G. E. (2014). Social determinants of health and health equity policy research: Exploring the use, misuse, and nonuse of policy analysis theory. *Social Science & Medicine, 108*, 147–155.

Ennis, S. R., Rios-Vargas, M., & Albert, N. G. (2011). *The Hispanic population 2010.* Retrieved from http://www.census.gov/prod/cen2010/briefs/c2010br-04.pdf

Evans, S. D., Sheffer, C. E., Bickel, W. K., Cottoms, N., Olson, M., Piti, L. P., ... Stayna, H. (2015). The process of adapting the evidence-based treatment for tobacco dependence for smokers of lower socioeconomic status. *Journal of Addiction Research & Therapy, 6*(1). doi: 10.4172/2155-6105.1000219.

Fairfield, K. M., Murray, K. M., Wierman, H. R., Han, P. K., Hallen, S., Miesfeldt, S., Trimble, E. L., ... Earle, C. C. (2012). Disparities in hospice care among older women dying with ovarian cancer. *Gynecologic Oncology, 125*(1), 14–18.

Falk-Raphael, A. R. (2001). Empowerment as a process of evolving consciousness: A model of empowered caring. *Advances in Nursing Science, 24*(1), 1–16.

Ferguson, L. A., & Pawlack, R. (2011). Health literacy: The road to improved health outcomes. *Journal for Nurse Practitioners, 7*(2), 123–129.

Finney-Brown, T. (2012). Metabolic and neurological consequences of maternal nutrition: A review. *Australian Journal of Herbal Medicine, 24*(13), 88–91.

Flaskerud, J. H., & Nyamanthi, A. M. (2000). Collaborative inquiry with low-income Latina women. *Journal of Health Care for the Poor and Underserved, 11*(3), 326–342.

Flaskerud, J. H., & Winslow, B. J. (1998). Conceptualizing vulnerable populations health-related research. *Nursing Research, 47*(2), 69–78.

Fleischer, N., Roux, A., Aazraqui, M., Spinelli, H., & De Maio, F. (2011). Socioeconomic gradients in chronic disease risk factors in middle-income countries: Evidence of effect modification by urbanicity in Argentina. *American Journal of Public Health, 101*(2) 294–301.

Flynn, L., Budd, M., & Modelski, J. (2008). Enhancing resource utilization among pregnant adolescents. *Public Health Nursing, 25*(2), 140–148.

Freudenberg, N., & Olden, K. (2010). Finding synergy: Reducing disparities in health by modifying multiple determinants. *American Journal of Public Health, 100*(S1), S25–S31.

Fyffe, D., Botticello, A., & Myaskovsky, L. (2011). Vulnerable groups living with spinal cord injury. *Topics in Spinal Cord Injury Rehabilitation, 17*(2), 1–9.

Galea, S., Tracy, M., Hoggatt, K. J., DiMaggio, C., & Karpati, A. (2011). Estimated deaths attributable to social factors in the United States. *American Journal of Public Health, 101*(8), 1456–1465.

Gelberg, L., Andersen, R., & Leake, B. (2000). The behavioral model for vulnerable populations: Application to medical care use and outcomes for homeless people. *Health Services Research, 34*(6), 1273–1302.

Gitterman, A. (Ed.). (2014). *Handbook of social work practice with vulnerable and resilient populations* (3rd ed.). New York, NY: Columbia University Press.

Gonzalez-Guarda, R. M., Peragallo, N., Vasquez, E. P., Urrutia, M. T., & Mitrani, V. B. (2009). Intimate partner violence, depression, and resource availability among a community sample of Hispanic women. *Issues in Mental Health Nursing, 30*(4), 227–236.

Gortmaker, S. L., Swinburn, B. A., Levy, D., Carter, R., Mabry, P. L., Finegood, D. T., ... Moodie, M. L. (2011). Changing the future of obesity: Science, policy, and action. *Lancet, 378*(9793), 838–847.

Hajat, S., Vardoulakis, S., Heaviside, C., & Eggen, B. (2014). Climate change effects on human health: Projections of temperature-related mortality for the UK during the 2020s, 2050s and 2080s. *Journal of Epidemiology & Community Health, 68*(7), 641–648. doi: 10.1136/jech-2013-202449.

Haley, D. F., Lucas, J., Golin, C. E., Wang, J., Hughes, J. P., Emel, L., El-Sadr, W., ... Hodder, S. L. (2014). Retention strategies and factors associated with missed visits among low-income women at increased risk of HIV acquisition in the US. *AIDS Patient Care & STDs, 28*(4), 206–217.

Hansen-Turton, T. (2012). *Nurse-managed health clinics provide badly needed primary care: But without funding, they and their patients are at risk*. Retrieved from http://www.rwjf.org/en/culture-of-health/2012/01/nurse-managed-health-clinics-provided-badly-needed-primary-carebut-without-funding-they-and-their-patients-are-at-risk.html

Hasnain-Wynia, R., Kang, R., Landrum, M. B., Vogeli, C., Baker, D., & Weissman, J. (2010). Racial and ethnic disparities within and between hospitals for inpatient quality of care: An estimation of patient-level hospital quality alliance measures. *Journal of Health Care for the Poor and Underserved, 21*(2), 629–648.

Heffner, K. L. (2011). Neuroendocrine effects of stress on immunity in the elderly: Implications for inflammatory disease. Neuroendocrine effects of stress on immunity in the elderly: Implications for inflammatory disease. *Immunology & Allergy Clinics of North America, 31*(1), 95–108.

Hilmers, A., Hilmers, D. C., & Dave, J. (2012). Neighborhood disparities in access to healthy foods and their effects on environmental justice. *American Journal of Public Health, 102*(9), 1644–1654.

Hiscock, R., Bauld, L., Amos, A., Fidler, J. A., & Munafo, M. (2012). Socioeconomic status and smoking: A review. *Annals of the New York Academy of Sciences, 1248*, 107–123.

Hiscock, R., Dobbie, F., & Bauld, L. (2015). Smoking cessation and socioeconomic status: An update of existing evidence from a national evaluation of English stop-smoking services. *Biomed Research International*, article ID 274056. Retrieved from http://www.hindawi.com/journals/bmri/2015/274056/

Hogan, V. K., Amamoo, M. A., Anderson, A. D., Webb, D., Mathews, L., Rowley, D., & Culhane, J. F. (2012). Barriers to women's participation in inter-conceptual care: A cross-sectional analysis. *BMC Public Health, 12*, 93.

Holt, J., Zabler, B., & Baisch, M. J. (2014). Evidence-based characteristics of nurse-managed health centers for quality and outcomes. *Nursing Outlook, 62*(6), 428–439.

Horowitz, A. M., Clovis, J. C., Wang, M. Q., & Kleinman, D. V. (2013). Use of recommended communication techniques by Maryland dental hygienists. *Journal of Dental Hygiene, 87*(4), 212–223.

Institute of Education Sciences, National Center for Education Statistics. (n.d.). *Children living in poverty*. Retrieved from nces.ed.gov/programs/coe/indicator_cce.asp

Institute of Medicine (IOM). (2003). *Unequal treatment: Confronting racial and ethnic disparities in healthcare*. Washington, DC: The National Academies Press.

Institute of Medicine (IOM). (2010). *For the public's health: The role of measurement in action and accountability*. Washington, DC: The National Academies Press.

Institute of Medicine (IOM). (2014). *Implications of health literacy for public health: Workshop summary*. Washington, DC: National Academies Press.

Jack, S. M., DiCenso, A., & Lohfeld, L. (2005). A theory of maternal engagement with public health nurses and family visitors. *Journal of Advanced Nursing, 49*(2), 182–190.

Jakubowski, M. (2011). Low-level environmental lead exposure and intellectual impairment in children—the current concepts of risk assessment. *International Journal of Occupational Medicine and Environmental Health, 24*(1), 1–7. doi: 10.2478/s13382-011-0009-z.

Jones, P., Winslow, B., Lee, J., Burns, M., & Esther-Zhang, X. (2011). Development of a caregiver empowerment model to promote positive outcomes. *Journal of Family Nursing, 17*(1), 11–23.

Kaiser Family Foundation. (2012, November 30). *Disparities in health and health care: Five key questions and answers*. Retrieved from http://kff.org/disparities-policy/issue-brief/disparities-in-health-and-health-care-five-key-questions-and-answers/

Kaiser Family Foundation. (2015). *Facts about the uninsured population*. Retrieved from kff.org/uninsured/fact-sheet/key-facts-about-the-uninsured-population/

Kanervisto, M., Vasankari, T., Laitinen, T., Heliovaara, M., Jousilahti, P., & Saarelainen, S. (2011). Low socioeconomic status is associated with chronic obstructive airway diseases. *Respiratory Medicine, 105*, 1140–1146.

Keeton, V., Soleimanpour, S., & Brindis, C. D. (2012). School-based health centers in an era of health care reform: Building on history. *Current Problems in Pediatric & Adolescent Health Care, 42*(6), 132–158.

Knickman, J. R., & Kovner, A. R. (Eds.). (2015). *Jonas & Kovner's health care delivery in the United States* (11th ed.). New York, NY: Springer.

Krewski, D., Westphal, M., Andersen, M. E., Paoli, G. M., Ciu, W. A. Al-Zoughool, M., ... Cote, I. (2014). A framework for the next generation of risk science. *Environmental Health Perspectives, 122*(8), 796–805.

Krieger, N., Koscheleva, A., Waterman, P. D., Chen, J. T., Beckfield, J., & Kiang, M. V. (2014). 50-year trends in US socioeconomic inequalities in health: US-born Black and White Americans, 1959–2008. *International Journal of Epidemiology*, 1294–1313. doi: 10.1093/ije/dyu047.

Krogstad, J. M., & Fry, R. (2014, April 24). *More Hispanics, Blacks enrolling in college, but lag in bachelor's degrees*. Retrieved from http://www.pewresearch.org/fact-tank/2014/04/24/more-hispanics-blacks-enrolling-in-college-but-lag-in-bachelors-degrees/

Kueny, A., Berg, J., Chowdhury, Y., & Anderson, N. (2011, May 13). Poquito a poquito: How Latino families with children who have asthma make changes in their home. *Journal of Pediatric Health Care*. doi: 10.1016/j.pedhc.2011.01.007.

Lee, K., Palacio, C., Alexandraki, I., Stewart, E., & Mooradian, A. (2011). Increasing access to health care providers through medical home model may abolish racial disparity in diabetes care: Evidence from a cross-sectional study. *Journal of the National Medication Association, 103*(3), 250–256.

Levine, M. E., Cole, S. W., Weir, D. R., & Crimmins, E. M. (2015). Childhood and later life stressors and increased inflammatory gene expression at older ages. *Social Science & Medicine, 130,* 16–22.

Liljestrand, J., & Sambath, M. R. (2012). Socioeconomic improvements and health system strengthening of maternity care are contributing to maternal mortality reduction in Cambodia. *Reproductive Health Matters, 20*(39), 62–72.

Loucks, E. B., Lynch, J. W., Pilote, L., Fuhrer, R., Almeida, N. D., Richard, H., … Benjamin, E. J. (2009). Life-course socioeconomic position and incidence of coronary heart disease: The Framingham Offspring Study. *American Journal of Epidemiology, 169*(7), 829–836.

Lubben, J., Gironda, M., Sabbath, E., Kong, J., & Johnson, C. (2015). *Social isolation presents a grand challenge for social work. Working paper no. 7.* Cleveland, OH: American Academy of Social Work and Social Welfare.

Madden, D. (2014). The relationship between low birth weight and socioeconomic status in Ireland. *Journal of Biosocial Science, 46*(2), 248–265.

Marek, K. D., Stetzer, F., Adams, S. J., Popejoy, L. L., & Rantz, M. (2012). Aging in place versus nursing home care: Comparison of costs to Medicare and Medicaid. *Research in Gerontological Nursing, 5*(2), 123–129.

Marmot, M., & Wilkinson, R. (Eds.). (2006). *Social determinants of health.* Oxford, UK: Oxford University Press.

Marmot, M., Ryff, C. D., Bumpass, L. L., Shipley, M., & Marks, N. F. (1997). Social inequalities in health: Next questions and converging evidence. *Social Science and Medicine, 44*(6), 901–910.

Martin-Gronert, M., & Ozanne, S. (2010). Mechanism linking early suboptimal nutrition and increased risk of type 2 diabetes and obesity. *The Journal of Nutrition, 140*(3), 662–666.

Maslow, A. (1987). *Motivation and personality* (3rd ed.). New York, NY: Addison-Wesley.

Mason, D. J., Jones, D. A., Roy, C., Sullivan, C. G., & Wood, L. J. (2015). Commonalities of nurse-designed models of health care. *Nursing Outlook, 63*(5), 540–553.

McAllister, M. (2010). Solution focused nursing: A fitting model for mental health nurses working in a public health paradigm. *Contemporary Nurse, 34*(2), 149–157.

Medline Plus. (2015). *How to write easy-to-read health materials.* Retrieved from https://www.nlm.nih.gov/medlineplus/etr.html

Mejdoubi, J., van den Haijkant, C. M., van Leerdam, F., Heymans, M. W., Crijnen, A. M., & Hirasing, R. A. (2015). The effect of VoorZorg, the Dutch Nurse-Family Partnership, on child maltreatment and development: A randomized controlled trial. *PLOS ONE, 10*(4), e0120182. doi: 10.371/journal.pone.0120182.

Mejdoubi, J., van den Haijkant, C. M., van Leerdam, F., Heymans, M. W., Hirasing, R. A., & Crijnen, A. M. (2013). Effect of nurse home visits vs. usual care on reducing intimate partner violence in young high-risk pregnant women: A randomized controlled trial. *PLOS ONE, 8*(10), e78185, 1–12.

Merletti, F., Galassi, C., & Spadea, T. (2011). The socioeconomic determinants of cancer. *Environmental Health, 10*(Suppl. 1), S7.

Michimi, A., & Wimberly, M. C. (2010). Associations of supermarket accessibility with obesity and fruit and vegetable consumption in the conterminous United States. *International Journal of Health Geographics, 9*(49), 1–14. doi: 10.1186/1476-072X-9-49.

Michimi, A., & Wimberly, M. C. (2015). The food environment and adult obesity in US metropolitan areas. *Geospatial Health, 10*(2), 368. doi: 10.4081/gh.2015.368.

Missildine, K., Varnell, G., Williams, J., Grover, K., Ballard, N., & Stanley-Hermanns, M. (2009). Comfort in the eye of the storm: A survey of evacuees with special medical needs. *Journal of Emergency Nursing, 35*(6), 515–520.

Monsen, K., Radosevich, D., Kerr, M., & Fulkerson, J. (2011). Public health nurses tailor interventions for families at risk. *Public Health Nursing, 28*(2), 119–128.

Montez, J. K., & Berkman, L. F. (2014). Trends in the educational gradient of mortality among US adults aged 45 to 84 years: Bringing regional context. *American Journal of Public Health, 104*(1), e82–e90.

Montez, J. K., & Zajacova, A. (2013). Trends in mortality risk by education level and cause of death among US white women from 1986 to 2006. *American Journal of Public Health, 103*(3), 473–479.

Naska, A., Katsoulis, M., Trichopoulos, D., & Trichopoulou, A. (2011). The root causes of socioeconomic differentials in cancer and cardiovascular mortality in Greece. *European Journal of Cancer Prevention, 21*(5), 490–496. doi: 10.1097/CEJ.0b013e32834ef1be.

Neumayer, E., & Plümper, T. (2015). Inequalities of income and inequalities of longevity: A cross-country study. *American Journal of Public Health, 106*(1), 160–165.

Nguyen, B. T., Cheng, Y. W., Snowden, J. M., Esakoff, T. F., Frias, A. E., & Caughey, A. B. (2012). The effect of race/ethnicity on adverse perinatal outcomes among patients with gestational diabetes mellitus. *American Journal of Obstetrics & Gynecology, 207*(4), 322e1–322e6.

Non, A. L., Roman, J. C., Gross, C. L., Gilman, S. E., Loucks, E. B., Buka, S. L., & Kubzansky, L. D. (2016). *Early childhood social disadvantage is associated with poor health behaviors in adulthood.* Annals of Human Biology.

Nurse-Family Partnership. (2011a). *Locations.* Retrieved from http://www.nursefamilypartnership.org/locations

Nurse-Family Partnership. (2011b). *Proven effective through extensive research.* Retrieved from http://www.nursefamilypartnership.org/proven-results

Nurse-Family Partnership. (2011c). *Evidence-based policy and program impact.* Retrieved from http://www.nursefamilypartnership.org/assets/PDF/Fact-sheets/NFP_Evidence-Based-2014pdf.aspx

Nurse-Family Partnership (NFP). (2015, April 15). *US Congress extends funding for the bipartisan-supported federal home visiting program.* Retrieved from http://www.nursefamilypartnership.org/NFP/media/Press-Release/NFP_Congress_MIECHV.pdf?ext=.pdf

O'Mahony, S., McHenry, J., Snow, D., Cassin, C., Schumacher, D., & Selwyn, P. A. (2008). A review of the barriers to utilization of the Medicare hospice benefits in urban populations and strategies for enhanced access. *Journal of Urban Health, 85*(2), 281–290.

Office of Disease Prevention and Health Promotion. (2015a). *Maternal, infant, and child health.* Retrieved from www.healthypeople.gov/2020/leading-health-indicators/2020-lhi-topics/Maternal-Infant-and-Child-Health/data

Office of Disease Prevention and Health Promotion. (2015b). *2020 topics and objectives—Objectives A-Z.* Retrieved from www.healthypeople.gov/2020/topics-objectives

Olds, D. L., Eckenrode, J., Henderson, C. R., Jr., Kitzman, H., Powers, L, Cole, R., … Luckey, D. (1997). Long-term effects of home visitation on maternal life course and child abuse and neglect. Fifteen-year follow-up on a randomized trial. *Journal of the American Medical Association, 278*(8), 637–643.

Olds, D. L., Kitzman, H. J., Cole, R. E., Hanks, C. A., Arcoleo, K. J., Anson, E. A., … Stevenson, A. J. (2010). Enduring effects of prenatal and infancy home visiting by nurses on maternal life course and government spending: Follow-up of a randomized trial among children at age 12 years. *Archives of Pediatric and Adolescent Medicine, 164*(5), 419–424.

Olds, D. L., Kitzman, H., Knudtson, M. D., Anson, E., Smith, J. A., Cole, R. (2014). Effect of home visiting by nurses on maternal and child mortality: Results of a 2-decade follow-up of a randomized clinical trial. *Journal of the American Medical Association Pediatrics, 168*(9), 800–806. doi: 10.1001/jamapediatrics.2014.472.

Ornstein, K., Smith, K., Foer, D., Lopez-Cantor, M., & Soriano, T. (2011). To the hospital and back home again: A nurse practitioner-based transitional care program for hospitalized homebound people. *Journal of the American Geriatrics Society, 59*(3), 544–551.

Ortega, L. (2016). Patient empowerment for dual eligible: Teaching the most vulnerable health plan members to manage their health. *Professional Case Management, 21*(1), 53–56.

Palmer, J. L., Langan, J. C., Krampe, J., Krieger, M., Lorenz, R. A. Schneider, J. K., … Lach, H. W. (2014). A model of risk reduction for older adults vulnerable to nursing home placement. *Research & Theory for Nursing Practice, 28*(2), 162–192.

Paul, I. M., Beiler, J. S., Schaefer, E. W., Hollenbeak, C. S., Alleman, N., Sturgis, S. A., …Weisman, C. S. (2012). A randomized trial of single home nursing visits vs. office-based care after nursery/maternity discharge. *Archives of Pediatric and Adolescent Medicine, 166*(3), 263–270. doi: 10.1001/archpediatrics.2011.198.

Pew Research Center. (2015, September 26). *Total fertility rate for population estimates and projections, by race-Hispanic origin and generation: 1965–1970; 2015–2020; 2060–2065.* Retrieved from http://www.pewhispanic.org/2015/09/28/modern-immigration-wave-brings-59-million-to-u-s-driving-population-growth-and-change-through-2065/9-26-2015-1-30-23-pm-2/

Rantz, M. J., Phillips, L., Aud, M., Popejoy, L., Marek, K. D., Hicks, L. L., … Miller, S. J. (2011). Evaluation of aging in place model with home care services and registered nurse care coordination in senior housing. *Nursing Outlook, 59*(1), 37–46.

Raphael, D. (2003). A society in decline. In R. Hofrichter (Ed.), *Health and social justice: Politics, ideology, and inequity in the distribution of disease* (pp. 59–88). San Francisco, CA: Jossey-Bass.

Rawlett, K. (2011). Analytical evaluation of the health belief model and the vulnerable populations conceptual model applied to a medically underserved, rural population. *International Journal of Applied Science and Technology, 1*(2): 15–21.

Roundtable on Health Literacy, Board on Population Health and Public Health Practice, Institute of Medicine, & The National Academies of Sciences, Engineering, and Medicine. (2015). *Health literacy: Past, present, and future: Workshop summary*. Washington, DC: National Academies Press.

Sadana, R., & Blas, E. (2013). What can public health programs do to improve health equity? *Public Heath Reports, 128*(Suppl. 3), 12–20.

Salem, B. E., Nyamathi, A. M., Brecht, M. L., Phillips, L. R., Mentes, J. C., Sarkisian, C., & Leake, B. (2013). Correlates of frailty among homeless adults. *Western Journal of Nursing Research, 35*(9), 1128–1152.

Scott, T. N. (2009). Utilization of the natural helper model in health promotion targeting African American men. *Journal of Holistic Nursing, 27*(4), 282–292.

Shi, L., & Stevens, G. D. (2011). *Vulnerable populations in the United States* (2nd ed.). San Francisco, CA: Jossey-Bass.

Shi, L., Stevens, G., Lebrun, L., Faed, P., & Tsai, J. (2008, November). Enhancing the measurement of health disparities for vulnerable populations. *Journal of Public Health Management and Practice,* s45–s52.

Shin, D. S., Kim, C. J., & Choi, Y. (2016). Effects of an empowerment program for self-management among rural older adults with hypertension in South Korea. *Australian Journal of Rural Health, 24*(3), 213–219. doi: 10.1111/ajr.12253.

Springer, P., Black, M., Martz, K., Deckys, C., & Soelberg, T. (2010). *Somali Bantu refugees in southwest Idaho: A community and cultural assessment*. Presentation at the Western Institute for Nursing. Abstract retrieved from http://www.nursinglibrary.org/vhl/handle/10755/157369

Stein, J. A., Andersen, R. M., Robertson, M., & Gelberg, L. (2012). Impact of hepatitis B and C infection on health services utilization in homeless adults: A test of the Gelberg-Andersen behavioral model for vulnerable populations. *Health Psychology, 31*(1), 20–30.

Strehlow, A., & Gongwa, M. (2005). *Innovative models of practice in vulnerable populations: Administrative perspective of the vulnerable populations model*. Presentation at the Western Institute for Nursing. Abstract retrieved from http://www.nursinglibrary.org/vhl/handle/10755/157991

Stremikis, K., Berenson, J., Shih, A., & Riley, P. (2011, August). *Health care opinion leaders' views on vulnerable populations in the U.S. health system*. Retrieved from http://www.cdc.gov/mmwr/pdf/other/su6203.pdf

Sumner, L., Wong, L., Schetter, C., Myers, H., & Rodriguez, M. (2012). Predictors of posttraumatic stress disorder symptoms among low-income Latinas during pregnancy and postpartum. *Psychological Trauma: Theory, Research, Practice, and Policy, 4*(2): 196–203. doi: 10.1037/a0023538.

Trivedi, A. N., Nsa, W., Hausmann, L., Lee, J. S., Ma, A., Bratzler, D. W.,… Fine, M. J. (2014). Quality and equity of care in U.S. hospitals. *The New England Journal of Medicine, 371,* 2298–2308.

Trupin, L., Katz, P. P., Balmes, J. R., Chen, H., Yelin, E. H., Omachi, T., & Blanc, P. D. (2013). Mediators of the socioeconomic gradient in outcomes of adult asthma and rhinitis. *American Journal of Public Health, 103*(2), e31–e38.

U.S. Census Bureau. (2008). *An older and more diverse nation by mid-century*. Retrieved from http://www.census.gov/ewsroom/releases/archives/population/cb08-123.html

U.S. Census Bureau. (2011). *2010 census shows America's diversity*. Retrieved from https://www.census.gov/2010census/news/releases/operations/cb11-cn125.html

U.S. Department of Health & Human Services (USDHHS). (2011). *Home visiting evidence of effectiveness: Implementing NFP*. Retrieved from http://homvee.acf.hhs.gov/Implementation/3/Nurse-Family-Partnership-NFP—Program-Model-Overview/14

U.S. Department of Health and Human Services. (2014). *Federal poverty guidelines for FFY 2015*. Retrieved from www.liheapch.act.hhs.gov/profiles/povertytables/FY2015/popstate.htm

U.S. Department of Health and Human Services (USDHHS). (2016). *About Healthy People 2020*. Retrieved from http://www.healthy-people.gov/2020/About-Healthy-People

U.S. Department of Health and Human Services (USDHHS). (n.d.). *Determinants of health*. Retrieved from http://www.healthypeople.gov/2020/about/DOHAbout.aspx

Wang, S., Quong, J., Kanaya, A., & Fernandez, A. (2011). Asian Americans and obesity in California: A protective effect of bicultur-alism. *Journal of Immigrant and Minority Health, 13*(2), 276–283.

Whitehead, M. & Dahlgren, G. (2006). *The concepts and principles for tackling social inequalities in health: Levelling up, Part 1*. Copenhagen, Denmark: WHO/EURO.

Williams, D. R., & Mohammed, S. A. (2013). Racism and health I: Pathways and scientific evidence. *American Behavioral Scientist, 57*(8), 1152–1173. doi: 10.1177/0002764213487340.

Wolf, M. S., Wilson, E. A. H., Rapp, D. N., Waite, K. R., Boccini, M. V., Davis, T. C., & Rudd, R. E. (2009). Literacy and learning in health care. *Pediatrics, 124*(Suppl. 3), s275–s281.

World Bank. (2015). *Overview*. Retrieved from www.worldband.org/en/topic/poverty/overview

World Health Organization. (2016a). *Health Impact Assessment (HIA): The determinants of health*. Retrieved from http://www.who.int/hia/evidence/doh/en/

World Health Organization. (2016b). *What are social determinants of health?* Retrieved from http://www.who.int/social_determinants/sdh_definition/en/

Wu, T. Y., Jen, M. H., Bottle, A., Liaw, C. K., Aylin, P., & Majeed, A. (2011). Admission rates and in-hospital mortality for hip fractures in England 1998 to 2009: Time trends study. *Journal of Public Health, 33*(2), 284–291.

Yang, S., Platt, R. W., Dahhou, M., & Kramer, M. S. (2014). The population-based interventions widen or narrow socioeconomic inequalities? The case of breastfeeding promotion. *International Journal of Epidemiology, 43*(4), 1284–1292.

Yarnell, J. W., Patterson, C. C., Arveiler, D., Amouyel, P., Ferrieres, J., Woodside, J. V., … Ducimetière, P. (2012). Contribution of lifetime smoking habit in France and Northern Ireland to country and socioeconomic differentials in mortality and cardiovascular incidence: The PRIME study. *Journal of Epidemiology and Community Health, 66*(7), 599–604. doi: 10.1136/jech.2010.123943.

Zarzaur, B., Croce, M., Fabian, T., Fisher, P., & Magnotti, L. (2010). A population-based analysis of neighborhood socioeconomic status and injury admission rates and in-hospital mortality. *Journal of the American College of Surgeons, 211*(2), 216–223.

Zerwekh, J. (2000). Caring on the ragged edge: Nursing persons who are disenfranchised. *Advances in Nursing Science, 22*(4), 47–61.

Clients with Disabilities and Chronic Illnesses

"I choose not to place 'DIS,' in my ability."

—*Robert M. Hensel* (1969–, Disability Advocate)

KEY TERMS

Activity
Activity limitations
American Sign Language
Americans with Disabilities
  Act
Assistive devices and
  technology

Body functions
Body structures
Braille
Built environment
Chronic disease
Disability
Environmental factors

Functioning
Handicaps
Impairments
Participation
Participation restrictions
People with disabilities
Personal factors

Secondary conditions
Universal design

LEARNING OBJECTIVES

Upon mastery of this chapter, you should be able to:

- Discuss the national and global implications of disability and chronic illness.
- Describe the economic, social, and political factors affecting the well-being of individuals with disabilities and chronic illness.
- Provide an example of primary, secondary, and tertiary prevention practices for disabled individuals.
- Describe the Americans with Disabilities Act.
- Discuss the benefits of universal design for all persons.

At some point in our lives, many or even most of us will be diagnosed with a chronic illness or develop some type of disability. We may be fortunate enough to be diagnosed early and treated promptly for our health conditions and receive sufficient and effective disease and symptom management. But on the other hand, we might become temporarily incapacitated, become unable to manage our daily lives, and require assistance from others. In these situations, we will hope that a swift recovery will assist us to resume our normal activities. Currently, over 53 million persons report living with some sort of disability in the United States (Courtney-Long et al., 2015). This represents approximately 22% of the population and includes 13% of people reporting mobility issues, 10.6% of people reporting cognitive disabilities, 6.5% of people reporting disabilities that inhibit independent living, 4.6% of people reporting vision deficits, and 3.6% of people reporting self-care deficit disabilities. In 2015, one of every five adults in the United States had been doctor-diagnosed with arthritis, mostly commonly osteoarthritis. With population growth and an aging population, by 2030, the number of adults with arthritis is expected to increase to 67 million (Centers for Disease Control and Prevention [CDC], 2016).

In addition to the human burden of disability and chronic illness, the related financial costs of direct medical care and associated indirect costs had significant impact on public and private payers of health and social insurance. A 2011 report (Anderson, Wiener, Finkelstein, & Armour, 2011) found that national disability-associated health care expenditures were $397.9 billion in 2006, or 26.7% of all U.S. national spending for health. Individuals with disabilities have higher health care costs because they have more chronic conditions, and secondly, they have poorer health status that requires more health care services. It is difficult to separate the costs of disability from the costs of chronic conditions, because it is often challenging to identify which occurred first (Smith, Molton, & Jensen, 2016). But it is clear that reducing both types of costs will be facilitated by improved health promotion and preventive services, as well as by expanding coordinated care and targeted disease management programs (Kyounghae et al., 2016).

Healthy People 2020 document details the continued impact of chronic and disabling diseases and conditions on Americans. For example, arthritis remains the leading cause of disability in the United States, with a direct impact on approximately 43 million individuals, including more than 20% of the adult population (Office of Disease Prevention and Health Promotion [ODPHP], 2016). Asthma is a national health concern for all ages, especially for those under 18 years of age, and represents one of the four most common causes of chronic illness in children. Of particular concern are health disparities in asthma morbidity and mortality, particularly for low-income and minority populations (ODPHP, 2016). The prevalence of chronic kidney disease (CKD) and end-stage kidney disease (ESKD) continues to increase; diabetes is the most common cause of kidney failure. Treatment of CKD and ESKD is expensive, with nearly 25% of the Medicare budget needed to treat Americans with these two diseases (ODPHP, 2016). Back pain impacts 80% of all Americans at some time in their lives; at any point in time, three to four percent of the population is temporarily disabled because of back pain. Chronic back pain has diverse risk factors, including age, fitness level, race, ethnicity, and occupation. Among those 50 years and older, 16.5% are estimated to have osteoporosis and have risk factors for additional serious injury or death following a potential fall (ODPHP, 2016). Addressing the complex and interrelated issues of disability and chronic illness is vital to the well-being of affected individuals and families and ultimately crucial to the financial health of the nation and its health care delivery systems.

This chapter discusses important and necessary health promotion and preventive efforts at every level. Although the treatment of chronic conditions has long been a mainstay of health care in the United States and globally, much less attention has been paid to health promotion approaches required to prevent, maintain, and improve overall well-being of individuals with chronic conditions and those at risk for these conditions. In addition, too little attention has been directed toward health promotion approaches for those with physical or psychological disabilities.

This chapter begins with an overview of disabilities and chronic illnesses, followed by a discussion of current national and global trends in addressing these issues. The various organizations that focus on improving the well-being of those affected by chronic and disabling conditions, the impact on their families, and the role of the community/public health nurse in addressing the related needs of individuals, families, and aggregates are discussed. The benefits of universal design and issues of easy access for all ages and abilities are introduced.

PERSPECTIVES ON DISABILITY, CHRONIC ILLNESS, AND HEALTH

Do you know someone living with a disability? Have you cared for a patient living with a disability? What have you learned about their lives? What does the word *disability* mean to you? Do you have thoughts or images that come to mind when you think about **disability** as it applies to an individual person? Disabilities may be congenital, developed early in life, or developed later in life. This can be a chronic condition or acquired through things like trauma (Krahn, Walker, & Correa-de-Araujo, 2015). Although in the past, people living with disabilities may have been invisible to most because they were often "shut-in" their family's home or institutionalized in a long-term state facility, today, those who face added physical challenges in their daily lives now emphasize their abilities, over what was viewed in the past as their incapacities, inabilities, or handicaps, and studies show that those with disabilities are able to engage in positive health behaviors when motivation is internal (Wilroy, Knowlden, & Birch, 2016).

The negative connotations embedded in public perceptions about disability evoke the prevalent societal views and stereotypes faced daily by **people with disabilities**. The negative views and blaming remarks that can be directed toward persons living with disabilities have been challenged by those living with disabilities, as well as their families, their allies, and their advocates. New and more positive approaches continue to emerge that view individuals and their needs from a more person-centered, holistic standpoint. The diverse personal narratives of those living with disabilities emphasize the individual circumstances and unique responses to disability, and social support and potential inclusive care for the individual have a positive impact on engaging those with disabilities in settings such as work (Cook, Foley, & Semeah, 2016).

The separate, but related, concept of **chronic disease** or chronic illness is any disease process that is prolonged, does not resolve spontaneously, and is rarely cured completely (Goodman, Posner, Huang, Parekh, & Koh, 2013). Chronic illness and disability-related needs differ from one individual to another and may differ from day to day or over time for one individual. An individual's needs may require different degrees or modes of accommodation. Chronic diseases may require regular self-care to avoid exacerbations and increased risks of complications, which could pose a significant burden in terms of mortality, morbidity, and personal and societal cost.

Because chronic diseases may be and are increasingly preventable, individuals living with a disability must be included in clinical and population health strategies to prevent acquisition of additional chronic diseases or threats to their health (Mahmoudi & Meade, 2015; Reichard, Gulley, Rasch, & Chan, 2015). In the landmark U.S. Surgeon General's *Call to Action to Improve the Health and Wellness of Persons with Disabilities* placed the health of persons living with disabilities equal in importance to the health of the nation, and today, disability remains a priority for the nation reflected in *Healthy People 2020* (ODPHP, 2016).

International Classification of Functioning, Disability, and Health

The *International Classification of Functioning, Disability, and Health* (ICF) supports the more positive, emerging approaches to understanding chronic and disabling conditions (World Health Organization [WHO], 2001). Although dated, this is the relevant guide to classification of disability worldwide. The ICF replaced the outdated *International Classification of Impairments, Disabilities, and Handicaps (ICIDH)*. The significant shift in the classification's title and framework concretely reflects the profound shifts in professional thought that led to removal of concepts such as **impairments** and **handicaps**. In what remains the current version of the ICF, "disability" serves as a broad term for impairments, activity limitations, and participation restrictions. Disability is linked to "**functioning**," a term that encompasses all body functions, activities, and participation (WHO, 2001).

The ICF (WHO, 2001) is a universal classification system using standardized language that views the domains of health from a holistic viewpoint. It takes into account body functions and structures, activities and participation, environmental factors, and personal factors. This multidimensional approach supports a complex evaluation of an individual's circumstances in terms of functioning, disability, and health. Through combining the "medical model" of health and health care for disabled persons with the "social model," the ICF provides a biopsychosocial approach for assessing people with disabilities. Its approach emphasizes that no two people with the same disease or disability have the same level of functioning: diseases and disabilities are conditions, not persons. Yet, a client may be referred to inappropriately as "the paraplegic" or "the amputee," rather than by the given name. This type of disrespectful designation or stereotype should be avoided: a disease or disability is something one has, not something one is. The individual context and status of each person must be identified as a first step.

The key aims of the ICF are the following:

- Provide a scientific basis for understanding and studying health and health-related states, outcomes, and determinations
- Establish a common language for describing health and health-related states to improve communication between different users such as health care workers, researchers, policy makers, and the public, including people with disabilities
- Permit comparison of data across countries, health care disciplines, services, and time
- Provide a systematic coding scheme for health information systems (WHO, 2001, p. 5)

Contributing to these emerging perspectives, the following concepts and related definitions further clarify the ICF view of health:

- **Body functions** are the physiologic functions of body systems and include psychological functions.
- **Body structures** are anatomic parts of the body such as organs, limbs, and their components.
- *Impairments* are problems in body function or structure, such as a significant deviation or loss.
- **Activity** is the execution of a task or action by an individual.
- **Participation** is involvement in a life situation.
- **Activity limitations** are difficulties an individual may have in executing activities.
- **Participation restrictions** are problems an individual may experience when involved in life situations.
- **Environmental factors** make up the physical, social, and attitudinal environments in which people live and conduct their lives (WHO, 2002a, p. 10).

- **Personal factors** are the features of an individual's background, life, and living that are not part of a health condition or health status, such as gender, race, age, other health conditions, fitness, lifestyle habits, upbringing, coping styles, social background, education, profession, past and current experience, overall behavior pattern and character style, individual psychological assets, and other characteristics—which may play a role in disability at any level.

For public health nursing practice, application of the ICF reinforces that disability and disease are additional factors to be considered in planning and implementing a care plan for individual clients and for population groups in the community. For individual clients, the ICF guides and facilitates assessment across a wide range of variables. Although two individuals may have the same apparent disability, such as a below-the-knee amputation, their health status and personal well-being can be quite different. One may have a more positive outlook, one may have more social supports than the other, or one may suffer more than the other from additional health issues that complicate rehabilitation. The public health nurse must always consider the totality of the situation, including the biologic, psychological, sociocultural, and environmental realms of the whole person.

Figure 26–1 depicts the interactions among the various components of the ICF, in relation to evaluation and assessment of clients with disabilities. It can also serve as a useful model for public health nursing practice in the overall assessment of people with disabilities.

The World Health Reports

The World Health Report (WHR) 2002: Reducing Risks, Promoting Healthy Life (WHO, 2002b) document heightened the standard for addressing global health. The World Health Organization challenged the global community to increase the focus on unhealthy behaviors that can ultimately lead to chronic disease, disability, and early mortality. Although infectious diseases and malnutrition require continuing surveillance because of their ongoing impact on populations in many parts of the world, WHO has stressed that these are not the only threat. Lifestyle choices are also one of the key contributors to morbidity and mortality levels in both affluent and poor countries. In heightening

the focus on unhealthy lifestyle choices, the 2002 report underscored a twofold purpose: to quantify the most important risks to health and to assess the cost-effectiveness of interventions designed to reduce those risks. The World Health Organization's overall goal was to help all governments lower health risks and increase healthy life expectancy within their country (WHO, 2002b). A high priority was to target interventions at local, national, regional, and international levels.

The *WHR 2002* (WHO, 2002b) emphasized that health care providers worldwide should broaden their clinical and population health practices, rather than continue a narrow focus on acute illness. Changes in lifestyles and behaviors that have key impacts on increasing healthy years of life should be emphasized. Some of the health risks detailed in 2002, as well as in the 2009 WHO report, highlight factors that are the direct result of economic poverty. Other factors result from excesses, especially among some populations in more affluent countries. The ten leading health risks identified by the WHO are (1) underweight; (2) unsafe sex; (3) high blood pressure; (4) tobacco consumption; (5) alcohol consumption; (6) unsafe water, sanitation, and hygiene; (7) iron deficiency; (8) indoor smoke from solid fuels; (9) high cholesterol; and (10) obesity (WHO, 2002b, 2009). Across the globe, these ten health risks contribute to more than one third of all deaths and a significant proportion of disability. Half of these risk factors—tobacco and alcohol consumption, high blood pressure, high cholesterol, and obesity—are directly related to lifestyle and behavioral choices (WHO, 2009). The 2011 report noted the importance of service delivery, technology and continued research, along with use of evidence-based practice in designing and evaluating services (WHO and The World Bank, 2011).

Given the vital link between nutrition and health, nutritional imbalances can contribute to severe chronic illness, disability, and premature death. Of the leading 10 health risks (above), five are directly related to consumption: underweight, hypertension, iron deficiency, high cholesterol, and obesity (WHO, 2009). The worldwide prevalence of adult overweight is estimated at 1.9 billion, including 600 million adults classified as obese. Being overweight increases the risk of coronary heart disease, stroke, diabetes, musculoskeletal disorders, and some types of cancer (WHO, 2016).

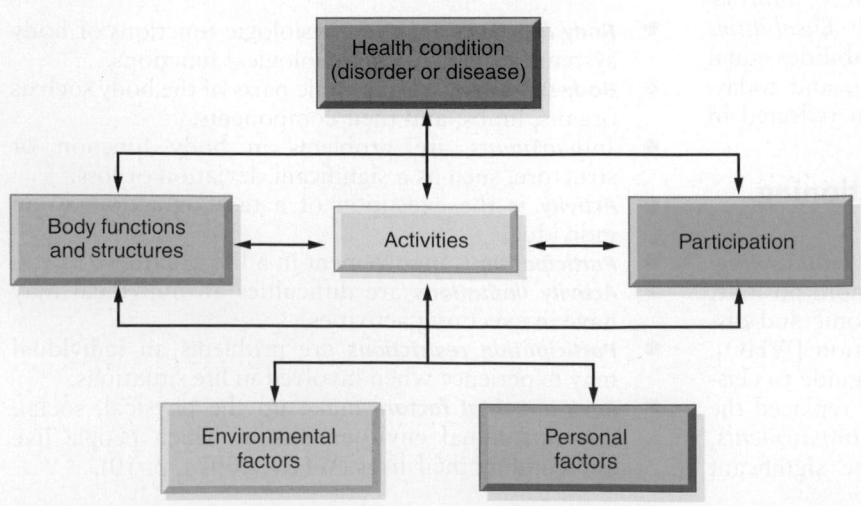

FIGURE 26–1 Model of functioning and disability. (From the World Health Organization (WHO). (2001). *ICF introduction.* Geneva, Switzerland: Author.)

In stark contrast to global patterns of overweight and obesity, an estimated 103 million children under 5 years of age (18%) were underweight in 2013 in developing countries, even though the number of affected children decreased 11% between 1990 and 2010 (WHO, 2016). In developing countries in 2011, an estimated 35% of all deaths in children 5 years of age and younger had underweight as an underlying cause (WHO, 2016). For underweight children who survive, malnutrition and deficits of important nutrients can lead to a wide array of preventable disabilities. For example, the leading cause of acquired blindness in children is vitamin A deficiency, and the leading cause of mental retardation and brain damage is iodine deficiency (Andersen, Olsen, & Laurberg, 2015; Stevens et al., 2015).

The health outlook for these at-risk populations would dramatically improve if national and local governments would make minimal strides toward improving the health of their citizens. Governments must take a proactive role in addressing the preventive health care needs of their citizens (Display 26–1). A shift away from the narrow focus on curative services for the most high-risk individuals, and a recentering on preventive interventions for the general population is essential (Moore, 2013). For decades, public health professionals have stressed that the main focus should be on primary and secondary prevention. As difficult as it has been in the United States to implement a shift in emphasis from treatment to health promotion efforts, it will be interesting to see if advocacy, education, and global health interventions can rebalance efforts between primary and secondary prevention against tertiary prevention. Preventing chronic disease and limiting disabilities are vital to improving global health. Although the cost of health care treatment is high, total costs are disproportionally higher when the human burden leading to lost productivity and decreased quality of life is considered. The adage "an ounce of prevention is worth a pound of cure" applies to these burdens as well.

The United Nations Convention on the Rights of Persons with Disabilities

An estimated 1 billion people across the globe (15% of the worldwide population) live with disabilities, with between 110 and 190 million (2.2% to 3.8%) people 15 years and older having significant difficulties in functioning (WHO, 2016). Factoring in the over 2 billion family members affected by disability, the WHO stressed that almost one third of the world population is directly impacted by disabilities. The sheer magnitude of this issue and the recognition that people with disabilities are a developmental challenge that is significantly overlooked across the world led to the 2006 United Nations (UN) Convention on the Rights of Persons with Disabilities (CRPD). To date, 160 countries have signed the Convention or its Optional Protocol (United Nations [UN], 2016). This document remains the standard for considering the rights of those with disabilities, regardless of age, race, gender, or other demographic considerations.

Specific principles of the UN Convention on the Rights of Persons with Disabilities (UN, 2016, para. 4) include the following:

- Respect for inherent dignity and individual autonomy, including the freedom to make one's own choices and independence of persons

- Nondiscrimination
- Full and effective participation and inclusion in society
- Respect for difference and acceptance of persons with disabilities as part of human diversity and humanity
- Equality of opportunity
- Accessibility
- Equality between men and women
- Respect for evolving capacities of children with disabilities and respect for the right of children with disabilities to preserve their identities

The U.S. National Council on Disability (NCD) has advocated for U.S. ratification of the Convention to provide leadership in the arena of disabilities and disability advocacy (NCD, 2014). Although the U.S. Congress passed legislation in support of the UN Convention on the Rights of Persons with Disabilities in 2009, this positive effort proved symbolic, because the effort fell short of the needed step to ratify the Convention. This happened because only Congress can ratify treaties. Wishing to take a concrete step that would be visible to other nations, President Barack Obama publicly signed the United Nations Convention on the Rights of Persons with Disabilities Proclamation. In doing so, he recalled his father-in-law's battle with disability secondary to multiple sclerosis and the beneficial contributions of the Americans with Disability Act (White House, 2009). By mid-2012, the U.S. Senate was still discussing the Convention's ratification (McCain, 2012). In mid-2016, despite a wide variety of successful legislation and program development at the national level in the United States (see Table 26–1), the United States has been unable to ratify the United Nations Convention on the Rights of Persons with Disabilities Proclamation. Many reasons are cited as to why this document has not been ratified, and supporters and opponents continue to heavily debate the ratification.

The World Report on Disability

In 2011, the WHO and the World Bank reassessed global progress on disability since the 2006 *Convention on the Rights of Persons with Disabilities* (UN, 2016). The *Convention* provided guidance to governments globally, that it was their responsibility to improve the lives of individuals and families living with disability. Citizens of every country must and need to participate in their country's development. People living with disabilities must advocate for the removal of barriers that prevent their full participation in their communities, including access to health, education, employment, transportation, and information services. To assure full participation of people with disabilities in their communities, stakeholders in each country—and globally—must establish an inclusive world characterized by enabling environments, rehabilitation and support services, adequate social protection, and relevant policies, programs, standards, and legislation (WHO and World Bank, 2011).

Specific recommendations of the 2011 *World Report on Disability* directed governments to

- Enable access to all mainstream systems and services
- Invest in specific programs and services for people with disabilities

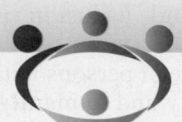

DISPLAY 26–1 BETTER HEALTH FOR PEOPLE WITH DISABILITIES

Better health for people with disabilities

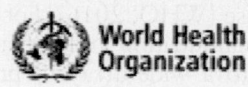
World Health Organization

Over 1 BILLION
people globally experience disability

1 in 7 people

People with disabilities have the same general health care needs as others

But they are:

2x more likely to find health care providers' skills and facilities inadequate

3x more likely to be denied health care

4x more likely to be treated badly in the health care system

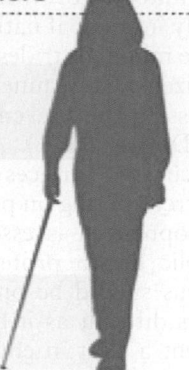

1/2 of people with disabilities cannot afford health care

They are:

50% more likely to suffer catastrophic health expenditure

These out-of-pocket health care payments can push a family into poverty

---

Rehabilitation and assistive devices can enable people with disabilities to be independent

200 MIL people need glasses or other low-vision devices and do not have access to them

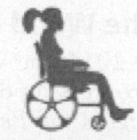

70 MIL people need a wheelchair. Only 5–15% have access to one

360 MIL people globally have moderate to profound hearing loss

Production of hearing aids only meets:

10% of global need **3%** of developing countries' needs

Making all health care services accessible to people with disabilities is achievable and will reduce unacceptable health disparities

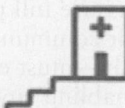

remove physical barriers to health facilities, information and equipment

make health care affordable

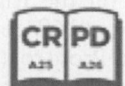
CRPD

train all health care workers in disability issues including rights

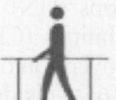

invest in specific services such as rehabilitation

Source: World report on disability: www.who.int/disabilities/world_report

WHO. (n.d.). *Disability and rehabilitation: Advocacy material.* Retrieved from http://www.who.int/disabilities/facts/Infographic_en_pdf.pdf?ua=1.

Table 26-1 Disability Rights Laws

Law	Summary	Contact
Americans with Disabilities Act (ADA)	Prohibits discrimination in (1) employment, (2) state and local government, (3) public accommodations, commercial facilities, transportation, and telecommunications	(1) U.S. Equal Opportunity Commission (2) Civil Rights Division (3) U.S. Department of Justice (USDOJ) (4) Office of Civil Rights, Federal Transit Administration
Telecommunications Act of 1996	Telecommunication equipment and services are accessible	Federal Communications Commission (FCC)
Fair Housing Act (amended 1988)	Prohibits housing discrimination	U.S. Department of Housing and Urban Development (HUD)
Air Carrier Access Act	Prohibits discrimination in air transportation by domestic and foreign carriers	U.S. Department of Transportation (DOT)
Voting Accessibility for the Elderly and Handicapped Act of 1984	Requires polling places to be physically accessible for federal elections	USDOJ, Civil Rights Division
National Voter Registration Act of 1993	"Motor Voter Act"—makes it easier to vote by increasing low registration rates by minorities and persons with disabilities	USDOJ, Civil Rights Division
Civil Rights of Institutionalized Persons Act (CRIPA) 1997	Right to receive care in the least restrictive setting	USDOJ
Individuals with Disabilities Education Act	Make available free public education in the least restrictive environment for all children with disabilities	U.S. Department of Education, Office of Special Education Programs
Rehabilitation Act	Prohibits discrimination in all federal programs or programs receiving federal financial assistance	(1) Employer's Equal Employment Opportunity Office (2) U.S. Department of Labor, Office of Federal Contract Compliance Programs (3) USDOJ
Architectural Barriers Act	Buildings constructed or altered with federal funds must meet federal accessibility standards.	U.S. Architectural and Transportation Barriers Compliance Board

From U.S. Department of Justice, Civil Rights Division, Disability Rights Section. (2009). *A guide to disability rights law*. Retrieved from http://www.ada.gov/cguide.htm

- Adopt a national disability strategy and plan of action
- Involve people with disabilities
- Improve human resource capacity
- Provide adequate funding and improve affordability
- Increase public awareness and understanding
- Improve disability data collection
- Strengthen and support research on disability (WHO and World Bank, 2011)

Citizens of every country, including Americans at every level, can become engaged in translating the recommendations of the *World Report on Disability* into action. Even though government at every level must play a significant part, operationalizing the *World Report* affords important roles for service providers, academic institutions, the private sector, communities, and especially people with disabilities and their families (The Arc, n.d.).

Healthy People 2020

In the United States, *Healthy People* is the most influential series of planning documents that seek to address health promotion and disease prevention as a basis for improving the health of all Americans (ODPHP, 2016). *Healthy People* strives toward a vision of a society in which all people live long, healthy lives. Through its clearly delineated, science-based, and measurable objectives, the decennial *Healthy People* has had far-reaching influences on national and state health initiatives, health care policy, research priorities, and funding since its first efforts in 1979. The evolving American perspectives on disability and on chronic illness have been reflected in the changing focus of the Healthy People series. Following the decades influenced by *Healthy People 1990* and *Healthy People 2000*, *Healthy People 2010* provided guidance during the 2000s, and *Healthy People 2020* guided public health interventions in the 2010s (ODPHP, 2016).

The four overarching goals of the current *Healthy People 2020* are to

- Attain high-quality, longer lives free of preventable disease, disability, injury, and premature death
- Achieve health equity, eliminate disparities, and improve the health of all groups
- Create social and physical environments that promote good health for all
- Promote quality of life, healthy development, and healthy behaviors across all ages (U.S. Department of Health & Human Services [USDHHS], 2016, para. 5)

A comparison among Healthy People plans since its inception underscores the emergence of new approaches to both identifying priority areas and planning to improve the health of individuals with disabilities and chronic illness. In *Healthy People 2000*, only one priority area was devoted to disability and chronic illness. The priority "Diabetes and Chronic Disabling Conditions" emphasized diabetes, with only limited attention to the broader range of other disabilities, including asthma, CKD, arthritis, deformities or orthopedic impairments, mental retardation, peptic ulcer disease, visual and hearing impairments, and overweight (USDHHS, 2016).

The development of *Healthy People 2010* (implemented 2001 to 2011) reflected the accelerating interest in addressing the health promotion and disease prevention needs of those living with disabilities. In this light, *Healthy People 2010* defined disability as a barrier for those with a heath condition to interacting with their environment (ODPHP, 2016). Individuals with disabilities were classified as those with activity limitations that prevent them from interacting successfully with their environment or the perception that the individual cannot react without difficulties within their environment (ODPHP, 2016). *Healthy People 2010* focused directly on disability and chronic illness in the section "Disability and Secondary Conditions," with frequent attention to these topics across almost all the focus areas of *Healthy People 2010*. In terms of disability and chronic illness, *Healthy People 2010* increased the emphasis on conditions expected to take a future toll on the nation's health in the coming years, as well highlighted conditions expected to become an economic burden to the nation and for individual Americans and their families.

One of the most influential aspects of the decade of *Healthy People 2010* was to promote a change in thinking within the health care community about the health promotion and disease prevention needs of people with disabilities. This shift was essential to remedy the lack of existing health promotion and disease prevention activities for this population. The previous degree of neglect of health promotion and disease prevention for people with disabilities led to an increase in the number and extent of secondary conditions, and this is a great concern, especially considering the impact on the medical, social, emotional, mental, family, or community problems that a person with a disability may experience (Froehlich-Grobe, Jones, Businelle, Kendzor, & Balasubramanian,

2016). Approaching the health needs of disabled persons from the traditional standpoint of asking what medical, rehabilitative, or long-term care is needed failed to reduce illness or improve the overall well-being of the disabled or chronically ill. In fact, misconceptions about those with disabilities and chronic illness impeded progress in this area. Examples of misconceptions include the following: (a) all people with disabilities have poor health or may have chronic pain, (b) those with disabilities should be treated as different and special, (c) public health activities need to focus only on preventing disability, (d) people with disabilities are similar, (e) there is no need for a clear definition of "disability" or "people with disabilities" in public health practice, and (f) environment does not play a significant role in the disability process (Together We Rock, n.d.).

Increased national attention to the needs of the disabled has improved and should continue to do so as the needs specific to disabled persons are seen as less specific to that population and more universal to all Americans. This changing focus in public perspectives on disability and health is clearly evident in the definition of health promotion used in *Healthy People 2010* to create healthy lifestyles and environments (USDHHS, 2016). It is important to note that *Healthy People 2020* does not list this as a separate component because the purpose of *Healthy People 2020* is to focus on health promotion (Bolin et al., 2015).

Implementation of *Healthy People 2010* led to improved documentation of the lack of parity between disabled and nondisabled populations for several *Healthy People* objectives, including (a) leisure-time physical activity, (b) use of community support programs, and (c) receipt of clinical preventive services. For example, people with disabilities reported engaging in some type of leisure-time physical activity less frequently than any other group, even less frequently than those with low rates of physical activity compared to the general population, such as individuals 65 years of age and older, as well as low-income persons. People with disabilities also have challenges in relation to additional *Healthy People 2010* objectives, including an increased likelihood of being overweight, increased adverse effects from stress, and reduced user rates for preventive services such as receiving tetanus boosters, Pap tests, breast examinations, and mammograms. Halfway between *Healthy People 2010* and *Healthy People 2020*, the 2005 *Midcourse Review* analyzed changes since implementation of *Healthy People 2010*. It recognized the issue with accommodations for those with disabilities in disaster management and disaster settings (USDHHS, 2016). Two objectives moved further away from their 2010 targets. A 7% increase occurred in the proportion of adults who expressed that negative feelings were impacting their lives—32% in 2003 versus the 28% level reported in 1997. Secondly, in relation to employment, the proportion of adults with disabilities who were employed dropped between 1997 and 2003. As during the recession of 2001, there was a further disproportionate impact on adults with disabilities of the economic instability beginning in 2008, resulting in decreased progression toward the employment goals for 2010 (USDHHS, 2006).

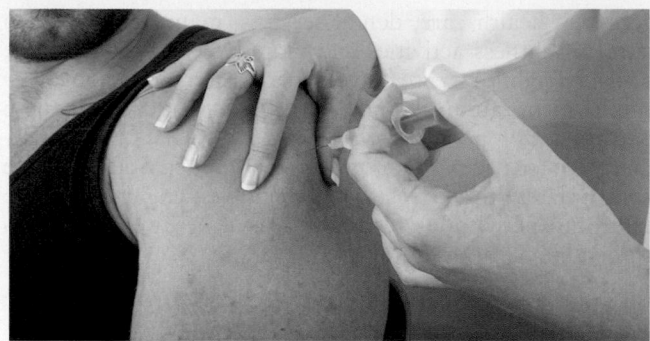

Preventive services, like immunizations, are sometimes forgotten among the disabled population.

Healthy People 2020 was released in late 2011, based on an extensive review of recent and evolving research and national surveys and public and professional reviews and input (Fielding, Kumanyika, & Manderscheid, 2013). In *Healthy People 2020*, the

section "Disability and Health" further strengthens *Healthy People*'s approach to disability to emphasize the principles of health promotion and disease prevention for those currently experiencing disabilities and/or chronic illnesses. Rather than narrowly defining individuals with disabilities and/or chronic illnesses through their limiting conditions, *Healthy People 2020* developers understand that individuals with disabilities and/or chronic illnesses have the potential to meet and exceed health promotion and disease prevention goals set for the nation's population as a whole. This approach is consistent with the multifaceted national goal of improving parity across all groups and among all individuals. For example, the goal of "Disability and Health" in *Healthy People 2020* is to engage those with disabilities of all ages to maintain the optimal state of health and prevent chronic conditions so that the highest quality of life can be maintained (ODPHP, 2016). Twenty main objectives were identified across four broad categories, including (1) systems and policies, (2) barriers to heath care, (3) environment, and (4) activities and participation (see Table 26–2).

Table 26–2 *Healthy People 2020:* Disability and Health—Objectives

Systems and Policies

- DH-1 Increase the number of population-based data systems used to monitor *Healthy People 2020* objectives that include in their core a standardized set of questions that identify people with disabilities.
- DH-2 Increase the number of Tribes, States, and the District of Columbia that have public health surveillance and health promotion programs for people with disabilities and caregivers.
- DH-3 Increase the proportion of U.S. master of public health (M.P.H.)-granting programs that offer graduate-level studies in disability and health.

Barriers to Health Care

- DH-4 Reduce the proportion of adults with disabilities aged 18 years and older who experience delays in receiving primary and periodic preventive care due to specific barriers.
- DH-5 Increase the proportion of youth with special health care needs whose health care provider has discussed transition planning from pediatric to adult health care.
- DH-6 Increase the proportion of people with epilepsy and uncontrolled seizures who receive appropriate medical care.
- DH-7 Reduce the proportion of older adults with disabilities who use inappropriate medications.

Environment

- DH-8 Reduce the proportion of adults with disabilities aged 18 years and older who experience physical or program barriers that limit or prevent them from using available local health and wellness programs.
- DH-11 Increase the proportion of newly constructed and retrofitted U.S. homes and residential buildings that have visitable features.
- DH-12 Reduce the number of people with disabilities living in congregate care residences.

Activities and Participation

- DH-13 Increase the proportion of adults with disabilities aged 18 years and older who participate in leisure, social, religious, or community activities.
- DH-14 Increase the proportion of children and youth with disabilities who spend at least 80% of their time in regular education programs.
- DH-15 Reduce unemployment among people with disabilities.
- DH-16 Increase employment among people with disabilities.
- DH-17 Increase the proportion of adults with disabilities who report sufficient social and emotional support.
- DH-18 Reduce the proportion of with disabilities adults aged 18 years and older who report serious psychological distress.
- DH-19 Reduce the proportion of people with disabilities aged five and older who in the previous 3 months experience nonfatal unintentional injuries that require medical care.
- DH-20 Increase the proportion of children with disabilities, birth through age 2 years who receive early intervention services in home or community-based settings.

From U.S. Department of Health and Human Services. (2016). *Healthy people 2020, topics and objectives: Disability and health objectives.* Retrieved from https://www.healthypeople.gov/2020/topics-objectives/topic/disability-and-health/objectives

These objectives reflect a growing emphasis on holistic approaches that recognize that life satisfaction is just as important to human health and well-being as are preventive services (ODPHP, 2016). It also indicates a growing realization that healthy life-years for persons with disabilities equate to decreased health costs at local, state, and national levels, just as they do for persons without disabilities. See Table 26–2 for objectives.

Plans for the next decade of Healthy People, *Healthy People 2030*, began in March 2016, under the supervision of the U.S. Department of Health and Human Services (USDHHS), Office of Disease Prevention and Health Promotion (ODPHP). Work on *Healthy People 2030* will review, revise, and establish disease prevention and health promotion objectives for the Nation for 2020 to 2030 (Federal Register, 2016; ODPHP, 2016). Many additional research and health organizations will participate in developing *Healthy People 2030*.

The health of people with disabilities is influenced by many social and physical factors. Using the ICF and the WHO principles of action for addressing health determinants, *Healthy People 2020* identified three areas for public health action. These areas, with accompanying suggested applications, are listed below:

1. Improve the conditions of daily life by
   - Encouraging communities to be accessible so all can live in, move through, and interact with their environment
   - Encouraging community living
   - Removing barriers in the environment using both physical universal design concepts and operational policy shifts

2. Address the inequitable distribution of resources among people with disabilities and those without disabilities by increasing
   - Appropriate health care for people with disabilities
   - Education and work opportunities
   - Social participation
   - Access to needed technologies and assistive supports

3. Expand the knowledge base and raise awareness about determinants of health for people with disabilities by increasing
   - The inclusion of people with disabilities in public health data collection efforts across the lifespan
   - The inclusion of people with disabilities in health promotion activities
   - The expansion of disability and health training opportunities for public health and health care professionals (ODPHP, 2016, para. 5)

HEALTH PROMOTION AND PREVENTION NEEDS OF THE DISABLED AND CHRONICALLY ILL

Misconceptions Impede Improvement

The emphasis on "secondary conditions" in *Healthy People 2010* has been replaced in *Healthy People 2020* with a concern for health disparities for people with disabilities. Compared with people without disabilities, people with disabilities are more likely to experience difficulties

accessing health care, dental services, mammograms, Pap tests, and fitness activities and more likely to use tobacco, be overweight or obese, have hypertension, and have lower employment rates (ODPHP, 2016). Key to addressing these barriers is for people with disabilities to have an opportunity to participate in public health activities, receive appropriately timed health interventions, engage with the environment without restrictions, and be able to participate in life without limitations (ODPHP, 2016).

Missed Opportunities by Health Care Providers or Missed Opportunities to Affect Quality of Life

All of us, whether healthy, disabled, or chronically ill, require basic elements to maintain health, including clean air and water, a safe place to live, sunshine, exercise, nutritious food, socialization, and the opportunity to be successful in life's pursuits. As self-evident as these health-promoting elements may seem, for the millions of persons who deal with disability, chronic disease, or both, such basic needs may too often take second place to other issues. It is equally problematic that health promotion and disease prevention measures, most notably at the primary and secondary levels, are often nonexistent or lacking. The CDC is making an effort to reduce health disparities among the disabled population. Surveillance, or use of surveys, helps to determine the needs and problems experienced, and research programs help to prevent the development of **secondary conditions**. Secondary conditions may include mental, emotional, social, medical, or family/community issues that may be experienced as a result of having a disabling condition. For instance, inadequate transportation was reported by 31% of disabled adults compared with only 13% of adults without disabilities; poverty is also a concern, as 26% of disabled adults report an annual income of under $15,000 compared to 9% of those without disabilities (CDC, n.d.). Programs in 16 states work to improve health outcomes and quality of life for this population.

The issue of missed opportunities in health promotion and prevention is depicted in Figure 26–2. The focus of the health care delivery system is increasingly skewed toward secondary and tertiary prevention efforts, and limited emphasis is placed on the health promotion

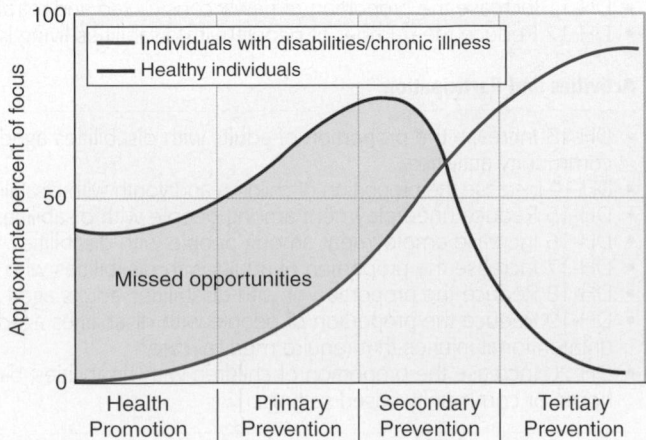

FIGURE 26–2 Difference in client focus between individuals with and without a chronic illness or disability.

and primary prevention needs of the population. Although this is a concern for all persons, it is of particular importance for persons with disabilities and chronic illnesses because they are more likely to have these needs ignored altogether. As Figure 26–2 shows, an entire area of issues may be addressed with a basically healthy person but not with a disabled or chronically ill individual. Some areas of secondary and tertiary prevention unique to persons with disabilities or chronic illnesses may be completely ignored. This nonreceipt of health-promoting or preventive education or actions vital to the health and well-being of those with disabilities or chronic illnesses is a grave concern (CDC, n.d.; Kung, Tsai, & Li, 2012). For example, issues such as sexuality are often not explored with the disabled or chronically ill. This skewed view of the lifestyles, behaviors, and needs of the disabled as "different" from those of the "able-bodied" is a clear example of lack of understanding by health professionals and the public alike and leads directly to health disparities between the able-bodied and the disabled populations.

It is likely that disability or chronic illness serves as the presenting reason for an individual's encounter with the health care community, including the public health nurse. As a result, the disability or illness often drives the selection of prevention efforts to the possible exclusion of other, equally important health issues. For example, for an individual with a primary diagnosis of type 2 diabetes, secondary prevention efforts often center on that disease (e.g., screening for diabetic retinopathy, peripheral neuropathy). The need to refer the client for a Pap test or a baseline mammogram may be overlooked. Likewise, the treatment plan may include a consultation with a dietitian but fail to address the basic needs for leisure-time activities, regular physical activity, a varied and interesting diet, fresh air and sunshine, and socialization—all of which may help prevent the development of depression, a common result of chronic illness. Display 26–2 offers several examples of missed opportunities in the areas of primary and secondary prevention. It is of particular concern to the practice of community/public health nursing

---

DISPLAY 26–2 MISSED OPPORTUNITIES

Example 1

A 60-year-old woman, blind since birth, self-sufficient, and active all of her life, has developed severe arthritis. She encounters a health care system that far too often focuses on her "disabilities" and not her "abilities." The focus is placed squarely on her tertiary health promotion needs, often at the expense of health-promoting or lifestyle-enhancing needs. The result is a failure to recognize that the "disability" of arthritis is likely no less and no more an issue for her than for a sighted person. She receives the same medication therapy as does a sighted person but may not be offered a physical therapy program because of her disability. Her need for physical therapy is no less important, but locating an appropriate, safe, and easily accessible program requires some additional work on the part of her provider. At issue is that options potentially discussed with a sighted person are more apt to be omitted completely, which may negatively affect the client's overall health and well-being.

Example 2

A 20-year-old man with learning disabilities, who is employed at a local factory, receives a regularly scheduled physical examination with a new provider. He lives in a congregate care facility, which is an out-of-home facility that provides housing for people with disabilities in which rotating staff members provide care for 16 or more adults or any number of children/youth younger than 21 years of age. It excludes foster care, adoptive homes, residential schools, correctional facilities, and nursing facilities (U.S. Department of Health and Human Services [USDHHS], 2016). The major finding of the examination is that he is due for a tetanus booster and should also begin the series for hepatitis

A, because he lives in a high-risk area of the western United States. He takes the referral slip and leaves the office. One year later, at his regularly scheduled visit, it becomes clear that he never received his immunizations. Apparently, he didn't know what he was supposed to do with the paper, because he has difficulty reading, and he had no idea where to go to get his "shots." The primary prevention elements were provided, but clearly not in a manner appropriate for this individual. With additional explanation and follow-up, perhaps the outcome would have been quite different.

Example 3

A 34-year-old woman, who has been severely obese since the birth of her last child (4 years ago), has not had a gynecologic examination since that birth. She is aware of the need to have regular examinations, yet she cannot bring herself to make an appointment. The reason is that she knows she will have to be weighed, and this terrifies her, especially because it is done in an open area where others can see. She finally gets the courage to call for an appointment and tells the clerk that she does not want to be weighed. The clerk's response is less than helpful, and she is essentially told that it is "policy." She makes the appointment but does not keep it. This situation could have been handled in a compassionate manner, recognizing the painful experience that weighing is for many individuals and suggesting alternatives, one of which could have been simply to bypass the scales until after the interview and examination. At that point, the woman may have been more amenable to the measurement and a more discrete area could have been offered. In this case, the opportunities to provide primary, secondary, and tertiary prevention were lost.

that the broad range of health promotion and prevention needs of all clients be addressed.

Iezzoni, Kurtz, and Rao (2015) documented the risk of missed opportunities for clinical preventive services among disabled women. Women with disabilities were less likely to receive routine mammograms compared to women without disabilities. Further, women with disabilities were less likely to receive routine cervical cancer screenings, and this is more disparate in rural settings (Horner-Johnson, Dobbertin, & Iezzoni, 2015). In light of the *Healthy People 2020* guidelines, these studies indicate a need to focus concerted efforts for improving preventive health screenings and services for those with disabilities. Specific lifestyle risk factor behaviors in those with disabilities were identified in several studies (McPherson, Keith, & Swift, 2014; An, Andrade, & Chiu, 2015). Study findings suggest that adults with disabilities with accompanying activity limitations and use of assistive devices may be at increased risk for poor lifestyle behaviors related to weight and physical activity. On the other hand, these same adults have lower use of alcohol consumption and increased vaccination rates than the nondisabled respondents. With the challenges faced by those with disabilities to maintain employment, it is vital that health care providers screen for lifestyle behavioral risks in all routine health care visits. A large population study in Taiwan revealed that only 15.8% of disabled adults ($n = 785,746$) over a 2-year time period used preventive health services that had been available through the public health department for many years (Kung et al., 2012). These studies suggest the need for ongoing attention to the health promotion needs of vulnerable individuals, as well as the value of identifying and taking every opportunity to address those needs.

Health Care Disparities and Discrimination

Individuals living with disabilities, and their families and advocates, have embraced concerns about the type and quality of the health-related services and the referral process. There are also concerns about the care received being appropriate to individual circumstances. This can result in increased illness and disability, as well as potentially decreased quality or length of life. It is important to consider the impact that access to care can have in the continuum of health. When considering the risk for unmet care in those with disabilities versus those without disabilities, the inability to access medical, dental, and prescription drug care is between 57% and 85% higher in those with disabilities (Mahmoudi & Meade, 2015). This is magnified in females, those without health insurance, and those living near or at the poverty level.

Additional disparities may exist in services received by those with chronic illness and disabilities. In children with cerebral palsy, vaccination rates were found to be lower (Greenwood, Crawford, Walstab, & Reddihough, 2013). In this population, protection from vaccine-preventable disease is vitally important and represents the difference between maximum health and complications from their increased vulnerability. Cody and Lerand (2013) noted that vaccination disparities occur because of many factors but cited that provider and parental attitudes toward disabled children can be a barrier to compliance

with vaccination recommendations. Human papillomavirus is a sexually transmitted vaccine-preventable disease, and it is important to consider providing those with disabilities with the same health protection as nondisabled counterparts. Reducing disparities between those with disabilities and those without disabilities provides an opportunity for maximal health of those with disabilities, as well as the general U.S. population.

When an individual receives unequal, inappropriate, or limited services compared with those received by others, this is categorized as discrimination. Although the difference in treatment can be due to a lack of understanding of the needs of disabled persons, it is nonetheless discriminatory. Even when such bias is not intentional, it can dramatically affect the health of clients and must be addressed through provider education and health policy requirements. The good news is that the incidence of unequal and inappropriate practices can be reduced with education and training of health care providers, agency staff, and insurance carriers. A crucial aspect of community/public health practice is to ensure that those individuals with disabilities or chronic illnesses are afforded the best possible care, treatment options, and opportunities to improve their health—the same options made available to nondisabled persons and those who do not suffer from chronic illness (Brolan et al., 2012).

Health promotion and primary, secondary, and tertiary prevention activities are essential aspects of quality care for all persons. Those with disabilities require specialized attention to needs resulting from or related to their disabilities, yet they also require the same attention to health and well-being as the rest of the population (Kung et al., 2012). PHNs are in a prime position to advocate needed changes for those with disabilities and chronic illnesses. Such changes can include increased attention to health promotion and disease prevention needs, accessible and appropriate delivery of those services, and specialized treatment plans that incorporate the latest knowledge of a specific illness or disability (see Perspectives: Student Voices).

CIVIL RIGHTS LEGISLATION

Policies such as *Healthy People 2020* are important elements in addressing the health and overall needs of people with disabilities and chronic diseases in the United States. Although it has a great deal of influence on the direction and type of programs initiated, health policies alone cannot assure that individuals with disabilities will find and receive needed services and accommodations. An act of legislation is vital to ensure that every individual's rights are protected and that there is legal recourse to secure needs that have been denied. As is often true for other issues of equality, legislation is only one of many steps that must be taken. The struggle to achieve civil rights for disabled persons in this country has gained momentum and continues to seek the influence and public attention that will improve the health and lives of those having disabilities, handicaps, and chronic illnesses. The **Americans with Disabilities Act (ADA)** was signed into law in 1990 to protect the civil liberties of the many Americans living with disabilities (Massey, 2015). This legislation was the result of a long and difficult struggle. Individuals with disabilities

PERSPECTIVES STUDENT VOICES

For as long as I can remember, I have wanted to work with children. When I was finally accepted into the nursing program, I was so disappointed when I learned that we would only have 7 weeks in our pediatric rotation. Then, I found out about an opportunity to work with children at a school in my community health practicum—I thought that was great. I just knew I'd be giving immunizations, physical assessments, and performing hearing checks. Then I found out that I would actually be working with school-aged children with disabilities and their parents in a special after-school health promotion program. The nurse I was assigned to asked me to come in before the program started so that she could fill me in on the program and my role. It actually sounded great, and I was confident that I could handle this. Then she asked me something that made me worried; she asked if I had ever worked with a child who used a wheelchair, or had a continuous insulin pump, or had seizures. I told her that I had some experience in the hospital and that I was sure that I would be prepared for any health care issues that might

occur. "You misunderstand," she said, "that's not what I meant. Have you *ever gotten to know a child* with a disability?" I really hadn't, and it suddenly made me a bit worried. She explained to me that many people don't treat children with disabilities just like any other child. They also don't always know how to talk to the parents about their child. She suggested that one way to give me a bit of information was to go home and do some reading and look at some Web sites she recommended. The National Organization on Disability (http://www.nod.org/) had a great feature called "Disability Etiquette Tips" that I have already found to be a big help with the kids and their parents. She also directed me to the Easter Seals Disability Web site (http://www.easter-seals.com), which has a great deal of information on programs that are currently available for children and adults. I even learned that this organization used to be called the National Society for Crippled Children—I'm really glad they changed the name.

Eileen S.

and their advocates made their voices heard by repeatedly demanding an end to inferior treatment and lack of equal protection under the law, which have impeded their daily lives. The ADA has set the standard for a number of subsequent laws that, together with pre-ADA legislation, have become a broad spectrum of protections for people with disabilities. These laws are listed in Table 26–1 and cover a variety of issues, including telecommunications, architectural barriers, and voter registration.

The ADA was written to protect those with disabilities by prohibiting any form of discrimination in the realm of employment, government, public accommodations, transportation, telecommunications, and commercial facilities (Edie, 2016). This federal law protects those with a disability, which is defined as a physical or mental impairment that substantially limits one or more major life activities with documentation of the impairment or being thought of to have the impairment (Kanter, 2015). The ADA does not list specific diagnoses, but instead, the ADA focuses on the impact the disability has on daily living. This includes things like the ability to care for self, perform manual tasks, see, hear, eat, sleep, walk, stand, lift, bend, speak, breathe, learn, read, concentrate, think, communicate, and work. This impacts the function of the immune system, normal cell growth, digestive, bowel, bladder, neurological, brain, respiratory, circulatory, endocrine, and reproductive functions (Chen, 2015). Despite this specificity, there remains a broad range of interpretations and legal challenges with respect to who is actually covered by the ADA.

In addition to the uncertainty about who is actually protected by the ADA, there can also be confusion about who is required to comply with the provisions of the Act and what specific remedial actions are necessary. The ADA currently applies to all employers with 15 or more employees (including religious organizations), and

all activities of state and local governments irrespective of their size. Public transportation, businesses that provide public accommodation, and telecommunications entities are also required to provide access for individuals with disabilities. It is important to note that the ADA does not override federal and state health and safety laws. However, successful legal challenges to those statutes have been made when they were clearly outdated or when it could be argued that the public safety was not actually at risk in a specific situation. Yet considerable gray areas exist in the application of the ADA, leaving open the prospect of challenges by those who are subject to the law and those who are protected by it (U.S. Department of Labor [USDOL], n.d.a).

Employers may hire the most qualified candidate of their choosing, provided that an individual's disability is not a factor; employers may also fire a disabled individual if the employee doesn't meet job requirements after appropriate accommodations have been made, and it is not related to the disability. Employees may also be terminated if their disability "poses a direct threat to health or safety" of others in the workplace (USDOL, n.d.a, para. 23). Individuals who believe that their legal rights under the ADA have been violated may seek remedy by filing a lawsuit or submitting a complaint to one of four federal offices, depending on the specific type of alleged violation: (1) the USDOJ, Civil Rights Division; (2) any U.S. Equal Employment Opportunity Commission field office; (3) the Office of Civil Rights, Federal Transit Administration; or (4) the Federal Communications Commission. The process for filing a complaint is not a simple task, and many seek the assistance of attorneys, legal aid societies, or various private organizations, some of which are discussed later in this chapter (see Display 26–3).

The ADA includes provisions and safeguards regarding employment (e.g., reasonable accommodations,

---

DISPLAY 26-3 OFFICE OF CIVIL RIGHTS: COMPLIANCE WITH ADA

The responsibility of the U.S. Department of Justice, Office of Civil Rights (OCR), is to investigate complaints of alleged violations of the Americans with Disabilities Act (ADA). An example of one of those complaints involved a 22-year-old Connecticut woman with cerebral palsy. She had been placed in a nursing home because of changes in her living situation and health care status, but wanted to move back into the community. The OCR intervened to ensure that the woman secured appropriate housing and that counseling and intensive case management services were in place when she moved back into the community. Another example involved a man with traumatic brain injury (TBI) who was told he must remain in a hospital when he requested home health care services.

OCR intervened and secured physical, occupational, and speech therapy for the client, as well as physical modifications needed for his home. A 32-year-old quadriplegic man had lived independently in his own apartment with a health aide's assistance, but suddenly lost his apartment and was transferred against his will to a facility. He was able to get a wheelchair accessible apartment, but could not get health aide services. OCR intervened on his behalf and secured a personal care assistant so that he could live in his new apartment. Without the protection afforded under the ADA, the outcome could have been much different.

Source: USDHHS, Office for Civil Rights. (2006, September). *Delivering on the promise: OCR's compliance activities promote community integration.* Retrieved from http://www.hhs.gov/civil-rights/for-individuals/special-topics/community-living-and-olmstead/compliance-activities-promote-integration/index.html

---

discrimination based solely on disability), public services (e.g., opportunity to participate, technology accessibility), and public accommodations (e.g., design standards, reasonable modifications, service animals, tax credits/deductions). Telecommunications services must also provide telecommunications relay services, closed captioning, and equal access for disabled individuals to emergency services. The ADA also prohibits "retaliation and coercion" (Disability.gov, n.d., para. 16). The ADA Amendments Act of 2008 overturned some court rulings, broadening and clarifying the ADA definition of disability.

The National Council on Disability discovered in the years following legislative changes that many federal agencies charged with protecting the civil rights of disabled persons were limited by insufficient funding and a lack of coherent and unifying national strategies. The NCD recommended clarification of the basis for evaluating agency performance to improve the intended full expression of the law. The 2008 study, *The Impact of the Americans with Disabilities Act: Assessing the Progress Toward Achieving the Goals of the ADA* by the NCD, continued to find that many people with disabilities, businesses, and employers still did not understand the requirements of the ADA in relation to employment. And Americans with disabilities continued to face barriers to becoming economically self-sufficient. But the NCD also found many areas for optimism: public transportation was more accessible, especially for wheelchair users. Ramps and sidewalks had been made more accessible, although full access still lagged. Access in public accommodations continued to improve, as did public attitudes toward those with disabilities. Many people with disabilities perceived improved quality of life, which they attributed to the ADA (NCD, 2008b).

In a yearly progress report, *National Disability Policy: A Progress Report*, the importance of accurate statistical data collection and reporting in order to address program effectiveness and policy development

was discussed. Civil rights were addressed, in relation to court decisions weakening the ADA, and technology accessibility, as well as voting and improvements made by the U.S. Department of Justice in protecting institutionalized individuals with disabilities. The report also called for "genetic nondiscrimination" legislation to ensure rights of the disabled in regarding privacy, confidentiality, and potential adverse selection in health insurance, employment, and housing because of one's disability (NCD, 2008a, p. 59). Recommendations included educational accommodations, especially for standardized testing, technology accessibility in schools and universities, and better monitoring of private schools' Individuals with Disabilities Education Act (IDEA) compliance. Health recommendations included mental health parity in health insurance, and improvement in programs and services from the CDC and the Centers for Medicare and Medicaid. In the area of employment, it was recommended that substantially more research and a thorough "examination of the issues" be supported (p. 139).

The 2014 progress report highlighted the gains made in education but encouraged further improvements to meet "the unique learning needs…for students with disabilities" (NCD, 2014, p. 10). The area of employment was a significant concern, as technology, workplace culture, and transportation represent potential barriers. The report also called for the U.S. Department of Labor to end the subminimum wage for disabled employees, and addressed the need for better engagement and "system refinement" in state Medicaid systems (p. 10). The employment gap for disabled individuals is 42.8%, and the income gap is $6,000 annually. Recommendations also included support for ratifying the Conventions on the Rights of Persons with Disabilities (CRPD), mentioned earlier in this chapter. Also, the shortage of community-based mental health services profoundly affects this population, and recommendations were made for more resources in this area and for veterans with mental health issues (NCD, 2014).

PERSPECTIVES
VOICES FROM THE COMMUNITY

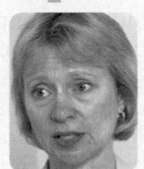

"I was always such an active and healthy person, so when I was diagnosed with multiple sclerosis, it hit me like a ton of bricks. Here I was with two small children and I was only 30 years old; it just wasn't fair. Some days are good, and some days are just awful. I finally broke down and applied for one of those disabled parking stickers. The doctor had to approve it, and he said it was a good thing to help me save my energy for the important things, like taking care of my family. I hated to use it, but I was just getting so tired. It is so frustrating to see the looks on people's faces when I park in the handicapped parking areas near the door. I know I don't look like I'm sick. I just hate those looks—I can hear them saying under their breath, "She can't be sick … I'll bet that sticker is for a family member and she's just abusing it—how lazy!" If I weren't so tired I'd park in the regular parking places."

Pat N, Tampa, Florida

It is important to those with disabilities, their families, and the professionals who serve them that a structure is in place to provide protection under the ADA, but a law does not prevent discrimination, nor does the existence of a structure such as the ADA provide immediate remedies. The most challenging aspect of providing services for persons with disabilities is to alter the perceptions and misunderstandings of others about people with disabilities (Yee, 2016). The perspective of one community member offers one such example (see Perspectives: Voices from the Community).

Currently, the NCD focuses its policy initiatives on civil rights, cultural diversity, education, emergency management, employment, financial management and incentives, health care, housing, international issues, long-term services and support, technology, transportation, and youth issues (2014). This organization provides tool kits for parents of those with disabilities, deinstitutionalization, and disability in Indian country. It is important to note that the policy and advocacy for those with disabilities is maintained through this organization as part of its charge run through the federal government.

FAMILIES WITH A DISABLED OR CHRONICALLY ILL MEMBER

The Family's Role in Advocacy

Families that include a member with a chronic illness or disability face many challenges. They are required to navigate a health care system that they may know little about and with which they often feel at odds. They serve as advocates for their family member in need (whether child, spouse, or parent) and may become exhausted or frustrated with their efforts, especially if they have been less than successful in achieving their goals. Many are forced to ask for or demand assistance from health care agencies, social services, or transportation sources to achieve the level of care needed by the family member

(Brolan et al., 2012). Many are required to open their home to others (e.g., community/public health nurses, social workers) to access the services. Families may also have little understanding of what services they are entitled to because of language barriers, difficult agency policies, or disjointed service delivery.

The PHN is usually not the first health care professional that the family encounters. They may already have been through a lengthy struggle to receive assistance. In these circumstances, the nurse may be confronted with a frustrated family, reluctant to trust yet another health care provider. Nurses must earn the trust and confidence of the family by practicing consistency, following through with promised actions, and always being truthful. Not all problems that the family faces can be remedied, and even for problems that do have solutions, time and effort may be needed to obtain the desired result.

The Impact on Families

Caring for a family member who is disabled, whether it is a child or an adult, is stressful. High levels of anxiety, stress, depression, and illness are often reported in families of disabled children (Dykens, 2015). Families caring for a member with epilepsy and intellectual disabilities report unsettled family dynamics, emotional and physical burdens, and practical concerns such as finances, the nonstop responsibility for caregiving and coordination of care, social isolation, and difficulty showing equal attention to all family members because of the increased needs of a disabled family member. However, they also note positive aspects of care, including family closeness and showing an example to other family members of caring behaviors and altruism (Thompson, Kerr, Glynn, & Linehan, 2014). In a study of parents of deaf and hard-of-hearing children, it is important to note that parental involvement and support is an essential aspect of the process for mitigating disabilities in this group (Lam-Cassettari, Wadnerkar-Kamble, & James, 2015). Parents who participated in a family-focused psychosocial video intervention program geared toward guiding them in proper communication with their child improved parental sensitivity, structuring, nonhostility, child responsiveness, and child involvement. This also improved parental self-esteem and a more connected parent–child relationship. It is important for nurses to support the family unit, not just the disabled patient. Nurses should be especially cognizant of the needs of families of children with disabilities and their unique needs. This was echoed in a study where parent–child interaction therapy was used to support the relationship between children with autism and their parents. By supporting the parents and the disabled child, parents were able to use appropriate interventions to support the child (Sheperis, Sheperis, Monceaux, Davis, & Lopez, 2015).

Hamilton, Mazzucchelli, and Sanders (2015) also examined parental support for children with disabilities. In the adolescent years, the needs of the disabled child dramatically shift from needs as a child as parenting styles that worked at a younger age were no longer effective. Parents report struggling to understand the needs and making accommodations for the transitions of their adolescent children, and this frustration leads to increased stress and feelings of grief. The study suggested that a targeted, evidence-based parenting program should be tailored toward this special population. Nurses should be prepared to provide parenting support and referrals to parental support groups and educational programs that can assist the parents in providing the best care possible to their disabled children.

Nurses should also be aware of the physical needs of parents caring for disabled children. In a study by McCann, Bull, and Winzenberg (2015), the researchers noted that parents report sleep deprivation as a direct result of the child's illness. Based on the particular disability, parents reported varying amounts of sleep deprivation, but at the core of the research is the need for parents to be especially vigilant while their children are sleeping. This can result in failing health among parents, and nurses should consider the amount and quality of sleep in order to assure that parents of disabled children are able to provide the care that is needed.

Geographic differences were noted in a large-scale study of children with special health care needs. Regional differences were found in access to mental health care, genetic counseling, specialist care, and physical/occupational therapy, for instance, in the West, and respite care, vision and dental care services were lacking in the South (Fulda, Johnson, Hahn, & Lykens, 2013). Also, for families with a disabled child, access to locations is an important consideration. For those with a physical disability, for example, a family may want to vacation at the beach. For those children who are wheelchair bound, this may not be a possibility for the family, or the child may be excluded while the other family members enjoy the location. Dickson (2016) reports that a city offered disabled access to the beach, but even this intervention was still problematic for complete access to this recreational pastime. Despite the ADA, many locations remain isolated from those with physical and mental disabilities creating a challenge for families that are trying to engage the disabled child and keep them included as part of the family. Even at home, when modifications are made to accommodate to improve access for a disabled child, families report dissatisfaction with the process, and a need to be inclusive with the family at all phases of the remodeling process was noted. Morgan, Boniface, and Reagon (2016) indicated that without family involvement in this process, the adaptations to improve access may not be utilized, and families may have a negative perception of their home.

Access to resources related to financial support is an important issue. In fact, the Disability Tax is a model that addresses the high cost of care of the disabled (Shick, 2015). The cost of care of a disabled child is high and is a financial burden to families as they navigate paying for obvious costs, such as doctor and hospital bills, diagnostic testing, medical treatments, and prescription medicines (Price & Oliverio, 2016). However, the cost of care is more than just the obvious costs. The cost of care of a disabled child may include 24-hour supervision for activities of daily living, and this does not end for many disabled children at the age of 18, rather the cost of care for a disabled child often requires a lifetime of services. Therapy, health care professionals, financial planners, support group facilitators, educational advocates, special education attorneys, and other professionals may be required for care. Whiting (2014a) found that parents of children with complex health needs identified that people, processes, and resources are the most important support needs. For instance, families may need a tracking or alarm system to ensure the safety of a disabled child who wanders; special equipment, such as wheelchairs, special vans, medical transportation, orthopedic devices, therapeutic beds, and lifting equipment, may be required, and this may need to be purchased multiple times as the child outgrows existing devices. Indirect costs can include medication changes, nutritional supplements, special diets, sensory considerations, and respite care—all of which can burden families with disabled children. While *Healthy People 2020* directly addresses obstacles to obtaining **assistive devices and technologies** in objective 10, under Disability and Health, it may still be problematic. This objective states that people with disabilities should be able to obtain assistive devices, technology and accessibility services, and service animals (ODPHP, 2016). This can be more difficult for children with disabilities, and advocates are often needed. This may be especially true in the school setting (see Chapters 22 and 30).

With repeated changes in available equipment, financing, and technology, it is little wonder that families struggle to find the best alternatives. Just because a technology exists does not mean that it can be obtained. The insurance carrier, whether private or governmental, will often set limits on which products can be obtained or which brands are acceptable. The overriding issue of financing is no small hurdle. It is often left up to the family to learn about options and legal rights through a process of trial and error. Interventions by the community/public health nurse can greatly reduce the burden on the family. With so many product lines available online, the nurse can assist families to weigh and select among options, especially for families with limited access or experience with the Internet. It is equally helpful for the nurse to intervene with insurance providers if coverage of equipment is not easily obtained or to seek sources of funding for the equipment from private agencies. Referring families to community groups or charitable organizations that provide specific assistance can be very helpful. Other families experiencing similar struggles can provide their experience and links to needed services and self-help/support groups. In addition, the community/public health nurse can provide expertise on available community resources and referral processes. Families that are just beginning to adjust to having a child with a disability or a complex health problem identify the "impact" of the diagnosis and the "need for help and support" as very important factors as they process the information and move forward. They often refer to the experience as a battle, and PHNs should consider this when working with these clients (Whiting, 2014b, p. 26).

Respite care is another resource of great importance for families of the disabled and the chronically ill. It was most often cited as an unmet need by parents of disabled children in a qualitative study by Whiting (2014a). Because it can be emotionally draining to meet the daily needs of a relative or friend who cannot perform self-care, in this situation, caregivers are at risk for related fatigue and stress. It is also important to recognize the effect of the situation on noncaregivers in the family, particularly nondisabled siblings of a disabled child. When focus is placed on the needs of one family member, other children may feel that their own needs are not as important, which can lead to behavioral and health-related problems. Respite care can be provided for the family member with disability, in the home or through admission to a hospice facility. Respite offers needed relief to families and allows for uninterrupted attention to the nondisabled children. Respite care may also be provided free of charge by a charitable organization or reimbursed by the health insurance provider. Sometimes families are able, and choose to, pay directly for hospice care. Whatever the source, respite care can be vital to the family's health and should be a considered a priority in the overall treatment plan of families of the disabled and chronically ill (see Using the Nursing Process).

The issue of employment is generally of great significance to families of the disabled and chronically ill, as employment options may be quite limited when a family member has special needs. The family may have to remain in a particular location to access needed health and social services, reducing the possibility of increased earning potential at a different location or in another field of employment. Family members who are working may choose less favorable employment options because the position is convenient or has more flexible hours. For instance, a person may take a part-time position at a local convenience store that does not pay particularly well in preference to a higher-paying, full-time factory position, because the store is close to home and allows for frequent adjustments in schedule. Baillargeon, Bernier, and Normand (2011) found in a study of almost 4,000 caregivers that parents of those most severely restricted in performing daily activities were more likely to report being unable to get childcare services and having to work fewer hours or quitting jobs in order to care for children with impaired psychological functions.

Having a chronically ill family member can mean that working individuals must take time off from work.

USING THE NURSING PROCESS WITH VULNERABLE POPULATIONS

Assessment

Anna Lopez is a mother of three children aged 2 to 9 years old. The eldest, Ernesto, was diagnosed with severe Down's syndrome at birth. He is confined to a wheelchair, requires total care, and remains at home with his mother and younger siblings, who are not yet in school. Anna's husband works long hours as a computer repairman for a large company. They have health insurance, but it does not cover additional expenses, such as day care for Ernesto. The family has done very well in providing for Ernesto's needs, and they receive periodic visits from you, the community health nurse, to evaluate his condition and check on the feeding tube used for his nourishment. Physically, Ernesto is stable, but you notice that Anna has slowly become more withdrawn at the visits and rarely offers information, even though she continues to respond to questions appropriately. She also seems less engaged with her other children and only occasionally smiles at them.

Nursing Diagnoses

1. At risk for depression related to ongoing caregiver demands and lack of respite care
2. At risk for altered health status due to limited focus on self-care needs

Plan/Implementation

• **DIAGNOSIS 1**
The community health nurse will discuss with Mrs. Lopez the need for a thorough physical assessment, including an evaluation for depression. The community health nurse will contact the insurance provider and charitable groups to seek day care/respite options for Ernesto. If unavailable, local community organizations will be contacted for other types of appropriate referrals. In addition, the need for more frequent visits to the family will be discussed with the insurance carrier to address the needs of the mother as caregiver.

• **DIAGNOSIS 2**
The community health nurse will discuss with Mrs. Lopez the nurse's concerns about her overall physical and mental health, some self-care options that may improve Mrs. Lopez' well-being, and possible improvements in nutrition, physical activity, leisure-time options, and adjustment of family schedule to accommodate more free time for self-care for Ms. Lopez.

Evaluation

Mrs. Lopez was at first very reluctant to make an appointment for an evaluation, but after thinking it over for a week and discussing it with her husband, she did so. Her husband was relieved that she had suggested the appointment, because he was growing increasingly concerned over her withdrawal but did not know how to bring up the subject. The family physician referred Mrs. Lopez to a psychologist for evaluation of the depression. The insurance carrier agreed to increase home visits on a short-term basis but did not have a respite care option available for Ernesto. Fortunately, a local faith-based community group was able to provide limited but appropriate assistance to the family. The group identified several members who had raised children with similar disabilities and who were willing to stay with Ernesto and the other children once a week for 4 hours. This allowed Mrs. Lopez some free time to make appointments with her psychologist, shop, or visit friends. After several months, Mrs. Lopez has begun to smile more and seems much more relaxed at the home visits. The children are all doing fine, and the respite care is expected to continue for at least the next 6 months. The community health nurse continues to emphasize to Mrs. Lopez the need for ongoing attention to her own self-care need.

Although some legal protections are provided under the Family and Medical Leave Act of 1993, it does not apply in all situations. For instance, it is only available in companies with more than 50 employees and is most often used for birth and care of a newborn or newly adopted child or for temporary care of a family member with a serious health problem (spouse, parent, child). More importantly, it allows only for time off; it does not mandate that employers continue a salary during those periods (USDOL, n.d.b). Family members may have to choose between taking unpaid time off and continuing to work while dealing with the needs of the family member as best they can. Some individuals choose to work part-time or not to work at all so that they can care for family members (Baillargeon et al., 2011). At a time when many families have two wage earners to help meet financial commitments, families engaged in caregiving may have to rely on only one income. Limitations in income are particularly challenging, considering the myriad needs of those who are disabled or chronically ill, needs that may not be covered by any insurance.

There are many financial programs to help individuals with disabilities and families caring for those with disabilities. Programs include Temporary Assistance for Needy Families (TANF) and Social Security's Supplemental Security Income (SSI). Families receiving financial and other assistance from TANF also face work-related pressures. The 1996 welfare reform legislation, the Personal Responsibility and Work Opportunity Reconciliation Act, introduced regulations that often impact families with a chronically ill child, especially those families living in poverty. Those now receiving TANF have a 5-year lifetime limit on receipt of benefits (and states may opt to reduce years of eligibility further), institution of work requirements, and elimination of entitlement to cash benefits (USDHHS, 2016; Wen, 2014). Those with disabilities and families caring for those with disabilities often are unaware of eligible programs and confusion about the rules and regulations of each program. Some SSI recipients manage their own money, but others cannot. Concern about how "financial capability assessments" are made, or judging when a beneficiary is not capable of managing their own benefits, has given rise to calls for reforms in that area (Appelbaum, Birkenmaier, & Norman, 2016, p. 704). Another concern is that the SSI program has grown substantially, whereas the number of disabled children on TANF rolls has decreased. Wen (2014) reports that SSI numbers have almost doubled since 2012, as broader disability classifications were accepted, and it now disburses more money than welfare programs largely because benefits are higher and continue longer and rules are more flexible. About 60% of children on SSI now have speech delays, depression, learning disorders, and autism spectrum disorder as well as ADHD. However, Ghosh and Parish (2015) noted that families of disabled children on SSI experienced significant hardships compared to families receiving SSI without disabilities, indicating a need to revise the policies around SSI.

Falk (2016) explored the relationship between welfare status and health. The researcher noted that families receiving Temporary Aid to Needy Families (TANF) often were eligible for many programs and that the different policies and requirements are difficult for families to navigate. While some families that receive TANF have children with disabilities and are eligible for other support programs, there is a need to establish policies that can offer guidance for these families to maximize the support and benefits obtained.

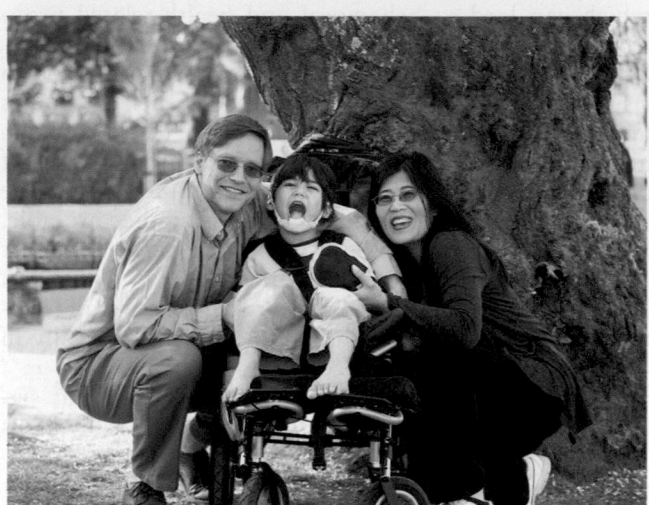

Public health nursing support for families with disabled children can be critical in helping them access resources and services.

Caregiver health needs and mental health status are another area of concern for families who must provide for a disabled or chronically ill family member. The mental health of the mother as caregiver is documented to be an area of concern, and the expression of depression in this population is concerning (In Sook & Hyun Sook, 2015; Yamaoka et al., 2015). While research often focuses on the mental health of the mother as caregiver, a line of research exploring paternal mental health when caring for a child with an intellectual disability is growing. This research supports that the child's behavior problems, father's daily stress, low parenting satisfaction, and childcare needs are the biggest predictor for father mental health difficulties (Giallo et al., 2015). A study exploring family health of parents caring for a child with disabilities indicated that parent caregivers who experienced activity restriction and low social support and those families in the lowest quartile of monthly expenditure were more likely to experience psychological distress (Yamaoka et al., 2015). It is important for nurses to provide detailed information about the child's health needs, disease, disability, medical services available, and social support available to meet the needs of the disabled child to decrease parental mental health stress and disorders. Recognizing that caregivers within a family are at increased risk for poor health outcomes, it is important that the PHN select appropriate interventions to address the health needs of all family members.

Families may suffer from financial difficulties, poor physical or mental health, and a variety of other challenges. For instance, a classic study on loss of family income related to having a child with autism spectrum disorder found an average decrease in annual income of 14% for these families (Montes & Halterman, 2008). Families are often ill prepared to deal with the complicated systems that must be accessed to obtain needed care. The PHN is in an optimal position to interpret those systems to the families and to advocate for the needed care, services, and equipment. The nurse must view the family holistically, recognizing additional needs that may develop as a result of the situation currently faced, and include an assessment of caregiver and family work patterns when caring for families with a disabled or chronically ill family member.

Disabled individuals may also seek employment, and a number of them have difficulties finding jobs. However, for those who do gain employment, benefits to their mental health have been demonstrated in research studies. Milner, Krnjacki, Butterworth, Kavanagh, and LaMontagne (2015) found that like those with no disabilities, disabled individuals show "significant mental health benefits" when "psychosocial job quality" was good (p. 104).

ORGANIZATIONS SERVING THE NEEDS OF THE DISABLED AND CHRONICALLY ILL

The impact of civil rights legislation would not have been achieved without the chorus of voices from advocates who deal on a daily basis with the issue of disability—the individuals themselves, their families, coworkers, employers, and advocates. Much of the credit for the legislative successes belongs to advocacy groups. This section provides an overview of some of the advocates for disabled and chronically ill individuals and their families. In addition to serving these specific populations, they also provide others opportunities to learn more about the lives and struggles of disabled persons. Each of the organizations noted offers a wide range of information, much of which can be accessed online. These organizations provide nurses with a starting point for exploring specific topics pertinent to practice. As clients and families may also be accessing online content through personal or public Internet access, it is important for nurses to prescreen and make recommendations to clients and families about reliable and accurate sites.

Government

The NCD is a small, independent federal agency tasked with making recommendations to the President, the U.S. Congress, and other federal agencies about issues facing Americans with disabilities. The NCD staff is led by 15 presidential and senate appointees. In 1986, the NCD recommended that Congress enact a civil rights law for people with disabilities and provide the initial draft legislation, which led to the passage of the ADA in 1990. NCD currently fulfills its advisory roles regarding disability policies, programs, procedures, and practices that enhance equal opportunity by gathering stakeholders to create recommendations and direct appropriate steps, review relevant data sources, network and collaborate with other groups regarding the appropriate direction, create solutions to problems, and provide tools for implementation (NCD, n.d.).

Private

Many private organizations—local, national, and international—address a variety of disabilities and chronic diseases. Many of the better-known organizations such as the American Heart Association and the American Cancer Association are discussed in other chapters of this book and therefore are not covered here (see Chapters 23 and 24). This discussion includes examples of groups that deal most directly with disability and chronic illness.

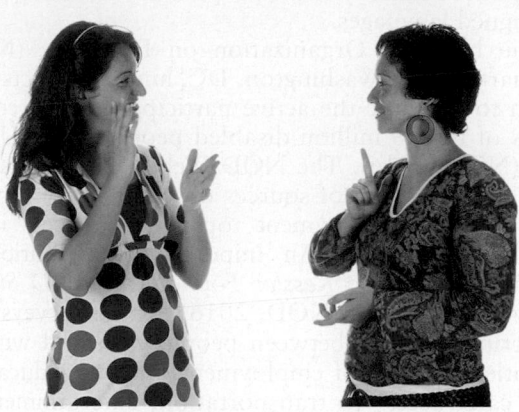
A conversation in sign language.

The National Association of the Deaf (NAD), headquartered in Washington, DC, is a private, nonprofit organization established in 1880. As the oldest U.S. organization serving the deaf community, it serves to protect and promote the rights of all deaf Americans, including civil, human, and linguistic rights (NAD, 2016). NAD's Vision 2020 Strategic Plan detailed the organization's beliefs and decade-focused goals, including ensuring that American Sign Language is at the core of all that are hard of hearing or deaf. NAD's programs include advocacy, captioned media, certification of American Sign Language (ASL) professionals and interpreters, legal assistance, and policy development and research. ASL uses precision hand movements to communicate without using any verbal or auditory-type communication (Fink, 2016). Display 26–4

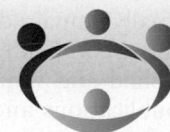

DISPLAY 26–4 SIGN LANGUAGES IN BRIEF

- Sign language is the use of "handshapes" and gestures to communicate ideas or concepts.
- **American Sign Language** is a unique language with its own rules of grammar and syntax.
- American Sign Language is primarily used in America and Canada and is the natural language of the deaf community; in Britain, British Sign Language (BSL) is used.
- Sign languages are not universal.
- International Sign Language (Gestuno) is composed of vocabulary signs from various sign languages for use at international events or meetings to aid communication.
- Systems of Manually Coded English (i.e., Signed English, Signing Exact English) are not natural languages but systems designed to represent the translation of spoken language word for word.

ASL University. (n.d.). *International sign language (Gestuno)*. Retrieved from http://www.lifeprint.com/asl101/pages-layout/gestuno.htm
CDC. (2014). *Manually coded English (MCE)*. Retrieved from http://www.cdc.gov/ncbddd/hearingloss/parentsguide/building/manual-english.html
National Institute on Deafness and Other Communication Disorders. (2015). *American sign language*. Retrieved from https://www.nidcd.nih.gov/health/american-sign-language

offers a brief summary of the purpose and use of ASL and other signed languages.

The National Organization on Disability (NOD) headquarters is in Washington, DC, and NOD acts on a mission to facilitate the active participation and contributions of the 56 million disabled people in the United States (NOD, 2016). The NOD Web site connects visitors to a rich variety of sources on community involvement, economic/employment topics, and access issues (http://www.nod.org/). An important contribution of NOD is the periodic *Kessler Foundation/NOD Survey by Harris Interactive* (NOD, 2016). These surveys seek to describe the gaps between people with and without disabilities in terms of employment, income, education, health care, access to transportation, entertainment or going out, socializing, attending religious services, political participation/voter registration, life satisfaction, and trends. Although improvements in all indicators have been demonstrated over the 24-year period of survey activity, progress is described as both slow and modest. The NOD has many programs to promote employment and created the Disability Employment Tracker to encourage companies to support the hiring and retention of those with disabilities (NOD, 2016).

The American Council of the Blind was founded in 1961 and has a current mission to work toward improving quality of life, security, equality, and independence for all visually impaired and blind people (American Council of the Blind, 2013). Services noted by the organization include information and referral, scholarship assistance, public education, and industry consultation, as well as governmental monitoring, consultation, and advocacy. Some of the major issues currently being pursued by the organization include improved education and rehabilitation for the blind and increased production and use of reading materials for the blind and visually impaired. The American Council of the Blind recognizes companies that work toward increasing access for blind and visually impaired individuals and provides publications and resources, policy advocacy, and forums for issues that concern the needs of this population.

Guide Dogs for the Blind is a nonprofit charitable organization established to train and make available guide dogs for the visually impaired, especially in the western United States. Its mission is to work toward improved mobility to individuals that would benefit from the partnership with a dog. This volunteer-driven organization works to train and nurture dogs to provide these services to qualified individuals (Guide Dogs for the Blind, 2015). Both the dogs and services are free (with an adoption fee), and the organization relies substantially on donations. It currently has two training sites, one in California and one in Oregon, with puppy raisers located throughout the Western states. The organization can be reached through its Web site (http://welcome.guidedogs.com).

The National Federation of the Blind (NFB) works toward equality and integrating the blind into society. Founded in 1940, its objective is to remove legal, economic, and social discrimination. It also works to educate the public about new concepts concerning blindness and to highlight promoting the achievement of blind people based on talents and capacities as they function to their fullest abilities (National Federation of the Blind, 2016). Citing

---

DISPLAY 26–5 WHAT IS BRAILLE?

Braille takes its name from Louis Braille, an 18-year-old blind Frenchman who created a system of raised dots on paper for reading and writing by modifying a system used on board sailing ships for night reading. The six raised dots of each Braille "cell" vary to form palpable letters and punctuation. Persons experienced in Braille can read at speeds of 200 to 400 words per minute, comparable to print readers. Braille text can be written (1) by hand with a slate and stylus, (2) with a Braille writing machine, or (3) with specialized computer software and a Braille-embossing device attached to the printer.

Source: National Federation of the Blind. (n.d.). *Braille–What is it? What does it mean to the blind?* Retrieved from http://www.nfb.org/images/nfb/Publications/fr/fr15/Issue1/f150113.html
More information about Braille is available at: http://nfb.org/search/node/braille

---

the need for assistance to the more than 1.1 million children and adults in the United States who are blind, the organization provides public education, information and referral, and support for increased availability of materials in Braille (Display 26–5).

The oldest organization devoted to eliminating barriers for the blind and visually impaired is the American Foundation for the Blind (AFB), founded in 1921. The AFB advocates for the visually impaired through increased funding at the federal and state levels in areas such as rehabilitation research for older, visually impaired persons; improved literacy for the visually impaired, including use of Braille and assistive technology; improved employment opportunities; and increased accessibility of technology. In addition, AFB houses the Helen Keller Archives, which contain her correspondence, photographs, and various personal items and documents (AFB, 2016).

The Obesity Society seeks to increase the science-based knowledge related to obesity regarding the causes, consequences, prevention, and treatment (Obesity Society, 2016). The organization addresses such issues as the need for attention to the impact of obesity on death and disability and for increased research, improved insurance coverage, and elimination of discrimination and mistreatment of people with obesity. The Society's Web site (http://www.obesity.org/home) offers informational literature ranging from obesity as a global health problem to treatment of obesity-related disability.

With growing awareness that HIV/AIDS has become a chronic condition for most individuals affected, their long-term needs are gaining increased attention. Hundreds of Web sites and organizations are available to provide information, assistance, and support. One Web site (http://www.thebody.com/; *The Body: The Complete HIV/AIDS Resource* [The Body, n.d.]) offers state-by-state links to a variety of Internet and print resources. The site also includes resources in Canada and specific sites for American Indians and Alaskan Natives.

Begun in the aftermath of World War I, the Disabled American Veterans organization has provided free services to military veterans seeking to obtain benefits for service-related injuries (Disabled American Veterans, n.d.). The organization is not a government agency and receives no federal funds, instead providing services through membership dues and public contributions. The mission of the organization is to help disabled veterans build better lives for themselves and their families. With the growing number of military injuries resulting from the Iraq and Afghanistan conflicts, the organization finds its service delivery even more stretched. The volunteers provide transportation to Veterans Administration (VA) medical facilities and provide ongoing service at VA hospitals, clinics, and nursing homes.

Universal Design

For those living with a disability or chronic disease and their family members, the issue of access is of utmost importance. As noted earlier, the cost to a family to accommodate the needs of a disabled person can be enormous. Considering that as the U.S. population ages, more and more of us will have need of accessibility in housing, business, and recreation in order to remain active and healthy as long as possible. In the concept of universal design, accessibility has been extended toward making tools, houses, and workplaces accessible to all. The cost of building our environments in a way that promotes access for all can be far less than the cost of remodeling those environments after the fact.

Universal design is the purposefully created environments so that things can be accessible by all without the need for modifications. The term "universal design" has been attributed to Ron Mace, founder of the Center for Universal Design, based out of North Carolina State University. Mace, who had suffered from polio as a child, died suddenly in 1998 leaving behind a long legacy of advocacy on behalf of accessibility in design (Center for Universal Design, 2016). Universal design is at the core of the ADA, and the important relationship between these two is important to note as inclusiveness and reduction of barriers to access are considered (Hums, Schmidt, Bocak, & Wolff, 2016). It is important to note that universal design is for all people, and research focusing on universal design has been instrumental in improving the quality of life of visually impaired individuals (Huang & Chiu, 2016) and disabled older adults (Mustaquim, 2015).

The issue of accessibility is not new. The ADA, as discussed earlier, addresses issues of access in employment, governmental building, and public accommodations. The Fair Housing Accessibility Guidelines, effective beginning in 1991, provide for design and construction of multifamily dwellings (four or more units) in accordance with accessibility requirements (United States Department of Housing and Urban Development [USDHUD], n.d.). The specific provisions include the following (Fair Housing Accessibility First, n.d.):

- Public use and common use portions of the dwellings are readily accessible to and usable by persons with handicaps.
- All doors within such dwellings that are designed to allow passage into and within the premises are sufficiently wide to allow passage by persons in wheelchairs.

- All premises within such dwellings contain the following features of adaptive design:
  1. An accessible route into and through the dwelling
  2. An accessible building entrance that is connected to accessible public transit stop route, as well as accessible parking, loading zones, public sidewalks, and streets
  3. Light switches, electrical outlets, thermostats, and other environmental controls in accessible locations (see Fig. 26–3)
  4. Reinforcements in bathroom walls to allow later installation of grab bars
  5. Usable kitchens and bathrooms such that an individual in a wheelchair can maneuver about the space (see Fig. 26–4)

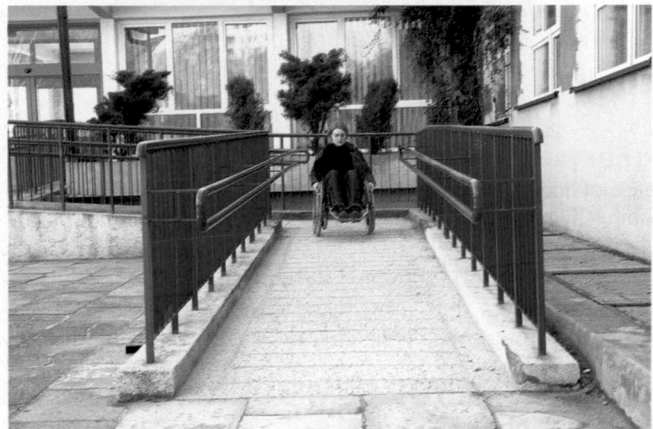

Ramps are needed for those using wheelchairs in order to gain access to buildings.

Universal design incorporates access, but access does not necessarily imply universal design. The design of a community's built environment and its impact on individuals plays a role in the overall health and well-being of those living there. Universal design and access play a key role in this discussion, but the importance of accessible design is more far-reaching. According to the CDC, the **built environment** creates a health environment and health places whereby the quality of life for all, regardless of disability status, is adequate to live, work, play, learn, and worship. This can be achieved through a variety of choices that are healthy, available, accessible, and affordable to all (CDC, 2015).

For those with existing disabilities, assuring ease of access to all types of recreation and exercise options is of paramount importance. For those who may develop disabilities or chronic illnesses, having the opportunities for healthy participation in physical activity may forestall or prevent the development of illness. For the community, having an environment that promotes rather than restricts a healthy lifestyle can be economically advantageous (see Fig. 26–5). Even schools have a role to play (CDC, 2015). Building new schools away from residential areas decreases opportunities for exercise and after-school activities. As parents are increasingly forced to drive their children to school, the children remain sedentary, the pollution from cars is increased, and the risk of automobile accidents increases. Community design is a complicated and evolving issue, but the point remains: a healthier

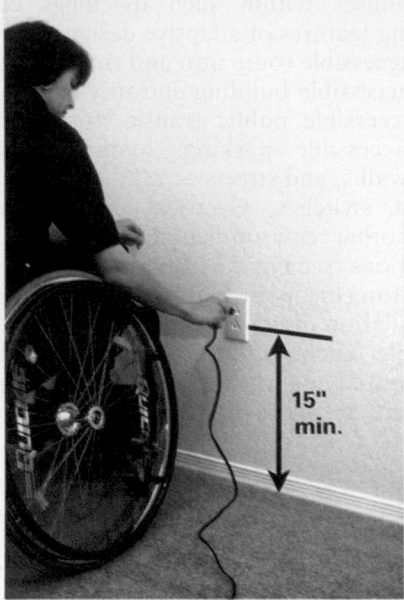

FIGURE 26–3 Recommended height of electrical outlet for ease of access for wheelchair-seated person. (From CDC Image Library. Retrieved from http://phil.cdc.gov/Phil/quicksearch.asp)

population may be achieved with attention to the environmental barriers that impede healthy lifestyles for all persons, including those with chronic or disabling conditions.

THE ROLE OF THE COMMUNITY/PUBLIC HEALTH NURSE

This chapter has discussed a number of areas in which the PHN plays a key role. It is important to review those roles in the context of the individual, the family, and the community. Chapter 3 first examined the broad spectrum of roles that the professional nurse assumes within the community (i.e., clinician, educator, advocate, manager, collaborator, leader,

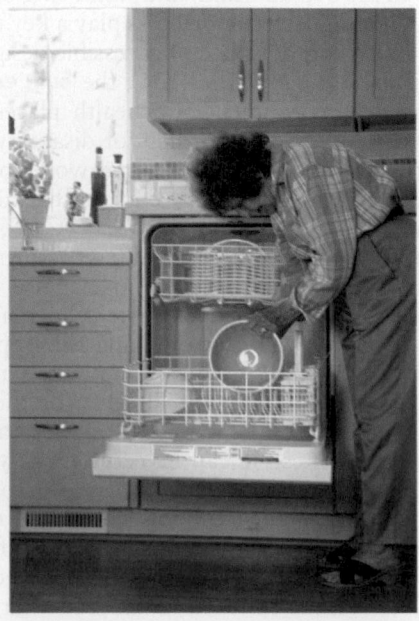

FIGURE 26–4 Universally designed raised dishwasher. (CDC Image Library. Retrieved from http://phil.cdc.gov/Phil/quicksearch.asp)

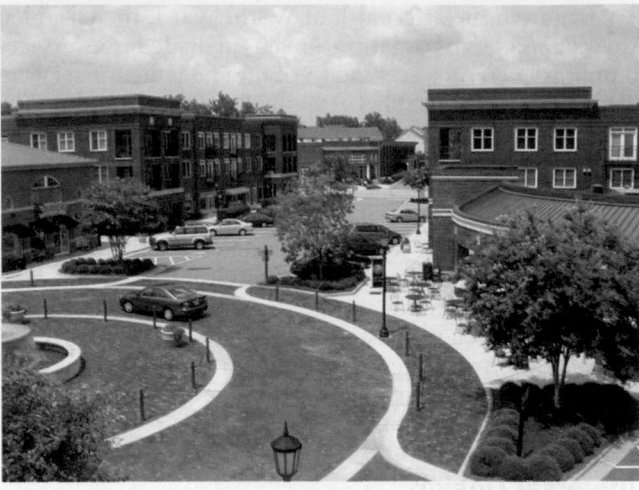

FIGURE 26–5 Planned, mixed-use development with curb cuts, well-marked crossings, sidewalks, and accessible commercial and public spaces (Source: Center for Universal Design. CDC Image Library).

researcher). It is helpful to review those roles and think about their application to disabled and chronically ill clients, their families, and the communities in which they live.

Consider an example of the variety of roles and multilevel practice that the PHN assumes with respect to a 55-year-old female client who uses a wheelchair. The client has difficulty obtaining a gynecologic examination because of the lack of accessible examination tables at the local clinic; as a result, she has not had an examination for more than 20 years. Recognizing the need for a complete examination, the public health nurse arranges with the clinic to find appropriate alternatives that will aid the client in receiving the needed examination, possibly by ensuring that additional personnel are provided (advocate role, individual level).

Because this solution is temporary and less than optimal, the nurse contacts a number of clinics in neighboring communities and finds one that has appropriate equipment for people who have difficulty transferring to a standard examination table. Unfortunately, this clinic is 1 hour away. The nurse then contacts a number of other community/public health nurses and discovers that they also have a significant number of women clients with this problem who have not received a gynecologic examination in many years (research role, community level).

Through a coordinated effort with a local transportation company and the clinic, the nurse is able to arrange a twice-yearly gynecologic screening program for women in the community who require special accommodations (advocate and coordinator roles, community level). Information sheets that discuss the need for annual gynecologic examinations and advertise the program are distributed to area public health nurses, employers, and health clinics (educator role, community level). Data collection on examinations provided over the next few years shows a 65% increase in the number of women with special needs who have received a gynecologic examination within the past year (research role, community level).

This is not an uncommon scenario in the practice of community/public health nursing. Often, the needs of an individual may open the door to areas of concern for many in a community and provide a basis for intervention that can benefit a larger population. Just as for nursing practice in general, the role of the public health nurse with respect to disabilities and chronic illness requires a broad and holistic practice. The complexity of issues surrounding these conditions requires creativity, tenacity, honesty, and, most of all, knowledge. Public health nurses who are informed about the issues that affect the disabled and chronically ill at local, state, and national levels are prepared to offer assistance to their clients and to their communities. Knowledge and advocacy for the civil rights of people living with disabilities, handicaps, and chronic diseases are crucial for nurses serving as their advocates (Mafuba & Gates, 2015).

The issues facing individuals and families with disabilities require strong and sustained efforts to achieve results. Although successes at the individual level are laudable, the extent to which the health and well-being of those affected are improved must be the ultimate goal. Public health nursing is in a prime position to initiate and support efforts to improve the health status of those populations. We can either leave the issues to other professionals or use our expertise and long history of caring for those less fortunate to make major and lasting changes. It is up to us. See an example of one PHN's experience with an individual who became disabled very late in life (From the Case Files: Annie's Story).

It is important for PHNs to consider population health among the disabled. As Grady (2011) reminds us, our U.S. population is living longer, is suffering multiple chronic illness and disabilities, and needs nurses trained to meet the requirements of this aging population. Population health promotion and prevention of secondary disabilities is also a public health concern across age groups and conditions (Ouellette-Kuntz, Cobigo, Balogh, Wilton, & Lunsky, 2015). Community-based interventions that help support disabled populations with self-management skills, improve health behaviors, and prevent secondary disabilities have been shown to be popular and can result in cost savings as well as improved health outcomes (Ravesloot et al., 2016). See Population-Focus.

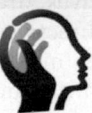

From the Case Files **I**

Annie's Story

Annie married young and had a couple of kids, but ended up divorced and supporting them on her own. She eventually married the love of her life, but he died from medical complications during a routine procedure. She worked very hard and had made a good living on her own. Her children were grown when she met her third husband. She was 80 when he died, and she continued to work at her business and taking care of her many rental properties. She worked most days, was fiercely independent, and was generally in good health.

This is where I enter the story. I met Annie at a community event and we hit it off instantly. She was interested in my work as a PHN, and I enjoyed working with seniors and hearing their life stories. Annie certainly had an interesting one. Hearing I was a nurse, she talked to me about her osteoporosis and having broken an arm and an ankle. She was still jet skiing with friends and family into her 80s, and she drove her large RV to scenic spots—often traveling alone (except for her beloved dog, Emily). She lived alone, too, in a large two-story house on a golf course. She also liked to golf, refusing to use a golf cart, and enjoying the exercise. She exemplified what I wanted to be when I reached my "golden years." She was happy, energetic, positive, and generally healthy (no hypertension, arthritis, or diabetes) and had many friends and colleagues who cared about her. Her kids lived out of state, but she talked with them often and visited when she could. She was well known in the community and loved by all who got to know her.

When Annie turned 90, she slipped and fell getting out of the shower. She broke her hip and lay on her back unable to get up or even to roll over onto her stomach. She was there for 5 days before being discovered. She lived in a desert area, and the air is very dry. The air conditioning was on, but it wasn't very cool on the second level. She had bowel movements and urinated while on the floor, and scooted on her back to get to some toilet paper and attempted to clean herself. She prayed—a lot. She said she knew that there was a God who was listening to her. She worried for her little dog, but she had done something that morning she didn't usually do. She had filled Emily's water dish with extra water. Each time Emily would drink water, she would go over to Annie and lick her mouth with her moist tongue. Annie lost track of time and felt like this ordeal would go on forever. The fall happened on Friday morning of a holiday weekend, but on the fifth day after her fall, she didn't show up for work at her business raising concern. Her colleagues called emergency personnel and they broke into her house, finding her lying naked on the floor. She was so embarrassed, and she told the young paramedics that she was sorry for "giving them that mental picture for life." Amazingly, her sense of humor was still there.

Annie spent a long time in the hospital, dealing with her fractured pelvis, dehydration, and an electrolyte imbalance, among other things. I went to see her, but this vibrant, independent woman was very confused and "different." She was transferred to three different skilled nursing facilities and was never able to return to her beautiful home. She had planned for her life to end independently—living in one of her smaller houses, maybe with some part-time help. It was so difficult for her to end up in a "nursing home." What happened to her on that floor in those 5 days caused so much damage to her heart and her body, as well as to her spirit, that she ended up in a downward spiral. She died in a nursing home shortly before her 93rd birthday.

Annie had lived a very long life in good health and thought that she could continue to do so until "something gave out." This is an example to me that we are all just a quick fall or an accident away from being disabled. If it could happen to Annie, it could happen to any of us!

Nell, PHN

POPULATION-FOCUS ON ADVANCE DIRECTIVES

Advance directives are a very personal and individual matter. Whenever you or I go into the hospital or surgery center for a procedure, we are usually asked by an admitting nurse or clerk if we have an advance directive (no matter our age or health status). How many people actually answer in the affirmative? Autonomy is a hallmark of ethical thought (see Chapter 4). We believe that people should be able to choose for themselves and have their choices respected; hence, the right to leave the hospital against medical advice (AMA). Therefore, we wait for patients to express their preference about advance directives (or the choice to have none).

Have you ever considered this from a population perspective? When someone does not choose a plan for end-of-life care, the option by default generally becomes full medical treatment and lifesaving measures to delay death, despite the futility of the pending outcome. Often, this causes needless suffering and is costly in terms of manpower and resources. But, do individuals truly understand their options? Can we offer better explanations of the alternatives? Behavioral economists explain that people are not always good at systematically looking at best evidence in order to make decisions. We rely on what others think or on rules of thumb because we are often faced with "decision fatigue." We are programmed to avoid loss and seek immediate rewards. Taking this into consideration, and the knowledge that terminal patients want comfort and quality of life at the end of life, researchers gave participants three options: (1) advance directives for comfort-oriented care (where life might be shorter), (2) advance directives for a longer life (where there might be more pain and suffering), and (3) no directives. Because of the way choices were structured, twice as many people chose the option with comfort as the goal over the other two choices. They termed this "choice architecture," as this reframing of the choices to draw attention to outcomes helps to "nudge" people toward their definitive goals (Hostetter & Klein, 2013, para. 17).

The argument could be made that evidence supports advance directives for comfort-oriented care, but is it ethical to influence behavior in this way? The elderly are a growing population, and the lack of advance directives does lead to more economic burden on the healthcare system. Population-focused initiatives are needed to educate the elderly about advance directives and the potential outcomes of the choices they make. Can you think of creative ways of addressing this issue on a population level?

Hostetter, M., & Klein, S. (2013, June–July). In focus: Using behavioral economics to advance population health and improve the quality of health care services. *Quality Matters*. Retrieved from http://www.commonwealthfund.org/publications/newsletters/quality-matters/2013/june-july/in-focus

SUMMARY

The issues of disability and chronic illness are of growing importance in public health and to community/public health nursing, both nationally and internationally. Through the efforts of the WHO, the international community has been challenged to provide increased attention to health promotion and disease prevention. Even in less developed countries, behavioral patterns linked to excesses in consumption (overweight and tobacco/alcohol use) have an impact on the quality and quantity of healthy years of life. The health promotion and disease prevention needs of the disabled and chronically ill must be given the same emphasis as the needs of those who are not disabled or ill.

The aging of the U.S. population and the rise in lifestyle-related illnesses such as diabetes and obesity are often linked with increasing rates of disability. Prevention of disability and disease is emphasized in *Healthy People 2020*, and it alerts Americans over the decades about the need to give serious attention to health-promoting and disease prevention activities. *Healthy People* has placed increasing focus on health promotion and disease prevention needs of those with disabilities and chronic illness. It is no longer acceptable that these individuals receive care solely for tertiary health needs. Research has shown that when health-promoting (lifestyle) issues are addressed with these clients, the rates of secondary conditions are reduced, including medical, social, emotional, mental, family, and community problems. Disabilities and chronic conditions are not universally debilitating, and the overall well-being and health of these individuals must be a priority.

Legislation is but one step toward equality for those affected by disabilities and chronic illnesses. The IDEA and ADA secured many improvements in accessibility and specific legal protections for the disabled, but it is only the beginning. Discrimination can occur at many levels; some is hurtful and intentional, but most results from misunderstanding of the needs and desires of disabled persons and their families. This may even occur in relation to the provision of health care because of lack of education. Improvement can be found only with increased community education programs for professionals and the public that target the myths and misunderstandings about those with disabilities and chronic illnesses.

The next time you have difficulty opening a door that is unusually heavy or struggle to open the lid of a jar or feel that you were treated differently than someone else in the receipt of services, take a moment to think. Think about the challenges, struggles, and pain that face so many citizens. Consider the impact of universal design at improving your life or the life of a family member or friend. Although many argue against improving accessibility of city streets and sidewalks because of the expense, those same people may one day find that they, too, are faced with trying to master a curb that is just a bit too high.

Public health nurses are in a prime position to advocate for the health needs of the disabled and chronically ill. With a long history of serving those who are most vulnerable, public health nurses can help make needed changes at the individual, family, and community levels. Although it is often easier to focus on the needs of the individual, those needs are most often shared by many others, thus making it a population-level concern. Nurses have long recognized the need to collaborate with other professionals in reaching the goal of improved health care for their clients; this continues to be an important aspect of successful efforts on behalf of the disabled and the chronically ill. It will take the concerted efforts of many to implement the changes necessary to improve the lives of those most affected, their families, and the communities in which they live.

ACTIVITIES TO PROMOTE **CRITICAL THINKING**

1. Interview an individual with a disability (e.g., hearing, vision, mobility) about the challenges that he or she has faced in interactions with nondisabled persons and in everyday activities.
2. Search the Web for sites related to disabled individuals and read some of the personal stories posted there. Discuss with a classmate how you might feel if you suddenly found yourself in these circumstances. How would you cope and adjust?
3. Take an inventory of your house or apartment and make a list of modifications you would need to make if you were abruptly confined to a wheelchair. Would you even be able to stay in your current residence (e.g., are you living in a building with only stairs to your second floor apartment)? What resources are available in your community to assist disabled individuals and families?
4. As part of your regular clinical assignment in community health clinical working with clients and families who are either disabled or have a chronic illness, assess how often you or other PHNs have addressed health promotion activities (e.g., healthy eating, physical activity, leisure-time activities) with those clients. Does the public health department have any outreach services for disabled clients to encourage them to get routine preventive services? Ask some of your clients with disabilities and chronic illnesses about their experiences and feelings about preventive services.
5. Review your family history for chronic health conditions. Are you at risk? If so, what have you done to reduce your risk over the past 12 months? Can any of these chronic health conditions lead to impaired visual, hearing, or motor functions?
6. Using the public health nursing roles of clinician, educator, advocate, manager, collaborator, and leader, research and record specific examples of the roles that PHNs assume in relation to disabilities and chronic illnesses. Take note of each role that you participate in or observe while completing your clinical experience. If you cannot find examples of the various roles at each level, interview a PHN during your clinical experience and find examples of how the nurse performs activities in each of those roles. You will most likely find that while addressing a single issue with a client, the public health nurse serves in a variety of roles and at different levels.

REFERENCES

American Council of the Blind. (2013). *Frequently asked questions*. Retrieved from http://www.acb.org/node/16

American Foundation for the Blind (AFB). (2016). *About us: Leading the vision loss community*. Retrieved from http://www.afb.org/section.aspx?FolderID=1

An, R., Andrade, F., & Chiu, C. (2015). Overweight and obesity among U.S. adults with and without disability, 1999–2012. *Preventive Medicine Reports, 2*, 419–422. doi: 10.1016/j.pmedr.2015.05.001.

Andersen, S. L., Olsen, J., & Laurberg, P. (2015). Foetal programming by maternal thyroid disease. *Clinical Endocrinology Oxford, 83*(6). doi: 10.1111/cen.12744.

Anderson, W. L., Wiener, J. M., Finkelstein, E. A., & Armour, B. S. (2011). Estimates of national health care expenditures associated with disability. *Journal of Disability Policy Studies, 21*(4), 230–240.

Appelbaum, P. S., Birkenmaier, J., & Norman, M. (2016). Improving Social Security's financial capability assessments. *Psychiatric Services, 67*(7), 704–706.

Baillargeon, R. H., Bernier, J., & Normand, C. L. (2011). The challenges faced by caregivers of children with impairments of psychological functions: A population-based cross-sectional study. *Canadian Journal of Psychiatry, 56*(10), 614–620.

Bolin, J. N., Bellamy, G. R., Ferdinand, A. O., Vuong, A. M., Kash, B. A., Schulze, A., & Helduser, J. W. (2015). Rural Healthy People 2020: New decade, same challenges. *Journal of Rural Health, 31*(3), 326–333. doi: 10.1111/jrh.12116.

Brolan, C. E., Boyle, F. M., Dean, J. H., Taylor-Gomez, M., Ware, R. S., & Lennox, N. G. (2012). Health advocacy: A vital step in attaining human rights for adults with intellectual disability. *Journal of Intellectual Disability Research, 56*(11), 1087–1097.

Center for Universal Design. (2016). *About the center: Ronald L. Mace*. Retrieved from https://www.ncsu.edu/ncsu/design/cud/about_us/usronmace.htm

Centers for Disease Control and Prevention (CDC). (n.d.). *CDC promoting the health of people with disabilities*. Retrieved from https://www.cdc.gov/ncbddd/disabilityandhealth/pdf/aboutdhprogram508.pdf

Centers for Disease Control and Prevention (CDC). (2015). *CDC's built environment and health initiative*. Retrieved from https://www.cdc.gov/nceh/information/built_environment.htm

Centers for Disease Control and Prevention (CDC). (2016). *Addressing the nation's most common cause of disability: At a glance, 2015*. Retrieved from http://www.cdc.gov/chronicdisease/resources/publications/aag/arthritis.htm

Chen, L. (2015). Disability as a constraint: The barriers approach to understanding disability under the ADA. *Review of Litigation, 34*(1), 157–185.

Cody, P. J., & Lerand, S. J. (2013). Original study: HPV vaccination in female children with special health care needs. *Journal of Pediatric and Adolescent Gynecology, 26*, 219–223. doi: 10.1016/j.jpag.2013.03.003.

Cook, L. H., Foley, J. T., & Semeah, L. M. (2016). Research paper: An exploratory study of inclusive worksite wellness: Considering employees with disabilities. *Disability and Health Journal, 9*, 100–107. doi: 10.1016/j.dhjo.2015.08.011.

Courtney-Long, E. A., Carroll, D. D., Zhang, Q. C., Stevens, A. C., Griffin-Blake, S., Armour, B. S., & Campbell, V. A. (2015). Prevalence of disability and disability type among adults—United States. *Morbidity and Mortality Weekly Report, 64*(29), 777–783.

Dickson, T. (2016, June 28). Jekyll under fire over beach access for disabled 2 access points offered, but synthetic mats stop short of hard sand. *Florida Times-Union*. Retrieved from http://jacksonville.com/news/georgia/2016-06-27/story/jekyll-island-working-improving-beach-access-disabled-amid-criticism#

Disability.gov. (n.d.). *Americans with Disabilities Act (ADA)*. Retrieved from https://www.disability.gov/americans-disabilities-act/

Disabled American Veterans. (n.d.). *Mission statement*. Retrieved from https://www.dav.org/learn-more/about-dav/mission-statement/

Dykens, E. M. (2015). Family adjustment and interventions in neurodevelopmental disorders. *Current Opinion in Psychiatry, 28*(2), 121–126.

Edie, A. (2016). Twenty-five years of the Americans with Disabilities Act. *Creative Nursing, 22*(2), 135–138. doi: 10.1891/1078-4535.22.2.135.

Fair Housing Accessibility First. (n.d.). *Requirements*. Retrieved from http://www.fairhousingfirst.org/fairhousing/requirements.html

Falk, G. (2016). Temporary Assistance for Needy Families (TANF): Size and characteristics of the cash assistance caseload. *Congressional Research Service: Report, 1*. Retrieved from https://www.fas.org/sgp/crs/misc/R43187.pdf

Federal Register. (2016, March 17). *Announcement of establishment of the secretary's advisory committee on national health promotion and disease prevention objectives for 2030 and solicitation of nominations for membership*. Retrieved from https://www.federalregister.gov/articles/2016/03/17/2016-06016/announcement-of-establishment-of-the-secretarys-advisory-committee-on-national-health-promotion-and

Fielding, J. E., Kumanyika, S., & Manderscheid, R. W. (2013). A perspective on the development of the Healthy People 2020 framework for improving U.S. population health. *Public Health Reports, 35*(1), 1–24.

Fink, K. (2016). Deaf American Sign Language (ASL) users and the challenges faced in neuroscience. *Canadian Journal of Neuroscience Nursing, 38*(1), 34–35.

Froehlich-Grobe, K., Jones, D., Businelle, M. S., Kendzor, D. E., & Balasubramanian, B. A. (2016). Research paper: Impact of disability and chronic conditions on health. *Disability and Health Journal*. doi: 10.1016/j.dhjo.2016.04.007.

Fulda, K. G., Johnson, K. L., Hahn, K., & Lykens, K. (2013). Do unmet needs differ geographically for children with special health care needs? *Maternal Child Health Journal, 17*(3), 505–511.

Ghosh, S., & Parish, S. L. (2015). Deprivation among U.S. children with disabilities who receive Supplemental Security Income. *Journal of Disability Policy Studies, 26*(3), 173. doi: 10.1177/1044207314539011.

Giallo, R., Seymour, M., Matthews, J., Gavidia-Payne, S., Hudson, A., & Cameron, C. (2015). Risk factors associated with the mental health of fathers of children with an intellectual disability in Australia. *Journal of Intellectual Disability Research, 59*(3), 193–207. doi: 10.1111/jir.12127.

Goodman, R. A., Posner, S. F., Huang, E. S., Parekh, A. K., & Koh, H. K. (2013). Defining and measuring chronic conditions: Imperatives for research, policy, program, and practice. *Preventing Chronic Disease, 10*, 120239. doi: 10.5888/pcd10.120239.

Grady, P. A. (2011). Advancing the health of our aging population: A lead role for nursing science. *Nursing Outlook, 59*, 207–209.

Greenwood, V. J., Crawford, N. W., Walstab, J. E., & Reddihough, D. S. (2013). Immunisation coverage in children with cerebral palsy compared with the general population. *Journal of Paediatrics & Child Health, 49*(2), E137. doi: 10.1111/jpc.12097.

Guide Dogs for the Blind. (2015). *Our mission*. Retrieved from http://www.guidedogs.com/site/PageServer?pagename=about_overview_mission

Hamilton, A., Mazzucchelli, T. G., & Sanders, M. R. (2015). Parental and practitioner perspectives on raising an adolescent with a disability: A focus group study. *Disability & Rehabilitation, 37*(18), 1664–1673. doi: 10.3109/09638288.2014.973969.

Hensel, R. M. (2016). *The official Robert M. Hensel website*. Retrieved from http://roberthensel.webs.com/myquotes.htm

Horner-Johnson, W., Dobbertin, K., & Iezzoni, L. I. (2015). Disparities in receipt of breast and cervical cancer screening for rural women age 18 to 64 with disabilities. *Women's Health Issues, 25*(3), 246–253. doi: 10.1016/j.whi.2015.02.004.

Huang, P., & Chiu, M. (2016). Integrating user centered design, universal design and goal, operation, method and selection rules to improve the usability of DAISY player for persons with visual impairments. *Applied Ergonomics, 52*, 29–42. doi: 10.1016/j.apergo.2015.06.008.

Hums, M. A., Schmidt, S. H., Novak, A., & Wolff, E. A. (2016). Universal design: Moving the Americans with Disabilities Act from access to inclusion. *Journal of Legal Aspects of Sport, 26*(1), 36–51.

Iezzoni, L. I., Kurtz, S. G., & Rao, S. R. (2015). Trends in mammography over time for women with and without chronic disability. *Journal of Women's Health, 24*(7), 593–601. doi: 10.1089/jwh.2014.5181.

In Sook, C., & Hyun Sook, R. (2015). Factors affecting depression in mothers of children with disabilities. *Child Health Nursing Research, 21*(1), 46–54. doi: 10.4094/chnr.2015.21.1.46.

Kanter, A. S. (2015). The Americans with Disabilities Act at 25 years: Lessons to learn from the convention on the rights of people with disabilities. *Drake Law Review, 63*(3), 819–883.

Krahn, G. L., Klein Walker, D., & Correa-de-Araujo, R. (2015). Persons with disabilities as an unrecognized health disparity population. *American Journal of Public Health, 105*(S2), S198–S206.

Kung, P. T., Tsai, W. C., & Li, Y. H. (2012). Determining factors for utilization of preventive health services among adults with disabilities in Taiwan. *Research in Developmental Disabilities, 33*(1), 205–213.

Kyounghae, K., Choi, J. S., Eunsuk, C., Nieman, C. L., Jin Hui, J., Lin, F. R., ..., Hae-Ra, H. (2016). Effects of community-based health worker interventions to improve chronic disease management and care among vulnerable populations: A systematic review. *American Journal of Public Health, 106*(4), e3–e28. doi: 10.2105/AJPH.2015.302987.

Lam-Cassettari, C. C., Wadnerkar-Kamble, M. B., & James, D. M. (2015). Enhancing parent–child communication and parental self-esteem with a video-feedback intervention: Outcomes with prelingual deaf and hard-of-hearing children. *Journal of Deaf Studies & Deaf Education, 20*(3), 266–274. doi: 10.1093/deafed/env008.

Mafuba, K., & Gates, B. (2015). An investigation into the public health roles of community learning disability nurses. *British Journal of Learning Disabilities, 43*(1), 1–7.

Mahmoudi, E., & Meade, M. A. (2015). Research paper: Disparities in access to health care among adults with physical disabilities: Analysis of a representative national sample for a ten-year period. *Disability and Health Journal, 8,* 182–190. doi: 10.1016/j.dhjo.2014.08.007.

Massey, W. (2015, July 24). *The ADA at 25: What's next for disability rights?* Retrieved from http://www.cnn.com/2015/07/24/living/ada-25-anniversary-disability-rights-feat/

McCain, J. (2012, May 25). *Press release: Bipartisan group of senators announce support for disability treaty.* Retrieved from http://www.mccain.senate.gov/public/index.cfm?FuseAction=PressOffice.PressReleases&ContentRecord_id=84b3c564-d49f-0cf5-7742-9ff158d8ef7e&Region_id=&Issue_id=

McCann, D., Bull, R., & Winzenberg, T. (2015). Sleep deprivation in parents caring for children with complex needs at home: A mixed methods systematic review. *Journal of Family Nursing, 21*(1), 86–118. doi: 10.1177/1074840714562026.

McPherson, A. C., Keith, R., & Swift, J. A. (2014). Obesity prevention for children with physical disabilities: A scoping review of physical activity and nutrition interventions. *Disability & Rehabilitation, 36*(19), 1573–1587.

Milner, A., Krnjacki, L., Butterworth, P., Kavanagh, A., & LaMontagne, A. D. (2015). Does disability status modify the association between psychosocial job quality and mental health? A longitudinal fixed-effects analysis. *Social Science Medicine, 144,* 104–111.

Montes, G., & Halterman, J. S. (2008). Association of childhood autism spectrum disorders and loss of family income. *Pediatrics, 121*(4), e821–e826.

Moore, M. H. (2013). *Recognizing public value.* Cambridge, MA: Harvard University Press.

Morgan, D. J., Boniface, G. E., & Reagon, C. (2016). The effects of adapting their home on the meaning of home for families with a disabled child. *Disability & Society, 31*(4), 481. doi: 10.1080/09687599.2016.1183475.

Mustaquim, M. M. (2015). A study of universal design in everyday life of elderly adults. *Procedia Computer Science, 67,* 57–66. doi: 10.1016/j.procs.2015.09.249.

National Association of the Deaf (NAD). (2016). *About us.* Retrieved from http://www.nad.org/about-us

National Council on Disability (NCD). (n.d.). *About us.* Retrieved from https://www.ncd.gov/about

National Council on Disability (NCD). (2008a). *Finding the gaps: A comparative analysis of disability laws in the United States to the United Nations Convention on the Rights of Persons with Disabilities (CRPD).* Retrieved from www.ncd.gov/publications/2008/May122008

National Council on Disability (NCD). (2008b). *National disability policy: A progress report.* Retrieved from https://www.ncd.gov/rawmedia_repository/ea8e79b7_17db_427b_a838_19030deb107e.pdf

National Council on Disability (NCD). (2014). *National disability policy: A progress report.* Retrieved from https://www.ncd.gov/progress_reports/10312014

National Federation of the Blind. (2016). *What is the National Federation of the Blind?* Retrieved from http://nfb.org/who-we-are

National Organization on Disability (NOD). (2016). *About: 30 years in the making.* Retrieved from http://www.nod.org/about/

Obesity Society. (2016). *About The Obesity Society (TOS).* Retrieved from http://www.obesity.org/about

Office of Disease Prevention and Health Promotion (ODPHP). (2016). *Healthy People 2020: Disability and health.* Retrieved from https://www.healthypeople.gov/2020/topics-objectives/topic/disability-and-health

Ouellette-Kuntz, H., Cobigo, V., Balogh, R., Wilton, A., & Lunsky, Y. (2015). The uptake of secondary prevention by adults with intellectual and developmental disabilities. *Journal of Applied Research on Intellectual Disabilities, 28*(1), 43–54.

Price, M. S., & Oliverio, P. (2016). The costs of raising a special needs child after divorce. *American Journal of Family Law, 30*(1), 25–31.

Ravesloot, C., Seekins, T., Traci, M., Boehm, T., White, G., ..., Monson, J. (2016). Living well with a disability, a self-management program. *MMWR Supplement, 65*(1), 61–67.

Reichard, A., Gulley, S. P., Rasch, E. K., & Chan, L. (2015). Diagnosis isn't enough: Understanding the connections between high health care utilization, chronic conditions and disabilities among U.S. working age adults. *Disability and Health Journal, 8*(4), 535–546. doi: 10.1016/j.dhjo.2015.04.006.

Sheperis, C. C., Sheperis, D., Monceaux, A., Davis, R. J., & Lopez, B. (2015). Parent–child interaction therapy for children with special needs. *Professional Counselor: Research & Practice, 5*(2), 248–260. doi: 10.15241/cs.5.2.248.

Shick, S. (2015). *The disability tax: The hidden burden people with disabilities and chronic illnesses face every day.* Roundtable presentation at the 110th Annual Meeting of the American Sociological Association, Chicago, IL.

Smith, A. E., Molton, I. R., & Jensen, M. P. (2016). Research paper: Self-reported incidence and age of onset of chronic comorbid medical conditions in adults aging with long-term physical disability. *Disability and Health Journal, 9,* 533–538. doi: 10.1016/j.dhjo.2016.02.002.

Stevens, G. A., Bennett, J. E., Hennocq, Q., Lu, Y., De-Regil, L. M., Rogers, L., ..., Ezzati, M. (2015). Articles: Trends and mortality effects of vitamin A deficiency in children in 138 low-income and middle-income countries between 1991 and 2013: A pooled analysis of population-based surveys. *The Lancet Global Health, 3,* e528–e536. doi: 10.1016/S2214-109X(15)00039-X.

The Arc. (n.d.). *Public policy and legal advocacy: Policy issues affecting people with disabilities.* Retrieved from http://www.thearc.org/what-we-do/public-policy

The Body. (2012). *The complete HIV/AIDS resource.* Retrieved from http://www.thebody.com/

Thompson, R., Kerr, M., Glynn, M., & Linehan, C. (2014). Caring for a family member with intellectual disability and epilepsy: Practical, social and emotional perspectives. *Seizure, 23*(10), 856–863.

Together We Rock. (n.d.). *Common myths and misconceptions about disability.* Retrieved from http://static1.squarespace.com/static/565dec2de4b0475ab00625b6/t/56cbc06a62cd94fc4bc447b3/1456193645073/Myths+and+Misconceptions+-+Accessible+Format+-+Jan+27%2C+2016.pdf

United Nations. (2016, May 30). *Treaty collection: Chapter IV: Human rights—Convention on the Rights of Persons with Disabilities.* Retrieved from https://treaties.un.org/Pages/ViewDetails.aspx?src=IND&mtdsg_no=IV-15&chapter=4&lang=en

U.S. Department of Health and Human Services (USDHHS). (2006). *Progress toward Healthy People 2010 targets: Disability and secondary conditions.* Retrieved from http://www.healthypeople.gov/2010/data/midcourse/html/focusareas/fa06progresshp.htm

U.S. Department of Health and Human Services (USDHHS). (2016). *Healthy People 2020: About Healthy People.* Retrieved from http://www.healthypeople.gov/2020/about/default.aspx

U.S. Department of Housing and Urban Development. (n.d.). *Fair housing accessibility guidelines.* Retrieved from http://portal.hud.gov/hudportal/HUD?src=/program_offices/fair_housing_equal_opp/disabilities/fhefhag

U.S. Department of Labor (USDOL). (n.d.a). *Employers and the ADA: Myths and facts.* Retrieved from https://www.dol.gov/odep/pubs/fact/ada.htm

U.S. Department of Labor (USDOL). (n.d.b). *The Family and Medical Leave Act.* Retrieved from https://www.dol.gov/whd/regs/compliance/1421.htm

Wen, P. (2014, August 28). *Aid to disabled children now outstrips welfare: As SSI expands, debate intensifies.* Retrieved from https://www.bostonglobe.com/metro/2014/08/27/cash-distributed-under-ssi-for-children-now-exceeds-welfare/ek0peSWTLJ00YId0CONFYI/story.html

White House. (2009, July 24). *Remarks by the president on signing the U.N. Convention on the Rights of Persons with Disabilities Proclamation.* Retrieved from http://www.whitehouse.gov/the-press-office/remarks-president-rights-persons-with-disabilities-proclamation-signing

Whiting, M. (2014a). Support requirements of parents caring for a child with disability and complex health needs. *Nursing Children and Young People, 26*(4), 24–27.

Whiting, M. (2014b). What it means to be a parent of a child with a disability or complex health need. *Nursing Children and Young People, 26*(5), 26–29.

Wilroy, J. D., Knowlden, A. P., & Birch, D. A. (2016). Comparing exercise motivations for each stage of change among people with a physical disability: A pilot study. *Palaestra, 30*(1), 43–48.

World Health Organization (WHO). (2001). *International classification of functioning, disability and health.* Geneva, Switzerland: Author.

World Health Organization (WHO). (2002a). *Towards a common language for functioning, disability, and health.* Retrieved from http://www.who.int/classifications/icf/icfbeginnersguide.pdf?ua=1

World Health Organization (WHO). (2002b). *World health report: Reducing risks, promoting healthy life.* Geneva, Switzerland: Author.

World Health Organization (WHO). (2009). *Global health risks: Mortality and burden of disease attributable to major risks.* Retrieved from http://www.who.int/healthinfo/global_burden_disease/global_health_risks/en/index.html

World Health Organization (WHO). (2016). *What's disability to me? Personal narratives.* Retrieved from http://www.who.int/disabilities/en/

World Health Organization and the World Bank. (2011). *World report on disability: Summary.* Retrieved from http://www.who.int/disabilities/world_report/2011/report/en/

Yamaoka, Y., Tamiya, N., Moriyama, Y., Sandoval Garrido, F. A., Sumazaki, R., & Noguchi, H. (2015). Mental health of parents as caregivers of children with disabilities: Based on Japanese Nationwide Survey. *PLoS One, 10*(12), e0145200. doi: 10.1371/journal.pone.0145200.

Yee, S. (2016). *Where prejudice, disability, and "disabilism" meet.* Retrieved from http://dredf.org/news/publications/disability-rights-law-and-policy/where-prejudice-disability-and-disabilism-meet/

thePoint: Everything You Need to Make the Grade!

thePoint® Visit http://thePoint.lww.com/Rector9e for selected readings, study aids for all learning styles, and more!

Behavioral Health in the Community

"Mental health and mental disorders are not opposites, and mental health is not just the absence of mental disorder."

—*World Health Organization*

"Addiction is a primary, chronic disease of brain reward, motivation, memory, and related circuitry. Dysfunction in these circuits leads to characteristic biological, psychological, social, and spiritual manifestations."

—*American Society of Addiction Medicine*

KEY TERMS

Addiction
Alcohol-related disorders
At-risk alcohol use
Behavioral health
Community mental health

Community mental health centers
Community mental health nurse
Craving
Intoxication

Mental health
Mental health care system
Recovery
Relapse
Screening
Self-stigma

Serious mental illness (SMI)
Social stigma
Structural stigma
Substance-related disorders
Tolerance

LEARNING OBJECTIVES

Upon mastery of this chapter, you should be able to:

● Discuss the incidence and prevalence of mental illness and substance use in the United States.
● Identify the *Healthy People 2020* objectives for reducing substance use and addressing mental health needs.
● Describe the role of the community health nurse across the continuum of care individuals and populations with mental and substance-related disorders.
● Implement individual-, community-, and policy-level interventions to promote behavioral health and recovery.

This chapter provides an overview of **behavioral health**, a term used to refer to both mental health and substance use. A comprehensive approach to behavioral health recognizes a continuum of care, from promotion to prevention, treatment, and recovery. Community health nursing practice with a focus on individual-, community-, and policy-level interventions is discussed. The community health nurse has a key role in working with individuals, families, and communities to promote optimal behavioral health and thereby decrease the prevalence and incidence of mental and substance-related disorders. See Display 27–1: Behavioral Health Terminology.

DEFRAGMENTING HEALTH CARE

Over the past several years, efforts have been undertaken to bridge the separate systems of care for persons with mental disorders, substance use disorders, and primary health. These changes are particularly relevant for community health nurses who have public health knowledge and skills to address the needs and problems of communities and vulnerable populations (see Chapter 1). Community health nurses, from their perspective of community-based and population-focused practice, understand that the communities in which people live and work have a profound influence on the collective health and well-being of the population.

The fragmented mental health service delivery system was identified by the president's New Freedom Commission on Mental Health (TPNFCMH, 2003) as a major impediment to the provision of quality mental health care. A person with medical, mental health, and substance use concerns moves between separate systems to receive needed care and among multiple health care providers within those systems. The best outcome can be promoted by integrating behavioral health and medical care for people with multiple health care needs. The shift to both improving and integrating behavioral and medical care has been facilitated by the Affordable Care Act (ACA) of 2014, the Mental Health Parity and Addiction Equity Act (MHPAEA) of 2008, and health coverage offered through Medicaid Expansion and the Marketplace requiring provision of mental health and substance use disorder benefits. Integrative care, according to the Agency for Health Care Research and Quality, "is derived from a practice team of primary care and behavioral health clinicians, working together with patients and families, using a systematic and cost-effective approach to provide patient-centered care for a defined population" (Peek & National Integration Academy Council, 2013, p. 2). The field of community health nursing has an integral role in assuming responsibility as a full professional partner in integrated care for the health of the community.

In considering the health of the community, it is important to keep in mind the continuum of health to illness. The World Health Organization (2014) defines **mental health** as "a state of well-being in which every individual realizes his or her own potential, can cope with the normal stresses of life, can work productively and fruitfully, and is able to make a contribution to her or his community" (p. 1). Behavioral, biological, and environmental mechanisms are linked to various human responses, such as anxiety, depression, and substance use. Community health nurses can intervene at three levels of prevention taking measures to keep illness or injuries from occurring (primary prevention), to detect and treat existing health problems at the earliest possible stage when a disorder or impairment is already present (secondary prevention), and to reduce the severity of a health problem to minimize disability, restore or preserve function, and promote recovery efforts (tertiary prevention).

Several documents address the need for prevention and treatment of mental health disorders, such as *Healthy People 2020* (U.S. Department of Health and Human Services [USDHHS], 2016b), *Mental Illness Surveillance Among Adults in the United States* (Centers for Disease Control and Prevention [CDC], 2011), and the classic *Report of the Surgeon General on Mental Health*, submitted by David Satcher (USDHHS, 1999). This 1999 report on mental health was the first Surgeon General's report ever published on the topic of mental health and mental illness. That report concluded that mental disorders are among the most prevalent and costly conditions and that effective treatments can reduce their prevalence and decrease their adverse effect on other health conditions.

The health care goals addressed within *Healthy People 2020* (USDHHS, 2016b) are relevant to community mental health nursing (see Tables 27–1 to 27–3). The overall goal for mental health and mental disorders is to improve mental health through prevention and by ensuring access to appropriate, quality mental health services. Only one of the indicators (MHMD11.1) met the target, and that was for a single year in 2013. A decrease in all indicators is needed to fully meet the targets. According to the 2014 progress report, from 2006 to 2010, the suicide rate increased about 7%, from 11.3 per 100,000 people (age adjusted) to 12.1, moving away from the *Healthy People 2020* target of 10.2 per 100,000 people. Additionally, between 2008 and 2012, the percentage of adolescents aged 12 to 17 reporting having had a major depressive episode in the past 12 months increased about 10%, from 8.3% to 9.1%, moving away from the *Healthy People 2020* target of 7.5% (Department of Health and Human Services Office of Disease Prevention and Health Promotion, 2014). Nearly a decade and a half later after the 1999 Surgeon General's Report and several years since *Healthy People 2020* was launched, the Substance Abuse and Mental Health Services Administration (SAMHSA, 2013a) reported that not all people are receiving treatment and not all people receive the appropriate type or adequate quantity or quality of care. Thus, greater efforts are needed to address the behavioral health needs of the nation.

DISPLAY 27–1 BEHAVIORAL HEALTH TERMINOLOGY

- **Addiction:** A complex neurobehavioral disorder characterized by impaired control, compulsive use, and repetition despite the consequences (Merlo, Wandler, & Gold, 2014).
- **Alcohol-related disorders:** A category of alcohol-induced disorders including a pattern of alcohol use leading to clinically significant impairment or distress (alcohol use disorder), **intoxication** (i.e., clinically significant problematic behavioral or psychological changes that develop during or shortly after alcohol ingestion), withdrawal (problematic behavioral change with physiological and cognitive concomitants that is due to the cessation of or reduction in heavy and prolonged alcohol use), and other alcohol-induced mental disorders (symptom profiles resemble independent mental disorders as describe in the *DSM*) (APA, 2013).
- **At-risk alcohol use:** Any level of alcohol consumption that increases the risk of harm to a person's health or well-being or that increases the risk of harm to others. The thresholds, listed below, are based on population studies among healthy adults (21 years and older) and are a starting point for evaluating risk in individuals. Various health conditions and activities may warrant lower levels or no alcohol consumption at all (Finnell, Mitchell, & Savage, in press).
  - Within a short period of time (i.e., 2 hours), which typically brings the average adult's blood alcohol concentration above 0.08 g/dL (also considered binge alcohol use) for the following is:
    - Women (healthy $\geq$ 21 years): consuming more than 3 drinks within a 2-hour period
    - Men (healthy $\geq$ 21 to 65 years): consuming more than 4 drinks within a 2-hour period
    - Men (healthy > 65 years): consuming more than 3 drinks within a 2-hour period
  - In a single day:
    - Women (healthy $\geq$ 21 years): consuming more than 3 drinks a day
    - Men (healthy $\geq$ 21 to 65 years): consuming more than 4 drinks a day
    - Men (healthy > 65 years): consuming more than 3 drinks a day
  - In a week:
    - Women (healthy $\geq$ 21 years): consuming more than 7 drinks a week
    - Men (healthy $\geq$ 21 to 65 years): consuming more than 14 drinks a week
    - Men (healthy > 65 years): consuming more than 7 drinks a week
- **Behavioral Health:** A term used to refer to both mental health and substance use. A comprehensive approach to behavioral health recognizes a continuum of care, from promotion to prevention, treatment, and recovery.

- **Community mental health:** A field of practice that seeks to promote the mental health of the community by preventing mental disorders and addressing the needs of persons with a mental disorder.
- **Community mental health centers (CMHCs):** Facilities that provide comprehensive, publicly funded services to the mentally ill population.
- **Community mental health nurse:** An individual whose practice is centered on the mental health needs of the populations served.
- **Mental health care system:** The collective programs designed for anyone with a mental illness. These programs may include treatments, services, or other types of supports, such as housing, employment, or disability benefits through government, private nonprofit, or private for-profit systems.
- Mental health: As defined in *Healthy People 2020*, mental health is "a state of successful performance of mental function, resulting in productive activities, fulfilling relationships with other people, and the ability to adapt to change and cope with challenges" (U.S. Department of Health and Human Services [USDHHS], 2016, para. 2).
- **Mental disorders:** "Health conditions that are characterized by alterations in thinking, mood, and/or behavior that are associated with distress and/or impaired functioning. Mental disorders contribute to a host of problems that may include disability, pain, or death" (USDHHS, 2016, para. 3).
- **Recovery:** A process of change through which individuals improve their health and wellness, live a self-directed life, and strive to reach their full potential (http://www.samhsa.gov/recovery).
- **Relapse:** Continued use of a substance after a period of abstinence. Return to heavy alcohol, tobacco, or drug use after a period of abstinence or moderate use (Douaihy, Daley, Marlatt, & Donovan, 2014).
- **Serious mental illness (SMI):** As defined by SAMHSA, "adults aged 18 or older who currently or at any time in the past year have had a diagnosable mental, behavioral, or emotional disorder (excluding developmental and substance use disorders) of sufficient duration to meet diagnostic criteria specified within DSM-IV (APA, 1994) that has resulted in serious functional impairment, which substantially interferes with or limits one or more major life activities" (SAMHSA, 2014).
- **Substance-related disorders:** Encompassing 10 separate classes of drugs that, taken in excess, have in common direct activation of the brain reward system, producing such an intense activation that normal activities may be neglected. This system is involved in the reinforcement of behaviors and the production of memories (APA, 2013).
- **Screening:** A mechanism used to detect health risks or problems using an established measure (i.e., psychometrically sound questionnaire such as the

(continued)

DISPLAY 27-1 BEHAVIORAL HEALTH TERMINOLOGY (*Continued*)

Alcohol Use Disorders Identification Test) or method (i.e., laboratory test such as drug toxicology using breath, blood, urine, hair).

- **Tolerance:** A need for markedly increased amounts of alcohol or drug to achieve intoxication or the desired effect or a markedly diminished effect with the continued use of the same amount of alcohol or drug (APA, 2013)

American Psychiatric Association. (2013). *Diagnostic and statistical manual of mental disorders* (5th ed.). Arlington, VA: Author.

Douaihy, A., Daley, D. C., Marlatt, G. A., & Donovan, D. M. (2014). Relapse prevention: Clinical models and intervention strategies. In R. Ries, D. Fiellin,

S. Miller, & R. Saitz (Eds.), *The ASAM principles of addiction medicine* (5th ed., pp. 991–1007). Philadelphia, PA: Wolters Kluwer.

Finnell, D.S., Mitchell, A., & Savage, C.L. Kane, I., Kearns, R., Poole, N., ... Coulson, S. (2015). Alcohol screening a brief intervention: A self-paced program for nurses. *Addiction Science in Clinical Practice, 10*(Suppl. 2), 018.

Merlo, L. J., Wandler, K., & Gold, M. S. (2014). Co-occurring addiction and eating disorders. In R. Ries, D. Fiellin, S. Miller, & R. Saitz (Eds.), *The ASAM principles of addiction medicine* (5th ed., pp. 1418–1432). Philadelphia, PA: Wolters Kluwer.

Substance Abuse and Mental Health Services Administration (SAMHSA). (2014). *Results from the 2013 National Survey on Drug Use and Health: Summary of national findings (NSDUH Series H-48, HHS Publication No. [SMA] 14-4863)*. Rockville, MD: Author.

U.S. Department of Health & Human Services (USDHHS). (2016). *Healthy People 2020: Mental health and mental disorders*. Retrieved from https://www.healthypeople.gov/2020/topics-objectives/topic/mental-health-and-mental-disorders

Table 27-1 *Healthy People 2020—Summary of Objectives for Mental Health and Mental Disorders (MHMD)*

Goal: Improve mental health through prevention and by ensuring access to appropriate, quality mental health services

Number	Objective
Mental Health Status Improvement	
MHMD-1	Reduce the suicide rate
MHMD-2	Reduce suicide attempts by adolescents
MHMD-3	Reduce the proportion of adolescents who engage in disordered eating behaviors in an attempt to control their weight
MHMD-4	Reduce the proportion of persons who experience major depressive episodes (MDEs)
MHMD-4.1	Reduce the proportion of adolescents aged 12 to 17 years who experience MDEs
MHMD-4.2	Reduce the proportion of adults aged 18 years and older who experience MDEs
Treatment Expansion	
MHMD-5	Increase the proportion of primary care facilities that provide mental health treatment onsite or by paid referral
MHMD-6	Increase the proportion of children with mental health problems who receive treatment
MHMD-7	Increase the proportion of juvenile justice facilities that screen admissions for mental health problems
MHMD-8	Increase the proportion of persons with serious mental illness (SMI) who are employed
MHMD-9	Increase the proportion of adults with mental health disorders who receive treatment
MHMD-9.1	Increase the proportion of adults aged 18 years and older with SMI who receive treatment
MHMD-9.2	Increase the proportion of adults aged 18 years and older with MDEs who receive treatment
MHMD-10	Increase the proportion of persons with co-occurring substance abuse and mental disorders who receive treatment for both disorders
MHMD-11	Increase depression screening by primary care providers
MHMD-11.1	Increase the proportion of primary care physician office visits where adults 19 years and older are screened for depression
MHMD-11.2	Increase the proportion of primary care physician office visits where youth aged 12 to 18 years are screened for depression
MHMD-12	Increase the proportion of homeless adults with mental health problems who receive mental health services

From U.S. Department of Health and Human Services (USDHHS). (2016). *Healthy People 2020: Mental health & mental disorders objectives*. Retrieved from http://www.healthypeople.gov/2020/topicsobjectives2020/objectiveslist.aspx?topicId=28

Table 27–2 *Healthy People 2020—Summary of Objectives for Substance Abuse*

Goal: Reduce substance abuse to protect the health, safety, and quality of life for all, especially children

Number	Objective
Policy and Prevention	
SA-1	Reduce the proportion of adolescents who report that they rode, during the previous 30 days, with a driver who had been drinking alcohol
SA-2	Increase the proportion of adolescents never using substances
SA-3	Increase the proportion of adolescents who disapprove of substance abuse
SA-4	Increase the proportion of adolescents who perceive great risk associated with substance abuse
SA-5	(Developmental) Increase the number of drug, driving while impaired (DWI), and other specialty courts in the United States
SA-6	Increase the number of states with mandatory ignition interlock laws for first and repeat impaired driving offenders in the United States
Screening and Treatment	
SA-7	Increase the number of admissions to substance abuse treatment for injection drug use
SA-8	Increase the proportion of persons who need alcohol and/or illicit drug treatment and received specialty treatment for abuse or dependence in the past year
SA-9	(Developmental) Increase the proportion persons who are referred for follow-up care for alcohol problems, drug problems after diagnosis, or treatment for one of these conditions in a hospital emergency department (ED)
SA-10	Increase the number of level I and level II trauma centers and primary care settings that implement evidence-based alcohol screening and brief intervention (SBI)
Epidemiology and Surveillance	
SA-11	Reduce cirrhosis deaths
SA-12	Reduce drug-induced deaths
SA-13	Reduce past month use of illicit substances
SA-14	Reduce the proportion of persons engaging in binge drinking of alcoholic beverages
SA-15	Reduce the proportion of adults who drank excessively in the previous 30 days
SA-16	Reduce average annual alcohol consumption
SA-17	Decrease the rate of alcohol-impaired driving (0.08 + blood alcohol content [BAC]) fatalities
SA-18	Reduce steroid use among adolescents
SA-19	Reduce the past-year nonmedical use of prescription drugs
SA-20	Decrease the number of deaths attributable to alcohol
SA-21	Reduce the proportion of adolescents who use inhalants

From U.S. Department of Health and Human Services (USDHHS). (2016). *Healthy People 2020: Substance abuse.* Retrieved from http://www.healthypeople.gov/2020/topicsobjectives2020/objectiveslist.aspx?topicId=40

Despite advances in health coverage for mental health and substance use treatment and efforts undertaken to integrate behavioral and primary health care, stigma continues to be a major barrier to treatment. Stigma is manifest at the self, social, and structural levels:

- **Self-stigma** is a subjective experience characterized by negative feeling about one's self or maladaptive behavior resulting from one's own experiences, perceptions, or anticipation of negative reactions (Livingston & Boyd, 2010).

Table 27–3 *Healthy People 2020—Summary of Objectives for Tobacco (Selected)*

Goal: Reduce illness, disability, and death related to tobacco use and secondhand smoke exposure

Number	Objective
Tobacco Use	
TU-1	Reduce tobacco use by adults
TU-2	Reduce tobacco use by adolescents
TU-3	Reduce the initiation of tobacco use among children, adolescents, and young adults
TU-4	Increase the smoking cessation attempts by adult smokers
TU-5	Increase recent smoking cessation success by adult smokers
TU-6	Increase smoking cessation during pregnancy
TU-7	Increase smoking cessation attempts by adolescent smokers
Health Systems Changes	
TU-8	Increase the comprehensive Medicaid insurance coverage of evidence-based treatment for nicotine dependency in states and the District of Columbia
TU-9	Increase tobacco screening in health care settings
TU-10	Increase tobacco cessation counseling in health care settings
Social and Environmental Changes	
TU-11	Reduce the proportion of nonsmokers exposed to secondhand smoke
TU-14	Increase the proportion of smoke-free homes
TU-17	Increase the Federal and State tax on tobacco products

From U.S. Department of Health and Human Services (USDHHS). (2016). *Healthy People 2020: Tobacco use*. Retrieved from http://www.healthypeople.gov/2020/topicsobjectives2020/objectiveslist.aspx?topicId=40

- Public or **social stigma** is a phenomenon of large social groups endorsing stereotypes about and acting against a group that is stigmatized, such as persons with mental disorders (Corrigan, Kerr, & Knudsen, 2005).
- **Structural stigma** refers to institutional rules, policies, and procedures that restrict rights or opportunities for members of stigmatized groups (Corrigan et al., 2005; Corrigan, Roe, & Tsang, 2011).

A systematic review found limited evidence for empirically evaluated interventions for substance use–related stigma (Livingston, Milne, Fang, & Amari, 2012). Despite the limited evidence to reduce stigma, community health nurses can help mitigate stigma by leading primary prevention strategies such as educational interventions enhanced by facilitated interactions between the public and persons who live with stigmatized health conditions. Programs that focus on educating nurses and other health care providers about mental and substance use disorders are also needed, given the limited content in formal curricula. For example, a survey study of nursing schools identified a mean of 11.3 hours of alcohol-related content; a gap signifying that nurses may not have the knowledge and competencies to care for this population

(Savage, Dyehouse, & Marcus, 2014). Teaching providers and the public about the neurobiological basis of these disorders may help to dispel attitudes toward and beliefs about persons with these disorders (Finnell & Nowzari, 2013). The terminology used relative to these stigmatizing health conditions also matters. The language that is used should respect the worth and dignity of all persons, that is, people-first language (Broyles et al., 2014). Language frames what the individual thinks and how they can be affected (i.e., self-stigma) and what the public thinks and promotes (i.e., social stigma) and informs the rules, policies, and procedures of institutions (i.e., structural stigma). Community health nurses can model the use of people-first language, such as the person with depression or the person who is at risk because of alcohol use.

INCIDENCE AND PREVALENCE OF MENTAL DISORDERS, SUBSTANCE USE, AND SUBSTANCE USE DISORDERS

Mental and substance use disorders are a worldwide problem. The World Health Organization measures burden of disease using the disability-adjusted life years (DALYs). This metric combines years of life lost (YLLs) because of premature mortality and YLLs because of time lived in states of less than full health. Findings from the most recent Global Burden of Disease Study were released in 2012. Mental and substance disorders were the fifth leading causes of disease burden in 2010 (Whiteford et al., 2013).

Suicide, defined as deaths caused by intentional, self-inflicted poisoning or injury, was the 13th leading cause of YLLs worldwide in 2010 (Lozano et al., 2012; Wang et al., 2012). When suicide is taken into account as a risk factor, mental and substance use disorders were responsible for two thirds of the suicide burden in 2010, elevating them to the third leading disease category of global burden in 2010. In developed countries, suicides are the largest source of intentional injury burden (Ferrari et al., 2014; World Health Organization [WHO], 2014). According to the CDC (2015), suicide was the 10th leading cause of death for all ages in 2013. Males take their lives at nearly four times the rate of females, with firearms being the most commonly used method among males (56.9%). Females are more likely than males to have suicidal thoughts and the most common method for suicide for females is poisoning. Among U.S. students in grades 9 to 12, 17.0% seriously considered attempting suicide in the previous 12 months, 13.6% made a plan, 8% attempted suicide, and 2.7% made an attempt that required medical attention (CDC, 2015).

Three large surveys, supported by the Department of Health and Human Services, provide national prevalence estimates of diagnosable mental illness. These surveys include the National Comorbidity Survey Replication (NCR-R), the National Comorbidity Survey Replication Adolescent Supplement (NCS-A), and the National Survey on Drug Use and Health (NSDUH). The NSDUH is a primary source of information on the use of illicit drugs, alcohol, and tobacco among U.S. citizens aged 12 years or older. Prevalence data for mental illness in the United States varies depending on the survey and methodology used. A 2015 report by Bagalman and Napili (2015) summarizes prevalence data from the three different surveys. For the NCR-R survey administered in 2001 to 2003, estimates of mental illness among adults were reported to be 26.2% and 32.4%, and when substance use disorders were excluded, the 12-month prevalence of mental illness was 24.8% among adults. The 12-month prevalence of SMI was estimated to be 5.8%. Using NCS-A data gathered from 2001 to 2004, the 12-month prevalence of mental illness among adolescents was 40.3% with SMI estimated to be 8.0% among this age group. Based on the NSDUH survey, the estimated 12-month prevalence of mental illness, excluding substance use disorders, was 18.5% among adults aged 18 or older with SMI estimated to be 4.2% among adults. Estimates of mental illness for adolescents aged 12 to 17 are not reported from the NSDUH survey (Han, Hedden, Lipari, Copello, & Kroutil, 2015). Regardless of the statistical caveats, a large proportion of the population is impacted.

Depression, bipolar disorder, schizophrenia, panic disorder, alcohol, and drug use were among the top 20 leading causes of disability according to the most recent study by the World Health Organization. Depression was also the one of the leading cause of DALYs, with the burden of depression 50% higher for females than males. Among women 15 to 44 years, depression is the leading cause of disease burden in both high-income and low- and middle-income countries. Compared with males, females were also noted to have a higher burden from anxiety disorders (WHO, 2008).

In 2013, about 24.6 million Americans surveyed with the NSDUH had used an illicit drug during the past month. This is about 9.4% of the population aged 12 years or older, a rate slightly higher than 8.9% reported in 2010. Across age groups, illicit drug use decreased slightly among youths aged 12 to 17 from the previous surveys (9.6% to 11.6% in 2002 and 2007) to 8.8% in 2013. Among adults aged 50 to 64, illicit drug use increased from 2.7% in 2002 to 6% in 2013. Results for illicit drug use among other aged groups (18 to 25 and adults aged 26 or older) in 2 to 13 were similar to rates in previous years (SAMHSA, 2014).

Among the illicit drugs, marijuana was the most commonly used (80.6% of those currently using illicit drugs) in 2013, with an increase from 5.1 million in 2005 to 2007 to 8.1 million persons in 2013 (SAMHSA, 2014). Cocaine use estimates of 1.5 million in 2013 were similar to those in 2012 (1.7 million) and 2009 (1.4 million). Heroin use in 2013 (681,000) was similar to the number in 2012 (669,000) and 2009 (582,000). Concerning, however, is that heroin use, even when it is not sustained, has been shown to predict a 3- to 4-fold excess risk of dying prematurely (Lopez-Quintero et al., 2015).

Methamphetamine use in the early 1990s was primarily a problem in the Western United States; however, the use has spread across the United States. In 2014, almost 569,000 people in the United States ages 12 and up reported using methamphetamines in the past month (Center for Behavioral Health Statistics and Quality, 2015). The most recent financial report from the RAND Corporation noted that methamphetamine abuse cost the nation approximately $23.4 to $48.3 billion in 2005 (Nicosia, Pacula, Kilmer, Lundberg, & Chiesa, 2009). Injuries, as a result of the illegal manufacture of methamphetamine, are also a major concern because its production can cause fires, explosions, injuries, and environmental contamination. A recent study examined injuries from methamphetamine-related chemical incidents in five states. A total of 1,325 meth-related chemical incidents were reported in the five states from 2001 to 2012 with 16% of injuries occurring in children. The percentage of injured persons who went to a hospital increased over time, from 75% (2001 to 2004), to 86% (2005 to 2007), to 90% (2008 to 2012) (Melnikova, Orr, Wu, & Christensen, 2015).

The rise in the nonmedical use of prescription opioids is also of concern. In the 2013 NSDUH survey, the percentage of persons aged 12 or older who used prescription drugs nonmedically in the past month was 2.5%, similar to the percentages in 2012 (2.7%) and 2010 (2.4%). However, among this age group who used pain relievers nonmedically in the past 12 months, 53% reported that they obtained the drug from a friend or relative for free and 10.6% brought the drug from a friend or relative. Other means of obtaining the prescription drug was from one physician (21.2%), from a drug dealer or stranger (4.6%), or about 0.1% purchased from the Internet (SAMHSA, 2014).

In the 2013 NSDUH Survey, more than half (52.2%) of Americans aged 12 or older reported current alcohol use, similar to the rate in 2012 (52.1%). Alcohol use among those aged 12 to 17 was 11.6% in 2013. This underage population reported obtaining alcohol by purchasing it (7.8%) or giving money to someone else to purchase it (20.5%). Among this age group who did not pay for alcohol, 36.6% got it from an unrelated person aged 21 or older; 24.5% from a parent, guardian, or other adult family member; and 16.4% from another person younger than 21 years old (SAMHSA, 2014). The Centers for Disease Control and Prevention (CDC, 2014b) reports that about 2 in 3 high school students who drink do so to the point of intoxication, that is, they binge drink (defined as having five or more drinks in a row), typically on multiple occasions. The NSDUH Survey defined binge use as having five or more drinks on the same occasion on at least 1 day in the 30 days prior to the survey (SAMHSA, 2014). From the NSDUH data, nearly one quarter (22.9%) of persons aged 12 or older reported binge alcohol use in 2013, with youth binge rates of 6.2%, lower than those in 2012 (12.9%). A growing concern is alcohol use among the older adult population with alcohol accounting for more than 21,000 deaths among adults 65 or older each year in the United States, and from the NSDUH Survey, 41.7% of people aged 65 and older reported current alcohol use with 9.1% reporting binge use (CDC, 2013; SAMHSA, 2014).

Social inequalities are associated with increased risk of many common mental disorders. A review of 115 studies conducted in low- and middle-income countries sought to explain the relationship between poverty and common mental disorders. In community-based studies, over 70% reported positive associations between a variety of poverty measures and common mental disorders, and 6% reported negative associations (Lund et al., 2010). Disparities are also evident in access to and receipt of mental health care. Using data from the National Health Interview Survey 2010 to 2013, researchers compared non-Hispanic Black and Hispanic men with non-Hispanic White men on mental health symptoms and mental health treatment utilization. Racial and ethnic differences were observed only for men aged 18 to 44 with non-Hispanic Black and Hispanic men nearly 30% less likely than non-Hispanic White men to have daily feeling of anxiety or depression. Among men aged 18 to 44 who had anxiety or depression, non-Hispanic Black and Hispanic men (26.4%) were less likely than non-Hispanic White men (45.4%) to have used mental health treatment. The disparity in treatment utilization was associated with lack of health insurance coverage (Blumberg, Clarke, & Blackwell, 2015).

There is a 13- to 30-year reduction in life expectancy for persons with SMI; the vast majority of deaths are due to physical illness. A review of the literature examined the association between physical illnesses and schizophrenia, bipolar disorder, and major depressive disorder. Researchers identified many physical disorders (e.g., obesity, diabetes, cardiovascular disease, viral diseases, respiratory tract diseases, metabolic syndrome, cancer, musculoskeletal diseases, urological, male/female genital diseases and pregnancy complications, stomatognathic diseases) that are more prevalent in individuals with SMI. The authors note that modifiable lifestyle factors and psychotropic medication side effects, as well as poor access to and quality of received health care contribute to the morbidity and mortality for persons with SMI (Hert et al., 2011).

Data from the 2007 National Health Interview Survey was used to compare sociodemographic and health characteristics, health care utilization, and participation in government assistance programs among adults with and without SMI. Over 2% of adults reported having a diagnosis of an SMI. Compared with their counterparts, those with SMI were younger, less educated, more likely to be poor and to live alone, and less likely to work. Further, 36% of adults with SMI reported having spent at least 24 hours either homeless or incarcerated during their lifetime, in contrast to 5% of other adults reporting that experience (Pratt, 2012). The homeless population with SMI faces many challenges. A descriptive study of mostly males in a state-operated mental health transitional shelter identified that 60.8% had a prior episode of homelessness and half had a history of incarceration. More than one third (36.5%) had a history of physical, sexual, or verbal/emotional abuse, and 23.0% had experienced adverse events in childhood. Co-occurrence of substance use disorders, mental disorders, and chronic medical illness was common; 36.5% had one or more diagnosis from each category. High rates of substance use disorders (44.6%) and chronic medical illnesses (82.4%) were noted (Viron, Bello, Freudenreich, & Shtasel, 2014).

Age influences the patterns of mental disorders in the community. Using data from the NCS-A survey of 10,123 adolescents aged 13 to 18 years in the United States, researchers found that anxiety disorders were the most common condition (31.9%), followed by behavior disorders (19.1%), mood disorders (14.3%), and substance use disorders (11.4%). The median age of onset was earliest for anxiety (6 years), followed by behavior disorders (11 years), mood disorders (13 years), and substance use disorders (15 years). Attention deficit/hyperactivity disorder (ADHD) is thought to be more common in boys than girls with estimated ratios ranging between 2:1 and 9:1 (Merikangas et al., 2010; Rucklidge, 2010). Prevalence estimates of ADHD vary depending on the person reporting symptoms for diagnostic evaluation, what instrument is used, and when more than one informant is used, as well as how the information is combined. A systematic review and meta-analysis was conducted using 175 unique studies including a majority conducted within school populations (74%) and 10% using a whole population approach. The overall pooled prevalence of ADHD was 7.2% (Thomas, Sanders, Doust, Beller, & Glasziou, 2015). ADHD can persist into adulthood, though is often underdiagnosed and untreated. ADHD prevalence in the adult population is 2.5% to 5% worldwide. In the United States, the most recent large-scale prevalence study noted 4.4% of adults have ADHD; however, other researchers note that adult ADHD is often underdiagnosed (Fayyad et al., 2007; Ginsberg, Quintero, Anand, Casillas, & Upadhyaya, 2014; Kessler et al., 2006; Simon, Czobor, Bálint, Mészáros, & Bitter, 2009).

Autism spectrum disorder (ASD) is a neurodevelopmental disorder that typically manifests early in development, often before the child enters grade school. ASD is characterized by persistent deficits in social communication and social interaction (American Psychiatric Association [APA], 2013). In 2014, the CDC reported that 1 in 68 children have been diagnosed with ASD and that it is almost five times more common among boys (1 in 42) than among girls (1 in 189). Considered to be chronic and permanent in conditions, data from the 2011 Survey of Pathways to Diagnosis and Services were used to better understand the path to diagnosis for children with ASD. The study by Blumberg et al. (2015) suggests that some children may be diagnosed with ASD though their symptoms (e.g., developmental delays, problems with attentional flexibility) may not meet diagnostic criteria. There may be variability in the quality of screening and evaluation leading to imprecise diagnosing (CDC, 2014a; Fenikile, Ellerbeck, Filippi, & Daley, 2014). Thus, rates of ASD need to be viewed with caution.

Asperger's syndrome has been absorbed into the diagnosis of ASD in the current fifth edition of the *Diagnostic and Statistical Manual* (APA, 2013). This disorder is marked by social interaction and verbal difficulties as well as difficulties with nonverbal communication. The prevalence of ASD is not well established, and while no studies have yet been conducted to determine the incidence of Asperger's syndrome in adult populations, studies of children with the disorder suggest that their problems with socialization and communication continue into adulthood (National Institute of Neurological Disorders and Stroke, 2015).

For American adults, according to the National Institute of Mental Health, the 12-month prevalence rate of anxiety is 18.1% of the U.S. adult population with women being 60% more likely than men to experience an anxiety disorder over their lifetime. On average, the lifetime prevalence rate for anxiety in people ages 18 to 59 years is 32%. The 12-month prevalence rate of mood disorders is 9.5% of the U.S. adult population with women 50% more likely than men to experience a mood disorder over their lifetime. On average, the lifetime prevalence rate for mood disorders for persons ages 18 to 59 years is about 23%. The 12-month prevalence for schizophrenia, a chronic, severe, and disabling mental disorder, is 1.1% of the U.S. adult population, with men and women affected equally (NIMH, n.d.).

Older adults tend to have lower rates of frequent mental distress compared with other age groups. According to the National Institute of Mental Health, adults 60 years or older have a 15.3% lifetime prevalence rate for an anxiety disorder and an 11.9% lifetime prevalence rate for a mood disorder (NIMH, n.d.). The Federal Interagency Forum on Aging-Related Statistics (2012) reported that men had higher suicide rates than women, with the largest difference occurring at age 85 and above (43 deaths per 100,000 for men compared with 3 per 100,000 for women). From the same report, non-Hispanic White men over age 85 had the highest rate of suicide overall at 47 deaths per 100,000. National prevalence estimates of Alzheimer's disease and other age-related cognitive impairment in older adults are lacking, likely because of the use of various measures or instruments to screen and assess for these disorders/conditions, but also because of differences in definitions and criteria used.

Mental and substance use disorders affect families, for whom support is available and accessible. Founded in 1979, the National Alliance on Mental Illness (NAMI) serves to provide advocacy, education, and support for persons affected by mental disorders. A survey conducted by NAMI assessed the experiences of 2,720 people living with mental disorders and their families who had private health insurances. The survey results identified a number of barriers that people with mental and substance use disorders encounter in their efforts to obtain quality care, including finding providers, accessing prescription medications, high out-of-pocket costs, and lack of access to information needed for informed decision making related to health plans (NAMI, 2015). Additional family-focused programs include classics such as:

- Community Reinforcement and Family Training (CRAFT), designed for families who were trying to encourage their family member to go into treatment. A 12-session structured program is available (Smith & Meyers, 2007), as is a CRAFT self-help book (Meyers & Wolfe, 2004).
- Free and easily accessible mutual support groups provide support for friend and families of persons with alcohol problems such as Al-Anon (www.al-anon.org), based on the twelve-step model, and Learn to Cope, Inc., a peer-led support network that offers support, education, recourses, and hope for families affected by mental and substance use disorders (www.learn2cope.org).
- Family psychoeducation is a means to provide information about mental disorders and learn problem-solving, communication, and coping skills. The Substance Abuse and Mental Health Services Administration (SAMHSA) provides an evidence-based family psychoeducation kit that is accessible at http://store.samhsa.gov/product/Family-Psychoeducation-Evidence-Based-Practices-EBP-KIT/SMA09-4423.

Cost of Mental and Substance Use Disorders

In addition to the human costs of mental and substance use disorders, the economic costs are also substantial. In describing the burden of mental, neurological, and substance use disorders, researchers point out that the total economic output lost to these disorders globally was about $8.5 trillion; if unabated, the cost will double by 2030. Further, the economic costs attributable to alcohol use and alcohol use disorders alone are about 1.3% to 3.3% of the gross domestic product of high- and middle-income countries (Patel et al., 2015). Despite evidence-based treatments focusing on prevention and early intervention, inpatient treatment accounts for a high proportion of the costs. In 2012, for example, 8.6 million inpatient stays in the United States involved at least one mental disorder or substance use disorder diagnosis, accounting for 32.3% of inpatient stays. Further, among stays with one of these disorders, 13.9% lacked insurance; this is more than two times greater than that among the 6% of stays without those diagnoses (Heslin, Elixhauser, & Steiner, 2015).

The Patient Protection and Affordable Care Act (PPACA) and the MHPAEA of 2008 are two sentinel pieces of legislation helping to reform health care. In analyzing data from a national survey of commercial health plans after the implementation of the MHPAEA, Horgan et al. (2015) concluded that the law had the intended effect of eliminating the quantitative limitations that applied only to behavioral health care without eliminating behavioral health coverage. This study provides support that the main goals of MHPAEA are being realized for increasing access to behavioral health services and ensuring equity with general medical services. Further promise lies with the implementation of integrated medical and behavioral health care. Melek, Norris, and Paulus (2014) suggest that a savings of $40 to $50 billion dollars annually could be realized with such integration, surpassing what is currently spent on mental health care in the United States.

Promotion, Prevention, Treatment, and Recovery for Mental and Substance Use Disorders

The Institute of Medicine (IOM) commissioned an investigation on mental health interventions that resulted in the development of the IOM "protractor" depicting a continuum of care as prevention, treatment, and recovery (Mrazek & Haggerty, 1994). The model, shown in Figure 27–1, explicitly includes promotion as a key component. This model provides a systematic framework for community health nurses to view the nature and degree of risk faced by persons with behavioral health issues as diagnosable disorders. Promotion strategies reinforce the entire continuum of behavioral health services. Promotion is aimed at supporting behavioral health and assisting individuals in withstanding challenges they encounter across the continuum.

Prevention strategies include three distinctions: universal, selective, and indicated as different levels of risk characterized by Gordon (1983) in a classic article on prevention. *Universal prevention* includes those strategies delivered to broad populations wherein the benefits outweigh the costs and risks for everyone. Examples of

this include public health campaigns related to suicide prevention, legislation related to impaired driving, and minimum age for purchase of alcohol.

Selective strategies are indicated when a person's risk of becoming ill is elevated. Through detection of risk, vulnerable subgroups of individuals can be identified. As a result, programs and practices can be provided to reduce the risk. An example of a selective strategy would be a program to address binge alcohol consumption among college students. Selective strategies for depression among adolescents include school-based, cognitive–behavioral, and family-based intervention programs (Gladstone, Beardslee, & O'Connor, 2011).

Indicated strategies address specific risk conditions, focusing efforts on individual risk factors or behaviors that put individuals at high risk for developing a behavioral disorder. Examples of indicated strategies include personalized normative feedback, an approach for reducing alcohol consumption among college students and the use of acceptance and commitment therapy in reducing suicidal ideation and depression among veterans (Dotson, Dunn, & Bowers, 2015; Walser et al., 2015).

Case identification entails the ability to correctly identify those individuals who have a behavioral disorder with minimal false positives. Thus, it is important to have measures with a high degree of sensitivity and specificity. Relevant optimal measures are presented later in this chapter. Yet, case identification will have limited benefit if there are no effective treatments in place.

Greater understanding of the mechanisms that underlie behavioral disorders (e.g., genetics, biological, behavioral, environmental) has resulted in established evidence-based treatments. A wide variety of pharmacological, psychotherapeutic, and social interventions have been established. For example:

- Antipsychotic, antidepressant, anxiolytic, and mood stabilizer medications are used to treat various mental disorders (Stahl, 2013).
- Medications used for alcohol use include those that produced adverse effects when alcohol is consumed (e.g., disulfiram) and those that modify the neurotransmitter systems that mediate alcohol reinforcement (e.g., naltrexone, acamprosate) (Myrick, Kranzler, Ciraulo, Saxon, & Jaffe, 2014).
- The principle opioid medications are those that act as μ-opioid receptor antagonists (e.g., naloxone and naltrexone), full agonist (e.g., methadone), partial agonist (e.g., buprenorphine), and the nonopioid α_2 adrenergic agonists (e.g., clonidine) (Stein & Kosten, 2014).
- Pharmacologic interventions for tobacco dependence include nicotine replacement therapy (e.g., gum, lozenge, nasal spray, nasal inhaler, patch), reuptake inhibitor of both norepinephrine and dopamine (i.e., bupropion), and partial nicotine agonist/antagonist (i.e., varenicline) (Hurt, Ebbert, Hays, & McFadden, 2014).

There are a number of evidence-based psychotherapies with procedures defined in manuals and efficacy established as single treatment or in combination with pharmacotherapy (Weissman, 2015). Although a wide variety of these interventions have a major role in the

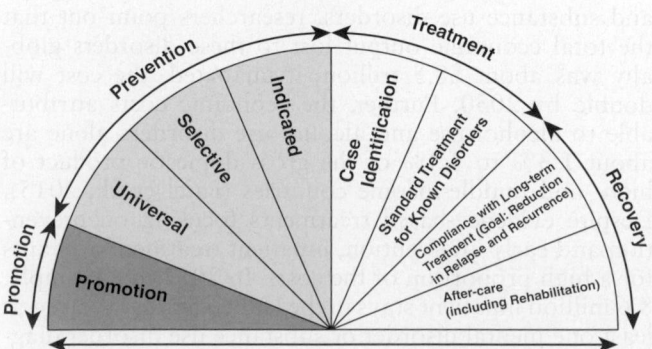

FIGURE 27–1   Behavioral health continuum of care model. (From Substance Abuse and Mental Health Services Administration (SAMHSA). (2015). *Prevention of substance abuse and mental illness*. Retrieved from http://www.samhsa. gov/prevention.)

treatment of mental and substance use disorders, a report from the IOM states that they are not used routinely in clinical practice or taught in educational programs preparing health professionals to deliver them. Further, no standard system is in place to ensure that the psychosocial interventions delivered to patients/consumers are effective. Despite the availability of treatments and efforts to increase access to treatment though the PPACA, only 39% of the 45.9 million adults with mental health disorders used mental health services in 2010 (England, Butler, & Gonzalez, 2015). In 2014, among the 4.1 million people in the United States aged 12 or older that received substance use treatment in the past year, the majority (2.2 million) reported receiving treatment though self-help groups. Outpatient treatment was the next highest modality for treatment, either in a rehabilitation facility (1.7 million) or mental health center (1.2 million). About 1.1 million received inpatient treatment in a rehabilitation or hospital setting (Han, Hedden, Lipari, Copello, & Kroutil, 2015).

In 2014, about 22.5 million people in the United States aged 12 or older needed substance use treatment, but only 11.6% received treatment at a specialty substance use treatment facility. Thus, the needs of 88.4% of this subgroup of the U.S. population, who warrant indicated strategies, were not addressed. Reasons for not receiving substance use treatment included not ready to stop using, no health coverage and could not afford, and not knowing where to go for treatment (Han et al., 2015). Community health nurses can have a significant role in removing such barriers to treatment.

Recovery is the final component of the Behavioral Health Continuum of Care Model. In their systematic review on personal recovery, Leamy, Bird, Le Boutillier, Williams, and Slade (2011) summarize personal recovery with the acronym CHIME (connectedness, hope, optimism about the future, identify, meaning in life, and empowerment). These aspects are aligned with SAMHSAs' guiding principles of recovery that focus on promoting a high-quality and satisfying life in the community for all people. Community health nurses can engage in partnership with individuals in supporting and promoting recovery goals, monitoring progress toward and recognizing movement away from goals, tailoring support, and supporting transitions throughout the recovery process. Community health nurses can engage in recovery movements, calling attention in order to educate the public on how stigma, including associated stigma, impedes help seeking and treatment participation (Ricci & Dixon, 2015; Yarborough, Yarborough, Janoff, & Green, 2015).

Substance Use and the Community Health Nurse

A survey of schools of nursing identified that about 11 hours of alcohol-related content was included in baccalaureate nursing curricula. Further, <10% required student competency in strategies to detect risk that would prompt the need for further indicated actions, such as brief interventions (BIs) (Savage et al., 2014). This gap in the curricula of BSN programs carries serious implications, in that nurses may not have the requisite understanding of alcohol and other drugs. Reductions in substance use (including tobacco) are 2 of the 44 focus areas in *Healthy People 2020*. See Table 27–2 for a list of substance abuse objectives. The goal is to "reduce substance abuse to protect the health, safety, and quality of life for all, especially children" (USDHHS, 2016a, para. 1). Among the 21 objectives listed are reducing the consequences of use, reducing actual use, reducing risk factors associated with harmful use, increasing access to treatment, and supporting policy initiatives.

The community health nurse plays a vital role in developing successful prevention and treatment programs related to substance use in a community. These prevention programs should be aligned with the Behavioral Health Continuum of Care Model previously discussed. The community health nurse focuses on the target population. For instance, *Monitoring the Future* is a yearly survey of drug and alcohol use among 8th, 9th, and 12th graders. Existing data such as these help determine the magnitude of the problem. Given a defined target geographic area, local health departments may have county-specific prevalence rates. The *Healthy People 2020* objectives related to substance use (Table 27–2) and tobacco use (Table 27–3) provide target benchmarks that can be used by the community health nurse in planning and developing prevention programs.

Whether providing individual-, community-, or policy-level interventions for substance use, the community health nurse must begin with a basic understanding of alcohol and other drugs; signs of use, intoxication, and withdrawal; and associated health risks. This understanding can help the community health nurse select an effective strategy (i.e., universal, indicated, targeted) that meets the particular needs of the population, subgroup, or individual. Table 27–4 lists some of the most commonly used substances.

Detecting Risk and Intervening

This section discusses the use of **screening** in behavioral health as a means for identification of mental health issues and substance use and providing early intervention. The U.S. Preventive Services Task Force, for over a decade, has recommended screening and *brief intervention* to reduce alcohol use by adults (USPSTF, 2015; Whitlock, Polen, Green, Orleans, & Klein, 2004). Given recommendations and mandates from multiple federal agencies and large health care organizations, nurses have been called upon to actively engage in integrating this health initiative into practice (American Public Health Association [APHA], 2008; Finnell et al., 2014). Given their major roles as clinician, educator, advocate, manager, collaborator, leader, and researcher, community health nurses can be instrumental in helping to reduce the harms associated with alcohol and other drug use through the use of the strategies described below. The section that follows discusses how to screen for risk for mental disorders, alcohol, drug, and tobacco use and, based on the evidence, what interventions are recommended based on the identified risk.

Screening is the presumptive identification of an unrecognized disease or defect by the application of tests, examinations, or other procedures that can be applied rapidly. Table 27–5 lists established measures for screening

(*Text continues on page 981*)

Table 27–4 Substances Commonly Used

Substance	Facts	Signs of Use	Possible Health Risks
Alcohol			
Standard drink contains about 14 g of pure alcohol (about 0.6 fluid ounces or 1.2 tablespoons)	A small, water-soluble molecule that is rapidly absorbed into the bloodstream from the stomach, small intestine, and colon. Metabolized primarily by enzymatic pathways; small amounts are excreted through the lungs as vapor.	Acutely acts as central nervous system depressant. When blood levels are rising, a period a disinhibition often occurs and signs of behavioral arousal are common (e.g., relief of anxiety, increased talkativeness, feelings of confidence and euphoria, enhanced assertiveness). As blood levels increase, there are impairments in judgment and reaction time, increased emotional outbursts, and ataxia. At higher blood levels, alcohol acts as a sedative and hypnotic, but quality of sleep is often reduced after alcohol intake.	A carcinogen associated with 44% of some cancers. A teratogen contributing to increased risk of fetal alcohol spectrum disorders, which include physical, behavioral, and learning disabilities. Negative effects on many body systems (e.g., central nervous system, cardiovascular, immune, gastrointestinal, hepatic, hematopoietic). In patients with sleep apnea, alcohol increases the frequency and severity of apneic episodes and the resulting hypoxia.
Cannabis			
Hashish (hash, herb, kif) Hashish oil (hash oil, honey) Marijuana (grass, weed, dope, ganja, reefer, pot, Acapulco gold, Thai sticks)	Synthesized from the hemp plant, *Cannabis sativa*. Tetrahydrocannabinol (THC) is the major psychoactive ingredient in cannabis. Binds to cannabinoid receptors in the brain. Inhalation produces the most rapid onset. Marijuana and hash may also be taken orally via food products with slower onset of effect and slower offset of action. Tolerance and physical dependence can develop. Sinsemilla is a highly potent form of marijuana.	Relaxation and euphoria Altered perceptions of time and space Hallucinations or anxiety attacks with use of highly potent cannabis (sinsemilla)	Major effects on respiratory system. Complex effects on immune system, with host resistance impaired by THC administration. Increases heart rate, produces orthostatic hypotension, may worsen congestive health failure, and increases hypertension Deleterious effects in patients with liver disease Marijuana can disrupt the female reproductive system and induce galactorrhea. In male animals (effects in human are unclear), disrupts reproductive function, reducing the secretion of testosterone and sperm production, motility, and viability
Nonalcohol Sedative Hypnotics			
Barbiturates (downers, barbs) Benzodiazepines (Valium, Librium, tranquilizers) Chloral hydrate (knockout, Mickey Finn) Glutethimide (Doriden) Methaqualone (Quaalude, Ludes) Other depressants (Equanil, Miltown, Noludar, Placidyl, Valmid)	Depressants act on major neurotransmitter systems in the brain. Benzodiazepines exert clinical effects trough the Gamma-aminobutyric acid (GABA) receptor, leading to the sedative, anticonvulsant, hypnotic, and amnestic effects of the drug. Barbiturates and sedative–hypnotic drugs have similar action, but different binding affinities to the GABA receptors.	Produce effects on a continuum from sedation to obtundation. Barbiturates have a greater risk for respiratory depression than do benzodiazepines. High doses of benzodiazepines—ataxia and impaired gag reflex	Mild withdrawal: anxiety, headache, insomnia, dysphoria, tremor, muscle twitching Severe withdrawal: autonomic dysfunction, nausea, vomiting, depersonalization, derealization, delirium, hallucinations, illusions, agitation, grand mal seizures

	Description	Effects
Hallucinogens Lysergic acid diethylamide (LSD) Phencyclidine (PCP, angel dust) Mescaline and peyote (Mesc, buttons, cactus) Psilocybin (mushrooms) Amphetamine variants (MDMA/Ecstasy, MDA/love drug, TMA, DOM, DOB, PMA, STP, 2.5-DMA) PCP analogues (PCE, PCPy, TCP) Other hallucinogens (bufotenine, ibogaine, DMT, DET)	Hallucinogens are psychedelic, mind-altering drugs that affect a person's perception, feelings, thinking, self-awareness, and emotions. A "bad trip" may result in the user's experiencing panic, confusion, paranoia, anxiety, unpleasant sensory images, feelings of helplessness, and loss of control. A "flash back" is a reoccurrence of the original drug experience without taking the drug again.	Dilated pupils, increased body temperature, heart rate, and blood pressure; sweating; loss of appetite; sleeplessness; dry mouth; tremors; hallucinations; disorientation; confusion; paranoia; violence; euphoria; anxiety; and panic Agitation; extreme hyperactivity; psychosis; convulsions; mental or emotional problems; death
Inhalants Amyl nitrate (poppers, snappers) Butyl nitrate (rush, bolt, bullet) Chlorohydrocarbons (aerosol sprays, cleaning fluids) Hydrocarbons (solvents, airplane glue, gasoline, paint thinner) Nitrous oxide (laughing gas, whippets)	Breathable chemicals that can be self-administered as gases or vapors. Products can be gases, liquids, aerosols, or, in some cases, solids. Toxicologic effects of the compounds differ. Subdivisions of abused inhalants include (1) volatile alkyl nitrates, (2) nitrous oxide, and (3) solvents, fuels, and anesthetics. Once inhaled, solvents rapidly enter the brain and distribute to lipid-containing membranes within the CNS.	A diverse array of acute effects, depend on the produced used. These effects may be euphoria and light-headedness; excitability; loss of appetite; forgetfulness; weight loss; sneezing; coughing; nausea and vomiting; lack of coordination; bad breath; red eyes; sores on nose and mouth; delayed reflexes; decreased blood pressure; flushing (skin appears to be reddish); headache; dizziness; and violence. CNS depression, respiratory problems, or suffocation, which may lead to death Neurotoxicity Irritation of the eyes, nose, and mouth; localized skin rash Inflammation of the lungs Effects on major organ systems (i.e., liver, kidney) Use during pregnancy—decreased fertility, spontaneous abortions, adverse effects on infant (low birth weight, facial and other physical abnormalities, microcephaly, delayed neurologic and physical maturation), fetal solvent syndrome
Opioids Heroin (H, harry, junk, brown sugar, smack) Morphine and synthetic compounds (oxycodone, codeine, meperidine, pentazocine, hydromorphone, hydrocodone, methadone, levo-alpha-acetyl, buprenorphine)	Narcotics are composed of opiates and synthetic drugs. Opioids refer to all compounds, natural and synthetic, functionally related to opium derived from poppies and endogenous opioid neuropeptides chemically developed to produce the effects of opiates. Act primarily on the brain's mu opioid receptor, which mediates both analgesic and rewarding effects of opioid compounds as well as their effects on many systems in the body (e.g., hypothalamic–pituitary–adrenal axis, immune, gastrointestinal, and pulmonary).	Acute opioid overdone: stupor or coma, respiratory depression, pinpoint pupils Cough, nausea, vomiting Euphoria; restlessness and lack of motivation; drowsiness; lethargy; decreased pulse rate; constricted pupils; flushing (skin appears to be reddish); constipation; nausea and vomiting; needle marks on extremities; skin abscess at injection sites; shallow breathing; watery eyes; and itching CNS: depression of the mental status, depression of respiratory activity, suppressed gag reflex, generalize seizures Pulmonary: frothy, pink bronchial secretions, cyanosis, rales, bronchospasm Cardiovascular: orthostatic hypotension, mild tachycardia, with IV use—bacterial endocarditis, venous thrombosis, septic pulmonary emboli, emboli of cornstarch and talc (additives) to the retina, lungs, kidney, and liver, with high doses of methadone—prolongation of QT interval and torsades de pointes Gastrointestinal: nausea, vomiting, slowing of GI motility (constipation and fecal impaction)

(continued)

Table 27-4 Substances Commonly Used (Continued)

Substance	Facts	Signs of Use	Possible Health Risks
			Renal: rhabdomyolysis, glomerulonephritis. Musculoskeletal: muscle rigidity of chest and abdominal wall, with IV use—osteomyelitis, septic arthritis, polymyositis, fibrous myopathy. Infectious diseases: injection—transmission of IVE, hepatitis B, hepatitis C, cellulitis, skin and neck abscesses, endocarditis, botulism. Fetal and neonatal: premature births; stillbirth, and acute infections among newborns, neonatal abstinence syndrome

Steroids

Substance	Facts	Signs of Use	Possible Health Risks
Anabolic–androgenic (roids, juice, D-ball)	Compounds that possess anabolic or tissue-building effects. The acceleration of physical development is what makes steroids appealing to athletes and young adults. Anabolic–androgenic steroids are chemically related to the male sex hormone testosterone. Steroids are injected directly into the muscle or taken orally.	Sudden increase in muscle and weight; increase in aggression and combativeness; violence ("roid rage"); hallucinations; jaundice; purple or red spots on body, inside mouth, or nose; swelling of feet or lower legs (edema); tremors; and bad breath. For women: breast reduction, enlarged clitoris, facial hair and baldness, deepened voice. For men: enlarged nipples and breasts, testicle reduction, enlarged prostate, baldness	Acne; high blood pressure; liver and kidney damage; heart disease; increased risk of injury to ligaments and tendons; bowel and urinary problems; gallstones and kidney stones; liver cancer. For men: impotence and sterility. For women: menstrual problems. For users who share or use unsterile needles to inject steroids: hepatitis, tetanus, AIDS

Cocaine, Amphetamines, and Other Stimulants

Substance	Facts	Signs of Use	Possible Health Risks
Amphetamines (uppers, pep pills); Cocaine (coke, flake, snow); Crack (rock); Ephedra; Khat; Methamphetamines (ice, crank, crystal); Methylphenidate (Ritalin); Phenmetrazine (Preludin, Preludes); Other stimulants (Adipex, Cylert, Didrex, Ionamin, Melfiat, Plegine, Sanorex, Tenuate, Tepanil, Prelu-2)	Stimulants include both naturally occurring plant alkaloids (e.g., cocaine, ephedra, khat) and synthetic compounds (e.g., amphetamines, methylphenidate). Smoked stimulants are rapidly absorbed through the lungs and reach the brain in 6 to 8 s, followed by a rapid decline in effect. IV administration produces brain effect in 4 to 7 min. Intranasal and oral stimulants have slower absorption and onset of effect (30 to 45 min).	Intense pleasurable feeling; increased energy, alertness, and sociability; elation or euphoria; and decreased fatigue, need for sleep, and appetite. Increased pulse rate, blood pressure, and body temperature; insomnia; loss of appetite; sweating; dry mouth and lips; bad breath; disorientation; apathy; hallucinations; irritability; and nervousness	Cardiovascular: increased heart rate, blood pressure, and systemic vascular resistance. Pulmonary: acute and chronic pulmonary toxicity (smoked); cough, shortness of breath, wheezing, chest pain, hemoptysis, exacerbation of asthma. Gastrointestinal: reduced gastric motility and delayed gastric emptying. Endocrine: decreased (acute cocaine use) or increased (chronic cocaine use) plasma prolactin levels

Head and neck: chronic rhinitis, perforated nasal septum and nasal collapse, oropharyngeal ulcers, osteolytic sinusitis (intranasal cocaine use); gingival ulceration and erosion of dental enamel (oral cocaine use); corneal ulcers (smoked cocaine)

Immune: vasculitic syndromes

Sexual function: erectile dysfunction or delayed or inhibited ejaculation (men); irregular menses (women)

Reproductive, fetal, and neonatal: reduced sperm count and motility; prenatal exposure—vaginal bleeding, abruption placenta, placenta previa, premature rupturing of membranes, decreased head circumference, low birth weight, tremulousness, irritability, poor feeding, and autonomic instability

Sources:

Balster, R. L. (2014). The pharmacology of inhalants. In R. Ries, D. Fiellin, S. Miller, & R. Saitz (Eds.), *The ASAM principles of addiction medicine* (5th ed., pp. 267–276). Philadelphia, PA: Wolters Kluwer.

Borg, L., Buonora, M., Butelman, E. R., Ducat, E., Ray, B. M., & Kreek, M. J. (2014). The pharmacology of opioids. In R. Ries, D. Fiellin, S. Miller, & R. Saitz (Eds.), *The ASAM principles of addiction medicine* (5th ed., pp. 135–150). Philadelphia, PA: Wolters Kluwer.

Ciraulo, D. A., & Knapp, C. M. (2014). The pharmacology of nonalcohol sedative hypnotics. In R. Ries, D. Fiellin, S. Miller, & R. Saitz (Eds.), *The ASAM principles of addiction medicine* (5th ed., pp. 117–134). Philadelphia, PA: Wolters Kluwer.

Gorelick, D. A., & Baumann, M. H. (2014). The pharmacology of cocaine, amphetamines, and other stimulants. In R. Ries, D. Fiellin, S. Miller, & R. Saitz (Eds.), *The ASAM principles of addiction medicine* (5th ed., pp. 151–179). Philadelphia, PA: Wolters Kluwer.

Lukas, S. E. (2014). The pharmacology of anabolic-androgenic steroids. In R. Ries, D. Fiellin, S. Miller, & R. Saitz (Eds.), *The ASAM principles of addiction medicine* (5th ed., pp. 277–293). Philadelphia, PA: Wolters Kluwer.

Passie, R., & Halpern, J. H. (2014). The pharmacology of hallucinogens. In R. Ries, D. Fiellin, S. Miller, & R. Saitz (Eds.), *The ASAM principles of addiction medicine* (5th ed., pp. 235–255). Philadelphia, PA: Wolters Kluwer.

Welch, S. P., & Malcolm, R. (2014). The pharmacology of marijuana. In R. Ries, D. Fiellin, S. Miller, & R. Saitz (Eds.), *The ASAM principles of addiction medicine* (5th ed., pp. 217–234). Philadelphia, PA: Wolters Kluwer.

Woodward, J. J. (2014). The pharmacology of alcohol. In R. Ries, D. Fiellin, S. Miller, & R. Saitz (Eds.), *The ASAM principles of addiction medicine* (5th ed., pp. 100–116). Philadelphia, PA: Wolters Kluwer.

Table 27–5 Screening Tools

Measure	Description	Source
Adapted-SAD PERSONS (sex, age, depression or affective disorder, previous attempt, ethanol drug abuse, rational thinking loss, social supports lacking, organized plan, negligent parenting, significant family stressors, suicidal modeling by parents or siblings, school problems)	10-item scale for suicide risk	Juhnke, G. A. (1996). The adapted-SAD persons: A suicide assessment scale designed for use with children. *Elementary School Guidance & Counseling, 30*(4), 252–258.
Alcohol Use Identification Test: 1–3 (U.S.)	3-item scale to identify alcohol consumption that is in excess of recommended guidelines	Babor, T. F., Higgins-Biddle, J. C., Dauser, D., Burleson, J. A., Zarkin, G. A., & Bray, J. (2006). Brief interventions for at-risk drinking: Patient outcomes and cost-effectiveness in managed care organizations. *Alcohol and Alcoholism, 41*(6), 624–631.
AUDIT (U.S.)	10-item scale to identify persons likely to be at risk, those at risk because of excessive alcohol use, those who have already experienced problems related to alcohol use, and those who may have an alcohol use disorder	See above.
Beck Depression Inventory	21-item measures characteristic attitudes and symptoms of depression	Beck, A. T., Ward, C. H., Mendelson, M., Mock, J., & Erbaugh, J. (1961). An inventory for measuring depression. *Archives of General Psychiatry, 4*, 561–571.
Brief Psychiatric Rating Scale (BPRS)	16-item scale screening for schizophrenia or other psychotic disorder	Overall, J. E., & Gorham, D. R. (1962). The brief psychiatric rating scale. *Psychological Reports, 10*(3), 799–812.
Center for Epidemiologic Studies Depression Scale (CES-D) (10 and 20 item versions)	10-item or 20-item screen for current depressive symptomatology related to major or clinical depression in adults and children	Radloff, L. S. (1977). The CES-D scale a self-report depression scale for research in the general population. *Applied Psychological Measurement, 1*(3), 385–401.
Cornell Scale for Depression in Dementia	19-item using information from patient and nursing staff interviews	Alexopoulos, G. S., Abrams, R. C., Young, R. C., & Shamoian, C. A. (1988). Cornell scale for depression in dementia. *Biological Psychiatry, 23*(3), 271–284.
Drug Abuse Screening Test (DAST)	10-item measure to determine the extent of drug use	Skinner, H. A. (1982). The drug abuse screening test. *Addictive Behaviors, 7*(4), 363–371.
Edinburgh Postnatal Depression Scale	10-item measure for coping with life changes of pregnancy and childbirth	Cox, J. L., Holden, J. M., & Sagovsky, R. (1987). Detection of postnatal depression. Development of the 10-item Edinburgh Postnatal Depression Scale. *The British Journal of Psychiatry, 150*(6), 782–786.
Generalized Anxiety Disorder	7-item screening tool for anxiety	Spitzer, R. L., Kroenke, K., Williams, J. B., & Löwe, B. (2006). A brief measure for assessing generalized anxiety disorder: The GAD-7. *Archives of Internal Medicine, 166*(10), 1092–1097.
Geriatric Depression Scale	15-item yes/no screening for depression in older adults	Burke, W. J., Roccaforte, W. H., & Wengel, S. P. (1991). The short form of the Geriatric Depression Scale: A comparison with the 30-item form. *Journal of Geriatric Psychiatry and Neurology, 4*(3), 173–178.
Patient Health Questionnaire-9 (PHQ-9) PHQ-2	9-item screen for depression in adults First 2 items from PHQ-2	Kroencke, K., Spitzer, R., & Williams, J. (2001). The PHQ-9: Validity of a brief depression severity measure. *Journal of General Internal Medicine, 16*(9), 606–613.
Primary Care Posttraumatic Stress Disorder (PC-PTSD)	4-item screen for post-traumatic stress disorder	Hanley, J., & Brasel, K. (2013). Efficiency of a four-item posttraumatic stress disorder screen in trauma patients. *Journal of Trauma and Acute Care Surgery, 75*(4), 722–727.

mental health problems, alcohol, and other drugs. From an apparently well population, screening tests separate persons who potentially have or are at increased risk for a disease from those who probably do not have the disease. A positive screening test result should be followed by a comprehensive assessment and, if indicated, evaluation to determine if a mental or substance-use disorder is present. Treatment should be initiated when a diagnostic determination has been made.

Given the stigma associated with these disorders, it is important to spend time addressing your role and, as with any conversations related to health, seeking permission to engage in the screening process and describing what will be done. The community health nurse needs to be cognizant that his/her beliefs and attitudes toward persons with mental and substance use disorders sets the stage for interactions with and the provision of interventions including recovery support for a person with one or more of these disorders. A government panel examining a tool to measure stigma found about only about one quarter of U.S. adults agreed that people are caring and sympathetic to people with mental illness (Kobau, DiIorio, Chapman, & Delvecchio, 2010). Community health nurses are in key positions to model therapeutic relationships with the vulnerable populations.

Behavioral health occurs along a continuum of care, from promotion to prevention, treatment, and recovery. The severity of symptoms associated with a mental disorder is variable, as are the symptoms that may never manifest as a diagnosable disorder. Similarly, substance use occurs across a continuum, from low risk to at risk to a possible substance use disorder. When developing a screening program to detect mental health and substance use, the community health nurse should be prepared to provide interventions or be able to refer persons whose screening results suggest that referral to specialty services is indicated. Therefore, a program should have links to clinically appropriate treatment services for persons across the continuum. Thus, the community health nurse should be knowledgeable of community agencies that provide mental health and substance abuse treatment. To ensure linkages to care, it is important to know the treatment capacity of the community where screening programs are being conducted. See Chapter 12.

MENTAL HEALTH DISORDERS: SCREENING, INTERVENTION, AND REFERRAL TO TREATMENT

The incidence and prevalence of mental and substance use disorders points to the importance of universal screening. For example, the National Depression Screening Day is an example of a community-level approach to screening. Resources and supplies, such as a comprehensive kit of materials, promotional information, media campaign, training, and technical assistance, are available by visiting the mental health screening Web sites (see Internet Resources found on thePoint).

Screening Questions/Surveys

Standardized surveys and measures should be used because they are evidence-based tools for detecting risk. Table 27–5 lists commonly used screening measures for anxiety, depression, and posttraumatic stress disorder. (Note that some measures are publically available for use, whereas others may require permission or fee for use.) The severity of risk is based on the scores and their interpretation for the particular measure.

Intervention

The immediate priority for the community health nurse is to ensure safety for an individual who is at risk to self or others. It may be imperative to contact emergency services in order to ensure that the individual receives immediate and specialized care. Given the range of mental health problems and disorders, and the range of mild to severe symptomatology, referral to mental health specialists for further assessment and diagnostic evaluation is warranted (Hall, Wren, & Kirby, 2014).

Referral to Treatment

Emergency, inpatient, and outpatient levels of treatment are available for individuals with mental health disorders. A principle of treatment is to ensure adequate care in the least restrictive environment. Inpatient mental health settings provide evaluation and treatment of acute mental disorders. Inpatient mental health treatment accounts for almost 60% of all admissions to general hospitals with a length of stay in most settings from 5 to 10 days. Partial hospitalization programs are designed to prevent relapse and prevent hospital admission while providing active treatment 4 to 5 days a week until such time as the individual is stabilized and level of functioning improves (Maree, 2013). Outpatient services are provided in an ambulatory care setting such as a mental health clinic, hospital outpatient department, community health center, or practitioner's office. SAMHSA provides a behavioral health treatment services locator on their website (https://findtreatment.samhsa.gov/), an online source of treatment facilities in the United States or U.S. territories.

ALCOHOL USE SCREENING, INTERVENTION, AND REFERRAL TO TREATMENT

The National Alcohol Screening Day is an annual event that provides information about alcohol and health as well as free, anonymous screening. The National Drug and Alcohol Facts Week is an activity specifically focused on bringing alcohol information for teens across communities (National Institute on Drug Abuse, 2016). Community health nurses can engage in these activities, reaching a population in which alcohol and drug use peaks across the lifespan.

Screening Questions/Surveys

Alcohol screening questions are based on knowledge of a standard drink. A standard drink in the United States is any drink that contains about 14 g of pure alcohol (about 0.6 fluid ounces or 1.2 tablespoons). Figure 27–2 provides a graphic depicting typical alcoholic drinks and standard drink sizes. It is important to know that the NIAAA recommends no more than four standard drinks a day *and* no more than 14 standard drinks a week for healthy males ages 21 to 64. No more than three standard drinks a day *and* no more than seven standard drinks a week are

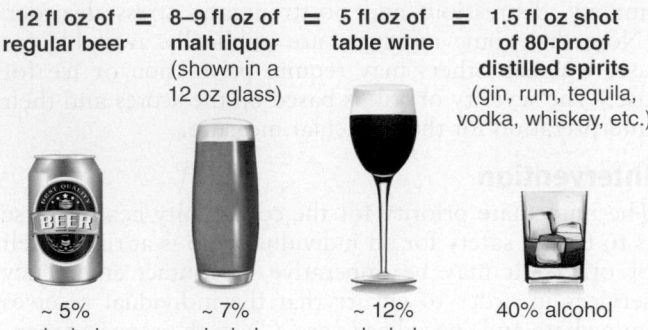

**12 fl oz of = 8–9 fl oz of = 5 fl oz of = 1.5 fl oz shot
regular beer   malt liquor   table wine   of 80-proof
                 (shown in a   distilled spirits
                 12 oz glass)   (gin, rum, tequila,
                                                 vodka, whiskey, etc.)**

~ 5%   ~ 7%   ~ 12%   40% alcohol
alcohol   alcohol   alcohol

The percent of "pure" alcohol, expressed here as alcohol by volume (alc/vol), varies by beverage.

FIGURE 27–2 What is a standard drink? Note: The percent of "pure" alcohol, expressed here as alcohol by volume (alc/vol), varies by beverage. Although the "standard" drink amounts are helpful for following health guidelines, they may not reflect customary serving sizes. In addition, although the alcohol concentrations listed are "typical," there is considerable variability in alcohol content within each type of beverage (e.g., beer, wine, distilled spirits) (NIAAA, n.d., para. 4). (From National Institute on Alcohol Abuse & Alcoholism (NIAAA). (n.d.). *What is a standard drink?* Retrieved from http://www.niaaa.nih.gov/alcohol-health/overview-alcohol-consumption/what-standard-drink.)

recommended for healthy females and for healthy males over age 65 (NIAAA, 2015b) (Fig. 27–3).

The single-question alcohol screen has a sensitivity of 82% and specificity of 79%; the single question, "How many times in the past year have you had five (men) or four (women or patients over age 65) drinks or more in a day?" makes it easy to ask within the context of collecting other health information. A positive score of one or more triggers the need for a further screening for harm and possible alcohol use disorder. Given the known risks of alcohol to the developing fetus, any alcohol use reported by persons who are pregnant is considered a positive

screen and constitutes at-risk alcohol use. Additionally, alcohol consumption under the age of 21 years is also considered to place the person at risk because the brain is still developing. The thresholds for alcohol consumption are based on population studies among healthy adults 21 years and older. Various health conditions and activities may warrant lower levels or no alcohol consumption at all (Fagbemi, 2011; Smith, Schmidt, Allensworth-Davies, & Saitz, 2009).

The Alcohol Use Disorders Identification Test (AUDIT) (see Table 27–5) is a 10-item screening instrument that includes questions about alcohol consumption during the past year, symptoms of alcohol use disorders, and alcohol-related problems or harm. Each response has a corresponding score and, when all 10 items are added together, results in a score ranging from 0 to 46. Scores ranging from 0 to 7 suggest abstinence or drinking below low-risk level. Scores from 8 to 15 suggest alcohol use in excess of recommended limits. Scores 16 and above suggest alcohol use above the recommended limits as well as the experience of alcohol-related harm (Rubinsky, Kivlahan, Volk, Maynard, & Bradley, 2010; Saunders, Aasland, Babor, De la Fuente, & Grant, 1993). The AUDIT-C is a three-item shorter form of the AUDIT screening tool (Fagbemi, 2011).

Underage alcohol use is also a concern, leading the American Academy of Pediatrics to recommend alcohol screening for all young teenagers. The CRAFFT (see Table 27–5) has been established to accurately screen for alcohol and other drug problems. A cutoff score of 2 has been found to be highly predictive of substance use disorder (Knight, Sherrit, Harris, Gates, & Chang, 2003; NIAAA, 2015c).

Biologic Screenings for Alcohol

Alcohol markers are not feasible for use in a community-based screening program because of the cost and the problems with obtaining biologic specimens. Andresen-Streichert et al. (2015) provided a review of various

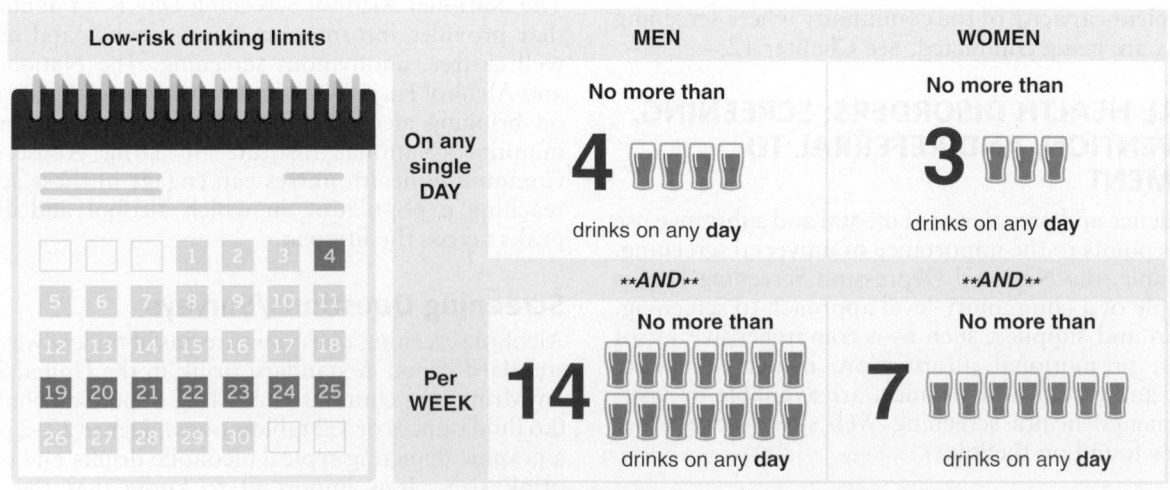

Low-risk drinking limits

	MEN	WOMEN
On any single DAY	No more than **4** drinks on any **day**	No more than **3** drinks on any **day**
	AND	****AND****
Per WEEK	No more than **14** drinks on any **day**	No more than **7** drinks on any **day**

To stay low risk, keep within BOTH the single-day AND weekly limits.

FIGURE 27–3 Low-risk drinking limits. (From National Institutes of Health (NIH). (2015). *Rethinking drinking: Alcohol and your health.* Retrieved form http://pubs.niaaa.nih.gov/publications/RethinkingDrinking/Rethinking_Drinking.pdf.)

specimens used to detect ethanol use. Direct detection of ethanol in blood or breath assesses the intake of alcohol during the preceding 10 to 12 hours. Ethyl glucuronide (EtG) is a metabolic product of ethanol that is detectable in the urine or hair. Specifically, EtG can be found in the urine for up to 80 hours after alcohol consumption and allows the detection of even small amounts of ethanol ingested. A segment of scalp hair of 1 cm reflects alcohol consumption over approximately 1 month (Andresen-Streichert et al., 2015). Phosphatidylethanol (PEth), carbohydrate-deficient transferrin (CDT), glutamyltransferase, aspartate aminotransferase, and alanine aminotransferase are alcohol markers that can be measured using blood samples. In comparing these alcohol markers and correlating with data from alcohol diaries, Walther et al. (2015) found that PEth had the highest sensitivity of all biomarkers studied. Further, PEth was the biomarker with the best correlation to self-reported alcohol consumption (Walther et al., 2015).

Intervention

A negative alcohol screen (i.e., 0 for the single question and/or a score < 4 for the AUDIT) is an opportunity for the community health nurse to have a conversation about the gender- and age-related alcohol consumption limits. Information about the standard drink size (Fig. 27–2), consumption limits (Fig. 27–3), and health risks (Table 27–4) can be provided with reinforcement and encouragement to maintain low-risk alcohol use.

A BI is warranted for individuals with a positive alcohol screen and AUDIT score of 4 to 13. The BI is a short conversation (5 to 15 minutes) with the individual who is reporting harms associated with alcohol use that is above the recommended limits. The BI is a nonconfrontational and patient-centered approach to at-risk alcohol use. With this approach, the nurse engages in a motivational discussion raising awareness of alcohol-related consequences and motivating a patient toward behavior change (APHA, 2008; Sullivan & Fleming, 1997). Helpful resources for conducting a BI include:

- *Helping Patients Who Drink Too Much: A Clinicians Guide* (NIAAA, 2015a) available at http://www.niaaa.nih.gov/guide and *Planning and Implementing Screening and Brief Intervention for Risky Alcohol Use: A Step-by-Step Guide for Primary Practices* (CDC, 2014c) available at http://www.cdc.gov/ncbddd/fasd/documents/alcoholsbiimplementationguide.pdf.
- In addition to the information identified above for those with a negative alcohol screen, the booklet *Rethinking Drinking: Alcohol and Your Health* (NIAAA, 2015b) is an additional resource for individuals who are thinking about changing their alcohol use. This booklet can be downloaded from http://pubs.niaaa.nih.gov/publications/RethinkingDrinking/Rethinking_Drinking.pdf.
- In collaboration with the American Academy of Pediatrics, NIAAA (2015c) developed *Alcohol Screening and Brief Intervention for Youth: A Practitioner's Guide*. Screening measures for this population are included in the guide, which is available at http://pubs.niaaa.nih.gov/publications/Practitioner/YouthGuide/YouthGuide.pdf.

Community health nurses should not be hesitant to engage in these conversations with individuals who are at risk because of alcohol use. According to the CDC (2014b), only one in six adults reported that they discussed their alcohol use with a health care provider and only 17% of women who were pregnant talked about their alcohol use. These BIs are consistent with community health nursing practice that involves health teaching. But this is much more than simply giving information to individuals; it is to promote a behavior change for healthier practices.

Referral to Treatment for Alcohol

Individuals with an AUDIT score of 14 and above warrant referral for further assessment and evaluation for specialty treatment. The community health nurse should engage in conversation with the individual, again using a nonconfrontational and patient-centered approach, providing feedback about the results of the AUDIT and information about the harms associated with continued alcohol use. A menu of support options can be provided, such as those included in the *Rethinking Drinking* booklet mentioned above (NIAAA, 2015b). In the motivational discussion, the community health nurse should work toward negotiating a plan that includes referral to specialty treatment. Thus, the PHN should be aware of services available in the community and how to access those services:

- SAMHSA's Behavioral Health Treatment Services Locator (https://findtreatment.samhsa.gov/) can be helpful in identifying alcohol-related treatment in a community.
- Alcoholics Anonymous also has a Web site listing contact numbers for AA groups within and outside the United States at http://www.aa.org/pages/en_US/find-aa-resources and also provides information about online AA meetings at http://aa-intergroup.org/.

SCREENING FOR DRUG USE INCLUDING PRESCRIPTION MEDICATION FOR NONMEDICAL REASONS

A single question for screening for drug use is, "How many times in the past year have you used an illegal drug or used a prescription medication for nonmedical reasons?" (Smith, Schmidt, Allensworth-Davies, & Saitz, 2010). Nonmedical reasons can be qualified with the explanation, "because of the experience or feeling it caused." The sensitivity for this screening question is 100% and the specificity is 74%. Any response greater than zero indicates a positive screen, meaning that the individual is at risk because of drug use. Follow-up questions are used to assess impact and whether substance use is serious enough to warrant a substance use disorder diagnosis. Additional information should be obtained about the specific drug(s) being used, frequency and quantity, and the negative impacts. A Boston University study found that for study participants, 88% of those who were alcohol dependent and 97% of those who were drug dependent could be identified by the use of a single screening question (Saitz, Cheng, Allensworth-Davies, Winter, & Smith, 2014).

The 10 questions in the Drug Abuse Screening Test (Skinner, 1982; Yudko, Lozhkina, & Fouts, 2007) provide additional information about the negative impacts and harms associated with drug use. The total "yes" responses are summed in order to obtain an overall score. A score of 0 reflects no use of drugs. A score of 1 and above indicates a level of risk that should be further assessed by a substance use specialist. This screening tool is widely used and can be found online from various sources (Counselling Resource, 2014).

Biologic Screening for Drug Use

Laboratory testing is not recommended for universal screening. Sources commonly used for drug testing include urine and blood. Other sources are oral fluid, sweat, hair, and meconium. Initial procedures for drug testing usually entail a urine immunoassay. Urine can be collected easily and noninvasively. However, urine specimens are easily adulterated or substituted. A positive test is based on a defined concentration of a component of the drug in a specimen (Warner & Lorch, 2014).

Interventions for Drug Use

Overall, there is fair evidence that people who reduce or stop drug use have a lower risk of negative health outcomes, at least those from trials conducted among treatment populations (Polen, Whitlock, Wisdom, Nygren, & Bougatsos, 2008). There are mixed results of studies on BIs for drug use. Saitz (2015) calls for well-designed studies of interventions that show efficacy, that are feasible, and that retain effectiveness in practice. A recent trial by Bogenschutz et al. (2014), among persons using drugs who were recruited from emergency departments, suggests that a BI with two boosters was not more efficacious than minimal screening. Thus, the data on BIs for drug use problems is limited. At a minimum, community health nurses should provide information about drug use treatment and support for reduction or stopping drug use.

Given the escalating number of overdoses associated with opioids, efforts have quickly been undertaken to expand naloxone access to those who may be at risk for overdose. Naloxone hydrochloride is a pure opioid antagonist that can effectively reverse the effects of opioid intoxication and overdose. Community health nurses can lead efforts to promote naloxone rescue measures. With the United States accounting for 99% of the world's hydrocodone consumption and one-quarter billion opioid prescriptions per year, this inexpensive life-saving treatment can avert some of the damage from opioid overdose (Humphreys, 2015). SAMHSA (2013b) is a leader in addressing this significant health concern detailed in their *Opioid Overdose Toolkit*, accessible at https://store.samhsa.gov/shin/content/SMA13-4742/Overdose_Toolkit_2014_Jan.pdf.

Referral to Treatment for Drug Use

As discussed in relation to alcohol use, the community health nurse should be aware of services available in the community and how to access those services:

- The SAMHSA Behavioral Health Treatment Services Locator (https://findtreatment.samhsa.gov/) provides such information.
- The Narcotics Anonymous Web site (https://www.na.org/) provides information on locating meetings.

TOBACCO SCREENING, INTERVENTION, AND REFERRAL TO TREATMENT

The U.S. Preventive Services Task Force (USPSTF, 2009) recommends screening and providing BIs for tobacco use as part of standard routine health care for adults and women who are pregnant. The U.S. Department of Health Services clinical practice guideline provides information about screening and interventions that can be provided based on the individual's willingness to quit or not. It is recommended that all patients be asked if they use tobacco and, if so, asked, "Do you want to quit?" (Fiore, Jaen, Baker, et al., 2009, p. iv).

The five major components for treating tobacco use and dependence (5 As) are "Ask" about tobacco use, "Advise" to quit, "Assess" willingness to make a quit attempt, "Aid" the person in quitting, and "Arrange" for follow-up (Agency for Healthcare Research & Quality [AHRQ], 2012, para. 2). Community health nurses are encouraged to adopt the 5As as part of their standard care to address this major health problem in the United States and globally. Strategies for various populations are provided in the AHRQ (2015) clinical practice guideline, including those who are willing to quit, those unwilling to quit, those who have recently quit, and specific populations (e.g., LGBT, persons with medical conditions, persons with HIV).

COMMUNITY- AND POPULATION-BASED INTERVENTIONS

Community interventions move beyond single interventions and outcomes at individual levels of health behavior change. Starting with a specific framework helps planners identify why and how the intervention will work. Two theoretical frameworks used in community/public health science are *process theory* and *effect theory*. These are both part of the Model of Program Theory and used to plan, deliver, and evaluate the program (Issel, 2013). In relation to behavioral health, process theory helps the community health nurse identify the resources and structure needed to develop, implement, and evaluate the program. Effect theory provides the rationale for why the intervention will work.

Process Theory: Component of Program Theory

Three components comprise process theory: (1) an organizational plan that includes information on personnel and resources to be used (e.g., fiscal, information technology, supplies), (2) a service utilization plan that specifies how the program will reach its targeted client population (e.g., social marketing, screening procedures, logistics of availability/access), and (3) specifications of their outputs (e.g., expected outcomes). These components are continually developed throughout the process and each affects the other (Issel, 2013).

Effect Theory: Component of Program Theory

The challenge for the community health nurse in developing interventions related to behavioral health is the fact that behavior management is needed for both mental and substance use issues or disorders. Effect theory is a useful framework for developing behavioral health interventions. Effect theory encompasses the theories of causal/determinant forces, intervention mechanisms, and outcome to impact (Issel, 2013). The causal theory is an explanation of the process that currently underlies the health problem and includes relevant components directly responsible for the health problem. The intervention theory explains how the intervention alters the causal factors, describing how the program actually works. The impact theory helps explain how the outcomes lead to impacts, which is how the immediate outcomes of the program lead to long-term changes to the health problem (Issel, 2013).

Once the framework has been selected, the community health nurse conducts a community assessment drawing on primary and secondary sources such as community members. Community health nurses can utilize other data such as vital statistics or census data to develop additional insights about the health needs of the community. National sources, such as the NSDUH, can provide national and state-level estimates on the use of tobacco products, alcohol, illicit drugs (including nonmedical use of prescription drugs) and mental health in the United States. See Chapter 15 on community assessment.

The next step is to analyze the data and develop a diagnosis of the community's needs, the community responses, and expected outcomes. The health-planning phase entails designing an orderly, detailed series of specific goals and objectives. Implementing the plan for promoting the health of the community involves engaging others in the action and encouraging their ownership, sense of responsibility, and autonomy. Engaging representatives of target populations in community coalitions in various interventions has been associated with noted improvements in health status and reduction in disparities in racial and ethnic minority populations (Anderson, Adeney, Shinn, Krause, & Safranek, 2015). Evaluation occurs throughout the process, but is often seen as the final step in determining the effectiveness of the service for the community. See Chapter 12.

A case example is provided to illustrate the process of developing a smoking cessation program for mothers in a rural county (see From the Case Files I).

When using effect theory to design a prevention program for behavioral health, a good place to start is to identify the specific health problem and then the desired health problem impact and health problem outcome. As the program is developed, the community health nurse starts by identifying the antecedent factors that led to behavioral health problems. This provides a clear rationale for why the intervention should provide the desired impact.

Policy-Based Interventions

Not-for-profit, private for-profit, and governmental agencies play crucial roles in community health care. The provision of health care to the population requires multidisciplinary approaches that are driven by monetary reimbursements based on health care problems. Local governments may institute community mental health care policies relative to administrative processes or procedural mechanisms. Policies at the community or state levels aim to ensure the rights of individuals and public safety. Thus, cities or counties with appropriate jurisdiction over a geographic area develop policies and guidelines necessary to encourage mental health program development and implementations that address the needs of the community population.

Depending on each county, certain rules or regulations apply. It is important to learn about the community agencies and interrelationships to other county service providers to ensure the coordination of care. At the local level are freestanding programs that focus on support for individuals, families, the indigent, or the homeless. Funding may come from charitable organizations or from local governments through grant monies obtained from periodic requests for proposals (RFPs) or requests for applications (RFAs) issued by the local governing body. Other governmental agencies have roles in mental health by encouraging employee wellness in the workplace or through rules and regulations that encourage employers to provide benefits, such as mental health insurance, bereavement leave, or stress leave. The incidence of violence in the workplace has necessitated policy initiatives, resulting in business community development of strategic plans and educational programs to address these issues (Occupational Safety & Health Administration [OSHA], 2015).

Mental Health Policy and Research

The WHO 2013–2020 Mental Health Action Plan (WHO, 2013) outlines the following objectives:

1. To strengthen effective leadership and governance for mental health
2. To provide comprehensive, integrated, and responsive mental health and social care services in community-based settings
3. To implement strategies for promotion and prevention in mental health
4. To strengthen information systems, evidence, and research for mental health (p. 10)

The action plan relies on six principles and approaches: (1) universal health coverage, (2) human rights, (3) evidence-based practice, (4) life course [lifespan] approach, (5) multisector approach, and (6) empowerment of persons with mental disorders and psychosocial disabilities (WHO, 2013, p. 10). Thus, the focus is to act, unite, and empower people and countries to promote health and well-being, as well as to improve the quality of care for persons with mental disorders.

Although there is a clear need for mental health services, the proportion of people who need, but do not receive, care is especially high in low- and middle-income countries. These countries also have fewer health care professionals than required to deliver mental health and substance use interventions to everyone who needs them (Baingana, al'Absi, Becker, & Pringle, 2015). Globally, nurses represented the most prevalent professional group working in the mental health sector. Thus, there is a clear need to build capacity of nurses prepared to address mental health needs. Further, Pike, Susser, Galea, and Pincus (2013) state that this increased human capacity needs to be deployed in integrated community care settings

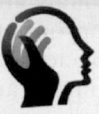

From the Case Files I

Smoking Cessation Program for Mothers in a Rural County

You have been working in the public health department well-child clinic in a rural Appalachian county and noticed that more than one third of the mothers you are seeing are smokers and that their babies seem to be smaller than the babies of moms who do not smoke. When you mention smoking to individual mothers, they tell you they want to stop, but just are not able to. You are interested in putting together a smoking cessation program. You decide to use Issel's (2013) effect theory as a framework for building your intervention. That is, you consider the relationships among health antecedents, causes of health problems, program interventions, and health effects. You are convincing in getting the county to fund the program. What data do you need before you begin to look at interventions (see Strategy 1 below)? What data can you get using existing databases, and what data will you need to collect yourself? Once you have reviewed the data, you decide that you want to include smoking cessation as part of well-baby visits for all mothers who are current smokers. What do you need to do before you put together the program (see Strategy 2 below)? After you have gathered all this information, what final piece is needed before you present your proposal to your public health department (see Strategy 3 below)? If you are able to implement the program what immediate impact do you expect to have and what long-term outcomes are you hoping for?

Strategies

1. Preliminary data needed:
   a. Low-birth-weight rates compared to state and national rates. (Available vital statistics public health data.)
   b. Low-birth-weight rates for smokers versus nonsmokers in your county, compared with the state and the nation. (Protected vital statistics public health data that will need approval from the state for you to access and analyze.)
   c. Comparison of asthma rates in children in your county with smoke-free homes versus homes with a parent

smoking. (Available survey data using prior studies, but may not be current. Will most likely need to conduct a survey at the county level. Check with state public health department for state-level data.)
   d. County tobacco use rates based on gender and age, and trends among adolescent girls in your county schools compared to state and national rates. (Available public health survey data at state and national levels. May need to conduct a survey at the county level.)
2. A review of the evidence related to smoking cessation interventions with women of childbearing age. Were any of the studies conducted with Appalachian women? Will you need to make some adjustments to interventions that work based on culture? Are there possible economic constraints for this population in relation to pharmacologic interventions? Are the time frames reasonable in your setting?
3. You need to do an analysis of the cost to implement the program, complete a cost–benefit projection, have clear program goals and objectives, and formulate a plan to evaluate the effectiveness of the program.

The desired health impact refers to the immediate impact expected from the program. For example, if the health problem is heavy episodic (binge) alcohol consumption among college students, a logical approach may be to institute an alcohol screening program. For such a program, the immediate *impact* for the program may be that 25% of students are screened and 75% of those who require a BI and/or a referral for further assessment receive those interventions. However, the desired *outcome* of the program is an overall reduction in heavy episodic alcohol consumption on campus over a specified time period—for instance, the next 2 years. Remember that not all desired impact is related to change. The goal may be to stabilize, prevent, or maintain a health state or problem. Having a clear understanding of what a behavioral program can actually accomplish and what long-term goal it hopes to achieve prior to implementing the program will provide a clearer picture of how to proceed with the program.

---

beyond the stand-alone mental health hospital and integrated into primary health care systems.

Substance Use Policy

Alcohol and other drugs are a substantial threat to the public good. As such, drug policy should aim to promote the public good by improving individual and public health, neighborhood safety, and community and family cohesion and by reducing crime. Researchers reviewed evidence that can be used to inform decision making about drug policies related to supply control, methods to control pharmaceutical drugs, prevention programs,

and health and social services for persons with drug use. A key message is that the effectiveness of these various strategies is unknown or additional research is needed. What is concerning is that programs that have widespread use, such as the Drug Abuse Resistance Education (DARE), according to meta-analyses show that the program is ineffective (Strang et al., 2012). Thus, it is important that community health nurses implement and evaluate evidence-based programs, rather than promoting programs that have widespread popularity.

Given the increase in fatal poisonings, most of which are caused by drug overdose, recent efforts have been directed to reversing opioid overdose. As of September 2015, 43 states and the District of Columbia have passed laws to increase access to naloxone. These laws are intended to increase naloxone prescribing and distribution, to increase pharmacy naloxone access, and to encourage overdose witnesses to summon emergency responders. Although these laws increase layperson access to this medication that can reverse overdose morbidity and mortality, barriers exist in terms of cost and status as a prescription medication (e.g., not an over-the-counter medication), among others things (Davis & Carr, 2015). In their role as advocates, community health nurses can take an active role in helping to remove these barriers.

Communities can set policies that restrict both alcohol availability and consumption; this is done by controlling the number of alcohol outlets, regulating the current outlets, and setting laws that will allow the community to close problem outlets. These measures are implemented through policies related to zoning and the licensing of establishments that sell alcohol. Another measure has been to require responsible alcohol-service training for bartenders. Other examples include keg registration, stricter enforcement of underage sales of alcohol and tobacco, and controlling alcohol outlet density. Major efforts in relation to tobacco consumption in public areas have resulted in a drastic restriction of locations where tobacco users can smoke outside of their own home. In one case in Washington, DC, a judge banned smoking in a private home in response to a lawsuit brought by the homeowner's neighbor (Mendoza, 2015). In California, 69 cities have banned smoking in multiunit apartments, condominiums, and public housing complexes (Center for Tobacco Policy & Organizing, 2015).

ROLE OF THE COMMUNITY MENTAL HEALTH NURSE

The nurse's role in community mental health is multifaceted involving advocacy, education, case management, collaboration, and community involvement; this has been evident throughout the chapter. The access and use of epidemiologic data to better understand and serve the population with behavioral health issues or disorders is vital. This means identifying their incidence and prevalence of, examining the causes and risk factors associated with these disorders, and identifying and addressing the needs of people with mental and substance use disorders (see Chapter 7 on Epidemiology).

Advocacy

An important part of the nurse's role is *advocacy*. As an advocate, the nurse seeks to increase client access to behavioral health services, to reduce stigma and promote improved public understanding of this population, and to improve services in community mental health (Barry, McGinty, Pescosolido, & Goldman, 2014). The advocacy role requires being politically involved by serving on decision-making boards and committees, lobbying for legislative changes, and helping to influence mental health policy development that will better serve this population. Membership in state and national nursing organizations can be helpful in establishing collaborative partnerships

to benefit the mentally ill. Membership in the National Alliance on Mental Illness (NAMI, 2011), or other advocacy groups, can also effect positive change (see Chapter 13 for more information on advocacy and policy making).

In any of these venues, the vision and expertise of the community mental health nurse can be useful to advocate for enhancing existing services, developing new services, and increasing access for the mentally ill to all services. Community health nurses can also work to confront media portrayals of behavioral disorders that are stereotypical, negative, and provide an unfavorable or inaccurate view.

Education

Another aspect of the nurse's role is *education*. The community mental health nurse teaches clients individually and in groups about their health conditions. Nurses can be instrumental in providing information about the neurobiological base of mental and substance use disorders, treatments, and self-management strategies such as taking medications consistently in order to promote optimal level of functioning in the community (Finnell & Ditz, 2007; Finnell & Nowzari, 2013). The nurse also teaches the public through community education programs and has an educational role with caregivers, family and community members, and health care decision-makers by providing information for service planning (see Chapter 11 for more on health education).

Case Management

Case management for persons with SMIs is also part of the community mental health nurse's role. This role includes screening, assessment, care planning, arranging for service delivery, monitoring, reassessment, evaluation, and discharge. Case management is often offered within the context of a community mental health center (CMHC). Case management helps the person with an SMI to access services and live as independently as possible (Townsend, 2015).

The nurse's role also involves *case finding and referral*. This means early identification of persons with mental disorders who are in need of treatment and referral of those persons to the appropriate resources for treatment. The purpose of this role is secondary prevention, because early identification and treatment help to ameliorate the severity of the mental disorder and promote a speedier recovery (Townsend, 2015). See Perspectives: Voices from the Community.

Collaboration

Finally, the nurse's role includes *collaboration*. Whether serving individual clients, groups, or populations, the nurse is part of the larger community mental health team and works in collaboration with many people to accomplish the goals of community mental health. The composition of the team—made up of clients, psychiatric nurses, physicians, social workers, nutritionists, epidemiologists, psychologists, health planners, and many more—is diverse and varies depending on the community health nurse's work setting. Collaboration allows for a pooling of professional expertise that enhances the quality and effectiveness of services for persons with mental and substance use disorders (Townsend, 2015).

PERSPECTIVES
VOICES FROM THE COMMUNITY

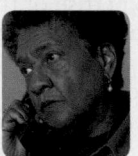

I have been a nurse for a long time. Even though I don't work in behavioral health nursing, per se, I have had many experiences throughout the years related to both mental health and substances. When I was a student in the 1970s, I remember doing a rotation in a locked mental health facility and feeling that it was just a "revolving door." Now, there are so many medications available that can quickly address symptoms, and prevention and early intervention are the focus. Then, the same patients came back over and over again, and all staff could offer them was counseling, a few medications (mostly Thorazine), and electroconvulsive therapy (ECT). They had a "rubber room"—a padded room where they would place patients who were dangerous to themselves or others. It seemed so futile to me, at the time.

Years later, a close friend I had known since childhood was hospitalized for a suicide attempt. She had always been charming and outgoing, often talking excitedly about things and using her hands to punctuate her thoughts. She seemed to have boundless energy and there was nothing she couldn't do. I was shocked to learn that she had been suffering from a terrible depression and had tried to overdose on prescription medications. She was subsequently diagnosed with bipolar disorder and began a long road to recovery with many medication changes and years of hard work in therapy with a very kind, patient counselor. Her marriage didn't survive and her children suffered

during her so-called crazy years, but she made it through to the other side and learned a lot from her experience. I learned a lot from that "personal" experience with mental illness.

I have also worked with many public health clients who have battled various types of mental illness (often postpartum depression, or eating disorders with new moms or teens), as well as bipolar disorder and schizophrenia among drug users and homeless individuals. I have seen firsthand the problem of alcohol and substance use disorders (not only alcohol and illicit drugs, but misuse of prescription medications or huffing glue and aerosols). I have struggled to help them and their families find resources or advocated on their behalf with landlords, the school system, or law enforcement, as their illnesses led to problems in all areas of their lives.

*Although I am not a mental health nurse practitioner, I feel that I have some understanding of the problems in the community, with families, and with individual clients. I realize the responsibility I have to reinforce with my students the human side of mental illness and substance abuse and to break through the fears they experience in order to help them look at the client in a different way. Brain chemistry is a powerful thing—people cannot just "will" themselves to be more cheerful/less depressed or to stop **craving** heroin (or chocolate, for that matter). Seeing each client as an individual and joining with them to address their issues is the best approach—that's community health nursing!*

Lori, Community Health Nursing Professor

SUMMARY

Behavioral health is a key component in the health of a community. Three of the top ten leading health indicators from *Healthy People 2020* are closely linked to behavioral health issues: tobacco use, substance use, and mental health (see Display 27–2). Objectives, health indicators, and target outcomes for tobacco, illegal substances, and alcohol use guide the PHN in program planning. In every community in the United States and the world, behavioral health directly or indirectly affects every other indicator of health. Unabated, mental and substance use disorders overburden the medical, social, economic, and criminal justice systems of communities and governments. Community health nurses are critical in addressing the needs of individuals who are among the most stigmatized in society. Community health nurses have a primary role in addressing the full continuum—from promotion to prevention to treatment to recovery for persons with mental and substance use disorders.

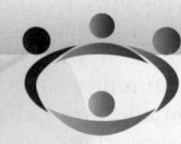

DISPLAY 27–2 *HEALTHY PEOPLE 2020* LEADING HEALTH INDICATORS

Top 10 Health Indicators

1. Physical activity
2. Overweight and obesity
3. Tobacco use
4. Substance abuse
5. Responsible sexual behavior
6. Mental health
7. Injury and violence
8. Environmental quality
9. Immunization
10. Access to health care

Treatment related to behavioral health at the community level begins with a community assessment in order to establish a community diagnosis, followed by intervention that can address the specific public health issue identified in the diagnosis. The community health nurse can use *Healthy People 2020* objectives as a starting point in the development of an intervention.

The community health nurse must incorporate behavioral health in the assessment, planning, and developing of community health interventions and in the evaluation of outcomes. With this comes the need for administrative, managerial, or supervisory support with commitment not only from a philosophical perspective but from a resource perspective as well. Success comes with a unified approach to mental health and substance use, requiring application of research and utilization of best practice models across the behavioral health continuum.

ACTIVITIES TO PROMOTE CRITICAL THINKING

1. As a community health nurse, you have been asked to design and present a 2-hour program on suicide prevention to the entire student body of the local high school. This activity is representative of which level of prevention? What are some of the considerations involved in planning this program to promote optimal success? How might you measure the effectiveness of this intervention?

2. You are part of a multidisciplinary team whose goal is to identify families in your city who are at risk for crisis (e.g., single parent, divorced, pregnant adolescents, unemployed) and develop a set of interventions. How would you locate these families? What interventions would be appropriate to meet their needs? What level of prevention would you be targeting? What might be the most effective methods of reaching them?

3. You have met a few elderly men in your area who live alone and are widowed, and you have heard that there are others. Assuming your advocacy role in community mental health, you decide to take some action to ensure that their needs are being met. How would you determine the risks and needs for this group? What interventions would be appropriate to meet their needs?

4. Select a problem that places people at risk for mental disorders (e.g., child abuse and neglect, drug abuse) and search the Internet to learn all you can about it. What is the incidence and prevalence of this problem? What interventions are most effective in addressing it? What can be done to prevent it? With a small group of students, brainstorm ideas for primary and secondary interventions.

5. Search for local treatment facilities and resources for alcohol and drug abuse clients. Call a few of them to inquire about cost, access, and types of assistance available. How many people can they serve? How does this compare to the numbers of reported alcohol and drug users in your area? Is there a waiting list? Where else can clients go when there are no more spaces available in your area?

6. Talk with a community/public health nurse working in your community. Ask questions about the available data used to assess the problems of substance abuse and mental health in the area. Ask his or her opinion on the accuracy of the data. Are adequate resources available? How does the nurse advocate on behalf of these clients?

REFERENCES

Agency for Healthcare Research & Quality (AHRQ). (2012). *Five major steps to intervention (the "5 A's")*. Retrieved from http://www.ahrq.gov/professionals/clinicians-providers/guidelines-recommendations/tobacco/5steps.html

Agency for Healthcare Research & Quality (AHRQ). (2015). *Treating tobacco use and dependence: 2008 update*. Retrieved from http://www.ahrq.gov/professionals/clinicians-providers/guidelines-recommendations/tobacco/index.html

American Psychiatric Association. (2013). *Diagnostic and statistical manual of mental disorders* (5th ed.). Arlington, VA: Author.

American Public Health Association (APHA) & Education Development Center, Inc. (2008). *Alcohol screening and brief intervention: A guide for public health practitioners*. Washington, DC: National Highway Traffic Safety Administration, U.S. Department of Transportation.

Anderson, L. M., Adeney, K. L., Shinn, C., Krause, L. K., & Safranek, S. (2012). Community coalition-driven interventions to reduce health disparities among racial and ethnic minority populations. *The Cochrane Library*. Retrieved from http://www.cochrane.org/ CD009905/PUBHLTH_community-coalition-driven-interventions-to-improve-health-status-and-reduce-disparities-in-racial-and-ethnic-minority-populations

Andresen-Streichert, H., Rothkrich, G., Vettorazzi, E., Mueller, A., Lohse, A., Frederking, D., ... Sterneck, M. (2015). Determination of ethyl glucuronide in hair for detection of alcohol consumption in patients after liver transplantation. *Therapeutic Drug Monitoring, 37*(4), 539–545.

Bagalman, E., & Napili, A. (2015). *Prevalence of mental illness in the United States: Data sources and estimates. Congressional Research Service*. Retrieved from https://www.fas.org/sgp/crs/misc/R43047.pdf

Baingana, F., al'Absi, M., Becker, A. E., & Pringle, B. (2015). Global research challenges and opportunities for mental health and substance-use disorders. *Nature, 527*(7578), S172–S177.

Barry, C. L., McGinty, E. E., Pescosolido, B. A., & Goldman, H. H. (2014). Stigma, discrimination, treatment effectiveness, and policy: Public views about drug addiction and mental illness. *Psychiatric Services, 65*(10), 1269–1272.

Blumberg, S. J., Clarke, T. C., & Blackwell, D. L. (2015). Racial and ethnic disparities in men's use of mental health treatments. *NCHS Data Brief, No. 206*, 1–8.

Blumberg, S. J., Zablotsky, B., Avila, R. M., Colpe, L. J., Pringle, B. A., & Kogan, M. D. (2015). Diagnosis lost: Differences between children who had and who currently have an autism spectrum disorder diagnosis. *Autism, 20*(7), 783–795.

Bogenschutz, M. P., Donovan, D. M., Mandler, R. N., Perl, H. I., Forcehimes, A. A., Crandall, C., ... Douaihy, A. (2014). Brief intervention for patients with problematic drug use presenting in emergency departments: A randomized clinical trial. *JAMA Internal Medicine, 174*(11), 1736–1745.

Broyles, L. M., Bifnswanger, I. A., Jenkins, J. A., Finnell, D. S., Faseru, B., Cavaiola, A., ... Gordon, A. J. (2014). Confronting inadvertent stigma and pejorative language in addiction scholarship: A recognition and response. *Substance Abuse, 35*(3), 217–221.

Center for Behavioral Health Statistics and Quality. (2015). *Behavioral health trends in the United States: Results from the 2014 National Survey on Drug Use and Health (HHS Publication No. SMA 15-4927, NSDUH Series H-50)*. Retrieved from http://www.samhsa.gov/data/

Center for Tobacco Policy & Organizing. (2015). *Smoke-free housing policies*. Sacramento, CA: American Lung Association in California.

Centers for Disease Control and Prevention (CDC). (2011). Mental illness surveillance among adults in the United States. *Morbidity and Mortality Weekly Report (MMWR), 60*(Suppl.), S1–S29. Retrieved from http://www.cdc.gov/mmwr/pdf/other/su6003.pdf

Centers for Disease Control and Prevention (CDC). (2013). *The state of aging & health in America 2013*. Atlanta, GA: Centers for Disease Control and Prevention, U.S. Department of Health and Human Services. Retrieved from http://www.cdc.gov/features/agingand-health/state_of_aging_and_health_in_america_2013.pdf

Centers for Disease Control and Prevention (CDC). (2014a). *Autism spectrum disorder, data and statistics*. Atlanta, GA: Centers for Disease Control and Prevention, U.S. Department of Health and Human Services. Retrieved from http://www.cdc.gov/ncbddd/autism/data.html

Centers for Disease Control and Prevention (CDC). (2014b). *Fact sheets—Age 21 minimum legal drinking age*. Atlanta, GA: Centers for Disease Control and Prevention, U.S. Department of Health and Human Services. Retrieved from http://www.cdc.gov/alcohol/fact-sheets/minimum-legal-drinking-age.htm

Centers for Disease Control and Prevention (CDC). (2014c). *Planning and implementing screening and brief intervention for risky alcohol use: A step-by-step guide for primary care practices*. Atlanta, GA: Centers for Disease Control and Prevention, National Center on Birth Defects and Developmental Disabilities.

Centers for Disease Control and Prevention (CDC). (2015). *Suicide: Fact at a glance*. Atlanta, GA: Centers for Disease Control and Prevention, U.S. Department of Health and Human Services. Retrieved from http://www.cdc.gov/ViolencePrevention/pdf/Suicide-DataSheet-a.pdf

Corrigan, P. W., Kerr, A., & Knudsen, L. (2005). The stigma of mental illness: Explanatory models and methods for change. *Applied and Preventive Psychology, 11*(3), 179–190.

Corrigan, P. W., Roe, D., & Tsang, H. W. (2011). *Challenging the stigma of mental illness: Lessons for therapists and advocates*. Malden, MA: John Wiley & Sons.

Counselling Resource. (2014). *Drug Abuse Screening Test (DAST)*. Retrieved from http://counsellingresource.com/quizzes/drug-testing/drug-abuse/

Davis, C. S., & Carr, D. (2015). Legal changes to increase access to naloxone for opioid overdose reversal in the United States. *Drug and Alcohol Dependence, 157*, 112–120.

Department of Health and Human Services, Office of Disease Prevention and Health Promotion. (2014). *Healthy People 2020 leading health indicators: Mental health*. Retrieved from http://www.healthypeople.gov/sites/default/files/HP2020_LHI_Mental_Hlth_0.pdf

Dotson, K. B., Dunn, M. E., & Bowers, C. A. (2015). Stand-alone personalized normative feedback for college student drinkers: A meta-analytic review, 2004 to 2014. *PLoS One, 10*(10), e0139518.

England, M. J., Butler, A. S., & Gonzalez, M. L. (2015). *Psychosocial interventions for mental and substance use disorders: A framework for establishing evidence-based standards*. Washington, DC: National Academies Press.

Fagbemi, K. (2011). What is the best questionnaire to screen for alcohol use disorder in an office practice? *One-Minute Consult, 78*(10), 649–651.

Fayyad, J., De Graaf, R., Kessler, R., Alonso, J., Angermeyer, M., Demyttenaere, K., ... Jin, R. (2007). Cross-national prevalence and correlates of adult attention–deficit hyperactivity disorder. *The British Journal of Psychiatry, 190*(5), 402–409.

Federal Interagency Forum on Aging-Related Statistics. (2012). *Older Americans 2012: Key indicators of well-being*. Washington, DC: U.S. Government Printing Office. Retrieved from http://www.aging-stats.gov/agingstatsdotnet/Main_Site/Data/2012_Documents/Docs/EntireChartbook.pdf

Fenikile, T. S., Ellerbeck, K., Filippi, M. K., & Daley, C. M. (2014). Barriers to autism screening in family medicine practice: A qualitative study. *Primary Health Care Research and Development, 16*(4), 356–366.

Ferrari, A. J., Norman, R. E., Freedman, G., Baxter, A. J., Pirkis, J. E., Harris, M. G., ... Whiteford, H. A. (2014). The burden attributable to mental and substance use disorders as risk factors for suicide: Findings from the Global Burden of Disease Study 2010. *PLoS One, 9*(4), e91936.

Finnell, D. S., & Ditz, K. A. (2007). Health diaries for self-monitoring and self-regulation: Applications to individuals with serious mental illness. *Issues in Mental Health Nursing, 28*(12), 1293–1307.

Finnell, D. S., & Nowzari, S. (2013). Providing information about the neurobiology of alcohol use disorders to close the 'referral to treatment gap'. *Nursing Clinics of North America, 48*(3), 373–383.

Finnell, D. S., Nowzari, S., Reimann, B., Fischer, L., Pace, E., & Goplerud, E. (2014). Screening, brief intervention, and referral to treatment (SBIRT) as an integral part of nursing practice. *Substance Abuse, 35*(2), 114–118.

Fiore, M.C., Jaen, C.R., Baker, T.B., et al. (2009). *Treating tobacco use and dependence: 2008 update. Quick reference guide for clinicians*. Rockville, MD: U.S. Department of Health and Human Services. Public Health Service.

Ginsberg, Y., Quintero, J., Anand, E., Casillas, M., & Upadhyaya, H. P. (2014). Underdiagnosis of attention-deficit/hyperactivity disorder in adult patients: A review of the literature. *The Primary Care Companion for CNS Disorders, 16*(3), PCC.13r01600. doi: 10.4088/PCC.13r01600.

Gladstone, T. R., Beardslee, W. R., & O'Connor, E. E. (2011). The prevention of adolescent depression. *Psychiatric Clinics of North America, 34*(1), 35–52.

Gordon, R. S., Jr. (1983). An operational classification of disease prevention. *Public Health Reports, 98*(2), 107.

Hall, A., Wren, M., & Kirby, S. (Eds.). (2014). *Care planning in mental health: Promoting recovery* (2nd ed.). Hoboken, NJ: Wiley Blackwell.

Han, B., Hedden, S. L., Lipari, R., Copello, E. A. P., & Kroutil, L. A. (2015). *Receipt of services for behavioral health problems: Results from the 2014 National Survey on Drug Use and Health*. Rockville, MD: Substance Abuse and Mental Health Services Administration. Retrieved from http://www.samhsa.gov/data/sites/default/files/NSDUH-DR-FRR3-2014/NSDUH-DR-FRR3-2014/NSDUH-DR-FRR3-2014.pdf

Hert, M., Correll, C. U., Bobes, J., Cetkovich-Bakmas, M., Cohen, D., Asai, I., ... Leucht, S. (2011). Physical illness in patients with severe mental disorders. I. Prevalence, impact of medications and disparities in health care. *World Psychiatry, 10*(1), 52–77.

Heslin, K. C., Elixhauser, A., & Steiner, C. A. (2015). *Hospitalizations involving mental and substance use disorders among adults, 2012: Statistical Brief #191*. Rockville, MD: Agency for Health Care Policy and Research. Retrieved from http://www-ncbi-nlm-nih-gov.ezp.welch.jhmi.edu/books/NBK310986/pdf/Bookshelf_NBK310986.pdf/

Horgan, C. M., Hodgkin, D., Stewart, M. T., Quinn, A., Merrick, E. L., Reif, S., ... Creedon, T. B. (2015). Health plans' early response to federal parity legislation for mental health and addiction services. *Psychiatric Services, 67*(2), 162–168.

Humphreys, K. (2015). An overdose antidote goes mainstream. *Health Affairs, 34*(10), 1624–1627.

Hurt, R. D., Ebbert, J. O., Hays, J. T., & McFadden, D. D. (2014). Pharmacologic interventions for tobacco dependence. In R. Ries, D. Fiellin, S. Miller, & R. Saitz (Eds.), *The ASAM principles of addiction medicine* (5th ed., pp. 811–822). Philadelphia, PA: Wolters Kluwer.

Issel, L. M. (2013). *Health planning and evaluation: A practical, systematic approach for community health* (3rd ed.). Burlington, MA: Jones & Bartlett Learning.

Kessler, R. C., Adler, L., Barkley, R., Biederman, J., Conners, C. K., Demler, O., Faraone, S. V., ... Zaslavsky, A. M. (2006). The prevalence and correlates of adult ADHD in the United States: Results from the National Comorbidity Survey Replication. *American Journal of Psychiatry, 163*(4), 716–723.

Knight, J. R., Sherrit, L., Harris, S. K., Gates, E. C., & Chang, G. (2003). A comparison of the AUDIT, POSIT, CAGE, and CRAFFT. *Alcoholism: Clinical and Experimental Research, 27,* 67–73.

Kobau, R., DiIorio, C., Chapman, D., & Delvecchio, P. (2010). Substance Abuse and Mental Health Services Administration/CDC Mental Illness Stigma panel members. Attitudes about mental illness and its treatment: Validation of a generic scale for public health surveillance of mental illness associated stigma. *Community Mental Health Journal, 46*(2), 164–176.

Leamy, M., Bird, V., Le Boutillier, C., Williams, J., & Slade, M. (2011). Conceptual framework for personal recovery in mental health: Systematic review and narrative synthesis. *The British Journal of Psychiatry, 199*(6), 445–452.

Livingston, J. D., & Boyd, J. E. (2010). Correlates and consequences of internalized stigma for people living with mental illness: A systematic review and meta-analysis. *Social Science & Medicine, 71*(12), 2150–2161.

Livingston, J. D., Milne, T., Fang, M. L., & Amari, E. (2012). The effectiveness of interventions for reducing stigma related to substance use disorders: A systematic review. *Addiction, 107*(1), 39–50.

Lopez-Quintero, C., Roth, K. B., Eaton, W. W., Wu, L. T., Cottler, L. B., Bruce, M., & Anthony, J. C. (2015). Mortality among heroin users and users of other internationally regulated drugs: A 27-year follow-up of users in the Epidemiologic Catchment Area Program household samples. *Drug and Alcohol Dependence, 156,* 104–111. pii: S0376-8716(15)01624-5. doi: 10.1016/j.drugalcdep.2015.08.030.

Lozano, R., Naghavi, M., Foreman, K., Lim, S., Shibuya, K., Aboyans, V., ... Cross, M. (2012). Global and regional mortality from 235 causes of death for 20 age groups in 1990 and 2010: A systematic analysis for the Global Burden of Disease Study 2010. *The Lancet, 380*(9859), 2095–2128.

Lund, C., Breen, A., Flisher, A. J., Kakuma, R., Corrigall, J., Joska, J. A., ... Patel, V. (2010). Poverty and common mental disorders in low and middle income countries: A systematic review. *Social Science & Medicine, 71*(3), 517–528.

Maree, E. G. (2013). Hospital-based psychiatric nursing care. In G.W. Stuart (Ed.), *Principles and Practice of Psychiatric Nursing* (10th ed., pp. 639–667). St. Louis, MO: Elsevier Mosby.

Melek, S. P., Norris, D. T., & Paulus, J. (2014). *Economic impact of integrated medical-behavioral healthcare, implications for psychiatry.* Arlington, VA: APA.

Melnikova, N., Orr, M. F., Wu, J., & Christensen, B. (2015). Injuries from methamphetamine-related chemical incidents—five states, 2001–2012. *MMWR. Morbidity and Mortality Weekly Report, 64*(33), 909–912.

Mendoza, J. (2015, March 11). Judge blocks DC man from smoking in his home...at least for a while. *The Christian Science Monitor.* Retrieved from http://www.csmonitor.com/USA/USA-Update/2015/0311/Judge-blocks-DC-man-from-smoking-in-his-own-home-at-least-for-a-while

Merikangas, K. R., He, J. P., Burstein, M., Swanson, S. A., Avenevoli, S., Cui, L., ... Swendsen, J. (2010). Lifetime prevalence of mental disorders in US adolescents: Results from the National Comorbidity Survey Replication–Adolescent Supplement (NCS-A). *Journal of the American Academy of Child and Adolescent Psychiatry, 49*(10), 980–989.

Meyers, R. J., & Wolfe, B. L. (2004). *Get your loved one sober: Alternatives to nagging, pleading, and threatening.* Center City, MN: Hazelden.

Mrazek, P. J., & Haggerty, R. J. (Eds.). (1994). *Reducing risks for mental disorders: Frontiers for preventive intervention research.* Committee on Prevention of Mental Disorders, Division of Biobehavorial Sciences and Mental Disorders. Washington, DC: National Academy Press.

Myrick, H., Kranzler, H. R., Ciraulo, D. A., Saxon, A. J., & Jaffe, J. H. (2014). Medications for use in alcohol rehabilitation. In R. Ries, D. Fiellin, S. Miller, & R. Saitz (Eds.), *The ASAM principles of addiction medicine* (5th ed., pp. 713–726). Philadelphia, PA: Wolters Kluwer.

National Alliance on Mental Illness (NAMI). (2011). *How you can help: Become a member.* Retrieved from http://www.nami.org/Template.cfm?section=Take_Action

National Alliance on Mental Illness (NAMI). (2015). *A long road ahead: Achieving true parity in mental health and substance use care.* Arlington, VA: Author.

National Institute of Mental Health (NIMH). (n.d.). *Transforming the understanding and treatment of mental illnesses: What is prevalence?* Retrieved from http://www.nimh.nih.gov/health/statistics/prevalence/index.shtml

National Institute of Neurological Disorders and Stroke. (2015). *Asperger Syndrome fact sheet. (NIH Publication No. 13-5624).* Rockville, MD: Author. Retrieved from http://www.ninds.nih.gov/disorders/asperger/detail_asperger.htm

National Institute on Alcohol Abuse and Alcoholism (NIAAA). (2015a). *Helping patients who drink too much: A clinician's guide.* Retrieved from http://pubs.niaaa.nih.gov/publications/Practitioner/CliniciansGuide2005/clinicians_guide.htm

National Institute on Alcohol Abuse and Alcoholism (NIAAA). (2015b). *Rethinking drinking: Alcohol and your health.* Retrieved from http://pubs.niaaa.nih.gov/publications/RethinkingDrinking/Rethinking_Drinking.pdf

National Institute on Alcohol Abuse and Alcoholism (NIAAA). (2015c). *Alcohol screening and brief intervention for youth: A practitioner's guide.* Retrieved from http://pubs.niaaa.nih.gov/publications/Practitioner/YouthGuide/YouthGuide.pdf

National Institute on Drug Abuse. (2016). *National drug and alcohol facts week.* Retrieved from https://www.drugabuse.gov/news-events/public-education-projects/national-drug-alcohol-facts-week

Nicosia, N., Pacula, R. L., Kilmer, B., Lundberg, R., & Chiesa, J. (2009). *The economic cost of methamphetamine use in the United States, 2005* (No. MG-829-MPF/NIDA). Santa Monica, CA: RAND Health.

Occupational Safety & Health Administration (OSHA). (2015). *Guidelines for preventing workplace violence for healthcare and social service workers.* Retrieved from https://www.osha.gov/Publications/osha3148.pdf

Patel, V., Chisholm, D., Parikh, R., Charlson, F., Degenhardt, L., Dua, T., Ferrari, A., ... DCP MNS Author Group. (2015). Addressing the burden of mental, neurological, and substance use disorders: Key messages from Disease Control Priorities, 3rd edition. *Lancet, 387*(10028), 1672–1685. doi: 10.1016/S1040-6736(15)00390-6.

Peek, C. J., & National Integration Academy Council. (2013). *Lexicon for behavioral health and primary care integration: Concepts and definitions developed by expert consensus* (AHRQ Publication No. 13-IP001-EF). Rockville, MD: Agency for Healthcare Research and Quality.

Pike, K., Susser, E., Galea, S., & Pincus, H. (2013). Towards a healthier 2020: Advancing mental health as a global health priority. *Public Health Review, 35,* 1–23.

Polen, M. R., Whitlock, E. P., Wisdom, J. P., Nygren, P., & Bougatsos, C. (2008). *Screening in primary care settings for illicit drug use: Staged systematic review for the United States Preventive Services Task Force. Evidence Synthesis No. 58, Part 1.* (Prepared by the Oregon Evidence-based Practice Center under Contract No. 290-02-0024; AHRQ Publication No. 08-05108-EF-s). Rockville, MD: Agency for Healthcare Research and Quality.

Pratt, L. A. (2012). Characteristics of adults with serious mental illness in the United States household population in 2007. *Psychiatric Services, 63*(10), 1042–1046.

Ricci, B., & Dixon, L. (2015). What can we do about stigma? *Psychiatric Services, 66*(10), 1009–1009.

Rubinsky, A. D., Kivlahan, D. R., Volk, R. J., Maynard, C., & Bradley, K. A. (2010). Estimating risk of alcohol dependence using alcohol screening scores. *Drug and Alcohol Dependence, 108*(1), 29–36.

Rucklidge, J. J. (2010). Gender differences in attention-deficit/hyperactivity disorder. *Psychiatric Clinics of North America, 33*(2), 357–373.

Saitz, R. (2015). Commentary on Gelberg et al. 2015: Alcohol and other drug screening and brief intervention–evidence in crisis. *Addiction, 110*(11), 1791–1793.

Saitz, R., Cheng, D. M., Allensworth-Davies, D., Winter, M. R., & Smith, P. C. (2014). The ability of single screening questions for unhealthy alcohol and other drug use to identify substance dependence in primary care. *Journal of Studies on Alcohol and Drugs, 75*(1), 153–157.

Saunders, J. B., Aasland, O. G., Babor, T. F., De la Fuente, J. R., & Grant, M. (1993). Development of the alcohol use disorders identification test (AUDIT). WHO collaborative project on early detection of persons with harmful alcohol consumption-II. *Addiction, 88,* 791–791.

Savage, C., Dyehouse, J., & Marcus, M. (2014). Alcohol and health content in nursing baccalaureate degree curricula. *Journal of Addictions Nursing, 25*(1), 28–34.

Simon, V., Czobor, P., Bálint, S., Mészáros, Á., & Bitter, I. (2009). Prevalence and correlates of adult attention-deficit hyperactivity disorder: Meta-analysis. *British Journal of Psychiatry, 194*(3), 204–211.

Skinner, H. A. (1982). The drug abuse screening test. *Addictive Behaviors, 7*(4), 363–371.

Smith, J. E., & Meyers, R. J. (2007). *Motivating substance abusers to enter treatment: Working with family members.* New York, NY: Guilford Press.

Smith, P. C., Schmidt, S. M., Allensworth-Davies, D., & Saitz, R. (2009). Primary care validation of a single-question alcohol screening test. *Journal of General Internal Medicine, 24*(7), 783–788.

Smith, P. C., Schmidt, S. M., Allensworth-Davies, D., & Saitz, R. (2010). A single-question screening test for drug use in primary care. *Archives of Internal Medicine, 170*(13), 1155–1160.

Stahl, S. M. (2013). *Essential psychopharmacology. Neuroscientific basis and practical applications* (4th ed.). New York, NY: Cambridge University Press.

Stein, S. M., & Kosten, T. R. (2014). Pharmacologic interventions for opioid dependence. In R. Ries, D. Fiellin, S. Miller & R. Saitz (Eds.), *The ASAM principles of addiction medicine* (5th ed., pp. 735–758). Philadelphia, PA: Wolters Kluwer.

Strang, J., Babor, T., Caulkins, J., Fischer, B., Foxcroft, D., & Humphreys, K. (2012). Drug policy and the public good: Evidence for effective interventions. *The Lancet, 379*(9810), 71–83.

Substance Abuse and Mental Health Services Administration (SAMHSA). (2013a). *Behavioral Health, United States, 2012* (HHS Publication No. [SMA] 13-4797). Rockville, MD: Author.

Substance Abuse and Mental Health Services Administration (SAMHSA). (2013b). *SAMHSA opioid overdose prevention toolkit* (HHS Publication No. [SMA] 13-4742). Rockville, MD: Author.

Substance Abuse and Mental Health Services Administration (SAMHSA). (2014). *Results from the 2013 National Survey on Drug Use and Health: Summary of national findings (NSDUH Series H-48, HHS Publication No. [SMA] 14-4863).* Rockville, MD: Author.

Sullivan, E., & Fleming, M. (1997). *A guide to substance abuse services for primary care clinicians: Treatment Improvement Protocol (TIP) series 24.* Rockville, MD: DHHS Publication.

The President's New Freedom Commission on Mental Health. (2003). *Achieving the promise: Transforming mental health care in America.* Retrieved from http://www.nami.org/Template.cfm?Section=Policy&Template=/ContentManagement/ContentDisplay.cfm&ContentID=16699

Thomas, R., Sanders, S., Doust, J., Beller, E., & Glasziou, P. (2015). Prevalence of attention-deficit/hyperactivity disorder: A systematic review and meta-analysis. *Pediatrics, 135*(4), e994–e1001.

Townsend, M. C. (2015). *Psychiatric mental health nursing: Concepts of care in evidence-based practice* (8th ed.). Philadelphia, PA: F. A. Davis Company.

U.S. Department of Health and Human Services (USDHHS). (1999). *Mental health: A report of the surgeon general.* Substance Abuse and Mental Health Services Administration, Center for Mental Health Services, National Institutes of Health, National Institute of Mental Health. Rockville, MD: Author.

U.S. Department of Health and Human Services (USDHHS). (2016a). *HealthyPeople.gov: Substance abuse overview.* Retrieved from https://www.healthypeople.gov/2020/topics-objectives/topic/substance-abuse

U.S. Department of Health and Human Services (USDHHS). (2016b). *HealthyPeople.gov: 2020 topics and objectives.* Retrieved from http://www.healthypeople.gov/2020/topicsobjectives2020/default.aspx

U.S. Preventive Services Task Force (USPSTF). (2009). Counseling and interventions to prevent tobacco use and tobacco-caused disease in adults and pregnant women: U.S. Preventive Services Task Force reaffirmation recommendation statement. *Annals of Internal Medicine, 150*(8), 551–555.

U.S. Preventive Services Task Force (USPSTF). (2015). *Alcohol misuse: Screening and behavioral counseling interventions in primary care.* Retrieved from http://www.uspreventiveservicestaskforce.org/Page/Document/UpdateSummaryFinal/alcohol-misuse-screening-and-behavioral-counseling-interventions-in-primary-care

Viron, M., Bello, I., Freudenreich, O., & Shtasel, D. (2014). Characteristics of homeless adults with serious mental illness served by a state mental health transitional shelter. *Community Mental Health Journal, 50*(5), 560–565.

Walser, R. D., Garvert, D. W., Karlin, B. E., Trockel, M., Ryu, D. M., & Taylor, C. B. (2015). Effectiveness of acceptance and commitment therapy in treating depression and suicidal ideation in veterans. *Behaviour Research and Therapy, 74*, 25–31.

Walther, L., Bejczy, A., Löf, E., Hansson, T., Andersson, A., Guterstam, J., … Isaksson, A. (2015). Phosphatidylethanol is superior to carbohydrate-deficient transferrin and γ-glutamyltransferase as an alcohol marker and is a reliable estimate of alcohol consumption level. *Alcoholism: Clinical and Experimental Research, 39*(11), 2200–2208.

Wang, H., Dwyer-Lindgren, L., Lofgren, K. T., Rajaratnam, J. K., Marcus, J. R., Levin-Rector, A., … Murray, C. J. (2012). Age-specific and sex-specific mortality in 187 countries, 1970–2010: A systematic analysis for the Global Burden of Disease Study 2010. *The Lancet, 380*(9859), 2071–2094.

Warner, E., & Lorch, E. (2014). Laboratory diagnosis. In R. Ries, D. Fiellin, S. Miller, & R. Saitz (Eds.), *The ASAM principles of addiction medicine* (5th ed., pp. 332–343). Philadelphia, PA: Wolters Kluwer.

Weissman, M. M. (2015). The Institute of Medicine (IOM) sets a framework for evidence-based standards for psychotherapy. *Depression and Anxiety, 32*, 787–789.

Whiteford, H. A., Degenhardt, L., Rehm, J., Baxter, A. J., Ferrari, A. J., Erskine, H. E., … Vos, T. (2013). Global burden of disease attributable to mental and substance use disorders: Findings from the Global Burden of Disease Study 2010. *The Lancet, 382*(9904), 1575–1586.

Whitlock, E. P., Polen, M. R., Green, C. A., Orleans, T., & Klein, J. (2004). Behavioral counseling interventions in primary care to reduce risky/harmful alcohol use by adults: A summary of the evidence for the US Preventive Services Task Force. *Annals of Internal Medicine, 140*(7), 557–568.

World Health Organization (WHO). (2008). *The global burden of disease: 2004 update.* Geneva, Switzerland: Author.

World Health Organization (WHO). (2013). *Mental health action plan 2013–2020.* Retrieved from http://apps.who.int/iris/bitstream/10665/89966/1/9789241506021_eng.pdf?ua=1

World Health Organization (WHO). (2014). *Strengthening our response.* Retrieved from http://www.who.int/mediacentre/factsheets/fs220/en/#

Yarborough, B. J. H., Yarborough, M. T., Janoff, S. L., & Green, C. A. (2015). Getting by, getting back, and getting on: Matching mental health services to consumers' recovery goals. *Psychiatric Rehabilitation Journal, 39*, 97–104. http://dx.doi.org/10.1037/prj0000160

Yudko, E., Lozhkina, O., & Fouts, A. (2007). A comprehensive review of the psychometric properties of the Drug Abuse Screening Test. *Journal of Substance Abuse Treatment, 32*(2), 189–198.

Working with the Homeless

"We have come dangerously close to accepting the homeless situation as a problem that we just can't solve."

—Linda Lingle (1953), American Politician

KEY TERMS

Chronically homeless
Continuum of care
Deinstitutionalization
Doubled up

Homelessness
Housing first
Point-in-time counts
Period prevalence counts

Single room occupancy
  (SRO) housing
Survival sex
Trauma informed care (TIC)

Unaccompanied youth
Unsheltered (hidden)
  homeless

LEARNING OBJECTIVES

Upon mastery of this chapter, you should be able to:

- Define the concept of homelessness.
- Describe the demographic characteristics of the homeless living in the United States.
- Discuss factors predisposing persons to homelessness.
- Examine the effects of homelessness on health.
- Compare and contrast the unique challenges confronting selected subpopulations within the homeless community.
- Analyze the extent and adequacy of public and private resources to combat the problem of homelessness.
- Assess your beliefs and values toward homelessness.
- Propose community-based nursing interventions to facilitate primary, secondary, and tertiary prevention in addressing the problem of homelessness.

What was once considered unthinkable in a prosperous nation is now an expected occurrence in towns and cities across the United States. Drive through an inner city or suburban community on any given day, and you will see people on street corners holding signs "Hungry and homeless." Where is the public outcry in response to this scene? Has the American conscience been anesthetized to this form of human suffering? Or is the need simply too overwhelming and the problems too far reaching to mount an effective campaign to prevent such a tragedy?

The purpose of this chapter is to define the concept of homelessness, examine the factors contributing to homelessness, analyze the major issues confronting the homeless, and examine the role of the community health nurse in addressing the needs of the homeless.

The McKinney-Vento Homeless Assistance Act (Title 42 of the U.S. Code) defines as homeless a person who lacks a fixed, regular, adequate nightly residence including supervised public or private shelters that provide temporary accommodations. Homeless individuals may also reside in institutional settings providing temporary shelter or in public or private places that are not designed for or used as a regular sleeping accommodation for human beings (e.g., cars, parks, campgrounds). Incarcerated individuals are not considered homeless under this definition (McKinney-Vento Homeless Assistance Act, 1987).

The education subtitle of the McKinney-Vento Homeless Assistance Act expands on the definition of **homelessness** when addressing homeless children and youth. The Act includes as homeless those children who share housing with others because of economic hardship or loss of housing, are abandoned in hospitals, are awaiting placement in foster care, or are living in motels, trailer parks, or camping grounds (National Center for Homeless Education [NCHE], 2012).

The U.S. Department of Housing and Urban Development (USDHUD, 2015) defines homeless people as those living on the streets, in vehicles, in shelters or parks, and in transitional housing; unaccompanied youth and families with children are defined as homeless under other federal statutes. Although this definition may be appropriate for the urban homeless who are more likely to live on the street or in shelters, persons living in rural areas tend to cohabit with relatives or friends in overcrowded, substandard housing (American Institutes for Research [AIFR], 2014; Housing Assistance Council [HAC], 2014). Table 28–1 outlines selected *Healthy People 2020* goals that relate to the homeless population.

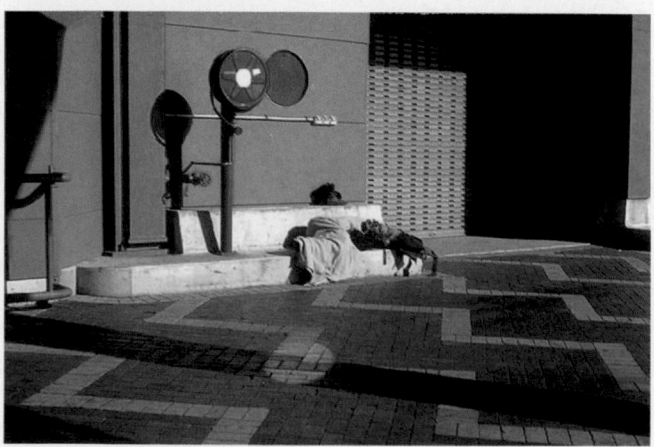

Homeless individuals often struggle to find shelter.

SCOPE OF THE PROBLEM

It is difficult to estimate the number of people who are homeless because homelessness is a temporary condition. Rather than trying to count the number of homeless people on a given night, or **point-in-time counts**, it may be more prudent to gauge the number of people who have been homeless over a longer time frame such as over the course of a year, or **period prevalence counts** (USDHUD, 2015; National Coalition for the Homeless [NCH], 2011a).

It is also difficult to locate and account for homeless people. Most estimates of homelessness are based on the number of people served in shelters or soup kitchens or the number of people who can easily be located on the streets. People who spend time at places that are difficult to reach (e.g., cars, campgrounds, caves, boxcars, wooded areas) are considered "**unsheltered**" or "**hidden**" **homeless**. Many people are unable to access shelters because of overcrowding and limited capacity. In rural areas, there are fewer housing options and resources for the homeless. As a result, people may be forced to live temporarily with friends or family (a practice known as "**doubling up**"). While still experiencing homelessness, these individuals are not always counted in homeless statistics or considered eligible for homeless services (AIFR, 2014; HAC, 2014; NCH, 2011a).

The USDHUD, in its *Annual Homeless Assessment Report to Congress*, publishes the latest counts of homelessness nationwide. In 2015, on a single night in January, there were an estimated 564,708 sheltered and unsheltered homeless people across the nation. Overall, the number of homeless decreased by 31% since 2007, with the number of people in unsheltered locations in 2015 at estimated at 30.6% and the number of homeless veterans decreasing by 1%. Nearly two thirds (64%) of homeless are individuals. The remaining one third (36%) comprised families with children (USDHUD, 2015). Because of the transient nature of homelessness and the difficulty involved in locating and counting the homeless, it

Table 28–1	Selected *Healthy People 2020* Objectives Related to Homelessness
MHMD-12	Increase the proportion of homeless adults with mental health problems who receive mental health services
HIV-23 (Developmental)	Reduce the proportion of persons with an HIV diagnosis receiving HIV services who were homeless or unstably housed in the 12-mo measurement period
Related Access to Care Objectives	
AHS-2 (Developmental)	Increase the proportion of insured persons with coverage for clinical preventive services
AHS-3	Increase the proportion of persons with a usual primary care provider
AHS-5	Increase the proportion of persons who have a specific source of ongoing care
AHS-6	Reduce the proportion of persons who are unable to obtain or delay in obtaining necessary medical care, dental care, or prescription medicines
AHS-7 (Developmental)	Increase the proportion of persons who receive appropriate evidence-based clinical preventive services
AHS-8 (Developmental)	Increase the proportion of persons who have access to rapidly responding prehospital emergency medical services
AHS-9.1 (Developmental)	Reduce the proportion of all hospital ED visits in which the wait time to see an ED clinician exceeds the recommended time frame

U.S. Department of Health & Human Services (USDHHS). (2016). *Healthy People 2020: Topics and objectives*. Retrieved from http://www.healthypeople.gov/2020/topicsobjectives2020/default

is unlikely that researchers will ever be able to estimate the exact magnitude of homelessness in America (NCH, 2011a).

There is a direct relationship between poverty and homelessness. In general, homelessness is decreasing due, in part, to the strides made over recent years to increase federal funding for homeless prevention and assistance programs. Funding for these federal programs is at its highest level in history. Despite improvements in employment and in the economy, however, those in poverty, living with friends and family, and paying over half their income for housing continue to be at risk for homelessness. Housing programs for the homeless have removed many homeless people from off the streets, but the lack of affordable housing continues to present formidable challenges to eliminating homelessness (National Alliance to End Homelessness [NAEH], 2014, 2015d).

In 2014, The U.S. Conference of Mayors Task Force on Hunger and Homelessness reported its survey findings of 25 cities across the nation. The survey revealed that, over the past year, the total number of homeless across the cities surveyed had increased by only 1%. The number of homeless families had increased by 3%. Lack of affordable housing, unemployment, poverty, and low-wage jobs contributed to the rise in homelessness among families (U.S. Conference of Mayors, 2014).

Demographics

Poverty is directly linked to homelessness. Demographic groups more likely to be poor are also at greater risk of becoming homeless.

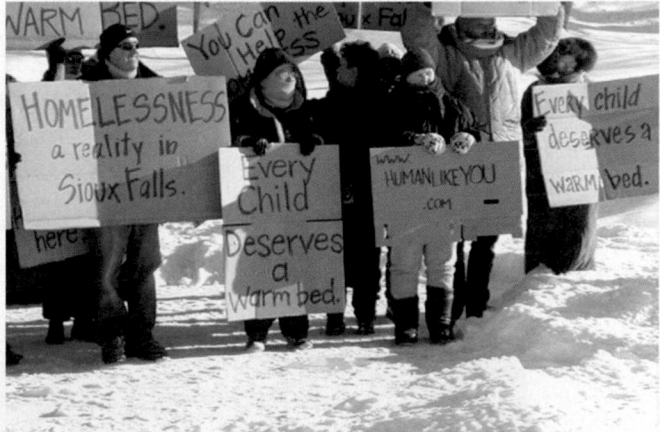

Raising awareness about homelessness is an important step in seeking community solutions.

Age

In 2015, 68% of all sheltered homeless persons were adults over 24. About 10% were between 18 and 24 and nearly 22.6% were under 18 years of age. Among the unsheltered homeless, 82.6% are over 24 and 7.7% are under 18 years of age (USDHUD, 2015).

Gender

The majority of homeless individuals are unaccompanied adult men. Single homeless adults are more likely to be male. Approximately 60% of sheltered homeless adults are men and 39.7% are women; about 2% identify as transgender (USDHUD, 2015).

Ethnicity

The racial and ethnic makeup of the homeless population varies based upon geographic location. Nationally, approximately 44.8% of the sheltered homeless are White, non-Hispanic, whereas approximately 45.9% are African American and 19.9% are Hispanic. African Americans represent the largest minority group in shelter situations, but among the unsheltered, that drops to 27.98%, whereas non-Hispanic Whites comprise 58.6% of the total and Hispanics remain steady at 20.1%. Five states have over 50% of the American homeless population, with 21% residing in California, 16% in New York, 6% in Florida, 4% in Texas, and 4% in Massachusetts (USDHUD, 2015). See Display 28–1.

Families

Families with children represented 36.5% of the homeless population in the United States in 2015. Approximately 60% of homeless people in families are children under 18 years of age. Nearly 9 in 10 homeless people in families reside in shelters. About 6% of homeless people in families are considered chronically homeless, but there were 2,308 fewer chronically homeless in 2015 than in 2014. The number of homeless people in families has declined by 12% since 2007 (USDHUD, 2015).

Although 60% of homeless families with children are made up of women or girls, the average homeless family household is comprised of three people. African American families with children represent 51% of sheltered families, and 55% of unsheltered families

are White. New York had 26% of the total homeless families with children population (also a 9% one-year increase), and California had 11% in 2015. During recessions and periods of economic decline, more two-parent families and families headed by single fathers are likely to become homeless. Because organizations serving homeless families are generally geared to serving single women with children, it may be difficult for intact families and families headed by men to access shelter (USDHUD, 2015).

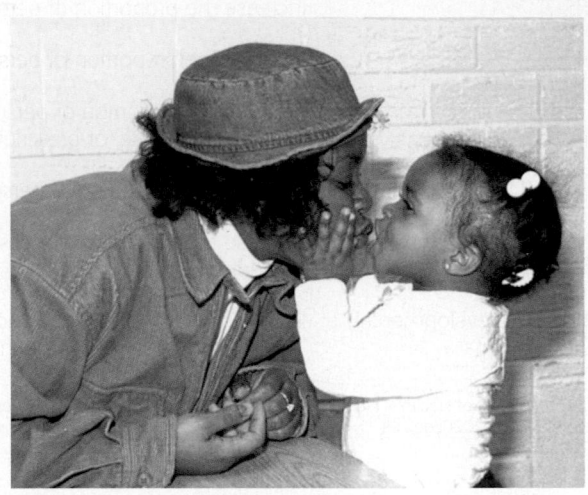

Over 36% of the U.S. homeless population in 2015 were families with children.

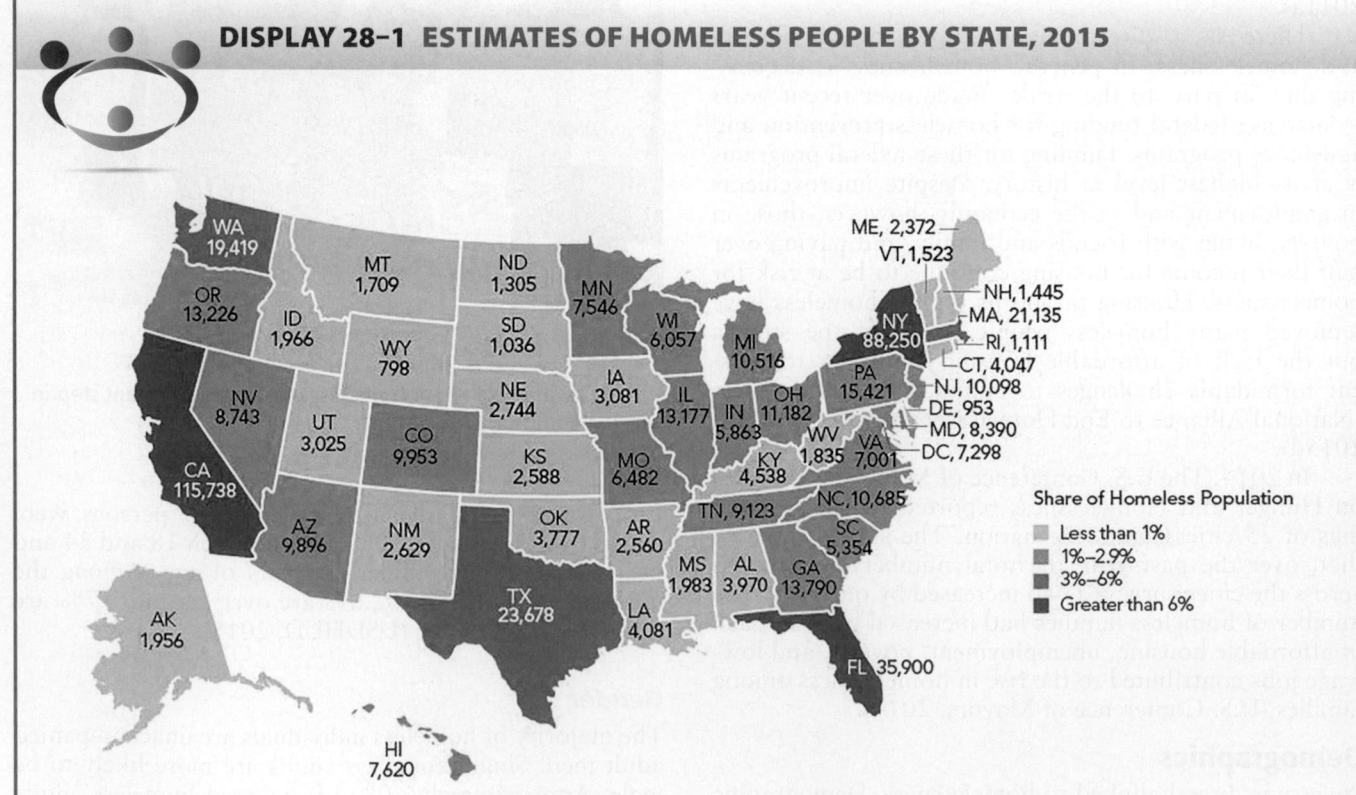

DISPLAY 28–1 ESTIMATES OF HOMELESS PEOPLE BY STATE, 2015

WA 19,419
OR 13,226
MT 1,709
ND 1,305
MN 7,546
ME, 2,372
VT, 1,523
ID 1,966
SD 1,036
WI 6,057
NH, 1,445
MA, 21,135
WY 798
IA 3,081
MI 10,516
NY 88,250
RI, 1,111
CT, 4,047
NV 8,743
NE 2,744
IL 13,177
IN 5,863
OH 11,182
PA 15,421
NJ, 10,098
DE, 953
UT 3,025
CO 9,953
KS 2,588
MO 6,482
KY 4,538
WV 1,835
VA 7,001
MD, 8,390
DC, 7,298
CA 115,738
AZ 9,896
NM 2,629
OK 3,777
AR 2,560
TN, 9,123
NC, 10,685
SC 5,354
MS 1,983
AL 3,970
GA 13,790
TX 23,678
LA 4,081
AK 1,956
FL 35,900
HI 7,620

Share of Homeless Population
- Less than 1%
- 1%–2.9%
- 3%–6%
- Greater than 6%

Retrieve from https://www.hudexchange.info/resources/documents/2015-AHAR-Part-1.pdf (p. 12).
Source: U.S. Department of Housing & Urban Development (USDHUD). (2015). *The 2015 annual homeless assessment report to Congress.* Retrieved from https://www.hudexchange.info/resources/documents/2015-AHAR-Part-1.pdf.

Contributing Factors

Persons are predisposed to homelessness because of a complex array of factors that result in individuals having to choose between necessities of daily living. Scarce resources limit choices. What would you do if you had to choose between eating and buying your child's medication? Housing consumes a huge portion of one's income and is often the first asset to be lost. Many families find they are only a paycheck away from homelessness. See What Do You Think?

Poverty

In 2013, more than 45 million people (or 14.5% of the U.S. population) were living in poverty. Approximately 20% of children under 18 live in poverty. Poverty rates are highest among single female head of households (DeNavas-Walt & Proctor, 2014). Factors impacting poverty include declining wages, loss of jobs that offer security and carry benefits, an increase in temporary and part-time employment, erosion of the true value of the minimum wage, a decline in manufacturing jobs in favor of lower-paying service jobs, globalization and outsourcing, and a decline in public assistance. As wages drop, the potential to secure adequate housing diminishes (NCH, 2011b).

Compounding the problem is a lack of affordable housing—particularly **single room occupancy (SRO) housing** (or housing units intended to be occupied by one person)

and limited funding for housing assistance. For example, a household seeking to rent a two-bedroom apartment in Florida is estimated to need to earn an average of at least $19.35 per hour; in California, it is estimated at $25.65 per hour (National Low Income Housing Coalition, 2016). An interactive map of all 50 states is available at http://www.nlihc.org/oor. This figure for Florida is more than two times the federal minimum wage of $7.25, and it is over three times that for the California estimate. A family of four with one full-time minimum-wage earner is 17% below the poverty line. In his 2014 State of the Union Address, President Barrack Obama asked Congress to raise the minimum wage to $10.10 an hour (White House, 2014). Some politicians and business owners have also supported this idea (Correa, 2016). But, it remains unchanged at $7.25, although 29 states and the District of Columbia (D.C.) have higher minimum-wage levels (the highest is $10.50 in D.C.). Two states (Georgia and Wyoming) have lower minimum rates of $5.15 per hour (United States Department of Labor, 2016).

When rental costs increase and the number of available low-rent units decline, the housing gap widens. Moreover, federal support for housing assistance is unable to keep pace with the high demand for housing. As a result, many persons must pay high rents to obtain shelter. This situation leads to overcrowding and substandard housing.

Because the demand for housing assistance exceeds federal housing assistance resources, there are often long waiting lists. Wait lists may close when demand for housing exceeds the supply of subsidized units available for occupancy (NCH, 2014; USDHUD, n.d.).

Lack of Affordable Health Care

In the absence of affordable health care coverage, a serious illness or disability can lead to job loss, savings depletion, and even eviction. Nearly half of individuals experiencing homelessness in the United States suffer from substance abuse disorders (United States Interagency Council on Homelessness [USICH], 2013d). One third of sheltered homeless persons have a chronic substance abuse issue, and over one quarter report a severe mental illness (U.S. Conference of Mayors, 2014).

In 2013, 42 million Americans (13.4% of the population) were without health care coverage (Smith & Medalia, 2014). Individuals with income levels below the poverty line comprise 27% of the uninsured population. The Affordable Care Act has expanded Medicaid coverage to millions of previously uninsured people and has provided tax credits to other low-income individuals, making health care more affordable for many low-income families (Kaiser Family Foundation, 2014).

The uninsured are less likely to receive preventive care or care for chronic health conditions. They are more at risk for preventable hospitalizations and missed diagnoses. Nearly half of all bankruptcies in the United States are due, in part, to medical debts (Kaiser Family Foundation, 2014). Those who are able to qualify for medical assistance may be reluctant to seek employment, fearing termination of benefits. Many others have limited insurance coverage that requires higher co-pays or deductibles and does not cover major catastrophic illnesses. A catastrophic adverse health event can plunge one into a homeless condition. See Chapter 6 for more on health care economics and insurance coverage.

What do *you* think?

Many of us ask why there are so many homeless, and why they choose not to use shelters. Richard Tripp, an author who was formerly among the homeless population, gives these reasons: (a) lack of beds/overcrowding (most places require you to stand in line for hours each day in order to secure a space at night; if you have a job, you can't always get in line early enough for a bed), (b) contagious illnesses (e.g., bedbugs, tuberculosis, hepatitis) are common and those who are contagious cannot be given separate quarters, (c) having your shoes stolen (theft is not an uncommon thing in shelters; good-fitting shoes are vital to survival), (d) not being allowed to bring your pet dog or cat with you (most shelters do not permit pets, so many homeless individuals choose to sleep outside with their animals), (e) exclusion of those using alcohol or drugs (even though, in some shelters, drug dealers are active), (f) some faith-based shelters compel their clients to listen to religious messages or sermons (this may conflict with their own beliefs, or they may feel coerced).

1. What do you think might be other reasons an individual would choose to sleep outside rather than in a homeless shelter?
2. How could some of these issues be effectively addressed?
3. How does your city address these issues and the overall problem of homelessness?

Adapted from Tripp, R. *Ten reasons the homeless would rather freeze than go to a shelter*. Retrieved from http://www.coppinc.com.

In a study of 300 homeless people at a day shelter, nurse researchers found 43% of them describing a serious and/or chronic health problem and 53% a significant mental health problem. Almost half revealed having a substance abuse disorder. Those with more serious health problems had some insurance and perceived better access to health care than those without insurance. This access, however, was less than they expected, and a longer duration of homelessness was associated with having insurance. They called for more research and better-matched services for this vulnerable population (Weber, Thompson, Schmiege, Peifer, & Farrell, 2013).

Employment

Low-income wage earners may hold jobs with nonstandard work arrangements. Temporary employees, day laborers, independent contractors, and part-time employees are examples of work arrangements that tend to pay lower wages, offer little or no benefits, and have less job security. For persons with little or no job skills, it is virtually impossible to compete for jobs that offer a living wage. Barriers to employment among the homeless include lack of education and job skills; lack of transportation, daycare, or other supportive services; lack of access to technology; and disabilities that make it difficult to pursue or retain employment. To overcome homelessness and maintain employment, one must not only obtain a job that pays a living wage but must also have access to supportive services such as child care and transportation (NCH, 2012c).

Domestic Violence

Domestic violence is a major cause of homelessness among women. For victims of domestic violence, the choice is often between living in an abusive situation or leaving and facing life on the streets. Those living on the streets face assaults and rape and often seek to appear invisible in order to evade this (Colorado Coalition for the Homeless, 2012). Fifteen percent of homeless adults in cities surveyed by the U.S. Conference of Mayors were victims of domestic violence (U.S. Conference of Mayors, 2014). Victims of domestic violence are often isolated from social support networks and financial resources, rendering them especially vulnerable. They may lack a steady income or a stable employment record and often suffer from anxiety, depression, panic disorder, or substance abuse disorders. Women who are victims of domestic violence may lack the resources needed to become independent and escape an abusive environment. A major challenge facing homeless service providers of domestic violence victims is the need to ensure a safe and secure environment and to protect client confidentiality (NAEH, 2015a).

Mental Illness

The U.S. Conference of Mayors (2014) estimates that, among its 25 cities surveyed across the nation, severe mental illness is reported by 28% of homeless adults. **Deinstitutionalization** (being released from institutions into the community), limited access to services, difficulty carrying out essential activities of daily living, and difficulty maintaining stable relationships contribute to the number of severely mentally ill persons represented in the homeless population (NCH, 2012m).

Poor mental health adversely affects an individual's ability to make sound judgments, solve problems effectively, and make wise decisions. Persons with mental illness may neglect to take the necessary precautions to avoid or reduce their risk of illness. Some mentally ill persons self-medicate their disturbing symptoms using street drugs, placing them at increased risk of addictions and diseases transmitted through injection drug use. Mental illness and substance abuse are often comorbid conditions that, coupled with poor physical health, make it especially difficult to secure employment and safe, affordable housing (NCH, 2012m).

Addictions Disorders

Rates of alcohol and drug abuse are disproportionately high among the homeless. Nearly half of all individuals experiencing homelessness and 70% of homeless veterans have substance abuse disorders (USICH, 2013d). One study of Skid Row homeless in Los Angeles found marijuana, crack, and alcohol to be the most frequently used substances (Rhoades et al., 2011). This makes it more difficult for them to access shelters that require abstinence for admission (Donley & Wright, 2012; USICH, 2013d).

For persons already at risk for homelessness, the behaviors associated with an addictive disorder can create instability and jeopardize family and employment support nets. The combination of substance abuse, job loss, and family breakdown often results in homelessness, especially if social support or government assistance/programs are not available. This may be further complicated with someone having little education or job skills and criminal justice system incarceration (Mago et al., 2013). Once homeless, persons may resort to drugs or alcohol to dull the pain of being homeless and ease the feelings of hopelessness that accompany such a desperate state. They may also turn to chemical substances in an attempt to self-medicate the disturbing symptoms of an untreated mental illness. Approximately half of all mentally ill homeless individuals have co-occurring substance abuse disorders (USICH, 2013d).

Although some homeless individuals may desire treatment to overcome their addictions, they often encounter obstacles that undermine their recovery and prevent them from obtaining the treatment they need. Limited access to care and lack of community resources make it difficult if not impossible to receive the services needed to achieve a successful recovery. Many shelters require sobriety to access services (USICH, 2013d). There may be long waiting lists for addictions treatment, and homeless people who do not have a phone and are difficult to locate may be dropped from the waiting list. Lack of transportation and lack of documentation needed to access programs (i.e., birth certificates, social security cards) further exacerbate the problem. Denial of Supplemental Security Income (SSI) or Social Security Disability Insurance (SSDI) to persons with substance abuse–related disabilities creates a huge barrier to achieving recovery support, proper medical care, and housing and income assistance. Moreover, the federal programs targeting homelessness, mental health, and addictions services lack the extent of funding necessary to exert an impact that could effectively address this problem on a national level (NCH, 2012o).

Additional Variables

Additional variables impacting homelessness include personal or financial crisis, natural disasters, or personal choice. For example, natural disasters may displace previously independent and self-sufficient individuals and families, rendering many homeless and in need of emergency shelter (Davidson, 2013). See more on disasters and their aftermath in Chapter 17.

Homeless Subpopulations

Although many of the struggles facing the homeless are universal, there are subpopulations within the homeless community that are uniquely vulnerable. Often, these groups face additional burdens because of their special needs and challenges.

Homeless Men

Approximately 63% of sheltered homeless adults are men (USDHUD, 2014). The majority of homeless men are single adults. Homeless men are more likely to be employed than their homeless female counterparts. However, they usually hold temporary, low-wage jobs that offer little security. They are also more likely than homeless women to have uncontrolled substance abuse issues (NCH, 2012o).

Some men find themselves in a cycle of intermittent homelessness as they move back and forth between prisons, treatment centers, shelters, temporary housing, and the streets. Other men are at risk for becoming **chronically homeless**. A chronically homeless adult is someone who has been homeless for long periods of time or has experienced repeated episodes of homelessness. These individuals have a diagnosed disability such as mental illness, substance abuse, or a chronic medical condition and have been homeless for at least a year or have experienced at least four episodes of homelessness in the past 3 years. Fifteen percent of the homeless population in the United States are chronically homeless (NAEH, 2015b). In 2015, the *Annual Homeless Assessment Report* to Congress recorded over 83,170 chronically homeless individuals in its point-in-time count (a 31% decline since 2007). Almost two thirds of these individuals were unsheltered or characterized as living on the street or in places not fit for human habitation (USDHUD, 2015).

Homeless men are more likely to be treated with disdain than other homeless subgroups. Some people perceive the homeless male as largely to blame for his plight, believing that he is able bodied and should be able to work. Moreover, homeless men may not suffer from disabilities severe enough to warrant eligibility for health and social services. Often health and social programs give priority to women and children, and there are estimates of 84% of the hidden homeless being males (Chalabi, 2013).

Homeless Women

Women, as single parents, lead most homeless families in the United States. About 90% of those women have experienced a minimum of one severely stressful traumatic event; for many of them, this began during childhood (AIFR, 2014). Domestic violence is a major cause of homelessness among women. Lack of affordable housing forces many women to choose between living in an abusive home and facing an uncertain life on the streets. Domestic violence victims often have poor credit and employment records because of the disruption caused by family violence. If violence is discovered in the home, landlords may evict tenants, forcing the family onto the streets (NCH, 2012a). They often have few job skills that lead to

low-paying often only intermittent jobs, inadequate child care, and limited social supports; this was exacerbated during and immediately following the economic downturns of great recession (AIFR, 2014). See Population-Focus. Once homeless and on the street, a woman faces the risk of greater abuse. Moreover, the potential for exposure to violence and sexual assault on the streets increases the risk for sexually transmitted infections and traumatic injuries (Colorado Coalition for the Homeless, 2012).

Homeless Children

One in every 30 children (2.5 million) in the United States are homeless, an increase of nearly 8% nationally. Poverty, lack of affordable housing, domestic violence, economic recession impacts, the challenges of being a parent, and racial disparities contribute to the growing trend in family homelessness (AIFR, 2014). Nearly half of all homeless children in the United States are under 6 years of age (National Center on Family Homelessness [NCFH], 2014). Unaccompanied homeless children and youth are more likely to be unsheltered than unaccompanied youth with 51% of **unaccompanied youth** under age 18 residing in unsheltered locations (USDHUD, 2015). These children are living in places that are dangerous and often difficult to access by service providers.

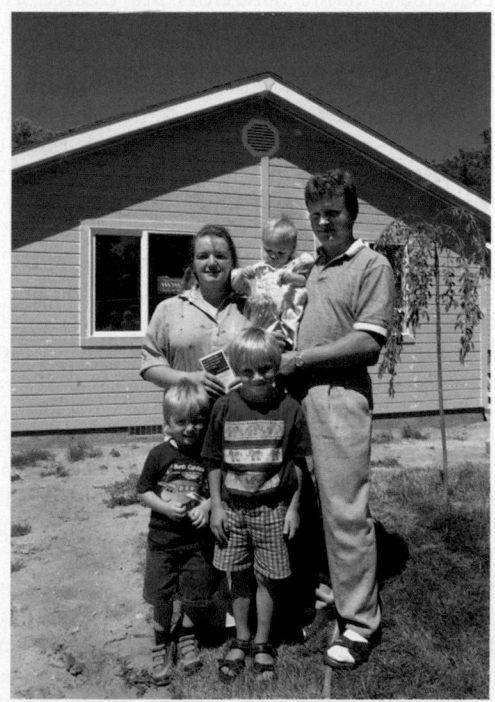

Lack of affordable housing, poverty, domestic violence, and the recent economic recession are factors leading to homelessness, especially increased numbers of homeless children.

The majority of homeless children and youth live in shelters, share housing with friends or relatives, or live in motels or campgrounds. Over 96% of homeless children under age 18 live in families (USDHUD, 2015). It is estimated that about 75% of homeless children and their families live with relatives or friends, "doubled up," especially in rural areas; they are often missed in surveys of the homeless (AIFR, 2014). When compared to their housed counterparts, homeless children are more

POPULATION-FOCUS
TENT CITIES AND SOLUTIONS FOR THE HOMELESS

After the Great Recession of 2007 to 2008, tent cities began springing up across many larger cities in the United States, some of them with mutually determined codes of conduct and social structures. These temporary communities were a similar phenomenon to the shantytowns of the Great Depression, and some cities responded with police action to clear them out or with legislation making it illegal for homeless to congregate in large numbers (Herring, 2015; National Law Center on Homelessness & Poverty [NLCHP], 2014). Cities have sometimes also sought means of controlling food sharing with the needy/homeless by passing laws to restrict the use of public property or to force agencies to meet stringent food–safety regulations (NLCHP, 2014; Stoops, 2014).

Imagine a world where it is illegal to sit down. Could you survive if there were no place you were allowed to fall asleep, store your belongings, or to stand still? Homeless people, like all people, must engage in activities such as sleeping or sitting down in order to survive. Yet in communities across the nation, these harmless, unavoidable behaviors are treated as criminal activity under laws that criminalize homelessness (NLCHP, 2014, p. 7).

The NCH, in its most recent report (2010), researched several of these large tent cities in an effort to better understand the problems facing this vulnerable population. In a good-sized tent city in Sacramento, California (n = 97), they found that a majority of the inhabitants were individuals (63%), and 37% were families. Three quarters of them were males, 23% were female, and 2% were transgender individuals. Most were between the ages of 35 and 45, and 65% had been homeless for over a year. Fifty-five percent of them had disabilities of some sort (e.g., problems walking, schizophrenia/other mental illness, PTSD, COPD, hepatitis C, back injuries), and 24% had been to an emergency room within the last 6 months. Three fourths of them had no insurance, and 19% were veterans. About 45% of them had some type of benefit income (24% general assistance/welfare, 11% SSI, 10% other).

When asked about willingness to go into an overflow winter shelter, only 33% said that they would do so. Of the majority who would not, 30% indicated an interest if the shelter provided some private space for couples or individuals, 22% were interested if there was some type of outdoor activity or open recreational space, 21% were agreeable if they were given more sleep time, and others wanted places to store their belongings or kennel their pets overnight. Sixty-five percent were willing to be sheltered if they could be placed on a waiting list for more permanent housing within a 2 to 3 month period, and 22% expressed an interest in alcohol/drug recovery housing. Reasons for not wanting to be placed in a homeless shelter included no pets allowed, not being able to make the 3 pm deadline for beds, no private showers/privacy/comfort/strict rules, no freedom/too many people, couples are unable to stay together, problem with transportation, no wheelchair access, and having to wake up too early every morning.

In California, tent cities in Sacramento, Fresno, Albany, and Ontario have been cleared out and demolished. But, in Seattle, Washington, two tent cities located in church parking lots have been maintained for a decade. Austin, Texas, put large tents, microhomes, and RVs on 27 acres of donated land and rents them at a low cost. This project also features communal garden, bees, chickens, and an outdoor cinema (Herring, 2015). Salt Lake City, Utah, established a goal to end homelessness in 10 years time. Their Housing First project has led to a 91% decrease in the city's homeless population. Even the most difficult, chronically homeless have been placed in affordable housing. One example is a 54-year-old chronically homeless man, who has lived outside for 5 or more years and who presently lives in a wooded area near a freeway. He calls it his "park" and has created a "fence" surrounding his makeshift tent. He became homeless after a back injury and has problems with alcohol and drug use and reports having had a stroke. Outreach workers say he has few remaining teeth and his speech is difficult to understand. He is now getting housing through the Housing First program and does not have to demonstrate sobriety before qualifying. He will pay either 30% of his income or $50/month (depending on which is greater). Because estimated annual costs to government (e.g., emergency room visits, incarceration) are between $30,000 and $50,000/person annually, the state saw an opportunity to help the homeless and more responsibility deal with government budgets. Although there is still limited housing in the state, each week, homeless people are placed in housing and supported by visits with outreach workers. So far, it seems to be working (McEvers, 2016).

1. Have you seen tent cities like this? What were your resultant feelings and emotions?
2. What do you think could be done to address some of the issues raised by the homeless population in this tent city? Debate the issue with classmates.
3. How could PHNs be involved in helping to design feasible population-focused interventions?

Herring, C. (2015, December). *Tent City, America*. Retrieved from https://placesjournal.org/article/tent-city-america/

McEvers, K. (2016, February 1). *Utah reduced chronic homelessness by 91 percent: Here's how*. Retrieved from http://www.npr.org/2015/12/10/459100751/utah-reduced-chronic-homelessness-by-91-percent-heres-how

National Coalition for the Homeless. (2010, March). *Tent cities in America: A Pacific Coast report*. Retrieved from http://nationalhomeless.org/wp-content/uploads/2014/06/Tent-Cities-Report-FINAL-3-10-10.pdf

National Law Center on Homelessness & Poverty (NLCHP). (2014). *No safe place: The criminalization of homelessness in U. S. cities*. Retrieved from https://www.nlchp.org/documents/No_Safe_Place

Stoops, M. (Ed.). (October, 2014). *Food-sharing report: the criminalization of efforts to feed people in need*. Washington, DC: National Coalition for the Homeless.

likely to become ill, to go hungry, and to suffer from emotional and behavioral disorders. They are also more likely to experience developmental delays and to suffer from learning disabilities. Children in homeless families are more likely to experience parental separation, either by being placed in foster care or by being placed in the care of friends or relatives. More than 25% of homeless children have witnessed violent acts (Child Trends Data Bank, 2015; NAEH, 2015b; NCFH, 2015). The effect of traumatic stress among homeless families experiencing domestic violence leads to depression, fear, and aggressive and antisocial behavior (NCH, 2012o; NCFH, 2011).

Education is compromised when one is homeless. Homeless children are more than twice as likely to repeat grades in school as other children and are more likely to drop out or be suspended or expelled (Child Trends Data Bank, 2015). During the 2011 to 2012 academic year, over 1.1 million school-age children and adolescents were enrolled in U.S. schools (NLCHP, 2014). Barriers to education include transportation to and from the shelter, lack of academic and medical records required for registration, unstable living arrangements necessitating multiple moves, and urgent needs for food and shelter that take priority over education (NCH, 2012b).

Homeless children are more likely to get sick than other children. Although acute and chronic health problems are more severe in homeless children, these children are less able to access medical and dental care. Asthma, hyperactivity/inattention disorders, and behavioral problems are more prevalent in homeless children than in the general population (Child Trends Data Bank, 2015). See Chapter 22 for more on school-aged children and adolescent.

Homeless Youth

The exact numbers of homeless youth is elusive. McKinney-Vento data are only collected on children and adolescents present in schools (AIFR, 2014). Factors contributing to youth homelessness include physical and sexual abuse, family addiction, parental neglect, strained relationships, or family financial crises that lead to family separation because of inadequate shelter, housing, or child welfare resources. Foster care placement is associated with homelessness among youth. Moreover, some youth who are discharged from residential or foster care with inadequate housing or income support end up homeless (NCH, 2012k). A study conducted in the Southwestern United States examined youth perceptions of barriers and facilitators to use of homeless shelters. Ha, Narendorf, Santa Maria, and Bezette-Flores (2015, p. 25) found attitude and access barriers (e.g., shame, pride, adverse staff attitudes, "restrictive shelter rules," and other adverse conditions). Facilitators included supportive staff/others, shelters' reaching out to other services to assist them, and having a particular condition (e.g., pregnancy). Further, an examination of homeless youth's experience with primary care services in Australia found that a variety of approaches to delivery of care and available services were accessed and that street-based clinics, which were linked to case management and counseling services, had the most impact on substance abuse and mental health outcomes for this population (Dawson & Jackson, 2013). Barriers included poor attitudes of health care providers, lack of knowledge about services, unwelcoming environments,

and costs of care. The researchers highlighted the need for public health nurses to collaborate with community and social workers in order to better serve this population.

Homeless adolescents may have difficulty accessing emergency shelters because of shelter policies that prohibit older youth from the facility or because of a lack of bed space. Because of lack of education or job training skills, many resort to prostitution or **survival sex** (exchanging sex for food, shelter, or other basic necessities). As a result, homeless youth are at higher risk for HIV, hepatitis, and sexually transmitted infections. Homeless youth also suffer disproportionately from anxiety, depression, malnutrition, conduct disorders, posttraumatic stress, and low self-esteem (NCH, 2012k).

It is not uncommon for homeless youths to be arrested for running away, breaking curfews, or being without supervision. As young people age out of the foster care system, they find themselves on the street with inadequate support systems and little opportunity for housing or employment (NCHE, 2012).

Homeless Families

Poverty and the lack of affordable housing place families at risk of becoming homeless. Declining wages, changes in welfare programs, unstable employment, domestic violence, substance abuse, and a struggling economy have all contributed to the rise in family homelessness.

Homelessness often breaks up the family unit. Families may be separated by shelter policies that prohibit admission to older boys or men. Sometimes, parents are forced to leave their children with family or friends or to place them in foster care to shelter them from becoming homeless (Child Trends Data Bank, 2015; NCH, 2012h). One North Carolina study of homeless shelter policies found that most shelters mandated that children be kept under constant supervision by parents, and many required random alcohol and drug testing, along with set bedtimes for children and sometimes for adults. No input from homeless residents was sought in policy setting, and their feelings of empowerment and self-esteem are most likely further diminished in shelters without any type of shared governance (Spriggs, 2013).

A child is at greater risk for homelessness if his father becomes injured or ill, experiences a job loss, has a substance abuse issue, or becomes involved with the criminal justice system. Fifty percent of fathers of homeless children are unemployed, and 43% have problems with drugs or alcohol. Homeless children are at a high risk of being placed in foster care, and a personal history of foster care predicts family homelessness during adulthood. To assist homeless families, attention must be focused on promoting affordable housing; supporting education, job training, and child care for parents; promoting access to school; expanding violence prevention and treatment services; and preventing unnecessary separation of families (NCFH, 2014; NCH, 2012h).

Homeless Veterans

According to the *2015 Annual Assessment Report to Congress*, 11% of homeless adults were veterans, and 34% of them were in unsheltered locations compared to 28% of total homeless adults. Over 90% of homeless veterans are males, and there were 4% fewer homeless veterans than in the previous year (USDHUD, 2015). In 2009, the U.S. Department of Veterans Affairs established a goal to end homelessness by 2015. Targeted funding of veteran assistance programs such as the HUD-VA supportive housing program, which provides permanent housing and treatment services to homeless veterans, along with programs funding community-based transitional housing and supportive services to low-income veterans have helped to reduce the rate of homelessness among the veteran population. Larger numbers of younger veterans of the Iraq and Afghanistan wars and projected cuts in defense spending, however, create new challenges for combating homelessness among veterans (U.S. Conference of Mayors, 2014).

Female homeless veterans represent 9% of the homeless veteran population (USDHUD, 2015). They are more likely to be married and have serious psychiatric illnesses but less likely to be employed or have addiction disorders than their homeless male counterparts. There is no difference in rates of mental illness or addictions between veteran and nonveteran homeless women (NCH, 2012j). See Perspectives.

The U.S. Department of Veteran Affairs (VA) administers programs that provide long-term care, emergency shelter, 2-year transitional housing, group homes, and work therapy for homeless veterans. These programs provide case management, residential treatment, and other services to homeless veterans and improve housing, employment, and access to care for the homeless veteran population. Unfortunately, the programs are often unable to keep pace with existing needs (NCH, 2012j).

The Rural Homeless

Homeless people in rural areas are more likely to be working families who are homeless for the first time. They are less likely to be on government assistance programs. Because there are fewer shelters in rural areas, they are also less likely to live in shelters or in the streets, and more likely to live in cars, substandard housing, or "doubled up" with friends and family. As a result, they may not be considered "homeless" for reporting purposes. Higher rates of homelessness may be found in rural areas than in large cities (AIFR, 2014). Moreover, the communities in which they live may not be able to access as much federal funding, because the statistics do not adequately reflect the magnitude of the problem. Families with single mothers and children comprise the largest segment of the rural homeless population. Native Americans and migrant workers are more likely to be among the rural homeless. Like urban homelessness, rural homelessness is largely a result of poverty and lack of affordable housing. Although housing costs are lower in rural areas, incomes are also lower (National Advisory Committee on Rural Health and Human Services, 2014; NCH, 2012n).

Homelessness in rural areas may be precipitated by structural or physical housing problems that force families to relocate to safer, but more expensive, housing. In addition, the lack of job opportunities, the distance between low-income housing and job sites, the lack of transportation, rising rents, geographic isolation, and lack of resources compound the problem. To address the needs of the rural homeless, the definition of homelessness needs to be expanded to include people living in temporary or substandard housing (NCH, 2012n).

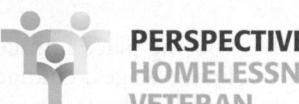

PERSPECTIVES
HOMELESSNESS FOR ONE FEMALE VETERAN

I am a female veteran, recently discharged from active duty service during which I was deployed to Iraq. I am now homeless. I am one of thousands of veterans who sleep on the streets of America every night. I did not know that I was at risk for homelessness when I joined the military; in fact, I thought a military career or enlistment would help me be successful in life. I did not know that women veterans are three to four times more likely to become homeless than nonveteran women. Or, that posttraumatic stress disorder (PTSD) is twice as likely to be diagnosed in women as in men. Considering that 14% of all deployed military personnel to Iraq and Afghanistan are women, I guess I should have known this was a possibility for me. But, I was not prepared for what happened to me. I am also a victim of sexual trauma, which is a trigger for PTSD, and this has profoundly impacted my ability to return to a normal life as a veteran. Now, I never feel safe and I am not able to trust anyone or anything. I am afraid to fall asleep in a shelter, and I am frightened to fall asleep in my car. I am exhausted, both from the constant fear and anxiety, as well as from the seemingly impossible effort it takes to obtain the basic resources necessary to survive. I know you look at me and wonder why I am in this position. I am sure that you don't understand why I do not seem to be able to change my situation. Believe me, I have tried.

Sarah, Veteran

1. *What resources are available in the community for homeless female veterans?*
2. *Are there barriers to accessing these resources for certain veterans?*
3. *What are some of the common assumptions and stereotypes circulating in your community about homeless veterans?*
4. *What would you want to include in your assessment in order to identify risks and to implement treatment planning for homeless veterans like Sarah?*
5. *In the above example, what health issues and risks might be critical for this homeless female veteran?*

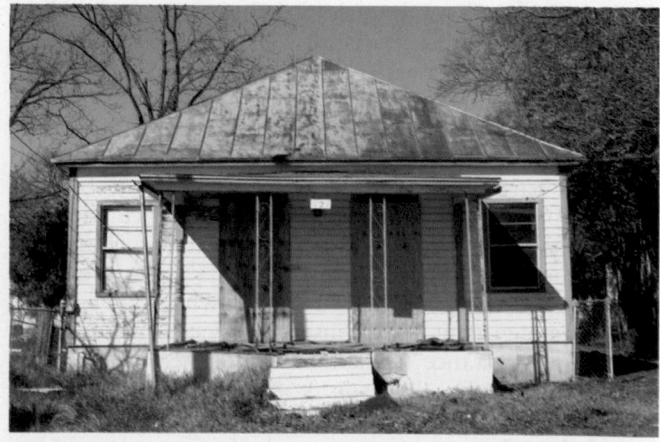

Rural housing may be structurally unsound or substandard.

The Older Homeless

Only 3.5% of sheltered homeless individuals were 62 or over in 2013 (USDHUD, 2014). Although the percentage of elderly individuals in shelters is low, it has increased over recent years from just over 4% in 2007 to over 5% in 2013 (USDHUD, 2014). The percentage of individuals aged 51 to 61 who are housed in shelters also increased from nearly 19% in 2007 to 25% in 2013 (USDHUD, 2014). It is expected to continue to rise, from 44,172 in 2010 to 58,772 in 2020—a 33% increase. And, the average age of sheltered individual homeless has been rising (National Health Care for the Homeless Council [NHCHC], 2013).

Two pathways for homelessness among the elderly have been identified. One is that chronically homeless individuals are an aging population and may be coming off the streets into shelters as their health further deteriorates, thus leading to increased numbers. Secondly, newly homeless individuals, who have never experienced housing issues, are now finding themselves without housing because of poverty, excessive cost of housing, job loss, and problems with physical health as well as mental health issues. In some cases, loss of social support systems is instrumental (NHCHC, 2013). Many older people live on a fixed income, and this restricted income renders them more vulnerable to unexpected financial crisis and even homelessness. Isolation also contributes to homelessness. Many older people live alone and lack a support network. Some researchers define the "older homeless" as homeless persons 50 and older because of the declining physical health that accompanies street living (NCH, 2012i). Because of health issues and homelessness, they may use emergency departments (EDs) more often. Brown and Steinman (2013) found that about one third of visits to the ED by homeless individuals were for those over age 50, and these individuals often came by ambulance and were admitted. Alcohol use in the elderly homeless population is not uncommon, but drug abuse is less common than in the general homeless population (NHCHC, 2013). Because older persons tend to distrust crowds at shelters and clinics, they are more likely to stay on the streets. They are prone to criminal victimization and suffer from a variety of health conditions including chronic diseases and functional disabilities. The Social Security benefits to which many are entitled are inadequate to cover housing costs. They may also encounter difficulties applying for benefits (NCH, 2012i). Planning for end-of-life care is very difficult with this population, but providing one-on-one counseling and assistance in this area has been helpful in completing advance directives (NHCHC, 2013).

Lesbian, Gay, Bisexual, Transgender Homeless

Lesbian, gay, bisexual, and transgender (LGBT) persons often struggle to locate shelters that accept them. They are sometimes required to identify themselves as a particular gender. Transgender individuals may be turned away from shelters or subjected to physical, sexual, or verbal abuse. It is estimated that 20% of homeless youth are LGBT, although some cities have noted rates of LGB youth to range from 12% to 35% and possibly 7% identifying as transgender. These youth are over seven times more likely to experience sexual violence. They also commit suicide at much higher rates than their heterosexual homeless counterparts, with some estimates as high as 62% versus 29% for those who identify as heterosexual youth. Shelter staff may not be trained in working with the LGBT population, and discrimination does occur (NAEH, 2016; NCH, 2012l). Ream and Forge (2014) describe their work with homeless LGBT youth in New York City and the oft-cited narratives of being thrown out of their homes by family who could not accept their LGBT lifestyles, struggling on the streets with sex work and hard drug use, the risks of HIV/AIDS, and suicide. However, they note that this does not reflect the majority of this population and that "trauma, discrimination in foster care and shelters, structural barriers to exiting homelessness, and emerging adult development" are the more common issues (p. 7). LGBT-specific shelters and transitional living programs are needed for this vulnerable population, but even though they are present there, not enough capacity exists to serve all who need these services.

HEALTH CARE AND THE HOMELESS

Homeless persons are three to four times more likely to die prematurely than their housed counterparts (NHCHC, 2011a). Acute and chronic health problems are prevalent among the homeless population. Chronic health conditions such as HIV/AIDS, diabetes, hypertension, addictions, and mental disorders require ongoing monitoring and are often difficult to treat in a population that is transient and lacks stable housing (NHCHC, 2015; NCH, 2012f). It is difficult for the homeless to adhere to complex treatment regimens. For example, where would a homeless person find a refrigerator to store insulin? Where would someone keep supplies for dressings? How could someone with no access to transportation keep regular appointments with health care providers? How does a homeless person keep track of multiple appointment dates? How is a shelter resident that is receiving the typical shelter diet high in carbohydrates, fats, and sodium able to adhere to a low-salt or diabetic diet? Where can a homeless person receive home health care if they are not allowed to stay in shelters during the day?

Many homeless people expend their time and energy trying to meet basic survival needs. Health care may take a back seat to finding food, clothing, or shelter. High cost and limited access to health care, as well as negative experiences with the health care system, can also result in avoidance or delays in seeking treatment (NCH, 2012f; NHCHC, 2011a). However, a large-scale study of 1,163 homeless adults demonstrated that their self-reports of visits to ambulatory care clinics, EDs, and hospitalizations are "quite accurate," especially visits to the ED and when they are hospitalized (Hwang, Chambers, & Katic, 2016, p. 282).

Frost bite, leg ulcers, and upper respiratory tract infections result from chronic exposure to adverse environmental conditions. The homeless are also at higher risk of trauma and criminal victimization including muggings, beatings, and rape. When one is homeless, it is difficult to maintain adequate nutrition or personal hygiene or to have access to basic first aid (NCH, 2012f, 2012g, 2012e). Communicable diseases such as TB,

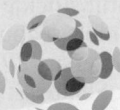

EVIDENCE-BASED PRACTICE

How do we engage homeless persons to use primary care services and to keep their medical appointments? McInnes et al. (2014) conducted a pilot study to determine the feasibility and cost-effectiveness of using mobile phone text messaging among homeless veterans frequenting an urban Veteran's Administration (VA) medical center. A purposive sample of 21 homeless individuals who owned a mobile phone and were knowledgeable in text messaging was obtained. Surveys were completed prior to and following the 8-week text messaging intervention. A semistructured interview was conducted following the intervention to evaluate the usefulness of texting as a communication device for enhancing medical appointment adherence. Patients received monetary incentives (store vouchers) for completing the surveys and participating in the interviews. The effectiveness of the intervention was determined by comparing the cost of transmitting text messages to the cost of patient cancellations, no show appointments, and ED visits.

The study found that participants reported high levels of satisfaction with the text messaging system.

Appointment cancellations were reduced by 30% and no shows were reduced by 19%. There was a statistically significant reduction in ED visits post intervention and a borderline significant reduction in hospitalizations. The potential cost savings to the entire VA system, assuming the program was implemented on a national level, was $2.3 to $115.7 million.

What creative outreach approaches might the CHN develop to improve medical appointment adherence and reduce unnecessary and costly ED visits? What new technologies or communication devices might be used to enhance outreach efforts? How can creative approaches be used to improve, not only health care delivery, but the delivery of other supportive services? How might the CHN use research evidence to make a case for funding technologies that enhance communication and service delivery in the homeless population?

McInnes, D., Petrakis, A., Gifford, A., Rao, S., & Houston, T. (2014). Retaining homeless veterans in outpatient care: A pilot study of mobile phone text message appointment reminders. *American Journal of Public Health*, 104(54), s588–s594.

HIV, hepatitis, and other infections threaten not only the homeless but also the public in general.

Poverty, substance abuse, poor nutrition, and coexisting medical and psychiatric illnesses also predispose the homeless to severe oral health problems. Persons with poor access to dental treatment and preventive services have higher rates of oral disease. Poor oral health is also associated with lower levels of education and income (USDHHS, 2016). A national study of homeless adult health care needs revealed 41% requiring dental health care (Baggett, O'Connell, Singer, & Rigotti, 2010). A study of 120 homeless families found that almost half of the children had dental caries and that 43% of those families were able to get dental care when shelter-based care was provided (DiMarco, Ludington, & Menke, 2010). In an evaluation of Health Care for the Homeless programs, homeless participants reported that their dental care treatment needs were being met, and this was similar among those who were not homeless (Zur & Jones, 2014).

Persons with HIV/AIDS are at higher risk of homelessness, because HIV-related illness can impact job stability. Moreover, health care costs associated with treating the illness can exact an enormous financial burden on a low-income family. Insufficient funds to adequately house the poor with HIV/AIDS may also contribute to homelessness among HIV-infected individuals. Substance abuse and sexual exploitation among the homeless increase the risk of HIV infection. Moreover, it is difficult to maintain adherence to complex HIV/AIDS medication regimens without access to good food, bathrooms, refrigeration, and clean water (NCH, 2012g).

Health Care for the Homeless is a model for homeless health care developed through a 19-city demonstration project funded by the Robert Wood Johnson Foundation and the Pew Memorial Trust. In 1987,

federal legislation (the McKinney Homeless Assistance Act) was passed that authorized federal funding for these programs. Grants are awarded to community-based organizations that deliver high-quality health care to homeless populations. Health Care for the Homeless projects can be found across the nation to address significant gaps in health care delivery for this vulnerable group in society (NHCHC, 2011b). In one study of a comparison of unmet needs among homeless and nonhomeless populations receiving care at Health Care for the Homeless programs, homeless patients reported similar rates of both medical and dental care treatment needs being met. However, they were significantly more likely to have an unmet need for mental health counseling than nonhomeless counterparts; and they had fewer problems accessing treatment for substance use disorders. Zur and Jones (2014) concluded that these programs should continue to have funding and should increase their capacity and the scope of their services. See Evidence-Based Practice.

RESOURCES TO COMBAT HOMELESSNESS

Both public and private sectors have promoted a variety of initiatives to address the problem of homelessness. These initiatives are intended to impact homelessness on the local, state, and national level and to insure a coordinated, comprehensive, and systematic approach to addressing the problem of homelessness.

Public Sector

The McKinney-Vento Homeless Assistance Act (PL100-77) was the first and only major piece of federal legislation intended to address the problem of homelessness on a national level. This landmark legislation act, passed by Congress in 1987, originally consisted of 15 programs to address the major, pressing needs of the homeless. These needs included emergency shelter, transitional housing, job training, primary health care, education, and housing (National Association for the Education of Homeless Children and Youth, 2015; NCH, 2006). The current act has been amended four times in an effort to expand its scope and strengthen its impact. In particular, the amendments made to the act in 1990 represented significant milestones in advocating for the needs of the homeless. These amendments included the creation of the Shelter Care Plus program, which provided for housing assistance for persons with disabilities, mental illness, AIDS, and drug and alcohol addiction. Another amendment created a demonstration program within the Health Care for the Homeless program to provide primary care and outreach to at-risk and homeless children. In addition, the Community Mental Health Services Program was amended and retitled: the Projects for Assistance in Transition from Homelessness (PATH). Finally, the amendments made in 1990 strengthened access to public education for homeless children and youth. For example, states were required to provide grant funding to local educational institutions to insure access to a free, appropriate education for homeless youth and children (National Association for the Education of Homeless Children and Youth, 2015; NCH, 2006).

Over the years, congress has appropriated funding to enable implementation of this federal legislation. The extent of federal funding has fluctuated over the years. In recent years, some of the programs have been repealed or restructured in an effort to contain costs. Although homeless advocates acknowledge that the act was an important step in addressing homelessness, the lack of adequate funding over recent years threatens its impact on a national level. Moreover, some homeless advocates feel that the legislation focuses more on emergency measures to address the crisis of homelessness rather than on promoting a proactive agenda to address the causes of homelessness, such as lack of good paying jobs with benefits and the lack of access to affordable health care (Homeless Hub, 2015; NCH, 2006). In Massachusetts, the number of homeless families increased 71% between 2007 and 2012. Short-term rental subsidy vouchers were developed to meet the needs of this population. After 2 years of vouchers along with supportive services to assist families in maintaining their rental homes without further subsidies, it was found that only one quarter were able to do so. Twenty percent moved in with friends/family members, 21.8% obtained a permanent housing subsidy, 23.6% were lost to follow-up, and 9% returned to homeless shelters, highlighting the need for more permanent solutions such as timelier integration of support services and "targeted workforce development" (Meschede & Chaganti, 2015, p. 85).

The USDHUD oversees a number of programs that provide supportive housing for elderly, low-income, and disabled persons. The department also funds programs to build, buy, or rehabilitate affordable housing units for rent or ownership (NCH, 2012d). In many communities, housing is based on a **continuum of care** model where programs are developed to assist persons to transition from emergency to transitional to permanent housing. Emergency shelters provide temporary overnight shelter,

whereas transitional housing provides up to 24 months of housing and supportive services. Rapid rehousing programs provide short-term rental assistance and supportive services, whereas permanent housing provides long-term housing and supportive services (USDHUD, 2013, 2016). In recent years, a **Housing First** philosophy has guided much of the publicly funded housing initiatives (NAEH, 2015c). In a Housing First approach, housing is viewed as an immediate priority. The goal of Housing First is to end homelessness by providing stable, permanent housing as soon as possible and to provide supportive services to enable people to maintain their housing (NAEH, 2015e; USICH, 2013c). Housing or supportive services are not contingent upon adherence to rigid rules or policies or to the maintenance of sobriety (USICH, 2013c). See the previous feature on tent cities and successful approaches to Housing First.

The Homeless Emergency Assistance and Rapid Transition to Housing (HEARTH) Act of 2009 increased funding for McKinney-Vento programs, which provide emergency, transitional, and permanent housing and supportive services to the homeless and provide resources to local school districts to coordinate services for homeless children (NCFH, 2014). On March 23, 2010, President Barak Obama signed federal health care reform legislation into law that extends health insurance coverage and gives states the option to expand Medicaid coverage to low-income individuals regardless of disability or family status. This legislation enables homeless individuals in many states to secure health care coverage (USICH, 2013b). See Chapter 6.

Another significant milestone in federal initiatives to reduce homelessness occurred when the federal government adopted the goal of ending chronic homelessness in 10 years. To meet this goal, annual funding was appropriated to create new permanent supportive housing. These resources helped to stimulate the production of housing. Many communities followed the lead of the federal government and developed their own 10-year plans (Burt, 2006; McEvers, 2016). In 2010, the U.S. Interagency Council on Homelessness published the nation's first comprehensive federal strategic plan to prevent and end homelessness. The document, entitled *Opening Doors*, outlined a comprehensive and ambitious plan aimed at eliminating homelessness on a national level. The goals of the plan included ending chronic homelessness in 10 years; preventing and ending homelessness for families, youth, and children in 10 years; preventing and ending homelessness among veterans in 5 years; and establishing a path to end all types of homelessness (USICH, 2010).

Table 28–2 summarizes the nine titles of the McKinney-Vento Act.

Table 28–3 presents selected federally sponsored programs for addressing the needs of the homeless.

Private Sector

The private sector has made a concerted effort to organize communities in the battle against homelessness by forming coalitions, alliances, and memberships that champion the causes of the homeless. These organized efforts are carried out at the national, state, and local

Table 28-2 McKinney-Vento Homeless Assistance Act Titles I to IX

Title I	Statement of findings by congress and definition of homelessness
Title II	Establishes the Interagency Council on Homelessness, a council comprised of 15 heads of federal agencies to address the needs of homeless populations
Title III	Authorizes the Emergency Food and Shelter Program, administered by the Federal Emergency Management Agency (FEMA)
Title IV	Authorizes the emergency shelter and transitional housing programs administered by the Department of Housing and Urban Development (HUD) including the Emergency Shelter Grant Program, the Supportive Housing Demonstration Program, Supplemental Assistance for Facilities to Assist the Homeless, and Section 8 Single Room Occupancy Moderate Rehabilitation
Title V	Requires federal agencies to make available federal land and buildings for states and local governments to use to assist the homeless
Title VI	Authorizes programs to provide health care services to the homeless, including Health Care for the Homeless program, Community Mental Health Services Block Grant Program, and two demonstration programs providing substance abuse and mental health treatment services to the homeless
Title VII	Authorizes the Adult Education for the Homeless Program, the Education of Homeless Children and Youth Program (administered by the Department of Education), the Job Training for the Homeless Demonstration Program (administered by the Department of Labor), and the Emergency Community Services Homeless Grant Program (administered by the Department of Health and Human Services)
Title VIII	Amends the Food Stamp Program to facilitate access by the homeless and expands the Temporary Emergency Food Assistance Program (administered by the Department of Agriculture)
Title IX	Extends the Veterans Job Training Act

Source: National Coalition for the Homeless. (2006). *McKinney-Vento Act*. Retrieved from http://www.nationalhomeless.org/publications/facts/McKinney.pdf

Table 28-3 Federally Sponsored Programs for the Homeless

The U.S. Interagency Council on Homelessness	The U.S. Interagency Council on Homelessness coordinates the federal response to homelessness and creates a national partnership with public and private sectors to reduce and end homelessness in the United States. The Council is responsible for reviewing the effectiveness of federal initiatives and programs to assist the homeless, promoting better coordination of services between programs, and informing state and local governments and private sector organizations about sources of federal homeless assistance (USICH, 2013a).
Substance Abuse and Mental Health Services Administration	The Center for Mental Health Services, a center of the federal Substance Abuse and Mental Health Services Administration (SAMHSA), supports states in facilitating access to mental health services and supports outreach and case management for the homeless mentally ill (SAMHSA, 2014).
Center for Mental Health Services	The Center for Mental Health Services operates the Homelessness Resource Center, which provides resource information and information on the latest research and best practices for addressing the problem of homelessness (SAMHSA, n.d.a, SAMHSA, n.d.b).
Projects for Assistance in Transition from Homelessness (PATH)	PATH is a grant program created under the McKinney Act to provide treatment and supportive services to persons with severe mental illnesses, including those who are homeless or at risk of becoming homeless. The grants support outreach, mental health and substance abuse treatment, and rehabilitation for the severely mentally ill (SAMHSA, 2004).
Health Care for the Homeless (HCH)	The HCH program (a provision of the McKinney Act) awards grants to community-based organizations that seek to provide quality, accessible health care to the homeless. The HCH program is administered by the U.S. Department of Health and Human Services (USDHHS). HCH projects are required to provide primary health care, substance abuse services, emergency care, outreach, and housing assistance. Many HCH projects also provide dental care, mental health treatment, supportive housing, and other services (NCH, 2012f).
The U.S. Department of Housing and Urban Development (HUD)	HUD provides funding for supportive housing for low-income families as well as low-income individuals with disabilities and low-income elderly. Funds can be used for housing development or rental assistance (to cover the difference between what a resident can afford to pay and the cost to operate the project). Grants are also provided to public housing agencies to rehabilitate or replace dilapidated public housing structures. Persons applying for public housing face a long waiting period, sometimes up to as long as 10 y (NCH, 2012d).
The White House Office of Faith-Based and Neighborhood Partnerships	The White House Office of Faith-Based and Neighborhood Partnerships promotes partnerships with faith-based and community organizations to more effectively serve individuals, families, and communities in need. This office provides information on federal grants that are available to faith-based and community organizations to address the needs of the homeless (USDHHS, 2014).

Table 28–4 Private Sector Initiatives to Combat Homelessness

National Coalition for the Homeless (NCH)	The National Coalition for the Homeless is the nation's oldest advocacy and direct service organization for the homeless. The coalition is comprised of a national network of people who are currently experiencing or who have experienced homelessness, activists and advocates, community-based and faith-based service providers, and others who are interested in its mission. The mission of the coalition is to prevent and end homelessness while ensuring the immediate needs of the homeless are men and their civil rights protected. See http://nationalhomeless.org.
The National Center on Family Homelessness (NCFH)	The National Center on Family Homelessness seeks to prevent and end family homelessness by advancing knowledge gained from research, programs, trainings, and collaborations with homeless shelter and service providers. The organization seeks to raise awareness of the causes and effects of homelessness and to inform local, state, and national solutions for the problem of homelessness. See http://www.family homelessness.org.
National Coalition for Homeless Veterans	The National Coalition for Homeless Veterans is a 501(c)(3) nonprofit organization that provides resource and technical assistance to service providers and local, state, and federal agencies that provide assistance to homeless veterans. The coalition advocates for the needs of homeless veterans and for increased funding for federal homeless veteran assistance programs. See http://www.nchv.org.
National Alliance to End Homelessness (NAEH)	The National Alliance to End Homelessness seeks to end homelessness by advocating for policies that promote solutions to homelessness, providing technical assistance to local communities, and advancing data and research on best practices and solutions for combating homelessness. See http://www.endhomelessness.org.
Commission on Homelessness and Poverty, American Bar Association	This commission is committed to educating the public and the legal community about the issue of poverty and homelessness and trains members of the legal community on how best to advocate for those in need. The commission also advocates for public policies that protect and provide for the needs of the poor and homeless. See http://www.americanbar.org/groups/public_services/homelessness_poverty/about_us.html.
National Low-Income Housing Coalition	The National Low-Income Housing Coalition is dedicated to establishing housing stability and expanding the supply of low income housing in America. A major priority of the coalition is to promote public policy that provides funding for housing for extremely low-income people. See http://www.nlihc.org.

level to positively impact the problem of homelessness in communities across the nation. Table 28–4 presents a list and description of selected resources in the private sector to combat homelessness.

ROLE OF THE COMMUNITY HEALTH NURSE

Community health nurses maintain a long tradition of providing care to vulnerable populations and play a vital role in addressing the health needs of the homeless. Settings for care include shelters, clinics, soup kitchens, churches, community centers, social service agencies, and even the streets.

Trust is an essential ingredient in the development of a therapeutic relationship with the homeless. A caring, consistent relationship is more likely to engage people who are homeless and get them into treatment. It is sometimes difficult to establish trust with clients who have experienced negative encounters with the health care system. Often, limited resources, inadequate access to care, or prejudicial views can intensify these negative emotions. As with other vulnerable populations, the homeless struggle with feelings of powerlessness, loss of control, and low self-esteem. Victim blaming is common. Some members of society perceive the homeless as responsible

for their own fate. It is not uncommon to hear people speak about the homeless in derogatory terms or to suggest that the solution to the problem of homelessness is to simply "get a job."

Behaviors that would ordinarily be considered lawful in the privacy of one's home become criminal activity when they are exhibited in public. For example, the homeless can be arrested for loitering, sleeping, urinating, or drinking alcohol in public. These behaviors can trigger a criminal record, thereby, jeopardizing future employment or housing opportunities (NLCHP, 2014). In all 50 states, men may be incarcerated for failing to pay child support (Carmon, 2015). Consider a man who is laid off from a low-wage job. He is unable to pay child support and is arrested. His violation generates a criminal record and compromises his ability to secure employment in the future. He becomes trapped in a cycle of poverty and homelessness that is difficult to escape.

To effectively address the multifaceted problems associated with homelessness, a comprehensive and holistic approach is needed. As such, the community health nurse is responsible for implementing primary, secondary, and tertiary preventive measures to prevent homelessness or to assist those who are homeless to obtain needed services. See Using the Nursing Process.

USING THE NURSING PROCESS

Sheila Hendricks, a public health nurse for the Manchester City Health Department, and her colleagues were brainstorming ideas for how to reach the growing population of homeless women and children in their jurisdiction. They arranged a meeting with the director of a local rescue mission in the area. The mission provided emergency shelter to 100 homeless women and children each night. The women were allowed to remain at the shelter for 30 days provided they actively sought employment, social services, or educational opportunities. Families typically left during the day to seek jobs or other forms of assistance and returned in the evening for shelter. The community health nurses negotiated with the rescue mission to establish an on-site nursing clinic twice a week that would provide health education, screenings, and referrals on a drop in basis. The hours of clinic operation were 4 PM to 8 PM to accommodate client schedules.

Assessment

After the clinic was in operation for 2 weeks, the following priority health issues began to emerge:

Inadequate maternal and child nutrition

Lack of primary health care services for women and children (i.e., immunizations, screenings, treatment for upper respiratory tract infections, dermatological problems, asthma, hypertension)

Depression

High rate of reported sexually transmitted infections and HIV because of history of violence, survival sex, and injection drug use

Untreated addiction disorders

Plan

The following diagnoses were developed (in order of priority):

Impaired access to health and social services related to lack of insurance, scarce community-based resources, and lack of transportation

Ineffective family coping related to untreated addictions, mental health issues, and history of intimate partner violence

At risk for injury related to untreated addictions and mental health disorders, history of intimate partner violence, and hazards of street life

Altered nutrition less than body requirements related to lack of resources to purchase nutritious foods, addictions disorders, and chronic health issues

After assessing priority needs and establishing relevant diagnoses, the nurses developed a plan of care for this population. The priority goal was to promote access to care by linking clients to essential health and social services. The rationale for establishing this goal as a top priority was that if clients were able to access needed services, the other diagnoses could potentially be addressed (i.e., need for counseling, health care, housing, education).

Implementation

A nurse practitioner was engaged from the health department to provide primary care services to the women and children at the shelter including screening and treatment for sexually transmitted infections and treatment of common acute and chronic health conditions. Conditions requiring more extensive follow-up were referred to the local federally funded Health Care for the Homeless clinic. A social worker from the local social service agency was recruited to visit the mission on a monthly basis to assist clients to apply for housing and public assistance programs. Clients were referred to the local community mental health center for counseling related to addictions and violence issues. The nurses conducted health education programs and one-on-one counseling on topics such as parenting, coping, healthy eating, basic hygiene, and safety. They also offered health screenings for blood pressure, diabetes, HIV, and tuberculosis and provided referrals to the health department clinic for cancer screenings (i.e., mammograms, colorectal screening).

Evaluation

After the clinic had been in operation for 90 days, preliminary evaluation data revealed the following:

Sixty-five women and 28 children had frequented the clinic over the past 3 months. All 65 women received health promotion teaching and a resource packet for further reference.

Eighty percent of clients who required referrals to outside agencies were successful in accessing care.

Twenty-five women and 15 children were under the care of the nurse practitioner for acute or chronic health conditions.

Ten cases of latent TB infection were identified through TB testing, and these clients were referred to the City Health Department TB clinic for follow-up treatment.

Seven abnormal PAP smears were identified, and eight clients were diagnosed with sexually transmitted infections.

Fifteen clients were found to be HIV positive. Clients with positive screenings were referred to the City Health Department or the local Health Care for the Homeless Clinic where treatment was initiated.

Forty women applied for social service benefits. Most of these clients are still awaiting the receipt of benefits.

Primary Prevention

Primary prevention includes advocating for affordable housing, employment opportunities, and better access to health care to prevent the downward spiral into homelessness. Strategies for preventing homelessness may include financial counseling to assist clients to better manage their money; assistance in locating sources of legal or financial aid to prevent eviction, such as loans or grants for emergency funds to help pay for rent and utilities; and assistance in accessing social services and temporary housing or health care to avoid a housing, health, or family crisis (Anderson & McFarlane, 2015; NLCHP, 2014).

What do *you* think?

Every nurse encounters new situations with prior assumptions, biases, and preunderstandings. When considering work with the homeless, it is important to clarify one's own beliefs and values about poverty, homelessness, addictions, and mental disorders. What has been your experience with the homeless? Have you ever observed a homeless individual asking for money or holding up signs at a busy intersection? What thoughts and feelings do encounters such as these provoke? Have you ever volunteered at a soup kitchen or food pantry, fed a group of homeless people, or donated food or clothing? Have you had the opportunity to get to know a homeless individual? Do you have a personal experience with homelessness or poverty? If so, how has it affected your understanding of what it means to be poor or homeless?

It may be helpful to interview people who work with the homeless or to visit clinics, shelters, or other settings where the homeless congregate or access services. How are homeless people treated? What is a typical day like for someone who is homeless? How often do homeless persons hear their names? How often are they looked in the eye when addressed by others? How often are they touched in a way that is therapeutic, respectful, and affirming? By reflecting on your personal values and by allowing yourself to get closer to the people and places that are a part of the experience of homelessness, you will gain a deeper understanding of the homeless condition and be better equipped to serve those suffering from homelessness.

Health education that addresses primary prevention may focus on positive parenting skills, violence prevention, anger management, coping skills, healthy eating, or principles of basic hygiene. Immunization programs will help to prevent communicable disease in this high-risk population. Counseling victims of intimate partner violence and helping them to locate safe shelter can also aid in the prevention of homelessness (Anderson & McFarlane, 2015). Addictions treatment

is also important to prevent the likely consequences of untreated addiction (e.g., death, incarceration, institutionalization, homelessness).

Secondary Prevention

The focus of secondary prevention measures is on the early detection and treatment of adverse health conditions. This requires a thorough assessment of client needs including the need for housing, health care, education,

PERSPECTIVES
A PHN'S HOLISTIC APPROACH TO HOMELESSNESS

I got a referral from our communicable disease coordinator, regarding a homeless client with a lesion on his lower leg (wound botulism). I quickly learned that he had a long history of drug abuse, suicide attempts (13 known), and repeated hospitalizations for this wound. He was discharged from the hospital each time because he had no insurance, and he was also misdiagnosed. I finally located him living on a friend's property in a disheveled travel trailer with a leaky roof and broken windows. It was a rainy week, during the winter months, and he and his small dog were trying to keep warm and dry. He used the oven for heat and a nearby field as his bathroom. His only relatives lived out of state, and he dumpster dived for food. He ate food from expired cans, when he could find them. He knew about the local food lunch program and health care at our county clinic, but he was seldom able to utilize these services, because of lack of transportation and difficulties with ambulation related to his leg wound.

As a PHN, your view of the patient is holistic and goes beyond the diagnosis. My PHN partner and I did the following:

- *Reviewed his wound care.*
- *Assisted him in getting his medication, with money from the local Coordinating Council and Ministerial Association.*

- *Referred his case to two churches who provided him with assistance from their food pantries and a Pizza Hut gift card for his birthday (to cheer him up).*
- *Obtained tarps for his trailer, and a sleeping bag from a local service group.*
- *Assisted him with a disability application.*
- *Connected him to a mobile mental health unit that we are assigned to weekly for mental health assessment and drug diversion; we also updated his immunizations.*
- *After the final diagnosis from the CDC was confirmed, we arranged for transport to another hospital for treatment, as the patient refused to go back to the original hospital that had misdiagnosed him and kept discharging him.*

I remember that after I graduated with my BSN, someone asked me why I was leaving the recovery room to go into public health nursing. At that time, I told the person "I didn't want my varicose veins popping out of my support hose before I retired." But, I love public health nursing and am so glad that I made this choice. And, as I am planning my retirement, I can truly say, "It's been quite a ride"!

Susan, District PHN

PERSPECTIVES
A NURSE'S VIEWPOINT ON WORKING WITH THE HOMELESS

When I first decided to visit the homeless men's shelter, I was scared to death. Here I was, a veteran nurse with over 20 years experience in community health, and I was afraid. But, I thought to myself—afraid of what? I couldn't tell you. I suppose I harbored the stereotypes and negative images that most of us associate with homeless addicts. I remember passing this shelter years ago, looking out at the men hanging out on the street corner, and thinking to myself "Please God, don't let my car break down!" I remember thinking "I would never step foot in a place like that."

Well, I believe God has a sense of humor. He was equipping me for a work I could not have ever imagined. My views about homelessness were challenged to the core when I peered into the faces of those men, heard their stories, and began to feel their pain. Theirs were stories of broken lives and lost hope but also of courage in the

face of suffering and the will to survive in the midst of great adversity. These men were as diverse as their stories. They were from all walks of life. They possessed incredible gifts and talents. They were musicians, artisans, businessmen, writers, and poets. They had families who loved them and families who left them. Left because they could not continue to watch them die a little each day and be destroyed themselves in the process.

So here I am. Doing what I can to bring hope and healing. The irony is I came to bring hope and yet I am the one who is being healed. Healed in the broken areas of my life. Healed in my narrow view of life and my internal prejudices. I am so grateful to God for giving me this unique opportunity. It is a great privilege to serve these men.

Rita, age 42

---

social services, and employment. Clients will also benefit from secondary prevention measures such as screening for communicable and chronic diseases (e.g., hepatitis, TB, STI, HIV, hypertension, diabetes, cancer).

Barriers to accessing services and the extent of community resources available to the homeless also need to be assessed (Anderson & McFarlane, 2015; NLCHP, 2014; Zur & Jones, 2014). Resources such as shelters, soup kitchens, medical clinics, social service agencies, and supportive housing should be readily accessible to the homeless population. Hauff and Secor-Turner (2014) interviewed staff from shelters and health services serving

a homeless population. Shelter staff was most concerned with barriers to appropriate care, health need/problems, and lack of medical respite/support services. Health service providers echoed those concerns to some degree with health needs/barriers to management of care, discharge planning issues, and the need for support/respite services. The researchers described the need for better training of health service providers about the homeless and cultural competencies. They also noted the need for training in **Trauma-Informed Care (TIC)**, a homeless service delivery model that recognizes the traumatic experience of homelessness as well as some of the traumatic events

---

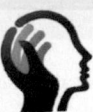

From the Case Files

Faith-Based Outreach

As a faith community nurse working in a large church congregation, you are invited to develop an outreach program to minister to the needs of an inner-city mission that is receiving financial support from the church. You begin by visiting the mission to conduct a needs assessment of its residents and to identify priority health issues. The shelter operates as a faith-based, nonprofit organization and is dedicated to serving the needs of homeless men with addictions. The shelter provides emergency overnight services and operates a 1-year residential faith-based addictions recovery program. Approximately 300 homeless male addicts frequent the shelter daily. Staff and residents have expressed concerns regarding a recent outbreak of boils among residents.

Assessment data reveal the following issues:

Approximately 80% of clients have a history of injection drug use.

Clients sleep in dormitory-style accommodations and share bathroom facilities.

An on-site barbershop operated by the residents provides haircuts for a nominal fee.

Clients have access to a small recreational area with donated exercise equipment.

Laundry services are available and residents take their clothing to the laundry on alternative days where it is washed. Laundry is typically washed in cold water and at times the laundry runs out of detergent.

Questions:

What additional data would you wish to gather to address the outbreak of boils at the shelter? How would you collect this data?

What host, agent, and environmental factors may have contributed to the outbreak of boils?

Discuss appropriate nursing interventions to address the outbreak. Consider the following levels of prevention: primary, secondary, and tertiary.

What advocacy role might the CHN play in addressing this issue?

that led to live on the streets. TIC is based on the need for staff to be aware of and understand trauma, along with the resolve to use strengths-based interventions and skill building with homeless clients in an effort to help them regain some control in their lives.

Lack of transportation can be a major barrier to accessing care. Some programs have responded to this need by adopting mobile health vans that provide care on street corners and in neighborhoods (Gibson, Ghosh, Morano, & Altice, 2014). Clinics have also been established in shelters to facilitate client access, and nurses often manage clinics (see Chapter 31). Nursing students also play an important role in promoting access to care for the homeless (Asgary, Garland, Jakubowski, & Sckell, 2014; Bowker, Weg, & Hansen, 2013). In a study of homeless and marginally housed adults in Connecticut, 51% reported that they had used some type of primary care in the previous 2 years. Those that had used primary care services were found to have also had regular visits with community health nurses, and this was a statistically significant association (Zhuo, Khoshnood, & Forster, 2015).

The community health nurse should also consider the role of faith-based communities in providing physical and spiritual support to the homeless. Many places of worship have responded to the crisis of homelessness by offering food, shelter, counseling, medical care, and social services within the context of the faith community. Clinics have been built within faith communities to promote access to care See From the Case Files.

Tertiary Prevention

Tertiary preventive measures attempt to limit disability and to restore maximum functioning. The goal is to provide rehabilitative care and support to clients who are already experiencing the consequences of homelessness. Often, homeless individuals suffer from chronic health conditions that have gone untreated for long periods of

---

LEVELS OF PREVENTION PYRAMID

SITUATION: Promoting health and preventing illness among homeless male addicts

GOAL: To apply the three levels of prevention to avoid adverse health conditions, promptly diagnose and treat disorders, and assist homeless male addict population to maintain or regain optimal health

TERTIARY PREVENTION

- Provide case management of chronic health conditions.
- Advocate for expansion of counseling, rehabilitative services, and addictions treatment programs for the homeless.
- Advocate for supportive and transitional housing to enable homeless residents with addictions disorders to successfully transition back into the community.

SECONDARY PREVENTION

Early Diagnosis and Treatment

- Conduct mass screenings for diseases commonly found in homeless male population (TB, HIV, hepatitis, prostate cancer, colorectal cancer).
- Develop programs for health screening and early diagnosis and treatment in the community that are culturally sensitive and accessible to the homeless (i.e., mobile vans, faith community, or shelter-based clinics).

PRIMARY PREVENTION

Health Promotion and Education	Health Protection
• Support employment and job training opportunities that assist clients to obtain jobs with livable wages and benefits. • Advocate through housing coalitions and legislative efforts to promote affordable housing, employment opportunities, and better access to health care. • Develop culturally sensitive health education programs that promote healthy coping, positive parenting, communication and relationship building, mental health, and injury and illness prevention. • Promote programs that offer counseling and support to prevent continued high-risk behaviors as a result of untreated addiction.	• Advocate for legislation to protect citizens from environmental toxins and industrial wastes common to low-income areas. • Provide immunization services to prevent communicable disease transmission. • Counsel clients on proper nutrition, exercise, and basic hygiene to promote healthy lifestyles and prevent disease transmissio. • Advocate for funding for nutrition programs for the homeless and for homeless shelters that would allow for the purchase of nutritious foods.

time. This neglect in attending to health needs results in significant disease morbidity. Treating complications of advanced disease, providing rehabilitative care, and offering counseling and support are important tertiary preventive strategies. Rae and Rees (2015) asked homeless adults in the United Kingdom about their perceptions of health care needs and their experiences in receiving care. They often recognized that they needed health care, but did not place a high priority on getting care. Further, many obstacles to care were shared with the researchers in this qualitative study (e.g., poor public attitudes toward them, bad experiences with health care personnel, difficulty finding a physician). Many felt that they received substandard care, but others reported positive experiences with care. A U.S. study found lower health care expenses for homeless individuals after they moved into supportive housing (Wright, Vartanian, Hsin-Fang, Royal, & Matson, 2016).

Case Management

At each level of prevention, the community health nurse functions as a case manager and coordinator of care to insure seamless delivery of services as people transition from one level of care to another. It is often difficult for the homeless to keep track of multiple appointments, negotiate the bureaucracy of multiple agencies and services, or maintain communication with providers through follow-up phone calls, letters, or visits. With no permanent address or phone, homeless clients encounter obstacles to adhering to recommendations

---

QSEN: Quality and Safety Education for Nurses

Quality improvement—Use data to monitor the outcomes of care processes and use improvement methods to design and test changes to continuously improve the quality and safety of health care systems.

Knowledge—Describe strategies for learning about the outcomes of care in the setting in which one is engaged in clinical practice.

Recognize that nursing and other health professions students are parts of systems of care and care processes that affect outcomes for patients and families.

Skills—Seek information about outcomes of care for populations served in care setting.

Attitudes—Appreciate that continuous quality improvement is an essential part of the daily work of all health professionals.

It is likely that you evaluate the quality of the care given to your patients in the acute care setting every day you are in a patient care environment. Biomarkers such as improvements in blood pressure and Hgb A1C levels, reduction in pain, or changes in function such as improvement in activities of daily living may serve as indicators of success when measuring the effectiveness of one's nursing interventions. But how is success measured when one is caring for large and diverse population groups such as the homeless?

To measure change in this context, one must first define what is meant by "success." For example, what are the markers for success when working with a population of homeless teen mothers? What about a population of veterans with decade-long histories of active addiction? Literature reviews, surveys, or focus groups may help point to measures of success. Interviews with key stakeholders also provide insight as to the most important measures for evaluating program effectiveness in a population.

Nelson et al. (2012) examined the impact of a work-skills program on employment and life domains among 638 homeless clients in New England. Data were tracked from program inception to 6 months following graduation. Assessment measures included data on general health status, housing, employment, self-esteem, self-efficacy, income level, and general work-skills such as workplace technology, basic literacy, communication, and social networking. Data revealed that the program resulted in improvements in work and life skills that were associated with improved self-esteem and self-efficacy. These improvements, in turn, increased the probability of securing stable housing in the future. Tyler et al. (2014) evaluated the impact of an interdisciplinary community-based intervention on hepatitis C knowledge among homeless adults. The authors found that the nurse case managed intervention, an approach that engaged key stakeholders, outreach workers, community organizations, and the homeless, predicted the greatest gain in HCV knowledge.

In considering measures for evaluating program success, one must also consider the context in which the program is being implemented and the philosophical perspectives and values systems of participants. For example, Lashley (2013) explores the tension between sacred and secular ways of knowing when evaluating programs for the homeless in a faith-based context. Critics may contend that faith-based interventions for the homeless cannot be fully understood through a secular lens. Even the idea that a spiritually based experience can be objectively measured may be perceived as offensive. Despite these concerns, research and evidence-based practice continue to be successfully integrated into faith-based ministries to improve patient outcomes. Community-based participatory research, which involves the community as a full partner in the research process, is an effective paradigm for engaging populations in outcomes-based program improvement (Lashley, 2013).

1. How might you engage a target population to actively participate in the evaluation process?
2. What outcomes do you believe are most important to track when caring for homeless populations?

Lashley, M. (2013). Creating a culture for evidence-based practice in the faith community. *Journal of Christian Nursing, 30*(3), 158–163.

Nelson, S., Gray, H., Maurice, I., & Shaffer, H. (2012). Moving ahead: Evaluation of a work-skills training program for homeless adults. *Community Mental Health Journal, 48*, 711–722.

Tyler, D., Nyamathi, A., Stein, J., Koniak-Griffin, D., Hodge, F., & Gelberg, L. (2014). Increasing hepatitis C knowledge among homeless adults: Results of a community-based, interdisciplinary intervention. *The Journal of Behavioral Health Services & Research, 41*(1), 37–49.

to follow up on test results or to notify their provider if symptoms persist or worsen. An Australian quality improvement project was conducted to examine how community-based palliative care services might be more effectively provided among a homeless population. MacWilliams, Bramwell, Brown, and O'Connor (2014, p. 83) reported that the "complex psychosocial and medical needs" of the homeless population, along with their inconsistent, unsafe, and often unreachable settings for care posed challenges. Also, their lack of social support and difficulty complying with treatment protocols (often because of substance abuse and mental health issues) make them especially challenging as a population. However, researchers noted that they needed to explore creative ways to meet the needs of this population who require "flexible, compassionate, and coordinated" care (p. 83). The community health nurse can help to bridge these gaps in service delivery and promote more effective adherence to therapeutic regimens.

Advocacy

Advocacy is a vital dimension of the community health nurse's role in working with the homeless. Advocacy entails working with different sectors of the community (including public officials, service providers, and persons living in the community) to develop innovative models for responding to the crisis of homelessness. Advocacy creates the broader system-wide changes needed to end homelessness (NCH, 2013). The community health nurse acts as an advocate at each level of prevention to effect positive change. For example, the nurse may advocate for mental health and substance abuse services to promote mental health and prevent homelessness (primary prevention). Alternatively, he or she may advocate for legislation to fund supportive housing, health care, or social services to benefit the homeless chronically mentally ill (tertiary prevention). The CHN can also assume an advocacy role by becoming involved in local, state, or national coalitions or organizations devoted to protecting the rights of the homeless or by speaking out on legislation that impacts the homeless (NCH, 2013).

SUMMARY

Rising poverty and lack of affordable housing have led to a dramatic rise in homelessness. Poverty, lack of housing, domestic violence, mental illness, addictions, personal crisis, and natural disasters are factors that may predispose persons to homelessness.

Homeless families represent the fastest growing segment of the homeless population. Acute and chronic health problems plague the homeless. Conditions such as HIV/AIDS, diabetes, hypertension, addictions, and mental disorders are prevalent among the homeless and are difficult to treat because of the challenges associated with being homeless.

Both the public and private sectors have launched concerted efforts to combat the problem of homelessness through the passage of federal legislation (most notably the McKinney-Vento Homeless Assistance Act) and through the formation of national, state, and local coalitions and alliances to champion the cause of the homeless. There is still much to be done.

Community health nurses maintain a long and distinguished tradition of providing care to the marginalized and underserved. As such, they play a vital role in addressing the needs of the homeless in society. At the core of community nursing practice is the development of a trusting relationship. The community health nurse needs to examine his or her values and presuppositions regarding poverty and homelessness to be more effective in rendering care that is respectful, compassionate, and nonjudgmental.

The community health nurse delivers primary, secondary, and tertiary preventive measures to prevent homelessness or to assist those who are homeless to obtain needed services. Primary prevention includes advocating for affordable housing, employment opportunities, and improved access to health care to prevent the downward spiral into homelessness. Secondary prevention includes screening for communicable and chronic diseases and promoting access to affordable health care and social services. Tertiary prevention includes rehabilitative and supportive care and counseling.

The community health nurse also serves as a case manager to coordinate care and to assist clients to negotiate the bureaucracy of multiple agencies and services. Finally, the CHN acts as an advocate to promote the rights of the homeless and to speak out on legislation impacting homelessness.

ACTIVITIES TO PROMOTE **CRITICAL THINKING**

1. Reflect in writing on the meaning of "home." Share your reflections with classmates. How similar are your responses?
2. Interview a homeless person regarding the most difficult choices he or she has had to make. What were the conditions surrounding these choices?
3. Volunteer to work at a soup kitchen or homeless shelter. Observe carefully the faces, sounds, attitudes, and activities. What is it like there? What would it be like to receive rather than give service?
4. Access the state information for American Institutes for Research (2014) document on homelessness available in the references. Look up your state to determine the number of homeless children, those at risk for homelessness, and your state's policy and planning regarding housing for the homeless population. How does your state compare to other states? Consider how you might address these issues in a letter or visit to your local state legislator.
5. Perform a windshield survey in a low-income community. What resources are lacking? Where is the nearest bank, school, grocery store, health clinic? What are the conditions of the roads, homes, and other buildings? How do you feel as you drive through the community? What do you think it would be like to live there?
6. Given that veterans make up 11% of the total population of homeless individuals and that problems may follow their return to civilian life, what might be the relationship between health and community integration in the population of veterans who are discharged following deployment to the Middle East?

   Access articles on reintegration of veterans: Sherman, M. D., Larson, J., & Borden, L. M. (2015). Broadening the focus in supporting reintegrating Iraq and Afghanistan veterans: Six key domains of functioning. *Professional Psychology: Research and Practice, 45*(5), 355–365.

   What is meant by community reintegration and how does this apply to the veteran population? What are the different dimensions of functioning that are involved in community participation? How might dysfunction in these dimensions impact the health of veterans, families, and communities?

REFERENCES

American Institutes for Research (AIFR). (2014). *America's youngest outcasts: A report card on child homelessness.* Retrieved from http://www.air.org/sites/default/files/downloads/report/Americas-Youngest-Outcasts-Child-Homelessness-Nov2014.pdf

Anderson, E., & McFarlane, J. (2015). *Community as partner: Theory and practice in nursing* (7th ed.). Philadelphia, PA: Wolters Kluwer Health/Lippincott Williams & Wilkins.

Asgary, R., Garland, V., Jakubowski, A., & Sckell, B. (2014). Colorectal cancer screening among the homeless population of New York City shelter-based clinics. *American Journal of Public Health, 104*(7), 1307–1313.

Baggett, T. P., O'Connell, J. J., Singer, D. E., & Rigotti, N. A. (2010). The unmet health care needs of homeless adults: A national study. *American Journal of Public Health, 100*(7), 1326–1333.

Bowker, D., Weg, B., & Hansen, E. (2013). Nontraditional clinical sites: Working with those who are the homeless. *Nurse Educator, 38*(4), 139–140.

Brown, R. T., & Steinman, M. A. (2013). Characteristics of emergency department visits by older versus younger homeless adults in the United States. *American Journal of Public Health, 103*(6), 1046–1051.

Burt, M. (2006). *Testimony related to provisions of s. 1801, The Community Partnership to End Homelessness Act of 2005.* Retrieved from http://webarchive.urban.org/UploadedPDF/900937_burt_033006.pdf

Carmon, I. (2015, April 9). *How falling behind on child support can end in jail.* Retrieved from http://www.msnbc.com/msnbc/how-falling-behind-child-support-can-end-jail#56748

Chalabi, M. (2013, May 7). *The other gender divide: Where men are losing out.* Retrieved from http://www.theguardian.com/news/datablog/2013/may/07/men-gender-divide-feminism

Child Trends Data Bank. (2015). *Homeless children and youth: Indicators on children and youth.* Retrieved from http://www.childtrends.org/wp-content/uploads/2015/01/112_Homeless_Children_and_Youth.pdf

Colorado Coalition for the Homeless. (2012). *Policy brief: The characteristics of homeless women.* Retrieved from http://www.coloradocoalition.org/!userfiles/TheCharacteristicsofHomelessWomen_lores3.pdf

Correa, R. (2016, January 12). *A business owner's call to raise the minimum wage.* Retrieved from https://blog.dol.gov/2016/01/12/a-business-owners-call-to-raise-the-minimum-wage/

Davidson, K. A. (2013, May 16). *Natural disasters displaced 32.4 million people in 2012, IDMC study shows.* Retrieved from http://www.huffingtonpost.com/2013/05/15/idmc-natural-disasters-displaced-people_n_3280854.html

Dawson, A., & Jackson, D. (2013). The primary health care service experiences and needs of homeless youth: A narrative synthesis of current evidence. *Contemporary Nurse, 44*(1), 62-75.

DeNavas-Walt, C., & Proctor, B. (2014). *U.S. Census Bureau current population reports: Income and poverty in the United States: 2013.* Washington, DC: U.S. Government Printing Office. Retrieved from http://www.census.gov/content/dam/Census/library/publications/2014/demo/p60-249.pdf

DiMarco, M. A., Ludington, S. M., & Menke, E. M. (2010). Access to and utilization of oral health care by homeless children/families. *Journal of Health Care for the Poor & Underserved, 21*(2), 67–81.

Donley, A. M., & Wright, J. D. (2012). Safer outside: A qualitative exploration of homeless people's resistance to homeless shelters. *Journal of Forensic Psychology Practice, 12,* 288–306.

Gibson, B., Ghosh, D., Morano, J., & Altice, F. (2014). Accessibility and utilization patterns of a mobile medical clinic among vulnerable populations. *Health and Place, 28,* 153–166. doi: 10.1016/j.healthplace.2014.04.008.

Ha, Y., Narendorf, S. C., Santa Maria, D., & Bezette-Flores, N. (2015). Barriers and facilitators to shelter utilization among homeless young adults. *Evaluation and Program Planning, 53,* 25–33.

Hauff, A. J., & Secor-Turner, M. (2014). Homeless health needs: Shelter and health service provider perspective. *Journal of Community Health Nursing, 31*,103–117.

Homeless Hub. (2015). *Causes of homelessness.* Retrieved from http://homelesshub.ca/about-homelessness/homelessness-101/causes-homelessness

White House. (2014). *A year of action: Program report on raising the minimum wage.* Retrieved from https://www.whitehouse.gov/sites/default/files/doc/rr

Housing Assistance Council (HAC). (2014). *Rural homelessness.* Retrieved from www.ruralhome.org/sct-initiatives/mn-rural-homelessness/

Hwang, S. W., Chambers, C. & Katic, M. (2016). Accuracy of self-reported health care use in a population-based sample of homeless adults. *Health Services Research, 51*(1), 282–301.

Kaiser Family Foundation. (2014). *Key facts about the uninsured population.* Retrieved from http://kff.org/uninsured/fact-sheet/key-facts-about-the-uninsured-population/

MacWilliams, J., Bramwell, M., Brown, S., & O'Connor, M. (2014). Reaching out to Ray: Delivering palliative care services to a homeless person in Melbourne, Australia. *International Journal of Palliative Nursing, 20*(2), 83–88.

Mago, V. K., Morden, H. K., Fritz, C., Wu, T., Namazi, S., Geranmayeh, P., ... Dabbaghian, V. (2013). Analyzing the impact of social factors on homelessness: A fuzzy cognitive map approach. *BMC Medical Informatics and Decision Making, 13*, 94. doi: 10.1186/1472-6947-13-94.

McEvers, K. (2016, February 1). *Utah reduced chronic homelessness by 91 percent: Here's how.* Retrieved from http://www.npr.org/2015/12/10/459100751/utah-reduced-chronic-homelessness-by-91-percent-heres-how

McKinney-Vento Homeless Assistance Act. (1987). *U. S. Congress, Public Law 100-77.* Retrieved from http://www.gpo.gov/fdsys/pkg/STATUTE-101/pdf/STATUTE-101-Pg482.pdf

Meschede, T., & Chaganti, S. (2015). Home for now: A mixed-methods evaluation of a short-term housing support program for homeless families. *Evaluation and Program Planning, 52*, 85–95.

National Advisory Committee on Rural Health and Human Services. (2014). *Homelessness in rural America.* Retrieved from http://www.hrsa.gov/advisorycommittees/rural/publications/homelessnessrural-america.pdf

National Alliance to End Homelessness (NAEH). (2014). *The state of homelessness in America 2014.* Retrieved from http://www.endhomelessness.org/library/entry/the-state-of-homelessness-2014

National Alliance to End Homelessness (NAEH). (2015a). *Domestic violence.* Retrieved from http://www.endhomelessness.org/pages/domestic_violence

National Alliance to End Homelessness (NAEH). (2015b). *Fact sheet: Chronic homelessness.* Retrieved from http://www.endhomelessness.org/library/entry/fact-sheet-chronic-homelessness1

National Alliance to End Homelessness (NAEH). (2015c). *Housing first.* Retrieved from http://www.endhomelessness.org/pages/housing_first

National Alliance to End Homelessness (NAEH). (2015d). *The state of homelessness in America 2015.* Retrieved from http://www.endhomelessness.org/library/entry/the-state-of-homelessness-2015

National Alliance to End Homelessness (NAEH). (2015e). *Youth.* Retrieved from http://www.endhomelessness.org/pages/youth

National Alliance to End Homelessness (NAEH). (2016). *LGBTQ youth.* Retrieved from http://www.endhomelessness.org/pages/lgbtq-youth

National Association for the Education of Homeless Children and Youth. (2015). *The McKinney-Vento Act and school fees.* Retrieved from http://www.naehcy.org/sites/default/files/pdf/School%20fees.pdf

National Center for Homeless Education (NCHE). (2012). *Increasing access to higher education for unaccompanied homeless youth: Information for colleges and universities.* Retrieved from http://center.serve.org/nche/downloads/briefs/higher_ed.pdf

National Center on Family Homelessness (NCFH). (2011). *The characteristics and needs of families experiencing homelessness.* Retrieved from http://www.familyhomelessness.org/media/306.pdf

National Center on Family Homelessness (NCFH). (2014). *America's youngest outcasts. A report card on child homelessness.* Retrieved from http://www.homelesschildrenamerica.org/mediadocs/282.pdf

National Center on Family Homelessness (NCFH). (2015). *Children.* Retrieved from http://www.familyhomelessness.org/children.php?p=ts

National Coalition for the Homeless (NCH). (2006). *McKinney-Vento Act.* Retrieved from http://www.nationalhomeless.org/publications/facts/McKinney.pdf

National Coalition for the Homeless (NCH). (2011a). *How many people experience homelessness?* Retrieved from http://www.nationalhomeless.org/factsheets/How_Many.html

National Coalition for the Homeless (NCH). (2011b). *Why are people homeless?* Retrieved from http://www.nationalhomeless.org/factsheets/why.html

National Coalition for the Homeless (NCH). (2012a). *Domestic violence and homelessness.* Retrieved from http://www.nationalhomeless.org/factsheets/domestic.html

National Coalition for the Homeless (NCH). (2012b). *Education of homeless children and youth.* Retrieved from http://www.nationalhomeless.org/factsheets/education.html

National Coalition for the Homeless (NCH). (2012c). *Employment and homelessness.* Retrieved from http://www.nationalhomeless.org/factsheets/employment.html

National Coalition for the Homeless (NCH). (2012d). *Federal housing assistance programs.* Retrieved from http://www.nationalhomeless.org/factsheets/federal.html

National Coalition for the Homeless (NCH). (2012e). *Hate crimes and violence against people experiencing homelessness.* Retrieved from http://www.nationalhomeless.org/factsheets/hatecrimes.html

National Coalition for the Homeless (NCH). (2012f). *Health care and homelessness.* Retrieved from http://www.nationalhomeless.org/factsheets/health.html

National Coalition for the Homeless (NCH). (2012g). *HIV/AIDS and homelessness.* Retrieved from http://www.nationalhomeless.org/factsheets/hiv.html

National Coalition for the Homeless (NCH). (2012h). *Homeless families with children.* Retrieved from http://www.nationalhomeless.org/factsheets/families.html

National Coalition for the Homeless (NCH). (2012i). *Homelessness among elderly persons.* http://www.nationalhomeless.org/factsheets/elderly.html

National Coalition for the Homeless (NCH). (2012j). *Homeless veterans.* Retrieved from http://www.nationalhomeless.org/factsheets/veterans.html

National Coalition for the Homeless (NCH). (2012k). *Homeless youth.* Retrieved from http://www.nationalhomeless.org/factsheets/youth.html

National Coalition for the Homeless (NCH). (2012l). *LGBT homeless.* Retrieved from http://www.nationalhomeless.org/factsheets/lgbtq.html

National Coalition for the Homeless (NCH). (2012m). *Mental illness and homelessness.* Retrieved from http://www.nationalhomeless.org/factsheets/Mental_Illness.html

National Coalition for the Homeless (NCH). (2012n). *Rural homelessness.* Retrieved from http://www.nationalhomeless.org/factsheets/rural/html/

National Coalition for the Homeless (NCH). (2012o). *Substance abuse and homelessness.* Retrieved from http://www.nationalhomeless.org/factsheets/addiction.html

National Coalition for the Homeless (NCH). (2013). *How you can help end homelessness.* Retrieved from http://www.nationalhomeless.org/want_to_help/index.html

National Coalition for the Homeless (NCH). (2014). *Take a number: The long wait for rental assistance.* Retrieved from http://nationalhomeless.org/take-a-number-the-long-wait-for-rental-assistance/

National Health Care for the Homeless Council (NHCHC). (2011a). *Health care for the homeless program.* Retrieved from http://www.nhchc.org/wp-content/uploads/2011/09/HCHFactSheetMay2011.pdf

National Health Care for the Homeless Council (NHCHC). (2011b). *Homelessness and health: What's the connection?* Retrieved from http://www.nhchc.org/wp-content/uploads/2011/09/Hln_health_factsheet_Jan10.pdf

National Health Care for the Homeless Council (NHCHC). (2013). *Aging and housing instability: Homelessness among older and elderly adults.* Retrieved from http://www.nhchc.org/wp-content/uploads/2011/09/infocus_september2013.pdf

National Health Care for the Homeless Council (NHCHC). (2015). *What is the relationship between health, housing, and homelessness?* Retrieved from https://www.nhchc.org/faq/relationship-health-housing-homelessness/

National Law Center on Homelessness & Poverty (NLCHP). (2014). *No safe place: The criminalization of homelessness in U. S. cities.* Retrieved from https://www.nlchp.org/documents/No_Safe_Place

National Low Income Housing Coalition. (2016). *Out of reach 2015: U.S. statistics.* Retrieved from http://www.nlihc.org/oor

Rae, B. E., & Rees, S. (2015). The perceptions of homeless people regarding their healthcare needs and experiences of receiving health care. *Journal of Advanced Nursing, 71*(9), 2096–2107.

Ream, G. L., & Forge, N. R. (2014). Homeless lesbian, gay, bisexual, and transgender (LGBT) youth in New York City: Insights from the field. *Child Welfare, 93*(2), 7–22.

Rhoades, H., Wenzel, S. L., Golinelli, D., Tucker, J. S., Kennedy, D. P., Green, H. D., & Zhou, A. (2011). The social context of homeless men's substance use. *Drug and Alcohol Dependence, 118,* 320–325.

Smith, J., & Medalia, C. (2014). *U.S. Census Bureau current population reports: Health insurance coverage in the United States 2013.* Washington, DC: U.S. Government Printing Office. Retrieved from http://www.census.gov/content/dam/Census/library/publications/2014/demo/p60-250.pdf

Spriggs, H. F. (2013). *An analysis of North Carolina homeless shelter policies: Potential for fracturing the integrity of help-seeking homeless families (Unpublished doctoral dissertation).* Greensboro, NC: University of North Carolina.

Substance Abuse and Mental Health Services Administration (SAMHSA). (n.d.a). *Homelessness Resource Center: About us.* Retrieved from http://homeless.samhsa.gov/about.aspx

Substance Abuse and Mental Health Services Administration (SAMHSA). (2004). *PATH legislation: Public Health Service Act Part C: Projects for Assistance in Transition from Homelessness.* Retrieved from http://pathprogram.samhsa.gov/Resource/PATH-Legislation-Public-Health-Service-Act-Part-C--Projects-for-Assistance-in-Transition-from-Homelessness-48766.aspx

Substance Abuse and Mental Health Services Administration (SAMHSA). (2014). *Who we are.* Retrieved from http://www.samhsa.gov/about-us/who-we-are/offices-centers/cmhs

Substance Abuse and Mental Health Services Administration (SAMHSA). (n.d.b). *Homelessness Resource Center facts.* Retrieved from http://www.nrchmi.samhsa.gov/Channel/View.aspx?id=18

U.S. Conference of Mayors. (2014). *Hunger and homelessness survey: A status report on hunger and homelessness in America's cities.* Retrieved from http://www.usmayors.org/pressreleases/uploads/2014/1211-report-hh.pdf

U.S. Department of Health and Human Services (USDHHS). (2014). *The Center for Faith-Based and Neighborhood Partnerships.* Retrieved from http://www.hhs.gov/partnerships/index.html

U.S. Department of Health and Human Services (USDHHS). (2016). *Healthy People 2020: Oral health.* Retrieved from http://www.healthypeople.gov/2020/topics-objectives/topic/oral-health

U.S. Department of Housing and Urban Development (2016). *Homeless prevention and rapid rehousing program.* Retrieved from http://portal.hud.gov/hudportal/HUD?src=/recovery/programs/homelessness

U.S. Department of Housing and Urban Development (n.d.). *Housing choice vouchers fact sheet.* Retrieved from http://portal.hud.gov/hudportal/HUD?src=/program_offices/public_indian_housing/programs/hcv/about/fact_sheet

U.S. Department of Housing and Urban Development (USDHUD). (2013). *Expanding opportunities to house individuals and families experiencing homelessness through public housing (PH) and housing choice voucher (HCV) programs.* Retrieved from http://portal.HUD.gov/hudportal/documents/huddoc?id=PIH2013-15HomelessQAs.pdf

U.S. Department of Housing and Urban Development (USDHUD). (2014). *The 2013 annual homeless assessment report to Congress.* Retrieved from https://www.hudexchange.info/onecpd/assets/File/2013-AHAR-Part-2.pdf

U.S. Department of Housing and Urban Development (USDHUD). (2015). *The 2015 annual homeless assessment report to Congress.* Retrieved from https://www.hudexchange.info/resources/documents/2015-AHAR-Part-1.pdf

U.S. Department of Labor. (2016). *Consolidated state minimum wage update table.* Retrieved from http://www.dol.gov/whd/minwage/america.htm

U.S. Interagency Council on Homelessness (USICH). (2010). *Opening doors: Federal strategic plan to prevent and end homelessness.* Retrieved from http://usich.gov/resources/uploads/asset_library/Opening%20Doors%202010%20FINAL%20FSP%20Prevent%20End%20Homeless.pdf

U.S. Interagency Council on Homelessness (USICH). (2013a). *About USICH.* Retrieved from http://usich.gov/about_us/

U.S. Interagency Council on Homelessness (USICH). (2013b). *The Affordable Care Act's role in preventing and ending homelessness.* Retrieved from http://usich.gov/usich_resources/fact_sheets/ACA/

U.S. Interagency Council on Homelessness (USICH). (2013c). *Housing first.* Retrieved from http://usich.gov/usich_resources/solutions/explore/housing_first/

U.S. Interagency Council on Homelessness (USICH). (2013d). *Substance abuse.* Retrieved from http://usich.gov/issue/substance_abuse/

Weber, M., Thompson, L., Schmiege, S. J., Peifer, K., & Farrell, E. (2013). Perception of access to health care by homeless individuals seeking services at a day shelter. *Archives of Psychiatric Nursing, 27*(4), 179–184.

Wright, B. J., Vartanian, K. B., Hsin-Fang, L., Royal, N., & Matson, J. K. (2016). Formerly homeless people had lower overall health care expenditures after moving into supportive housing. *Health Affairs, 35*(1), 20–27.

Zhuo, S., Khoshnood, K., & Forster, S. H. (2015). Assessing impact of community health nurses on improving primary care use by homeless/marginally housed persons. *Journal of Community Health Nursing, 32*(3), 161–169.

Zur, J., & Jones, E. (2014). Unmet need among homeless and non-homeless patients served at Health Care for the Homeless programs. *Journal of Health Care for the Poor and Underserved, 25*(4), 2053–2068.

thePoint: Everything You Need to Make the Grade!

thePoint® Visit http://thePoint.lww.com/Rector9e for selected readings, study aids for all learning styles, and more!

Issues with Rural, Migrant, and Urban Health Care

"No city should be too large for a man to walk out of in a morning."

—Cyril Connolly (1903–1974), British Critic

"Globalization is exposing new fault lines—between urban and rural communities, for example."

—Ban Ki-moon, United Nations Secretary General

KEY TERMS

Built environment
Critical access hospitals
Federally qualified health centers
Frontier area
Ghettos
Health professional shortage areas (HPSAs)

In-migration
Medically underserved areas (MUAs)
Medically underserved population
Metropolitan statistical area
Micropolitan statistical area
Migrant farmworkers

Migrant streams
Out-migration
Patterns of migration
Population density
Rural
Rural health clinics
Seasonal farmworkers
Social justice

Telehealth
Urban
Urban health
Urbanized area (UA)
Urban cluster (UC)
Urban health penalty
Urban planning

LEARNING OBJECTIVES

Upon mastery of this chapter, you should be able to:

- Define the terms *rural, frontier, migrant,* and *urban*.
- Discuss the population characteristics of rural residents.
- Describe five barriers to health care access for rural clients.
- Describe the migrant lifestyle.
- Identify at least three health problems common to migrant workers and their families.
- Discuss barriers and challenges to migrant health care.
- Identify common health disparities found among rural and urban populations.
- Propose intervention strategies at the aggregate or community level to assure a healthier *built environment* in both rural and urban areas.
- Explain the concept of *social justice* and how it relates to public health nursing in rural and urban areas.
- Compare and contrast the challenges and opportunities related to rural and urban community health nursing practice.

About half of the population live in what is known as the suburbs, but the remainder live in one of two diametrically opposed areas: rural or urban. There is a good chance that many of you reading this book live either in very densely populated, bustling urban areas or in sparsely populated, somewhat isolated rural areas. Public health nursing in urban and rural areas requires not only general public health nursing knowledge and skills but also a unique understanding of how these distinctive environments affect the health of the populations living there. Where you live can and does markedly affect your health outcomes, with rural and urban areas having distinctive problems and issues, as described in a seminal 2002 article by van Dis (2002). These differences are much more than just the ability to shop at "Wal-Mart versus Pottery Barn" (p. 108). Both rural and urban clients have health disparities and disadvantages, although they may be dissimilar in nature (Anderson, Saman, Lipsky, & Lutfiyya, 2015).

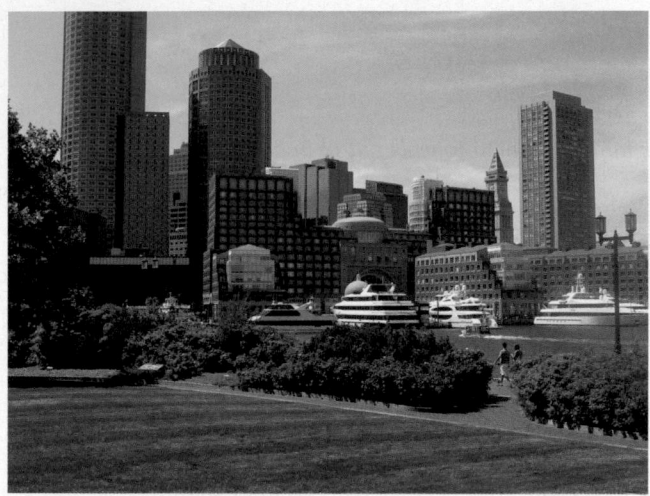

Boston Park Harbor. (Source: USA.gov.)

Rural nursing practice offers many opportunities. Nurses are respected community members—their judgment and opinions count. Rural nurses are key members of the health care team. They can make a difference in the lives of their neighbors, friends, and community. Rural PHNs often struggle with helping clients gain access to quality health care and the inherent transportation problems found in isolated areas. The challenges are many, but the rewards are great.

Urban PHNs often specialize in particular areas of interest. They deal with different types of problems, such as homelessness, overcrowding, bioterrorism threats, and violent crime. They are often called upon to advocate for their most vulnerable clients, and they develop collaborative relationships with other professionals. Urban community health nursing can also be very rewarding and satisfying.

This chapter addresses the special health needs and concerns of rural, migrant, and urban clients and the ways in which a community health nurse can address those needs. After reading the chapter, you may come to appreciate the many advantages that rural nurses enjoy and consider rural nursing as a practice choice or you may find that being a PHN in an urban area offers you more opportunities for specialization and networking. Either way, your contributions can improve the health of populations living at both extremes.

DEFINITIONS AND DEMOGRAPHICS

Depending on one's geographic location, professional discipline, agency or institutional affiliation, or other frame of reference, the term *rural* has different and specialized meanings. Moreover, rural populations and characteristics have changed significantly over many years. These differences and their implications are described in this chapter.

Definitions of "Rural"

The term *rural* means different things to different people. It is helpful to be aware of the precise meaning of the term as it is used in a particular agency, community, or piece of legislation because differences in semantics can affect public policy regarding rural communities. For example, federal dollars are often distributed to communities based on rural or urban status.

The U.S. government provides several definitions of rural. These can seem confusing and complicated, but it is important to understand the terms and how they are used in federal programs and grant funding. The U.S. Census Bureau (2015) classifies **urban** areas as densely developed land that includes commercial, residential, and any other nonresidential areas and recognizes rural areas as including "all population, housing, and territory not included within an urban area" (para. 1). Two types of urban areas are described—an **urbanized area (UA)** or an **urban** cluster (**UC**). A UA consists of densely settled territory with a population of at least 50,000 people. A UC has a population <50,000 but more than 2,500 (U.S. Census Bureau, 2015). Past descriptions have relied on a specific measure of density. **Population density** refers to the number of persons per square mile—urban areas are much more densely populated than rural areas. Some counties may include both rural and urban designations, as these designations do not follow municipal boundaries but rather denote population density (like the dense grouping of buildings that you might notice from an airplane).

A consideration in urban areas is the term *megacity*; this is an urban center with over 10 million residents. New York and Los Angeles are characterized as megacities, as are London, Tokyo, Rio de Janeiro, and others around the world (Hayes, 2011). Public health problems are intensified with larger population areas; issues with communicable disease, poverty, inadequate housing, and unemployment become even more magnified with larger populations. Since the 2000 Census, the U.S. Office of Management and Budget (OMB) reclassified the United States into metropolitan and micropolitan statistical areas. This nomenclature identifies a **metropolitan statistical area** as a core-based statistical area (CBSA) associated with at least one UA that has a minimum population of 50,000. **Micropolitan statistical areas** are CBSAs associated with at least one UC of no <10,000 and no more than 50,000 people (U.S. Census Bureau, 2013). Both

metropolitan and micropolitan statistical areas comprise the central county or counties containing the core, and also included are adjacent outlying counties that have a high degree of social and economic integration with the central county (based on the number of people who commute to work). With such a broad definition, micropolitan statistical areas can include both rural and urban areas. Before 2003, the OMB defined urban and rural in terms of metropolitan and nonmetropolitan counties. By making these changes, the number of people living in what used to be considered nonmetropolitan areas decreased.

The U.S. Department of Agriculture (USDA) rural–urban continuum examines metropolitan and nonmetropolitan areas on the basis of counties, and this provides different data apart from census reports. Nonmetropolitan areas have some type of combination that includes "open countryside," rural towns (<2,500 people), and urban areas (2,500 to 49,999 people) (See Fig. 29–1). State and federal agencies recognize county-level jurisdictions and governments and depend upon employment, income, and population data that are available on an annual basis (USDA, 2013). Many states have offices of rural health or other agencies dealing with issues specific to rural populations.

For the purposes of this chapter, **rural** is defined as *communities with fewer than 10,000 residents and a county population density of <1,000 persons per square mile*. This definition of rural is arbitrary because rural clients do not merely consider population density or community size when

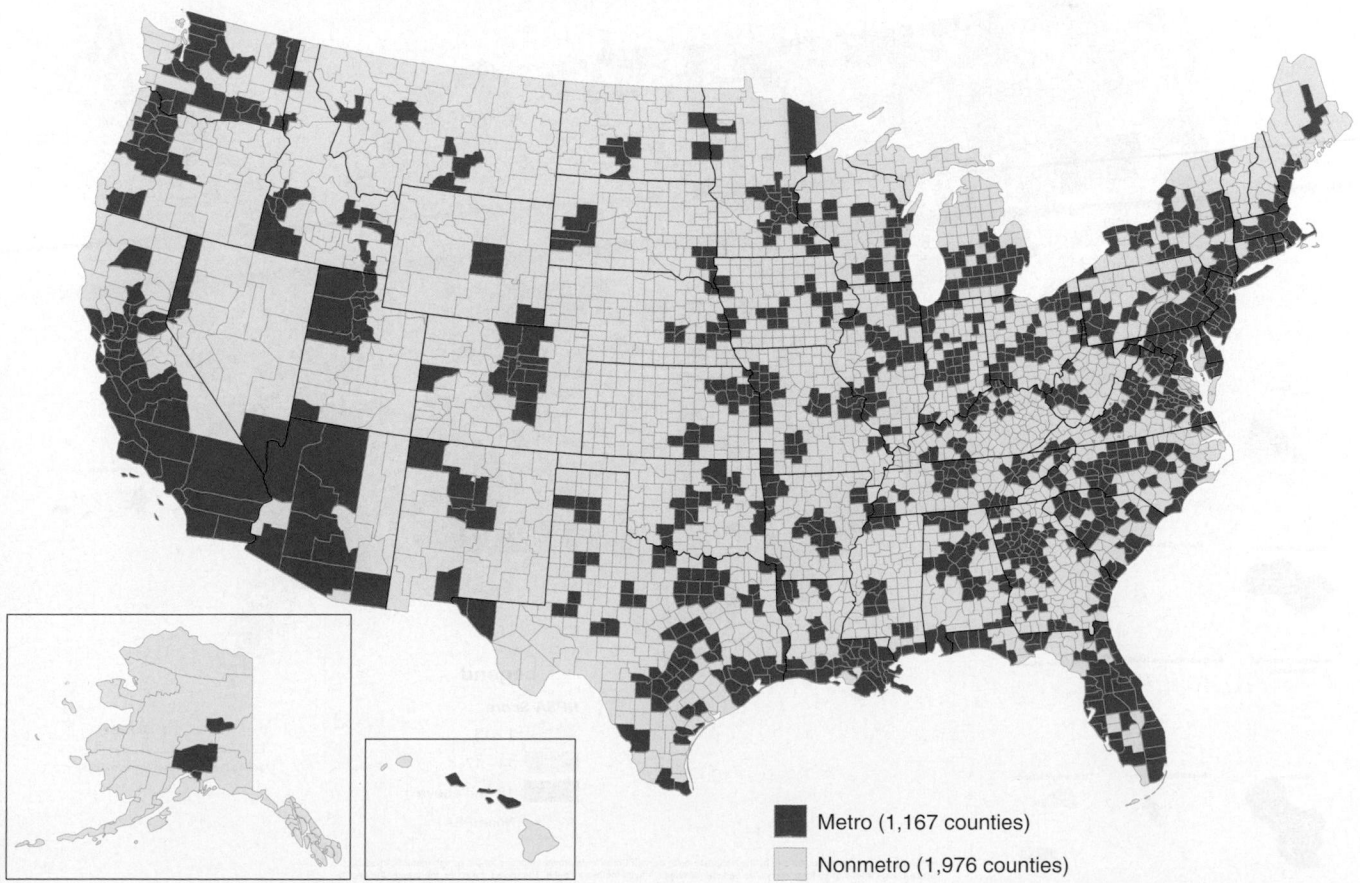

Metro (1,167 counties)

Nonmetro (1,976 counties)

FIGURE 29–1 Metro and nonmetro counties, 2013. (Retrieved from http://www.ers.usda.gov/media/1103491/metrononmetro.png.)

defining their *ruralness*. They have a multitude of reasons for defining their community as rural, such as distance from a large city, major occupations in the area (e.g., agriculture), or number of students in the local schools. If you have access to a small community, ask some of the residents the reasons why they consider their community to be urban or rural.

The term **frontier area** is used to designate sparsely populated rural places that are isolated from population centers and services, but specific definitions vary (Rural Assistance Center [RAC], 2012). A common definition of a "frontier and remote area" (FAR) is one with six or fewer persons per square mile, but others include not only population density but also distance and travel time to market service areas. For instance, 60 mi. or 60 minutes of driving on paved roads to the nearest 75-bed (or greater) hospitals could constitute a frontier area. The USDA (2015) has developed FAR codes, based upon urban–rural census data and delineated by ZIP codes. There are four levels of FAR codes; level one includes a good number of people living far from city areas where higher-level goods are available (e.g., regional airport hubs, stores with major household appliances, advanced medical care), whereas level four includes fewer people with a more significant level of remoteness (e.g., access to stores selling gas or groceries, basic medical care).

The other two levels may also have access to movie theaters, car dealerships, and clothing stores. This is helpful to researchers and public health agencies in determining rural–urban status and designing programs to meet specific needs. Rural–urban commuting area (census data) is also used to designate remote areas (RAC, 2012). It is estimated that 3 million people (4% of population) live in frontier areas that comprise 56% of the U.S. land areas. States with more than 10% of their population in a frontier area include Idaho, Nebraska, Maine, Arkansas, Oklahoma, Alaska, Arizona, Montana, Wyoming, New Mexico, Colorado, North Dakota, and South Dakota (National Center for Frontier Communities, 2014).

Health issues of concern to rural areas may be of even greater concern to frontier areas. Sparsely populated areas may be less able to attract health care professionals. The term **health professional shortage areas (HPSAs)** is used to identify urban or rural geographic areas, population groups, or facilities with chronic shortages of medical, dental, or mental health professionals. The federal government determines which areas are HPSAs. As of 2015, there were 15,557 in the United States. Over 59 million people live in areas that have been designated as HPSAs for primary care, representing about 60% of need met (Fig. 29–2). Over 90.3 million live in mental health

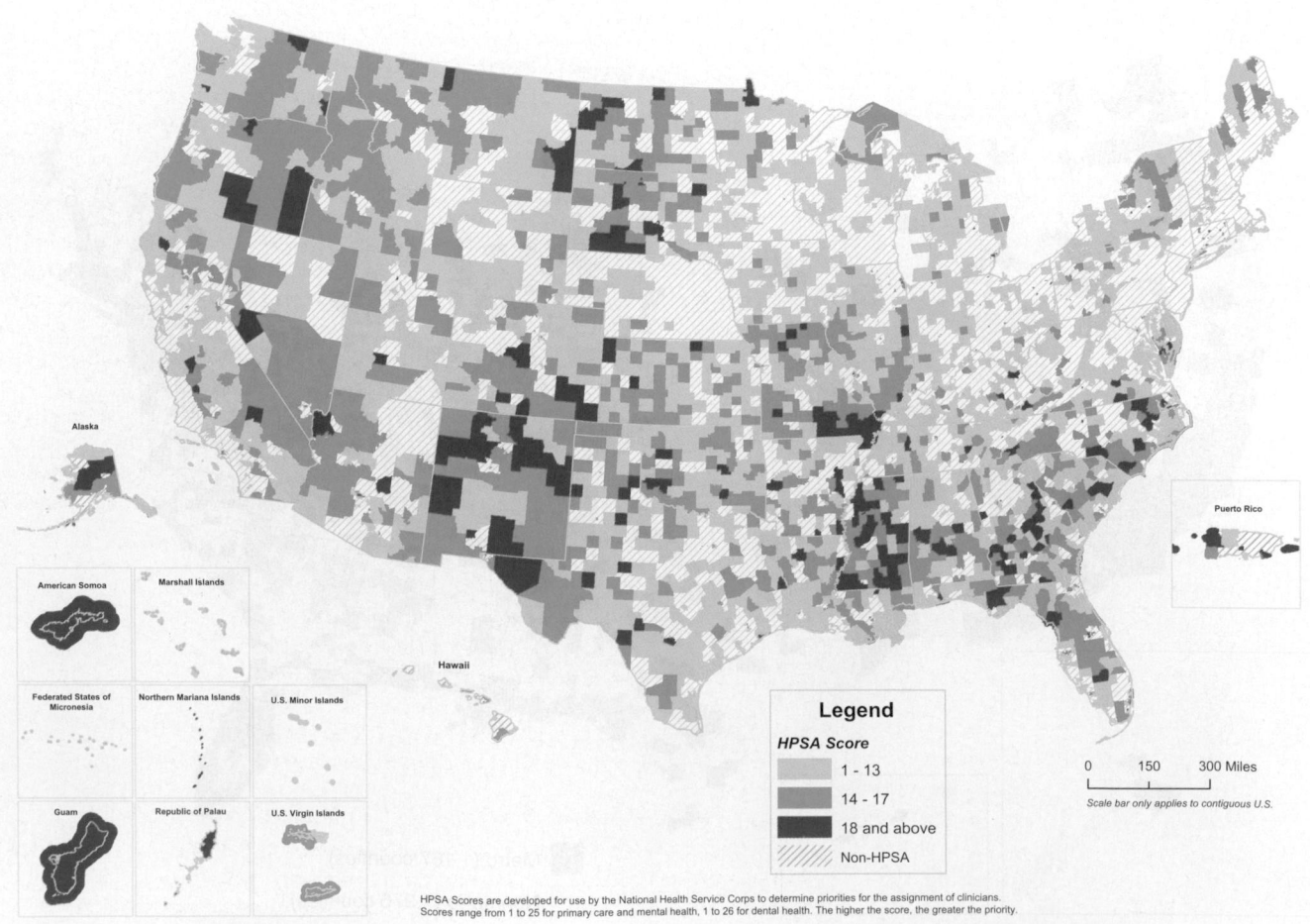

FIGURE 29–2 Health professional shortage area, primary care, 2016. (Retrieved from http:// datawarehouse.hrsa.gov/ExportedMaps/HPSAs/HGDWMapGallery_BHPR_HPSAs_PC.pdf.)

HPSAs, and 47.4 million are in areas with shortages of dentists (Health Resources and Services Administration [HRSA], 2015). In **medically underserved areas (MUAs)**, residents experience a shortage of health services; these areas are determined by the federal government using a score based on the shortage of primary care physicians, high infant mortality rates, high percentage of the population living below the poverty level, and a high proportion of residents over age 65. A **medically underserved population** (MUP) includes those with economic and cultural/linguistic barriers to primary health care services (HRSA, n.d.a).

Population Statistics

The number of persons living in urban areas of the United States tripled since the mid-1800s, to almost 60 million in 2000, and grew 10.8% from 2000 to 2010. About 75% of the total population can be found in urban areas (Gorski, 2011). California, Arizona, and Texas showed the largest growth in suburbs of large metropolitan cities. During the same period, rural population growth was 4.5% with 46% to 60% of rural counties losing residents. An all-time high of 51% of the population live in the suburbs. Only 16% of the U.S. population is characterized as rural, the lowest ever. The primary cause for this shift is thought to be children leaving home for larger cities with better employment opportunities. Rural areas are caught in a vicious cycle, because of individuals moving away to find jobs and businesses reluctant to relocate to rural areas because of a smaller pool of potential workers. Great Plains states are at risk of losing the most population and with growth of non-white populations, with Appalachia, West Texas, Arkansas, and Mississippi also losing substantial portions of their populations (Barcus & Simmons, 2013; Nusca, 2011).

Poverty and joblessness are common among rural Americans. The average per capita income is significantly lower in rural versus urban areas, and the percentage of the population living below the poverty level is higher in rural areas (Gorski, 2011). Jobs in rural America are changing, with agriculture, fishing, and forestry declining; at the same time, government, manufacturing, and service jobs are increasing (Council of Economic Advisors, n.d.). More involuntary part-time employment is also found among rural workers (29% females, 27% males), and states with a high proportion of rural population often don't provide unemployment benefits for these workers (Glauber, 2013). Rural residents are more likely to work for small companies that pay lower wages and don't offer health insurance; there are also more unemployed workers (Gorski, 2011). Even with employer penalties that came with health care reform and the expected move to reduce employee workloads below the 30-hour threshold, this did not occur across the board (Dougherty, 2011). While an estimated one million workers between ages 19 and 64 may be affected by some employers dropping work hours below the threshold to avoid penalties associated with health care reform, the number of workers characterized by involuntary part-time employment have not increased in industries or occupations where workers aren't affected by health reform mandates (Even & MacPherson, 2015). Rural areas have high rates of

uninsured and public insurance coverage (e.g., Medicaid, Medicare). There is also a higher percentage of elderly and those living in poverty, along with higher rates of chronic illness (about half have one chronic illness or more) and more rural residents reporting poor to fair health (Seright & Winters, 2015). Rural residents are less likely to receive recommended preventive services, and they make fewer visits to health care providers. They also have fewer physicians (10% of total), and there is continuous concern about physician recruitment in rural areas of the United States and other countries beyond what incentives (e.g., scholarships, forgivable loans) can offer (Fuchs & Jotkowitz, 2012). Specialized medical care is rarely found in rural areas. Of the 2,000 rural hospitals, 75% of them have 50 or fewer beds; most are designated *critical access hospitals* (CAHs) as they have 25 or fewer beds (Agency for Healthcare Research and Quality [AHRQ], 2012; Gale, 2010; Gorski, 2011). CAHs must provide 24-hour emergency care, with either MD on site or RN on site with MD on call and able to arrive within 30 minutes. They must also have 25 beds maximum and be over 35 mi from the next hospital or 15 mi if the terrain is difficult (Seright & Winters, 2015). Also, the quality and staffing levels of rural nursing homes, as determined by national survey inspection data, are below that of those in urban areas. Higher rates of contractures and lower staffing levels, along with structural and operational problems of rural facilities, accounted for most of the disparity (Bowblis, Meng, & Hyer, 2013). James (2014, p. 2122) denotes a "rural mortality penalty" that has existed for over 20 years, reversing the prior trend for higher urban mortality rates in the 19th and early 20th century because of high levels of infectious disease and water/sewage contamination.

Rural areas have a slightly higher fertility rate than urban areas (Johnson & Lichter, 2012). However, this population growth related to births (termed *natural increase*) is offset by the loss of rural youth moving to more urban areas for education, jobs, and marriage (Nusca, 2011). This has been characterized as leading to a "brain drain" from rural areas, often leaving older adults or those with less education and income remaining.

Birth rates in rural and urban areas are declining slightly overall, while there is an inflow of older adults and an already aging population (Environmental Protection Agency [EPA], 2014).

Changing Patterns of Migration

Population changes in rural areas are usually related to natural increase through births or through **out-migration**, the process of residents moving out of rural communities and into urban places (EPA, 2014). When America was a more rural country, there was more natural increase than out-migration, which caused continued growth in the rural population. In the 1970s, the proportion of births decreased, but many people moved into rural communities, resulting in an increase in population there. During the 1980s, the population trends shifted, when most rural areas lost population to out-migration as a result of economic recession and a serious farming crisis. During the first half of the 1990s, the population trend in rural communities changed to **in-migration**, an increase in residents moving into rural communities from urban places. White-collar workers were affected by changing technologies, and many young professionals with families elected to live in more rural settings. Since the beginning of the 21st century, more rural counties have experienced out-migration, and rural towns in some areas have disappeared; this trend has slowed but continued overall (Kilkenny, 2010; USDA, 2016). The lack of in-migration is related to a decrease in retirees moving to rural areas along with problems recruiting professionals and managers for local manufacturing companies. Poverty and low quality of life are also causative factors (USDA, 2013). Because of the boom in energy-related employment, Montana and North Dakota have had more in-migration (USDA, 2014). Some rural areas with few natural amenities, such as mild winters and forest areas, have also experienced out-migration, but others with beautiful landscapes, desirable climates, or proximity to tourist areas (e.g., ski slopes, lakes, beaches, national parks) have experienced more growth, and there has also been some remigration with former residents moving back to raise families in more rural environments (McGranahan Cromartie, & Wojan, 2010). Because of the boom in energy-related employment, areas in Montana and North Dakota have had more in-migration, along with some counties in Arkansas, Louisiana, Pennsylvania, and Texas (USDA, 2014).

Population trends have many implications for the health services needed by rural people. The patterns of rural migration change like shifting sand, adding to the challenge of planning resources for rural communities.

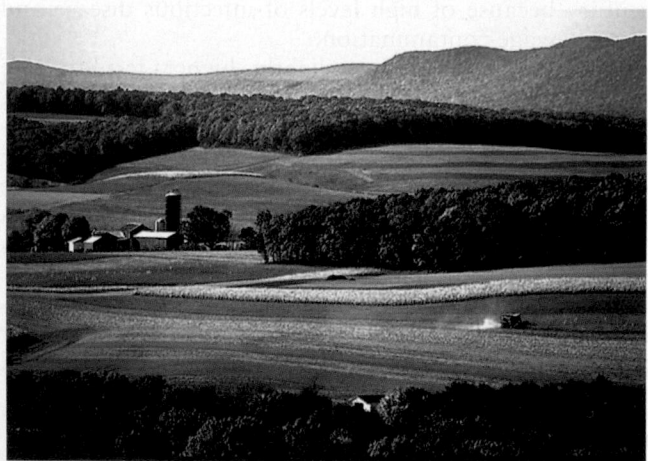

A farm in rural Pennsylvania. (Source: USDA, Agricultural Research Service.)

POPULATION CHARACTERISTICS

The following information is meant to describe, not stereotype, rural clients. Each rural community is unique, as are its residents. The PHN must determine whether the population characteristics discussed fit a specific rural community. The nursing student who plans to practice in the international arena will need to seek out relevant information about the specific rural population to be served. A rural culture is often very different from that found in larger cities (Eisenhauer, Hunter, & Pullen,

2010), and it is important to spend time in rural areas and to learn from our clients.

Age and Gender

Approximately 22.8% of women over age 18 live in rural areas (American Congress of Obstetricians and Gynecologists [ACOG], 2014). The proportion of females age 35 and over is higher in rural areas than in urban areas, or even the United States as a whole. Those females below age 18 (17.5%) and above age 65 (14.6%) comprise the largest percentages in rural areas, but urban areas have more females in the 18- to 34-year range (Maternal Child Health Bureau, 2011). Changes in age distribution for both males and females over three decades reveal net losses of those below age 20, and similar gains for those between the ages of 20 to 49 and over 65 in both rural and urban populations. Little change is noted for both rural and urban populations in the age group 50 to 64 (Council of Economic Advisors, n.d.). Elderly persons, those age 65 and older, are the fastest growing population in the United States in every location, including rural America.

Population trends have a direct relationship to the kinds of health services that are needed in rural communities. Growing families with young children need maternity, pediatric, and family health medical services, along with dental care and mental health services. They also can benefit from health promotion and disease prevention activities. The elderly, on the other hand, need health care to manage increased number of chronic health conditions. Rural communities need to provide access to nursing homes and rehabilitative services, as well as to hospitals, clinics, and health promotion programs that serve the elderly and the entire community.

Race and Ethnicity

Rural areas have historically had less racial diversity than urban areas. However, that is rapidly changing. Racial and ethnic groups have historically been concentrated in certain areas of the country—for example, Blacks in the rural South and American Indians in the rural Southwest and West, as well as Mexican Americans in the border states of the Southwest (McGranahan et al., 2010). Rapid Hispanic growth areas are found in the Midwest and Southeast (see Fig. 29–3) as well as the Great Plains (Barcus & Simmons, 2013). California, Texas, and Florida are home to 55% of the U.S. Hispanic population, with 14.4 million living in California. Other states experiencing growth include Illinois, New York, New Jersey, Colorado, Arizona, and Georgia (Brown & Lopez, 2013). The Hispanic population reached 55 million in 2014, but growth has slowed dropping from an annual average increase of 4.8% between 1995 and 2000 to 2.2% from 2010 to 2014. The median age for Hispanics is younger than other ethnic and racial groups, but it has been slowly rising; in 2000, it was 26; in 2010, it was 27; and it is now estimated at 29 years compared to 43 for non-Hispanic Whites, 34 for non-Hispanic Blacks, and 36 for Asians (Krogstad, 2015).

Higher birth rates led to faster growth of this population, and this could signal a need for changing health policies and practices. For instance, in rural counties with a high elderly population and established caseloads of

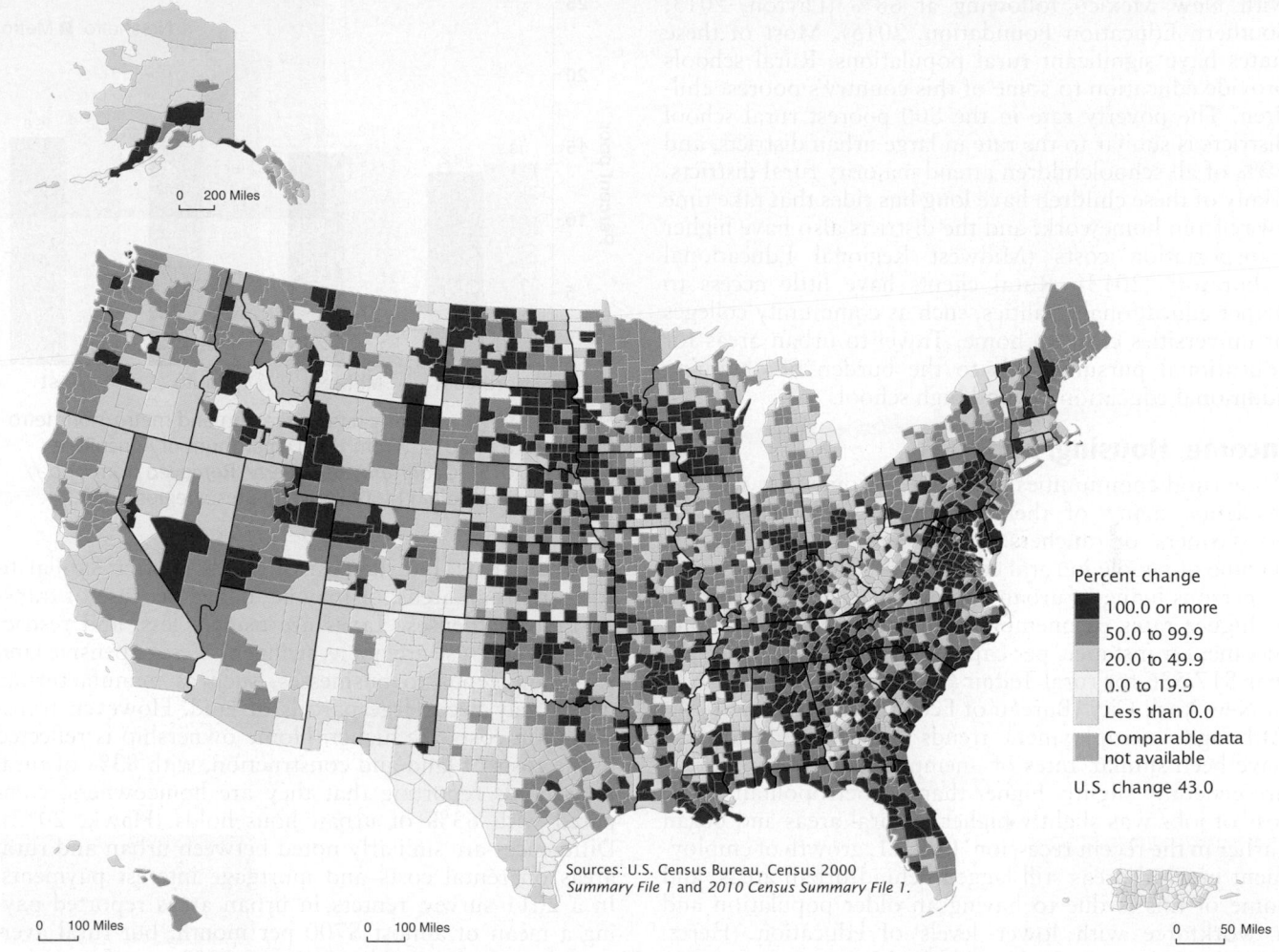

Percent change

- 100.0 or more
- 50.0 to 99.9
- 20.0 to 49.9
- 0.0 to 19.9
- Less than 0.0
- Comparable data not available

U.S. change 43.0

Sources: U.S. Census Bureau, Census 2000
Summary File 1 and *2010 Census Summary File 1.*

FIGURE 29–3 Percent change in Hispanic or Latino population by county: 2000 to 2010.

chronic disease patients, an influx of younger Hispanic populations may require a shift in policies and resources to include more pediatric and obstetric care. Almost half of rural counties lacked an obstetrician in 2010, and some states have no mother/infant tertiary care centers. Because of this, Wyoming approves out-of-state providers and reimbursement for transport and care when deemed medically necessary (ACOG, 2014). All of these changes influence geographic patterns of health status.

Education

Rural clients in the United States have historically had lower educational attainment than those in urban areas. However, the gap has closed for high school completion. By 2012, 12% of urban versus 14% of rural working age adults had less than a high school education, but rural areas had a greater proportion of those with a high school education. The gap for those with college degrees was much wider (32% of urban vs. 18 % of rural working age adults), and 12% of urban versus 6% of rural had advanced degrees (USDA, 2014). In the United States, while high school graduation overall rates rose to 81% for White students, Hispanics had a 76%, and African American students a 68% rate of graduation (Moskowitz,

2014). Some studies have shown urban–rural differences overall, but Jordan, Kostandini, and Mykerezi (2012) found dropout rates to be similar and noted that many ethnic differences were more likely due to peer influences and "some location attributes" (p. 18). Some educational researchers note that Hispanic students begin with a disadvantage, as their parents often do not speak English and have low levels of education (e.g., 41.3% of mothers had less than high school education). They are also often more likely to attend "hypersegregated schools" (e.g., majority of students are non-white), and as a group, they often perform below other ethnic and racial groups throughout their K to 12 schooling (Bouie, 2016). Only 9% of 25- to 29-year-olds completed a bachelor's degree in 2012, but approximately 18% enrolled in college during the 2011 to 2012 school year (Krogstad & Fry, 2014).

Lower levels of education are associated with poverty, especially in rural areas. In 2013, for the first time in five decades, the majority of public school children live in low-income homes. This is evidenced by 51% of them being eligible for free or reduced lunches; the highest percentages (above 50%) are in the southern states, along with California, Nevada, Utah, Kentucky, and West Virginia. Mississippi had the highest percentage at 71%, with New Mexico following at 68% (Layton, 2015; Southern Education Foundation, 2015). Most of these states have significant rural populations. Rural schools provide education to some of this country's poorest children. The poverty rate in the 800 poorest rural school districts is similar to the rate in large urban districts, and 19% of all schoolchildren attend majority rural districts. Many of these children have long bus rides that take time away from homework, and the districts also have higher transportation costs (Midwest Regional Educational Laboratory, 2013). Rural clients have little access to higher educational facilities, such as community colleges or universities close to home. Travel to urban areas for educational pursuits adds to the burden of obtaining additional education beyond high school.

Income, Housing, and Jobs

Some rural communities are home to some very wealthy residents, many of them landowners, business owners, farmers, or ranchers. On the average, however, the income of people in rural communities is lower than that of persons living in urban communities. This is reflected in higher rates of unemployment and lower per capita income; for instance, per capita personal income in 2013 was $17,536 for rural Telfair County, GA, but $121,632 in New York City (Bureau of Economic Analysis, 2014). Although unemployment trends over the past decade have been similar, rates of unemployment in rural areas are generally slightly higher than in metropolitan areas; loss of jobs was slightly higher in rural areas and began earlier in the recent recession. In 2011, growth of employment in rural areas still lagged behind urban areas, and some of this is due to having an older population and a workforce with lower levels of education (Hertz, Kusmin, Marré, & Parker, 2014). Mean rates of unemployment in rural counties with lower educational attainment were 2 percentage points higher than in those with higher rates (Economic Research Service [ERS], 2016). Also, many residents of rural areas are underemployed or only seasonally employed because of the nature of agriculture or other industries (Jensen, Mattingly, & Bean, 2011). Persistent poverty, defined as 20% or more of the population living in poverty for over 30 years, is more common in rural counties than in urban ones. Of the 386 counties with this designation, 340 of them are in nonmetropolitan areas, and a large number are in the South (USDA, 2011). More rural children live in poverty than those in urban areas (24% vs. 15%), and poverty among rural non-Whites is also higher than for children living in large cities (49% Blacks, 37% Hispanics vs. 41%, 35% Whites), according to Jensen and colleagues (2011). Also, the percentage of working poor in rural areas is higher than in urban areas (Glasgow & Berry, 2013). In 2009, about 11% of poor families living in rural areas reported receiving Temporary Aid to Needy Families (TANF) income, whereas 14% of poor urban families received income from TANF (Jensen et al., 2011).

See Figure 29–4, Poverty rates by residence.

Living in a rural area, however, has a number of economic advantages. The cost of land is lower than in urban areas; therefore, housing costs are also lower. The median cost of homes in remote rural areas is less than

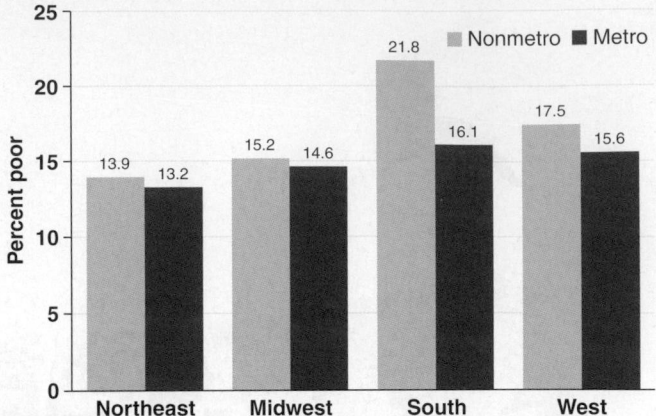

FIGURE 29–4 Poverty rates by region and metro/nonmetro status, 2010 to 2014. (From U.S. Department of Agriculture (USDA). (2015). *Geography of poverty*. Retrieved from http://ers.usda.gov/media/114604/povertyratesbyregion.png.)

in urban areas, but the cost of goods is often similar to costs in urban areas, or may be higher, because of transportation expenses. Taxes are usually less, and restrictions on land use are not as stringent. Less expensive land is advantageous to businesses, such as manufacturing, which may need large parcels of land. However, transportation costs are higher. Home ownership is reflected in the costs of land and construction, with 83% of rural households reporting that they are homeowners, compared with 63% of urban households (Hawk, 2013). Differences are similarly noted between urban and rural areas on rental costs and mortgage interest payments. In a 2011 survey, renters in urban areas reported paying a mean of almost $700 per month, but rural average rent was reported at around $350 monthly. Urban households are twice as likely to rent than rural ones, and the total household budget reflects high housing costs in both area households, 34.1% in urban versus 28.5% in rural (Hawk, 2013). Rental units in rural areas represent over 28% of total available housing. Although rural housing costs for the most part are lower, 47% of rural renters are considered "cost burdened" with over half of these renters paying over 50% of their monthly income on rental housing (Hawk, 2013, p. 2). Most low-income housing in rural areas consists of single-family homes, not large apartment complexes, and manufactured homes comprise 12% of rental units (over twice the overall housing rate). Almost 43% of rural renters are in single-family homes. Older housing is also common, and units are often substandard and in need of repair. Often because of high rates of poverty, those owning homes in rural areas live in houses that are old and need significant repairs. The highest small town and rural rental rates are found in Hawaii (39%), California (37.4%), Rhode Island (34.6%), and Alaska (34.3%), whereas Texas, California, North Carolina, and Ohio had the largest number of small town and rural renter–occupied units (Housing Assistance Council [HAC], 2013).

Some government assistance is available to help low-income renters. Section 515, the USDA loan program for rental homes for low-income individuals, provides over 400,000 affordable rental houses. The USDA

What do *you* think?

HELP FOR AILING HOMES

Many rural homes are rundown and in need of repair. Because building and construction are not always prevalent in rural areas, it is difficult for homeowners to find assistance. For instance, one woman inherited a family home built in 1949 but could not keep up with routine repairs. At first, the water pump broke and she hauled water from outside, then the heating quit working, and she began burning kindling and wood in her wood-burning stove. She had to use laundry and shower facilities at neighbors' or friends' homes. Eventually, the wind tore off a good portion of the roof. In searching for assistance, the homeowner had difficulty finding an agency that would help her repair her home. There were some programs for purchasing homes, but she didn't want to assume more debt. Eventually, she found an agency that provides assistance for rural residents. They helped her salvage her home so that she could remain there. In this case, the outcome was positive, but some individuals become frustrated and give up—living with family or friends or becoming homeless (often living in cars or camping out).

From White, G. B. (2015, January 28). Rural America's silent housing crisis. *The Atlantic*. Retrieved from http://www.theatlantic.com/business/archive/2015/01/rural-americas-silent-housing-crisis/384885/

offers rent subsidies to low-income elderly or disabled residents of multifamily housing units through Section 521. Section 8, a rental voucher program administered by the U.S. Department of Housing and Urban Development (HUD), is targeted to very low–income families who can choose from privately owned rental housing (HAC, 2013; USDHUD, 2016b). However, funds for this program are limited and applicants may wait several years for approval. Both rent subsidy programs supplement participants' rental costs above 30% of their income. HUD's Healthy Homes Program, created in 1993 to decrease childhood lead exposure, has expanded priorities to include radon, asbestos, allergens, mold/moisture, pest/pesticides, drinking water contamination, injury/fire hazards, and indoor air quality (Ashley, 2015). HUD has provided grant funding for demonstration projects with nurses, environmental specialists, and community workers targeting conditions in the home related to asthma and other conditions (Polivka, Chaudry, Crawford, Bouton, & Sweet, 2011). See Chapter 9.

The United States is unique in that it feeds its population with a small proportion of workers committed to food production and still is able to export food products to the rest of the world. Although many people equate farming with rural life, <1% of nonmetropolitan employment is directly related to agricultural farmworkers (ERS, 2015). When compared with urban areas, rural

communities typically offer fewer job options. Types of rural work, such as crop agriculture, manufacturing, and forestry, vary by locale, and these employment opportunities have been diminishing along with concomitant decreases in population and the shift from a goods-based to a service-based economy. Two thirds of all rural employment is now in the service sector, often in jobs that assist retirees. Although there is more manufacturing in the South, manufacturing has decreased overall, whereas health and social service sector jobs have increased substantially. White-collar jobs have increased; examples of white-collar occupations include professional, management, and sales, as well as technical/administrative support, but hands-on occupations (e.g., construction trades, assembly/production, repair/maintenance) are often more common in rural areas (Florida, 2012).

Although the use of the Internet for commerce is now very common in urban and suburban areas, the *rural digital divide* still exists. In 2013, 70% of urban households and 73% of suburban households reported having broadband Internet access, but only 62% of rural households did. When smartphones with Internet connection are added to the mix, the percentages for urban and suburban areas each rise by 10%; the increase for rural areas is only 8%, largely because of access and older demographics (Zickuhr, 2013). Roughly 72% of Americans currently use broadband; many in rural areas find it either nonexistent or too expensive (Zickuhr, 2013). The benefits of broadband services apply not only to wider employment opportunities but also to job retraining, education, and medicine (e.g., telehealth). A national survey of U.S. households found that rural residents had less access to the Internet (59.7% vs. 69.4%), and overall use was lower for non-white respondents and those without a medical condition (Wang, Bennett, & Probst, 2011b). Where broadband Internet services are readily available, higher-skilled remote workers could remain in rural areas while still providing high-tech services to clients across the country, thus potentially reducing the out-migration of young adults.

RURAL HEALTH ISSUES

Population-level differences in health between rural and urban areas are commonly noted (Anderson et al., 2015). Health concerns of populations in rural areas are related to the environment, occupations, injuries, and distance from health care providers. Environment issues particularly relate to agriculture and the health risks that accompany farming and other rural lifestyles.

Agriculture and Health

Although farming is not characteristic of all rural areas where agricultural production occurs, both direct and indirect effects on health can exist. In an important classic book about this sponsored by the Institute of Medicine (Merchant, Coussens, & Gilbert, 2006), it is noted that pesticides and fertilizers can affect water, air, and soil, and dust created from plowing for crops can affect the air quality. For instance, an "estimated 70% of antibiotics are used for nontherapeutic purposes in intensive livestock production," placing workers at risk for developing antibiotic-resistant infections (p. 4). Occupational exposures to windblown soil, organic dust, pesticides, mycotoxins, ammonia, animal dander, and hydrogen sulfite are only some of the air quality issues in rural areas (Lee, Mulay, Diebolt-Brown, & Lackovic, 2010). In Iowa, for instance, it is estimated that for every pound of corn harvested, 2 lb of soil are "exported" (p. 7). Livestock growth-producing agents, along with radon, pesticides, and fertilizers, can contaminate ground water (Blake, 2014). Kasner and associates (2012) found an "overrepresentation of females among farmworker illness and injury cases" among females that did not handle pesticides but were often working on nut and fruit crops and exposed to off-target drift of pesticides (p. 571). They noted that, while females were at increased risk for acute injury and illness related to pesticides, the male farmworkers had higher total absolute numbers with these illness and injuries. Lee and colleagues (2011) examined Occupational Health and Safety Administration (OSHA) databases and found almost 3,000 cases of illnesses related to drift of agricultural pesticides in a study of 11 states. They noted that 47% had work exposures, and 9 out of 10 had a fairly low severity of illness. Fourteen percent of the exposures were found in children under the age of 15. Most often (45%), the cause was fumigant soil applications and 24% with applications by air (e.g., crop dusters). Fumigants are commonly used on agricultural crops such as strawberries, potatoes, melons, tomatoes, grapes, peanuts, cotton, and tobacco (Dow AgroSciences, 2015). Lawsuits have been filed in California, Delaware, Florida, Hawaii, and Missouri against Monsanto over its popular herbicide, Roundup, with its active ingredient now thought to be a "probable human carcinogen" (Gillam, 2016, para. 8).

Many rural residents depend on their own well water for drinking, and water quality is monitored only sporadically by well owners and then usually only for nitrates and coliform bacteria (Lee et al., 2010). About 30% of rural residents obtain drinking water from very small water systems, without the monitoring and regulations associated with large urban water suppliers. Testing of small water systems should be done at regular intervals in order to get a true picture of water quality (Wedgworth et al., 2015).

Agricultural-related morbidity and mortality are relatively high. Agriculture (grouped together with fishing and forestry) now ranked above mining in the rate of fatal occupational injuries (26.8 vs. 19.8 per 100,000) in 2010. When examining rates for specific occupations, farmers/ranchers were 41.4 per 100,000 in 2010, behind fishermen, loggers, and aircraft pilots. Occupational incidents, such as off-road tractor overturn, increased 4% between 2009 and 2010 (U.S. Department of Labor, 2011). By 2013, agriculture was still in the top 10 occupations with the highest death rates (Smith, 2013). Tractor rollover accidents are very common and often involve older tractors (average farm tractor age is >25 years) without rollover protective structures (ROPS) (Murphy et al., 2010). Tractor injuries make up about 33% of all deaths, and farm children are at higher risk for injuries than hired farmworkers, and preschool and older male adolescents have the highest risk for fatalities from injuries (Wright, Marlenga, & Lee, 2013).

It is estimated that 33,000 injuries to children are farm related, and approximately 100 of them are fatal. Of the fatal injuries to youth, 23% were machinery related (often tractors), 19% were vehicle related (including ATVs), and drowning was to blame in 16% of fatalities. Most fatalities (34%) were in the 16- to 19-year age group (Occupational Health & Safety Administration [OSHA], n.d.). Farming injuries can result from tractor rollovers, suffocations in grain bins, exposure to harmful substances, falls, fires or explosions, accidents with other farm equipment, and on- or off-road collisions. Some injuries result in permanent disability, and worker training programs to recognize hazards and prevent injuries are rare in rural areas. A study reviewing government databases for nonfatal occupational injuries and illnesses in agriculture found significant undercounts. Leigh, Du, and McCurdy (2014) found that 73.6% of crop farm incidents and 81.8% of animal farm incidents were missed, because of the government's exclusion of small farm employees, farmers, and family members in their surveys. See Display 29–1 for two examples of common agricultural accidents.

Out of total farming operations, family farms account for 97.6%, and they represent 85% of all farm production (MacDonald, 2014). About 91% of farm families have a member working off the farm. Almost 36% of farmers and spouses with off-farm employment worked in management or professional occupations; other common areas of employment include construction, manufacturing, education, and health care (Brown & Weber, 2013). This contributes to the time spent in travel and its attendant problems. Because of the lack of mass transit, rural commuting increases air pollution and the incidence of injury or death from traffic accidents.

The Built Environment in Rural Areas: Relationship to Health

Even with the advances of medicine and genomics, and the staggering percentage of our gross domestic product (GDP) spent on health care, scientists feel that we will not be able to significantly improve our overall health and quality of life without addressing how we plan our living spaces.

Substantial scientific evidence gained in the past decade has shown that various aspects of the built environment can have profound, directly measurable effects on both physical and mental health outcomes, particularly adding to the burden of illness among ethnic minority populations and low-income communities (Frost et al., 2010; Hansen, Umstattd Meyer, Lenardson, & Hartley, 2015). Lack of sidewalks, bike paths, and recreational areas in some communities discourages physical activity and contributes to obesity; in those low-income areas that do have such amenities, the threat of crime keeps many people inside. Income segregation—the practice of housing the poor in discrete areas of a city—has also been linked with obesity and adverse mental health outcomes. Low-income and/or ethnic minority communities—already burdened with greater rates of disease, limited access to health care, and other health disparities—are also the populations living with the worst built environment conditions. The stress of housing insecurity has

DISPLAY 29–1 AGRICULTURAL ACCIDENTS

Farm Tractor Accident

In the old days before mechanical equipment, a farmer might be injured by one of his horses or mules, or accidently stabbed with a pitchfork. Today, tractors are involved in the majority of injuries and deaths. ROPS, or a roll cage over the tractor seat, can save lives; they were standard

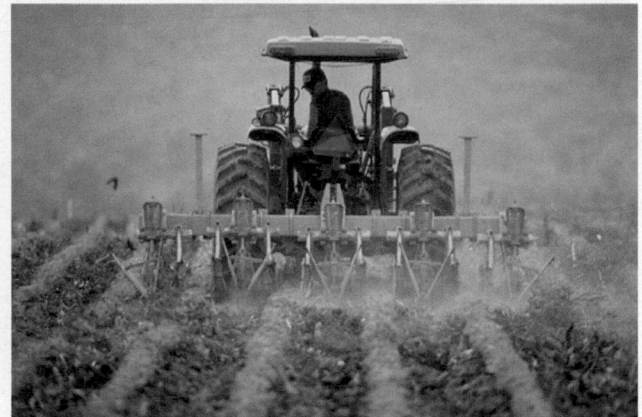

on every tractor manufactured in the country since 1985 (1959 in Sweden). If a farmer uses the seat belt and the tractor equipped with ROPS turns over, there is a good chance that he will survive the accident. Sadly, many farmers don't use seat belts, and many use older tractors without ROPS protection. There are many potential hazards on farms (e.g., falling bales of hay, heat stroke, dangerous equipment like hay balers, choppers, combines), but tractor rollovers and children falling from tractors are much too common and can often be prevented.

Death on the Farm

Agricultural deaths are not uncommon, as Tim Smith, an Iowan and fourth-generation farmer knows well. He almost died 26 years ago in a farm accident when as manure-pumping equipment caught his jeans and almost pulled his leg from his body. He was flown to a hospital and considers himself lucky to have his leg and his life. Tim reports that in his county with a population under 17,000, five people have died from agricultural-related accidents in the last 4 years. Some died from tractor rollovers and others in grain bins (from suffocation and crushing). Farmers face dangers of being gored by bulls, being electrocuted (as tall farm equipment hits overhead power lines), or being overcome by deadly fumes (often from manure pits on dairy farms), among other things. Just a few months ago, Tim says that two workers who were scooping silage (animal feed) from a wagon were injured. One worker's sweatshirt got caught in the beater mechanism and he became tangled in the machinery in an instant and flipped over onto his back. He had severe cuts and had to be airlifted to a hospital where doctors were able to save his life only because one of the cuts narrowly missed his femoral artery. In manure pit incidents, four members of the same family died (farmer, wife, two daughters) as they rushed to aid a farmhand who had fallen into the pit. They all died quickly after falling/climbing into the pit. But many die from exposure to the fumes and pass out, slipping into the manure slurry and drowning. Janna Swanson, a city girl who married a farmer, had no clue about the dangerous work of agriculture. Now, she worries all the time.

Source: Hirsch, J. (2014, June 16). *Death on the farm: Agricultural jobs are the most dangerous in the world. Why aren't we talking about it?* Retrieved from http://modernfarmer.com/2014/06/farm-deaths/. (Photo source: USDA Agricultural Research Service)

---

been associated with poor health status, poor mental health, and more limitations to daily activity (Stahre, VanEenwyk, Siegel, & Njai, 2015).

The **built environment** consists of the development of housing, highways, shopping areas, and other man-made features added to the natural environment. As populated areas expand, stresses are placed on natural habitats, water supplies, and air quality. The built environment is inextricably related to health.

Urban sprawl is a concern in some rural areas, as people move from urban centers to more suburban environments. Urban encroachment into agricultural areas creates problems with air and water pollution, access to health care, and heat islands. *Heat islands* occur when green areas are exchanged for asphalt, resulting in temperature and ecosystem changes that can extend to more rural areas (Trivedi et al., 2015; U.S. Environmental Protection Agency [EPA], 2011). Ozone levels are often highest just outside the city, because "ozone is formed relatively slowly by the action of sunlight on oxides of

nitrogen and hydrocarbons" (p. 72). Urban sprawl also causes problems with water pollution and the availability of water. Encroachment of housing areas into natural habitats or farmlands can lead to wider human exposure to pesticides, herbicides, and other hazards such as mosquito-borne illnesses. Mass transit is not often available in suburban areas and almost never found in rural areas. Opportunities for health-promoting behaviors are often more limited in rural areas. Deteriorating (or no) sidewalks can be a barrier to walking in rural areas. Exercise or fitness facilities, bike paths, jogging trails, and other incentives for physical activity are also often lacking in rural communities. Trivedi and colleagues (2015) examined data from a large national survey and found that rural adults were 1.19 times more likely to be obese when compared to urban adults. The prevalence was 35.6% in rural residents versus 30.4% for urban residents, and that difference was also found for both males and females (37.7% vs. 32.5%; 33.4% vs. 28.2%). Rural adults reported lower fiber and fruit intake, higher intake of sweetened drinks, and having no time for leisure activity than their urban counterparts (38.8% vs. 31.8%). Also, exercise levels were lower among rural adults than for those in urban areas (Trivedi et al., 2015). Obesity is prevalent in rural areas, and the physical environment, along with diet, plays a role in this epidemic (Lenardson, Hansen, & Hartley, 2015). Eating out, especially at buffets, fast-food restaurants, and cafeterias, instead of cooking at home, as well as not participating in physical activity have been associated with higher rates of obesity (Lenardson et al., 2015).

Rural roads are another concern because they are often narrow, without streetlights, and poorly maintained. More fatalities occur on rural roads and highways. While 19% of the country's population lived in rural areas in 2012, 54% of all road fatalities occurred there (National Highway & Traffic Safety Administration, 2015). Speeding, failure to use safety restraints, and alcohol are common causes of fatal crashes in rural areas. Over half of fatal crashes occurred during daylight hours in rural areas; the opposite is true in urban areas. Fifty-five percent of all fatal alcohol-related crashes occurred in rural areas, and 65% of rural occupant deaths in pickup trucks were not using restraints. Also, because time to trauma centers is much longer in rural versus urban areas, of all drivers who died en route to the hospital, 68% were from rural areas (National Highway Traffic Safety Administration, 2014). The majority of first responders in rural areas are volunteers (National Rural Health Association [NRHA], 2015). Slow-moving farm equipment traveling on rural roads, along with speeding and failure to use safety restraints, are often fatal conditions for drivers in rural areas. Researchers in North Dakota implemented a pilot program in two rural counties to "heighten awareness and safety on rural roads," but their interventions yielded "little effect on overall seat belt use" (Huseth, Vachal, Benson, & Lofgren, 2011, para. 1).

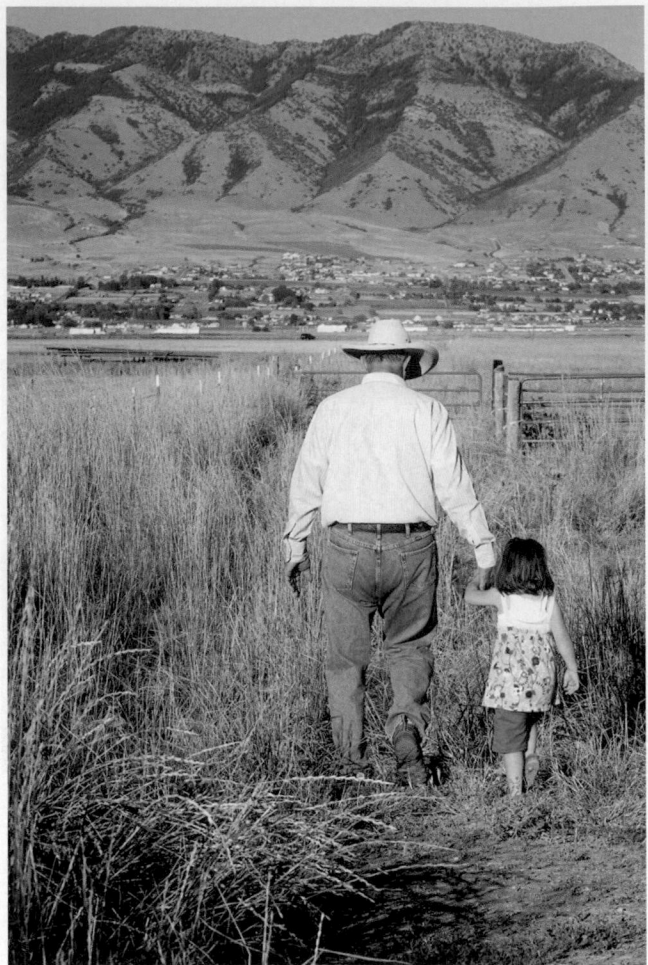

Life in a rural area may seem idyllic, but there are some significant risks of a rural lifestyle. (Private author photo with permissions of Tamara Harris, Tobey Roos, & Richard Wosnik.)

Self, Home, and Community Care

Historically, self-management of health care problems has been the most common way for rural people to cope with illness. This can be viewed as a type of strength, or it may be seen as a limitation. Mental health professionals note that the values held by those living in rural areas often include self-sufficiency, a high regard for privacy and autonomy (Smalley, Warren, & Rainier, 2012b). Rural residents are often viewed as hardworking, traditional, hardy, self-reliant, and resistant to accepting help or services from outside agencies regarded by them as welfare-type programs. Many rural clients are considered individualistic, independent, and resourceful. They often take care of illnesses or injuries on their own or have a supportive network to help them get their health needs met. Small communities commonly have strong social networks, but this type of familiarity may lead to problems with privacy and confidentiality, as well as stigma regarding mental health or substance abuse treatment. It can also exert a protective factor, as rural participants in one study reported better perceptions of physical and mental health, and less depressive symptoms, when they were more "socially connected" (Galloway & Henry, 2014, p. 43).

Because cost, travel, weather, and distance are barriers to obtaining health services from formal health care providers, rural clients may employ a variety of folk treatments and home remedies before consulting a nurse or a physician; such clients tend to visit providers at a much later stage than do people in urban areas. A cross-sectional study, examining rural and urban differences on 2013 County Health Rankings found that those living in rural counties had poor health outcomes overall and statistically significant differences in morbidity factors, health behavior, physical environment, and clinical care (Anderson et al., 2015). Rural residents put off getting care because of problems with transportation (10% vs. 5%) and cost (25% vs. 14%) at higher levels than urban counterparts in a study examining veteran's health (Spoont et al., 2011). They are also less likely to receive home health or palliative care services and physical therapy visits at home. They are also more likely to report poor or fair health (one in three adults), to have chronic diseases such as diabetes, and to die from heart disease than are residents of urban areas (AHRQ, 2011; O'Connor & Wellenius, 2012). One large-scale study found that rural residents pay more for medications than urban residents, but consistently significant differences were found between rural and urban health care expenditures (Lee, Jiang, Phillips, & Ohsfeldt, 2014b). Rural residents, however, receive care in a less timely manner than urban residents and utilize physicians who are more likely to provide care that is outside their specialty areas. Compared with hospitals that are less rural, CAHs have been found to have significantly higher patient mortality rates and worse processes of care for patients having heart failure, acute MIs, and pneumonia (Joynt, Harris, Orav, & Jha, 2011). A longitudinal cohort study from Canada noted that rural patients recently diagnosed with heart failure had fewer physician office visits in the first year, higher rates of hospitalization, and more ED visits (Gamble et al., 2011).

The low population density in rural areas makes service delivery more difficult, especially for those with special health needs such as the elderly, the disabled, and others (AHRQ, 2011). In rural Iowa, medical oncologists have served rural patients in outreach clinics for more than 20 years (Gruca, Nam, & Tracy, 2014). While insurance rates in rural areas are problematic, the greater treatment barriers when living in an isolated area are geography and lack of adequate transportation; poverty and unemployment are also big factors. In one example from Northern California, a few residents of the tiny, isolated town of Hayfork catch a ride 30 mi through winding mountain roads to a clinic in Mad River (Hernandez, 2015).

Suicide rates in rural areas, especially the rural West, can be as much as three times those in urban areas. Young rural males have been found to have almost double the rates of suicide compared to those in urban areas; firearm suicides are most common at 51.1%, with hanging/suffocation at 33.9% (Wallis, 2015). Female rural youth rates for suicide are less than rural males but are higher than rates for young urban females. Over twice the rate of anxiety and depression has been found in rural women, as opposed to urban women (Smalley et al., 2012b). A study of rural Midwest women found that 36.4% reported being depressed; self-report and depression screening were congruent 76.8% of the time, indicating that the women generally correctly identified their depressive symptoms (Groh, 2012). Military veterans, and those still on active duty, are more prone to higher levels of depression than their civilian counterparts. Dittrich et al. (2015) researched a national database for veterans with depressive symptoms and noted that those living in rural areas were more likely to Hispanic or multiracial, unemployed, and over age 65 or to have some type of health service deficit (e.g., uninsured, lack of routine medical exams, deferring medical care because of cost). In another study, less than half of rural community clinics or primary care settings accurately diagnosed depression in their patients; and over 85% of the rural population resides in a mental HPSA (Smalley, Warren, & Klibert, 2012a). This is another area where rural health care is lacking.

Home health care (HHC) is particularly difficult in sparsely populated areas, for both patients and nurses. Locating addresses in very rural areas often takes additional skills. (See Display 29–2 for the story of a home health nurse trying to locate a client's home.) The benefits of HHC are worthwhile; it allows people to stay at

---

DISPLAY 29–2 LOCATING A RURAL HOME HEALTH CLIENT

The following written (verbatim) directions were given by a discharge planner to a case manager (home care nurse) when making a referral for Mary, a 67-year-old woman who lived 37 mi from the hospital:

> Drive on the gravel road east of town until you get to the third set of mailboxes. Then, turn left; drive up the road until you see the old church; cross the broken bridge toward the river. Mary lives on the third farm. Her house has some trees and a fence around it (p. 222).

It took the home health nurse over 2 hours to drive about 30 mi on the narrow country roads after the morning rain. The nurse had to stop four times to ask residents for additional directions and hints for finding Mary's house. It was finally located, hidden in a large group of trees. The total travel time for this visit was about 4 hours.

From Bushy, A. (2003). Considerations for working with diverse rural client systems. *Lippincott's Case Management, 8*(5), 214–223.

---

home, supports their hardiness, and compensates for the long distance between home and formal health care. An examination of rural and urban HHC patients revealed that rural patients were more ill and had more risk factors for hospitalization and generally poorer health overall. Living in a rural area was correlated with higher odds (1.16) of being in a serious or fragile condition and also higher likelihood of receiving respiratory treatments (21.1% rural vs. 14.6% urban); there is a greater prevalence of smoking among rural residents (15.5% vs. 11.9%). Also, 29.8% of rural residents were more likely than urban residents (26.7%) to have surgical wounds that required further care (Probst & Bhavsar, 2014).

Access to Acute Care

Rural hospitals have a high risk for financial problems and closures, thus leaving rural patients stranded without services nearby and forcing them to drive long distances for inpatient care. The Medicare Rural Hospital Flexibility Program encouraged states to form rural health networks, improve emergency medical services, and improve the financial performance of rural hospitals by designating them CAHs. **Critical access hospitals** are rural hospitals, located a minimum of 35 mi from the next hospital or 15 mi if the terrain is mountainous or the only routes are on secondary roads (RAC, n.d.). One intention of this designation was to reduce the number of rural hospital closures by providing cost-based Medicare reimbursements, which differ from the prospective payments given to larger hospitals. Most CAHs are nonprofit, have limited lengths of stay and bed capacity, and are heavily dependent on Medicare and Medicaid funding (Holmes & Pink, 2011). Higher Medicare reimbursement rates are given to CAHs, but expected decreases in

Medicare payments to all hospitals over the next decade are a source of concern (Spencer, 2013). However, even though urban and rural Medicare patients receive similar amounts of care, quality of care is not always comparable to urban areas (Stensland, Akamigbo, Glass, & Zabinski, 2013). Lower-quality follow-up care after discharge was noted among rural Medicare clients and this has implications for reimbursement rates as hospitals are penalized for some readmissions (Toth et al., 2015). And "the digital divide between urban and rural hospitals that are adopting electronic health records and using the technology effectively is widening" (Sandefer, Marc, & Kleeberg, 2015, p. 1).

Major Health Problems

Among major health problems affecting individuals in rural areas are cardiovascular disease (CVD), diabetes, and human immunodeficiency virus (HIV). Geography, economics, and rural lifestyle factors may account for the higher rate of these major health problems.

Cardiovascular Disease

When it comes to CVD, geography may play a role. Geographic concentrations of CVD and other diseases vary from one rural location to the next, possibly related to inadequate health care, distance from care, environmental exposures, infectious disease in the area, and other factors. These multidimensional elements interact in such a way to cause cardiovascular mortality statistics to vary among regions and ethnic groups. However, one recent national cohort study found "geographic variation in inflammatory biomarkers among otherwise healthy women that cannot be completely attributed to traditional clinical risk factors or lifestyle characteristics" (Clark, Coull, Berkman, Buring, & Ridker, 2011, para. 3).

CVD is a leading cause of death in the United States (1 in 7 deaths), and the total direct and indirect costs of CVD and stroke were estimated at over $320.1 billion in 2015 (American Heart Association, 2015). Mortality because of heart disease is highest in the South, especially following the path of the Mississippi River (Bolin & Bellamy, 2015). Regional variations have been noted in prevalence of CVD and stroke, as well as heart failure readmissions (Cook & Lauer, 2011). Studies have found increased stroke mortality in the South (stroke belt), and many researchers are focusing on the possible underlying risk factors related to geographical variations. One group of researchers wanted to better understand the effect of length of time living in the stroke belt and age at first exposure. Howard and colleagues (2013) studied almost 25,000 residents who were stroke free at initial survey and later had strokes and found that the "risk of stroke was significantly associated with proportion of life" in the stroke belt (p. 1655). They used a proportional hazards model to determine the association of stroke incidence and with their "indices of exposure" (e.g., born in stroke belt, current residence, years in stroke belt during specific age ranges). Those individuals who were lifelong residents of the stroke belt had the strongest association with risk of stroke, but living in that area during childhood was the most predictive of future stroke, when adjusting for risk factors (p. 1655). Davis, Gebreab, Quarells,

and Gibbons (2014) examined social determinants (e.g., stress, racial discrimination, socioeconomic status [SES]) of cardiovascular health (e.g., risk factors of diabetes, high cholesterol, hypertension, obesity) among black and white women in the stroke belt (defined as urban) and stroke buckle (defined as rural). They noted that black women overall had poorer cardiovascular health than white women in both rural and urban areas (odds ratio 2.68 for rural and 2.92 for urban). White women who reported high levels of daily stress were found to have poorer cardiovascular health than those who reported lower levels of stress (odds ratio 2.85). They concluded that risk reduction measures should be tailored to specific populations in the South, targeting low-SES black women and white women with high stress levels. In a study of the predictors of uncontrolled hypertension in the stroke belt, researchers found that blacks were more likely than whites to have uncontrolled blood pressure (both systolic and diastolic). They noted that not correctly taking medications, age, and race were significant predictors of uncontrolled systolic blood pressure. Interventions could be targeted to address hypertension management in blacks and older adults in an effort to control hypertension and help prevent strokes (Dave et al., 2013). Other researchers have focused attention outside the stroke belt and noted racial and urban–rural disparities with stroke mortality. Mortality from strokes is higher among blacks and residents of rural areas (Sergeev, 2011). An Australian study also found urban–rural differences, with increased odds of death following strokes for patients treated in rural hospitals (Cadilhac Kilkenny, Longworth, Pollack, & Levi, 2011). After implementation of a Rural Stroke Project in rural hospitals (e.g., stroke units, aspirin within 24 hours of ischemic stroke, team health assessment within 48 hours, adherence to care plans, clinical coordinators), more patients were discharged home and care was improved (Cadilhac et al., 2013).

Rural areas usually have less high-tech health care equipment available, which may affect outcomes for patients with cardiovascular emergencies. Being within 60 minutes of a Primary Stroke Center (PSC) can determine outcome for many patients. Mullen and associates (2014) noted that 65.8% of Americans had that access (87% being in major cities, 59% in minor cities, and only 9% in suburbs/1% rural areas). They also noted that PSC access was generally lower in the stroke belt (44% inside vs. 69% outside) and that non-Whites and Hispanics were more likely to have access than Whites (77% vs. 62%, 78% vs. 64%). Demographics were only meaningfully associated with access in smaller cities, not major cities and suburbs. Less access was found in smaller cities with lower levels of education, income, health care resources/utilization, and higher numbers of uninsured along with Medicare/Medicaid eligible individuals. PHNs can advocate for better access to care and promote healthy lifestyle choices as well as population-targeted interventions to reduce stroke and CVD.

Rural residents may ignore early cardiovascular symptoms and give little heed to preventive interventions such as exercise and low-fat diets. A small study of women in rural Midwest states found that the participants had problems identifying symptoms associated with heart attacks in women, especially when they had no prior exposure. This may lead to delays in seeking treatment, but the women also were reluctant to call for help because of privacy concerns, thinking that an ambulance wouldn't get to them in time, and they did not want to ask relatives for help; researchers concluded that rural women may need educational programs and better information in order to seek assistance in a timely manner (Jackson & McCulloch, 2014). Other risk factors, such as smoking and poverty, affect cardiovascular health. Adults in rural counties are most likely to smoke and use smokeless tobacco, and they are more likely to be in the presence of smokers at home and work (Vander Weg, Cunningham, Howren, & Cai, 2011). Rural residents are also more likely to be obese than urban counterparts (Trivedi et al., 2015). Lee et al. (2014a) found a higher prevalence of prediabetes in both blacks and whites living in the stroke belt than those living outside it. Also, prediabetes prevalence was higher for blacks independent of where they live. Rates of diabetes are higher in rural areas; this also plays a part in higher CVD morbidity and mortality (Bolin & Bellamy, 2015). A study of health risk behaviors of insured and uninsured patients using a rural health clinic found that the majority of all patients regularly ate fried foods, did not eat the daily recommended servings of vegetables or fruits, drank high-calorie beverages, and did not regularly exercise (Smalley et al., 2012a). Uninsured patients also were more likely to text and talk on cell phones while driving, drink alcohol, have unprotected sex, and not seek necessary medical care in a timely manner.

Diabetes

Rural populations are disproportionately affected by diabetes and CVD (8.6% and 38.8%, respectively); the prevalence is generally greater in rural areas, and this is even more pronounced among Hispanics and Blacks. Causes for these differences are not always well understood but may be due to poverty, tobacco use, and greater incidence of obesity in rural populations, all of which put them at a higher risk for chronic illness (O'Connor & Wellenius, 2012). Rural areas have been cited as promoting obesity on a population level because of fewer opportunities for walking, as residents spend a great deal of time commuting to work or driving to essential services, and rural residence was positively correlated with BMI, distance to retail food, and commute times, among other things (Calancie et al., 2015). Lower physical activity rates and greater barriers to physical activity are commonly found in rural populations, as opposed to populations living in urban settings (Bolin & Bellamy, 2015).

Rural populations also face greater barriers in diagnosis, treatment, and follow-up care. Some compliance issues with prescribed medication regimens may relate to the lack of health insurance and low-income levels in rural areas but could also be due to lower health literacy and education levels. Other problems with accessing care may involve transportation and weather. A lack of access to quality health care services has been a long-standing problem for rural Americans. The lack of appropriate services, such as certified diabetes educators or endocrinologists, is also common in rural America; expensive, up-to-date technologies requiring technical expertise are not readily available in most rural areas (Patel, Darling, Samuels, & McClellan, 2014). The U.S. Department of Health and Human Services and the United Nations have both identified rural residence as a potential barrier to better health outcomes (Sparks, 2012). Because of the significant difference in access to health care, Douthit, Kiv, Dwolatzky, and Biswas (2015) cite a need for an ongoing effort at reform to improve services, recruit health care professionals, and train them specifically for service in rural areas, as well as increasing health insurance coverage and focusing more on health promotion.

Anderson et al. (2015), in a comparison study of people living in rural counties versus nonrural counties, found that rural residents had statistically lower scores in areas such as clinical care, morbidity factors, and general health behavior. Many factors facing rural populations create barriers to engaging in preventive services (Weaver & Gjesfjeld, 2014). For instance, a classic study by Krishna, Gillespie, and McBride (2010) highlighted the extreme complications encountered by rural residents who often have to travel great distances to access services for diabetes care, such as basic follow-up with podiatrists for diabetic foot care, ophthalmologists for retinal health, and nutritionists and health educators, as well as routine laboratory blood tests, to guide lifestyle choices. Maez, Erickson, and Naumuk (2014, p. 1) found that "nutritional patient education, motivational counseling and lifestyle modifications" were the most important factors in promoting better outcomes for rural clients. Harvey and Janke (2014) found that a chronic disease management program, using weekly group sessions, initiated positive changes in behavior among a group of rural clients. Multiple strategies were found to be effective in a systematic review of rural diabetes care (Ricci-Cabello, Ruiz-Perez, Rojas-Garcia, Pastor, & Gonçalves, 2013). PHNs, especially in rural and frontier areas, often provide follow-up for diabetic clients who may be unable to regularly access their health care providers because of problems with distance or transportation. Home visits to check on their diet/exercise, blood glucose monitoring, and foot care are important safeguards for this population. Also, interventions targeted to behavior change can be helpful.

Human Immunodeficiency Virus Infection

Human immunodeficiency virus or HIV, the virus that causes acquired immunodeficiency syndrome (AIDS), was first identified among the urban U.S. population in the early 1980s. The Centers for Disease Control and Prevention (CDC) estimates that more than 1.1 million U.S. residents have HIV, and 34,247 were diagnosed with AIDS in 2009. In 2012, almost 1.2 million people were living with AIDS in the United States (CDC, 2015). About 5% to 8% of all HIV cases in the United States were among rural populations in the early 1990s, with 56,209 diagnosed with AIDS by 2007. In the South, there are rising incidences of new cases and deaths from AIDS; in 2009, 68% of new cases were in the rural South. In 2009, the Northeast reported the highest rate of persons per 100,000 living with an AIDS diagnosis (248.7), followed by the South (169.5), the West (133.6), and the Midwest (77.2) (CDC, 2012). A study examining HIV prevalence, level of urbanization, and poverty found that racial and ethnic differences in HIV prevalence were still evident, after controlling for poverty in rural areas; this was not the case in more urban areas, where racial and ethnic differences in HIV prevalence were not significant in high-poverty areas (Vaughan, Rosenberg, Shouse, & Sullivan, 2014).

Also, 50% of rural AIDS cases are among African Americans, and young African American women are the fastest growing group infected through heterosexual exposures. In all racial/ethnic groups in rural areas, men have the highest rate of AIDS at 9.1 per 100,000 (almost three times that of women), and more than 50% are exposed through sexual contact with men. Injection drug use accounts for 20% of male AIDS cases, and over 50% of rural HIV infections are only diagnosed within the year after advancing to AIDS. While there have been no significant differences between rural and urban populations in numbers of sexual partners, rates of unprotected sex, and being tested for HIV, rural residents were found to be less likely to change sexual behaviors or condom use in response to the AIDS epidemic (Rural Center for AIDS/STD Prevention, n.d.). Rural HIV patients were slower to adopt novel HIV therapy than urban counterparts in a Veterans' Administration study of raltegravir (Ohl et al., 2013).

Early diagnosis and treatment of HIV/AIDS are issues that must be faced by all rural communities. Physicians, nurses, and other health practitioners need to be educated about the changing face of the disease. Barriers to access among rural California HIV-infected women were similar to those noted for other health care issues: lack of transportation, problems navigating the health care system, physical health issues (Sarnquist et al., 2011). Depression is linked to lower medication adherence in HIV-positive women, and this has implications for rural care (Tyer-Viola et al., 2014). Because relatively few cases of HIV/AIDS may be present in any one rural community, specialized services are often not available, and it can be a challenge to stay up-to-date with the newest treatment protocols (National Rural Health Association [NRHA], 2016). Each state health department has resource persons who can provide information to health professionals in rural communities about the HIV/AIDS epidemic and current treatment protocols. A study of HIV testing and other treatment services in rural counties in the South found that 53% of health departments responding to the survey provided HIV testing, and 48% had HIV treatment sites. Clients had to travel an average of 50 mi to reach these services, which was considered a barrier, but facilitators included rapid HIV testing, integrating HIV testing into other services, and establishment of free/easily accessible HIV testing services (Sutton, Anthony, Vila, McLellan-Lemal, & Weidle, 2010). Communities must determine the burden of disease and tailor services to their population while at the same time providing education and case finding. For example, a study examining social service needs of HIV patient in Alabama found that case management, financial assistance, and help getting medical care were the most common needs. Women often needed help finding child care, and those scoring in the highest 25% required assistance with more than

basic needs, but also legal and medical needs, as well as substance use treatment (Stewart, Phillips, Walker, Harvey, & Porter, 2011). A study of HIV-positive women in California found that 45.3% of those interviewed had problems traveling to appointments, 32.8% had physical problems that prevented them from traveling, 31.2% had no transportation, and 25% cited difficulty in navigating the health care system (Sarnquist et al., 2011).

Increased community awareness may be accomplished through faith-based organizations or by having local coaches or radio personalities raise the issue of HIV/AIDS; after-school service learning programs for youth may be helpful in reducing adolescent sexual risk-taking behaviors. Free HIV testing made available where rural populations gather (e.g., regional athletic events, colleges, health centers, church congregations) or high-risk groups gather (e.g., adult or gay bookstores, bars) can be effective. Testing incoming and outgoing prisoners, and providing condoms, can also reach a high-risk population. Many health departments offer services through Ryan White CARE Act grant funding; these may include comprehensive care clinics or PHN case management services, as well as education/prevention.

It may be difficult for a person to seek diagnosis or treatment from a rural health practitioner. Confidentiality is an issue of concern, as is lack of anonymity. People with HIV/AIDS may fear the stigma of HIV/AIDS and the rejection that is often associated with it. They may have concern for their jobs or their position in the community if their diagnosis is divulged, and they frequently fear that health care workers will break confidentiality rules (NRHA, 2016). Instead, rural people may choose to seek out HIV/AIDS testing through an urban health care facility where they know no one. Returning to the community can be devastating because of the lack of needed support services and the fear of sharing their diagnosis with others.

Another issue that may arise is that of urban residents with rural roots who return to their home communities as their illness worsens. These people seek family support and can overwhelm their caregivers, especially if the caregivers do not seek support for themselves. Community health nurses are in a good position to assist families with any health issues and can offer to facilitate connections to other social, spiritual, financial, and health care providers. A recent study of HIV-positive women found that satisfaction with social support and coping that focused on managing HIV disease were the best predictors of adherence to medication regimens (Tyer-Viola et al., 2014). In addition, it is important for health care providers to develop interventional strategies aimed at improving quality of life while screening patients for HIV-related symptoms and depression (Vyavaharkar, Moneyham, Murdaugh, & Tavakoli, 2012). Adherence to the treatment plan was lower in patients experiencing adverse effects, thus management of these side effects is vital (Al-Dakkak et al., 2013). It is important to continue HIV/AIDS treatment even if the viral load becomes undetectable, as this is a sign that the medications are working. If patients stop taking their medications, the virus will start reproducing again and the viral load will increase (AIDS.gov, 2016).

Access to Health Care

Insurance, Managed Care, and Health Care Services

Health insurance in today's market is costly, especially for individual purchasers. Some people, therefore, forego health insurance for themselves and their families. As noted earlier, rural workers are less likely to be offered health insurance through their employers, often because they are either self-employed or because of the size or type of employers (AHRQ, 2012). Depending on their income, people may or may not be eligible for Medicaid or State Children's Health Insurance Programs (S-CHIPs). Even people who are eligible for government health assistance may not apply because of their belief that it is a sign of weakness to accept a handout. Thompson (2015) reported on farmers in Kansas and their reaction to the Affordable Care Act (ACA). Most farmers are self-employed and were often unable to pay for individual insurance or had preexisting conditions that prevented them from being eligible for insurance. One insurance agent noted that 60% to 70% of farmers still purchase through individual markets and most are in their late 50s. Because farming is considered dangerous work and many of them have some preexisting health problem, they pay higher premiums than most people. Many were uninsured and a few depended on spouses' health insurance through their employers. Since the ACA was enacted, a good number of farmers "now have health insurance for the first time in 40 years," despite being political conservatives and probably never voting for a Democrat in their life (para. 22). While some younger farmers feel that rates are too high, he goes on to explain that most farmers understand that many of their neighbors have been uninsured for a long time and that health care reform provides an opportunity for them to finally get health insurance.

Historically, a traditional fee-for-service model delivered health care in rural and urban communities (see Chapter 6). However, that is changing, and it is challenging for rural providers to deliver the cost-effective, complex health care that rural persons need via solo or small group practices. Rural patients often utilize family practice clinics. The managed care model, which attempts to control costs and improve health care delivery, has slowly diffused into rural communities. One reason for the sluggishness is that rural practitioners are reluctant to become part of organizations that negotiate to reduce their payments, as many of them already see a disproportionate number of Medicaid and uninsured patients that impact their bottom line. Another reason is the low population density, making this type of health care insurance less profitable. However, more states are moving to Medicaid managed care models, and Medicare offers this option to beneficiaries. This puts rural residents at a disadvantage, as they may have poor access to services because of distance and travel time.

Building provider networks in rural communities is both time- and effort-intensive because rural providers are often inexperienced with managed care organizations (MCOs). The federal government provides support for **rural health clinics** in areas designated as underserved and nonurban; differences in effectiveness and efficiency have been noted in larger clinics versus smaller clinics (Ortiz & Wan, 2012; RAC, n.d.). These clinics have served rural clients for more than 30 years, and they are an important source of health care. However, in a study of rural health clinics and their perceptions of the ACA's Accountable Care Organization (ACO) model, researchers found that almost half of respondents had very little knowledge of ACOs (Ortiz, Bushy, Zhou, & Zhang, 2013). While a majority of clinic respondents felt that ACOs could improve patient safety and quality, many were concerned about having adequate funding to upgrade technology and were concerned about potential regulatory and legal barriers. These are valid concerns, as Bradley (2013) notes. Despite the cost savings expected with ACO's more integrated health care delivery model, the high costs for initial technology upgrades, and the potential for small rural providers to be overtaken by larger consolidated groups, in rural areas, this component of health care reform may be problematic. Some grant funding targeted to implementation of the ACA in rural areas is available (National Advisory Committee on Rural Health & Human Services, 2011). See Chapter 6.

Other specialized *migrant clinics* may also be located in rural areas with large migrant worker populations. Many of these are **federally qualified health centers** that provide care to underserved populations through Medicare, Medicaid, or a sliding fee scale (RAC, n.d.). Because only 9% of physicians work in rural areas (where 21% of the population resides), midlevel practitioners, such as physician assistants (PAs) and nurse practitioners (NPs), are often employed in these clinics (AHRQ, 2012). Also, specialists are most often found in metropolitan areas; rural areas are devoid of most of the smaller specialty physicians, and the population has difficulty accessing these services. For instance, 90% of geriatric specialists are found in urban areas, along with a greater proportion of internal medicine physicians. Family physicians are more evenly distributed between urban and rural areas (Peterson, Bazemore, Bragg, Xierali, & Warshaw, 2011).

Rural areas are characterized by a lack of core health care services (e.g., primary care, hospital care, emergency medical services, long-term care, mental health and substance abuse counseling services, dental care, public health services). A national survey of CEOs from rural hospitals found that over 75% reported physician shortages, most commonly family practice (58.3%) and internal medicine (53.1%). Other shortages were noted for physicians specializing in psychiatry, general surgery, neurology, pediatrics, cardiology, and OB-GYN. Over 73% reported shortages of registered nurses, and over half needed pharmacists. Thirty-five percent reported a need for NPs (MacDowell, Glasser, Fitts, Nielsen, & Hunsaker, 2013). In a comparative study of rural and urban primary care physicians, Weigel, Ullrich, Shane, and Mueller (in press) found those working in rural areas provided care to more patients per physician than their urban counterparts, as well as a wider variety of services. Population health services in rural areas may be covered by a combination of public health departments, physicians in private practice, and local hospitals, as well as various community agencies. In some rural or frontier areas, state health departments may offer services, as no local infrastructure may be present. Many rural residents depend heavily on public health department services.

Seventeen percent of local health departments (LHDs) serve small towns (populations under 10,000), and 44% serve communities with populations between 10,000 and 49,999. These LHDs are less likely than larger health departments to provide environmental health services, but they often provide many of the other services (e.g., primary prevention, health services, epidemiology/surveillance) found in larger health departments (National Association of County and City Health Officials, 2014). Many rural public health agencies are small and isolated, with a need for connections with other agencies in the region or state. PHNs serve in a variety of capacities—often wearing many hats. The highest level of education for many PHNs is an associate degree, which generally doesn't include public health content in the curriculum (NRHA, 2011). Rural public health departments generally have lower public funding for programs and services and must guard against fragmentation of resources/programs. They also experience difficulty competing against urban agencies in access to grant funding and recruiting specialized staff. Transportation costs and adequate provision of a variety of services are other issues faced by rural public health departments, and all of these issues affect the health of the populations served. However, one study comparing willingness to respond to emergency situations revealed that rural health department workers were significantly more likely to respond than urban

workers (Barnett et al., 2012). In all response scenarios provided (weather related, pandemic influenza, radiological "dirty" bomb, anthrax), rural workers were more willing to respond and report to the health department; the lowest response from both groups was found for a "dirty" bomb scenario (78.7% rural, 73% urban).

Barriers to Access

In rural areas, numerous access barriers to health care exist. The physical distance between place of residence and location of health care services can be considerable. Weather and geographical barriers may also be a factor. Rural clients may be referred to a distant urban medical center for cancer therapy or other sophisticated care. Members of the population may be frustrated if they travel to a faraway site for care and do not have their problem resolved. Rural clients must be advised before they travel to make sure that the health care provider is not behind schedule or unable to see them; see From the Case Files I for a hard lesson learned by one PHN student.

Transportation barriers can hinder access to health care services and are especially common among low-income and vulnerable populations (Syed, Gerber, & Sharp, 2013). Transportation can also be an issue, especially for people who do not drive or who lack dependable vehicles. Almost 33% have transportation disadvantages, with those earning between $20,000 and $50,000 spending 30% of their income on a car and the costs related to driving it (American Public Health Association [APHA],

---

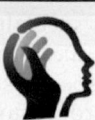 **From the Case Files I**

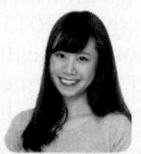

A Lesson in Rural Transportation

I live in a relatively large city of 450,000 people. When I started my community health nursing rotation, I was assigned to a rural county public health department in an adjoining county over 50 mi from my house. To make matters worse, when I got there for my first clinical day, my professor told me that I was assigned to see clients in an isolated community another hour away from the health department! There was nothing but farmland between the county seat and this small, forgotten oil town. This small town didn't even have sidewalks, much less a fast-food restaurant! After I got over my frustration about traveling such long distances, I began to visit some of my families and started to actually enjoy my time with them. They were so appreciative and open to my suggested interventions. I really seemed to be making a difference. One older gentleman, Armando, was a diabetic who spoke very little English. He lived with his wife of 50 years, who spoke almost no English. Their children had moved away in order to go to school and get better jobs. His diabetes was not well controlled, and the rural health clinic FNP suggested that he see a specialist (actually an

internist) in the county seat. I helped him make arrangements with the doctor for an early afternoon visit and made sure that he could catch the county bus that ran between the smaller communities and the county seat. When I came back for a follow-up visit the next week, I was shocked to learn that Armando's appointment had been pushed back to 4:30 PM because of the doctor's involvement in hospital emergencies, and by the time Armando was finished with his appointment, the county bus service had ended. Armando, with no money and no one to call for a ride, began walking back to his home—over 52 mi away! About halfway home, a farm truck driver gave him a lift to the large cotton farm a few miles from his home. You can imagine my horror and embarrassment when I learned of this ordeal. I never realized how difficult it was for rural people to get to their medical appointments. I always had a car and could drive wherever my gas budget could take me. I thought that the bus would not be a problem, but I learned my lesson. Now, I make sure that the physician's office understands the patient's circumstances and the importance of getting them back to the bus stop in time to make the last bus.

Andrea, Senior Nursing Student

n.d.a). Unpredictable weather adds to potential barriers for rural clients. Snow, ice, wind, flash floods, and rain can make travel dangerous, even over short distances. Parents may decide not to risk driving on poorly maintained roads to get their children immunized or to have their own hypertension evaluated. Elderly people may choose to delay health care when long travel times, especially in isolated rural areas, are involved. Rural populations have disproportionately high injury mortality rates, much of which is due to motor vehicle accidents (APHA, n.d.a).

According to a classic study by Branas, McKenzie, and Williams (2005), almost 47 million rural Americans do not have access to either level I or level II trauma centers within an hour's driving time, leaving them at higher risk for death from injuries. However, almost 43 million urban Americans are able to access trauma centers (level I or level II) within an hour's time. There is a noted mortality benefit of direct trauma center transport, and regional trauma systems can provide a population-based approach to provide urgent care (Haas et al., 2012). Hsia and Shen (2011a) found that 31% of those in rural areas had difficulty accessing trauma centers within one hour of driving time, and certain vulnerable populations are at an even greater risk of poor access to health care services. A good number of hospital trauma centers have closed since 2001, with a negatively disproportionate affect for rural residents (Hsia & Shen, 2011b). Inadequate phone service, dead zones in cell coverage, and the lack of adequate numbers of board-certified emergency physicians on staff are all problems frequently encountered in rural areas (Bolin & Bellamy, 2015). However, Lipsky et al. (2014) examined differences in survival among rural and urban trauma patients after implementation of the Model Rural Trauma Project. They noted, after statistical correction for differences among the 1,122 patients, that rural mortality was not significantly different from that for urban patients.

Limited choice of health care providers is a barrier for some rural residents. Fewer physicians, nurses, dentists, and other providers work in rural areas (AHRQ, 2012). Those with special needs often must travel to urban medical centers to get required care. One seminal study of disabled adults noted that they found their local rural physicians to be less familiar with their conditions, thus requiring these disabled patients to "teach" their health care provider. They also described rural public transportation as often unreliable and inaccessible (Iezzoni, Killeen, & O'Day, 2006). A literature review revealed that rural residents have diverse types of disabilities yet have barriers to accessing needed care. Children/adolescents, mentally ill, working adults, the elderly, and those with HIV/AIDS were populations of interest, and rural health care providers were often found to be lacking in training and experience necessary to treat some of the more complex medical needs of these clients. The authors also noted the need for regional specialized care services, telehealth, better training and networking for local primary care physicians, and the use of case managers and trained local paraprofessionals to bridge the gap in care (Lishner, Richardson, Levine, & Patrick, n.d.). As Medicare payments to primary care physicians are reduced and often late, there is a real threat to rural disabled and elderly clients, as some physicians either limit the number of Medicare clients they will serve or close their offices in rural areas. As mentioned earlier, concerns about confidentiality or provider expertise sometimes cause clients to seek care from even more distant providers, but as the options for health care continue to shrink, rural clients may have few choices available locally. Those persons with disabilities who are also uninsured (more common in rural populations) have significantly more access barriers to care than those without disabilities (Iezzoni, Frakt, & Pizer, 2011).

New Approaches to Improve Access

The *Healthy People 2020* document mandates improvements in access, health education, health screening, immunizations, and disease morbidity for the United States. Creative ways of delivering these and other services to rural clients need to be explored. Access to care is a social justice issue: clients who live in rural areas should receive quality health care, regardless of where they choose to live.

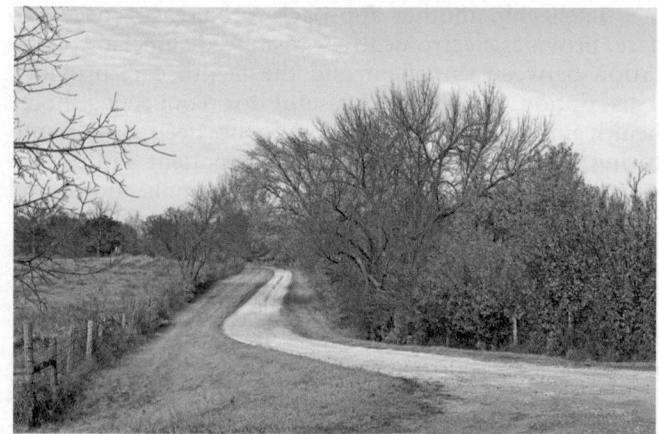

A country road, often without street signs and sometimes difficult to locate.

Faith-based nursing has been a staple in rural areas, as well as with some urban communities, but is gaining momentum as more formal interventions are developed, for instance, mental health promotion for rural Latino immigrants (Stacciarini et al., 2016). Even informal support from other church members and friends may provide a compassionate environment for needed behavioral changes such as healthy diet and increased physical activity (Kegler et al., 2012). Church communities may also provide assistance and relief to caregivers in rural areas, especially when more formal services are unavailable or geographically distant (Greene, Perkins, Scott, & Burt, 2011). See more on faith-based nursing in Chapter 31.

One approach that has been successful in numerous rural areas is the use of *mobile clinics*. These clinics bring health care providers to remote places for health screenings, immunizations, dental care, mental health visits, and other services. Mobile health clinics are frequently staffed by NPs and can improve access to health care for low-income residents. They often are available to residents on evenings and weekends and offer culturally sensitive and bilingual outreach, as well as care for uninsured clients. They may be helpful in overcoming access problems for vulnerable populations (Isler, Miles, Banks, & Corbie-Smith, 2012).

School-based clinics can improve access for schoolchildren (and sometimes their families) but may be less prominent in rural areas (see more on school-based clinics in Chapter 30). Only 27% are in rural areas and 16% in suburban areas, with the majority in urban areas. These clinics provide available, community-based, affordable, and culturally acceptable care to well and sick children. Often, grant-supported, school-based clinics facilitate the receipt of health education and primary care by children who are otherwise without easy access to health services (National Conference of State Legislatures, 2011). A study by Bains, Franzen, and White-Fresé (2014) revealed that Latino and African American male adolescents, who generally seek mental health services and obtain care at lower levels than White adolescent males, were more likely to access these services at school-based health centers because of the accepting nature of services there. See more in Chapter 30.

Telehealth, another approach to increasing access to care, provides electronically transmitted clinician consultation between the client and the health care provider. This option is especially useful for connecting home health nurses with their patients who need close monitoring at home. It is also useful for patient and professional health education, public health applications, and health administration. Specialty health care also may be accessed, with patients and providers connected via two-way audiovisual transmission over telephone lines or the Internet, thus obviating the need for patients to leave their residences. Streaming media, video conferencing, and store-and-forward imaging are just some of the applications commonly utilized (HRSA, n.d.b). Clients can also be assessed quickly by interactive communication from physician offices, hospitals, and other sites. Rural American Indians and Alaska Natives found cancer support groups offered through this technology to be helpful (Doorenbos et al., 2010). Telehealth technology may decrease visits to emergency departments and hospitalizations, if early assessment and intervention can be provided, and telehealth has been used to manage rural heart failure patients to decrease hospital readmission rates (Graves, Ford, & Mooney, 2013). Telehealth interventions for speech–language services to rural children and one systematic review of the use of technology with underserved clients acknowledged the effectiveness of the use of various methods of technology in promoting health and improving outcomes (Fairweather, Lincoln, & Ramsden, 2016; Montague & Perchonok, 2012). McIllhenny, Guzic, Knee, Demuth, and Roberts (2011) found that a nurse educator coaching clients to access to a Web portal with diabetes-related health education resources could be useful in providing diabetes care to a rural population. Physical therapists provided physical therapy sessions to veterans through home video technology and noted significant physical improvement along with cost savings of over \$1,151 and travel time of over 46 hours (Levy, Silverman, Huanguang, Geiss, & Omura, 2015). Grants and other funding are available to promote

the use of this technology (HRSA, n.d.b). Rural hospitals in a health care profession shortage area that employ hospital-to-hospital telemedicine services can qualify for Medicare reimbursement; over 50% of all U.S. hospitals now use some type of telehealth, with many larger systems having telehealth networks (Kutscher, 2014). See Chapter 10.

Healthy People 2020 Goals

The four overarching goals of *Healthy People 2020* are to:

1. Attain high-quality, longer lives free of preventable disease
2. Achieve health equity, eliminate disparities, and improve the health of all groups
3. Create social and physical environments that promote good health for all
4. Promote quality of life, healthy development, and healthy behaviors across all life stages (USDHHS, 2016b, para. 5)

Because of the unique health issues facing rural America, *Rural Healthy People 2020*, a rural-oriented document was developed (Bolin & Bellamy, n.d.). Using surveys, literature reviews, and other methods of data collection and analysis, top priorities for rural health were identified. The original *Rural Healthy People 2010* document also highlighted current knowledge on rural health and identified best practices, and it called for further research on rural health promotion (Bellamy, Bolin, & Gamm, 2011). Certainly, there are data to substantiate continued problems with access to health care and insurance, as well as emergency services, in rural areas. And there is a higher rate of CVD and diabetes, along with obesity and tobacco use among rural populations (NRHA, n.d.). The *Healthy People 2020* document notes specific differences in oral health and social determinants of health related to geography. A national survey (*n* = 688) conducted between 2010 and 2011 listed the initial top ten priorities for *Rural Healthy People 2020*, with access to quality health services as the most important priority (Bolin & Bellamy, n.d.). However, funding cuts prevented the broadened surveys first proposed, and the authors launched a second Web-based survey in 2012, that at 1,214 respondents. Again, access to quality health services was the first priority chosen, with nutrition and weight status, diabetes, mental health/disorders, substance abuse, heart disease/stroke, physical activity/health, older adults, maternal–child health, and tobacco use making up the top ten priorities (Bolin & Bellamy, 2015; Bolin et al., 2015). A large longitudinal study of maternal and infant health in Maine revealed that access to prenatal care, along with pregnancy care and outcomes, was similar for rural and urban women over an 11-year period (Harris, Aboueissa, Baugh, & Sarton, 2015). Rural mothers had higher BMIs prior to pregnancy and were generally younger, less well educated, unmarried, and living in low-income households. They were also more likely to smoke, but less likely to drink alcohol, and were not often sure of their pregnancies until later than urban mothers, but they still accessed prenatal care at similar times (Harris et al., 2015).

Access to quality care is linked to availability of health insurance. Rural residents, when compared to urban counterparts, have higher rates of uninsured, higher out-of-pocket costs, and higher proportions of emergency room visit costs; they are also less likely to be covered through group health insurance or managed care plans and less likely to have prescription drug coverage (Bolin & Bellamy, 2015). Also, insurance instability (gaps in coverage) is correlated with increased use of emergency rooms, and this is particularly significant for rural residents who often have less access (Fields, Bell, Moyce, & Bigbee, 2015). Because of lower rates of insured rural residents, their preventive health care is often lacking (e.g., lower rates of mammograms, colonoscopies, vision exams). Also, around 65% of primary care professional shortages occur in rural counties. Rural residents are also less likely than urban residents to have a usual source of primary care, and this is especially true in the 18- to 44-year-old age group (Bolin & Bellamy, 2015).

Problems more commonly seen in rural areas include oral health and cigarette and smokeless tobacco use. Sixty percent of rural counties are considered professional shortage areas for dental health, and more dentists are over age 55 in rural areas (42% vs. 38% in urban). Rural populations are less likely to have an annual dental examination. They are also more likely to have tooth or gum disease, often because of higher rates of cigarette and smokeless tobacco use, and they are more likely to use the emergency room because of dental caries than urban residents (Bolin & Bellamy, 2015; Kronkosky Charitable Foundation, 2011). Smoking prevalence in rural areas is higher than in urban areas, and smokeless tobacco use is twice or three times higher in rural areas (Bolin & Bellamy, 2015; Borders & Booth, 2007; Kronkosky Charitable Foundation, 2011). Over one fourth of rural pregnant women smoke during their pregnancy, compared to 11.2% of urban women (Bolin & Bellamy, 2015).

Alcohol dependence is more common in rural than suburban or urban areas, and one study found that current and lifetime rates of alcohol, tobacco, and illicit drug use were significantly higher for rural adolescents than for their urban complements (Coomber et al., 2011). Some studies show that overall prevalence of illicit drug use is similar, but access to substance abuse services is better in urban areas. Methamphetamine use is often prevalent in rural areas because "cooking" is easier because of availability of ingredients such as anhydrous ammonia (farm fertilizer) and remote, isolated locations (Oser et al., 2011). Prescription opioid use and abuse is increasingly becoming a public health crisis across the United States. Nonmedical abuse of prescription opioids is often concentrated in rural areas (e.g., Alaska, Kentucky, Oklahoma, West Virginia) and is best addressed on macro, local, and micro levels (e.g., overall drug availability, family/peer stressors, genetic vulnerability/psychiatric morbidity). In 2006, it was the cause of 37% of all poisoning deaths, but in nonmetropolitan counties, there was a threefold increase; there are also more nonmedical than medical opioid users in rural areas (Keyes, Cerda, Brady, Havens, & Galea, 2014). Depression is often associated with opioid drug abuse among rural residents, as is the number of medical comorbidities (e.g., CVD, diabetes, chronic renal disease); better screening is needed before these powerful medications are prescribed, as the potential for abuse is high (Kapoor & Thorn, 2014). Also, newer and less addictive types of pain control are needed (Dryden, 2016). The vast majority (80%) of rural residents live in counties without detoxification facilities and primary care practitioner in rural areas often lack sufficient training to effectively screen for substance use (Bolin & Bellamy, 2015; Kronkosky Charitable Foundation, 2011).

Children in rural areas are at greater risk for death and disability because of the lack of pediatric emergency services (Bolin & Bellamy, 2015). Children with special needs who live in a rural area are often lacking needed services to promote health and prevent illness. Research has also demonstrated that rural residence is a risk factor for overweight and obesity in children (Davis, Bennett, Befort, & Nollen, 2011). Rural areas also frequently have deficient physical education programs in schools, but residents have greater inactivity and calorie consumption (Bolin & Bellamy, 2015; Kronkosky Charitable Foundation, 2011).

Cancer disparities are found in rural populations. For example, cervical cancer rates for rural women are statistically higher than for Caucasian and Black women living in urban areas (Evans, Cole, & Norris, 2015). Survival rates for cervical cancer are also lower in nonmetropolitan areas, especially so for rural black women who had a 50.8% 5-year survival rate compared with 60.2% for those in metropolitan areas (Singh, 2012). Rural women are less likely to receive screening mammograms and Pap smears than urban women. Rural populations also have a lower proportion of colonoscopies to screen for colorectal cancer. Further, most rural physicians are trained as generalists, therefore not trained to perform colonoscopies (Evans et al., 2015). Rural PHNs need to consider the *Healthy People 2020* objectives and *Rural Healthy People 2020* priority areas as guides for improving the health status of clients in rural communities.

MIGRANT HEALTH

You may not have seen migrant workers, yet you are a direct beneficiary of their labor. Have you ever thought about the people who harvest the fruits and vegetables that you eat? What would happen to the complex system of agricultural production and distribution if workers were not available to pick crops at peak harvest times? Have you ever thought about who they are, where they come from, where they live, or what their health is like? A common question among Americans who have never worked with migrant populations is "Why are they here?" and the answer is often a case of simple economics. Whatever your political, social, or ethical views on this subject, migrant workers and their families often cross paths with PHNs and we need to understand them in order to effectively provide care. See What Do You Think?

Migrant farmworkers are an integral part of the farming community in the United States and across the world. The agricultural industry relies heavily on migrant workers to harvest the almost endless array of fresh produce that appears year-round in supermarkets across

What do *you* think?

There are many critics of undocumented migrant workers. Some feel that it is their willingness to work for low wages keeps overall wages lower for everyone working in agriculture. Others feel that migrants are taking jobs away from Americans. The United Farmworkers, an agricultural worker union, introduced the *Take Our Jobs* program in 2010 to address these issues. Unemployed Americans were invited to work in the fields along with migrant farmworkers, but very few accepted this invitation; those that did attempt it had a difficult time keeping up with the grueling pace of work. Stephen Colbert, a television show host and comedian, picked beans and packed corn as part of the challenge, and filmed some of his workday experiences for his late-night show. He also gave testimony to Congress on the need for better wages, living conditions, and visa programs for these workers. What do you think about the issue?

From Lerner, A. (2011). *Migrant labor, immigration, and food production.* Retrieved from http://find.galegroup.com/gic/infomark.do?&source=gale&idigest=a24509ee707e3735cde6db3e17c5304e&prodId=GIC&userGroupName=bhs&tabID=T001&docId=CX1918600173&type=retrieve&version=1.0

the United States as fresh, frozen, and canned fruits and vegetables. It is estimated that the cost of vegetables (e.g., tomatoes) would most likely increase by 25% to 40% if migrant farmworkers were not readily available to pick crops in a timely manner (Lerner, 2011). More than 3 million seasonal and migrant farmworkers provide labor for the $28 billion vegetable and fruit crops of the United States (National Center for Farmworker Health [NCFH], 2012b). Many of these workers are unauthorized or illegal immigrants to the United States, often from Mexico. A study of Canadian migrant workers, a country with a seasonal agricultural worker program offering higher wages and shorter time periods away from home and family (up to 8 months), found that 100% of those leaving Mexico on their first entry into Canada were legal temporary workers. In contrast, only 18% of those leaving for the United States were entering legally as workers with an H-2A (work program) visa (Massey & Brown, 2011). The vast majority entered this country in an unauthorized manner. Because Canada recruited temporary workers from Mexico under a formal agreement, their workers were over age 18 (usually 22 to 45 years), had agricultural experience, and had no prior criminal records. Mexico also stipulated that they have some education (third to ninth grade) and be in a stable relationship (married or common law). Because of this program, with benefits to both countries as well as the temporary workers, Canada has a low proportion of workers becoming permanent residents and a more "circular flow" with repeat migrations. With the H-2A visa, there are restrictions against farmworkers changing employers, and this could affect their work safety climate (Arcury et al., 2015c). In the

United States, undocumented workers often stay for longer periods of time because of "tighter controls on border crossing making repeated migrations more difficult than before 9/11" (Massey & Brown, 2011, p. 119).

Despite their importance to American agriculture, migrant workers are not often visible members of our society. They go unnoticed beyond the fringes of the camps and farms to which they travel in order to pursue their livelihood. Most come to the United States from other countries (72%), and of those, about 68% are from Mexico. Most have been in the United States 10 years on average. The average age is 36 years, 78% are males, and 35% stated that they spoke no English. The average level of completed education was the eighth grade (NCFH, 2012b). Approximately 42% of farmworkers are considered migrant (traveling 75 mi to obtain farm jobs), and many travel to multiple farm sites within a year. Most (34%) worked in fruit and nut crops, and 69% find employment through family and friends. Only 6% are salaried, with the majority paid low hourly wages or by the piece. California, Florida, Texas, North Carolina, Michigan, Washington, Tennessee, and Oregon currently have the highest number of migrant farmworkers (NCFH, 2012b). They come with the hope of bettering their impoverished lives. Some are legal residents, but most are undocumented aliens and live in fear of deportation. All endure backbreaking, menial labor for low wages and are often deprived of basic rights to safe working conditions, adequate sanitation/housing, health care, and a quality education for their children. See From the Case Files II.

Migrant Farmworkers: Profile of a Nomadic Population

Maintaining a low public profile, migrant workers are, for the most part, marginalized from mainstream society. They remain unseen, unheard, poorly understood, and excluded from many programs that provide health care assistance for low-income people. The migrant worker is a kind of disenfranchised person, for whom no one wants to take responsibility. Yet the needs of these workers are great. They are plagued with different, more complex, and more frequent health problems than the general population (Arcury & Quandt, 2011; Migrant Clinician's Network, 2016). Common ailments include infectious diseases (e.g., TB, parasites), gastrointestinal disorders, dermatitis because of pesticide exposure, emotional distress and depression, vision and eye problems, cancer, and chronic illnesses, such as asthma, bronchitis, diabetes, and hypertension. They are plagued by poverty, poor nutrition, substandard housing conditions, extended working hours, and grueling, often unsafe, working conditions. Their demographics, socioeconomic conditions, and lifestyle resemble those of a Third World country despite the fact that they live and work in one of the most prosperous nations on Earth. Although migrant families are in dire need of health resources, various economic, cultural, and language barriers prevent this aggregate from accessing available health services. Poverty, frequent mobility, low literacy, and language and cultural barriers impede farmworkers access to cost-effective health care and social services (NCFH, 2012b).

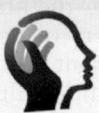

From the Case Files II

A Case of Active TB in a Rural Community

As the PHN in a rural community, I received many types of referrals for families including maternal child, older adults, child abuse, or communicable disease cases. The small public health district office where I worked was staffed with one nurse and one aide, and we hosted clinics for immunizations, well-child care, and family planning. It was located in a small agricultural town of approximately 20,000 people, with a very large Hispanic- and Spanish-speaking population. One day I was summoned to the main office, approximately 30 mi away, to respond to a new active tuberculosis (TB) case. A 20-year-old Hispanic male was a patient in the county hospital and he was on respiratory isolation. I picked up the case file from my supervisor and we discussed the plan of action. When the patient was released, he would return to live in the small community that I covered. I would need to examine his living conditions and his contacts.

I first visited Gregorio in the county hospital. I spent time interviewing him, donning an N95 mask, and educated him about who I was, as well as the reason for my visit. Gregorio explained that he, along with other men from his home country of Chiapas, Mexico, had taken an arduous journey to come to our area in order to find work. He could no longer stand the pain in his chest and his brothers decided to drop him off at the hospital. He provided his address and the names of his brothers with whom he lived or visited with regularly, as well as most of the names of the other men with whom he worked. There were 20 names in total that were close contacts and needed follow-up. I explained to Gregorio that I would be his nurse when he was released from the hospital and that I would be helping him receive treatment for TB.

The next day, the Public Health Aide and I traveled to Gregorio's home address. It must have seemed very strange to have a nurse and an aide knock on the door of a male household of agricultural workers. Many of the men did not receive health care in their home country. They were very welcoming, and with the assistance of Gregorio's older brother, we began to complete the contact investigation. They lived in a 2-bedroom home, without furniture, and each man took a spot on the floor to sleep at night. One by one, each was interviewed for TB risk assessment and a TB skin test was placed. On return to the home in 2 days, skin tests were read and those who had positive tests were referred to the community health center for chest x-rays. Many of the men had not yet been successful in obtaining work and had no income. The County Public Health Officer (a physician) intervened to ensure that appropriate treatment would be received. The large number of close contacts and the difficulty in arranging transportation from the rural community necessitated that the Health Officer come to the rural district office to hold a TB clinic so that each close contact could be evaluated. The men could walk approximately 1 mi to the public health office to meet with the MD. The men seemed a bit bewildered regarding our very intensive efforts to get them into health care. However, they were very cooperative, and no other close contacts were found to have active TB, but many were prescribed treatment for latent TB infection (LTBI).

Gregorio was hospitalized until he was no longer communicable, and he was picked up by the public health medical investigator to return home. By this time, some men had found work in the fields and had made other living arrangements. I had to find the new addresses where they had moved in order to ensure compliance with LTBI treatment. When I showed up at the homes of the contacts that had moved, they were neither pleased nor unhappy to see me, but they were cooperative.

Gregorio and his brothers stayed in the original home. The county public health department instituted daily Direct Observed Therapy (DOT) and assisted with transportation to medical appointments. Gregorio was cooperative with the plan of care and enjoyed the company of the public health staff including the PHNs, aides, medical investigators, and DOT workers. Five days a week, Gregorio had a visitor to assess his needs and oversee his medications. At times, this included support through food baskets and other community resources when work could not be found. In addition, we made DOT scheduling considerations for late afternoons during times when Gregorio was working, as this was highly important to him so that he could work and get paid.

Over the year that Gregorio was on treatment, he understood that we cared for his well-being and wanted to prevent him from having more serious complications. Without public health interventions, his untreated TB could have created a serious public health threat in this small community. However, because public health was present, the outcomes were such that Gregorio was able to live productively and contribute to the stability of his brothers' household, as well as that of his more family back in his home country.

Judy H. Pedro, MSN, RN, APHN-BC

Migrant workers live and work in areas where health care practitioners are generally in short supply. In a large national study of farmworkers, only 52% had used U.S. health care services within the last 2 years, and barriers include lack of health insurance, fear of immigration consequence, low English proficiency, and access to transportation (Hoerster et al., 2011). Among Latino immigrants, common barriers include communication problems, difficulty proving financial eligibility, and long waiting periods for gaining access to health care services (Cristancho, Peters, & Garces, 2014). They often used traditional cultural remedies (e.g., herbal medications, traditional healers) and often blended both traditional and U.S. health care practices (Jostad-Laswell, Guendelman, & Castañeda, 2013). An 18-month ethnographic study of indigenous Triqui migrant workers followed them from Oaxaca, Mexico, to central California and onto the northwest area of Washington as they harvested crops. Interviews were conducted with them and the health care providers who worked in the clinics serving them. The researcher (Holmes, 2009, p. 873) found that "social and economic factors in health care and subtle cultural factors... keep medical professionals from seeing the social determinants of suffering," and this leads them to inadvertently blame the patients. Additional barriers include limited transportation, prejudice because of immigrant status, mistreatment because they are "undocumented," lack of time-efficient health care delivery methods, increasing cost of health care, and needed services not being offered (NCFH, 2012b, 2015).

Historical Background

Both historically and internationally, farmers have rarely been able to permanently employ the large workforces needed to harvest their crops. Throughout the 19th century, however, the small, family-owned farms typical in the United States got through the harvest by using schoolchildren, neighbors, and local day laborers. As time went by, this became more and more difficult to accomplish. During the decade ending in 1929, over half a million Mexicans migrated to the United States, many drawn to work in seasonal agriculture. With the Great Depression, many of the small, independently run farms went bankrupt, and citizens were concerned about scarce employment opportunities. Because of this, state and federal governments were lobbied by civic groups to "round up Mexican Americans indiscriminately ... and to 'repatriate' them to Mexico" (University of California, 2012, para. 5.). Within a few years, the outbreak of World War II caused an increased need for food production and additional workers, as many U.S. workers joined the military. To keep abreast of the demand for produce, the larger surviving farms turned to migrant labor for help. The Emergency Labor Program—known as the Bracero Program—was enacted in 1942 to permit temporary Mexican immigration to provide needed workers for American agriculture and industry (University of California, 2012). Between 1942 and 1964, more than 4 million Mexican workers participated in this program, leaving their families behind and coming to work in Californian fields. When this program ended, workers continued to cross the border to seek employment, often bringing along their families. Employers hired needed undocumented workers from Mexico, as well as Central and South America. The 1986 Immigration Reform and Control Act created sanctions for employers who hired undocumented workers and made them responsible for checking documents and eligibility for potential employees (National Agricultural Law Center, n.d.).

Living apart from society, the plight of migrant farmworkers was largely ignored until exposure on a 1960 television documentary—Edward R. Murrow's *Harvest of Shame*—created a national outcry. This led to the passage of the Migrant Health Act of 1962, which addressed the specific health needs of migrant workers for the first time in U.S. history. This act authorized delivery of primary and supplementary health services to migrant farmworkers (NCFH, n.d.). Federally funded migrant health clinics serve areas in the United States where significant number of migrant farmworkers gather. In 2010, 165 migrant clinics served more than 863,000 seasonal and migrant farmworkers and members of their families, a number far below the estimated 3+ million farmworkers thought to be in this country. Eligibility for services at the clinics includes being principally employed in agricultural labor for the prior 24 months (Farmworker Justice, 2016). Services may be provided seasonally, on a temporary basis, or year-round. Staffing usually includes doctors, nurses, NPs, PAs, outreach workers, social workers, and dental and pharmacy workers, along with health educators. Transportation may also be a component in some areas. Primary and preventive health care services are provided to migrant workers and their families throughout more than 500 clinic sites. However, funding is often inadequate, and many clinics are not sufficiently staffed or operated to meet the health needs of migrant farmworkers and their dependents. Most migrant health centers receive funding from a variety of sources, including Medicaid in some instances. Additionally, although these clinics exist throughout the United States, large geographic regions are not served well or at all. Other services, such as *promotora programs* that employ Hispanic lay health workers or nursing voucher programs providing NP services at participating clinics and nurse referrals to specialists, are available in some areas (Fiandt, Doeschot, & Lanning, 2010; Molokwu, Penaranda, Flores, & Shokar, in press; Wright et al., 2015). Migrant workers in areas without migrant clinics or other targeted services must rely on LHDs and emergency rooms for health care, or they may simply go without needed care.

In 1964, the U.S. Department of State initiated the H2 Temporary Guest Worker Program. In 2010, a total of 55,721 H-2A visas were granted to migrant farmworkers (NCFH, 2012b). The current H-2A program for temporary agricultural workers permits employers to file paperwork, demonstrating a need for temporary workers that cannot be met by U.S. workers, and then, workers from approved countries can apply for a visa. It allows them to work for up to 1 year in the United States, and they may bring spouses and children under age 21 under a companion visa program (H-4) that does not permit them to work (U.S. Department of Homeland Security, 2012). Only a small percentage of workers and employers utilize this program, approximately 1% in the last national survey. More recently, approximately 48% of migrant farmworkers were described as unauthorized to work in the United States, 33% were U.S. citizens, and 26% have been in the United States <4 years (NCFH, 2012b).

Demographics

Because migrant farmworkers constitute a mobile population with shifting composition, it is difficult to precisely determine their number or origins. Estimates of the number of migrant workers vary also because of the influx of illegal and undocumented workers. A large number of seasonal and migrant farmworkers reside in the United

States, and 33% are U.S. citizens, and others have permanent resident status. Most of the estimated 3 million migrant (42%) and seasonal (58%) farmworkers tend to be either newly arrived immigrants, with few connections, or established legal residents with limited opportunities and skills, who rely on farm labor for survival (NCFH, 2012b). In addition to male workers, who make up the majority, you may also see mothers bring infants and young children to work with them, and the children spend their days strapped to their mother's back or playing among the pesticide-laden fields.

Seasonal farmworkers generally live in one geographic location and are temporarily employed in agriculture, whereas **migrant farmworkers** meet that classification while moving to find agricultural work throughout the year, usually from state to state, and establishing temporary residences (Migrant Clinicians Network, 2016). Some live apart from their families, forming groups of single men; others travel with their entire families. The average migrant farmworker spends from June to September doing seasonal harvesting, with about 8 weeks on the road traveling from farm to farm for work, and is then unemployed unless other work, such as hauling or canning, is found. Days begin before dawn and work continues for 12 hours or longer. Farmworkers cannot be paid for overtime, as federal laws exclude this category of work, and 14 states don't require workers' compensation (Barbassa, 2010; NCFH, 2012b). The main reason migrant workers immigrate is to find work, and most migrant farmworkers end up in areas where they already have social networks, such as family or acquaintances from their own areas of Mexico or other countries (Cohen, 2010; Rose, 2013).

Migrant farmworkers have the potential to receive compensation below minimum wage standards. Although most are paid by the hour, 11.7% receive piece-rate pay. Eight out of ten migrant farmworkers live below the U.S. poverty line (NCFH, 2010). Since 2000, Latino migrant farmworkers have had a median annual income of around $10,000 (Lerner, 2011). Families working in the cotton fields of Texas and other states report working long hours, and children as young as 11 may work alongside adults (Coursen-Neff, 2011). The Fair Labor Standards Act of 1938 (FLSA) was amended in 1978 to mandate minimum wage for workers on large farms but has never been changed to provide overtime pay for farmworkers. Farmworkers paid at a per-piece rate may earn as little as 40 cents for a bucket of tomatoes or sweet potatoes, therefore needing to pick approximately 2 tons of produce (125 buckets) to earn 50 dollars (Student Action Farmworkers [SAF], 2011–2016).

Migrant Streams and Patterns

Migrant farmworkers usually have their permanent residence, or *home base*, in states with a traditionally high number of immigrants, like California, Texas, Florida, Washington, Oregon, and North Carolina (SAF, 2011–2016). From their home base, they move to locations where each new crop is ready for harvest. As they follow the harvest seasons of agricultural crops, migrant farmworkers move from place to place, usually along predetermined routes called **migrant streams** (Fig. 29–5). Some migrant farmworkers are multigenerational; that is, their families have been farmworkers for several generations, traveling the same streams for many years. It is very common for farmworkers and other foreign workers to send money back home to family members; total migrant and foreign worker remittances constitute large sums of money and provide significant support for families in other countries, like Mexico, China, India, and the Philippines (Tomlinson, 2013). Of farmworkers in the United States, 75% were born in Mexico and 60% live apart from their immediate family members. Immigrant farmworkers often leave their home country to seek a better life for their families (SAF, 2011–2016).

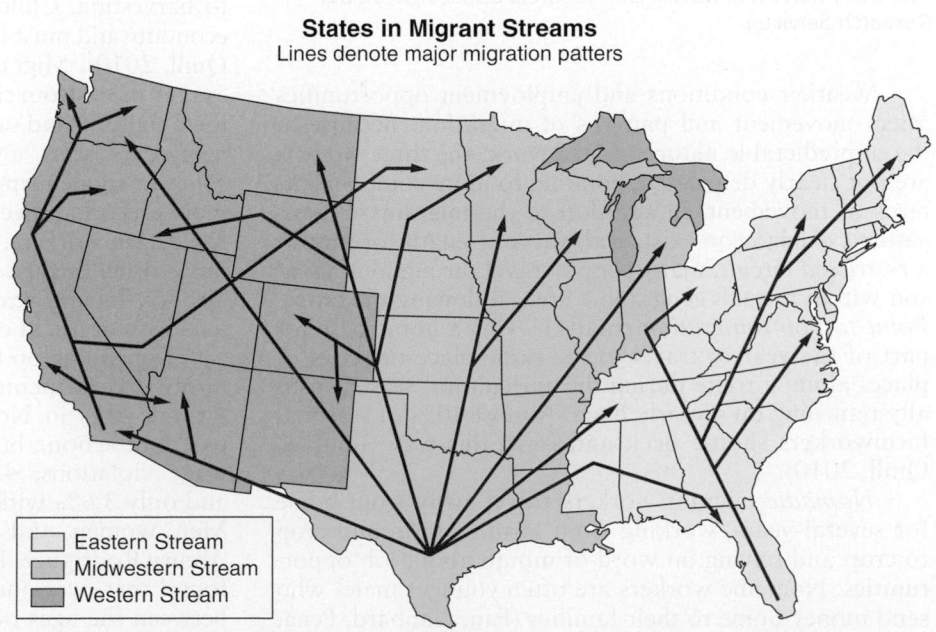

States in Migrant Streams
Lines denote major migration patters

Eastern Stream
Midwestern Stream
Western Stream

FIGURE 29–5 Migrant streams. (Source: Migrant Head Start Program, USHDHUD [same—unchanged].)

Three principal streams formulate the agricultural routes that migrant laborers follow. The *eastern stream* originates in Florida, where most of their time is spent, and extends up the East Coast through North Carolina, Tennessee, Kentucky, Virginia, and other states east of the Mississippi, as far as north as Ohio, New Jersey, New York, Connecticut, Massachusetts, New Hampshire, Vermont, and Maine. The *midwestern stream* begins in southern Texas or northern Mexico and fans out across the United States, ending in the Northwestern and Midwestern states bordering Canada, both east and west of the Mississippi. The *western stream* originates in California and moves up the West Coast to all western states and from central California into North Dakota per a seminal article by Formichelli (2008). California, Florida, and Texas are regarded as *sending states*, as they are often home states with long growing seasons where migrant streams begin and end. Male workers may travel with the crops and leave their families in these home states (USDHUD, 2016a). Workers move from areas with cotton, tree fruits and nuts, and vegetable crops to other areas where they harvest cherries, watermelons, cantaloupes, or potatoes.

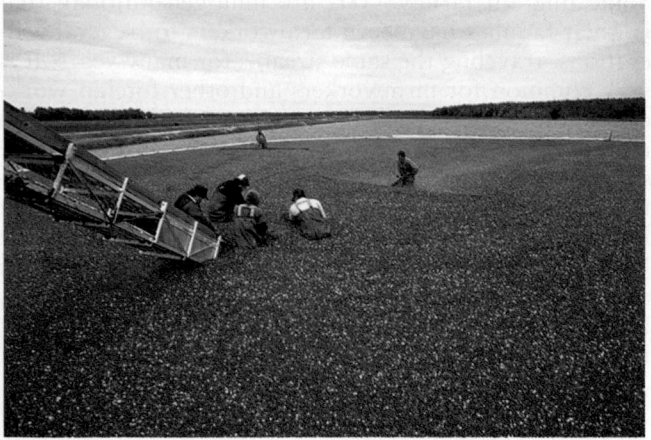

Cranberry harvest in New Jersey. (Source: USDA, Agricultural Research Service.)

Weather conditions and employment opportunities affect movement and patterns of migration. Because of the unpredictable nature of farmwork, the three streams are not clearly delineated, pointing to more complex patterns of movement. In addition to the migrant streams, **patterns of migration** exist, with varying lengths of stay. In a *restricted circuit*, many people travel throughout a season within a small geographic area, following the crops. *Point-to-point migration* entails leaving a home base for part of the year to travel to the same place or series of places along a route during the agricultural season, usually returning on a yearly basis. Almost 40% of seasonal farmworkers shuttle back and forth this way (Loue & Quill, 2010).

Nomadic migrant workers travel away from home for several years, working from farm to farm and crop to crop and relying on word of mouth about job opportunities. Nomadic workers are often younger males who send money home to their families (Fan, Gabbard, Pena,

& Perloff, 2014; Loue & Quill, 2010). Some of these workers eventually settle in the areas to which they have migrated, whereas others return to their home base. A given ethnic group usually follows its own particular stream and pattern of migration. New growth states, like Utah, Minnesota, Wisconsin, Nebraska, Kansas, Tennessee, and Arkansas, have seen immigrant populations increase. Some migrant workers find work in service sector jobs and others labor in construction or landscaping, thus ending their need to constantly move with the crops. Overall, the migration rate of farmworkers has dropped from 53% in 1998 to 23% in 2009, thought to be due to economic, institutional, and governmental changes (e.g., stricter U.S. border enforcement, improved Mexican economy), in both the United States and Mexico (Fan et al., 2014). Married men, not living with their families, are more likely to migrate than those living with their families, often because of the need to send money back home. This drop in migrant labor has implications for American farmers, as they find it more difficult to find sufficient laborers during peak planting and harvesting periods and may need to pay higher wages that ultimately result in higher consumer prices for agricultural products (Fan et al., 2014).

Migrant Lifestyle

To understand the health needs of migrant farmworkers and their families, it is important to understand their lifestyle. Migrant workers and their families endure a transient and uncertain life, with long hours, stressful working conditions, low wages, and poor health care. Substandard housing, unsafe working conditions, and language barriers make life even more difficult (USDHUD, 2016a).

Migrant workers must confront the vagaries of an unpredictable world. Migrants typically remain in an area for only 6 to 8 weeks, working the fields 6 days a week from sunrise to sunset. Depending on weather and crop conditions, work may be plentiful 1 week and virtually gone the next. Because yearly income must be earned during the harvest season, all family members contribute to harvesting. Children are essential to the core group's economy and must help in the fields and at home (Loue & Quill, 2010). Migrant workers often drive night and day as they move from crop to crop. Typically, they travel with their children and only their most essential possessions, in aging cars, vans, and trucks. Occasionally, van loads of *solos*, or single men, migrate together. Their status is even more precarious because they lack family support systems. Male farmworkers, single or away from their families, more often engage in risk-taking behaviors of drinking alcohol, having sex with commercial sex workers, and inconsistent use of condoms (Rhodes et al., 2010).

Depending on the economy and the crop, a migrant farmworker's income varies widely. A study of migrant farmworkers in North Carolina found that 90% were paid by the hour, but 18.3% of all farmworkers reported wage violations: 45.3% of those without H-2A visas and only 3.6% with H-2A visas (Robinson et al., 2011). Men, women, and older children all work in the fields. Arcury Rodriguez, Kearney, Arcury, and Quandt (2014b) found that over one quarter of youth farmworkers were between the ages of 10 and 13, and 39.1% were 14- to

15-year-olds. Over 34% were 16- to 17-year-olds, and 78.2% of the study participants working in tobacco, sweet potato, and berry crops were born in the United States. Over 55% of them were paid piece rate, rather than hourly wages, and almost 22% had problems getting their correct pay. Because inexpensive child care is seldom available, mothers often leave very young children alone playing in fields, where they are exposed to sun, chemicals, and dangerous machinery. Sometimes, children are brought to the fields and left in cars or in cardboard boxes. Often, a teenage girl or the mother of an infant may remain in the camp to babysit all the children; she is usually stranded there, because all available cars are used to take workers to the fields. There are Head Start and Migrant Head Start programs in many areas, but they can only provide services to a minority of children needing them.

Migrant laborers learn about employment opportunities from recruiters, farm labor contractors, and crew leaders, as well as from other migrants. About 33% of California farmworkers and 20% of those nationwide are usually employed through farm labor contractors (University of California, 2012). Migrant farmworkers may travel in crews or groups and are often employed by farm labor contractors (an individual who serves as the mediator between workers and the farmer). These contractors may also provide transportation, housing, and meals for the workers and may also supervise their work in the fields. The farmer usually pays the labor contractor, who, in turn, pays the workers (National Agricultural Law Center, n.d.). This can be viewed as a way for farmers to remove themselves from the responsibility of paying minimum wages to workers, providing worker's compensation, meeting legal responsibilities (e.g., state and federal worker safety rules), and preventing union organizing because they employ the contractor, not the individual workers. Owners may also ignore abuses, because they are not directly employing workers. The labor contractor may underreport hours of workers, or piecework, and harassment can often occur. An unscrupulous crew leader can withhold payment and keep the migrant workers in constant debt. There is often no recourse, as access to legal counsel is rare and legal aid programs funded by the federal government are prohibited from providing services to undocumented workers, and workers generally don't speak out about injustices because of fear and feelings of hopelessness. One remarkable exception is a multimillion-dollar judgment awarded to five farmworkers "kept in virtual indentured servitude by their contractors" at an organic farm supplying the upscale supermarket chain, Whole Foods. The contractors charged "smuggling fees, rent, and cleaning charges" that left workers with only $2 out of their $7 hourly wage. They were threatened with violence and the contractors carried guns to ensure compliance (Goldstein, Howe, & Tamir, 2010, p. 3).

Female migrant farmworkers comprise about 21% of the agricultural workforce in this country, and they face the same occupational hazards (e.g., respiratory, skin, and infectious diseases; pesticide exposure/illness; musculoskeletal disorders; injuries) including reproductive health problems (Habib & Fathallah, 2012).

They also endure the lack of a stable home and social isolation, discrimination and fear, and the added difficulties of child-rearing and housekeeping while living a nomadic lifestyle. Despite the moves and difficulty with health care coordination, the health network providing pregnancy care to migrant women reports that 97% of those followed had babies born at the target birth weight (Migrant Clinicians Network [MCN], 2013).

Migrant Hero

César Chavez founded the National Farm Workers Association (NFWA; later changed to United Farm Workers [UFW]), the first union in agricultural labor history to successfully organize migrant farmworkers. As a child, he traveled with his family to harvest crops, but they rarely had enough food to eat and often lived in shacks. Work was frequently scarce, wages were low, and labor contractors cheated the family out of the money they earned. Moving to California during the Great Depression, the family became part of the migrant community. Chavez attended as many as 65 different schools and dropped out of school upon completing eighth grade, to help support his family by working full-time in the fields.

Chavez organized many successful strikes and boycotts, the most famous one being the boycott of California grapes as a protest against the indiscriminate use of spraying by growers. This boycott lasted for longer than 5 years, and on two occasions, he fasted as a protest against the use of agricultural pesticides. His efforts united people who, as individuals, had no significance in the power structure. His legacy is an example of how people can unite to build power together. He achieved great recognition, although he never had the financial trappings of success (Bardacke, 2011). Throughout his life, he ignored personal hardships to continue the struggle with union victories and losses.

Health Risks of Migrant Workers and Their Families

A community with varied and profound health needs complicated by disease and social isolation, migrant farmworkers and their families are at risk. Migrant workers, often paid piecework, labor at a fast pace, largely without breaks, in order to take advantage of the short growing season (Connor, Layne, & Thomisee, 2010; Lerner, 2011). Because seasonal earnings must last the entire year, the migrant farmworker generally avoids or delays seeking health care until illness becomes debilitating. Immediate treatment is generally only sought when a worker is "completely debilitated," if a pesticide exposure has occurred, or a work supervisor has been notified (Thierry & Snipes, 2015, p. 178). Migrant farmworkers and their families suffer illnesses caused by poor nutrition, a lack of resources to seek care early in the disease process, and infectious diseases because of overcrowding and poor sanitation. A study on food security among U.S. farmworker households noted that about half were consistently in a food secure state, but 29% were in a transient state of food security; seasonal versus migrant status and having proper immigration documents versus being undocumented were predictive of food security (Ip et al.,

2015). Another study found that 62.83 % of migrant workers surveyed in Georgia were food insecure, and those without H-2A visas were almost three times more likely than those with visas to be without sufficient food (Hill, Moloney, Mize, Himelick, & Guest, 2011). National statistics on migrant seasonal workers are sparse, with much of the data regional and only sporadically collected. Some of the statistics include the following:

- The life expectancy of a migrant worker is lower than the general population, with high rates of poverty, reduced access to health care, and an inverse and increasingly powerful relationship between stressors (e.g., problems speaking English, legal status, discrimination) and mental/physical health among Mexican workers (Williams, 2012; Williams & Sternthal, 2010).
- Migrant farmworkers are more likely to come from a country with higher rates of TB (e.g., Mexico 14.2/100,000 vs. United States 3.6/100,000 cases of TB in 2010). Farmworkers are six times more likely to develop active TB over their lifetime than other workers (Hernández-Garduño, Mendoza-Damián, Garduño-Alanis, & Ayón-Garibaldo, 2015; NCFH, 2013b).
- Migrant children are often delayed for immunizations and have an increased incidence of TB; intestinal parasites and infections; nutritional deficiencies and malnutrition; skin, respiratory tract, and ear infections; dental problems; and pesticide and lead exposure (American Academy of Pediatrics, 2014; SAF, 2011–2016). Almost one third of preschool migrant/seasonal farmworker children were reported to be food insecure, yet obesity was also present in these children and adults (Borre, Ertle, & Graff, 2010; Hernandez, Reesor, Alonso, Eagleton, & Hughes, 2015).
- Migrant workers have high rates of work-related conditions, such as musculoskeletal injuries, heat stress, eye injuries, hearing loss, and skin diseases, because of equipment use and exposure to chemicals, dust, and sun (Habib & Fathallah, 2012; Quandt, Schulz, Talton, Verma, & Arcury, 2012). A study of migrant youth, ages 10 to 17, found 54% reporting musculoskeletal injuries and almost 61% having a traumatic injury (Arcury et al., 2014b). Migrant children are often exposed to heat and sun, musculoskeletal injuries, pesticides, and hazardous tools and machinery (NCFH, 2012a). Their employers are often seen as demanding and their work is sometimes dangerous. Yet, they are generally unwilling to report injuries or even complain to employers because of fear of deportation or firing. A mind-set that they must endure bad work environments as a temporary, but necessary, condition of their work life in the United States is not uncommon; they may feel that "they are undeserving of health care" (Willen, 2012, p. 807). They often continue to work while injured or ill because of perceived difficulty leaving work and pervasive *no work, no pay* employment situations (Arcury et al., 2012a; Gleeson, 2010; Hoerster et al., 2011).

Although training in occupational safety is common for many jobs, it is not always done with agricultural workers. Many Latino migrant and seasonal workers have developed an informal "occupational safety information exchange," including pesticide safety, as a way to alert new workers to occupational dangers (Spears, Summers, Spencer, & Arcury, 2012). In 2011, the U.S. Department of Health and Human Services reported that federally grant-funded health centers provided services to 803,933 farmworkers for the following reasons: dental exams, diabetes mellitus, child immunizations, hypertension, flu vaccine, contraception, fluoride treatments, and Pap tests (NCFH, 2012b).

Occupational Hazards

The hazards of agricultural employment, coupled with limited legal protection, jeopardize the health of the migrant farmworker. As mentioned earlier, agriculture (grouped with forestry and fishing) ranks in the top 10 job categories with the highest occupational death rates (Smith, 2013). Falls, cuts, muscle strains and sprains, and repetitive motion injuries (e.g., carpal tunnel syndrome) commonly afflict migrant laborers. Migrant and seasonal farmwork typically requires stooping, long hours working in wet clothes, working with sometimes contaminated soil and water, climbing, carrying heavy loads, and exposure to the sun and the elements. Failure to perform these activities on a rigid timetable dictated by seasons and weather can result in crop loss. For instance, a shortage of workers resulted in a $1 million loss for an asparagus farmer in Michigan (Schmidt, 2012). This urgency compels farmworkers to labor in all weather conditions, including extreme heat or cold, rain, bright sun, and high humidity.

It is difficult to reach this population in order to gain a full picture of their injuries but musculoskeletal injuries (e.g., back and shoulder pain, numbness/pain in hands), respiratory illnesses (because of molds, various types of dust, pesticide exposure), skin and eye problems (caused by sunburns, rashes, calluses, eye trauma/irritation), infectious diseases (because of crowded, unsanitary conditions), injuries and fatalities (because of hazardous tools, machinery), and exposure to heat and sun (e.g., heat exhaustion, heat stroke, and pesticide exposures are common concerns (NCFH, 2013a). An interesting finding is that farmworkers with H-2A visas had fewer reports of musculoskeletal pain compared to manual laborers not working in agriculture in one North Carolina study (Tribble, Summers, Chen, Quandt, & Arcury, 2015).

In a small study of migrant workers, the incidence rate for work-related eye injuries was 23.8/10,000 worker years compared to a national incidence rate of 6.9 in 2009. Eye injuries (from tree branches, tools, or irritants) can cause serious problems and are seldom reported to employers. Treatment, if any, is often delayed, and penetrating or open wounds were common (Quandt et al., 2012). Extreme cold can lead to frostbite, and overexposure to the sun may result in heat stroke; farm laborers are more often at risk for these conditions. Some plants, like tobacco, pineapples, and garlic, release chemicals that are irritants or can be toxic to farmworkers who come in close contact with them.

Pesticide Exposure

Migrant farmworkers are at greater risk for pesticide poisoning when fields are sprayed or during initial re-entry into the field. Many migrant camps are located within large open fields or on the periphery of cropland. Overhead pesticide sprayings then endanger not only those at work in the fields but also those in the camp. If fields are not posted with warning signs, mass poisoning of farmworkers can occur: thousands of rural residents, in addition to farmworkers, have been poisoned by pesticide drift. One study of almost 3,000 cases of agricultural pesticide drift in 11 states found 47% of participants had work exposures and 14% were children under age 15. Soil fumigants comprise 45% of pesticide poisonings, and 24% are related to aerial applications (Advocate Precautionary Principle, 2011). Two nurses, who as children worked alongside their families in the fields, recalled: "as the planes sprayed the fields, you could feel the drifts" and when the spray mixed with the early morning dew "the pesticide residue would be on your clothes and your skin—it looked like a white film" (Formichelli, 2008, para. 15).

Contaminated water sources in the field enhance the absorption and spread of pesticides and organic compounds. EPA standards that bar entry to sprayed fields for at least 24 hours are often ignored. Pesticides can drift from the fields to contaminate food, yards, or children playing nearby. Children are at greater risk for pesticide-induced illnesses because of their higher metabolic rate, greater surface absorption, still developing organs, and possibility for chronic long-term exposure (Rauh et al., 2011). It is estimated that thousands of farmworkers suffer pesticide poisoning each year, but exact counts are not possible because of inadequate surveillance systems and reluctance of farmworkers to report injuries (Farmworker Justice, n.d.). Surveillance systems are only in place in 11 states; the Sentinel Event Notification System or Occupational Risk (SENSOR) is a means of reporting pesticide-related injuries as well as other occupational illnesses and injuries (National Institute for Occupational Safety & Health, 2012). Some farmworkers, primarily those without H-2A visas, were less likely to be provided pesticide safety equipment and often were not notified when pesticides were applied (Robinson et al., 2011). Reporting of pesticide-induced morbidity and mortality is not required in every state. California has the oldest pesticide surveillance system in the United States, beginning in 1971 (California Department of Pesticide Exposure, 2013).

But, even with reporting laws, many cases are never recognized because workers do not seek medical care. Pesticide burns and rashes often go untreated because of lack of education about the dangers of pesticides and lack of available services. Migrant workers are often unaware of the hazards of pesticides. Arcury et al. (2010) found that a large number of migrant farmworkers had multiple detections for several pesticide and herbicide urinary metabolites. In a later study, Arcury et al. (2014a) noted that farmworkers had consistently greater levels of lifetime and residential exposure to pesticides than nonfarmworkers and that among both groups, education level was inversely related to lifetime pesticide exposure. An Eastern Washington state study, comparing farmworker adults and children with nonfarmworker adults and children living in close proximity to farmland, found organophosphate metabolite concentrations (urine and house dust) significantly higher among those working in the fields and their children. However, even those adults and children just living near farmland had metabolites present. Researchers found a 20% decrease in metabolite concentration for every mile of distance from

farmland (Coronado et al., 2011). Pesticide drift has been shown to result in elevated levels of active compounds in both indoor air and house dust in homes near agricultural application areas. Houses closer to agricultural herbicide applications had significantly elevated levels of herbicides in house dust than in homes that were further away (Shelton & Hertz-Picciotto, 2015). Orchard air-blast applications of pesticides, along with wind direction, can influence pesticide drift from crops into agricultural residences; potential exposures can be analyzed through screening tests (Burns, Cohen, & Lunchick, 2015; U.S. Environmental Protection Agency, 2014).

Even though it may be required of health care providers to report pesticide poisoning, it is often misdiagnosed because the symptoms can mimic those of viral infections or heat-related illness. Symptoms of pesticide exposure include sore throat, runny nose, headache, fatigue, red/swollen/watery eyes, drowsiness, itchy skin, abdominal pain, and nausea or vomiting. More severe symptoms may include sweating, salivation, blurred vision or pinpoint pupils, fever, severe thirst, muscle twitching, or weakness and incontinence (especially with organophosphate or carbamate exposures). Finally, with the most severe exposures, seizures, respiratory depression, and unconsciousness or coma can occur. There are over 19,000 pesticide products registered with the EPA and more than one thousand active ingredients. Biomarkers, or signs of a specific chemical's presence in the body, are important in definitively proving exposures; however, chemical companies are not currently required to provide this information (Huber, 2011).

Only a few categories of pesticides account for more than half of the cases of acute illness; these include inorganic compounds, carbamates, pyrethroids, and organophosphates. Although the impact of acute pesticide poisoning is widely recognized, little is understood about the long-term effects of the repeated low-level exposures to which migrant farmworkers are constantly subjected. The Florida Department of Health lists the chronic effects of long-term pesticide exposure as birth defects, cancers, blood disorders, neurological problems, and reproductive issues. Extreme exposure can lead to loss of consciousness, coma, or death (NCFH, 2013a). Several studies showed that entire families are at risk for pesticide exposure because of drift from nearby areas, poor handwashing

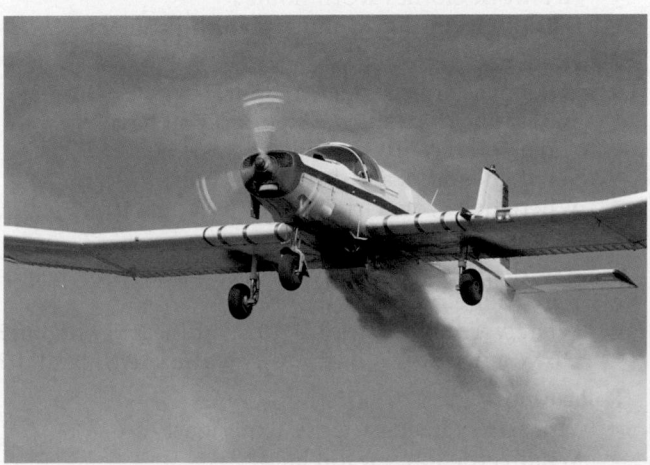

Low-flying crop duster spreads pesticide on fields.

facilities, and bringing pesticides home on clothing (Quandt et al., 2010). Numerous studies have examined the link between exposure to pesticides and various neurologic problems and cancer—most often with organophosphate-based pesticides. Some pesticides have been suspected of leading to depression, suicidal ideation, and other psychological distress (Bienkowski, 2014). Some evidence of an association between pesticide exposure and the incidence of diabetes has been found (Diabetologia, 2015). Non-Hodgkin's lymphoma, leukemia, prostate cancer, sarcomas, and multiple myelomas have been associated with organophosphates, herbicides, and insecticides (Cockburn et al., 2011). Prenatal exposure to organophosphate pesticides has been significantly associated with slightly decreased intellectual development (Bouchard et al., 2011). Today, it is more common for farmworkers to be exposed to "nonpersistent" pesticides that are metabolized in the body within days (NCFH, 2013a).

A large body of supportive research has indicated a link between Parkinson's disease, other neurologic disorders, and pesticide exposure, and some specific pesticides (e.g., ziram, paraquat) have been implicated (Van der Mark et al., 2012; Wang et al., 2011a). Display 29–3, Environmental Exposure History, is a helpful assessment tool for community health nurses working with migrant and seasonal workers to use to determine pesticide exposure. When a client presents with symptoms that may be suggestive of pesticide exposure, mnemonic prompts may help to clarify common symptoms (see Display 29–4).

Pesticide exposure can be a single event, may occur multiple times, or can even be continuous. Health effects are thought to be a function of the frequency of exposure and the dose. Most migrant workers come into contact with pesticides through their work. However, exposure to pesticides does not affect only those working in the

---

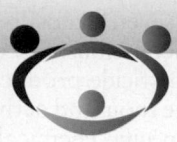

DISPLAY 29–3 ENVIRONMENTAL EXPOSURE HISTORY

Do an Exposure History to:
- Identify current or past exposures
- Reduce or eliminate current exposures
- Reduce adverse health effects

Taking an Exposure History: Questions to Consider

Use the **I PREPARE** mnemonic:

I–Investigate potential exposures
- Have you ever felt sick after coming in contact with a chemical, pesticide, or other substance?
- Do you have any symptoms that improve when you are away from your home or workplace?

P–Present work
- Are you exposed to solvents, dusts, fumes, radiation, loud noise, pesticides, or other chemicals?
- Do you know where to find Material Data Safety Sheets on chemicals that you work with?
- Do you wear personal protective equipment?
- Are work clothes worn home?
- Do coworkers have similar health problems?

R–Residence
- When was your residence built?
- What type of heating system do you have?
- Have you recently remodeled your home?
- What chemicals are stored on your property?
- Where does your drinking water come from?

E–Environmental concerns
- Are there environmental concerns in your neighborhood (e.g., air, water, soil)?
- What types of industries or farms are near your home?
- Do you live near a hazardous waste site or landfill?

P–Past work
- What are your past work experiences?
- What is the longest job held?

- Have you ever been in the military, worked on a farm, or done volunteer or seasonal work?

A–Activities
- What activities and hobbies do you and your family engage in?
- Do you burn, solder, or melt any products?
- Do you garden, fish, or hunt?
- Do you eat what you catch or grow?
- Do you use pesticides?
- Do you engage in any alternative healing or cultural practices?

R–Referrals and resources (use these key referrals and resources)
- Agency for Toxic Substances and Disease Registry: www.atsdr.cdc.gov
- Association of Occupational and Environmental Clinics: www.aoec.org
- Environmental Protection Agency: www.epa.gov
- Material Safety Data Sheets: www.hazard.com/msds
- Occupational Safety and Health Administration: www.osha.gov
- LHDs, environmental agencies, and poison control centers

E–Educate (a checklist)
- Are materials available to educate the patient?
- Are alternatives available to minimize the risk of exposure?
- Have prevention strategies been discussed?
- What is the plan for follow-up?

Source: Agency for Toxic Substances & Disease Registry. (n.d.). *Environmental exposure history*. Retrieved from http://www.atsdr.cdc.gov/asbestos/site-kit/docs/IPrepareCard.pdf
Practice Case Studies Available From: Agency for Toxic Substances & Disease Registry. (2015). *ASTDR case studies in environmental medicine: Taking an exposure history*. Retrieved from http://www.atsdr.cdc.gov/csem/exphistory/docs/exposure_history.pdf

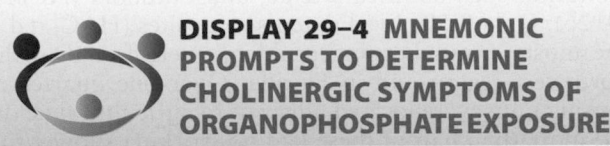

DISPLAY 29–4 MNEMONIC PROMPTS TO DETERMINE CHOLINERGIC SYMPTOMS OF ORGANOPHOSPHATE EXPOSURE

SLUDGE	DUMBBELS
Salivation	Defecation
Lacrimation	Urination
Urination	Miosis
Defecation	Bronchorrhea
Gastric secretions	Bradycardia
Emesis	Emesis
	Lacrimation
	Salivation/seizures/sweating

The four most acute symptoms: bradyarrhythmias, bronchospasm, muscle weakness, and bronchorrhea

Sources: Clark, R. F. (2007). Pesticides. In R. S. Hoffman, L. S. Nelson, M. A. Howland, N. A. Lewin, N. E. Flomenbaum, & L. R. Goldfrank (Eds.). *Goldfrank's toxicological emergencies* (pp. 817–872). New York, NY: McGraw-Hill Medical.
Robey, W. C., III & W. J. Meggs. (2004). Insecticides, herbicides, rodenticides. In J. E. Tintinalli, G. D. Kelen, and J. S. Stapczynski (Eds.). *Emergency medicine: A comprehensive study guide* (pp 1134–1143). New York, NY: Mc Graw-Hill.
Utah Poison Control Center. (2006). Organophosphate poisoning. *Utox Update*, 8(2), 1–4.

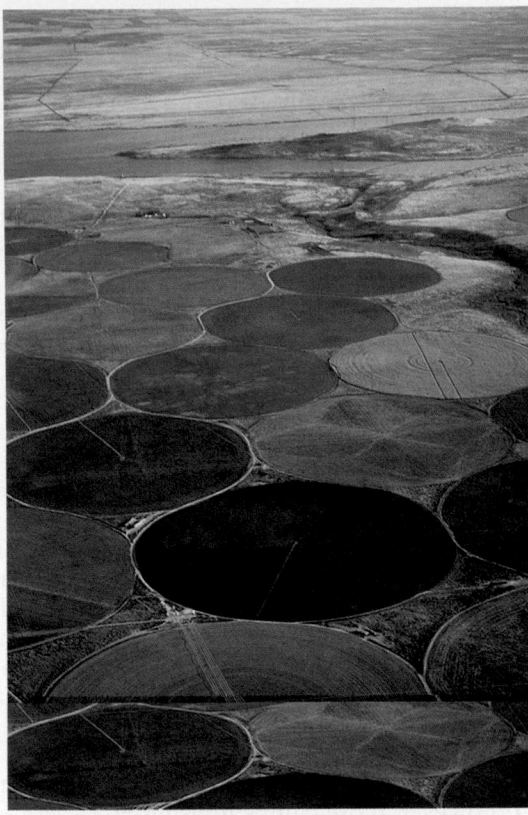

Fields in Eastern Oregon. (Source: USDA, Agricultural Research Service.)

fields. "Most farmworker housing is contaminated with a broad range of pesticides," and this exposes not only workers but also their families to pesticide-related risks. "Most workers and family members have absorbed measurable doses of pesticides" according to a seminal study by Arcury and Quandt (2009, p. 103). Organophosphates decrease the levels of acetylcholinesterase, found in nerve endings, and can be absorbed through the skin, inhaled, or ingested. Most workers have metabolites present, and farmwork and housing close to agricultural fields are common factors associated with exposure. Drifts from sprayed fields and residues on farmworker clothing, shoes, tools, and skin, as well as food brought from the fields, are all potential sources of exposure. Vehicles can also become contaminated, as can carpets and furniture. Contaminated clothing should be kept in separate hampers and laundered separately; workers need to be encouraged to leave boots and shoes outside their homes and to change clothing and shower before eating and playing with their children. Substandard housing is also a factor.

Agricultural fields are usually located in isolated areas on the outskirts of rural communities. While in these isolated fields, migrant workers often are not provided with sanitation facilities or fresh drinking water. The Occupational Safety and Health Administration (OSHA) mandates field sanitation (at least one toilet and handwashing station) and fresh drinking water for each agricultural establishment employing 11 or more hand-labor workers on any given day (OSHA, 2011).

Substandard Housing and Poor Sanitation

Quality of housing affects farmworker health, and more comparative studies are needed (Arcury et al., 2015a; Arcury, Jacobs, & Ruiz, 2015b; Quandt et al., 2015). Formal demographic data on farmworker housing are often lacking. One cohort study of a farmworker population in Mendota, California (MICASA), employed door-to-door enumeration in a rural agricultural community. Almost 10% of the dwellings were classified as "back houses or unofficial dwellings," thought to have been missed during the last census (Stoecklin-Marois, Hennessy-Burt, & Schenker, 2011, p. 291). A survey of growers about migrant health and nutrition in the Midwest found that the median migrant camp had 23 seasonally employed residents (for 10 weeks up to 6 months), with 7 accompanying children. No consistency was reported in kitchen appliances, and most owners had little information about migrant health services. Also, they reported that migrant laborers had restricted access to fresh produce for meals and children did not have easy access to public play areas but mostly used open fields (Kilanowski, 2012). In a classic article by Cole and Crawford (1991), a vivid example of one migrant camp in Alabama highlighted workers living in a converted chicken house. An upper portion of the wall had been removed for ventilation, creating easy access for insects and birds. A dirt floor, a single light bulb, and two portable toilets located a distance away were some of the other features. Two sinks in a common living area provided the only water for the almost 60 people who lived in the chicken house. Many did not have mattresses, and because the workers were harvesting potatoes, potato baskets conveniently served as the only furniture. Such living situations still exist today. Living with 13 other workers in a three-bedroom home in Watsonville, California, a female farmworker remarked, "We have to put up with this because we can't afford anything else" (Holden, n.d., p. 40). A description of dorm-style rooms in Immokalee, Florida, revealed "the shower has filthy, crumbling concrete walls—the kind that won't come clean...(and) a metal sink held by a rotting plywood counter, and the toilet often backs up, so the tiny room reeks of sewage" (p. 41).

Migrant farmworkers move frequently and often have great difficulty securing adequate housing. In the past, many growers or owners provided housing to migrant workers and their families. This practice has now become much less common, and only limited numbers of government-sponsored housing units are available for migrant workers. Housing conditions may actually be considered hazardous in some areas, and employer-owned labor camp regulations are much less stringent than Section 8 housing standards (Summers, Quandt, Talton, Galván, & Arcury, 2015; Vallejos, Quandt, & Arcury, 2009). Many migrant farmworker camps have ongoing violations. One study found a range of 4 to 22 per camp, with the mean number of total violations at 11.4; however, those camps housing H-2A visa workers and those examined early in the season had fewer violations (Arcury, Summers et al., 2012). In another study, GIS mapping was used to determine the differences between visible and hidden farm labor camps in North Carolina (Summers et al., 2015). Almost 38% of the camps were hidden, and hidden camps were substantially larger and more likely to have barracks-type housing. Historically, employer-owned farm labor camps were often infested with pests and had structural damage and insufficient bathing facilities. Researchers noted that hidden camps perpetuate social isolation and the potential for substandard housing.

When private housing is available, it is often only offered at prices that outpace worker's wages. Data are scant, but a large survey of migrant workers in the eastern, Midwestern, and western migrant streams conducted by the HAC revealed that over 50% of all housing units surveyed were overcrowded (only 3% of U.S. households are and 44% of mobile homes were substandard). Almost one quarter of units surveyed had at least one broken appliance or fixture, and 11% had no working stove. Between 13% and 39% of housing is owned by employers, and for those lucky enough to find employer-owned housing, over half of those units were offered without charge. Agricultural employers most commonly own single-family homes (39%) and apartments (14%), but workers and their families also are housed in barracks or dormitories, in motels, and in mobile homes (Holden, n.d.; HAC, n.d.). Forty-two percent of farmworkers lived in single-family homes and 21% in apartments; fifteen percent lived in mobile homes and the same proportion in duplex/triplex housing. About 4% lived in dorms/barracks, and 2% lived in motels. Approximately 2% reported living conditions not meant for human habitation such as in cars tents, and outdoors (NCFH, 2012b). Only 0.5% lived in tents/campsites (HAC, n.d.). The most serious housing problems were found in the Northwest region and in Florida. Over one quarter of housing units were located adjacent to agricultural fields, and more than half of these had no working shower/tub or washing machine—or both (HAC, n.d.).

Families with children occupied 65% of both severely substandard and moderately substandard units (HAC, n.d.). Structural problems, such as holes in the roof (15%), sagging frames or roofs (22%), or damage to foundations (15%), were common. Broken glass or window screens were noted in 36% of units, and peeling external paint was found in over 40% of units (Holden, n.d.; HAC, n.d.). Evidence of water damage was found in 29% of units, and 9% had exposed wiring. An examination of 183 North Carolina migrant farmworker camps in 2010 revealed 11.4 mean housing violations, with a range from 4 to 22 (Arcury et al., 2012b). Bathroom violations were most common, and camps housing workers without H-2A visas or posted state inspection certificates, or those examined later in the migrant season, had more violations. An example with serious consequences is Jensen Farms, a Colorado cantaloupe grower, who was fined for substandard housing provided to migrant workers in their fields and packing facility. The owner of Jensen Farms also owned the Gateway Motel, used for migrant housing during harvesting season, where workers each paid $25 per week for space in overcrowded rooms without beds (and no laundry facilities). The owner claimed that he was an "innkeeper" and did not fall within the purview for migrant and seasonal worker housing laws, but he was found out of compliance and fined $4,250. In 2011, Jensen Farms shipped out *Listeria*-contaminated cantaloupes that resulted in "the deadliest outbreak of food-borne illness in nearly 100 years" (Flynn, 2012, para. 2). Although unsanitary worker housing may not be directly related to the outbreak, this may be just another indication of overall carelessness that led to unsafe farming practices.

Substandard housing is not the only concern. Crowding is also a problem, as many farmworkers, unable to find sufficient numbers of rental units, share housing—sometimes paying per-person costs. One of the few studies on migrant housing found that Minnesota seasonal vegetable workers' construction trailer barracks, housing 15 to 20 single migrant workers, rented for $90 per month per person. The California Migrant Housing Authority reported two-bedroom housing units available for $345/month (Migrant Housing, n.d.). In the HAC study, almost one third of migrant workers paid rental costs that were in excess of 30% of their gross incomes—defined as a housing cost burden (HAC, n.d.). The costs led to further crowding, as families doubled up to save expenses. When housing cannot be found, workers and families may have to resort to paying rent to live in garages, barns, sheds, or chicken coops, or they may be forced to stay in their cars. One Michigan farmer with 65 acres of blueberries describes the migrant workers he has employed for 7 to 9 weeks of every year for the past 25 years as "the hardest workers I know," stating that "we would not be here if it wasn't for the migrant workforce." Each year, around 90,000 migrant workers come to Michigan, but employer-provided housing only can accommodate about 22,000 of them (Schmidt, 2012, para. 3). More permanent, though seasonally occupied, housing is needed to accommodate these workers.

Migrant Family Health

Migrant workers have higher rates of obesity than season farmworkers, and females are more likely to be obese and have diabetes than males. However, males were more likely to smoke than females (Castañeda, Rosenbaum, Holscher, Madanat, & Talavera, 2015). Despite often working among fruit and vegetable crops, migrant families often have difficulty procuring food and maintaining a sufficient supply. The lack of food supplies was often due to limited access to resources and isolation, but parents attempted to sacrifice in order to feed their children, and when eligible utilize government food sources (Quandt, Grzywacz, Trejo, & Arcury, 2014). Because of frequent moves, migrant children are often educationally, socially, and physically disadvantaged; many migrant parents have an eighth grade education or less and the majority of migrant children who meet criteria for special services at school are actually receiving them (Habib & Fathallah, 2012; Waldman, Cannella, & Perlman, 2010). The children have "some of the lowest socioeconomic and educational indicators," and their parents are frequently viewed by school personnel as difficult to reach and not involved in their children's education (Jasis & Marriott, 2010, p. 126). One explanation for their lack of participation is their extended work hours, beginning early in the morning and ending long after school hours. But some programs have been successful in reaching out to migrant parents. A community-based adult education program that improved migrant parents' self-actualization and promoted changes in interactions between parents and school personnel also led to improved school outcomes for migrant children; the process of engaging Latino immigrant families includes encouraging participation, leadership development, and organizing activities (Jasis & Marriott, 2010; Jasis & Ordoñez-Jasis, 2012). Migrant education programs, especially with Mexican American resource teachers as role models, have also been helpful.

Migrant children are often called upon by their families to stay home from school to work, care for younger children, or attend to other household chores. They may feel socially estranged, be constantly moving, and have difficulty finding health-promoting recreational activities and have difficulty assimilating (Portes & Rivas, 2011). A large seminal California study found significantly higher odds of developmental risk among children of undocumented Mexican parents but not for children of documented Mexican parents (Ortego et al., 2009). This may indicate stressors related to immigration status. There has been a 45-fold increase in the number of undocumented workers taken into custody by the U.S. Immigration and Customs Enforcement (ICE) agency between 2001 and 2007. And highly publicized ICE raids have led migrant parents to withdraw their children from Migrant Head Start programs, noticeably decreasing enrollments across the country and further placing migrant children

at risk for academic problems (Mather & Parameswaran, 2012). Connor, Layne, and Hilb (2014) note that despite the many trials facing migrant children, they show great strength and resilience that helps them face their challenges.

A survey of over 2,000 migrants (ages 12 to 65) found an increased risk for depressive symptoms among returning migrants and anxiety and depressive symptoms among migrant relatives (Familiar, Borges, Orozco, & Medina-Mora, 2011). A program available for migrant farmworkers or their children is CAMP, the College Assistance Migrant Program, serving about 2,000 students annually (U.S. Department of Education, 2015).

The children of migrant farmworkers receive only fragmented health care. Common health problems of migrant children include general poor nutrition, anemia, vitamin A deficiency, increased risk for respiratory and ear infections, dental problems, lead and pesticide poisoning, intestinal parasites, skin infections, TB, and delayed development (American Academy of Pediatrics, 2014). Migrant farmworker children (ages 0 to 16) in Georgia were assessed and found to have a higher prevalence of obesity and stunting than nonmigrant children; among the 6- to 12-year-old group, migrant children had higher prevalence of elevated blood pressures, and elevated blood pressures were found in older migrant teens (Nichols, Stein, & Wold, 2014). Another study found that migrant boys were more likely to be obese than girls, and hypertension and anemia were more prevalent among obese migrant children (Gonzalez, Billings, Shin, Rosenbaum, & Song, 2013). Lack of awareness that minor symptoms, such as diarrhea or fever, may indicate a more serious underlying problem can cause delays in seeking medical attention, as can poverty and a lack of health insurance. An earache is minor, but it can lead to a major problem, such as deafness, if left untreated.

Studies on the impact of Head Start enrollment on migrant children's health outcomes revealed that higher rates of health treatments were obtained for those attending one or more years and for lower rates of obesity for those attending Migrant Head Start program for multiple years (Lee & Pond, 2015; Lee & Song, 2015).

A systematic review of migrant children and adolescents compared with nonmigrant counterparts did not find a significant difference in behavioral or emotional problems (Belhadj Koulder, Koglin, & Petermann, 2015). Migrant adolescents are less likely to abuse substances when they first arrive, but the likelihood increases as they remain in this country and is higher for second-generation Hispanics (The Future of Children, 2011). Overall, they are less likely to graduate from high school, because their education is often interrupted. Globally, children between the ages of 7 and 14 who live in a rural setting are less likely to attend school but more likely to work. Also, migration causes educational interruption and difficulty "catching up." The average level of education completed was the eighth grade (NCFH, 2012a). Stress from acculturation, poor working conditions, deficient social support, and poor family functioning have been associated with greater anxiety and depressive symptoms among farmworkers (Winkelman, Chaney, & Bethel, 2013). Research on children whose parents have been arrested, detained, and/or deported has found increased economic and social instability leading to parental depression and poor cognitive and behavioral outcomes for children (Chaudry et al., 2010; Migration Policy Institute, 2015). The situation becomes even more complicated when one parent of legal children is born in the United States and is a legal citizen and the other is not; approximately 4.5 million children live in mixed status families (Brabeck, Lykes, & Hunter, 2014).

Mixed methods research by Winkelman et al. (2013) showed that about 25% of migrant farmworkers experienced stress, depression, or anxiety in their lifetime from sources such as (1) physical stress because of working conditions; (2) psychological stress because of family situations, work environment, documentation status, and lack of resources; (3) depression because of separation from family; and (4) use of both positive and negative coping mechanisms to deal with stress and depression. Acculturative stress, workload, and depression have been found among migrant workers in other countries, such as Korea (Lee, Ahn, Miller, Park, & Kim, 2012). This study by Winkelman et al. (2013) suggests that stress and depression are significant mental health issues among Latino migrant farmworkers because of a lack of permanent employment and continued work uncertainty. Behaviors used to cope with stress included (1) watching TV (75%), (2) sleep (73.3%), (3) family support (66.7%), (4) listening to music (56.7 %), (5) humor (50%), and (6) prayer (48.3%). Negative coping behaviors used by migrant farmworkers included (1) smoking or use of tobacco products (16.7%), (2) eating unhealthy foods (16.7%), (3) playing the lottery (15%), (4) drinking alcohol (15%), and (5) gambling (11.7%).

Display 29–5 lists some stressors from the Hispanic Stress Inventory evaluation tool. Social isolation factors ranked slightly lower, but being away from friends and family was often mentioned. In this study of farmworkers, migrating mostly from Mexico, almost 42% met the classification as depressed, and over 18% had anxiety levels consistent with impaired functioning. The researchers concluded that social isolation had a stronger potential effect on anxiety, whereas poor working conditions were associated more with depression. The need for migrant workers to congregate in neighborhoods with others from their cultural background is an attempt to counter this social isolation. When surrounded by others who share their culture and speak their language, and when they can find familiar music, television, entertainment, and food, it helps to allay feelings of anxiety and depression. It is easy to understand why many migrant workers in specific migrant streams originate from the same states or communities in Mexico or other countries; it is an attempt to hold onto some semblance of their social networks as they migrate to the United States (Loue & Quill, 2010).

Alcohol use has been noted to be common among male migrant workers, and the stressors migrant farmworkers face related to their employment and acculturation put them at a higher risk for drug and alcohol abuse, as well as other high-risk behaviors. Arcury et al. (2016) compared interview data from male Latino migrant farmworkers and Latino nonfarmworkers in North Carolina and found that 48.5% of farmworkers reported heavy episodic drinking in the past 3 months; 23.8% admitted that this behavior was frequent. However, no significant differences were noted between the two groups regarding behavior related to alcohol consumption. Stress and being a farmworker, however, were significant factors for being at risk for alcohol dependence; reduced risk was noted for farmworkers who were married. Drugs and alcohol may be used as a means of coping with separation from family and social isolation.

Problems with substance abuse may also be associated with violence. Respondents with higher stress levels also reported greater interpersonal violence and depression (Kim-Godwin, Maume, & Fox, 2014). Aggression

---

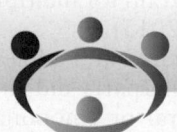

DISPLAY 29–5 EXTRAFAMILIAL AND INTRAFAMILIAL STRESSORS FOR HISPANIC ADULTS

Common Extrafamilial Stressors

Difficult interactions with others because of not being able to speak English

Feeling an expectation to work harder because of being a Latino

Feeling pressures to learn English

Difficulty finding work I want to do because I am Latino

Forced to take low-paying jobs

Continually concerned with quality of my work so that others do not consider me lazy

Being treated badly because of my poor English

Difficulty getting promotions or salary increases because I am Latino

Not having sufficient income to support my family

Common Intrafamilial Stressors

Conflicts among my family members

Physical violence among my family members

Serious arguments among my family members

Children have too liberal ideas about sexuality

Children talk about leaving home

Children receive bad school reports or grades

Spouse and I disagree about how to raise our children

Children do not respect my authority as I think they should

Adapted from Cavazos-Rehg, C., Zayas, L., Walker, M., & Fisher, E. (2006). Evaluating an abbreviated version of the Hispanic Stress Inventory for Immigrants. *Hispanic Journal of Behavioral Sciences, 28*, 498–515.

at migrant farm labor camps was often tied to alcohol use and was more common as the work season progressed; while acts of aggression were prevalent among male migrant workers, the frequency was low (Kraemer-Diaz et al., in press). In a San Diego, California study of intimate partner violence (IPV) among farmworkers, researchers found that 16% of women interviewed, and 32% of males reported victimization, perpetration, or both (Duke & Cunradi, 2011). Male drinking and female impulsivity were significant correlates to IPV. Although research on migrant children and violence is almost nonexistent, one classic article reported that 46% of children have witnessed some form of violence, 20% had witnessed a shooting, and 11% had witnessed a murder (Triantafillou, 2003). Many migrant families come from areas where violent crime levels (e.g., murder rates) are high, and gang activity, along with domestic violence, are widespread (Thale, 2014). In a classic study conducted in Texas border counties, verbal abuse was the most frequently reported form of IPV (72%). Only 22% reported knowledge of a shelter where they could go to gain assistance (Kugel et al., 2009). While health care provider screening for IPV increases the rates of identification, many providers do not effectively screen (Wilson, Rappleyea, Hodgson, Hall, & White, 2014; Wilson et al., in press). One large California study of migrant farmworkers found a 5% prevalence of being a victim of personal violence within the past year. Males experienced violence in workplaces, or other public settings, whereas over 80% of self-reported violence reported by females was the result of violence (Villarejo et al., 2010). Research on domestic violence among this vulnerable population is scant, but more than 1,000 battered farmworker women in a multicenter study were interviewed and researchers identified the typical profile as:

- Childbearing age (15 to 40)
- Hispanic
- Afraid of their partner
- Married or living with partner
- Drug or alcohol use by partner

The overall incidence was 20.6%. Fifty percent of abused women were pregnant at the time of the abuse (MCN, n.d.). Nationally, just over 35% of women report sexual, physical abuse, or stalking by an intimate partner during their lifetime (Black et al., 2011). See Chapter 20 for a more complete discussion of domestic/IPV. What makes farmworker domestic violence so significant is the fact that these women often experience language barriers, do not have adequate access to health care, live isolated lives with little social support, and fear deportation if they report the abuse—all factors that lead them to endure their violent situation in silence. One example is a migrant woman, who shared a one-room dwelling with her husband, infant, and five single men. Her husband became increasingly violent and unpredictable. He began to beat her and the baby, and she was unable to predict what would initiate a violent attack. She finally fled when one of the men living with them also began beating her. She attributed the aggressive behavior to the powerlessness felt by the men. The Violence Against Women Act of 1994 affords protection for undocumented battered

women and children by allowing them to seek legal immigration status without the help of their abusers (Migrant Clinician's Network, n.d.). PHNs must be aware of these issues and what resources are available in the community (see Levels of Prevention Pyramid).

Infectious Diseases

As noted earlier, TB is a common infectious disease among farmworkers. Some studies find that farmworkers are six times more likely to develop active TB over their lifetime than other workers, with 48.8 cases per 100,000 detected among agricultural workers seen at migrant health centers in 2011; this is higher than the rate for nonagricultural workers at all health centers at 33.1 cases per 100,000 (NCFH, 2013b). Because of their migrant patterns, it is difficult to complete treatment regimens. Because of frequent moves, poor access to health care, and social isolation, it is often difficult for migrant farmworkers to be accurately diagnosed and treated. Many factors may prevent them from successfully completing a treatment regimen, and language barriers, along with cultural differences, may preclude them from fully understanding the impact of their disease on themselves and others. For instance, a Mexican migrant worker may be diagnosed with TB in California and begin treatment there but may move to Washington state to pick cherries and run out of medication before completing treatment. Moving back to California for summer work, he may again start treatment but may travel home to Mexico during the winter, only to be reinfected by an older, untreated member of his extended family.

Migrant workers are at greater risk of HIV infection for many of the same reasons. Albarrán and Nyamathi (2011) found that Mexican migrant workers were at higher risk for HIV infection because of limited health care access, multiple sexual partners, low levels of condom use, injection practices, and men having sex with men. They also note that there is now a higher prevalence of HIV found in rural areas of Mexico, as workers bring the infection back to their homes. HIV-positive status may be misunderstood and, because of stigmatization and fears of deportation, may be purposely hidden from health officials. Estimated HIV rates are reported to be between 2.6% and 13%, depending on geographic area and personal risk factors like drug abuse; however, accurate national prevalence rates are almost impossible to attain (NCFH, 2011). High-risk behaviors, such as sex while under the influence of alcohol and drugs, sex with commercial sex workers, inconsistent use of condoms, performing sex works, and sex with a male partner, were increased in male migrant farmworkers, elevating their risk for HIV/AIDS (Sanchez et al., 2012). A larger proportion of male migrant farmworkers reported condom use after migration to the United States, demonstrating an increase in preventative measures; this is an encouraging report, as overall, loneliness has been negatively associated with condom use in a study of rural men having sex with men (Hubach et al., 2015; Sanchez et al., 2012). There is a great need for more effective outreach and education strategies (Hernandez, Mata, Vasquez, & Martinez, 2014). Other infectious diseases (e.g., hepatitis, enteric diseases, parasites) may commonly afflict

LEVELS OF PREVENTION PYRAMID

SITUATION: Domestic violence in the migrant population. Research is scant; however, informal discussions occur among women and health care providers. Outreach workers sometimes possess lists of men who are abusive and their victims. Although the migrant lifestyle and experience are difficult for the entire family, women and children suffer most from family violence that the migrant way of life promotes. Isolation and subjugation to a patriarchal system usually prohibit migrant women from seeking help if they are abused. Fear of consequences and difficulty expressing negative views about husbands prevent women from speaking out (Migrant Clinician's Network, n.d.).
GOAL: Using the three levels of prevention, negative health conditions are avoided, promptly diagnosed, and treated, and/or the fullest possible potential is restored.

TERTIARY PREVENTION

Rehabilitation	Primary Prevention	
	Health Promotion and Education	*Health Protection*
• Promote family rehabilitation, with or without abuser in the home. • Encourage ways to eliminate or reduce social and geographic isolation among vulnerable women.	• Alleviate stressors of the migrant lifestyle, such as overcrowding and substandard living conditions. • Provide emotional support and educate on what constitutes abuse. • Promote self-esteem to the point where a woman can take control of her situation.	• Encourage women to contact health care providers as they migrate. • Encourage women to find appropriate lay community outreach workers for support. • Encourage migrant women to unite and create an environment that allows them to speak up and out while supporting one another against abuse.

SECONDARY PREVENTION

Early Diagnosis	Prompt Treatment
• Promptly identify an abused woman—through self-identification or by other family members or professionals—and remove her from the dangerous situation.* • Keep communication lines open, be culturally sensitive, and examine for injuries.	• Secure the victim in a safe battered women's shelter. • Assist victim to regain self-esteem.

*Secondary prevention is difficult because of limited financial resources, lack of transportation, no nearby friends or relatives for support, language barriers (e.g., non–English speaking), and limited safe shelters for battered women in rural areas.

PRIMARY PREVENTION

Health Promotion and Education	Health Protection
• Create awareness of the harsh living conditions that migrant families endure. • Advocate for improved and safe living conditions on state and national levels. • Provide adequate housing that eliminates overcrowding and offers privacy.	• Train bilingual and bicultural lay migrant women on the issues of spousal abuse and help them form support groups. • Provide opportunities for women and men to improve self-esteem that will change attitudes toward each other.

The World Health Organization (2014) addressed the health sector's role in migrant IPV prevention, and the following lists are recommendations for the policy, health system, health facility, and health care provider levels of care.

At the health policy and health system levels
1. Promote social participation in the design of health policy.
2. Strengthen coordination between the health system and other sectors.
3. Develop a multisectoral approach.
4. Promote evidence-based policy-making.
5. Identify objectives and indicators for monitoring and evaluation.

LEVELS OF PREVENTION PYRAMID (Continued)

At the health facility level

6. Address and prevent institutional discrimination.
7. Identify and address access barriers.
8. Address language and cultural barriers to health services.
9. Address administrative and practical barriers.
10. Identify relevant program adaptations that respond to health needs of migrant and ethnic minority women facing IPV.
11. Develop systems for organizational learning relating to IPV among migrant and ethnic minority women.
12. Explore opportunities for prevention activities within primary care.

At the health provider level

1. Engage in training to better understand the IPV vulnerability of migrant and ethnic minority women.
2. Know the legal implications of health services work with regard to IPV.
3. Become familiar with research literature on health provider bias and discrimination in medical decision-making with respect to migrant and ethnic minority women.
4. Create and participate in networks of health care professionals to address IPV with migrant and ethnic minority women during medical encounters.
5. Share best practices and engage in program coordination with organizations that work directly with migrant and ethnic minority women experiencing IPV.

World Health Organization. (2014). *Preventing and addressing intimate partner violence against migrant and ethnic minority women: the role of the health sector.* Retrieved from http://www.euro.who.int/__data/assets/ pdf_file/0018/270180/21256-WHO-Intimate-Partner-Violence_low_V7.pdf

---

migrant workers, often because of inadequate sanitation and hygiene facilities.

Economic Barriers and Limited Health Resources

Most migrant workers are unable to qualify for basic health and disability benefits such as Workers' Compensation, Social Security, occupational rehabilitation, and disability compensation because of undocumented status. One California survey found that between 27% of male and 11% of female migrant workers had been paid Workers' Compensation claims over the course of their work history, with about 40% of undocumented migrant workers having any knowledge of this program even though there is universal coverage (Kresge Foundation, 2012; Villarejo et al., 2010). Federal legislation passed in 2006 requires proof of U.S. citizenship (e.g., passport, birth certificate) when applying for or renewing Medicaid coverage, so undocumented workers are generally unable to qualify (Farmworker Justice, n.d.). As a group, migrant farmworkers have more difficulty accessing Medicaid than any other population.

Medicaid benefits have little value in the face of constant mobility, because they are not transferable from state to state. On one hand, although the low income of migrant workers meets the guidelines for state medical assistance, few families remain in one state long enough for the 30-day residency requirement. On the other hand, farmworker families may not qualify for Medicaid because, during certain months of the year, they earn more than the state's poverty limits. Ironically, migrant workers suffer from preventable and treatable diseases covered under Medicaid, but they are frequently unable to obtain treatment. Some undocumented workers may be eligible for emergency Medicaid—a very limited benefit (Farmworker Justice, n.d.).

Although many are eligible for public programs such as food stamps, S-CHIP, and the Women, Infants, and Children (WIC) program, migrant farmworkers as a whole generally do not participate. They may fear immigration penalties or be totally unaware of the available benefits. Some are eligible for Social Security benefits but do not possess the ability to process their claim (NCFH, 2012b). Workers who do not have valid Social Security numbers, but still have taxes withheld from their wages, are estimated to contribute $7 billion in Social Security taxes and about $1.5 billion in Medicare taxes.

Some think that undocumented workers are a drain on the U.S. economy and illegal immigration is a hot-button topic. However, a substantial amount of research demonstrates that immigrants generally pay more money into the system than they extract from it. While they may earn better wages, it may come at a high personal cost. A large, longitudinal study of Mexican migrant farmworkers noted that those returning to live in Mexico have a higher prevalence of obesity, smoking, heart disease, and mental health disorders than nonmigrants. Researchers posit that migrant workers discard more traditional nutrition patterns for unhealthy behaviors (e.g., consumption of fast food, overeating), possibly because of their increased income level. Also, the stress of migration (e.g., discrimination, fear) may be associated with increased levels of depression and anxiety. They may also be returning home to Mexico for family support and to seek medical treatment for health problems (Ullmann, Goldman, & Massey, 2011). Researchers surveyed 186 unauthorized and temporary migrant workers returning to Tijuana, Mexico, and found that 71% were uninsured in the United States, but 42% did use some health care services while there. However, approximately 11% did not seek needed medical care (Martinez-Donate et al.,

2014). Others have noted that increased access to "culturally-specific mental health services, especially in rural areas" is needed (Garcia, Gilchrist, Vazquez, Leite, & Raymond, 2011, p. 500).

Whatever your viewpoint on this issue, it is important to the public's health that basic health care services be available to vulnerable populations. Continued efforts must be made to conduct research assessing risks and hazards, especially those of pesticide exposure. Many government publications document the despair and isolation of migrant workers, yet very little has been done to address the living and working environments that contribute to diminished health. Although migrant workers are a mobile population and difficult to study, they represent an important, integral part of our economy; infectious disease among this population increases health risks for all (Flynn, 2012; NCFH, 2012b).

Unique Methods of Health Care Delivery and Primary Prevention

Because migrant health centers do not adequately meet the health needs of the entire migrant community, several innovative methods of health care delivery have been developed and implemented by community health nurses.

Mobile health vans staffed with bilingual community health nurses and lay workers can travel directly to migrant camps and are an effective strategy for outreach health screening and education. By going to migrant camps and delivering care where the clients live and work, especially during nonwork hours such as evenings and weekends, community health nurses increase health access and overcome barriers of culture and lack of child care. Although migrant families receive only fragmented acute care, a nurses' outreach team can succeed in encouraging migrant farmworkers to prevent illness with immunizations, good nutrition, and healthy lifestyles. A viable alternative to traditional medical clinics, the mobile nursing clinic provides primary care to an underserved population through health promotion, disease prevention, and early treatment. In Georgia, a mobile health clinic reported the most common diagnoses as back pain, high blood pressure, and musculoskeletal and GI problems, along with eye and skin problems (Luque et al., 2012).

Mobile dental vans also provide services to migrant worker's children, often with arrangements made through school nurses and dental care provided by dental schools or through partnerships (Luque & Castañeda, 2013). Migrant workers suffer from dental problems at a rate higher than the national average and one California study found that 36% of men had dental caries, 30% had broken or missing teeth, and 18% had gingivitis (Villarejo et al., 2010). Another California survey noted that 36% of male and 29% of female farmworkers reported having dental cavities (Kresge Foundation, 2012). Migrant farmworkers were reported to have low levels of knowledge about oral cancer risk factors and signs/symptoms and to be less likely to seek preventive care (Dodd, Schenck, Chaney, & Padhya, 2016). For migrant children, over 87% of those accessing a mobile dental clinic had untreated caries (Mulligan, Seirawan, Faust, & Habibian, 2010). Migrant preschoolers were found to have overall low-quality diets, with fewer than recommended levels of vegetables, fruits, and whole grains in one study (Quandt et al., 2016).

Promotoras (i.e., lay community outreach workers), or *doulas* (i.e., usually trained childbirth assistants), have promoted health in migrant communities (Lucio et al., 2011). Some programs use *doulas* to provide classes on childbirth and other perinatal subjects in an interactive manner; these provide extensive case management services along with the traditional duties of childbirth coach. Because *doulas* and *promotoras* are generally members of the migrant community, they are readily accepted. Some *promotoras* teach parenting classes to avert child neglect/abuse; others may work with special populations to deter domestic violence or substance abuse or promote breast-feeding (Blanco, 2011). Some deal with interventions and education to control hypertension, and others facilitate early screening and treatment for cancer (Nuno, Martinez, Harris, & Garcia, 2011). One program in a rural area on the United States–Mexico border showed statistically significant improvement in reports of mammograms (two times more likely with the educational intervention from *promotoras*), and there was an even stronger result for those who had not had either mammograms or Pap smears at baseline or within the last year (Nuno et al., 2011). Some *promotoras* migrate with workers and families to provide year-round support and resources. In the United States prior to the Affordable Care Act, many migrants had only limited access to health care (Ingleby, Chiarenza, Deville, & Kotsioni, 2012).

Information Tracking Systems

Mobility impedes continuity of care, and the inadequate system of medical record keeping for the migrant population is particularly frustrating and challenging. Data information systems are vital components for monitoring the health status of individual farmworkers as they migrate. Furthermore, these data are essential for generating research and follow-up care as well as long-range health planning. They also help justify appropriation of monies to migrant health agencies. The MCN has instituted several tracking systems. *TBNet* promotes the completion of TB treatment among migrant populations, and *Diabetes Track II* is geared toward those with diabetes and helps with monitoring and control. *CAN-Track* is a system for coordination of cancer care, and the newest tracking system, *Prenatal Health Network Project*, offers greater continuity for pregnant migrant women. *Heart Fax* is another system of tracking for those with CVD.

Migrant children are susceptible to medical "feast or famine" and may be either over- or undertreated simply because their medical histories are unknown to current providers. One now defunct method for tracking the health status of migrant school-age children was through the Migrant Student Record Transfer System (MSRTS), a computerized system that collected and maintained health and academic records for migrant children. School nurses collected data on migrant children about personal and family history; immunization status; visual, auditory, and dental problems; nutritional status; and general physical condition. The U.S. Department of Education (2014) now offers Migrant Student Information Exchange (MSIX) that permits states to transfer health and educational information on migrant students. However, the ability to track these children in the migratory lifestyle from work location to work location is often inconsistent. Early intervention for migrating children is not always feasible, but it can greatly improve outcomes.

MiVIA ("my way" in Spanish) is putting health records online and making them available to migrant workers and their health care providers. Workers get a photo identification card, and their records can be accessed only by the use of a personal password. They can access their medical files, medications, a medical reference guide (bilingual), and other resources, such as local clinics and doctors, public transportation, and housing online, no matter their location (Hou, 2010; MiVIA, 2013). The program began in California's wine country but is spreading to more distant locations.

THE ROLE OF COMMUNITY HEALTH NURSES IN CARING FOR A MOBILE WORKFORCE

Beyond barriers to health care, such as lack of health services, language, and cultural impediments, inadequate to nonexistent transportation, financial strains, under-insurance, and questionable residency status, which are by themselves formidable obstacles, the migrant lifestyle is fraught with challenges. Because of the insecurity and instability inherent in a mobile lifestyle, long-term health goals are difficult to establish and long-term follow-up of any chronic illness is doubtful. Nonetheless, PHNs provide much-needed services using community resources, innovative thinking, tenacity, and sensitivity.

Strategies for improving the health status and resource use of migrant workers and their families include:

- Improving existing services
- Advocating and networking
- Practicing cultural sensitivity
- Using lay personnel for community outreach
- Utilizing unique methods of health care delivery
- Employing information tracking systems

Community health nurses are the major providers of migrant health services and have a crucial role in the development and management of interventions. In response to the growing need for available, accessible, and affordable health care for farmworker families, nurses are called on not only to understand the migrant lifestyle but also to help migrant families overcome the barriers to health care (see Perspectives: Voices From the Community).

An aggregate at risk, migrant workers suffer higher frequency of illness, more complications, and more long-term debilitating effects. Exacerbated by a magnitude of environmental and work stressors, the health of migrant families is also compromised by limited access to health care, mobility, language and cultural barriers, low educational levels, and few economic and political resources. Because migrant health needs are largely manageable within community settings, community health nurses are ideal health providers. Implementing health education at migrant camps, training lay health workers, and

providing clinic hours to accommodate late workdays are successful interventions. Learning the language of the migrant workers and their unique cultures is also helpful in reaching this population. PHNs must advocate for the health of migrant workers, who have very little economic or political power, and also guide them through the complexities of a changing health care system.

In the past, male migrant workers traveled primarily in organized crews; now, they may travel in family units with women and children. Added attention must be given to family members exposed to the hazards of the migrant lifestyle. Even as many migrant workers settle into communities, the cycle of poverty continues as other workers arrive from impoverished countries. With a paucity of health resources, the PHN is sometimes the only health provider who can and will care for this population.

Providing care for migrant workers presents a challenge, requiring nurses to be innovative and to go beyond the boundaries of traditional health services (see Using the Nursing Process). Although many resources and programs exist to help migrant families, the needs are still overwhelming. By aligning with the goals of *Healthy People 2020* to improve the health of one of the most underserved populations, the community health nurse will also be improving the health of the nation as a whole.

COMMUNITY HEALTH NURSING IN RURAL AREAS

The Health Resources and Services Administration (HRSA) completed the last national public health workforce study in 2012, and no PHN to population ratio was reported. However, local public health workforce data for three states were collected: Georgia, New Mexico, and New York. Urban public health worker ratios were respectively reported at 41, 16, and 30 per 100,000 people. Rural public health worker ratios were 216, 111, and 96, respectively (HRSA, 2013). It is difficult to estimate the total number of PHNs and to provide accurate estimates of those working in rural areas (Washington State Nurses Association, 2011). PHNs, though, make up 12% to 20% of the public health workforce, second only to administrative/clerical personnel at 18% to 23% (HRSA, 2013). No average age was provided; however, the average age of PHNs was reported at 46.6 years in 2005. Most rural nurses working in the community are thought to have little education in public health, as the associate degree in nursing is often accepted by health departments in rural areas (Knudsen & Meit, n.d.). Working urban nurses with a BSN numbered 51%, whereas only 36% of those working in rural areas had a baccalaureate degree, in the most recent comparison study (Rural Health Research Center, 2007). However, rural areas promote a broad scope of PHN practice, as these nurses deal with a wide variety of issues—immunizations, home health, school nursing, maternal–child health, emergency preparedness, as well as communicable disease/epidemiology. While no differences were found in regard to education level, overall perception of competency was associated with years of professional practice experience in one seminal study of rural and frontier PHNs (Bigbee, Otterness, & Gehrke, 2010). Highest levels of competency were reported in

"I spoke with one of my students after clinical last week, and she told me about her work this semester with a 35-year-old single mother of two who had been discharged from the hospital following a lupus flare-up. The student felt that her client was a devoted mother, but she let her 8- and 12-year-old children stay home from school to help with family farm tasks in order to make ends meet. After weekly visits with her client for almost 2 months, she told me—I was finally able to get her to trust me enough to help her trust others. She has reached out to her neighbors and asked for help and they are more than willing to lend a hand. Now, her children can return to school and go back to being children instead of day laborers! I told her that sometimes, it takes a strong person to reach out for help and that she is a strong woman!

—Kevin, Nursing Faculty Member, faith-based college, Western Massachusetts

I was having a conversation with students about how to "break the ice" when making home visits to families who have never had home health services. One student mentioned that at the beginning of the semester, she was afraid that her shyness would be her downfall. But in the week that followed, it occurred to her that the best way to establish trust with anyone is to express an interest in answering questions they have before you pose your own. The student now makes it a habit to ask every patient the three things they would like her to know about them that will help her to personalize their care. During week 8 of the clinical semester, the student stated—This was a real "icebreaker" and my patients have been much more open to listening and learning from me once I listen and learn about them!

—Betsy, Community Health Nursing Instructor, Northern California School of Nursing

"First of all, a nurse should expect the unexpected. Because of the migratory way of life…clients do not always know where they will be next week or next month. Therefore, we must understand that they do not always have their medical records, immunization records, or income records. Hours are very irregular, depending on what time the workers get in from the fields and what time the shifts are. Because of the distances we travel, we work anywhere from 8 to 12 hours a day. The most rewarding part of the job is bringing health services to the underserved and uninsured. The people are so gracious and appreciative of whatever services we provide."

—J. S., RN, Michigan

"Since farmworkers come to our area for only 4 months of the year, it is rare that I care for a migrant woman through her entire pregnancy. I may diagnose her pregnancy, I may see her for three or four prenatal visits, or I may meet her only once before she goes into labor and delivers her baby. I struggle with the desire to make a difference in a short period of time and with the disappointment of not being able to follow through."

—C. K., CNM, RN, Pennsylvania

"Be warm and interested in the whole family. If you do not speak Spanish or Creole, work with translators who understand how you work. Use translators as…vehicles to get the information out and in. Eye contact and touch are crucial. Learning to be clinically relevant as well as competently utilizing a translator is an art and takes time and experience to hone. Learning some phrases or some of the most frequently asked questions in the language of the farmworker should be encouraged. Even the attempt to speak the patients' language will build trust and confidence. These harvesters of the nation's food are very bright and resourceful people who travel great distances and undergo severe deprivation in order to work. The nobility of this pursuit is getting short shrift in the press and legislative bodies today, but the sheer enormity of the service [that] this group of oppressed people do for the rest of us needs to be acknowledged and honored by the clinicians who will provide primary health care to them and theirs."

—W. H., RN, Michigan

"I worked as a Head Start nurse for many years in an agricultural area of California. One of my assignments was a state/county migrant farm labor housing project. I was asked to make a home visit to check on a 4-year-old who hadn't come to preschool in a few days. When I arrived at the family's duplex, I found the sixth grader there, caring for all five of her younger siblings, including the 4-year-old and an 8-month-old baby. When I asked why she was home with all of the children, she guardedly informed me (after some coaxing) that her parents had been picked up in a raid at the tree farm where they worked and had been taken back to Mexico. The children were now alone, with no family nearby. I worked with a nun at Catholic Social Services to provide care for the children until the parents returned to the United States so that the children, who were all U.S. citizens, would not be placed in foster care. The parents had not been allowed to contact their children before being placed on the bus to Mexico, but other workers, who were not undocumented, had seen them go and told the children about their plight. It was heartbreaking to see the fear in their eyes. I quickly went to work looking for resources for them. A nun from Catholic Social Services stayed with the children until the parents returned and helped them with food."

—Holly, Head Start Nurse, California

"I'm dealing right now with Hispanic women, migrant workers, who do not have any access to prenatal care, none whatsoever. What I'm doing is creative financing, a lot of begging, a lot of pleading, a lot of being nice to people I don't even want to be nice to because it means that much to me for them to get help. So I find myself in situations that are sometimes uncomfortable, but nonetheless, I do it because I feel that as a nurse that's my job. Having been a farmworker myself, I would want someone to do that for my mother, and they did."

—Unidentified female nurse, Idaho Falls, Idaho

"I was appalled and dismayed by the comments of one of my students on the course discussion board. When discussing at-risk populations in urban and rural centers, the point was made that a diagnosis of HIV often imposed an additional barrier for residents who were trying to get themselves and their loved ones out of poverty and into safer and healthier living situations. One student responded that the diagnosis was a result of—'irresponsible choices and these patients need to own their own behaviors.' This spurred further discussion about the need for all health care professionals to self-reflect on a regular basis to assess for the presence of prejudices and biases that may impact our care. Although these were difficult discussions, I believe that this student was able to turn an incidence of bias into an exemplar of a teachable moment."

—Maggie, novice PHN faculty member from a large state university in the Southwest

USING THE NURSING PROCESS WHEN WORKING WITH MIGRANT FAMILIES

Background Data and Assessment

Tom Reynolds is a community health nurse in central Montana. He has three migrant camps in his service area that are homes for primarily Mexican residents. The men primarily work in strenuous construction jobs–masonry, landscaping, and in agriculture, cherry orchards, dairy farm, and ranches. The women work as housekeeping staff in private homes, motels, and hotels in the area. One evening, he made it a point to stop by one of the camps that he could catch up with residents and assess any health concerns that need to be addressed. At the end of a three-week period, Tom had made a conscious effort to meet with the residents in each of the three camps. The feedback from these informal conversations assisted Tom in the formulation and implementation of a nursing plan of care targeting the health promotion needs of this unique population of residents.

Nursing Diagnoses

1. Alteration in family health status secondary to language, transportation barriers, and health literacy barriers.
2. Fear related to risks of deportation and separation from family members.
3. At risk for occupational and situational injury, illness, and stress because of extended work hours and poverty-level living conditions.

Plan and Implementation

Tom researched funding options for a demonstration project that was sponsored by the LHD. The Director of the Health Department agreed to support the project for 6 months if Tom could find matching funds for the project from a local foundation, recruit the personnel he needed, and the results were positive.

Tom was able to recruit three other community health nurses, one of whom was bilingual and familiar with the cultural values and practices of the migrant workers. In addition, Tom reached out to the university's undergraduate nursing program and the community health instructor agreed to utilize the three camps as clinical sites for the upcoming semester. The nurses, students, and staff social worker from the public health department coordinated weekly evening and weekend visits to each of the three camps. The teams completed a family assessment for each family: established a health record, completed a community-based assessment for each of the three camps, administered immunizations, assisted with arranging transportation to and from medical appointments, and enrolled families in the Women, Infants, and Children Supplemental Food Program (WIC). In addition, the teams completed short teaching sessions on topics such as oral care, hand hygiene, family planning, and infant safety.

The students were inspired by Tom's energy and they asked to utilize this experience to develop their Capstone Projects that centered on meeting an unmet need of the unique group of residents. The local farmworkers heard about all of the activities at the camp and they began to organize food and clothing drives to assist the residents in meeting the challenges of the warm Montana summers and very snowy winters.

Evaluation

The evaluation of the interventions was so positive that the program became a permanent service of the health department. In the months that followed, a NP was added to the team and a volunteer dentist who provided on-site oral care and evaluations. With optimal health and a decrease in issues related to health disparities, several families were able to leave the camps and establish a permanent home in the local community.

---

the areas of culture, communication, and leadership/systems, whereas lower levels of competency were noted for basic public health, finances, policy/program planning, and analytic assessment in another classic study of PHN rural and frontier one-nurse offices (Bigbee, Gehrke, & Otterness, 2009). Rural health departments are often lacking in technological and communication systems, but there is an even greater need for reliable communication capability and training opportunities for rural PHNs who provide the majority of care in rural and frontier communities (Knudsen & Meit, n.d.). Place, MacLeod, John, Adamack, and Lindsey (2011) found that a Rural Nursing Certificate Program was well received despite technological and distance obstacles. Advanced nursing degrees are also offered through the use of distance technologies, making them more accessible to rural nurses (Rutledge, Haney, Bordelon, Renaud, & Fowler, 2014).

Working in a Rural Community

Rural community health nurses most often grew up in rural areas or lived for a time in small communities. They frequently have extended family there. Rural PHNs

are active members of their community and are highly respected professionals. The need for registered nurses in rural areas is rated at approximately 74% nationally. In addition, rural areas demonstrate a significant shortage of health care professionals including physicians, nurses, physical therapists, occupational therapists, and pharmacists (MacDowell et al., 2013).

The rural community health nurse plays many roles:

1. *Advocate*: Assists rural clients, families, and populations in obtaining the best possible care
2. *Coordinator/case manager*: Connects rural clients with needed health and social services, often assisting with information on transportation
3. *Health teacher*: Provides education to individuals, families, or groups on health promotion or other health-related topics (e.g., prepared childbirth, parenting, diabetes maintenance, home safety)
4. *Referral agent*: Makes appropriate connections between rural clients and urban service providers
5. *Mentor*: Guides new community health nurses, nursing students, and other nurses new to the rural community

6. *Change agent/researcher*: Suggests new approaches to solving patient care or community health problems based on research, professional literature, and community assessment

7. *Collaborator*: Seeks ways to work with other health and social service professionals to maximize outcomes for individual clients and the community at large

8. *Activist*: With a deep understanding of the community and its population, takes appropriate risks to improve the community's health

See From the Case Files III for a day in the life of a rural PHN.

Rural PHNs have the opportunity to use autonomy in daily practice. Nurses must rapidly assume independent and interdependent decision-making roles because of the small workforce and large workload. For nurses who live and work in rural areas, resources are limited and demands are many. These health care professionals are highly visible, stating "As a nurse, you are kind of in a fishbowl....people know who the nurses are and you will be approached in various places for advice and information" (Zibrik, MacLeod, & Zimmer, 2010, p. 25). This visibility in the rural community can make confidentiality a preservation of client anonymity challenging. The role of the PHN is similar to being "a specialist in general nursing" (Zibrik et al., 2010). Rural PHNs

learn to prioritize tasks quickly and work efficiently with others to get the job done. Referrals to other rural providers are facilitated because providers frequently know one another. The rural community health nurse has an advantage over urban nurses in that the rural health care system is smaller and easier to influence and change, but specialization is seldom possible and long-distance travel is generally a necessity (Cant, Birks, Porter, Jacob, & Cooper, 2011).

Rural PHNs may experience the challenge of physical isolation from personal and professional opportunities associated with urban areas. Rural nurses may also feel isolated in their clinical practices because of the scarcity of professional colleagues. See From the Case Files IV for examples from nurses working in frontier areas.

The rural community health nurse often receives a salary that is lower than that of urban nurses in comparable positions (Knudsen & Meit, n.d.). However, there are benefits to rural nursing. Housing costs are usually lower than in larger cities, and long commutes to and from work on congested highways are often avoided, although rural driving can be hazardous. As a place to live and raise a family, rural communities offer a slower pace of life, open spaces, and friendly atmosphere. The smaller system of health care in a rural community can be advantageous to the PHN. It may be easier to understand the system and initiate planned change. There are many

---

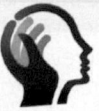 *From the* **Case Files** **III**

A Day in the Life of a Rural PHN

Lisa S. arrives at Sampson County Public Health Department in rural North Carolina. She reviews the seven case files of the patients and families that have been assigned to her caseload for the day and begins her work. Prior to leaving the office, she contacts the Director of the Senior Center to confirm that she will be able to speak at the Alzheimer's and Dementia Caregiver Support Group next week about safety proofing home settings when a loved one has a progressive dementing illness (*health promotion/primary prevention educator*). Then, she calls the family of a hospitalized patient (*care coordinator/case manager*) to assist in the coordination of the discharge of their family member. At 11:00, Lisa makes a home visit to the O'Brien family. Mr. O'Brien explains that he does not understand the process of applying for Meals on Wheels and he can't get anyone at any agency to call him back. Lisa gives Mr. O'Brien an informational handout with telephone numbers, addresses, and Web site information so that he or his daughter can contact the appropriate agency (*referral agent*) and even calls her friend from church who works at the office to let him know that the family may need some special attention to navigate the process (*advocate*). At lunch, Lisa runs into the physical therapist

and they discuss concerns about the hospitalized individual with whom Lisa spoke with earlier in the day (*collaborator*). Both question whether the family will be able to manage the care needed for the patient with only minimal outside support. After lunch, Lisa returns to her office for a staff meeting and discusses an update to the electronic medical record (EMR) (*change agent/researcher*) that she is recommending for implementation by all disciplines within the department. At the same meeting, she agrees to work with a graduate public health nursing student during his rural practicum (*mentor*). That evening, as a concerned member of the local community, Lisa participates in a meeting at the town hall about issues related to the growing numbers of opioid overdoses within the local community. She addresses the group, giving them data and expresses concern (*activist*), then volunteers to lead a task force that will examine the issue and propose a plan for a "Prescription Give-Back Day" that would allow residents to turn in old/unused prescriptions at the health department offices. It is quite apparent that PHNs working in rural settings take on many roles during the course of a typical workday. As a nursing student working in a rural community, you may have the opportunity to "try on" many of these roles and demonstrate your creativity, compassion, and skills.

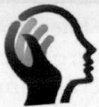

From the Case Files IV

Frontier Nursing, Then and Now

As described in Chapter 2, Mary Breckinridge founded the Frontier Nursing Service in 1925, with nurse–midwives providing care to clients in their own homes. Nurses traveled by horseback and on foot into the sparsely populated hollows of Kentucky (Stone, 2011). Today, NPs working in nurse-managed clinics in rural Appalachian communities in Virginia were interviewed about their practices, in a classic study by Caldwell (2007), and spoke about their connections to the people and communities they serve. One said, "Here you get to know the whole family and that is rewarding…you know what is important to them… what their worries and concerns are….so you probably get closer to your patient in this area than you might outside here. It becomes an extended family, which is very rewarding" (p. 76).

Another NP described a man with severe COPD who visited her clinic. He was also a patient of another area provider, but when the NP examined the man, she noticed the gauze 4 × 4 he had on the back of his neck and inquired about it. The man said he "cut himself shaving." The NP pressed the man to see the wound and found that he had "cancer with the bone exposed," describing it as "the most awful thing that I had ever seen in my life. I could put my fist in there. And you could see his carotids pulsating." She told the patient how serious this was

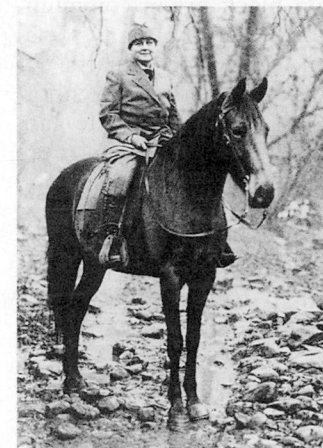
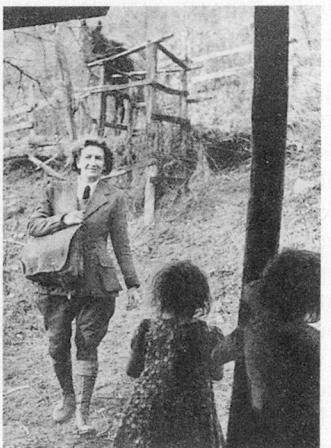

and arranged for a plastic surgeon to see him right away. He had a total neck resection and recovered completely. She reflected, "What if I had accepted his story about the sore and it being all right? It was not what he was coming to see me for…I look at more than just the chief complaint" (p. 77).

For these nurses, isolation was considered a positive aspect of their professional practice. It encouraged connection and caring relationships with their patients (Stone, 2011).

---

possibilities to enhance rural nursing practice, including continuing education through distance learning or at satellite campuses, partnerships with larger medical centers, and invitations to clinical experts to provide on-site workshops (Place et al., 2011). Grants can be written to facilitate these endeavors, and private sponsors may be approached to provide assistance. Given a smaller, more manageable community, it may be easier for PHNs to organize collaborations between private and public agencies, as well as key stakeholders within the community; collaboration is a cornerstone of public health nursing in any setting (Keller, Stroschein, & Schaffer, 2011).

However, many rural areas find it difficult to recruit nurses and need to more effectively advertise their benefits (Prengaman, Bigbee, Baker, & Schmitz, 2014). When RN to population ratios are high in both rural and urban areas, years of potential life lost and rates of poor health are significantly improved, as well as rates of teen births and mammography; however, this association was shown to improve even more as the level of rurality increased demonstrating the importance of adequate nurse staffing in all areas (Fields, Bigbee, & Bell, in press).

URBAN HEALTH

Urban health considers those characteristics of the environment as they relate to the health of the population living within large cities. According to Vlahov, Boufford,

Pearson, and Norris (2010), the factors responsible for the health of urban residents reflect three broad themes: the physical environment, the social environment, and access to health and social services. As opposed to rural areas, there may be less of a feeling of community connectedness in urban life, along with lower overall levels of trust and weaker family and community ties. Connectedness has been shown to be a protective factor, especially for adolescent risk behaviors. Inner-city neighborhoods are often observed to have "high unemployment levels, lack of educational and jobs skills, broken families, alcohol and drug abuse, and low incomes conducive to the growth of street gangs and their culture of violence" (Vlahov et al., 2010, p. 195). Community involvement and social networks, often deficient in densely populated areas, are components of social capital (discussed in Chapter 25), and community participation, social trust, and sense of belonging were significantly associated with positive health outcomes, such as mental and physical health (Ryff et al., 2015). Population turnover, racial/ethnic diversity, and poverty in urban cities are thought to contribute to the "lowered ability of individuals and communities to control crime, vandalism, and violence" (de Snyder, Friel, Fotso, & Khadr, 2011, p. 1183). Urban communities may be marked by negative social support, such as that found associated with drugs and gangs. Moreover, the social exclusion stems from the high concentration of poverty in central cities as well as high stress levels from violence and social isolation (Vlahov et al., 2010). Urban communities are made up of multiethnic and diverse racial communities, and these groups are often socially and economically separate from what one might believe to be mainstream urban communities. Poverty, especially within black urban communities, has remained stable over time despite many social programs to address poverty and jobs; recent analysis of the socioeconomic quality of racial and ethnic neighborhoods found some narrowing of this black–white gap, as more whites live in poorer neighborhood and more blacks live in neighborhood with less poverty (Firebaugh & Farrell, 2016; Lewis et al., 2013). Urban areas have been associated with *food deserts*, or areas with few or only small stores, and food insecurity has been found in urban families spending more than 30% of their income on private, rather than public, housing (Kirkpatrick & Tarasuk, 2011; Walker, Block, & Kawachi, 2012). Both housing and food are more expensive in large cities. Hodson (2016) notes that we are currently experiencing the largest urban growth period in history, with over half of the world's population living in cities. Even more growth is expected; thus, it is important to examine the health of urban dwellers.

In 2000, the Johns Hopkins University founded the Urban Health Institute as a means to bolster support among an inner-city population. This interface between the university and the Baltimore community was created to improve the health and well-being of the residents of East Baltimore (Johns Hopkins University, 2016). Its mission is to promote evidenced-based interventions to solve local as well as national, health problems encountered in urban America. The New York Academy of Medicine (2016) has organized the Institute of Urban Health to promote research that improves the health and well-being of urban populations and decreases health disparities by studying the social, biologic, and environmental influences on health. The academy sponsors the *Journal of Urban Health,* a publication that focuses on population-based research with low-income, disadvantaged populations living in urban areas. But how did the health of these urban communities evolve to such a state that targeted efforts are now required? It began in the 1800s.

History of Urban Health Care Issues

Urban living has a long and checkered history in the United States. Arriving immigrants increased population density, especially in the large Eastern and Midwestern cities. Millions of immigrants arrived in the United States between the mid-1800s and the early 1900s. Because most had some family or distant relatives who had arrived here earlier, they made their ways to where these people lived, hoping to receive temporary shelter while they sought work (Dolkart, 2008). Many came with large families and roomed with other large European and Eastern European families in tenements. Others came alone or as a nuclear family without close ties to others already living here. Nonetheless, they gathered in **ghettos**, thickly populated sections of cities inhabited predominantly by members of the same minority group. This enabled them to be with people from their homeland—people who knew the same language and the same ways (Bial, 2002). The 1893 World's Columbian Exposition in Chicago introduced the "city beautiful" concept of replacing crumbling urban cities and tenements with more classical buildings and parks/lakes to address the crime and social problems of the day (Pain, 2016).

As time went on, many families left ghetto communities and found housing in smaller towns or in the beginnings of suburbs. As described in the classic work by Minetor (2010), the Irish left New York City in the early 20th century; then Blacks, coming from the South, moved in. Many Black families later left for outlying suburban areas, and Puerto Rican families moved in. Today, Haitian and Middle Eastern families inhabit some of the same neighborhoods. After 100 years, many of the same buildings continue to provide less than optimal shelter for a new group of immigrants. Although ghetto living provides a sense of belonging, for many, it is temporary because it engenders more negatives than positives. Children and grandchildren of the original immigrants seek different lives for themselves, away from the urban areas that are often riddled with crime, unsafe housing, and disease. Others, because of poverty, drugs, or fear of being homeless, remain in urban slum areas.

In a classic position paper, the American College of Physicians used the term **urban health penalty** to describe the "concentration of economic decline, job loss, and major health problems" afflicting inner-city populations experiencing health problems when healthier and wealthier residents moved to the suburbs, leaving poverty zones of economic and physical deterioration that act as determinants of health (1997, p. 485). As discussed earlier, that health penalty is now more prevalent in rural areas. An urban health penalty has historically been associated with large cities because of economic inequalities that often prevented subpopulations of poor from having the basic quality of life found in mainstream society (Vlahov et al., 2010). These unhealthy environments were thought to lead to inequality in health. However, more careful statistical analysis of population size and the death counts of four major diseases found both an urban health penalty when looking at total counties and an urban health advantage when examining subgroups, noting that there is a tipping point that must be considered (Choi, Lee, & Chang, 2015).

Who has been responsible for addressing the needs of these communities over the last hundred or more years? Who has been, or should have been, addressing the needs evolving among the urban communities? Two connected disciplines, urban planning and public health, have addressed these issues from the 19th century to the present. **Urban planning** worked to improve the welfare of individuals and communities by creating more healthful, efficient, attractive, and equitable places. The activities of urban planners often include addressing the community's needs related to diversification of the transportation system, housing, reducing air pollution and greenhouse gases, street network design, and built environment site design; in some large cities, these tasks are handled by separate departments that do not often interface with environmental or public health (Nieuwenhuijsen, 2016).

Public health, of course, is directed at improving human well-being through assessing and ensuring the delivery of services at the community level. Together, these disciplines both addressed the needs of the identified vulnerable populations. Initially, during the late 19th and early 20th centuries, these two systems were linked in promoting health by facilitating physical activity through the creation of green space. They also designed cities to be less vulnerable to contagions (Owens, 2016). They joined together in preventing infectious diseases by ensuring healthful drinking water and sewage systems. They also protected the community from exposure to hazardous substances related to industry by monitoring land uses and instituting zoning ordinances (Boarnet & Takahashi, 2011). During the middle of the 20th century, the focus of planning and public health agencies drifted apart, partly because of their successes in limiting injury and health risk caused by inappropriate mixing of land use. The target of public health agencies shifted from investigating ways to improve the infrastructure to a focus on germ theories and immunizations, challenges that were easier for physicians to address than changing environments. On the other hand, urban planning switched its energy to aiding economic development with large transportation and infrastructure (Viel, Hägi, Upegui, & Laurian, 2011). At about the same time, Rachel Carson's book *Silent Spring*, published in 1962, described the effects of pesticides on wildlife and the eventual effects on human health, thus initiating the *environmental justice movement* and focusing environmental health professionals largely on toxic chemical exposures. See Chapter 9.

According to Boarnet and Takahashi (2011), the disciplines of urban planning and public health are collaborating once again, working together to improve transportation and air quality and addressing national health issues such as injury prevention, physical activity, health care access, energy use, and greenhouse gas emissions, along with disaster preparation and response. A Canadian example brought agencies together, led by a land use/transportation consultant, to build a sustaining and collaborative relationship between agencies and local government and to prioritize land use and transportation planning while keeping in mind the built environment in order to better align with population health goals (Miro et al., 2014). This team effort is a natural partnership when addressing such concerns as physical activity and the provision of safe and accessible spaces, for instance. Several studies demonstrated a positive association between the built environment and physical activity. Land use mix, "connectivity," population density, and neighborhood design were also determinants of physical activity (McCormack & Shiell, 2011). These factors are significant in reaching the *Healthy People 2020* objectives directed at the prevention of chronic disease, injury prevention, and health promotion. Leaders at the CDC are concerned with factors that affect people and their environments and support efforts that address the improvement of both physical and social environments as related to places to live, work, and play. The CDC's *Healthy Places* describes the components involved: interaction between environment and health, poorly planned growth leading to sprawl and increased used of vehicles,

and healthy community design that promotes health and well-being (2016).

The World Health Organization's Healthy Cities movement emphasizes health in planning and policy development. It encompasses economic and urban development and considers health inequality and urban poverty, as well as the vulnerable populations living in urban areas (World Health Organization, 2012) (see Chapter 1 for more on Healthy Cities). Health care reform also offers opportunities to address urban health issues, especially related to health care access. Policy development to address the unique challenges of urban areas is part of public health advocacy for urban PHNs and other public health officials. And the move toward quality health care in the public health system will positively affect the health of all populations, including urban residents (Honoré et al., 2011).

Urban communities must be given the opportunity to participate, particularly in activities that focus on change at the community and systems levels of prevention and public health practice. An example is the building of coalitions among key neighborhood stakeholders and agencies, as well as the individuals and families residing in those neighborhoods. Tapping into already existing neighborhood networks can facilitate health promotion efforts through capacity building and common goals that develop through collaborative partnerships. Such interventions reflect many of the key public health nursing interventions, as demonstrated in Chapter 14 through the use of the Minnesota Wheel and other models.

The *Healthy People 2020* document addresses societal determinants of health that include both physical and social environments. Notwithstanding the complexity of urban areas, particularly in large metropolitan cities, health promotion efforts and a focus on healthier environments are key components of this national health effort. Reduction of inequalities in the physical environment (e.g., transportation, parks, healthy food access) and the social environment (e.g., crime) can lead to improvement in key health indicators and aid in meeting the goals and objectives of *Healthy People 2020* (Secretary's Advisory Committee on Health Promotion and Disease Prevention Objectives for 2020, 2016). Urban development, transportation, housing, education, and agriculture must be addressed, as well as health promotion and disease prevention, in order to affect substantive change. Research and data collection are important to guide our progress.

Emerging Issues in Access to Health Services

Access to health care in the United States is regarded as "unreliable" because many people do not receive the appropriate and timely care they need. The U.S. health care system, which was already overwhelmed, has faced an even greater influx of patients because health care reform was fully implemented in 2014; this was when 32 million Americans obtained health insurance for the first time (U.S. Department of Health & Human Services [USDHHS], 2016a). Health care issues that should be monitored over the next decade include (1) increasing and measuring access to appropriate, safe, and effective care, including clinical preventive services; (2) decreasing disparities and measuring access to health care for diverse populations, including racial and ethnic minorities and older adults; and (3) increasing and measuring access to safe long-term and palliative care services and access to quality emergency care (USDHHS, 2016a).

Urban Populations and Health Disparities

The majority of the world's populace now lives in cities, which is a change from long-held rural dominance. Along with urban living, other global challenges including economic globalization, climate change, financial difficulties, food and energy insecurities, armed conflicts, and changing patterns of diseases (Friel et al., 2011a). The greatest growth of large cities around the world is among less-wealthy nations, where urban slums are developing at a rapid rate (Ieri, 2015; Vlahov et al., 2010). Depending upon the classification used, more than one third of the U.S. population lives in central cities. This is the highest number since 1950 (Mather, Pollard, & Jacobsen, 2012). However, suburbs of metropolitan areas had the fastest growth, especially in the West and the South; over half of the populace lives in *suburban areas*. More than 84% of the U.S. population lives in what are characterized as central-city or metropolitan areas (Mather et al., 2012).

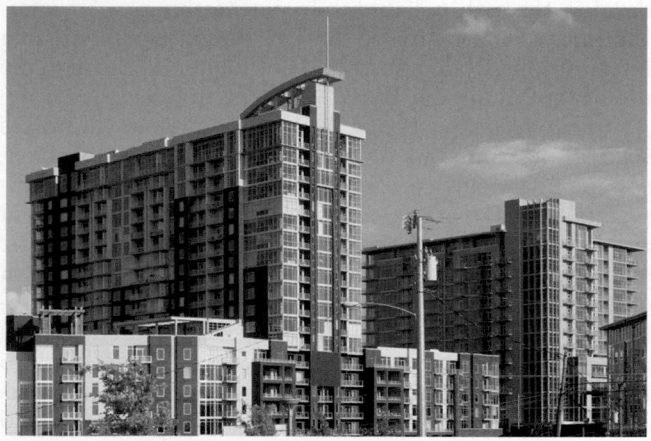

An example of urban housing.

Although some metropolitan areas have recorded substantial population losses in central-city areas (e.g., Pine Bluff, AR, at 5.53%; Farmington, NM, at 4.81%; and Johnstown, PA, 4.14%), others exhibited substantial population growth (The Villages, FL, at 22.4%; Midland, TX, at 13.85%; Austin, TX, at 13.23%; and Odessa, TX, at 12.23%) between 2010 and 2014 (Demographia, 2012; Wikipedia, 2016).

One example of how changes in population can adversely affect large cities can be found in Detroit, Michigan. Between the 2000 and 2010 censuses, the population dropped 25% (or 237,500 people) to the lowest level since 1910. This is a lower proportion than the 29% population loss experienced by New Orleans because of Hurricane Katrina. However, the total number of people was much less in New Orleans (only 140,000). The dramatic losses in Detroit pulled down the numbers for the state of Michigan, and it was the only U.S. state to show

a net population loss. Auto and other industrial losses, combined with large numbers of home foreclosures, are thought to be at the root of the problem. Population loss leads to a smaller tax base and a greater proportion of poor residents, yet the city had the same maintenance expenses for sewers, water lines, and streets (Seelye, 2011). With the loss of jobs, many people moved to the suburbs, and unemployment and welfare rates increased in Detroit. The poverty rate jumped from 10.4% in 2000 to 17% in 2010 (Davis, 2012).

Historically, movement to the suburbs began with the housing boom and highway expansion occurring after WWII. People moved from large cities to more suburban areas, and shopping malls and schools followed. Cars became even more essential, because public transportation did not always extend into suburban areas thereby leading to long commute times and traffic congestion. Although not all suburban areas have remained attractive and vital, an income gap persists between city and suburban residents. Poverty is two times greater in large central cities than in corresponding suburban areas (18.8% vs. 9.4%), but in total population, there were 1 million more suburban poor in 2005. By 2012, 59 of the top 95 metropolitan areas in the United States found the majority of their region's poor located in the suburbs. In addition, this demonstrated an increase in 93 of 95 metropolitan areas between 2000 and 2012 (Kneebone, 2014). This is indicative of a "suburbanization of poverty" (p. 12). Poverty rates were highest in metropolitan areas in the Midwest and South, and almost half of all large cities had significant increases in poverty rates. Only about one third of suburban areas recorded poverty rate increases.

Today, the declining urban situation is not confined to a few large cities. To achieve the vision of creating "social and physical environments that promote good health for all" as an overarching goal of the *Healthy People 2020* document, more must be done to promote health and prevent disease in urban areas (USDHHS, 2016b, para. 5). The primary reason for health disparities, as mentioned in Chapter 25, is the disproportionate burden of certain health and social problems among different populations—in this instance, urban areas. Environmental exposure to air pollution contributes to illness and mortality including heart disease, cancer, and respiratory diseases. Consumer products (e.g., fast food, alcohol, tobacco) are more readily available in urban and low-income areas and have been shown to be significant health risks that contribute to health disparities (Freudenberg, & Olden, 2011). Other environmental issues, such as extreme heat events where temperatures rise and lead to climate-related deaths, may amplify public health stressors and primarily affect vulnerable populations. When examining urban form and its relationship to this weather phenomenon, Stone, Hess, and Frumkin (2010) found an increase in annual extreme heat events between 1956 and 2005, with more than twice the number of events in sprawling metropolitan areas when compared with compact metro regions; urban planners are urged to consider construction limits in order to help with thermal regulation (Wu & Lung, 2016). Urban cities are often heat islands because of fewer green spaces and a larger proportion of asphalt. Extreme heat events not only lead to increased ED visits for heat-related illness, they can lead to increased hospitalizations for those with asthma and other chronic conditions, as well as death for elderly and other vulnerable populations (Matte et al., 2016; Soneja et al., 2016; Winquist, Grundstein, Chang, Hess, & Sarnat, 2016). Cities provide interventions such as extreme heat warnings and cooling centers, but not all residents avail themselves of these services (Hess, McCowell, Luber, 2012). Canadian researchers (Bélanger et al., 2016) interviewed almost 3,500 people in 1,647 buildings in disadvantaged areas across nine of the largest cities to determine their perception of adverse health effects of urban heat. Those with negative health impacts relied more on adaptation methods (e.g., eating iced foods, visiting air conditioned places, taking showers to cool down, turning off appliances), indicating that these measures were more reactive in nature. As with rural areas, the built environment greatly impacts urban neighborhoods.

Friel et al. (2011a, p. 861) show that "social patterning in health outcomes within and between cities," suggesting that urban physical environments, social environments, and living conditions are causing health changes. Urban health equity depends on political empowerment of the people to strongly represent their interests and needs in order to challenge unfair distribution of resources. Further, with most of the world living within the built environment, this poses a major opportunity to improve urban health and equity (APHA, n.d.b; Friel et al., 2011a). Poor social conditions and health inequalities have been recognized in urban areas around the world. Urban slums in low- and some middle-income countries provide social exclusion for many living in poverty and threaten development (de Snyder et al., 2011). In this country, overcrowding and poor-quality housing have been found to have a direct relationship with poor mental health, developmental delay, and even to shorter stature (Vlahov et al., 2010). Inadequate urban housing and neighborhood disorder are related to poor-quality sleep among Latino adults (Chambers, Pichardo, & Rosenbaum, 2016). Prenatal exposure to particulate matter (diesel fuel, perchloroethylene) has been shown to affect math scores when the children reach third grade; researchers suggest "individual pollutants may additively impact health" (Stingone, McVeigh, & Claudio, 2016, p. 144). Urban housing and neighborhoods have been linked to childhood asthma morbidity. Indoor area pollutants (e.g., nitrogen dioxide, particulate matter) have been associated with asthma symptoms in children, and reduction of indoor allergens and pollutants has shown improvements in asthma symptoms (Matsui, 2014). Adamkiewicz et al. (2014) demonstrated that urban indoor environments in multifamily housing units were very common; over 50% of those tested had 3 or more exposures to problems such as pests, mold, ventilation, or combustion and noted that cumulative exposure could be linked to poor health.

In addition to concerns about housing, hazardous waste landfill sites are often located in or near urban areas. Air pollution and noise exposure, often associated with large inner cities, have been linked to asthma, cardiovascular death, hypertension, ischemic heart disease, and hearing impairment (Vlahov et al., 2010). Also, Ard (2015) examined industrial air toxins over a 9-year period and found that African Americans were consistently exposed more often than Whites and Hispanics even though air toxins decreased overall during that time; income level was not a protective factor for them. In Flint, Michigan, following pollution of their water system, soil lead data show higher lead values in the metropolitan city center, and seasonal blood lead variations indicate that resuspension of lead dust may be to blame (Laidlaw et al., 2016). See Chapter 9 for more on environmental health.

Continued exposure to higher sound levels found in large cities can lead to noise-induced hearing loss as well as decreased levels of work performance, among other things (Recio, Linares, Banegas, & Diaz, 2016). Significantly lower psychomotor speed and reduced working memory were found in a sample of healthy adults when subjected to urban noise levels (Wright, Peters, Ettinger, Kuipers, & Kumari, 2016). Lead poisoning and hazards related to asthma have been more often reported in older, larger cities (Maring, Singer, & Shenassa, 2011).

A national study found that traffic-related air pollution (measured by nitrogen dioxide levels) was significantly associated with small for gestational age births and lower birth weights and may be a source of air pollution related to poor pregnancy outcomes in Canada (Stieb et al., 2016). Another study examined the effects of long-term air pollution exposure on survival rates for acute myocardial infarctions (Chen et al., in press). Researchers concluded 12.4% of deaths could have been prevented if the lowest measured concentration of ambient fine particulate matter in urban areas had been consistently achieved over the study period.

The risk for major depressive disorder has also been shown to increase as exposure to particulate matter increased; this was true in the general population but was even more highly significant in people with chronic diseases (Kim et al., in press). Suicide rates in New York City have declined from 8.1 per 100,000 to 4.8 per 100,000 and remained stable through 2006 (Nandi et al., 2012). While global data have often suggested that urban residents have better health on average than their rural counterparts, this benefit is truly only greater for those at the high end of the income scale. This only magnifies the disparities in urban areas between rich and poor or the social gradient. A more current view is that those living in urban slums, often in megacities outside the United States, have health outcomes that are either similar to or worse than those of their rural neighbors (Friel et al., 2011a; Vlahov, 2015; Vlahov et al., 2011). Using the social determinants of health, researchers in Toronto, Canada, modeled both short- and long-term interventions (Mahamoud, Roche, & Homer, 2013). The Rockefeller Foundation funds two projects that will further examine ways to improve urban health equity and develop a global research agenda, as well as identify better ways of measuring and evaluating population health in urban settings (Friel, Vlahov, & Buckley, 2011b).

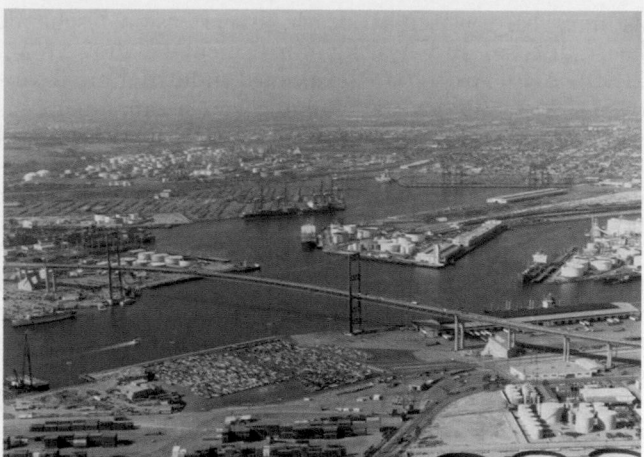

Air pollution is a common problem in metropolitan areas, as seen in this view of San Pedro in Los Angeles County. (Source: California Department of Transportation.)

Violence is often associated with large metropolitan cities. The U.S. Department of Justice (Langton & Truman, 2015) revealed that the overall rate of violent crime was 20.1 per 1,000 in 2014, not significantly different from the previous year. The rate of violent crime in metropolitan areas is over two times that reported in nonmetropolitan (rural) areas: 410.3 versus 188.1 per 100,000. Cities outside metropolitan areas have higher rates of property crimes than both urban and rural areas, although vehicle thefts were highest in urban areas (U.S. Department of Justice, Office for Victims of Crime, n.d.). Kneebone and Raphael (2011) note that, with community diversification, the association between community demographics (e.g., race/ethnicity) and crime significantly weakened. For example, Black or Hispanic population density associated with property crime or violent crime was significantly reduced or almost disappeared. Over a four-decade period, Parker and Stansfield (2015) found that increased population diversity in U.S. cities contributed to declining homicide rates; racial differences were noted with growing Hispanic presence in Black areas leading to lower Black homicide rates, but no differences were found in White homicide rates. Black and Hispanic growth rates, however, have been shown to strongly affect socioeconomic changes in urban areas, decreasing the per capita income growth rate and increasing poverty rates (Park, 2011).

Social disorganization theory is thought to predict relationships between delinquency rates and neighborhood social structures and processes (e.g., poverty, residential instability, overcrowding), and one study of Chicago neighborhoods found that individual-level risk factors (e.g., lack of adult supervision, individual/peer alcohol use, depression) were a more consistent predictor of physical aggression than neighborhood factors baseline levels of aggression were taken into account (Jennings, Maldonado-Molina, Reingle, & Komro, 2011). They also cited previous research on programs such as Head Start, residential relocation efforts, and neighborhood supervision of teen peer groups as having shown some effectiveness in dealing with individual risk factors; they

further noted the need for interventions that address multiple causal factors.

Among youth, Latinos/Hispanics are disproportionately represented among youth gangs, and substance use and sales are gang-related activities. Gang violence and bullying are making its way onto social media sites (Patton et al., 2014), and a study of over 16,000 adolescents found that those reporting being bullies or having been bullied were at greatest risk of becoming involved in violence, having academic problems, and using multiple substances (Bradshaw, Waasdorp, Goldweber, & Johnson, 2013). Individuals who are exposed to urban violence may develop PTSD, and a study examining health-related quality of life among those with PTSD who were exposed to urban violence found that they had higher levels of anxiety and depression, more childhood traumas, and more new trauma experiences (Pupo, Serafim, & deMello, 2015). Supportive family members were shown to be associated with lower reported involvement with violence during adolescence. While those living in low-resource urban areas may not be able to avoid witnessing violence, having one supportive parent had significantly less violence involvement, and those with a supportive mother only or two supportive parents had a significant inverse correlation with violence involvement (Culyba et al., in press).Van Dommelen-Gonzalez, Deardorff, Herd, and Minnis (2015) chose as positive deviance framework to study the relationship between positive peer networks associated with aspirations for college, along with frequent marijuana/alcohol use, among gang-affiliated youth in San Francisco. Having close friends with plans to attend 4-year colleges was positively related to lower frequency of alcohol/marijuana use. How adolescents perceive their communities can also influence behaviors and health. A Baltimore study found that girls perceived vacant homes and few recreational facilities as having an influence on sexual health, but boys felt there was more of an influence on violence and drugs (Mmari et al., 2014). Mmari, Marshall, Lantos, and Blum (in press) noted that adolescent trust of authority (e.g., institutions) was lacking, as over half of the study participants did not trust police and a good percentage had no trust in any type of authority. Levels of trust were found to correlate with risk behaviors.

Inner cities are often thought to be places with low-income residents living in large, poorly maintained government housing projects. Dilapidated housing in central cities exposes residents to cracks in walls and ceilings, peeling paint, broken windows, leaking pipes, and pests such as cockroaches and rats. There is often limited access to adequate rental properties, and rent is often higher in large cities, making it difficult for low-income residents to find adequate housing. Nationwide, about one third of households live in rentals, but 43% of rental properties are in central cities. Most rental property in this country (80%) is considered private, with landlords not receiving any government subsidies. Rents in large metropolitan areas rose 9% between 2000 and 2005, but household incomes of renters fell 5% during that time period. As the recession began in 2008, "rent-to-income ratios were higher than they had been" since the early days of the Depression (DiPasquale, 2011, p. 58). Vacancy rates in

2009 peaked at 10.6%, and rents declined across the country (DiPasquale, 2011). However, Dewan (2014) reports that median rents in 90 cities were over 30% of the gross median income; no more than 30% of one's household income is considered to be affordable rent. In Chicago, the average rental percentage increased from 21% to 31%, and New Orleans reported 35%, from a low of 14%. Miami rent is now 43% of the typical household income, despite efforts to increase the number of apartment buildings. Apartment vacancy rates are now very low, and rents will most likely continue upward.

Low-income housing, when available, is often plagued with construction and maintenance problems and is characterized by crowding, poor quality, high population density, and attendant health problems. Over 1.3 million U.S. households are located in public housing. Over one third of rental housing was built before 1960, and owners of multifamily rental properties that have lost tenants and income may scrimp on maintenance that decreases property values even more (DiPasquale, 2011). Gielen et al. (2012) examined low-income urban housing quality and found that 99% of 246 homes studied failed on HUD's housing quality standards. Heating and cooling, walls/ceilings/floors, and sanitation/safety issues were areas with the highest failure rates. Homelessness is more prevalent in urban areas than in rural areas, and some of the community-level determinants include high rent levels, lower level of home ownership, high-poverty levels, aging population, a growing Hispanic population, and proportion of recently moved or single-person households (Boozer, 2014). Byrne, Munley, Fargo, Montgomery, and Culhane (2013) estimate a 15% to 39% increase in homelessness for every $100 increase in rent in metro, suburban, or rural areas. See Chapter 28 for more on the homeless and promising interventions.

Urban poor are often forced to live in neighborhoods that do not facilitate outdoor activity or have markets that provide healthy foods, such as fresh fruits and vegetables. A walk through most urban corner markets reveals that they do not always offer low-fat dairy products or fresh produce but generally do their best business selling lottery tickets, liquor, sodas, and cigarettes. A study of urban food environments and residents' shopping behaviors noted that healthful food inventory scores were lowest for convenience or corner stores, but these were the most common type of retail food outlet (78.6%). Almost 95% of participating residents did "primary food shopping" at chain supermarkets with higher scores, but most shopped at a store further from their home in order to find healthier foods (Cannuscio et al., 2013, p. 606). Distance to store and the price of food items were both found to be positively correlated with obesity (Ghosh-Dastidar et al., 2014). In New York City, it is estimated that only half of residents consume two or more servings of fruits and vegetables daily, and typical interventions aimed at increasing consumption are not likely to be effective in neighborhoods with low education levels (Li, Zhang, & Pagán, 2016).

In a Philadelphia study of patients with high hospital utilization (≥3 inpatient admissions within 12 months; ≥6 chronic illnesses), 30% were found to be food insecure, and 25% were marginally food insecure (Phipps,

Singletary, Cooblall, Hares, & Braitman, in press). In the past 30 days, 40% were concerned that their food would run out, 17.5% said that they did not eat for a full day, and 10% reported being hungry and not eating some or all of the time. Food insecurity can have negative impacts on health, especially for those with chronic conditions. In a qualitative study of San Francisco area individuals with HIV/AIDS, participants discussed living on insufficient food supplies and being hungry, as well as having concerns about the potential poor health effects of eating a "cheap diet" (Whittle et al., 2015, p. 154). Some reported having to use socially and personally unacceptable means of getting food (e.g., trading sex for food, depending on friends/family/charities). High rents related to gentrification of their neighborhoods were cited as a cause of their food insecurity.

Alcohol availability is higher in areas with greater concentrations of lower-income minority residences and the concentration of liquor stores and other alcohol outlets in disadvantaged communities has been found to contribute to increased alcohol consumption, especially among teens, in a systematic review of 26 studies (Bryden, Roberts, McKee, & Petticrew, 2012). In a study of California cities, adolescents had a greater increase in past-year use of alcohol and heavy drinking when higher levels of adult drinking were also found. Bar density was also associated with higher levels of past-year use of alcohol (Paschall, Lipperman-Kreda, & Grube, 2014). Youth exposed to higher-density levels of alcohol outlets were found to be at risk for both recent heavy alcohol use and lifetime alcohol use (Shih et al., 2015). Restricting the number of alcohol outlets in urban areas and making it more difficult for youth to enter clubs and bars are important to addressing this problem. In a study of national survey data on alcohol consumption, Jones-Webb and Karriker-Jaffe (2013) found that significantly more individuals from disadvantaged neighborhoods reported negative consequences from drinking alcohol than those in higher-income areas. Being a resident of an African American neighborhood was associated with increased liquor consumption and more negative consequences from drinking. The researchers called for an examination of tax policies and advertising practices in minority neighborhoods that support the easy availability of alcohol and problem drinking.

Urban substance abuse follows a similar pattern as rural, except that those admitted for treatment are more often Black and Hispanic, rather than White, and more often unemployed with no reported primary source of income; a greater proportion of those in urban areas use heroin and cocaine, whereas those in rural areas have higher percentages of alcohol, marijuana, and nonheroin opioid use (Substance Abuse and Mental Health Services Administration, 2012). As drug use increases, financial resources decrease (Ompad et al., 2012). A Baltimore study of 3,245 injection drug users (former, current) over a 22-year period found that 57% were incarcerated at least once and that incarceration was positively related to subsequent injection drug use among those who were former, not current, users in this largely African American sample (90%). Genberg, Astemborski, Vlahov, Kirk, and Mehta (2015) also reported that 29% of their participants were females and about one third were HIV positive. Weiss et al. (2014) reported on outcomes of the Cessation of Heroin: A Neighborhood Grounded Exploration (CHANGE) study and noted that those heroin users wanting to stop and who are successful use a combination of approaches: treatment, strategies to avoid heroin triggers, engaging in some type of alternative activity (e.g., support groups, faith-based practices, exercise), and motivations (e.g., wanting a better quality of life and relationships, fear of incarceration, illness, or death).

Drug overdose deaths are becoming a national epidemic, rising from 9 to 15 per 100,000 between 2003 and 2014 (Park & Bloch, 2016). Heroin deaths quadrupled between 2002 and 2013; heroin use increased 63% overall, and there was a 50% increase among men (Fox, 2015). For women, the numbers doubled. It is no longer urban poor who are addicted; heroin has made its way into the suburbs and higher-income white populations. Analgesic (not heroin) overdose deaths occur in higher-income, less unequal neighborhoods than heroin overdose deaths (Cerdá et al., 2013). An interesting study of a particular opioid receptor gene (OPRM1) found that those individuals with a particular allele (118G) had over five times greater odds of suffering respiratory or cardiac arrest with acute drug overdose (Manini, Jacobs, Vlahov, & Hurd, 2013). The Food and Drug Administration (2015) approved a nasal spray form of Narcan, to make it more easily accessible as a lifesaving measure for opioid drug overdoses. Other interventions are needed to address this problem in urban areas and across this country (see Chapter 27).

Sociologists Wilson and Kelling first proposed the *broken window theory* in 1982, noting that if a broken window goes unrepaired, soon more windows are broken, and this sends a powerful message to residents that no one cares. A classic research study by Keizer, Lindenberg, and Steg (2008) tested this theory in six-field experiments where neighborhoods, characterized by broken windows, litter, unreturned shopping carts, and graffiti, were studied. They found that when residents see others violating social norms or rules (e.g., disorderly or petty criminal behavior), they are then more likely to also violate norms and rules and that this is a cause for the spread of disorder. Gau, Corsaro, and Brunson (2014) studied the causal path of broken window theory and found that fear is the result of disorder, partially because of poor neighborhood cohesion and lower expectations for social control. Welsh, Braga, and Bruinsma (2015) note that the theory is helpful in measuring neighborhood disorder and in developing interventions to address the problems related to it. Research has demonstrated that crime and safety were more significant predictors, walkability measures, in a study of behaviors affecting mental health outcomes and health status of low-income urban women (DeGuzman, Merwin, & Bourguignon, 2013).

Population density, complexity, and racial/ethnic diversity are associated with urban areas. Central cities are often home to a large proportion of poor people and those from different racial and ethnic groups. Less than half of all Hispanics lived in the top ten metropolitan areas in 2005, with 22% living in Los Angeles and New York. These two large cities are also home to 27% of the Asian population, with 56% living in the top 10 metro

areas. Over the past 15 years, there has been significant movement of blacks to Southern metropolitan areas, but movement to other areas (e.g., Las Vegas, Phoenix, Sacramento, Minneapolis) has also occurred. In the 21st century, America has evolved into a metropolitan nation with >8 out of 10 Americans living in metropolitan areas of varying sizes. Between 2000 and 2010, the fastest growing cities included Las Vegas, NV; Raleigh, NC; Cape Coral, FL; and Provo, UT. Conversely, the cities with the greatest rates of decline included New Orleans, LA; Youngstown, OH; Detroit, MI; and Cleveland, OH. During the latter part of the decade, though, there were major shifts that occurred because of the economy and the housing market collapse (Frey, 2012).

Urban poor have health problems characterized by accidental and violent injuries, as well as noncommunicable diseases and chronic stress (Kliewer & Lepore, 2015; Maxmen, 2016). In a classic comparison of neighborhood characteristics in the Multi-Ethnic Study of Atherosclerosis, researchers found that distinct neighborhood features, not associated with race or ethnicity, had health modifying effects. Increased levels of smoking, depression, and not walking for exercise were found in less socially cohesive neighborhoods, whereas individuals living in neighborhoods with the fewest problems had less smoking, depression, and drinking (Echeverria, Diez-Roux, Shea, Borrell, & Jackson, 2008). As noted in Chapter 25, poverty makes a significant difference in health status. Gilster (2014) found an association between neighborhood stressors and depressive symptoms in low-income, non-white neighborhoods in Chicago. Neighborhood factors were also associated with inner-city school children performance on math and reading tests and behavioral problems and being held back in school (Kim, Mazza, Zwanziger, & Henry, 2014). Neighborhood disadvantage and disorder (drug activity, violent crime) have been related to the rapid transition from no drug involvement to problem drug use (Reboussin et al., 2015). Neighborhood poverty has been associated with HIV diagnosis in a New York City study (Wiewel et al., 2016). Goldsmith and Blakely (2010) note that political and economic forces, especially for poor city dwellers, generate poverty. Working class urban residents no longer can find industrial jobs, and a concerted effort to improve conditions in urban America is needed in the form of urban policy development.

Over the past 25 years, cities and their suburbs have become more alike, and the demographic and health profiles that were previously uniquely urban are now shared by "edge cities" and suburbs populated by poor and minority families. Political power has shifted to more affluent suburban areas, where the tax base and spending practices are greater, at the expense of these cities. Monies that once came to cities to support new resources have also declined. Hanlon (2012) studied 5,000 U.S. "inner-ring" suburbs, many early suburban areas of large metropolitan cities. These developed just prior to or immediately after WWII and are often considered to be very similar in composition. She found, however, that this was not the case and that many were sliding into decline with higher levels of poverty, foreclosures, and significant fiscal problems.

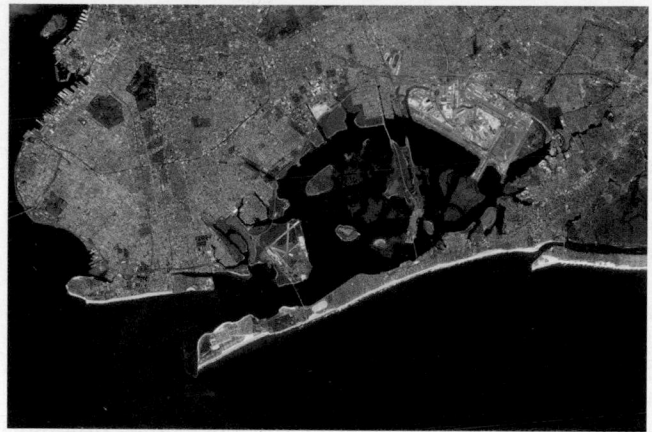

This aerial view of New York City shows Central Park and other green areas interspersed among densely populated areas, an example of good urban planning. (Source: National Aeronautics & Space Administration.)

Urban health disparities present a challenge that can be addressed only by the joint effort of public health and urban planning bodies. Coalitions of public health professionals, planners, builders, and architects, along with transportation engineers and government officials, are needed to promote healthy, sustainable communities (Boarnet & Takahashi, 2011). There is a move to make cities and their suburbs *sustainable communities*. These are seen as healthy places where both natural and historic resources are protected, employment is available, urban sprawl is contained, neighborhoods are safe, air pollution is minimized, lifelong learning is promoted, health care and transportation are easily accessible, and all citizens have the opportunity to improve their quality of life. A federal collaborative program, the Partnership for Sustainable Communities (n.d.), is a nonprofit organization that helps American cities become more socially, economically, and environmentally sustainable while focusing on land use planning, affordable housing, community development, energy use, and transportation.

As with all good plans, the sustainable development plan requires that the recipient of the planning be involved. Democratizing the practice of urban planning is vital to its success. Communities that have been victimized through ineffective planning must be included in the decision-making process. This process will require the inclusion of the practical experience that residents bring to the table, alongside expert input. However, to ensure equitable participation and to level the discussions, the community must have access to all the necessary resources, such as technical, medical, legal, and financial assistance, and crowdsourcing, health portals, and Web-based tools may be helpful (Gottlieb, Hoehndorf, Dumontier, & Altman, 2015; Jiao et al., 2015; Wong et al., 2015). The health of communities must be addressed from all levels of environmental impact (individual, community, and systems), and population health in the urban setting must be studied (Gottlieb et al., 2016). Data must be included from the various environments, such as homes, workplaces, schools, and community spaces. These approaches then bring such action in line with what is often referred to as *environmental justice* or the marriage of environmental health and civil rights (Walker,

2012). A framework to ensure such justice requires that all individuals and communities have the right to work, play, and live in environments that are safe and healthy. It also requires that polluters are punished and required to provide compensation for damages and/or renovation.

Community Health Nursing in an Urban Setting

Urban public health nursing can be very rewarding, and many nurses are drawn to urban areas where salaries are higher and opportunities for advancement or additional education greater. In urban areas, there are a larger number of nurses, more schools of nursing, and more intensive recruitment efforts than in rural areas, although inner-city areas, much like rural settings, can have problems filling PHN vacancies. While there were 41,290 PHNs working at local, state, and federal levels in 2012, it is difficult to determine how many work primarily in urban settings (Public Health Foundation, 2013). However, RN workforce studies reveal a higher rate of nurses (934.8 vs. 852.7 per 100,000 population) and a greater proportion of nurses with a BSN (46.6% vs. 33.9%) in urban areas when compared with rural areas (HRSA, 2013).

PHN practice is population-focused care that requires unique knowledge, competencies, and skills. PHN roles have always extended beyond sick care, also encompassing advocacy, health education, community organization, as well as political and social reform (Kulbok et al., 2012). Contemporary public health nursing also involves collaboration with both community agencies and community members as equal partners. Primary prevention (health promotion) is a major focus. PHNs have a key role of working with populations to improve health and social conditions of vulnerable populations (Kulbok et al., 2012). These nurses practice in diverse settings such as community nursing centers, home health agencies, housing developments, local and state health departments, neighborhood centers, churches, schools, and worksites. PHNs can develop sustainable programs and build community capacity for health promotion in collaboration with community members. By utilizing a community-based participatory research (CBPR) model, PHNs can collaborate with community members, leaders, and stakeholders to identify resources and solutions to problems. Specific public health roles include advocates, collaborators, educators, partners, policy-makers, and researcher (Kulbok et al., 2012).

Bond, Jones, Ompad, and Vlahov (2013) report on the interest of faith-based organizations in working with LHDs to provide influenza vaccination programs (60% were interested in providing on-site vaccinations, and 16.5% had contacted LHDs). This collaboration may be especially helpful with black congregations, as other studies have shown low interest and vaccination rates among this population (Vlahov, Bond, Jones, & Ompad, 2012). A seminal study by Schulte (2000) demonstrated that urban PHNs create connections through caring processes and an underlying sense of regard for their clients as human beings. Community health nurses collaborate with their clients to develop their facility for long-term health promotion and improvement of their quality of life. Their ultimate goal is to empower clients to be self-sufficient. The centrality of caring is noted in the following PHN comment:

"Public health nursing is more than a job.... When I'm out there, I care about the people, about what happens to them. I don't think I'd make a really good PHN if I didn't care. You get results if they know you care—they're willing to make some change. If they don't think you care at all about them, why should they take a risk for you? I think public health nursing is all about caring about people" (p. 8).

This type of caring is typical of public and community health nursing in all settings, including urban and rural health departments (Keller et al., 2011).

There are many points at which the community health nurse can make a difference in people's lives. Nurses provide services in deteriorating urban areas, with those living in poverty in all settings, and among all vulnerable populations. Nurses first need to assess themselves for their attitudes and preconceptions. Although access to care can be improved for many low-income people in urban areas, many clients simply need an advocate. Our ability to envision solutions and join together with clients aids us in helping to create a healthier environment for our clients (Fullilove & Cantal-Dupart, in press). The urban communities, and the poor or vulnerable people living in them, need strengthening and interventions that can be initiated by PHNs using the nursing process as a guide. See Chapter 25.

Self-Assessment

Confronting poverty and caring for vulnerable people from diverse backgrounds, whether in rural or urban areas, necessitate reflective assessment of one's own assumptions and beliefs. Because poverty may be prevalent over a lifetime, a good number of nursing students have personal or family experience of living in poverty. However, because the stigma is so great and faultfinding so pervasive in American society, acknowledging and reflecting on this experience may well be painful. In contrast, because poverty is so hidden and frequently denied, some nursing students have lived apart from any knowledge of the human experience of poverty. They may have come to believe many of the negative stereotypes about poor people. Nursing students and practicing nurses need to ask such questions as "How have my judgments been shaped? How can I open myself to caring for those from whom most of society turns away?"

We learn from one another's stories. First, learn from your classmates, friends, and neighbors who are courageous enough to tell you their own experiences of living in poverty. Ask them and listen intently. Then, let your clients teach you. One honor that nurses have is the opportunity to work with people from all walks of life. During your clinical experiences in community health, you are particularly likely to meet impoverished, vulnerable individuals and families living outside the mainstream. And you can join with them to empower them by helping to build skills and confidence and connecting them to resources. See From the Case Files V about experiences of students through the eyes of their professors.

Improving Access

Even with ACA and government-sponsored health insurance and services, extensive barriers prevent many people from accessing services. The community health nurse serves as an advocate and bridge for families who need to gain access. Barriers to access associated with the clients themselves include reluctance to seek coverage because of feelings of powerlessness; being unaware that such services exist or are worthwhile; lacking resources such as a telephone, transportation, or fare for children who need to go along because no babysitter is available; being illiterate; and preoccupation with meeting survival needs and competing life priorities instead of health needs.

Barriers associated with applying for health insurance include a system that is unfriendly and complicated. Paperwork is overwhelming and may be returned for correction; presentation of paid utility bills or other statements that are not often saved may be required. Informative materials may be too difficult to understand; programs may seek to restrict enrollments by restricting information. The process may require a car, a phone, and appointments at inconvenient times. Also, service interruptions are not uncommon, as wages vary over time. Wait times for reinstatement may be long. The nurse can intervene as a coach and guide, interpreting the system to the client and the client to the system. Likewise, nurses can serve as change agents to improve the system whenever possible.

Strengthening Communities

We are all connected. All of us as citizens have a stake in preventing the adverse hardships of poverty and ill health. All of society pays to support community members that do not contribute, to house those who are incarcerated, and to ignore the vulnerable. This weakens us. We fear crime in our homes, schools, businesses, and communities in general. Society, as a whole, is impacted when adults are incapable of providing nurturing environments for their children. And the alienation of many groups in society erodes our sense of community as a nation.

The common good is enhanced by strengthening community resources, including investing in people of historically low status, developing and strengthening ties within families and among people involved in neighborhood mutual support, and redeveloping neighborhood resources (Latkin, German, Vlahov, & Galea, 2013; see Chapter 13). Whenever possible, the PHN voices support of economic redevelopment of neighborhoods to enhance schools, housing, and employment. The nurse can also work to promote subsidized carpools, school-to-work transition programs, and inner-city economic development programs. Reflecting community priorities and needs as well as focusing on population health are two examples of cornerstones of public health nursing (Keller et al., 2011).

Many caution well-intentioned professionals to beware when seeking solutions to vulnerability through the use of service programs alone. For instance, a whole population of people can become defined in terms of their problems instead of their strengths. In addition, citizens acting to help themselves within their community can be weakened when they are seen as clients requiring professional services. Also, being dependent on multiple human services often has a disabling effect, reducing self-worth, and leads to feelings of powerlessness.

Because human service interventions can have negative as well as positive effects, it is important to consider

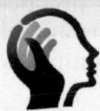

From the Case Files V

Examples from Community Health Nursing Instructors

- Ann, a nursing faculty member at a small Roman Catholic college, had a one-to-one postclinical conference with a student and relays this conversation. The student had made many visits to an African American teen mother of two thriving children. The young mother lived in a dangerous housing project, and, although she locked him out of her second-floor apartment, her abusive boyfriend had been known to climb up the drainage pipe and over the porch roof. Sometimes, he forced open a window and beat her. The mother worked every day at a fast-food establishment; her grandmother took care of the children. After a couple of months of weekly visits, the student exclaimed, "When I read her chart, I saw her as an immoral girl—a slut—and I expected her to be a loser. Now, I can't believe what I've learned about how strong she is. She just keeps fighting for herself and for her kids to survive! She's a great mom and I told her so!"

- Another faculty member, Sharon, who taught community health nursing in a Midwestern school of nursing was having an informal discussion with a student who related her experience of trying to get comfortable making home visits with low-income young women. She was making brave attempts at home visits to a pregnant woman, about her age, living in the deteriorating outskirts of a major city. She thought she had established rapport and was making headway developing trust with the client. One day, the client asked the student, with concern in her voice, if she had "broken off her engagement." The flustered student then had difficulty explaining the absence of her engagement ring, which she had never mentioned, but the client had obviously noticed. During the previous week, she had suddenly realized she was wearing this special ring in marginal neighborhoods and thought it best to leave it at home. Of course, she thought that she had to fabricate another reason to tell the client but felt badly for being so judgmental when the client was identifying with the student and believed they had something in common.

- Lynn, a new public health nursing faculty member from a large state university in the West, was shocked and repulsed by the comment of one of her students during lecture one day. When discussing vulnerable populations in urban centers and rural areas, the point was made that poverty can be a generational phenomenon and that many of our clients may find it difficult to dig out of this circumstance. Social justice was discussed, along with the need for PHNs to become social activists in order to change political and socioeconomic factors that keep the status quo. One student, a Hispanic female from a middle-class family, spoke up stating "they should all get jobs at McDonalds." This spurred further discussion about population-focused versus individual-focused interventions and approaches and the need for all of us to be aware of our prejudices and stereotypical viewpoints.

---

whether more community agencies are the answer to resolving community hardship. Community health planning should seriously consider an organizing process that builds community and that focuses on developing neighborhood competence to solve problems and create solutions for itself (see the discussion of community development in Chapter 15).

SOCIAL JUSTICE AND PUBLIC HEALTH NURSING

Justice is concerned with treating people fairly. *Distributive justice* refers to the justified distribution of burdens and benefits throughout society (see Chapter 4 for a discussion of distributive justice). In the United States, the marketplace largely determines the distribution of goods and services. Although equality is claimed as a social ideal, dramatic inequities are accepted as being determined by the law of the marketplace. In contrast, community health nursing is grounded in commitment to a just distribution of primary goods for all members of society (Falk-Raphael & Betker, 2012). The founder of American public health nursing, Lillian Wald (1915/1971), was in the forefront of social reform movements emphasizing just allocation of resources for the immigrant and poor laborer. At the start of the 21st century, PHNs have inherited her legacy but are we living up to it?

Social justice occurs when a society provides for the overall health and well-being of all people by treating people fairly. It involves an equal societal bearing of burdens and reaping of benefits, and it is a widely held view that social justice is the foundation of public health nursing (Drevdahl, 2013). Community health nurses who practice social justice have broad and holistic views of health; they have strong convictions that health care is a basic human right and that improving the health of communities is an example of social justice. For instance, PHNs concerned with social justice will include socially marginalized and vulnerable populations (e.g., prisoners, undocumented aliens) in their influenza pandemic planning processes. Not to do so would constitute discrimination and would be morally indefensible (Rosoff & DeCamp, 2011). Social justice ensures the distribution of resources that benefits marginalized populations and holds in check the self-interest of more privileged populations. Impartiality is the goal.

PHNs must have a heightened sense of the value of cultural, racial, and socioeconomic differences and awareness that these differences are often turned into discrimination in health care services and policies. They must be determined to extend the bonds of community so that everyone has a firm place to stand and is equally entitled to health care services with a high standard of care for all.

Where is nursing's role within the concept of social justice? Social justice can be both an individual- and a population-based concept, but it is through the population lens that PHNs must focus their greatest attention. Urban health nursing directs its practice to the systems and community- or population-based level, at which both political and economic solutions must be considered. Although most nurses in urban settings continue to provide service on the individual level, nurses should step back and analyze their practice and synthesize recommendations for a plan of action at the level of community planning to better address the needs of the city or neighborhood (Kulbok, Thatcher, Park, & Meszaros, 2012).

Therefore, although day-to-day practice usually includes individual services, the overall planning for change and improvement must occur from the perspective of the population level. From this level of practice, the construct of *person* incorporates the population level of aggregates, institutions, communities, states, and nations—not solely the individual. The concept of the *environment* at the individual level is often associated with physical and psychosocial influences. With a population focus, it incorporates economic and political structures that can influence health or illness and addresses community and global systems that must be utilized to initiate change and solutions.

Like the other constructs, *health* is expanded to include a population focus that recognizes sociopolitical influences. By acknowledging the health issues encountered at the individual as well as the population level, the urban nurse can incorporate interventions that address the more dynamic societal level. In order to combine critical caring theory with public health nursing practice, PHNs contribute to creating "supportive and sustainable physical, social, political, and economic environments" (Falk-Raphael & Betker, 2012, para. 1).

Nursing practice requires cultural and racial competence in order to advocate for the diverse communities served by nursing. The standards of practice for culturally competent care are based on the framework of social justice. It is through the application of social justice and culturally competent care that inequalities in health outcomes may be decreased (Douglas et al., 2011). This should lead to an enhancement of the practice and research needed to contribute solutions for addressing health disparities in all settings.

The urban nursing profession must focus, much like public health nursing, on including both primary and secondary prevention—not only at the local or community level but also include the state, national, and international levels—to enact change for the common good. The role of advocate in these practice settings must include not only the individual level but also the community or population and systems levels. Examples of such actions would include advocating for adequate funding of government health systems, such as Medicare and Medicaid, and helping to ensure that all communities are safe and healthy environments in which to live and work. To connect all populations to fair and just, systems requires that health care is accessible, affordable, available, and sustainable and that it is distributed both impartially and equitably, without any regard to personal advantage. Good health not only should belong to those who are blessed with the means of paying for health care, education, and safe working environments but should be a benefit for all of us living together on this planet.

SUMMARY

Rural clients are a unique aggregate. Community health nurses are key to ensuring the delivery of appropriate health services to this population. There are numerous definitions of the term *rural*. In this chapter, rural is defined as communities with fewer than 10,000 residents and a county population density of fewer than 1,000 people per square mile. Between the 2000 and 2010 censuses, urban population growth was about twice than in rural areas. The elderly are a rapidly growing population in rural communities. Rural areas often have less diversity than urban cities, but that is changing in many areas. Rural clients generally have lower educational levels than urban clients, due in part to less access to higher education and lower-paying jobs. Income levels and housing costs are frequently lower than in larger cities.

Rural Healthy People 2020 initiative identifies national goals applicable to rural communities. Many at-risk populations live in these communities, where there are often fewer employment opportunities, a lack of adequate housing, and limited access to health and social services. Rural elders may have more limited alternatives for housing if they can no longer live alone. Mental health services are inadequate, even though the need may be great. Numerous risks are associated with agriculture. The community health nurse can help this population identify hazards and practice injury prevention.

A PHN needs to engage in community assessment of the rural area as a part of orientation. It is helpful to identify the strengths of the community. Rural clients are frequently resourceful and often have a supportive network of people to meet their needs.

Access to health care is an important issue in rural communities. Health insurance may not be easily available, but some progress has been made through the Affordable Care Act. Barriers to access include distance, weather, transportation, and limited choice of providers. Some ways to improve access

in these communities are school-based clinics, mobile health vans, faith-based nursing initiatives, and use of the latest technologies. University-sponsored nursing centers that could serve rural populations should be expanded.

Migrant farmworkers are an integral part of the farming community in the United States and across the world; however, they are rarely visible members of our society. As members of a community with varied and profound health needs complicated by disease, social isolation, and occupational hazards such as pesticide exposure and working with dangerous farm equipment, they also endure substandard housing and poor sanitation, and migrant farmworkers and their families often live in high-risk environments. Migrant children are often educationally, socially, and physically disadvantaged. Because migrant health centers do not adequately meet the health needs of the entire migrant community, several innovative methods of health care delivery have been developed and implemented by community health nurses, including mobile health vans and information tracking systems.

Rural PHNs are key members of the professional community. Their roles include advocate, coordinator/case manager, health teacher, referral agent, mentor, change agent/researcher, collaborator, and activist. Community health nurses have challenges and opportunities related to their clinical practices. Confidentiality and personal/professional boundary issues may exist. Salaries for rural nurses may be lower than for nurses in urban areas. But rural community health nurses are highly respected individuals who make a difference in the communities they serve.

Urban health issues have existed for hundreds of years in the United States, and they continue today. Many disenfranchised and minority groups call inner cities home. Air pollution, poverty, discrimination, substandard housing, crime, substance abuse, and social disorganization often characterize life in urban settings. The built environment is an important consideration in urban as well as rural settings and can contribute to greater health risks. Some large cities have had marked decreases in population and significant problems with unemployment, although more people around the world live in urban areas now than in rural areas.

Although nursing services may often be delivered at the individual level, the true impact on health must be addressed at the community or population level, as well as the system level. Key to recognizing the potential impact for improvement in existing health disparities is the acceptance of a social justice orientation that will empower nurses to address the required changes needed within the existing social, political, and economic systems.

ACTIVITIES TO PROMOTE **CRITICAL THINKING**

1. Search for six recent articles in both rural and urban newspapers relating to access to health care or quality of care. After summarizing the content, identify barriers to access that are common to both, and those that are different. What are the main themes relating to health and access to care?

2. Discuss with your clinical group the common characteristics of rural, migrant, and urban clients. How can the PHN be better prepared to meet their unique needs? What are some specific challenges facing the PHN working in a rural area? In an urban area?

3. Describe some of the benefits of rural public health nursing. Do the same for urban public health nursing.

4. Compare and contrast health, living, and working concerns between migrant workers and recent immigrants. Discuss how many recent immigrants from places such as Asia, Russia, or the Middle East experience the same hardships as migrant workers do. How does a nomadic lifestyle affect and differentiate the needs of migrant workers and recent immigrants?

5. If you are from a rural area, interview a peer who was raised in an urban setting (or vice versa). Compare your experiences with family, school, friends, entertainment, etc.

6. Search the Internet for examples of community needs assessment from both rural and urban areas. What are the main findings of each? How do planned interventions differ? How are they similar?

7. Debate with a classmate the need for ready access to specialist medical care and sophisticated diagnostic equipment in all communities. Is this feasible? If not, how can services best be made available to urban and rural clients?

8. Search YouTube for videos related to rural public health nursing, migrant workers, urban health, social justice, or other topics described in this chapter. Discuss key points with your clinical group and highlight the major issues.

REFERENCES

Adamkiewicz, G., Spengler, J. D., Harley, A. E., Stoddard, A., Yang, M, ... Sorensen, G. (2014). Environmental conditions in low-income urban housing: Clustering and associations with self-reported health. *American Journal of Public Health, 104*(9), 1650–1656.

Advocate Precautionary Principle. (2011, June 8). *NIOSH study confirms pesticide drift hazards posed by chemical pesticide applications*. Retrieved from http://appprecautionaryprinciple.wordpress.com/2011/06/08/niosh-study-confirms-pesticide-drift-hazards-posed-by-chemical-pesticide-applications/

Agency for Healthcare Research and Quality (AHRQ). (2011). *National health care disparities report, 2010*. Retrieved from http://www.ahrq.gov/qual/nhdr10/Chap10a.htm

Agency for Healthcare Research and Quality (AHRQ). (2012). *Primary Care Workforce Facts and Stats: Overview*. Retrieved from http://www.ahrq.gov/research/pcworkforce.htm

AIDS.gov. (2016). *Changing or stopping treatment*. Retrieved from www.dids.gov/hiv-aids-basics/just-diagnosed-with-hiv-ais/treatment-options/changing-stopping-treatment/index.html

Al-Dakkak, I., Patel, S., McCann, E., Gadkari, A., Prajapati, G., & Maise, E. M. (2013). The impact of specific HIV treatment-related adverse events on adherence to antiretroviral therapy: A systematic review and meta-analysis. *AIDS Care: Psychological, Socio-medical Aspects of AIDS/HIV, 25*(4), 400–414.

Albarrán, C. R., & Nyamathi, A. (2011). HIV and Mexican migrant workers in the United States: A review applying the vulnerable populations conceptual model. *Journal of the Association of Nurses in AIDS Care, 22*(3), 173–185.

American Academy of Pediatrics. (2014). Providing care for immigrant, migrant, and border children. *Pediatrics, 131*, e2028.

American College of Physicians. (1997). Inner-city health care. *Annals of Internal Medicine, 126*(6), 485–490.

American Congress of Obstetricians and Gynecologists (ACOG). (2014). *Committee on healthcare for underserved women: Health disparities in rural women*. Retrieved from http://www.acog.org/Resources-And-Publications/Committee-Opinions/Committee-on-Health-Care-for-Underserved-Women/Health-Disparities-in-Rural-Women

American Heart Association. (2015). *Heart disease and stroke statistics—at-a-glance*. Retrieved from https://www.heart.org/idc/groups/ahamah-public/@wcm/@sop/@smd/documents/downloadable/ucm_470704.pdf

American Public Health Association (APHA). (n.d.a). *At the intersection of public health and transportation: Promoting healthy transportation policy*. Retrieved from http://www.apha.org/NR/rdonlyres/43F10382-FB68-4112-8C75-49DCB10F8ECF/0/TransportationBrief.pdf

American Public Health Association (APHA). (n.d.b). *Get the facts: Public health and equity*. Retrieved from www.apha.org/~/media/files/pdf/topics/apha_public_health_equity.ashv

Anderson, T. J., Saman, D. M., Lipsky, M. S., & Lutfiyya, M. N. (2015). A cross-sectional study on health differences between rural and non-rural U.S. counties using the County Health Rankings. *BMC Health Services Research, 15*(1), 441. doi: 10.1186/s129113-015-1053-3.

Arcury, T. A., & Quandt, S. A. (2009). Pesticide exposure among farmworkers and their families in the Eastern United States: Matters of social and environmental justice. In T. A. Arcury & S. A. Quandt (Eds.), *Latino farmworkers in the Eastern United States* (pp. 103–129). New York, NY: Springer. doi: 10.10007/978-0-387-88347-2_5.

Arcury, T. A., Grzywacz, J. G., Talton, J. W., Chen, H., Vallejos, Q. M., Galván, L., ... Quandt, S. A. (2010). Repeated pesticide exposure among North Carolina migrant and seasonal farmworkers. *American Journal of Industrial Medicine, 53*(8), 802–813.

Arcury, T. A., & Quandt, S. A. (2011). Living and working safety: Challenges for migrant and seasonal farmworkers. *North Carolina Medical Journal, 72*(6), 466–470.

Arcury, T. A., O'Hara, H., Grzywacz, J. G., Isom, S., Chen, H., & Quandt, S. A. (2012a). Work safety climate, musculoskeletal discomfort, working while injured, and depression among migrant farmworkers in North Carolina. *American Journal of Public Health, 102*(S2), S272–S278.

Arcury, T. A., Weir, M., Chen, H., Summers, P., Pelletier, L. E., Galván, L., ... Quandt, S. A. (2012b). Migrant farmworker housing regulation violations in North Carolina. *American Journal of Industrial Medicine, 55*(3), 191–204.

Arcury, T. A., Nguyen, H. T., Sumers, P., Talton, J. W., Holbrook, L. C., Walker, F. O., ... Quandt, S. A. (2014a). Lifetime and current pesticide exposure among Latino farmworkers in comparison to other Latino immigrants. *American Journal of Industrial Medicine, 57*(7), 776–787.

Arcury, T. A., Rodriguez, G., Kearney, G. D., Arcury, J. T., & Quandt, S. A. (2014b). Safety and injury characteristics of youth farmworkers in North Carolina: A pilot study. *Journal of Agromedicine, 19*(4), 354–363.

Arcury, T. A., Gabbard, S., Bell, B., Casanova, V., Flocks, J. D., Swanberg, J. E., & Wiggins, M F. (2015a). Collecting comparative data on farmworker housing and health: Recommendations for collecting housing and health data across places and time. *New Solutions, 25*(3), 287–312.

Arcury, T. A., Jacobs, I. J., & Ruiz, V. (2015b). Farmworker housing quality and health. *New Solutions, 25*(3), 256–262.

Arcury, T. A., Summers, P., Talton, J. W., Nguyen, H. T., Chen, H., & Quandt, S. A. (2015c). Job characteristics and work safety climate among North Carolina farmworkers with H-2A visas. *Journal of Agromedicine, 20*(1), 64–76.

Arcury, T. A., Talton, J. W., Summers, P., Chen, H., Laurienti, P. J., & Quandt, S. A. (2016). Alcohol consumption and risk for dependence among male Latino migrant farmworkers compared to Latino non-farmworkers in North Carolina. *Alcoholism: Clinical & Experimental Research, 40*(2), 377–384.

Ard, K. (2015). Trends in exposure to industrial air toxins for different racial and socioeconomic groups: A spatial and temporal examination of environmental inequality in the U.S. from 1995 to 2004. *Social Science Research, 53*, 375–390.

Ashley, P. J. (2015). HUD's Healthy Homes Program: Progress and future directions. *Journal of Environmental Health, 78*(2), 50–53.

Bains, R. M., Franzen, C. W., & White-Fresé, J. (2014). Engaging African-American and Latino adolescent males through school-based health centers. *Journal of School Nursing, 30*(6), 411–419.

Barbassa, J. (2010, June 25). Farmworkers challenge the jobless: Try our jobs. *San Francisco Chronicle*. Retrieved from http://www.sfgate.com/cgi-bin/article.cgi?f=/c/a/2010/06/25/BALT1E4KUR.DTL

Barcus, H. R., & Simmons, L. (2013). Ethnic restructuring in rural America: Migration and the changing faces of rural communities in the Great Plains. *The Professional Geographer, 65*(1), 130–152.

Bardacke, F. (2011). *Trampling out the vintage: Cesar Chavez and the two souls of the United Farm Workers*. Brooklyn, NY: Verso Books.

Barnett, D., Thompson, C., Errett, N., Semon, N., Aderson, M., Ferrell, J., ... Links, J. M. (2012). Determinants of emergency response willingness in the local public health workforce by jurisdictional and scenario patterns: A cross-sectional survey. *BMC Public Health, 12*, 164. Retrieved from http://www.biomedcentral.com/1471–2458/12/164

Bélanger, D., Abdous, B., Valois, P., Gosselin, E., & Sidi, A. L. (2016). A multilevel analysis to explain self-reported adverse health effects and adaptation to urban heat: A cross-sectional survey in the deprived areas of 9 Canadian cities. *BMC Public Health, 16*, 144.

Belhadj Koulder, E., Koglin, U., & Petermann, F. (2015). Emotional and behavioral problems in migrant children and adolescents in American countries: A systematic overview. *Journal of Immigrant & Minority Health, 17*(4), 1240–1258.

Bellamy, G. R., Bolin, J. N., & Gamm, L. D. (2011). Rural Healthy People 2010, 2020 and beyond: The need goes on. *Family & Community Health, 34*(2), 182–188.

Bial, R. (2002). *Tenement: Immigrant life on the Lower East Side*. New York, NY: Houghton Mifflin Company.

Bienkowski, B. (2014). Pesticide use by farmers linked to high rates of depression, suicides. *Environmental Health News*. Retrieved from http://www.environmentalhealthnews.org/ehs/news/2014/oct/pesticides-depression

Bigbee, J. L., Gehrke, P., & Otterness, N. (2009). Public health nurses in rural/frontier one-nurse offices. *Rural and Remote Health, 9*, 1282.

Bigbee, J. L., Otterness, N., & Gehrke, P. (2010). Public health nursing competency in a rural/frontier state. *Public Health Nursing, 27*(3), 270–276.

Black, M. C., Basile, K. C., Breiding, M. J., Smith, S. G., Walters, M. L., Merrick, M. T., ... Stevens, M. R. (2011). *The National Intimate Partner and Sexual Violence Survey (NISVS): 2010 summary report*. Retrieved from http://www.cdc.gov/violenceprevention/pdf/nisvs_report2010-a.pdf

Blake, S. B. (2014). Spatial relationships among dairy farms, drinking water quality, and maternal-child health outcomes in the San Joaquin Valley. *Public Health Nursing, 31*(6), 492–499.

Blanco, C. E. (2011). Promotoras: A culturally sensitive intervention for Hispanic breastfeeding women. *Journal of Obstetric, Gynecologic, & Neonatal Nursing, 40*(s1), s19.

Boarnet, M. G., & Takahashi, L. M. (2011). Interactions between public health and urban design. In T. Banerjee & A. Loukaitou-Sideris (Eds.), *Companion to urban design* (pp. 198–207). New York, NY: Routledge.

Bolin, J. N., & Bellamy, G. (n.d.). *Rural Healthy People 2020.* Retrieved from http://www.srph.tamhsc.edu/centers/srhrc/images/rhp2020#rhp2020

Bolin, J. N., & Bellamy, G. (Eds.). (2015). *Rural Healthy People 2020.* College Station, TX: Texas A & M Health Science Center School of Public Health, Southwest Rural Health Research Center.

Bolin, J. N., Bellamy, G. R., Ferinand, A. O., Vuong, A. M., Kash, B. A., ... Helduser, J. W. (2015). Rural Healthy People 2020: New decade, same challenges. *Journal of Rural Health, 31*(3), 326–333.

Bond, K. T., Jones, K., Ompad, D. C., & Vlahov, D. (2013). Resources and interest among faith based organizations for influenza vaccination programs. *Journal of Immigrant & Minority Health, 15*(4), 758–763.

Boozer, C. (2014, March 11). *Community-level determinants of homelessness.* Retrieved from http://chicagopolicyreview.org/2014/03/11/community-level-determinants-of-homelessness/

Borders, T., & Booth, B. (2007). Rural, suburban, and urban variations in alcohol consumption in the United States: Findings from the National Epidemiologic Survey on Alcohol & Related Conditions. *Journal of Rural Health, 23*(4), 314–321.

Borre, K., Ertle, L., & Graff, M. (2010). Working to eat: Vulnerability, food insecurity, and obesity among migrant and seasonal farmworker families. *American Journal of Industrial Medicine, 53*(4), 443–462.

Bouchard, M. F., Chevrier, J., Harley, K. G., Kogut, K., Vedar, M., Calderon, N., & Eskenazi, B. (2011). Prenatal exposure to organophosphate pesticides and IQ in 7-year old children. *Environmental Health Perspectives, 119*(8), 1189–1195.

Bouie, J. (2016). *Still separate and unequal: Why American schools are becoming segregated again.* Retrieved from http://www.slate.com/articles/news_and_politics/politics/2014/05/brown_v_board_of_education_60th_anniversary_america_s_schools_are_segregating.html

Bowblis, J. R., Meng, H., & Hyer, K. (2013). The urban-rural disparity in nursing home quality indicators: The case of facility-acquired contractures. *Health Services Research, 48*(1), 47–69.

Brabeck, K. M., Lykes, M. B., & Hunter, C. (2014). The psychosocial impact of detention and deportation on U.S. migrant children and families. *American Journal of Orthopsychiatry, 84*(5), 496–505.

Bradley, E. (2013). Accountable Care Organizations antitrust guidelines will not save rural providers. *Journal of Legal Medicine, 34,* 295–311.

Bradman, A., Salvatore, A. L., Boeniger, M., Castorina, R., Snyder, J., Barr, D. B., ... Eskenazi, B. (2009). Community-based intervention to reduce pesticide exposure to farmworkers and potential take-home exposure to their families. *Journal of Exposure Science & Environmental Epidemiology, 19,* 79–89.

Bradshaw, C. P., Waasdorp, T. E., Goldweber, A., & Johnson, S. L. (2013). Bullies, gangs, drugs, and school: Understanding the overlap and the role of ethnicity and urbanicity. *Journal of Youth & Adolescence, 42*(2), 220–234.

Branas, C., McKenzie, E., & Williams, J. (2005). Access to trauma centers in the United States. *Journal of the American Medical Association, 293,* 2626–2633.

Brown, A., & Lopez, M. H. (2013, August 29). Ranking Latino populations in the states. Retrieved from http://www.pewhispanic.org/2013/08/29/ii-ranking-latino-populations-in-the-states/

Brown, J. P., & Weber, J. G. (2013). *The off-farm occupations of U.S. farm operators and their spouses.* Retrieved from http://www.ers.usda.gov/media/1187209/eib-117.pdf013

Bryden, A., Roberts, B., McKee, M., & Petticrew, M. (2012). A systematic review of the influence on alcohol use of community level availability and marketing of alcohol. *Health & Place, 18*(2), 349–357.

Bureau of Economic Analysis. (2014, November 20). *Local area personal income, 2013.* Retrieved from http://www.bea.gov/newsreleases/regional/lapi/lapi_newsrelease.htm

Burns, C. J., Cohen, S. Z., & Lunchick, C. (2015). Neurodevelopmental disorders and agricultural pesticide exposures. *Environmental Health Perspectives, 123*(4), A79.

Byrne, T., Munley, E. A., Fargo, J. D., Montgomery, A. E., & Culhane, D. P. (2013). New perspectives on community-level determinants of homelessness. *Journal of Urban Affairs, 35*(5), 607–625.

Cadilhac, D. A., Kilkenny, T., Longworth, M., Pollack, M., & Levi, C. R. (2011). Metropolitan-rural divide for stroke outcomes: Do stroke units make a difference? *Internal Medicine Journal, 41*(4), 321–326.

Cadilhac, D. A., Purvis, T., Kilkenny, M. F., Longworth, M., Mohr, K., Pollack, M., ... Levi, C. R. (2013). Evaluation of rural stroke services: Does implementation of coordinators and pathways improve care in rural hospitals? *Stroke, 44,* 2848–2853.

Calancie, L., Leeman, J., Jilcott Pitts, S. B., Kettel Khan, L., Fleishhacker, S., Evenson, K. R., ... Ammerman, A. (2015). *Nutrition-related policy and environmental strategies to prevent obesity in rural communities: A systematic review of the literature, 2002-2013.* Retrieved from https://www.cdc.gov/pcd/issues/2015/14_0540.htm

Caldwell, D. R. (2007). Bloodroot: Life stories of nurse practitioners in rural Appalachia. *Journal of Holistic Nursing, 25,* 73–79.

California Department of Pesticide Exposure. (2013). *Pesticide illness surveillance program.* Retrieved from http://www.cdpr.ca.gov/docs/whs/pisp.htm

Cannuscio, C. C., Tappe, K., Hillier, A., Buttenheim, A., Karpyn, A., & Glanz, K. (2013). Urban food environments and residents' shopping behaviors. *American Journal of Preventive Medicine, 45*(5), 606–614.

Cant, R., Birks, M., Porter, J., Jacob, E., & Cooper, S. (2011). Developing advanced rural nursing practice: A whole new scope of responsibility. *Collegian, 18*(4), 177–182.

Castañeda, S. F., Rosenbaum, R. P., Holscher, J. T., Madanat, H., & Talavera, G. A. (2015). Cardiovascular disease risk factors among Latino migrant and seasonal farmworkers. *Journal of Agromedicine, 20*(2), 95–104.

Centers for Disease Control and Prevention (CDC). (2012). *HIV and AIDS in the United States by geographic distribution.* Retrieved from http://www.cdc.gov/hiv/pdf/statistics_geographic_distribution.pdf

Centers for Disease Control and Prevention (CDC). (2015). *HIV/AIDS.* Retrieved from www.cdc.gov/hiv/basics/statistics.html

Centers for Disease Control and Prevention (CDC). (2016). *Healthy places.* Retrieved from http://www.cdc.gov/healthyplaces/

Cerdá, M., Ransome, Y., Keyes, K. M., Koenen, K. C., Tardiff, K., & Gala, S. (2013). Revisiting the role of the urban environment in substance use: The case of analgesic overdose fatalities. *American Journal of Public Health, 103*(12), 2252–2260.

Chambers, E. C., Pichardo, M. S., & Rosenbaum, E. (2016). Sleep and the housing and neighborhood environment of urban Latino adults living in low-income housing: The AHOME study. *Behavioral Sleep Medicine, 14*(2), 169–184.

Chaudry, A., Capps, R., Pedroza, J. M., Castaneda, R. M., Santos, R., & Scott, M. M. (2010). *Facing our future: Children in the aftermath of immigration enforcement.* Washington, DC: The Urban Institute.

Chen, H., Burnett, R. T., Copes, R., Kwong, J. C., Villeneurve, P. J., ... Tu, J. V. (2016). Ambient fine particulate matter and mortality among survivors of myocardial infarction: Population-based cohort study. *Environmental Health Perspectives, 124*(9), 1421–1428.

Choi, S. B., Lee, Y. J., & Chang, Y. S. (2015, November 2). An empirical fact of urban health advantage vs. urban health penalty—scaling analysis of death count in four major disease categories. *Social Science Research Network.* Retrieved from http://dx.doi.org/10.2139/ssrn.2685480

Clark, C. R., Coull, B., Berkman, L. F., Buring, J., & Ridker, P. M. (2011). Geographic variation in cardiovascular inflammation among healthy women in the Women's Health Study. *PLoS ONE, 6*(11), e27468.

Cockburn, M., Mills, P., Zhang, X., Zadnick, J., Goldberg, D., & Ritz, B. (2011). Prostate cancer and ambient pesticide exposure in agriculturally intensive areas in California. *American Journal of Epidemiology, 173*(11), 1280–1288.

Cohen, J. H. (2010). Oaxacan migration and remittances as they relate to Mexican migration patterns. *Journal of Ethic and Migration Studies, 36*(1), 149–161.

Cole, A., & Crawford, L. (1991). Implementation and evaluation of the health resource program for migrant women in the Americus, Georgia area. In A. Bushy (Ed.), *Rural nursing* (Vol. 1, pp. 364–374). Newbury Park, CA: Sage Publications.

Connor, A., Layne, L. P., & Hilb, L. E. (2014). A narrative literature review on the health of migrant farm worker children in the USA. *International Journal of Migration, Health and Social Care, 10*(1), 1–17.

Connor, A., Layne, L., & Thomisee, K. (2010). Providing care for migrant farm worker families in their unique sociocultural context and environment. *Journal of Transcultural Nursing, 21*(2), 159–166.

Cook, N. L., & Lauer, M. S. (2011). The socio-geography of heart failure: Why it matters. *Circulation: Heart Failure, 4,* 244–245.

Coomber, K., Toumbourou, J. W., Miller, P., Staiger, P. K., Hemphill, S. A., & Catalano, R. F. (2011). Rural adolescent alcohol, tobacco, and illicit drug use: A comparison of students in Victoria, Australia, and Washington State, United States. *Journal of Rural Health,* 27(4), 409–415.

Coronado, G. D., Holte, S., Vigoren, E., Griffith, W. C., Barr, D. B., Faustman, E., & Thompson, B. (2011). Organophosphate pesticide exposure and residential proximity to nearby fields: Evidence for the drift pathway. *Journal of Occupational & Environmental Medicine,* 53(8), 884–891.

Council of Economic Advisors. (n.d.). *Strengthening the rural economy: The current state of rural America.* Retrieved from https://www.whitehouse.gov/administration/eop/cea/factsheets-reports/strengthening-the-rural-economy/the-current-state-of-rural-america

Coursen-Neff, Z. (2011, November 17). *Child farmworkers in the United States: A "worst form of child labor."* Retrieved from http://www.hrw.org/news/2011/11/17/child-farmworkers-united-states-worst-form-child-labor

Cristancho, S., Peters, K., & Garces, M. (2014). Health information preferences among Hispanic/Latino immigrants in the U.S. rural Midwest. *Global Health Promotion,* 21(1), 40–49.

Culyba, A. J., Ginsburg, K. R., Fein, J. A., Branas, C. C., Richmond, T. S., Miller, E., & Wiebe, D. J. (in press). Examining the role of supportive family connection in violence exposure among male youth in urban environments. *Journal of Interpersonal Violence,* pii: 0886260516646094.

Dave, G. J., Bibeau, D. L., Schulz, M. R., Aronson, R. E., Ivanov, L. L., Black, A., & Y Spann, L. (2013). *Journal of Clinical Hypertension (Greenwich),* 15(8), 562–569.

Davis, A. M., Bennett, K. J., Befort, C., & Nollen, N. (2011). Obesity and related health behaviors among urban and rural children in the U.S.: Data from the National Health and Nutrition Examination Survey 2003-2004 and 2005-2006. *Journal of Pediatric Psychology,* 36(6), 669–676.

Davis, K. D. (2012, January 26). Governmental fragmentation in metropolitan Detroit. *McNair Scholars Research Journal,* 4(1), article 4.

Davis, S. K., Gebreab, S., Quarells, R., & Gibbons, G. H. (2014). Social determinants of cardiovascular health among black and white women residing in Stroke Belt and Buckle regions of the South. *Ethnicity & Disease,* 24(2), 133–143.

DeGuzman, P. B., Merwin, E. I., & Bourguignon, C. (2013). Population density, distance to public transportation, and health of women in low-income neighborhoods. *Public Health Nursing,* 30(6), 478–490.

Demographia. (2012). *U.S. major metropolitan area population: 2000–2010.* Retrieved from http://www.demographia.com/db-2010usmet.pdf

de Snyder, V., Friel, S., Fotso, J. C., & Khadr, Z. (2011). Social conditions and urban health inequities: Realities, challenges and opportunities to transform the urban landscape through research and action. *Journal of Urban Health,* 88(6), 1183–1193.

Dewan, S. (2014, April 14). In many cities, rent is rising out of reach of middle class. *New York Times.* Retrieved from http://www.nytimes.com/2014/04/15/business/more-renters-find-30-affordability-ratio-unattainable.html?_r=0

Diabetologia. (2015, September 15). *Analysis of 21 studies shows exposure to pesticides is associated with increased risk of developing diabetes.* Retrieved from https://www.sciencedaily.com/releases/2015/09/150915211340.htm

DiPasquale, D. (2011). Rental housing: Current market conditions and the role of federal policy. *Cityscape: A Journal of Policy Development & Research,* 13(2), 57–70.

Dittrich, K. A., Lutfiyya, N., Kucharyski, C. J., Grygelko, J. T., Dillon, C. L., Hill, T. J., … Huot, K. L. (2015). A population-based cross-sectional study comparing depression and health service deficits between rural and non-rural U.S. military veterans. *Military Medicine,* 180(4), 428–435.

Dodd, V. J., Schenck, D. P., Chaney, E. H., & Padhya, T. (2016). Assessing oral cancer awareness among rural Latino migrant workers. *Journal of Immigrant & Minority Health,* 18(3), 552–560.

Dolkart, A. (2008). *Biography of a tenement house in New York City: An architectural history of 97 Orchard Street.* Chicago, IL: Center for American Places.

Doorenbos, A. Z., Eaton, L. H., Haozous, E., Towle, C., Revels, L., & Buchwald, D. (2010). Satisfaction with telehealth for cancer support groups in rural American Indian and Alaska Native communities. *Clinical Journal of Oncology Nursing,* 14(6), 765–770.

Dougherty, C. (2011, April 11). Population leaves heartland behind. *Wall Street Journal.* Retrieved from http://online.wsj.com/article/SB10001424052748704843404576251150723518240.html?mod=WSJ_hp_MID

Douglas, M. K., Pierce, J. U., Rosenkoetter, M., Pacquiao, D., Callister, L. C., Hattar-Pollara, M., … Purnell, L. (2011). Standards of practice for culturally competent nursing care: 2011 update. *Journal of Transcultural Nursing,* 22(4), 317–333.

Douthit, N., Kiv, S., Dwolatzky, T., & Biswas, S. (2015). Exposing some important barriers to health care access in the rural USA. *Public Health,* 129(6), 611–620.

Dow AgroSciences. (2015). *Products & applications.* Retrieved from http://www.dowagro.com/en-US/soil/Products

Drevdahl, D. J. (2013). Injustice, suffering, difference: How can community health nursing address the suffering of others? *Journal of Community Health Nursing,* 30(1), 49–58.

Dryden, J. (2016, February 3). Scientists more effectively control pain by targeting nerve cell's interior. *Brain in the News,* 23(3), 1–2.

Duke, M. R., & Cunradi, C. B. (2011). Measuring intimate partner violence among male and female farmworkers in San Diego County, CA. *Cultural Diversity & Ethnic Minority Psychology,* 17(1), 59–67.

Echeverria, S., Diez-Roux, A. V., Shea, S., Borrell, L. N., & Jackson, S. (2008). Associations of neighborhood problems and neighborhood social cohesion with mental health and health behaviors: The Multi-Ethnic Study of Atherosclerosis. *Health & Place,* 14(4), 853–865.

Economic Research Service (ERS). (2015). *Farm labor: Background.* Retrieved from http://www.ers.usda.gov/topics/farm-economy/farm-labor/background.aspx

Economic Research Service (ERS). (2016). *Rural America at a glance,* 2015 edition. Retrieved from http://www.ers.usda.gov/media/1952235/eib145.pdf

Eisenhauer, C. M., Hunter, J. L., & Pullen, C. H. (2010). Deep roots support new branches: The impact of dynamic, cross-generational rural culture on older women's response to formal healthcare. *Online Journal of Rural Nursing and Health Care,* 10(1), 48–59.

Evans, D. V., Cole, A. M., & Norris, T. E. (2015). Colonoscopy in rural communities: A systematic review of the frequency and quality. *Rural and Remote Health,* 15, 3057. Retrieved from www.rrh.org.av.publishedarticles/article_print_3057.pdf

Even, W. E., & MacPherson, D. A. (2015, September). *The Affordable Care Act and the growth of involuntary part-time employment.* Retrieved from http://dx.doi.org/10.2139/ssrn.2653995

Fairweather, G. C., Lincoln, M. A., & Ramsden, R. (2016, April). Speech-language pathology teletherapy in rural and remote educational settings: Decreasing service inequities. *International Journal of Speech-Language Pathology,* 1–11.

Falk-Raphael, A., & Betker, C. (2012). Witnessing social injustice downstream and advocating for health equity upstream: "The trombone slide" of nursing. *Advances in Nursing Science,* 35(2), 98–112.

Familiar, I., Borges, G., Orozco, R., & Medina-Mora, M. E. (2011). Mexican migration experiences to the US and risk for anxiety and depressive symptoms. *Journal of Affective Disorders,* 130(1–2), 83–91.

Fan, M., Gabbard, S., Alves Pena, A., & Perloff, J. M. (2014). *Why do fewer agricultural workers migrate now?* (IRLE Working Paper No. 117-14). Retrieved from http://irle.berkeley.edu/workingpapers/117-14.pdf

Farmworker Justice. (n.d.). *The dangers of pesticides for farmworkers.* Retrieved from http://www.fwjustice.org/pesticide-safety

Farmworker Justice. (2016). Migrant health centers. Retrieved from https://www.farmworkerjustice.org/content/migrant-health-centers

Fiandt, K., Doeschot, C., & Lanning, J. K. (2010). Characteristics of risk in patients of nurse practitioner safety net practices. *Journal of the American Academy of Nurse Practitioners,* 22, 474–479.

Fields, B. E., Bell, J. F., Moyce, S., & Bigbee, J. L. (2015). The impact of insurance instability on health service utilization: Does non-metropolitan residence make a difference? *Journal of Rural Health,* 31(1), 27–34.

Fields, B. E., Bigbee, J. L., & Bell, J. F. (2016). Associations of provider-to-population ratios and population health by county-level rurality. *Journal of Rural Health,* 32(3), 235–244.

Firebaugh, G., & Farrell, C. R. (2016). Still large, but narrowing: The sizable decline in racial neighborhood inequality in metropolitan America, 1980-2010. *Demography,* 53(1), 139–164.

Florida, R. (2012, April 6). *America's urban-rural work divide.* Retrieved from http://www.citylab.com/work/2012/04/americas-urban-rural-work-divide/1651/

Flynn, D. (2012, January 21). Jensen Farms owner fined for shoddy worker housing. *Food Safety News*. Retrieved from http://www.foodsafetynews.com/2012/01/civil-fine-imposed-on-eric-jensen-over-shoddy-migrant-housing/

Food and Drug Administration. (2015, November 18). *FDA moves quickly to approve easy-to-use nasal spray to treat opioid overdose*. Retrieved from http://www.fda.gov/NewsEvents/Newsroom/PressAnnouncements/ucm473505.htm

Formichelli, L. (2008). A harvest of hope. *Minority Nurse*. Retrieved from http://minoritynurse.com/immigrant-health/harvest-hope

Fox, M. (2015, July 7). *Heroin deaths quadruple across U.S.* Retrieved from http://www.nbcnews.com/health/health-news/heroin-deaths-quadruple-across-us-n388006

Freudenberg, N., & Olden, K. (2011). *Getting serious about the prevention of chronic disease. Public Health Research, Practice, and Policy*, 8(4), A90. Retrieved from http://www.cdc.gov/pcd/issues/2011/jul/10_0243.htm

Frey, W. H. (2012). *Population growth in metropolitan America since 1980: Putting the volatile 2000s in perspective*. Retrieved from http://www.brookings.edu/~/media/research/files/papers/2012/3/20-population-frey/0320_population_frey.pdf

Friel, S., Akerman, M., Hancock, T., Kumaresan, J., Marmot, M., Melin, T., & Vlahov, D. (2011a). Addressing the social and environmental determinants of urban health equity: Evidence for action and a research agenda. *Journal of Urban Health: Bulletin of the New York Academy of Medicine*, 88(5), 860–874.

Friel, S., Vlahov, D., & Buckley, R. M. (2011b). No data, no problem, no action: Addressing urban health inequity in the 21st century. *Journal of Urban Health*, 88(5), 858–859.

Frost, S. S., Goins, R. T., Hunter, R. H., Hooker, S. P., Bryant, L. L., Kruger, J., & Pluto, D. (2010). Effects of the built environment on physical activity of adults living in rural settings. *American Journal of Health Promotion*, 24(4), 267–283.

Fuchs, I., & Jotkowitz, A. (2012). Reversing the brain drain: the role of medical schools. *American Journal of Bioethics*, 12(5), 42–43.

Fullilove, M. T., & Cantal-Dupart, M. (2016). Medicine for the city: Perspective and solidarity as tools for making urban health. *Journal of Bioethical Inquiry*, 13(2), 215–221.

Gale, J. A. (2010). *Rural America: A look beyond the images*. Retrieved from https://www.chausa.org/publications/health-progress/article/september-october-2010/rural-america-a-look-beyond-the-images

Galloway, A. P., & Henry, M. (2014). Relationships between social connectedness and spirituality and depression and perceived health status of rural residents. *Journal of Rural Nursing & Health Care*, 14(2), 43–79.

Gamble, J., Eurich, D., Ezekowitz, J., Kaul, P., Qua, H., & McAlister, F. (2011). Patterns of care and outcomes differ for urban versus rural patients with newly diagnosed heart failure, even in a universal healthcare system. *Circulation: Heart Failure*, 4(3) 317–323.

Garcia, C. M., Gilchrist, L., Vazquez, G., Leite, A., & Raymond, N. (2011). Urban and rural immigrant Latino youths' and adults' knowledge and beliefs about mental health resources. *Journal of Immigrant & Minority Health*, 13, 500–509.

Gau, J. M., Corsaro, N., & Brunson, R. K. (2014). Revisiting broken window theory: A test of the mediation impact of social mechanisms on the disorder-fear relationship. *Journal of Criminal Justice*, 42, 579–588.

Geiger, C. T. (2009). *Educational leaders and migrant populations: Policies and issues in the state of Florida*. Doctoral dissertation, University of Florida. Retrieved from http://etd.fcla.edu/UF/UFE0024877/geiger_c.pdf

Genberg, B. L., Astemborski, J., Vlahov, D., Kirk, G. D., & Mehta, S. H. (2015). Incarceration and injection drug use in Baltimore, Maryland. *Addiction*, 110(7), 1152–1159.

Ghosh-Dastidar, B., Cohen, D., Hunter, G., Zenk, S. N., Huang, C., Beckman, R., & Dubowitz, T. (2014). Distance to store, food prices, and obesity in urban food deserts. *American Journal of Preventive Medicine*, 47(5), 587–595.

Gielen, A. C., Shields, W., McDonald, E., Frattaroli, S., Bishai, D., & Ma, X. (2012). Home safety and low-income urban housing quality. *Pediatrics*, 130(6), 1053–1059.

Gillam, C. (2016, May 6). *What killed Jack McCall? A California farmer dies and a case against Monsanto takes root*. Retrieved from http://www.huffingtonpost.com/carey-gillam/what-killed-jack-mccall-a_b_9852216.html

Gilster, M. E. (2014). Neighborhood stressors, mastery, and depressive symptoms: Racial and ethnic differences in an ecological model of the stress process in Chicago. *Journal of Urban Health*, 91(4), 690–706.

Glasgow, N., & Berry, E. H. (Eds.). (2013). *Rural aging in 21st century America*. New York, NY: Springer.

Glauber, R. (2013, Summer). *Wanting more but working less: Involuntary part-time employment and economic vulnerability* (Issue Brief No. 64). Durham, NH: Carsey Institute.

Gleeson, S. (2010). Labor rights for all? The role of undocumented immigrant status for worker claims making. *Law & Social Inquiry*, 35(3), 561–602.

Goldsmith, W., & Blakely, E. (2010). *Separate societies: Poverty and inequality in U.S. cities* (2nd ed.). Philadelphia, PA: Temple University Press.

Goldstein, B., Howe, B., & Tamir, I. (2010). *Weeding out abuses: Recommendations for a law-abiding farm labor system*. Retrieved from http://www.fwjustice.org/files/immigration-labor/weeding-out-abuses.pdf

Gonzalez, A., Billings, L., Shin, D., Rosenbaum, R., & Song, W. (2013). Health disparities in migrant and seasonal farmworker children in Michigan. *Journal of the Academy of Nutrition and Dietetics*, 113(9), A74–A80.

Gorski, M. S. (2011). *Advancing health in rural America: Maximizing nursing's impact*. Retrieved from http://campaignforaction.org/sites/default/diles/rural-health-nursing-gorski.pdf

Gottlieb, A., Hoehndorf, R., Dumontier, M., & Altman, R. B. (2015). Ranking adverse drug reactions with crowdsourcing. *Journal of Medical Internet Research*, 17(3), e80.

Gottlieb, L., Glymour, M. M., Kersten, E., Taing, E., Hagan, E., Vlahov, D., & Adler, N. E. (2016). Challenges to an integrated population health research agenda: Targets, scale, tradeoffs and timing. *Social Science & Medicine*, 150, 279–285.

Graves, B. A., Ford, C. D., & Mooney, K. D. (2013). Telehealth technologies for heart failure disease management in rural areas: An integrative review. *Online Journal of Rural Nursing & Health Care*, 13(2), 56–83.

Greene, M., Perkins, M. M., Scott, K., & Burt, C. (2011). State responsibilities to support rural caregiving: The Georgia example. In R. C. Talley, K. Chwalisz, & K. C. Buckwalter (Eds.), *Rural caregiving in the United States: Research, practice, policy* (pp. 213–231). New York, NY: Springer Science.

Groh, C. J. (2012). Depression in rural women: Implications for nurse practitioners in primary care settings. *Journal of the American Association of Nurse Practitioners*, 25, 84–90.

Gruca, T. S., Nam, I., & Tracy, R. (2014). Trends in medical oncology outreach clinics in rural areas. *Journal of Oncology Practice*, 10(5), e313–e320.

Haas, S., Stukel, T. A., Gomez, D., Zagorski, B., De Mestral, C., Sharma, S.V., … Nathens, A. B. (2012). The mortality benefit of direct trauma center transport in a regional trauma system: A population-based analysis. *Journal of Trauma & Acute Care Surgery*, 72(6), 1510–1517.

Habib, R. R., & Fathallah, F. A. (2012). Migrant women farm workers in the occupational literature. *Work*, 41, 4356–4362.

Hanlon, B. (2012). *Once the American dream: Inner-ring suburbs of the metropolitan United States*. Philadelphia, PA: Temple University Press.

Hansen, A. Y., Umstattd Meyer, M. R., Lenardson, J. D., & Hartley, D. (2015). Built environments and active living in rural and remote areas: A review of the literature. *Current Obesity Reports*, 4(4), 484–493.

Harris, D. E., Aboueissa, A. M., Baugh, N., & Sarton, C. (2015). Impact of rurality on maternal and infant health indicators and outcomes in Maine. *Rural & Remote Health*, 15(3), 1–17.

Harvey, I. S., & Janke, M. (2014). Qualitative exploration of rural focus group members' participation in the chronic disease self-management program, USA. *Rural & Remote Health*, 14(4), 1–13.

Hawk, W. (2013). Expenditures of urban and rural households in 2011. *Beyond the Numbers: Prices & Spending*, 2(5). Retrieved from http://www.bls.gov/opub/btn/volume-2/expenditures-of-urban-and-rural-households-in-2011.htm

Hayes, J. C. (2011). Megacities. *Public Health Nursing*, 28(3), 201–202.

Health Resources and Services Administration (HRSA). (n.d.a). *Shortage designation: Health professional shortage areas and medically underserved areas/populations*. Retrieved from http://www.hrsa.gov/shortage/mua/

Health Resources and Services Administration (HRSA). (n.d.b). *Telehealth*. Retrieved from http://www.hrsa.gov/telehealth/default.htm

Health Resources and Services Administration (HRSA). (2013, July). *Public health workforce enumeration, 2012*. Retrieved from http://www.phf.org/resourcestools/Documents/UM_CEPHS_Enumeration2012_Revised_July_2013.pdf

Health Resources and Services Administration (HRSA). (2015). *Designated health professional shortage areas statistics.* Retrieved from https://ersrs.hrsa.org/ReportServer?/HGDW_Reports/BCD_HPSA/BCD_HPSA_SCR50_Smry_HTML&rc:Toolbar=false

Hernandez, D. (2015). An uphill battle: Health care on the other side of the mountain. *Rural Roads, 13*(2), 7–10.

Hernandez, K., Mata, H., Vasquez, E. P., & Martinez, J. (2014). Community outreach along the U.S./Mexico border: Developing HIV health education strategies to engage rural populations. *Online Journal of Rural Nursing and Health Care, 14*(1). doi: http://dx.doi.org/10.14574/ojrnhc.v14i1.302

Hernandez, D. C., Reesor, L., Alonso, Y., Eagleton, S. G., & Hughes, S. O. (2015). Household food insecurity status and Hispanic immigrant children's body mass index and adiposity. *Journal of Applied Research on Children, 6*(2). Retrieved from http://digitalcommons.library.tmc.edu/childrenatrisk/vol6/iss2/14/

Hernández-Garduño, E., Mendoza-Damián, F., Garduño-Alanis, A., & Ayón-Garibaldo, S. (2015). Tuberculosis in Mexico and the USA, comparison of trends over time 1990-2010. *Tuberculosis and Respiratory Diseases, 78*(3), 246–252.

Hertz, T., Kusmin, L., Marré, A., & Parker, T. (2014, October 6). *Rural employment in recession and recovery. Amber Waves.* Washington, DC: USDA.

Hess, J. J., McCowell, J. Z., Luber, G. (2012). Integrating climate change adaptation into public health practice: Using adaptive management to increase adaptive capacity and build resilience. *Environmental Health Perspectives, 120*(2), 171–179.

Hill, B. G., Moloney, A. G., Mize, T., Himelick, T., & Guest, J. L. (2011). Prevalence and predictors of food insecurity in migrant farmworkers in Georgia. *American Journal of Public Health, 101*(5), 831–833.

Hiott, A., Grzywacz, J., Davis, S., Quandt, S. A., & Arcury, T. A. (2008). Migrant farmworker stress: Mental health implications. *Journal of Rural Health, 24*(1), 32–39.

Hodson, R. (2016). Urban health and well-being. *Nature, 531*(7594), s49.

Hoerster, K. D., Mayer, J. A., Gabbard, S., Kronick, R. G., Roesch, S. C., Malcarne, V. L., & Zuniga, M. L. (2011). Impact of individual-, environmental-, and policy-level factors on health care utilization among US farmworkers. *American Journal of Public Health, 101*(4), 685–692.

Holden, C. (n.d.). *Migrant health issues: Housing.* Monograph No. 8. Buda, TX: National Center for Farmworker Health.

Holmes, M., & Pink, G. (2011, April). *Risk of financial distress among critical access hospitals: A proposed model.* Retrieved from http://www.flexmonitoring.org/documents/PolicyBrief20_Strategies.pdf

Holmes, S. M. (2009). The clinical gaze in the practice of migrant health: Mexican migrants in the United States. *Social Science & Medicine, 74*(6), 873–881.

Honoré, P. A., Wright, D., Berwick, D. M., Clancy, C. M., Lee, P., Nowinski, J., & Koh, H. K. (2011). Creating a framework for getting quality into the public health system. *Health Affairs, 30*(4), 737–745.

Hou, S. I. (2010). Health literacy, e-health, and communication: Putting the consumer first. *Health Promotion Practice, 11*(3), 303–306.

Housing Assistance Council (HAC). (n.d.). *Farmworkers.* Washington, DC: Author. Retrieved from http://www.ruralhome.org/storage/documents/farmoverview.pdf

Housing Assistance Council (HAC). (2013). *Rental housing in rural America. Rural Research Note.* Washington, DC: Author.

Howard, V. J., McClure, L. A., Glymour, M. M., Cunningham, S. A., Kleindorfer, D. O., Crowe, M., ... Lackland, D. T. (2013). Effect of duration and age of exposure to the Stroke Belt on incident stroke in adulthood. *Neurology, 80*(18), 1655–1661.

Hsia, R. Y., & Shen, Y. C. (2011a). Possible geographical barriers to trauma center access for vulnerable patients in the United States: An analysis of urban and rural communities. *Archives of Surgery, 146*(1), 446–452.

Hsia, R. Y., & Shen, Y. C. (2011b). Rising closures of hospital trauma centers disproportionally burden vulnerable populations. *Health Affairs, 30*(10), 1912–1920.

Hubach, R. D., Dodge, B., Li, M. J., Schick, V., Herbenick, D., Ramos, W. D., ... Reece, M. (2015). Loneliness, HIV-related stigma, and condom use among a predominantly rural sample of HIV-positive men who have sex with men (MSM). *AIDS Education & Prevention, 27*(1), 72–83.

Huber, B. (2011, June 18). *Will the EPA help farmers fight pesticide poisoning?* Retrieved from http://grist.org/industrial-agriculture/2011-06-22-public-health-advocates-urge-epa-to-require-pesticide-makers/

Huseth, A., Vachal, K., Benson, L., & Lofgren, M. (2011). *Pilot study to assess sustained and multifaceted traffic activity on North Dakota's rural roads.* Retrieved from http://ntl.bts.gov/lib/45000/45300/45379/MPC11–233.pdf

Ieri, V. (2015, May 5). *Urban slums a death trap for poor children.* Retrieved from http://www.ipsnews.net/2015/05/urban-slums-a-death-trap-for-poor-children/

Iezzoni, L., Killeen, M., & O'Day, B. (2006). Rural residents with disabilities confront substantial barriers to obtaining care. *HSR: Health Services Research, 41*(4), 1258–1275.

Iezzoni, L., Frakt, A., & Pizer, S. (2011). Uninsured persons with disability confront substantial barriers to health care services. *Disability and Health Journal, 4*(4), 238–244.

Ingleby, D., Chiarenza, A., Deville, W., & Kotsioni, I. (Eds.). (2012). Inequalities in healthcare for migrants in ethnic minorities. *COST Series on Health and Diversity* (Vol. 2). Antwerp, Belgium: Garant Publishing.

Ip, E. H., Saldana, S., Arcury, T. A., Grzywacz, J. G., Trejo, G., & Quant, S.A. (2015). Profiles of food security for US farmworker households and factors related to dynamic of change. *American Journal of Public Health, 105*(10), e42–e47.

Isler, M. R., Miles, M., Banks, B., & Corbie-Smith, G. (2012). Acceptability of a mobile health unit for rural HIV clinical trial enrollment and participation. *AIDS and Behavior.* doi: 10.10997/s10461-012-0151-z.

Jackson, M. N. G., & McCulloch, B. J. (2014). Heart attack symptoms and decision-making: The case of older rural women. *Rural & Remote Health, 14*(2), 1–13.

James, W. L. (2014). All rural places are not created equal: Revisiting the rural mortality penalty in the United States. *American Journal of Public Health, 104*(11), 2122–2129.

Jasis, P., & Marriott, D. (2010). All for our children: Migrant families and parent participation in an alternative education program. *Journal of Latinos and Education, 9*(2), 126–140.

Jasis, P. M., & Ordoñez-Jasis, R. (2012). Latino parent involvement: Examining commitment and empowerment in schools. *Urban Education, 47*(1), 65–89.

Jennings, W. G., Maldonado-Molina, M. M., Reingle, J. M., & Komro, K. A. (2011). A multi-level approach to investigating neighborhood effects on physical aggression among urban Chicago youth. *American Journal of Criminal Justice, 36*(4), 392–407.

Jensen, L., Mattingly, M. J., & Bean, J. A. (2011, Summer). *TANF in rural America: Informing re-authorization* (Policy Brief No. 19). Durham, NH: Carsey Institute. Retrieved from http://scholars.unh.edu/cgi/viewcontent.cgi?article=1145&context=carsey

Jiao, Y., Bower, J. K., Im, W., Basta, N., Obrycki, J., Al-Hamdan, M. Z., ... Hood, D. B. (2015). Application of citizen science risk communication tools in a vulnerable urban community. *International Journal of Environmental Research & Public Health, 13*(1), 11.

Johns Hopkins University. (2016). *Urban Health Institute: About us.* Retrieved from http://urbanhealth.jhu.edu/about_us/

Johnson, K. M., & Lichter, D. T. (2012). Rural natural increase in the new century: America's demographic transition. *International Handbook of Rural Demography, 3*, 17–34.

Jones-Webb, R., & Karriker-Jaffe, K. J. (2013). Neighborhood disadvantage, high alcohol content beverage consumption drinking norms, and drinking consequences: A mediation analysis. *Journal of Urban Health, 90*(4), 667–684.

Jordan, J. L., Kostandini, G., & Mykerezi, E. (2012). Rural and urban high school dropout rates: Are they different? *Journal of Research in Rural Education, 27*(12), 1–21.

Jostad-Laswell, A., Guendelman, S., & Castañeda, X. (2013). *Traditional, contemporary, and alternative medicine in Mexican-origin populations.* Retrieved from https://hiaucb.files.wordpress.com/2014/04/traditional-complementary-and-alternative-medicine.pdf

Joynt, K. E., Harris, Y., Orav, E. J., & Jha, A. K. (2011). Quality of care and patient outcomes in critical access rural hospitals. *Journal of the American Medical Association, 306*(1), 45–52.

Kapoor, S., & Thorn, B. E. (2014). Healthcare use and prescription of opioids in rural residents with pain. *Rural & Remote Health, 14*(3), 1–12.

Kasner, E. J., Keralis, J. M., Mehler, L., Beckman, J., Bonnar-Prado, J., Lee, S. J., ... Calvert, G. M. (2012). Gender differences in acute pesticide-related illnesses and injuries among farmworkers in the United States, 1998-2007. *American Journal of Industrial Medicine, 55*(7), 571–583.

Kegler, M. C., Escoffery, C., Alcantara, I. C., Hinman, J., Addison, A., & Glanz, K. (2012). Perceptions of social and environmental support for healthy eating and physical activity in rural Southern churches. *Journal of Religion and Health, 51*(3), 799–811.

Keizer, K., Lindenberg, S., & Steg, L. (2008). The spreading of disorder. *Science, 322*(5908), 1681–1685.

Keyes, K. M., Cerda, M., Brady, J. E., Havens, J. R., & Galea, S. (2014). Understanding the rural-urban differences in nonmedical prescription opioid use and abuse in the United States. *American Journal of Public Health, 104*(2), e52–e59.

Keller, L. O., Strohschein, S., & Schaffer, M. A. (2011). Cornerstones of public health nursing. *Public Health Nursing, 28*(3), 249–260.

Kilanowski, J. F. (2012). Midwest growers' mail survey of contributors to migrant health and nutrition. *Journal of Agromedicine, 17*(4), 377–385.

Kilkenny, M. (2010). Urban/regional economics and rural development. *Journal of Regional Science, 50*(1), 449–470.

Kim, K. N., Lim, Y. H., Bae, H. J., Kim, M., Jung, K., & Hong, Y. C. (2016). Long-term fine particulate matter exposure and major depressive disorder in a community-based urban cohort. *Environmental Health Perspectives, 124*(10), 1547–1553.

Kim, S., Mazza, J., Zwanziger, J., & Henry, D. (2014). School and behavioral outcomes among inner city children: Five-year follow-up. *Urban Education, 49*(7), 835–856.

Kim-Godwin, Y. S., Maume, M. O., & Fox, J. A. (2014). Depression, stress, and intimate partner violence among Latino migrant and seasonal farmworkers in rural southeast North Carolina. *Journal of Immigrant Minority Health, 16*, 1217–1224.

Kirkpatrick, S., & Tarasuk, V. (2011). Housing circumstances are associated with household food access among low-income urban families. *Journal of Urban Health, 88*(2), 284–296.

Kliewer, W., & Lepore, S. J. (2015). Exposure to violence, social cognitive processing, and sleep problems in urban adolescents. *Journal of Youth & Adolescence, 44*(2), 507–517.

Kneebone, E., & Raphael, S. (2011, May). *City and suburban crime trends in metropolitan America.* Retrieved from https://gspp.berkeley.edu/assets/uploads/research/pdf/p66.pdf

Kneebone, E. (2014). *Confronting suburban poverty in America.* Retrieved from http://ag.purdue.edu/programs/hhs/efnep/Conferences/KeynoteAddress-ConfrontingSurburbanPovertyinAmerica.pdf

Knudsen, A., & Meit, M. (n.d.). *Public health nursing: Strengthening the core of rural public health* (Policy Brief). Kansas City, MO: National Rural Health Association.

Kraemer-Diaz, A. E., Weir, N. M., Isom, S., Quandt, S. A., Chen, H., & Arcury, T. A. (2016). Aggression among male migrant farmworkers living in camps in Eastern North Carolina. *Journal of Immigration & Minority Health, 18*(3), 542–551.

Kresge Foundation. (2012). *Health-related inequities among hired farm workers and the resurgence of labor-intensive agriculture.* Retrieved from http://kresge.org/sites/default/files/Health-farm-worker-whitepaper.pdf

Krishna, S., Gillespie, K. N., & McBride, T. M. (2010). Diabetes burden and access to preventive care in the rural United States. *Journal of Rural Health, 26*(1), 3–11.

Krogstad, J. M. (2015, June 25). *Hispanic population reaches record 55 million, but growth has cooled.* Retrieved from http://www.pewresearch.org/fact-tank/2015/06/25/u-s-hispanic-population-growth-surge-cools/

Krogstad, J. M., & Fry, R. (2014, April 24). *More Hispanics, Blacks enrolling in college, but lag in bachelor's degrees.* Retrieved from http://www.pewresearch.org/fact-tank/2014/04/24/more-hispanics-blacks-enrolling-in-college-but-lag-in-bachelors-degrees/

Kronkosky Charitable Foundation. (2011, January). *Rural healthcare research brief.* Retrieved from http://www.kronkosky.org/research/Research_Briefs/Rural%20Healthcare%20January%202011.pdf

Kugel, C., Retzlaff, C., Hopfer, S., Lawson, D., Daley, E., Drewes, C., & Freedman, S. (2009). Familias con Voz: Community survey results from an intimate partner violence (IPV) prevention project with migrant workers. *Journal of Family Violence, 24*(8), 649–660.

Kulbok, P. A., Thatcher, E., Park, E., & Meszaros, P. S. (2012). Evolving public health nursing roles. *Online Journal of Issues in Nursing, 17*(2). Retrieved from www.me-scape.com/viewarticle/772434

Kutscher, B. (2014). Wiring in rural patients. *Modern Healthcare, 44*(10), 1–20.

Laidlaw, M. A., Filippelli, G. M., Sadler, R. C., Gonzales, C. R., Ball, A. S., & Mielke, H. W. (2016). Children's blood lead seasonality in Flint, Michigan and soil-sourced lead hazard risks. *International Journal of Environmental Research & Public Health, 13*(4), e358.

Langton, L., & Truman, J. (2015). *Criminal victimization, 2014.* Retrieved from http://www.bjs.gov/content/pub/press/cv14pr.cfm

Latkin, C. A., German, D., Vlahov, D., & Galea, S. (2013). Neighborhoods and HIV: A social ecological approach to prevention and care. *American Psychologist, 68*(4), 210–224.

Layton, L. (2015, January 16). Majority of U.S. public school students are in poverty. *The Washington Post.* Retrieved from https://www.washingtonpost.com/local/education/majority-of-us-public-school-students-are-in-poverty/2015/01/15/df7171d0-9ce9-11e4-a7ee-526210d665b4_story.html

Lee, H., Ahn, H., Miller, A., Park, C. G., & Kim, S. J. (2012). Acculturative stress, workload-related psychosocial factors, and depression in Korean-Chinese migrant workers in Korea. *Journal of Occupational Health, 54*, 206–214.

Lee, K., & Pond, D. (2015). The impact of Head Start enrollment duration on migrant children's health outcomes. *Social Work in Health Care, 54*(10), 869–891.

Lee, K., & Song, W. (2015). Effect of enrollment length in Migrant Head Start on children's weight outcomes. *Health & Social Work, 40*(2), 142–150.

Lee, L. T., Alexandrov, A. W., Howard, V. J., Kabagambe, E. K., Hess, M. A., McLain, R. M., ... Howard, G. (2014a). Race, regionality, and pre-diabetes in the Reasons for Geographic and Racial Differences in Stroke (REGARDS) study. *Preventive Medicine, 63*, 43–47.

Lee, S. J., Mehler, L., Beckman, J., Diebolt-Brown, B., Prado, J., Lackovic, M., Waltz, J., ... Calvert, G. M. (2011). Acute pesticide illnesses associated with off-target pesticide drift from agricultural applications: 11 states, 1998-2006. *Environmental Health Perspectives, 119*(8), 1162–1169.

Lee, S. J., Mulay, P., Diebolt-Brown, B., & Lackovic, M. J. (2010). Acute illnesses associated with exposure to fipronil—surveillance data from 11 states in the United States, 2001–2007. *Clinical Toxicology, 48*(7), 737–744.

Lee, W. C., Jiang, L., Phillips, C. D., & Ohsfeldt, R. L. (2014b). Rural-urban differences in health are expenditures: Empirical data from US households. *Advances in Public Health,* Article ID 435780.

Leigh, J. P., Du, J., & McCurdy, S. A. (2014). An estimate of the U.S. government's undercount of nonfatal occupational injuries and illnesses in agriculture. *Annals of Epidemiology, 24*(4), 254–259.

Lenardson, J. D., Hansen, A., & Hartley, D. (2015). Rural and remote food environments and obesity. *Current Obesity Reports, 4*(1), 46–53.

Lerner, A. (2011). *Migrant labor, immigration, and food production.* Retrieved from http://find.galegroup.com/gic/infomark.do?&source=gale&idigest=a24509ee707e3735cde6db3e17c5304e&prodId=GIC&userGroupName=bhs&tabID=T001&docId=CX1918600173&type=retrieve&version=1.0

Levy, C. E., Silverman, E., Huanguang, J., Geiss, M., & Omura, D. (2015). Effects of physical therapy delivery via home video telerehabilitation on functional and health-related quality of life outcomes. *Journal of Rehabilitation Research & Development, 52*(3), 361–320.

Lewis, K. M., Schure, M. B., Bavarian, N., DuBois, D. L., Day, J., Ji, P., ... Flay, B. R. (2013). Problem behavior and urban, low-income youth: A randomized controlled trial of positive action in Chicago. *American Journal of Preventive Medicine, 44*(6), 622–630.

Li, Y., Zhang, D., & Pagán, J. A. (2016). Social norms and the consumption of fruits and vegetables across New York City neighborhoods. *Journal of Urban Health, 93*(2), 244–255.

Lipsky, A. M., Karsteadt, L. L., Gaushe-Hill, M., Hartmans, S., Bongard, F. S., Cryer, H. G., ... Lewis, R. J. (2014). A comparison of rural versus urban trauma care. *Journal of Emergencies, Trauma, and Shock, 7*(1), 41–46.

Lishner, D. M., Richardson, M., Levine, P., & Patrick, D. (n.d.). *Access to primary health care among persons with disabilities in rural areas: A summary of the literature.* Retrieved from http://www.amsa.org/programs/barriers/access.pdf

Loue, S., & Quill, B. E. (Eds.). (2010). *Handbook of rural health.* New York, NY: Kluwer Academic/Plenum Publishers.

Lucio, R. L., Zuniga, G. C., Seal, Y. H., Garza, N., Mier, N., & Trevino, L. (2011). Incorporating what *promotoras* learn: Becoming role models to effect positive change. *Journal of Community Health, 37*(5), 1026–1031.

Luque, J. S., & Castañeda, H. (2013). Delivery of mobile clinic services to migrant and seasonal farmworkers: A review of practice models for community-academic partnerships. *Journal of Community Health, 38*(2), 397–407.

Luque, J. S., Reyes-Ortiz, C., Marella, P., Bowers, A., Panchal, V., Anderson, L. & Charles, S. (2012). Mobile farm clinic outreach to address health conditions among Latino migrant farmworkers in Georgia. *Journal of Agromedicine, 17*(4), 386–397.

MacDonald, J. M. (2014, March 4). *Family farming in the United States.* Retrieved from http://www.ers.usda.gov/amber-waves/2014-march/family-farming-in-the-united-states.aspx#.VzNol2Mqhwg

MacDowell, M., Glasser, M., Fitts, M., Nielsen, K., & Hunsaker, M. (2013). A national view of rural health workforce issues in the USA. *Rural Remote Health, 10*(3), 1531.

Maez, L., Erickson, L., & Naumuk, L. (2014). Diabetic education in rural areas. *Rural & Remote Health, 14*(2), 1–7.

Mahamoud, A., Roche, B., & Homer, J. (2013). Modeling the social determinants of health and simulating short-term and long-term intervention impacts for the city of Toronto, Canada. *Social Science & Medicine, 93*, 247–255.

Manini, A. F., Jacobs, M. M., Vlahov, D., & Hurd, Y. L. (2013). Opioid receptor polymorphism A118G associated with clinical severity in a drug overdose population. *Journal of Medical Toxicology, 9*(2), 148–154.

Maring, E. F., Singer, B. J., & Shenassa, E. (2011, April). Healthy homes: A contemporary initiative for extension education. *Journal of Extension, 49*(2), article 2FEA9.

Martinez-Donate, A. P., Zhang, X., Rangel, M. G., Hovell, M., Simon, N. J., Amuedo-Dorantes, C., ... Guendelman, S. (2014). Healthcare access among circular and undocumented Mexican migrants: Results from a pilot survey on the Mexico-US border. *International Journal of Migration & Border Studies, 1*(1), 57–108.

Massey, D. S., & Brown, A. E. (2011). New migration stream between Mexico and Canada. *Migraciones Internacionales, 6*(1), 119–144.

Maternal Child Health Bureau. (2011). *Population characteristics: Rural and urban women. Women's Health USA 2011.* Retrieved from http://www.mchb.hrsa.gov/whusa11/popchar/downloads/pdfs/103ruw.pdf

Mather, M., Pollard, K., & Jacobsen, L. A. (2012). *First results from the 2010 Census.* Retrieved from http://www.prb.org/Publications/ReportsOnAmerica/2011/census-2010.aspx

Mather, S., & Parameswaran, G. (2012). School readiness for young migrant children: The challenge and the outlook. *International Scholarly Research Network, 2012.* Article ID 847502. doi: 10.5402/2012/847502.

Matsui, E. C. (2014). Environmental exposures and asthma morbidity in children living in urban neighborhoods. *Allergy, 69*(5), 553–558.

Matte, T. D., Lane, K., & Ito, K. (2016). Excess mortality attributable to extreme heat in New York City, 1997–2013. *Health Security, 14*(2), 64–70.

Maxmen, A. (2016). Stress: The privilege of health. *Nature, 531*(7594), s58–s59.

McCormack, G. R., & Shiell, A. (2011). In search of causality: A systematic review of the relationship between the built environment and physical activity among adults. *International Journal of Behavioral Nutrition and Physical Activity, 8*, 125. Retrieved from http://www.ijbnpa.org/content/8/1/125

McGranahan, D., Cromartie, J., & Wojan, T. (2010, November). *Nonmetropolitan outmigration counties: Some are poor, many are prosperous.* Washington, DC: USDA Economic Research Service. ERR-107.

McIllhenny, C. V., Guzic, B. L., Knee, D. R., Demuth, B. R., & Roberts, J. B. (2011). Using technology to deliver healthcare education to rural patients. *Rural & Remote Health, 11*(4), 1–11.

Mejia, O. L., & McCarthy, C. J. (2010). Acculturative stress, depression, and anxiety in migrant farmwork college students of Mexican heritage. *International Journal of Stress Management, 17*(1), 1–20.

Merchant, J., Coussens, C., & Gilbert, D. (2006). *Rebuilding the unity of health and the environment in rural America.* Washington, DC: National Academies Press.

Midwest Regional Educational Laboratory. (2013, May). *Relationship between bus ride and academic achievement & rural student experiences on buses.* Retrieved from http://www.relmidwest.org/sites/default/files/RDR2013_05_QP8665692_Length%20of%20Bus%20Ride_web.pdf

Migrant Clinicians Network (MCN). (n.d.). *Monograph series: Domestic violence in the farmworker population: Resources for clinicians.* Retrieved from http://www.migrantclinician.org/files/resourcebox/DVMonograph.pdf

Migrant Clinicians Network (MCN). (2013). *2012 year in review for Health Network.* Retrieved from http://www.migrantclinician.org/files/HealthNetworkYearInReview2012_English.pdf

Migrant Clinicians Network (MCN). (2016). *The migrant/seasonal farmworker.* Retrieved from http://www.migrantclinician.org/issues/migrant-info/migrant.html

Migrant Housing. (n.d.). *Migrant center housing.* Retrieved from www.stancoha.org/Migrant.htm

Migration Policy Institute. (2015, September 21). *Deportation of a parent can have significant and long-lasting harmful effects on child well-being, as a pair of reports from MPI and the Urban Institute detail.* Retrieved from http://www.migrationpolicy.org/news/deportation-parent-can-have-significant-and-long-lasting-harmful-effects-child-well-being-pair

Minetor, R. (2010). *A guided tour through history: New York immigrant experience.* Guilford, CT: Morris Book Publishing, LLC.

Miro, A., Perrotta, K., Evans, H., Kishchuk, N. A., Gram, C., Stanwick, R. S., & Swinkels, H. M. (2014). Building the capacity of health authorities to influence land use and transportation planning: Lessons learned from the Healthy Canada by Design CLASP project in British Columbia. *Canadian Journal of Public Health, 106*(Suppl. 1), s40–s52.

MiVIA. (2013). *Connecting patients and clinicians nationwide: Welcome to MiVIA.* Retrieved from https://www.mivia.org

Mmari, K., Lantos, H., Brahmbhatt, H., Delany-Moretlwe, S., Lou, C., Sangowawa, A., Acharya, R., & Sangowawa, A. (2014). How adolescents perceive their communities: A qualitative study that explores the relationship between health and the physical environment. *BMC Public Health, 14*, 349.

Mmari, K., Marshall, B., Lantos, H., & Blum, R. W. (2016). Who adolescents trust may impact their health: Findings from Baltimore. *Journal of Urban Health, 93*(3), 468–478.

Molokwu, J., Penaranda, E., Flores, S., & Shokar, N. K. (2015). Evaluation of the effect of a promotora-led educational intervention on cervical cancer and human papillomavirus knowledge among predominately Hispanic primary care patients on the US-Mexico border. *Journal of Cancer Education.* doi: 10:1007s13187-015-0938-5.

Montague, E., & Perchonok, J. (2012). Health and wellness technology use by historically underserved health consumers: Systematic review. *Journal of Medical Internet Research, 14*(3), e78. doi: 10.2196/jmir.2095.

Moskowitz, P. (2014, April 28). High school graduation rate hits 80 percent for first time. *Aljazeera America.* Retrieved from http://america.aljajeera.com/articles/2014/4/28/graduation-rates80.html

Mullen, M. T., Wiebe, D. J., Bowman, A., Wolff, C. S., Albright, K. C., Roy, J., ... Carr, B.G. (2014). Disparities in accessibility of certified primary stroke centers. *Stroke, 45*(11), 3381–3388.

Mulligan, R., Seirawan, H., Faust, S., & Habibian, M. (2010). Mobile dental clinic: An oral health care delivery model for underserved migrant children. *Journal of the California Dental Association, 38*(2), 115–122.

Murphy, D. J., Myers, J., McKenzie, E. A., Cavaletto, R., May, J., & Sorensen, J. (2010). Tractors and rollover protection in the United States. *Journal of Agromedicine, 15*(3), 249–263.

Nandi, A., Prescott, M. R., Cerdá, M., Vlahov, D., Tardiff, K. J., & Galea, S. (2012). Economic conditions and suicide rates in New York City. *American Journal of Epidemiology, 175*(6), 527–535.

National Advisory Committee on Rural Health and Human Services. (2011). *Reducing health disparities in rural America: Key provisions in the Affordable Care Act. Policy Brief.* Retrieved from https://www.apa.org/pi/ses/resources/webinars/rural-america.pdf

National Agricultural Law Center. (n.d.). *Labor—an overview.* Retrieved from http://nationalaglawcenter.org/overview/labor/

National Association of County & City Health Officials. (2014). *2013 National profile of local health departments.* Retrieved from http://nacchoprofilestudy.org/wp-content/uploads/2014/02/2013_National_Profile021014.pdf

National Center for Farmworker Health (NCFH). (n.d.). *Migrant health center legislation.* Retrieved from http://www.ncfh.org/?pid=186

National Center for Farmworker Health (NCFH). (2010). *A profile of migrant health: 2010.* Retrieved from www.ncfh.org/fact-sheets-research.html

National Center for Farmworker Health (NCFH). (2011). *HIV/AIDS farmworker factsheet.* Retrieved from http://www.ncfh.org/docs/fs-HIV_AIDS.pdf

National Center for Farmworker Health (NCFH). (2012a). *Child labor in agriculture*. Retrieved from www.ncfh.org/uploads/3/8/6/8/38685499/fs-child_labor.pdf

National Center for Farmworker Health (NCFH). (2012b). *Facts about farmworkers*. Retrieved from http://www.ncfh.org/uploas/3/8/6/8/38685499/fs-facts_about_farmworkers.pdf

National Center for Farmworker Health (NCFH). (2013a). *Farmworkers occupational health and safety*. Retrieved from www.ncfh.org/uploads/3/8/6/8/38685499/fs-occ_health.pdf

National Center for Farmworker Health (NCFH). (2013b). *Tuberculosis*. Retrieved from http://www.ncfh.org/uploads/3/8/6/8/38685499/fs-what_is_tb.pdf

National Center for Farmworker Health (NCFH). (2015). *Farmworkers' health fact sheet*. Retrieved from www.ncfh.org/uploads/3/8/6/8/38685499/fs-nawshealthfactsheet.pdf

National Center for Frontier Communities. (2014). *2010 update: Frontier maps*. Retrieved from http://frontierus.org/maps

National Conference of State Legislatures. (2011, October). *States implement health reform: School-based health centers*. Retrieved from http://www.ncsl.org/portals/1/documents/health/HRSBHC.pdf

National Highway Traffic Safety Administration. (2014, July). *Traffic safety facts 2012 data: Rural/urban comparison*. Washington, DC: Author.

National Highway & Traffic Safety Administration. (2015, July). *Traffic safety facts 2013 data: Rural/urban comparison*. Retrieved from http://www-nrd.nhtsa.dot.gov/Pubs/812181.pdf

National Institute for Occupational Safety & Health. (2012). *Pesticide illness & injury surveillance: SENSOR-pesticides program*. Retrieved from http://www.cdc.gov/niosh/topics/pesticides/overview.html

National Rural Health Association (NRHA). (n.d.). *Rural health issues: Implications for Rural Healthy People 2020*. Kansas City, MO: Author.

National Rural Health Association (NRHA). (2011, January). *Public health nursing: Strengthening the core of rural public health. NRHA policy brief*. Retrieved from http://www.ruralhealthweb.org/index.cfm?objectid=320C9967-3048-651A-FEAEB48180B4AD37

National Rural Health Association (NRHA). (2015). *What's different about rural health care?* Retrieved from http://www.ruralhealthweb.org/go/left/about-rural-health/what-s-different-about-rural-health-care

National Rural Health Association (NRHA). (2016). *Rural HIV/AIDS Resource Center*. Retrieved from http://www.ruralhealthweb.org/go/left/programs-and-events/programs-and-events-overview/rural-hiv/aids-resource-center/rural-hiv/aids-resource-center

New York Academy of Medicine. (2016). *Institute for Urban Health*. Retrieved from http://www.nyam.org/institute-urban-health/

Nichols, M., Stein, A. D., & Wold, J. L. (2014). Health status of children of migrant farm workers: Farm Worker Family Health Program, Moultrie, Georgia. *American Journal of Public Health*, *104*(2), 365–370.

Nieuwenhuijsen, M. J. (2016). Urban and transport planning, environmental exposures and health—new concepts, methods and tools to improve health in cities. *Environmental Health*, *15*(Suppl. 1), 38.

Nuno, T., Martinez, M. E., Harris, R., & Garcia, F. (2011). A *promotora*-administered group education intervention to promote breast and cervical cancer screening in a rural community along the U.S.-Mexico border: A randomized controlled trial. *Cancer Causes and Control*, *22*(3), 367–374.

Nusca, A. (2011, July 28). *Rural U.S. population lowest in history, demographers say*. Retrieved from http://www.smartplanet.com/blog/smart-takes/rural-us-population-lowest-in-history-demographers-say/17982

Occupational Safety & Health Administration (OSHA). (n.d.). *Youth in agriculture*. Retrieved from https://www.osha.gov/dsg/topics/agriculturaloperations/youngworkers.html

Occupational Safety & Health Administration (OSHA). (2011). *Agricultural operations standards: Field sanitation*. Retrieved from http://www.osha.gov/pls/oshaweb/owadisp.show_document?p_table=STANDARDS&p_id=10959

O'Connor, A., & Wellenius, G. (2012). Rural-urban disparities in the prevalence of diabetes and coronary heart disease. *Public Health*, *126*(10), 813–820.

Ohl, M., Lund, B., Belperio, P. S., Goetz, M. B., Rimland, D., Richardson, K., ... Vaughan-Sarrazin, M. (2013). Rural residence and adoption of a novel HIV therapy in a national, equal-access healthcare system. *AIDS Behavior*, *17*, 250–259.

Ompad, D. C., Nandi, V., Cerdá, M., Crawford, N., Galea, S., & Vlahov, D. (2012). Beyond income: Material resources among drug users in economically disadvantaged New York City neighborhoods. *Drug & Alcohol Dependence*, *120*(1–3), 127–134.

Ortego, A. N., Horwitz, S. M., Fang, H., Kuo, A., Wallace, S. P., & Inkelas, M. (2009). Documentation status and parental concerns about development in young U.S. children of Mexican origin. *Academic Pediatrics*, *9*(4), 278–282.

Ortiz, J., Bushy, A., Zhou, Y., & Zhang, H. (2013). Accountable care organizations: Benefits and barriers as perceived by rural health clinical management. *Rural & Remote Health*, *13*(2), 1–13.

Ortiz, J., & Wan, T. H. (2012). Performance of rural health clinics: An examination of efficiency and Medicare beneficiary outcomes. *Rural & Remote Health*, *12*(1), 1–12.

Oser, C., Leukefeld, C., Staton-Tinall, M., Duvall, J., Garrity, T., Stoops, W., ... Booth, B. (2011). Criminality among rural stimulant users in the United States. *Crime Delinquency Journal*, *57*(4), 600–621.

Owens, C. (2016, January 29). *Reconnecting urban planning and public health*. Retrieved from https://nextcity.org/daily/entry/urban-planning-public-health-collaborating

Pain, S. (2016). The rise of the urbanite. *Nature*, *531*(7594), 550–551.

Park, C. (2011). Relationship between the growth of ethnic groups and southeastern conditions in U.S. metropolitan areas. *Korean Journal of Policy Studies*, *26*(2), 121–136.

Park, H., & Bloch, M. (2016, January 19). How the epidemic of drug overdose deaths ripples across America. *The New York Times*. Retrieved from http://www.nytimes.com/interactive/2016/01/07/us/drug-overdose-deaths-in-the-us.html?_r=0

Parker, K. F., & Stansfield, R. (2015). The changing urban landscape: Interconnections between racial/ethnic segregation and exposure in the study of race-specific violence over time. *American Journal of Public Health*, *105*(9), 1796–1805.

Partnership for Sustainable Communities. (n.d.). *About us*. Retrieved from https://www.sustainablecommunities.gov/mission/about-us

Paschall, M. J., Lipperman-Kreda, S., & Grube, J. W. (2014). Effects of the local alcohol environment on adolescents' drinking behaviors and beliefs. *Addiction*, *109*(3), 407–416.

Patel, K., Darling, M., Samuels, K., & McClellan, M. (2014, December 5). *Transforming rural health care: High-quality, sustainable access to specialty care*. Retrieved from http://healthaffairs.org/blog/2014/12/05/transforming-rural-health-care-high-quality-sustainable-access-to-specialty-care/

Patton, D. U., Hong, J. S., Ranney, M., Patel, S., Kelley, C., Eschmann, R., & Washington, T. (2014). Social media as a vector for youth violence: A review of the literature. *Computers in Human Behavior*, *35*, 548–553.

Peterson, L. E., Bazemore, A., Bragg, E. J., Xierali, I., & Warshaw, G. A. (2011). Rural-urban distribution of the U.S. geriatrics physician workforce. *Journal of the American Geriatrics Society*, *59*(4), 699–703.

Phipps, E. J., Singletary, S. B., Cooblall, C. A., Hares, H. D., & Braitman, L. E. (2016). Food insecurity in patients with high hospital utilization. *Population Health Management*. doi: 10.1089/pop.2015.0127.

Place, J., Macleod, M., John, N., Adamack, M., & Lindsey, A. E. (2011). "Finding my own time": Examining the spatially produced experiences of rural RNs in the rural nursing certificate program. *Nursing Education Today*, *32*(5), 581–587.

Polivka, B. J., Chaudry, R. V., Crawford, J., Bouton, P., & Sweet, L. (2011). Impact of an urban healthy homes intervention. *Journal of Environmental Health*, *73*(9), 16–20.

Portes, A., & Rivas, A. (2011). The adaptation of migrant children. *Future of Children*, *21*(1), 219–246.

Prengaman, M. P., Bigbee, J. L., Baker, E., & Schmitz, D. E. (2014). Development of the Nursing Community Apgar Questionnaire (NCAQ): A rural nurse recruitment and retention tool. *Rural & Remote Health*, *14*(1), 1.

Probst, J. C., & Bhavsar, G. P. (2014, October). *Differences in case-mix between rural and urban recipients of home health care*. Retrieved from http://rhr.sph.sc.edu/report/(12-3)Differences_in_case-mix.pdf

Public Health Foundation. (2013). *Public health workforce enumeration 2012*. Retrieved from http://www.phf.org/resourcestools/Documents/UM_CEPHS_Enumeration2012_Revised_July_2013.pdf

Pupo, M. C., Serafim, P. M., & deMello, M. F. (2015). Health-related quality of life in posttraumatic stress disorder: 4 years follow-up study of individuals exposed to urban violence. *Psychiatry Research*, *228*(3), 741–745.

Quandt, S. A., Brooke, C., Fagan, K., Howe, A., Thornburg, T. K., & McCurdy, S. A. (2015). Farmworker housing in the United States and its impact on health. *New Solutions*, 25(3), 263–286.

Quandt, S. A., Chen, H., Grzywacz, J. G., Vallejos, Q. M., Galvan, L., & Arcury, T. A. (2010). Cholinesterase depression and its association with pesticide exposure across the agriculture season among Latino farmworkers in North Carolina. *Environmental Health Perspectives*, 18(5).

Quandt, S. A., Grzywacz, J. G., Trejo, G., & Arcury, T. A. (2014). Nutritional strategies of Latino farmworker families with preschool children: Identifying leverage points for obesity prevention. *Social Science & Medicine*, 123, 72–81.

Quandt, S. A., Schulz, M. R., Talton, J. W., Verma, A., & Arcury, T. A. (2012). Occupational eye injuries experienced by migrant farmworkers. *Journal of Agromedicine*, 17(1), 63–69.

Quandt, S. A., Trejo, G., Suerken, C. K., Pulgar, C. A., Ip, E. H., & Arcury, T. A. (2016). Diet quality among preschool-age children of Latino migrant and seasonal farmworkers in the United States. *Journal of Immigrant & Minority Health*, 18(3), 505–512.

Qenani-Petrela, E., Mittelhammer, R., & Wandschneider, P. (2008). Permanent housing for seasonal workers? A generalized peak load investment model for farm worker housing. *Journal of Agricultural and Applied Economics*, 40(1), 151–169.

Rauh, V., Arunajadai, S., Horton, M., Perera, F., Hoepner, L., Barr, D. B., & Whyatt, R. (2011). Seven-year neurodevelopmental scores and prenatal exposure to chlorpyrifos, a common agricultural pesticide. *Environmental Health Perspectives*, 119(8), 1196–1201.

Reboussin, B. A., Green, K. M., Milam, A. J., Furr-Holden, D. M., Johnson, R. M., & Ialongo, N. S. (2015). The role of neighborhood in urban Black adolescent marijuana use. *Drug & Alcohol Dependence*, 154, 69–75.

Recio, A., Linares, C., Banegas, J. R., & Diaz, J. (2016). Road traffic noise effects on cardiovascular, respiratory, and metabolic health: An integrative model of biological mechanisms. *Environmental Research*, 146, 359–370.

Rhodes, S. D., Bischoff, W. E., Burnell, J. M., Whalley, L. E., Walkup, M. P., Vallejos, Q. M., … Arcury, T. A. (2010). HIV and sexually transmitted disease risk among male Hispanic/Latino migrant farmworkers in the Southeast: Findings from a pilot CBPR study. *American Journal of Industrial Medicine*, 53(10), 976–986.

Ricci-Cabello, I., Ruiz-Perez, I., Rojas-Garcia, A., Pastor, G., & Gonçalves, D. C. (2013). Improving diabetes care in rural areas: A systematic review and meta-analysis of quality improvement interventions in OECD countries. *PLOS One*. doi: 10.1371/journal.pone.0084464.

Robinson, E., Nguyen, H. T., Isom, S., Quant, S. A., Grzywacz, J. G., Chen, H., & Arcury, T. A. (2011). Wages, wage violations, and pesticide safety experience by migrant farmworkers in North Carolina. *New Solutions*, 21(2), 251–268.

Rose, M. (2013, June 3). *Qaxacan immigration to Poughkeepsie*. Retrieved from http://pages.vassar.edu/hudsonvalleyguidebook/2013/06/03/oaxacan-immigration-to-poughkeepsie/

Rosoff, P. M., & DeCamp, M. (2011). Preparing for an influenza pandemic: Are some people more equal than others? *Journal of Health Care for the Poor & Underserved*, 22(3 Suppl.), 19–35.

Rural Assistance Center. (n.d.). *CAH frequently asked questions*. Retrieved from http://www.raconline.org/ info_guides/hospitals/cahfaq.php#whatis

Rural Assistance Center. (2012). *Frontier frequently asked questions*. Retrieved from http://www.raconline.org/topics/frontier/frontierfaq.php

Rural Center for AIDS/STD Prevention. (n.d.). *HIV/AIDS in rural America: Challenges and promising strategies*. Retrieved from http://www.indiana.edu/~aids/factsheets/factsheet23.pdf

Rural Health Research Center. (2007, October). *Changes in the rural registered nurse workforce from 1980–2004*. Retrieved from http://depts.washington.edu/uwrhrc/uploads/RHRC%20FR115%202Pager.pdf

Rutledge, C. M., Haney, T., Bordelon, M., Renaud, M., & Fowler, C. (2014). Telehealth: Preparing advanced practice nurses to address needs in rural and underserved populations. *International Journal of Nursing*, 11(1), 1–9.

Ryff, C. D., Miyamoto, Y., Boylan, J. M., Coe, C. L., Karasawa, M., Kan, C., … Kitayama, S. (2015). Culture, inequality, and health: Evidence from the MIDUS and MIDJA comparison. *Culture & Brain*, 3(1), 1–20.

Sanchez, M. A., Hernandez, M. T., Hanson, J. E., Vera, A., Magis-Rodriguez, C., Ruiz, J. D., … Lemp, G. F. (2012). The effect of migration on HIV high-risk behaviors among Mexican migrants. *Journal of Acquired Immune Efficiency Syndrome*, 61, 610–617.

Sandefer, R. H., Marc, D. T., & Kleeberg, P. (2015, Spring). Meaningful use attestations among US hospitals: The growing rural-urban divide. *Perspectives in Health Information Management*, 1–10.

Sarnquist, C. C., Soni, S., Hwang, H., Topol, B. B., Mutima, S., & Maldonado, Y. A. (2011). Rural HIV-infected women's access to medical care: Ongoing needs in California. *AIDS Care*, 23(7), 792–796.

Schulte, J. (2000). Finding ways to create connections among communities: Partial results of an ethnography of urban public health nurses. *Public Health Nursing*, 17(1), 3–10.

Schmidt, M. (2012, February 1). *Port Sheldon Township migrant worker housing causes conflict*. Retrieved from http://www.hollandsentinel.com/news/x715341972/Port-Sheldon-Township-migrant-worker-housing-causes-conflict

Secretary's Advisory Committee on Health Promotion and Disease Prevention Objectives for 2020. (2016). *Healthy People 2020: Secretary's advisory committee*. Retrieved from https://www.healthypeople.gov/2020/about/history-development/Secretary's-Advisory-Committee

Seelye, K. Q. (2011, March 22). Detroit census confirms a desertion like no other. *The New York Times*. Retrieved from http://datadrivendetroit.org/wp-content/uploads/2011/03/NYTimes_3_22_11.pdf

Sergeev, A. V. (2011). Racial and rural-urban disparities in stroke mortality outside the stroke belt. *Ethnicity & Disease*, 21(3), 307–313.

Seright, T. J., & Winters, C. A. (2015). Critical care in critical access hospitals. *Critical Care Nurse*, 35(5), 62–67.

Shelton, J. F., & Hertz-Picciotto, I. (2015). Neurodevelopmental disorders and agricultural pesticide exposures: Shelton and Hertz-Picciotto respond. *Environmental Health Perspectives*, 123(4), A79–A80.

Shih, R. A., Mullins, L., Ewing, B. A., Miyashiro, L., Tucker, J. S., Pedersen, E. R., … D'Amico, E. J. (2015). Associations between neighborhood alcohol availability and young adolescent alcohol use. *Psychological & Addictive Behaviors*, 29(4), 950–959.

Singh, G. K. (2012). Rural-urban trends and patterns in cervical cancer mortality, incidence, stage, and survival in the United States, 1950-2008. *Journal of Community Health*, 37(1), 217–223.

Smalley, K. B., Warren, J. C., & Klibert, J. (2012a). Health risk behaviors in insured and uninsured community health center patients in the rural US South. *Rural & Remote Health*, 12(4), 1–8.

Smalley, K. B., Warren, J. C., & Rainer, J. P. (Eds.). (2012b). *Rural mental health: Issues, policies, and best practices*. New York, NY: Springer Publishing.

Smith, J. (2013, August 22). *America's ten deadliest jobs*. Retrieved from http://www.forbes.com/sites/jacquelynsmith/2013/08/22/americas-10-deadliest-jobs-2/#14bae2c15095

Soneja, S., Jiang, C., Fisher, J., Upperman, C. R., Mitchell, C., & Sapkota, A. (2016). Exposure to extreme heat and precipitation events associated with increased risk of hospitalization for asthma in Maryland. *Environmental Health*, 15, 57.

Southern Education Foundation. (2015). *A new majority research bulletin: Low income students now a majority in the nation's public schools*. Retrieved from http://www.southerneducation.org/Our-Strategies/Research-and-Publications/New-Majority-Diverse-Majority-Report-Series/A-New-Majority-2015-Update-Low-Income-Students-Now

Sparks, P. J. (2012). Rural health disparities. In L. J. Kulcsár & K. J. Curtis (Eds.), *International Handbook of Rural Demography* (Vol. 3). Netherlands: Springer.

Spears, C. R., Summers, P. Y., Spencer, K. M., & Arcury, T. A. (2012). Informal occupational safety information exchange among Latino migrant and seasonal farmworkers. *Journal of Agromedicine*, 17(4), 415–420.

Spencer, A. (2013, October 29). *Closer look at critical access hospitals*. Retrieved from http://www.centerforhealthjournalism.org/fellowships/projects/closer-look-critical-access

Spoont, M., Greer, N., Su, J., Fitzgerald, P., & Rutks, I. (2011). *Rural vs. urban ambulatory health care: A systematic review*. Washington, DC: Department of Veterans Affairs.

Stacciarini, J. M., Vacca, R., Wiens, B., Loe, E., LaFlam, M., Pérez, A., & Locke, B. (2016). FBO leaders' perceptions of the psychosocial contexts for rural Latinos. *Issues in Mental Health Nursing*, 37(1), 19–25.

Stahre, M., VanEenwyk, J., Siegel, P., & Njai, R. (2015). Housing insecurity and the association with health outcomes and unhealthy behaviors, Washington state, 2011. *Preventing Chronic Disease*, 12, 140511. Retrieved from http://www.cdc.gov/pcd/issues/2015/14_0511.htm

Stensland, J., Akamigbo, A., Glass, D., & Zabinski, D. (2013). Rural and urban Medicare beneficiaries use remarkably similar amounts of health care services. *Health Affairs, 32*(11), 2040–2046.

Stewart, K. E., Phillips, M. M., Walker, J. F., Harvey, S. A., & Porter, A. (2011). Social services utilization and the need among a community sample of persons living with HIV in the rural South. *AIDS Care, 23*(3), 340–347.

Stieb, D. M., Chen, L., Hystad, P., Beckerman, B. S., Jerrett, M., Tjepkema, M., ... Dugandzic, R. M. (2016). A national study of the association between traffic-related air pollution and adverse pregnancy outcomes in Canada, 1999-2008. *Environmental Research, 148*, 513–526.

Stingone, J. A., McVeigh, K. H., & Claudio, L. (2016). Association between prenatal exposure to ambient diesel particulate matter and perchloroethylene with children's 3rd grade standardized test scores. *Environmental Research, 148*, 144–153.

Stoecklin-Marois, M. T., Hennessy-Burt, T. E., & Schenker, M. D. (2011). Engaging a hard-to-reach population in research: Sampling and recruitment of hired farm workers in the MICASA study. *Journal of Agricultural Safety & Health, 17*(4), 291–302.

Stone, S. (2011). News from the frontier. *Frontier Nursing Service Quarterly, 87*(1), 5–8.

Stone, B., Hess, J. J., & Frumkin, H. (2010). Urban form and extreme heat events: Are sprawling cities more vulnerable to climate change than compact cities? *Environmental Health Perspectives, 118*(10), 1425–1428.

Student Action Farmworkers (SAF). (2011–2016). *U.S. farmworker factsheet.* Retrieved from saf-unite.org/content/united-states-farmworker-factsheet

Substance Abuse and Mental Health Services Administration. (2012). *Treatment Episode Data Set: The TEDS report.* Retrieved from http://archive.samhsa.gov/data/2k12/TEDS_043/TEDSShortReport043UrbanRuralAdmissions2012.htm

Summers, P., Quandt, S. A., Talton, J. W., Galván, L., & Arcury, T. A. (2015). Hidden farmworker labor camps in North Carolina: An indicator of structural vulnerability. *American Journal of Public Health, 105*(12), 2570–2575.

Sutton, M., Anthony, M., Vila, C., McLellan-Lemal, E., & Weidle, P. (2010). HIV testing and HIV/AIDS treatment services in rural counties in 10 Southern states: Service provider perspectives. *Journal of Rural Health, 26*(3). 240–247.

Syed, S. T., Gerber, B. S., & Sharp, L. K. (2013). Traveling towards disease: Transportation barriers to health care access. *Journal of Community Health, 38*, 976–993.

Thale, G. (2014, June 17). *The plight of migrant children at the border highlights need to invest in Central America.* Retrieved from http://www.wola.org/commentary/the_plight_of_migrant_children_at_the_border_highlights_need_to_invest_in_central_america

The Future of Children. (2011, Spring). *Immigrant children.* Princeton, NJ: Author.

Thierry, A. D., & Snipes, S. A. (2015). Why do farmworkers delay treatment after debilitating injuries? Thematic analysis explains if, when, and why farmworkers were treated for injuries. *American Journal of Industrial Medicine, 58*(2), 178–192.

Thompson, B. (2015, March 26). *Some farmers warming up to the Affordable Care Act.* Retrieved from http://harvestpublicmedia.org/article/some-farmers-warming-affordable-care-act

Tomlinson, S. (2013, January 31). *Revealed: How immigrants in America are sending $120 billion to their struggling families back home.* Retrieved from http://www.dailymail.co.uk/news/article-2271455/Revealed-How-immigrants-America-sending-120-BILLION-struggling-families-home.html

Toth, M., Holmes, M., Van Houtven, C., Toles, M., Weinberger, M., & Silberman, P. (2015). Rural Medicare beneficiaries have fewer follow-up visits and greater emergency department use postdischarge. *Medical Care, 53*(9), 800–808.

Tribble, A. G., Summers, P., Chen, H., Quandt, S. A., & Arcury, T. A. (2015). Musculoskeletal pain, depression, and stress among Latino manual laborers in North Carolina. *Archives of Environmental & Occupational Health, 30*, 1–8.

Trivedi, T., Liu, J., Probst, J., Merchant, A., Jhones, S., & Martin, A. B. (2015). Obesity and obesity-related behaviors among rural and urban adults in the USA. *Rural Remote Health, 15*(4), 3267.

Triantafillou, S. A. (2003). North Carolina's migrant and seasonal farmworkers. *North Carolina Medical Journal, 64*(3), 129–131.

Tyer-Viola, L. A., Corless, I. B., Weibel, A., Reid, P., Sullivan, K. M.; International Nursing Network for HIV/AIDS Research. (2014).

Predictors of medication adherence among HIV-positive women in North America. *Journal of Obstetrical, Gynecological, & Neonatal Nurses, 43*(2), 168–178.

Ullmann, S. H., Goldman, N., & Massey, D. S. (2011). Healthier before they migrate, less healthy when they return? The health of returned migrants in Mexico. *Social Science & Medicine, 73*, 421–428.

University of California. (2012). Hispanic Americans: Migrant workers and Braceros (1930s–1964). Retrieved from http://www.calisphere.universityofcalifornia.edu/calcultures/ethnic_groups/subtopic3b.html

U.S. Census Bureau. (2013). *Metropolitan and micropolitan statistical areas main.* Retrieved from http://www.census.gov/population/metro/

U.S. Census Bureau. (2015). *Geography: Urban and rural classification.* Retrieved from http://www.census.gov/geo/www/ua/2010urbanruralclass.html

U.S. Department of Agriculture (USDA). (2011). *Rural income, poverty, and welfare: Poverty geography.* Retrieved from http://ers.usda.gov/Briefing/IncomePovertyWelfare/povertygeography.htm#graph

U.S. Department of Agriculture (USDA). (2013). *Rural overview.* Retrieved from http://www.ers.usda.gov/topics/rural-economy-population/rural-classifications.aspx

U.S. Department of Agriculture (USDA). (2015). *Frontier and remote area codes.* Retrieved from http://www.ers.usda.gov/data-products/frontier-and-remote-area-codes.aspx

U.S. Department of Agriculture (USDA). (2016). *Population & migration: Overview.* Retrieved from http://www.ers.usda.gov/topics/rural-economy-population/population-migration.aspx

U.S. Department of Education. (2014). *Migrant Student Records Exchange Initiative.* Retrieved from http://www2.ed.gov/admins/lead/account/recordstransfer.html

U.S. Department of Education. (2015). *Migrant education—College Assistance Migrant Program.* Retrieved from http://www2.ed.gov/programs/camp/index.html

U.S. Department of Health & Human Services (USDHHS). (2016a). *Access to health services.* Retrieved from https://www.healthypeople.gov/2020/topics-objectives/topic/Access-to-Health-Services

U.S. Department of Health & Human Services (USDHHS). (2016b). *Healthy People 2020: About healthy people.* Retrieved from https://www.healthypeople.gov/2020/About-Healthy-People

U.S. Department of Homeland Security. (2012). *H-2A temporary agricultural workers.* Retrieved from http://www.uscis.gov/portal/site/uscis/menuitem.eb1d4c2a3e5b9ac89243c6a7543f6d1a/?vgnextoid=889f0b89284a3210VgnVCM100000b92ca60aRCRD&vgnextchannel=889f0b89284a3210VgnVCM100000b92ca60aRCRD

U.S. Department of Housing & Urban Development (USDHUD). (2016a). *Common questions about migrant/farmworkers.* Retrieved from http://portal.hud.gov/hudportal/HUD?src=/states/florida/working/farmworker/commonquestions

U.S. Department of Housing & Urban Development (USDHUD). (2016b). *Housing choice vouchers fact sheet.* Retrieved from http://portal.hud.gov/hudportal/HUD?src=/topics/housing_choice_voucher_program_section_8

U.S. Department of Labor. (2011, August 25). *National census of fatal occupational injuries in 2010 (preliminary results).* Retrieved from http://www.bls.gov/news.release/pdf/cfoi.pdf

U.S. Department of Justice, Office for Victims of Crime. (n.d.). *2013 NCVRW resource guide.* Retrieved from http://victimsofcrime.org/docs/default-source/ncvrw2014/urban-rural-crime-statistics-2014.pdf?sfvrsn=2

U.S. Environmental Protection Agency (EPA). (2011). *Basic information: What is an urban heat island?* Retrieved from http://www.epa.gov/heatisld/about/index.htm

U.S. Environmental Protection Agency (EPA). (2014). *The changing face of rural & small town America.* Retrieved from http://www2.epa.gov/sites/production/files/2014-06/documents/ref_herman_081612.pdf

Vallejos, Q. M., Quandt, S. A., & Arcury, T. A. (2009). The condition of farmworker housing in the eastern United States. In T. A. Arcury, & S. A. Quandt (Eds.), *Latino farmworkers in the eastern United States* (pp. 37–67). New York, NY: Springer Science.

Van der Mark, M., Brouwer, M., Kromhout, H., Nijssen, P., Huss, A., & Vermeulen, R. (2012). Is pesticide use related to Parkinson disease? Some clues to heterogeneity in study results. *Environmental Health Perspectives, 120*, 340–347.

van Dis, J. (2002). Where we live: Health care in rural vs. urban America. *Journal of the American Medical Association, 87*(1), 108.

Van Dommelen-Gonzalez, E., Deardorff, J., Herd, D., & Minnis, A. M. (2015). Homies with aspirations and positive peer network ties: Associations with reduced frequent substance use among gang-affiliated Latino youth. *Journal of Urban Health*, 92(2), 322–337.

Vander Weg, M. W., Cunningham, C. L., Howren, M. B., & Cai, X. (2011). Tobacco use and exposure in rural areas: Findings from the Behavioral Risk Factor Surveillance System. *Addictive Behaviors*, 36(3), 231–236.

Vaughan, A. S., Rosenberg, E., Shouse, R. L., & Sullivan, P. S. (2014). Connecting race and place: A county-level analysis of White, Black, and Hispanic HIV prevalence, poverty, and level of urbanization. *American Journal of Public Health*, 104(7), e77–e84.

Viel, J. F., Hägi, M., Upegui, E., & Laurian, L. (2011). Environmental justice in a French industrial region: Are polluting industrial facilities equally distributed? *Health & Place*, 17(1), 257–262.

Villarejo, D., McCurdy, S. A., Bade, B., Samuels, S., Lighthall, D., & Williams, D. (2010). The health of California's immigrant hired farmworkers. *American Journal of Industrial Medicine*, 53, 387–397.

Vlahov, D. (2015). A pivotal moment for urban health. *Cadernos de Saúde Pública*, 31(Suppl. 1). Retrieved from http://dx.dooi.org/10.1590/0102-311XPE01S115

Vlahov, D., Agarwal, S. R., Buckley, R. M., Caiaffa, W. T., Corvalan, C. F., Ezeh, A. C., ... Watson, V. J. (2011). Roundtable on urban living environment research (RULER). *Journal of Urban Health*, 88(5), 793–857.

Vlahov, D., Bond, K. T., Jones, K. C., & Ompad, D. C. (2012). Factors associated with differential uptake of seasonal influenza immunizations among underserved communities during the 2009-2010 influenza season. *Journal of Community Health*, 37(2), 282–287.

Vlahov, D., Boufford, J. I., Pearson, C., & Norris, L. (Eds.). (2010). *Urban health: Global perspectives*. San Francisco, CA: John Wiley & Sons, Inc.

Vyavaharkar, M., Moneyham, L., Murdaugh, C., & Tavakoli, A. (2012). Factors associated with quality of life among rural women with HIV disease. *AIDS Behavior*, 16, 295–303.

Wald, L. (1971). *The house on Henry Street*. New York, NY: Dover Publications. (Original work published 1915)

Waldman, H. B., Cannella, D., & Perlman, S. P. (2010). Migrant farm workers and their children. *Exceptional Parent*, 40(11), 52–53.

Walker, G. (2012). *Environmental justice: Concepts, evidence, and politics*. New York, NY: Routledge.

Walker, R. E., Block, J., & Kawachi, I. (2012). Do residents of food deserts express different food buying preferences compared to residents of food oases? A mixed-methods analysis. *International Journal of Behavioral Nutrition & Physical Activity*, 9, 41.

Wallis, L. (2015). Rural youths commit suicide almost twice as often as urban counterparts. *American Journal of Nursing*, 115(6), 15.

Wang, A., Costello, S., Cockburn, M., Zhang, X., Bronstein, J., & Ritz, B. (2011a). Parkinson's disease risk from ambient exposure pesticides. *European Journal of Epidemiology*, 26(7), 547–555.

Wang, J. Y., Bennett, K., & Probst, J. (2011b). Subdividing the digital divide: Differences in Internet access and use among rural residents with medical limitations. *Journal of Medical Internet Research*, 13(1), e25.

Washington State Nurses Association. (2011). *Public health and public health nursing. Position paper*. Seattle, WA: Author.

Weaver, A., & Gjesfjeld, C. (2014). Barriers to preventive services use for rural women in the southeastern United States. *Social Work Research*, 38(4), 225–234.

Wedgworth, J. C., Brown, J., Olson, J. R., Johnson, P., Elliott, M., Grammar, P., & Stauber, C. E. (2015). Temporal heterogeneity of water quality in rural Alabama water supplies. *Journal--American Water Works Association*, 107(8), e401–e415.

Weigel, P. A., Ullrich, F., Shane, D. M., & Mueller, K. J. (2016). Variation in primary care service patterns by rural-urban location. *Journal of Rural Health*, 32(2), 196–203.

Weiss, L., Gass, J., Egan, J. E., Ompad, D. C., Trezza, C., & Vlahov, D. (2014). Understanding prolonged cessation from heroin use: Findings from a community-based sample. *Journal of Psychoactive Drugs*, 46(2), 123–132.

Welsh, B. C., Braga, A. A., & Bruinsma, G. (2015). Reimagining broken windows: From theory to policy. *Journal of Research in Crime and Delinquency*, 52(4), 447–463.

Whittle, H. J., Palar, K., Hufstedler, L. L., Seligman, H. K., Frongillo, E. A., & Weiser, S. D. (2015). Food insecurity, chronic illness, and gentrification in the San Francisco Bay area: An example of structural violence in United States public policy. *Social Science & Medicine*, 143, 154–161.

Wiewel, E. W., Bocour, A., Kersanske, L. S., Bodach, S. D., Xia, Q., & Braunstein, S. L. (2016). The association between neighborhood poverty and HIV diagnoses among males and females in New York City, 2010-2011. *Public Health Reports*, 131(2), 290–302.

Wikipedia. (2016). *List of metropolitan statistical areas*. Retrieved from https://en.wikipedia.org/wiki/List_of_Metropolitan_Statistical_Areas

Willen, S. S. (2012). Migration, "illegality," and health: Mapping embodied vulnerability and debating health-related deservingness. *Social Science & Medicine*, 74(6), 805–811.

Williams, D. R. (2012). Miles to go before we sleep: Racial inequalities in health. *Journal of Health & Social Behavior*, 53(3), 279–295.

Williams, D. R., & Sternthal, M. (2010). Understanding racial-ethnic disparities in health: Sociological contributions. *Journal of Health and Social Behavior*, 51(S), S15–S27.

Wilson, J. B., Rappleyea, D. L., Hodgson, J. L., Brimhall, A. S., Hall, T. L., & Thompson, A. P. (2015). Healthcare providers' experiences screening for intimate partner violence among migrant and seasonal farmworking women: A phenomenological study. *Health Expectations*. doi: 10.1111/hex.12421.

Wilson, J. B., Rappleyea, D. L., Hodgson, J. L., Hall, T. L., & White, M.B. (2014). Intimate partner violence screening among migrant/seasonal farmworker women and healthcare: A policy brief. *Journal of Community Health*, 39(2), 373–377.

Winkelman, S. B., Chaney, E. H., & Bethel, J. W. (2013). Stress, depression, and coping among Latino migrant and seasonal farmworkers. *International Journal of Environmental Research in Public Health*, 10, 1815–1830.

Winquist, A. Grundstein, A., Chang, H. H., Hess, J., & Sarnat, S. E. (2016). Warm season temperatures and emergency department visits in Atlanta, Georgia. *Environmental Research*, 147, 314–323.

Wong, M., Wolff, C., Collins, N., Guo, L., Meltzer, D., & English, P. (2015). Development of a web-based tool to collect and display water system customer service areas for public health action. *Journal of Public Health Management and Practice*, 21(Suppl. 2), s44–s49.

Wright, B., Damiano, P. C., & Bentler, S. E. (2015). Implementation of the Affordable Care Act and rural health clinic capacity in Iowa. *Journal of Primary Care & Community Health*, 6(1), 61–65.

Wright, B. A., Peters, E. R., Ettinger, U., Kuipers, E., & Kumari, V. (2016). Moderators of noise-induced cognitive change in healthy adults. *Noise Health*, 18(82), 117–132.

Wright, S., Marlenga, B., & Lee, B. C. (2013). Childhood agricultural injuries: An update for clinicians. *Current Problems in Pediatric and Adolescent Health Care*, 43(2), 20–44.

World Health Organization. (2012). *Healthy cities*. Retrieved from http://www.euro.who.int/en/what-we-do/health-topics/environment-and-health/urban-health/activities/healthy-cities

Wu, C. D., & Lung, S. C. (2016). Application of 3-D urbanization index to assess impact of urbanization on air temperature. *Scientific Reports*, 6, 24351.

Zibrik, K. J., MacLeod, M. L., & Zimmer, L. V. (2010). Professionalism in rural acute-care nursing. *Canadian Journal of Nursing Research*, 42(1), 20–36.

Zickuhr, K. (2013, August 26). *Home broadband 2013*. Retrieved from http://www.pewinternet.org/2013/08/26/home-broadband-2013/

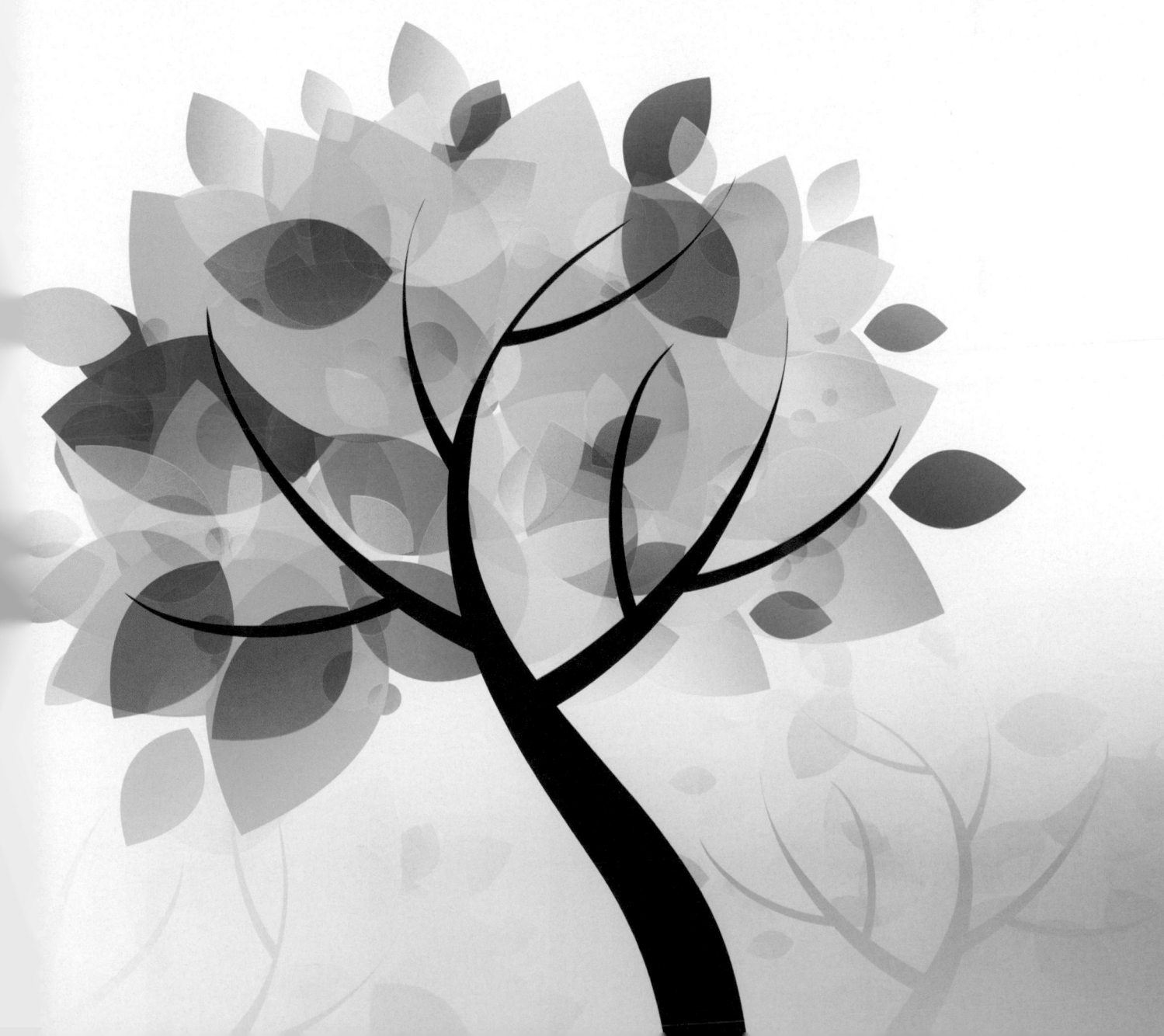

SETTINGS FOR COMMUNITY HEALTH NURSING

8

SETTINGS FOR COMMUNITY HEALTH NURSING

Public Settings for Community Health Nursing

"A [community nurse] must first nurse. She must be of yet higher class and yet of fuller training than that of a hospital nurse because she has no hospital appliances at hand at all and because she has to take notes on the case for the doctor who has no one but her to report to him."

—Florence Nightingale, 1876 (as cited in Edgecomb, 2001)

KEY TERMS

Block grant funding
Correctional nurses
Indian Health Services (IHS)
Individualized education
  plans (IEPs)

Individualized health plans
  (IHPs)
Local health departments
  (LHDs)
Public health nurse (PHN)

School nurse
School nurse practitioners
School-based health centers
  (SBHCs)
Section 504 plans

U.S. Public Health Service
  Commissioned Corps

LEARNING OBJECTIVES

Upon mastery of this chapter, you should be able to:

- Explain the focus of the nursing process and how public health nurses (PHNs) and other nurses working in the publicly funded sector use it to provide care in their communities.
- Describe how federal, state, and local public health infrastructures influence the population's health.
- Evaluate the potential benefits of school-based health centers (SBHCs) and discuss possible parental or community objections.
- Compare and contrast common roles and functions of PHNs, school nurses, and correctional nurses.

Many nursing students are not aware of the vast employment opportunities available outside the hospital in publicly funded settings. This chapter discusses several of these publicly funded health settings and the opportunities nurses can garner, particularly in services such as public health nursing, school nursing, or correctional nursing. This chapter is a practical explanation of the work of these nurses in the public sector.

Although each of these nursing opportunities differs greatly, they have several characteristics in common. First, community nurses who work in a setting supported through public funds (e.g., taxpayer-funded) still use the nursing process, but their client is a population or group of people, rather than an individual. Second, emphasis is placed on prevention of disease or disability. Third, community nurses employed in publicly funded settings work with a variety of people, usually vulnerable populations. They must be able to network and collaborate with other agencies and disciplines. For example, a nurse working in a correctional facility often collaborates with mental health workers and correctional officers. A nurse working in the public setting has many opportunities to be an advocate for individuals and the community and may serve on regional task forces or advisory boards. In addition, PHNs focus on population-based care. Nurses may perform individual care, especially correctional nurses; however, most of the focus is placed on the population as client. Finally, nurses who work in the public setting must be autonomous, flexible, creative thinkers who are self-directed and able to prioritize and use the nursing process to make educated decisions and plan care for their respective populations. Nurses who work in public settings must have the highest level of nursing, communication, problem-solving, and intellectual skills.

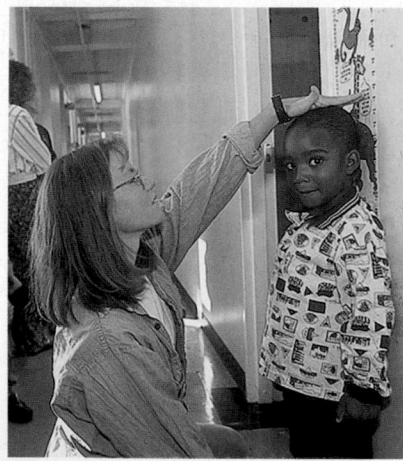

Nurses working in the public sector generally need to be very self-directed, autonomous, and creative thinkers.

PUBLIC HEALTH NURSING

A **public health nurse (PHN)** is a nurse who works to promote and protect the health of an entire population (American Nurses Association [ANA], 2013a). The 2012 data specify the highest enumeration estimate of 516,193 workers comprising the U.S. public health workforce (University of Michigan Center of Excellence in Public Health Workforce Studies, 2013). This workforce consists of epidemiologists, nurses, environmentalists, laboratory professionals, nutritionists, dental workers, social workers, and other health care providers.

Looking at public health from a nursing perspective, approximately 7.8% of all registered nurses (RNs) work in public/community health settings (Health Resources and Services Administration [HRSA], 2010). Public or community agencies are the third largest employer of RNs, after hospitals (employing 62.2% of nurses) and ambulatory care (employing 10.5% of nurses). However, with the struggle to find adequate access to health care, along with its increased costs, more nursing care is being performed in a public or community setting. Unfortunately, you may not know of these wonderful employment opportunities available in the public sector. This section describes the role and opportunities for RNs at the local, state, and federal levels of government. The focus will be on governmental agencies, because these agencies employ the majority of PHNs.

Education

The ANA (2013b) recommends that an entry-level PHN should have a bachelor's degree in nursing. This is important because baccalaureate programs provide additional training in public health and leadership. Some states, such as California, require nurses to take additional classes and obtain certification beyond a bachelor's degree if the BSN program does not offer specific content (e.g., child abuse, public health didactic, and practicum). PHNs working with specific populations, or in administration, should hold a master's degree. A PHN with a master's degree in community/public health nursing may take a national certification examination offered by the American Nurses Credentialing Center (2015). Many, but not all, master's programs offer dual nursing and public health degrees. The emphasis on national certification is due to an ever-increasing need to keep the population protected from health threats, such as bioterrorism (especially after September 11, 2001), emerging diseases (e.g., pandemic flu), or natural disasters (e.g., hurricanes, earthquakes).

Key Functions of the PHN in the Public Setting

Public health nursing practice consists of many areas of expertise, including:

- Focusing on the health of populations
- Reflecting the needs and priorities of the community
- Requiring caring relationships with individuals, families, communities, and systems
- Being grounded in cultural sensitivity, compassion, social justice, and a belief in the worth of all people (e.g., vulnerable populations)
- Encompassing all aspects of health (e.g., physical, emotional, mental, social, spiritual, and environmental)
- Using strategies to promote health that are motivated by epidemiologic evidence
- Involving individual, as well as collaborative, strategies to achieve results
- Knowing that Nurse Practice Act provides authority for independent action (Keller, Strohschein, & Schaffer, 2011)

In brief, the role of the PHN is to focus on the health of the public. PHNs combine their nursing and clinical knowledge of disease and the human response to it, along with public health skills, in order to accomplish their goals (ANA (2013b); Swider, Krothe, Reyes, & Cravetz, 2013). They apply the nursing process, not only with individuals but also with populations. PHNs are a critical link between data tracking (e.g., epidemiology) and clinical understanding of a disease or condition (Kroelinger, Kasenhagen, Barradas, & Ali, 2012; McCulloch & Prieto, 2008). PHNs use the data to prioritize their interventions to stop the spread of diseases, such as measles, and also to intercede with other concerns (e.g., childhood obesity). For example, PHNs may develop a campaign for children to wear bike helmets after an increase of fatal head injuries is noted in their area. A key emphasis of the PHN is prevention, and a key focus is educating and empowering the community. Several other differences exist between PHNs and nursing in general (see Table 30–1 for a comparison). In 2010, the Quad Council (comprised of the Association of Community Health Nurse Educators/ ACHNE, the Association of State and Territorial Directors of Nursing/ASTDN, the PHN Section of the American Public Health Association/APHA, and the American Nurses Association's Congress on Nursing Practice and Economics/ ANA) developed the Quad Council Competencies for Public Health Nurses as a tool in education and for agencies in orienting new public health nurses (Swider et al., 2013).

PHNs may focus on a population that is a geographic community (e.g., a state or municipality) or a focus group (e.g., adolescents or the elderly) spanning all socioeconomic levels. To accomplish this, PHNs often work with individuals or families at highest risk, and their motive is to improve, protect, and promote the health of the entire population. One of the goals that characterize PHNs, and differentiate their goals from those of other specialty disciplines, is achieving the greatest good for the majority of people (ANA, 2013b). See Chapter 13 for an

Table 30–1 Comparing Public Health and General Nursing

Public Health Nursing	General Nursing
Population based	Individual based
Grounded in social justice	Grounded in a relationship of caring
Focuses on the greater good	Focuses on individual good (patient)
Health promotion and disease prevention	Restoration of health and function
Utilize and organize community resources	Manage resources at hand
Seek out clients in need	Take care of clients who come to them
Commitment to the community as a whole	Commitment to individual patient

Adapted from *Cornerstones of Public Health Nursing* (Minnesota Department of Health, 2007).

in-depth discussion of social justice. This requires priority planning and a basic knowledge of the community. It can also create ethical dilemmas for PHNs who may have personal and passionate issues that they would like to pursue, but which may not be the top priority for the majority of community members.

For example, many issues exist in a community. In one community, one child may have been hit by a car while riding his bike without a helmet, while at the same time, in the same community, there may be 10 births to teen moms, 20 instances of drug overdose, and an outbreak of pertussis. The PHNs in that community must prioritize which issue to address first by deciding which issue impacts the most people and what interventions will help the population thrive (ANA, 2013b). Because each community is different, once all factors are taken into account, the priorities will vary among communities. Hence, *assessment* is a critical component of public health and a key tool for the nurses who work in the public sector (ANA, 2013b; Institute of Medicine [IOM], 1988; Turnock, 2016). See Display 30–1.

Another way public health nursing differs from other areas in nursing is that PHNs must actively seek out and identify potential problems and situations (ANA, 2013b). Nurses who work in a hospital setting address the issues

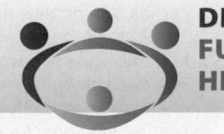

DISPLAY 30–1 THREE CORE FUNCTIONS OF PUBLIC HEALTH (IOM, 1988)

1. Assessment
2. Assurance
3. Policy development

that come to them. If a nurse works in the intensive care unit (ICU) of a hospital, she will work with her assigned patient load. PHNs, on the other hand, are out in the community identifying the problems, not waiting for problems to come to them. For example, PHNs may participate in visits to childcare centers to note any safety hazards, ensure that rules and regulations are being followed, and that children are properly immunized. These visits are part of the priority of *assurance* identified by the IOM (1988) and Turnock (2016), noted in Display 30–1.

PHNs cannot perform all these activities alone. They need to collaborate with other partners and optimally use often limited resources. PHNs are in a unique situation because they work with their populations (i.e., clients) and with others to find the best solutions for a situation or problem. For instance, PHNs may notice an increase in the number of measles cases in their community. They may then work with families to identify where and how the children were exposed to the disease and with local health care providers to provide treatment and vaccinations for those at highest risk of exposure to and damage from measles. PHNs also work with school nurses and other school personnel to exclude from school attendance those children who are not adequately immunized against measles. This helps decrease the spread and potential harm because of measles. PHNs educate a variety of groups, such as parent–teacher associations (PTAs) and city or school officials, as to how

measles spreads, what can be done to treat the disease, and the importance of herd immunity in protecting the public. Education thus empowers each group to be part of the solution. Finally, PHNs can work with public health officials to develop a policy for all new school entrants to receive a second booster of measles vaccine. *Policy development* is the third critical component of public health identified by the IOM (1988) and Turnock (2016). See Display 30–1.

PUBLIC HEALTH FUNDING AND GOVERNMENTAL STRUCTURES

PHNs can work at any and all levels of government. Hence, it is important to understand the organizational structure, communication, and funding streams between the federal, state, and local levels of government (see Chapter 6 for more on the structure of the public health system). At each level, all three branches of the government are involved in public health, although often the legislative and executive branches play the most important roles, and this discussion focuses on these areas.

The legislative branch (meaning Congress, state legislatures, or local councils) mandates laws or policies and decides how much of the funding in its jurisdiction will be appropriated to public health. Much of the work for public health is carried out in the executive branch of government (Fig. 30–1). Because state and local

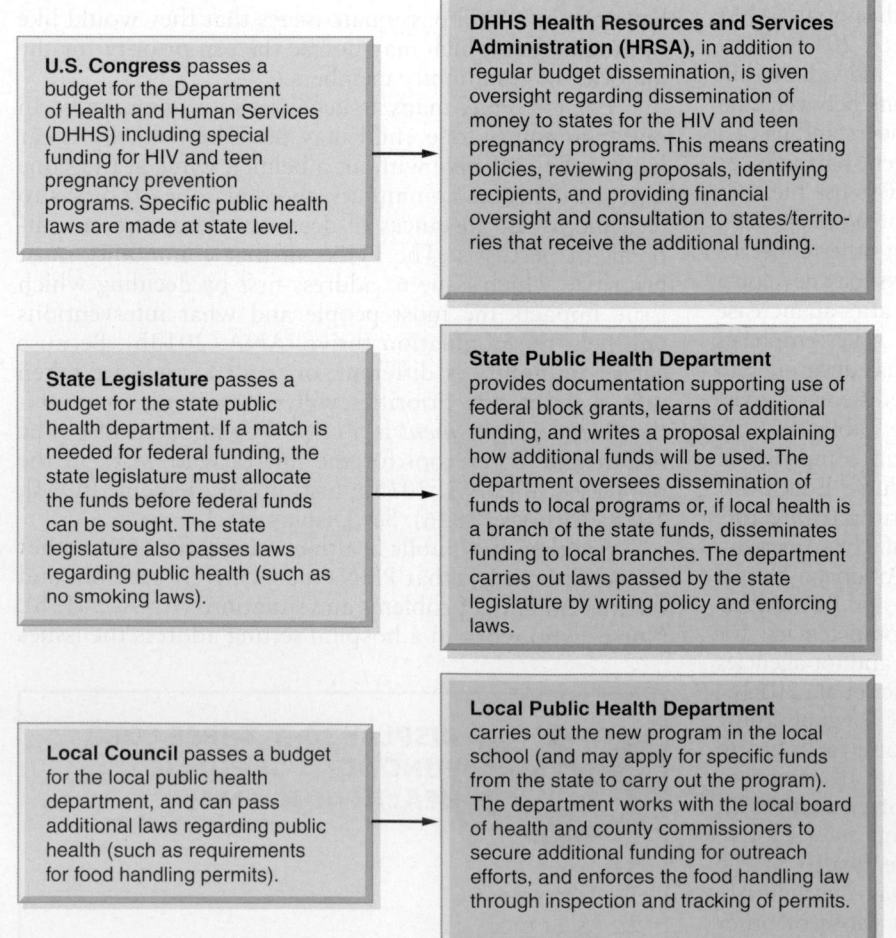

U.S. Congress passes a budget for the Department of Health and Human Services (DHHS) including special funding for HIV and teen pregnancy prevention programs. Specific public health laws are made at state level.

DHHS Health Resources and Services Administration (HRSA), in addition to regular budget dissemination, is given oversight regarding dissemination of money to states for the HIV and teen pregnancy programs. This means creating policies, reviewing proposals, identifying recipients, and providing financial oversight and consultation to states/territories that receive the additional funding.

State Legislature passes a budget for the state public health department. If a match is needed for federal funding, the state legislature must allocate the funds before federal funds can be sought. The state legislature also passes laws regarding public health (such as no smoking laws).

State Public Health Department provides documentation supporting use of federal block grants, learns of additional funding, and writes a proposal explaining how additional funds will be used. The department oversees dissemination of funds to local programs or, if local health is a branch of the state funds, disseminates funding to local branches. The department carries out laws passed by the state legislature by writing policy and enforcing laws.

Local Council passes a budget for the local public health department, and can pass additional laws regarding public health (such as requirements for food handling permits).

Local Public Health Department carries out the new program in the local school (and may apply for specific funds from the state to carry out the program). The department works with the local board of health and county commissioners to secure additional funding for outreach efforts, and enforces the food handling law through inspection and tracking of permits.

FIGURE 30–1 Examples of government organization in relation to public health.

organizations can be set up in a variety of ways, nurses need to contact local health departments (LHDs) for specifics. Public health services are delivered by centralized (28%), decentralized (37%), or combined authority (35%) of local, state, and federal government agencies or nongovernmental organizations (Hyde & Shortell, 2012).

Federal Agencies

The federal government oversees national policy and funding, provides expertise, and sets a national agenda (Shi & Johnson, 2014). Several federal organizations are part of the executive branch that oversees the health of the nation. The main organization involved with public health is the Department of Health and Human Services (DHHS), which is overseen by the Secretary of Health and Human Services. The Secretary of DHHS is appointed by the President and is a member of the President's cabinet. Within DHHS are many agencies, including eight that specifically impact public health (U.S. Department of Health and Human Services [USDHHS], 2015). Table 30–2 provides additional detail regarding these eight agencies. Other federal agencies that also impact public health include the Environmental Protection Agency (EPA), the Department of Homeland Security, the Department of Agriculture, the Department of Education, and the Department of Veterans Affairs.

These various organizations receive funding and directives from the Congress (i.e., the legislative branch of the federal government) as part of the DHHS budget process. It is the prime responsibility of DHHS and other agencies to ensure that legislative mandates are followed, policies carried out, and funds appropriately disseminated. State health entities receive a large portion of funds as part of **block grant funding**. These funds are lumped together to pay for some general use that states have identified (see Chapter 6 for more detailed information). *Healthy People 2020* and state needs assessments help set priorities for state funding. For example, the maternal and child health (MCH) block grants received by states are then used for reproductive health, child health, and immunizations. States with LHDs also disseminate a portion of these funds to the local level. In addition, state and

Table 30–2   Agencies within Department of Health and Human Services

Agency	Headquarters	Responsibility and Bureaus
Health Resources and Services Administration (HRSA)	Rockville, Maryland	Medically underserved—includes Medicare/Medicaid, HIV/AIDS, maternal and child, health professions, primary health care
Indian Health Services (IHS)	Rockville, Maryland	Provides health services for Native Americans (including Alaskan Natives)
Centers for Disease Control and Prevention (CDC)	Atlanta, Georgia	Health surveillance and prevention of disease and bioterrorism
National Institutes of Health (NIH)	Bethesda, Maryland	Medical research
Food and Drug Administration (FDA)	Rockville, Maryland	Ensures safety of food, medication, medical procedures, and equipment
Substance Abuse and Mental Health Services Administration (SAMHSA)	Rockville, Maryland	Oversees prevention, diagnosis, and treatment for mental health and substance abuse
Agency for Toxic Substances and Disease Registry (ATSDR)	Atlanta, Georgia	Protects public from environmental exposures
Agency for Health Care Research and Quality (AHRQ)	Rockville, Maryland	Includes research on health care quality and effectiveness
Center for Medicaid/Medicare Services (CMS)	Baltimore, Maryland	Provides oversight of the Medicare program, the federal portion of the Medicaid program and State Children's Health Insurance Program, the Health Insurance Marketplace
Agency for Children and Families (ACF)	Washington, District of Columbia	Promotes the economic and social well-being of families, children, individuals, and communities
Administration for Community Living (ACL)	Washington, District of Columbia	Increases access to community support and resources for the unique needs of older Americans and people with disabilities
U.S. Public Health Service Commissioned Corps	Rockville, Maryland	An elite team of 6,500 health care professionals working in several federal agencies protecting, promoting, advancing the health, and well-being of the nation

Source: http://www.hhs.gov/about/agencies/hhs-agencies-and-offices/index.html
Turnock, B. J. (2016). *Essentials of public health: What it is and how it works* (6th ed.). Burlington, MA: Jones & Bartlett Learning.

local tax dollars are used to supplement various programs (Knickman & Kovner, 2015). Thus, the political leanings of state and local officials can strongly influence local health initiatives.

State Agencies

The U.S. Constitution bestows states with the responsibility to safeguard the health of their citizens (Turnock, 2016). Much of public health is overseen at a state level. However, the structure of where public health fits into the executive branch of state government varies. More than half of the states have an independent state-level public health agency; another third of the states are part of a "super agency" that may include human services and other state programs (Madamala, Sellers, Beitsch, Pearsol, & Jarris, 2011; Shi & Johnson, 2014). The governor appoints a commissioner, or leading health official, to oversee public health and serve as a member of the governor's cabinet. These cabinet members are usually medical doctors, appointed by the governor. In recent years, state directors have also included social workers (e.g., Michigan) and public health professionals (e.g., Arkansas). In 2007, Governor Phil Bredesen appointed Susan Cooper, RN, MSN, as the first nurse to serve as public health commissioner for the state of Tennessee. The first nurses appointed to director of state offices of public health were Barbara Sabol and Gloria Smith in the states of Kansas and Michigan (Feldman, 2012).

The purpose of state agencies is to carry forth regulations and policies determined by the federal government. Examples of these programs are the Medicaid, Medicare, and State Children's Health Insurance Programs (SCHIPs). Many of these programs may have specific federal requirements, but they also allow states the ability to personalize the programs to fit the state's individual needs. An example of such a program is the MCH block grant, which provides funding and guidelines for the states. However, states determine which programs (e.g., reproductive health or children's health) will be funded and how they will be implemented. See Chapter 21.

Another example of federal leadership is the *Healthy People 2020* document that provides goals for a variety of health outcomes. States can use these outcomes, or develop additional performance measures, according to state characteristics and needs. In addition, the state agency is influenced by the state legislative body, which oversees the state budget and can pass laws specific to the state. Each state is different because of varying needs, cultures, and political environments. Examples of public health laws at a state level include immunization requirements for school entrance, seat belt safety laws, and regulations regarding parental rights concerning birth control and abortion services for teens. Other health policies that influence public health include laws to quarantine persons with communicable diseases, especially during times of outbreaks. State laws must be in place outlining legal jurisdiction of containing and reporting communicable disease; such laws often need to be updated as new threats occur. This was recently exemplified during the early 2000s when smallpox became a bioterrorist threat. State laws allowing persons to be quarantined for smallpox had expired, and new laws had to be passed in order to prepare for potential outbreaks. Without these laws in place, public health officials and law enforcement do not have the power and authority required to maintain the health of the public (Turnock, 2016).

Local Public Health

Local health departments (LHDs) carry out state laws and policies (Turnock, 2016). They provide the most direct, immediate care of the population (Shi & Johnson, 2014). For example, they may provide immunization clinics, track and treat cases of tuberculosis (TB) and other communicable diseases, and provide education on a variety of subjects (e.g., HIV/AIDS, smoking cessation). They often carry out programs with funding from federal and state agencies. For instance, federal funding to address asthma may be obtained through the state agency, and local agencies may organize an educational program on asthma triggers in a local business where many community members work. State and local agencies do not work alone in such endeavors, however. Collaboration is very important in addressing the public health needs of a community. Public health agencies work with private organizations, hospitals, nonprofit groups, universities, and government agencies that oversee food and housing to meet citizens' needs.

LHDs work with state health departments, some independently and some as dependent branches of the state agency. The size and services offered by a local agency also differ depending on state laws, structure, and wealth (Turnock, 2016). A total of 61% of LDHs serve communities of 50,000 or less population. Most (68%) are county agencies, but 20% are city or town agencies. Almost 77% of LHDs are locally governed, most often a local board of health. The majority of LHDs collaborate with other community agencies: 67% on emergency preparedness and 47% on community assessment/planning. Over 60% of LHDs in the United States have fewer than 25 employees. Along with clerical/administration personnel, registered nurses are the most common occupation found in LHDs at 96%. The number of LHDs per state can vary dramatically. For example, Delaware has only 2 LHDs, California has 61, and Massachusetts has the most with 329 (NACCHO, 2014). Nearly all LHDs (96%) employ nurses, who make up 19% of the total public health workforce at the local level (NACCHO, 2014).

NURSING ROLES IN LOCAL, STATE, AND FEDERAL PUBLIC HEALTH POSITIONS

Nurses can work in a variety of capacities at the various levels of government, which may cover most aspects of public health (Shi & Johnson, 2014; Turnock, 2016). Generally speaking, nurses who work at the local level of public health tend to provide direct service care. For example, they often administer immunizations, monitor patients with TB, provide education to school groups, provide cancer screenings, and track communicable disease rates. Local PHNs are the eyes and ears of their communities. Many PHNs working at the local level, especially in rural or small public health departments, may have a variety of responsibilities. For instance, a PHN may be a full-time employee whose time could be split into 50% cancer screening; 25% with the Women, Infants, and Children (WIC) program; and 25% on Medicaid outreach

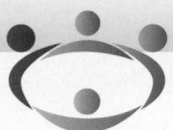

DISPLAY 30–2 A TYPICAL DAY IN THE LIFE OF A PUBLIC HEALTH NURSE

8:00 AM Staff reproductive health clinic. Provide counseling regarding family planning services, as well as breast and other cancer screenings.

10:30 AM Make a home visit to a mother and baby who is not thriving. Conduct an examination of the baby and assess the living situation. Assist the mother regarding breast-feeding, nutrition, newborn care, and parenting.

12:30 PM Attend a lunch meeting of a newly formed coalition that is concerned about the increased rate of teen pregnancy in the city. Provide community statistics as well as firsthand knowledge of teens participating in the Women, Infants, and Children (WIC) program and the Nurse-Family Partnership home visiting program. Offer information on how to approach the problem.

1:15 PM Respond to phone messages from local school nurses about possible round worm infection of preschoolers in one local school.

2:00 PM Investigate the case of a third grader who has TB. With the help of the school nurse, check immunization records of other students and staff. Contact the family to learn who else is exposed and at risk. Provide proper testing and education regarding the signs and symptoms of TB, the need for regular testing, and following the treatment regimen.

3:30 PM Staff cancer screening clinic performing Pap smears and providing counseling to women regarding risks of breast and cervical cancer. Follow up with patients from last week's clinic whose results were questionable.

4:45 PM Call environmental health sanitarian to discuss possible water system contamination at a farm labor camp and arrange for testing and follow-up.

5:00 PM Finish paperwork and head home.

(see Display 30–2 for an example of a PHN's day). PHNs also serve in administrative roles within agencies, as well, where they may oversee an entire bureau or program, for example, or serve as supervisors for a group of PHNs (Kulbok, Thatcher, Park, & Meszaros, 2012).

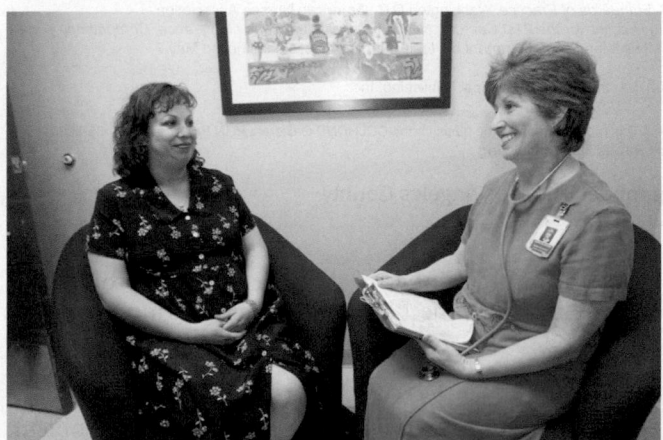

Public health nurses working for local health departments are the eyes and ears of their communities.

Within each of the governmental agencies, programs may be arranged according to a particular subject area. For example, a PHN may work in the cardiovascular disease program, overseeing cholesterol screenings and promoting physical health and nutrition. A PHN could also work in epidemiology, tracking diseases, or be part of a community emergency response team to prepare for a natural or manmade disaster. A PHN could also work in the immunization program, promoting and tracking the immunization requirements of school-age children. The nurse may also be in charge of day care licen-

sure requirements, traveling throughout the state and conducting inspections or writing policies. Or, the nurse could oversee a program to decrease sudden infant death syndrome (SIDS) in the state and track SIDS-related deaths. Thus, the variety of locations and programs are limitless for PHNs (Swider, Levin, & Kulbok, 2014). The following is a brief overview of some of the main roles of nurses working at state health department and LHD. Specific options and means by which PHNs serve as advocates and change agents to protect and promote the health of all are discussed, using the nursing process as an outline. Figure 30–2 provides a practical model of how PHNs use the nursing model and public health principles in their everyday functions.

Assess

An assessment of the situation is key to any nursing care. PHNs assess the situation in a variety of ways. They observe a great deal when they are in the community and when they conduct home visits. They also assess data to identify trends. Often, nurses work with other public health personnel when assessing and tracking data, although nurses may serve as specialists in epidemiology. For example, PHNs can use morbidity and mortality statistics to determine the leading causes of death nationally and locally. They can assess communicable disease rates to identify an outbreak before it becomes too widespread. They track how many people in the community are in compliance with immunizations to keep the herd immunity high and decrease the chance of outbreaks. PHNs use census data to determine population growth. As an example, global reports indicate that the number of individuals aged 60 years or older will grow from 841 million in 2013 to over 2 billion worldwide by 2050. Estimates indicate that in 2050, approximately 21.1% of the world's population will be over the age of 60 (United

Public Health Nursing Practice Model*

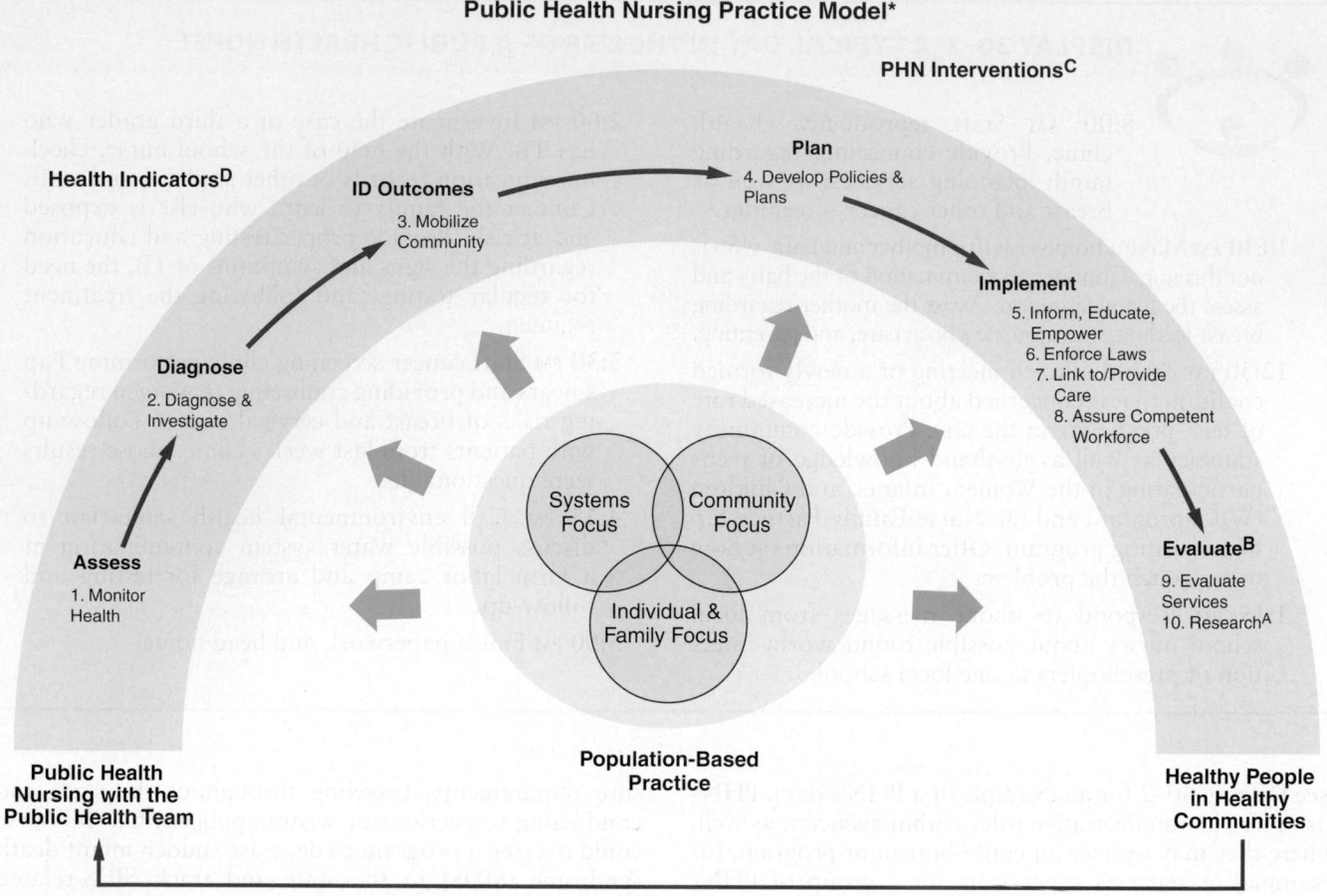

PHN Interventions[C]

Plan
4. Develop Policies & Plans

Health Indicators[D]

ID Outcomes
3. Mobilize Community

Implement
5. Inform, Educate, Empower
6. Enforce Laws
7. Link to/Provide Care
8. Assure Competent Workforce

Diagnose
2. Diagnose & Investigate

Systems Focus

Community Focus

Individual & Family Focus

Evaluate[B]
9. Evaluate Services
10. Research[A]

Assess
1. Monitor Health

Public Health Nursing with the Public Health Team

Population-Based Practice

Healthy People in Healthy Communities

References:
(A) Public Health Functions Steering Committee. (1994, Fall). *Public Health in America*. Retrieved May 7, 2001, from the World Wide Web: http://health.gov/phfunctions/public.htm
(B) Quad Council of Public Health Nursing Organizations. (2007). *Public Health Nursing: Scope & Standards of Practice*. Washington D.C.: American Nurses Association.
(C) Minnesota Department of Health, Public Health Nursing Section. (2000). *Public Health Nursing Practice for the 21st Century: National Satellite Learning Conference; Competency Development in Population-based Practice October 5, November 2, December 7, 2000*. St. Paul, MN: Minnesota Department of Health Nursing Section. Retrieved May 7, 2001, from the World Wide Web: http://www.health.state.mn.us/divs/chs/phr/material.htm
(D) U.S. Department of Health and Human Services. (2000). Healthy People 2010. (Vol. 1). McLean, VA: International Medical Publishing, Inc.

*Created by Los Angeles County DPH, Public Health Nursing with input from CCLHDND-Southern Region. This model serves as the basis for the CCLHDND California PHN Practice Model (05-2002).
© 2007 Los Angeles County DPH Public Health Nursing

FIGURE 30-2 Public health nursing model from Los Angeles County.

Nations, 2013). This is important in planning for future activities and resources. PHNs also use prevalence data to determine which ethnic groups are at higher risk than others. For example, PHNs at a county health department notice increased cases of TB. Upon further investigation, they learned that the greatest increases were within the immigrant Hispanic population. By using data and conducting an assessment, they were able to successfully target interventions for this population (Community Tool Box, 2016). See Chapters 12 and 15.

Environmental risks are important to the public's health and are often assessed by nurses. For example, a PHN conducting blood tests noticed that students living in a mining community had elevated blood lead levels. This assessment information forms the basis for the nurse's intervention. Each nurse must assess his or her own community, because each has specific characteristics and needs. A community positioned next to a factory that emits fumes will have different issues than a rural community 90 miles away from any industry. At the same

time, an outbreak of *Escherichia coli* in one town may identify a risk to the PHN in the neighboring town. See Chapter 9.

Diagnose

Assessment is key to diagnosing a situation or problem. For a PHN, diagnosis also includes identifying priorities for the many concurrent issues. Nurses who work in public settings may perform skin tests or simple blood work in public clinics to determine TB exposure, or risk of high blood pressure, or other conditions (see From the Case Files I). Other nurses utilize microscopes to identify cases of vaginitis and cervicitis. This could all occur on the same day.

As nurses diagnose individual needs, they apply this information and watch for increased or decreased rates (e.g., of disease or injury) among the population. For instance, a nurse working in a public health clinic may notice an increase in the number of people diagnosed with diabetes. The nurse further assesses the situation to

et al., 2011). World events have also placed additional emphasis on public health roles, including the global spread of TB, bioterrorism, pandemic influenza, and natural disasters (Madamala et al., 2011). Because of their nursing and epidemiologic skill, PHNs serve as critical members of emergency preparedness and response teams (Association of Public Health Nurses, 2014). The nursing and epidemiologic skills they use when tracking outbreaks of communicable diseases, such as TB, are easily transferable to the communicable agents of bioterrorism (e.g., smallpox, anthrax).

Plan and Implement

Once PHNs have diagnosed and prioritized the needs of their community, they develop and carryout plans to address those needs. Development of care plans is an important function for nurses. Many interventions require collaborating and working with other agencies. Education is also a key to many public health nursing interventions. However, education alone will not change behavior; thus, it is important to address the issue from many different angles, as well as at different levels. PHNs cannot solve all issues, but they can serve as advocates to influence those who can make the changes (Swider et al., 2013). The interventions are endless, but here are a few examples:

- Nurses conduct home visits to mothers at risk. They conduct family assessments to determine the level of psychological issues and education needed by the family regarding specific needs, such as responses to medication. They also help mothers receive needed psychological counseling by linking them to a local mental health agency.
- A community nurse working in risk management develops and teaches an education program about workplace safety and ergonomics. She develops policies regarding shift hours and heavy lifting.
- A school nurse serves as an advocate for a program that will assist children with special health care needs attend a clinic closer to home.
- A PHN develops a campaign for social media sites (e.g., Twitter, Facebook), television, radio, and local newspapers regarding the need to receive a flu shot. The nurse also includes incentives that target the elderly community who are at additional risk for developing complications from this illness.
- The community health nurse organizes a health clinic at local shelters providing foot care and screenings for blood pressure, diabetes, TB, and cholesterol, as appropriate.
- The school nurse works with schools to educate teens regarding birth control and the impact of teen pregnancy. She includes counseling regarding STDs. She works with the community to ensure that a variety of teen-focused activities are available for this population.
- The community outreach nurse conducts home visits to new mothers who need assistance with breastfeeding and newborn care. The nurse also contacts the housing authority to report hazardous conditions in the housing project she has visited.

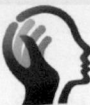

From the **Case Files** I

Tuberculosis (TB) Exposure (Compare Your Local Response With That Outlined Here)

As a public health nurse (PHN), you are alerted to a person who has an active TB case. He present into the health department for a chest x-ray after he failed his tuberculin skin test. The person has recently arrived by plane from another state. He stayed for a few weeks with family members in a small house but now lives with friends in a small apartment. When talking to the patient, you note that he coughs often and does not cover his mouth.

- As a PHN, what steps would you take to determine exposure?
- How will you determine who was exposed and will need to be tested?
- What questions can you ask to help determine when and how the patient was exposed to TB?
- What type of education will you provide to him?
- How can you ensure that the patient is compliant with medication treatment?
- Imagine that you are the school nurse of the patient's 8-year-old daughter who has also tested positive. What steps would you take?
- What would you do differently if you were a correctional nurse and the patient was an inmate?
- What are the ethical and legal issues related to TB?

    See example of a PHN caring for a new TB client in Chapter 29.

determine if it is a population need and also the degree of the problem. Another PHN may assist with newborn genetic testing. Nurses are in the perfect position to identify issues and trends early on. As more is known regarding genetic trends, the PHN can use this information to advocate policies and laws that will impact a particular population (Community Tool Box, 2016).

Constant assessment and diagnosis are tools by which PHNs identify critical situations and prioritize issues that must be addressed first. Several documents have helped PHNs prioritize issues. *Healthy People 2020*, a guide to identifying many of the nation's top priorities, is a valuable tool (USDHHS, 2016). See Display 30–3. Public health performance standards also assist nurses in prioritizing needs (Centers for Disease Control and Prevention [CDC], 2015f; Swider et al., 2013). The IOM (2015) has also identified a need for a greater focus on informatics and genomics in improving patient care and health research.

Improved medical technology has supplied immunizations that have decreased the rates of many communicable diseases. This led to the emergence of new issues and priorities for PHNs, specifically, injury prevention and the management of chronic diseases (Madamala

DISPLAY 30–3 *HEALTHY PEOPLE 2020*—PUBLIC HEALTH PRIORITIES

Healthy People 2020: Public Health
Healthy People 2020 provides the direction and goals for all public health nurses (PHNs). *Healthy People 2020* is used to guide prioritizing activities for PHNs. Specifically, PHNs focus on the ten leading indicators, which include:

- Access to health services
- Clinical preventive services
- Environmental quality
- Injury and violence
- Maternal, infant, and child health
- Mental health
- Nutrition, physical activity, and obesity
- Oral health
- Reproductive and sexual health
- Social determinants
- Substance abuse
- Tobacco

Healthy People 2020: Educational and Community-Based Programs (School Nursing)
One objective directly relates to school nurse staffing:

ECBP-5   Increase the proportion of the nation's elementary, middle, junior high, and senior high schools that have a nurse-to-student ratio of at least 1:750

Other objectives that school nurses can use to help prioritize activities include:

ECBP-2   Increase the proportion of elementary, middle, and senior high schools that provide comprehensive school health education to prevent health problems in the following areas: unintentional injury; violence; suicide; tobacco use and addiction; alcohol or other drug use; unintended pregnancy, human immunodeficiency virus (HIV)/acquired immune deficiency syndrome (AIDS), and sexually transmitted disease (STD) infection; unhealthy dietary patterns; and inadequate physical activity

ECBP-4   Increase the proportion of elementary, middle, and senior high schools that provide school health education to promote personal health and wellness in the following areas: handwashing or hand hygiene, oral health, growth and development, sun safety and skin cancer prevention, benefits of rest and sleep, ways to prevent vision and hearing loss, and the importance of health screenings and checkups

Healthy People 2020: Adolescent Health
AH-6   Increase the proportion of schools with a school breakfast program

Healthy People 2020: Disability and Health
DH-5   Increase the proportion of youth with special health care needs whose health care provider has discussed transition planning from pediatric to adult health care

DH-14   Increase the proportion of children and youth with disabilities who spend at least 80% of their time in regular education programs

Healthy People 2020: Environmental Health
EH-16   Increase the proportion of the nation's elementary, middle, and high schools that have official school policies and engage in practices that promote a healthy and safe physical school environment

Healthy People 2020: Family Planning
FP-8   Reduce pregnancy rates among adolescent females

FP-9   Increase the proportion of adolescents aged 17 years and under who have never had sexual intercourse

FP-12   Increase the proportion of adolescents who received formal instruction on reproductive health topics before they were 18 years old

Healthy People 2020: Immunization and Infectious Diseases
IID-10   Maintain vaccination coverage levels for children in kindergarten

IID-11   Increase routine vaccination coverage levels for adolescents

IID-12   Increase the percentage of children and adults who are vaccinated annually against seasonal influenza

IID-18   Increase the proportion of children under 6 years of age whose immunization records are in fully operational, population-based immunization information systems

Healthy People 2020: Injury and Violence Prevention
IVP-27   Increase the proportion of public and private schools that require students to wear appropriate protective gear when engaged in school-sponsored physical activities

Healthy People 2020: Mental Health and Mental Disorders
MHMD-2   Reduce suicide attempts by adolescents
MHMD-3   Reduce the proportion of adolescents who engage in disordered eating behaviors in an attempt to control their weight

Healthy People 2020: Nutrition and Weight Status
NWS-10   Reduce the proportion of children and adolescents who are considered obese

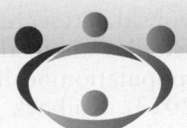

DISPLAY 30–3 *HEALTHY PEOPLE 2020—PUBLIC HEALTH PRIORITIES (Continued)*

NWS-15 Increase the variety and contribution of vegetables to the diets of the population aged 2 years and older

Healthy People 2020: Oral Health

OH-2 Reduce the proportion of children and adolescents with untreated dental decay

Healthy People 2020: Respiratory Diseases

RD-5 Reduce the proportion of persons with asthma who miss school or work days

Healthy People 2020: Substance Abuse

SA-3 Increase the proportion of adolescents who disapprove of substance abuse

Healthy People 2020: Tobacco Use

TU-2 Reduce tobacco use by adolescents

TU-3 Reduce the initiation of tobacco use among children, adolescents, and young adults

Healthy People 2020: Vision

V-2 Reduce blindness and visual impairment in children and adolescents aged 17 years and under

Healthy People 2020: **Correctional Nursing**

IID-27 Increase the percentage of persons aware that they have a hepatitis C infection

IID-29 Reduce tuberculosis (TB)

MHMD-7 Increase the proportion of juvenile residential facilities that screen admissions for mental health problems

MHMD-10 Increase the proportion of persons with co-occurring substance abuse and mental disorders who receive treatment for both disorders

SA-8 Increase the proportion of persons who need alcohol and/or illicit drug treatment and received specialty treatment for abuse or dependence in the past year

TU-13 Establish laws in states, District of Columbia, territories, and tribes on smoke-free indoor air that prohibit smoking in public places and worksites (13.13 correctional facilities)

From: USDHHS. (2016). *Healthy People 2020: Educational & community-based programs.* Retrieved from https://www.healthypeople.gov/2020/topics-objectives/topic/educational-and-community-based-programs/objectives
Adolescent Health: https://www.healthypeople.gov/2020/topics-objectives/topic/Adolescent-Health/objectives
Disability and Health: https://www.hcalthypeople.gov/2020/topics-objectives/topic/disability-and-health/objectives
Environmental Health: https://www.healthypeople.gov/2020/topics-objectives/topic/environmental-health/objectives
Family Planning: https://www.healthypeople.gov/2020/topics-objectives/topic/family-planning/objectives
Immunizations and Infectious Diseases: https://www.healthypeople.gov/2020/topics-objectives/topic/immunization-and-infectious-diseases/objectives
Injury and Violence Prevention: https://www.healthypeople.gov/2020/topics-objectives/topic/injury-and-violence-prevention/objectives
Mental Health and Mental Disorders: https://www.healthypeople.gov/2020/topics-objectives/topic/mental-health-and-mental-disorders/objectives
Nutrition and Weight Status: https://www.healthypeople.gov/2020/topics-objectives/topic/nutrition-and-weight-status/objectives
Oral Health: https://www.healthypeople.gov/2020/topics-objectives/topic/oral-health/objectives
Respiratory Diseases: https://www.healthypeople.gov/2020/topics-objectives/topic/respiratory-diseases/objectives
Substance Abuse: https://www.healthypeople.gov/2020/topics-objectives/topic/substance-abuse/objectives
Tobacco Use: https://www.healthypeople.gov/2020/topics-objectives/topic/tobacco-use/objectives
Vision: https://www.healthypeople.gov/2020/topics-objectives/topic/vision/objectives

- The PHN helps identify resources for families without insurance to ensure that well-child and adult screenings are performed regularly in order to reduce health care costs associated with illness.
- The school nurse organizes an immunization clinic at the local school after an outbreak of measles. The nurse also conducts classes at the school regarding communicable disease prevention and tobacco cessation.
- The PHN organizes a bicycle fair to educate the community regarding the need for bicycle helmets, in hopes of decreasing head injuries. She also works to develop public policy related to child car seat/booster seat usage and collaborates with local businesses in providing vouchers for discounts on child restraints for low-income parents.

- The nurse, who is a paid lobbyist, works to change laws regarding e-cigarettes.
- A nurse, who is an elected member of the state legislature, sponsors a bill to increase funding for school nurses.
- After a hepatitis outbreak at a local business, the nurse conducts an assessment of the business and provides education classes, as well as suggesting policy changes to help guard against future outbreaks.

The following interventions are based on evidence-based practice (see Chapter 4). Below are some examples of EBP in public health nursing:

- Media campaigns targeting specific populations have been successfully used to educate and promote healthy behavior (Atusingwize, Lewis, & Langley, 2015).

- Improving work-based health literacy through educational programs to improve musculoskeletal pain (Larsen et al., 2015).
- School-based program to increase physical activity among sedentary middle school girls (Robbins Pfeiffer, Maier, Lo, & Wesolek, 2012).
- Bike helmets (and legislation requiring helmet use) have been proven to be effective in decreasing head injuries (Walter, Olivier, Churches, & Grzebieta, 2011).

Evaluate

The world in which PHNs work is always changing. It is crucial to constantly evaluate programs and interventions to determine if goals are reached. For example, a nurse may visit childcare facilities or senior centers to ensure that laws regarding licensure are being followed. Evaluating is often equated with assessing. PHNs also can evaluate data to determine whether various rates (e.g., infant mortality or other health indicators) increase or decrease as a result of their interventions.

Another way that PHNs can determine if their interventions are effective is by becoming involved in research. The Quad Council supports research studies about the impact that PHNs have on improving population health and societal outcomes (Swider et al., 2013). Kulbock et al. (2012) describe the interrelatedness of the core competencies and evidence supporting PHN role expansion that can increase the health benefits of the population served.

PUBLIC HEALTH NURSING CAREERS

Nurses who work at the state and federal levels tend to have consultant, or oversight-type roles, and some nurses head programs that are specifically funded at the state and/or federal levels (e.g., HIV/AIDS, immunization programs). Some state-employed nurses may work in clinics for children with special health care needs. Some federally employed nurses may provide direct care through ambulatory care clinics. PHNs at all levels may also be called upon to help during a disaster or communicable disease outbreak. See Perspectives: PHN Nursing Instructor.

Among distinct opportunities at the federal level are those associated with the Department of Veterans Affairs and the U.S. Department of Health and Human

---

LEVELS OF PREVENTION PYRAMID

HEALTH ISSUE: Cervical cancer community setting

TERTIARY PREVENTION		
Rehabilitation	**Primary Prevention**	
	Health Promotion and Education	*Health Protection*
• Provide nursing support groups after hysterectomy and other treatment.		

SECONDARY PREVENTION	
Early Diagnosis	**Prompt Treatment**
• Promote regular Pap smears • Provide Pap smear and high-risk screening counseling at local health fairs	• Provide resources of medical services available for women diagnosed with cervical cancer

PRIMARY PREVENTION	
Health Promotion and Education	**Health Protection**
• Promote healthy lifestyle choices that will decrease risk of human papillomavirus (HPV) (use of condoms, decrease tobacco use, food containing vitamin C and beta carotene) • Provide HPV vaccine at appropriate age • Educate public on risks related to cervical cancer (HPV vaccine, multiple sex partners) • Educate women to get regular Pap smears	

Services (USDHHS, 2014d, 2015). Agencies headed by the USDHHS include the National Institutes of Health (NIH), the Indian Health Service, the Health Resources and Services Administration (HRSA), the Center for Medicaid/Medicare Services (CMS), U.S. Food and Drug Administration (FDA), the Administration for Community Living (ACL), the Substance Abuse and Mental Health Services Administration (SAMSHA), the Administration for Children & Families, and the Centers for Disease Control and Prevention (CDC).

PHNs in these agencies oversee and carryout the initiatives of *Healthy People 2020*, along with other program initiatives. Many of their functions are similar to those mentioned earlier. For example, they may oversee and develop programs, such as national surveys, that collect data used to determine priorities. Examples of these surveys include the Behavioral Risk Factor Survey (BRFS), the Youth Risk Behavior Survey (YRBS), and the National Health Interview Survey (NHIS). Federally employed PHNs at HRSA may review state funding proposals for projects and ensure that guidelines are met. They are a resource for state health department and LHD and often are called upon as consultants. Nurses working at the NIH may assist in conducting research, or work with legal and bioethics staff in evaluating the impact of research on participants, monitoring patients for adverse reactions, or coordinate care for specific groups of patients (NIH, 2016). In addition to these opportunities, PHNs may work as clinicians for the Indian Health Services (IHS), Federal Bureau of Prisons (BOP), and Immigration Customs and Enforcement within the Department of Homeland Security (DHS).

Indian Health Services

Indian Health Services (IHS) started from special relationships between the federal government and the Native American tribes. This relationship is based on information found in the Constitution (Article I, Section 8) and was started in 1787. Over time, other treaties, policies, and laws have influenced the present structure of the IHS. The main goal of IHS is to ensure that comprehensive, culturally acceptable personal and public health services are available and accessible to American Indian and Alaska Native people (IHS, 2015). IHS is responsible for providing health care to Native Americans (American Indians and Alaska Natives). The IHS provides services for members of 566 federally recognized Tribes, or 2.2 million American Indians and Alaska Natives in 170 IHS and tribally managed service units (IHS, 2015). Employment with the IHS allows a nurse to live in a variety of rural and urban settings and to work specifically with Native Americans, a vulnerable population. These nurses work and oversee health care services in clinics run by IHS. The clinics are usually focused on primary care and on general practice. They may work with patients who have diabetes, providing nutritional counseling and education; they may also provide immunizations, perform well-child examinations, or conduct HIV/AIDS screenings. Unique aspects of these jobs are that most clinics are located in remote areas of the country and face unique challenges. Some houses on Native American reservations may not have a telephone or consistent electricity, and these clients may have numerous special needs (IHS, 2015). This type of nursing is very challenging but can also be extremely rewarding.

Uniformed Public Health Nursing

The **U.S. Public Health Service Commissioned Corps** is a group of more than 6,500 specially trained public health members who serve their country with the goal of protecting and promoting the health of the nation. The Corps was established in 1798, as part of an act to treat sick seamen in Marine hospitals. Over the years, the Corps expanded to oversee the health of immigrants entering the country and to assist in preventing/treating communicable disease outbreaks. The U.S. Surgeon General, 2016 oversees the Commissioned Corps and supports the officers stationed in more than 20 federal agencies or departments across the nation, often in very remote areas, filling essential public health leadership and clinical service roles within the nation's federal government agencies (USDHHS, 2014a).

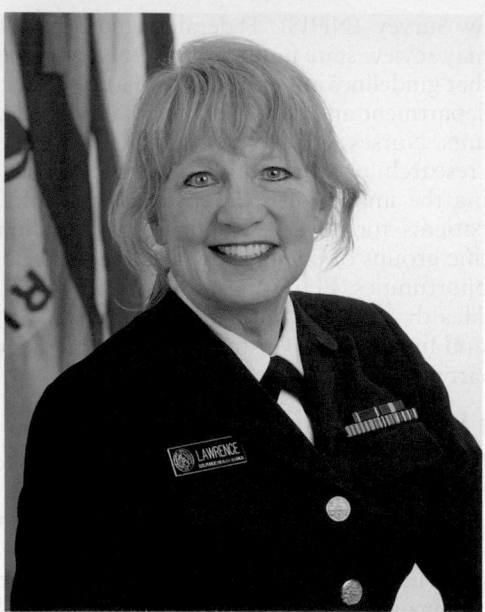

Nurses can serve in each of the seven uniformed services of the U.S. Department of Defense (e.g., Army, Navy, Marine, Air Force), U.S. Department of Homeland Security (Coast Guard), U.S. Department of Commerce (National Oceanic and Atmospheric Administration [NOAA] Commissioned Corps), and the U.S. Public Health Service Commissioned Corps (USPHSCC).

Nurses are an integral part of the Corps. They provide nursing care and health care leadership around the world. Their focus is on improving health for the entire community by providing care, conducting research, or reviewing new medications. These nurses work in a variety of federal agencies, many of them listed earlier. On a daily basis, they may perform tasks similar to civilian nurses. However, as commissioned officers, they can also be deployed to protect the nation's health. For example, USPHSCC nurses were some of the first on the scene to assist in the aftermath of the 2010 earthquake in Haiti. Nurses may also be deployed in the case of a widespread communicable disease outbreak. Their activities can be international as well, in providing expertise and support on global issues such as the Asian

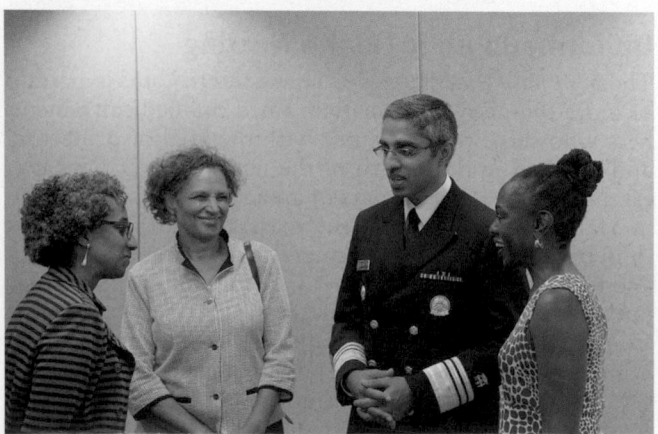

The U.S. Surgeon General, Vice Admiral Vivek H. Murthy, M.D., M.B.A., talking to staff.

tsunami or the worldwide spread of HIV/AIDS. A unique opportunity presented itself to the USPHS Commissioned Corps during the height of the Ebola Virus global epidemic. The President of the United States called upon the USPHS Commissioned Corps to deploy to West Africa to provide care to the health care workers who had been exposed to or infected with the Ebola virus (White House, 2014). Four teams of approximately 70 officers composed of clinicians (physicians, nurses, behavioral health specialists), pharmacists, infection control and laboratory officers, and administrative management personnel rotated to Liberia for 60 days at a time beginning in October 2014 (Lushniak, 2014). Upon the departure of these specially trained teams of PHS officers in May 2015, Liberia was declared Ebola-free. Concurrently, smaller teams of PHS officers served to combat the Ebola outbreak in Guinea and Sierra Leone and remained on site educating the community on Ebola treatment and prevention. President presented the USPHS Commissioned Corps with the Presidential Unit Citation, the highest award for a uniformed service, for their contributions in the fight against Ebola. For more information and a video on the presentation, visit the C-SPAN Web site (http://www.c-span.org/video/?328326-3/president-obama-meets-public-health-officials).

As commissioned officers, USPHSCC nurses are compensated with regular salaries based upon rank following the military pay system. In addition to a potential signing bonus, TRICARE health insurance, eligibility for veteran's benefits, and access to military base lodging and recreational facilities are available. Officers are supported with opportunities to further their education and advance their careers. Student tuition reimbursement and loan payment options are also available through select federal agencies (USDHHS, 2014c).

To qualify as a nurse in the Commissioned Corps, one must be a U.S. citizen, under age 44, able to pass a physical examination and security suitability clearance, possess a bachelor's or higher degree from an accredited nursing program, and hold a valid nursing license from one of the 50 states, the District of Columbia, Puerto Rico, Guam, or the U.S. Virgin Islands (USDHHS, 2014b). For more information on the USPHSCC, visit their Web site (www.usphs.gov).

School Nursing

School nurses save lives and assist in helping children so that they are able to learn and reach their greatest potential. School nursing is a specialized practice of professional nursing that advances the well-being, academic success, and lifelong achievement of students. School nurses are a link between the school, families, community, and health care stakeholders. These nurses (between 2.1% and 2.8% of RN population) are tasked with serving as advocates for health and healthy school environments (National Association of School Nurses [NASN], 2014e). In a qualitative study examining how school nurses provide health care to students, Rademacher (2012, p. 242) describes the school nurse "caring for" and "caring about" children's health needs and being motivated to assist students in achieving their best at school.

A **school nurse** works primarily with the students who attend the nurse's assigned schools, as well as with the families of those schoolchildren, members of the school staff and administration, health care providers, and other helping professionals within the school and community. In fall 2015, approximately 50.1 million students were expected to attend public elementary and secondary schools (National Center for Education Statistics, 2015). These children are the parents, workers, leaders, and decision-makers of tomorrow, and their future success depends in good measure on achieving their educational goals today. Their school success is intertwined, to some degree, with the state of their health (American School Health Association, n.d.; CDC, 2011). See Chapter 22.

Think back to your own elementary and secondary schooling. Did you have access to a school nurse? If so, how did that person influence your health and the health of your peers? If you did not have a school nurse, how do you think a school nurse might have improved your school environment or educational experience? The school nurse is a key provider of a variety of services.

History of School Nursing

Beginning in the mid-1800s and continuing through the early years of the 20th century, mandatory education was instituted in the United States. The early years included health services often conducted by "medical inspectors," usually physicians. In New York City, where communicable disease was rampant, inspectors sent notes home with children with the message "you are sick—go home" and citing the reason for their exclusion from school (Vessey & McGowan, 2006, p. 255). The reasons for exclusion were largely the contagious illnesses commonly found among the tenements and crowded slums of the growing city. However, parents often did not receive these notes, or couldn't read them, and because families lacked resources, most children were left untreated and simply remained out of school as truants. No efforts were made by medical inspectors to follow up on excluded children. Because these excluded children played with healthy children after school hours, the levels of contagious illness actually worsened (Vesey & McGowan, 2006). As noted in Woodfill and Beyrer's classic text (1991), the absentee children promoted the spread of various communicable diseases. In 1902, the practice of school nursing began when the New York Board of Education contracted with Lillian Wald's Henry Street Settlement to provide a PHN to work with the families and schools to facilitate the return of healthy children to school. The nurse was Lina Rogers. She made home visits to follow up on excluded children and was assisted by other Henry Street nurses in providing care, educating families about diseases and the need for hygiene, and working with other organizations to provide needed food, shoes, and clothing (Hawkins & Watson, 2010; Rollins, 2011; Vessey & McGowan, 2006). In the first month of the school nurse experiment, 98% of children previously excluded from school for medical reasons were treated and readmitted (Woodfill & Beyrer, 1991). Lina Rogers, who later married and was known the last name of Struthers, described her first school "dispensary" as an "unused stair closet" where she was unable to stand fully erect, but still provided treatment for skin and eye diseases, as well as draining ears (Struthers, 1917, p. 19). The board hired 12 more school nurses, and over the next few years, other cities

and states began hiring nurses to work in the schools. School nurses have historically advocated for hot lunches, breakfast programs, better social conditions, and the need for increased health education in schools and for families (Abrams, 2005; Rollins, 2011). See Chapter 2.

School nurses continue as a specialty branch of professional nursing that serves the school-age population. Approximately 61,000 to 70,000 RNs are working in elementary and secondary schools (K-12) currently (NASN, 2014e). However, according to the recent School Health Policies and Programs Study (SHPPS), the nationally recommended ratio of one school nurse for every 750 students has not been achieved at the elementary and middle/high school levels, with only 85.2% and 78.4%, respectively, reporting that they had a school nurse. However, about half of all schools reported having an RN for 30 or more hours per week, and around 60% of all schools had licensed practical nurses available and not RNs. Many schools still report having an insufficient amount of school nursing services (CDC, 2015g). Several school sites serving adolescent students provided a cell phone app to those interested in contacting school nurses with questions or concerns; they receive a return text with information on where to access information and resources, as well as a call from the nurse if it is during school hours. Students and school nurses have found this innovative approach helpful (Penfold, 2013).

School nurses deliver services to students from birth through age 21 years. They also work with students' families and the school community in regular and special education schools, as well as other educational settings (e.g., preschools, court, and other community schools). Studies show that having a school nurse present increases health and social services and improves absentee rates (Hill & Hollis, 2011). The role of the school nurse has expanded over the years, along with the increase in chronic conditions and challenges in accessing health care (Kennedy, 2014). It is estimated that 8% of children aged 3 to 17 years have a learning disability, about 9% have ADHD, and 14% have ever had an asthma diagnosis (Bloom, Cohen, & Freeman, 2012). Federal law requires school systems to provide care for children with disabilities. The Individuals with Disabilities Education Act (IDEA, 1975), the Rehabilitation Act of 1973, and Title II of the Americans with Disabilities Act all mandate equal educational opportunities for all students, including children with complex medical conditions. In 2012, 95% of 6- to 21-year-old students with disabilities were being educated in regular schools, and only 3% received services in a separate school (National Center for Education Statistics, 2016). Legislative mandates and technology that has allowed low-birth-weight babies to survive have led to a steady increase in the number of children with special health care needs attending school (American Academy of Pediatrics [AAP], 2016). It is now commonplace for children to attend school accompanied by feeding tubes, catheters, insulin pumps, glucose monitors, and ventilators. There is a growing population of adolescent and preadolescent children who are within 6 months of dying from chronic disease and are routinely attending school (NASN, 2014c).

According to Kennedy (2014, p. 7), over the past 15 years, the school nurse role has dramatically changed, as has the student population. "There are more immigrant students, more children living in poverty, more children likely to have food insecurity and poor health because of lack of access. And there are more students with chronic conditions who need support to manage their illness so they can stay in school. Schools can't afford *not* to have a school nurse" (Kennedy, 2014, p. 7). The lack of access to health care has added extra burdens on schools, and school nurses are often "the sole provider of access to health care" (Sonnenberg, 2013 para. 20). Also, children often come to school sick or miss additional days of school resulting from complications of illnesses that could have been easily treated in earlier stages. In 2012, 7% of U.S. children had no coverage for health insurance, and 4% had no usual source of health care. Some children access health care services only at school, and 12% made at least one visit to the ED, whereas 5% had two or more visits (Bloom, Jones, & Freeman, 2013). Results from the 2011–2012 National Health Survey indicate that 6.2% of children missed 11 days of school or more in the past year because of illness, and this was more of a problem in children with special health care needs as the proportion increased to 14.9% (CDC, 2013a; National Quality Measures Clearinghouse, 2013). Children from families of lower socioeconomic status were twice as likely to miss 11 days of school or more than were children from families with higher income levels (9% vs. 4%).

In their survey of almost 400 school nurses in 35 states, Krause-Parello and Samms (2011) found that school nurses "very frequently" worked with students having asthma (59.2%), allergies (58.7%), ADHD (52.7%), diabetes (29.6%), depression (13.5%), and seizure disorders (8.8%). Although asthma was the most common condition observed, only a little over 20% reported having asthma action plans for 100% of their students with asthma. Seasonal allergies were most common, followed by nut and dairy allergies.

School nurses spend a good deal of time on health promotion, and 87% in one survey saw a "direct correlation with student academic outcomes" and health-promoting activities (Krause-Parello & Samms, 2011, p. 34). Most school nurses promote self-care and safety education (87.8%), and 64.4% did environmental assessments of their schools. School nurses, administrators, teachers, parents, and community stakeholders are all vital in coordinated school health program and in developing health-promoting schools (Hung, Chiang, Dawson, & Lee, 2014). School wellness programs often incorporate education on healthy nutrition and increasing physical activity, for instance (Avery, Johnson, Cousins, & Hamilton, 2013). Walker (2014) reminds us that the school nurse is also a role model for wellness promotion, in addition to providing individual and group health education. Some of the health school nurse behaviors include drinking water, eating a healthy lunch in the teacher's lounge (often filled with unhealthy snacks), walking during recess or free time, eating healthy snacks (e.g., fresh fruit, vegetables), and limiting consumption of unhealthy foods and beverages.

School nurses are also involved in emergency preparedness and disaster planning. The National Association of School Nurses (NASN, 2014d), in their position statement on this issue, noted that school nurses are a crucial link between local public health agencies and emergency services. School nurse roles include prevention/mitigation, preparedness, response, and recovery; their role with special needs children is especially vital. Epidemics (e.g., influenza), weather-related emergencies (e.g., hurricanes, tornadoes, earthquakes, flooding), and other sudden crises (e.g., school shootings, terrorism) are all potential issues facing school nurses. The Federal Emergency Management Institute (a division of the Department of Homeland Security and the Federal Emergency Management Administration [FEMA]) offers training courses for school administrators, school nurses, and teachers to aid them in preparing for various emergencies (see Chapter 17). Additionally, school nurses must consider emergency evacuation plans, especially for disabled students, and determine the best way to reunite students with their families.

Key Roles of the School Nurse

The school nurse's main role is to provide both individual and population health care and coordination for school-age children and adolescents. School nurses utilize their knowledge of normal growth and development, social determinants of health, safety and health (including environmental health), and the educational system in providing services. They clearly understand the connection between health and learning and promote health among students, families, and staff. They provide case management for children with chronic illnesses (e.g., diabetes, asthma, severe allergies), immunization monitoring/access, and collaborate with parents, teachers, and psychologists in providing appropriate educational plans for students requiring special education services. They work with school staff to ensure a healthy and safe environment (e.g., nutrition, physical activity, playground safety). They also collaborate with community agencies (e.g., public health departments/other health agencies, charitable groups/service clubs), physicians, dentists, parent groups, and child protective services in order to meet students' and families' needs. They often conduct screenings and work with school staff to promote their health and wellness. School nurses may also work with school-based clinics to provide direct health care to children and their families. They are an integral leader in coordinated school health programs (AAP, 2016).

The National Association of School Nurses (NASN, 2016) describes the broad role of the school nurse as a "specialized practice of professional nursing that advances the well-being, academic success and lifelong achievement and health of students" (para. 8). The school nurse:

- Facilitates the normal development of students and promotes positive intervention outcomes
- Provides leadership in the areas of health promotion, safety, and a healthy school environment
- Provides high-quality health care and promotes early intervention for actual and potential student health problems
- Uses sound clinical judgment in the provision of case management for students
- Collaborates actively and professionally with others to promote student/family capacity for self-management and adaptation, as well as learning and self-advocacy (NASN, 2016)

Parents of schoolchildren cite first aid/emergency care, teacher education about special needs students, parent/school/health care provider communication, control/prevention of disease, and provision of medical treatments to special needs children or those with chronic illnesses as the most important roles and duties of the school nurse (Lineberry & Ickes, 2015). The partnership between school nurses and families is important for the child's health outcomes, and the use of problem-based communication strategies helps promote this collaboration (Mäenpää, Paavilainen, & Åstedt-Kuri, 2012).

Liaison with the Interdisciplinary School Health Team

School nursing services are part of a coordinated school health program that provides school health services, health education, and health promotion programs for faculty and staff (American School Health Association, n.d.). Although the school nurse plays a central role, collaboration with many other individuals is important. School nurses must be familiar with the education setting and work closely with teachers/aides, special education teachers/staff, principals, administrators, school office staff, health aides, psychologists, speech therapists, as well as parents and families. The Whole School, Whole Community, Whole Child (WSCC) model focuses on the child and emphasizes a school-wide approach and acknowledges learning, health, and the school as being a part and reflection of the local community (CDC, 2015a, 2015l). See Figure 30–3 for the WSCC Model. It includes 10 components:

- Health education
- Physical activity/education
- Nutrition services/environment
- Health services
- Counseling/social/psychological services
- Social/emotional climate
- Physical environment
- Employee wellness
- Family engagement
- Community involvement

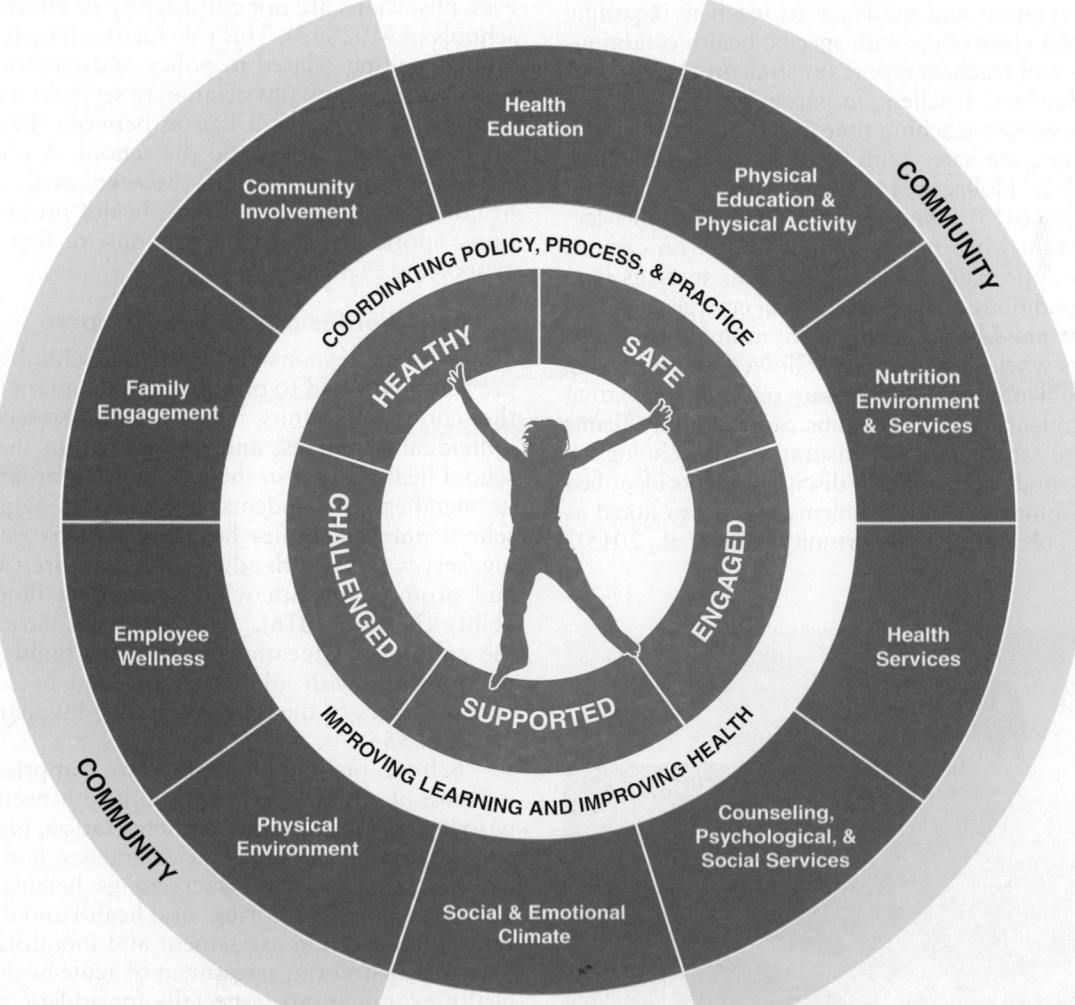

FIGURE 30–3 Whole School, Whole Community, Whole Child (WSCC) model. From Centers for Disease Control and Prevention. (2016). *Whole School, Whole Community, Whole Child.* Retrieved from http://www.cdc.gov/healthyyouth/wscc/

Positive Working Relationship with School Team Members

The school principal influences all phases of the school health program by promoting good school health through active support of the school's health services, participation in setting health-related policies, and tapping into community resources. The principal can reinforce positive efforts within the school, ranging from the health teaching in the classroom to the cleaning activities of the custodian. Because of the principal's influential position, it is absolutely essential for the nurse and principal to maintain a positive and cooperative working relationship. Studies have noted that parents, principals, teachers, and school staff have positive attitudes toward school nurses and find that having a school nurse present saves time for school administrators, teachers, and staff (Baisch, Lundeen, & Murphy, 2011; Lineberry & Ickes, 2015).

Teachers, whether they are involved in regular instruction, physical education, or special education, play a major role in school health. Because they spend the most time with students, their observations, health teaching, and personal health habits have a profound effect on student health and the quality of school health services. The school nurse and teachers must collaborate constantly, as the school nurse provides information and guidance to teachers regarding students in their classrooms with specific health conditions and concerns and teachers report on students' health concerns and behaviors. Teachers, in particular, feel that they have more classroom teaching time and that students with chronic illnesses are safer with school nurses on school grounds (Hill & Hollis, 2011. Biag, Srivastava, Landau, and Rodriguez (2015) found that teachers had higher levels of satisfaction when nurses were available on campus full time and appreciated nurses' help with students having chronic conditions, managing medical emergencies, and providing first aid when students were injured. They also found benefits when school nurses followed up on hearing and vision problems, making necessary referrals and getting services for students having problems. Student Study Teams (SSTs), where teachers, administrators, psychologists, school nurses, and others meet to discuss students identified as having learning or health problems, were also noted as an important collaborative opportunity (Biag et al., 2015).

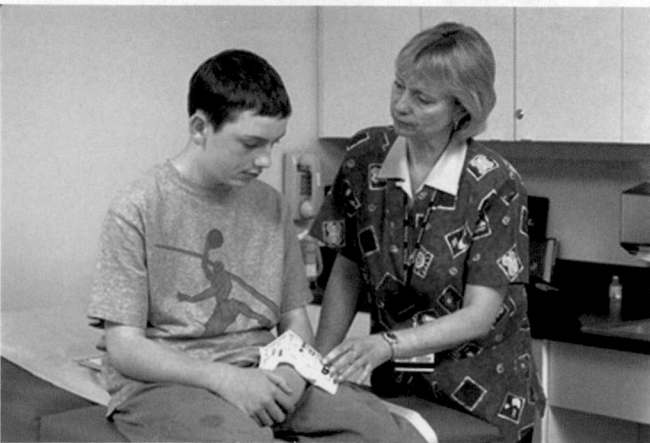

The school nurse is part of a team providing a coordinated school health program.

Other health team members, such as health educators, health coordinators, psychologists, audiologists, speech therapists, occupational therapists, physical therapists, counselors, health care providers, dentists, dental hygienists, social workers, security and juvenile justice personnel, health aides, and volunteers, may also be involved, depending on size and financial resources of the school. All team members, including students, parents, bus drivers, and custodians, have a specialized role complementary to that of the school nurse.

School-based health centers (SBHCs) provide an access to health care services for youth confronted with barriers to social determinants of health and are often sponsored or funded by public health departments, community health centers, or hospitals. They often provide care for children, and sometimes their families, who otherwise do not have access to health care. SBHCs "bring critical, developmentally appropriate services to children and adolescents where they spend most of their waking hours; at school" (Keeton, Soleimanpour, & Brindis, 2012, p. 132).

If the school system desires such services, a physician may work on a part-time consultative basis; however, physicians are not consistently or effectively used in schools (AAP, 2013). This role focuses largely on advising and consulting related to policy and medical–legal matters. A community physician may serve on a school advisory panel, acting as a liaison between the community, other health agencies, and the school. A physician or a nurse practitioner (NP) may become involved in student health appraisals, rescreenings, health problem interventions, sports physical examinations, or first aid support at sporting events.

Responsibilities of the School Nurse

The primary responsibilities of the school nurse are to prevent illness and to promote and maintain the health of the school community. The school nurse serves not only individuals, families, and groups within the context of school health but also the school as an organization and its membership (students and staff) as aggregates. The school nurse identifies health-related barriers to learning, serves as a health advocate for children and families, and promotes health while preventing illness and disability (NASN, 2016). "School nurses must understand the culture of education in order to build professional relationships with administrators and be seen as valuable members of the school team" (Maughan & Adams, 2011, p. 355).

School nursing activities are comprised of nursing care of children with special health needs, including nasogastric tube feedings, catheterization, insulin pumps, and suctioning; general and emergency first aid; vision, hearing, scoliosis, and TB screenings; height, weight, and blood pressure monitoring; oral health and dental education; immunization assessment and monitoring; medication administration; assessment of acute health problems; health examinations (especially for athletic participation or school entry); and referrals (DuChateau, Beversdorf, & Wolff, 2015; Jones & Boyd, 2011). School nurses also assess and are the frontline providers for identifying communicable diseases, such as outbreaks of influenza or meningitis. A systematic review of research on the impact of school nurses noted that fewer absences occurred when school nurses were present and that rates for immunization compliance were also improved (Lineberry & Ickes, 2015).

Medication administration is another common school nurse duty. In one study, 91.9% of school nurses reported giving ADHD medications, 88.8% gave bronchodilators, 88.6% gave over-the-counter (OTC) medications, 86% gave antibiotics, and almost 71% gave insulin. This study also found that medications may be given by school nurses (92.7%) and unlicensed assistive personnel (UAP; 31.9%), such as health aids or school clerks (Krause-Parello & Samms, 2011). Administrators, teachers, and others may also give medications depending upon state laws. For instance, only school nurses and physicians may administer medications in Massachusetts, but many other states (e.g., Pennsylvania, California) allow UAPs to give medications in the nurse's absence (Krause-Parello & Samms, 2011).

School nurses perform first aid, help students with inhalers and nebulizer treatments, and some may do gastric tube feedings and ventilator/tracheostomy care. They are responsible for documenting their care, but this can be difficult because of time constraints, educational regulations, and lack of a functional standardized data set or method of collection. A study by Johnson, Dewey Bergren, and Westbrook (2012) collected and evaluated data from six states. They found that most school nurses and school districts reported on staffing, risk management, case management, episodic care, and health promotion activities. However, applying existing data classification systems (NANDA, NIC, NOC) did not "adequately describe the scope of school nursing practice" (p. 103). They called for a nationally standardized school nursing/health database to improve care coordination and more efficient delivery of care to school-age children and youth.

Other duties of a school nurse may include training school staff in cardiopulmonary resuscitation (CPR), universal precautions and first aid, as well as overseeing the health and wellness of school staff members. They also participate in emergency planning and disaster drills, as well as school evacuation plans. Many of these activities may be performed concurrently (Sonnenberg, 2013). Lineberry and Ickes' (2015) systematic review noted four main areas of school nurse activity: (a) "health promotion and disease prevention," (b) "triage and treatment" of acute infectious diseases and injuries, (c) managing "chronic conditions," and (d) offering "psychosocial support" (p. 31). See Display 30–4 for a typical day in the life of a school nurse. Each school nurse must assess and prioritize how to address the specific needs in each individual school and determine the order. As you can see,

---

DISPLAY 30–4 A DAY IN THE LIFE OF A SCHOOL NURSE

6:00 AM This morning, I texted one of my nurses to make sure that she was going to be well enough to come to work. If she was still too sick to work, I would have had to get an early start contacting one of our two district nursing substitutes to see if they could cover again (nursing subs are rare gems within our profession).

8:00 AM At school, I stopped to say hello to the office staff, to see how they were doing, and to ask if they did anything fun since seeing them last. I have learned during my time with the district that it is vital for the office staff to like and respect you because they are the heart of each and every school. They know all of the students, including home and health issues, who the regulars are in the health room, when there are field trips, and anything else that may be important for me to know. They are also my health room assistants, because it is impossible for me, or my support nurses, to be present at each school all day, every day. I always carry a personal phone and a work phone to be easily reached when not on site.

8:15 AM As I walked into my office, I had a call from my support nurse at the high school. She updated me on a student having an allergic reaction to the latex that the science room was using for an experiment. There was enough of an exposure that the student was given her EpiPen and staff called 911. It was decided that the student would be removed temporarily from the classroom during the 6-day experiment, and arrangements would be made to make it safe for the student to return to the classroom at that time.

8:25 AM After that call, I had another nurse call asking about one of her diabetic students who wanted to begin participating in an after school program provided by the school. I asked her to send me the student's daily schedule for monitoring and treating his blood glucose (BG) levels as well as some history of his BG highs and lows. Fortunately, the support nurse and I had time in the coming week to put something together. A triage list is necessary in school nursing!

8:45 AM Finally, I was able to get caught up with my email. At one of my other elementary schools, we had an upcoming field trip for the 5th grade classes. I emailed all the teachers to request a day and time to do a basic med training before the big day and to answer any questions the teachers might have. One of the classes has a diabetic student in it so I also called the parents to see if one of them would be able to go on the trip as a chaperone and to care for their student. If they couldn't, a nurse would have to go. This would mean having one less support nurse for much of the day. I then checked in with my nurse that helps to cover three of my other elementary schools to see how she was doing and to send her a to-do list for the day.

10:45 AM Before checking on our two diabetics for their lunches, I had just enough time to print out

(continued)

DISPLAY 30–4 A DAY IN THE LIFE OF A SCHOOL NURSE (*Continued*)

a report that shows which students are noncompliant with their vaccinations. I then stopped by the lunchroom to see how one of the diabetic student's lunch went. His blood glucose numbers were high, but when he rechecked after recess, his blood glucose was on the way back down to normal range again. I made it back just as my younger diabetic walked into my office for her BG check. I love being able to have time to talk to my diabetic students because not only do I enjoy the conversation, I can also get an idea of how their week is going to go based on their experiences over the weekend, if they are sick, if they have any big plans coming up, etc. I can also pick up on when things are a little off. This diabetic student was acting a little more goofy than normal. I discovered that her blood glucose level was 71 and her dex had two arrows facing downward. Fortunately she was a few minutes late for her check so she was able to go straight to lunch. I walked her to the lunchroom so that I could see what she picked to eat for hot lunch. I always check her again after her lunch is complete to see how many carbohydrates she consumed for dosing her insulin.

11:30 AM Once back in the health room, a student came in very upset, clutching his arm. He had fallen off of the playground set and landed on his arm. My assessment revealed that his forearm was oddly shaped. It was clearly broken. While I assessed him, I had an office staff member call 911 and his parents to update them about the situation. Fortunately, it was not a compound fracture, and he still had sensation and capillary refill. Because we are not at a hospital, there are many things we do not have available to us when caring for patients in the schools. I improvised a splint, using my clipboard with an ice pack resting on his arm to help reduce swelling until the paramedics arrived.

11:35 AM To distract the student from the pain, I asked what educational show they liked, and loaded it up on my computer to distract him. The office staff completed the paperwork to report the injury and emailed me a copy.

11:35 AM My diabetic came in to have me check her food tray so that she could get her insulin dose. Usually, I go out to meet her but in this situation, I had her bring her tray to my office where I checked and dosed her.

11:45 AM After everyone left, I debriefed with the office staff about how things went, what they did well, and to answer any questions or concerns that they might have had.

12:00 PM I checked the immunization list to see who might be excluded from school for being noncompliant with vaccinations. I will determine which students will need reminder letters mailed home and prepare them for mailing.

1:00 PM A diabetic student came in again because her dex was alarming. When we checked her again, she was at 49. I gave her a juice and a snack while I called her mom to let her know what was happening. I had her stay with me for 15 minutes after she finished her snack and then retested her. She was up within range by her next check but, with her mom's permission, I gave her a protein snack to keep her going on the way home.

1:30 PM I checked in with my nurses. The nurse with the student using the EpiPen was able to find information about how to clean out the room for the student, and she let me know that the teachers had been informed of the situation, a report had been filed, and the family called saying the student was fine.

2:00 PM One of the teachers stopped in to see me. She had been sick for a while and was showing signs of pneumonia. She knew she was very sick, but she needed encouragement to go see her provider. Usually, people think that school nurses focus on just the students but in reality, we care for the adults as well. School staff and families rely on us to give health care advice.

3:00 PM It's the end of the school day! I only made a dent in my to-do list by the end of the day but, more importantly, the students were safe and we had all made it through another day. Things may be hectic at times but knowing that I am helping keep people safe and making them feel better when they are ill makes it all worthwhile.

Heather D., Lead Nurse, Spokane WA

---

there are a wide variety of activities involved in school nursing. This largely autonomous practice requires specific skills and training.

Education: Special Training and Skills of the School Nurse

School nurses operate from one of two administrative bases: the school system or the public health department. In most localities, public or private school systems or districts hire school nurses, and they maintain a specialized, school-based practice. Private schools and universities also hire school nurses (NASN, 2014f). In

this specialized role, the nurse can concentrate time and effort solely on the school health program and develop specialized skills in school health assessment and intervention. Today, with the emphasis on delivery of health care at community sites where clients spend most of their time (e.g., schools for children, the workplace for adults), the nurse whose specialty is school health care seems better prepared to meet the complex needs of the school-age population. In contrast, the school nurse who operates under the board of health's jurisdiction provides services to schools as one part of generalized public health nursing services to the community. The community health nurse working through the health department usually devotes only a portion of the workday to the school; she may have additional responsibilities, such as clinic nursing and home visits. This broader base allows contact with preschoolers and their families, provides a stronger knowledge of the community and its resources, and promotes integration of in-school and out-of-school care (Selekman, 2013).

Depending on the state of residence, a school nurse is usually an RN—frequently with additional education beyond the bachelor's degree in nursing, sometimes including a master's degree—that has primary responsibility for the health care of school-age children and school personnel in an educational setting. In some areas of the country, licensed practical nurses (LPNs) or licensed vocational nurses (LVNs) may be hired by school districts, but they must generally work under the supervision of an RN. *School nursing: Scope and standards of practice* (ANA & NASN, 2011) indicates that school nurses should, at minimum, possess a bachelor's degree. As the needs of school-aged populations become increasingly complex, some states require even more specialized training for school nurses. In California, for instance, school nurses are expected to hold a school health services credential. This credential is obtained through a postbaccalaureate program that includes course work in audiology, guidance and counseling, exceptional children, school health principles and practice, a practicum in school nursing, child psychology, and health curriculum development, in addition to other courses. However, most California school nurse credential programs are now available only as part of a master's degree program. A national certification is available as well (NASN, 2014a).

School nurse practitioners (SNPs) are RNs with advanced academic and clinical preparation (generally certification and a master's degree in nursing), along with a guided experience in physical assessment, diagnosis, and treatment, so that the SNP may provide primary care to school-age children. Many school districts see the advantage of having an SNP on staff, rather than using the limited services of a physician. Assessment, diagnosis, treatment, and referral of injuries, communicable diseases, or other health problems can be managed more efficiently by a NP who is educationally prepared to work holistically with the school-age population and is part of the educational setting. If this arrangement is impractical, an SNP who is available to school nurses for consultation or who is employed on a part-time basis can become the impetus for comprehensive school-based health services. Some school districts utilize SNPs to provide services to teachers and staff to promote wellness or to handle job-related injuries. Some research findings cite cost savings related to SNP services, as students and staff served by them experience fewer days of absenteeism (Kerr et al., 2011). As the population continues to become more diverse and the problems of children and their families grow in complexity, the school nurse with specialized training in school health, the education system, case management, and advanced practice nursing (e.g., NPs, clinical nurse specialists) becomes even more essential.

Functions of School Nursing Practice

The three main functions of school nursing practice are health services, health education, and promotion of a healthy school environment. Health services include caring for individual students who have chronic conditions or acute situations while at the same time thinking of the entire population and tracking trends (Rollins, 2011). For example, the school nurse observes an increase in the number of students diagnosed with asthma and investigates ways to help all students with asthma. One way of doing this may be to organize an *Open Airways* course (developed by the American Lung Association, 2016) to assist students in identifying triggers and managing their own care. The goal of this course would be to decrease student asthma attacks.

Health Services for Children with Chronic Conditions

Chronic health conditions are commonly considered to involve having medical needs that are greater than those usual for a child of similar age, or functional limitations, and to last longer than 3 months to a year (Crump et al., 2013). The number of children afflicted with chronic diseases is rising and is thought to affect over 5 million children and adolescents (Compas, Jaser, Dunn, & Rodriguez, 2012; Crump et al., 2013). Common chronic conditions include hay fever, sinusitis, dermatitis, tonsillitis, asthma, diabetes, seizure disorders, and hearing difficulties (Goodwin et al., 2013). In addition, acute illnesses such as stomachaches, headaches, colds, and flu are frequent complaints of school-age children. A retrospective cohort study of almost 23,000 children and adolescents found that having a chronic health condition was associated with lower English language and math performance, despite socioeconomic status or ethnicity. In this study, absences did not significantly change the low performance scores for children with chronic conditions; conditions such as autism, ADHD, and seizure disorders had the strongest associations (Crump et al., 2013). Although, reducing absenteeism is a common function for school nurses, and chronic absences have often been linked with chronic conditions like asthma and diabetes (Jacobsen, Meeder, & Voskuil, 2016). School nurses need to "develop and maintain a high level of clinical expertise" with these common chronic conditions of children and youth and may need additional resources in the case of neurological conditions, such as seizure disorders, brain cancers/injuries, and Tourette syndrome (Sprague-McRae & Rosenblum, 2013, p. 276). See Quality and Safety Education in Nursing (QSEN).

For students in special education programs, school nurses can coordinate **individualized education plans (IEPs)** with **individualized health plans (IHPs)** to develop health management goals for students. Medically fragile or technology-dependent students, who may require procedures such as suctioning or tube feeding, would have IHPs developed for *specialized physical health care procedures* (Galemore & Sheetz, 2015). School nurses utilize additional reference books and Web sites in order to keep up to date with current procedures (DuChateau et al., 2015). Because these students are often hospitalized, interrupting their education, the school nurse

QSEN: Focus on Quality for School Nurse Working with Student Returning to School After a Concussion			
QSEN Definition	**SN Knowledge**	**SN Skills**	**SN Attitudes and Judgment**
Patient-centered care: Recognize the student and parent as the source of control and full partner in providing compassionate and coordinated care based on respect for child's preferences, values, and needs.	Comprehension of pathology related to concussions, including symptoms/comorbid conditions, coping, complications, affect on academic functioning, pain control, and absences.	– Basic neurological assessments and baseline testing. – Symptom recognition, adaptive strategies. – Medical clearances, returning to sports.	– Expectations of time needed to return to full function or new state of functioning. – Encourage counseling and other services, if needed. – Recognize student and family connection to sport; discuss change to lower impact sport, and risks/long-term complications of repeated concussions.
Teamwork* and *collaboration: Function effectively within nursing and interprofessional teams, fostering open discussion, mutual respect, and shared decision making to achieve quality patient care.	Utilize effective communication with student, parents, teachers, coaches, neurologist and other professionals.	– Work closely with neurologist and school team to assist student in school reintegration, making up work, and gaining needed accommodations (e.g. rest breaks, reduced homework). – IEP, Section 504 plans, if needed.	– Be proactive in educating school team members about injury, be open to questions and strive for effective communication.
Evidence-based practice: Integrate best current evidence with clinical expertise and patient/family preferences and values for delivery of optimal health care.	Explain evidence regarding postconcussion syndrome, medications, sports safety, student health plan, where to find reliable evidence and practice guidelines.	Discuss variables that can affect a student's return to playing sports (e.g., previous concussions, severity of injury, expected time for recovery) and potential timetable. – Use evidence to update concussion plan.	– Rely on critically appraised current evidence and not personal examples or anecdotes. – Discuss the lack of evidence in some situations.
Quality Improvement: Use data to monitor outcomes of care processes and use improvement methods to design and test changes to continuously improve the quality and safety of health care systems.	Utilize national and other databases on head injuries, including information on types of sports involved, circumstances of injuries, prevention measures, and implications of negative outcomes.	– Work with school and district on developing a concussion database. – Educate school staff about student health issues. – Help to infuse new evidence into school sports program and academic practice standards.	– Work with students, parents, coaches, and trainers to encourage sports safety in schools. – Share information on potential for poor outcomes, and long-term financial/legal considerations.
Safety: Minimize risk of harm to patients and providers through both system effectiveness and individual performance.	Review safety principles on repeated concussions, serious sequelae (e.g., brain swelling, bleeding, sudden-impact disorders, sudden death).	– Utilize acute and continuing neurological assessment skills and teach coaches about initial concussion assessment/management. – Work with staff on PE modifications and using new technology to decrease injuries.	– Use change theory to promote a safety culture in schools, recognizing potential barriers. – Employ the use of personal stories from athletes who have had concussions.
Informatics: Use information technology to communicate, manage knowledge, mitigate error, and support decision-making.	Assert vigilance in following media coverage of concussions, current academic literature, and updated web sources.	– Promote computer literacy in locating resources, and communicating with parents/staff. – Use email and other electronic methods to provide information to staff and others.	– Teach others about reliable sources of information on the web. – Recommend caution when seeking information from unrecognized sources.

Case Western Reserve University. (2014). *QSEN graduate KSAs.* Retrieved from http://qsen.org/competencies/graduate-ksas/Rosenblum, R. K., & Sprague-McRae, J. (2014). Using principles of Quality and Safety Education for Nurses in school nurse continuing education. *Journal of School Nursing, 30*(2), 97–102.

needs to assist with transition planning. Collaboration with school psychologists and school and health team members is important to transition planning that is also needed as students move from elementary to middle school, from middle school to high school, and as they move out of public schools and on to other educational or job training settings (Finch, Finch, McIntosh, Thomas, & Maughan, 2015; NASN, 2015). School nurses develop individualized health plans (IHPs) to ensure that students with special needs (e.g., chronic conditions) have these needs met. If these students attend the regular classroom and do not fall under the IDEA, the plans may be known as **Section 504 plans**, named after the section of the Rehabilitation Act and the accompanying statute, the Americans with Disabilities Act (ADA), that specifically allows for school accommodations with this population. Some examples might include severe peanut allergies that lead to anaphylaxis, serious asthma complications, diabetes, or heart disease. Students are to be provided with a "free and appropriate public education" (FAPE), and some students may be covered under both IEPs and Section 504 plans (Zirkel, Granthom, & Lovato, 2012, p. 425). See Table 30–3 for a list of IEP eligible disabilities.

The five chronic conditions most often seen in school-age children are asthma, diabetes, seizures, severe food allergies, and attention deficit/behavioral disorders. A recent survey of New Jersey school nurses by Krause-Parello and Samms (2011) found that chronic conditions most often seen by the school nurse included allergies (87.3%), asthma (74.6%), ADHD (47.6%), diabetes (20.6%), and depression (9.5%). They also found that the most common procedures done by school nurses included first aid (98.4%), nebulizer treatments and inhalers (96.8% and 95.2%, respectively), along with wound care (90.5%), and glucose monitoring (87.3%). Urinary catheterizations, insulin injections, and gastrostomy tube feedings were less common, but were done by many school nurses.

ASTHMA. Asthma is often deemed the most common chronic disease of childhood. Although reports indicate that morbidity and mortality from asthma have stabilized in the past few years, in 2010, an estimated 17% of children aged 17 years and younger have been diagnosed with asthma (Sondick, Madans, & Gentleman, 2011). Non-Hispanic Blacks exhibit the highest asthma attack rates, and boys more often than girls reported an episode within the past year (Sondick et al., 2011). An estimated 10.5 million school days are missed annually because of asthma, the condition that is the leading cause of absences. Children with asthma also tend to show comorbidities, such as learning disabilities (Hauptman & Phipatanakul, 2015). School environmental factors (e.g., mold, allergens, indoor air quality) also exacerbate asthma symptoms in children and youth. Asthma management programs are useful in helping students manage symptoms and reduce asthma triggers. School nurses work with students, their families, and their doctors to develop an *asthma action plan* to control, prevent, or minimize untoward effects of acute asthma episodes. This can extend beyond the school into the students' homes. For instance, in Ohio, public health nurses collaborated with other professionals through a Healthy Homes Program Grant to perform housing control assessments, education, and interventions (e.g., home visits, education) in housing units. Results showed reduced asthma symptoms, fewer schools days and workdays missed, and the number of emergency room visits for asthma events were decreased (Polivka, Chaudry, Crawford, Bouton, & Sweet, 2011). A Healthy Homes program headed by public health nurses in Baltimore, Maryland, focused upon home assessments for environmental health risks (lead, asthma triggers, carbon monoxide, pesticide use, environmental tobacco smoke) as well as source of heating in the home. They also included educational sessions to review home environmental health risks and a targeted hazard reduction intervention (U.S. Department of Housing and Urban Development, 2015a, 2015b).

Peak flow meters can be used regularly to determine early signs of asthma problems. The activities of nurses acting as case managers have been found to decrease the number of ER visits and hospitalizations of school-age children with asthma (Toole, 2013). Noyes et al. (2013) found that a daily dose of preventive asthma medication, given while the child was at school, was both cost-effective and effective in reducing inner city children's symptoms. Monitoring asthma medications and teaching proper methods of inhaler use are also vital school nursing functions. It often falls to school nurses to ensure that proper protocols and training are in place.

DIABETES. Diabetes is another common chronic illness in young people: approximately 215,000 under age 20 have diabetes. This translates into 0.26% of youth having diabetes (National Diabetes Education Program, 2011), and experts now conclude that both type 1 and type 2 diabetes mellitus are found in school-age children. It is estimated that there are 13,600 newly found youth under the age of 20 annually diagnosed with type 2 diabetes (National Diabetes Education Program, 2011). Type 2 diabetes is rising almost exponentially in adolescents, leading some scientists to frame it as a major public health crisis caused largely by obesity, sedentary lifestyle, and the predisposition of certain ethnic groups to diabetes.

Table 30–3	Individuals with Disabilities Education Act (IDEA)

Thirteen Eligible Disabilities (Galemore & Sheetz, 2015, p. 86):
- Autism
- Deaf-blindness
- Deafness
- Emotional disturbance
- Hearing impairment
- Intellectual disability
- Multiple disabilities
- Orthopedic impairment
- Other health impairment
- Specific learning disability
- Speech or language impairment
- Traumatic brain injury
- Visual impairment, including blindness

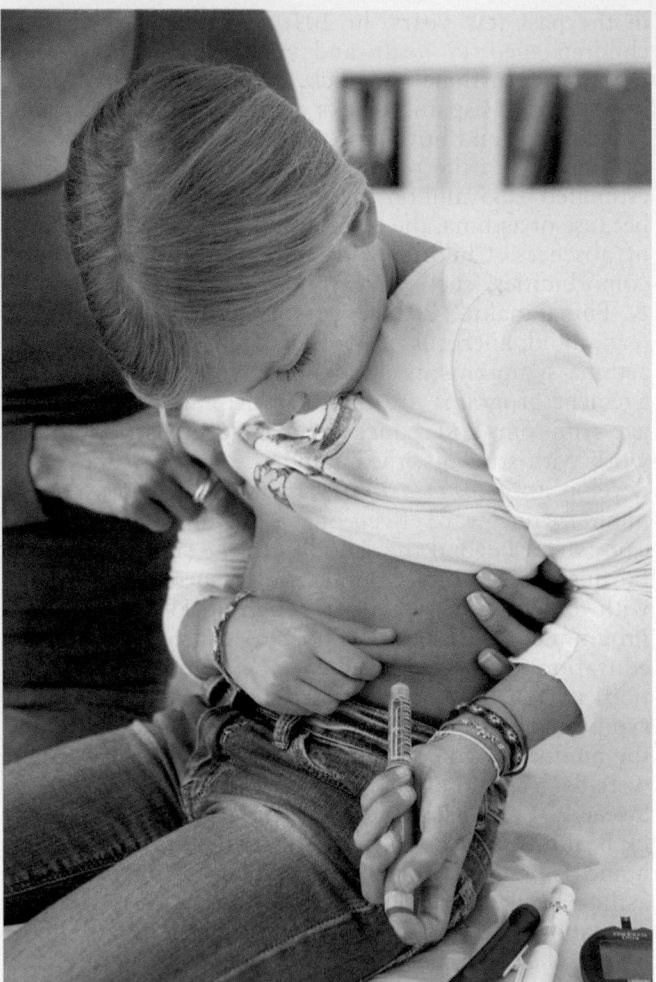

School nurse assisting a diabetic child with their insulin.

Working with families and health care providers, school nurses assess and develop a care plan for students with diabetes. School nurses work closely with the family to maintain confidentiality and at the same time ensure that the school is a safe environment for the child. A multidisciplinary team approach is needed, with family, school, and physician collaboration. Training for teachers and fellow classmates is also important. Teachers are often called upon to assist students with their insulin or food management. Younger children with type 1 diabetes, especially those who use insulin pumps, may need careful monitoring—something that is not always possible for the school nurse, who may not be present where and when problems arise. If the child has an insulin reaction, fellow students should be taught to quickly get a member of the school personnel (NASN, 2012b; National Institute of Diabetes and Digestive and Kidney Diseases, 2012). A current position of the American Diabetes Association (ADA) is that a *diabetes medical management plan* should be in place and that the "school nurse should be the primary coordinator and provider of care and should coordinate the training of an adequate number of school personnel" to assist in the care of children with diabetes (ADA, 2012, p. s78). However,

many school nurses do not feel comfortable delegating tasks such as administration of insulin or glucagon. See Chapter 13 for more on this issue.

Testing blood sugar and taking insulin at school can be frustrating and can cause children to feel singled out or different from their peers. One study found that adolescents with type 1 diabetes have significantly higher rates of depression than those without diabetes (Fritsch, Overton, & Robbins, 2011). Also, some schools do not permit blood sugar testing and insulin administration in classrooms, so that school health offices are often a place of refuge for diabetic students (Winsch, 2011). It is important for school nurses to understand each child's concerns and to alert teachers and school personnel to the signs and symptoms (as well as the treatment) of hypoglycemia. In addition to the obvious emergency health-related concerns for diabetic children, it can cause long-term health problems for children, though not generally for adults (National Institute for Health and Care Excellence, 2015). Pertinent to the school setting, a classic study showed that diabetes-related severe hypoglycemia does affect memory tasks (Hershey, Bhargava, Sadler, White, & Craft, 1999). Over time, memory deficits can affect learning and progress in school.

Type 2 diabetes cases have been rising, and school nurses can be instrumental in prevention measures and early identification. It is often found more frequently in Native American and Hispanic populations and less frequently among non-Hispanic Whites. Also, obesity is an independent risk factor, with close to a quarter of children and youth being obese. Visceral fat is associated with insulin resistance and impaired glucose tolerance, a pathology linked to type 2 diabetes. Culturally sensitive interventions that include increased physical activity and education on good nutrition, as well as behavior modification and ongoing methods of support (e.g., group meetings, phone/email reminders) were shown to be effective in a systematic review (Brackney & Cutshall, 2015). Individually tailored counseling for overweight children and families is thought to be more effective than general information about nutrition and exercise (Magnusson, Kjellgren, & Winkvist, 2012). School nurses should assess their school population and promote interventions that benefit at-risk students, as well as the general school population.

SEIZURE DISORDERS. Seizure disorders are not uncommon in the school-age population. Epilepsy is a disorder of the brain in which neurons sometimes give abnormal signals. A person who suffers from epilepsy may have comorbidities including autism, depression, and anxiety (Brooks-Kayal et al., 2013). For the majority of those diagnosed, seizures can usually be controlled with medication (e.g., antiepileptic drugs specific to the pediatric population), surgical treatment, or a special (e.g., ketogenic) diet (Epilepsy Foundation, 2014; National Institute of Neurological Disorders and Stroke, 2015).

It is important for school nurses to develop care plans to address seizure concerns during school hours. Care plans include monitoring medication compliance and teaching school staff about first aid measures for seizure victims. Children and adolescents with seizure disorders may feel embarrassed or be the victims of teasing or bullying. They may exhibit signs of school avoidance. Nurses need to work with these children and to teach all students about the disease process and the need for empathy and understanding. Similar to issues related to insulin administration for diabetic students, children with seizure disorders may have an emergency medication ordered by their physician (e.g., Diastat, midazolam, lorazepam, clonazepam). Prescribing providers and school nurses should be aware of the laws regarding the administration of seizure rescue medications, particularly as they pertain to unlicensed assistive personnel (Hartman, Devore, & Section on Neurology, Council on School Health, 2016). The Epilepsy Foundation (n.d.) has advocated for its use in schools, and school nurses are often caught between the rights of students and their parents and their state's nursing practice act.

FOOD ALLERGIES AND ANAPHYLAXIS. Another leading chronic condition found in school settings is severe food allergies that can lead to anaphylactic shock. Such severe allergies result in approximately 200,000 ER visits each year (Food Allergy Research & Education, 2016). Food allergies cause 30% to 50% of all anaphylaxis cases (Cianferoni & Muraro, 2012). Eight common foods account for 90% of severe food allergies. They are fish, shellfish, soy, milk, egg, wheat, peanuts, and tree nuts (e.g., cashews, walnuts). Many common foods and school supplies (e.g., play dough) can contain hidden allergens, and care must be taken to prevent exposure. School nurses coordinate and work with students and their families, along with school personnel, to raise awareness and enlist caution. They also work with families, and health care providers, to ensure that epinephrine via an autoinjector (EpiPen) is available for the child in case of emergencies. Epinephrine reverses the body's allergic reaction to the allergen, and timely intramuscular administration is the treatment of choice for anaphylaxis (Tiyyagura, Arnold, Cone, & Langhan, 2014). It is also used for beesting and other allergies, in addition to food allergies. Students are often allowed to carry an EpiPen on their person because reactions can occur very quickly (Elementary Teachers Federation of Ontario, 2015). School nurses should coordinate with teachers and lunchroom personnel to ensure that proper protocol is followed for allergic reactions. School personnel should be made aware of the food allergy, understand an anaphylactic reaction, and be able to verbalize or demonstrate how to use the EpiPen or other needed medication (NASN, 2012a). Chicago Public Schools has instituted a policy of stocking schools with EpiPens and authorizing school nurses to administer them if it is determined that the child is having an initial anaphylactic reaction. Citing a frightening statistics—that 25% of initial anaphylactic reactions in children occur during school hours—the Student Health and Wellness staff sought a remedy. Problems with implementation, however, include not having daily school nurse coverage in all schools due to budget issues; this is a common problem in school health (Zadikoff, Whyte, DeSantiago-Cardenas, Harvey-Gintoft, & Gupta, 2014).

BEHAVIORAL PROBLEMS AND LEARNING DISABILITIES. Other chronic childhood health problems are those of emotional, behavioral, and intellectual development.

These are not always easy to detect and measure, and they can be debilitating. Although these problems are not new, awareness and concern have increased as the rates of occurrence for other life-threatening childhood diseases have diminished. The National Institute of Mental Health (NIMH) reports that emotional and behavioral disorders affect 10% to 15% of children globally (Kid's Mental Health Portal, 2016). Problems such as oppositional defiant disorder, bipolar disorder, and early schizophrenia can affect the school-age population and is a concern to school nurses and staff (Pryjmachuk, Graham, Haddad, & Tylee, 2011; Riley, Ahmed, & Locke, 2016). The causes of emotional behavioral problems and learning disabilities appear to have genetic, environmental, and cultural influences. The number of children with learning disabilities in the lowest economic group is twice that in the highest group (Sondick et al., 2011). Children who were characterized as being in fair or poor health were almost five times as likely to have a learning disability and more than twice as likely to have attention deficit hyperactivity disorder (ADHD) as children with excellent, very good, or good health status (Sondick et al., 2011). High-risk children often come from families with a high incidence of child abuse (physical and sexual) and neglect. The number of children affected by parental drug use has surpassed that of children with disabilities caused by lead poisoning, another major contributor to developmental problems in children.

ADHD is a cluster of problems related to hyperactivity, impulsivity, and inattention. Approximately 6.4 million school-age children have been diagnosed with ADHD (National Center for Learning Disabilities, 2014). School nurses must be aware of the signs and symptoms and serve as an advocate for these children and their families. At each stage of development, those with ADHD are presented with distinct challenges. For example, children in elementary school may often have difficulty and conflict with peers, as well as problems organizing tasks. They may be more accident prone and may have more school-related problems, such as grade retention and suspension or expulsion. They often have problems with grooming and with handwriting, and they exhibit difficulty sleeping. ADHD is sometimes found with associated disorders, such as communication or language disorders and learning disabilities. It is estimated that as many as one third of children with learning disabilities also have ADHD (National Center for Learning Disabilities, 2014). Counseling and behavior therapy are often used with these children with a 70% to 80% success rate demonstrated by improved behavior (Substance Abuse Mental Health Services Agency, 2015).

Behavioral and emotional problems of school-age children can stem from many causes. School nurses can be alert to early symptoms and refer families for counseling. Collaboration is needed between the child's family, the school, and the child's health care provider to diagnose ADHD and effectively plan appropriate interventions and educational accommodations. Teacher confirmation of ADHD-related behaviors is very important. Numerous checklists and assessment tools are available, and school psychologists typically serve as a source for additional information and resources. School nurses can assist parents in recognizing the symptoms of ADHD and obtaining appropriate treatment and follow-up. A multimodal treatment approach may include stimulant medication, usually methylphenidate (Ritalin or Concerta), dextroamphetamine (Dexedrine), and amphetamine (Adderall), or antidepressants (such as Wellbutrin). Family and individual counseling, parent support groups, and training in behavior management techniques, as well as family education about the condition, are also essential features of this method of treatment. Not all children and adolescents respond to medication, and medication dosage must be carefully monitored and titrated. Research suggests that adopting a strengths-based assessment and treatment plan for students with ADHD has potential to provide a healthier educational experience that can reduce the risks of comorbid conditions associated with ADHD. Rather than focus on identifying and treating the deficits associated with ADHD, the strengths-based approach focuses on interventions that reinforce well-being and resilience (Climie & Mastoras, 2015). School nurses and community health nurses can work closely with school staff, parents, and physicians in determining the efficacy of treatment regimens.

Collaboration is needed between the child's family, the school, and the child's health care provider to diagnose ADHD and effectively plan appropriate interventions and educational accommodations. Teacher confirmation of ADHD-related behaviors is very important. Numerous checklists and assessment tools are available, and school nurses typically serve as a resource for additional information. School nurses in partnership with behavioral health providers can assist parents in recognizing the symptoms of ADHD and obtaining appropriate treatment and follow-up. A multimodal treatment approach may include stimulant medication, or antidepressants. School accommodations for learning problems and social skills training for the child with ADHD may be indicated. Family and individual counseling, parent support groups, and training in behavior management techniques, as well as family education about the condition, are also essential features of this method of treatment. Not all children and adolescents respond to medication, and medication dosage must be carefully monitored and titrated. School nurses can assist parents in this task. The main goal of medication for school-age children is academic improvement. If this does not occur, medication may need to be changed or discontinued. School nurses and community health nurses can work closely with school staff, parents, and physicians in determining the efficacy of treatment regimens (Chan, Fogler, & Hammerness, 2016).

MEDICATION ADMINISTRATION. Medication administration for a variety of conditions has historically been an important responsibility for school nurses (NASN, 2012c). In schools where a nurse is present every day, the nurse can personally oversee medication administration. Unfortunately, many nurses cover more than one school and so other school personnel (e.g., secretaries, health aides) may be tasked with overseeing medication administration. The majority of states have laws allowing teachers or health aides to administer medication. In these situations, school nurses should provide training and audit records to ensure that proper guidelines are followed. Multiple studies show that medication errors increase when school nurses cover multiple schools and unlicensed personnel assist in medication administration (Richmond, 2011). Problems commonly occur with omission of doses because students fail to come to the office for medication administration. This is especially problematic with students taking insulin or antidiabetic drugs, antibiotics, and medication for ADHD.

Another issue surrounding medication administration in the school setting is regarding delegation. Each state's individual nurse practice act provides rules on delegation of nursing tasks. School nurses must understand their own state's act and the legal implications regarding their decisions. School districts are responsible for including medication administration guidelines in their policies, and school nurses must comply with established guidelines. Recently, much discussion has occurred regarding the administration of Diastat gel in the school setting (ANA & NASN, 2011). Diastat gel is often administered rectally to stop the onset of cluster seizures. However, Diastat can decrease respirations as well. School nurses have the skills and experience to properly assess such occurrences, where lay personnel, even if trained in proper administration of the medication, do not. ANA & NASN (2011) supports only school nurses administering this medication, but parents and others have pushed the administration of Diastat by lay people (Kahn & Grasska, 2014).

In the case of insulin administration in schools, the American Nurses Association filed a lawsuit on behalf of California school nurses to prevent insulin administration by unlicensed personnel. There argument centered on the state's Nurse Practice Act and the need for licensed nurses to administer this medication (with dosage often checked by two nurses in hospital settings). However, the American Diabetes Association and others argued that not all schools have adequate school nurse coverage, and over one quarter of schools do not employ a licensed nurse. Two courts ruled on the side of the school nurses, but the California Supreme Court ultimately overturned those decisions, making it possible for unlicensed personnel to give medications, including insulin, with parental and medical permission (Balestra, 2012; Walsh & Lambert, 2013). The concept of "in loco parentis" instructs nurses, teachers, and school staff to provide care for the student in the parent's place and with their consent (Health & Welfare Committee, 2012, p. 13).

Health Services to Prevent Illness and Injury

School nurses emphasize prevention and focus many of their efforts on prevention of communicable disease (via immunizations) and of injuries.

IMMUNIZATIONS. Among schoolchildren, the incidence rates of measles (rubeola), rubella (German measles), pertussis (whooping cough), infectious parotitis (mumps), and varicella (chickenpox) have dropped considerably over the last several decades because of widespread immunization efforts, although these communicable diseases do still occur and sometimes with serious complications such as birth defects from rubella and nerve deafness from mumps. Although the number of reported cases of hepatitis A, measles, and meningococcal disease decreased from 2008 to 2009, cases of pertussis and mumps increased (Maternal and Child Health Bureau, 2013).

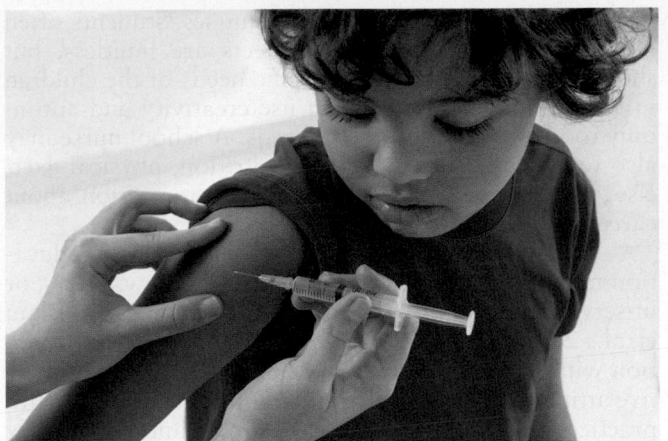

School nurses assist with immunization clinics.

Low immunization levels in many areas, particularly among poor populations, and increased disease rates signal the need for constant surveillance, outreach programs, and educational efforts. School nurses are deeply involved in each of these preventive activities. Health departments and schools often work collaboratively to provide immunization services. Compulsory immunization laws for school entrance, which vary among states, have enabled public health personnel to carry out these preventive services. All states require children to be vaccinated against certain communicable diseases as a condition for school attendance (CDC, 2015b). Statewide immunization information systems can be beneficial for schools, school nurses, and children and their families. School nurses, like public health nurses, may have access to not only viewing immunization records but also the ability to update them. This provides ready access for children and parents, as well as school nurses, to check immunization records, track those children whose immunizations are incomplete, and provide critical information during times of disease outbreaks. These systems also make it easier for school nurses to complete district and state immunization reports and work with public health agencies in providing necessary vaccines in a timely manner (Bobo, Etkind, Martin, Chi, & Coyle, 2013).

School nurses often oversee and ensure that children are in compliance with school entrance laws regarding immunizations. They may call parents directly when they note that the student is out of compliance. They may also arrange to help the student get immunized by facilitating appointments or, in some school districts, by directly providing the immunizations. Kaufman et al. (2013) studied randomized control trials to evaluate the effects of face-to-face interventions delivered to individual parents or groups of parents in order to provide information or education about early childhood vaccination. The data collected revealed that these strategies do not consistently improve either immunization rates or parent knowledge and understanding of vaccination. The Centers for Disease Control and Prevention provides information for National Immunization Awareness Month and provides a toolkit for school nurses and others to follow when developing successful immunization outreach programs in schools (CDC, 2016). School nurses can be effective

advocates in helping parents make decisions about vaccines (e.g., HPV for adolescents), especially when they have sufficient knowledge and recognize their role as an opinion leader (Rosen, Ashwood, & Richardson, 2016).

Many school districts require TB skin testing upon school entry, but not all states have policies regarding this. Some areas with a high proportion of school entries who have recently immigrated from high-TB countries and areas do require TB skin testing upon admission to school or when transferring in to a district from another area and may use interferon gamma release assay (IGRA) testing as well as skin testing (Flood, 2013). It is important for school nurses to work with their school districts in developing policies for TB screening and monitoring, as TB outbreaks in schools can affect large numbers of students (Galemore, 2016). School nurses work with public health agencies to identify and test contacts and refer them for treatment if necessary. Laboratories can also provide genotypic testing to determine in-school or out-of-school transmission (Williams et al., 2016). See Chapters 8 and 22 for more on TB testing, parental resistance to vaccines, and current immunization schedules for school-age children and adolescents.

SAFETY. School nurses are also involved in ensuring that injury prevention efforts are encouraged. Emphasis on a healthful physical environment includes proper selection, design, organization, operation, and maintenance of the school building and playground equipment. The Centers for Disease Control and Prevention estimate that there are more than 200,000 children treated in the emergency department every year for playground-related injuries (CDC, 2012).

About 67% of playground injuries involve falls or equipment failure, and the most common injuries are fractures (36%), abrasions/contusions (20%), and lacerations (17%), but concussions and other serious injuries can occur (National Program for Playground Safety, 2016). Custodial personnel assist in the maintenance of school grounds, but school nurses must be aware of conditions and make recommendations to remedy unsafe situations. As school nurses provide first aid treatment for playground injuries, they may observe trends (e.g., a high number of injuries where faulty playground equipment or other factors influence higher injury rates) and request action. When injury trends are noted, school nurses work with maintenance departments and administration to advocate change and prevent future injury. School nurses also assist with physical adaptations for students with special needs (e.g., ramps, electric doors); they work to ensure safety in and around schools, and they are mindful of visual, thermal, and acoustic factors in school buildings, as well as aesthetic values. Additionally, they promote sanitation and the safety of the school bus system, as well as food services.

Another area of growing concern is student safety after natural disasters or emergency situations. Recent earthquakes and potential bioterrorism events may impact schools or not permit children to return home at the end of a school day. School nurses are ideal persons to assist in disaster/emergency relief. Students do spend much of their time in school, and local schools are often designated as shelters in times of disasters (NASN, 2016). School nurses can assist in the development of emergency plans, as well as provide care and comfort to children and their families in times of emergencies.

Health Education and Health Promotion

Another main function of school nursing practice involves education and health promotion. This includes planned and incidental teaching of health concepts and health curriculum development. In some states, school nurses even teach the regular health classes. Education may be one-on-one to help a child obtain better control over asthma or to explain to a newly diagnosed diabetic student what is occurring in his body. As an educator, the school nurse may also teach an entire class regarding a student's severe food allergy or the need for proper hand hygiene. The school nurse explains in simple terms what allergies are and helps students understand that allergies are not contagious, what to do in the case of an allergic reaction, and the importance of not sharing foods that may contain potential allergens (NASN, 2016). The application of research is important in school nursing. See Evidence-Based Practice.

Because students trust school nurses, students often listen to them. Educational subjects are limitless, but should always apply to the specific needs of the children in the school. The nurse must use creativity and autonomy to identify and prioritize needs. A school nurse may also teach about basic first aid, nutrition, physical exercise, and seat belt safety, or provide information about careers in the health care professions.

In addition to lecture or verbal teaching, education may also be in the form of posters, e-newsletters, or in-service presentations for educators and parents (Islam et al., 2016). These activities integrate health information with students' daily living experiences to build positive attitudes toward health and to establish sound health practices that will carry forward into adulthood (Avery et al., 2013).

Screenings: Opportunities for Teaching

Most local school districts provide some type of health screening services, usually through the school nurse or local health care providers. Although the goal of all screening is to promote early intervention, screening also provides the school nurse many opportunities to teach

---

 **EVIDENCE-BASED PRACTICE FOR SCHOOL NURSING**

A review of the literature identified seven studies that investigated the impact of school-located influenza vaccination (SLIV) program on rates of absenteeism. Six of the articles compared schools that participated in SLIV programs with control schools. Results from all the studies indicated children who were vaccinated had fewer days of being absent.

Although school nurses often work with individual children, they also look at the school community as a whole and should conduct interventions that will benefit the school population. School nurses must also collect data and determine the effectiveness of their treatments. Finally, school nurses must also remember the goals of the institution in which they work (i.e., education) and strive to meet these goals (i.e., increased attendance) while at the same time protecting the public's health.

Reference

Hull, H. F., & Ambrose, C. S. (2011). The impact of school-located influenza vaccination programs on student absenteeism: A review of the U.S. literature. *Journal of School Nursing, 27*(1), 34–42.

Another example of evidence-based practice in school nursing involves a coordinated school health program intervention to increase physical activity and decrease BMI among minority children. The nurse researchers used a parallel group, randomized control design, and employed a community-based participatory research approach between the University of California, Los Angeles, and five underserved elementary schools. Randomization of schools occurred—to either a control group with general education, or Kids N Fitness intervention. Nurses, community health workers, and

physical education specialists conducted the weekly 90-minute sessions over a 6-week period that included nutrition and behavior modification, family involvement, and physical activity. All activities were culturally appropriate, and children's exercises included Salsa and Hip Hop dancing, soccer, and jumping rope. Parents were given information on problems that result from obesity in a support group atmosphere. Children and parents were then instructed on healthy food choices, portion control, and food labels and shopping tips. Baseline measurements (height, weight, BMI, waist circumference, resting BP) were gathered, following physical exam clearance by NPs, and were collected again at the end of the class sessions (4 months) and 12 months after the intervention. Questionnaires on nutrition and physical activity were also used over the same time intervals.

Significant results were found for participants ($n = 251$) between the two groups and over the time period for the study among those participating in the intervention. For boys, there was a decrease in TV viewing, and for girls, there were higher reports of daily physical activity, PE class attendance, and decreases in BMI at 12 months.

Reference

Wright, K., Giger, J. N., Norris, K., & Suro, Z. (2013). Impact of a nurse-directed, coordinated school health program to enhance physical activity behaviors and reduce body mass index among minority children: A parallel-group, randomized control trial. *International Journal of Nursing Studies, 50*(6), 727–737.

How could you use information from these studies to improve school nursing practice and the health of school-age children?

students and staff. Referral information resulting from screening results is usually given to parents, and school nurses may contact parents to encourage follow-through (CDC, 2015k; Krause-Parello & Samms, 2011). Children who are not present for school screenings may not receive the benefits of these screenings (e.g., homeschooled and private school students). School nurses often help to coordinate screening resources and benefits, and they often carry out additional screenings for students who were absent when mass screenings were held.

VISION. The 2014 SHPPS noted that 82.3% of reporting school districts offered vision screening (CDC, 2015). School nurses often oversee routine vision screenings at periodic intervals so that vision problems that can interfere with learning may be detected and treated early (e.g., nearsightedness, farsightedness, strabismus, amblyopia). School nurses also are involved in follow-up and referral. They often send emails or letters to parents, make phone follow-ups, and provide referrals and resources to ensure that corrective eyewear is obtained. Local Lions Clubs may be involved in paying for area optometrists to assist with and/or direct screenings, as well as to provide follow-up care (Mattey, Zein, O'Malley, & Haron, 2013).

HEARING. Hearing screenings were reported by 77.2% of districts, down from earlier surveys (CDC, 2015). These mass screenings are done to detect any serious hearing deficits that may be related to recurrent ear infections or noise-induced hearing loss (NIHL), often resulting from loud music, video games, or excessive exposure to noise. About 20% of school-aged children, aged 6 to 19, have some type of irreversible, permanent hearing damage (Hendershot, Pakulski, Thompson, Dowling, & Price, 2011). Some have a type of *sensorineural hearing loss*—or one that involves the inner ear or the nerves leading from the inner ear. It is permanent and cannot be surgically or medically corrected (American Speech-Language-Hearing Association, 2016). One national survey of school nurses indicated that about half of them saw a lack of educational programs addressing NIHL and noted the need to recommend programs and policies to address all types of hearing loss (Hendershot et al., 2011). Similar to vision screening, school nurses screen and refer students with suspected hearing problems to medical specialists (e.g., audiologists, physicians). School nurses can use the opportunity afforded by vision and hearing screenings to provide education to students and their parents about preventing problems such as noise-induced hearing loss.

OTHER HEALTH SCREENINGS. Height, weight, and sometimes blood pressure and cholesterol screenings are done on a regular basis to monitor normal growth and development and allow for early intervention with populations who are especially susceptible to hypertension and heart disease. In some areas, scoliosis screening is also done, frequently during middle school years or in fifth grade, to permit early detection and referral for medical intervention (e.g., bracing, surgery). One multistate survey found that almost 60% of school nurses reported conducting scoliosis screenings (Krause-Parello & Samms,

2011). Scoliosis may be congenital, but is often idiopathic, and the efficacy of school screening programs has been questioned; some evidence-based recommendations suggest that scoliosis screening should be discontinued (Jakubowski & Alexy, 2014). Literature reviews have not shown sufficient evidence to support screenings, but one population-based cohort study, conducted over a 10-year period, found "sustained clinical effectiveness in identifying patients with adolescent idiopathic scoliosis" that needed continued clinical observation, and the researchers advocated for routine screenings (Deurloo & Verkerk, 2015; Fong et al., 2015, p. 825).

In Texas, and some other areas of the country, *acanthosis nigricans* (hyperpigmentation from various causes, but sometimes a symptom of diabetes) screenings are being done to look for early markers of type 2 diabetes, especially in high-risk populations (Texas Department of Health Services, 2016).

Pediculosis (or head lice) in school-age children is a continual problem for school nurses. Between 6 and 12 million children aged 3 to 11 each year are estimated to be infected with head lice, and school nurses are often called upon to do "head checks" for pediculosis. Pediculicides (e.g., permethrin, pyrethrins, dimethicone) are helpful in killing lice, and school nurses often provide families with education on prevention and eradication methods (Ihde, Boscamp, Loh, & Rosen, 2015; Pontius, 2014). See Chapter 22 for a more in-depth discussion on head lice and treatment.

ORAL AND DENTAL HEALTH: TEACHING AND REFERRAL. Dental caries affect more than half of school-age children and are the most common chronic disease for that age group. In 2010, about 7% of children aged 2 to 17 years had unmet dental needs because the families could not afford dental care (Sondick et al., 2011). Approximately a quarter of U.S. children do not have dental insurance, either private or public (CDC, 2014). The percentage of children and adolescents aged 5 to 19 years with untreated tooth decay is twice as high for those from low-income families (25%) compared with children from higher-income households (11%) (Dye et al., 2012). School nurses can address dental health issues in a variety of ways. At a community level, they can educate the public about the benefits of dental fluoride treatments. They can advocate for fluoridation of drinking water, school-provided fluoride rinses or gels, and dental sealant programs. These are all cost-effective, proven methods of reducing dental caries in school-age children. At the classroom level, school nurses can provide dental education and provide toothbrushes, toothpaste, and floss to ensure that students are able to practice good dental hygiene habits. Local organizations and businesses often will donate such supplies. Many programs from the American Dental Association, the CDC, and other organizations provide resource materials. At an individual level, school nurses can assist in finding resources for those with no dental health insurance. Finally, school nurses can successfully educate parents, especially those who are immigrants or have different cultural beliefs, regarding the importance of oral and dental health (Hassmiller, 2016; Smith, Brach, & Horowitz, 2015; Swan, Barker, & Hoeft, 2010).

Dental screenings or clinics may be conducted to determine the incidence of dental caries, especially in elementary school children, and to encourage follow-up with local dentists for necessary restorations. At the time of the most recent national survey of schools, only 30.3% of districts reported performing some type of oral health screening (CDC, 2015). See Chapter 22.

Promotion of a Healthful School Environment

A third function of school nursing practice includes maintaining and promoting a healthful school environment. Promotion of healthful school living emphasizes planning a daily schedule for monitoring healthy classroom experiences, extracurricular activities, school breakfasts and lunches, emotional climate, discipline programs, and teaching methods. It also includes screening, observing, and assessing students to identify needs early and to report illegal drug use, bullying, suspected child abuse, and violations of environmental health standards (Patestos, Patterson, & Fitzsimons, 2014). Cyberbullying is another area where school nurses can provide education to students, parents, teachers, and school staff, as well as response to warning signs among school-age children and youth (Van Ouytsel, Walrave, & Vandebosch, 2015). Health promotion also involves the nurse in supporting the physical, mental, and emotional health of school personnel by being an accessible resource to teachers and staff regarding their own health and safety.

PROPER NUTRITION AND EXERCISE. Many factors can affect the school environment—heating, cooling, lighting, safe playgrounds, and policies and practices to limit bullying and social aggression or other forms of school violence. The school cafeteria and physical education activities can promote health or contribute to obesity and sedentary lifestyles.

OBESITY. Obesity rates have steadily increased for all children since the 1980s; the rates have doubled for children between ages 2 to 5 and adolescents (ages 12 to 19). Rates have tripled for those between ages 6 and 11 years. Approximately 17% (or 12.7 million) of children and adolescents aged 2 to 19 years are obese (CDC, 2015c). Obesity often begins in childhood and becomes a risk factor for cardiovascular disease and diabetes later in life. With the increase in child obesity rates, the number of children diagnosed with type 2 diabetes continues to rise, especially among youth of minority race/ethnicity. It is estimated that there are 13,600 newly diagnosed youth under the age of 20 diagnosed with type 2 diabetes annually (National Diabetes Education Program, 2011). In 2011–2012, the CDC (2015c) reported that the prevalence among children and adolescents was higher among Hispanics (22.4%) and non-Hispanic Blacks (20.2%) than among non-Hispanic Whites (14.1%).

As children become older, families have less impact on food choices, and peers begin to have more influence. Results of the 2013 YRBS indicate that very few high school students eat enough fruits and vegetables—of those surveyed only 22% had consumed more than three servings of fruit, and 16% had eaten a sufficient number of vegetables in the 7 days prior to being surveyed (CDC, 2013b).

School nurses should play an integral role in the prevention of overweight and obesity, as well as in addressing the health needs of overweight and obese students (NASN, 2013). Approximately 32% of youth are overweight or obese. Many factors contribute to this health issue: diet, lack of physical activity, genetics, family and social factors, culture, socioeconomic status, and media marketing (NASN, 2013). School nurses can provide education to students and families about healthy food and lifestyle choices and help families connect to resources in the community that will support the adoption of healthier lifestyles. A national survey found that 52.2% of school nurses reported screening for obesity, even though they noted that childhood obesity was a significant problem. Fewer than half of school nurses reported calculating and recording BMI measurements (Krause-Parello & Samms, 2011). Steele et al. (2011) studied school nurses' perceived barriers to counseling student and parents about weight problems. They found barriers related to the school nurse's knowledge and self-perceived competency, personal weight problems/role model, lack of time and support from school administration, prior negative experiences with families regarding school-based weight management programs, and the student's lack of motivation as well as ineffective interventions to address weight problems for all students. These barriers should be addressed and sound evidence-based interventions sought.

HOMELESSNESS AND HUNGER. Poor nutrition and obesity are not uncommon among adolescents, whose diets often consist of snacks with limited nutritional value interspersed among unhealthful meals. Homelessness and hunger can also have serious consequences, one being an impact on the academic performance of children. Irritability, lack of energy, and difficulty concentrating are only some of the problems that arise from skipped meals or consistently inadequate nutrition. Infection and illness (e.g., ear infections, asthma, bronchitis, gastroenteritis) that lead to loss of school days can affect academic progress and interfere with the acquisition of basic skills, such as reading and mathematics. Dental caries are frequent. Poor nutrition is frequently associated with poverty and hunger, but social pressure to be thin can also spark purposeful malnutrition. Homelessness and food insecurity can lead to overreliance on fast food and convenience stores, and lack of stable housing triggers stress and anxiety, which can lead to obesity. About 43% of homeless children in Baltimore were obese or overweight (Hindman & Mincemoyer, 2014). Dental caries are also much more common among homeless children than other low-income housed children (Chiu, DiMarco, & Prokop, 2013). See Chapters 22 and 28.

School nurses can help coordinate services for homeless children and advocate for better nutritional choices in the lunchroom and vending machines. This may include working for policy changes to limit soft drink sales in public schools. They can also teach all grade levels regarding proper nutrition, and they can educate students and parents alike about nutritious snacks in contrast to snacks with little food value, as well as provide information on community resources (e.g., food banks, health clinics, shelters). School nurses may also work with staff to provide nutrition and exercise programs, support groups, and collaborative efforts to assist families dealing with hunger and homelessness.

EATING DISORDERS. Eating disorders are another area of concern. Issues with body image and control are at the heart of *anorexia nervosa* and *bulimia nervosa*, common problems for adolescent girls. These diseases have emotional causes that pose complex challenges to treatment. School nurses must be aware of the signs and symptoms of eating disorders and be proactive in identifying students at risk, working collaboratively with other members of the mental health treatment service team to advocate for the child. Scoliosis screenings are an optimal time to also observe for eating disorders, as examination of the spine allows for visualization of the body core. School nurses can work with students to develop a healthier self-concept and identify outside treatment resources (National Eating Disorders Association, 2015).

ADOLESCENT HIGH-RISK BEHAVIORS. Mortality and morbidity rates for adolescents are low overall and demonstrate considerable improvement since the early 1900s. There are six categories of high-risk behaviors that are directly related to morbidity and mortality in youth and young adults: behaviors that lead to unintentional injury and violence, tobacco use, alcohol and drug use, sexual behaviors that lead to pregnancies and sexually transmitted infections, unhealthy dietary behaviors, and lack of physical activity (Kann et al., 2012). Many of the health problems faced by adolescents are a result of their own choices and high-risk activity (CDC, 2015i). For example, sexual activity, substance abuse, injury, and violence are all high-risk behaviors in which adolescents can choose to participate or not. The effects of such choices may not be discovered for many years. Suicide is a leading cause of death of adolescents, with boys more likely to die from suicide than girls (Kaslow, 2014). Within the last decade, a good number of states developed policies to address alcohol and drug use (increasing from 22% to 42%), STD prevention (up from 17.6% to 32%), suicide prevention (from 16% to 28%), and tobacco use (rising

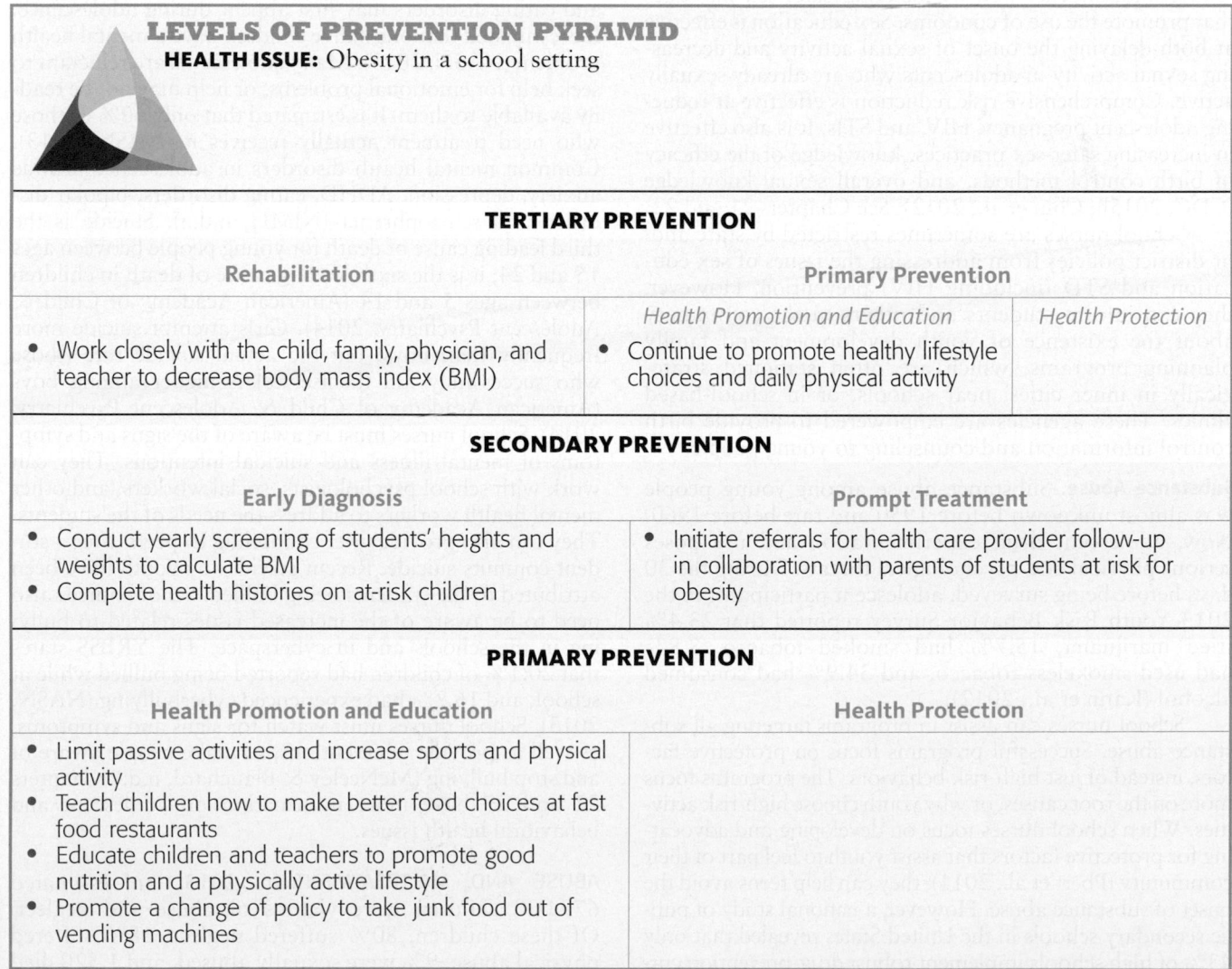

LEVELS OF PREVENTION PYRAMID

HEALTH ISSUE: Obesity in a school setting

TERTIARY PREVENTION

Rehabilitation	Primary Prevention	
	Health Promotion and Education	*Health Protection*
• Work closely with the child, family, physician, and teacher to decrease body mass index (BMI)	• Continue to promote healthy lifestyle choices and daily physical activity	

SECONDARY PREVENTION

Early Diagnosis	Prompt Treatment
• Conduct yearly screening of students' heights and weights to calculate BMI • Complete health histories on at-risk children	• Initiate referrals for health care provider follow-up in collaboration with parents of students at risk for obesity

PRIMARY PREVENTION

Health Promotion and Education	Health Protection
• Limit passive activities and increase sports and physical activity • Teach children how to make better food choices at fast food restaurants • Educate children and teachers to promote good nutrition and a physically active lifestyle • Promote a change of policy to take junk food out of vending machines	

from 19.6% to 40%), in an effort to address these behaviors (CDC, 2015d). See Chapter 22.

Sexual Activity: Teen Pregnancy and STDs. Sexual activity is a sensitive issue. However, the 2013 YRBS indicates that 46.8% of students surveyed reported they had had sexual intercourse, and 15.0% had had sexual intercourse with four or more partners in their lifetime (Kann et al., 2012). Each year, about half of new STD cases in the United States occur among those between the ages of 15 and 24 (CDC, 2015). The overall rates of syphilis, gonorrhea, chlamydia, human papillomavirus (HPV), and herpes simplex virus are climbing.

Providing STD services and HIV/AIDS education can be a daunting task. Young people with STDs are often afraid or embarrassed to seek help. Those who have been exposed to the HIV virus may not know that they are infected. Although in some communities the school-based clinic dispenses condoms, in other areas, school nurses may be restricted in what safer-sex products they can provide. However, nurses *can* provide teens with education and with information about resources that are available outside of school property. School nurses can promote, at the local and state level, the HPV vaccine that guards against cervical cancer. They can promote abstinence or delaying sexual initiation, as well as fostering safer-sex messages that promote the use of condoms. Sex education is effective at both delaying the onset of sexual activity and decreasing sexual activity in adolescents who are already sexually active. Comprehensive risk reduction is effective at reducing adolescent pregnancy, HIV, and STIs. It is also effective in increasing safer-sex practices, knowledge of the efficacy of birth control methods, and overall sexual knowledge (CDC, 2015h; Chin et al., 2012). See Chapters 21 and 22.

School nurses are sometimes restricted by state and/or district policies from addressing the issues of sex education and STD (including HIV) prevention. However, they can inform students and others in the community about the existence of youth development and family planning programs, which are often stationed strategically in inner cities, near schools, or in school-based clinics. These agencies are empowered to provide birth control information and counseling to young people.

Substance Abuse. Substance abuse among young people was almost unknown before 1950 and rare before 1960. Now, adolescent drug experimentation and use poses serious physical and psychological threats. During the 30 days before being surveyed, adolescent participants in the 2013 Youth Risk Behavior Survey reported that 23.4% tried marijuana, 15.7% had smoked tobacco, 8.8% had used smokeless tobacco, and 34.9% had consumed alcohol (Kann et al., 2012).

School nurses can assist in programs targeting all substance abuse. Successful programs focus on protective factors, instead of just high-risk behaviors. The programs focus more on the root causes, or why youth choose high-risk activities. When school nurses focus on developing and advocating for protective factors that assist youth to feel part of their community (Pbert et al., 2011), they can help teens avoid the onset of substance abuse. However, a national study of public secondary schools in the United States revealed that only 43% of high schools implement robust drug-prevention curricula (Catalano et al., 2012). See Chapters 22 and 27.

School nurses can also provide resources for smoking cessation and substance abuse programs. Pbert et al. (2011) found that school nurses are successful members of school smoking cessation programs. In addition to school-based education, programs of peer leadership and parental education/involvement and community-wide task forces have been developed to lobby for local legislation and strengthen community–school ties. School nurses can be advocates at a community level by lobbying the city council for tougher ordinances controlling advertising content and zoning (especially near schools). School nurses often work in conjunction with law enforcement officials, school district administrators, and other community agencies to ensure compliance with local regulations and prevent or delay tobacco use. Other groups, such as 4-H clubs, religious congregations, the Catholic Youth Organization, and Boy Scouts, use peer counseling to influence young people to assume responsibility for healthy lifestyles, with the goal of developing decision-making skills that lead to healthy lifestyle choices in adolescence and through adulthood. The school nurse participates in and supports existing programs in addition to counseling and referring young people who need help.

Mental Health Issues and Suicide. Depression, schizophrenia, and eating disorders may first appear during adolescence. It is estimated that one in five children have a mental health problem (NASN, 2013). Many adolescents are reluctant to seek help for emotional problems, or help may not be readily available to them. It is estimated that only 40% of those who need treatment actually receives it (NASN, 2013). Common mental health disorders in adolescence include anxiety, depression, ADHD, eating disorders, bipolar disorder, and schizophrenia (NIMH, n.d.a). Suicide is the third leading cause of death for young people between ages 15 and 24; it is the sixth leading cause of death in children between ages 5 and 14 (American Academy of Child & Adolescent Psychiatry, 2014). Girls attempt suicide more frequently than boys, but the actual suicide rate (those who successfully kill themselves) is higher among boys (American Academy of Child & Adolescent Psychiatry, 2014). School nurses must be aware of the signs and symptoms of mental illness and suicidal intentions. They can work with school psychologists, social workers, and other mental health workers to address the needs of the students. They can also provide grief counseling to peers after a student commits suicide. Recent suicides by youth have been attributed to the students being bullied. School nurses also need to be aware of the increased issues related to bullying in the schools and in cyberspace. The YRBSS states that 20.1% of children had reported being bullied while at school, and 16.2% had experienced cyberbullying (NASN, 2013). School nurses must watch for signs and symptoms, as well as provide interventions, to make people aware of and stop bullying (McNeeley & Blanchard, n.d.). Chapters 22 and 27 have more information on adolescent and behavioral health issues.

ABUSE AND MALTREATMENT. In 2013, an estimated 679,000 children were victims of abuse and neglect. Of these children, 80% suffered neglect, 18% suffered physical abuse, 9% were sexually abused, and 1,520 died (National Children's Alliance, 2014). Girls tended to be maltreated more often than boys. Black, non-Hispanic youth were also at greater risk. In 2014, the victim rate was reported to be 9.4 per 1,000 children with neglect and physical abuse being the most common (Agency for Children and Families, Children's Bureau, 2016). Child abuse prevention education programs can be found in many school districts as a primary preventive intervention. School nurses are required by law to report suspected or confirmed cases of abuse. In addition, school nurses can educate teachers and other school personnel regarding the signs and symptoms of abuse. Abuse can also include issues related to bullying and school violence (King, 2014). Early identification of abuse and intervention is critical for the safety of the child. The number of adverse childhood experiences related to child abuse is directly correlated with long-term health issues. Eisbach and Driessnack (2010) completed a small qualitative study of school nurses and pediatric/mental health practitioners that highlighted the difficulty nurses have in dealing with this issue and their frustration with reporting abuse that often leads to subsequent inaction by authorities. It is important to be well versed in subtle signs and symptoms of maltreatment and develop strong collaborative relationships with social service professionals. Signs that a child might be maltreated include reports of abuse, a sudden change in behavior, lack of medical treatment follow-through, learning problems of unknown etiology, child responses that are consistently guarded or compliant, and an avoidance of home or certain individuals (NASN, 2014b). For more information on health problems and issues concerning children and adolescents, see Chapter 22.

School-Based Health Clinics

Because of the complex and intertwined emotional, physical, and educational needs of school-age children and adolescents, a more comprehensive interdisciplinary approach to services is needed than the piecemeal approaches attempted previously. School nurses are able to do much to influence schoolchildren's health. However, often they need to refer the children to a health care provider. Yet, more parents are working and less available to take care of their children's health care needs during the day. School-based health centers (SBHCs) provide ready access to health care for large numbers of children and adolescents during school hours, reducing absences from school due to health care appointments. SBHCs provide a variety of services in a user-friendly manner at a convenient location.

In 2013–2014, there were 2,315 SBHCs in the United States; this figure is up 20% from the 2010–2011 *Census of SBHCs* (School-Based Health Alliance, 2014). These clinics are distributed in high schools (23.4%), middle schools (8.8%), and elementary schools (15.3%) and are generally established on school grounds (School-Based Health Alliance, 2014). Some clinics provide services only to schoolchildren, whereas others extend services to their families and to other neighborhood families with preschool-age children. Most centers are open full-time. Many SBHCs in middle schools and high schools offer abstinence counseling, pregnancy testing, sexually transmitted infection diagnosis and testing, and pap tests (School-Based Health Alliance, 2014).

SBHCs are staffed by interdisciplinary teams of helping professionals, paraprofessionals, and other staff and can include nurses, nurse practitioners, and social workers. Many hospitals, HMOs, and health departments are sponsors of these school clinics, because it is a cost-effective way to decrease visits to the emergency department and promote health, especially to underserved groups such as adolescents. They help meet the need for patient-centered medical homes, as outlined in the Affordable Care Act. Third-party billing, especially to access Medicaid funding, is increasingly more common among SBHCs, and private foundations have also been instrumental in providing financial and technical support. School nurses support the clinics by referring students who need additional attention. In some areas, school-linked health centers are utilized. These clinics are not on school property, but may be nearby or easily accessible through mass transit. Schools refer students to these centers and have established collaborative, working relationships that promote information sharing and support (Larson & Chapman, 2013).

Evaluation research has demonstrated that SBHCs are effective in increasing student access to health care. This is especially true for adolescents, who often are difficult to reach and do not willingly access health care. Onsite SBHC services are more appealing for adolescents, who have been shown to utilize substance abuse and mental health counseling services, as well as STD and family planning services (School-Based Health Alliance, n.d.). SBHCs also have been found to increase the use of contraception in sexually active teenage girls (Ethier et al., 2011).

School Nursing Careers

School nurses must be able to work autonomously. They need excellent communication skills and the ability to prioritize and collaborate with many others (professional and nonprofessional). The pay for school nurses depends on location and employer (health department or school district). In some places, the wage may be lower than acute care nurses, but the health insurance and benefits package are usually quite extensive (NASN, 2014f). School nurses are sometimes frustrated working in an educational setting, in which health may be a secondary priority, but their expertise is generally highly valued. Baisch et al. (2011) examined the value placed on school nursing services by school staff and found that school nurses were "considered vital to eliminating barriers to student learning and improving overall school health" (p. 74). School nurses save time for teachers and administrators, permitting them to focus on their job of educating students. They also found that school nurses positively influence management of student health concerns, student record accuracy, and student immunization rates. In addition, school nurses may become involved with other issues in the school, such as violence prevention, that extend beyond the traditional role of the nurse (King, 2014; Khubchandani, Telljohann, Price, Dake, & Kendershot, 2013).

Some schools of nursing find that their students can be helpful "school nurse extenders" in permitting school nurses to complete more screenings, referrals, and follow-ups for students (Rossman, Dood, & Squires, 2012, p. 734). Many nursing schools are utilizing schools as clinical sites, with school nurses as preceptors, in an effort to bring more new nurses into this specialty area. There are many positive reasons to work as a school nurse: school nurses generally do not work on weekends, many have contracts that give them the summer off, and the daily work schedule and holidays often coincide with those of the nurse's own school-age children, thus allowing a parent to be home with children during off-school hours (NASN, 2014e). Finally, for most of those employed as school nurses, it is a wonderful and rewarding experience to work with children whose eagerness and innocence can often refresh the soul. It is an opportunity to protect and heal our future leaders, who may become the ones who will eventually protect and heal the world. See Perspectives: School Nurse.

PERSPECTIVES
SCHOOL NURSE

A great aspect of being a school nurse is being able to work with many different people. I like being able to work with people who aren't necessarily sick but can benefit from my help. Additionally, school nurses must become familiar with resources and people in the community and surrounding areas. By making friends and connections in multiple facilities, occupations, and the like, school nurses can involve local resources as well as specific individuals in improving the population. That is an essential aspect to recognize: nurses shouldn't be alone in working with the community; they should involve as many people as possible, because community members should be active in improving their own area. Unfortunately, working as a school nurse takes a lot of effort and is time consuming. Even with the work that has been done at the school, it makes me wonder just how long our interventions will last. Unlike working in a hospital, where results come in just a few days, school nurses must work tirelessly for long periods of time to see the fruits of their labors. Resources aren't as readily available as they are for other types of nursing. Being a school nurse requires learning how to get funding for projects. School nurses often don't have models to work from, as each situation may be unique. They must be innovative, resourceful, and dedicated in order to stick with a project long enough for it to be beneficial to the population.

My overall opinion on working as a community nurse has changed over the past few weeks. Being a school nurse has been hard, but rewarding. I know several students in my semester who don't really consider community nursing to be truly nursing practice. I would beg to differ; school nursing is probably the epitome of what nursing was meant to be. It is focused on service and improving the health and well-being of the populace. Although nursing in the early days mainly dealt with fixing problems and injuries after they happened, everyone knows that an ounce of prevention is worth a pound of cure. Therefore, school nurses are doing the work that should benefit people the most. However, because their focus is on prevention, they seem to get little recognition for their work, because they are saving lives before they are endangered, they are saving teeth before they fall out, and they are saving families before they are lost. I believe their work is pivotal to the improvement of society.

Neil P., School Nurse

CORRECTIONAL NURSING

Nurses who work within the criminal justice system—correctional facilities, prisons, jails, detention centers, and substance abuse treatment programs—work with clients spanning a range of ages from juvenile to elderly, both male and female (ANA, 2013a). The facilities in which they work can hold just a few inmates or may house over 30,000 at one time. The United States has 25% of the world's prisoner population, but only 5% of the world's total population (Aufderheide, 2014). In 2010, there were 1,605,127 state and federal prisoners (rate: 497 per 100,000 U.S. residents), a decrease of 9,228 prisoners in 2009 (Guerino, Harrison, & Sabol, 2011). In 2014, about 1 in 36 adults was supervised through adult correctional systems, including probation and parole—the lowest rate since 1996 (Glaze, Kaeble, Minton, Tsoutis, & BJS Statisticians, 2015). The U.S. per capita rate of incarceration is the highest in the world, and approximately 15 million individuals are processed by the correctional system annually (Reznick, Comfort, McCartney, & Neilands, 2011). Tracking the number of nurses who work in correctional facilities is difficult. The last attempt, made in 2000, estimated the number to be 18,033 registered nurses working in corrections (Knox, 2013).

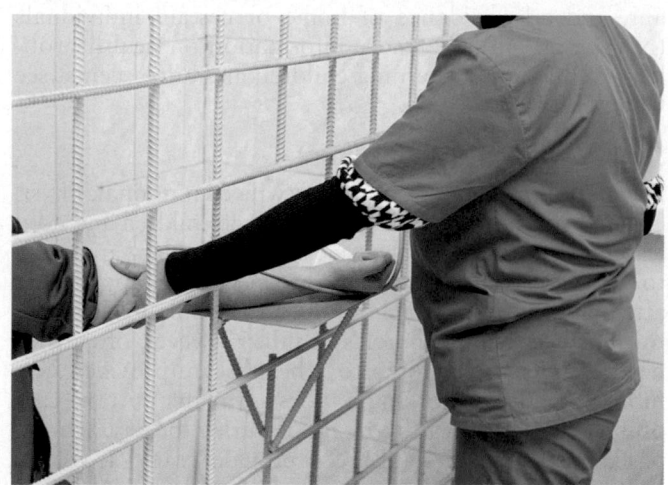

Correctional nurse taking an inmate's blood pressure.

History of Nursing in the Correctional Setting

Although the correctional system of prisons and jails has been around for a very long time, it historically provided minimal, if any, health care to inmates. Early nurses involved with prisoner and mentally ill populations included Dorothea Dix, who visited prisons around the country in the 19th century and found prisoners in chains, without proper sanitation, living conditions, nutrition, or clothing (ANA, 2013a). In the 1970s, Rena Murtha described the nurse at a large prison as the physician's slave, having little personal connection to patient/prisoners (ANA, 2013a). Prison was viewed as a punishment, and the inmates were seen as not deserving of care that was being paid from public dollars. The situation did not change until 1976, when the U.S. Supreme Court issued its decision regarding *Estelle v. Gamble*. The Supreme Court ruled that not providing medical services inflicted pain and denied inmates their Eighth Amendment rights. This decision led to major reforms in the correctional health system. Medical providers were hired and inmates' rights were established (Aufderheide, 2014; Schoenly, 2015). These rights included (American Bar Association, 2016):

- The right to access care and prompt medical treatment
- The right to professional judgment
- The right to care that is ordered
- The right to informed consent
- The right to refuse treatment
- The right to medical confidentiality

The American Correctional Health Services Association (n.d., para. 3) lists the following principles for correctional nurses and other health professionals:

- The inmate should be assessed as a client/patient at every "healthcare encounter."
- Treatment and procedures should only be administered after informed consent and medical diagnosis.
- Inmates have the right to refuse care, and involuntary care is only given when an immediate threat of danger to the inmate or others is present, or in cases of "grave disability."
- Privacy should be protected when possible (always for sound and when possible for sight).
- Health care should be provided to all inmates, without consideration of custody status.
- Providers should correctly identify themselves, as well as their professional certification or license and accompanying duties.
- Providers should not be a part of death penalty execution.
- Maintenance of the confidentiality for health care information and health records at all times (even during transport) should be ensured.
- Participation in research studies on prisoners should only be done after appropriate human subjects criteria have been met.

Although the right to access care or refuse it, the right to informed consent, and the right to confidentiality are considered basic, these are not always easily granted in correctional facilities. Courts have ruled that prisoners who refuse care may "create confusion and discord in the prison" and have permitted administrative decisions to overrule prisoner wishes (Dubler, 2014, p. 18). Confidentiality is tenuous, as correctional officers regularly observe prisoners and general population prisoners can often view inmates visiting some clinics (e.g., HIV/AIDS), leaving little doubt about their diagnosis. Strip/cavity searches and being present during forced takedowns, among other activities unique to this setting, provide new ethical dilemmas for health care professionals (Dubler, 2014).

Although the correctional health system is relatively new, it is under intense pressure from the courts to ensure that adequate and humane care is provided. Several lawsuits have occurred, and unsolved issues in the correctional health care setting continue to be highlighted. Some main issues regard the provision of ethically appropriate and timely patient care for inmates and provide adequate mental health treatment, prevent prisoner-on-prisoner violence, maintain sanitary and safe conditions, and stop inmate neglect and abuse. Ensuring that inmates' health needs are met—along with the growing number of inmates and the increasing intensity of their health concerns—has imposed a huge financial burden on systems that are already overtaxed. Funding for correctional health care derives from public tax dollars. Some have wondered if such care and expense should be given to incarcerated persons (Cohen, 2013). This is an ethical dilemma nurses working in correctional facilities must face every day. Keeping equipment up-to-date and avoiding shortcuts can also be challenging. In an attempt to decrease costs and save money, most states utilize managed care organizations to provide some services for inmates. Correctional Medical Services (2011) is the largest provider of prison health care in the nation. Some states are increasingly relying on private prison health care providers, or HMOs (Kutscher, 2013).

Many institutions have a house clinic, medical unit, or infirmary. However, these clinics do not have the capability to provide all the services inmates may need. For example, if imaging procedures, such as magnetic resonance imaging (MRI) or computed tomography (CT) scans, are needed or specialty consultations required, inmates must go to other sources outside of the prison or jail. In these instances, most corrections' facilities use managed health care systems. **Correctional nurses** work in on-site medical units housed in criminal justice facilities. These facilities can be local jails or may be at state and federal prison. The staff members in these units focus on the individual, immediate, and ambulatory care needs of the patients. They also attend to emergency needs and may help manage chronic conditions. They often provide screenings and preventive services. Larger facilities offer ambulatory and emergency care, mental health services, and subacute care units for short-term therapies (e.g., IV medications). As prisoners age, long-term care and end-of-life care must also be provided (Schoenly, 2015). Correctional nurses have the potential to assist inmates to obtain optimal health and thus save taxpayer dollars (International Association of Forensic Nurses, 2015).

The challenge of correctional nursing is to maintain the fundamental nature of nursing in a challenging environment that is not primarily focused on health care and to remain nonjudgmental toward clients (ANA, 2013a). Correctional nurses may face many ethical dilemmas surrounding ensuring patient basic privacy, but also maintaining personal safety. Today, correctional nurses work with a variety of clients, some of them potentially dangerous. Correctional nurses have for many years identified that there is a conflict between health care in prison and the aims of the prison administration (Powell, Harris, Condon, & Kemple, 2010). They may be instructed to avoid unnecessary touching of inmates, empathizing, engaging in conversations beyond medical care, and developing personal relationships with inmates; as well as referring to inmates by first name.

An estimated 6,851,000 persons (or 1 in 36 adults; 2.8% of the population) were under U.S. adult correctional system supervision during 2014; that represents a drop of over 52,000 from the previous year. The correctional population is comprised of both incarcerated adults and those in community supervision (parole or probation), and females represent about 22% of the total population but only 7% of the total prison population. The peak population was reached in 2007, with 7,399,600 adults in the U.S. adult correctional system. Texas, California, and Georgia have the highest total populations (Carson, 2015; Kaeble, Glaze, Tsoutis, & Minton, 2016). Demographically, inmates differ from the general population. First, inmates have all committed some type of crime, and 97% of those in state and federal prisons are serving more than 1 year, and over half (53.2%) are serving time for violent crimes. Thirteen percent of males and eleven percent of females in state prisons have been convicted of murder. Half of federal prison inmates are serving time for drug offenses. National statistics indicate a larger portion of Black (37%) and White (32%) than Hispanic (22%) male inmates in state and federal prisons. For female prisoners, Whites more than double the total number of Black prisoners and almost triple the number of Hispanic prisoners. The imprisonment rate for males is 890 per 100,000 U.S. residents, but for females, it is only 65. Many prison facilities are overcrowded, and some states have resorted to using private prisons to accommodate overcrowded conditions (Carson, 2015). In addition, the inmate population is drawn disproportionately from lower socioeconomic backgrounds when compared with the general public. This increases their chances of having a long trajectory of poorer access to health care and treatment. Statistics show a greater disproportion of inmates who are chronically ill and have infectious diseases than the nonincarcerated population (Carson, 2015).

Education and Skills Needed

The preferred educational level for correctional nurses is a bachelor's degree. The level of skill, judgment, and autonomy needed by nurses who work in corrections is supported and developed within baccalaureate education. Some institutions may require additional coursework in criminal justice, decision-making, assessment, and administrative skills. Master's level nurses (specifically NPs) also are working in corrections, providing primary health care to inmates. National certification, through the National Commission on Correctional Health Care as a certified correctional health professional (CCHP) or the American Correctional Association (ACA) as a certified correctional nurse (CCN), is available (ANA, 2013a; National Commission on Correctional Health Care, 2015).

Functions of Correctional Nurses

The prime responsibility of the correctional nurse is to restore and maintain the health of inmates by providing nursing care within correctional settings (ANA, 2013a). The work location does set correctional nurses apart as being the only nurses who enter their workplaces through metal detectors and grill gates and into a locked-down unit. Yet, the knowledge and skill set of a correctional nurse overlaps the knowledge and skill sets of many other nursing specialties.

Correctional nurses use public, community, and school health nursing skills, along with skills acquired from the ER, occupational health, mental health, orthopedics, and ambulatory care specialties. Like public, community, and school health nurses, correctional nurses are autonomous and must make decisions on their own. They track and screen for communicable diseases. They assist in setting up resources so that inmates who are released can continue getting medical treatment. They also educate inmates and promote healthful lifestyles among them. They collaborate with other health care professionals (e.g., physicians, dieticians, counselors) to provide appropriate services (Schoenly, 2015).

Correctional nurses often work in clinic settings, assisting the health care provider in assessing medical situations. They review sick call requests to determine what and if any action needs to be taken and by whom (nurse or physician). They may also oversee the medical unit beds that house patients who suffer from a variety of conditions (e.g., neurological trauma) requiring critical care or kidney disease requiring dialysis. They provide nursing care for inmates with uncontrolled diabetes, those with pneumonia needing IV antibiotics, inmates with mental health issues, or those undergoing withdrawal ("detox") from years of substance abuse (International Association of Forensic Nurses, 2015; Schoenly, 2015). They participate in administering medications, as many inmates receive a variety of medications. In addition, by law, inmates in most facilities must have a physical assessment within 14 days of admittance. Correctional nurses often perform these assessments. Correctional nurses also provide assessment and assistance in occupational safety issues and prenatal care with female inmates (Schoenly, 2015; Schoenly & Knox, 2013).

Finally, correctional nurses are called upon to assist in medical emergencies, anywhere in the facility, such as helping with an accident in a woodshop or evaluating an inmate too sick to leave his cell. If inmates need to go to a hospital or appointment outside the correctional facility, a correctional officer generally accompanies them, not the nurse. With so many responsibilities and the uncertainty of new issues, it is imperative for correctional nurses to prioritize their day (see Display 30–5). Because correctional facilities operate 24 hours a day, every day of the year, it is also vital that they also address emergency preparedness and disaster planning. *Continuity of operations plans* (COOP) are the operational guides used during disaster management in correctional facilities, and most also include Incident Command System (ICS) guidelines as outlined by the FEMA. The National Institute of Corrections publishes a guide for jail emergencies to assist correctional nurses in emergency preparedness. Taylor and Crianza (2011) provide vivid examples of natural disasters affecting a large jail system (over 10,000 inmates) and the need to plan for power, water, and telephone outages, as well as housing and moving prisoners under emergency conditions. In these situations, nursing and other staff are often asked to remain on-site for extended periods of time and while making arrangements for their own families.

Common Issues in Correctional Nursing

Correctional nurses address several common health problems among their population of interest. These concerns include mental health, drug abuse, and communicable

DISPLAY 30–5 A DAY IN THE LIFE OF A CORRECTIONAL NURSE

A day in my life depends on whether or not I am working at the infirmary or on the forensic unit. I will begin with the prison's infirmary.

Today, I worked in the infirmary. These are 12-hour day shifts, so I begin at 6 AM and end at 6:30 PM.

6:00 AM I take report from the night shift charge registered nurse (RN). Within our infirmary, we have both a medical side and a psychiatric side where report is given. Following report, I decide with the other nurses whether or not I am going to be responsible for the medical or psychiatric patients, or the walk-ins (acute/emergency care patients).

7:00 AM I take the medical side for the day, and set up the medications and then wait for the other nurse to set up his or her medications for the psychiatric in-patients. We usually do what we call "pill line" together. Following pill line, I return to the nursing station and do my charting.

8:30 AM Currently, we have a quadriplegic and paraplegic on our medical side who require a lot of personal care. We also have several patients with MRSA (methicillin-resistant *Staphylococcus aureus*) requiring fairly extensive dressing/packing changes along with IV antibiotics. I will have officers escort the MRSA patients out to a trauma bed in order for me to perform the dressing change and/or administration of IV antibiotics (usually vancomycin) that take 1 to 2 hours to complete. Following care, these inmates return to their medical cells, and I do my usual charting.

11:00 AM The quadriplegic and paraplegic inmates have call lights, so I have to attend to their needs when called. This may consist of feedings, diaper changes, and repositioning. Depending on the day, I will administer showers or bed baths for them. We also currently have an inmate with Parkinson's disease and comorbid psychiatric disorder and neuropathy, who also requires a great deal of care. We are not staffed for this type of care and try to get compassionate releases so that they can be sent to nursing homes. Luckily, we all help each other, so I get some assistance from the psychiatric staff.

12:45 PM Lunch when I can get it!

2:00 PM Even though I am responsible for the medical in-patients, I still might take a walk-in or two and do some of the "q30-minute checks" on the psychiatric side.

4:00 PM I attend to call lights and help other staff with their patients.

6:30 PM At the end of the day, I make sure that all my charting is done and then go on my way.

When I work on the forensic unit, my day is a bit different.

6:00 AM I take report from the night RN. On this unit I, along with our one LPN, am responsible for passing all the medications and performing all the blood sugars and insulin administrations for the diabetics in the morning, noon, and afternoon.

10:00 AM Charting, and doing some blood draws, along with giving some shots for those inmates on forced medications. I consider this unit more of a nursing management unit rather than a hands-on patient care unit. Begin mental health notes on B-section bottom tier inmates.

12:00 PM Passing medications, performing blood sugars, and administering insulin for diabetics. More charting and blood draws. I usually make sure that all the medications are current and check for any expired critical medications that might need reordering.

1:00 PM Lunch with staff.

2:00 PM I have to perform an extensive mental health note on all the inmates in the maximum-security unit of this building, which consists of 10 to 12 inmates on average. I then have to finish less extensive mental health notes on all the inmates in our B-section bottom tier, which consists of approximately 20 to 24 inmates. Following all my charting, I enter in all the diabetic care and scan all the medications passed on our electronic MAR (medication administration record).

5:00 PM Passing medications, performing blood sugars, and administering insulin for diabetics. More charting and blood draws. Continue with any mental health notes needing completion, entering the diabetic care, and scan all passed meds into MAR.

6:30 PM End of the day. Finish up any charting and head home.

Travis H., Correctional Nurse

diseases. As the inmate population grows, an increase in elderly and female inmates creates additional health concerns for correctional nurses. The following sections briefly describe some of these concerns, along with examples of what correctional nurses may do to address the issues facing them. See What Do You Think?

Mental Health Issues

States began to deinstitutionalize mentally ill, as they closed mental health hospitals during the 1960s and 1970s. The goal was to have them live more independent lives, but community treatment programs did not meet expectations, and some believe that many of these individuals ended up incarcerated—or just changing their institutionalization from mental health to prisons (Aufderheide, 2014; Swanson, 2015).

Mental health continues to be a major concern in correctional facilities (NIMH, n.d.b). Around 20% of prisoners have a serious mental illness, and 30% to 60% have a substance abuse disorder. Between 13.1% and 18.6% of state prison inmates have major depressive disorder, and between 2.1% and 4.3% have bipolar disorder, and about the same proportion have schizophrenia or another psychotic disorder (Aufderheide, 2014). In

What do *you* think?

During sick call today, your correctional nurse colleague notices that four to five inmates from the same housing unit have similar complaints—blurred vision, feeling sick, and some difficulty breathing. It is flu season—could that be the cause? You know that homemade alcohol is not uncommon in prisons and that it can be easily made from fermented fruit or other food waste. Prisoners call it moonshine, pruno, hooch, brew, raisin jack, and other names. You remember reading about a recent CDC report regarding several outbreaks of botulism in California, Utah, and Arizona prisons. Prisoners there had used potato peels, and the closed containers used to produce alcohol permitted the toxin to grow during fermentation. With no heat used to kill it, the bacteria grew and affected everyone who drank the brew. With botulism, it is most important to act quickly, as the toxin leads to nerve paralysis, and when it reaches the respiratory muscles, it can cause death. You talk with your colleague and decide to talk with the housing correctional officers and the patients for further information. I think it is better to be safe than sorry! What do you think?

Adapted from: Schoenly, L. (2016). *Botulism and prison brew*. Retrieved from http://correctionalnurse.net/?s=botulism

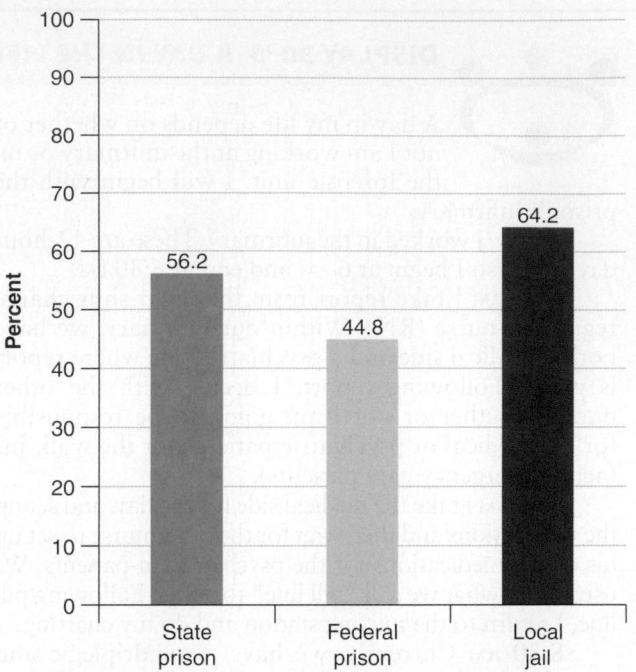

FIGURE 30–4 Inmates with 12-month mental health problems. From National Institute of Mental Health. (n.d.b). *Inmate mental health*. Retrieved from http://www.nimh.nih. gov/health/statistics/prevalence/inmate-mental-health.shtml

a 2011–2012 study of U.S. prisoners, 15% of state and federal inmates and 26% of local jail inmates reported serious psychological distress in the past 30 days (Beck, Berkofsky, Caspar, & Krebs, 2013). All but six states have more individuals with serious mental illness in at least one jail or prison than in the their largest state psychiatric facility, leading some to seriously question our society's ability to provide appropriate treatment for the mentally ill population (Swanson, 2015). One meta-analysis found a prevalence rate for traumatic brain injury (TBI) among the adult offender population to be 60%, whereas the general population's rate is only 8.5% (Shiroma, Ferguson, & Pickelsimer, 2012). See Figure 30–4 for a graph of inmates with mental health problems.

Reported incidents of sexual victimization are 4% for state and federal inmates and 3.2% for jail inmates during 2011–2012 (Beck et al., 2013). Perpetrators of sexual victimization are other inmates (2%) or facility staff (2.4%) or both (.4%) in state or federal institutions. For jail inmates, the proportions are 1.6%, 1.8%, and 0.2%, respectively. For inmate sexual abuse, rates are higher among female inmates, Whites versus Blacks, and those with college educations versus those not finishing high school. In instances of staff sexual victimization of inmates, rates were higher among male inmates, Blacks versus Whites, and for inmates aged 20 to 24 years (Beck et al., 2013). Over 6% of state and federal prison inmates with mental illness or psychological distress report sexual victimization, and those who report gay, lesbian,

or bisexual orientation had the highest rates; 12.2% of prisoners were victimized by other inmates, and 5.4% were victimized by staff (Beck et al., 2013). For inmates who had reported ever having mental health counseling, rates of inmate sexual abuse were three to four times higher than those who had not received counseling.

Mental illness also impacts suicide rates. Since 2000, suicide has been the leading cause of death in jails. In 2013, 334% of jail inmate deaths were due to suicide; this represents an increase of 14% over the previous year. The age of suicide victims was between 25 and 44 in 60% of jail suicides from 2000 to 2013, and the suicide mortality rate was 1.5 times higher for males than female inmates and higher for Whites than other racial/ethnic groups (Noonan, Rohloff, & Ginder, 2015). The rates for suicide are higher in local jails than in state or federal prisons: 40 for jails versus 16 for prisons per 100,000 people in 2012, compared to 13 per 100,000 for the total U.S. population (Kaste, 2015). Often, those incarcerated in local jails have not been in serious trouble with the legal system before this and suffer from "the shock of confinement" (Kaste, 2015, para. 2). For more on behavioral health, see Chapter 27.

Correctional nurses provide a good deal of mental health nursing care and assist in identifying undiagnosed conditions (Hoke, 2015). A postarrest diversion program, in which detainees are evaluated for mental health or substance abuse conditions, is highly effective as long as the resources are not diverted away from these programs (Mental Health America, Positions Statement 52, n.d.). The prearrest diversion programs train police officers to identify persons with mental illness have been successful in assisting with treatment and avoiding arrest.

Correctional nurses assist in multiple medication administrations per day to ensure that inmates receive the medications needed for their mental illnesses. They can also provide counseling regarding medication usage and assist inmates in understanding the side effects of their medication, which for some are many. Correctional nurses advocate for medication changes when they note severe side effects or a change in the mental status of inmates. Nurses can facilitate setting up medication support groups to allow inmates an opportunity to discuss concerns regarding their medications. They also can assist inmates in understanding the importance of taking their medication. As inmates prepare to leave the institution, correctional nurses assist in finding outpatient mental health clinics and other resources that will provide support and further treatment for the inmate. Finally, correctional nurses can provide education and training to other correctional workers regarding signs and symptoms of mental illness and the impact mental health has on decision making and the general health of a person (Schoenly, 2015). See Perspectives: Correctional Nurse.

Drug Abuse

Drug abuse by inmates is very high. Over 80% of local jail and state prison inmates have used an illegal drug; 55% did so within 30 days prior to their arrest. Cocaine, crack, methamphetamine, and heroin were the most commonly cited drugs of choice. About one third of state prison inmates were under the influence of illegal substances during their offense, and 16.5% admitted committing a crime in order to buy drugs. Substance

use is also linked to recidivism rates, with 68% of drug offenders being rearrested within 3 years of leaving prison (Belenko, Hiller, & Hamilton, 2013).

Drug Treatment Alternative to Prison (DTAP) program diverts drug offenders into long-term residential treatment rather than incarceration. If offenders successfully complete treatment, their sentence can be vacated, and program has garnered a 1-year retention rate of 76% and rearrests dropped 42% (Belenko et al., 2013). Other community-based supervision and treatment programs have demonstrated success, as have drug courts.

In jail or prison settings, drug education and counseling programs are offered to inmates and have shown good results, but longer, more intensive counseling is more effective than brief or intermittent efforts. Innovative programs like Jail In-Reach Intervention demonstrated significantly lower drug and alcohol use 12 months after program completion for female jail inmates. Other interventions, using journaling, community-based drug treatment follow-up, have also shown promise. In prison populations, with higher rates of personality disorders and psychological problems, poor impulse control, greater propensity for risk taking, higher cognitive deficits, and criminal thought patterns, it is critical to utilize evidence-based interventions targeted to the needs of this vulnerable population (Belenko et al., 2013). See Evidence-Based Practice.

Of the drug users in prison, 40% of state and 49% of federal inmates had participated in treatment programs, in the latest national sample of U.S. prisoners (Mumola & Karberg, 2007). Correctional nurses can help with referrals and also provide nursing care as patients withdraw from substances while in prison. Withdrawal can cause life-threatening symptoms that need immediate medical attention. In addition, correctional nurses can organize and provide support groups to assist inmates in staying sober and drug-free. They can advocate for the inclusion of Alcoholics Anonymous, Narcotic Anonymous, and Al-Anon services in the correctional facility. Counseling can be offered to assist inmates as they leave the facility, so that they do not return to prior bad habits if and when they return to areas where drug and alcohol use is rampant (Hoke, 2015; Schoenly, 2015). Returning to this environment increases their chances of returning to substance abuse, and inmates leaving prisons or jails need to be connected to outside resources.

Communicable Disease

In correctional facilities, communicable diseases can spread quickly. A large study of state and federal prisons noted that during the 2009–2010 influenza season, 79% of respondents reported some level of activity, whereas 53% reported an "outbreak" of H1N1 flu and seven deaths also occurred. Although 90% of those responding stated that they had developed some type of general disaster or influenza emergency plan before flu season, it was noted that "the lack of a consistent system of disease surveillance across prison facilities" (inmates and staff) made it difficult to determine a true baseline and quickly contain or prevent an outbreak (Potter, Schwartz, Blackmore, & May, 2011, p. 73). Many communicable diseases are of great concern in the correctional community such as TB, hepatitis C, and STDs including HIV/

PERSPECTIVES
CORRECTIONAL NURSE

The prison is, in my opinion, a very good place to work. I believe that every student should experience nursing within corrections. I have worked floor nursing before, and working at the prison is much better. Although it can get crazy and chaotic from time to time, the atmosphere is much more laid back. Nurses at the prison seem to have a lot more autonomy than do nurses at other facilities or companies. The prison offers nurses a chance to experience many different skills. You might not gain absolute proficiency in any one skill, but you will gain many skills, and you will become very good at many of them. The nice thing is that nurses come from many different backgrounds, and so they can and will certainly help you and teach you what they know to help with your own skill base. I guarantee that if you work at the prison, you will get to see and experience things that people in normal society will never get the opportunity to see. Come to the prison, and you will get to be a medical nurse, a psych nurse, a triage nurse, an orthopedic nurse, and you can get to do the medical/psychiatric intake screenings for all the new or parole violation inmates who come to the prison on a daily basis. There is probably more, but certainly keep your minds and options open for a great and secure career.

Travis H., Correctional Nurse

EVIDENCE-BASED PRACTICE

What Are the Research Priorities in Correctional Nursing?

Because correctional nursing research is sparse and only more recently being conducted, a three-round Delphi technique was used to poll expert correctional nurses, educators, administrators, and researchers to determine research priorities in that specialty field of nursing. The top five research priorities included:

- How to help correctional nurses develop critical thinking skills and determine which skills provide improved correctional nursing performance and patient outcomes.
- Determine correctional nursing's core competencies.
- Define excellent clinical judgment among correctional nurses.

- Which patient outcomes are most affected by correctional nursing care?
- Complete replication studies related to nurse education level in the correctional setting.

How can these priorities advance the profession of nursing in the correctional setting? What other research priorities should be considered?

How has research that has examined education level of nurses and patient outcomes in acute care settings demonstrated the benefits of the BSN? Do you feel that this might be replicated in the correctional setting?

Schoenly, L. (2015). Research priorities in correctional nursing practice: Results of a three-round Delphi study. *Journal of Correctional Health Care*, 2(4), 400–407.

LEVELS OF PREVENTION PYRAMID

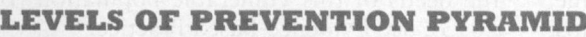

HEALTH ISSUE: Sexually transmitted disease (STD) in correctional facilities

TERTIARY PREVENTION

Rehabilitation	Primary Prevention	
	Health Promotion and Education	*Health Protection*
• Work closely with inmates and physician to decrease side effects of STD (i.e., cervical cancer)	• Continue to promote responsible sexual behavior	

SECONDARY PREVENTION

Early Diagnosis	Prompt Treatment
• Provide STD screening upon entering facility • Provide regular, routine STD screenings	• Provide treatment for inmates diagnosed with STDs • Promote facility policies that allow for STD screenings and early treatment

PRIMARY PREVENTION

Health Promotion and Education	Health Protection
• Teach inmates how STDs are transmitted and what can be done to stop transmission (condoms, other preventive measures) • Teach signs and symptoms of commonly occurring STDs • Teach that gonorrhea and chlamydia are often asymptomatic, and so routine screening is important for individuals at risk	

AIDS. The concern of communicable disease is not only for the health of the inmate with the disease, but the susceptibility of all inmates and ultimately the general public (if the inmate is released while still infected). Increased rates of these diseases are due to high-risk behaviors and increased rates of abusive behaviors, including rape, both before and during incarceration. Of special note is the fact that most U.S. prisons prohibit distribution of condoms or sterile injection equipment (Reznick et al., 2011).

A hallmark study, conducted by the RAND Corporation (2011), indicated that inmates were four times as likely to have active TB, nine to ten times as likely to have hepatitis C, and five times as likely to be infected with HIV as the general population. Maruschak, Berzofsky, and Unangst (2015) noted that in a 2011–2012 study of U.S. inmates, 21% of prisoners and 14% of jail inmates had hepatitis B or C, TB, or an STD (excluding HIV/AIDS). Testing for tuberculosis was done for 94% of prisoners, and 71% had HIV testing done since being incarcerated. For jail inmates, 54% had TB testing and 11% had HIV testing done. Six percent of prison inmates reported ever having TB, whereas only 0.5% of the general population reported this. The rate for local jail inmates is lower at 2.5% Total hepatitis was reported at 10.9% for prisoners and 0.1% for the general public. HIV/AIDS was reported by 1.3% of prisoners, and by only 0.1% of the general population (Maruschak et al., 2015). In 2012, data reported that the number of inmates living with HIV/AIDS was 20,449 in federal and 1,538 in state correctional facilities (CDC, 2012).

Inmates are at risk for hepatitis C because of the heavy IV drug use among prisoners. Tattooing is also problematic, as is the incidence of piercing and physical violence (Treloar, McCreedie, & Lloyd, 2015). Ten percent of prisoners reported having hepatitis C, and it was the most highly reported communicable disease in a recent survey (Maruschak et al., 2015). Internationally, it can be as high as 38%, and IV drug use is the greatest risk factor. Screening of high-risk populations can help reduce the spread of this virus, but is not always feasible (Zampino, Coppola, Sagnelli, DiCaprio, & Sagnelli, 2015).

TB is widespread among prisoners, and rates are much higher than in the general population. According to the World Health Organization, TB rates of inmates were 23 times higher than the general public for a variety of reasons (Baussano et al., 2010). Some have reported it as high as 50 times greater than national averages and noted that prisons are increasingly reservoirs of drug-resistant TB (O'Grady et al., 2011). Because many inmates are homeless and abuse alcohol and/or drugs, they are more susceptible to TB; to compound the problem, the closeness of living conditions in jails and prisons facilitates the quick spread of TB (Baussano et al., 2010). Prisoners are at a high risk of moving from latent TB infection to actual tuberculosis, and medication compliance is often low after inmates are discharged. A study in San Francisco found that the stream of TB-infected individuals released from incarceration changes, but there are high numbers of foreign-born individuals who may need to have interferon-gamma release assay testing in order to detect true infections because of the large proportion having

received bacillus Calmette-Guérin (BCG) vaccination in their countries of origin (White, Nelson, Kawamura, Grinsdale, & Goldenson, 2012).

Correctional nurses must track rates of communicable diseases and provide education regarding the spread and treatment of those diseases. They must provide data on the number of cases of reportable diseases to the state health department. Correctional nurses can provide preventative care by offering immunizations to inmates. In addition, they can provide the necessary treatment for TB, STDs, and other diseases and can assist in advocating for measures to decrease the spread of disease within correctional facilities. Correctional nurses can assist institutions by providing initial screenings upon arrival of inmates and periodic screening for certain diseases and surveillance of potential communicable diseases during sick call (National Commission on Correctional Health Care, 2016). The CDC (2015j, 2009) recommends routine opt-out screenings for HIV and other communicable screenings if at risk. However, screening based solely on risk may miss many inmates, and so routine screening and treatment of inmates for various communicable diseases may be beneficial and cost-effective.

For chronic communicable diseases, such as HIV/AIDS, correctional nurses can facilitate and organize peer educator groups. These have been found to be successful in educating inmates on HIV/AIDS, substance abuse, and low self-esteem. Others have demonstrated increased HIV testing in inmates and their female partners, along with better communication about HIV-related topics (Reznick et al., 2011). Successful programs also exist to assist inmates as they prepare for release. Correctional nurses can facilitate programs that empower inmates not to return to behaviors that increase their chance of contracting HIV and can also identify resources for inmates suffering from TB, so that they can continue their medication and treatment upon their release.

Future Trends

Because of advances in health care, longer prison terms, and more restrictive policies, inmates are older, sicker, and remain in prison longer than they did even 20 years ago. And historically, inmates have not taken good care of themselves. Hence, a 50-year-old inmate may have the health of a typical 65-year-old in the general public (ANA, 2013a; Schoenly, 2015). This surge in the inmate population is creating a lack of resources and beds for the aging inmate population.

Correctional nurses can increase efforts to empower inmates to take control of their health and can provide them with resources for health care access outside the prison, so that inmates will continue their care upon release. Correctional nurses can also be advocates and lobby state and federal legislatures to allocate funding for the additional resources needed within the prison system (Hoke, 2015).

The female inmate population is also increasing. In addition to women's reproductive health issues, females tend to have higher rates of diabetes, HIV, STDs, mental illness, drug abuse, and emotional issues (ANA, 2013a; Schoenly, 2015). Researchers have found that women in jail have a high risk of cervical cancer and increased rates of abnormal Papanicolaou (Pap) test results (Binswanger,

Mueller, Clark, & Cropsey, 2011). Correctional nurses can begin providing routine cervical and breast cancer screenings for female inmates. They can also provide counseling and emotional support. Researchers have suggested that women in prison need trauma-informed, gender-responsive treatment because of past trauma histories (Hayes, 2015; White, 2012). There has been a movement to provide trauma-informed care and gender-responsive programs (GRPs) to women in prison. However, a recent online national survey conducted by the National Institute of Corrections to assess the extent of such programmatic and policy develop concluded that despite widely expressed support for developing gender-responsive, trauma-informed correctional policies, "The degree to which policies adapted for women offenders are aligned with evidence-based literature and theories is unknown" (King & Foley, 2014 p. 3). Women in prison can experience retraumatization through prison practices such as strip searches, pat-downs, and the use of segregation (King & Foley, 2014), as well as sexual and other types of assaults by other inmates or correctional staff (Blackburn, Mullings, & Marquart, 2008). Although trauma-informed, gender-responsive treatment has become a new practice in the correctional setting, it has not been uniformly applied to correctional nursing. As Harner and Burgess (2011) stated,

> ...clinicians in correctional facilities have an opportunity to help ensure that incarcerated women leave jails and prisons in better physical and mental health than when they arrived. To that end, the provision of evidence-based, gender-responsive, and trauma-informed care in correctional settings must be our goal (p. 474).

Chronic disease, such as diabetes, cancer, heart disease, arthritis, cirrhosis of the liver, and asthma, is also increasing in the incarcerated population. About 40% of the 2011–2012 population of state/federal prisoners and jail inmates reported having a current chronic condition; hypertension was the highest reported chronic conditions at 30% of prisoners and 26% of inmates, with arthritis and asthma being the second and third most common chronic conditions. Females, rather than males, were more likely to report a chronic health condition, and older prisoners and inmates over age 50 were about twice to as likely to report a chronic condition as those aged 18 to 24 years. About one quarter of all prisoners and inmates reported multiple chronic conditions (Maruschak et al., 2015). Correctional nurses can facilitate chronic disease clinics to educate and empower inmates to better control their chronic conditions. To this end, correctional nurses need to conduct thorough family health histories, as many health conditions tend to have a genetic component and employ screenings to identify

conditions as soon as possible, so that early intervention can decrease complications and stop disease progression. They can follow up by promoting better nutrition and exercise habits and medication management.

Ethical and legal issues in correctional nursing often center on the patient (most often someone convicted of a crime, possibly involving violence). Caring for the patient is vital, but custody must also be maintained and safety is essential. Nurses must demonstrate nonjudgmental attitudes while at the same time ensuring protection from assault. Also, correctional workers (including nurses) may be subject to lawsuits brought by inmates for *deliberate indifference*, or perceived retaliation leading to an adverse action. For instance, this may include withholding health care that could lead to increased health problems in retaliation for the inmate filing grievances or formal complaints against the worker (Pont, Stöver, & Wolff, 2012). Incarceration may present as counterproductive to the health and well-being of the affected population. However, it does create a public health opportunity for providing screening, diagnosis, treatment, and postrelease linkage to care for members of a vulnerable population who may not seek or have access to services otherwise. Correctional nurses have an opportunity, to help reduce the burden of disease for communities by providing trilevel preventive health care pre-, intra-, and postincarceration (Macmadu & Rich, 2015).

CORRECTIONAL NURSING CAREERS

Correctional nurses must have good mental health and assessment skills. They must be able to communicate well and be strong nursing advocates and strong advocates for their clients. They work in an intense environment where their safety could be threatened, and they must deal with clients who may be noncompliant, combative, and manipulative. Correctional nurses must also be very flexible and knowledgeable about a variety of nursing specialties (Minority Nurse, 2016). Correctional nurses are also increasingly becoming Certified Correctional Health Care Professionals (National Commission on Correctional Health Care, 2015).

Salaries depend upon the state, although they tend to be generally higher than in other nursing fields. Moreover, correctional nurses usually receive extensive employee benefits and insurance packages as government employees. Correctional nurses have the ability to see recoveries from illnesses and injuries because they work with the same patients for a longer time than hospital-based nurses. Correctional nursing provides an opportunity to work with a vulnerable population and practice the true art and science of nursing. You use every nursing skill you have learned and advocate for a population that is in need. It can be a challenging, rewarding career. See Perspectives about the hiring process for new correctional nurses.

PERSPECTIVES
SUPERVISOR AND A DIRECTOR OF CORRECTIONAL NURSING ON HIRING NEW NURSES

Do you think you might like a job at a prison facility? A Director of Nursing and a Supervisor of Correctional Nursing provide some information on the interview process:

Before we hire new correctional nurses, we ask them to review the correctionalnurse.net blog (Schoenly, 2016) and the Correctional Nurse Manifesto (Schoenly, 2014). As part of the interview process, at the second interview, the nurse candidates have a facility-wide tour with a correctional supervisor and then another interview with the nursing team members. These represent the people with whom they will work; applicants ask questions and be questioned in order to make certain that they are suitable for the unique position of correctional nurse. The nurses who are hired receive civilian training and are assigned a preceptor. The process is designed to educate the candidate to the realities and complexities of correctional nursing. As the director notes, "No one dreams of going into correctional nursing, but once you are in, you are hooked because you realize the difference you can make."

The interview process follows the guidelines set forth by the ANA Correctional Nursing: Scope and Standards of Practice (2013) and the textbook Essentials of Correctional Nursing (Shoenly & Knox, 2013). This textbook provides crucial information such as the ethical, legal, and safety considerations of correctional nursing; common inmate-patient health care concerns and diseases; nursing care processes; and professional role and responsibilities. Also, unlike the nurses hired in the past, newer correctional nurses do provide health care education and health care clinics for chronic diseases on a regular basis. Because of the lack of an inpatient facility, 24-hour nursing care is not provided in some correctional facilities. When 24-hour nursing care is necessary, the inmates are transferred to a correctional facility where such coverage is available or to an acute care facility if more extensive care is required. In addition, the correctional officers are trained to follow procedure and call 911 during an emergency. There is a policy regarding distribution of medications in the prison setting. For example, red medications, such as psychiatric medications, insulin, and cardiac medications, are administered by the nurses; yellow medications, such as cholesterol medications and antibiotics, can be administered by correctional officers (at the supervisor's particular prison no medications are administered by officers, however); and green medications, such as Tylenol, ibuprofen, and some cardiac medications, are self-administered by the inmates.

Challenges to correctional nursing include the philosophy in the prison setting that "safety comes first," which could result in an inmate missing a sick call. Should this occur, however, their medical needs are taken care of as soon as it is safe and without compromise to their condition, according to both the supervisor and the director of nursing. Transportation for medical issues requiring care outside of the prison can be problematic as there may not be correctional staff available to provide the necessary transportation. Fortunately, this does not happen during emergencies, in which case 911 is called and correctional

officers are not involved in the transportation. One emergency that correctional nurses are occasionally faced with is suicide attempts; a situation that is always "scary" even if you have seen it happen before. This situation leads to a lock-down so that all resources can be focused on the suicidal inmate, who sometimes is found hanging and needs to be cut down and resuscitated.

The ability of correctional nurses to deliver medically appropriate care is hindered by the lack of access to preexisting medical records and history. Nurses must often rely on inmate self-reporting rather than a comprehensive medical history. Self-reporting is a far less reliable means for determining an inmate's risk factors and overall wellness. This may be one of the reasons that civil litigation by inmates, alleging medical negligence, is a weighty problem for all correctional agencies.

Aside from the organizational impediments that correctional nurses encounter that may contribute to inmate litigation over medical care is the additional challenge of finding nurses who hold bachelor or other advanced degrees in nursing to apply for vacant positions. Diploma or Associate degree programs fail to provide the level of training in community and public health, as well as psychiatric nursing that correctional nursing requires. Incarcerated populations present unique health needs that are generally not as pervasively distributed in general medical settings. A CNA HealthPro and Nurses Services Organization (2011) 5-year study on nurses' professional liability exposure reports higher claims indemnity payments for respondents who had only completed a nursing diploma program in comparison to those with a bachelor's or associate's degree. That is why the director of nursing is focusing on hiring BSN-prepared nurses.

The director of nursing also said, "Our goal is for them [inmates] to leave healthier. We have an incredible opportunity to improve the health of our population by returning our patients to the community healthier than when they came to us." She also commented "We are not here to be punitive. We are here to care." The Correctional Nurse Manifesto (Schoenly, 2014, p. 2) mandates that correctional nurses:

- *Treat inmates with the dignity and respect deserving of any patient.*
- *Work within my scope of practice at all times.*
- *Not become cynical to the health requests of my patient population.*
- *Hold myself and my peers to the professional boundaries of practice.*
- *Continually guard my own and other's physical and mental safety.*
- *Speak up when I see ill treatment of my patient population.*
- *Be a force for good in the community in which I work.*

—T. P., Supervisor of Correctional Nursing
—C. F., Director of Correctional Nursing

CNA HealthPro and Nurses Service Organization. (2011). *Understanding nurse liability, 2006–2010: A three-part approach.* Retrieved from http://www.nso.com/Individuals/Documents/RN-2010-CNA-Claims-Study(professional%20liability).pdf
Schoenly, L. (2014). *The correctional nurse manifesto.* Professional & Technical Kindle eBooks.
Schoenly, L. (2016). *Correctional nursing blog.* Retrieved from http://correctionalnurse.net

SUMMARY

Nurses who work in publicly funded settings are critical to the health and well-being of their communities. Public health nursing interventions are essential in keeping our nation healthy. They may not be as visible as hospital nurses, who interact with individual patients in the hospital, because PHNs often work from behind the scenes. Those who come in contact with them directly know of their worth, but much of the general population remains unaware of the role and the need for PHNs. PHNs deal with a number of issues including communicable diseases, chronic diseases, injuries, STDs, maternal child health, immunizations, and substance abuse. They work with all ages, ethnicities, socio-economic groups, and populations. Their emphasis is on health prevention and promotion. Some PHNs work in the uniformed public health service and in other branches of the military.

School nurses work with school populations including students, their families, and the school staff. They provide individual care and are the bridge between medical providers and schools. School nurses provide health care services, such as direct nursing care, first aid, and specialized health care for children with special needs. They also provide population health services and health protection measures such as immunizations and environmental assessments. Finally, school nurses provide health promotion activities including education, health screenings and referrals, immunizations, and staff wellness programs. School-based clinics are another means of providing care for the school population. Children and adolescents are important population groups for community health nurses because their physical and emotional health is vital to the future of our country and because they require guidance and direction.

Correctional nurses work with inmates in federal, state, or local facilities, including drug treatment and juvenile detention centers. They provide individual care in facility clinics and infirmaries while also identifying and developing programs to address major population health concerns of inmates, including mental illness, drug and alcohol abuse, and communicable diseases. The inmate population is growing older, staying longer, and suffering more from chronic disease. This, along with an increase in female inmates, brings additional challenges for correctional nurses.

All three nursing specialty areas impact the health of our communities. Because of the high level of nursing knowledge, communication skills, autonomy, and leadership needed for these nursing specialties, entry level should be at least a baccalaureate degree. Community nurses who work in public settings provide a valuable service needed to keep our nation healthy.

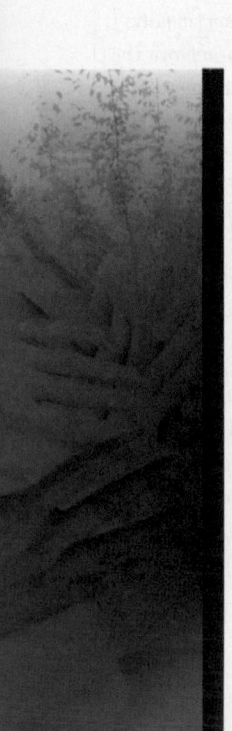

ACTIVITIES TO PROMOTE **CRITICAL THINKING**

1. As a correctional nurse, you deal with people from a variety of backgrounds, social classes, and past crimes. How can your values and attitudes toward criminal activity impact your treatment of inmates? Does social class, race, age, or gender make any difference in how you feel about them and interact with them as your clients?

2. One of the concerns expressed by correctional facility nurses is the antisocial and manipulative behavior of inmates, along with potential violence. How can a nurse working in a state prison effectively determine the health care needs of inmates?

3. Discuss possible methods of doing nutritional assessments in school-age children. What programs could be instituted to encourage healthier diets and increased exercise? What other factors might need to be considered? How could you, as a school nurse, work with schools and parents to increase physical activity and improve nutrition for school-age children and adolescents?

4. Go to this Web site (https://www.nhlbi.nih.gov/files/docs/public/lung/asthma_actplan.pdf) and print out a copy of the *Asthma Action Plan*. Discuss this with the parent of a school-age child or adolescent who has asthma. Has a school nurse or public health nurse ever gone over a plan with them? Have they ever been shown how to use a peak flow meter or correctly use an asthma inhaler? What methods have they used to control asthma triggers?

5. Describe potential areas of employment as a member of the U.S. Public Health Service. What types of care are rendered? In what areas of the country? What are benefits of this type of nursing career?

6. Most schools require that children entering school show proof of being fully immunized for a variety of communicable diseases. With a partner, discuss what would happen if schools no longer had this requirement. How else can immunizations be reinforced in the public?

7. Many prisoners suffer from mental illness. List types of programs and/or support groups that the nurse could provide for these inmates. What about inmates not formally diagnosed with a mental illness?

8. What do you think are the most significant ethical and legal issues involving correctional nursing? If possible, interview a correctional nurse and discuss this. Also, discuss what they most enjoy about their job, as well as their most significant concerns.

9. Debate the problems of mental illness and substance abuse in prisons. Are prisons and jails appropriate facilities for meeting the needs of these populations? Why or why not? If not, what other alternatives may be more effective?

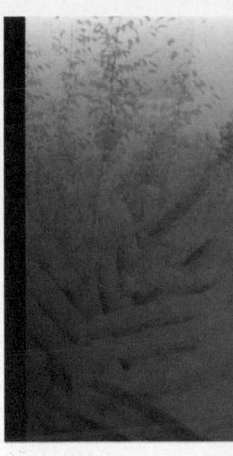

REFERENCES

Abrams, S. E. (2005). Changing times, changing needs, changing programs. *Public Health Nursing, 22*(3), 267–268.

Agency for Children and Families, Children's Bureau. (2016). *Child maltreatment report, 2014.* Retrieved from http://www.acf.hhs.gov/programs/cb/research-data-technology/statistics-research/child-maltreatment

American Academy of Child & Adolescent Psychiatry. (2014). *Fact sheet: Teen suicide.* Retrieved from http://www.aacap.org/page.ww?name=Teen+Suicide&section=Facts+for+Families

American Academy of Pediatrics (AAP). (2013). *Role of the school physician.* Retrieved from http://pediatrics.aappublications.org/content/131/1/178

American Academy of Pediatrics (AAP). (2016). *Policy statement: Role of the school nurse in providing school health services.* Retrieved from http://pediatrics.aappublications.org/content/pediatrics/early/2016/05/19/peds.2016-0852.full.pdf

American Bar Association. (2016). *Legal status of prisoners.* Retrieved from http://www.americanbar.org/publications/criminal_justice_section_archive/crimjust_standards_prisoners_status.html#23-1.1

American Correctional Health Services Association. (n.d.). *Mission & ethics statement.* Retrieved from http://www.achsa.org/mission-ethics-statement/

American Diabetes Association (ADA). (2012). Position statement: Diabetes care in the school setting. *Diabetes Care, 35*(Suppl. 1), S76–S80. Retrieved from http://www.diabetes.org/assets/pdfs/schools/ps-diabetes-care-in-the-school-and-daycare-setting.pdf

American Lung Association. (2016). *Open airways for schools.* Retrieved from http://www.lung.org/lung-health-and-diseases/lung-disease-lookup/asthma/asthma-education-advocacy/open-airways-for-schools/

American Nurses Association (ANA). (2013a). *Correctional nursing: Scope and standards of practice* (2nd ed.). Silver Spring, MD: Author.

American Nurses Association (ANA). (2013b). *Public health nursing: Scope and standards of practice.* Silver Spring, MD: Author.

American Nurses Association (ANA) and National Association of School Nurses (NASN). (2011). *School nursing: Scope and standards of practice* (2nd ed.). Silver Spring, MD: Author.

American Nurses Credentialing Center. (2015). *Public health nurse, advanced.* Retrieved from http://www.nursecredentialing.org/Certification/NurseSpecialties/AdvPublicHealth.aspx

American School Health Association. (n.d.). *About the American School Health Association: Core beliefs.* Retrieved from http://www.ashaweb.org/wp-content/uploads/2015/02/ASHA-Core-Beliefs-Combined_2.6.20152.pdf

American Speech-Language-Hearing Association. (2016). *Sensorineural hearing loss.* Retrieved from http://www.asha.org/public/hearing/Sensorineural-Hearing-Loss/

Association of Public Health Nurses. (2014). *The role of the public health nurse in disaster preparedness, response, and recovery.* Retrieved from http://www.achne.org/files/public/APHN_RoleOfPHNinDisasterPRR_FINALJan14.pdf

Atusingwize, E., Lewis, S., & Langley, T. (2015). Economic evaluations of tobacco control mass media campaigns: A systematic review. *Tobacco Control, 24*(4), 320–327.

Aufderheide, D. (2014). *Mental illness in America's jails and prisons: Toward a public safety/public health model.* Retrieved from http://healthaffairs.org/blog/2014/04/01/mental-illness-in-americas-jails-and-prisons-toward-a-public-safetypublic-health-model/

Avery, G., Johnson, T., Cousins, M., & Hamilton, B. (2013). The school wellness nurse: A model for bridging gaps in school wellness programs. *Pediatric Nursing, 39*(1), 13–17.

Baisch, M. J., Lundeen, S. P., & Murphy, M. K. (2011). Evidence-based research on the value of school nurses in an urban school system. *Journal of School Health, 81*(2), 74–80.

Balestra, M. (2012). Amicus brief supports administration of insulin to students only by licensed nurses. *Journal of Nursing Law, 15*(1), 27–32.

Baussano, I., Williams, B. G., Nunn, P., Beggiato, M., Fedeli, U., & Scano, F. (2010). Tuberculosis incidence in prisons: A systematic review. *PLoS Medicine.* Retrieved from http://www.plosmedicine.org/article/info:doi/10.1371/journal.pmed.1000381

Beck, A. J., Berkofsky, M., Caspar, R., & Krebs, C. (2013). *Sexual victimization in prisons and jails, reported by inmates, 2011–2012.* Retrieved from http://www.bjs.gov/content/pub/pdf/svpjri1112.pdf

Belenko, S., Hiller, M., & Hamilton, L. (2013). Treating substance use disorders in the criminal justice system. *Current Psychiatry Reports, 15*(11), doi: 10.1007/s11920-013-0414-z.

Biag, M., Srivastava, A., Landau, M., & Rodriguez, E. (2015). Teachers' perceptions of full- and part-time nurses at school. *Journal of School Nursing, 31*(3), 183–195.

Binswanger, I. A., Mueller, S., Clark, C. B., & Cropsey, K. L. (2011). Risk factors for cervical cancer in criminal justice settings. *Journal of Women's Health, 20*(12), 1839–1845. doi: 10.1089/jwh.2011.2864.

Blackburn, A. G., Mullings, J. L., & Marquart, J. W. (2008). Sexual assault in prison and beyond: Toward an understanding of lifetime sexual assault among incarcerated women. *The Prison Journal, 88*(3), 351–377.

Bloom, B., Cohen, R. A., & Freeman, G. (2012). Summary health statistics for U.S. children: National health interview survey, 2011. *Vital Health Statistics, 10*(254), 1–88.

Bloom, B., Jones, L. I., & Freeman, G. (2013). Summary health statistics for U.S. children: National health interview survey, 2012. *Vital Health Statistics, 10*(258), 1–81.

Bobo, N., Etkind, P., Martin, K., Chi, A., & Coyle, R. (2013). How school nurses can benefit from immunization information systems. *NASN School Nurse, 28*(2), 100–109.

Brackney, D. E., & Cutshall, M. (2015). Prevention of type 2 diabetes among youth: A systematic review, implications for the school nurse. *Journal of School Nursing, 31*(1), 6–21.

Brooks-Kayal, A. R., Bath, K. G., Berg, A. T., Galanopoulou, A. S., Holmes, G. L., Jensen, F. E., ... Scharfman, H. E. (2013). Issues related to symptomatic and disease-modifying treatments affecting cognitive and neuropsychiatric comorbidities of epilepsy. *Epilepsia, 54*(s4), 44–60.

Carson, E. A. (2015). *Prisoners 2014*. Retrieved from http://www.bjs.gov/content/pub/pdf/p14.pdf

Catalano, R. F., Fagan, A. A., Gavin, L. E., Greenberg, M. T., Irwin, C. E., Ross, D. A., & Shek, D. T. (2012). Worldwide application of prevention science in adolescent health. *Lancet*, *379*(9826), 1653–1664.

Centers for Disease Control and Prevention (CDC). (2009). *HIV testing implementation: Guidance for correctional settings*. Retrieved from http://www.cdc.gov/hiv/pdf/risk_Correctional_Settings_Guidelines.pdf

Centers for Disease Control and Prevention (CDC). (2011). *Health & academics data & statistics*. Retrieved from http://www.cdc.gov/healthyyouth/health_and_academics/data.htm

Centers for Disease Control and Prevention (CDC). (2012). *HIV in correctional facility fact sheet*. Retrieved from www.cdc.gov/hiv/resources/factsheets/pdf/correctional.pdf

Centers for Disease Control and Prevention (CDC). (2013a). *Summary health statistics for U.S. children: National health interview survey, 2012*. Retrieved from http://www.cdc.gov/nchs/data/series/sr_10/sr10_258.pdf

Centers for Disease Control and Prevention (CDC). (2013b). *Trends in the prevalence of obesity, dietary behaviors, and weight control practices*. Retrieved from http://www.cdc.gov/healthyyouth/data/yrbs/pdf/trends/us_obesity_trend_yrbs.pdf

Centers for Disease Control and Prevention (CDC). (2014). *National diabetes statistics report, 2014*. Retrieved from http://www.cdc.gov/diabetes/pubs/statsreport14/national-diabetes-report-web.pdf

Centers for Disease Control and Prevention (CDC). (2015a). *Adolescent and school health: Whole school, whole community, whole child*. Retrieved from http://www.cdc.gov/healthyyouth/wscc/index.htm

Centers for Disease Control and Prevention (CDC). (2015b). *Asthma-related missed school days among children aged 5–17 years*. Retrieved from http://www.cdc.gov/asthma/asthma_stats/default.htm

Centers for Disease Control and Prevention (CDC). (2015c). *Childhood overweight and obesity*. Retrieved from http://www.cdc.gov/obesity/childhood/

Centers for Disease Control and Prevention (CDC) (2015d). *Effective HIV and STD prevention programs for youth: Fact sheet*. Retrieved from http://www.cdc.gov/healthyyouth/sexualbehaviors/effective_programs.htm

Centers for Disease Control and Prevention (CDC). (2015e). *HIV among incarcerated populations*. Retrieved from http://www.cdc.gov/hiv/group/correctional.html

Centers for Disease Control and Prevention (CDC). (2015f). *National public health performance standards*. Retrieved from http://www.cdc.gov/od/ocphp/nphpsp/

Centers for Disease Control and Prevention (CDC). (2015g). *Results from the school health policies and practices study 2014*. Retrieved from http://www.cdc.gov/healthyyouth/data/shpps/pdf/shpps-508-final_101315.pdf

Centers for Disease Control and Prevention (CDC). (2015h). *STDs in adolescents and young adults*. Retrieved from http://www.cdc.gov/std/stats14/adol.htm

Centers for Disease Control and Prevention (CDC). (2015i). *Teens (ages 12–19)—Risk behaviors*. Retrieved from http://www.cdc.gov/parents/teens/risk_behaviors.html

Centers for Disease Control and Prevention (CDC). (2015j). *Sexually transmitted disease surveillance 2014*. Retrieved from http://www.cdc.gov/std/stats14/default.htm

Centers for Disease Control and Prevention (CDC). (2015k). *Vaccination laws*. Retrieved from http://www.cdc.gov/phlp/publications/topic/vaccinationlaws.html

Centers for Disease Control and Prevention (CDC). (2015l). *Whole school, whole community, whole child (WSCC)*. Retrieved from http://www.cdc.gov/healthyschools/wscc/index.htm

Centers for Disease Control and Prevention (CDC). (2016). *Recognizing national immunization awareness month (NIAM)*. Retrieved from http://www.cdc.gov/vaccines/events/niam.html

Chan, E., Fogler, J. M., & Hammerness, P. G. (2016). Treatment of attention-deficit/hyperactivity disorder in adolescents: A systematic review. *Journal of American Medical Association*, *315*(18), 1997–2008.

Chin, H. B., Sipe, T. A., Elder, R., Mercer, S. L., Chattopadhyay, S. K., Verughese, J., ... Community Preventive Services Task Force. (2012). The effectiveness of group-based comprehensive risk-reduction and abstinence education interventions to prevent or reduce the risk of adolescent pregnancy, Human Immunodeficiency Virus, and sexually transmitted infections: Two systematic reviews for the guide to community preventive services. *American Journal of Preventive Medicine*, *42*(3), 272–294.

Chiu, S., DiMarco, M. A., & Prokop, J. L. (2013). Childhood obesity and dental caries in homeless children. *Journal of Pediatric Health Care*, *27*(4), 278–283.

Cianferoni, A., & Muraro, A. (2012). Food-induced anaphylaxis. *Immunology & Allergy Clinics of North America*, *32*(1), 165–195.

Climie, E. A., & Mastoras, S. M. (2015). ADHD in schools: Adopting a strengths-based perspective. *Canadian Psychology*, *56*(3), 295–300.

Cohen, A. (2013). *One of the darkest periods in the history of American prisons*. Retrieved from http://www.theatlantic.com/national/archive/2013/06/one-of-the-darkest-periods-in-the-history-of-american-prisons/276684/

Community Tool Box. (2016). *Section 7. Ten essential public health services*. Retrieved from http://ctb.ku.edu/en/table-of-contents/overview/models-for-community-health-and-development/ten-essential-public-health-services/main

Compas, B. E., Jaser, S. S., Dunn, M. J., & Rodriguez, E. M. (2012). Coping with chronic illness in childhood and adolescence. *Annual Review of Clinical Psychology*, *8*, 455–480.

Correctional Medical Services. (2011). *CMS: Correctional Medical Services*. Retrieved from http://www.cmsstl.com/home.aspx

Crump, C., Rivera, D., London, R., Landau, M., Erlendson, B., & Rodriguez, E. (2013). Chronic health conditions and school performance among children and youth. *Annals of Epidemiology*, *23*, 179–184.

Deurloo, J. A., & Verkerk, P. H. (2015). To screen or not to screen for adolescent idiopathic scoliosis? A review of the literature. *Public Health*, *129*(9), 1267–1272.

Dubler, N. (2014). *Ethical dilemmas in prison and jail health care*. Retrieved from http://healthaffairs.org/blog/2014/03/10/ethical-dilemmas-in-prison-and-jail-health-care/

DuChateau, T. A., Beversdorf, S., & Wolff, M. (2015). Best practice at your fingertips: The WISHeS school nurse procedure website. *NASN School Nurse*, *30*(3), 172–178.

Dye, B. A., Xianfen, L., Beltrán-Aguilar, E. D. (2012). *Selected oral health indicators in the United States 2005–2008* (NCHS Data Brief, no. 96). Hyattsville, MD: National Center for Health Statistics, Centers for Disease Control and Prevention.

Eisbach, S., & Driessnack, M. (2010). Am I sure I want to go down this road? Hesitations in the reporting of child maltreatment by nurses. *Journal for Specialists in Pediatric Nursing*, *15*(4), 317–323. doi: 10.1111/j.1744-6155.2010.00259.x.

Elementary Teachers Federation of Ontario. (2015). *Epi-pen fact sheet and Sabrina's Law*. Retrieved from http://www.etfo.ca/ADVICEFORMEMBERS/PRSMATTERSBULLETINS/Pages/Epipen%20Fact%20Sheet%20-%20Sabrinas%20Law.aspx

Epilepsy Foundation. (2014). *Ketogenic diet*. Retrieved from http://www.epilepsy.com/learn/treating-seizures-and-epilepsy/dietary-therapies/ketogenic-diet

Epilepsy Foundation. (n.d.). *Diastat 101*. Retrieved from http://www.epilepsy.com/get-help/seizure-first-aid/responding-seizures/diastat-101

Estelle v. Gamble. No. 75-929 (U.S. Supreme Court, 1976).

Ethier, K. A., Dittus, P. J., DeRosa, C. J., Chung, E. Q., Martinez, E., & Kerndt, P. R. (2011). School-based health center access, reproductive health care, and contraceptive use among sexually experienced high school students. *Journal of Adolescent Health*, *48*(6), 562–565.

Feldman, H. (2012). *Nursing leadership: A concise encyclopedia* (2nd ed.). New York, NY: Springer Publishing.

Finch, M., Finch, W. H., McIntosh, C. E., Thomas, C., & Maughan, E. (2015). Enhancing collaboration between school nurses and school psychologists when providing a continuum of care for children with medical needs. *Psychology in the Schools*, *52*(7), 635–649.

Flood, J. (2013). *Recommendations for responding to shortage of TB skin test antigens*. Retrieved from https://www.cdph.ca.gov/programs/tb/Documents/TBCB-Antigen-Shortage.pdf

Fong, D. Y., Cheung, K. M., Wong, Y. W., Wan, Y. Y., Lee, C. F., Lam, T. P., ... Luk, K. D. (2015). A population-based cohort study of 394,401 children followed for 10 years exhibits sustained effectiveness of scoliosis screening. *Spine Journal*, *15*(5), 825–833.

Food Allergy Research & Education. (2016). *Facts and statistics*. Retrieved from https://www.foodallergy.org/facts-and-stats

Fritsch, S. L., Overton, M. W., & Robbins, D. R. (2011). The interface of child mental health and juvenile diabetes mellitus. *Pediatric Clinics of North America*, *58*(4), 937–954.

Galemore, C. A. (2016). Too busy for TB: Managing a case of tuberculosis disease in the school setting. *NASN School Nurse*, *31*(2), 83–89.

Galemore, C. A., & Sheetz, A. H. (2015). IEP, IHP, and Section 504 primer for new school nurses. *NASN School Nurse, 30*(2), 85–88.

Glaze, L., Kaeble, D., Minton, T., Tsoutis, A., & BJS Statisticians. (2015). *Correctional populations in the United States, 2014.* Retrieved from http://www.bjs.gov/index.cfm?ty=pbdetail&iid=5519

Goodwin, R. D., Robinson, M., Sly, P. D., McKeague, I. W., Susser, E. S., Zubrick, S. R., … Mattes, E. (2013). Severity and persistence of asthma and mental health: A birth cohort study. *Psychological Medicine, 43*(6), 1313–1322.

Guerino, P., Harrison, P. M., & Sabol, W. J. (2011). *Prisoners in 2010.* Retrieved from http://bjs.ojp.usdoj.gov/index.cfm?ty=pbdetail&iid=2230

Harner, H., & Burgess, A. W. (2011). Using a trauma-informed framework to care for incarcerated women. *Journal of Obstetric, Gynecological & Neonatal Nursing, 40,* 469–476.

Hartman, A. L., Devore, C. D., & Section on Neurology, Council on School Health. (2016). Rescue medicine for epilepsy in education settings. *American Academy of Pediatrics, 137*(1), e20153876.

Hassmiller, S. (2016). *Why school nurses are the ticket to healthier communities.* Retrieved from http://www.rwjf.org/en/culture-of-health/2016/05/why_school_nursesar.html

Hauptman, M., & Phipatanakul, W. (2015). The school environment and asthma in childhood. *Asthma Research & Practice, 1,* 12.

Hawkins, J. W., & Watson, J. C. (2010). School nursing on the Iron Range in a public health nursing model. *Public Health Nursing, 27*(6), 571–578.

Hayes, M. O. (2015). The life pattern of incarcerated women: The complex and interwoven lives of trauma, mental illness, and substance abuse. *Journal of Forensic Nursing, 11*(4), 214–222. doi: 10.1097/JFN.0000000000000092.

Health & Welfare Committee. (2012). *Administrative rules review.* Retrieved from http://adminrules.idaho.gov/legislative_books/2012/temporary/12S_TEMP_H&W.pdf

Health Resources and Services Administration (HRSA). (2010). *Findings from the 2008 national sample of Registered Nurses Survey: The registered nurse population 1980–2008.* Retrieved from http://bhpr.hrsa.gov/healthworkforce/rnsurveys/rnsurveyfinal.pdf

Hendershot, C., Pakulski, L. A., Thompson, A., Dowling, J., & Price, J. H. (2011). School nurses' role in identifying and referring children at risk of noise-induced hearing loss. *Journal of School Nursing, 27*(5), 380–389.

Hershey, T., Bhargava, N., Sadler, M., White, N. H., & Craft, S. (1999). Conventional versus intensive diabetes therapy in children with type 1 diabetes: Effects on memory and motor speed. *Diabetes Care, 22*(8), 1318–1324.

Hill, N. J., & Hollis, M. (2011). Teacher time spent on student health issues and school nurse presence. *Journal of School Nursing, 27*(6). doi: 10.1177/1059840511429684.

Hindman, J. L., & Mincemoyer, J. A. (2014). *School nurses: It's not just bandages anymore!* Retrieved from https://education.wm.edu/centers/hope/publications/infobriefs/documents/SchoolNurse2014.pdf

Hoke, S. (2015). Mental illness and prisoners: Concerns for communities and healthcare providers. *Online Journal of Issues in Nursing, 20*(1), Manuscript 3.

Hung, T. T., Chiang, V. C., Dawson, A., & Lee, R. L. (2014). Understanding of factors that enable health promoters in implementing health-promoting schools: A systematic review and narrative synthesis of qualitative evidence. *PLoS ONE, 9*(9), e108284.

Hyde, J. K., & Shortell, S. M. (2012). The structure and organization of local and state public health agencies in the U.S.: A systematic review. *American Journal of Preventive Medicine, 42*(5, Suppl. 1), s29–s41.

Ihde, E. S., Boscamp, J. R., Loh, J. M., & Rosen L. (2015). Safety and efficacy of a 100% dimethicone pediculicide in school-age children. *BMC Pediatrics, 15,* 70.

Indian Health Services (IHS). (2015). *IHS year 2015 profile fact sheet.* Retrieved from https://www.ihs.gov/newsroom/factsheets/ihsyear2015profile/

Individuals with Disabilities Education Act (IDEA). (1975). *20 U.S.C. §§ 1400 et. seq., as amended and incorporating the Education of All Handicapped Children Act (EHA), 1975, P.L. 94-142, and subsequent amendments; Regulations at 34 C.F.R. §§ 300–303* [Special education and related services for students, preschool children, and infants and toddlers].

Institute of Medicine (IOM). (1988). *The future of public health.* Washington, DC: National Academies Press.

Institute of Medicine (IOM). (2015). *Genomics-enabled learning health care systems: Gathering and using genomic information to improve patient care and research.* Retrieved from http://www.nap.edu/read/21707/chapter/1

International Association of Forensic Nurses. (2015). *Correctional nursing.* Retrieved from http://www.forensicnurses.org/?page=correctionalnursing

Islam, N. S., Patel, S., Wyatt, L. C., Sim, S. C., Mukherjee-Ratham, R., Chun, K., … Kwon, S. C. (2016). Sources of health information among select Asian American immigrant groups in New York City. *Health Communication, 31*(2), 207–216.

Jacobsen, K., Meeder, L., & Voskuil, V. R. (2016). Chronic student absenteeism: The critical role of school nurses. *NASN School Nurse, 31*(3), 178–185.

Jakubowski, T. L., & Alexy, E. M. (2014). Does school scoliosis screening make the grade? *NASN School Nurse, 29*(5), 258–265.

Johnson, K. H., Dewey Bergren, M., & Westbrook, L. O. (2012). The promise of standardized data collection: School health variables identified by states. *Journal of School Nursing, 28*(2), 95–107.

Jones, M. L., & Boyd, L. D. (2011). Interface with a community feeding team to address oral health of special needs children: A pilot project. *Journal of Dental Hygiene, 85*(2), 132–140.

Kaeble, D., Glaze, L., Tsoutis, A., & Minton, T. (2016). *Correctional populations in the United States, 2014.* Retrieved from http://www.bjs.gov/content/pub/pdf/cpus14.pdf

Kahn, M., & Grasska, R. (2014). *Navigating the new landscape for medication administration at schools.* Retrieved from http://www.schoolhealthcenters.org/wp-content/uploads/2014/03/Navigating-New-Landscape-for-Medication-Administration-at-Schools.pdf

Kann, L., Kinchen, S., Shanklin, S. L., Flint, K. H., Hawkins, J., Harris, W. A., … Zaza, S. (2012). Youth Risk Behavior Surveillance—United States, 2013. *MMWR Surveillance Summaries, 63*(4), 1–170.

Kaslow, N. (2014). *Suicidal behavior in children and adolescents.* Retrieved from https://www.apa.org/about/governance/president/suicidal-behavior-adolescents.pdf

Kaste, M. (2015, July 27). *The "shock of confinement": The grim reality of suicide in jail.* Retrieved from http://www.npr.org/2015/07/27/426742309/the-shock-of-confinement-the-grim-reality-of-suicide-in-jail

Kaufman, J., Synnot, A., Ryan, R., Hill, S., Horey, D, Willis, N., … Robinson, P. (2013). Face to face interventions for informing or educating parents about early childhood vaccination. *Cochrane Consumers and Education Group.* doi: 10.1002/1465 1858.CDO100038.Pub2.

Keeton, V., Soleimanpour, S., & Brindis, C. (2012). School-based health centers in an era of health care reform: Building history. *Current Problems in Pediatric & Adolescent Health Care, 42*(6), 132–158.

Keller, L. O., Strohschein, S., & Schaffer, M. A. (2011). Cornerstones of public health nursing. *Public Health Nursing, 28*(3), 249–260.

Kennedy, M. S. (2014). Every child deserves a school nurse. *American Journal of Nursing, 114*(9), 7. doi: 10.1097/01.NAJ.0000453729.20605.92.

Kerr, J., Price, M., Kotch, J., Willis, S., Fisher, M., & Silva, S. (2011). Does contact by a family nurse practitioner decrease early school absence. *Journal of School Nursing, 28*(1), 38–46. doi: 10.1177/1059840511422818.

Khubchandani, J., Telljohann, S., Price, J., Dake, J., & Kendershot, C. (2013). Providing assistance to the victims of adolescent dating violence: A national assessment of school nurses' practices. *Journal of School Health, 83*(2), 127–136.

Kid's Mental Health Portal. (2016). *Children's behavioral and emotional disorders.* Retrieved from http://www.kidsmentalhealth.org/childrens-behavioral-and-emotional-disorders/#ChildrensBehavioralandEmotionalDisorders

King, K. K. (2014). Violence in the school setting: A school nurse perspective. *Online Journal of Issues in Nursing, 18*(4), 1.

King E. & Foley, J. E. (2014). *Gender-responsive policy development in corrections: What we know and roadmaps for change.* Washington, DC: U.S. Department of Justice National Institute of Corrections.

Knickman, J. R., & Kovner, A. R. (Eds.). (2015). *Jonas & Kovner's health care delivery in the United States* (11th ed.). New York, NY: Springer Publishing Company.

Knox, C. (2013). *Do you wonder how many correctional nurses are out there?* Retrieved from http://bhpr.hrsa.gov/healthworkforce/reports/rnsurvey/rnss1.htm

Krause-Parello, C. A., & Samms, K. (2011). School nursing in a contemporary society: What are the roles and responsibilities? *Issues in Comprehensive Pediatric Nursing, 34*, 26–39.

Kroelinger, C. D., Kasenhagen, L., Barradas, D. T., & Ali, Z. (2012). Building leadership skills and promoting workforce development: Evaluation data collected from public health professionals in the field of maternal and child health. *Maternal Child Health Journal, 16*(2), 370–375.

Kulbok, P. A., Thatcher, E., Park, E., & Meszaros, P. S. (2012). Evolving public health nursing roles: Focus on community participatory health promotion and prevention. *OJIN: The Online Journal of Issues in Nursing, 17*(2), Manuscript 1. doi: 10.3912/OJIN.Vol17No02Man01.

Kutscher, B. (2013). *Rumble over jailhouse healthcare: As states broaden outsourcing to private vendors, critics question quality of care and cost savings.* Retrieved from http://www.modernhealthcare.com/article/20130831/MAGAZINE/308319891

Larsen, A. K., Holtermann, A., Mortensen, O. S., Punnett, L., Rod, M. H., & Jørgensen, M. B. (2015). Organizing workplace health literacy to reduce musculoskeletal plain and consequences. *BMC Nursing, 14*, 46. Retrieved from http://bmcnurs.biomedcentral.com/articles/10.1186/s12912-015-0096-4

Larson, S. A., & Chapman, S. A. (2013). Patient-centered medical home model: Do school-based health centers fit the model? *Policy & Politics in Nursing Practice, 14*(3–4), 163–174.

Lineberry, M. J., & Ickes, M. J. (2015). The role and impact of nurses in American elementary schools: A systematic review of the research. *Journal of School Nursing, 31*(1), 22–33.

Lushniak, B. (2014). *Update on the U.S. Public Health Service response to the Ebola outbreak: Surgeon General's perspectives.* Retrieved from http://www.surgeongeneral.gov/library/publichealthreports/#PAGE_4

Macmadu, A., & Rich, J. D. (2015). Correctional health is community health. *Issues in Science and Technology, 3*(1), 64–70.

Madamala, K., Sellers, K., Beitsch, L. M., Pearsol, J., & Jarris, P. E. (2011). Structure and functions of state public health agencies. *American Journal of Public Health, 101*(7), 1179–1186.

Mäenpää, T., Paavilainen, E., & Åstedt-Kuri, P. (2012). Family-school nurse partnership in primary school health care. *Scandinavian Journal of Caring Sciences, 27*(1), 195–202.

Magnusson, M. B., Kjellgren, K. I., & Winkvist, A. (2012). Enabling overweight children to improve their food and exercise habits—School nurses' counseling in multilingual settings. *Journal of Clinical Nursing, 21*, 2452–2460.

Maruschak, L. M., Berzofsky, M., & Unangst, J. (2015). *Medical problems of state and federal prisoners and jail inmates, 2011–2012.* Retrieved from http://www.bjs.gov/content/pub/pdf/mpsfpji1112.pdf

Maternal and Child Health Bureau. (2013). *Child health 2012: Vaccine preventable diseases.* Retrieved from http://mchb.hrsa.gov/chusa12/hs/hsc/pages/vpd.html

Mattey, B., Zein, W. M., O'Malley, D., & Haron, C. (2013). Preventing vision loss among students through eye safety and early detection. *NASN School Nurse, 28*(5), 233–236.

Maughan, E., & Adams, R. (2011). Educators' and parents' perception of what school nurses do: The influence of school nurse/student ratios. *Journal of School Nursing, 27*, 355–363.

McCulloch, J., & Prieto, J. (2008). Health protection and the role of the public health nurse. In L. Coles, & E. Porter (Eds.), *Public health skills: A practical guide for nurses and public health practitioners* (pp. 155–169). Malden, MA: Blackwell Publishing.

McNeeley, C., & Blanchard, J. (n.d.). *The teen years explained: A guide to healthy adolescent development.* Retrieved from http://www.jhsph.edu/research/centers-and-institutes/center-for-adolescent-health/_includes/_pre-redesign/Interactive%20Guide.pdf

Minority Nurse. (2016). *Correctional facility nursing.* Retrieved from http://www.mentalhealthamerica.net/positions/correctional-facility-treatment

Mumola, C. J., & Karberg, J. C. (2007). *Drug use and dependence, state and federal prisoners, 2004.* (NCJ 213530, page updated 2010). Retrieved from http://bjs.ojp.usdoj.gov/index.cfm?ty=pbdetail&iid=778

National Association of County and City Health Officers (NACCHO). (2014). *2013 national profile of local health departments study.* Retrieved from http://nacchoprofilestudy.org/wp-content/uploads/2014/02/2013_National_Profile021014.pdf

National Association of School Nurses (NASN). (2012a). *Allergy/anaphylaxis management in the school setting.* Retrieved from https://www.nasn.org/PolicyAdvocacy/PositionPapersandReports/NASNPositionStatementsFullView/tabid/462/ArticleId/9/Allergy-Anaphylaxis-Management-in-the-School-Setting-Revised-June-2012

National Association of School Nurses (NASN). (2012b). *Diabetes management in the school setting.* Retrieved from https://www.nasn.org/PolicyAdvocacy/PositionPapersandReports/NASNPositionStatementsFullView/tabid/462/smid/824/ArticleID/22/Default.aspx

National Association of School Nurses (NASN). (2012c). *Medication administration in the school setting.* Retrieved from https://www.nasn.org/PolicyAdvocacy/PositionPapersandReports/NASNPositionStatementsFullView/tabid/462/ArticleId/86/Medication-Administration-in-the-School-Setting-Amended-January-2012

National Association of School Nurses (NASN). (2013). *Mental health of students.* Retrieved from https://www.nasn.org/PolicyAdvocacy/PositionPapersandReports/NASNPositionStatementsFullView/tabid/462/ArticleId/36/Mental-Health-of-Students-Revised-June-2013

National Association of School Nurses (NASN). (2014a). *About us.* Retrieved from http://www.nasn.org/Default.aspx?tabid=57

National Association of School Nurses (NASN). (2014b). *Care of victims of child maltreatment: The school nurse's role.* Retrieved from http://www.nasn.org/PolicyAdvocacy/PositionPapersandReports/NASNPositionStatementsFullView/tabid/462/smid/824/ArticleID/639/Default.aspx

National Association of School Nurses (NASN). (2014c). *Do not attempt resuscitation (DNAR)—The role of the school nurse.* Retrieved from https://www.nasn.org/PolicyAdvocacy/PositionPapersandReports/NASNPositionStatementsFullView/tabid/462/smid/824/ArticleID/640/Default.aspx

National Association of School Nurses (NASN). (2014d). *Emergency preparedness and response in the school setting: The role of the school nurse.* Retrieved from https://www.nasn.org/PolicyAdvocacy/PositionPapersandReports/NASNPositionStatementsFullView/tabid/462/ArticleId/117/Emergency-Preparedness-and-Response-in-the-School-Setting-The-Role-of-the-School-Nurse-Revised-June

National Association of School Nurses (NASN). (2014e). *Frequently asked questions.* Retrieved from https://www.nasn.org/AboutNASN/FrequentlyAskedQuestions

National Association of School Nurses (NASN). (2014f). *Planning a career in school nursing?* Retrieved from https://www.nasn.org/RoleCareer/PlanningaCareerinSchoolNursing

National Association of School Nurses (NASN). (2015). Position statement: Transition planning for students with chronic health conditions. *NASN School Nurse, 30*(2), 125–127.

National Association of School Nurses (NASN). (2016) *Role of the school nurse position paper.* Retrieved from http://www.nasn.org/PolicyAdvocacy/PositionPapersandReports/NASNPositionStatementsFullView/tabid/462/ArticleId/87/Role-of-the-School-Nurse-Revised-2011

National Center for Education Statistics. (2015). *Fast facts: Back to school statistics.* Retrieved from http://nces.ed.gov/fastfacts/display.asp?id=372

National Center for Education Statistics. (2016). *Students with disabilities, inclusion of.* Retrieved from https://nces.ed.gov/fastfacts/display.asp?id=59

National Center for Learning Disabilities. (2014). *The state of learning disabilities: Facts, trends and emerging issues.* Retrieved from https://www.ncld.org/wp-content/uploads/2014/11/2014-State-of-LD.pdf

National Children's Alliance. (2014). *National statistics on child abuse.* Retrieved from http://www.nationalchildrensalliance.org/media-room/media-kit/national-statistics-child-abuse

National Commission on Correctional Health Care. (2015). *Certified correctional health care professional.* Retrieved from http://www.ncchc.org/cchp

National Commission on Correctional Health Care. (2016). *Screening, sick call, and triage.* Retrieved from http://www.ncchc.org/cnp-screening-sickcall-triage

National Diabetes Education Program. (2011). *Overview of diabetes in children and adolescents.* Retrieved from http://ndep.nih.gov//media/youth_factsheet.pdf

National Eating Disorders Association. (2015). *Get the facts on eating disorders.* Retrieved from https://www.nationaleatingdisorders.org/get-facts-eating-disorders

National Institute for Health and Care Excellence. (2015). *Diabetes (Type 1 and Type 2) in children and young people: Diagnosis and management.* London, England: Author. Retrieved from http://www.ncbi.nlm.nih.gov/books/NBK315806/

National Institute of Diabetes and Digestive and Kidney Diseases. (2012). *Helping the student with diabetes succeed: A guide for school personnel.* Retrieved from http://www.niddk.nih.gov/health-information/health-communication-programs/ndep/health-care-professionals/school-guide/Pages/publicationdetail.aspx

National Institute of Mental Health (NIMH). (n.d.a). *Child and adolescent mental health.* Retrieved from http://www.nimh.nih.gov/health/topics/child-and-adolescent-mental-health/index.shtml

National Institute of Mental Health (NIMH). (n.d.b). *Inmate mental health.* Retrieved from http://www.nimh.nih.gov/health/statistics/prevalence/inmate-mental-health.shtml

National Institute of Neurological Disorders and Stroke. (2015). *Curing the epilepsies: The promise of research.* Retrieved from http://www.ninds.nih.gov/disorders/epilepsy/epilepsy_research.htm#Section1_2

National Institutes of Health (NIH). (2016). *Nurse positions open at NIH.* Retrieved from https://jobs.nih.gov/nurses/

National Program for Playground Safety. (2016). *Injuries.* Retrieved from http://playgroundsafety.org/about

National Quality Measures Clearinghouse. (2013). *Missed school days: Number of school days missed in the past 12 months due to illness or injury.* Retrieved from https://www.qualitymeasures.ahrq.gov/content.aspx?id=47477#Section566

Noonan, M., Rohloff, H., & Ginder, S. (2015). *Mortality in local jails and state prisons, 2000–2013—Statistical tables.* Retrieved from http://www.bjs.gov/content/pub/pdf/mljsp0013st.pdf

Noyes, K., Bajorska, A., Fisher, S., Sauer, J., Fagnano, M., & Halterman, J. S. (2013). Cost-effectiveness of the School-Based Asthma Therapy (SBAT) program. *Pediatrics, 131*(3), e709–3717.

O'Grady, J., Maeurer, M., Atun, R., Abubakar, I., Mwaba, P., Bates, M., ... Zumia, A. (2011). Tuberculosis in prisons: Anatomy of global neglect. *European Respiratory Journal, 38*(4), 752–754.

Patestos, C., Patterson, K., & Fitzsimons, V. (2014). Substance abuse prevention: The role of the school nurse across the continuum of care. *NASN School Nurse, 29*(6), 310–314.

Pbert, L., Druker, S., DiFranza, J. R., Gorak, D., Reed, G., Magner, R., ... Osganian, S. (2011). Effectiveness of a school nurse-delivered smoking-cessation intervention for adolescents. *Pediatrics, 128*(5), 926–936. doi: 10.1542/peds.2011-0520.

Penfold, J. (2013). Students access school nurses through smartphone apps. *Primary Health Care, 23*(7), 8–9.

Polivka, B. J., Chaudry, R. V., Crawford, J., Bouton, P., & Sweet, L. (2011). Impact of an urban healthy homes intervention. *Journal of Environmental Health, 73*(9), 16–20.

Pont, J., Stöver, H., & Wolff, H. (2012). Dual loyalty in prison health care. *American Journal of Public Health, 102*(3), 475–480.

Pontius, D. J. (2014). Demystifying pediculosis: School nurses taking the lead. *Pediatric Nursing, 40*(5), 226–235.

Potter, R. H., Schwartz, R., Blackmore, J., & May, R. (2011). The impact of the H1N1 pandemic on US prisons: Results of a national survey. *Corrections Today, 73*(4), 73–74.

Powell, J., Harris, F., Condon, L., & Kemple, T. (2010). Nursing care of prisoners: Staff views and experiences. *Journal of Advanced Nursing, 66*(6), 1257–1265.

Pryjmachuk, S., Graham, T., Haddad, M., & Tylee, A. (2011). School nurses' perspectives on managing mental health problems in children and young people. *Journal of Clinical Nursing, 21,* 850–859.

Rademacher, P. A. (2012). *The nurse in the school health office: Exploring health care in a public school.* (Doctoral dissertation, University of Nebraska) Retrieved from http://digitalcommons.unl.edu/cgi/viewcontent.cgi?article=1140&context=cehsdiss

RAND Corporation. (2011). *Understanding the public health implications of prisoner reentry in California: State-of-the-state report.* Retrieved from http://www.rand.org/content/dam/rand/pubs/monographs/2011/RAND_MG1165.pdf

Rehabilitation Act of 1973, Section 504. (1973). *29 U.S.C. §794 et seq., Regulations at 34 C.F.R. §104.* Retrieved from https://www.disability.gov/rehabilitation-act-1973/

Reznick, O., Comfort, M., McCartney, K., & Neilands, T. (2011). Effectiveness of an HIV prevention program for women visiting their incarcerated partners: The HOME project. *AIDS Behavior, 15,* 365–375.

Richmond, S. L. (2011). Medication error prevention in the school setting: A closer look. *NASN School Nurse, 26*(5), 304–308.

Riley, M., Ahmed, S., & Locke, A. (2016). Common questions about oppositional defiant disorder. *American Family Physician, 93*(7), 586–591.

Robbins, L. B., Pfeiffer, K. A., Maier, K. S., Lo, Y. J., & Wesolek, S. M. (2012). Pilot intervention to increase physical activity among sedentary urban middle school girls: A two-group pretest-posttest quasi-experimental design. *Journal of School Nursing, 28*(4), 302–315.

Rollins, J. A. (2011). Every child deserves a school nurse. *Pediatric Nursing, 37*(5), 225–226.

Rosen, B. L., Ashwood, D., & Richardson, G. B. (2016). School nurses' professional practice in the HPV vaccine decision-making process. *Journal of School Nursing, 32*(2), 138–148.

Rossman, C. L., Dood, F. V., & Squires, D. A. (2012). Student nurses as school nurse extenders. *Journal of Pediatric Nursing, 27,* 734–741.

Schoenly, L. (2015). *The Wizard of Oz guide to correctional nursing: This isn't Kansas anymore, Toto!* Genesee, PA: Enchanted Mountain Press.

School-Based Health Alliance. (2014). *National census of school-based health centers.* Retrieved from http://www.sbh4all.org/school-health-care/national-census-of-school-based-health-centers/

School-Based Health Alliance. (n.d.). *Adolescents do not use the health care system enough.* Retrieved from http://www.sbh4all.org/school-health-care/health-and-learning/access-to-health-care/#one

Selekman, J. (2013). *School nursing: A comprehensive text* (2nd ed.). Philadelphia, PA: F. A. Davis Co.

Shi, L., & Johnson, J. A. (2014). *Novick & Morrow's public health administration principles for population-based management* (3rd ed.). Burlington, MA: Jones & Bartlett Learning.

Shiroma, E., Ferguson, P., & Pickelsimer, E. (2012). Prevalence of traumatic brain injury in an offender population: A meta-analysis. *Journal of Head Trauma & Rehabilitation, 27*(3), e1–e10.

Shoenly, L., & Knox, C. M. (Eds.). (2013). *Essentials of correctional nursing.* New York, NY: Springer Publishing Company.

Smith, W., Brach, C., & Horowitz, A. M. (2015). Poor oral health literacy: Why nobody understands you. *Access, 29,* 33–35.

Sondick, E., Madans, J. H., & Gentleman, J. F. (2011). *Summary health statistics for U.S. children: National health interview survey, 2010.* Retrieved from http://www.cdc.gov/nchs/data/series/sr_10/sr10_250.pdf

Sonnenberg, M. (2013). School nurses' duties expand with changing times. *USA Today.* Retrieved from http://www.usatoday.com/story/news/nation/2013/10/24/school-nurses-duties-expand-with-changing-times/3176657/

Sprague-McRae, J. M., & Rosenblum, R. K. (2013). Chronic neurological conditions in the classroom: A school nurse curriculum for sustaining a healthy learner. *Pediatric Nursing, 39*(6), 276–282.

Steele, R. G., Wu, Y. P., Jensen, C. D., Pankey, S., Davis, A. M., & Aylward, B. S. (2011). School nurses' perceived barriers to discussing weight with children and their families: A qualitative approach. *Journal of School Health, 81*(3), 128–137.

Struthers, L. (1917). *The school nurse: A survey of the duties and responsibilities of the nurse in the maintenance of health, physical perfection and the prevention of disease among school children.* New York, NY: G. P. Putnam's Sons.

Substance Abuse Mental Health Services Agency. (2015). *Treatments for mental disorders.* Retrieved from http://www.samhsa.gov/treatment/mental-disorders

Swan, M. A., Barker, J. C., & Hoeft, K. S. (2010). Rural Latino farmworker fathers' understanding of children's oral health. *Pediatric Dentistry, 32*(5), 400–406.

Swanson, A. (2015). *A shocking number of mentally ill Americans end up in prison instead of treatment.* Retrieved from https://www.washingtonpost.com/news/wonk/wp/2015/04/30/a-shocking-number-of-mentally-ill-americans-end-up-in-prisons-instead-of-psychiatric-hospitals/

Swider, S., Krothe, J., Reyes, D., & Cravetz, M. (2013). The Quad Council practice competencies for public health nursing. *Public Health Nursing, 30*(6), 519–536.

Swider, S. M., Levin, P. F., & Kulbok, P. (2014). *Quad Council of Public Health Nursing Organizations invitational forum on the role and future of nurses in public health: Final report.* Retrieved from http://www.achne.org/files/Quad%20Council/PHNInvitationalConferenceReportFINAL03102014.pdf

Taylor, R., & Crianza, S. G. (2011). Lessons learned: How Harris County jail prepares for disasters. *Corrections Today, 73*(4), 44–46.

Texas Department of Health Services. (2016). *Frequently asked questions: Implementation of laws on screening for type 2 diabetes (acanthosis nigricans screening bill)*. Retrieved from http://www.dshs.texas.gov/schoolhealth/organscreen.shtm?terms=acanthosis%20nigricans%20screening

Tiyyagura, G. K., Arnold, L., Cone, D. C., & Langhan, M. (2014). Pediatric anaphylaxis management in the prehospital setting. *Prehospital Emergency Care, 18*(1), 46–51.

Toole, K. P. (2013). Helping children gain asthma control: Bundled school-based interventions. *Pediatric Nursing, 39*(3), 115–124.

Treloar, C., McCreedie, L., & Lloyd, A. R. (2015). Acquiring hepatitis C in prison: The social organisation of injecting risk. *Harm Reduction Journal, 12*, 10. Retrieved from https://harmreduction-journal.biomedcentral.com/articles/10.1186/s12954-015-0045-2

Turnock, B. J. (2016). *Essentials of public health: What it is and how it works* (6th ed.). Burlington, MA: Jones & Bartlett Learning.

U.S. Department of Health and Human Services (USDHHS). (2014a). *U.S. Commissioned Corps of the U.S. Public Health Service: America's health responders*. Retrieved from http://www.usphs.gov/aboutus/

U.S. Department of Health and Human Services (USDHHS). (2014b). *U.S. Commissioned Corps of the U.S. Public Health Service: Applying to the Commissioned Corps*. Retrieved from http://www.usphs.gov/apply/apply.aspx

U.S. Department of Health and Human Services (USDHHS). (2014c). *U.S. Commissioned Corps of the U.S. Public Health Service: Nurse salary & benefits*. Retrieved from http://www.usphs.gov/profession/nurse/compensation.aspx

U.S. Department of Health and Human Services (USDHHS). (2014d). *Why a career at HHS?* Retrieved from http://www.hhs.gov/about/careers/

U.S. Department of Health and Human Services (USDHHS). (2015). *About Health and human services*. Retrieved from http://www.hhs.gov/about/agencies/hhs-agencies-and-offices/index.html

U.S. Department of Health and Human Services (USDHHS). (2016). *Healthy people 2020*. Retrieved from http://healthypeople.gov/2020/default.aspx

U.S. Department of Housing and Urban Development. (2015a). *Healthy homes demonstration grant program*. Retrieved from http://portal.hud.gov/hudportal/HUD?src=/program_offices/healthy_homes/hhi/hhd

U.S. Department of Housing and Urban Development. (2015b). *Healthy homes program. Abstracts by region*. Retrieved from http://portal.hud.gov/hudportal/HUD?src=/program_offices/healthy_homes/hhi/hhabstracts

U.S. Surgeon General. (2016). *Office of the US surgeon general*. Retrieved from http://www.surgeongeneral.gov/about/index.html

United Nations. (2013). *World population ageing 2013*. Retrieved from http://www.un.org/en/development/desa/population/publications/pdf/ageing/WorldPopulationAgeing2013.pdf

University of Michigan Center of Excellence in Public Health Workforce Studies. (2013). *Public health workforce enumeration, 2012*. Ann Arbor, MI: University of Michigan.

Van Ouytsel, J., Walrave, M., & Vandebosch, J. (2015). Correlates of cyberbullying and how school nurses can respond. *NASN School Nurse, 30*(3), 162–190.

Vessey, J., & McGowan, K. (2006). A successful public health experiment: School nursing. *Pediatric Nursing, 32*(3), 255–257.

Walker, J. R. (2014). Wellness promotion: School nurses as models of health. *NASN School Nurse, 29*(3), 18–129.

Walsh, D., & Lambert, D. (2013). *California Supreme Court OKs insulin shots by school staff*. Retrieved from http://www.sacbee.com/news/local/health-and-medicine/article2578449.html

Walter, S. R., Olivier, J., Churches, T., & Grzebieta, R. (2011). The impact of compulsory cycle helmet legislation on cyclist head injuries in new South Wales, Australia. *Accident Analysis & Prevention, 43*(6), 2064–2071. doi: 10.1016/j.aap.2011.05.029.

White, G. D. (2012). Gender-responsive programs in US prisons: Implications for change. *Social Work in Public Health, 27*(3), 283–300.

White, M. C., Nelson, R. W., Kawamura, L. M., Grinsdale, J., & Goldenson, J. (2012). Changes in characteristics of inmates with latent tuberculosis infection. *Public Health, 126*(9), 752–759.

White House. (2014). *Fact sheet: U.S. response to the Ebola epidemic in West Africa*. Retrieved from https://www.whitehouse.gov/the-press-office/2014/09/16/fact-sheet-us-response-ebola-epidemic-west-africa

Williams, B., Pickard, L., Grandjean, L., Pope, S., Anderson, S. R., Morgan, G., & Williams, A. (2016). The need to implement effective new entrant tuberculosis screening in children: Evidence from school 'outbreak'. *Journal of Public Health*. doi: 10.1093/pubmed/fdv186.

Winsch, B. J. (2011). *Taking the pulse of student health needs in America: The role of school nurses in improving student health and academics*. Retrieved from http://www.jefferson.k12.ky.us/Departments/Planning/ProgramEvaluation/WebMASTER_Updates_July2011/StudentHealthNeedsinAmerica62911_BW.pdf

Woodfill, M. M., & Beyrer, M. K. (1991). *The role of the nurse in the school setting: A historical perspective*. Kent, OH: American School Health Association.

Zadikoff, E. H., Whyte, S. A., DeSantiago-Cardenas, L., Harvey-Gintoft, B., & Gupta, R. S. (2014). The development and implementation of the Chicago Public Schools emergency EpiPen policy. *Journal of School Health, 84*(5), 342–347.

Zampino, R., Coppola, N., Sagnelli, C., DiCaprio, G., & Sagnelli, E. (2015). Hepatitis C virus infection and prisoners: epidemiology, outcome and treatment. *World Journal of Hepatology, 7*(21), 2323–2330.

Zirkel, P. A., Granthom, M. F., & Lovato, L. (2012). Section 504 and student health problems: The pivotal position of the school nurse. *Journal of School Nursing, 28*(6), 423–432.

thePoint: Everything You Need to Make the Grade!

thePoint® Visit http://thePoint.lww.com/Rector9e
for selected readings, study aids for all learning styles, and more!

Private Settings for Community Health Nursing

"To insure good health: eat lightly, breathe deeply, live moderately, cultivate cheerfulness, and maintain an interest in life."

—*William Londen*

KEY TERMS

Community collaboration
Comprehensive Primary Care Center
Education Resource Center (ERC)
Entrepreneurial nurse

Faith community nurse (FCN)
Federally Qualified Health Center (FQHC)
Nurse-led health centers/clinics (NLHCs)

Occupational and environmental health nurses
Occupational Safety and Health Administration (OSHA)

Request for proposal (RFP)
Safety-net health care provider
Sustainability
wellness centers

LEARNING OBJECTIVES

Upon mastery of this chapter, you should be able to:

- Describe the historical roots of nurse-led health centers.
- Identify the distinctiveness of various nurse-led health center models.
- Describe interventions that support *Healthy People 2020* goals.
- Describe funding sources for nurse-led health centers.
- Articulate the importance of sustainability for nurse-led health centers.
- Describe the evolution of faith community nursing.
- Describe and differentiate among the roles of the faith community nurse.
- Identify the steps for establishing a practice as a faith community nurse.
- Explain the role of the occupational and environmental health nurse and other members of the occupational health team in protecting and promoting workers' health and safety.
- Identify educational preparation for occupational and environmental health nurses.
- Recognize at least three adverse working conditions that impact health status.
- Discuss the opportunities for nurse entrepreneurship in community/public health practice.

Healthy People 2020: Improving the Health of Americans (U.S. Department of Health and Human Services [USDHHS], Centers for Medicare and Medicaid Services [CMS], 2016a) provides goals and clear objectives for promoting health and preventing disease for the next decade. The next 10 years will see unprecedented changes and challenges in the nation's health. As we ponder what those changes will be, the Healthy People initiative will continue to encourage collaborations across communities and sectors, empower individuals toward making informed health decisions, and measure the impact of prevention activities. Building on the Healthy People goals for the nation's health, there will be ever-increasing opportunities for community/public health nurses to make a difference in their communities. This chapter examines four distinct areas of practice in the community as potential options for your own professional road ahead. Each of these roles contributes in very tangible ways to improving the health of individuals, families, and the communities in which they live. National health care reform and global influences on community/public health nursing are included.

Chapter 30 discussed a wide variety of practice opportunities in the public sector. This chapter examines four unique private sector roles and practice environments available in the United States and in many other countries: nurse-led health centers (NLHCs), faith community nursing, occupational and environmental health nursing, and nurse entrepreneurship. Nurse-led (or nurse-managed) health centers offer the opportunity for more autonomous practice and present excellent learning venues for nursing students. Many such centers are connected to academic nursing programs. Faith community nursing, begun in the mid-1980s, has gained increasing attention in many religious communities. Although volunteers often hold faith-based positions, there are increasing opportunities for paid employment. Occupational and environmental health is a specialty health practice that focuses on the health and well-being of the working population, including both paid and unpaid positions, and therefore covers most of the country's working adults. This role provides the vital link between nursing and sound business practices. The nurse entrepreneur role offers new venues for meeting the health care needs in communities while providing challenging and autonomous practice. Each of these areas of practice offers community health nurses an avenue to address health disparities in their communities, increase years of healthy life, and provide holistic, client-centered care to meet the current and emerging health needs in their communities, as indicated in *Healthy People 2020*.

NURSE-LED HEALTH CENTERS

Nurse-led health centers/clinics (NLHCs), or nursing centers (sometimes referred to as nurse-managed health centers), are organizations that give vulnerable and/or underserved clients access to professional nursing services. Located in or near health professional shortage areas (HPSA) and medically underserved areas (MUA) in both urban and rural communities, NLHCs are found in convenient sites where people live, work, learn, and worship. A nurse executive with an advanced degree provides oversight. Traditionally, targets of service have been those who are least likely to be engaged in ongoing health care services for themselves and their family members. Currently, NLHCs serve population groups of all ages that are both uninsured and underinsured.

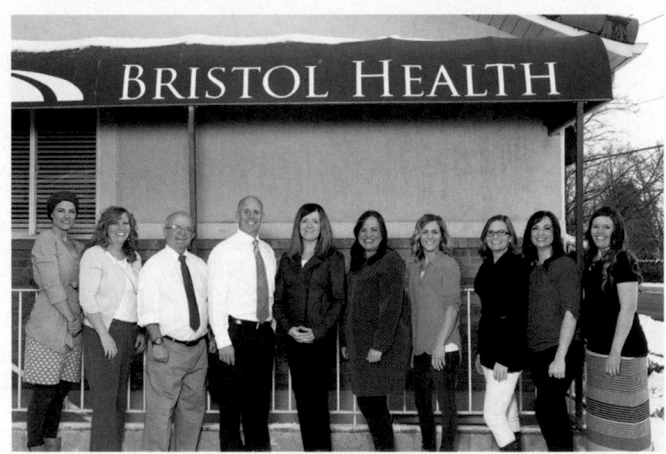

Historically, the most frequently cited definition of *nursing centers* is the one developed in the mid-1980s by the American Nurses Association Nursing Centers Task Force. Display 31–1 presents a modified version of this definition. However, with an amendment to Title III of the Public Health Service Act (42 U.S.C. 241 et seq.), the Nurse-Managed Health Clinic Investment Act of 2009 of the 111th Congress provides a more present-day definition of NMHCs. Display 31–2 presents this definition.

Although all NLHCs share the core elements of these definitions, they vary in their practice models. Services offered at NLHCs range from health promotion and wellness to conventional primary care (Hansen-Turton, 2012; Hansen-Turton, Miller, & Greiner, 2009). In this chapter, the terms NLHC, nurse-led health clinic, and nursing center are used interchangeably to describe this model of contemporary health care.

NLHCs represent a rising movement of health centers that have emerged as vital safety-net health care providers in America's health care delivery system (Hansen-Turton, Sherman, & King, 2015; Pohl, Tanner, Pilon, & Benkert, 2011). A **safety-net health care provider** is defined as a provider that by mandate or mission organizes and delivers a significant level of health care and other health-related services to the uninsured, Medicaid, and other vulnerable populations (Health Resources and Services Administration, 2013; Institute of Medicine [IOM], 2000).

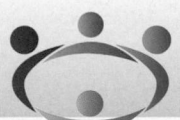

DISPLAY 31–1 DEFINITION OF NURSING CENTER

Nursing centers—sometimes referred to as community nursing organizations, nurse-managed centers, nursing clinics, and community nurse–managed health centers—are organizations that give clients and communities direct access to professional nursing services. Professional nurses in these centers diagnose and treat human responses to actual and potential health problems and promote health and optimal functioning among target populations and communities. The services provided in these centers are holistic, client centered, and affordable. Overall accountability and responsibility remain with the nurse executive/director. Nurse-managed health centers are not limited to any particular organizational configuration. Nurse-managed health centers can be freestanding businesses or may be affiliated with universities or other service institutions like home health agencies and hospitals. The primary characteristic of the organization is responsiveness to the health needs of populations. The nurse is responsible for all patient care and operations (Hansen-Turton, Sherman, & King, 2015).

Hansen-Turton, T., Sherman, S., & King, E. (2015). *Nurse-led health clinics: Operations, policy and opportunities.* New York, NY: Springer.

NLHCs differ from other public health agencies and tertiary medical care facilities. Although some services overlap, the distinctiveness of NLHCs is found in the community orientation of the nurse-managed centers. This model is depicted by *Lundeen's Comprehensive Community-Based Primary Healthcare Model* (Lundeen, 2005) where NLHCs are referred to as community nursing centers and are the central figure in this model of health care utilized at the University of Milwaukee, Wisconsin (see Fig. 31–1).

DISPLAY 31–2 DEFINITION OF NURSE-MANAGED HEALTH CLINIC

The term "nurse-managed health clinic" or "NMHC" means a nurse practice arrangement, managed by advanced practice nurses, that provides primary care or wellness services to underserved or vulnerable populations and is associated with a school, college, university, or department of nursing; federally qualified health center; or an independent nonprofit health or social services agency (Nurse-Managed Health Clinic Investment Act, 2009).

Nurse-Managed Health Clinic Investment Act of 2009, S.B. 1104/H.R. 2754, 111th Congress (2009).

Healthy People 2020

The groundbreaking publication of *Healthy People: The Surgeon General's Report on Health Promotion and Disease Prevention* (U.S. Department of Health, Education and Welfare, 1979) focused attention on the nation's health promotion and disease prevention activities. Three decades later, *Healthy People 2020* goals and objectives expand upon this health promotion and disease prevention initiative. The four main goals of *Healthy People 2020* are to attain high-quality, longer lives free of preventable disease, disability, injury, and premature death; achieve health equity, eliminate disparities, and improve the health of all groups; create social and physical environments that promote good health for all; and promote quality of life, healthy development, and healthy behaviors across all life stages (USDHHS, Office of Disease Prevention and Health Promotion, 2016a). Achieving *Healthy People 2020* goals requires a long-term commitment to **community collaboration** and partnerships among many diverse people and groups (Kinsey & Miller, 2016). NMHCs are an excellent venue to address identified Key Health Indicators to meet the goals of *Healthy People 2020*. Display 31–3 contains exemplars of *Healthy People 2020* Key Health Indicators that are applicable to NMHCs.

History of the Nurse-Led Model

Although today's NLHCs trace their roots to changes in national health care laws begun in the mid-1960s, the nursing model of holistic care that focuses on vulnerable populations and integrates primary care and public health dates back to the 19th century. Florence Nightingale's passion for at-risk populations, as well as her success related to health reform, provides a model for NLHCs today. Visionaries such as Lillian Wald, who founded the Henry Street Settlement, and Margaret Sanger, who initiated the first family planning clinic, are two examples of nurses providing holistic care to vulnerable populations (see Chapter 2). These nurse activists sought to resolve 20th century problems caused by immigration, urbanization, and industrialization in the United States (Judd & Sitzman, 2014; Wilson, Whitaker, & Whitford, 2012).

Since the late 1970s, in conjunction with the development of educational programs for nurse practitioners, faculties in schools of nursing have established NLHCs. Linkages have provided clinical sites for educating nurses at all levels and settings, as well as for faculty practice opportunities (Resick, Miller, & Leonardo, 2015). For example, one urban academic nursing center at Duquesne University School of Nursing in Pittsburgh, Pennsylvania, involves students and faculty in primary and secondary prevention services to the community. "Brown bag" medication review days, chair exercises, health fairs, safety assessments, nutrition education, computer classes, and health screenings are examples of services and special programs that undergraduate and graduate students have been engaged in for almost two decades. Currently, there are many nursing clinic sites across the city of Pittsburgh that work with older adults and vulnerable populations, providing both nursing and health science students with opportunities for community-based experiences (Duquesne University School of Nursing, 2015;

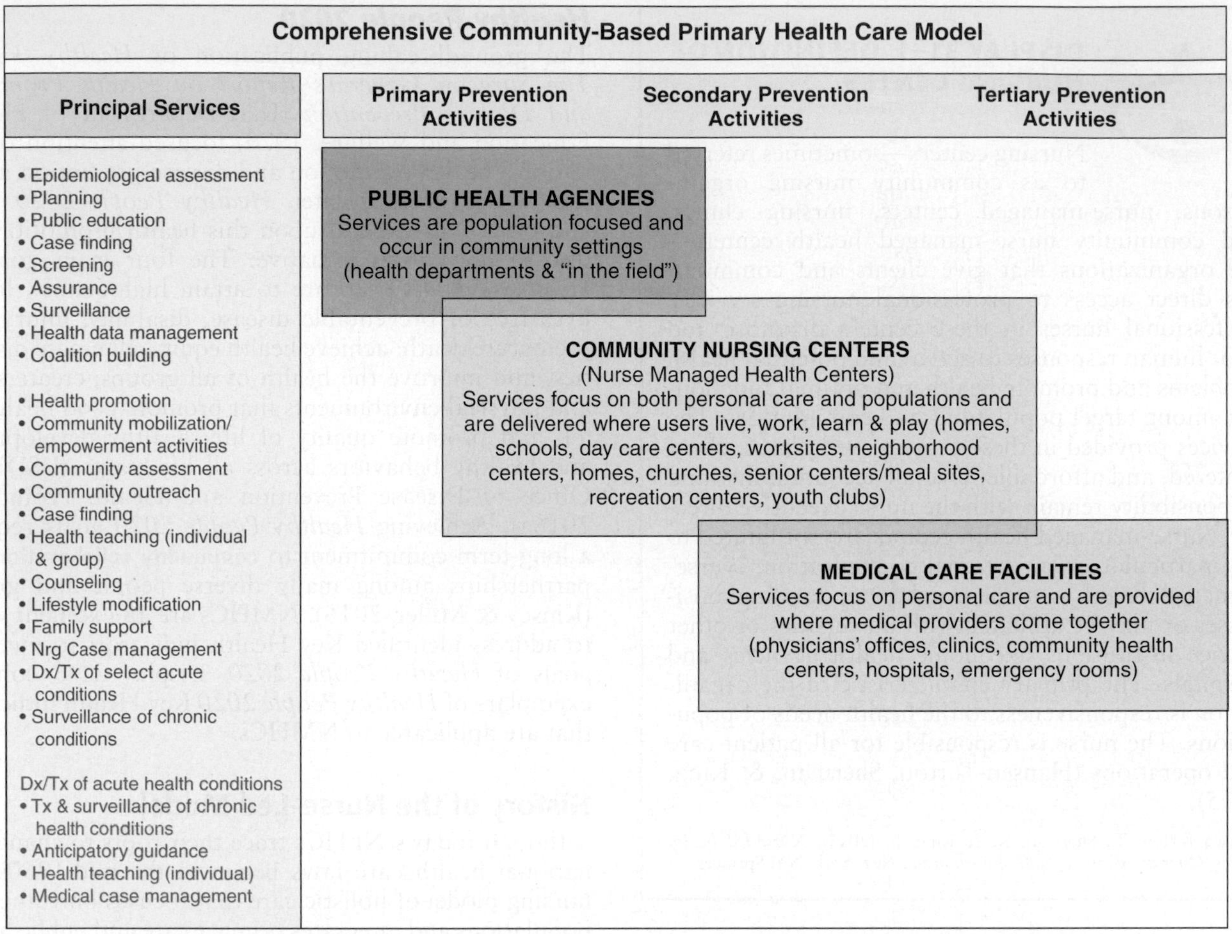

Comprehensive Community-Based Primary Health Care Model			
Principal Services	**Primary Prevention Activities**	**Secondary Prevention Activities**	**Tertiary Prevention Activities**
• Epidemiological assessment • Planning • Public education • Case finding • Screening • Assurance • Surveillance • Health data management • Coalition building • Health promotion • Community mobilization/ empowerment activities • Community assessment • Community outreach • Case finding • Health teaching (individual & group) • Counseling • Lifestyle modification • Family support • Nrg Case management • Dx/Tx of select acute conditions • Surveillance of chronic conditions Dx/Tx of acute health conditions • Tx & surveillance of chronic health conditions • Anticipatory guidance • Health teaching (individual) • Medical case management	**PUBLIC HEALTH AGENCIES** Services are population focused and occur in community settings (health departments & "in the field") **COMMUNITY NURSING CENTERS** (Nurse Managed Health Centers) Services focus on both personal care and populations and are delivered where users live, work, learn & play (homes, schools, day care centers, worksites, neighborhood centers, homes, churches, senior centers/meal sites, recreation centers, youth clubs) **MEDICAL CARE FACILITIES** Services focus on personal care and are provided where medical providers come together (physicians' offices, clinics, community health centers, hospitals, emergency rooms)		

FIGURE 31–1 Comprehensive community-based primary health care model. (From Lundeen, S. (1993, 2005). *Lundeen's comprehensive community-based primary health care model.* Milwaukee, WI: University of Wisconsin–Milwaukee College of Nursing, with permission.)

Hansen-Turton et al., 2009). Another academic nursing center at Florida Atlantic University began by providing diabetes care in 2012, but has expanded to a comprehensive health center with six nurse practitioners, three mental health providers, and two diabetes educators (Wood, 2015). Both undergraduate nursing and nurse practitioner students work at the center, and case management, chronic disease management, preventive health, and nutritional counseling

---

DISPLAY 31–3 *HEALTHY PEOPLE 2020* **SELECTED KEY HEALTH INDICATORS EXEMPLARS FOR NMHCS**

The Leading Health Indicators are organized under 12 topics. The *Healthy People 2020* Leading Health Indicators are

Access to Health Services
- Persons with medical insurance
  - Persons with a usual primary care provider

Clinical Preventive Services
- Adults who receive a colorectal cancer screening based on the most recent guidelines
- Adults with hypertension whose blood pressure is under control
- Adult diabetic population with an A1c value >9%
  - Children aged 19 to 35 months who receive the recommended doses of DTaP, polio, MMR, Hib, hepatitis B, varicella, and PCV vaccines

Environmental Quality
Injury and Violence
Maternal, Infant, and Child Health
Mental Health
Nutrition, Physical Activity, and Obesity
Oral Health
Reproductive and Sexual Health
Social Determinants
Substance Abuse
Tobacco

are provided to a diverse population. The center has federal, state, and private foundation grant funding. Today, NLHCs meet the traditional role of nurses who have historically provided compassionate health care focusing on the special needs of societies most vulnerable: the poor, the aged, those experiencing social injustice, and those living in geographic areas with limited or no access to adequate health care facilities (National Nursing Centers Consortium [NNCC], 2014). Unlike traditional health care venues that provide primary care and public health services, NLHCs include community participation in program development, implementation, and evaluation (NNCC, 2014). See From the Case Files I.

Nurse-Led Health Center Models

There are several types of nursing centers; each has an individuality of its own that reflects the community in which it is located and the particular services it offers (Hansen-Turton, Valdez, Ware, & King, 2015; Kinsey & Miller, 2016). Academic-based nursing centers, which are located within schools of nursing, are a common organizational structure. There are also hospital-based and freestanding community-based NLHCs that offer a mixture of primary care, health promotion, wellness, and disease prevention services (Hansen-Turton, Valdez, et al., 2015; Kinsey & Miller, 2016).

NLHCs meet requirements for **Federally Qualified Health Center (FQHC)** designation as defined in Section 330 of the Public Health Service Act. FQHCs are safety-net providers whereby the main purpose is to enhance primary care services in underserved rural and urban communities (USDHHS, Centers for Medicare and Medicaid Services [CMS], 2011). Hansen-Turton (2012) states that

---

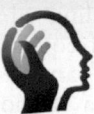 *From the* **Case Files** **I**

The RICHY Program: Interprofessional Primary Care and Wellness in the Community

In 2014, two local universities, the region's largest health network, and two community nonprofit organizations in Lehigh Valley Pennsylvania spearheaded what would become the Regional Integrated Collaborative for Healthy Youth (RICHY) program. The RICHY program provides an access point to primary care and wellness services for an at-risk population that is difficult to engage. This novel pilot program is believed to be the first of its kind in the country.

This collaboration resulted in the development and implementation of a unique interprofessional initiative targeting homeless, at risk for homelessness, or runaway teens, designed to meet three overarching goals: (1) to support these vulnerable pregnant and parenting women with health services for themselves and their babies, (2) to empower these women to become more active managers of their own care and that of their child, and (3) to educate them on how to best utilize the health care system, thereby reducing costs.

Using an integrated behavioral health model, family nurse practitioner students, graduate social work students, and undergraduate senior nursing students work at a residential housing complex with at-risk adolescent girls and young mothers and their babies. Graduate students working with the program are supervised by both university faculty and clinicians from the health network. Family nurse practitioner students provide primary care and preventive medical services on site. Graduate social work students provide ongoing behavioral health and social work support to the youth between visits as needed, increasing trust and follow-through with recommendations. Senior undergraduate nursing students in a clinical practicum that promotes the nurse-led wellness model provide primary prevention via education. The undergraduate nursing students anecdotally report that the RICHY project broadened their vision of how health care can be delivered in nontraditional settings.

During the first 6 months of the 12-month pilot program, data related to patient health literacy, patient activation, and utilization of the health care system reveal the following:

- Residents attended 41 visits to the Nurse Practitioner–Behavioral Health team during the first 6 months of the program; 78% of the visits focused on health management, which is a primary goal of the program.
- Use of the emergency department (ED) was minimal during the first 6 months. Adolescents went to the ED only one time; three ED visits occurred for young children of the residents; five ED visits were avoided by having access to the services provided through this initiative.
- Eight of the residents have become patients at the collaborating health network's family medicine community clinic, connecting them to a family medicine primary care practice. These eight individuals have engaged in 15 visits at the FHC across 5 months. All but one resident now has a designated primary care provider, either at FHC or elsewhere.
- Undergraduate nursing students conducted group education primary prevention sessions. All of the residents who attended these sessions reported positive feedback, noting that they learned new information about self-esteem and self-image, when to go to the ED or seek health care, signs of illness in young children, and healthy relationships.

The 12-month data report will help determine if this unique model can become self-sustaining once grant funds supporting it have ended. It will attempt to determine what the value of the program was to the mothers and the organizations involved, if better outcomes were realized for the patients, if decreased health care costs were seen, and how it might be possible to fund such a model in other communities.

Family & Youth Services Bureau. (2015, November 4). An onsite clinic builds healthy connections for homeless youth and their kids. Retrieved from http://ncfy.acf.hhs.gov/news/2015/11/onsite-clinic-builds-healthy-connections-homeless-youth-and-their-kids

NLHCs meet all of the requirements for FQHC designation, and funding to support them is vital to their existence. Health care reform legislation has helped with this funding. This is an especially important designation, as it enables NLHCs to qualify for many funding sources vital to service provision that would not be available without this designation. The specific requirements are that they:

- be located in an MUA or serve a medically underserved population
- have a nonprofit, tax exempt, or public status
- have a board of directors, a majority of whom must be consumers of the center's health services
- provide culturally competent, comprehensive primary care services to all age groups
- offer a sliding scale fee and provide services regardless of ability to pay

The variety of nursing center models currently being used and their organizational structures demonstrates the diversity of contemporary NLHCs. Display 31–4 describes the major types of centers (wellness centers, specialty nursing centers, and Comprehensive Primary Care Centers) along with the various organizational structures that influence their delivery models.

Funding for Nurse-Led Health Centers

As NLHCs vary in their models, so too are their methods of cost reimbursement, including the following: fee for service, sliding fees, contracts, grant support, third-party payments, and cost-based reimbursement (Hansen-Turton, 2012; Pilon & Hansen-Turton, 2015). Most nursing centers' operational and salary budgets entail a combination of these funding sources.

In **Comprehensive Primary Care Centers**, advanced practice nurses provide primary care services. Such services are usually reimbursable under Medicaid and managed care medical insurance plans. In **wellness centers**, public health nurses and other interdisciplinary team members provide a range of primary and secondary prevention strategies. These services are usually not reimbursed by insurance plans but are often covered by grants and contracts (Hansen-Turton, 2012; Resick et al., 2015). Additionally, foundation support and private donations from community organizations and members provide fiscal support for NMHC initiatives (see From the Case Files II).

It is important to distinguish between grants and contracts as funding sources for NLHCs. Funding organizations usually release guidelines regarding what initiatives they will fund. Grant guidelines are frequently termed **request for proposal (or RFP)**. Grants can be a source of initial start-up funding as well as a support for ongoing activities (Kinsey & Miller, 2016). A proposal submitted by the NLHC to the funding organization describes how the center would meet the goals and

---

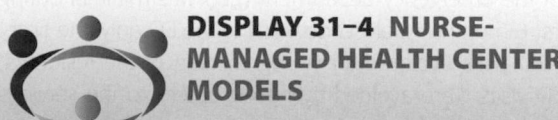

DISPLAY 31–4 NURSE-MANAGED HEALTH CENTER MODELS

Center Types
- Wellness Center: provides public health as well as health promotion and disease prevention programs, focus on primary and secondary prevention strategies
- Special Care Centers: provide programs that target specific health conditions such as HIV or diabetes
- Comprehensive Primary Care Center: provides traditional primary care and public health programs

Organizational Structure
- Academic Nursing Center: located within a School of Nursing
- Freestanding Center: independent center with its own governing board
- Subsidiary: part of a larger health care system, such as home health agencies, community centers, schools, and other venues
- Affiliated Center: legal partnership with a health care or human services organization

Adapted from Kinsey, K., & Miller, M. E. (2016). The nursing center: A model for nursing practice in the community. In M. Stanhope & J. Lancaster (Eds.), *Public Health Nursing: Population-centered health care in the community* (9th ed., pp. 455–475). St. Louis, MO: Elsevier.

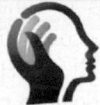 *From the* **Case Files** **II**

Ms. Jones is a 22-year-old mother of three small children who recently moved to an urban area. She brings her oldest child, age 6, to a local comprehensive primary care nurse-managed health clinic (NMHC) for school immunizations. During the course of the history and physical examination, the nurse practitioner becomes aware that this mother also has two younger children, aged two and three, at home. The family rents a small apartment in housing that was built in the mid-1950s. Ms. Jones reports that her mother (the children's grandmother) also resides with them. The grandmother is the childcare provider while Ms. Jones works as a local hair salon. The grandmother smokes 1.5 to 2 packages of cigarettes daily; Ms. Jones reports that she is a nonsmoker. Upon further questioning, the nurse practitioner learns that the 3-year-old child has a chronic cough and occasional wheezing. Ms. Jones also confides to the nurse practitioner that she recently missed two menstrual periods and is sexually active.

1. What are some possible health care needs of Ms. Jones? Her mother?
2. What screenings should be performed on Ms. Jones? Her mother?
3. What screenings should be performed on Ms. Jones' children?
4. What other interdisciplinary team members should be involved in this family's health care?
5. What are some possible referrals that would benefit this family?

objectives set by the funding organization. Outcomes, or the end results at a specific point in time, are increasingly becoming more important to funders. NLHCs must include measures to collect outcome data and project what outcomes will occur in their submitted proposals. Additionally, funders tend to view initiatives that include interagency collaboration in a more favorable manner. Partnering with one or more NLHCs or other community-based organizations is a strategy that provides additional strength to the proposal when it is under review by the funding organization.

Contracts are another source of funding for NLHCs. Contracts are awards for a legal procurement relationship between a funder and a recipient obligating the contractor to furnish a product or service defined in detail by the funder (National Institutes of Health, Office of Extramural Research, 2013). A contract has specific goals, objectives, and activities, as well as a time frame for which the activities are to be implemented and evaluated. Contracts are awarded on a noncompetitive basis and oftentimes are renewable when goals and objectives are met.

Managing the various funding streams that feed the personnel and operations budgets of an NLHC is an arduous task. To ensure that budgetary dollars are spent in the manner specified by the funding organization, meticulous record keeping and itemization of spending is another undertaking that the nurse executive or an operations coordinator of an NLHC must carry out. It is imperative that key personnel from the NLHC maintain precise records and submit accurate quarterly, semiannual, or annual reports as specified in the grant or contract award.

Sustainability of Nurse-Managed Health Clinics

Sustainability, or the ability to carry on services and health promotion activities when funding is no longer available, is one of the main challenges of NLHCs. The challenge of "sustainability" is a common dilemma that funders and grantees both face at the end of an initiative's funding period (Ely, 2015).

NLHCs have much to offer toward resolving the national health care crisis facing vulnerable populations who are uninsured or underinsured. However, without the ability to maintain fiscal sustainability, NLHCs may fail to reach their full potential for positively influencing the future of health care (Ely, 2015; Hansen-Turton, 2012). Financial sustainability in NLHCs is challenging. Administrative personnel from NLHCs must continually scan local, state, and federal avenues for grant opportunities to maintain, or expand, services (Pilon & Hansen-Turton, 2015).

In the past, funders were often confronted with the task to help organizations find and secure other resources, or extend their own financial support, to ensure the continuity of services. More recently, both public and private funders are stipulating that organizations describe detailed plans for sustainability after the award period ceases in their application submitted for funding. A seminal document by Cutler (2002, p. 23) proposes "critical sustainability questions" that can be used as a preliminary avenue of consideration for organizations such as NMHCs when completing a grant application for funding (see Display 31–5).

DISPLAY 31–5 CRITICAL SUSTAINABILITY QUESTIONS

When applying to a funding organization, applicants should consider the following questions:

1. Assuming acceptable results and assuming that the task will not be fully completed at the end of the grant period, is it expected that this initiative will continue beyond the period for which funding is available?
2. If so, what level of financial and other resources will be needed to continue?
3. What capacity-building measures are needed to make the initiative sustainable? How will these measures be implemented?
4. What is it about this initiative that is likely to attract interest and elicit support?
5. Who are the most likely future funders? (Be specific. If government, what level of government, what agency, what funding stream? If private, which foundation or other source?)
6. Is there a history of this entity supporting efforts (a) of this sort and (b) of this size?
7. Would success in this effort obviate the need to spend resources on something else, and could that money be diverted to this effort? How?
8. Who within the anticipated funding organization would have to decide to fund, through what processes?

Source: Cutler, I. (2002). *End games: The challenge of sustainability.* Baltimore, MD: Annie E. Casey Foundation Publisher.

National Organization: The National Nursing Centers Consortium

In 1996, because of interest from several nursing center directors, staff, and community members to address all aspects of operations and to provide ongoing collaboration and continuing education, the Regional Nursing Centers Consortium (RNCC) of Pennsylvania, New Jersey, and Delaware was established. In the short span of 5 years, nursing centers nationwide were contacting the RNCC with inquiries related to all aspects of operations, funding, and sustainability. It became rapidly evident that the RNCC needed to expand its service area to meet the needs of NLHCs around the nation. In 2001, The National Nursing Centers Consortium (NNCC) was formed to represent NLHCs nationwide. Headquartered in Philadelphia, Pennsylvania, with a second office in Washington, DC, the NNCC expanded in 2005 to include an international focus with the addition of an NMHC in Auckland, New Zealand. The vision, mission, and goals of the NNCC are found in Display 31–6.

Best Practices of Nurse-Led Health Centers

In contemporary health care, evidence-based practice is the process of making clinical decisions based upon the best available research evidence, clinical expertise, and

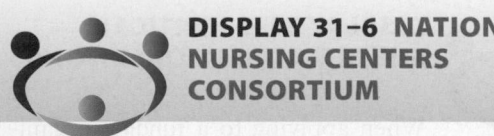

DISPLAY 31–6 NATIONAL NURSING CENTERS CONSORTIUM

Mission

To advance nurse-led health care through policy, consultation, programs, and applied research to reduce health disparities and meet people's primary care and wellness needs (para. 2).

Our Mission is Accomplished by

1. Providing national leadership in identifying, tracking, and advising health care policy development
2. Positioning nurse-managed health clinics as a recognized mainstream health care model
3. Fostering partnerships with people and groups who share common goals (para. 3)

Source: National Nursing Centers Consortium. (2014). *Who we are.* Retrieved from http://www.nncc.us/about-nncc/who-we-are

---

client preferences in the context of available resources (Melnyk & Fineout-Overholt, 2014). NLHCs implement evidence-based practice via best guidelines, or the application of the best available evidence to improve practice and systematic reviews have found that they provide effective services (IOM, 2011; Jakimowicz, Stirling, & Duddle, 2015; Schadewaldt & Schultz, 2011). Chapter 4 provides an extensive overview of evidence-based practice.

Biennially, the NNCC conducts a *Best Practice Conference* at varied national locations. This professional conference brings together nurses, staff members, funders, and political leaders to share best practices and participate in networking opportunities. Continuing education credits are available for attendance at scientific sessions. This is one example of how NLHCs set standards for quality improvement and promote professional growth among members.

Nursing Research and NLHCs

NLHCs provide research opportunities, for both primary prevention and wellness initiatives. Descriptive data have been collected about client demographics, types of service provided, funding methods, and sustainability efforts. The first national collection of quality measures for NLHCs compared with national ambulatory care benchmarks is now published (Barkauskas, Pohl, Tanner, Onifade, & Pilon, 2011). The quality measures in this report were for breast cancer screening, cervical cancer screening, diabetes care, hypertension management, and smoking cessation. These authors found that quality measure findings compared favorably with national benchmarks, with high quality demonstrated for chronic disease care management. They also reported that their experience with national data collection proved to be feasible. Additional studies with multisite NLHCs designed to measure variables such as psychosocial needs, accessibility and affordability of services, and quality of life indicators are warranted.

Role of Students in Nurse-Led Health Centers

Undergraduate and graduate students from many disciplines play a vital part in the activities of NLHCs. These disciplines include, but are not limited to, nursing, social work, mental health, dental, nutrition, speech–language–hearing science, and public health. When students engage in NLHC activities for their clinical experience, they become aware of the distinctiveness of nurse-managed centers from other health care delivery systems, the variety of models and organizational structures that exist, and are active participants in vital nursing center activities. Most often, students are engaged in primary and secondary prevention strategies via health education, outreach, immunization, and screening programs. Roles that students fulfill are similar to the roles of their staff mentors, such as advocate, case manager, change agent, educator, and referral agent. Faculty roles in NLHC academic models involve clinical supervision and mentorship of undergraduate and graduate students assigned to the nursing center for their clinical experience (see From the Case Files III).

Community Service Learning in Nurse-Led Health Centers

Additionally, schools of nursing and NLHCs are an excellent venue to conduct community service learning (CSL) projects with both undergraduate and graduate students. Using a "wall-less" concept of a nursing wellness center, undergraduate and graduate nursing students can participate in CSL activities in a variety of community settings. CSL activities provide opportunities for students to partner with key community agencies to help meet the needs of underserved and vulnerable populations (Resick et al., 2015). Benefits for students include academic

---

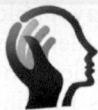

From the Case Files **III**

Public health nurses from an academic wellness NLHC and undergraduate student nurses are conducting blood pressure and glucose screenings at a church-sponsored health fair. This event is conducted on Sunday from 10 AM to 2 PM, before, during, and after church services. Approximately 50% of adults screened have hypertension and/or hyperglycemia. One African American male participant, who was asymptomatic, had severe hypertension (220/154) and was immediately transported to the nearest hospital for evaluation.

1. What are some feasible referrals that may have been made for those with abnormal screening results?
2. What types of primary prevention strategies may benefit those attendees who had normal screening results?
3. What is the rationale for conducting the health fair on a Sunday?
4. Why is it important for student nurses to be knowledge about the most current blood pressure guidelines?
5. In what ways do student nurses benefit from participating at a health fair?

growth, life skill development, civic engagement, and partnership with the larger community (Resick et al., 2015). Within NLHCs, broader implications of service learning include interpersonal, social, and moral development, as well as increased awareness of community, national, and global health problems (Sabo et al., 2015). One exemplar of a CSL project conducted at urban and rural schools is the "Safety Town" initiative. This CSL project entails educating preschool and early elementary school–aged children on indoor and outdoor safety for trauma prevention (Miller & Mest, n.d.). Qualitative feedback from nursing students reveals personal and professional growth regarding primary prevention in pediatric trauma in nontraditional clinical settings within the community.

Future Directions for NLHCs

In 2008, the IOM appointed a committee on the Robert Wood Johnson Foundation (RWJF) Initiative on the Future of Nursing. The purpose of this committee was to produce a report making recommendations for the future of nursing. This committee developed four key messages regarding the future of nursing: (1) nurses should practice to the full extent of their education and training; (2) nurses should achieve higher levels of education and training through an improved education system that promotes seamless academic progression; (3) nurses should be full partners, with physicians and other health care professionals, in redesigning health care in the United States; and (4) effective workforce planning and policy making requires better data collection and information infrastructure (IOM, 2011). NLHCs play a vital role in the transformation of the national health care system. The passage of the Affordable Care Act (ACA) in 2010 (see Chapters 1 and 13) and implementation strategies that were put into action in 2014, are relevant to activities conducted in NLHC models. Main areas of focus for health care reform are prevention and improving the quality of care. In NLHCs, advanced practice nurses lead interprofessional teams as critical safety-net providers in America's health care delivery system. Nurses in NLHCs are vital change agents as they partner with the community, interprofessional team members, and students to improve access to care and health outcomes (Jakimowicz et al., 2015). Continued expansion of the NLHC model in the next decade and beyond will meet key recommendations from the IOM report on nursing's future and the goals of the ACA (Wilson et al., 2012). See Perspectives for an example of an NLHC that meets the needs of the population served, provides continuity of care, and reduces the use of overcrowded and expensive ED services for routine health care.

FAITH COMMUNITY NURSING

Historical Background of Faith-Based Nursing

Faith community nursing is one of the newest nursing specialties and one of the oldest means of health care delivery. For hundreds of years, deaconesses, sisters, and lay members of religious communities have been involved in ministering to the sick. This tradition was revitalized through the efforts of Reverend Dr. Granger Westberg. As a hospital chaplain and Lutheran minister, Westberg (1990) observed a great need for preventive and holistic health services, especially among the underserved. He estimated that one third of the illnesses his patients experienced could have been prevented, or the severity reduced, by education and health promotion. To address these needs, he launched several church-based holistic health clinics in the 1970s, each staffed by a physician, nurse, and chaplain. These clinics provided health services to the underserved in the community for several years. The clinics eventually closed, but the experience led Reverend Westberg to recognize the unique ability of nurses to bridge the disciplines of medicine and religion and assist the client in understanding the physical and spiritual influences on health (Hickman, 2011).

Spurred by the positive impact of the church-based health clinics, Westberg initiated a pilot project in 1984 in which nurses provided holistic, preventive health care for six Christian congregations in the Chicago area. These nurses were called *parish nurses*. The surrounding communities recognized the beneficial influence of the parish nurses on the six congregations. Gradually, more and more churches sought to incorporate a parish nurse into their staff. The parish nursing movement soon spread outside of Christian religious institutions and beyond the borders of the United States to 22 other countries. The International Parish Nurse Resource Center (IPNRC, n.d.), formed in 1986, provides educational programs and resources for nurses who seek to practice as a parish nurse and for educators wishing to conduct training programs for parish nursing.

The Health Ministries Association (HMA), formed in 1989, was instrumental in developing the first *Scope and Standards of Parish Nursing Practice* (HMA, 2010). In the original standards, the term parish nurse was defined as "a registered professional nurse who serves as a member of the ministry staff of a faith community to promote health and wholeness of the faith community ..." (American Nurses Association [ANA]/Health Ministries Association [HMA], 1998, p. 1). The term faith community was defined as an "organization of families and individuals who share common values, beliefs, religious doctrine and faith practices ... such as a church, synagogue, or mosque ..." (ANA/HMA, 1998, p. 6). These definitions were carried over to the revised scope and standards, published in 2005, and the title of parish nurse was changed to **faith community nurse** (FCN), while the name of the specialty was changed to faith community nursing (ANA/HMA, 2005). Today, nurses who practice in a faith community may be referred to as FCNs, parish nurses, health ministry nurses, congregational nurses, or church nurses depending upon preference and the traditions of the faith community. No matter what title is used, a nurse who practices in a faith community should adhere to the *Faith Community Nursing: Scope and Standards of Practice, 2nd ed.* (ANA/HMA, 2012); the current definition of FCN is "a specialized practice of professional nursing that focuses on the intentional care of the spirit as part of the process of promoting holistic health and preventing or minimizing illness in a faith community" (p. 1).

What Do Faith Community Nurses Do?

Activities and interventions used by FCNs are as diverse as their faith communities. Authors have described key aspects of this specialty, which include meeting the emotional and spiritual support needs of the dying and serving

PERSPECTIVES
DENTON COMMUNITY HEALTH CLINIC: A NURSE-LED COMMUNITY CLINIC

In the fall of 2011, I realized that many of the low income or homeless had difficulty accessing health services. Other health organizations in our community, a city of 120,000 in northeast Texas, were promoting that the low-income or homeless population were "noncompliant" and did not care about their health. I had learned through volunteering that access to existing community health care resources presented many barriers. These barriers were minimal payment amounts that were too high, service hours that were not convenient to the low-income population, and pre-enrollment criteria that many could not meet. Most existing health care organizations required proof of income, proof of residency, and so on. The low-income population often has day jobs and income that may be high 1 week and nonexistent the next week. Many share a residence with others so that it is more affordable and so do not have a proof of residence. Hence, the low-income and/or homeless populations tend to use the hospital EDs for care.

Consequently, equipped with evidence-based knowledge about the low-income and homeless populations, with community health models such a Pender's Health Promotion Model (Pender, Murdaugh, & Parsons, 2011), and population health care frameworks (Bisognano & Kenney, 2012), I embarked in setting up a health clinic that didn't have those unrealistic requirements. Individuals needing health services simply have to fill out an income self-declaration, and if they have no proof, that is fine. There are two reasons for the declaration. First, it helps the staff determine what the person could afford based on their income, and second, it is a screening tool to identify people who may need to be hooked up to community resources. The low-income and homeless populations are very mistrusting of community health and social services. They live day by day. They have to focus on the here and now: Where will my next meal come from? Where will I shower? Where will I launder my clothes? Where will I sleep? Guided by the understanding that the low-income population has its own culture and very specific needs, the clinic was set up as a caring, compassionate, and supportive environment for this population. Research has shown that individuals are more likely to adopt health-promoting behaviors if they are able to develop relationships with role models (Calvert, Isaac, & Johnson, 2012; Cook-Craig, Ely, Flaherty, Dignan, & White, 2012). The staff at the clinic is trained to treat everyone in a nonjudgmental manner. When a patient does not show up for an appointment, the staff calls the individual within a couple of hours of the missed appointment—not to scold the patient, but rather to check and see if the patient is all right. At that time, the staff ascertains the reason for the missed appointment and encourages the individual to reschedule. The staff also educates the person to call the next time so

that we know he or she is fine. Consequently, the clinic has a very low rate of patients not showing up for appointments. Patients of the clinic state that they feel "listened to," even though the length of appointments is still only 20 minutes.

Based on the knowledge that this population has difficulty getting time off from work and has problems with lack of transportation in our community and that they work different schedules, the clinic set up its hours to offer early morning hours, lunch time hours, and evening hours. The clinic does not close for lunch, so that if someone can only call at lunch, the call will be answered. Another strategy to improve access is that the clinic provides not only medical care but also behavioral care, by providing medical follow-up for mental health illnesses as well as counseling and social services. The decision to implement these services within the clinic was made because individuals tend to open up more when a relationship is built over time. Hence, treatment for patients' depression, anxiety, and other behavioral health issues are better managed with the help of the counselors and social worker.

The clinic is the patient-centered medical home for this population. Because the providers and staff build a relationship with the patient and family, the clinic staff is able to coordinate care, offer support services, and help individuals strengthen their coping and problem-solving skills.

The outcomes of the clinic interventions in helping individuals learn to manage their chronic illnesses are that individuals are able to keep working, be productive members of society, and learn to seek health services at the clinic rather than use the more expensive hospital ED. Individuals who previously had uncontrolled diabetes are now better controlled and are able to articulate what they need to do to control their blood sugars. Individuals with uncontrolled blood pressure now monitor their own blood pressure and call when the blood pressure goes beyond a certain level. As a nurse, I find myself constantly advocating for patients, ensuring that their needs are being systematically assessed and that the proper interventions are put in place to ensure maximal health at a lower cost. It is a rewarding experience!

M. Alice Masciarelli, RN, DNP, FACHE, CPHQ
Executive Director, Denton Community Health Clinic, Denton, TX

Bisognano, M., & Kenney, C. (2012). Pursuing the Triple Aim: Seven innovators show the way to better care, better health, and lower costs. San Francisco, CA: John Wiley & Sons.
Calvert, W. J., Isaac, P., & Johnson, S. (2012). Health-related quality of life and health-promoting behaviors in Black men. Health & Social Work, 37(1), 19–27.
Cook-Craig, P., Ely, G., Flaherty, C., Dignan, M., & White, C. R. (2012). Seeking health advice from social networks in low-income urban neighborhoods. American Journal of Health Behaviors, 36(6), 723–735.
Pender, N., Murdaugh, C., & Parsons, M. A. (2011). Health promotion in nursing practice (6th ed.). Upper Saddle River, NJ: Pearson Education.

as an advocate for individuals who are hospitalized, living at home, or in long-term care facilities (Evans, 2011; Hickman, 2011; Van Dover & Pfeiffer, 2012; Ziebarth, 2014). FCNs are also well positioned to address health conditions associated with stigma or embarrassment such as sexually transmitted infections and HIV (Archibald & Newman, 2015; Stewart, Thompson, & Rogers, 2015)

and mental health issues (Caplan & Cordero, 2015; Singh et al., 2015). An FCN seeks to understand how religious beliefs and life transitions (e.g., marriage, divorce, birth, death, illness) impact on spiritual and mental health care (Anaebere & DeLilly, 2012). The ongoing and long-term nature of the FCN's relationship with the faith community is helpful for addressing highly personal and/or stigmatizing subjects as well as increasing awareness and promoting health through education.

FCNs have been instrumental in meeting the educational and health promotion needs of underserved and older adult populations. For example, faith-based approaches were based on scripture and included an exercise program called "Walk by Faith" and cancer screening programs "Ribbons of Faith" (Baltic et al., 2015). Other programs on healthy eating education are known as "Bread of Life" and "The Body is a Holy Temple." Many faith-based interventions address overweight and obesity among vulnerable populations: Elijo Salud is one example of an intervention to address poor eating habits among Hispanic youth (Oakley & Hoebeke, 2014), and Project TEACH (Transforming, Empowering, and Affecting Congregation Health) is another program working with obese Black women to improve their nutrition and exercise behaviors (Cooper, King, & Sarpong, 2015). Seton Health developed a program called "Defy Diabetes!" to identify adults at risk for diabetes, provide education to decrease risk, and improve the management of patients with diabetes. The FCN taught the courses and each session began and ended with prayer. Education was provided on nutrition, exercise, and the role prayer plays in stress relief. Observation and surveys concluded that participants developed awareness of their disease and adopted a healthier lifestyle (Sheehan et al., 2013). A randomized community trial of "Fit Body and Soul," a faith-based lifestyle intervention program to prevent diabetes among an African American population, showed a significant overall decline in fasting plasma glucose (almost 11 mg/dL) for those program participants identified as prediabetic versus an increase (4.22 mg/dL) for those receiving only health education over a 12-week period (Sattin et al., 2016). Participants also had significantly greater weight loss.

A review of parish nursing (FCN) literature from 2008 to 2012 found that FCNs from diverse geographic areas and faith traditions performed consistent interventions to address health concerns that were often aligned with national health priorities (Dandridge, 2014). In addition, many of the interventions, such as education, advocacy, and referral, were comparable to those used in traditional nursing practice. However, FCNs tended to engage in more health promotion interventions and to integrate spiritual and religious practices into their approaches. FCN services are growing and can provide cost-effective services to a range of populations, including those who may be more difficult to reach through more traditional health care venues (Yeaworth & Sailors, 2014). Holistic support offered by FCNs include actions that address physical, social, emotional, mental, and spiritual needs such as health education, counseling, referral to community agencies, advocacy on the client's behalf to meet needs and reduce complications, and coordinating care by mobilizing other members of the faith community to provide support such as prayer, visitation, meals, and transportation (Dandridge, 2014; Pappas-Rogich & King, 2014). Although the interventions used by FCNs may not emphasize providing direct physical care, such as medication administration, or other prescribed treatments, all registered professional nurses including FCNs share the use of the nursing process (ANA/HMA,

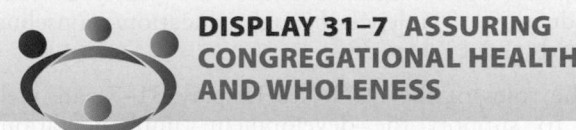

DISPLAY 31–7 ASSURING CONGREGATIONAL HEALTH AND WHOLENESS

Roles of the Faith Community Nurse

1. Health educator
2. Health counselor
3. Advocate
4. Referral agent
5. Developer of support groups
6. Coordinator of volunteers
7. Integrator of faith and health

Accountability

1. ANA scope and standards of nursing practice
2. ANA scope and standards of faith community nursing
3. Congregational standards
4. Institutional standards
5. ANA social policy statement
6. ANA code of ethics for nurses with interpretive statements
7. State nurse practice act
8. Patients rights

2012). For the FCN, implementation of a plan of care incorporates actions that fall within one or more of the seven roles of the FCN (see Display 31–7).

FCNs develop and implement a variety of health programs that address the health needs of their congregants. Many programs have been implemented that address the leading health indicators of *Healthy People 2020* such as physical activity, tobacco use, responsible sexual behavior, injury and violence, immunization, overweight and obesity, substance abuse, mental health, environmental quality, and access to health care (USDHHS, Office of Disease Prevention and Health Promotion, 2016a). Pappas-Rogich and King (2014) studied the role of FCNs and their support of *Healthy People 2020* objectives. A convenience sample of 247 FCNs completed an online survey linked to the International Parish Nurse Resource Center (IPNRC) Web site. Results indicate that most had an average of 15 years experience and were between age 51 and 71, and the majority (95%) was White. More of them were volunteers (68%), and 58% worked part time for 10 hours or less weekly. The parishioners they served were largely White (79%) and 79% of them were over the age of 65. They reported most often doing weekly health counseling and integrating health/faith. The most frequent monthly roles were health educator, making referrals, advocacy, and coordination of volunteers. Almost 40% stated that they never led support groups. The *Healthy People 2020* objectives that were most often implemented included the following:

● Promotion of physical activity (weekly; 33.5%)
● Promotion of good nutrition (monthly; 33.2%)
● Promotion of emotional health/well-being (monthly; 30.1%)

- Reduction/elimination of tobacco use (yearly; 29.8%)
- Reduction of violence through education/counseling (yearly; 30.1%) (p. 232)

The roles of the FCN (see Display 31–7) are well suited to support the development, implementation, and evaluation of these and other faith-based health programs.

Roles of the Faith Community Nurse

The goal of the FCN is "protection, promotion and optimization of health and abilities; prevention of illness and injury" and to respond "to suffering within the context of the values, beliefs, and practices of the faith community" (ANA/HMA, 2012, p. 3). Health promotion outcomes may be primary, directed at prevention of disease, illness, or injury; secondary, focused on early detection and appropriate intervention; or tertiary, concerned with promoting a sense of well-being when preventing or curing a condition may not occur. To achieve the goal of faith community nursing, seven diverse nursing roles are central to incorporate into practice (Dandridge, 2014).

Health Educator

A primary role of the FCN is as a health educator. Anaebere and DeLilly (2012) listed health education as the most common intervention in their study of parish nursing. Increasing awareness of health issues through health education is the foundation for health promotion and lifestyle changes. The FCN uses assessment skills to determine the health issues that may be present in the faith community and assesses the educational needs related to these issues. In the role of health educator, the FCN may provide individual and group education strategies such as providing health education materials, leading health education classes, or providing health screenings. The FCN may also develop educational displays or flyers, or write educational articles for the faith community newsletter or Web site.

Health Counselor

When education alone is not sufficient for empowering the individual to initiate a change or seek assistance, health counseling may be indicated. In the health counselor role, the nurse seeks to understand the individual's perceptions, fears, and barriers that prevent the person from taking action. The FCN may use a five-step health counseling process described as the five A's: ask, advise, assess, assist, and arrange (Agency for Healthcare Research and Quality, n.d.). Using this process, the FCN asks about the person's perceptions related to a specific health concern, advises the person about the health concern and the benefits of taking health-promoting actions, assesses the person's readiness to take action, offers assistance and guidance in planning ways to address the health concern, and arranges follow-up support. FCNs collaborated with a local hospital and pharmacists to promote better medication self-care in older adults (Shillam, Orton, Waring, & Madsen, 2013). They organized medication reviews during brown bag lunches and provided personal health counseling. Three months later, statistically significant results indicated that the older adult participants had decreased their total number of medications.

Advocate

The third role of an FCN is that of an advocate, helping individuals obtain needed services or care whether in the hospital, a long-term care facility, or at home. In the advocate role, the FCN uses knowledge of the health care system and awareness of safe and effective care practices to facilitate appropriate, timely intervention. Advocacy is indicated when dealing with vulnerable populations, such as older adults, children, or the homeless, who may not have the ability to speak for themselves or may lack the knowledge or awareness of what constitutes safe, effective care. FCNs have actively advocated for those with mental health problems, finding treatment sources and providing referrals and support (Anaebere & DeLilly, 2012).

Referral Agent

The role of referral agent involves several related aspects. First, the nurse needs to develop knowledge of community resources and contacts. Knowledge of what is available, how the service is accessed, eligibility criteria, and limitations of the service is essential. Next, the nurse networks with and develops collaborative relationships with community leaders and agencies that provide the services. Through networking with community agencies, the FCN becomes aware of and able to easily access a variety of community resources to support the client's physical, social, financial, emotional, or spiritual needs. The nurse is able to draw upon the relationships established with agency personnel to facilitate the eventual use of these resources, when needed. The final aspect of referral involves matching the needs of the individual or group to the services available. Thoughtful referral will assist and guide the client through the health care system and connect them with needed community resources. For instance, FCNs can be instrumental in ensuring improved vaccination rates for elderly and those with young children in their congregations and may seek collaborative arrangements with public health agencies (Pappas-Rogich, 2012), and a group of FCNs collaborated with public health staff to develop a toolkit for emergency preparedness and infection control (Reilly et al., 2011).

Developer of Support Groups

Receiving emotional support from persons who share similar experiences can provide strength, comfort, knowledge, and a sense of empowerment. When the FCN discovers a need for a support group that is not currently available in the community at large, the FCN may fulfill the role of developer of support groups. The FCN develops groups tailored to the faith community needs such as coping with loss and grief, cancer, caregiver stress, chronic illness, single parenting, addiction recovery, and more. The FCN may lead or facilitate the support groups or may train others to fulfill those positions. In one congregation, small groups were organized for workshops on sexuality (Cockroft, 2012). In another instance, telephone support groups were organized for homebound elderly members of a congregation; this effort seemed to help them with their movement and speech (Hayman, 2012).

Coordinator of Volunteers

The health ministry mission of a faith community typically includes a variety of services and activities to provide holistic support of the physical, social, emotional, mental, and spiritual needs of its members. Such a diverse array of services cannot be provided by the FCN alone. In the role of coordinator of volunteers, the FCN recruits, trains, and coordinates other members of the faith community. Volunteers provide or assist with a variety of services such as home, hospital, or long-term care visitations; respite care; assisting with transportation needs of homebound individuals; calling or sending cards to ill or injured members; and assisting with health screenings. Health ministry volunteers may include nurses, counselors, physical therapists, pharmacists, and other health care providers, as well as those with no health care background. Lay volunteers have been trained by FCNs to lead exercise groups or provide health education (Ellis & Morzinski, 2013; Reilly et al., 2011; Whisenant et al., 2013).

Integrator of Faith and Health

A distinctly unique role of the FCN is as integrator of faith and health. This role emphasizes the holistic relationship between physical, social, emotional, mental, and spiritual dimensions of the person. The FCN helps the person to improve health or enhance wellness by appreciating how the dimensions of the person are interconnected and by helping the person strengthen or support the weaker aspects, as needed. The FCN assesses community's strengths and health needs and incorporates an understanding of the connection between faith and health (Dandridge, 2014). Using opportunities to enhance the awareness of the interaction between faith and health is central to this role. Patients reported a renewal of their spiritual identity after receiving spiritual care from their FCN in a grounded-theory study by Van Dover and Pfeiffer (2012).

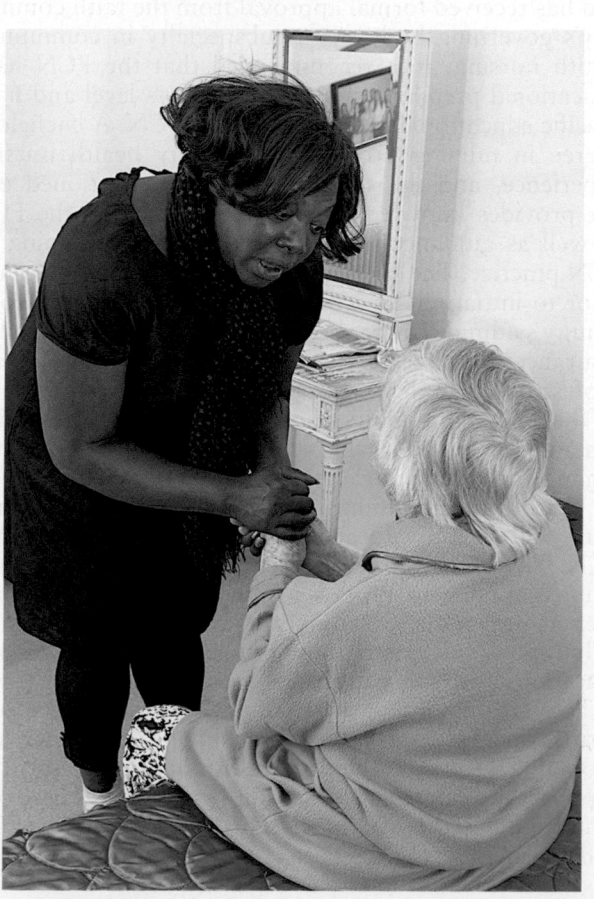

Faith Community Nursing Practice

Models of faith community nursing practice are diverse and may be categorized according to volunteer versus salaried positions with institutional versus faith-based sponsorship. The type of practice model adopted depends upon variables such as the number of faith community members served, the existing health ministry services in place, the faith community's governance structure and financial resources, and existing health care systems in the community at large. Early in the development of faith community nursing, FCNs were typically part-time volunteers who were members of the faith community they served. This voluntary, part-time status, coupled with the newness of faith community nursing practice, has resulted in limited research on faith community nursing. Nonetheless, studies that have been conducted have validated the effectiveness of FCNs and the programs they have implemented:

- Parent–child communication interventions on sex behaviors and cognitive outcomes for Black and Hispanic youth (Sutton, Lasswell, Lanier, & Miller, 2014)
- Faith-based lifestyle intervention to prevent diabetes among African Americans (Sattin et al., 2016)
- Faith-based healthy eating and physical activity intervention (Walk by Faith) to reduce weight and cancer risk among overweight and obese Appalachian adults (Baltic et al., 2015)
- HIV prevention in an Afro Caribbean faith-based community (Archibald & Newman, 2015)
- African American church-based HIV testing and linkage to care (Stewart et al., 2015)

There are growing trends in the types of FCN delivery models used today. In larger faith communities, one trend is to include the FCN as a salaried full- or part-time staff position. Smaller faith communities may join forces and pool resources to hire a full- or part-time FCN to serve multiple congregations. Another trend is the formation of partnerships with organizations such as universities or hospitals that agree to provide nursing services to the faith community. Partnerships with universities may involve individual faculty and student groups. For nursing faculty, faith community nursing can provide a flexible venue for part-time nursing practice that utilizes their skills in teaching and health promotion. The American Hospital Association (2012) reports on the success of a partnership between Methodist Le Bonheur Healthcare and the Congregational Health Network that has improved care transitions. In the 473 patients studied, their mortality rate was about half that of matched patients who were not enrolled in this collaborative service. Nursing students can be involved in providing service to faith communities by participating in service learning projects. The philosophy underlying service learning is that both parties benefit from the partnership; students learn and acquire needed skills, and faith communities obtain needed health education or health screenings (Sabo et al., 2015). A South African study examined the benefits to nursing students engaged in service learning within a faith community (du Plessis, Koen, & Bester, 2013). Students became more aware of cultural and religious factors with mental health patients they served, and the perception of their role and feelings of competence emerged over the time they participated in home visits. Families expressed feelings of growth and having experienced caring from the students.

Alegent Creighton Health of Omaha, Nebraska, recognized the financial benefits of a program that incorporated faith-based approaches. Data were collected on the cost savings accrued by the health system utilizing an FCN to transition patients from hospital to home and to care for them within their homes. The study indicated cost savings of $1,910,630 from 2005 to 2012 (Yeaworth & Sailors, 2014). Regardless of the model of practice utilized, integrating the FCN position into the faith community's organizational structure is recommended (Hickman, 2011). One way this integration can be provided is through the formation of a *health cabinet* or health and wellness committee within the faith community. The health cabinet was originally described by Reverend Westberg (1990) as a way to provide health ministry for a faith community that is interested in adding an FCN to its staff. The health cabinet includes members from the faith community who are interested in promoting and sponsoring health-related activities and programs for the faith community. Members may be nurses, other health care professionals, or persons with no health care background. The FCN functions as a member of the health cabinet and receives guidance and support from the cabinet in developing, promoting, and delivering programs and services to members of the faith community.

Becoming a Faith Community Nurse

The FCN practices community nursing with a high degree of independence and autonomy. Often, the FCN deals with clients experiencing complex health care situations who may have limited resources and extensive health-related needs. Recommended educational preparation for an FCN includes a bachelor's degree in nursing with community nursing experience as part of the program (ANA/HMA, 2012) and completion of additional education such as the 36-hour *Foundations of Faith Community Nursing* course offered through the IPNRC (IPNRC, n.d.). This course addresses the roles of the FCN and provides information on establishing, promoting, and maintaining an FCN practice. Participants gain experience in resolving complex client situations using scenarios and case studies.

Establishing a Faith Community Nursing Practice

Several steps are involved in creating an FCN position within a faith community. One of the first things to do is assess the community the nurse plans to serve, identifying the health needs of the faith community and the roles of the FCN that meet those needs. For example, a nurse might assess the demographics of the community and determine the most common health concerns and what education or health counseling needs the faith community may have. A needs assessment survey of the membership about health concerns, or topics of interest, may be conducted. Questions to explore include the following: Does the faith community need support groups for members who are experiencing the stress of illness, injury, or loss and grief? Do the members of the faith community need more information or assistance to access existing community resources? And, is there a need for health screening, respite care, or visitation for the sick or injured in their home, hospital, or long-term care facility?

Once the nurse has assessed the needs of the faith community, the next step is to identify how an FCN could help to meet those needs. The FCN uses this information to seek the support of the faith community members and staff, usually through visits with key members of the faith community, including the minister, past and present board members, and long-standing members. The nurse describes to these key members the roles of an FCN and how specific health needs of the faith community could be addressed by the services of an FCN and then solicits input from the staff and spiritual leaders of the faith community.

After key members and leaders of the faith community have verbalized support for adding an FCN to the organization's health ministry, the nurse seeks formal approval from the organization's governing body. The scope of services to be offered, time commitment expected, process of referral to the FCN, means of contacting the FCN, and other administrative aspects of the position should be negotiated before approval is finalized. The organization's bylaws, governing body, committee structure, and spiritual leader will play a part in the formal approval process and in determining where the FCN will fit in the organizational structure. The approval process may require a formal presentation of the nurse's proposal to the board members or to the faith community as a whole.

Launching an FCN practice should begin after the nurse has received educational preparation as an FCN and has received formal approval from the faith community's governing body. As a subspecialty in community health nursing, it is recommended that the FCN have educational preparation at the bachelor's level and have specific educational preparation as an FCN. A bachelor's degree in nursing provides community health nursing experience, and the foundation course mentioned earlier provides knowledge of the seven roles of the FCN as well as guidance in establishing and maintaining an FCN practice. The FCN must also have an active license. Prior to initiating services, the nurse and the faith community's administrator should assure that proper liability insurance is in effect. The FCN should carry individual professional liability insurance, and the administrator of the faith community should determine if the activities and services that will be provided are covered by the organization's insurance carrier.

If the faith community is not familiar with FCNs, the nurse will want to educate members about the roles of the FCN. The FCN can give presentations about faith community nursing to groups within the faith community, such as prayer circles, adult Sunday school, teen groups, pulpit talks, and existing support groups. During the presentations, the FCN can discuss specific activities that will be actively pursued, such as home or hospital visitations, formation of support groups, teaching health classes, and providing health screening, health counseling, spiritual support, and referral to community resources. These presentations will provide multiple benefits for both the FCN and the members of the faith community by allowing the nurse to establish relationships with members of the faith community and by allowing members to become familiar with the FCN and the services offered (Hickman, 2011).

In addition to providing presentations about faith community nursing to groups within the faith community, the nurse should consider other ways to inform members of the services provided. If the faith community publishes a newsletter or has a Web site, including a brief introduction to faith community nursing and providing some personal background and professional experience, information will be useful. The FCN may develop flyers and brochures that describe what an FCN does and the services offered. These materials may be distributed initially to new members and may be continually displayed on the community bulletin board. Business cards that provide the FCNs name, contact information, and outline FCN services may be distributed. The FCN may also write a monthly feature for the newsletter to provide health education and to keep the congregation informed of the services offered. These strategies and others will provide mechanisms for initial and ongoing marketing of the FCNs services to the faith community and can be useful tools for health promotion (Elwell, 2015).

Another aspect of preparation involves establishing community contacts and compiling information about community resources. The FCN should visit local health-related agencies, clinics, and hospitals and discuss services they provide and determine how these services may be accessed by FCN referral of faith community members. Information from community organizations, such as the March of Dimes, American Cancer Society, American Heart Association, and others, can provide health information and online resources for health promotion activities.

And finally, the FCN will need to decide on a method of documentation and record keeping. Documentation of the FCN activities and outcomes will provide ongoing evidence of the effectiveness of programs and interventions, which can be used to justify continuation of programs and services. The IPNRC (n.d.) offers resources regarding an electronic documentation system. Miller and Carson (2010) developed a system for documentation in faith community nursing that includes a daily activity log, a monthly activities report (developed from the daily logs), and individual interaction forms (when more in-depth interventions are needed or visits occur over several weeks/months). They note that a system of documentation must be "concise, require minimal time, and be formatted to facilitate tracking activity" so that both the congregation and community partners can quickly discern the FCN role and activities (p. 122) (see Display 31–8). Whatever method of documentation is used, the FCN will need to assure consistent documentation, confidentiality, and proper storage of the records.

OCCUPATIONAL AND ENVIRONMENTAL HEALTH NURSING

Business and industry provide another group of settings for community health nursing practice. **Occupational and environmental health nurses** work with employers to cultivate creative and business-appropriate health and safety

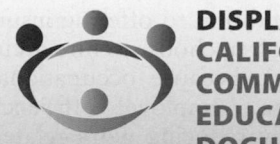

DISPLAY 31–8 NORTHERN CALIFORNIA FAITH COMMUNITY NURSE EDUCATION NETWORK DOCUMENTATION

Daily Activities Log

Can be a checklist that includes date, time spent, mileage, and specific activities or patient names (e.g., education programs, meetings, home visits, individual/group contacts, screenings, referrals) and assessment, interventions, and outcomes. Demographic categories are needed (e.g., age, ethnicity, gender), and NANDA, NIC, and NOC categories may be used to group the data for less complicated retrieval.

Monthly Activities Report

These are composed of aggregated data from daily activities logs and provide a summary of care provided by the FCN. Key categories such as individual or group contacts, specific problems, referrals made, programs given, meetings attended, work with volunteers, and program planning activities are grouped together, again using NANDA, NIC, and NOC classifications.

Individual Interaction Form

This is similar to other patient forms that request a health history, current status of health, contact information, and space for (or a checklist for common) NANDA, NIC and NOC information.

Adapted from Miller, S., & Carson, S. (2010). A documentation approach for faith community nursing. *Creative Nursing, 16*(3), 122–131.

programs. Program development must take into account the business' unique type of work, workforce demographics, and the work/community environments. The practice of occupational health nursing utilizes an interdisciplinary approach to advocate for the employee's right to have cost-effective, prevention-oriented health and safety programs.

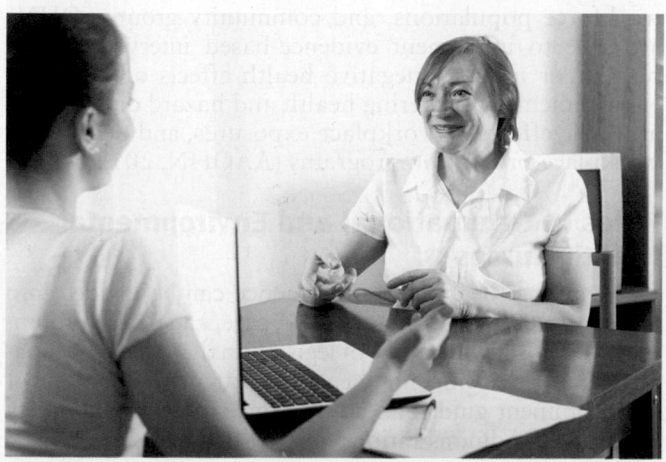

Organizations are expected to provide a safe and healthy work environment in addition to offering insurance for health care. Businesses often choose to hire occupational health nurses (OHNs), because occupational health programs help maximize employee efficiency and decrease costs by effectively reducing work-related injuries, disability claims, absenteeism, and improve employee health and safety. Present-day OHNs observe and assess workers' health status considering the workers job tasks and hazards. Using their specialized training, education, and experience, they use the nursing process to prevent occupational illness and injury. An additional and equally important responsibility is to help organizations maintain compliance with federal, state, and local laws, regulations, and guidelines for workplace health and safety (American Board for Occupational Health Nurses [ABOHN], 2012).

History of the Occupational and Environmental Health Nurse

Community health nurses have a long history of involvement in occupational health. Betty Moulder provided care for coal miners and families in Pennsylvania beginning in 1888 (American Association of Occupational Health Nurses [AAOHN], 2012). In 1895, the Vermont Marble Company hired Ada Mayo Stewart, said to be the first *industrial nurse* in the United States. Stewart provided care for employees and their families focusing on health promotion and disease prevention (Thompson, 2012). Early on, the profession primarily focused on providing infant and child health education to the employee families as well as the whole community. World War II showed a marked increase in employment of OHNs. In keeping with the changing times, the OHN's practice broadened to include comprehensive health and safety programs designed to prevent illness and injury for the U.S. workforce.

Although occupational and environmental health nursing has been in existence since the late 1800s, the Occupational Safety and Health Act of 1970 led to the proliferation of occupational health nursing employment in the United States. This important legislation established the **Occupational Safety and Health Administration (OSHA)** in the Department of Labor, to ensure a safe working environment for workers in the United States. In an effort to ensure business and industries meet OSHA standards, OHNs monitor the health status of individual workers, workforce populations, and community groups. OHNs are able to implement evidence-based interventions to prevent or mitigate negative health effects of the work environment by gathering health and hazard data, evaluating the effects of workplace exposures, and developing workplace prevention programs (AAOHN, 2012).

Roles of Occupational and Environmental Health Nurses

Occupational health nursing practice can be divided into three main categories: compliance, care, and health promotion. There is a wide range of legislation that guides occupational and environmental health nursing practice. Some of the prominent guidelines come from Occupational Safety and Health Administration (OSHA) U.S. statutes, Genetic

Information Nondiscrimination Act (GINA), Family Medical Leave Act (FMLA), Americans with Disabilities Act (ADA), Health Insurance Portability and Accountability Act (HIPAA), Department of Transportation, and U.S. Environmental Protection Agency (EPA). The following are a few examples of how regulatory guidance can influence an OHN's nursing practice:

- OSHA standards require training and hearing tests for employees who are exposed to loud noise at the workplace (29 CFR 1910.95).
- The Department of Transportation (n.d.) requires commercial drivers to pass a physical exam before they are allowed to drive and periodically throughout their driving career (49 CFR 391).
- The Americans with Disabilities Act (ADA) requires employers with 15 or more employees to make reasonable accommodations for persons with disabilities (ADA, 2000), and nurses are often part of the reasonable accommodation decision-making team.
- In health care settings, employee health nurses are instrumental in ensuring the institution's compliance with requirements for immunizations and tuberculosis testing (AAOHN, 2012).

The OHN is typically the first person to evaluate an injury that occurs in the workplace. In addition to providing first aid, larger occupational health clinics are moving toward a model that provides not only occupational health services but also case management and primary care (Mattaliano, 2013; Merrill et al., 2013). According to Workforce Management Data Bank, the primary reason employers establish an on-site clinic are to decrease health care costs, improve workers' quality, and improve the company's cost-effectiveness (Graeve, McGovern, Nachreiner, & Ayers, 2014; Moore & Moore, 2014). Comprehensive occupational worksite programs offer both health protection and health promotion services. After employees are injured or become ill at work, OHNs work to ensure a speedy and functional recovery, frequently helping employees work through the workers' compensation or insurance bureaucracy. Although some companies outsource case management for work-related injuries, many OHNs manage cases to ensure the employee's optimum recovery while helping to control costs.

It is in the best interest of both the injured/ill workers and employers to have employees return to the workplace as soon as possible. The National Safety Council estimates that more than 80 million lost work days are due to occupational injuries or illness (Presmanes, 2015). Additionally, the annual costs associated with employee injury or illness, including medical care and the decrease in productivity, come to $183.7 billion (National Safety Council, 2013). Occupational health and environmental nursing activities can assist employers to reduce the amount of time employees remain out of work because of illness and injury. See Display 31–9 Occupational and Environmental Health Nursing Care Plan.

In addition to addressing the health needs of the employees, it is important for the OHN to recognize the impact of the workplace on their own personal health. For instance, there are various causes of job stress for the occupational and environmental health nurse, and there

DISPLAY 31–9 OCCUPATIONAL AND ENVIRONMENTAL HEALTH NURSING CARE PLAN

Evelyn Robbins has been the occupational and environmental health nurse at ABC Metals for 4 years. She works with management, the company physician (who works at ABC Metals 2 days a week), union representatives, unit foremen, individual employees, and representatives from the community businesses and neighborhoods surrounding the plant. The company employs 400 workers—380 in manufacturing, primarily an assembly line making telephone electrical boxes, and 20 management and administrative staff.

Recently, 12 employees came to the worksite clinic complaining of hand injuries that had not occurred before. Mr. Robbins treated the wounds, reported the occurrences to the foremen involved, and reported the incidents to management. In addition, she wanted to explore the cause of these injuries so that they could be interrupted. She used the nursing process in her exploration.

Assessment

- Tour the areas where the incidents occurred.
- Inquire among the foremen to determine whether there was a change in routine, equipment, employee assignment, or product being manufactured.
- Ask injured employees what they were doing when the injury occurred.
- Reassess wounds for likenesses and differences, for example, was it the right or left hand and was it on the same part of the hand in each case?

Diagnoses

- Wounds occurred in factory areas where a new piece of equipment had been installed.
- Injured employees did not receive orientation to the equipment.

Plan

- Plan to work with foremen to provide an orientation for all employees who work with the new equipment.
- Plan an orientation program (with foremen, union representatives, and one employee from each unit in the factory) for all employees before working with new equipment in the future, to prevent further injuries.

Implementation

- Implement the orientation for employees who work with the new equipment.
- Initiate the orientation program as new equipment is introduced into the factory.

Evaluation

- Have there been any new equipment-related injuries in the factory?
- Has there been any change in general safety in the factory related to the increased focus on safety with new equipment?

---

may be related personal, professional, and employer factors. The nurse may experience role ambiguity because of a lack of professional preparation or inadequate orientation and continuing education. The corporate culture and leadership may foster work overload, not be supportive, and there may be limited career opportunities for the nurse. Like nurses working in acute care and other settings, occupational and environmental health nurses need to apply strategies to reduce job stress and potential job strain by modeling health-affirming choices, networking with other nurses and professional organizations in the community, and setting appropriate occupational health standards (Kamau, Medisauskaite, & Lopes, 2015).

Health Promotion Opportunities

OHNs play a vital role advocating health promotion and wellness programs for the workforce they serve. OHNs are in an ideal position to provide guidance, counseling, education, and coaching for employees who want to improve their health. Faced with high health care costs, many employers are turning to worksite health programs to help employees adopt healthier lifestyles and lower their risk of developing costly chronic diseases while improving worker productivity (AAOHN, 2012).

There is a link between healthy lifestyle and lower health care costs. Workplace wellness programs provide primary, secondary, and tertiary prevention services. Primary prevention examples include immunizations to protect employees against vaccine-preventable illness, safe lifting demonstrations, and postoffer assessments of preexisting limitations so that reasonable accommodations (per the ADA) can be made to prevent work-related injuries (Moore & Moore, 2014). Postoffer employment testing is a way to screen newly hired job candidates for their ability to complete all essential functions of their new job and to also screen for any preexisting conditions or injuries that may need to be accommodated before they are formally hired. It often includes physical demands analysis. Secondary prevention in the workplace setting often takes place as part of the medical surveillance process. OHNs do many screenings to gather data about the effects of workplace exposures and use the data to prevent occupational illnesses and injuries. Screenings can be based on OSHA standards, the U.S. Preventive Services Task Force (2014) recommendations, and/or other regulatory organizations. The Department of Transportation (DOT), the Mine Safety and Health Administration, and the Nuclear Regulatory Commission are some examples. Tertiary prevention aims to lessen the impact of a chronic illness or injury that has long-term effects. A worker may need to transition to a new job or do his or her existing job in a new or different way, and the OHN serves as a facilitator, advocate, or case manager to limit adverse health effects of the work environment.

Total Worker Health (TWH) is a national initiative designed to provide holistic approaches to employee wellness. TWH is defined as a strategy that integrates occupational safety and protection of health along with health promotion to prevent worker injury and illness and to improve worker well-being and health (National Institute for Occupational Safety and Health [NIOSH], 2015b). American workers spend a large part of their day at work. The workplace is now considered a social determinant of health; job-related factors include salary, the work environment, time spent at work, physical and psychological stress, employee/employer dynamics, and work–life balance. Activities that take place at the workplace, businesses, and industries all can affect the health and well-being of individual workers, families, and communities, and OHNs are often asked to organize workplace health promotion programs (Dombrowski, Snelling, & Kalicki, 2014). Figure 31–2 describes issues the nurse should consider when planning occupational health programs.

Although OHNs had been advocating healthy lifestyles for several decades, executives of American companies only recently began to recognize the value of having healthy workers. Research supports the link between

healthy lifestyle and lower health care costs indicating that healthy employees are less likely to be absent from work and more likely to be more productive when they are at work (Kowlessar, Goetzel, Carls, Tabrizi, & Guindon, 2011; Mattaliano, 2013; Merrill et al., 2013). Integrated approaches that address both physical and mental health have been found to be more effective; integrated approaches that deal with injury prevention, company cost saving, and occupational health and safety have shown less consistent results (Cooklin, Joss, Husser, & Oldenburg, in press). However, getting Americans to embrace a healthy lifestyle of physical activity, good nutrition, and sufficient rest is a challenge.

Because workers spend so much of their life at work (in both hours and years), it is important to develop a culture of health at the workplace. At every encounter with an employee, whether for an occupational health exam or an injury, the nurse has an opportunity to encourage healthy choices. OHNs are learning to become health coaches in an effort to assist individual employees improve their health. Health coaches use a variety of strategies and techniques to motivate individuals to set

Issues Relevant to Advancing Worker Well-being Through Total Worker Health®

Control of Hazards and Exposures
- Chemicals
- Physical Agents
- Biological Agents
- Psychosocial Factors
- Human Factors
- Risk Assessment and Risk Management

Organization of Work
- Fatigue and Stress Prevention
- Work Intensification Prevention
- Safe Staffing
- Overtime Management
- Healthier Shift Work
- Reduction of Risks from Long Work Hours
- Flexible Work Arrangements
- Adequate Meal and Rest Breaks

Built Environment Supports
- Healthy Air Quality
- Access to Healthy, Affordable Food Options
- Safe and Clean Restroom Facilities
- Safe, Clean and Equipped Eating Facilities
- Safe Access to the Workplace
- Environments Designed to Accommodate Worker Diversity

Leadership
- Shared Commitment to Safety, Health, and Well-Being
- Supportive Managers, Supervisors, and Executives
- Responsible Business Decision-Making
- Meaningful Work and Engagement
- Worker Recognition and Respect

Compensation and Benefits
- Adequate Wages and Prevention of Wage Theft
- Equitable Performance Appraisals and Promotion
- Work-Life Programs
- Paid Time Off (Sick, Vacation, Caregiving)
- Disability Insurance (Short- & Long-Term)
- Workers' Compensation Benefits
- Affordable, Comprehensive Healthcare and Life Insurance
- Prevention of Cost Shifting between Payers (Workers' Compensation, Health Insurance)
- Retirement Planning and Benefits
- Chronic Disease Prevention and Disease Management
- Access to Confidential, Quality Healthcare Services
- Career and Skills Development

Community Supports
- Healthy Community Design
- Safe, Healthy and Affordable Housing Options
- Safe and Clean Environment (Air and Water Quality, Noise Levels, Tobacco-Free Policies)
- Access to Safe Green Spaces and Non-Motorized Pathways
- Access to Affordable, Quality Healthcare and Well-Being Resources

Changing Workforce Demographics
- Multigenerational and Diverse Workforce
- Aging Workforce and Older Workers
- Vulnerable Worker Populations
- Workers with Disabilities
- Occupational Health Disparities
- Increasing Number of Small Employers
- Global and Multinational Workforce

Policy Issues
- Health Information Privacy
- Reasonable Accommodations
- Return-to-Work
- Equal Employment Opportunity
- Family and Medical Leave
- Elimination of Bullying, Violence, Harassment, and Discrimination
- Prevention of Stressful Job Monitoring Practices
- Worker-Centered Organizational Policies
- Promoting Productive Aging

New Employment Patterns
- Contracting and Subcontracting
- Precarious and Contingent Employment
- Multi-Employer Worksites
- Organizational Restructuring, Downsizing and Mergers
- Financial and Job Security

November 2015

Total Worker Health® is a registered trademark of the US Department of Health and Human Services

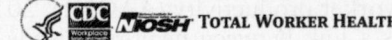

FIGURE 31–2   Relevant issues in Total Worker Health®.

and attain goals for lifestyle improvements. OHNs partner with communications professionals to craft compelling messages that encourage healthy choices, and they may provide consultation to upper management in order to help ensure that benefits packages reflect the company's desire for healthful personal practices. Additionally, the OHN is in a position to influence the type of food that is offered in the company's cafeteria as well as the selection of products available in vending machines (Miller, 2011).

The Occupational Health Team

OHNs work in a team environment with a variety of other professionals. Depending on the size of the company, the occupational health team may include a safety specialist, industrial hygienist, ergonomist, industrial or organizational psychologist, toxicologist, physical or occupational therapist, physician, lawyer, and employee assistance counselor. Human resources, management, security, and emergency response personnel are also part of the team. The employee is central to the team and is the reason for the team's existence.

Team collaboration is essential to the success of the occupational and environmental health program, and the OHN has a key role in ensuring adequate and appropriate communication among the members of the team. Establishing working relationships is paramount in the success of a functional and effective team (Draper, Ladou, & Tennenhouse, 2011; Thompson, 2012). Strong interpersonal relationship skills are extremely valuable in a team environment.

Finally, the occupational health team is not complete without the workers themselves. Employees can help identify problems and needs while contributing to decision-making about health programs. Their cooperation in implementing and evaluating programs is essential for an effective health protection and promotion effort.

Settings for Occupational and Environmental Health Nursing

Occupational and environmental health nursing may be one of the most challenging and rewarding nursing specialties, affording nurses the opportunity to establish long-term relationships with their clients and address issues across the wellness–illness continuum. Unlike nursing in acute care settings and public health departments, the employer's primary mission is not typically related to health or illness. Companies exist to make a profit; occupational health and safety professionals are employed to keep workers productive and to ensure compliance with state and federal health and safety requirements (AAOHN, 2012).

Some nurses select occupational health nursing because they are looking for a career change away from acute care nursing. Others find that rotating shifts and working weekends and holidays are not conducive to their desired lifestyle. Still others seek fulfillment through the establishment of more long-term relationships with their clients. On occasion, nurses can move straight into occupational health when they graduate from a BSN program. Nurses who move into occupational and environmental health from an acute care setting should expect a significant learning curve to feel comfortable in this nontraditional setting. Nurses who select the field of occupational health and safety encounter experiences that differ significantly from those found in an acute care setting. To make the adjustment, the nurse should be aware of the factors that make occupational health unique. Unlike hospitals or ambulatory care centers, the workplace is a non–health care institution in which production or service (not health care) is the primary goal. The occupational and environmental health nurse participates in the organization's goals through activities that contribute to the productivity of the workforce. In addition to learning the role of the occupational and environmental health nurse, the nurse needs to understand the parent company and become familiar with the employees' work environment and work tasks (AAOHN, 2012).

In many work settings, the occupational and environmental health nurse is the only health professional. In these situations, the nurse must have excellent assessment skills, not only for individuals but also for the working population served. Independent decision-making is critical. Nurses in occupational settings must also have strong communication skills, including listening, speaking, and writing. Models of practice differ depending on the philosophy and size of the company. Nurse-managed clinics are managed by registered nurses (or advance practice nurses) who employ or contract with other health professionals as needed (Thompson & Wachs, 2012). Nurse-managed clinics may utilize OHNs, a nurse practitioner or physician assistant, a physical therapist, a health educator, and a part-time occupational physician. A single-nurse unit is a common model of practice in many smaller companies. In a single-nurse unit, OHNs typically build strong networks of colleagues with whom they can discuss professional practice issues. Some companies use a medical model of practice, in that a physician determines clinic staffing and the department's approach to clinical practice. During the early 21st century, many companies in the United States began implementing primary care clinics as a method of controlling the cost of health care. Services in primary care clinics may be extended to dependents and retirees, and they typically offer urgent care services; they may also provide routine health examinations in addition to the usual occupational health services needed by an employer (Guidotti et al., 2013). One cost–benefit analysis of an on-site health clinic at a self-insured university found that it was more cost-effective than were off-site services for upper respiratory infections in full-time employees (McCaskill, Schwartz, Derouin, & Pegram, 2014).

Community-Based Occupational Health Nursing

OHNs work in a variety of settings. The manufacturing sector has a strong tradition of employing OHNs, but utility companies, mines, retail store chains (e.g., grocery, department, home improvement), hospitals, theme parks, banks, school systems, and government also employ OHNs. Because professional nurses have a variety of skill sets, they can care for injuries, manage disabilities, counsel employees who are troubled, help workers control their chronic diseases, and encourage high-level wellness (Burgel & Childre, 2012). Entrepreneurial nurses may set up an occupational health clinic in areas where many small businesses are located (e.g., industrial parks) and provide professional nursing services for employers that may not need a dedicated, full-time nurse (Harber, Alongi, & Su, 2014).

Agencies external to business and industry also provide occupational and environmental health nursing services. Historically, public health nurses from visiting nurse associations made home visits to sick employees and their families. In subsequent years, public health agencies provided part-time nursing services to small companies. These services included supervising the work environment, conducting health examinations, keeping records, disability management, emergency preparedness, teaching about and counseling on health issues, providing first aid, giving immunizations, and referring workers to community resources. More recently, occupational health nursing services have offered health screening and health promotion programs, and one study examining activity logs of a national sample of OHNs found that both management and clinical skills are routinely used and indirect client care is also common (Harber et al., 2014). The majority of the nurse participants were paid directly by their employers. Furthermore, occupational and environmental health nurse consultants based in state departments of health provide consultation and continuing education programs to nurses employed in occupational health settings.

Hospital-based occupational health programs, large medical–industrial health clinics, and insurance companies also provide occupational and environmental health nursing services. These services may be in the form of direct care (e.g., rehabilitation of an injured worker) or indirect care (e.g., consultation on implementing regulations regarding record keeping or compiling health statistics).

A continuing unmet need is attending to the health of workers in smaller companies. These companies tend to have more hazards because equipment and controls are often inadequate. They seldom, if ever, have a health professional on site. Attempts have been made by some communities to provide needed health protection services, but no sustained efforts exist. Community health nurses are in a position to accept this challenge and develop a system that will ensure ongoing service to this high-risk population.

Evidence-Based Practice and Educational Preparation

During the last two decades, a number of nursing education programs (primarily on the graduate level) have developed a specialty focus in occupational and environmental health. In addition, many continuing education programs provide occupational and environmental health nurses with updated information and skill training for identifying and assisting in the management of the physical, chemical, biologic, ergonomic, and psychosocial factors in the work environment that can affect worker health and safety. OHNs are the largest group of health professionals working in occupational health, and quality continuing education and more widespread graduate level educational programs are needed (McCullagh, 2012).

The National Institutes for Occupational Safety and Health (NIOSH), part of the Centers for Disease Control and Prevention (CDC), is an agency established by the Occupational Safety and Health Act of 1970 (Public Law

91-596). NIOSH is responsible for conducting research related to worker health and safety and for educating health and safety professionals to prepare them for evidence-based careers in occupational and environmental health and safety. NIOSH has established 18 university-based **Education Resource Centers (ERCs)** to fulfill that responsibility (NIOSH, 2015a). Many ERCs provide online courses, and scholarships are available.

Additionally, OHNs may become certified in this specialty field. The American Board for Occupational Health Nurses (ABOHN) is an independent nursing specialty certification board. Founded in 1972, ABOHN is an independent not-for-profit organization that sets professional standards and conducts occupational health nursing specialty certification. ABOHN is the sole certifying body for OHNs in the United States (ABOHN, 2014). This independent nursing specialty board has the stated purposes of (1) establishing standards and examinations for professional nurses in occupational health, (2) elevating and maintaining the quality of occupational health nursing services, (3) stimulating the development of improved educational standards and programs in the field of occupational health nursing, and (4) encouraging OHNs to continue their professional education (ABOHN, 2014).

The Effect of Work on Health

Workers in the United States generally spend more time at work than on any other activity except sleep. Thus, the work environment can have a significant impact on workers' health. Work can contribute to the well-being of employees, provided that they have good, supportive supervision (Modini et al., in press). However, the type of work that people engage in dictates the hazards they encounter. For instance, think about the work of hospital-based nurses. They encounter physical hazards, such as lifting patients in bed without mechanical lifting devices. There are biological hazards associated with blood and body fluids, as well as infectious diseases. Some nurses are at risk for chemical exposures, such as those associated with operating room gases or chemotherapy. Radiation hazards may exist when working with patients undergoing radiation therapy.

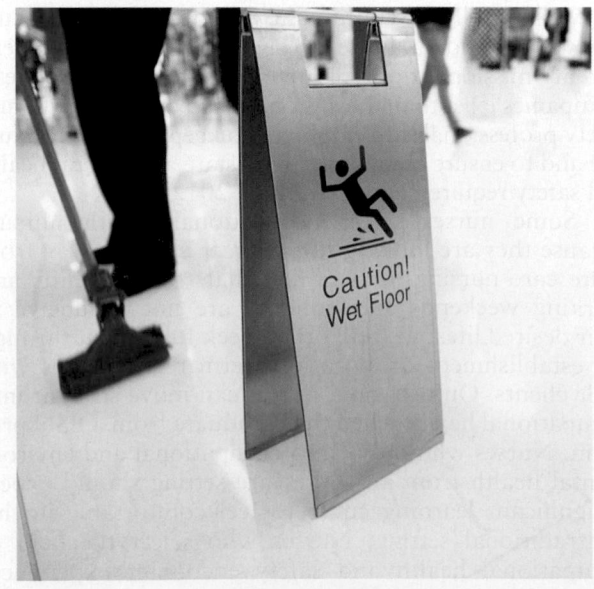

Hazardous substances can get into a person's body through inhalation, ingestion, or absorption or percutaneously. Although personal protective equipment (PPE) is available to workers, some may not use PPE consistently, or the equipment may not be entirely effective. Workers exposed to chemicals may not wash their hands sufficiently before eating or smoking, thus providing an opportunity for chemicals to get into their system through ingestion or inhalation.

Employees who work in awkward positions or who do repetitive tasks that use the same muscle groups are at risk for musculoskeletal disorders (MSDs). Stressing muscles and joints repeatedly can result in inflammation and pain and can lead to serious conditions that require physical therapy and/or surgery. Carpel tunnel syndrome is often associated with repetitive movements, like typing at a computer keyboard. Hegmann et al. (2016) conducted a large prospective cohort study to look at the relationship between carpel tunnel syndrome (or abnormal nerve conduction) prevalence and cardiovascular disease risk factors. They found that there was a strong significant relationship with odds ratios between 4.16 and 7.35 (for carpel tunnel and abnormal nerve conduction, respectively). It may be important to examine cardiovascular disease risk factors more closely among those employees with signs of nerve conduction problems.

Employees who compound a workplace exposure with off-work activities that use the same muscle groups in similar actions will accelerate or aggravate a problem. For instance, a mechanic may work on his own car in the evenings and on the weekend, so the muscles that are used every day never really get a chance to rest and recover. A research study examining the prevalence of musculoskeletal disorders (MSDs) among office workers found the highest number of MSDs noted in lower back (almost 50%) and neck (49%) areas (Piranveyseh et al., 2016). Researchers also looked at organizational factors, along with psychosocial and individual factors, and found that they were significantly associated with prevalence of MSDs.

Repeated exposure to loud noise can result in a high-frequency hearing loss (Council for Accreditation in Occupational Hearing Conservation, 2012; Kirchner et al., 2012). Such hearing losses are gradual; employees may not heed advice to wear hearing protection devices, which they may consider uncomfortable or annoying. High-frequency hearing loss diminishes an individual's ability to understand what others are saying, especially in a noisy environment such as a restaurant. Research shows that hearing losses can result in social isolation with resulting depression among the elderly (Ciorba, Bianchini, Pelucchi, & Pastore, 2012; Dawes et al., 2015; Mick, Kawachi, & Lin, 2014). A systematic review of research has demonstrated that repeated occupational exposure to loud noise is associated with increased levels of hypertension, and a smaller effect for noise and cardiovascular disease mortality was also noted (Skogstad et al., 2016).

Shift work, particularly rotating shift work, negatively impacts sleep and rest cycles (Takahashi, 2012). Insufficient sleep is associated with obesity and diabetes (Nakanishi-Minami, Kishida, Funahashi, & Shimomura,

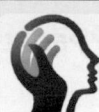

From the Case Files IV

The human resources director approaches the occupational health nurse regarding a situation he learned about from a manager in building 2. The manager reported that an employee has been acting out during the last 2 weeks, shouting at other employees. Additionally, the employee's work product has not met quality standards on several occasions during the same time period. Another employee told the manager that she heard the employee say that he was "fed up with everyone" and was going to "put an end to it."

1. What should the occupational health nurse do?
2. Who on the team should be involved with this situation?
3. What preventive measures could be put into place as part of the team's structure to be prepared to respond to situations like this?
4. What could you suggest as a primary intervention for these types of concerns?

2012). Low-paying jobs may drive workers to get a second or even a third job to make ends meet. Personal stressors or balancing work and family demands, plus employer expectations at work, can have an adverse effect on worker health (see from the Case Files IV). A systematic review of research on workplace mental health interventions found moderate evidence for effectiveness of these programs and their outcomes. Programs that included both physical and mental health interventions and multicomponent interventions had greater evidence of support (Wagner et al., 2016). Also, education to reduce the stigma associated with mental illness has also been shown to be effective in improving worker knowledge and promoting more supportive behavior toward peers with mental health issues (Hanisch et al., 2016).

Healthy People 2020

Occupational safety and health objectives are included in *Healthy People 2020*. The goal is to promote the health and safety of the U.S. workforce through prevention and early intervention. The intent of the 10 main objectives and eight sub-objectives is to prevent diseases, injuries, and deaths because of working conditions (USDHHS, Office of Disease Prevention and Health Promotion, 2016b). The occupational and environmental health nurse plays a crucial role in assisting businesses and employees to meet *Healthy People 2020* occupational safety and health objectives. See Display 31–10 *Healthy People 2020* Occupational Health and Safety Objectives.

Future Trends

The broad goal for occupational health professionals is to promote and maintain the highest level of physical, social, and emotional health for all workers. Occupational health and environmental nurses play a crucial role in making positive strides toward this goal

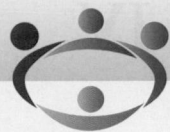

DISPLAY 31–10 *HEALTHY PEOPLE 2020* OCCUPATIONAL HEALTH AND SAFETY OBJECTIVES

OSH-1	Reduce deaths from work-related injuries.
OSH-1.1	Reduce deaths from work-related injuries in all industries.
OSH-1.2	Reduce deaths from work-related injuries in mining.
OSH-1.3	Reduce deaths from work-related injuries in construction.
OSH-1.4	Reduce deaths from work-related injuries in transportation/warehousing.
OSH-1.5	Reduce deaths from work-related injuries in agriculture, forestry, and fishing.
OSH-2	Reduce nonfatal work-related injuries.
OSH-2.1	Reduce work-related injuries in private sector industries resulting in medical treatment, lost time from work, or restricted work activity, as reported by employers.
OSH-2.2	Reduce work-related injuries treated in emergency departments (EDs).
OSH-2.3	Reduce work-related injuries among adolescent workers (15–19 yrs.).
OSH-3	Reduce the rate of injury and illness cases involving days away from work due to overexertion or repetitive motion.
OSH-4	Reduce pneumoconiosis deaths.
OSH-5	Reduce deaths from work-related homicides.
OSH-6	Reduce work-related assaults.
OSH-7	Reduce the proportion of persons who have elevated blood lead concentrations from work exposures.
OSH-8	Reduce occupational-related skin diseases/disorders among FT workers.
OSH-9	Increase the proportion of employees who have access to workplace programs that prevent or reduce employee stress.
OSH-10	Reduce new cases of work-related, noise-induced hearing loss.

Source: U.S. Department of Health and Human Services, Office of Disease Prevention and Health Promotion. (2016). *Healthy People 2020 topics and objectives: Occupational health and safety.* Retrieved from http://www.healthypeople.gov/2020/topics-objectives/topic/occupational-safety-and-health/objectives

by embracing evidence-based research and best practices. Presently, there is room for improvement toward fully realizing this goal. Productive working communities can be attained by the work of collaborative public health partnerships, private industry, occupational health professionals, government, establishments of higher learning, and the workforce joining together. Changes in U.S. businesses practices and the economic challenges experienced by workers over the last decade have required occupational and environmental health nursing practice to evolve. Downward economic trends, America's increasingly complex health care system, and health care reform will shape the future of occupational health nursing. *The Future of Nursing: Leading Change, Advancing Health* provides a comprehensive report focusing on future nursing practice and health care needs in the United States (IOM, 2011). The report notes three significant factors that will likely impact the future practice of OHNs:

1. Health care reform will significantly influence health care needs.
2. Meeting the increasing health care demand will require that nurses are allowed to practice to the full extent of their scope of practice.

3. Well-prepared nurses will need additional education and training to meet the demand for complexity and increasing volume.

Current occupational and environmental health nurse practice will continue to evolve to meet future needs. The focus is shifting from one-on-one health services to involving broader environmental, business, and research skills. The ACA has a focus on preventive care, and typically, a large portion of wellness activities are provided by RNs. Increases are projected in outpatient-focused care, and emerging models of care, such as the Primary Care Medical Home, are anticipated to influence the delivery of occupational health services. Occupational and environmental health nursing professionals will need extensive education in the areas of community health, social and psychological services, and general management in order to be successful (Spetz, 2014).

Educational training of OHNs has progressed in recent years. The need for nurses with advanced degrees will continue to grow to meet future demands (McCullagh, 2012). New strategies to expand funding, continuing education, certification, and educational opportunities to prepare the next generation of occupational health and environmental nurses remain a top priority. There are a wide range of skills and knowledge required to effectively provide comprehensive workplace wellness programs.

Standard OHN activities include the following:

1. Supervising care for emergencies and minor illnesses
2. Counseling employees about health risks
3. Following up with employees' workers' compensation claims
4. Performing periodic health assessments
5. Evaluating the health status of employees returning to work

Emerging occupational health nurse activities include the following:

1. Analyzing trends (health promotion, risk reduction, and health expenditures)
2. Developing programs suited to corporate needs
3. Recommending more efficient and cost-effective in-house health services
4. Determining cost-effective alternatives to health programs and services
5. Collaborating with others to identify problems and propose solutions

As we move further into the 21st century, occupational and environmental health nurses and management will share the goal of developing a healthy, productive, and profitable workplace. A healthy workplace consists of healthy and productive employees, and healthy employees mean lower health care costs. Lower costs result in an increased competitive edge and higher profits. Higher profits can make more resources available to support more programs and to improve employee health.

The occupational and environmental health nurse will particularly need skills in effective communication, leadership, change management, research, business acumen, and assertiveness. These tools will be crucial for effectively interpreting the OHN's role and promoting ideas. Success of programs developed by the OHN depends on establishment of positive working relationships with the other team members. Nurses involved in occupational health have a unique opportunity to help shape the health profile of the working population. An example of this type of effort was described in an article by Demko and Martin (2014), discussing the impact of mental health issues in the workplace. The OHN plays a significant role partnering with the employer and advocating on behalf of the employee. Early identification, coordinating treatment, possible absence from the workplace, and case management can all impact the employee's successful return to work. Occupational and environmental health nursing demands a great deal from the nurse. Individual needs in the workplace always compete for the nurse's time and take attention away from aggregate needs, often to the detriment of the latter. To maintain a proper focus on aggregate needs requires discipline and commitment—commitment based on a different mind-set and the realization that the health and productivity of workers are interrelated with the health of the community. The degree of the occupational nurse's influence depends on how the nurse defines the occupational and environmental health nurse role. Also, the nurse must be able to overcome the many obstacles found in the occupational setting, including restrictive company policies, misunderstanding of the nurse's role, and lack of time for innovative program development. The nurse's role in occupational health, therefore, varies considerably. It ranges from providing only emergency care for on-the-job injuries or illness to establishing comprehensive policies and programs covering health promotion, accident and disease prevention, and innovative care for disease and disability (Guzik, 2013).

NURSE ENTREPRENEUR IN COMMUNITY/PUBLIC HEALTH NURSING

As you have discovered throughout this chapter, the roles and responsibilities of nurses in the community often require skill with grant writing, agency and personnel management, collaboration both inter- and intraprofessionally, fiscal management, and agency promotion. The community/public health nurse often works within an agency or organization to address unmet needs in the community with the ultimate goal of enhancing service delivery. This is true for an FCN, a nurse in an NLHC, or an OHN. These positions are often nonexistent until the nurse is able to identify a need and take the necessary steps to start a stand-alone service or to develop a role within an existing agency. There is, however, a growing trend in nursing to seek a more independent practice in health care delivery and services through entrepreneurship. In 1986, Susan Hartley of the ANA posted a letter to the editor in the *American Journal of Public Health* requesting information on nurse entrepreneurs with the stated goal of "developing a list of nurse entrepreneurs as part of a continuing effort to describe the delivery of nursing services" and to "gather data and resource people to support lobbying efforts to achieve payment systems for nursing" (p. 1034). This brief request punctuates the growing recognition of the varied roles that nurses have and the impact of reimbursement on service delivery. As you think about your own career, can you envision yourself running a health care business, seeking a small business loan to start a venture, or having the courage to explore other professional options? Independent practice is not for everyone, and nurses are often socialized to view their role as working within a larger organization, a health department, a community clinic, and most often a hospital. At some point in your career, you may find yourself working with a nurse entrepreneur or becoming one yourself. The following discussion will give you a glimpse at the challenges and rewards of this journey.

Merriam-Webster (2015) defines an entrepreneur as "one who organizes, manages, and assumes the risks of a business or enterprise" (para. 1). By extension, an **entrepreneurial nurse** is one who is willing to take on that role within a health care or social context. Common examples of nurse entrepreneurs include legal consultants, forensic nurses, home health care agency owners, authors, and nurse consultants in a variety of areas. The National Nurses in Business Association (n.d.) offers membership and resources for those entrepreneurial nurses who are self-employed or small business owners. For the community/public health nurse, these and many other options offer the independence to provide services in perhaps a new and innovative way. For health care to continue to respond to the changing environment, the innovators are often the ones who have the courage to test those new methods. They may fail or fall short in those efforts, but they learn from both the success and challenges and are better positioned for a successful outcome.

Steps to Becoming a Nurse Entrepreneur

One of the first steps to becoming a nurse entrepreneur is to have an idea. It doesn't have to be a new idea or even a "big" idea, but it must address an unmet need within a community. Community/public health nurses are often the first to identify the challenges and needs within a community and to explore solutions. Very often, participation in professional organizations helps to identify health care issues that can be addressed by nurses. The common refrain—"why doesn't someone just (invent, build, provide, etc.)?"—can often be answered by a nurse. Nurses are problem solvers, and using the nursing process, they assess the situation, identify the problem, determine a course of action, and evaluate the results. This nursing skill can be leveraged for entrepreneurship (e.g., to start a new business venture, to develop a nonprofit agency, or to create educational tools for use by other health care professionals or the general public). Whatever the health care need, nurses can and do find the solutions. This was highlighted in a structured ethnographic study of nurse entrepreneurs in Canada (Wall, 2014). The study took place during a time of significant change and restructuring in Canada's health care system to reduce costs, and the participants chose to leave the system rather than remain in a "dysfunctional, demeaning, abusive, excessively demanding" situation (p. 516). Even though the nurses were engaged in a wide variety of activities (e.g., diabetic outreach business, alternative health care specialist, laser hair removal, occupational health nursing, corporate wellness consultant, project management, wound care specialist, health counseling), they had similar characteristics in common. They were different from other nurses in their quest for challenging experiences and need for change, as well as their tolerance for risk. They often thought "outside the box" and questioned routine hospital practices and procedures. The common strategies they used to effect their transformation into entrepreneurs included the following:

- Capitalizing on the enterprise culture (taking advantage of the instability of the system and increased market focus of Canadians)
- Used self-employment to re-establish services (some of their new businesses filled gaps in service caused by restructuring and reform, like diabetic foot care)
- Using entrepreneurship to broad the meaning of health care (they focused on caring and had a vision that extended beyond the hospital, like a corporate wellness business)
- Expanding professional jurisdiction (being self-employed nurses in Canada requires significant paperwork and oversight and many had to defend their scope of practice and jurisdiction)
- Preparing themselves for a preferred future (they used formal and informal methods to expand their education and training in preparation for their nontraditional roles)
- Reclaiming health services for nursing (project managers offered both business and nursing skills as opposed to solely nonnursing business degrees in administrative roles; diabetic foot care by RNs rather than currently employed lower paid, less skilled workers)
- Expanding the territory of nursing (laser hair removal was often done by dermatologists or estheticians; foot care could be provided by podiatrists)
- Building on the familiar (even though they were breaking new ground, they all relied on their nursing knowledge base and referred to professional standards and guidelines)
- Applying transferable nursing knowledge to new work (they used the nursing process to guide them in their various endeavors, such as holistic care plans, developing consulting guidelines; they used nursing's "people skills" like active listening and motivational interviewing in work with clients)
- Attending to professional standards (they used professional standards as a basis for developing policies and procedures in their new areas of nursing practice; they practiced within the guidelines of nursing's ethical principles; they sought out evidence-based research to guide their practices) (Wall, 2014, p. 517–521)

Even though they were excited with their new opportunities, they noted consequences (e.g., resistance from the public/other health care providers, regulatory issues/oversight). Some of them still consulted with large hospital systems and health care organizations, and hoped to influence change within those systems. Others found "a niche in the system" and responded to the needs of their consumers (p. 525). All of them sought to move beyond "profit-motivated and opportunistic" viewpoints of entrepreneurship and incorporate professionalism into their independent ventures (p. 526).

A past president of the NNBA, Patricia Bemis, offers a number of suggestions in the development of a business plan (2006). This plan is essential to starting a business, growing a business, and obtaining financial support. At the very minimum, the business plan should include the description of the business; marketing strategies; competitive analysis, design, and development plan; operations and management plan; and financial factors. Bemis also emphasizes the need for choosing a name and marketing format for promotional materials. She cautions that the "name of your business is not about creativity but is an integral component of your marketing strategy" (p. 1). The name should be easily spelled and pronounced, elicit a positive emotional response from the customer, and be short and to the point (see Display 31–11).

Opportunities

As the health care needs of the population demand newer, better, and less expensive solutions, nurse entrepreneurs are well positioned to address those needs. While there are many examples in your own communities of nurse entrepreneurship, the role of the community/public

---

DISPLAY 31–11 QUESTIONS TO CONSIDER: NURSE ENTREPRENEURSHIP

1. What are your goals (personal, business)? Do you have the determination and drive to succeed in business? Do you have the means to finance a business? Did you know that the average cost to start up a business is about $30,000 (Beesley, 2015)? What are your assets and potential monthly expenses, as well as your capital expenditures (e.g., property, vehicles, equipment)?

2. What are you interested in doing? Is there a market for this? Who is your target population? What industry trends may influence your success or failure? Who are your competitors?

3. Do you know someone with a successful business that can mentor you in this endeavor? Do you have friends and family who may be able to assist you at low or no cost (e.g., Web site design, business card design, accountant, attorney, business experts)?

4. Have you investigated the benefits of your local Chamber of Commerce, information/loan availability from the federal Small Business Administration (SBA), and any state or foundation grants/loans that may be available?

5. Do you know how to develop a business plan? Have you considered the type of business structure you may need (e.g., sole proprietorship, corporation)?

6. 6. Have you thought of a name for your business? How will you design your logo? What type of Web site design will you need? How will you decide on your business card and letterhead design? What types of brochures will you need?

7. How will you reach your target population (e.g., e-mails, Facebook, local advertising)?

Adapted from Leach-Baker, E. (2015). *Nurse incorporated: Turn your nursing passion into business profits. Game changing secrets every nurse starting and growing a business should know.* Raleigh, NC: Lulu Publishing Services. Beesley, C. (2015). *Blogs: Starting a business.* Retrieved from https://www.sba.gov/blogs/how-estimate-cost-starting-business-scratch

---

health nurse can serve as a strong base for meeting the health care challenges locally, nationally, and internationally. One example of a nurse entrepreneur is Nancy Dirubbo, a family nurse practitioner who first opened a New Hampshire women's health center in 1985. She offered patient-centered care and a patient-friendly environment that was designed with feedback from her patients. Always interested in new things, Dirubbo began investigating travel health and obtained certification in this specialty from the International Society of Travel Medicine. She also completed a DNP and decided to transition from the clinic to a new direct pay practice for those clients needing travel health services. Government programs and most private insurance companies do not cover travel health immunizations and visits. She began offering part-time services in the same building as her clinic, and developed clientele through word of mouth. She is actively engaged in CDC and WHO LISTSERVS and has not needed to advertise widely. She has a Web site (http://travelhealthnh.com), and is certified as a yellow fever center by the CDC. She planned for 3 to 5 years as a start-up period for her new business, and she offers comprehensive visits with patients, along with evidence-based education and immunizations. She discusses food safety and potential areas for risk and gives patients a take-home booklet with detailed information about their destination and the education/immunizations she provided during their visit (Clayton, 2015). See Perspectives: Nurse Entrepreneur.

Although the previous example seems unique, we are reminded that early nurses were often self-employed entrepreneurs. Whelan (2012) examined the history of private duty nursing in the United States and noted that most nurses in the early part of the 20th century were independent contractors serving private pay patients in their homes. At that time, hospital-based schools of nursing were most common, and hospitals took advantage of the free labor provided by student nurses who spent most of their time at the hospital. They rarely hired new graduates from these programs, so these new graduates had to find other means of making a living. They sought out patients in need of nursing services and provided this in patients' homes. At this time, most people wanted to be cared for at home and very few used hospitals. Private duty nurses lived in patient homes, working 24/7 until the illness was resolved or the patient died. In order to simplify this process, some enterprising nurses organized an infrastructure of private duty registries. Nurses and patients/families or physicians would contact the agencies (like an employment service), and connections were made for nursing services. The nurses paid a fee to the agency, and the family paid the nurse directly. In some instances, registries were able to place nurses in hospitals to care for patients or to fill an open position there. A few of them also offered sick room supplies and provided special diets. Most registries were nurse-run and nurse-owned, but some were affiliated with hospitals and professional nursing organizations. In 1915, an ANA committee located 40 central registries; in 1924, 75 registries were located (Whelan, 2012). New York City and Chicago had very large central registries. The New York registry closed during the Depression, and the Chicago registry, with innovative leadership and programs, remained open until 1980. By 1949, private duty nurses constituted only about 20% of the total U.S. nurse population. However, even today, hospitals rely on short-term, traveling nurses from various agencies, much like the per diem nurses during the middle decades of the 20th century to fill critical vacancies in acute care settings.

Gilliss (2011) notes that social entrepreneurship works toward good health outcomes for all, without

PERSPECTIVES
NURSE ENTREPRENEUR

As a newly graduated nurse practitioner, I was excited to step into the role in a small family practice clinic. I worked alongside a family physician who owned the clinic. The two of us worked together to establish office policies and procedures and to provide the best care for our patients. We took pride in the product we delivered because we made decisions that directly impacted patient care.

A few years later, a corporation bought out that small family practice clinic. This corporation had previously been a specialty clinic, but was expanding to include family practice clinics. Upon the sale of the clinic, the administrative decisions were made by people not only unfamiliar with our patients but unfamiliar with family medicine. They determined how many patients I should see, how long I should spend with each patient, and the services I should or should not provide. Nameless faces on the other end of phone trees addressed my patients' concerns, as the corporation centralized the call centers under the direction of corporate management.

I became frustrated with the dictates of others and the negative impact it had on my patients. This frustration led to my desire to make a change. I could not change the entire system, nor could I change medical staff, administrators, or the corporation. But, I could change my reality and sphere of influence and in turn help the individual patient. In seeking change, I looked to fill a need. I looked to find my niche.

My first entrepreneurial experience came when an owner of a manufacturing plant approached me about creating and running an on-site clinic for his employees. Together, the company owner and I talked about our vision of the clinic. I created a model where I could run the clinic by myself, with one medical assistant. Care was free to employees, and insurance companies were not involved. The owner of the manufacturing plant paid the overhead. This was a model unlike any other on-site medical clinic in the area.

A few years after starting the on-site clinic, I saw the lack of access my patients had to mental health care in my state. Again, I could not fix the entire problem or the broken system, but I could change my sphere of influence. There was a serious shortage of psychiatrists to manage psych meds, so I started a mental health clinic to provide better access to those in my community. This clinic, run by family practice nurse practitioners, provides medication management and psychotherapy to those without access to psychiatry. I rent space to psychologists who provide counseling, and I work with two other experienced NPs to manage medications and make referrals.

Both clinics I own and run are not traditional health care models. I became a nurse practitioner to help others and make a difference in the world. In order to truly make a difference, I assessed the needs in my community and did what I could to fill the gaps.

Kelly Wosnik, DNP, NP-C

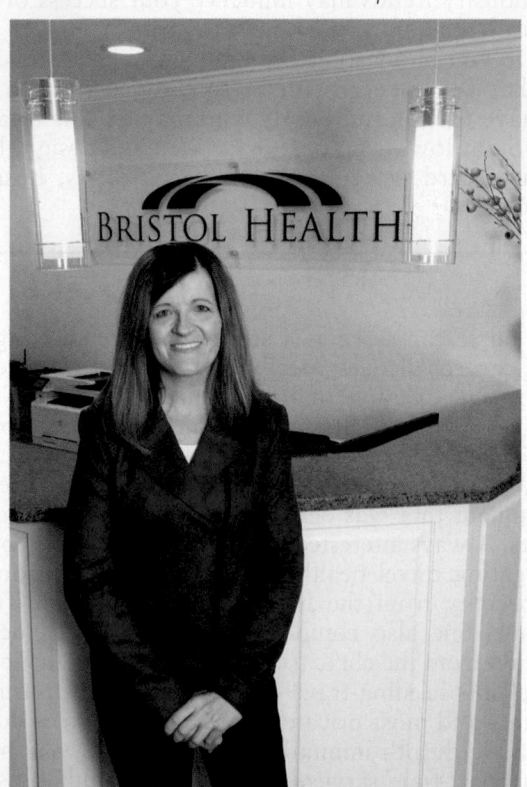

Can you think of something that may frustrate you and see where you might provide a much-needed service, like this nurse entrepreneur?

necessarily a profit motive, and that it brings us back to our nursing roots (e.g., Lillian Wald, Florence Nightingale). With health care reform, social entrepreneurship, as well as opportunities to implement innovative programs within public health and other agencies—"intrapreneurship"—can also flourish (Wilson et al., 2012). What is needed are nurses who enjoy a challenge and are willing to take risks in order to provide needed services and improve patient outcomes.

The opportunities are limitless for nurse entrepreneurship; the only missing piece is the nurse willing to take that leap, come up with an idea, explore the options, create a business plan, garner funding, and make a difference. Community/public health nurses are uniquely qualified to address the ever-growing challenges in our communities. As opportunities in one area of nursing practice recede, other avenues open up; the trick is to recognize those opportunities when they present.

SUMMARY

Healthy People 2020 document guides both public and private sector nursing practice well into the next decade. Community health nurses have a number of options available to them as they seek to address the myriad health issues facing our communities. For many, opportunities may present to assume roles in a variety of nontraditional settings, including NLHCs, faith community nursing, occupational and environmental health nursing, and nurse entrepreneurship. All four roles offer the community health nurse the opportunity to address health disparities in their communities, promote healthy lifestyles, and improve the overall health and well-being of their respective populations.

NLHCs represent a growing movement of health centers that have emerged as vital safety-net providers in America's contemporary health care delivery system. Various nursing center models exist and are located in MUA in urban and rural communities. Interdisciplinary teams of advanced practice nurses, social workers, substance abuse counselors, community health outreach workers, and students from varied disciplines provide services that generally focus on primary and secondary prevention strategies. Lundeen's Comprehensive Community-Based Primary Health Care Model demonstrates how NLHCs are distinct from public health agencies and medical care facilities. Funding sources for NLHCs include reimbursement from various organizations, sliding scale fees, grants, contracts, foundation support, and private support via gifts. Sustainability is an ongoing challenge in all NLHC models. An international organization to strengthen the capacity, growth, and development of NLHCs is the NNCC. NLHCs identify, develop, and share best practices. Nurse leaders and staff from NLHCs engage in sociopolitical activities to raise awareness of the outcomes generated by the nursing center model. These activities are implemented to raise awareness of the role of NLHCs in the health care system and to promote sustainability of the centers. Undergraduate and graduate students from various disciplines engage in all aspects of NLHC activities and augment the interdisciplinary team.

FCNs practice community nursing within a unique setting—a faith community. An FCN may provide services to a single faith community or may coordinate services for multiple communities. The FCN addresses the physical, social, emotional, mental, and spiritual needs of the faith community through the roles of health educator, health counselor, referral agent, advocate, developer of support groups, coordinator of volunteers, and integrator of faith and health.

Occupational and environmental health nursing applies the philosophy and skills of nursing, community, and environmental health to protect and promote the health of people in their workplaces. The occupational and environmental health nurse's role is evolving as business becomes more competitive and health care reform has been implemented. That expanded role will include analyzing current trends, recommending more cost-effective and innovative in-house health services, and collaborating with other members of the multidisciplinary occupational health team, including management, to develop appropriate programs. Occupational and environmental health nurses help companies remain competitive by promoting health and well-being in worker populations.

The nurse entrepreneur is not a new concept. Nurses have traditionally worked in private duty, as well as within existing agencies (hospitals, clinics, or health departments), yet many have sought the autonomy of providing health-related services independently, by starting a new business venture. As community/public health nurses gain experience and confidence in starting and developing health care programs, those same skills can be utilized to identify unmet community needs, develop a business plan, seek funding sources, and start an independent business. The FCN may market his services to a number of small faith communities, an NLHC may, in addition to providing grant-based services, begin marketing services to employees of local businesses, the OHN may recognize a growing need for health education materials that could be purchased by other industries, or the nurse may leverage their specially area skills to publish educational materials or start a nonprofit agency to meet community needs. The opportunities for nurse entrepreneurship are a growing and much needed area for community/public health nurses to explore.

Each of these professional practice areas provides a unique opportunity for community health nursing practice. Escalating health care costs, increasing numbers of uninsured and underinsured, and the many gaps in services experienced by so many in our communities present an unprecedented opportunity for community health nurses. The many unmet needs in our communities can be addressed but only if there are nurses willing to take the "road less traveled" as did Lillian Wald and the other pioneers of nursing. As you ponder your options for practice, consider the challenges and the many benefits of these and the many other practice areas in your community. Perhaps you cannot envision yourself in this type of service at this point in your career. A time may come, however, when you are afforded the chance to participate in your own faith community health education efforts—or refer a client to a NLHC—or possibly collaborate with an occupational and environmental health nurse to address an emerging health issue in your community. You may even find that starting your own business or nonprofit agency affords you the independence and challenge you seek in your career.

ACTIVITIES TO PROMOTE CRITICAL THINKING

1. You are practicing as a newly hired nurse in an NLHC. What assessments would you conduct to determine the needs for the local community that surrounds the clinic? What sources of data (qualitative and quantitative) would be useful to you during your assessment?
2. Based upon your findings in the previous question, what public policy issues are apparent in this community? How could you, as a nurse working in this NLHC, impact public policy in the future? What key legislators would you contact? How would you accomplish this?
3. Locate an NLHC in your community. Interview a public health nurse or a nurse practitioner employed there. Ask the nurse to describe the type of NLHC model he/she works in. Ask the nurse about **Best Practices** performed in his/her role. If you cannot locate an NLHC in your local community, search online via the National Nursing Centers Consortium's Web site, and e-mail the nurse listed as the contact person and ask him/her the questions found above. Alternately, you may want to search for an FQHC.
4. This chapter covers the role of the parish or faith community nurse (FCN). Search for information about this area of community health nursing in your community. Do you know an FCN? If so, plan to observe his or her practice for a few hours and explore what the role entails in this faith community.
5. Contact an FCN in your area and arrange to interview or shadow the nurse. Explore the services offered by FCNs in your area. Identify the knowledge and skills needed to function effectively in the role. Discuss the process the nurse used to establish his or her FCN practice. Determine if there is a local or regional professional association for FCNs in your area.
6. Conduct a literature search to discover health programs that have been developed and used by faith communities to address the leading health indicators identified in *Healthy People 2020*. What leading indicators have the most evidence of effective health programs? Which indicators have the least evidence of effective health programs? Evaluate which health program could be adapted for use in your community.
7. This chapter covers the role of the occupational and environmental health nurse. Search for information about this specialty area of nursing in your community. Do you know an occupational health nurse? If so, plan to observe his or her practice for a few hours and explore what the role entails in this organization.
8. Think about workers whom you see every day (grocery store checkers, hairdressers, firefighters, landscapers, utility linemen, etc.). What hazards are they exposed to? What are the potential health problems that they may have due to their work? What primary prevention efforts would be suitable for those workers?

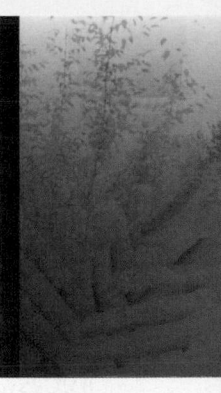

9. Select an employer close to where you live or go to school. The employer may be a municipal government, a school system, or a for-profit company. If you were to provide occupational health nursing services to the workers of that employer, what information would be important to obtain before providing services? How would you obtain that information? How would you identify risks to that population? What other health care or other professionals would you include in your team approach to health care at this site?

10. Think about your clinical experiences in community/public health nursing. Are their unmet needs in the community that could be addressed through a nurse-led business? What elements would you include in a business plan? Write a one-paragraph statement that you could present in obtaining a small business loan. Locate a nurse entrepreneur and discuss the challenges they met in starting their business; how were those addressed?

REFERENCES

Agency for Healthcare Research and Quality. (n.d.). *Five major steps to intervention*. Rockville, MD: U.S. Public Health Service. Retrieved from http://www.ahrq.gov/clinic/tobacco/5steps.htm

American Association of Occupational Health Nurses (AAOHN). (2012). *The occupational and environmental health nursing profession*. Retrieved from www.aaohninformationsheet_rev022012.pdf

American Board for Occupational Health Nurses (ABOHN). (2012). *Frequently asked questions*. Retrieved from http://www.abohn.org/faq.cfm

American Board for Occupational Health Nurses (ABOHN). (2014). *Who we are and what we do*. Retrieved from http://www.abohn.org/

American Hospital Association. (2012). *Engaging health care users: A framework for healthy individuals and communities*. Retrieved from http://www.aha.org/research/cor/content/engaging_health_care_users.pdf

American Nurses Association (ANA)/Health Ministries Association (HMA). (1998). *The scope and standards of parish nursing practice*. Washington, DC: American Nurses Publishing.

American Nurses Association (ANA)/Health Ministries Association (HMA). (2005). *Faith community nursing: Scope and standards of practice*. Silver Spring, MD: Nursesbooks.org.

American Nurses Association (ANA)/Health Ministries Association (HMA). (2012). *Faith community nursing: Scope and standards of practice* (2nd ed.). Silver Spring, MD: Nursesbooks.org.

Americans with Disabilities Act (ADA). (2000). *A guide for persons with disabilities seeking employment*. Retrieved from http://www.ada.gov/workta.htm

Anaebere, A. K., & DeLilly, C. R. (2012). Faith community nursing: Supporting mental health during life transitions. *Issues in Mental Health Nursing, 33*(5), 337–339.

Archibald, C. M., & Newman, D. (2015). Pilot testing HIV prevention in an Afro Caribbean faith-based community. *ABNF Journal, 26*(2), 43–49.

Baltic, R. D., Weier, R. C., Katz, M. L., Kennedy, S. K., Lengerich, E. J., Lesko, S. M., ... Paskett, E. D. (2015). Study design, intervention, and baseline characteristics of a group randomized trial involving faith-based healthy eating and physical activity intervention (Walk by Faith) to reduce weight and cancer risk among overweight and obese Appalachian adults. *Contemporary Clinical Trials, 44*, 1–10.

Barkauskas, V., Pohl, J., Tanner, C., Onifade, T., & Pilon, B. (2011). Quality of care in nurse-managed health centers. *Nursing Administration Quarterly, 35*(1), 34–43. doi: 10.1097/NAQ.0b013e3182032165.

Bemis, P. A. (2006). Nurse entrepreneur: Devise and implement a great game plan. *Alternative Journal of Nursing, 11*, 1–5.

Burgel, B. J., & Childre, F. (2012). The occupational health nurse as the trusted clinician in the 21st century. *Workplace Health & Safety, 60*(4), 143–150. doi: http://dx.doi.org/10.3928/21650799-20120328-24.

Caplan, S., & Cordero, C. (2015). Development of faith-based mental health literacy program to improve treatment engagement among Caribbean Latinos in the Northeastern United States of America. *International Quarterly of Community Health Education, 35*(3), 199–214.

Ciorba, A., Bianchini, C., Pelucchi, S., & Pastore, A. (2012). The impact of hearing loss on the quality of life of elderly adults. *Clinical Interventions in Aging, 7*, 159–163. doi: 10.2147/CIA.S26059.

Clayton, H. (2015). Change on the horizon. *Nursing News: New Hampshire, 39*(3), 10.

Cockroft, M. C. (2012). When the topic is sex: Facilitating parent child communication in the faith community. *Journal of Christian Nursing, 29*(3), 152–155.

Cooklin, A., Joss, N., Husser, E., & Oldenburg, B. (2016). Integrated approaches to occupational health and safety: A systematic review. *American Journal of Health Promotion*. doi: 10.4278/ajhp.141027-LIT-542.

Cooper, K. C., King, M. A., & Sarpong, D. F. (2015). Tipping the scales on obesity: Church-based health promotion for African American women. *Journal of Christian Nursing, 32*(1), 41–45.

Council for Accreditation in Occupational Hearing Conservation. (2011). Retrieved from http://www.caohc.org/index.php

Cutler, I. (2002). *End games: The challenge of sustainability*. Baltimore, MD: Annie E. Casey Foundation.

Dandridge, R. (2014). Faith community/parish nursing literature: Exciting interventions, unclear outcomes. *Journal of Christian Nursing, 31*(3), 100–106.

Dawes, P., Emsley, R., Cruickshanks, K. J., Moore, D. R., Fortnum, H., Edmondson-Jones, M., & Munro, K. J. (2015). Hearing loss and cognition: The role of hearing aids, social isolation and depression. *PLoS One, 10*(3), E0119616. doi: 10.1371/journal.pone.0119616.

Demko, M., & Martin, P. (2014). The added value an occupational health nurse brings to an organization. *Journal: The Official Publication of the Ontario Occupational Health Nurses Association, 33*(2), 13.

Dombrowski, J. J., Snelling, A. M., & Kalicki, M. (2014). Health promotion overview: Evidence-based strategies for occupational health practice. *Workplace Health & Safety, 62*(8), 342–349.

Draper, E., Ladou, J., & Tennenhouse, D. (2011). Occupational health nursing and the quest for professional authority. *NEW SOLUTIONS: A Journal of Environmental and Occupational Health Policy, 21*(1), 57–88. doi: 10.2190/NS.21.1.

du Plessis, E., Koen, M. P., & Bester, P. (2013). Exploring home visits in a faith community as a service-learning opportunity. *Nurse Education Today, 33*(8), 766–771.

Duquesne University School of Nursing. (2015). *Community-based health and wellness center for older adults*. Retrieved from http://www.duq.edu/academics/schools/nursing/about-the-school/school-of-nursing-centers/community-based-health-and-wellness-center-for-older-adults

Elwell, J. (2015). Practical health promotion: Weekly health tips for the faith community. *Journal of Christian Nursing, 32*(3), 174–178.

Ely, L. T. (2015). Nurse-managed clinics: Barriers and benefits toward financial sustainability when integrating primary care and mental health. *Nursing Economics, 33*(4), 193–202.

Ellis, J. L., & Morzinski, J. A. (2013). Training lay volunteers to promote health in central-city African American churches. *Journal of Christian Nursing, 30*(2), 112–116.

Evans, A. R. (2011). *Is god still at the bedside? The medical, ethical, and pastoral issues of death and dying*. Grand Rapids, MI: Eerdmans Publishing Co.

Gilliss, C. L. (2011). The nurse as social entrepreneur: Revisiting our roots and raising our voices. *Nursing Outlook, 59*, 256–257.

Graeve, C., McGovern, P., Nachreiner, N., & Ayers, L. (2014). Establishing the value of occupational health nurses' contributions to worker health and safety: A pilot test of a user-friendly estimation tool. *Workplace Health & Safety, 62*(1), 36–41. doi: http://dx.doi.org/10.3928/21650799-20131220-06.

Guidotti, T. L., Arnold, S., Lukcso, D. G., Green-McKenzie, J., Bender, J., Rothstein, M. A., ... Stecklow, M. (2013). *Occupational health services: A practical approach.* (2nd ed.). New York, NY: Routledge.

Guzik, A. (2013). *Essentials for occupational health nursing.* Ames, IA: Wiley-Blackwell.

Hanisch, S. E., Twomey, C. D., Szeto, A. C., Birner, U. W., Nowak, D., & Sabariego, C. (2016). The effectiveness of interventions targeting the stigma of mental illness at the workplace: A systematic review. *BMC Psychiatry, 16*(1), 1.

Hansen-Turton, T. (2012). *Nurse-managed health clinics provide badly needed primary care: But without funding, they and their patients are at risk.* Retrieved from http://www.rwjf.org/en/culture-of-health/2012/01/nurse-managed-health-clinics-provided-badly-needed-primary-carebut-without-funding-they-and-their-patients-are-at-risk.html

Hansen-Turton, T., Miller, M. E., & Greiner, P. (2009). *Nurse-managed wellness centers: Developing and maintaining your center. A National Nursing Center Consortium guide and toolkit.* New York, NY: Springer Publishing.

Hansen-Turton, T., Sherman, S. & King, E. (2015). *Nurse-led health clinics: Operations, policy and opportunities.* New York, NY: Springer.

Hansen-Turton, T., Valdez, B., Ware, J. & King, E. (2015b). Anatomy of a nurse-led clinic: An introduction to the model of care. In T. Hansen-Turton, S. Sherman, & E. King, *Nurse-led health clinics: Operations, policy and opportunities* (pp. 3–10). New York, NY: Springer, Chapter 1.

Harber, P., Alongi, G., & Su, J. (2014). Professional activities of experienced occupational health nurses. *Workplace Health & Safety, 62*(6), 233–242.

Hartley, S. (1986). Letters to the editor: Data requested on RN entrepreneurs. *American Journal of Public Health, 76*(8), 1034.

Hayman K. (2012). Teleclasses: Improve belonging, vitality, and health in church homebound. *Journal of Christian Nursing, 29*(4), 243–245.

Health Ministries Association (HMA). (2010). *About HMA.* Retrieved from http://www.hmassoc.org/about_us.php.

Health Resources and Services Administration. (2013). *Medicare part D and safety net providers.* Retrieved from http://www.hrsa.gov/medicare/modelcontract.htm

Hegmann, K. T., Thiese, M. S., Kapellusch, J., Merryweather, A. S., Bao, S., Silverstein, B., ... Drury, D. L. (2016). Association between cardiovascular risk factors and carpal tunnel syndrome in pooled occupational cohorts. *Journal of Occupational and Environmental Medicine, 58*(1), 87–93.

Hickman, J. S. (2011). *Fast facts for the faith community nurse: Implementing FCN/parish nursing in a nutshell.* New York, NY: Springer Publishing.

Institute of Medicine (IOM). (2000). *America's healthcare safety net: Intact but endangered.* Washington, DC: National Academies Press.

Institute of Medicine (IOM). (2011). *The future of nursing: Leading change, advancing health.* Washington, DC: National Academies Press.

International Parish Nursing Resource Center (IPNRC). (n.d.). *What Is the International Parish Nursing Resource Center?* Retrieved from http://www.churchhealthcenter.org/fcnhome

Jakimowicz, S., Stirling, C., & Duddle, M. (2015). An investigation of factors that impact patients' subjective experience of nurse-led clinics: A qualitative systematic review. *Journal of Clinical Nursing, 24*(1/2), 19–33.

Judd, D., & Sitzman, K. (2014). *A history of American nursing: Trends and eras* (2nd ed.). Burlington, MA: Jones & Bartlett Learning.

Kamau, C., Medisauskaite, A., & Lopes, B. (2015). Inductions buffer nurses' job stress, health, and organizational commitment. *Archives of Environmental & Occupational Health, 70*(6), 305–308.

Kinsey, K., & Miller, M. E. (2016). The nursing center: A model for nursing practice in the community. In M. Stanhope & J. Lancaster (Eds.), *Public health nursing: Population-centered health care in the community* (9th ed., pp. 455–475). St. Louis, MO: Elsevier.

Kirchner, L., Evenson, E., Dobie, R., Rabinowitz, P., Crawford, J., Kopke, R., & Hudson, T. (2012). *Occupational noise-induced hearing loss.* Retrieved from http://www.caohc.org/pdfs/ACOEM%20policies%20and%20position.pdf

Kowlessar, N. M., Goetzel, R. Z., Carls, G. S., Tabrizi, M. J., & Guindon, A. (2011). The relationship between 11 health risks and medical and productivity costs for a large employer. *Journal of Occupational and Environmental Medicine, 53*(5), 468–477.

Lundeen, S. (2005). *Lundeen's comprehensive community-based primary health care model.* Milwaukee, WI: Milwaukee College of Nursing.

Mattaliano, R. (2013). On-site Health Clinics = Increased Productivity. *Professional Case Management, 18*(5), 266–267. doi: 10.1097/NCM.0b013e31829e5711.

McCaskill, S. P., Schwartz, L. A., Derouin, A. L., & Pegram, A. H. (2014). Effectiveness of an on-site health clinic at a self-insured university: A cost-benefit analysis. *Workplace Health & Safety, 62*(4), 162–169. doi: 10.3928/21650799-20140305-01.

McCullagh, M. C. (2012). Occupational health nursing education for the 21st century. *Workplace Health & Safety, 60*(4), 167–176.

Melnyk, B. M., & Fineout-Overholt, E. (2014). *Evidence-based practice in nursing and healthcare: A guide to best practice* (3rd ed.). Philadelphia, PA: Lippincott Williams & Wilkins.

Merriam-Webster Online Dictionary. (2015). Entrepreneur. Retrieved from http://www.merriam-webster.com/dictionary/entrepreneur

Merrill R. M., Aldana, S. G., Pope, J. E., Anderson, D. R., Coberley, C. R., Grossmeier, J. J., Whitmer, R. W. (2013). HERO Research Study Subcommittee. Self-rated job performance and absenteeism according to employee engagement, health behaviors, and physical health. *Journal of Occupational and Environmental Medicine, 55*(1), 10–18.

Mick, P., Kawachi, I., & Lin, F. R. (2014). The association between hearing loss and social isolation in older adults. *Otolaryngology–Head and Neck Surgery, 150*(3), 378–384. doi: 10.1177/0194599813518021.

Miller, C. (2011). An integrated approach to worker self-management and health outcomes: Chronic conditions, evidence-based practice, and health coaching. *AAOHN Journal, 59*(11), 491–501.

Miller, S., & Carson, S. (2010). A documentation approach for faith community nursing. *Creative Nursing, 16*(3), 122–131.

Miller, M. E., & Mest, C. (n.d.). *My eyes were blind but now I see: Reflections from graduate nursing students about community service and learning and application to graduate nursing education.* Unpublished manuscript.

Modini, M., Joyce, S., Mykletun, A., Christensen, H., Bryant, B. A., Mitchell, P. B., & Harvey, S. B. (2016). The mental health benefits of employment: Results of a systematic meta-review. *Australasian Psychiatry, 24*(4), 331–336.

Moore, P. & Moore, R. (Eds.). (2014). *Fundamentals of Occupational and Environmental Health Nursing: AAOHN Core Curriculum* (4th ed.). Pensacola, FL: AAOHN.

Nakanishi-Minami, T., Kishida, K., Funahashi, T., & Shimomura, I. (2012). Sleep-wake cycle irregularities in type 2 diabetics. *Diabetology and Metabolic Syndrome, 4*(1), 18. doi: 10.1186/1758-5996-4-18.

National Institute for Occupational Safety and Health (NIOSH). (2015a). *NIOSH Education and Research Centers (ERCs).* Retrieved from http://www.cdc.gov/niosh/oep/erclist.html

National Institute for Occupational Safety and Health (NIOSH). (2015b). *What is total worker health?* Retrieved from http://www.cdc.gov/niosh/twh/totalhealth.html

National Institutes of Health, Office of Extramural Research. (2013). *Glossary and acronym list.* Retrieved from http://grants.nih.gov/grants/glossary.htm

National Nurses in Business Association. (n.d.). *About the NNBA.* Retrieved from https://nnbanow.com

National Nursing Centers Consortium (NNCC). (2014). *About nurse-managed care.* Retrieved from http://www.nncc.us/about-nurse-managed-care

National Safety Council. (2013). Injury facts. Retrieved from http://www.mhi.org/downloads/industrygroups/ease/technicalpapers/2013-National-Safety-Council-Injury-Facts.pdf

Nurse-Managed Health Clinic Investment Act of 2009, S.B. 1104/H.R. 2754, 111th Congress (2009).

Oakley, J., & Hoebeke, R. (2014). I choose health (Elijo Salud): Impacting youth through parish nursing. *Journal of Christian Nursing, 31*(4), 252–257.

Occupational Safety and Health Act (OSHA). (1970). *Occupational noise exposure.* Retrieved from http://osha.gov/pls/oshaweb/

owasrch.search_form?p_doc_type=STANDARDS&p_toc_level=1&p_keyvalue=1910

Pappas-Rogich, M. (2012). Faith community nurses: Protecting our elders through immunizations. *Journal of Christian Nursing, 29*(4), 232–237.

Pappas-Rogich, M., & King, M. (2014). Faith community nursing: Supporting Healthy People 2020 initiatives. *Journal of Christian Nursing, 31*(4), 228–234.

Pilon, B., & Hansen-Turton, T. (2015). Nurse-managed health centers and sustainability. In T. Hansen-Turton, S. Sherman, & E. King (Eds.), *Nurse-led health clinics: Operations, policy and opportunities* (pp. 67–82). New York, NY: Springer.

Piranveyseh, P., Motamedzade, M., Osatuke, K., Mohammadfam, I., Moghimbeigi, A., Soltanzadeh, A., & Mohammadi, H. (2016). Association between psychosocial, organization, and personal factors and prevalence of musculoskeletal disorder in office workers. *International Journal of Occupational Safety and Ergonomics, 13,* 1–19.

Pohl, J. M., Tanner, C., Pilon, B., & Benkert, R. (2011). Comparison of nurse managed health centers with federally qualified health centers as safety net providers. *Policy, Politics & Nursing Practice, 12*(2), 90–99.

Presmanes, G. T. (2015). Workers' compensation, return to work, and use of light duty work offers: An overview of programs throughout the United States. *Tort Trial & Insurance Practice Law Journal, 50*(3), 781–808.

Reilly, J. R., Hovarter, R., Mrochek, T., Mittelstadt-Lock, K., Schmitz, S., Nett, S., ... Behm, L. (2011). Spread the word, not the germs: A toolkit for faith communities. *Journal of Christian Nursing, 28*(4), 205–211.

Resick, L., Miller, M. E., & Leonardo, M. E. (2015). Overview of nurse-managed wellness centers and wellness programs integrated into nurse-managed primary care clinics. In T. Hansen-Turton, S. Sherman, & E. King (Eds.), *Nurse-led health clinics: Operations, policy and opportunities* (pp. 179–191). New York, NY: Springer.

Robert Wood Johnson Foundation (RWJF). (2008). *Health care spending as percentage of GDP.* Retrieved from http://www.rwjf.org/pr/product.jsp?id=45110

Sabo, S., de Zapien, J., Teuifel-Shone, N., Rosales, C., Bergsma, L., & Taren, D. (2015). Service learning: A vehicle for building health equity and eliminating health disparities. *American Journal of Public Health, 105*(S1), S38-S43.

Sattin, R. W., Williams, L. B., Dias, J., Garvin, J. T., Marion, L., Joshua, T. V., ... Narayan, K. M. (2016). Community trial of a faith-based lifestyle intervention to prevent diabetes among African-Americans. *Journal of Community Health, 41*(1), 87–96.

Schadewaldt, V., & Schultz, T. (2011). Nurse-led clinics as an effective service for cardiac patients: Results from a systematic review. *International Journal of Evidence-Based Healthcare, 9*(3), 199–214.

Sheehan, A., Austin, S. A., Brennan-Jordan, N., Frenn, D., Kelman, G., & Scotti, D. (2013). Defy diabetes! Impact on faith community/parish nurses teaching healthy living classes. *Journal of Christian Nursing, 30*(4), 244–247.

Shillam, C. R., Orton, V. J., Waring, D., & Madsen, S. (2013). Faith community nurses and brown bag events help older adults manage meds. *Journal of Christian Nursing, 30*(2), 90–96.

Singh, S. P., Brown, L., Winsper, C., Gajwani, R., Islam, Z., Jasani, R., ... Birchwood, M. (2015). Ethnicity and pathways to care during first episode psychosis: The role of cultural illness attributions. *BMC Psychiatry, 15*(1), 287. doi: 10.1186/s12888-015-0665-9.

Skogstad, M., Johannessen, H. A., Tynes, T., Mehllum, I. S., Nordby, K. C., & Lie, A. (2016). Systematic review of the cardiovascular effects of occupational noise. *Occupational Medicine, 66*(1), 10–16.

Spetz, J. (2014). How will health reform affect demand for RNs? *Nursing Economics, 32*(1), 42–44.

Stewart, J. M., Thompson, K., & Rogers, C. (2015). African American church-based HIV testing and linkage to care: Assets, challenges and needs. *Culture, Health & Sexuality, 11,* 1–13.

Sutton, M. Y., Lasswell, S. M., Lanier, Y., & Miller, K. S. (2014). Impact of parent-child communication interventions on sex behaviors and cognitive outcomes for black/African-American and Hispanic/Latino youth: A systematic review. *Journal of Adolescent Health, 54*(4), 369–384.

Takahashi, M. (2012). Prioritizing sleep for healthy work schedules. *Journal of Physiological Anthropology, 31*(1), 1–9. doi: 10.1186/1880-6805-31-6.

Thompson, M. (2012). Professional autonomy of occupational health nurses in the United States. *Workplace Health & Safety, 60*(4), 159–165. doi: 10.3928/21650799-20120328-23.

Thompson, M., & Wachs, J., (2012). Occupational health nursing in the United States. *Workplace Health & Safety, 60*(3), 127–133. doi: 10.3928/21650799-20120227-89.

U.S. Department of Health and Human Services (USDHHS), Centers for Medicare and Medicaid Services (CMS). (2011). *Federally Qualified Health Center: Rural health fact sheet series.* Retrieved from http://www.cms.gov/MLNProducts/downloads/fqhcfactsheet.pdf

U.S. Department of Health and Human Services (USDHHS), Office of Disease Prevention and Health Promotion. (2016a). *Healthy People 2020: Topics and objectives.* Retrieved from http://www.healthy-people.gov/2020/topics-objectives

U.S. Department of Health and Human Services (USDHHS), Office of Disease Prevention and Health Promotion. (2016b). *Healthy People 2020 topics and objectives: Occupational health and safety.* Retrieved from http://www.healthypeople.gov/2020/topics-objectives/topic/occupational-safety-and-health/objectives

U.S. Department of Health, Education, and Welfare. (1979). *Healthy People: The Surgeon General's report on health promotion and disease prevention.* Washington, DC: U.S. Government Printing Office.

U.S. Preventive Services Task Force. (2014). *Guide to clinical preventive services.* Retrieved from https://innovations.ahrq.gov/qualitytools/guide-clinical-preventive-services-2014

United States Department of Transportation (DOT). (n.d.). *Standards—49 CFR part 391.41: Physical qualifications for drivers.* Retrieved from https://www.fmcsa.dot.gov/regulations/title49/section/391.41

Van Dover, L., & Pfeiffer, J. (2012). Patients of parish nurses experience renewed spiritual identity: A grounded theory study. *Journal of Advanced Nursing, 68*(8), 1824–1833.

Wagner, S. L., Koehn, C., White, M. I., Harder, H. G., Schultz, I. Z., Williams-Whitt, K., ... Wright, M. D. (2016). Mental health interventions in the workplace and work outcomes: A best-evidence synthesis of systematic reviews. *International Journal of Occupational and Environmental Medicine, 7*(1), 1–14.

Wall, S. (2014). Self-employed nurses as change agents in healthcare: Strategies, consequences, and possibilities. *Journal of Health Organization and Management, 28*(4), 511–531.

Westberg, G. E. (1990). *The parish nurse: Providing a minister of health for your congregation.* Minneapolis, MN: Augsburg.

Whelan, J. C. (2012). When the business of nursing was the nursing business: The private duty registry system, 1900–1940. *Online Journal of Issues in Nursing, 17*(2), 1.

Whisenant, D., Cortes, C., & Hill, J. (2013). Is faith-based health promotion effective? Results from two programs. *Journal of Christian Nursing, 31*(3):188–193.

Wilson, A., Whitaker, N., & Whitford, D. (2012). Rising to the challenge of health care reform with entrepreneurial and intrapreneurial nursing initiatives. *Online Journal of Issues in Nursing, 17*(2), Manuscript 5.

Wood, D. A. (2015, July 13). *FAU's nurse-led health center cares for underserved.* Retrieved from https://news.nurse.com/2015/07/13/faus-nurse-led-health-center-cares-for-underserved/

Yeaworth, R. C., & Sailors, R. (2014). Faith community nursing: Real care, real cost savings. *Journal of Christian Nursing, 31*(3), 178–183.

Ziebarth, D. J. (2014). Discovering determinants influencing faith community nursing practice. *Journal of Christian Nursing, 31*(4), 235–239.

CHAPTER

32

Clients Receiving Home Health and Hospice Care

"People from all walks of life agree that someone who is sick deserves, in principle, compassion and care."

—*Paul Farmer,* American anthropologist and physician

KEY TERMS

Centers for Medicare and
  Medicaid Services (CMS)
Community-based long-term
  care
Compassion fatigue
Home health care

Homebound
Hospice
Medicaid
Medicare home health
  benefit
Medicare hospice benefit

Medicare prospective
  payment system
OASIS (Outcome and
  Assessment Information
  Set)
Palliative interventions

Potentially inappropriate
  medications
Visiting Nurse Associations

LEARNING OBJECTIVES

Upon mastery of this chapter, you should be able to:

● Summarize the history and contemporary circumstances of home health and hospice care.
● Describe Medicare standards for home health and hospice programs.
● Explain family caregiver burdens of providing home care.
● Explain how Medicare reimburses home health and hospice care.
● Describe essential characteristics of home health and hospice nursing practice.
● Identify unique challenges of infection control, medication management, fall prevention, use of technology, and nurse safety during home visits.
● Contrast the goals of home health care and hospice.
● Explain the gaps in home health care and hospice and the need for a coherent community-based long-term care program in the United States.

A home health nurse sits in an upscale condominium with a frail, elderly gentleman tethered to his home oxygen unit and suffering air hunger as he struggles to speak of the "good old days" when he was young, full of vigor, and taking on the world. During her next visit to a trailer park, she inspects an infected pressure sore that has become smaller and cleaner with each home visit, as the client's wife carefully follows through with wound care teaching. Next, she monitors the pulmonary and cardiac status of a patient newly discharged to his aging bungalow, detecting early signs of cardiac decompensation and treating them at home in close collaboration with his physician. At that same time, her hospice nurse colleague walks into family chaos with a mother in pain and vomiting at the end of her life and then leaves with everyone calm and the patient comfortable. These are the kinds of experiences that make up the daily lives of nurses who work with home care and hospice clients. Indeed, home health and hospice programs allow nurses to practice what some see as the very heart of compassionate and highly skilled nursing care. Home health care and hospice programs are expanding and are the work settings for more and more nurses. Almost 4% of RNs work in home health care settings (National Center for Nursing Workforce Analysis, 2013).

Home health care is discussed in the first section of this chapter, followed by an overview of hospice care. The reader is also referred to the discussions in Chapter 19 on working with families, Chapter 20 on violence in families, Chapter 24 on care of the older adult, and Chapter 26 on chronic illness.

OVERVIEW OF HOME HEALTH CARE

Historically, patients have been cared for in their homes by family members. In the first part of the 19th century, home care was preferred over hospital care. During the later part of the 19th century, private duty nursing was common, and Visiting Nurse Associations were established in many American cities (Buhler-Wilkerson, 2016). The need for health care at home continues to accelerate. Drastic changes in financing and more people living with complex illness have contributed to this trend. For example, early hospital discharges resulting from third-party payers' efforts toward cost containment have forced clients to return home quickly to recuperate from surgeries and severe illnesses. Likewise, a growing population survives and yet suffers from complex chronic and life-threatening illness that they struggle to manage at home. Advanced technologies such as telehealth monitoring, point of care devices, intravenous (IV) antibiotics, chemotherapy, total parenteral nutrition (TPN), dialysis, and mechanical ventilation are routinely provided and maintained in the client's home. As the population ages, and particularly now that the baby boomer generation is entering their elder years, home health nursing is challenged to respond. Professional home health care agencies seek to maximize the client's level of independence and to minimize the effects of existing disabilities through noninstitutional services. Professional home health services aim to decrease rehospitalization rates and prevent or delay institutionalization (National Association for Home Care and Hospice [NAHC], 2010). The NAHC Web site provides a variety of direct services to members, including the publication *Caring* and monthly newsletters.

This section explores the evolution of home health care in the United States; describes home health agencies, clients, and personnel; and examines Medicare criteria and documentation. Finally, the unique characteristics of home health nursing are explored.

HISTORY AND POLITICS OF HOME HEALTH

Throughout human history, family members have provided health care at home. In the United States, the earliest known organized effort to care for the sick poor at home was made by the Ladies Benevolent Society in Charleston, South Carolina, in 1813 (Buhler-Wilkerson, 2007). Later in the 19th century, it became possible for women to become nurses trained in the manner of Florence Nightingale, and wealthy women began to hire them as visiting nurses and to sponsor visiting nurse services. In 1893, Lillian Wald began home visiting in New York City and is famed for professionalizing visiting nursing. One of her most famous collaborations was with insurance companies for payment of home care services. When she retired in 1933, the staff of 265 visiting nurses saw more than 100,000 clients and made over 550,000 home visits (Visiting Nurse Service of New York, 2016). Between 1909 and 1952, 100 million home visits were made to the policyholders of Metropolitan Life Insurance Company. Then, as now, the need for cost containment and therefore quick discharge were in diametric opposition to nursing goals of providing needed care at the patient's side as long as needed (Buhler-Wilkerson, 2016).

In the 20th century, insurance companies began to see the benefit of providing care in homes, rather than hospitals. When Medicare went into effect in the 1960s, less expensive alternatives to hospital care were sought. Private home health agencies evolved from the demand to provide care for the chronically ill client in their home. In the later half of the 20th century, as hospitals became increasingly effective in providing acute care, more people survived to live with debilitating chronic illness and disability, and referral to home care was used to discharge those nonacute patients from the hospital. Payment for home health care visits via Medicare and health insurances has allowed the individuals to rehabilitate at home, and that has proven to increase patient satisfaction and therefore promote positive outcomes while being cost-effective (Buhler-Wilkerson, 2016).

The **Medicare home health benefit** was established with certain goals in mind. It was designed to provide intermittent home visits, in which nurses and therapists would provide services and instruct clients and families in self-care. Home health nursing was clearly differentiated from longer nursing shifts in which nurses stayed in the home for several hours at a time. The period of visiting was to be brief and provide direct skilled care just temporarily until patients and families could care for themselves. Neither health promotion nor long-term care was valued or reimbursed. Families were expected to manage long-term care alone. Whereas nurses had previously controlled their own practice, services under the new benefit were seen as extensions of medical care, with physicians certifying needed services for short-term treatment of sickness.

The number of Medicare-certified home care agencies grew rapidly until enactment of the Balanced Budget Act (BBA) of 1997, which sought explicitly to reduce federal payments for home health care. To achieve this, payment to providers was changed from reimbursement for each visit to the **Medicare prospective payment system** that determined Medicare payment rates based on patient characteristics and need for services. Most private pay insurance agencies followed suit and adopted the standards of the Medicare prospective payment system (PPS). It was felt that compliance with established standards of care would increase positive outcomes in a cost-effective manner. However, the adoption of the standards resulted in a closure of many of the nation's Medicare-certified home health agencies (over 3,000 immediately after the 1997 legislation). Because of standardized reimbursement rates, many Medicare-qualified patients, requiring intensive skilled and personal services, needed to become independent in providing their health care needs at home. As a result, the amount of patient rehospitalizations increased and positive health care outcomes decreased. This has necessitated the focus of the home health nurse to change from provision of care to education and training. The home health nurse is charged with the responsibility of educating the patient and family on specific techniques to address the health need. Visits to the patient home are primarily evaluative of the patient's progress (Buhler-Wilkerson, 2016). In 2012, there were 12,200 home health agencies (Centers for Disease Control and Prevention [CDC], 2015).

With enactment of the Patient Protection and Affordable Care Act, many provisions are currently and will likely continue over the next decade to impact the provision of home health care. Although many of the Medicare policies for home care are unchanged, the act includes a number of new programs that if well implemented, will have a positive impact on home care. For instance, supplemental payments for rural home care providers have been reinstated for 2010–2015. This was done to address the lower ratio of home care professionals in rural areas throughout the United States as compared to more urban areas (Centers for Medicare and Medicaid Services [CMS], 2015f). New innovations included in the act are two programs that directly impact the provision of care in the home (CMS, 2012d):

- *Community First-Choice Option* allows states to offer home- and community-based services to disabled people through Medicaid rather than institutional care in nursing homes.
- *Community Care Transitions Program* helps high-risk Medicare beneficiaries who are hospitalized avoid unnecessary readmissions by coordinating care and connecting patients to services in their communities.

Although the new provisions can enhance the capacity of agencies to provide care, as with any change, the new rules and regulations will undoubtedly be a challenge. One concerning aspect for home health care providers is the 2012 ruling by the U.S. Supreme Court (National Federation of Independent Business et al. vs. Sebelius, Secretary of Health and Human Services) that allows for states to opt out of the provision in the act to expand Medicaid services (Kliff, 2012). **Medicaid** services are provided primarily to low-income populations. With a growing percentage of payments for home health coming from Medicaid, this is obviously of concern to care providers and consumers of care. Home health care expenditures from Medicaid are expected to exceed Medicare payments in the coming years. How this shift in payment source and the limitation that many states may impose on Medicaid coverage is unknown at this time. The **Centers for Medicare and Medicaid Services (CMS)** oversee expenditures and policy implementation.

CMS and other government Web sites provide a wealth of information for the providers of care, as well as consumers (CMS.gov; healthcare.gov). Despite the challenges, the recognition of improved outcomes and cost savings associated with home care as opposed to hospitalization and skilled nursing facility (SNF) stays is encouraging. Stolee, Lim, Wilson, and Glenny (2011) conducted a systematic review to compare rehabilitation measures between home-based and inpatient rehabilitation for musculoskeletal disorders. Their findings supported home-based care with equal or improved outcomes in function, cognition, quality of life, and satisfaction with the intervention. The cost-effectiveness of home-based rehabilitation for older patients can be inferred by these findings. Home health care has been shown to be effective in decreasing long-term care and mortality, as well as reestablishing functional abilities in patients. Those agencies with positive work environments demonstrated lower rates of hospitalizations and higher rates of patient discharges to community settings when compared to those with inferior work environments (Jarrin, Flynn, Lake, & Aiken, 2014). The American Association for Homecare (2015) cites numerous studies comparing costs between the skills and equipment provided in homes versus institutions.

It is important to be aware that a distinct difference exists between professional and nonprofessional home care services provided to clients. Specialists with licenses, certifications, or specific qualifications provide professional home care. These professionals typically work for home care agencies with internal and external standards that guide the provision of their services. Nurses, social workers, physical therapists, occupational therapists, and home health aides are examples of professional home care practitioners. In contrast, there are home care organizations that provide nonprofessional home care and those who sell equipment for home care.

The National Association for Home Care and Hospice (NAHC) developed a code of ethics that serves as a guideline for agencies in assuring that patients and families are treated with a high standard of care and in an ethical manner. The code of ethics for home health agencies addresses:

- Patient Rights and Responsibilities
- Relationships to other Provider Agencies
- Responsibility to the National Association
- Fiscal Responsibilities
- Marketing and Public Relations
- Personnel
- Legislation
- Appeal process

(NAHC, 2016, para. 7)

HOME HEALTH AGENCIES

The mix of Medicare-certified home health care agencies includes voluntary nonprofits, hospital-based agencies, proprietary for-profit agencies, governmental agencies, or agencies not federally certified to provide care.

Voluntary nonprofit agencies traditionally have a charitable mission and are exempt from paying taxes. They are financed with nontax funds such as donations, endowments, United Way contributions, and third-party provider payments. If nonprofit agencies make any money, they reinvest it back into the agency. An unpaid board of directors frequently oversees voluntary agencies. They are considered community based because they provide services within a well-defined geographic location. Whereas in the past these agencies were assured of receiving almost all of the home care referrals in their community, the proliferation of other agencies has eroded their traditional base and put them in a competitive mode. The number of nonprofit home health agencies is diminishing across the country.

Hospital-based agencies comprise about 13% of Medicare-certified agencies (NAHC, 2010). A hospital may operate a separate department as a home health agency. It may be nonprofit or generate revenue for the hospital. The hospital's board of directors or trustees serves as the governing body for hospital-based agencies. The referrals to such hospital-based agencies usually come from the hospital staff, and the missions of the agency and the sponsoring hospital are similar. The same is true for rehabilitation and skilled-nursing facilities with home health departments.

For-profit proprietary agencies may be owned by individuals, but many are part of large, regional, or national chains that are administered through corporate headquarters. Proprietary agencies are expected to turn a profit on the services they provide, either for the individual owners or for their stockholders. They are required to pay taxes on profits generated. Although some participate in the Medicare program, others rely solely on "private-pay" clients (NAHC, 2010). In 2012,

over 78% of home health care agencies were for-profit (CDC, 2015).

Some city and county government agencies also provide home care services. They are created and empowered through statutes enacted by legislation. Services are frequently provided by the nursing divisions of state or local health departments and may or may not combine care of the sick with traditional public health nursing services, including health promotion, illness prevention, communicable disease investigation, environmental health services, and maternal–child care.

Many agencies providing services in the home remain outside the federal Medicare system that reimburses skilled nursing. These *noncertified* agencies are usually private and derive their funding from direct payment by the client or from private insurers. They may be governed by individual owners or by corporations. For instance, some agencies offer private duty shifts of registered nurses, licensed practical nurses, various therapists, or home health aides who are usually paid for out of pocket rather than reimbursed by insurance or Medicare. Other services include unskilled assistance in the home with homemaking or housekeeping. Some of these agencies provide live-in personal care. Other organizations provide *durable medical equipment* (DME), such as wheelchairs, commodes, beds, or oxygen. Additional services include high-technology pharmacy.

CLIENTS AND THEIR FAMILIES

The client in home health care is not only the individual patient but also the family and any significant others. The nurse must consider how the environmental, political, economic, cultural, and religious dimensions impact the client's illness and ability to meet the goals outlined in the plan of care.

Home care recipients are predominantly elderly patients with acute and chronic health needs. The medical diagnoses coincide with the morbidity rates of the region. Many have chronic conditions, which complicate acute conditions. In 2013, it was reported that approximately 12 million people in the United States require home care with the majority of them being women. The most common conditions were diabetes, heart failure, chronic skin ulcers, osteoarthritis, and hypertension (Harris-Kojetin, Sengupta, Park-Lee, & Valverde, 2013).

Individuals recovering from severe illness or living with debilitating chronic illness rely on family members or other sources of unpaid assistance. Almost 30% of the U.S. population provides informal caregiving for an adult family member or friend (National Alliance for Caregiving [NAC], 2012). Two thirds of these providers are women with an average age of 47, although people can become caregivers at any age. Frail elderly caregivers are especially vulnerable to deterioration of their own health because of their caregiving burden. Family caregiving tasks range from personal care such as bathing and feeding to sophisticated skilled care, including managing tracheostomies or IV lines. Primary caregivers are those who assume the daily tasks of care, whereas secondary caregivers assume intermittent responsibilities such as shopping or transportation. Formal caregivers are either volunteers or paid workers, whereas informal caregivers are either family members or those friends and neighbors with substantial relationships to the patient (NAC, 2014).

These informal caregivers assume a considerable physical, psychological, and economic burden in the care of their loved one at home. When layered on top of existing responsibilities, caregiver tasks compete for time, energy, and attention. As a result, caregivers often describe themselves as emotionally and physically drained and may very much need information about resources to assist them. Likewise, the economic cost of providing home care places a significant burden on informal caregivers. Out-of-pocket expenditures include medications, transportation, home medical equipment, supplies, and respite services. These costs may be nonreimbursable and are often invisible, but they are very real to families struggling to provide care on a fixed income. Although family members compassionately assume their responsibilities, their collective burden in our society as a whole is mounting. Home health nurses must continually assess the strain on caregivers as they seek to develop realistic plans of care.

HOME HEALTH CARE PERSONNEL

Nurses and home care aides are the largest number of home care employees (NAHC, 2010). Registered nurses and licensed practical nurses represent just under half of full time equivalent (FTE) positions in Medicare-certified agencies. Home care aides, physical therapy staff, occupational therapists, social workers, and administrative personnel comprise the rest of the home health team. The business and office personnel of a home health agency are critical to the agency's ability to deliver services to clients. Home health nurses must acquire an understanding of the financial aspects of their clients' care and provide this information to the agency staff, so that appropriate and full reimbursement can be obtained for the services provided.

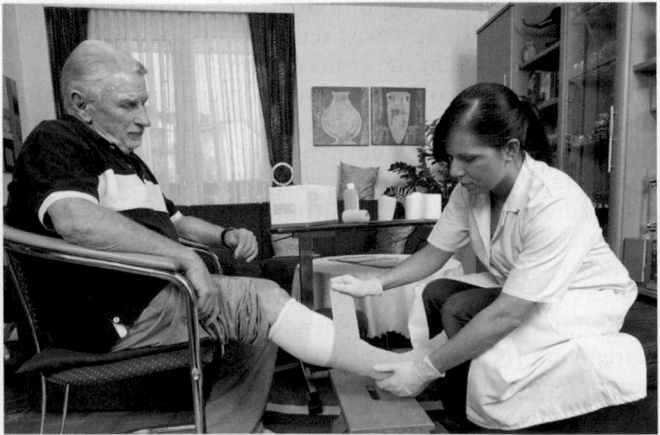

REIMBURSEMENT FOR HOME HEALTH CARE

Both corporate and governmental third-party payers, as well as by individual clients and their families, reimburse home health services. Corporate payers include insurance companies, health maintenance organizations (HMOs), preferred provider organizations (PPOs), and case-management programs. Government payers include Medicare, Medicaid, the military health system (TRICARE), and the Veterans Administration system. These governmental programs have specific conditions for coverage of services, which are often less flexible than those of corporate payers. For a general description of these reimbursement systems, see Chapter 6. The Medicare policies for home health programs set the precedent for all other reimbursement sources and are discussed below.

Medicare Criteria and Reimbursement

Medicare is the largest single payer for home care services in the United States and has set the standard in establishing reimbursement criteria for other payers. Therefore, it is essential that home care nurses seek to understand the complex Medicare home health requirements and rules for determining eligibility for home care services. It is important to acknowledge that a person may be in dire need of care at home, yet not meet eligibility standards for home health care under Medicare. There are five criteria that must all be met to be eligible for reimbursement by Medicare (Display 32–1). Consider the implications of these requirements. Documentation must justify that the plan of care is medically "reasonable and necessary." The person must be under the care of a physician. He or she must be "homebound" and in need of services that Medicare narrowly defines as "skilled." A person who is "homebound" must be confined to home except for visits to the physician, outpatient dialysis, adult day center, or outpatient chemotherapy and radiation therapy. "Skilled" services are restrictively defined and include selected aspects of nursing, physical therapy, or speech therapy. Home visits must be *intermittent* and time limited. Extensive documentation is required according to Medicare specifications (CMS, 2015c). All of these requirements are subject to contradictory interpretations, which can put an agency's reimbursement at risk.

The Medicare PPS pays an agency for a 60-day "episode of care." All services and many medical supplies must be provided under the payment amount adjusted to geographic location and determined by the patient's clinical and functional status at the start of care, as well as the projected need for services over the anticipated 60-day period (CMS, 2012b). When the patient is admitted, the patient is comprehensively assessed using a lengthy tool called the **Outcome and Assessment Information Set** (**OASIS**). Clinical, functional, psychological, and service scores are calculated from selected OASIS items. The stated purpose of OASIS is to "represent core items of a comprehensive assessment for an adult home care patient; and form the basis for measuring patient outcomes for purposes of outcome-based quality improvement" (CMS, 2012, para. 1). The updated version of this assessment tool is OASIS-C1, and it examines process as well as outcomes (CMS, 2015e). In the ongoing campaign to hold down the federal budget by diminishing health costs, home health care faces the ongoing threat of freezes or cuts in payment. These proposals overlooked the reality that home health care is a cost-effective alternative to hospital and nursing home care. As home health care is restricted to save money and reduce fraud, greater amounts will need to be spent for inpatient care

DISPLAY 32–1 MEDICARE HOME HEALTH ELIGIBILITY

1. The type of services and frequency provided must be reasonable and necessary. To determine whether this criterion is met, the client's current health status, medical record, and plan of care are evaluated. If a care plan has been ineffective with a client over a long period of time, continuation of that care plan would not be considered reasonable. Therefore, comprehensive documentation is essential to validate that the provided care was both reasonable and necessary.

2. The client must be **homebound**. This means that the client leaves the home with difficulty and only for medical appointments or adult day care related to the client's medical care.

3. The plan of care must be entered onto specific Medicare forms. The forms require very specific information regarding the client's diagnosis, prognosis, functional limitations, medications, and types of services needed. The home health nurse often has the primary responsibility for ensuring that the forms are completed appropriately.

4. The client must be in need of a skilled service. In the home setting, skilled services are provided only by a nurse, physical therapist, or speech therapist. *Skilled nursing services* include skilled observation and assessment, teaching, and performing selected procedures requiring nursing judgment.

5. Services must be intermittent and part-time.

---

when people cannot cope in the absence of health care assistance at home (see Perspectives: Voices From the Community).

It is a Medicare requirement that patients receiving home health care must be recertified every 60 days. This recertification includes a detailed assessment (OASIS) that validates the need for skilled care within the home and the fact the patient cannot easily receive care from other sources. A face-to-face visit made with a comparison of progress from the initial assessment to the present must be made, and this can be done by the patient's physician, a nurse practitioner, a clinical nurse specialist, or a certified nurse midwife or physician assistants who work under the supervision of a physician. A determination of continued visits is then made based upon the objective data obtained (CMS, 2015b).

PERSPECTIVES
VOICES FROM THE COMMUNITY

It is vital to develop an expanded vision about the health care needs of frail elders and the kinds of services that are needed in the community. Sometimes, after nurses have been working in Medicare home health for a while, they may begin to identify more with the Medicare guidelines than with their patients. Too often, I have heard experienced home health nurses say about a patient living with severe chronic illness, "She doesn't deserve services. She doesn't have skilled needs." In contrast, I would hope knowledgeable nurses would say to families and decision makers, "She needs and deserves services, but the Medicare home health benefit will not pay for them. Our agency cannot continue to provide care because of the limits imposed on us. We'll do everything possible to find help for her, but resources are limited." This kind of insight leads to patient advocacy, development of community networks, and becoming outspoken about needed changes in health policy. Visiting nurses witness the struggles of chronically ill people living at home; we must not abandon them.

—*Beth L., Nursing Instructor*

Medicare Documentation

Initially, every patient must be assessed using the OASIS tool, which determines reimbursement, is integral to agency surveys and certification, and collects information used to measure quality. OASIS assessment combines objective data gathered by the nurse combined with subjective data gathered from the patient and family to determine optimal functional outcomes for the patient. Selected quality outcomes are measured, and data are released on the CMS Web site (CMS, 2015a), which is accessed as "Home Health Compare" (http://www.medicare.gov/). Display 32–2 identifies selected quality measures. Note that the expectation is that of improving function, not simply stabilizing function, and consider the implications of this standard for very disabled patients.

The nurse also completes the Medicare plan of care at admission, and the physician must sign this. It is then used to assess agency compliance with Medicare and state requirements. Obviously, great pains must be taken to assure accuracy. All follow-up services must match the plan of care. Likewise, OASIS identified needs and plan of care services must match (CMS, 2015b).

HOME HEALTH NURSING PRACTICE

The practice of home health nursing has roots in community/public health nursing (see Chapters 2 and 3). The nurse provides home health nursing care to acute, chronic, and terminally ill clients of all ages in their homes while integrating public health nursing principles that focus on the environmental, psychosocial, economic, cultural, and personal health factors affecting a client's and family's health status and well-being. Home health is a unique field of nursing practice that requires a synthesis of public health nursing principles with the theory and practice of medical/surgical, geriatric, mental health, and other nursing specialties. The official journal of the Home Healthcare Nurses Association (HHNA, 2012), *Home Healthcare Nurse*, is the primary source of up-to-date nursing knowledge in this rapidly changing field of practice.

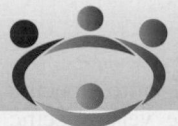

DISPLAY 32–2 COMPARE HOME HEALTH CARE PROVIDERS

The Medicare.gov Web site offers information for consumers about the quality of home health care agencies. It includes data on how frequently best practices are used in patient care and if patients improved in relation to certain aspects of care. It also includes patient feedback about recent home health agency experiences.

You and/or your clients can go to: https://www.medicare.gov/homehealthcompare/search.html and enter your ZIP Code (or city, state), and you can see a list of all agencies and the services provided by each (that meet certain criteria). You may select agencies for comparison, and general information is provided, along with the quality patient care information and results of patient surveys. For quality patient care, star ratings are used to denote summaries of 9 out of 29 quality measures, with 4 or 5 stars indicating better performance than other agencies. Star rankings of one or two indicate below-average performance. Most agencies nationwide fall within 3 or 3.5 stars. Survey results include percentages related to how often care was given in a professional manner, how well the team communicated with clients, if they discussed pain, medications, and home safety with clients, how the client rates their overall care from this agency, and would they recommend the agency to family/friends. Overall percentages can be graphed for comparison with state and national averages.

The effective home health nurse must

- Deliberately build trust
- Sense "where people are" and suspend judgment
- Develop a connection at the first visit
- Develop "giant antennae" to detect cues in the home
- Keep the focus on patient care, despite persistent distractions during home visits
- Help people solve their own problems
- Keep priorities fluid
- Determine how to keep the unstable client safe until the next visit
- Thoughtfully maintain boundaries between personal and professional life
- "Make do" with limited supplies
- Face immense challenges with time management and paperwork demands
- Be vigilant about personal safety in neighborhoods and homes
- Continue the development of skills in clinical assessment and care coordination
- Provide effective teaching for patients and families

According to the American Nurses Association (ANA) *Scope and Standards of Practice for Home Health Nursing* (2014), home health nursing goes beyond providing skilled nursing care in the home; it requires the ability of the nurse to coordinate a broad variety of services and professional caregivers in order to manage patients' complex health problems. See Display 32–3 for an abbreviated look at the standards of practice.

Nursing Practice During the Home Visit

The practice competencies of home health nurses can be illustrated with the Home Health Nursing Caregiving Wheel (Fig. 32–1).

Locating the Client and Getting Through the Door

The first step in making a home visit is finding where the person lives, which might involve telephone instructions, or a global positioning system (GPS) unit. For most home health nurses, locating clients involves driving their own cars to the home. Sometimes, nurses drive agency cars, and occasionally transportation may involve a bus, subway, boat, or airplane. Directions and household identification can be unclear. In rural areas, tracking down clients can involve vague instructions involving barns, bridges, trees, and other colorful local landmarks (see From the Case Files for an example). When families are unstable, clients may not be staying in households designated on the nurse's paperwork. They may have moved in with relatives or friends or be back home alone despite major care needs. Locating is especially challenging when neighbors or even family members are not cooperative, for whatever reason.

Even when the wheels stop at the correct household, there is the challenge of getting through the closed door and making the connection. *Always remember that you are a guest in the home.* Respect and attentive listening are the foundation for establishment of trust between the client and nurse. Agendas must be laid aside initially as the nurse focuses on the concerns and realities of both client and family. Assumptions and stereotypes are overturned in the process of discovering how clients live, what they believe, and who comprises their family and community. The nurse must take into account the spiritual, cultural, and developmental, as well as environmental, realms of the client in order to be able to develop individualized plans of care to promote health.

The home health nurse is aware that the client is the driver of the plan of care. To have effective outcomes, the nurse must develop a therapeutic relationship in which the client identifies the desired outcomes. This approach provides increased cooperation between the nurse and client in establishing interventions to reach the desired outcome. The nurse must emphasize positives to the extent possible, rather than telling people what they are doing wrong and need to change. Autonomy should be respected, and the family should be empowered by actions recognizing that they are in charge of their lives. At the same time, the nurse must be up front and truthful regarding the medical and nursing problems that need resolution. For example, a nurse might say, "You might lose your foot if we cannot work together to figure out a plan of care that you can live with. Let's think together about what we can do to prevent it." The nurse, the patient, and family must work together to establish mutually agreed-upon goals. (See Chapters 10 and 25 for more information on communication, collaboration, contracting, and effective approaches for developing effective nurse–client partnerships.)

DISPLAY 32–3 EXAMPLES OF STANDARDS OF PRACTICE FOR HOME HEALTH NURSING

Clinical roles of the home health nurse include patient educator, clinical care/case manager, and patient advocate. Standards of practice in this specialty area of nursing encompass:

- Assessment (including family dynamics, knowledge of caregivers, patient values/goals/health beliefs)
- Diagnosis (including validation of diagnosis with patient/family, actual and potential risks, health barriers)
- Outcomes identification (including collaboration with patient/family to identify goals, consideration of cultural, ethical, and personal beliefs and values)
- Planning (including collaborating with patient/family on an individualized plan of care, strategies to address health promotion and restoration, prevention of injury/illness, pain relief/palliative care, interprofessional collaboration regarding care, planning for transitions to and from home health care)
- Implementation (including collaboration on implementing plan of care, engaging patients in disease management, use of evidence-based practice interventions, providing holistic care, utilizing health care technologies and community resources, integrating complementary practices with traditional approaches, promoting problem solving behaviors in patients/families)
- Coordination of care (including collaborating with team members, helping patients/families recognize alternative care options when plan of care no longer meets patient needs, works closely with patients/families during care transitions)
- Health Teaching & Health Promotion (including developmentally and culturally sensitive health promotion/teaching that promotes patient engagement with self-care, utilizes information and health care technologies as appropriate)
- Consultation (including synthesizing evidence, clinical data and theory, involves patients/families in determining role responsibilities and in making decisions, offers education to the team of health care workers)
- Evaluation (including ongoing and systematic outcomes evaluation, engages the team and the patient/family to participate in evaluation process, evaluates patient progress toward short-term goals/objectives, uses evaluation to redesign plan of care, provides results of evaluation to patient/family and health care team members)
- Ethics (including practicing within the ANA [2015] *Code of Ethics for Nurses with Interpretive Statements*)
- Education (including continuing professional education)
- Evidence-Based Practice & Research (including use of current findings to guide clinical nursing practice, sharing research findings with health care team members/peers)
- Quality of Practice (including documentation, participation in quality improvement initiatives, collecting quality-related data, updating guidelines/procedures to improve quality of nursing practice and patient care outcomes)
- Communication (including assessment of patient preferences/literacy/language skills, communicating effectively with interprofessional team members)
- Leadership (including development of conflict resolution and communication skills, serving as a preceptor for new colleagues, participation on agency committees)
- Collaboration (including partnering with others to promote change, helps build consensus, applying negotiation skills and group process techniques with patients/families/health care team, builds teamwork)
- Professional practice evaluation (including evaluation of own practice and identification of strengths/areas needing professional growth, offers feedback to peers on performance)
- Resource utilization (including resources available to patient/family in implementing plan of care, delegates to team members when appropriate, advocates for enhancement of nursing practice through use of technology and additional resources, helps patient/family find services needed for care and cost/benefits/risks of decisions)
- Environmental health (including understanding of risks related to management of supplies (e.g., syringes, needles, medications, waste), assessment of home and neighborhood for unsafe/unsanitary conditions, works to reduce environmental risks that affect health of patient/family, promotes health communities)

Adapted from American Nurses Association. (2014). *Scope and standards of practice: Home health nursing.* (2nd ed.). Silver Spring, MD: Author.

Hub of the Family Caregiving Wheel: Promoting Self-Management

Home health nursing involves home visits to promote independence rather than dependence on the home health team. Lasting health improvement is only possible when the home health nurse works with the client/family to make decisions that are truly their own. Although financial incentives push home health nurses to minimize the number of visits and duration of service, pressuring a client or family to adopt the agency agenda denies any sense of partnership and can backfire, resulting in nonadherence to the therapeutic regimen. This can place a client in a no-win situation.

Every effort is made to develop capacity for independent self-care, so that the home team can safely withdraw. Obviously, this is quite appropriate for those recovering from an episode of acute illness. The challenge

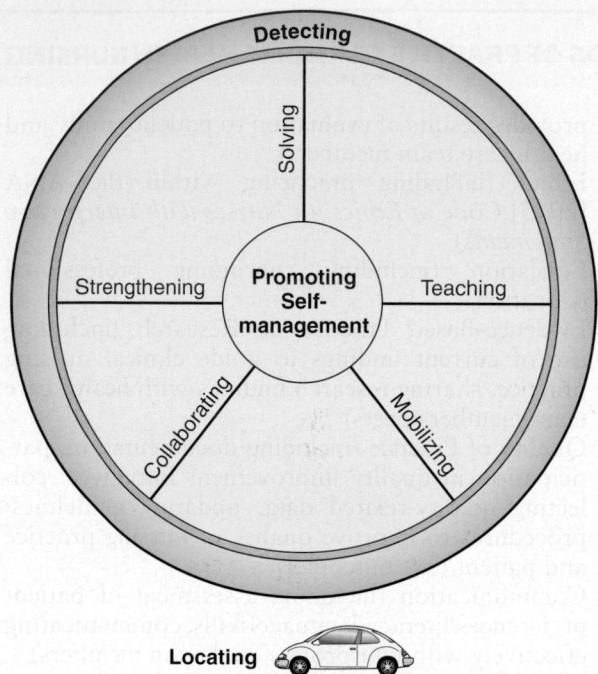

FIGURE 32–1 Home health nursing caregiving wheel.

to the home health nurse is often assisting the severely chronically ill client be able to adapt in the community to be safe and functional. Coordination with other professionals must often be instituted to provide comprehensive quality care. This may include social workers, clergy, physical therapists occupational therapists, as well as mental health professionals. Because regulations require that the client make progress toward the outcomes, the nurse must often limit or terminate visits when measurable progress is not being made. This may lead to rehospitalization or the inability to provide self-care. Currently, no governmental program assures long-term care for those people unable to care for themselves. The home health nurse must utilize interprofessional collaboration to agency social workers to mobilize resources to care after the agency leaves.

Rim of the Home Health Caregiving Wheel: Detecting

Nurses in the home are challenged by an extraordinarily complex environment with much to investigate and frequently many distractions to ignore. Detecting is an all-encompassing, continuing assessment process as the nurse seeks to understand the client's health in the context of home. The nurse keeps her ears and eyes "wide open." Who lives in the home? How do they interact? Who are the caregivers, and how do they care? What is the relevance of culture and religion in the life of the household? How does the physical environment impact patient safety and security? Can the bathroom tub be used? The questions are endless. The OASIS format provides the baselines for the first visit, and then the nursing assessment broadens with each visit as the nurse continually widens his or her lens to take it all in. Home visits reveal discoveries that can never be imagined in clinic or hospital settings. Take for example the client whose refrigerator no longer chills

---

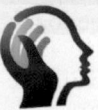 *From the* **Case Files**

Locating the Client's Home

"You can't miss our place," Diane had reassured me on the phone. I slowed in front of the decrepit Sunrise Motel, its roof partially collapsed, and reviewed my notes. I was supposed to turn right on the unmarked gravel road just after the abandoned motel and continue until the road ended. I proceeded slowly through an evergreen tunnel past an old blue truck body, resting belly up. A little girl, perhaps 5 years old, came from around the truck and joined two grade-school-aged boys playing Frisbee in a clearing. I asked them where Diane Quimby lived, and they pointed around a curve in the road. In a moment, I came to a stop near a large wooded area and a metal shed with smoke coming out of a crooked metal pipe in the roof. I knocked. No answer. I heard dialogue from "General Hospital" coming from inside. I knocked again and shouted, "Hello! It's the nurse." "Come on in!" a loud voice responded.

I pushed open the door. There was no knob. Illuminated by one weak lamp, I could just make out a round face with wire rim glasses and a long gray-blond braid. Here was Diane, sitting on a sagging sofa facing a TV tray and watching television. I could see a wooden table in the corner, three mismatched dining chairs, and a couple of cots against the wall. The air was hazy with the smell of wood smoke.

Diane invited me to pull up a chair. "How are you doing? I am here to see how I can assist you". I began. Diane had unstable, insulin-dependent diabetes and high blood pressure. In June, surgeons had removed her gangrenous left foot with an amputation that ended just below the left knee. Now, there was an infection in the wound that had not healed despite extended use of antibiotics.

During the course of the visit, I learned that Diane had no tub or shower for bathing. She also had no money for dressings and no supplies. Because Diane's vision was impaired, her 9-year-old grandson was doing the dressing changes. Until the latest surgery, Diane worked as a cook in a local board and care home for frail elders. She was 68 years old and had Medicare coverage. I learned that Diane was the legal guardian for two grandchildren, ages 5 and 9.

Apply the nursing process to comprehensively identify and prioritize nursing diagnoses and propose interventions. Use the Home Health Nursing Caregiving Wheel to guide your care planning.

and whose impaired vision prevents awareness of the expanding family of roaches in the kitchen. Upon each visit the nurse is assessing:

- Client safety: Is the client in a safe environment where the outcome can be reached? Are there safety devices available for client safety? Are essential services (food, power, water, housing, security) available and sufficient for the client to function safely independently in the home?
- Supportive, knowledgeable caregivers: Are the caregivers attentive, knowledgeable, and willing to provide care to the client in the absence of the nurse? Is the caregiver competent in providing care?
- Material resources: Does the client have the necessary material resources to support the interventions? Are the medications, dressings, and supplies accessible? Does the patient have the financial support to obtain the equipment?

Spokes of the Home Health Caregiving Wheel: Collaborating, Mobilizing, Strengthening, Teaching, Solving Problems

Home health nursing competencies that radiate from the hub and contribute to promotion of self-care and family care include *collaborating* with multiple team members and *mobilizing resources* in the community that can sustain the client after discharge. The home health care nurse usually is the coordinator of all other home health team members. Working with the social worker, the nurse proposes needed connections with community services. Likewise, *strengthening* involves development of self-management or family caregiving ability. People learn that they can give injections, manage IV lines, safely take complex drug regimens, provide rehabilitation for loved ones after stroke, and perform countless other skills that they do not believe possible until a nurse shows them and they discover that they can do it themselves.

The home health nurse is constantly *teaching* clients and/or family caregivers through concrete explanation, discussion, and modeling behavior. Teaching facts is no assurance of behavior change and improved management of a health problem. Underlying factors influencing health behavior must be diagnosed and addressed. Health coaching, also called *motivational interviewing, is useful. The* principles of adult learning highlight that adults must be involved and see some self-benefit in order to learn. Instead of telling people what to do, this involves asking people how they would like to change—for instance, "What worries you the most?" Those concerns and relevant feelings must be validated, and the nurse leads the person to consider options for change. The solution develops through a mutual, participatory process. Ultimately, people are responsible for their own health decisions (see Chapter 11).

Finally, home health nursing competency requires flexibility and creativity in *solving* health care problems and the challenges of everyday living. All outcomes of care can be achieved only by adapting to the skills and resources available in the home. Although people of all socioeconomic backgrounds present with severe health problems requiring home health nursing, many families live on the margins. The home health nurse must often be creative in obtaining supplies and adjusting to conditions in the home. For example, how do patients and families with no running water wash their hands before providing care, such as dressing changes? This may lead the home health nurse to contact social agencies in order to provide services or teach the patient and family the use of alcohol-based gels to clean their hands. The home health nurse must be nonjudgmental, but work with the patient and family to help them understand the need to keep areas clean.

Home Health Nursing Case Management

The home health nurse is the case manager for each client and responsible for coordination of the other professionals and paraprofessionals involved in the client's care.

The nurse plans the frequency and duration of visits. Will home visits be made twice weekly, once weekly, or every day? For how long will visits continue? As the care is provided and the client's condition improves, the home health nurse determines whether the frequency of visits should be reduced or whether the client can be discharged.

The home care nurse is the primary contact with the client's physician, collaborating on the initial plan of care, reporting changes in the client's condition, and securing changes in the plan of care. The nurse conducts case conferences among team members to share information, discuss problems, and plan actions to affect the best possible outcomes for the client. Medicare mandates such case conferences every 60 days in home care. The nurse case manager also supervises the paraprofessionals, such as home health aides, who also serve the homebound client. The definition of homebound involves two considerations: (1) it takes extraordinary effort for the client to leave their home and receive care and (2) that they need physical assistance or the use of medical equipment (e.g., walkers, wheelchairs, crutches) in order to leave their home (Medicare Interactive, n.d.).

The home health nurse must know who is going to pay for services from the first visit to the time of discharge from the agency. If the client does not have a source of payment for the care that is needed, the agency must determine whether the client will receive the care free of charge or at a reduced rate. Many agencies have a sliding fee scale, which means that the charge for the services is based on the client's ability to pay.

Selected Nursing Challenges in the Home

Working in the home immerses the nurse in challenges unlike anything encountered in controlled institutional environments. Some of these include infection control, medication safety, fall risk, technology at home, and nurse safety.

Infection Control

Home health nurses frequently need to work with the family to prevent infection in clients who are debilitated and may be immunocompromised; in addition, many are now dwelling at home with invasive medical devices that make them especially vulnerable to infection. Likewise, nurses are challenged to consider how to protect the home health care team, family, and community from a client with contagious disease. In such cases, all people living in the home will need instruction. Some households have inadequate facilities to control disease transmission. There may be no access to running water, no heating unit to boil equipment, or inadequate facilities to dispose of contaminated equipment. These conditions necessitate the development of creative solutions to control infection.

Complexities of the home environment require the nurse to carefully consider exactly how microorganisms are likely to exit the body, how might they be transmitted, and how are they likely to enter the body of another individual. Households cannot be organized like hospital units with isolation rooms. The nurse must decide when gloves are absolutely essential, when protecting clothing with a gown is needed, when a mask should be worn, and what environmental surfaces are likely to be contaminated and must be scrupulously cleaned. How should soiled tissues or dressings, dishes, and laundry be handled? What is realistic and can actually be carried out by client and family? As in the hospital environment, hands are the main method of transmission of contagion, and hand hygiene is the main intervention that must be emphasized. In a study of 423 home health nurses, almost 6% reported having been diagnosed with a multiple-drug-resistant organism acquired on their jobs, and almost 80% of nurses report that their agency does not have an infection control specialist on staff (Kenneley, 2012).

To guide the nurse, home health agencies have adapted infection control policies and procedures based on the Centers for Disease Control and Prevention's (CDCs) isolation precautions for health care settings each agency setting up their own specific policy and procedure based upon the standard (Siegel, Rhinehart, Jackson, Chiarello, & Healthcare Infection Control Practices Advisory Committee, 2011).

Medication Safety

Home health nurses assume major responsibility for medication safety. The home health client taking multiple medications is at particular risk of multiple errors in self-administration, including incorrect medication, dose, time, interval, or route. Often, doses are missed or doubled. Clients may discontinue a drug or not complete the full course. Sometimes, the drug or drugs ordered are inappropriate considering the patient's condition at home.

The home presents risks of medication errors that are different from those found in hospital or nursing home. Every visiting nurse has stories of finding drawers and cupboards filled with multiple prescriptions from various physicians, some current and some outdated for many years. Polypharmacy becomes very obvious in the home setting. Clients often have received prescriptions from multiple sources for similar drugs. Also, well-meaning friends often share their prescriptions with the attitude that it "helped them." Clients taking at least one potentially inappropriate medication were found to be at greater risk when they received Medicare or Medicaid-provided services (Bao, Shao, Bishop, Schackman, & Bruce, 2011). Using data from the 2007 National Home and Hospice Care Survey, 38% of elderly home health clients were taking one or more potentially inappropriate medications, and the risk for polypharmacy showed

a correlated increase (Bao et al., 2011). **Potentially inappropriate medications** (PIM) are those that senior citizens should avoid due to either their ineffectiveness or because the potential adverse effects overshadow the proposed benefits; they also should be avoided if other, safer drugs are available (Bao et al., 2011). Additional findings from the Bao et al. study included an increased risk of exposure to potentially inappropriate medications when clients were admitted to home health care from a nursing home or other subacute facility, rather than community admission. This not only supports the need for home care but improvements to discharge planning from skilled nursing facilities.

Even if the client is well organized and taking every drug prescribed, those prescriptions may have originated from several providers over time and may have contradictory side effects. Sometimes, medication errors at home include failure to clearly reconcile hospital or nursing home orders with home discharge orders. Although weekly medication organizers can helpfully put medications in order, they can also confuse new or impaired users. Distraction, visual impairment, forgetfulness, depression, and cognitive impairment are common causes of unintentional medication noncompliance. The home health nurse investigates how the medication is taken by reviewing and reconciling the current list of medications and having the patient explain and demonstrate the process he goes through. Intervention requires clear and repeated instruction, updating the medication list, charting or diagramming the schedule for medication taking, and assuring that the client or caregiver knows how to use the medication box. See Chapter 24 for more on medication issues with older adults.

Some of the reasons for intentional noncompliance are knowledge deficit, unacceptable side effects, no immediately obvious consequence when the drug is stopped, resistance to authority, perception of personal weakness if needing medication, and prohibitive cost (Gottlieb, 2016). Health insurance plans with restrictive formularies, high copayments, and limited incomes have been associated with lower levels of medication compliance (Iuga & McGuire, 2014). The home health nurse seeks to nonjudgmentally elicit reasons and mutually work out solutions that help clients manage medications at home and prevent intensive medical interventions.

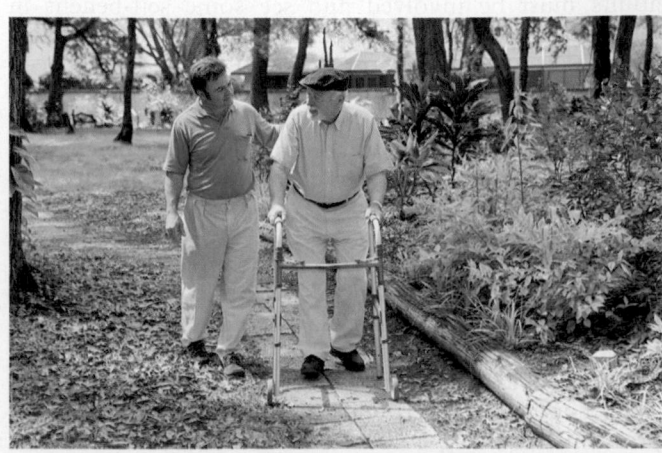

Risk of Falling

Falls are a serious issue especially for the elderly. Estimates are that one in three adults 65 years and older will fall each year, and 250,000 are hospitalized for hip fractures (CDC, 2015). Physiological risk factors include orthostatic hypotension and cardiac dysrhythmias, dizziness, neurologic and musculoskeletal effects on gait and balance, urinary urgency, impaired hearing or vision, alcohol or drug abuse, and medication effects impairing alertness, balance, urinary frequency, and blood pressure. Clients should be observed as they move through their home and carry out activities of daily living. It is important to investigate factors that obstruct movement or threaten balance. The nurse in the home should inspect sidewalks, stairs, and surfaces outside the home; floor, rugs, electrical cords, stairs, lighting, and clutter inside the home; kitchen safety; and bathroom features including grab bars and a raised seat for the toilet and safety modifications for the bathtub. Common home modifications, such as eliminating throw rugs and loose mats and the use of nonslip bath mats, have a significant protective effect. Display 32–4 lists teaching guidelines to prevent falls. See Chapter 24 for more on fall prevention in the home.

Technology at Home

Home health nurses teach patients and their family to manage a wide array of complex technologies. Home regimens often require mini-intensive care units. In the past, the average home had a limited capacity for technology; medication was swallowed, and food and fluid were consumed with the aid of fork and spoon. Now, the IV needle has evolved into venous access devices,

and plastic IV fluid bags can be stacked in the refrigerator and hung from the arm of a lamp. The household becomes home to dialysis, ventilators, isolation suites, enteric and IV nutrition, and vasopressors—the list goes on. Nurses teach clients and families to manage it all; we become the guardians and advocates of complex regimens that require multiple nursing visits. Paradoxically, our primary mission is to be protectors and advocates for the well-being of client and family. Consider the human impact when the machines and the sickbed become the center of household activities (Munck, Sandgren, Fridlund, & Martensson, 2012). Also, medical devices have caused injuries and deaths, so careful instructions on use in the home and oversight are needed (Swayze & Rich, 2012). Home health nurses have the unique position of being able to assess the client in their own environment and determine the impact of their health condition on their desired lifestyle. Sometimes, we can foster dialogue with clients and families to consider the benefits and burdens of continuing technologies. Consider four reasons why technology may be inappropriate: (1) the technology is not achieving a therapeutic purpose, (2) the therapeutic purpose can be met more simply, (3) complications of the intervention outweigh benefits, and (4) the resulting quality of life does not justify the technology. See Perspectives: Home Health Nursing.

Recent information technologies being adopted by home health care agencies significantly improve quality of client care. These include medical records available instantly on the nurse's laptop or tablet and daily telemedicine monitoring of electrocardiogram, blood pressure, oxygen saturation, and other vital measures. This is known as telehealth because objective measurements of the patient's current health status can be transmitted electronically to a home health agency or physician office. These assessments can be monitored, and the patient plan of care may be altered based on the analysis. Determination of face-to-face visits from the home health nurse or the physician is often based on the change in the plan of care. For example, a patient with the medical diagnosis of congestive heart failure is showing an increase in blood pressure and weight; this may warrant an immediate visit so that medications may be adjusted and a subsequent hospital visit may be avoided. As the results of one study cautioned (Shea & Chamoff, 2012), health care providers may overestimate the value of telemedicine in self-care for chronic conditions. The findings of the study support using explicit goals and intensions with clients and to individualize instructions provided. Essentially, frequency of contact did not mean quality communication. See Chapter 10 for more on technology in the community.

Nurse Safety

Nurses and other health care workers experience higher rates of workplace violence when compared with other types of work (Gross, Peek-Asa, Nocera, & Casteel, 2013). Home health nurses face risks not only dealing with driving to their client's homes but also because of environmental hazards: the nurses must be constantly aware of personal safety and surroundings. Client homes

---

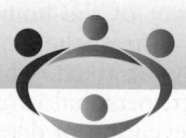

DISPLAY 32–4 TEACHING TO PREVENT FALLS

- Encourage the client to
  Get exercise to strengthen leg muscles and improve balance
  Be aware of effects and side effects of medications
  Have vision checked regularly
  Eliminate hazards at home

Steps for home safety
Remove things that you can trip over (books, papers shoes, throw rugs).
Install handrails and lights on all staircases.
If using throw rugs, secure them with double-sided tape to prevent slipping.
Put grab bars inside and next to the tub or shower as well as the toilet.
Use nonslip mats in the bathtub and on shower floors.
Improve the lighting in the home.
Wear shoes both inside and outside the home.

Adapted from Centers for Disease Control and Prevention. (n.d.). *Preventing falls among older adults*. Retrieved from https://www.cdc.gov/Features/OlderAmericans

PERSPECTIVES
HOME HEALTH NURSING

I have worked in home health for about 15 years. I started in the hospital on a pediatrics unit and later moved to home health. Recently, I have been working with medically fragile children who are discharged home but who still need more intensive care than can be provided by the families (e.g., premature infants; children with either cardiac, neurological, or respiratory problems; those on ventilators or with feeding tubes). The child or infant may need daily treatments and careful monitoring, and their physician requests medically necessary services from the home health agency. As a pediatric home health nurse, I provide skilled nursing care for set periods of time (up to 24 hours/day). A nurse is always available on call, and we develop close relationships with our families. We often check in with them by phone between visits and help parents adjust to the "tubes and wires" or other technology needed by their infant or child. Sometimes, parents send us a note with their preemie's "first day of school" photo. It is uplifting to see these fragile newborns looking like any other kindergartener. I really love my job!

Ava, Pediatric Home Health Nurse

Adapted from Hand to Hand. (2016). What does a pediatric home health provider do? Skilled nursing care at home. Retrieved from http://handtohold.org/resources/meet-the-provider/what-does-a-pediatric-home-health-provider-do-skilled-nursing-care-at-home/

DISPLAY 32–5 SAFE HOME VISITS

- Carry a cell phone.
- Be sure the agency knows your itinerary.
- Clarify directions before travel. Use GPS and client directions to the home.
- Make joint visits or request security escort if safety is threatened. Discuss plan for discontinuance of visits with supervisor when there is strong evidence of personal danger.
- Call to schedule the visit, and do not go into the home without invitation.
- Dress simply without expensive jewelry. Do not carry large amounts of cash. Keep wallet or purse locked in the trunk of your car during the visit.
- Wear an agency badge.
- Follow family directions about how to get by in their neighborhood and when to come in or leave their home. Patients and families usually have a desire to protect their nurse.

are uncontrolled environments, unlike acute care hospital settings, and nurses may face instances of family violence, illegal drug activity, or weapons may be present. The surrounding neighborhood also may pose risks of violence, car theft, vandalism, and robbery. Many home health organizations and their nurses work closely with local law enforcement agencies to identify the wisest process for visiting dangerous neighborhoods and isolated rural areas. Every home health care agency should have a carefully developed program to assure the safety of personnel traveling to homes, and training on how to predict aggressive behaviors, diffuse threatening circumstances, along with methods of self-protection if threats escalate. One study of California home health and hospice agencies found that only 55% of the 40 participants reported formal workplace violence prevention programs in place, even though state guidelines for this were recommended 20 years earlier (Gross et al., 2013). For those having programs, more emphasis was placed on pet dangers than on potential dangers of patient history of violence or mental illness, guns, and substance abuse. Surrounding community threat assessment was generally not included. Only 15% of participating agencies provided employee training on prediction of aggression and violence. Very few gave trainings on diffusion of threats or methods for self-protection. Nurses making home visits were seldom members of the safety committees that oversaw these programs and policies. If the personal safety of the nurse is in jeopardy, then the client may be discharged from the agency's care if other arrangements

cannot be made. Display 32–5 lists practices for safe home visiting.

THE FUTURE OF CARE IN THE HOME

In conclusion, it can be seen that present-day Medicare home health care intervenes during brief episodes of acute medical trouble, relies on family at home as caregivers, and is expected to get in and out of the home as inexpensively as possible. Consider instead the true needs of the frail elderly or severely disabled who require prolonged psychosocial support, personal care, housekeeping, promotion of health, prevention of deterioration, and early detection of medical problems. In other words, they need case management that extends over months and years. For this to happen, the United States must continue to develop a **community-based long-term care** system. Home health nurses will play a pivotal role in that system. The primary role of the home health nurse will be education and advocacy for the client. Some baby boomers will be able to afford these services by paying out of their own pockets for a network of elder management services. Most baby boomers will need the development of a national community-based long-term care benefit. The Affordable Care Act is one step in that direction, but two programs provided in the act, the Community First Choice Option and the Community Care Transitions Program, do not provide for the long-term care so often required (CMS, 2015f). They are, however, a step in the right direction. *Healthy People 2020* provides a number of objectives *scattered throughout the document* that support the health and well-being of home health clients and their caregivers (USDHHS, 2016).

OVERVIEW OF THE HOSPICE MOVEMENT

Although science and technology have advanced in the world of health care, death is ultimately inevitable for all of us. The contemporary circumstances of death in America are often dehumanizing; most people die in hospitals and long-term care institutions, surrounded by strangers. Uncertainty and denial often prevail during the final stage of life because prognoses are uncertain, and many serious illnesses are now treated aggressively until the last breath. The battle against the "evil" of death seems to be the primary emphasis, with patient, family, and professionals wanting to believe that it is possible to win the final struggle. In the twenty-first century, fatal conditions have been turned into expensive chronic illnesses. Too often, discomfort is not relieved, and treatment causes further suffering. And as the period of disability extends and the body deteriorates, social isolation develops. The modern preoccupation with action, productivity, and beauty has little interest in the process of dying. In dramatic contrast to the dehumanization of death, the **hospice** movement has developed to humanize the end-of-life experience and provide palliative care. **Palliative interventions** relieve suffering without curing underlying disease. The hospice movement has emphasized four major changes in end-of-life care: (1) care should encompass body, mind, and spirit; (2) death should be discussed and not considered off-limits; (3) medical technology should be used only when absolutely necessary; and (4) clients should be actively involved in discussions about treatment decisions. Table 32–1 contrasts home health with hospice. This section explores the evolution of hospice care in the United States, describes hospice agencies, and examines Medicare criteria for hospice reimbursement. It concludes with an exploration of the unique characteristics of hospice nursing practice.

EVOLUTION OF HOSPICE CARE

In medieval Europe, hospices were refuges for the sick and dying. The contemporary hospice movement originated in England, where a physician, Dame Cicely Saunders, founded St. Christopher's Hospice in 1967. Dr. Saunders was credentialed as a nurse, social worker, and physician, and she developed a unique program based both on compassion and skillful relief of physical discomfort through around-the-clock analgesics administered by mouth. It had been previously assumed that only injections, administered sparingly, could be used for terminal pain control. In 1974, the first hospice in the United States was established in Branford, Connecticut. Florence Wald, who was then Dean of the Yale School of Nursing, led this movement. Because even in the 1970s, there was concern about saving money by keeping less critical patients out of the hospital and shortening hospital stays, and hospices in the United States came to focus on providing care in the home. To that end, Congress established the permanent **Medicare hospice benefit** in 1986, with the intention of keeping people at home, yet receiving comprehensive services that are less expensive than hospitalization (National Hospice and Palliative Care Organization, 2015).

Hospice characteristics have changed over time. Initially, nearly all clients suffered from terminal cancer; presently, people with a variety of end-stage diseases are served. Heart and pulmonary diseases, AIDS, Alzheimer's, renal failure, amyotrophic lateral sclerosis (ALS) and

Table 32–1 Contrasts Between Home Health and Hospice

Hospice	Home Health
Emphasis is on quality of life and comfort.	Emphasis is on rehabilitation, physiological stabilization, and adaptation.
Focus is on health of whole family.	Focus is on health of client.
Plan of care is guided by client choice.	Plan of care is determined by medical need and client choice.
Nurse is case manager until death.	Nurse is case manager until home health discharge.
Client chooses how to live last days.	Priority is given to correcting physiologic imbalances.
Intermittent visits increase in frequency as death becomes imminent.	Intermittent visits decrease in frequency as client stabilizes.
Nurses are expert in symptom control.	Symptom control is domain of physician with some nurses having expertise.
Sedatives and opioids are expertly adjusted to eliminate suffering.	Sedatives and opioids are used hesitantly to reduce suffering.
End-of-life disease course is managed to avoid crises.	End-of-life problems tend to be seen as medical crises.
Goal is for symptoms at end of life to be managed at home if possible.	Client is brought to hospital for unmanaged symptoms.
Spiritual care is focus of whole team.	Spiritual needs are met by own clergy.
Survivors have bereavement support.	No bereavement support is provided.

other neurological conditions, along with serious strokes, are all potential diagnoses for hospice care (Cummings, 2013). Many diseases that were once quick death sentences have now become chronic, life-limiting diseases. Palliative care, to ease pain and suffering and improve quality of life, can be offered in earlier stages of illness, along with continuing medical treatments. With prognoses difficult to predict and denial of death by the patient and family a continuing issue, some hospice referrals are now made very late in the disease process. Brief hospice stays make it difficult to significantly help families and clients prepare for death. With highly reliable Medicare payment, for-profit hospices have expanded and are competing in many communities for the hospice market share. They grew by 128% between 2001 and 2008; nonprofit hospices only grew by 1% during that time. Many have used aggressive marketing campaigns, and there is a consensus that most serve a higher percentage of patients that require less expensive care, leading to better profit margins (Bouchard, 2011). There is concern that the original purpose of hospice may be lost when profit motives abound. And, a study of hospice expansion found the mean length of hospice stay increased from 72.1 to 92.6 days during roughly the same time period that for-profit hospice growth occurred. Larger Medicare spending was noted, not offset by reduced hospital spending. Explanations for this included poor prognostication in patients, for instance, with Alzheimer's leading to longer hospice experiences and fewer end-of-life hospital expenses (Gozalo, Plotzke, Mor, Miller, & Teno, 2015).

HOSPICE SERVICES AND REIMBURSEMENT

As in home health care, Medicare has determined the way services are provided. The Medicare hospice benefit requires that a client who has a prognosis of 6 months or less must sign up for the comfort-focused hospice benefit and waive regular Medicare health services, except for conditions unrelated to their terminal illness. This mandates that the client acknowledges a terminal prognosis and chooses comfort care instead of life-extending care from a Medicare-approved hospice. When this choice is made, the hospice coordinates care in all settings, functioning both as clinical and financial case manager. The government pays a flat rate to the hospice for each day the patient receives care. There are four payment levels: (1) routine home care with intermittent visits, (2) continuous home care when the patient's condition is acute and death is near, (3) inpatient hospital care for symptom relief, and (4) respite care in a nursing home to relieve family members (CMS, 2015d).

Hospices coordinate home care and direct inpatient care if needed. The emphasis is on palliation, with a focus on physical, psychosocial, and spiritual comfort. A strong emphasis is placed on caring for the entire family. The hospice team includes nurses, physicians, home health aides, physical and occupational therapists, social workers, volunteers, palliative medication and medical equipment specialists, and bereavement counselors. Staff members meet regularly to explore together the challenges of assuring comfort at the end of life. A nurse or physician is available on-call 24 hours a day/7 days a week (CMS, 2015d).

Trained volunteers fill an important need in hospice care. They act as companions to the client when the family must be somewhere else or is away for short respite. They run errands for family members, shop, organize hot meals prepared by friends and neighbors, provide childcare, and perform other services as needed.

HOSPICE AND PALLIATIVE CARE NURSING PRACTICE

The nurse's role is central in the hospice interdisciplinary team. The hospice/palliative care nurse functions as case manager and visits the client more frequently than other members of the team. Nurses work in close collaboration with physicians in the development of a plan of care to assure management of symptoms. This plan of care changes rapidly as the end of life nears. In addition to home visits focusing on palliation and interdisciplinary planning, hospice nurses rotate through 24-hour call 7 days a week to assure continuous availability by telephone and visits for emergent problems reported by client or family. Hospice nursing competencies and challenges are similar to those described for home health nurses, with the added expertise needed to relieve physical and emotional suffering of terminally ill clients and their families. The American Nurses Association (ANA) and the Hospice and Palliative Nurses Association (HPNA) (2014) have established standards of practice for hospice and palliative nursing. Certification of hospice and palliative nursing is available. Palliative care nursing addresses the continuum of patient illness and provides both effective pain management and support, as the patient either prepares for continued life-prolonging treatments or a peaceful and dignified death. It is centered on patients and families, generally begins with life-threatening illness, and ends with family bereavement care. An overview of palliative care nursing standards encompasses the same general standards as home health nursing standards, with specific competencies delineated (e.g., comfort care, suffering and symptom palliation, support of patient/family throughout illness course, reaffirmation of goals with families during regularly scheduled family meetings, care coordination with interdisciplinary team members).

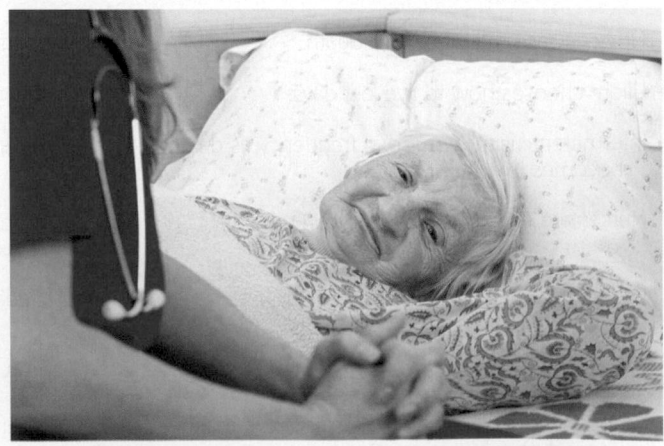

Hospice caregiving can be illustrated as a tree, strongly rooted in the process of nurses deliberately practicing self-care for themselves (Fig. 32–2). This tree has been drawn to explain the expert competencies of hospice

SPEAKING TRUTH

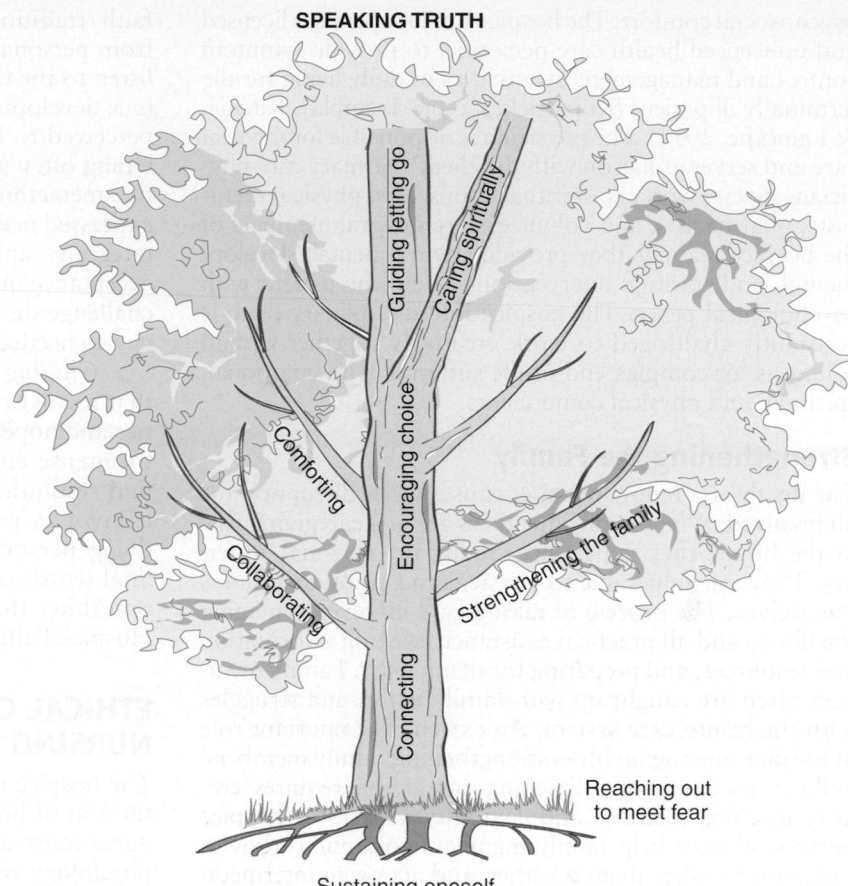

FIGURE 32–2 The hospice caregiving tree.

nurses who were interviewed to capture the essence of their practice, as described by Zerwekh (1995, 2006). Each of the hospice nursing practices visualized by the tree diagram is briefly summarized below.

Roots of Hospice Nursing: Sustaining Oneself

Effective hospice nurses understand that to care for others, they must care for themselves. Without strong healthy roots, the tree will not thrive. *Sustaining oneself* requires deliberate effort to maintain one's own physical, emotional, and spiritual well-being. Knowing oneself, identifying sources of stress, and learning how to care for self are important. Expert hospice nurses keep themselves healthy by maintaining a balance between giving and receiving, letting go of predetermined agendas and idealistic hopes to achieve more than is humanly possible, being emotionally open and clear, and deliberately replenishing themselves to restore their energy. Hospice nurses are constantly giving of themselves and embracing the suffering of their clients. This makes them particularly vulnerable to "compassion fatigue" and burnout (Harris & Griffin, 2015; Slocum-Gori, Hemsworth, Chan, Carson, & Kazanjian, 2011; Wentzel & Bryziewicz, 2014).

The Trunk Reaching Upward: Connecting, Speaking Truth, and Encouraging Choice

Rooted in self-care, hospice nurses practice *connecting*, which refers to the centrality of relationships in providing hospice care. The hospice nurse seeks to understand the emotional and spiritual distress common to the end of life,

particularly the progressive experience of loss after loss. Guided by that understanding, hospice nurses emphasize attentive listening to understand each individual's unique story. This requires quieting your own thoughts to truly hear what is being expressed. Sometimes, listening involves simply being present in the moment, paying attention. Having heard the client's story, it is important for hospice nurses to speak honestly when other professionals and family feel obliged to keep being cheerful and positive. Hospice nurses openly seek to speak truthfully about many issues that can be painful to discuss. *Speaking truth* is visualized as encircling the entire top of the caregiving tree. Hospice nurses bring up difficult subjects, so that the client is freed to speak about his greatest fears and concerns. Sometimes, it leads to joint problem solving and *encouraging choice* through informed decision-making (Monsen, Radosevich, Kerr, & Fulkerson, 2011). After truth has been discussed and the client has made a decision, the hospice nurse often advocates for client wishes against the resistance of various authorities. Remember that these are the final decisions in a dying person's life.

Collaborating

Interdisciplinary teamwork is an essential branch on the tree. Hospice team members communicate around the table and are constantly consulting each other, as well as family caregivers (Wittenberg-Lyles et al., 2013). The hospice interdisciplinary team members share information and work interdependently. The hospice nurse coordinates the plan of care and day-to-day efforts to provide physical and psychosocial comfort. The hospice nurse supervises licensed and unlicensed health care personnel to provide symptom control and management of activities of daily living for the terminally ill patient (Kilpatrick, Lavoie-Tremblay, Ritchie, & Lamothe, 2011). The physician is responsible for medical care and serves as liaison with the client's primary care physicians. Social workers, spiritual counselors, physical therapists, pharmacists, and volunteers are integral members of the hospice team as they provide environmental, developmental, and spiritual interventions to aid the patient with psychological peace. The hospice interdisciplinary team is constantly challenged to work creatively together to find solutions for complex end-of-life suffering with emotional, spiritual, and physical components.

Strengthening the Family

The death of a family member causes great disruption for all involved. When family members are in a caregiving role in the home, they experience significant personal suffering. They are vulnerable to physical and emotional illness themselves. The process of taking care involves managing the illness and all practical assistance, seeking information and resources, and preparing for death itself. Family members often are caught up with family issues and struggles with the health care system. An extremely important role in hospice nursing involves strengthening family members' abilities as caregivers. Teaching caregiving requires creative teaching methods and flexibility. Often, the hospice nurse is able to help family members communicate with each other, gather them together, and act as an intermediary if necessary (Mandel & Savoy, 2011).

Comforting

Hospice nurses develop extensive expertise in pain and symptom management. Contemporary medical/surgical nursing textbooks discuss the essentials in this field, and advanced knowledge is developed through experience, continued education, and reading. Display 32–6 lists fundamental palliative principles, and Display 32–7 identifies four important components of pain relief.

Spiritual Practice and Letting Go

As death draws near, spiritual needs intensify, with the final search for meaning, reconciliation, hope, and transcendence beyond the limits of human lived experience (Dillon, Roscoe, & Jenkins, 2012). This is a developmental milestone as well as a spiritual and physical journey. The effect of the journey on the client is also impacted by the environmental and cultural habits and customs the client has experienced through their lifetime. Spirituality is in essence learned behavior and is individually defined by the client (Richardson, 2014). In a multisite study of quality of life for advanced cancer patients being treated with palliative radiation, researchers found that those who used religious and spiritual coping reported improved quality of life on all outcome measures. They also noted that the majority of patients (85%) wanted nurses to attend to their spiritual concerns (Vallurupalli et al., 2012). Hospice nurses recognize spiritual distress and practice spiritual caring interventions that include respect for beliefs and spiritual practices and fostering reconciliation if there is a problem with estrangement from family, friends, and

faith tradition. The nurse must remain objective, free from personal beliefs and customs, while they attentively listen to the client and promote life review. Although this is a developmental milestone in the client's life is often perceived to be stressful for the client, and the act of listening often gives them psychological peace. In a qualitative metaethnography, Dillon et al. (2012) uncovered the expressed need of African Americans for hospice care that integrates and emphasizes spiritual support, not merely acceptance or tolerance. Both research studies cited above challenge the hospice nurse to support that spiritual journey so needed by the dying and their family members.

Guiding letting go is a truly unique nursing practice that involves helping the client to let go of former activities and hopes, including life itself. This involves listening to intense emotions and helping the person and family find resolution (Raingruber & Wolf, 2015). Sometimes, it involves participating in a vigil at the bedside of the dying person and encouraging loved ones to say their final words of farewell. It is this action that often is that one thing that gives the client peace. See Perspectives: Hospice/Palliative Care Nursing.

ETHICAL CHALLENGES IN HOSPICE NURSING

The hospice nurse confronts striking ethical challenges at the end of life. As an advocate for the client, the hospice nurse must integrate their own knowledge of the pathophysiology of the disease process with the physiological needs of the dying client while accounting for the psychological and cultural needs of the client and family (Storch, 2015). As client advocates, we, as nurses, must be aware of the ethical challenges surrounding the dying experience. Wide-ranging issues include respect or disregard for client autonomy, relief or disregard for client suffering, and avoidance of killing at the very end of life (Fernandes, 2015). The hospice nurse needs to develop their own knowledge of nursing and medical ethics in order to question the ethical implications of interventions and to advocate for client and family. An example of this is the widely held belief in hospice care that dehydration enhances client comfort. Cohen, Torres-Vigil, Burbach, de la Rosa, & Bruera (2012) conducted a phenomenological study with 84 caregivers and 85 clients regarding the issue of hydration of advanced-cancer patients receiving hospice care. Their findings revealed that patients and their families viewed fluids as enhancing comfort, dignity, and quality of life. Physiologically, as nurses, it is understood that often this is not the case. These findings support the need to tailor individual care based on specific patient needs and family preferences (Cohen et al., 2012). They challenge the hospice nurse to embrace ongoing professional development in order to keep abreast of best practice modalities.

Ethical unrest in the client, family, as well as the nurse is best addressed through the institutional ethics board. This board consists of various disciplines specializing in health care, ethics, legal, and spiritual care. When the nurse is unsure of the ethical ramifications of decisions by the client or family, it is their obligation to bring the case before the board following the procedures of the institution. See Chapter 4 for more on ethics.

EVIDENCE-BASED PRACTICE
Nurses and Compassion Fatigue

Do you wonder how hospice nurses sustain compassionate practice as they work day in and day out with suffering patients who always die? Expert hospice nurses embrace the suffering of the client and family and become susceptible to compassion fatigue. **Compassion fatigue** is often viewed as secondary stress. It is the stress felt by the caregiver from exposure to a traumatization. Nurses often describe this as overload. Although signs of compassion fatigue are individualized, they often include exhaustion and a reduced ability to express empathy for the client. This may result in withdrawal by the nurse emotionally from the client and family, as well as the role of nurse. One study, conducted at a nonprofit hospice in Texas, found that the exposure to "chronic bereavement" experienced by hospice nurses often led to sleep problems and symptoms of depression (Carter, Dyer, & Mikan, 2013, p. e368). Others have noted the spiritual, physical, and mental exhaustion that is part of the cost of caring and the need to set boundaries, take care of themselves through exercise, hobbies, and reflection or sharing stories (Melvin, 2012; Slocum-Gori, Hemsworth, Chan, Carson, & Kazanjian, 2011).

Staying healthy as a hospice nurse requires a high level of self-awareness. The nurse must be aware of the signs and symptoms that they may have a tendency to exhibit. Symptoms are individualized based on how the nurse adapted to stress in the past. Often they are subject to developmental, spiritual, cultural, and environmental influences. Recognition of the symptoms allows the hospice nurse to institute stress-relieving activities early in the process. According to the Compassion Fatigue Awareness Project (2013), some symptoms that a nurse may experience include

- Isolating oneself; poor self-care (appearance, hygiene)
- Repressed emotions; apathy; mentally/physically exhausted
- Always finding blame with others; many complaints about job/administration
- Substance abuse; compulsive behaviors (e.g., eating, spending, gambling)
- In debt; legal problems; recurrent flashbacks/nightmares; chronic health problems
- Problems concentrating; feeling preoccupied; denies problems

Compassion fatigue can affect an agency, if enough nurses suffer from the problem and nothing is done to assist them. It can cause problems between nurses and administrators, lead to high turnover and absenteeism, and lead to self-perpetuation. Organizations may exhibit these symptoms:

- Poor teamwork; high absentee rates; continually changing coworker relationships
- Challenging/breaking agency rules; aggression among staff members
- Poor task/assignment completion; unable to meet deadlines; lack of flexibility
- Negative feelings toward management; reluctance toward change
- Poor vision of future; not able to believe that improvements can be made
    (Compassion Fatigue Awareness Project, 2013)

Compassion fatigue is not isolated to hospice nurses. A review of the literature will show that nurses score higher for compassion fatigue and burnout than many other professions. Those nurses who are both professional and family caregivers (e.g., RN daughter caring for failing mother) are at special risk for compassion fatigue (Ward-Griffin, St-Amant, & Brown, 2011). Often it is noted that caregivers experiencing compassion fatigue are unable to identify it in themselves. What ways can you identify compassion fatigue in others? What recommendations can you make to reduce compassion fatigue for yourself?

Sources:

Carter, P. A., Dyer, K. A., & Mikan, S. Q. (2013). Sleep disturbance, chronic stress, and depression in hospice nurses: Testing the feasibility of an intervention. *Oncology Nursing Forum, 40*(5), e368–e373.

Harris, C., & Griffin M. (2015). Nursing on empty: Compassion fatigue signs, symptoms and system interventions. *Journal of Christian Nursing, 32*(2), 80–87.

Mandel, M., & Savoy, E. (2011). Research on supporting patients and family caregivers with palliative and end-of-life care. *Home Healthcare Nurse, 29*(3), 148–154.

Melvin, C. S. (2012). Professional compassion fatigue: What is the true cost of nurses caring for the dying? *International Journal of Palliative Nursing, 18*(12), 606–611.

Slocum-Gori, S., Hemsworth, D., Chan, W., Carson, A., & Kazanjian, A. (2011). Understanding compassion satisfaction, compassion fatigue, and burnout: A survey of the hospice palliative care workforce. *Palliative Medicine, 27*(2), 172–178.

Ward-Griffin, C., St-Amant, O., & Brown, J. B. (2011). Compassion fatigue within double duty caregiving: Nurse-daughters caring for elderly parents. *Online Journal of Issues in Nursing, 16*(1), 4.

THE FUTURE OF HOME HEALTH AND HOSPICE

Given a rapidly expanding population of elders living longer with challenging chronic illnesses, home health and hospice care in the home will soon need to transform into a community-based long-term care system that doesn't discharge after an acute episode or admit only at the very end of life. In response to out-of-control medical inflation, federal and state governments have sought to hold down expenses in all areas, including restrictions on home health and hospice care. However, costs keep rising in step with technologic and pharmacologic innovation and marketing. Containing costs will eventually force a shift in services from expensive institutional and high technology interventions to community-based home services.

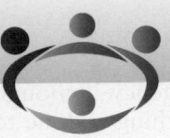

DISPLAY 32–6 Fundamentals of Palliative Care

- Make no assumptions about what is wrong.
- Believe the patient's report of symptoms.
- Relieve discomfort to the extent that the patient chooses and finds acceptable.
- Investigate the biologic, psychosocial, and spiritual dimensions of discomfort.
- Anticipate symptoms, and relieve them before they occur again.
- Use nursing and complementary (integrative) interventions.
- Become an expert in the use of palliative medication.
- Continually evaluate the effectiveness of interventions.
- Choose the least complex and most manageable interventions that patients and families can manage themselves at home.
- Never give up. Persist in trying different palliative strategies.

The entire model for service provision in the home must change to a health care delivery system that continuously serves those living with disabling and terminal illness to maximize well-being at home, anticipate and prevent crises, and minimize emergent and inpatient interventions. Hospice care is focused on symptom

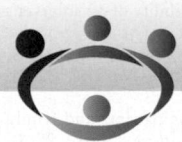

DISPLAY 32–7 Essential Components of Pain Relief

1. Continually assess the extent of pain and the relief afforded by interventions.
2. Schedule analgesics around the clock to maintain continuous blood levels and prevent the return of pain.
3. Use the least invasive route for analgesic administration, with oral as first choice.
4. Follow the World Health Organization (2016) three-step ladder:

   Step 1 for mild pain: Nonopioid (acetaminophen or NSAID) plus adjuvant such as corticosteroid, antidepressant, anxiolytic, or anticonvulsant

   Step 2 for persisting pain: Opioid and nonopioid and/or adjuvant

   Step 3 for moderate to severe pain: Strong opioid and nonopioid and/or adjuvant

Source: World Health Organization. (2016). *WHO's cancer pain ladder for adults.* Retrieved from www.who.int/cancer/palliative/painladder/en
Note: WHO also offers guidelines for persisting pain in children: www.who.int/medicines/areas.quality_safety.guide_perspainchild/en/

PERSPECTIVES
HOSPICE/PALLIATIVE CARE NURSING

When I graduated from nursing school, I went directly into the intensive care unit. I loved it! I enjoyed the challenge of working intensely with one or two patients, as well as the supportive work environment with my close-knit group of colleagues. With marriage and children (my first pregnancy resulted in twins), the 12-hour shifts and full-time schedules were more difficult to balance with family life. At first, I dropped down to working one weekend a month. But, with our growing family, it seemed that I would not be able to remain in the ICU. I talked to a friend and learned about our hospital's hospice agency; she enjoyed working there, and I thought I would give it a try. It was a perfect fit for me and for our four boys. People always think of hospice/palliative care as depressing, but I find it to be very fulfilling. I think about it as "joining with a family" at their most vulnerable time. The patients let you in, sharing very personal things about their life with you, and they are grateful for your assistance at this time of transition. It can be a very spiritual experience, and I consider it a privilege to be able to share this time with my patients and their families. The only difficult cases for me are the children; our agency doesn't have a large pediatric hospice, but it is beginning to expand. It is difficult for parents to lose a child, as one would expect. I remember coming home after a long night with a family whose young child lost his long battle with cancer and hosting my 2-year-old's birthday party with family and friends. I couldn't help but think about the contrast—my happy, healthy toddler and the loss of a young boy to cancer. But, I know that I made a difference for that family and child; I am honored to be a hospice/palliative care nurse.

Jessica, Hospice RN

management, not curative interventions. Care revolves around maintenance of quality of life, not necessarily quantity. Clients in hospice care, under Medicare regulations, receive care for symptom management. If care is needed for other health conditions not related to the terminal diagnosis, care is received under their original Medicare benefit. Hospice services should be based on client choice and the reality of a terminal diagnosis. The physician must sign a declaration stating that the terminal diagnosis, if it follows the normal course of the disease process, will cause death in a finite period of time (6 months or less). A sustainable, affordable approach to care in the home requires ongoing case management to coordinate and manage resources with incentives that control cost while assuring quality of life and comfort. The hospice nurse becomes a coordinator of an interprofessional team of health care, spiritual, and community resources. Team members often include volunteers, who, after training, become involved with respite care for the family. Determination of the team members is defined in collaboration with the client and family to allow them independence and minimize the disruption to their

POPULATION-FOCUS
HOSPICE CARE FOR CHILDREN

Although it may be difficult for a family to accept hospice care for their terminally ill child, there is increasing evidence showing that a pediatric palliative care program reduces stress and worry for caregivers. Also, because medical care is received in a stress-free setting, the quality of life as well as length of life may be increased (Gans et al., 2015). Hospice plays an important role in supporting the child and family in the areas of medical, social, spiritual, and psychological support. The value of this service and underutilization justify research in this area. The National Hospice and Palliative Care Organization is committed to care of the child and family who can benefit from hospice care. They provide professional resources and education, as well as patient education information.

Children with life-threatening illnesses are hospitalized more often and spend more days in the hospital than those whose diseases are not life threatening. Communication between the health care team and education of health care workers can often eliminate these hospitalizations (Nageswaran, Radulovic, & Anania, 2014).

Sanchez Varela et al. (2012) also explored the barriers to the use of hospice by children. In this North Carolina study of hospice organizations, the researchers used quantitative methods to determine the factors contributing to underutilization of hospice services. Factors included lack of trained pediatric nurses, pediatric pharmacy, pediatrician consultation, coordination of care, as well as inconsistent communication between care providers. Other factors of importance were limited referrals and the wishes of the family to continue with curative therapy, which could preclude qualification for hospice services.

Although the studies were conducted in separate countries, similar needs emerged from both studies. Most important to nursing practice is the limited access to ongoing education and the lack of consistent professional experiences with these children and their families. Both of these factors were seen as contributing to underutilization of services. What can be inferred from these findings is that efforts to maintain a trained hospice workforce with specialized skill in working with children, ongoing opportunities to develop and maintain skills, and wider use of hospice in this population are needed. The identified value of hospice services and the findings of these studies support ongoing research into methods to increase use of these services and the infrastructure to create and maintain a trained workforce.

Do you think most nurses working in hospitals are aware of hospice and palliative care services for children? What could you do to help communicate the availability and effectiveness of hospice services for children with life-threatening illnesses?

References

Gans, D., Hadler, M., Chen, X., Wu, S., Dimand, R., Abramson, J., ... Kominski, G. (2015). Impact of a pediatric palliative care program on the caregiver experience. *Journal of Hospice & Palliative Nursing, 17*(6), 559–565. doi: 10.1097/NJH.00000000000203.

Nageswaran, S., Radulovic, A., Anania, A. (2014). Transitions to and from the acute inpatient care setting for children with life-threatening illness. *Pediatric Clinic of North America, 61*(4), 761–783.

Sanchez Varela, A. M., Deal, A. M., Hanson, L. C., Blatt, J., Gold, S., & Dellon, E. P. (2012). Barriers to hospice for children as perceived by hospice organizations in North Carolina. *American Journal of Hospice & Palliative Medicine, 29*(3), 171–176.

individual lifestyle. Although inpatient hospices do exist, the goal of the hospice nurse is to keep the client in their home environment for as long as possible. There is evidence that palliative care may prolong life, and there is a call to make services more available in all settings (e.g., nursing homes, hospitals, homes) in order to provide equitable care for all and to augment the palliative care workforce (Meier, 2011). Nurses, nurse practitioners, and home visiting physicians will need to have the diagnostic and therapeutic resources to monitor physiologic status and intervene in the home. Telehealth and home monitoring will be essential. The focus must change from doing everything possible to prolong physiologic survival to promoting meaningful and comfortable lives. Nurses will have an active role in this process.

The Institute of Medicine (2015) report, *Dying in America: Improving Quality and Honoring Individual Preferences Near the End of Life*, gives direction for needed changes that put the requirements of patients and families first. The report encourages policy changes and serves as a charge for all of us to advocate for improved social, spiritual, and psychological support and care for those of us nearing the end of our lives. As health care providers, we need to strive to provide compassionate, quality-centered, evidence-based care that is consistent with the wishes of our patients and their families.

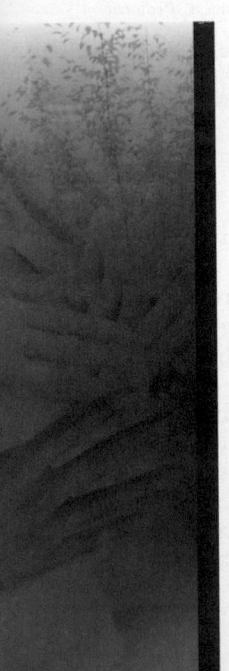

SUMMARY

Community/public health nurses have an important role in working with clients who receive home care or hospice services. As the population continues to age, the need for nurses to work with older adults where they live, as they are discharged from acute care settings earlier and earlier and, if they are terminally ill, during their final months and days, will only increase. Services are also needed for clients across the lifespan.

Many types of home care agencies exist: voluntary, proprietary, hospital based, official, homemaker, and hospice. Both formal and informal caregivers provide service. Professional staff members, such as nurses, social workers, therapists, and certified nursing assistants, work in collaboration with family members and, in some situations, with friends and neighbors.

Hospice is a newer concept in the United States, but has a longer history in England. Medicare covers hospice care without the restrictions experienced by nonhospice home care clients. Hospice and palliative care programs provide holistic care to clients during the last months of life. Many programs are home based, and they may be offered by a home health agency. In addition to in-home hospices, inpatient hospices exist; these can be located in a freestanding building, in an area of a SNF, or in a section of an acute care facility. The focus of hospice care is not historically aimed at cure, and it employs holistic caregiving practices that involve family members, professionals, and volunteers.

The nurse provides direct physical nursing care both in home health care and with hospice clients. In addition, the nurse teaches clients, family members, and volunteers; supervises; collaborates with team members; and case manages. Nurse assessment of clients to determine health status and eligibility for additional services as well as service as a client advocate occur with both groups of clients. Determining the frequency and duration of services occurs in home care. With both home care and hospice clients, the nurse must become familiar with the requirements of documentation to promote continuity of care and ensure reimbursement.

ACTIVITIES TO PROMOTE **CRITICAL THINKING**

1. Search the Internet for home health and hospice agencies in your city or town. Select two agencies and compare the employment opportunities of each (one nonprofit and one for-profit). How do these job descriptions and the published pay ranges compare to hospitals in your area? What are the benefits of working in home health and hospice? Will the agency hire new graduates, or do they require prior acute care experience?

2. John S., age 58 years, was recently diagnosed with liver cancer following years of heavy alcohol consumption. At the urging of his physician, his wife contacted the local hospice agency for assistance. You have been assigned this case. When you arrive at John's house, his wife tells you that he refuses to see you and is continuing to drink alcohol. She is very distressed and begins to cry. How would you handle this situation? What are some of the issues inherent in this case?

3. Review your personal health insurance policy or that of a family member. What coverage, if any, is provided for home health or hospice care? What restrictions are stated in the coverage—total reimbursement, source of care, or length of service? Do you think this will be adequate to meet your or your family member's needs when these services may be needed? What other options might be available to help defray the cost of this type of care?

4. Interview a home health nurse to find out the most rewarding part of their job. What things are problematic? Ask about a typical case and home visit. How does this compare to your experiences in your community health nursing clinical course? Do you feel that home health nursing might be something you will consider in the future?

5. Interview a nurse working in hospice and palliative care. Have them describe their most memorable cases. Ask if they have noticed signs of compassion fatigue among colleagues. Discuss the signs and symptoms listed in this chapter, and compare with those your interviewee mentions. What do they feel is most rewarding about their work? Consider if this specialty might be a good fit for you.

6. Compare and contrast the roles and functions of home health nurses and those working in hospice/palliative care with acute care (hospital) nursing. What are the main similarities? What differences do you notice?

REFERENCES

American Association for Homecare. (2015). *Cost effectiveness of homecare*. Retrieved from https://www.aahomecare.org/issues/cost-effectiveness-of-homecare\

American Nurses Association (ANA). (2014). *Scope and standards of practice: Home health nursing* (2nd ed.). Silver Spring, MD: Author.

American Nurses Association (ANA). (2015). *Code for nurses with interpretive statements*. Washington, DC: Author.

American Nurses Association (ANA) and Hospice and Palliative Nurses Association (HPNA). (2014). *Scope and standards of practice: Palliative nursing, an essential resource for hospice and palliative nurses*. Silver Spring, MD: Author.

Bao, Y., Shao, H., Bishop, T. F., Schackman, B. R., & Bruce, M. L. (2011). Inappropriate medication in a national sample of U.S. elderly patients receiving home health care. *Journal of General Internal Medicine, 27*(3), 304–310.

Bouchard, S. (2011). *Concerns raised about increase in for-profit hospice care*. Retrieved from http://www.healthcarefinancenews.com/news/concerns-raised-about-increase-profit-hospice-care

Buhler-Wilkerson, K. (2007). No place like home: A history of nursing and home care in the U.S. *Home Healthcare Nurse, 25*(4), 253–259.

Buhler-Wilkerson, K. (2016). *Caring for the sick at home*. Retrieved from http://www.nursing.upenn.edu/nhhc/Pages/HomeCare.aspx

Centers for Disease Control and Prevention (CDC). (2015). *Important facts about falls*. Retrieved from http://www.cdc.gov/homeandrecreationalsafety/falls/adultfalls.html

Centers for Medicare and Medicaid Services (CMS). (2012). *Background: OASIS*. Retrieved from https://www.cms.gov/Medicare/Quality-Initiatives-Patient-Assessment-Instruments/OASIS/Background.html

Centers for Medicare and Medicaid Services (CMS). (2015a). *Home health quality initiative*. Retrieved from https://www.medicare.gov/HomeHealth Compare/...Quality-MeasuresList.html

Centers for Medicare and Medicaid Services (CMS). (2015b). *Home health PPS*. Retrieved from https://www.cms.gov/Medicare/Medicare-Fee-for-Service-Payment/HomeHealthPPS/index.html?redirect=/homehealthpps/

Centers for Medicare and Medicaid Services (CMS). (2015c). *Medicare home health benefit*. Retrieved from https://www.medicare.gov/Pubs/pdf/02154.pdf

Centers for Medicare and Medicaid Services (CMS). (2015d). *Medicare hospice benefits*. Retrieved from https://www.medicare.gov/Pubs/pdf/02154.pdf

Centers for Medicare and Medicaid Services (CMS). (2015e). *OASIS-C1 data sets*. Retrieved from https://www.cms.gov/Medicare/Quality-Initiatives-Patient-Assessment-Instruments/HomeHealthQualityInits/OASIS-C1-DataSets.html

Centers for Medicare and Medicaid Services (CMS). (2015f). *Patient protection and affordable care act*. Retrieved from https://www.www.medicare.gov/...affordable-care-act/affordable-care-act.html

Cohen, M. Z., Torres-Vigil, I., Burbach, B. E., de la Rosa, A., & Bruera, E. (2012). The meaning of parenteral hydration to family caregivers and patients with advanced cancer receiving hospice care. *Journal of Pain and Symptom Management, 43*(5), 855–865.

Compassion Fatigue Awareness Project. (2013). *Recognizing compassion fatigue*. Retrieved from www.compassionfatigue.org/pages/symptoms.html

Cummings, K. (2013). *End of life and hospice care*. Retrieved from http://www.takingcharge.csh.umn.edu/conditions/end-life-and-hospice-care

Dillon, P. J., Roscoe, L. A., & Jenkins, J. J. (2012). African Americans and decisions about hospice care: Implications for health message design. *Howard Journal of Communication, 23*, 175–193. doi: 10.1080/10646175.2012.667724.

Fernandes, J. (2015). Assisted dying is a threat to the ethics of palliative nursing. *International Journal of Palliative Nursing, 21*(9), 421–422.

Gans, D., Hadler, M., Chen, X., Wu, S., Dimand, R., Abramson, J., ... Kominski, G. (2015). Impact of a pediatric palliative care program on the caregiver experience. *Journal of Hospice & Palliative Nursing, 17*(6), 559–565. doi: 10.1097/NJH.00000000000203.

Gottlieb, H. (2016). *Medication nonadherence: Finding solutions to a costly medical problem*. Retrieved from http://www.medscape.com/viewarticle/409940_4

Gozalo, P., Plotzke, M., Mor, V., Miller, S. C., & Teno, J. M. (2015). Changes in Medicare costs with the growth of hospice care in nursing homes. *New England Journal of Medicine, 372*, 1823–1831.

Gross, N., Peek-Asa, C., Nocera, M., & Casteel, C. (2013). Workplace violence prevention policies in home health and hospice agencies. *Online Journal of Issues in Nursing, 18*(1), Manuscript 1.

Harris, C., & Griffin, M. (2015). Nursing on empty: Compassion fatigue signs, symptoms and system interventions. *Journal of Christian Nursing, 32*(2), 80–87.

Harris-Kojetin, L., Sengupta, M., Park-Lee, E., & Valverde, R. (2013). *Long-term care services in the United States: 2013 overview*. Retrieved from http://www.cdc.gov/nchs/data/nsltcp/long_term_care_services_2013.pdf

Home Healthcare Nurses Association (HHNA). (2012). *About HHNA*. Retrieved from http://www.hhna.org/About/

Institute of Medicine. (2015). *Dying in America: Improving quality and honoring individual preferences near the end of life*. Washington, DC: National Academies Press.

Iuga, A. O., & McGuire, M. J. (2014). Adherence and health care costs. *Journal of Risk Management and Healthcare Policy, 7*, 35–44.

Jarrin, O., Flynn, L., Lake, E. T., & Aiken, L. H. (2014). Home health agency work environments and hospitalizations. *Medical Care, 52*(10), 877–883.

Kenneley, I. (2012). Infection control in home healthcare. *Home Healthcare Nurse, 30*(4), 235–245.

Kilpatrick, K., Lavoie-Tremblay, M., Ritchie, J. A., & Lamothe, L. (2011). Advanced practice nursing, health care teams, and perceptions of team effectiveness. *Health Care Management, 30*(3), 215–226.

Kliff, S. (2012, June 28). The Supreme Court surprise: Medicaid ruling could reduce coverage. *The Washington Post*. Retrieved from https://www.washingtonpost.com/news/wonk/wp/2012/06/28/the-supreme-court-surprise-medicaid-ruling-could-reduce-coverage/

Mandel, M., & Savoy, E. (2011). Research on supporting patients and family caregivers with palliative and end-of-life care. *Home Healthcare Nurse, 29*(3), 148–154.

Medicare Interactive. (n.d.). *What homebound means*. Retrieved from http://www.medicareinteractive.org/page2.php?topic=counselor&page=script&script_id=2

Meier, D. E. (2011). Increased access to palliative care and hospice services: Opportunities to improve value in health care. *Millbank Quarterly, 89*(3), 343–380.

Monsen, K., Radosevich, D., Kerr, M., & Fulkerson, J. (2011). Public health nurses tailor interventions for families at risk. *Public Health Nursing, 28*(2), 119–128.

Munck, B., Sandgren, A., Fridlund, B., & Martensson, J. (2012). Next-of-kin's conceptions of medical technology in palliative homecare. *Journal of Clinical Nursing, 21*, 1868–1877.

Nageswaran, S., Radulovic, A., & Anania, A. (2014). Transitions to and from the acute inpatient care setting for children with life-threatening illness. *Pediatric Clinics of North America, 61*(4), 761–783. doi: 10.1016/j.pxl.2014.04.008.

National Alliance for Caregiving (NAC). (2012). *About Alliance research*. Retrieved from http://www.caregiving.org/research/about-our-research

National Alliance for Caregiving (NAC). (2014). *Definitions*. Retrieved from https://www.caregiver.org/definitions-0

National Association for Home Care and Hospice (NAHC). (2010). *Basic statistics about home care*. Retrieved from http://www.nahc.org/assets/1/7/10HC_Stats.pdf

National Association for Home Care and Hospice (NAHC). (2016) *Code of ethics*. Retrieved from http://www.nahc.org/about/code-of-ethics

National Center for Nursing Workforce Analysis. (2013). *The U.S. nursing workforce: Trends in supply and education*. Retrieved from http://bhpr.hrsa.gov/healthworkforce/reports/nursingworkforce/nursingworkforcefullreport.pdf

National Hospice and Palliative Care Organization. (2015). *History of hospice care*. Retrieved from http://www.nhpco.org/history-hospice-care

Raingruber, B., & Wolf, T. (2015). Nurse perspectives regarding the meaningfulness of oncology nursing practice. *Clinical Journal of Oncology Nursing, 19*(3), 292–296.

Richardson, P. (2014). Spirituality, religion and palliative care. *Annals of Palliative Medicine, 3*(3), 150–159.

Sanchez Varela, A. M., Deal, A. M., Hanson, L. C., Blatt, J., Gold, S., & Dellon, E. P. (2012). Barriers to hospice for children as perceived by hospice organizations in North Carolina. *American Journal of Hospice & Palliative Medicine, 29*(3), 171–176. doi: 10.1177/1049909111412580.

Shea, K., & Chamoff, B. (2012). Telehomecare communication and self-care in chronic conditions: Moving toward a shared understanding. *Worldviews on Evidence-Based Nursing, 9*(2), 109–116. doi: 10.1111/j.1741-6787.2012.00242.x.

Siegel, J. D., Rhinehart, E., Jackson, M., Chiarello, L., & Healthcare Infection Control Practices Advisory Committee. (2011). *2007 Guideline for isolation precautions: Preventing transmission of infectious agents in healthcare settings.* Atlanta, GA: Centers for Disease Control and Prevention. Retrieved from http://www.cdc.gov/hicpac/2007IP/2007ip_part4.html

Slocum-Gori, S., Hemsworth, D., Chan, W., Carson, A., & Kazanjian, A. (2011). Understanding compassion satisfaction, compassion fatigue, and burnout: A survey of the hospice palliative care workforce. *Palliative Medicine, 27*(2), 172–178.

Stolee, P., Lim, S. N., Wilson, L., & Glenny, C. (2011). Inpatient versus home-based rehabilitation for older adults with musculoskeletal disorders: A systematic review. *Clinical Rehabilitation, 26*(5), 387–402. doi: 10.1177/0269215511423279.

Storch, J. (2015). Ethics in practice: At end-of-life—part 1. *Canadian Nurse, 111*(6), 20–21.

Swayze, S. C., & Rich, S. E. (2012). Promoting safe use of medical devices. *Online Journal of Issues in Nursing, 17*(1). doi: 103912/OJIN.Vol17No01PPT01.

U.S. Department of Health and Human Services (USDHHS). (2016). *About Healthy People 2020.* Retrieved from http://healthypeople.gov/2020/about/default.aspx

U.S. Supreme Court. (2012). *National Federation of Independent Business et al. v Sebelius, Secretary of Health and Human Services.* Retrieved from http://www.supremecourt.gov/opinions/11pdf/11-393c3a2.pdf

Vallurupalli, M., Lauderdale, K., Balboni, M. J., Phelps, A. C., Block, S. D., Ng, A. K., … Balboni, T. A. (2012). The role of spirituality and religious coping in the quality of life of patients with advanced cancer receiving palliative radiation therapy. *Journal of Supportive Oncology, 10*(2), 81–87.

Visiting Nurse Service of New York. (2016). *100 years in the community.* Retrieved from http://www.vnsny.org/community/our-history/100-years-in-the-community/

Wentzel, D., & Bryziewicz, P. (2014). The consequence of caring too much: Compassion fatigue and the trauma nurse. *Journal of Emergency Nursing, 40*(1), 95–97.

Wittenberg-Lyles, E., Oliver, D. P., Kruse, R. L., Demiris, G., Gage, L. A., & Wagner, K. (2013). Family caregiver participation in hospice interdisciplinary team meetings: How does it affect the nature and content of communication? *Health Communication, 28*(2), 110–118.

World Health Organization. (2016). *Cancer: WHO's pain ladder for adults.* Retrieved from http://www.who.int/cancer/palliative/painladder/en/

Zerwekh, J. (1995). High-tech home care for nurses. *Home Healthcare Nurse, 13*(1), 9–14.

Zerwekh, J. (2006). *Nursing care at the end of life.* Philadelphia, PA: F.A. Davis.

thePoint: Everything You Need to Make the Grade!

thePoint® Visit http://thePoint.lww.com/Rector9e for selected readings, study aids for all learning styles, and more!

INDEX